Compliments of
Karen Kinsail
AMGEN.

2nd edition
CANCER CHEMOTHERAPY HANDBOOK

Robert T. Dorr, PhD
Associate Professor of Pharmacology
Director, Pharmacology Program
Arizona Cancer Center
Tucson, Arizona

Daniel D. Von Hoff, MD
Professor of Medicine
University of Texas Health
 Sciences Center at San Antonio
Director of Institute for Drug Development
Cancer Therapy and Research Center
San Antonio, Texas

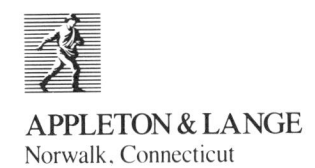

APPLETON & LANGE
Norwalk, Connecticut

Notice: The authors and the publisher of this volume have taken care to
make certain that the doses of drugs and schedules of treatment are correct
and compatible with the standards generally accepted at the time of
publication. Nevertheless, as new information becomes available, changes in
treatment and in the use of drugs become necessary. The reader is advised to
carefully consult the instruction and information material included in the
package insert of each drug or therapeutic agent before administration.
This advice is especially important when using new or infrequently used drugs.
The publisher disclaims any liability, loss, injury, or damage incurred as
a consequence, directly or indirectly, of the use and application of any of
the contents of this volume.

Copyright © 1994 by Appleton & Lange
Simon & Schuster Business and Professional Group

All rights reserved. This book, or any parts thereof, may not be used or
reproduced in any manner without written permission. For information,
address Appleton & Lange, 25 Van Zant Street, East Norwalk, Connecticut 06855.

94 95 96 97 98 / 10 9 8 7 6 5 4 3 2 1

Prentice Hall International (UK) Limited, *London*
Prentice Hall of Australia Pty. Limited, *Sydney*
Prentice Hall Canada, Inc., *Toronto*
Prentice Hall Hispanoamericana, S.A., *Mexico*
Prentice Hall of India Private Limited, *New Delhi*
Prentice Hall of Japan, Inc., *Tokyo*
Simon & Schuster Asia Pte. Ltd., *Singapore*
Editora Prentice Hall do Brasil Ltda., *Rio de Janeiro*
Prentice Hall, *Englewood Cliffs, New Jersey*

Cancer chemotherapy handbook / [edited by] Robert T. Dorr, Daniel D.
  Von Hoff. —2nd ed.
    p. cm.
  Rev. ed of: Cancer chemotherapy handbook / Robert T. Dorr, William
L. Fritz. c1980.
  Includes index.
  ISBN 0-8385-1036-1
  1. Cancer—Chemotherapy—Handbooks, manuals, etc.
  2. Antineoplastic agents—Handbooks, manuals, etc. I. Dorr, Robert
T. II. Von Hoff, Daniel D.
  [DNLM: 1. Antineoplastic Agents—handbooks. 2. Neoplasms—drug
therapy—handbooks. 3. Immunotherapy—handbooks. QZ 39 C2148
1993]
RC271.C5D67 1993
616.99'4061—dc20
DNLM/DLC
for Library of Congress   93-3504

Acquisitions Editor: Julia L. White
Production Editor: Karen W. Davis
Production Assistant: Jennifer Szakonyi
Interior design by Janice Barsevich Bielawa

ISBN 0-8385-1036-1

PRINTED IN THE UNITED STATES OF AMERICA

Contributors

Ronald N. Buick, PhD
Vice President of Research
Ontario Cancer Institute
Toronto, Ontario

Robert T. Dorr, PhD
Associate Professor of Pharmacology
Director, Pharmacology Program
Arizona Cancer Center
Tucson, Arizona

Suzanne Fields, PharmD
Director, Investigational Drug Section
Cancer Therapy and Research Center
San Antonio, Texas

Amy J. Galpin, PharmD
Research Fellow
St. Jude Children's Research Hospital
Memphis, Tennessee

Barbara Carlile Holmes, RN, MSN, OCN
Oncology Nursing Consultant
PhD Candidate
University of Texas at Austin
Austin, Texas

Rebecca Johnson Irvin, PharmD
Clinical Assistant Professor
College of Pharmacy
University of Texas at Austin
Austin, Texas
Clinical Assistant Professor
Department of Pharmacology
University of Texas Health Sciences
  Center at San Antonio
San Antonio, Texas

James M. Koeller, MS
Clinical Associate Professor of Pharmacy
University of Texas at Austin
Austin, Texas
University of Texas Health Sciences Center
  at San Antonio
San Antonio, Texas

John G. Kuhn, PharmD
Professor of Pharmacy
College of Pharmacy
University of Texas at Austin
Austin, Texas
University of Texas Health Sciences Center
  at San Antonio
San Antonio, Texas

J. Patrick McGovren, PhD
Associate Director of Cancer Research
Pharmaceutical Research and Development
The Upjohn Company
Kalamazoo, Michigan

Suzanne A. Miller, RN
Oncology Nurse Consultant
Los Gatos, California

Daniel D. Von Hoff, MD
Professor of Medicine
University of Texas Health Sciences Center
  at San Antonio
Director of Institute for Drug Development
Cancer Therapy and Research Center
San Antonio, Texas

Contents

Preface ix

Acknowledgments xi

Part I: Pharmacologic Considerations in Cancer Chemotherapy 1

Chapter 1: Cellular Basis of Chemotherapy 3
Ronald N. Buick

Chapter 2: Pharmacologic Principles 15
J. Patrick McGovren

Chapter 3: Hypercalcemia of Malignancy 35
Amy J. Galpin
Rebecca Johnson Irvin
John G. Kuhn

Part II: Chemotherapy Administration and Nursing Considerations 55

Chapter 4: Administration of Cancer Chemotherapy Agents 57
Barbara Carlile Holmes

Chapter 5: Alternative Routes of Chemotherapy Administration 95
James M. Koeller
Suzanne Fields

Chapter 6: Pharmacologic Management of Vesicant Chemotherapy Extravasation 109
Robert T. Dorr

Chapter 7: Legal Implications for the Nurse Involved in the Administration of Cytotoxic Agents 119
Suzanne A. Miller

Part III: Drug Monographs 129
Robert T. Dorr
Daniel D. Von Hoff

Acivicin 131
Aclarubicin 135
Acodazole 140
Acronycine 143
Adozelesin 146
Alanosine 148
Aldesleukin 150
Allopurinol Sodium 161
Altretamine 166
Aminoglutethimide 170
Amonafide 175
Ampligen 180
Amsacrine 182
Androgens 189
Anguidine 194
Aphidicolin Glycinate 197
Asaley 200
Asparaginase 201
5-Azacitidine 209
Azathioprine 212
Bacillus Calmette-Guérin (BCG) 216
Baker's Antifol (Soluble) 219
Beta-2'-Deoxythioguanosine 222
Bisantrene HCl 224

Bleomycin Sulfate 227
Busulfan 236
Buthionine Sulfoximine 241
BWA 773U82 248
BW 502U83·HCl 251
BW 7U85 Mesylate 253
Caracemide 254
Carbetimer 257
Carboplatin 259
Carmustine 267
Chlorambucil 275
Chloroquinoxaline Sulfonamide 279
Chlorozotocin 280
Chromomycin A$_3$ 284
Cisplatin 286
Cladribine 298
Corticosteroids 302
Corynebacterium parvum 309
CPT-11 314
Crisnatol 316
Cyclocytidine 318
Cyclophosphamide 319
Cytarabine 332
Cytembena 341
Dabis Maleate 342
Dacarbazine 343
Dactinomycin 349
Daunorubicin HCl 355
Deazauridine 365
Dexrazoxane 367
Dianhydrogalactitol 372
Diaziquone 375
Dibromodulcitol 380
Didemnin B 384

Diethyldithiocarbamate 387
Diglycoaldehyde 391
Dihydro-5-Azacytidine 393
Doxorubicin 395
Echinomycin 416
Edatrexate 419
Edelfosine 423
Eflornithine 425
Elliott's B Solution 431
Elsamitrucin 433
Epirubicin 434
Esorubicin 439
Estramustine Phosphate 443
Estrogens 446
Etanidazole 451
Ethiofos 453
Etoposide 459
Fadrazole 472
Fazarabine 474
Fenretinide 476
Filgrastim 479
Finasteride 484
Flavone Acetic Acid 485
Floxuridine 489
Fludarabine Phosphate 495
5-Fluorouracil 500
Fluosol® 515
Flutamide 518
Gallium Nitrate 521
Gemcitabine 524
Goserelin Acetate 527
Hepsulfam 529
Hexamethylene Bisacetamide 531
Homoharringtonine 536

Hydrazine Sulfate	540
4-Hydroxyandrostenedione	543
Hydroxyurea	545
Idarubicin HCl	551
Ifosfamide	558
Interferon Alfa	564
Interferon Beta	582
Interferon Gamma	585
Interleukin-1, Alpha and Beta	589
Interleukin-3	595
Interleukin-4	601
Interleukin-6	605
4-Ipomeanol	609
Iproplatin	613
Isotretinoin	617
Leucovorin Calcium	624
Leuprolide Acetate	630
Levamisole	634
Liposomal Daunorubicin	637
Liposome Encapsulated Doxorubicin	639
Lomustine	644
Lonidamine	650
Maytansine	654
Mechlorethamine Hydrochloride	657
Melphalan	662
Menogaril	673
Merbarone	678
6-Mercaptopurine	680
Mesna	685
Methanol Extraction Residue of Bacillus Calmette-Guérin	689
Methotrexate	692
N-Methylformamide	705
Mifepristone	708
Mitoguazone	711
Mitomycin-C	717
Mitotane	726
Mitoxantrone Hydrochloride	730
Monocyte/Macrophage Colony-Stimulating Factor	735
Nabilone	741
Nafoxidine	744
Neocarzinostatin	746
Octreotide Acetate	750
Ormaplatin	754
Oxaliplatin	758
Paclitaxel	761
Pala	768
Pentostatin	774
Piperazinedione	780
Pipobroman	783
Pirarubicin	784
Piritrexim	788
Piroxantrone Hydrochloride	791
PIXY-321	794
Plicamycin	797
Porfimer Sodium	801
Prednimustine	805
Procarbazine	809
Progestins	815
Pyrazofurin	821
Razoxane	825
Sargramostim	829
Semustine	837
Spirogermanium	841
Spiromustine	844
Streptonigrin	847
Streptozocin	850

Sulofenur	856
Suramin Sodium	859
Tamoxifen	866
Taxotere	875
Tegafur	878
Teniposide	882
Terephthalamidine	889
Teroxirone	891
Thioguanine	893
Thiotepa	898
Thymidine Injection	905
Tiazofurin	911
Topotecan	914
Toremifene	920
Tretinoin	922
Trifluoperazine Hydrochloride	930
Trifluridine	932
Trimetrexate	933
Tumor Necrosis Factor	939
Uracil Mustard	945
Vinblastine Sulfate	946
Vincristine Sulfate	951
Vindesine	957
Vinorelbine	966
Vinzolidine	969
Yoshi 864	973
Zorubicin	975

Appendices 979

1. Nomogram for Determination of Body Surface Area from Height and Weight—Adults 981
2. Nomogram for Determination of Body Surface Area from Height and Weight—Children ... 982
3. Formula for Estimation of Creatinine Clearance (CrCl) Using Serum Creatinine (Cr_s) 983

Index 985

Preface

The production of this second edition has been a long odyssey. The intervening 13 years have witnessed both the commercialization of many "investigational" drugs listed in the first edition, as well as the explosive growth of biotechnology agents for cancer treatment and support. There were 83 drug monographs in the first edition and 181 in this second edition. We have also included some chemopreventive agents in this edition. Because of the large number of such new anticancer agents, less space in the second edition is devoted to ancillary therapy or general toxicities. Instead, the individual drug monographs have been strengthened. An emphasis has also been made to include new recombinant proteins that have shown clinical promise for use in treating cancer or cancer drug side effects.

The information in the monographs includes many nonstandard experimental therapies and, in some cases, dosing schemes that are still being defined. Therefore, the reader is cautioned not to use this handbook as a sole source of cancer drug information and to consult primary references for current drug dosing or toxicity considerations.

Robert T. Dorr, PhD
Daniel D. Von Hoff, MD

Acknowledgments

This work is dedicated to my family, who made numerous sacrifices to allow me to complete the second edition. My wife Cindy has been a constant support as have been my children Kerry and Bobby. I also have to thank my mother Lorena B. Dorr who continually pushed my brother Bill and me towards higher educational goals. I only wish my father Lt. Col. William R. Dorr, Jr, USMC could have lived to see this. Such is the price of our freedom.

    Without the assistance of my secretary Ann Barrett this book could not have been completed. Her tireless efforts are greatly appreciated.

Robert T. Dorr, PhD

I dedicate this book to my mother and dad Stanley and Mary Anna Von Hoff, who spent long hours shaping my intellect and and giving me a great start in life. I would also like to dedicate this book to my loving wife Ann and my fantastic children Paul, Jane, and Carol, all of whom made sacrifices to help complete this book.

    I would like to acknowledge the assistance of the fine people who helped by typing the drafts of the chapters. These include Dot Bandy, Adelaida Garcia, Jennifer Klaus, PharmD, Brenda Oldham, Julia Perkins, and Cathy Robledo.

Daniel D. Von Hoff, MD

Part I

Pharmacologic Considerations in Cancer Chemotherapy

Chapter 1

Cellular Basis of Chemotherapy

Ronald N. Buick

Cancer is a disease of cells characterized by loss of the normal controlling mechanisms that maintain tissue organization. Comparisons have been made of tumor and normal tissue equivalent from which can be summarized the basic features of cancer cells:

1. Uncontrolled cell proliferation
2. Decreased cellular differentiation
3. Inappropriate ability to invade surrounding tissue
4. Ability to establish new growth at ectopic sites

Tumors increase in size because they contain a population(s) of cells that is expanding as a result of cell division. Unlike cells in normal renewing tissues, tumor cells apparently fail to respond to homeostatic control mechanisms underlying the cellular birth and death process.

Over the last few decades, cell kinetic techniques have allowed an understanding of tumor growth in relation to the proliferation of individual cells. It has been established that the proportion of proliferating cells and their rate of proliferation are characteristic of an individual tumor. Furthermore, in keeping with the origin of tumors in renewing tissues, nonproliferating cells are common and there is frequently a very high rate of cell death.

Concepts relating to the progress of cells through the cell cycle, the growth kinetics of tumors, normal tissue models of cell population dynamics and cell death, and the biochemical mechanisms of drug interactions (and resistance) are key to the definition of effective chemotherapeutic regimens, and form the basis of this chapter.

THE CELL CYCLE

Our present understanding of the cell cycle derives from experiments using [^{3}H]thymidine autoradiography and flow cytometry, which have determined that DNA synthesis takes place in a specific period of the life span of a dividing cell: the S phase. The period (gaps) between DNA synthesis and cell division (mitosis, M phase) are termed G_1 and G_2. The duration of individual phases of the cycle varies considerably from cell type to cell type and also between cells within a single tumor: M, 0.5 to 1 hour; G_1, highly variable; S, 10 to 20 hours; G_2, 2 to 10 hours. Mitosis and S phase were shown to be usually well-defined and time-conserved phases. G_2 was somewhat variable in length, whereas G_1 was highly variable in length. Later research showed that this G_1 variance was mostly the result of another "phase," G_0, wherein the cell was not actively committed to division (or was "out" of the cycle). This has allowed for the development of a circular pictorial model (see Fig 1.1) with clockwise progression through a cell cycle. This concept depends on the events between the birth of a new cell and its subsequent division being ordered as a series of unique biochemical events (Pardee 1989). In this diagram the relative times/phases are given representative dimensions and the relationships between proliferating and nonproliferating cells and cell death are portrayed.

Chemotherapeutic drugs have been classified with respect to their effects on cells as measured by cell survival assays in relation to drug dose (Fig 1.2). For many drugs, including some alkylating agents, cell survival is exponentially related to dose; the

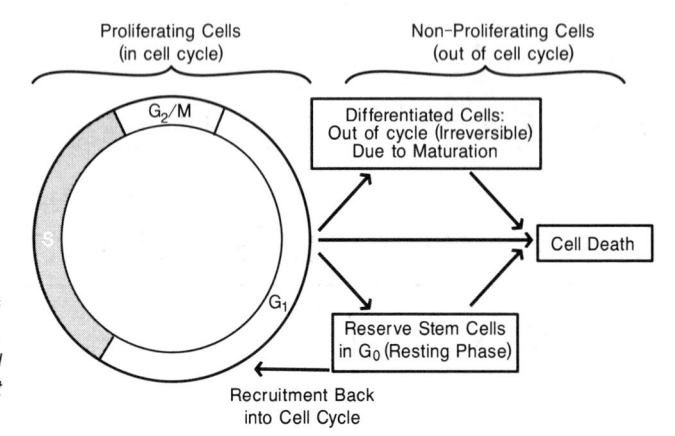

Figure 1.1. Model for the distribution of cells to phases of the cell cycle and the relationship between proliferating, nonproliferating, and dying cells. (From Tannock IF. Cell kinetics and chemotherapy: A critical review. Cancer Treat Rep. 1978;62:1117–1133. Adapted with permission.)

slope of the survival curve is related to the rate of cell proliferation. These agents exert their toxic effects irrespective of cell cycle state (non-cell cycle phase specific). On the other hand, for certain agents, survival curves show a plateau after a low-dose exponential region. This pattern of cell survival is typical of agents that are now known to act primarily at one phase of the cell (cell cycle phase specific), for example, antimetabolites and tubulin-binding agents such as methotrexate, cytarabine, and vincristine. Cell cycle phase-specific agents, in general, depend on the production of some type of unique biochemical blockade of a particular reaction(s) occurring in a single phase of the cell cycle.

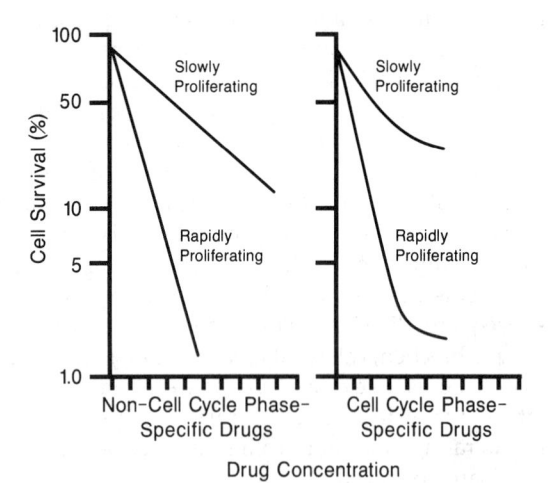

Figure 1.2. Theoretical cell survival curves for rapidly and slowly proliferating cells subsequent to a short exposure to drugs that are not cell cycle specific and drugs that are active in one phase of the cell cycle. (From Tannock IF, Hill RT, eds. The Basic Science of Oncology. New York: Pergamon Press; 1992. Adapted with permission.)

Many antimetabolites exert their lethal effects only on cells that are actively synthesizing DNA, whereas methotrexate and doxorubicin have maximum toxicity in S phase, but also have some activity during other phases of the cycle. Vincristine and vinblastine are known to disrupt formation of the mitotic spindle, leading to arrest of cells in mitosis (lethality, however, occurs when cells are in S phase, when mitotic spindle formation is initiated). Bleomycin acts mainly in G_2 phase in some cells, but with no specificity in other cells. Table 1.1 is a partial list of drugs classified on the basis of cell cycle specificity.

As the relative specificity of phase-targeted agents results in partly synchronized cell populations after treatment, these agents can achieve a greater overall cell kill when applied in multiple repeated fractions scheduled to take advantage of the cyclical accumulation of phase-sensitive cells. Although this principle is well established in animal tumor models, the wide spread in cell cycle times in human tumors renders this difficult to achieve clinically.

GROWTH KINETICS OF TUMORS AND NORMAL TISSUES

Tumor growth can be determined by measuring tumor volume as a function of time. Such estimations have been difficult to perform for human tumors because few tumors can ethically be left untreated, the time available for measurement is likely a small proportion of the tumor life, and measurements have been restricted to relatively few sites, for example, superficial metastases or lung metastases

TABLE 1.1. CELL CYCLE (PHASE)-SPECIFIC DRUGS

S phase dependent
    Antimetabolites
        Cytarabine (Ara-C®, Cytosar-U®, Aracytidine®)
        Doxorubicin (Adriamycin®, Adriacin®, Adriblastina®)
        5-Fluorouracil (Efudex®, Fluoroplex®, Fluorouracil Injection®)
        6-Mercaptopurine (Purinethol®)
        Methotrexate (Methotrexate Sodium®, Mexate®, Rheumatrex®)
        6-Thioguanine (Tabloid® brand, Lanvis®)
        Hydroxyurea (Hydrea®, Litalir®)
        Prednisone (Deltasone®, Decortin®, Meticortin®)
        Procarbazine (Matulane®, Natulan®)
        Diglycoaldehyde
M phase dependent
    Vinca alkaloids*
        Vincristine (Oncovin®, Vincasar®)
        Vinblastine (Velban®, Velbe®, Velsar®)
Colchicine derivatives
    Trimethylcolchicinic acid
Podophyllotoxins
    Etoposide (VP-16-213®, VePesid®)
    Teniposide (VM-26®, Vehem®, Vumon®)
G_2 phase dependent
    Bleomycin (Blenoxane®)
G_1 phase dependent
    Asparaginase (Elspar®)
    Diglycoaldehyde (also in early S phase)
    Corticosteroids

*Have greatest effects in S phase and possibly late G_2; cell blockade or death, however, occurs during early mitosis

measured on radiographs. A number of generalizations can, however, be made; (1) Tumor growth is exponential, at least over part of its life history. (2) There is a wide variation in growth rate among tumors, even those of the same histology; representative doubling times for lung metastases of common tumors are 2 to 3 months. (3) There is a tendency for childhood tumors and chemotherapy-sensitive tumors (eg, testicular carcinoma, lymphoma) to grow more rapidly than unresponsive tumors (eg, colon cancer). For a detailed review of the literature in this field, the reader is referred to the work of Steel (1977).

Explanation of the heterogeneity in growth rates of human tumors depends on knowledge of the fates and potentials of individual tumor cells. For this reason a variety of cell kinetic and tissue culture approaches have been developed including thymidine autoradiography and flow cytometry-based procedures and clonogenic assays designed to track the influence of individual cells on tumor growth. As the chemotherapeutic sensitivity of a tumor may be influenced by the population of cells in active cell cycle, by the heterogeneity of rate of cell cycle progression, and by the growth potential (clonogenicity) of individual cells, a detailed discussion is warranted of the terms and definitions in the field of cell kinetics.

Cell Cycle Times

The use of labeled thymidine has provided a unique marker with which to investigate the life history of individual cells in tissues. Because thymidine is incorporated specifically into proliferating cells, proportions of replicating cells can be quantitated by autoradiography. An alternate technique involving incorporation of the thymidine analog 5-bromodeoxyuridine (5-BrdU) has been developed. When this precursor is used by replicating cells, 5-BrdU-substituted DNA can be detected by antibody-based techniques. The proportion of labeled cells in the tissue a short interval (usually 1 hour) after injection of [^{3}H]thymidine or 5-BudR into an animal or patient is called the labeling index (LI). If all cells in the population were proliferating at an equivalent rate the LI would be related to the ratio of the time of S phase (T_S) to total cell cycle time (T_c). Estimation of the cell cycle time and the duration of individual phases of the cell cycle often utilizes the percentage labeled mitoses (PLM) method. Serial biopsies are taken at intervals after a [^{3}H]thymidine injection and the proportion of labeled mitoses is estimated. The passage of labeled cells that were initially in S phase through the M phase leads to waves of labeled mitoses with a width of T_s and a separation of T_c.

Growth Fraction

Growth fraction is the term used to describe the overall proportion of proliferating cells in a given population. It is computed from a knowledge of cell cycle phase durations, which allows calculation of the proportion of proliferating cells in DNA synthesis. A comparison of this number with the LI (the proportion of all cells in DNA synthesis) provides the growth fraction. Growth fraction has proven to be a useful indicator of overall sensitivity to cycle-dependent chemotherapeutic agents.

Cell Loss

The doubling time (T_D) of tumor growth rarely is as rapid as would be expected from the growth fraction and cell cycle times. Many of the cells produced during the growth of a tumor are subsequently lost, possibly through necrosis, metastases, or differentiation. The cell loss factor is described as

$$1 - \frac{\text{potential doubling time}}{\text{actual doubling time}}.$$

Cell Proliferation in Normal Tissues

The application of similar cell kinetic techniques to normal tissues allows the classification of tissues by proliferation rate (Fig 1.3). It is of interest that the side effects of chemotherapy (eg, mucositis, myelosuppression, sterility) occur in tissues that are rapidly proliferating, reflecting the greater toxicity of chemotherapeutic agents to proliferating cells. Such tissues are known to rely on stem cell renewal processes for expansion and maintenance of short-lived differentiated cells (Potten et al 1979, Wright and Alison 1984). In such tissues, cell production is balanced by cell loss to provide for tissue homeostasis. Considerable evidence suggests that, under normal conditions, stem cells are less likely to be in cycle than those cells in the expanding population. Thus, stem cells of normal tissues may be regarded as being in a privileged state with respect to susceptibility to cell-cycle-specific chemotherapeutic agents.

Considerable detailed knowledge has been accumulated concerning the cellular organization of hematopoietic tissue. In particular, knowledge is now available on the molecules that regulate lineage-specific cell production (the colony-stimulating factors). The molecular cloning and expression of these molecules have allowed their use in vivo (Clark and Kamen 1987). The ability to overcome drug-induced myelosuppression promises to vastly improve the therapeutic ratio of drugs limited by bone marrow toxicity.

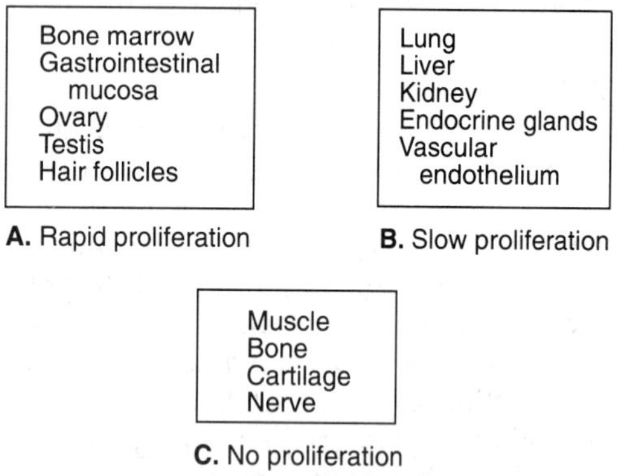

Cell Proliferation in Human Tumors

Cell kinetic techniques have been applied to human tumors either through rare in vivo administration of [^{3}H-]thymidine or 5-BrdU or, more commonly, through incubation of fresh biopsies with [^{3}H-]thymidine in vitro. Representative LI values for several types of solid tumor and leukemia are listed in Table 1.2. Typical values of LI for common solid tumors are 2 to 8%, whereas in lymphomas cell proliferation is more rapid. It is of interest to compare these values with the LI of a rapidly renewing epithelial tissue such as intestinal mucosa ($\approx$ 16%). Likewise, typical values of LI in acute leukemias (5–11%) are lower than those in the myeloid precursors in normal bone marrow (30–70%). Accumulation of tumor cells, even in acute leukemia, is therefore not due to an increased rate of proliferation. Rather, there is defective maturation that causes the rate of cell proliferation to exceed the rate of cell death or removal from the population.

In a few circumstances serial biopsies from leukemias or superficial solid tumors have allowed an estimation of cell cycle parameters (T_c and T_s) by PLM methodology. Mean values of T_c and T_s for acute leukemia and solid tumors tend to be rather similar (60 and 20 hours, respectively), despite widely different rates of growth. It follows from these statements of low LI values and relatively rapid T_c and T_s that most human tumors have a low ($\approx$ 20%) growth fraction. This, of course, could con-

A. Rapid proliferation
Bone marrow
Gastrointestinal mucosa
Ovary
Testis
Hair follicles

B. Slow proliferation
Lung
Liver
Kidney
Endocrine glands
Vascular endothelium

C. No proliferation
Muscle
Bone
Cartilage
Nerve

Figure 1.3. Classification of tissues by rate of proliferation: **A.** Renewal tissues, rapid proliferation, labeling index (LI) > 5%. **B.** Slowly proliferating, expanding tissues, LI < 1%. **C.** Nonproliferative tissues. *(From Tannock IF, Hill RT, eds. The Basic Science of Oncology. New York: Pergamon Press; 1992. Adapted with permission.)*

TABLE 1.2. REPRESENTATIVE VALUES OF THE LABELING INDEX OBTAINED FROM STUDIES OF HUMAN TUMOR BIOPSIES

Type of Tumor	Mean or Median Labeling Index
Breast	2
Colon	3
Lung/larynx	8
Lymphoma	30
Squamous cell carcinoma (various sites)	8
Acute myelogenous leukemia (bone marrow)	5–11
Acute lymphoid leukemia (bone marrow)	4–12

tribute to the relative resistance of many slow-growing human tumors to cycle-active therapy.

Computation from typical LIs (2–8%) suggests that common human tumors could have a potential doubling time of approximately 20 days; however, typical actual volume doubling times are 2 to 3 months. The apparent discrepancy can be accounted for by a cell loss factor, which approaches 80 to 90% for many common tumors; that is, 80 to 90% of new cell production is subsequently lost from the growing tumor mass.

The preceding results have shown that proliferating cells in human tumors may cycle quite rapidly, although no more so than cells in normal renewal tissues. The rate of volume growth of tumors is typically quite slow based on a large population of nonproliferating cells and a high rate of cell death. Unrestrained cell proliferation is not, therefore, a common hallmark of tumors. Rather, tumors appear to represent caricatures of normal renewal tissues (Pierce et al 1978) in which a defect in homeostasis leads to an imbalance in the rates of cell production and cell loss.

STEM CELL CONCEPT APPLIED TO TUMORS

Two general theories have been proposed about carcinogenesis in renewing tissues. First, a carcinogenic event might occur in a differentiated cell of a particular tissue, rendering that cell proliferative although still able to organize tissue-specific differentiation. The acquisition of proliferative features in a differentiated cell necessitates the concept of "dedifferentiation," but there is no convincing evidence that this may occur. An alternative theory proposes that tumors arise from carcinogenic events occurring in the stem cells of a particular tissue (Mackillop et al 1983). The properties of stem cells are such that it is not necessary to assume "dedifferentiation" as a mechanism of tumor induction. Rather, it is proposed that the changes associated with the carcinogenic insult cause a defect in the control of the normal stem-cell functions, self-renewal and differentiation.

Much evidence supports the validity of stem cell mechanisms in the initiation and growth of human tumors (Selby et al 1983). First, the monoclonal origin of tumors that contain cells from multiple lineages of differentiation (eg, chronic myelogenous leukemia) is consistent with the cell of origin being a stem cell. Second, tissue-specific differentiation is a distinguishing feature of many human tumors, and evidence exists to support the ability of human tumor cells to differentiate in vivo and in vitro; in many tumors an inverse relationship has been observed between indices of cell proliferation and differentiation. Third, experience with radiation therapy suggests that in many human tumors, only a small proportion of tumor cells have the capacity to regenerate the tumor after subcurative therapy. These conclusions are based on knowledge of the quantitative radiation sensitivity of human cells and the fact that relatively small doses of radiation can achieve permanent local control of large skin, breast, and cervical tumors (Bush and Hill 1975). These results can be explained if the proportion of stem cells in such tumors was approximately 1 in 1000, as only stem cells would need to be sterilized to achieve cure.

The stem cell model has major implications for the treatment of human tumors (Fig 1.4). When the aim of treatment is cure or long-term control, then therapy must be directed toward eradication of stem cells, as only these cells maintain the potential to regenerate the tumor population (Mackillop et al 1983). If stem cells represent a small subpopulation of the total cells in some tumors, as suggested by the results of treatment with radiotherapy, then short-term changes in tumor volume may not reflect the effects of treatment on stem cells.

A common method for measuring stem cell properties involves placing the cells in an environment in which they may express their potential to generate a large number of progeny, that is, a colony-forming assay. The degree to which colony-forming assays in culture reflect the stem cell nature of cell populations in tumors is controversial (Selby et al 1983). A number of attempts have been made to use such procedures to gain productive information concerning tumor chemotherapeutic response (eg Salmon et al 1978), but as yet there has been little evidence of impact on therapy outcome.

MODELS OF TUMOR GROWTH AND CHEMOTHERAPY EFFECTS

Gompertzian Model

When tumor growth is plotted against time on semilogarithmic scales, growth curves are convex upward and flatten out with time; that is, in most cases growth rate decreases with time. This relationship

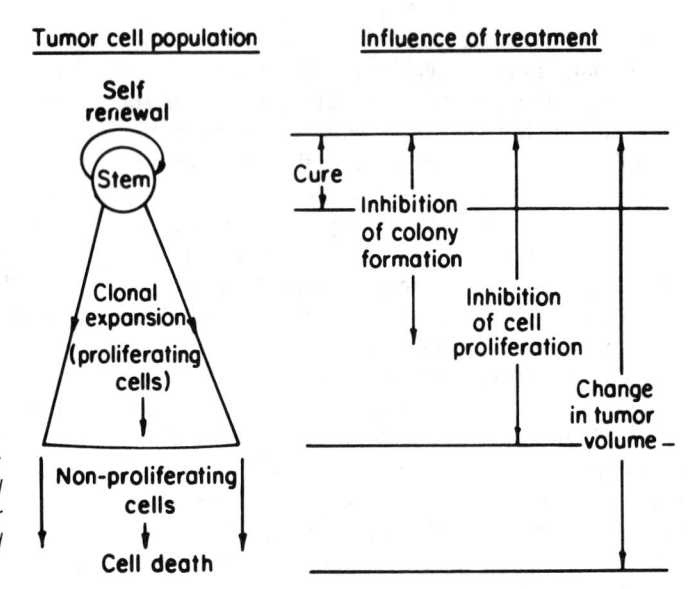

Figure 1.4. Implications of the stem cell model for cancer treatment. *(From Mackillop WJ, Ciampi A, Till JE, Buick RN. A stem cell model of human tumor growth. J Natl Cancer Inst. 1983;70:9–16. Adapted with permission.)*

has been found to be accommodated by the Gompertz equation. Gompertz was a German insurance actuary who described the relationship of an individual's age to expected time of death by means of an asymmetric sigmoidal curve.

Figure 1.5 demonstrates several current chemotherapy principles plotted against a Gompertz tumor growth curve. Also noted is the rather large tumor cell burden required to produce clinical symptomatology. The outcome of two treatment regimens is outlined. In each case, the treatment is equally effective, producing a 2-log tumor cell reduction. Only with the more frequently given regimen, however, is total eradication possible. In reality, such consecutive 2-log reductions are not consistently achievable. Thus, initial therapy for many solid tumors involves primarily other modalities (eg, surgery and irradiation) to achieve bulk tumor reduction. Then adjuvant chemotherapy and/or immunotherapy are optimally added to eradicate micrometastatic (subclinical) tumor masses. The same general principle is followed in

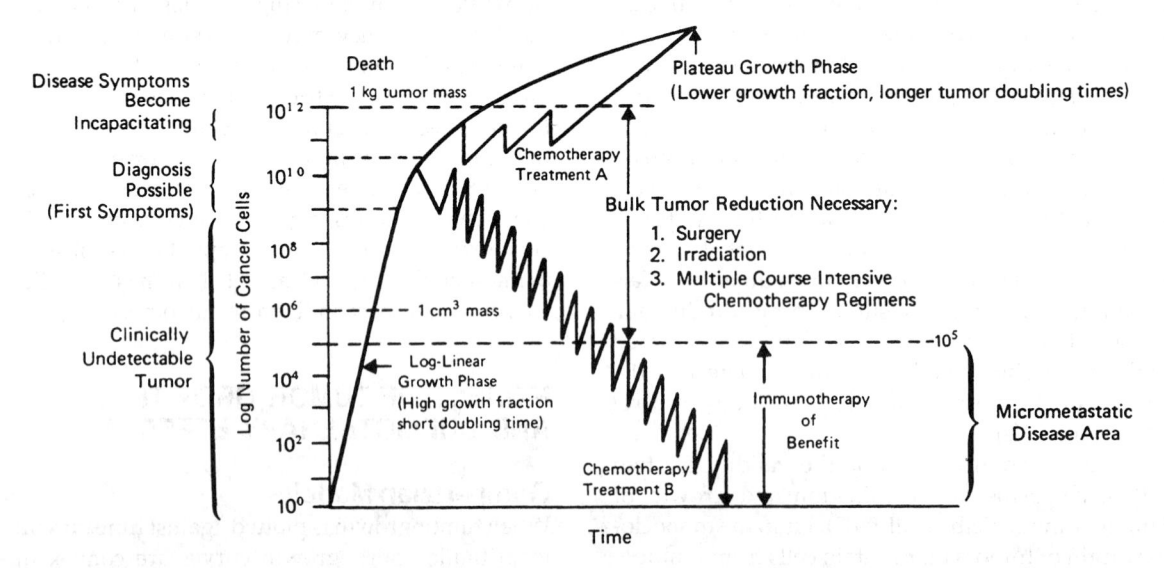

Figure 1.5. Gompertzian kinetics tumor growth curve: relationship to symptoms, diagnosis, and various treatment regimens.

hematologic malignancies, wherein an intensive "induction" chemotherapy regimen is used to provide bulk tumor reduction, perhaps producing a remission. This is then followed with less intensive consolidation and remission maintenance doses of chemotherapy to provide control for subclinical tumor burdens.

Cell-Kill Hypothesis

The fundamental kinetic consideration in cancer chemotherapy is the "cell-kill" hypothesis, derived from detailed studies in animal tumor systems. Basically, the effects of cancer chemotherapy on tumor cell populations follow first-order kinetic principles. This simply means that the number of cells killed by a particular agent or combination of drugs is proportional to one variable, the dose used. (For this purpose, relative sensitivity is not considered, and the growth rate is assumed constant.) Importantly, the proportion of tumor cells killed is a constant percentage of the total number of cells present. In other words, chemotherapy kills a constant proportion of cells, not a constant number of cells. Furthermore, chemotherapy follows an exponential or log-kill model. Particular treatments, then, may be said to have a specific exponential or "log-kill" potential. For example, a log-kill of 2 reduces a theoretical human tumor burden of 10^9 cells to 10^7 cells. Although this represents 99% reduction, at least 10,000,000 viable cells (10^7) are left. A log-kill of 3 would impart a 99.9% reduction, but would leave 1,000,000 (10^6) cells remaining in this same example. The fractional reductions possible with cancer chemotherapy, therefore, can theoretically never completely reduce tumor populations to zero.

This traditional cell-kill model of Skipper and Schabel (Schabel 1975) is based primarily on exponentially growing laboratory tumors such as L-1210 murine leukemia. An alternative to the constant first-order log-kill hypothesis proposed by Norton and Simon (1977) holds that clinical tumor regressions as a result of chemotherapy are probably best explained by the relative growth fraction present in the tumor at the time of treatment. Thus, very small and large tumors are less responsive than those of intermediate size, where the Gompertzian growth fraction is maximal. Log cell kills in this model occur only at times of maximal tumor growth fraction.

Although this model has not been directly confirmed clinically, it does explain some clinical observations of chemotherapy responses in large and small tumors in humans. Certainly, further work is necessary in this area to validate these models or to suggest alternatives.

SELECTIVITY OF ANTICANCER DRUGS

There is a common belief that cancer chemotherapy generally produces nonselective cell killing on normal as well as cancerous tissues. Although this belief is somewhat true for agents such as mechlorethamine (Mustargen®, HN2®) and carmustine (BCNU®) the majority of anticancer drugs act more against tumor than normal tissues. For example, in a sensitive lymphoma the effect on tumor cells can be more than 10,000 times greater than that on normal bone marrow cells.

The hormonal agents are probably the best examples of truly selective anticancer agents; however, the selectivity for the cytotoxic chemotherapy agents appears to inversely follow cell cycle specificity. Therefore, the non-cell cycle phase-specific agents tend to be less selective. These agents, such as mechlorethamine, carmustine, and other nitrosoureas, tend to produce much more toxic effects on normal bone marrow.

In addition to the hormones, a few other anticancer drugs kill cancer cells by taking advantage of unique biochemical differences. Most agents are effective at key enzymatic sites with equal potential activities in normal and neoplastic cells. The enzyme asparaginase takes advantage of the relative deficiency in some leukemic cells of aspartic acid synthetase. At high concentrations uptake of methotrexate by cancer cells is apparently selective. This uptake can be experimentally enhanced by vincristine or asparaginase and inhibited by aminoglycosides and cephalosporin antibiotics. Prostatic tumors and tumors rich in acid can somewhat selectively activate the hormone diethylstilbestrol phosphate (DES®, Stilbestrol®) intracellularly.

Much research needs to be done in the search for drugs that can exploit the unique biochemical differences between normal and neoplastic cells. Tumor drug selectivity must still be based largely on differences in the cell kinetics of normal and neoplastic cell lines. Even though the cell-kill hypothesis probably explains a portion of drug selectivity, there certainly are other mechanisms involved. In addition, normal systems can theoretically withstand greater cellular losses to chemotherapy than can tumors, even though the proportions killed in both might be identical. Overall, the more responsive tumors are those with large growth fractions.

Tissue-type drug sensitivity is recognized for some anticancer agents. The antimetabolite 5-fluorouracil is more active on cancers arising from endodermal tissues such as neoplasms of the gastrointestinal tract and the breast. With dacarbazine (DTIC®, DTIC-Dome®) there is some selective action for melanoma cells. Bleomycin is active against epithelial tumors (eg, squamous cell cancers of lung and cervix).

DRUG RESISTANCE

The acquisition of resistance to chemotherapeutic drugs, a well-documented clinical phenomenon, presents a major obstacle to effective therapy. Underlying molecular and cellular mechanisms are not totally understood but represent an extremely active area of investigation. Drug resistance involves cellular selection; populations of drug-resistant cells may be inherently produced by clonal evolution (Nowell 1976) or mutation, perhaps under the influence of a mutagenic cytotoxic agent. At the molecular level there appear to be a number of major mechanisms by which drug resistance can be acquired (Table 1.3). For a review see Fox and Fox (1984). Intracellular effects that bring about drug resistance are often secondary to cellular adaptation to altered enzyme levels or properties. The most studied example relates to methotrexate resistance; in cell culture systems, drug resistance in this case can be attributed to increased intracellular levels of the enzyme dihydrofolate reductase (Schimke 1984). Alkylating agents and cisplatin (Platinol®, Cisplatyl®, Neoplatin®) induce cell death by binding to DNA and causing crosslinks and breakage of DNA strands. Cells may be resistant to these drugs through a number of mechanisms, including decreased cellular uptake, reduced drug activation, and increased inactivation of alkylating species; however, a major determinant of resistance to alkylating agents appears to be the capacity for repair of lesions in DNA. Resistance to antimetabolite drugs may derive from a number of mechanisms. These include impaired drug transport into cells, overproduction or reduced affinity of the molecular target, stimulation of alternative biochemical pathways, and impaired activation or increased catabolism of the drug.

TABLE 1.3. PROBABLE MECHANISMS ASSOCIATED WITH RESISTANCE TO COMMONLY USED ANTICANCER DRUGS

Mechanism	Drug
Increased efficiency of DNA repair	Cisplatin, cyclophosphamide, melphalan, mitomycin-C, mechlorethamine, nitrosoureas
Decreased cellular uptake or increased efflux of drugs	Actinomycin, daunorubicin, doxorubicin, melphalan, 6-mercaptopurine, methotrexate, mechlorethamine, vincristine, vinblastine
Increased levels of "target" enzyme	Methotrexate
Alterations in "target" enzyme	5-Fluorouracil, 6-mercaptopurine, methotrexate, 6-thioguanine
Decreased drug activation	Cytarabine, doxorubicin, 5-fluorouracil, 6-mercaptopurine, 6-thioguanine
Increased drug breakdown	Bleomycin, cytarabine, 6-mercaptopurine
Alternative biochemical pathways	Cytarabine

From Tannock IF, Hill RT, eds. The Basic Science of Oncology. New York: Pergamon Press; 1992. Adapted with permission.

There is a considerable body of evidence that many types of drug resistance are generated by genetic mechanisms. In tissue culture, drug-resistant cells can be generated at a frequency consistent with known rates of genetic mutation. Mutagenic agents (such as ethylmethanesulfonate) increase the frequency of generation of drug-resistant cells. This may be of significance clinically, as many chemotherapeutic agents are themselves mutagenic. Further evidence derives from the ability to transfer drug-resistant phenotypes to drug-sensitive cells by transfer of DNA in vitro. This phenomenon may have clinical relevance if drug resistance can be transferred to repopulating bone marrow cells in autologous rescue situations.

Genetic changes underlying drug resistance can be based on point mutation or gene amplification. Resistance based on an altered gene product resulting from a point mutation(s) would be expected to occur in single cells at a single step. The frequency of resistant cells would be expected to be independent of the concentration of drug used for selection, and once selected, the mutation should be stable. Although such mechanisms are common in tissue culture cell circumstances (eg, mutations in

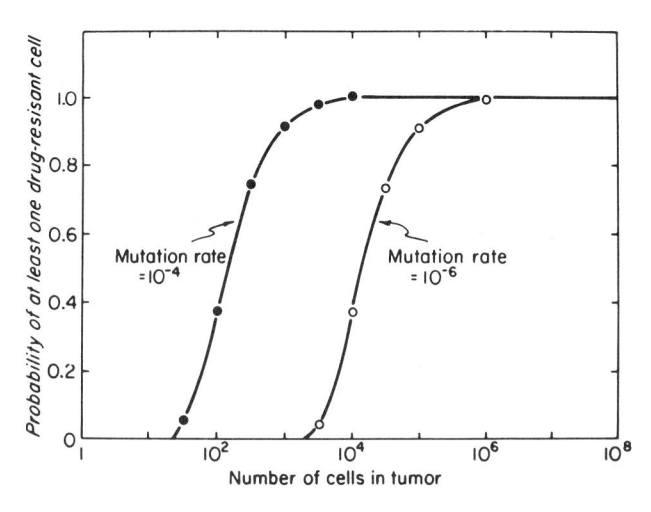

Figure 1.6. Theoretical relationship between tumor growth and acquisition of drug-resistant clones based on mutation rate. Probability that at least one drug-resistant cell/tumor increases to unity over a relatively short period in life history of a tumor. (From Goldie JH, Coldman AJ. The genetic origin of drug resistance in neoplasms: Implications for systemic therapy. Cancer Res. 1984;44:3643–3653. Adapted with permission.)

the HPRT gene), their significance for human tumor responses to therapy are not clear.

In contrast to point mutation, gene amplification appears to occur in a stepwise manner and is influenced by the concentration of the selecting drug. Evidence suggests that gene amplification may play a role in clinical drug resistance (eg, overproduction of P-glycoprotein; see later text). There is wide speculation that conditions of chemotherapy treatment may facilitate gene amplification through mutational effects or cell cycle progression delay.

The potential appearance of drug-resistant mutants among tumor cell populations has important implications for planning optimal chemotherapy. Goldie and Coldman (1984) have demonstrated that the probability of at least one drug-resistant cell being present in a tumor population is dependent on tumor size (Fig 1.6). On the basis of assumptions concerning rates of mutation to drug resistance and the number of cell divisions required to generate clinically detectable tumors, it is suggested that drug resistance will impact treatment of all human tumors. This implies a greater chance of cure if therapy is begun early, when the total burden of tumor cells is low. The Goldie–Coldman model also predicts a better therapeutic effect when different schedules of two equally effective and non-cross-resistant drugs are alternated, rather than given sequentially, as this minimizes the emergence of cell populations that are resistant to both drugs.

MULTIPLE DRUG RESISTANCE

An important aspect of drug resistance relates to the fact that cells selected for resistance to one of a group of drugs often show cross-resistance (Table 1.4) to each of the other drugs in the group (for review, see Bradley et al 1988). Many of the drugs within a group might have quite different chemical structures, but most of them are derived from natural products. Resistance was demonstrated to be based on reduced uptake of the selecting drug or other cross-resistant agents. The molecular basis for this form of drug resistance has been shown to be based on the overexpression of a membrane glycoprotein (gp170) termed *P-glycoprotein*. Overexpression is frequently associated with gene amplification, and the degree of resistance correlates with the

TABLE 1.4. FAMILY OF DRUGS ASSOCIATED WITH CROSS-RESISTANCE AND EXPRESSION OF P-GLYCOPROTEIN

Colchicine (ColBENEMID®)	Melphalan (Alkeran®, Sarcoclorin®) (weaker association)
Dactinomycin (actinomycin D; Cosmegen®)	Podophyllotoxin
Daunorubicin (daunomycin; Cerubidine®)	Puromycin (Stylomycin®)
Doxorubicin (Adriamycin®, Adriacin®, Adriblastina®)	Vinblastine (Velban®, Velbe®, Velsar®)
Emetine	Vincristine (Oncorin®, Vincasar®)
Etoposide (VP-16-213®, VePesid®)	Vindesine (Eldisine®)

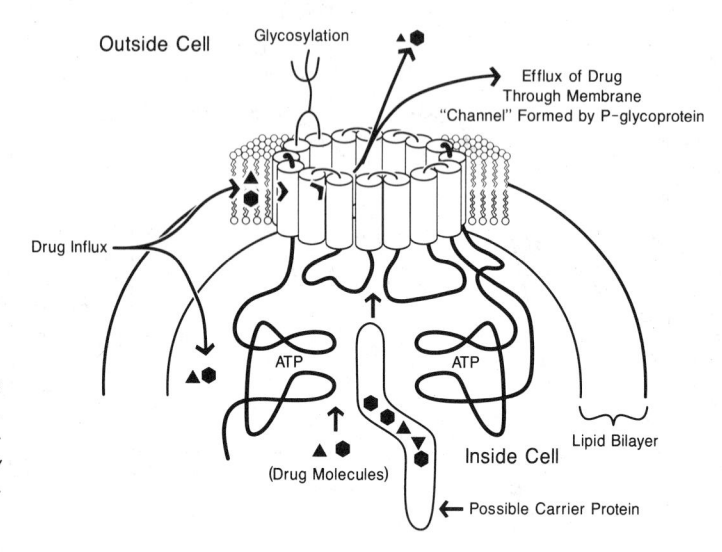

Figure 1.7. Model of the P-glycoprotein molecule as a channel-forming ATP-dependent export pump. (From Endicott JA, Ling V. The biochemistry of P-glycoprotein-mediated drug resistance. Annu Rev Biochem. 1989;58:137–171. Adapted with permission.)

amount of P-glycoprotein expressed in the cell membrane. CDNA cloning work has shown that a family of P-glycoproteins are encoded by related genes. Drug resistance can be induced in drug-sensitive cells by gene transfer. The recent elucidation of the putative structure of the molecule (Fig 1.7) implies a role as a drug efflux pump (Endicott and Ling 1989).

Recent evidence has shown the utility of knowledge of P-glycoprotein overexpression in soft tissue sarcoma of childhood (Chan et al 1990). It will be important to seek methods to reverse the phenomenon. Preliminary evidence suggests that drugs that inhibit calcium influx (eg, verapamil), drugs that inhibit the calcium-binding protein calmodulin, and other drugs that tend to stabilize membranes (eg, quinidine) all tend to restore partial sensitivity without alerting the drug sensitivity of normal tissues.

DRUG SENSITIVITY VERSUS TUMOR KINETICS AND HISTOLOGY

Mean kinetic parameters and overall tumor responsiveness to chemotherapy were tabulated from Charbit et al (1971) (Table 1.5). As discussed previously, considerable variability exists from one tumor to the next, yet these data, though general, are helpful in relating tumor histology and kinetic behavior to anticancer drug sensitivity.

In addition, DeVita et al (1975) related apparent responsiveness to chemotherapy to tumor type and grouped tumors into four categories (Table 1.6). Tumors in group I are highly chemosensitive, whereas tumors in group IV are much less responsive. As improved drug treatment programs become available and more tumor types must be considered as responsive, these lists are changing.

With the classification of DeVita et al placed

TABLE 1.5. RELATIONSHIP BETWEEN KINETIC PARAMETERS AND RELATIVE CHEMOTHERAPEUTIC SENSITIVITY

Histologic Type	Doubling Time (d)	Labeling Index (%)	Growth Fraction (%)	Drug Sensitivity
Embryonal tumors (testis)	27	30	90	+++
Malignant lymphomas	29	29	40–90	++
Mesenchymal sarcomas	41	4	11	−
Squamous cell carcinomas	58	8	25	+
Adenocarcinomas	83	2	6	±

TABLE 1.6. CLASSIFICATION OF TUMORS ACCORDING TO GENERAL SENSITIVITY TO CHEMOTHERAPY

Group I	Group II
Cancers in Which Drugs Have Been Responsible for Some Patients Achieving a Normal Life Span	*Cancers in Which Responders to Chemotherapy Have Demonstrated Improvements in Survival*
Acute leukemia in children	Ovarian carcinoma
Hodgkin's disease	Breast carcinoma
Histiocytic lymphoma	Adult acute leukemias
Skin cancer	Multiple myeloma
Testicular carcinoma	Endometrial carcinoma
Embryonal carcinoma	Prostatic cancer
Rhabdomyosarcoma	Lymphocytic lymphomas
Ewing's sarcoma	Neuroblastoma
Wilms' tumor	Adrenal cortical carcinoma
Burkitt's lymphoma	Malignant insulinoma
Retinoblastoma	Stomach cancer
Choriocarcinoma	Cervical cancer

Group III	Group IV
Cancers Responsive to Drugs for Which Clinically Useful Improvements in Survival of Responders Have Not Been Clearly Demonstrated	*Cancers Only Marginally Responsive or Unresponsive to Chemotherapeutic Agents*
Head and neck cancers	Hypernephroma
Gastrointestinal cancer	Bladder carcinoma
Central nervous system cancer	Cancer of the esophagus
Endocrine gland tumors	Epidermoid carcinoma of the lung
Malignant melanoma	Pancreatic carcinoma
Malignant carcinoid tumors	Hepatocellular carcinoma
Osteogenic sarcomas	Thyroid carcinoma
Soft tissue sarcomas	

From DeVita VT, Young RC, Canellos Gp. Combination versus single agent chemotherapy: A review of the basis for selection of drug treatment of cancer. *Cancer.* 1975;35:98–110. Modified with permission.

into historical perspective, there would not have been any advanced cancers listed under group I 20 to 30 years ago. Thus, the dramatic advances of chemotherapy involving multiple drug combinations and augmented patient support capabilities have occurred over a relatively short period of medical history. This has provided for an accelerating shift of tumors in each category toward more chemosensitive classifications. An increase in life span for greater number of patients is now conceivable.

REFERENCES

Bradley G, Juranka PF, Ling V. Mechanisms of multidrug resistance. *Biochim Biophys Acta.* 1988;**948**:87–128.

Bush RS, Hill RP. Biologic discussion augmenting radiation effects and model systems. *Laryngoscope.* 1975;**85**(7):1119–1133.

Chan HSL, Thorner PS, Haddad G, Ling V. Immunohistochemical detection of P-glycoprotein: Prognostic correlation in soft tissue sarcoma of childhood. *J Clin Oncol.* 1990;**8**:689–704.

Charbit A, Malaise EP, Tubiana M. Relation between the pathological nature and the growth rate of human tumors. *Eur J Cancer.* 1971;**7**:307–315.

Clark SC, Kamen R. The human hematopoietic colony-stimulating factors. *Science.* 1987;**236**:1229–1237.

DeVita VT, Young RC, Canellos GP. Combination versus single agent chemotherapy: A review of the basis for selection of drug treatment of cancer. *Cancer.* 1975;**35**:98–110.

Endicott JA, Ling V. The biochemistry of P-glycoprotein-mediated drug resistance. *Annu Rev Biochem.* 1989;**58**:137–171.

Fox BW, Fox M, eds. *Antitumor Drug Resistance.* Berlin: Springer-Verlag; 1984.

Goldie JH, Coldman AJ. The genetic origin of drug resistance in neoplasms: Implications for systemic therapy. *Cancer Res.* 1984;**44**:3643–3653.

Mackillop WJ, Ciampi A, Till JE, Buick RN. A stem cell model of human tumor growth. *J Nat Cancer Inst.* 1983;**70**:9–16.

Norton L, Simon R. Tumor size, sensitivity to therapy, and design of treatment schedules. *Cancer Treat Rep.* 1977;**61**:1307–1317.

Nowell PC. The clonal evolution of tumor cell populations. *Science.* 1976;**194**:23–28.

Pardee AB. G$_1$ events and regulation of cell proliferation. *Science.* 1989;**246**:603–608.

Pierce GB, Shike R, Fink LM. *Cancer: A Problem of Developmental Biology.* Englewood Cliffs, NJ: Prentice-Hall; 1978.

Potten CJ, Schofield R, Lathja LG. A comparison of cell replacement in bone marrow and three regions of surface epithelium. *Biochim Biophys Acta.* 1979;**560**:281–299.

Salmon SE, Hamburger AW, Soehnlen BS, et al. Quantitation of differential sensitivity of human tumor stem cells to anticancer drugs. *N Engl J Med.* 1978;**298**:1321–1327.

Schabel FM Jr. Concepts for systemic treatment of micrometastases. *Cancer.* 1975;**35**:15–24.

Schimke RT. Gene amplification, drug resistance and cancer. *Cancer Res.* 1984;**44**:1735–1742.

Selby P, Buick RN, Tannock I. A critical appraisal of the "human tumor stem cell assay." *N Engl J Med.* 1983;**308**:129–134.

Steel GG. *Growth Kinetics of Tumours: Cell Population Kinetics in Relation to the Growth and Treatment of Cancer.* Oxford: Clarendon Press; 1977.

Tannock IF. Cell kinetics and chemotherapy: A critical review. *Cancer Treat Rep.* **62**:1117–1133.

Tannock IF, Hill RT, eds. *The Basic Science of Oncology.* New York: Pergamon Press; 1992.

Wright N, Alison M. *The Biology of Epithelial Cell Populations.* Oxford: Clarendon Press; 1984.

Chapter 2

Pharmacologic Principles

J. Patrick McGovren

This chapter summarizes information on the mechanisms of action of the marketed and group C cytotoxic and hormonal anticancer drugs and on the clinical pharmacologic and toxicologic characteristics shared by agents of similar mechanism. A separate chapter addresses the immunotherapeutic agents. The individual drugs are discussed in detail in the drug monographs in Part III.

Cancer chemotherapeutic agents are classified in this chapter by their currently accepted mechanisms of action into five categories:

1. *DNA-interactive agents, which alter DNA structure and interfere with its template functions*
2. *Antimetabolites, structural mimics of natural metabolites that disrupt nucleic acid synthesis either by fraudulent incorporation into DNA or RNA or by inhibition of normal precursor biosynthesis or polymerization*
3. *Tubulin-interactive drugs, which poison the cellular machinery for mitotic cell division*
4. *Hormonal agents, which inhibit the growth of endocrine-responsive neoplastic tissues directly through specific receptor interactions or indirectly through modulation of endogenous hormone metabolism*
5. *Miscellaneous drugs, which do not fit the other classes*

Table 2.1 categorizes the commercially available anticancer drugs by their mechanisms and lists their major uses, either singly or in combination with other drugs.

DNA-INTERACTIVE AGENTS

The broad category of DNA-interactive agents includes the alkylating agents (eg, cisplatin, cyclophosphamide, carmustine); the DNA strand-breakage agent bleomycin; the intercalating topoisomerase II inhibitors (eg, dactinomycin and doxorubicin); the nonintercalating topoisomerase II inhibitors etoposide and teniposide; and the DNA minor groove binder plicamycin.

Alkylating Agents

The alkylating agents form covalent chemical adducts with cellular DNA, RNA, and protein molecules and also with small molecules such as amino acids and glutathione. DNA is considered to be the most important therapeutic target of this class of drugs. Both enzymatic (metabolic) and nonenzymatic (chemical) activation steps are involved in the generation of alkylating intermediates. Alkylation occurs when electrophilic drug molecules, or their chemical or metabolic products, react covalently with nucleophilic atoms in cellular constituents, such as the amino, carboxyl, phosphate, and sulfhydryl groups in nucleic acids, proteins, amino acids, or glutathione (Fig 2.1). The nitrogen atom at the 7-position (N-7) in the purine base guanine of DNA is highly nucleophilic. *N*-7-Guanine is the site in DNA most frequently alkylated by nitrogen mustards, nitrosoureas, and cisplatin. Other sites in DNA (ie, *O*-6-guanine, *N*-3-cytosine) may also react with

TABLE 2.1. CANCER CHEMOTHERAPY DRUGS AND THEIR MAJOR USES AS SINGLE AGENTS OR IN COMBINATION[a]

Mechanism of Action/Drug	Approved Indications	Other Uses
DNA-Interactive Agents		
Alkylating agents		
Nitrogen mustards		
• Chlorambucil	CLL,[b] malignant lymphoma, Hodgkin's disease	Choriocarcinoma, ovarian ca
• Cyclophosphamide	ALL, CLL, malignant lymphoma, Hodgkin's disease, AML, multiple myeloma, mycosis fungoides, neuroblastoma, ovarian ca, retinoblastoma, breast ca	Small cell and non-small cell lung ca, rhabdomyosarcoma
• Ifosfamide	Testicular ca	
• Mechlorethamine	Hodgkin's disease, malignant lymphoma, CML, CLL, bronchogenic ca, mycosis fungoides	
• Melphalan	Multiple myeloma, ovarian ca	Breast ca
• Uracil mustard	CML, CLL, malignant lymphoma, Hodgkin's disease, mycosis fungoides	
Aziridine		
• Thiotepa	Bladder tumors, breast ca, ovarian ca	
Methanesulfonate ester		
• Busulfan	CML	
Nitrosoureas		
• Carmustine	Brain tumors, multiple myeloma, Hodgkin's disease, and malignant lymphomas	Non-small cell lung ca
• Lomustine	Brain tumors, Hodgkin's disease	
• Streptozocin	Metastatic islet cell ca of pancreas	Carcinoid tumor, Hodgkin's disease, colorectal ca
Platinum complexes		
• Cisplatin	Testicular ca, ovarian ca, bladder ca	Cervical ca, non-small cell lung ca
• Carboplatin	Ovarian ca	
Bioreductive alkylator		
• Mitomycin	Adenocarcinoma of stomach and pancreas	Breast ca
Suspected alkylators		
• Procarbazine	Hodgkin's disease	Malignant lymphomas, mycosis fungoides, brain tumors, small cell lung cancer
• Dacarbazine	Melanoma, Hodgkin's disease	Soft tissue sarcoma, neuroblastoma
• Altretamine	Ovarian ca	Non-small cell lung ca
DNA strand-breakage agent		
• Bleomycin	Malignant lymphomas, Hodgkin's disease, squamous ca of head and neck, oral cavity, skin, genitals	Renal ca, soft tissue sarcomas
DNA topoisomerase II inhibitors		
Intercalators		
• Amsacrine	AML	
• Dactinomycin	Wilms' tumor, rhabdomyosarcoma, Ewing's sarcoma, trophoblastic tumors, testicular ca	Kaposi's sarcoma
• Daunorubicin	AML, ALL	CML
• Doxorubicin	Breast ca, ovarian ca, bladder ca, bronchogenic ca, thyroid ca, gastric ca, soft-tissue and osteogenic sarcomas, neuroblastoma, Wilms' tumor, malignant lymphomas and Hodgkin's disease, ALL, AML	Ewings' tumor, head and neck ca, cervical and vaginal ca, ca of testes, prostate, and uterus, multiple myeloma

Mechanism of Action/Drug	Approved Indications	Other Uses
• Idarubicin	ANLL	
• Mitoxantrone	AML	Breast ca
Nonintercalators		
• Etoposide	Testicular ca, small cell lung ca	Non-small cell lung ca, malignant lymphomas and Hodgkin's disease
• Teniposide	AML	
DNA minor groove binder		
• Plicamycin	Testicular ca	
Antimetabolites		
Folate antagonist		
• Methotrexate	Trophoblastic neoplasms, AML, ALL, breast ca, head and neck cancer, squamous cell and small cell lung ca, malignant lymphomas	
Purine antagonists		
• Fludarabine phosphate	CLL	
• Mercaptopurine	ALL, AML, CML	
• Pentostatin	Hairy cell leukemia	
• 6-Thioguanine	ALL, AML, CML	
Pyrimidine antagonists		
• Azacitidine	AML	
• Cytarabine	AML	
• Floxuridine	Regional chemotherapy of head and neck ca, brain tumors, liver, gallbladder, biliary tract ca	
• Fluorouracil	Ca of colon, rectum, breast, stomach, pancreas	
Tubulin-Interactive Agents		
• Vinblastine	Malignant lymphomas, Hodgkin's disease, mycosis fungoides, testicular ca, Kaposi's sarcoma, choriocarcinoma, breast ca	
• Vincristine	AML, ALL, Hodgkin's disease, malignant lymphomas, neuroblastoma, rhabdomyosarcoma, Wilms' tumor	Sarcomas, small cell lung ca, brain medulloblastoma, multiple myeloma, breast ca, renal ca, Kaposi's sarcoma
• Paclitaxel	Ovarian ca	Breast ca
Hormonal Agents		
Estrogens		
• Chlorotrianisene	Prostatic ca	
• Conjugated estrogens	Breast ca, prostatic ca	
• Dienestrol		Prostatic ca
• Diethylstilbestrol	Breast ca, prostatic ca	
• Estradiol	Breast ca, prostatic ca	
• Ethinyl estradiol	Breast ca, prostatic ca	
Androgens		
• Fluoxymesterone	Breast ca	
• Methyltestosterone	Breast ca	
• Testosterone	Breast ca	

(*continued*)

TABLE 2.1. CANCER CHEMOTHERAPY DRUGS AND THEIR MAJOR USES AS SINGLE AGENTS OR IN COMBINATION[a] (continued)

Mechanism of Action/Drug	Approved Indications	Other Uses
Hormonal Agents (*cont.*)		
Progestins		
• Hydroxyprogesterone caproate	Endometrial ca	Breast ca
• Medroxyprogesterone acetate	Endometrial ca, renal ca	
• Megestrol	Endometrial ca, breast ca	
Adrenal corticosteroids		
• Dexamethasone		(ALL, CLL, CML [blast crisis], lymphomas, Hodgkin's disease, multiple myeloma, breast ca)
• Hydrocortisone		
• Methylprednisolone		
• Prednisolone		
• Prednisone		
LH-RH agonists		
• Leuprolide acetate	Prostatic ca	
• Goserelin acetate	Prostatic ca	
Antihormonal agents		
Antiestrogen		
• Tamoxifen	Breast ca	Endometrial ca
Antiadrenal		
• Aminoglutethimide	Adrenal ca	Breast ca
• Mitotane	Adrenal ca	Breast ca
Antiandrogen		
• Flutamide	Prostatic ca	
Miscellaneous Agents		
• Asparaginase	ALL	Lymphosarcoma, CML, AML, CLL
• Hydroxyurea	Melanoma, CML, ovarian ca, head and neck ca	

[a] References: McEvoy GK, ed. *AHFS Drug Information*, Bethesda, MD: American Society of Hospital Pharmacists, 1991, and *Physicians' Desk Reference*, Oradell, NJ: Medical Economics, 1991.
[b] Abbreviations used: ca, carcinoma; AML, acute myelocytic leukemia; CML, chronic myelocytic leukemia; ALL, acute lymphocytic leukemia, CLL, chronic lymphocytic leukemia; ANLL, acute nonlymphoblastic leukemia.

these or other drugs. The relationship between the various DNA alkylation targets of chemotherapeutic drugs and different biochemical effects is poorly understood. There is some evidence from DNA repair studies that O-6-guanine alkylation by nitrosoureas may be more important to cytotoxicity than the more frequent N-7-guanine reaction.

Alkylation of DNA has a number of important biochemical and cellular consequences. First, structural alteration of DNA bases may activate enzymatic DNA repair processes. Attempted repair of alkylated DNA may lead to single-strand breaks if the adducts are excised but not subsequently filled in or ligated. Second, the two strands of the DNA helix may become crosslinked by covalent reaction of a bifunctional drug molecule with two bases on the same or opposite strands (intra- or interstrand cross-linking) (see Fig 2.1). Interstrand crosslinking of DNA strands may be a particularly important action of cisplatin, the nitrogen mustards, and the nitrosoureas, based on good correlations between cytotoxic activity and extent of interstrand adduct formation. Monofunctional adducts and intrastrand crosslinks are, however, far more numerous than interstrand crosslinks and also contribute to overall effects. In addition, compounds capable of only monoadduct formation can be cytotoxic and tumor selective. Third, alteration of DNA base structures by alkylation can cause miscoding during DNA replication, leading to genetic mutations (eg, abnormal base pairing).

DNA mutations, crosslinking or monoadduct formation, and strand breakage interfere with cellular replication of DNA, transcription of RNA, and

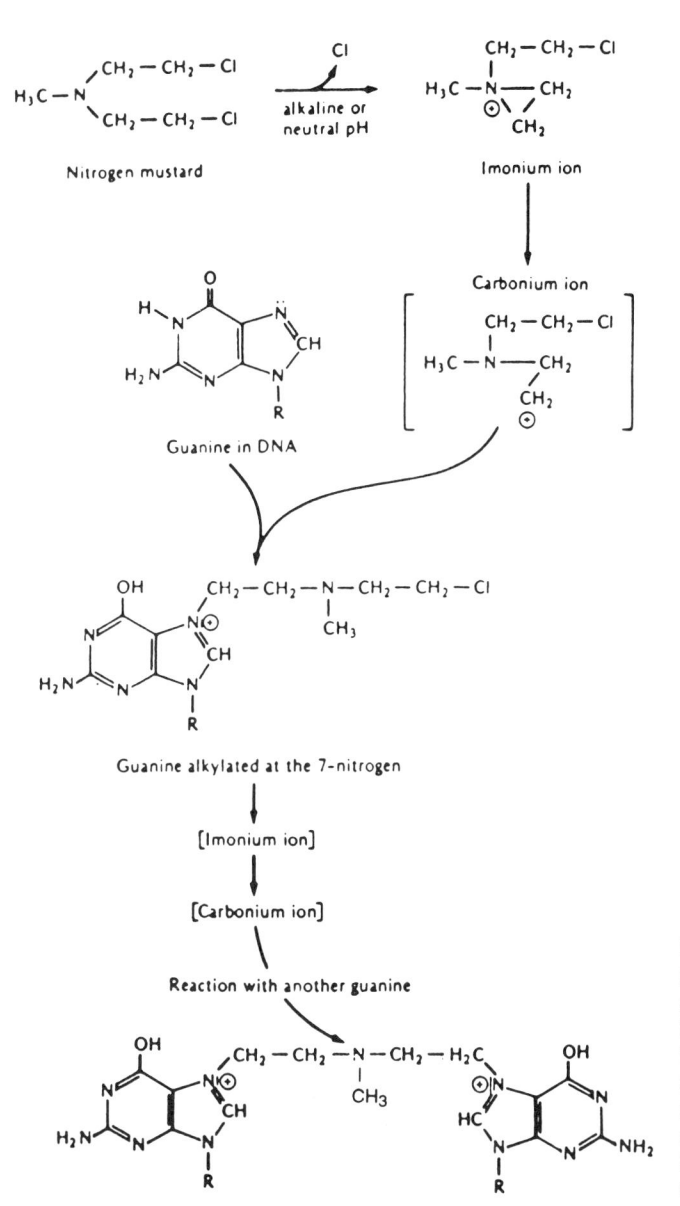

Figure 2.1. Mechanism by which nitrogen mustard becomes covalently bonded to the 7-nitrogen atoms of two guanines. In solution, the drug forms a reactive cyclic intermediate that reacts with the N-7 of a guanine residue in DNA to form a covalent linkage. The second chloromethyl arm can then cyclize and react with nucleophilic groups, such as a second guanine moiety in an opposite DNA strand or in the same strand. Reactions between DNA and RNA and between DNA and protein can also occur. *(From Pratt WB, Ruddon RW. The Anticancer Drugs. New York: Oxford University Press; 1979:66. Reprinted with permission.)*

translation into protein. The precise molecular mechanisms by which alkylating agent-induced DNA lesions poison critical processes such as DNA replication and lead to cell death are, however, poorly understood. One interesting laboratory finding is that transcriptionally active regions of DNA are more likely to be alkylated. In addition to cytotoxic effects and mutagenesis, teratogenesis and carcinogenesis are also potential cellular consequences of alkylation.

Intracellular reaction of alkylating drugs with the tripeptide glutathione has been postulated as a major means of detoxification. Tumor cell resistance to this class of drugs is thought to be mediated by efficient glutathione conjugation or by enhanced enzymatic DNA repair processes.

The various alkylating drugs are subdivided according to their chemical structures and mechanisms of covalent bonding.

Bischloroethylamines, Thiophosphoramide, Busulfan.

The oldest or "classic" alkylating agents, the nitrogen mustards or bischloroethylamines, were serendipitous discoveries arising from chemical warfare. Research into this type of molecules was stimulated by the compound dichloroethyl sulfide (sulfur mustard), which was first synthesized during the mid nineteenth century and subsequently used as a chemical weapon during World War I for its vesicant properties on the skin, lungs, and eyes. The mustards were also noted to produce atrophy of lymphoid and myeloid tissues, an observation that led, in the early 1940s, to exploration of their use in treating lymphomas and leukemias. Subsequently, these agents and structurally related compounds were found to be useful in the treatment of a variety of neoplasms. Today there are three chemical subgroups of this type in use. They are the bischloroethylamines, including cyclophosphamide (Cytoxan®, Neosar®), ifosfamide (IFEX®, Cyfos®, Holoxan®), melphalan (Alkeran®), uracil mustard, mechlorethamine (Mustargen®), and chloroambucil (Leukeran®, Amboclorin®); the aziridine thiophosphoramide (triethylene thiophosphoramide); and the alkyl sulfonate busulfan (Myleran®, Mytosan®, Misulban®). The bischloroethylamines and thiophosphoramide produce highly reactive carbonium ions, whereas busulfan appears to react by nucleophilic displacement. The chemical stability of these agents ranges from that of mechlorethamine, which is highly unstable in aqueous solution, to that of cyclophosphamide and ifosfamide, which are quite stable in solution, and require metabolic activation before alkylation can occur.

Thiophosphoramide, busulfan, and the nitrogen mustards are cell cycle phase nonspecific (ie, they kill both resting and dividing cells) and may be used effectively in treating some tumors with a small growth fraction. Effects are most pronounced, however, on normal and tumor cells that are rapidly dividing and that may not be able to repair DNA damage before initiating a new round of DNA synthesis.

The major toxic effects associated with this category of alkylating agents are related to their cytotoxic effects. The normal tissues most affected are those with a rapid growth rate: the hematopoietic system, the gastrointestinal tract, and the gonads. Nausea and vomiting are seen with the administration of most of these drugs, particularly with intravenous use. This may be the result of an effect on the chemoreceptor trigger zone in the medulla of the brain, rather than toxicity to the gastrointestinal tract. The myelosuppression is primarily a leukopenia, which usually reaches a nadir in 10 to 14 days and recovers in about 1 month. Busulfan and chlorambucil have slightly more prolonged myelosuppressive effects. This bone marrow depression is responsible for the most serious complications of therapy, which are increased potential for bleeding episodes, as a result of thrombocytopenia, and for infection, as a result of leukopenia. Anemia from depressed erythrocyte production occurs less frequently. Local tissue necrosis can occur if these drugs extravasate from the venous injection site. Cyclophosphamide and ifosfamide cause cystitis, which is thought to be related to the compound acrolein formed as a metabolic by-product of drug activation of the alkylating species, phosphoramide mustard. Cystitis can be prevented by hydration or by coadministration of the agent sodium 2-mercaptoethanesulfonate (mesna; Mesnex®) which, on hydrolysis to mercaptan in the urine, chemically inactivates acrolein and alkylating metabolites of cyclophosphamide and ifosfamide.

Nitrosoureas.

Development of nitrosourea-type compounds as anticancer drugs was based on results of screening experiments showing that molecules containing the nitroso functionality had activity in mouse tumor models. Structure–activity studies then showed that chloroethyl analogs of nitrosoureas were superior in the preclinical tumor models. The nitrosoureas in common clinical use include carmustine (BiCNU®), lomustine (CCNU®, Cee NU®), and streptozocin (streptozotocin; Zanosar®). Chemical decomposition of carmustine and lomustine in solution yields two highly reactive intermediates, chloroethyl diazohydroxide and isocyanate. The former further decomposes to yield the alkylating chloroethyl carbonium ion, and the latter reacts extensively with amino groups, forming carbamoylated proteins. The alkylating activity leads to interstrand DNA crosslinks, which are believed to mediate the antitumor effects; the carbamoylating activity is associated with toxic side effects. Like other alkylating agents, the nitrosoureas appear to kill cells equally well in all phases of the cell cycle. Inhibition of DNA synthesis occurs. These agents are metabolized rapidly to bioinactive compounds, which may undergo enterohepatic circulation prior to excretion in the urine. Carmustine and lomustine are lipid-soluble and cross the blood–brain barrier into the central nervous system. Streptozocin is a naturally occurring nitrosourea-containing analog of glucose; it is produced in cultures of *Streptomyces achromogenes*. Streptozocin is specifically taken up into β cells of the islets of Langerhans, making the drug particularly useful in the therapy of metastatic pancreatic islet cell carcinoma.

The major adverse reaction encountered with most nitrosoureas is dose-dependent depression of the hematopoietic system, which is quite delayed in onset and duration with respect to reactions to the other classes of alkylating agents. The white blood cell nadir occurs 3 to 5 weeks after treatment and lowered counts may persist for several more weeks. Severe nausea and vomiting may also be dose-limiting. With streptozocin, renal toxicity, rather than myelosuppression, is dose-limiting. Streptozocin nephrotoxicity is cumulative and may be life-threatening.

Platinum Complexes. Cisplatin (Platinol®) was the first inorganic compound to be used in the treatment of human malignancies. The cytotoxic activity of platinum complexes was discovered serendipitously when laboratory workers noted that bacterial cell division was inhibited in an electric field generated between platinum electrodes. Chemical analysis showed that this inhibition was due to a hydrolysis product of the platinum electrode, *cis*-diamminedichloroplatinum or cisplatin, which was then synthesized and shown to increase the life span of tumor-bearing mice. Cisplatin subsequently was shown to be efficacious in several forms of human cancer (see Table 2.1). In the presence of low chloride concentrations in solution (such as intracellularly), the two chloride atoms in cisplatin are displaced by two water molecules, yielding an aquated complex which can react bifunctionally with DNA, RNA, or protein molecules to form crosslinked species. DNA/platinum adduct formation (or platination, commonly referred to as *alkylation*) is thought to be the cytotoxic event. Both intrastrand and interstrand DNA crosslinks are formed, with the intrastrand guanine–platinum–guanine adduct being the most numerous. There is evidence that interstrand cisplatin–DNA adducts, though less frequent, are most important in antitumor action. Exposure of cells to cisplatin causes inhibition of DNA synthesis. In general, cytotoxicity appears to be cell cycle phase independent, but some types of cells may be more sensitive in the G_1 phase. Cisplatin and several products of cisplatin chemical breakdown in body fluids are largely excreted in the urine over 24 to 48 hours. Toxic effects associated with cisplatin administration include renal damage (which is preventable with mannitol diuresis); nausea and vomiting, which can be severe; and peripheral neuropathy. Myelosuppression (leukopenia and thrombocytopenia) is moderate at the usual clinical doses. A second-generation platinum complex, carboplatin (Paraplatin®), appears to have a lower potential for causing nephrotoxicity, neurotoxicity, and emesis but is significantly more myelosuppressive. Tumor cell resistance to platinum complexes is thought to result from decreased cellular uptake of drug, elevated intracellular levels of protective nucleophiles like glutathione, or enhanced ability of cells to repair DNA interstrand crosslinks.

Bioreductive Alkylator. Mitomycin-C (Mutamycin®) is a member of a group of cytotoxic antibiotics isolated from the fermentation broth of *Streptomyces caespitosus*. Like other alkylating agents, mitomycin-C is thought to kill cells by crosslinking DNA after conversion of the parent drug molecule to a reactive electrophilic species. Metabolic activation of mitomycin-C in cells is complex and is initiated by enzymatic reduction at the quinone moiety. Alkylation occurs at adenine and guanine bases in DNA and results in single-strand breakage and DNA synthesis inhibition. The process of DNA adduct formation by activated forms of mitomycin-C is referred to as bioreductive alkylation. Clinically, myelosuppression is delayed and cumulative, as seen with the nitrosoureas. Renal failure is another important potential side effect, as is local tissue necrosis on injection site extravasation.

Suspected Alkylating Agents: Procarbazine, Dacarbazine, Altretamine. Procarbazine (Matulane), dacarbazine (DTIC-Dome®), and altretamine (Hexalen®) are structurally unrelated agents requiring metabolic activation to exert cytotoxic effects. All three are believed to act via alkylation; however, the chemical intermediates responsible for biological activity have not been precisely characterized and thus the mechanism of action is not as well understood as for the other alkylating agents. This is particularly true for altretamine, for which the biochemical basis for antitumor activity is poorly understood.

Procarbazine is a synthetic hydrazine-type compound discovered in an analog screening program originally targeted at discovery of monamine oxidase inhibitors. Multistep metabolism in vivo appears to be mediated by liver cytochrome P450 enzymes and generates species that can act as methylating agents. Studies with radiolabeled drugs have shown transfer of the label to DNA, RNA, protein, and phospholipids. In addition procarbazine may also be converted to free radical species, but it is not clear that these contribute to antitumor activity. Cellular effects are manifested as inhibition of DNA and RNA synthesis and alterations in chromosomal structure. Procarbazine appears to be most toxic to cells in the G_1 phase of the cell cycle.

Dacarbazine was synthesized as a potential antimetabolite analog of a purine precursor and shown to have therapeutic activity in experimental mouse tumor systems; however, subsequent investigations showed that it does not act as an antimetabolite. Rather, dacarbazine's activity is believed to be related to a DNA methylating species, methyldiazonium ion, formed through metabolism by liver microsomal enzymes. Dacarbazine appears to kill cells nonspecifically with respect to cell cycle and to inhibit DNA, RNA, and protein synthesis.

Altretamine (hexamethylmelamine) is a chemical analog of a known alkylating molecule, triethylenemelamine, and studies with radiolabeled compound have shown binding of radioactive species to cellular macromolecular fractions. The structure of a metabolite that could alkylate and presumably be responsible for cytotoxic effects has not yet been elucidated.

Procarbazine, dacarbazine, and altretamine have relatively mild bone marrow toxicity compared with other alkylating agents and antitumor drugs. For this reason they are frequently used in combination with other agents because they often can be administered at full therapeutic doses. The three compounds share nausea and vomiting as a frequently occurring side effect. Procarbazine causes both central and peripheral neurotoxicity. Ingestion of alcohol may cause disulfiram-like reactions in procarbazine-treated patients. Procarbazine also retains some monoamine oxidase inhibitor properties, and hypertension may be observed in combination with certain drugs or tyramine-containing foods. Altretamine may cause reversible peripheral neuropathy on prolonged administration.

DNA Strand-Breakage Agent: Bleomycin

Bleomycin (Blenoxane®) is a mixture of glycopeptides produced by *Streptomyces verticillis*. The predominant compound in the mixture is known as bleomycin A_2, which is a metal complex containing chelated Cu(II). Cu(II)–bleomycin is inactive, but becomes active when Fe(II) is exchanged for Cu(II) in the biological environment. The Fe(II)–bleomycin complex produces single- and double-strand breaks and various types of chromosomal lesions in cellular DNA. The DNA strand-breakage activity of bleomycin is due to intercalation of its bithiazole ring adjacent to guanine–cytosine base pairs, followed by catalytic production by the bound metal–drug complex of free radicals from molecular oxygen. The highly reactive oxygen metabolites (presumed to be superoxide or hydroxyl radical) then diffuse to and cleave the DNA backbone. Bleomycin's catalytic properties have led to its being characterized as a small-molecular-weight form of ferrous oxidase. DNA synthesis is inhibited. Cells in G_2 phase are selectively killed by bleomycin. The drug slows progression through S phase and blocks progression at $G_2 + M$. In cancer patients, bleomycin has minimal toxicity to bone marrow, making it very useful in combination chemotherapy regimens containing myelosuppressive drugs. Sites of bleomycin toxicity include the skin and the lungs, which may be relatively deficient in a drug-inactivating enzyme known as bleomycin hydrolase. The lung toxicity of bleomycin is cumulative and irreversible and can lead to extensive interstitial fibrosis and death.

Topoisomerase II Inhibitors

One aspect of the dynamic three-dimensional arrangement of chromosomal DNA in cells is its "topologic state," which refers to the highly ordered twisting and winding of a DNA double-strand molecule around itself. The topoisomerases constitute one of several groups of enzymes that regulate the topologic state of DNA by unwinding or unlinking coiled DNA double-strand molecules. Topoisomerases are thought to play critical roles in the regulation of DNA replication and transcription. Topoisomerases act on DNA by breaking and rejoining one or both strands of the phosphodiester backbone. Topoisomerase I catalyzes the relaxation of supercoiled DNA by transiently severing one of the two DNA strands, forming a "swivel." Topoisomerase II mediates the passage of one double-strand DNA segment through another by formation of a temporary "gate" through both strands of one segment. Drugs that inhibit topoisomerases bind to and trap the covalent complex formed between DNA and the enzyme and, thus, indirectly cause the formation of protein-associated single- or double-strand DNA breaks. Topoisomerase II is now thought to be an important biochemical target of a group of structurally diverse anticancer drugs, including several that also interact with DNA more directly by intercalation between base pairs. A model for topoisomerase II action and inhibition by drugs is shown in Figure 2.2. Currently, no marketed drugs are known to act through topoisomerase I; however, topotecan and irinotecan, two semisynthetic analogs of the plant natural product and topoisomerase I inhibitor camptothecin, are under clinical investigation. It is doubtful that either the drug-induced DNA strand breaks or the inhibition of topoisomerase function is directly lethal to cells, as the extent to which drug–topoisomerase–DNA complexes are formed does not necessarily correlate quantitatively with cytotoxicity. Rather, formation of such complexes appears to block other critical functions such as DNA replication or to trigger as yet unknown mechanisms that mediate cell death.

Intercalating Topoisomerase II Inhibitors. The intercalators in current clinical usage include dactinomycin (Cosmegen®); the anthracycline antibiotics doxorubicin (Adriamycin®), daunorubicin (Cerubidine®), and idarubicin (Idamycin®); the synthetic anthracenedione mitoxantrone (Novantrone®); and the acridine derivative amsacrine (*m*-AMSA®, Amsidine®). DNA intercalators may mediate their antitumor and toxic effects through several possible mechanisms. These molecules bind to double-helical DNA by interposing their planar ring structures between stacked DNA base pairs, leading to conformational distortions. All clinically used intercalating drugs have also been shown to be inhibitors of topoisomerase II. The relationship between DNA intercalation and inhibition of topoisomerase II is poorly understood at present, as nonintercalating compounds such as teniposide and etoposide may also be potent topoisomerase II inhibitors. To complicate the picture further, the intercalating drugs all contain quinone moieties, which make them substrates for cellular oxidation–reduction reactions, leading to the formation of highly reactive free radicals which can damage DNA and other macromolecules. The relative contribution of intercalator-mediated free radical metabolism to the antitumor effects of this class of drugs is unknown; however this biochemical action is thought to be involved in the cardiotoxicity associated with anthracycline therapy, as myocardial cells appear to have a lower capacity to detoxify oxygen free radicals than cells in other tissues. It may be that intercalation (with its consequent DNA distortion), inhibition of topoisomerase II, and free radical formation all contribute in vivo to the antitumor efficacy of this class of agents. There may be a different balance of effects associated with different molecules, leading to their individual therapeutic and toxicologic profiles.

Dactinomycin was the first approved antitumor drug of natural origin. It is a fermentation product of *Streptomyces parvulus* and consists of two cyclic polypeptide chains linked to a planar phenoxazone ring, which is believed to intercalate be-

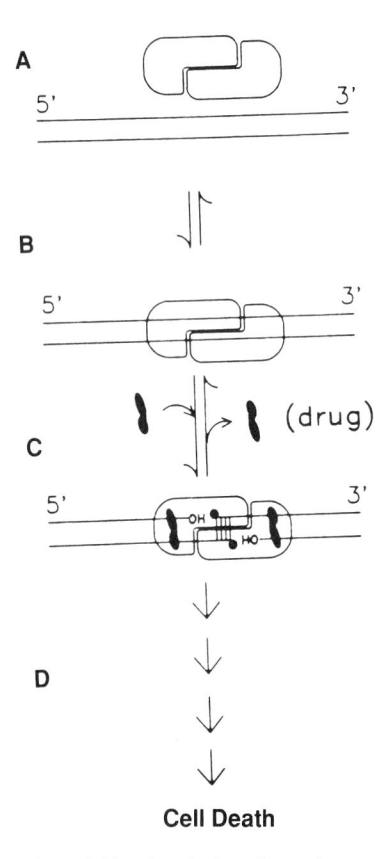

Figure 2.2. A model for drug-induced, topoisomerase II-mediated DNA cleavage and cell death. **A.** Unbound DNA topoisomerase II and substrate DNA. **B.** Reversible formation of a noncleavable complex between topoisomerase II and DNA. **C.** Reversible formation of a drug-induced cleavable complex containing topoisomerase II, DNA, and intercalative topoisomerase II-targeting antitumor drug. **D.** Processing of the cleavable complex by cellular functions resulting in cell death. (From Bodley AL, Liu LF. Topoisomerases as novel targets for cancer chemotherapy. Bio/Technology. 1988;6:1315–1319. © 1988 Bio/Technology. Reprinted with permission.)

tween adjacent guanine–cytosine base pairs in DNA. Characteristic biochemical actions of dactinomycin include the inhibition of the chain elongation step of DNA-directed RNA synthesis and the production of DNA single-strand breaks, the latter possibly mediated by free radicals. Hematologic toxicity, nausea and vomiting, and oral mucosal ulceration are dose-limiting for dactinomycin.

Doxorubicin and daunorubicin, antibiotics isolated from cultures of *Streptomyces peucetius* var. *caesius* and *Streptomyces coeruleorubidus*, respectively, are members of the chemical class known as anthracyclines. Idarubicin is a synthetically prepared analog of daunorubicin. Doxorubicin is generally considered to be the most active antitumor agent ever discovered, with life-extending or palliative activity in a broad spectrum of disease types (see Table 2.1). Daunorubicin's indications are the acute leukemias. Daunorubicin, which is very close in structure to doxorubicin, has not been as extensively evaluated in solid tumor therapy. Idarubicin appears to be superior to daunorubicin in the treatment of acute nonlymphocytic leukemia and, in addition, is orally active. All three compounds are DNA intercalators, inhibitors of topoisomerase II, and substrates for cellular oxidation–reduction leading to free radical intermediates. In addition to myelosuppression (the acute dose-limiting toxic effect), nausea and vomiting, and alopecia seen with other intercalators, chronic use of any anthracycline can potentially cause a characteristic, cumulative, dose-related, and irreversible cardiomyopathy which culminates in lethal congestive heart failure. This unusual toxic effect limits the total dose of these agents that can be administered on a chronic basis, even to responding patients. Another important toxic effect of the anthracycline compounds is tissue necrosis, which occurs on accidental extravasation of drug into tissues surrounding the intravenous injection site. Metabolism of doxorubicin, daunorubicin, and idarubicin is a major pathway of elimination. The major metabolites are know to possess cytotoxic activity.

Mitoxantrone is a synthetic DNA intercalator and topoisomerase II inhibitor of the anthracenedione chemical type. This drug was developed after certain anthraquinone-containing dyes were noted to be active in mouse tumor systems. Mitoxantrone is used to treat leukemia and breast cancer. Studies of free radical formation in mitoxantrone-treated cells suggest that use of this particular compound should incur a much lower incidence of clinical cardiotoxicity compared with the anthracycline drugs, and clinical results support this hypothesis.

Amsacrine is an antileukemic chemical derivative of the DNA-intercalating dye acridine. It is an inhibitor of topoisomerase II and may also lead to the formation of oxygen free radicals and DNA damage. Amsacrine may also alkylate cellular macromolecules through a free radical metabolic intermediate known as *m*-AQDI. As with the other DNA-intercalating free radical generators, there is some risk of cardiotoxicity.

Nonintercalating Topoisomerase II Inhibitors. Etoposide (VePesid®) and teniposide are semisynthetic derivatives of podophyllotoxin, a natural product isolated from the May apple or mandrake plant. Although not used clinically, podophyllotoxin is an antimitotic agent that binds to tubulin; however, its clinically useful derivatives (known as epipodophyllotoxins) do not affect microtubular assembly at pharmacologically relevant concentrations. Rather, they appear to act as non-DNA-binding inhibitors of topoisomerase II, trapping the enzyme–DNA complex and stabilizing the DNA double-strand breaks. Etoposide and teniposide differ only slightly in chemical structure. Maximum cell killing occurs late in S or in G_2 phase. Cells are prevented from progressing beyond G_2. The epipodophyllotoxins cause dose-limiting leukopenia. In addition, nausea and vomiting (more extensive after oral than after intravenous administration), alopecia, and peripheral neuropathy occur in many treated patients.

Multidrug Resistance. Laboratory studies have shown that certain tumor cell lines made resistant to one agent are resistant to a number of other mechanistically unrelated agents. This phenomenon, known as multidrug resistance (MDR), has led to elucidation of a mechanism of tumor cell resistance possibly relevant to human cancer. Multidrug-resistant cells are resistant to a number of the intercalating and nonintercalating topoisomerase II inhibitors, in addition to the tubulin-interactive drugs vinblastine and vincristine. These agents are natural products or analogs thereof and are relatively large, hydrophobic molecules. Such molecules appear to be substrates for a molecular efflux pumping system located in the cell membrane and mediated by the P-glycoprotein (permeability glycoprotein or P170). P-glycoprotein appears to be expressed not only in cultured tumor cell lines, but also in a number of nonneoplastic human tissues, such as colon, small intestine, adrenal gland, kidney, and liver. The P-glycoprotein and the MDR phenotype may constitute a natural cellular defense mechanism against potentially toxic xenobiotics ingested in food. Evidence is accumulating that malignant cells in epithelial solid tumors in humans may express or overexpress P-glycoprotein and this may at least partially explain the common clinical observation of tumor resistance to a broad range of mechanistically unrelated drugs.

DNA Minor Groove Binding Agent: Plicamycin

Plicamycin (mithramycin, aureolic acid; Mithracin®) is an antitumor antibiotic isolated from fermentations of *Streptomyces plicatus*. It is believed to kill cells by binding to DNA and inhibiting macromolecular synthesis, particularly of RNA; however, its mode of DNA interaction is different from those of the alkylating agents and intercalators and may involve tight noncovalent binding to the DNA minor groove. The binding of plicamycin to DNA is dependent on the presence of divalent cations such as magnesium. A strong binding preference for DNA sequences containing guanine–cytosine base pairs is exhibited. In addition to antitumor applications, plicamycin is used clinically at lower doses to treat hypercalcemia associated with malignancy or Paget's disease of bone. This effect appears to be related to prevention of bone resorption by osteoclasts. Plicamycin has a range of toxic effects, including nausea and vomiting, hemorraghic diathesis, and renal and hepatic damage.

ANTIMETABOLITES

The antimetabolites are structural analogs of naturally occurring metabolites. They interfere with the normal synthesis of nucleic acids by falsely substituting for biosynthetic precursors or other intermediates in metabolic pathways. Some purine and pyrimidine antimetabolites are incorporated into DNA and RNA. The antimetabolites exert their major cytotoxic activity during the DNA synthesis or S phase of the cell cycle. Because of this, they are generally most effective against tumors that have a high growth fraction. This group of drugs is subdivided into the folate antagonists, the purine antagonists, and the pyrimidine antagonists. Antimetabolite mechanisms of action are illustrated in Figure 2.3.

Folate Antagonists

Methotrexate is the 4-amino-4-deoxy-*N*-methyl analog of folic acid and is the principal folate antagonist used clinically. Methotrexate exerts its cytotoxic effect by binding tightly to the enzyme dihydrofolate reductase, thereby blocking the reduction of folate to its active form, N^5, N^{10}-methylene tetrahydrofolate, a carrier of one-carbon groups used in purine and thymidylate synthesis. Synthesis of thymidine and purine is stopped, thus arresting DNA and RNA synthesis; however, only small quantities of dihydrofolate reductase are required to maintain adequate levels of the reduced folate pool. For maximal cytotoxic effect, the intracellular levels of methotrexate must be sufficiently high to bind essentially all of the dihydrofolate reductase. Methotrexate normally enters the cell through an active, carrier-mediated cell membrane transport system which it shares with leucovorin. When this transport system is functional in tumor cells, adequate intracellular levels of methotrexate can easily be achieved. Some tumors lack or have reduced transport capabilities. In such tumors, very high extracellular levels of methotrexate are required to effect transport into the cells by a passive mechanism. Such high levels can be achieved by means of "high-dose" regimens, which also improve drug penetration into tumor "sanctuary" sites such as the testis and central nervous system. The toxic effects of very high doses of methotrexate can be reversed clinically by "rescue" of normal cells, which retain the folate transport capability, by administration of reduced folates such as folinic acid and calcium leucovorin (also called citrovorum factor).

Methotrexate is eliminated predominantly as the unchanged drug but a small fraction is conjugated intracellularly to one or more glutamate molecules. The polyglutamated forms of methotrexate have prolonged biochemical effects either because of their lengthy retention within cells or because of higher affinity for dihydrofolate reductase or other enzymes such as thymidylate synthetase that do not interact with methotrexate itself.

Methotrexate is a cell cycle phase-specific agent that is most toxic to cells in S phase. Resistance is thought to develop as a consequence of either decreased cellular uptake or overexpression of dihydrofolate reductase.

Effective doses of methotrexate produce bone marrow depression with a nadir at 1 to 2 weeks. Damage to the gastrointestinal endothelium is frequent and results in symptoms ranging from mild

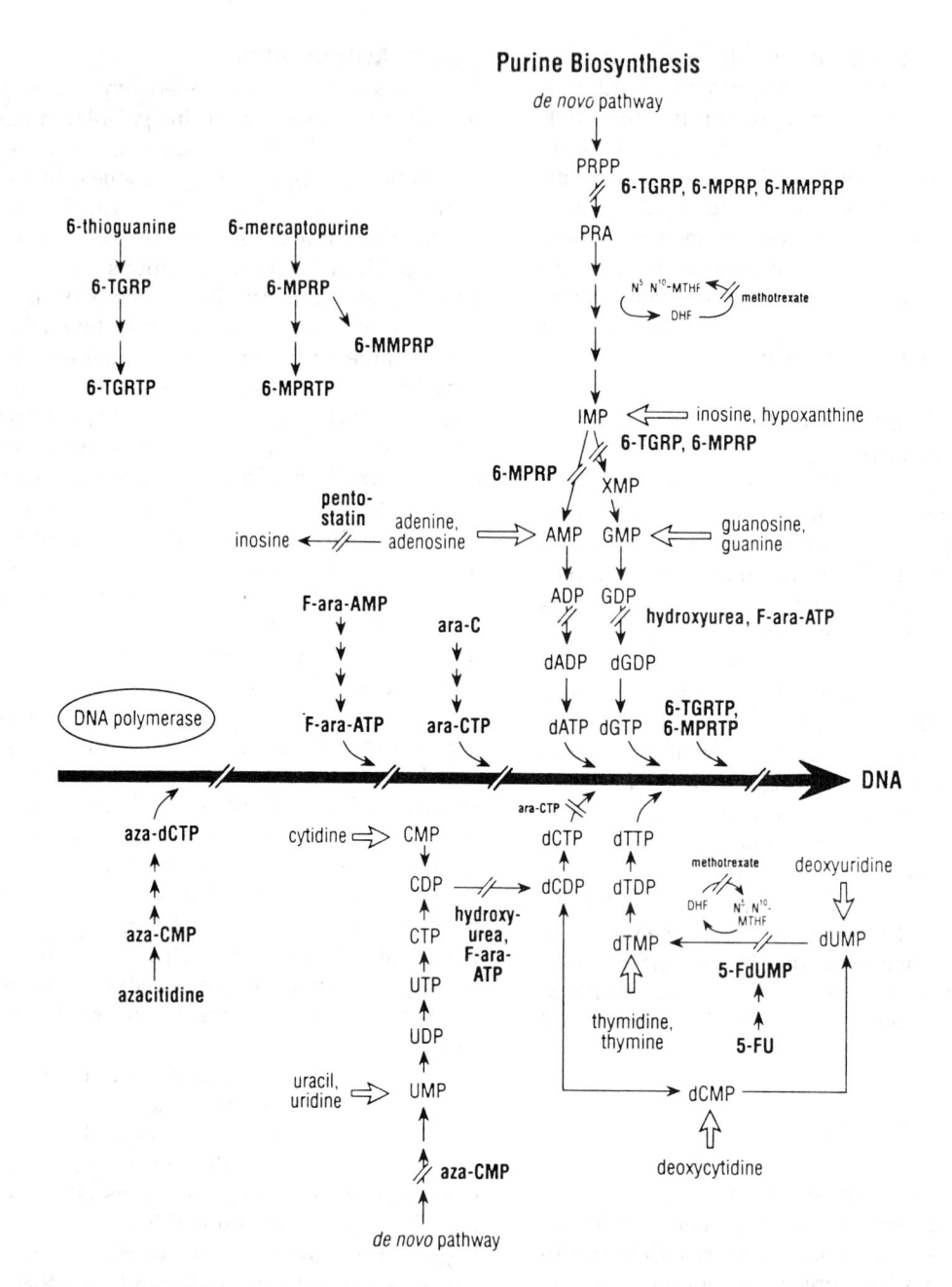

Figure 2.3. Biosynthetic pathways to purine and pyrimidine DNA precursors and sites of action of antimetabolites and hydroxyurea. Salvage pathways are indicated by open arrows. Drugs are printed in boldface. Blocked pathways are indicated by interrupted solid arrows. d, deoxyribose; A, G, C, T, U, X, and I, adenosine, guanosine, cytosine, thymidine, uridine, xanthosine, and inosine; MP, DP, and TP, mono-, di-, and triphosphate; DHF, dihydrofolate; N^5, N^{10}-MTHF, N^5, N^{10}-methylene tetrahydrofolate; PRPP, 5-phosphoribosyl-1-pyrophosphate; PRA, 5-phosphoribosylamine; aza-CMP, 5-azacytosine monophosphate; aza-dCTP, 2′-deoxy-5-azacytosine triphosphate; 5-FU, 5-fluorouracil; 5-FdUMP, 5-fluro-2′-deoxyuridine monophosphate; F-ara-AMP, fludarabine or arabinosyl-2-fluoroadenine monophosphate; F-ara-ATP, arabinosyl-2-fluoroadenine triphosphate; ara-C, cytarabine or arabinosyl cytosine; ara-CTP, arabinosylcytosine triphosphate; 6-TGRP and 6-TGRTP, 6-thioguanine ribosyl monophosphate and triphosphate; 6-MPRP and 6-MPRTP, 6-mercaptopurine ribosyl monophosphate and triphosphate; 6-MMPRP, 6-methylmercaptopurine ribosyl monophosphate. (From Chabner BA, Myers CE. Clinical pharmacology of cancer chemotherapy. In: DeVita VT Jr, Hellmann S, Rosenberg SA, eds. Cancer, Principles and Practice of Oncology, Philadelphia: JB Lippincott; 1985:350. Redrawn with permission.)

diarrhea and mucositis to severe ulcers and bleeding. Hepatotoxicity, central nervous system abnormalities, and skin rash may also occur.

Purine Antagonists

6-Mercaptopurine (Purinethol®) and thioguanine are S phase-specific cytotoxic analogs of the natural purines hypoxanthine and guanine, respectively. 6-Mercaptopurine and 6-thioguanine have the hydroxyl group on the 6-position of the purine ring substituted with a sulfhydryl group.

6-Mercaptopurine acts as a false metabolite because of its close chemical similarity to the purine hypoxanthine. Free 6-mercaptopurine is not active. It must first be metabolized to the nucleotide, which then fraudulently competes with similar nucleotides for the enzymes responsible for the conversion of phosphoribosyl pyrophosphate to phosphoribosylamine and of inosinic acid to adenine and xanthine nucleotides. In addition, the nucleotide triphosphate metabolite of 6-mercaptopurine is incorporated into DNA. 6-Mercaptopurine can also be metabolized to 6-methyl mercaptopurine ribotide (6-MMRP), which is itself a potent inhibitor of purine synthesis. 6-Mercaptopurine thus interferes with synthesis of both DNA and RNA. 6-Thioguanine also acts as a false metabolite. Again, the free intact drug is not pharmacologically active. 6-Thioguanine is activated to the nucleotide form and then substitutes for the corresponding guanine nucleotide, thus blocking purine synthesis.

There appear to be no significant differences in the indications or efficacy of 6-thioguanine compared with 6-mercaptopurine. The use and toxic effects are identical, and the two drugs are cross-resistant. Allopurinol (Zyloprim®), when given concomitantly with 6-mercaptopurine, may significantly block its metabolism by xanthine oxidase, necessitating a reduction to one-fourth to one-third normal dosage. This drug interaction is not a problem with 6-thioguanine, however, because its major means of detoxification is methylation. The major dose-limiting toxic effect of 6-mercaptopurine and 6-thioguanine is myelosuppression consisting primarily of leukopenia with lesser effects on platelets and red blood cells. Gastrointestinal distress is common and liver damage may occur.

Pentostatin (2'-deoxycoformycin; Nipent®) is an analog of the purine nucleoside adenosine. Pentostatin blocks conversion of adenosine to inosine by the enzyme adenosine deaminase. This results in cellular accumulation of adenosine, which appears to be selectively toxic to certain types of T lymphocytes. This action appears to be the basis for the marked activity of pentostatin in the treatment of hairy cell leukemia. Toxic effects of pentostatin include neutropenia and increased risk of infection unrelated to myelosuppression, in addition to renal and central nervous system effects, skin rash, nausea and vomiting, conjunctivitis, and lethargy.

Fludarabine phosphate (arabinosyl-2-fluoroadenine monophosphate, F-ara-AMP; Fludara®) is a monophosphorylated fluoro-derivative of the fraudulent nucleoside Ara-A. Although Ara-A has antitumor properties, it is not useful in cancer treatment because of rapid metabolism to an inactive form by adenosine deaminase. Blockage of Ara-A metabolism by coadministration of pentostatin to decrease clearance and increase tumor cell exposure has been investigated clinically; however, pentostatin has a spectrum of toxic effects which add to those of Ara-A (see earlier text). The fluoro- analog of Ara-A was found to be a poor substrate for the enzyme and to be cleared slowly enough to exert useful antitumor effects. Biochemically, fluoro-Ara-A inhibits DNA polymerase α and ribonucleotide reductase in addition to being incorporated into DNA. Fludarabine, which is the monophosphate derivative of fluoro-Ara-A, was prepared to confer water solubility and convenience of formulation. In vivo, fludarabine is rapidly metabolized by phosphatases to fluoro-Ara-A, which is then rephosphorylated intracellularly to the active species. Fludarabine appears to be useful in the treatment of chronic lymphocytic leukemia. Its dose-limiting toxic effect is myelosuppression. Neurotoxicity, which may be severe, irreversible, or lethal, has been observed but appears to be controllable at antileukemic doses when the drug is administered by continuous infusion.

Pyrimidine Antagonists

Fluorouracil, first synthesized in 1957, is a classic example of a successful rationally designed drug. Its development was based on observations that rat tumor cells used uracil more efficiently than normal tissues, suggesting that fraudulent uracil analogs might be selectively toxic. Fluorouracil is first metabolized to the nucleotide 5-fluorouridine-5'-triphosphate (5-FUTP), which is incorporated into RNA, disrupting RNA metabolism. FUTP is also converted to 5-fluoro-2'-deoxyuridine 5'-monophosphate (5-FdUMP), which binds covalently to thymidylate synthetase. By inhibiting this enzyme, the conversion of deoxyuridine monophosphate (dUMP) to deoxythymidine monophosphate (dTMP) (thymidylate) is blocked and DNA synthesis is inhibited. Fluorouracil is more toxic to dividing than to resting cells but does not show phase-specific toxicity, possibly because synthesis of both RNA and DNA is affected. Fluorouracil is catabolized in the liver by dihydrouracil dehydrogenase. Fluorouracil causes myelosuppression which reaches a nadir in 1 to 2 weeks. In addition nausea, anorexia, stomatitis, and alopecia occur. Neurotoxicity may also be seen.

In laboratory studies, the efficacy of fluorouracil appears to be enhanced by combination treatment with the reduced folate leucovorin, and this approach is currently the subject of large-scale clinical trials in patients with solid tumors. Supplementation of cellular reduced folate pools by administration of leucovorin is thought to increase the binding of FdUMP to thymidylate synthetase through formation of a reduced folate–FdUMP–synthetase ternary complex, thereby increasing the duration of fluorouracil-mediated DNA synthesis inhibition.

Recently, improved survival has been observed in colon cancer patients in phase III trials receiving combination treatment with fluorouracil and levamisole (Ergamisol®), an anthelmintic compound with some immunostimulant properties and very little toxicity. Whether this therapeutic synergism is related to the immune effects of levamisole or to unknown mechanisms of biochemical modulation is not clear.

Floxuridine (5-fluoro-2′-deoxyuridine; FUDR®), the chemically prepared nucleoside of 5-FU, is used as an alternative to 5-FU in continuous regional intraarterial infusion therapy of cancer. Floxuridine is more soluble than fluorouracil, allowing administration of smaller volumes by means of portable infusion pumps. Floxuridine undergoes rapid metabolism to 5-FU.

Clinically used analogs of cytidine include cytarabine (Cytosar-U®) and azacitidine (5-azacytidine). The active form of cytarabine is the nucleotide triphosphate ara-CTP, which competes with deoxycytidine for DNA polymerase, thereby inhibiting DNA synthesis. Ara-CTP is also incorporated into DNA. Cytarabine is metabolized by cytidine deaminase in the liver, granulocytes, and gastrointestinal tract to uracil arabinoside, an inactive compound. Total body clearance of drug is very rapid. Cytarabine is therefore administered at conventional doses by prolonged continuous infusion to increase the probability of killing tumor cells not initially in S phase. In recent years, the use of "high-dose" cytarabine regimens (1–3 g/m^2 infused over 1–3 hours and repeated every 12 hours for 4 to 12 doses) has been explored in acute myelogenous leukemia patients who are refractory to conventional cytarabine doses and other therapeutic approaches. The intent of high-dose therapy is to enhance the retention of the active species, ara-CTP, by leukemic cells. Cytarabine can cross the blood–brain barrier, and, under steady-state conditions, levels of drug in cerebrospinal fluid approach 60% of plasma levels, presumably as a result of the negligible levels of cytidine deaminase in the cerebrospinal fluid.

The mechanism of action of azacitidine is not as well established. The nucleotide monophosphate (aza-CMP) inhibits orotidylate decarboxylase, blocking pyrimidine biosynthesis. The reduced deoxynucleotide triphosphate metabolite (aza-dCTP) is incorporated into RNA and, to a lesser extent, into DNA. Although azacitidine is most active in S phase, it appears to have some activity in all phases of the cell cycle. Azacitidine inhibits synthesis of DNA, RNA, and protein. Also, even though some cross-resistance with the other cytidine analog exists, it is not complete. These facts suggest an additional mechanism of action not present with cytarabine. In experimental systems, azacitidine has caused differentiation of malignant cells, possibly mediated by inhibition of DNA methylation. This property led to clinical trials of azacitidine for induction of fetal hemoglobin synthesis in patients with β-thalassemia.

The toxic effects of cytarabine and azacytidine are similar to those of the other pyrimidine antagonists and include myelosuppression and gastrointestinal effects. High-dose cytarabine regimens are associated with a significant incidence of cerebral and cerebellar neurotoxicity.

TUBULIN-INTERACTIVE AGENTS

The vinca alkaloids vincristine (Oncovin®) and vinblastine (Velban®) were isolated from the periwinkle plant, *Vinca rosea*, which has a long history of use in folk medicine. Although quite similar chemically and mechanistically, vincristine and vinblastine have markedly different clinical activities (see Table 2.1) and toxicities. Both vincas appear to act by binding to specific sites on tubulin, a protein that polymerizes to form cellular microtubules. Microtubules are critical structural units involved in a number of cellular activities, including formation of the mitotic spindle. Binding of vincristine or vinblastine to tubulin inhibits microtubule formation. The structure of the mitotic spindle depends on a dynamic balance between microtubule formation and dissolution. Inhibition of tubulin polymerization into microtubules by drugs leads to disappearance of the spindle apparatus. Consistent with these effects, the vinca alkaloids block the progression of cells beyond the metaphase of mitosis; however, mitosis is not the most drug-sensitive phase. The drugs appear to kill cells in all phases, with late S phase being most sensitive. Other biochemical effects of the vincas have been demonstrated, such as inhibition of RNA and DNA synthesis; however, the antitumor effects are believed to result primarily from the interaction with tubulin.

Vinblastine and vincristine exhibit similar pharmacokinetics in cancer patients. Both drugs are extensively metabolized but the metabolites have not been well characterized. As noted earlier, there is a marked difference in the toxicity profiles of vincristine and vinblastine. Vinblastine's dose-limiting toxic effect is myelosuppression, with leukopenia being more pronounced than thrombocytopenia. Vincristine's dose-limiting adverse effect is neurotoxicity, with peripheral neuropathy occurring very frequently. Vincristine has relatively mild hematologic effects, making it useful in combination regimens. Both drugs are irritating to local tissues if extravasated and can cause necrosis. Both also cause nausea and vomiting. Resistance to vincristine and vinblastine may be mediated by tubulin mutations or by increased drug efflux from tumor cells (see discussion of Multidrug Resistance under Topoisomerase II Inhibitors).

Paclitaxel (Taxol®) is a complex diterpene product which is isolated from various yew (*Taxus*) species or prepared semisynthetically from biosynthetic precursors. Paclitaxel has a unique mechanism of action, blocking cells in mitosis by overstabilizing microtubules rather than by inhibiting microtubule assembly. The plasma levels that are achievable in cancer patients have been shown to induce the formation of aberrant microtubules in cultured cells. Paclitaxel binds with high affinity to microtubules, preferring a specific site on the β-subunit of tubulin. Paclitaxel does not bind to unpolymerized tubulin dimers. Due to its insolubility, paclitaxel is formulated with high concentrations of the surfactant Cremophor EL. In initial clinical trials, the formulated drug was associated with a high incidence of hypersensitivity reactions, some of which were life-threatening. It is not established whether these reactions were due to the surfactant or to the drug itself. Schedule modifications (infusion over 6 or 24 hours) and use of a prophylactic premedication regimen have reduced the incidence of hypersensitivity reactions substantially. The dose-limiting toxicity is neutropenia. Paclitaxel also induces peripheral neuropathy and disturbs cardiac rhythm in some patients. Clearance of paclitaxel is predominantly by metabolism and biliary excretion (of unchanged drug and metabolites). A semisynthetic analog, taxotere, is currently in clinical trials. Taxotere appears to share many of paclitaxel's properties but is slightly more potent.

HORMONAL AGENTS

A number of human tumors arise from tissues normally sensitive to hormonal growth controls. In their more differentiated forms, such tumors retain hormone receptors. Therapy of these hormonally sensitive tumors involves endocrine ablation (removal of a particular hormone-secreting tissue that stimulates tumor growth) or the administration of natural or synthetic hormonal substances that downregulate tumor growth. Chemically, many of these substances are natural steroids or steroidal derivatives. Some are synthetic nonsteroid hormone-like compounds, and a few are pharmacologic antagonists or antihormonal entities. A few unusual drugs block critical biochemical steps in certain tissues (eg, the adrenal gland) and interrupt hormone synthesis. Common treatment programs involve the administration of naturally occurring, biologically antagonistic steroidal compounds. Examples include the use of estrogens in androgen-sensitive prostatic carcinomas, the use of progestins in endometrial tumors, and the use of androgens in breast cancers. The adrenal glucocorticoids appear to retard lymphocytic cellular proliferation selectively. Table 2.1 includes common therapeutic uses of the hormonal agents. Hormonal therapies, in general, lack direct cytotoxicity and, therefore, offer little curative potential. Rather, they offer significant palliation with a low liability of significant toxicity.

Tissues in which hormonally sensitive tumors arise require specific hormones for optimal growth and function. The exact pharmacologic mechanisms for hormonal effects on growth and development are incompletely understood. A general pattern involves modulation of metabolism at subcellular (nuclear or cytoplasmic) levels by the binding of hormones to specific receptor proteins. Steroid–cellular interactions (Fig 2.4) appear to be mediated by steroid entry into cells followed by binding to specific cytoplasmic proteins (receptors); translocation (along with transformation) of the drug–receptor complex to the nuclear chromatin; binding of the receptor–steroid complex to DNA and stimulation of transcription of specific genes; and synthesis of specific proteins involved in cellular growth control. Clinical applications are therefore directed to blocking the receptor proteins with a competitive antagonist (eg, the antiestrogenic drug tamoxifen), thereby depriving the cell of a natural hormonal growth stimulant, or administering compounds that have biologically antagonistic properties (eg, estrogens in prostate cancer). The usual biologic consequence of hormonal therapy is a decrease in the growth fraction of the responding tumor, resulting in more cells in the G_0 or resting phase.

It is believed that one key to success with hormonal therapy resides in the presence or absence of sufficient numbers of receptors (steroid-binding proteins) in the tumor. For example, in a general (unselected) population of patients with breast cancer treated without knowledge of receptor status, responses to endocrine therapy would occur in about one third. If treatment were restricted to patients in whom receptors were present (as determined by measurement of estrogen receptor content in a tumor biopsy), the chances for a therapeutic response would be improved at least twofold. Much effort has been spent on learning how to use receptor information to enhance response rates. For example, the presence of both estrogen and progesterone receptors in breast tumors increases the probability of response. This is because progesterone receptor production is estrogen-induced and the presence of progesterone receptors implies the presence of functional estrogen receptors.

Other clinical factors (eg, rate of disease progression and sites of involvement) must be considered when contemplating endocrine therapy. Guidelines have been developed in particular patient populations thought likely to benefit. More slow-growing, well-differentiated tumors are more likely to respond (eg, recurrent breast cancer with a long disease-free interval after mastectomy). Certain sites of disease (skin, lymph nodes, bone) are more likely to respond than others (liver, bone marrow, brain). Clinical responses to hormonal treatment may be delayed in onset, and thus the patient should be stable and observed on hormonal therapy for several weeks before discontinuing treatment as having failed. As noted earlier, biologic antagonism

Figure 2.4. Model of steroid hormone action. After entering the cell (**1**), the steroid binds (**2**) in a stereospecific, noncovalent manner to a soluble protein receptor (*R*) located in the cytoplasm and thus forms a steroid–receptor complex (*RS*). The complex then undergoes a temperature-dependent transformation (**3**) to a form (*RS^n*) capable of binding to acceptor sites in the cell nucleus (**4**). The association of the *RS^n* complex with chromatin in some way causes the synthesis of specific mRNAs (**5**) and consequent new protein synthesis (**6**). The newly synthesized proteins produce the cellular alterations that mediate the gross physiologic effect. *(From Pratt WB. The mechanism of glucocorticoid action in fibroblasts. J Invest Dermatol 1978;71:24–35. © by Williams & Wilkins. Reprinted with permission.)*

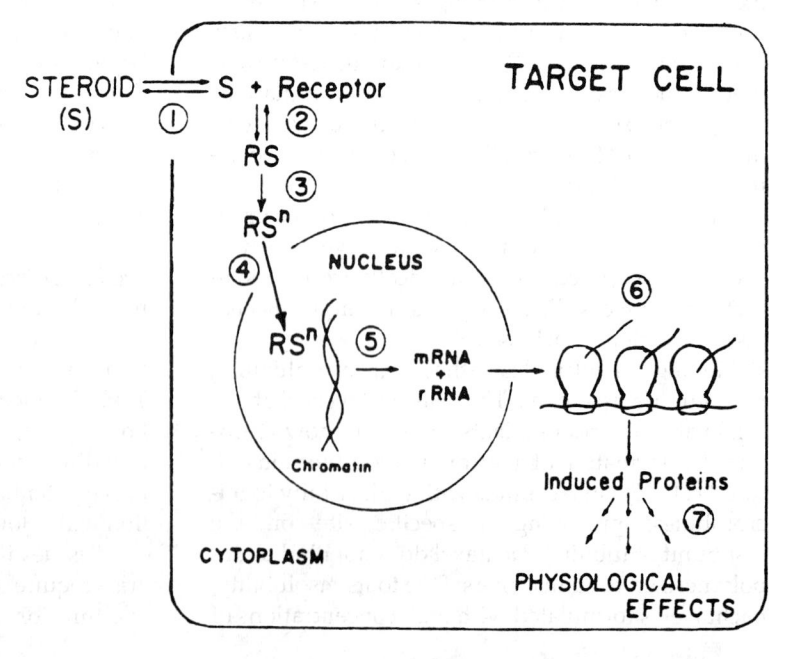

is a basic concept for most hormonal therapies, with the notable exception of estrogen use in postmenopausal breast cancer.

The side effects of hormonal therapy are generally tolerable and usually relate to extensions of the normal actions of pharmacologic doses of steroids (eg, fluid retention). Another example is androgen-induced hirsutism, deepening of the voice, and increased libido.

The corticosteroid hormones that are active in lymphocytic proliferations also apparently require specific receptor interactions. These are believed to be common in lymphoid tumors, wherein a high incidence of response is clinically characteristic. Here the pharmacologic mechanism appears to involve decreased utilization of cellular energy caused by an impairment of glucose transport or phosphorylation. A direct cytotoxic effect on lymphocytes, however, has also been observed.

Overall, the responses to hormonal therapy can be dramatic and prolonged. The steroid hormones offer some of the most specifically tumor-directed activities of any agents used in chemotherapy. They also do not add to myelosuppression and generally have minimal side effects. In some exquisitely sensitive tumors, single-agent hormonal therapy can offer long and easily tolerated disease palliation. Eventual hormonal resistance is, however, common and usually denotes a loss of the hormonally dependent growth characteristic.

Estrogens

Estrogens offer significant disease palliation in patients with advanced prostatic cancer. These effects may be mediated by a direct effect on prostate tissue as well as through suppression of adrenal luteinizing hormone secretion. Estrogens are also beneficial, through unknown mechanisms, in a small proportion of patients with advanced carcinoma of the breast. In addition to the antitumor effects previously described, estrogens have a variety of other diverse pharmacologic actions.

Agents available include the natural steroids estradiol (Emcyt®, Estrace®, Estraderm®) and conjugated estrogens and the natural steroid derivative ethinyl estradiol (Brevicon®, Demulen®, Levlen®). Synthetic nonsteroidal compounds with potent estrogenic activity are most often used in cancer therapy, however. This category includes diethylstilbestrol (DES®, Stilbestrol®) chlorotrianisene (TACE®), and dienestrol (Ortho Dienestrol Cream®).

In prostate cancer patients relatively low estrogen doses are efficacious. Indeed, in controlled studies, 1 mg diethylstilbestrol was as effective as higher doses that appeared to accelerate cardiovascular disease. Estrogen use in breast cancer is indicated in postmenopausal patients only. Common side effects include gynecomastia in men (which may be prevented by prophylactic, low-dose breast irradiation) and vaginal bleeding and breast tenderness in women. In premenopausal breast cancer patients, estrogens can exacerbate disease symptoms. Other considerations for estrogen use in breast cancer patients include the possibility of edema from sodium retention and potential worsening of impaired cardiovascular function or acute hypercalcemia on initial estrogen therapy. The latter occurs most often in patients with bone involvement. Male patients will often report some degree of physiologic feminization, which can be disconcerting and sometimes leads to discontinuation of therapy by the patient.

In treating breast cancer, estrogen therapy should be continued for at least 3 months before switching to alternate treatments; however, most patients will respond within 1 to 2 months of initiation of treatment. Paradoxically, some patients will respond on withdrawal of estrogen. Pharmacologically, estrogens are well absorbed orally. They are inactivated in the liver but are enterohepatically recycled. Although the natural products appear to be rapidly eliminated in the urine as glucuronide conjugates, the synthetic agents can be biotransformed to active compounds (eg, chlorotrianisene) and are more slowly degraded and eliminated.

Progestins

Progestins are compounds related to the natural human steroid progesterone, which is produced by the placenta and corpus luteum. The progestins used to treat metastatic endometrial breast carcinomas include hydroxyprogesterone caproate (Delalutin®, Hydroxon®, Pro-Depo®), medroxyprogesterone (Cycrin®, Depo-Provera®, Provera®), and megestrol (Megace®).

The exact biochemical mechanism for the antitumor effect is not well known. From other steroid models, the presence of specific receptors is thought to be required for activity. Although there can be direct feedback effects on pituitary and/or hypothalamic growth control mechanisms, a direct, local, biologically antagonistic growth effect may be most responsible for disease regression. Some progestins have definite antiestrogen effects.

As with most steroid derivatives, progestins are

metabolized in the liver and excreted partially in the urine. The large pharmacologic doses commonly used are usually well tolerated. Side effects include occasional liver function abnormalities, mild fluid retention, and, rarely, acute hypercalcemia in patients with bony metastases. Anabolic effects of progestins may be useful in support of the cachectic patient.

Androgens

Androgens are derivatives of testosterone, the natural male sex hormone, which is produced primarily by testicular Leydig cells. Compounds useful in anticancer therapy are testosterone (cypionate [Andro-Cyp®], enanthate [Andro L.A.®], and propionate [Androlan]) itself or synthetic derivatives of testosterone such as fluoxymesterone and methyltestosterone (Android-10®, Estratest®, Testred®). Clinical effects are most often observed in breast cancer patients with either demonstrated steroid receptors or a history of prior response to other endocrine manipulations. In all cases the presence of specific receptors is probably required for activity. The exact biochemical mechanism of the antitumor effect, however, is unknown. Paradoxically, estrogens and androgens are not completely antagonistic, and mutual receptor site competition has not been observed. Other biologic actions of androgens include stimulatory effects on the bone marrow, increasing red cell mass, and on the fibrinolytic and immune response systems, as well as the characteristic anabolic effects, with retention of nitrogen, potassium, phosphorus, and calcium.

Androgens are usually well tolerated but can produce nausea and vomiting. Other side effects include virilization, mild fluid retention, and hypercalcemia (rarely on initiation). In a very small percentage of patients an acute tumor "flare" may occur with sudden increase in bone pain for those breast cancer patients with skeletal metastases. Androgens can also cause abnormalities of liver function and, rarely, jaundice. Cholestatic (obstructive) jaundice is well documented and, on occurrence, requires immediate discontinuation of the drug. Androgens can also have profound psychologic effects ("steroid rage").

Corticosteroids

Corticosteroids are synthetic compounds derived from the natural adrenal hormone cortisol (hydrocortisone). There are diverse pharmacologic activities of these agents, but individual compounds differ chiefly in their duration of effect and in their relative mineralocorticoid (aldosterone-like) salt-retaining activity. Some of the effects include stimulation of carbohydrate storage, anti-insulin effects, rising blood glucose, protein catabolic effects, aldosterone-like activity, increasing salt and water retention, depressive activity on eosinophils and lymphocyte proliferation, enhanced gastric acid secretion, increased muscle and bone catabolism, nervous system effects, and, importantly, suppressive actions on immunologic tissue inflammatory responses. Corticosteroids are often combined with other agents in cancer treatment, as bone marrow suppression is not augmented. The anti-inflammatory activity and euphoria produced by high doses can be beneficial for some patients; however, euphoria can progress to "steroid psychosis," necessitating dosage reduction or discontinuation. Corticosteroids are useful in the primary combination chemotherapy of both acute and chronic lymphocytic leukemias, in both Hodgkin's and non-Hodgkin's lymphomas, in myelomas, and in a few breast cancers. Selective binding to lymphoid elements probably occurs as a result of specific corticosteroid receptors in lymphoid tumors. The specific cellular mechanism that acts to halt DNA synthesis appears to be mediated by inhibition of glucose transport or phosphorylation. This may then lead to a decrease in available intracellular energy. The agents are known to retard mitotic division. Cellular protein synthesis is also inhibited, and both normal and abnormal lymphoid elements are depressed. Other therapeutic uses in cancer patients include a weak antihypercalcemic effect and suppression of the inflammatory edema of bony and/or brain metastases.

The compound most often used in cancer therapy is prednisone (Deltasone®), a synthetic compound closely related to hydrocortisone. Prednisone retains some mineralocorticoid activity and has a relatively short duration (3–4 hours) of pharmacologic effects. Other adrenal corticosteroids include the natural compound hydrocortisone and other synthetic analogs, dexamethasone (Decadron®), methylprednisolone (Medrol®), and prednisolone. In contrast to prednisone, the methylprednisolone derivative and other synthetic congeners lose the salt-retaining properties entirely and the relative potency and duration of effect are greatly increased. For example, dexamethasone has 30 times the anti-inflammatory potency of hydrocortisone (milligram per milligram) and is devoid of salt-retaining action. Its duration of action probably exceeds 24 hours, although the parent compound is cleared more rapidly.

There are both oral and injectable esters of most major corticosteroids. These are usually well tolerated and can often promote a feeling of euphoria along with mild stimulation of appetite. Long-term complications include the production of a Cushingoid state, hypertension, diabetes, and osteoporosis. A sometimes devastating complication is profound immunosuppression which may lead to a serious infection, often by opportunistic and uncommon pathogens. Peptic ulceration has also been observed with long-term corticosteroid use. Other metabolic side effects may include hypokalemia and sodium and fluid retention, depending on the compound selected. Psychosis is possible while on or when discontinuing high-dose therapy. A "flulike" steroid withdrawal syndrome for the chronic user may also progress to acute adrenal insufficiency.

Luteinizing Hormone-Releasing Hormone Agonists

Luteinizing hormone-releasing hormone (LH-RH) agonists (also known as gonadotropin-releasing hormone [Gn-RH] agonists) are used primarily in the treatment of prostatic cancer. Synthetic LH-RH agonists, such as leuprolide acetate (Lupron®) and goserelin acetate (Zoladex®), prevent the biosynthesis of steroids in the testes and thereby remove the androgenic stimulation for prostate tissue growth. The initial effect of drug treatment is an increased testosterone level resulting from enhanced release of LH. With continued treatment, the pituitary gland becomes desensitized as a result of a drop in the number of Gn-RH receptors. Pituitary release of LH into blood is thereby inhibited and, eventually, estrogen and androgen synthesis in the glands is shut down. The initial surge in testosterone may result in disease flare in some patients. Gn-RH agonists appear to be as effective and better tolerated than diethylstilbestrol in treatment of patients with prostatic carcinoma, particularly with respect to cardiovascular complications of estrogen therapy. Combinations of LH-RH agonists with antiandrogenic agents such as flutamide have been employed.

Antihormonal Agents

The broad category of antihormonal agents contains the antiestrogenic compound tamoxifen (Nolvadex®), the antiandrogen flutamide (Eulexin®), and the antiadrenal agents mitotane (Lysodren®) and aminoglutethimide (Cytadren®). Tamoxifen is a nonsteroidal compound that acts by competitively blocking the access of natural estrogens to their specific cell membrane receptors. Its use is theoretically limited to endocrine-derived tumors expressing the estrogen receptor. Responses noted in patients with estrogen receptor-negative tumors may be an artifact of false-negative receptor analyses. However, recent laboratory studies suggest that tamoxifen may activate "programmed cell death" in estrogen-receptor-negative breast carcinoma cells by unknown mechanisms. Tamoxifen has good oral activity and is relatively well tolerated. Side effects include "menopause-like" reactions, such as hot flashes and mild nausea and vomiting. Increased bone pain with a local "flare" of disease may occasionally dictate discontinuation. Overall side effects are both mild and rare and tamoxifen represents a very useful form of hormonal therapy.

Flutamide is a nonsteroidal androgen antagonist that blocks binding of testosterone and dihydrotestosterone to the androgen receptor. It is frequently used in combination with estrogen or LH-RH agonist therapy of prostate carcinoma.

The antiadrenal compounds include the DDT insecticide analog mitotane and aminoglutethimide, a compound once used as an anticonvulsant. Mitotane is used in the treatment of inoperable adrenal tumors. Mitotane is selectively toxic, through unknown mechanisms, to normal and cancerous adrenal tissues, inducing atrophy and necrosis and resulting in adrenal steroid synthetic shutdown. Mitotane can thus control the symptoms related to excess hormone production. Its principal side effects are central nervous system and gastrointestinal disturbances and skin rash.

Aminoglutethimide was originally tested as an anticonvulsant but was noted to cause symptoms of adrenal insufficiency. This was shown to be caused by inhibition of mitochondrial function with blockade of all classes of steroid hormone synthesis (mineralocorticoids, glucocorticoids, and sex steroids). The drug acts by inhibiting the enzymatic conversion of cholesterol to pregnenolone. In advanced breast cancer patients, aminoglutethimide is sometimes successfully used to produce a "medical adrenalectomy." Concomitant therapy with hydrocortisone is necessary to block a compensatory increase in pituitary adrenocorticotropin secretion, which would override the aminoglutethimide inhibition of adrenal hormone production. Hydrocortisone is used rather than dexamethasone because aminoglutethimide induces metabolism of the latter corticoid. Most patients experience side effects, usually limited to gastrointestinal and dermatologic toxicities and mild central nervous system effects.

MISCELLANEOUS DRUGS

Hydroxyurea (Hydrea®) is a compound of very simple structure that is useful in the treatment of chronic myelogenous leukemia. It appears to act primarily through inhibition of the enzyme ribonucleotide reductase, which plays a central role in DNA synthesis by catalyzing the conversion of ribonucleotides to deoxyribonucleotides (see Fig 2.3). Synthesis of RNA and protein is not affected. As expected from its biochemical target, hydroxyurea is most toxic to cells that are actively synthesizing DNA. The drug blocks cellular progression at or near the G_1–S interface. The major adverse effects are bone marrow depression, gastrointestinal upset, and, rarely, dermatologic reactions and renal impairment.

Asparaginase (Elspar®) is an enzyme used as a cancer therapeutic agent. Most normal cells possess the ability to synthesize the amino acid asparagine. Some tumor cells, such as those in acute lymphoblastic leukemia, do not possess this ability and require exogenous asparagine. The enzyme asparaginase converts asparagine to nonfunctional aspartic acid and deprives the tumor cell of this crucial amino acid, thereby blocking protein synthesis. Side effects encountered with the clinical use of this agent include pancreatic and hepatic damage, cerebral dysfunction, and protein synthesis inhibition leading to clotting disorders. As asparaginase is a biologic product obtained from *Escherichia coli* or *Erwinia*, allergic reactions are frequently encountered.

REFERENCES

Bodley AL, Liu LF. Topoisomerases as novel targets for cancer chemotherapy. *Bio/Technology*. 1988;**6**:1315–1319.

Chabner B. *Pharmacologic Principles of Cancer Treatment*. Philadelphia: WB Saunders; 1982.

Chabner BA, Myers CE. Clinical pharmacology of cancer chemotherapy. In: DeVita VT Jr, Hellman S, Rosenberg SA, eds. *Cancer, Principles and Practice of Oncology*. Philadelphia: JB Lippincott; 1985:349–395.

Deuchars KL, Ling V. P-glycoprotein and multidrug resistance in cancer chemotherapy. *Semin Oncol*. 1989; **16**:156–165.

Howell A, Wakeling AE. Steroid and peptide hormone and growth factors. In: *Cancer Chemotherapy and Biological Response Modifiers*, Annual 9. Amsterdam: Elsevier; 1987:121–133.

Howell A, Wakeling AE. Steroid and peptide hormones and growth factors. In: *Cancer Chemotherapy and Biological Response Modifiers*, Annual 10. Amsterdam: Elsevier; 1988:117–128.

McEvoy GK, ed. *AHFS Drug Information*. Bethesda, MD: American Society of Hospital Pharmacists; 1991.

Pratt WB, Ruddon RW. *The Anticancer Drugs*. New York: Oxford University Press; 1979.

Rowinsky, EK, Onetto, N, Canetta, RM, Arbuck, SG. Taxol: The first of the taxanes, an important new class of antitumor agents. *Semin. Oncol*. 1992;**19**:646–662.

Sutherland DJ. Hormones and cancer. In: Tannock IF, Hill RP, eds. *The Basic Science of Oncology*. New York: Pergamon Press; 1987:204–222.

Weiss GR, Arteaga CL, Brown TD, et al. New anticancer agents. In: *Cancer Chemotherapy and Biological Response Modifiers*, Annual 9. Amsterdam: Elsevier; 1987:93–120.

Weiss GR, Arteaga CL, Brown TD, et al. New anticancer agents. In: *Cancer Chemotherapy and Biological Response Modifiers*, Annual 10. Amsterdam: Elsevier; 1988:85–116.

Chapter 3

Hypercalcemia of Malignancy

Amy J. Galpin, Rebecca Johnson Irvin, John G. Kuhn

Hypercalcemia is estimated to occur in 10 to 20% of all cancer patients and is described as the most common metabolic emergency in this population. Although nearly 90% of hypercalcemia cases may be attributed to either malignancy (35%) or primary hyperparathyroidism (54%), malignancy remains the most common cause of emergent hypercalcemia in the hospitalized population. Hypercalcemia-induced symptoms may also significantly compromise the patient's quality and duration of remaining life.

The incidence of hypercalcemia varies for different malignancies. It rarely occurs in such common tumors as colorectal or lung cancer of small cell histology, yet frequently is associated with breast cancer, multiple myeloma, and squamous cell neoplasms (eg, of the lung, and head and neck). In contrast, uncommon tumors that demonstrate consistent associations with hypercalcemia include parathyroid carcinoma, cholangiocarcinoma, and vasoactive intestinal peptide (VIP)-producing tumors. Hypercalcemia frequently occurs in association with advanced-stage disease, with survival averaging less than 1 year following the initial hypercalcemic episode (often less than 3 months). Nevertheless, for many tumors, correlations are poor between the severity of hypercalcemia and the stage of disease, extent of bony involvement, or survival.

CALCIUM HOMEOSTASIS AND PHYSIOLOGIC REGULATION OF BONE METABOLISM

Ionized calcium influences several important physiologic and cellular processes, including secretion of neurohumors and other cellular products, stabilization of membranes and maintenance of neuromuscular excitability, coupling of excitation to contraction, and facilitation of blood coagulation and mineralization of newly formed bone. In view of the potential impact of aberrant levels, extracellular calcium levels are tightly maintained within a "normal" range corresponding to a total serum calcium value of 8.5 to 10.5 mg/dL (2.1 to 2.6 mmol/L). Most laboratories report measured values as total serum calcium, which reflects the sum of ionized (unbound), nonionized (protein-bound), and complexed (diffusible) forms of calcium. Ionized calcium is the physiologically active species. Therefore, it is important to correct reported total values for alterations in the unbound (ionized) fraction. Abnormalities in acid–base status or in serum protein content may falsely "lower" (eg, acidosis or hypoalbuminemia) or "elevate" (eg, alkalosis or myeloma paraproteinemia) and total serum calcium values. Clinically useful formulas, listed in Table 3.1, have been developed to "correct" for hypoalbuminemia. Direct measurement of ionized calcium may be useful in detecting subtle or false elevations of calcium; however, this is not readily available in most laboratories and offers little advantage over monitoring total serum calcium in routine clinical practice.

Although the combined extracellular fluid (ECF) and soft tissue compartments contain only 1% of total body calcium, the ECF serves as a central exchange pool, between the gut, kidney, and bone. These organs are respectively responsible for calcium entry, excretion/reabsorption, and storage. Calcium flux between these regulatory sites is controlled largely by three hormones: parathyroid hormone (PTH), calcitriol, and calcitonin. Net calcium

TABLE 3.1. SERUM CALCIUM LEVELS

Total serum calcium (8.5–10.5 mg/dL) exists in three forms

1. Protein-bound: 50% (nonionized, inactive)
   a. Reported total Ca^{2+} corrected for hypoalbuminemia

   corrected Ca^{2+} = measured Ca^{2+} + 0.8 (4.0 − albumin)
   or corrected Ca^{2+} = (measured Ca^{2+} − albumin) + 4

   b. Abnormal elevation of serum protein (multiple myeloma paraproteins) may "falsely" increase value
2. Complexed diffusible form: 5–15% (nonionized, inactive)
   a. Complexed to citrate, bicarbonate, phosphate
3. Free, ionized calcium: 40–50% (active)
   a. Normal value: 4–5 mg/dL
   b. Protein binding and therefore free fraction altered by acid–base status (acidosis increases free fraction, alkalosis decreases)

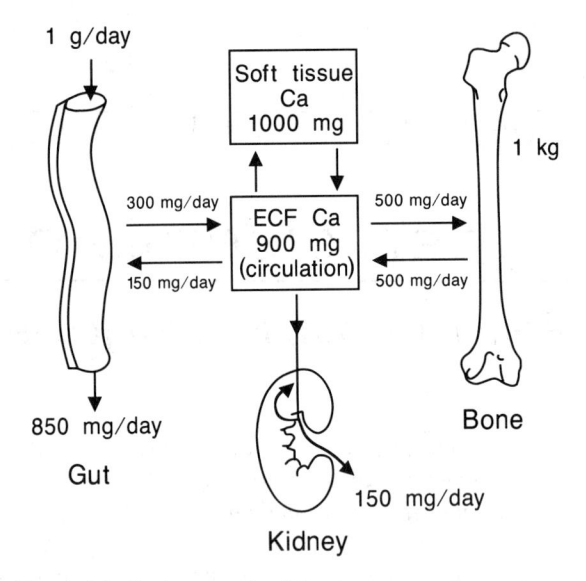

Figure 3.1. Exchanges of calcium between major regulatory organs. ECF, extracellular fluid. *(From Mundy GR. Treatment of hypercalcemia due to malignancy. In: Mundy GR, ed. Calcium Homeostasis: Hypercalcemia and Hypocalcemia. 2nd ed. New York: Oxford University Press; 1990:2. Reprinted with permission.)*

absorption from the gastrointestinal tract (15–70%) is enhanced by calcitriol. Renal calcium reabsorption occurs largely in the proximal tubule (65%) and the loop of Henle (25%) and is positively linked to sodium and fluid reuptake. States promoting sodium retention, such as volume depletion, therefore tend to reduce urinary clearance of calcium. Fine-tuning of calcium excretion (10%) occurs in the distal tubule, where calcium reabsorption is promoted by PTH and calcitriol (convoluted tubule) and inhibited by pharmacologic doses of calcitonin.

Bone serves as a repository for 99% of the body's calcium. The processes of bone formation and resorption are coupled, such that calcium exchange in and out of bone are normally equal, impacting minimally on overall calcium balance. When imbalances arise, however, net calcium fluxes between the bone and ECF may assume a specific "direction," compensating for dietary deficits, unusual losses, or retention for skeletal growth (Fig 3.1).

Table 3.2 details the regulation of calcium homeostasis by the "calcitropic" hormones PTH, calcitriol, and calcitonin. Because calcium metabolism is closely linked to bone and phosphate turnover, numerous other hormones and cytokines affecting these processes may indirectly impact calcium metabolism. The importance of normal or abnormal states of interaction between hormones which regulate skeletal integrity and calcium homeostasis is not entirely clear.

REGULATION OF BONE REMODELING: RESORPTION AND FORMATION

Bones are continuously being remodeled by the coupled processes of resorption and formation. The bone-forming unit, the osteon, consists of a central nutrient canal (the Haversion canal), osteoclasts, osteoblasts, and osteocytes (osteoblasts that have been interred into bone). Bone turnover occurs asynchronously, in multiple discrete foci, throughout the skeleton, but is collectively greatest at endosteal surfaces, in metaphyseal areas, or in areas of bone growth or healing.

The osteoclast appears to be the final common effector cell of bone resorption. Osteoclasts are derived from hematopoietic precursors similar to that of a mononuclear phagocyte, which later undergo fusion into multinuclear giant cells (Fig 3.2). The point at which osteoclast differentiation diverges from other hematopoietic cell lineages, and the influence of endogenous or exogenously administered hematopoietic growth factors on osteoclast differentiation, is currently unknown. Osteoclasts initiate resorptive activity by podosomal adhesion along the ruffled cell border, to areas of inorganic mineralization. These podosome membranes form a

TABLE 3.2. NORMAL HORMONAL REGULATION OF CALCIUM

Hormone	Stimulus	Effect	Outcome	Feedback
Parathyroid hormone	↓ Serum calcium (↑ Phosphate)	↑ Bone resorption (osteoblast–osteoclast) ↑ Distal tubule calcium reabsorption ↑ Formation of 1,25-(OH$_2$)-vitamin D$_3$ ↑ Renal loss of phosphate	↑ Serum calcium ↓ Phosphate	Magnesium plays "permissive role" ↑ Serum calcium ↑ Calcitriol?
Calcitriol (1,25-dihydroxy-vitamin D$_3$)	↑ Parathyroid hormone ↓ Phosphorus	↑ Gut absorption of calcium phosphate ↑ Bone turnover (mineralization and resorption) ↑ Tubular resorption of calcium phosphate	↑ Serum calcium ↑ Phosphate	↑ Phosphorus
Calcitonin	↑ Serum calcium	↓ Bone resorption by osteoclast	↓ Phosphate ↓ Serum calcium	Short-term control of serum calcium

sealed zone extracellularly, into which hydrogen ions are secreted. Local pH is consequently reduced to 5.5, which solubilizes hydroxyapatite crystal, leads to bone demineralization, and generates free calcium for entry into the ECF pool. Proteases are also released, which hydrolyze the demineralized bone matrix proteins.

Osteoblasts, arising from stromal or fibroblastic lineages, are responsible for the synthesis and mineralization of osteoid. Osteoblasts deposit a matrix of unmineralized bone proteins in the vicinity of previous osteoclastic resorption which include osteocalcin (bone Gla protein), osteonectin, type I collagen, and bone-modulating proteins (BMPs). Min-

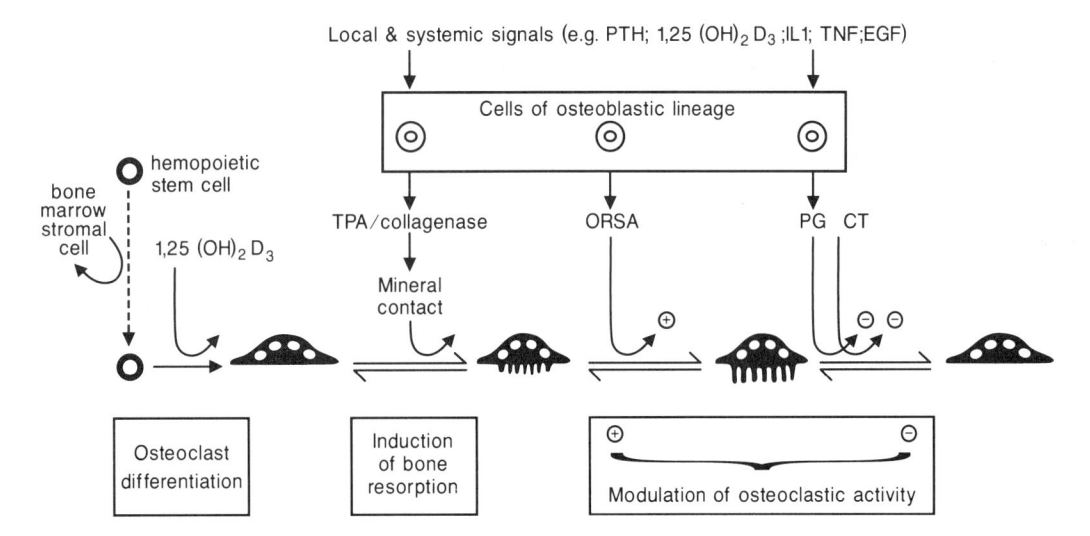

Figure 3.2. Diagrammatic representation of the mechanism of regulation of osteoclastic differentiation and function. Among systemic regulators, only calcitonin (CT) acts directly on osteoclasts. All the agents so far tested that stimulate bone resorption in organ culture act primarily on cells of the osteoblastic lineage. These cells are able to initiate and subsequently modulate osteoclastic resorption. PTH, parathyroid hormone; IL-1, interleukin-1; TNF, tumor necrosis factor; EGF, epidermal growth factor; PG, prostaglandin; TPA, tissue plasminogen activator; ORSA, osteoclast resorption stimulation activity. *(Chambers TJ. Regulation of bone resorption. In: Russell RGG, Kanis JA, eds. Tumor-Induced Hypercalcemia and Its Management. London: Royal Society of Medicine Services Ltd: 1991:2. Reprinted with permission.)*

eralization of the osteoid occurs as calcium and phosphate are precipitated at the osteoid surface in the form of immature hydroxyapatite complexes which gradually "ripen" in crystal size and strength. Calcitriol indirectly enhances bone formation by ensuring that adequate concentrations of calcium and phosphate are present at the bone interface. In addition to synthesizing osteoid, osteoblasts appear to influence bone mineralization by producing regulatory enzymes, such as alkaline phosphatases or by incorporating regulatory BMPs into the matrix.

Even in many states of heightened bone turnover, new bone formation balances resorption, in both quantity and location. Although bone resorption precedes bone formation, most factors found to promote osteoclastic resorption, in vitro, are dependent on the presence of osteoblastic cell types. This suggests that an intracellular messenger system exists between osteoblasts and osteoclasts. Even within the realm of resorption, control of osteoclasts may be exerted at various levels: production/differentiation of osteoclasts, initiation of resorption, and modulation of ongoing resorption activity. For example, osteoblasts permit osteoclasts access to mineralized bone for subsequent bone remodeling to begin. The generation of osteoclasts appears to require calcitriol. The hematopoietic growth factors granulocyte–macrophage colony-stimulating factor [GM-CSF], M-CSF, G-CSF have been suggested both to promote and to inhibit osteoclast recruitment or differentiation. These factors and other cytokines, collectively termed osteoclast-activating factors (OAFs), may require osteoblastic intermediaries to modulate osteoclast functions. Table 3.3 lists hormonal and cytokine factors thought to influence bone turnover.

PATHOGENESIS OF HYPERCALCEMIA IN MALIGNANCY

Even in cancer patients, nonmalignant factors may exacerbate 10 to 25% of hypercalcemic episodes. Table 3.4 lists possible etiologies that should be included in the differential diagnosis of hypercalcemia. In hypercalcemia of malignancy (HCM), the abnormalities of calcium homeostasis appear to be, in decreasing order of pathogenic importance: the bone, the kidney, and occasionally the gut.

Increased bone resorption is probably necessary to induce, but not maintain, a hypercalcemic state. In HCM, bone resorption still appears to be mediated primarily by osteoclasts, but in cancers associated with osteolytic lesions, destruction of bone directly by tumor may also contribute. Osteoclast activation may be heightened by humoral factors such as parathyroid-related peptide (PTHrP), released systemically by tumor cells. In response to tumor stimuli, normal host cells can indirectly promote bone resorption by producing cytokines which

TABLE 3.3. AGENTS THAT MAY ACT DIRECTLY OR INDIRECTLY ON OSTEOCLASTS OR OSTEOBLASTS

	Hormones	Cytokines	Drugs and Other Agents
Osteoclasts			
Activators of bone resorption	PTH, thyroxine, 1,25-(OH)$_2$-vitamin D$_3$	PGE$_2$, TGF-α, GM-CSF, M-CSF, IL-3, TNF-α and -β, EGF, PTHrP	Retinoids, heparin, phorbol esters, mellitin, β-endotoxin
Inhibitors of bone resorption	Calcitonin	IFN-γ, TGF-β	Bisphosphonates, gallium salts colchicine, plicamycin, protease inhibitors
Osteoblasts			
Activators of bone formation	PTH, insulin, anabolic steroids, thyroxine	Somatomedin, TGF-β, prostaglandins	Phosphate, fluoride
Inhibitors of bone formation or mineralization	Glucocorticoids		Aluminum salts, phenytoin, glucocorticoids, bisphosphonates (eg, etidronate at high doses)

PTH, parathyroid hormone; PG, prostaglandin; TGF, transforming growth factor; IL, interleukin; GM, granulocyte–macrophage; CSF, colony-stimulating factor; TNF, tumor necrosis factor; EGF, epidermal growth factor; IFN, interferon; PTHrP, parathyroid hormone-related protein; IGF, insulin-like growth factor.
From Russell RGG, Kanis JA, eds. Tumor-Induced Hypercalcemia and Its Management. London: Royal Society of Medicine Services Ltd; 1991. Adapted with permission.

TABLE 3.4. MNEMONIC FOR THE DIFFERENTIAL DIAGNOSIS OF HYPERCALCEMIA

Vitamins A and D	**T**hiazides, lithium, and
Immobilization	other drugs
Thydrotoxicosis	**R**habdomyolysis, renal
Addison's disease	failure
Milk-alkali syndrome	**A**IDS
Inflammatory disorders	**P**aget's, total parenteral
Neoplastic-related disease	nutrition, and parathyroid
Sarcoidosis	disease

From Allan P. Unusual causes of hypercalcemia. Endocrinol Metab Clin North Am. 1989;18:753–763. Adapted with permission.

activate osteoclasts (eg, IL-1, TNF-B, IL-6, GM-CSF). If osteoclast-activating mediators are released locally, the associated clinical syndrome is characterized by discrete bone lesions, whereas if released systemically to act at distant sites, the corresponding syndrome tends to be one of diffuse osteopenia (or a mixed pattern). The classification of proposed osteoclast activators is not strictly "local" or "systemic," because some mediators may be active at either level, depending on the underlying malignancy (Fig 3.3). Because production or elevation of these cytokines does not always result in hypercalcemia, it is likely that a combination of variables or synergism between factors is necessary to produce HCM.

Recent focuses on the structure and function of PTHrP reveals a peptide sharing chromosomal and structural homologies with endogenous immunoreactive PTH. Evidence is mounting that PTHrP is an important mediator of hypercalcemia in several malignancies, although it is in normal tissues at various stages of development, implying other physiologic roles. The biologic activity of PTHrP is attributed to the first 34 amino acids of the $-NH_2$ terminus. PTHrP binds to PTH receptors, producing responses similar to those observed with PTH: increased bone turnover, renal phosphate wasting and enhanced calcium reabsorption in association with elevated nephrogenous cyclic adenosine monophosphate (cAMP), and promotion of calcitriol production. Immunoreactive assays that are able to distinguish between PTH and PTHrP should soon become clinically available, aiding in the differential diagnosis of HCM and hyperparathyroidism.

The kidney is normally able to increase calcium excretion roughly fivefold; however, in the face of massive skeletal calcium mobilization, renal compensatory capacities are overwhelmed. Renal calcium excretion may also be blunted as a result of fixed renal insufficiencies (nephrotoxin-, disease-, or myeloma-induced), sepsis, or hypercalcemia-induced impairments of renal function (nephrocalcinosis or chronic interstitial nephritis). Volume depletion will further impair renal response and hemoconcentrate calcium levels.

In hypercalcemia of malignancy, the impact of gut-related factors is usually negligible. For most patients, intestinal calcium entry is reduced, as a result of either appropriate homeostatic decreases in PTH and calcitriol production or reduced dietary intake.

Three subgroups of patients with HCM have been described by Mundy (1990): "humoral " HCM, HCM associated with "osteolytic metastases," and "hematologic" HCM. These distinctions are somewhat arbitrary in that they share considerable overlap, whether categorized by pathophysiology, clinical characteristics, underlying malignancy, or suggested clinical management.

"Humoral hypercalcemia of malignancy" is associated with solid tumors in the absence of obvious bone metastases (eg, non small-cell lung cancer, renal carcinoma). Production of PTHrP appears to be an important factor which promotes generalized osteoclast activation and renal calcium reabsorption. Unlike states of excess endogenous PTH, calcitriol production is minimal, and bone formation appears suppressed, possibly due to additional

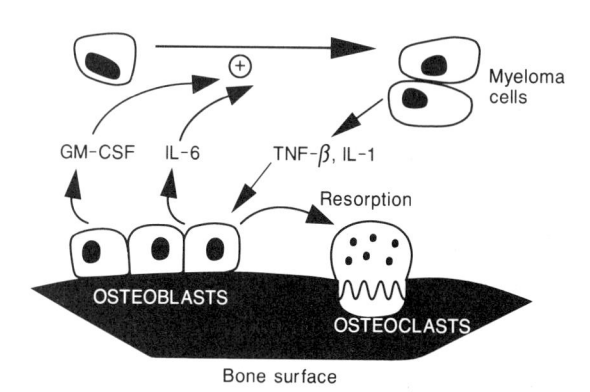

Figure 3.3. Possible interactions between myeloma and bone. GM-CSF, granulocyte–macrophage colony-stimulating factor; IL, interleukin; TNF, tumor necrosis factor. (From Russell RGG. Cytokines and growth factors as regulators of bone metabolism, and their relation to cancer. In: Russell RGG, Kanis JA, eds. Tumor-Induced Hypercalcemia and Its Management. London: New York, Royal Society of Medicine Services Ltd; 1991:19. Reprinted with permission.)

osteoblast-inhibiting factors. Appropriately, endogenous PTH levels are reduced. A diffuse osteopenic state predominates; however, local pathologic fractures are a potential complication.

The syndrome of "hypercalcemia and osteolytic metastases" features solid tumors with clincally identifiable bone metastases (eg, breast cancer, multiple myeloma). Focal destruction of bone is mediated by direct tumor invasion or by local release of OAFs. The degree of hypercalcemia, does not necessarily correlate with the extent of bony destruction; therefore, other variables such as reductions in urinary calcium excretion are probably also important. The third category of "hematologic malignancies" includes primarily multiple myeloma and lymphomas. Leukemia is rarely associated with hypercalcemia. Identifiable bone lesions are invariably present in myeloma, but may not be detected in the other hematologic malignancies. Proposed pathologic mechanisms are heterogenous: OAFs are probably active at both the local and systemic levels and calcitriol may be elevated in lymphomas. Elevations in calcitriol are noted in approximately 50% of lymphomas linked to the human T-lymphotropic virus I (HTLV-I) virus (adult T-cell) and B-cell and Hodgkin's lymphomas; however, hypercalcemia is uncommon, implying that other factors are important. Hypercalcemia in Hodgkin's disease occurs almost exclusively in those with high-grade or bulky abdominal disease. Elevations of 1,24-hydroxyvitamin D, in the absence of PTHrP, have been noted in a few solid tumors, such as small cell lung cancer patients. In myeloma, disease-related renal impairment and the production of TNF-β (formerly, lymphotoxin), in conjunction with IL-6, appear to be important cofactors that promote hypercalcemia.

CLINICAL FEATURES OF HYPERCALCEMIA IN MALIGNANCY

Hypercalcemia-induced symptoms can be insidious, nonspecific, or easily attributed to other patient factors that are frequently present. Timely recognition and institution of specific management for hypercalcemia mandate a high index of suspicion for those patients at greatest risk of becoming hypercalcemic. Patients vary considerably in their tolerance of a given calcium level. In general, the severity of hypercalcemic symptoms parallels not only the absolute calcium level, but also patient age and the rate and magnitude of the rise in calcium. Patients experiencing gradual or long-standing elevations of calcium, such as those with primary hyperparathyroidism, may be only mildly symptomatic at calcium levels that would otherwise induce significant symptoms if developed acutely. Underlying patient conditions will also influence the threshold at which HCM becomes symptomatic or life-threatening. At a serum calcium of less than 12 mg/dL, the majority of patients are only mildly symptomatic. With serum calcium levels above 13.5 mg/dL, most (>90%) patients are appreciably symptomatic. Potentially fatal events, such as cardiac arrythmias and severe obtundation, are infrequent below calcium levels of 15 to 16 mg/dL.

Many of the symptoms of hypercalcemia reflect the deranged function of calcium in its physiologic role. Hence, major findings involve the cardiovascular, gastrointestinal, renal, and neurologic systems (Table 3.5). Renal function, an important compensator in calcium elevation, is also reduced. The inhibitory effect of calciuria on renal free water reabsorption leads to polyuria and dehydration. Anorexia, nausea, vomiting, and altered mental status further impair efforts to maintain oral hydration. These compounding factors contribute toward progres-

TABLE 3.5. CLINICAL MANIFESTATIONS OF HYPERCALCEMIA

Neurologic
Depression, irritability, sleep disorders
Lethargy, confusion, stupor, coma
Muscle weakness, hypotonia
Absent deep tendon reflexes
Decreased auditory acuity

Gastrointestinal
Anorexia, vomiting, gastric atony
Constipation/diarrhea
Acute pancreatitis (rare)

Cardiovascular
Shortening QT interval
Broadening T wave
Heart block, asystole
Ventricular arrhythmias
Synergism with digoxin

Renal
Polyuria, polydipsia
Dehydration
Decreased glomerular filtration rate, nephrocalcinosis

sive volume depletion, ECF contraction, and the promotion of sodium retention, which blunts renal calcium excretion. In turn, the elevation of calcium is perpetuated. Patients may demonstrate only a few to occasionally several of the clinical symptoms associated with hypercalcemia.

Some generalizations can be stated, contrasting the symptomatology of HCM and primary hyperparathyroidism (PHP). Although serum calcium levels of 13 to 17 mg/dL can be consistent with both etiologies, values in the range 17 to 22 mg/dL are linked more often to PHP than to HCM alone. With the exception of retroperitoneal tumors, hypercalcemia as the presenting symptom of occult malignancy is rare. Subtle psychopathologic and cognitive changes occur in more than 50% of those with PHP. These manifest as emotional lability, nightmares, and personality or cognitive changes. In contrast, neurologic findings resulting from HCM will usually progress in an obvious fashion, as the calcium rises. Although nerve deafness, ataxia, and visual scotomas have been reported in association with HCM, focal neurologic findings are uncommon. Electroencephalographic abnormalities may mimic patterns consistent with diffuse cerebral metastases that persist for several weeks after serum calcium levels and mental status have normalized. Constipation is more frequently associated with chronic hypercalcemia, whereas anorexia and vomiting are more commonly seen with an acutely rising calcium. Pancreatitis has only rarely been reported as a complication of HCM and is usually associated with PHP. Nephrocalcinosis and metastatic calcification are usually limited to situations where the serum calcium is above 18 mg/dL or the serum phosphate is also elevated (eg, renal dysfunction, milk-alkali syndrome, or hypervitaminosis D).

MANAGEMENT OF HYPERCALCEMIA OF MALIGNANCY

General Approaches

Management of the hypercalcemic cancer patient requires an individualized approach, in formulating both therapeutic goals and a treatment plan, particularly for patients with advanced disease and brief estimated periods of survival or for those afflicted significantly by additional morbidities. The decision *even to treat* hypercalcemia should be made in accord with patient or family wishes regarding extension of survival or quality of life. Initially, the clinician must determine the urgency and level of care warranted and institute several general support measures. The following patient variables should be assessed in defining the level of therapeutic aggression: extent of underlying disease and potential response to antineoplastic therapy, serum calcium level, severity or acuity of symptoms, and other disease states or drugs that increase the risk of detrimental sequelae from hypercalcemia. At a corrected serum calcium below 13 to 13.5 mg/dL (3.1 to 3.3 mmol/L), aggressive measures are reserved for patients with significant symptoms. Asymptomatic patients may be managed less urgently. At corrected serum calcium values above 13.5 to 14 mg/dL (3.25 to 3.5 mmol/L), immediate calcium-lowering measures are instituted, regardless of symptomatology.

Iatrogenic factors contributing to HCM (eg, thiazide diuretics, calcium, or calcitriol supplements) should be eliminated if possible. Until serum calcium can be lowered, measures to provide symptomatic relief of nausea, vomiting, constipation, and bone pain are warranted, although hypercalcemic patients may be unusually sensitive to the sedating or psychotropic effects of antiemetics or narcotics. Efforts to increase mobilization may help in reducing bone resorption; however, this may be dangerous in obtunded patients or in those with osteolytic disease or accompanying bone metastases. If congruent with patient and familial wishes, treatment of the underlying malignancy may be undertaken. Because hypocalcemic benefit is neither immediate nor always proportional to reductions in tumor burden, clinical stabilization and more rapidly acting calcium-lowering measures are often necessary prior to embarking on antitumor therapies.

Available calcium-lowering therapies in HCM target the major points of disturbance of calcium homeostasis previously identified: bone, kidney, and gut. Mechanisms by which calcium might be lowered include inhibition of calcium mobilization via bone resorption (preferably at a final common pathway, eg, the osteoclast), enhancement of renal calcium excretion, antagonism of calcitriol-sensitive intestinal calcium absorption, expansion of extracellular volume (direct dilution), and tumor-ablative therapy. Extracorporeal removal, by exchange with calcium-poor peritoneal or hemodialysis baths, may be appropriate in patients with renal failure or in emergent situations. Because HCM is usually multifactorial or the primary disturbance may not be completely reversible, calcemic control may be best achieved by combining modalities that facilitate compensatory responses (eg, excretion), as well as attempting to correct specific aberrations (eg, resorption or osteolysis).

"Conventional" recommendations for the management of hypercalcemia have used a stepwise approach based on the urgency of care deemed necessary and the relative efficacies and toxicities of available calcium-lowering therapies. Unfortunately, rational evaluation of the relative efficacy for many previous "standards" has been made difficult by the paucity of objective data available from controlled trials. Prior to the late 1980s, a large number of clinical trials in hypercalcemia were flawed as enumerated recently by Warrell (1988). Frequent downfalls included inadequate sample sizes (increasing the chance of type II errors), failure to clearly differentiate between reported calcium values as "total" and "corrected," lack of clearly defined outcomes such as "normocalcemia" and "duration of normocalcemia," lack of double-blinded assessments for subjective outcome criteria, and failure to account separately for the effects of hydration and/or tumor-ablative therapies. Although more recent clinical trials testing newly available calcium-lowering agents (particularly gallium nitrate and various bisphosphonates) have improved vastly in design, such potential faults should be remembered in any rigorous evaluation of trials in hypercalcemia. In addition, the increasing availability of outpatient and sophisticated home intravenous therapies and nursing support has caused the traditional separation between "inpatient" and "outpatient" approaches to become less structured.

Restoration of Extracellular Volume and Saline Diuresis. The majority of hypercalcemic patients will present in moderate to severe ECF volume depletion, with deficits averaging 2 to 4 L but occasionally reaching 5 to 10 L. Failure to restore volume will impair renal calcium excretion, perpetuating the pathophysiologic and symptomatic cycle of HCM. Volume repletion will provide not only an immediate dilutional effect, which may modestly reduce serum calcium (0.5–2 mg/dL), but will also partially relieve symptoms. As the glomerular filtration rate is restored, urinary calcium excretion will be facilitated by increases in sodium and calcium delivery to the proximal and distal tubules, followed by decreased fractional reabsorption of calcium (and sodium) at both sites. Improvement, at least to baseline renal function and calcium excretion, may lag 12 to 48 hours behind initial volume repletion. Ultimate reductions in serum calcium following volume repletion and continued diuresis collectively range from 1 to 3 mg/dL. The nadir occurs 24 to 48 hours after maximal improvement of renal function; however, continued diuresis may allow for further decreases in serum calcium. Approximately 20% of moderately hypercalcemic patients may reach normal serum calcium values following volume repletion and saline diuresis alone. This improvement is usually temporary unless adequate hydration is maintained and/or additional measures are instituted. Aggressive utilization of saline diuresis may be limited by poor cardiopulmonary reserves, fixed renal impairment, hypoalbuminemia, and electrolyte disturbances. Loop diuretics may be cautiously employed to counter volume overload. It is *imperative* that intravascular volume depletion be avoided. Thiazide diuretics are contraindicated because of their inhibitory effects on calcium excretion. Significant free water deficits may exist at the onset of a hypercalcemic episode or following saline diuresis, not only because calciuria impairs free water retention, but also because diuretics enhance hypotonic urinary losses. Provision of adequate free water is an important aspect of volume management.

Clinical Use and Dosing. Initial saline administration rates average 2.5 to 6 L daily, or an amount required to restore estimated volume deficits may be given over the initial 24 hours. In those without pre-existing renal impairment, a reasonable goal at 24 to 48 hours is a urine output of at least 2 L/d. Subsequent adjustments are guided by intakes versus outputs (I/Os), weight, and cardiovascular and clinical tolerance. To produce a forced saline diuresis, continued infusion rates of 150 to 250 mL/h are employed. Loop diuretics should be used only as needed to correct volume overload (eg, 20–80 mg IV furosemide at 6-hour intervals). Electrolyte replacement should be anticipated (especially K, Mg) and adequate urine flow must be established prior to aggressive supplementation. The initial 24-hour management plan for all hypercalcemic patients should include correction of volume deficits and reestablishment of renal calcium excretion. This is usually accomplished prior to the institution of other calcium-lowering therapies. The new "baseline" serum calcium at 24–28 hours is used to base further therapeutic decisions. Depending on the severity of hypercalcemia at presentation, it may be appropriate to institute additional measures in tandem with or before completing volume repletion.

Diuretic-Induced Calciuresis. Although loop diuretics inhibit calcium reabsorption in the loop of Henle and facilitate urinary calcium excretion, controlled studies demonstrating clinically significant effects have used a furosemide dosage ranging from 80 to 200 mg IV every 1 to 2 hours. At these doses, tremendous urinary volume and electrolyte losses necessitate intensive care monitoring and hourly fluid and electrolyte replacement. In most cases, the limited calcium-lowering benefit does not warrant the significant risk posed to the patient. In contrast, a consistent calciuric effect from the furosemide doses typically used for volume management has not been systematically demonstrated. Published clinical comparisons of the calciuric effect from furosemide versus the other loop diuretics, bumetanide or ethacrynic acid, are currently not available.

Calcitonin. Calcitonin is produced endogenously by the parafollicular tissue ("C cells") of the thyroid gland, and appears to be the sole regulatory hormone that actively mediates short-term decreases in serum calcium. Release of calcitonin is prompted by increases in serum calcium and gastrointestinal peptides (gastrin, glucagon, and secretin). Under normal conditions, the hypocalcemic effects of calcitonin are thought to result primarily from inhibition of osteoclastic bone resorption; however, the inhibition of distal renal tubular reabsorption, and possibly the intestinal absorption, of calcium may become important in pathologic conditions (eg, hypercalcemia) or when calcitonin is administered exogenously in pharmacologic doses. Calcitonin receptors have been located on osteoclasts. Osteoblasts do not appear to have calcitonin receptors. These receptor-mediated actions appear to involve decreased osteoclast formation, contraction of the resorpting ruffled cytoplasmic membrane, and breakdown of osteoclasts into mononuclear cells. Declines in serum calcium (1–3 mg/dL) are dose-dependent and become apparent within 6 to 8 hours of a calcitonin dose. Calcium nadirs are reached within 9 to 12 hours of a single dose or within 24 to 48 hours with repeated doses. Response may also depend on the underlying malignancy. Reported response rates range from 0 to 50%. Fewer than 30% of moderately hypercalcemic patients will normalize serum calcium following calcitonin therapy. Impressions perpetuated in the literature suggest that myelomas and epidermoid tumors respond more frequently to calcitonin than do nonepidermoid tumors. In contrast, the hypercalcemia of renal carcinoma and small cell lung cancer is anecdotally stated to be recalcitrant to calcitonin. In addition to its calcium-lowering effects, calcitonin may provide relief of bone pain in those patients with widespread or localized resorptive processes. Whether the analgesic benefit is due to direct effects or results from reduced bone resorption has not been clearly determined.

The calcium-lowering effects of calcitonin are short-lived, lasting less than 24 hours after a single dose. Despite repeated dosing, tachyphylaxis is usually apparent within 3 to 7 days. This "escape" phenomenon has been attributed to receptor downregulation, which limits the hormone's regulatory influence on calcium homeostasis or bone turnover. In the setting of HCM, loss of activity at the renal tubule may have the greatest impact. The purported ability of glucocorticoids to amplify or prolong calcitonin efficacy is believed to reflect enhancement or preservation of renal calcitonin responses. Antibody formation to nonhuman forms of calcitonin has also been hypothesized as a mechanism of calcitonin resistance, and in theory might be deterred by glucocorticoids as well. This theory has not, however, been clearly demonstrated to be clinically relevant, nor can it account for tachyphylaxis to nonantigenic "human" forms of calcitonin.

Numerous methods to abrogate tachyphylaxis from calcitonin's hypocalcemic effects have been espoused by various authors. Largely on the basis of anecdotal experience, controlled data documenting consistent benefit are minimal. Although short-term dose escalations may temporarily overcome resistance, intermittent dosing schedules that allow for drug "holidays" (eg, 5 days "on," 2 days "off") may allow for enough receptor upregulation to maintain chronic responsiveness. As previously alluded to, combination with glucocorticoids may preserve either the overall or the calciuric response to calcitonin. Most of the reported successes using this combination have been in patients with myeloma or hematologic malignancies, where glucocorticoids and calcitonin appear to be uniquely suited. The minimal necessary glucocorticoid dosage is ill-defined, as is the agent of choice and the dosing schedule. Listed values have generally ranged from 30 to 75 mg daily of prednisone equivalent or 100 mg of hydrocortisone succinate every 6 hours IV. At these doses, the potential toxicities of chronic use may be of concern for patients with longer anticipated survivals. In limited studies the combination of calcitonin with other calcium-lowering agents appears to result in additive rather than synergistic or antagonistic effects. Early use of calcitonin in combination with agents having a delayed onset allows for induction of a rapid, albeit modest and temporary, decline in serum calcium until more effective and lasting hypocalcemic agents become active.

Calcitonin is generally well tolerated, producing mild nausea (25%), abdominal cramps, and flushing as its most frequent adverse effects. Allergic rashes or other allergic-type responses occasionally develop with the salmon product, and patients with a history of salmon or fish allergy should receive the recommended intradermal test dose. The negative predictive value of the test dose is relatively low and is no substitute for close monitoring and continued awareness of the potential for development of later allergic responses. Calcitonin is not known to produce significant organ toxicities, and may be used safely in patients with renal or cardiac dysfunction, prior to full volume repletion.

Clinical Use and Dosing. The form of calcitonin most widely used in the United States has been a salmon-derived product intended for intramuscular or subcutaneous use. Dosage recommendations for salmon calcitonin have generally ranged from 4 to 8 IU/kg every 6 to 12 hours, although the calcitonin dose and interval most likely to optimize the magnitude and duration of calcium-lowering benefit have not been systematically studied. Intramuscular administration may be more effective for volume-depleted patients until tissue perfusion is restored or when higher doses requiring large injection volumes (eg, 2–3 mL) are used. Unfortunately, intramuscular administration is painful and cumbersome for outpatient or chronic use. In Europe, the salmon product has also been used intravenously, but the relative safety of this route versus intramuscular/subcutaneous administration has not been clearly defined (Mosekilde et al 1991). A recombinant engineered "human" form of calcitonin is commercially available, but this product is approved only for use in Paget's disease and data regarding its use for HCM are scarce. Human calcitonin appears to have biologic potency similar to or less than that of the salmon product and may be administered intravenously as well as subcutaneously or intramuscularly. Its extremely short kinetic half-life may limit its utility in HCM. Experimental calcitonin dosage forms have included intranasal and rectal formulations. Although these routes have been well tolerated and effective in other metabolic bone disorders, their efficacy in HCM has not been explored and commercial availability remains a problem.

Glucocorticoids. Aside from their controversial use to prolong the effects of calcitonin, glucocorticoids may independently provide calcium-lowering benefit in a limited number of HCM syndromes. Although high-dose glucocorticoids may have nonspecific calciuric, antiresorptive (via osteoclast and ultimately osteoblast inhibition), and inhibitory effects on intestinal calcium absorption, they do not predictably attenuate hypercalcemia in the majority of patients with primary hyperparathyroidism or malignant humorally mediated (PTHrP) or osteolytic syndromes. Although generally ineffective, glucocorticoids will improve calcemic control in a small number of patients with solid tumors. Responses are more likely in patients with hematologic malignancies and in syndromes associated with excess calcitriol (eg, iatrogenic intoxication or granulomatous disorders). Glucocorticoids may also provide analgesia for metastatic or osteolytic bone pain; however, long-term use may ultimately worsen skeletal integrity, in addition to presenting the usual chronic glucocorticoid toxicities. The time frame, magnitude, and duration of benefit in steroid-responsive patients are poorly defined.

Clinical Use and Dosing. Reported doses, largely empirically derived, have ranged from 30 to 80 mg/d for prednisone, 10 to 40 mg/d for dexamethasone, and 100 to 400 mg/d for hydrocortisone. Which agent possesses the greatest calcium-lowering efficacy has not been clearly established. Many patients with hematologic malignancies may already be receiving glucocorticoids as part of their chemotherapeutic or antiemetic regimen. Chronically induced steroid toxicities are of less concern in patients having brief life expectancies (eg, 3–6 months). Metabolic derangements, ulcerogenesis, and increased risk for certain infections may be valid short-term concerns, particularly in those undergoing cytotoxic therapy or exhibiting additional risk factors. Glucocorticoids are most prudently employed as a second-line measure for patients with lymphoproliferative disorders or myeloma.

Plicamycin (Mithramycin). Although active against some embryonal cell tumors, plicamycin has relinquished its role as an antineoplastic to one of "salvage" therapy for a limited number of testicular cancers. Inhibition of DNA-dependent RNA synthesis presumably forms the basis for its antiproliferative effect against tumor cells and osteoclasts. Calcium lowering results from subsequent inhibition of bone resorption, resulting from interference with either the function or the formation of osteoclasts from precursors, rather than from appreciable reductions in tumor burden. The actions of plicamycin on other bone cells, for example, osteoblasts, and any indirect effects on resorptive coupling are not well described. Plicamycin is one of the more effective agents for those hypercalcemic syndromes generated primarily by osteoclastic resorption. Declines in serum calcium usually exceed 2 to 3 mg/dL, producing normocalcemia in roughly 80% of moderately to severely hypercalcemic patients. Calcium usually begins to fall within 12 to 24 hours, and maximal decreases are observed 24 to 96 hours (usually 36 to 72 hours) after dosing. Calcemic control frequently lasts between 3 and 9 days, but occasionally endures for weeks. Some patients exhibit abrupt and exaggerated rebounds in serum calcium on the recurrence of hypercalcemia.

Because of its potential to produce serious toxic effects plicamycin has usually been reserved as a second- or third-line hypocalcemic agent. The risk for adverse effects is less at the doses used for calcium-lowering and include thrombocytopenia, coagulopathy (even in the absence of thrombocytopenia or hypoprothrombinemia), nausea, hepatotoxicity (in 20%, a transient transaminase elevation of ill-defined clinical significance), nephrotoxicity (proteinurea, elevation of serum creatinine), and bone marrow suppression. Since renal excretion is the primary route of elimination, dose reduction has been suggested in patients with renal dysfunction. This will not only reduce the risk of further renal damage, but may decrease the severity of the aforementioned toxic effects.

Clinical Use and Dosing. Although a loose dose–response relationship exists, adequate calcium reductions can usually be achieved using doses one fifth to one tenth of those used for antineoplastic purposes. Numerous recommendations are encountered; most regimens employ an initial dose of 15 to 25 µg/kg. This dose may be repeated if the observed response is inadequate (anticipated to be maximal by 48–96 hours) or on a recurrent rise in serum calcium. Less commonly, daily infusions for up to 5 days may be given, although the greater dose intensity may increase the risk of adverse sequelae. Chronic or "maintenance" schedules have generally been discouraged. Although the drug may be given as a slow IV push over 10 minutes, slower administration (eg, over 4 to 6 hours) may reduce infusion-related nausea. As plicamycin is a vesicant, prolonged peripheral infusions require dilution in a large volume (eg, 500–1000 mL) of fluid. Smaller volumes may be used in patients having central venous access or receiving the drug as an IV push. Because less toxic agents with similar efficacy are available, plicamycin is currently reserved as a third- or fourth-line agent. Except in refractory cases, its use in patients with significant hepatic or renal dysfunction, thrombocytopenia, or other bleeding disorders is contraindicated.

Gallium Nitrate. Gallium is a group IIIa transitional metal. In the 1970s, the activity of gallium nitrate (Ganite) against various cancers was explored by the National Cancer Institute (NCI). Because therapeutic results were generally disappointing, efforts toward developing gallium as an antineoplastic were largely abandoned. During initial phase I and II studies, hypocalcemia and nephrotoxicity were frequently noted to be dose-limiting toxic effects of gallium. The present clinical focus has been on the use of gallium as an antiresorptive and calcium-lowering agent.

Gallium is taken up into areas of new bone mineralization or remodeling by adsorption onto the forming surfaces of hydroxyapatite crystal. The resulting crystalline structure is improved in calcium content and integrity and demonstrates greater resistance to dissolution by acid media such as that induced by osteoclasts. Although the rates of both hydroxyapatite formation and dissolution are slowed by gallium, its net effect on bone turnover is to enhance retention of bone mineral content, protein, and density. Unlike aluminum, gallium does not appear to induce osteomalacia by "poisoning" the hydroxyapatite crystal, nor does gallium induce obvious alterations in osteoclast or osteoblast formation, morphology, or viability. In culture, gallium renders bone resistant against osteoclastic resorption, whether stimulated by cytokines or indirectly by PTH. Thus, despite preliminary data suggesting that osteoclast function may be inhibited, gallium is believed to act primarily by physicochemical rather than cellular mechanisms. The incorporation of gallium into bone requires exposure to threshold gallium concentrations (1 μg/mL) for a minimum of 24 hours and delays the onset of calcium-lowering effect. As bone becomes stabilized against osteoclastic resorption, initial declines in serum calcium are also dependent on the ongoing elimination of calcium and the simultaneous inhibition of its further release from bone.

In dose ranging and comparative trials, continuous 5- to 7-day intravenous infusions of gallium have promoted decreases in serum calcium of at least 2 mg/dL in roughly 94% of those receiving 200 mg/m^2/d, compared with 83% of patients at the 100 mg/m^2/d dosage level. At 200 mg/m^2/d, mean drops in serum calcium approximate 3 to 4 mg/dL. In patients with posthydration-corrected calcium levels above 12 mg/dL, this dose has been adequate to restore normocalcemia in 75 to 92%. The reported mean durations of normocalcemia, induced by a 5-day course of gallium, have ranged between 6 and 10 days. Serum calcium begins to fall 24 to 72 hours after the start of infusion, and nadirs at 5 to 10 days. Differential response rates to gallium have not been noted between major tumor histologies, although several trials have excluded lymphoma patients because of the potential antitumor effect. In well-designed trials comparing gallium with calcitonin (Warrell et al 1988) or gallium with etidronate (Warrell et al 1991), gallium proved statistically superior to calcitonin and etidronate with respect to mean drop in serum calcium, percentage of patients achieving normocalcemia, and duration of normocalcemia. Calcitonin peaked in full effect more rapidly than gallium, but then exhibited subsequent loss of calcium-lowering efficacy which was surpassed by gallium after 72 hours. In these trials, calcitonin and etidronate demonstrated lower response rates than in earlier less rigorous trials. It should be remembered that "normocalcemia," defined as a corrected serum calcium less than 10.5 mg/dL, may be an outcome criterion that does not correlate well with symptomatic scales of benefit. As of 1992, there were no published studies that directly compared gallium with pamidronate.

Pharmacokinetics. The oral absorption of gallium nitrate is poor and this route of administration has not been clinically pursued for HCM. Although clinical trials in Paget's disease have demonstrated chronic subcutaneous dosing of gallium to be effective and well tolerated, published pharmacokinetic data comparing the intravenous and subcutaneous routes are not available. Gallium appears to be extensively distributed into tissue compartments. Its distribution half-life is roughly 1 hour, followed by a prolonged terminal half-life ranging from 24 to more than 124 hours. The recommended dose of 200 mg/m^2/d yields steady-state serum levels ranging from 0.9 to 2.4 μg/mL, which meet or exceed the suggested threshold for hypocalcemic effects. Gallium is renally excreted intact. Following single short infusions, urinary excretion approaches 50% within 24 hours and accounts for 90% of an administered bolus dose at 5 days. Cumulative urinary excretion data following prolonged infusions are not currently available.

Adverse Effects. Nephrotoxicity is dose-limiting at more than 300 to 400 mg/m^2/d, particularly when given by bolus infusion. At currently recommended doses, the overall clinical incidence of nephrotoxicity is only 12.5%. The HCM population has a relatively high background incidence of mild to moderate renal dysfunction, and true worsening due to gallium occurs almost exclusively in patient subsets having such risk factors as posthydration serum creatinine above 2.5 mg/dL, concurrent or recent aminoglycoside use, or urine output less than 2000 mL/d. Gallium should be discontinued if serum creatinine rises above 2.5 mg/dL or urine output drops. Other untoward but usually mild effects include asymptomatic hypocalcemia (calcium decreases to 6.5–8 mg/dL in 36–45% of patients), hypophosphatemia (occasionally requiring oral supplementation), mild decreases in serum bicarbonate (consistent with respiratory alkalosis), and delayed decline in blood pressure associated with peripheral edema. Toxic effects characteristic at the higher antineoplastic doses but rare at antihypercalcemic doses include anemia, magnesium wasting, mild granulocytosis, pulmonary infiltrates, pleural effusion, acute optic neuritis, tinnitus, and loss of visual acuity.

Clinical Use and Dosing. Assuming a posthydration-corrected calcium of 12 mg/dL or greater, the usual recommended dose for patients with significant symptoms is 200 mg/m^2/d as a continuous intravenous infusion, for 5 to 7 days. For those who are only mildly symptomatic, reduction to 100 mg/m^2/d is suggested. Should an early or exaggerated response occur (ie, normalization of serum calcium within 5 days), administration of gallium should be halted and calcium and phosphate should be closely monitored in anticipation of further declines. Although reported mean durations of normocalcemia range from only 6 to 10 days, calcemic control may extend for up to 3 weeks. Unfortunately, dosing guidelines for repeat courses or chronic maintenance have not been developed. Although continuous intravenous infusions of gallium in large volumes of normal saline or D5W are recommended, alternative routes of administration are currently being evaluated in ongoing clinical trials. Such alternatives would not circumvent the need to maintain adequate oral or parenteral hydration. Gallium shows promise as a general antiresorptive, with potential applications in numerous metabolic diseases of bone.

Bisphosphonates. Pyrophosphates are endogenous inhibitors of calcium phosphate precipitation. The antiresorptive bisphosphonates are analogs of pyrophosphate, in which the oxygen of the natural P—O—P pyrophosphate backbone has been replaced by carbon, to yield P—C—P (Fig 3.4). The resulting moiety is rendered stable to the natural degradation processes which inactivate pyrophosphate. Two bisphosphonates have become available in the United States, etidronate (Didronel®), and pamidronate (Aredia®). In Europe, a third agent, clodronate, is also in use. Aledronate, risendronate, and BM21-0955 represent a few of the "third"-generation bisphosphonates currently in clinical trials. Trends in the development of new agents are toward increasing the antiresorptive potency and improving the tolerance or efficacy of oral formulations. Side-chain manipulations not only appear to increase antiresorptive potency, but also have the potential to alter metabolic, pharmacokinetic, and toxicity profiles.

Bisphosphonates were initially thought to exert their inhibitory effects at a common "distal" step in resorptive processes in a physicochemical manner similar to gallium. These agents adsorb avidly onto solid-phase calcium phosphate and inhibit crystal dissolution and crystal growth. The drug concentrations required to produce these effects in vitro are much greater than those usually attained in vivo, bringing the clinical importance of these actions into question.

Current theory attributes the antiresorptive efficacy of pamidronate, and probably other bisphosphonates, to inhibitory effects on the osteoclast. Suggested mechanisms include (1) morphologic changes, such as reducing the surface membrane resorptive area, or interfering with podosomal attachment to bone; (2) functional changes, such as reducing the production or release of lysosomes, protons, lactate-mediated energy, or interactions with other regulatory cell lineages (osteoblasts or the exquisitely bisphosphonate-sensitive monocyte–macrophage lineages); or (3) reduction of osteoclast formation, differentiation, or recruitment. Inhibition of osteoclast resorption occurs at much lower bisphosphonate concentrations than physicochemical influences on mineralization, suggesting that structure–activity relationships are separable. The net effect of each bisphosphonate on bone mineral retention, therefore, is a function not only of the relative inhibition of hydroxyapatite dissolution and formation, but also of how this ratio is offset or augmented by decreases in osteoclastic resorption. Differences occur between the various bisphosphonates in the balance and selectivity of effects on mineralization versus resorption.

Because bisphosphonates, like gallium, do not appear to directly alter renal or gut elimination of calcium, hypercalcemics most likely to respond are those in whom osteolysis or bone resorption is the major pathophysiologic factor. In contrast, hypercalcemics whose renal calcium reabsorption is inappropriately high (eg, PTH or PTHrP-mediated HCM) may be somewhat refractory to measures that are purely antiresorptive. Some patients appear to respond to pamidronate initially, but then lose calcemic control despite continued bisphosphonate therapy. It is not known whether this results from true osteoclast resistance, decreased incorporation of pamidronate into bone, or secondary responses that otherwise alter calcium homeostasis.

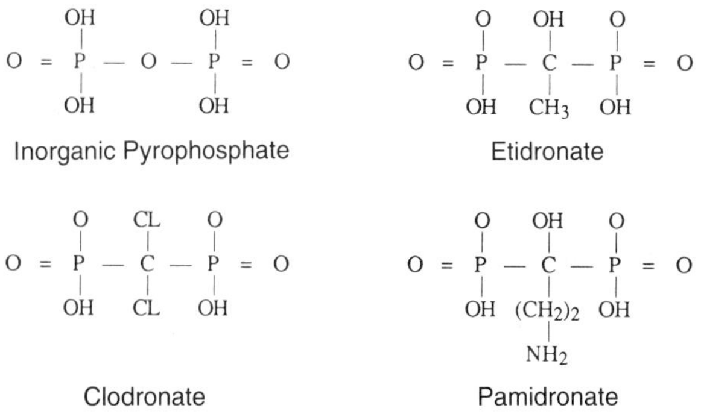

Figure 3.4. Structures of pyrophosphate and three currently available biophosphonates.

Studies have demonstrated similar responses to pamidronate and clodronate when administered as multiple "low-dose" daily infusions. There is still debate over whether a true drug concentration "threshold" does exist and whether the dose–response curve exhibits a predictable plateau. In general, pamidronate and clodronate will produce calcium declines of 3 to 4 mg/dL or greater. Reductions produced by etidronate rarely exceed 2 to 3 mg/dL. Calcium levels begin to drop 24 to 72 hours following the initiation of bisphosphonate therapy and reach a nadir in 4 to 9 days. The onset of calcium reduction for pamidronate and clodronate is more rapid than for etidronate; however, this may reflect current dosing practices. The reported percentage of patients normalizing serum calcium also varies widely with bisphosphonate and dose. Response rates for a 3- to 5-day course of intravenous etidronate range from 24 to 60%, but are generally higher following a 5- to 7-day course of therapy. Pamidronate, in one dose ranging study, normalized serum calcium in a dose-dependent fashion: 30-, 60-, and 90-mg infusions over 24 hours produced "complete responses" (defined as a serum calcium less than 10.5 mg/dL) in 40, 61, and 100% of patients, respectively (Ciba-Geigy, data on file). The overall complete response rate (CR) was 68%. In this study, duration of CR (Ca < 10.5 mg/dL) and median time to relapse (Ca > 12 mg/dL) were also dose-dependent, averaging 4, 5, and 6 days (duration of CR) and 0, 6, and 11 days (to relapse). These results are in fair agreement with data from other studies using 30- to 60-mg doses.

Reported durations of response to pamidronate range from 1 to 10 weeks, with an average response of 2 to 3 weeks. Etidronate provides less durable responses, averaging only 1 to 7 days, and clodronate averaging 10 to 14 days. Subsequent oral "maintenance" therapy may extend calcemic control. The oral formulation for etidronate is usually ineffective for inducing responses, but may prolong or maintain responses following an intravenous course.

A study in patients having post-hydration-corrected serum calcium levels above 12 mg/dL compared pamidronate (60 mg as a single 24-hour infusion) and etidronate (7.5 mg/kg IV daily for 3 days). Complete response was defined as normocalcemia (serum Ca < 10.5 mg/dL), partial response (PR) as a 15% or greater decline in baseline serum calcium, and combined total response rate (TR) as the sum of CR and PR. Pamidronate produced a CR of 70% and a combined TR of 97%, versus 41% (CR) and 65% (TR) for etidronate. Durations of response were 7 and 5 days, respectively (Gucalp et al. 1992).

Pharmacokinetics. Bisphosphonates have poor oral bioavailability, ranging from 1 to 10% for etidronate, but approaching 2 to 3% with pamidronate and clodronate. Absorption occurs in the small intestine and increases with the size of the dose. Food, especially dairy products or antacids, decrease bisphosphonate absorption. Bisphosphonates are rapidly cleared from the plasma by nonrenal (skeletal uptake) and renal elimination.

Reported plasma distribution half-lives range from 0.8 to 3 hours for pamidronate and 0.2 to 2 hours for clodronate. Following the avid skeletal uptake of the bisphosphonates, plasma levels rapidly fall below the limits of assay detection, making estimates of terminal half-lives and skeletal retention difficult. By the use of ^{14}C-labeled compound in murine systems, the skeletal retention half-lives for clodronate and pamidronate were found to be approximately a year. Skeletal uptake and retention of the bisphosphonates are probably a function of skeletal turnover rates and influenced by osteolytic processes. Leyvraz et al (1992) found a direct correlation between the degree of bone involvement and body retention of pamidronate. The mean body retention of pamidronate was 51% in patients with fewer than five bone metastases compared with 76% in patients with more than 15 metastases. Thirty to forty percent of a dose of pamidronate or etidronate is renally excreted, whereas 75% of clodronate is recovered unchanged in the urine.

Adverse Effects. Very few serious adverse effects have thus far been associated with the bisphosphonates. Rapid administration (less than 2 hours) could theoretically induce renal damage, by the precipitation of bisphosphonate–calcium complex in the kidney. Transient drops in ionized calcium might also induce hypotension. The actual incidence of these adverse effects in clinical practice is not well documented, although worsening of renal function has been noted in a small percentage of patients with elevated baseline serum creatinines receiving etidronate. In patients with serum creatinines of 5.0 mg/dL or greater, etidronate is contraindicated, and pamidronate should be used with caution. Adequate hydration is a necessary precaution for etidronate administration and a prudent prerequisite to use of pamidronate. Etidronate has been associated with an altered (metallic) taste sensation, hyperphosphatemia (possibly as a result of interference with renal phosphate excretion), occasional worsening of renal function, gastrointestinal intolerance to high oral doses, and osteomalacia or rickets-like syndromes with chronically high doses (eg, longer than 2 to 3 months). Pamidronate and other aminobisphosphonates may induce a "first-dose" response consisting of a mild temperature elevation (1–2°C), beginning 24 to 48 hours after the initial oral or intravenous dose and lasting 24 to 72 hours. Transient leukopenia (lymphocytes), decreases in serum zinc, and an increase in C-reactive protein and possibly interleukin-6 or -1 release suggest an acute phase response. Pamidronate is a venous irritant. When given orally at doses above 300 to 600 mg/d, oral ulceration, nausea, vomiting, diarrhea, and abdominal pain are frequent. Moderate to significant hypophosphatemia is not uncommon with pamidronate and clodronate. Supplementation with potassium and magnesium is occasionally required. Concerns over the leukemogenic potential of clodronate resulted in its withdrawal from U.S. development, but have not been substantiated in European studies.

Dosing and Clinical Use. Numerous dosing regimens employed for all three bisphosphonates have yielded efficacy rates with considerable overlap. Although this allows some flexibility in dosing guidelines, potential correlations between dose and efficacy are obscured. The following equivalent cumulative effective doses have been proposed: etidronate (1500 mg IV), clodronate (600 mg IV), pamidronate (45–60 mg IV), alendronate (10 mg), BM21.0995 (1 mg).

Etidronate is given in multiple IV doses of 7.5 mg/kg/d as a 2-hour or longer infusion in at least 250 mL of volume. Maintenance oral therapy with doses of at least 15 to 20 mg/kg/d may allow continued calcemic control. In general, calcemic control on oral etidronate maintenance endures less than 1 month, and gastrointestinal intolerance to effective doses may be considerable.

Intravenous pamidronate dosing schedules have included 15 to 45 mg/d for 1 to 6 days and 15 to 90 mg as a single dose. Multiple low-dose daily infusions have been supplanted by the use of single infusions ranging from 30 to 90 mg. Recent studies supporting dose-dependent responses have led to dosing guidelines based on posthydration calcium levels: 60 mg for serum calcium of 12 to 13.5 mg/dL, and 90 mg for values above 13.5 mg/dL. Other clinicians have elected not to exceed 60 mg on any initial dose, providing or adjusting subsequent doses should the initial response prove inadequate. The manufacturer recommends administration as a single infusion over 24 hours; however, a wide range of more rapid infusion rates (over 4–24 hours) have been employed clinically without obvious adverse effects. Maximal infusion rates of 7.5 to 15 mg/hour have also been suggested, as has a minimal infusion time of 2 hours for all doses. Infusion rates may be limited by peripheral venous irritation. Therefore, a dilution volume of 1000 mL or a maximum concentration of 15 mg/125 mL (= 0.12 mg/mL) is recommended. Patients receiving the drug centrally should be tolerant of more concentrated solution. Dosing guidelines for augmentation of an inadequate initial response, hypercalcemic relapse, or prophylactic maintenance have not been systematically determined. Redosing is not recommended prior to 7 days from initial therapy or after a cumulative initial dose of 90 mg. For previously hypercalcemic patients with adequate initial responses, remission might be maintained by repeating a dose at the first sign of rising calcium. The manufacturer recommends that repeat doses be given "in a manner similar to the initial dose."

Although some studies have based pamidronate dose on weight (0.5–1.5 mg/kg), adult doses are generally not adjusted for weight or body habitus (eg, obesity). Pediatric dosing guidelines are not available. Oral pamidronate in doses of 1200 mg/d for 5 days appears to provide similar efficacy and systemic delivery of pamidronate as doses of 30 mg/d IV × 5 days. Oral doses of 150 to 500 mg/d pamidronate have been used as a maintenance regimen for calcemic control. Oral formulations of pamidronate are currently available investigationally in Europe, and although seemingly effective over a wide dosing range, gastrointestinal intolerance and mucosal irritation are frequent dose-limiting toxic effects.

Clodronate has also been studied, for antihypercalcemic purposes, in a wide range of doses, including 300 mg IV/d × 2 to 5 days, 500 mg IV × 1 to 3 days, 600 mg IV × 1, 800 to 3200 mg/d PO for various lengths of time. Oral therapy for induction or maintenance of normocalcemia, by limited initial data, appears to be better tolerated and clinically more feasible than that for pamidronate or etidronate.

Miscellaneous Measures

Phosphates (Oral and Intravenous). Inorganic intravenous phosphates are thought to lower serum calcium acutely by increasing the calcium phosphate ion product above the limits of solubility, driving calcium (as calcium phosphate) into tissues. Calcium begins to decline within minutes, and peak effects are seen within 12 to 24 hours. The reduction in serum calcium is dependent on the degree to which calcium phosphate solubility is exceeded. This is a function of phosphate dose, administration rate, and baseline calcium. Although a portion of this calcium phosphate is deposited into bone, the majority is precipitated into organs, blood vessels, and soft tissues. Life-threatening complications of metastatic calcification caused by calcium phosphate include renal failure and acute hypotension secondary to rapid drops in ionized calcium levels. Because of these potential dangers, the use of intravenous phosphate in the context of hypercalcemia is discouraged. Only truly refractory patients or patients with hypophosphatemia should be considered for phosphate therapy. The time frame and magnitude of response to oral phosphate are variable. In responsive patients, calcium may decline for a week or so after commencing therapy. Except in the setting of chronic hyperparathyroidism, long-term calcemic control is usually not maintained by phosphate alone.

Clinical Use and Dosing. Intravenous phosphates have been given in doses ranging from 10 to 75 mmol/d, over 12 to 24 hours. Precautions regarding potassium content and venous irritation are necessary when using potassium phosphate as the phosphate salt. Oral phosphate may be given in doses of 1 to 3 g daily. Diarrhea is dose limiting, and single doses greater than 500 mg (10–15 mmol or roughly 5 mL of oral phosphosoda) should be avoided. Although chronic oral phosphate may be useful in some disorders of metabolism, this form of therapy is reserved for truly hypophosphatemic patients requiring supplementation (serum phosphate < 1–1.5 mmol/L). Recipients should be well hydrated and be monitored for acute or chronic declines in renal function.

Prostaglandin Synthesis Inhibitors. Prostaglandins, particularly those of the "E" series, have been implicated as local mediators of bone resorption, acting either directly to stimulate osteoclasts or indirectly to alter the release or activity of other lymphokines and OAFs. In turn, this may facilitate the establishment of bony metastases and further enhance osteolytic processes. Despite the proposed pathogenetic role of prostaglandins in hypercalcemia and promising initial clinical results, clinical trials with prostaglandin E inhibitors in hypercalcemia have been disappointing. The onset and magnitude of calcium decline are variable and predictive clinical features or diagnostics are not available that might identify the occasional responder.

Clinical Use and Dosing. The majority of published experience has been with indomethacin (150 mg/d) or anti-inflammatory doses of aspirin. Not uncommonly, NSAIDs produce side effects (renal impairment, platelet inhibition, and ulcerogenicity), nonsteroidal anti-inflammatory drugs (NSAIDs) are best reserved for hypercalcemics having other therapeutic indications (eg, bone pain). Volume repletion and adequate renal perfusion should be ensured prior to instituting NSAID therapy. Prophylaxis of other toxic effects such as ulcerogenesis should be considered.

Ethiofos. Originally studied as an antineoplastic, ethiofos (amifostine WR-2721) is now under study as a sulfhyrdryl-donating chemo- and radioprotectant, which also induces hypocalcemia in a significant number of normocalcemic recipients. Proposed mechanisms for its calcium-lowering effects include the inhibition of PTH secretion or activity at the renal tubule, inhibition of non-PTH-mediated renal calcium reabsorption, and osteoclastic inhibition. Following short infusions, a transient decline in serum calcium occurs which lasts less than 24 hours. Although animal studies modeling states of excess PTH or PTHrP suggest improved results with continuous infusion (eg, subcutaneously), clinical studies of chronic use have not have conducted. Mild adverse effects are frequent and include nausea, vomiting, somnolence, hypotension (asymptomatic), and sneezing. Further development of this agent as an antihypercalcemic in malignancy will probably be limited because of its modest benefit and requirement for continuous dosing.

MANAGEMENT APPROACHES TO HYPERCALCEMIA OF MALIGNANCY

Despite recent advances, our understanding of the pathophysiologic factors leading to hypercalcemia of malignancy is incomplete. Hence, our approach to managing the hypercalcemic remains somewhat "generalized," targeting the major common aberrations noted in calcium homeostasis: accelerated release of calcium from bone, impaired or inadequate renal calcium excretion, and occasionally excessive calcitriol activity. Individualization of therapy is based on the severity of hypercalcemia (after correcting values for hypoalbuminemia), patient and caregiver goals, patient risks contraindicating the use of specific therapies, and identifiable aberrations of calcium homeostasis. Iatrogenic and nonmalignant factors exacerbating hypercalcemia should be sought out and eliminated. Although therapy of the underlying malignancy remains the truly definitive therapy for HCM, this may not provide immediate calcium-lowering benefit, nor may it be feasible or desired.

Patients who are severely symptomatic or present with a serum calcium greater than 13.5 to 14 mg/dL warrant aggressive calcium-lowering measures. In those with less severe symptoms or calcium levels (12–13.5 mg/dL), less urgent therapies may suffice. Hydration with saline is a universal initial measure which may improve symptoms and restore mild hypercalcemics to the point of self-regulation. In those with adequate cardiovascular and renal function, enhancement of renal excretion by continued saline diuresis may promote another 1 to 2 mg/dL decline in serum calcium. Modest doses of loop diuretic may be necessary to prevent volume overload, but intravascular volume depletion should be avoided. Following 24 hours of volume repletion, most patients still require additional measures to correct or prevent the recurrence of hypercalcemia.

Calcitonin remains a "first-line" agent in selected populations: those with hematologic malignancies and severe hypercalcemia requiring immediate calcium reduction. Calcitonin may be safely employed prior to full volume repletion and in patients with renal or cardiac dysfunction.

Additional measures can be instituted at the 24–48 hour reassessment to improve and extend calcemic control. Pamidronate is the therapeutic mainstay at this point because of its efficacy and ease of administration. Although roughly equivalent in efficacy, gallium presents greater risk of nephrotoxicity and therefore is reserved by most clinicians as a "third-line" agent. Plicamycin may offer a slightly faster onset in calcium reduction than pamidronate, but is considered a third- or fourth-line agent because of its toxicity profile. Limited use of plicamycin may be within acceptable risk margins for refractory patients without contraindications. Because antiresorptive agents require 24 to 72 hours to produce initial declines in serum calcium, it may be appropriate to institute these agents in tandem with "first-line" measures. Pamidronate offers the greatest margin of safety in patients whose renal function has not been fully restored. In patients in whom exaggerated renal calcium reabsorption is the primary contributor to the development of hypercalcemia, maximal antiresorptive measures still may not achieve calcemic control. The combined use of antiresorptives has not been systematically studied. As general antiresorptives, pamidronate and gallium may provide additional benefit in terms of reducing bone pain and fracture rates and inhibiting progression of bony metastases.

Glucocorticoids may be useful in those with hematologic malignancies and in a small fraction of solid tumor patients. Oral phosphates may be helpful in moderate hypercalcemia, but are generally reserved for patients with low serum phosphates having adequate renal function. The use of "maintenance" doses of pamidronate, given as a short infusion on an outpatient basis, appears more promising for prophylactic use than to maintain normocalcemia with oral etidronate; however, dosing guidelines are not currently available. The development of effective and tolerated oral bisphosphonates should greatly facilitate chronic management of hypercalcemia. Alternative dosing methods for gallium may increase the utility of this drug in the chronic management of hypercalcemia.

REFERENCES

Adams JS. Vitamin-D metabolite-mediated hypercalcemia. *Endocrinol Metab Clin North Am.* 1989;**18**:765–778.

Allan P. Unusual causes of hypercalcemia. *Endocrinol Metab Clin North Am.* 1989;**18**:753–763.

Bajorunas OR. Clinical manifestations of cancer-related hypercalcemia. *Semin Oncol.* 1990;**17**(suppl 5):516–525.

Bilezikian JP. Management of acute hypercalcemia. *N Engl J Med.* 1992;**326**:1196–1203.

Binstock ML, Mundy GR. Effect of calcitonin and glucocorticoids in combination on the hypercalcemia of malignancy. *Ann Intern Med.* 1980;**93**:269–272.

Body JJ, Pot M, Borkowser A, et al. Dose–response study of aminohydroxypropylidene bisphosphonate in tumor associated hypercalcemia. *Am J Med.* 1987;**92**:957–963.

Bonjour JP, Rizzoli R. Clodronate in hypercalcemia of malignancy. *Calcif Tissue Int.* 1990;**46**(suppl):20–25.

CIBA-GEIGY Corporation. Data on file. A multi-center, randomized parallel, double-blind trial using a single infusion of 30, 60, or 90 mg APD in hypercalcemia of malignancy. 1989; *Protocol 01.*

Coleman RE. Bisphosphonate treatment of bone metastases and hypercalcemia of malignancy. *Oncology.* 1991;**5**:55–62.

Coleman RE, Rubens RD. APD for the treatment of hypercalcemia of malignancy (HCM): A comparison of different doses and schedules of administration. *Br J Cancer.* 1989;**60**:448.

Delmas PD. Biochemical markers of bone turnover for the clinical assessment of metabolic bone disease. *Endocrinol Metab Clin North Am.* 1990;**90**:1–18.

Filton AF, McTavish D. Pamidronate: A review of its pharmacological properties and therapeutic efficacy in resorptive bone disease. *Drugs.* 1991;**41**:289–318.

Green LM, Donehower RC. Hepatic toxicity of low doses of mithramycin in hypercalcemia. *Cancer Treat Rep.* 1984;**68**:1379–1381.

Gucalp R, Ritch PS, Wiernik PH, et al. Comparative study of pamidronate disodium and etidronate disodium in the treatment of cancer-related hypercalcemia. *J Clin Oncol.* 1992;**10**:134–142.

Hasling C, Urwin GH, Mosekilde L. Etidronate disodium in the management of malignancy-related hypercalcemia. *Am J Med.* 1987;**82**(suppl 2A):51–54.

Hosking DJ. Assessment of renal and skeletal components of hypercalcemia. *Calcif Tissue Int.* 1990;**46**(suppl):511–519.

Hosking DJ, Stone MD, Foote IW. Potentiation of calcitonin by corticosteroids during the treatment of hypercalcemia of malignancy. *Eur J Clin Pharmacol.* 1990;**38**:37–41.

Insogna KL. Humoral hypercalcemia of malignancy: The role of parathyroid hormone-related protein. *Endocrinol Metab Clin North Am.* 1989;**18**:794–797.

Krakoff IH, Newman RA, Goldberg RS. Clinical toxicologic and pharmacologic studies of gallium nitrate. *Cancer.* 1979;**44**:1722–1727.

Leyvraz S, Hess U, Flesch G, et al. Pharmacokinetics of pamidronate in patients with bone metastases. *J NCI.* 1992;**84**:788–792.

Mallette LE. Regulation of blood calcium in humans. *Endocrinol Metab Clin North Am.* 1989;**18**:601–610.

Morton AR, Cantrill JA, Criag AE, et al. Single dose-versus daily intravenous aminohydroxy-propylidene bisphosphonate (APD) for the hypercalcemia of malignancy. *Br Med J.* 1988;**296**:811–814.

Mosekilde L, Ericksen ET, Charles P. Hypercalcemia of malignancy: Pathophysiology, diagnosis and treatment. *Crit Rev Onco Hematol.* 1991;**11**:1–27.

Muggia FM. Overview of cancer-related hypercalcemia: Epidemiology and etiology. *Semin Oncol.* 1990;**17**(suppl 5):3–9.

Mundy GR, ed. *Calcium Homeostasis and Hypocalcemia.* 2nd ed. New York: Oxford University Press; 1990.

Ralston SH, Gardner MD, Jinkins AS, et al. Malignancy associated hypercalcemia: Relationship between mechanisms of hypercalcemia and response to antihypercalcemic therapy. *Bone Mineral.* 1987;**2**:227–242.

Ralston SH, Patel V, Fraser WD, et al. Comparison of three intravenous bisphosphonates in cancer-associated hypercalcemia. *Lancet.* 1989;**2**:1180–1182.

Ringenberg QS, Ritch PS. Efficacy of oral administration of etidronate disodium in maintaining normal serum calcium levels in previously hypercalcemic patients. *Clin Ther.* 1987;**9**:1–7.

Ritch PS. Treatment of cancer-related hypercalcemia. *Semin Oncol.* 1990;**17**(suppl 5):26–33.

Russell RGG, Kanis JA, eds. *Tumor-Induced Hypercalcemia and Its Management.* London: Royal Society of Medicine Services Ltd; 1991.

Sawyer N, Newstead C, Drummond A. Fast (4 hr) or slow (24 hr) infusions of pamidronate disodium (APD) as single shot treatment of hypercalcemia. *Bone Mineral.* 1990;**9**:122–128.

Schalff RAB, Hall TG, Bar RS. Medical treatment of hypercalcemia. *Clin Pharmacol.* 1989;**8**:108–121.

Singer FR, Fernandez M. Therapy of hypercalcemia of malignancy. *Am J Med.* 1987;**82**(suppl 2A):534–541.

Singer FR, Ritch PS, Lad TE, et al. Treatment of hypercalcemia of malignancy with intravenous etidronate. *Arch Intern Med.* 1991;**151**:471–476.

Slayton RE, Shnider BI, Elias E, et al. New approach to the treatment of hypercalcemia: The effect of short-term treatment with mithramycin. *Clin Pharmacol Ther.* 1971;**12**:833–837.

Stevenson JC, Evans IMA. Pharmacology and therapeutic use of calcitonin. *Drugs.* 1981;**21**:257–272.

Thiebaud D, Jaeger PH, Jacquet AF, et al. Dose-response in the treatment of hypercalcemia of malignancy by a single infusion of the bisphosphonate AHPrBP. *J Clin Oncol.* 1988;**6**:762–768.

Todd PA, Filton A. Gallium nitrate: A review of its pharmacological properties and therapeutic potential in cancer related hypercalcemia. *Drugs.* 1991;**42**:261–273.

Warrell RP. Questions about clinical trials in hypercalcemia. *J Clin Oncol.* 1988;**6**:759–761.

Warrell RP, Alcock NW, Bockman RS. Gallium nitrate inhibits accelerated bone tumor in patients with bone metastasis. *J Clin Oncol.* 1987;**5**:292–298.

Warrell RP, Israel R, Frisone M, et al. Gallium nitrate for

acute treatment of cancer-related hypercalcemia. *Ann Intern Med.* 1988;**108:**669–674.

Warrell RP, Murphy WP, Schulman P, et al. A randomized double blind study of gallium nitrate compared to etidronate for acute control of cancer-related hypercalcemia. *J Clin Oncol.* 1991;**9:**1467–1475.

Warrell RP, Skelos A, Alcock NW, et al. Gallium nitrate for acute treatment of cancer-related hypercalcemia: Clinicopharmacological and dose response analysis. *Cancer Res.* 1986;**46:**4208–4212.

Yates AJP, Jerums GJ, Murray RML, et al. A comparison of single and multiple intravenous infusion of APD in the treatment of hypercalcemia of malignancy. *Aust NZ J Med.* 1987;**17:**387–391.

Part II

Chemotherapy Administration and Nursing Considerations

Chapter 4 □ □ □ □ □

Administration of Cancer Chemotherapy Agents

Barbara Carlile Holmes

The administration of chemotherapy is a specialized area of care requiring skillful and knowledgeable professional practice. The responsibility for this administration has shifted throughout the years. During the early years of chemotherapy administration, circa 1950s, the physician was the only health care professional to perform this procedure (Hilkemeyer 1982, Lind and Bush 1987). Professional registered nurses have now assumed the majority of the responsibility involved in the actual delivery of chemotherapeutic agents, as well as the development of policies, procedures, and national standards for safe administration (Burke et al 1991).

Not only are the schedule, method, and route of administration of chemotherapy greatly varied, but so are the health care settings in which chemotherapy administration occurs. These can include the hospital, the outpatient/ambulatory facility, and the home. It is imperative that the clinician who administers chemotherapy have a thorough knowledge of the drugs; their modes of administration, dissemination, and elimination; the technical skills of venipuncture and the accessing and management of vascular access devices; and knowledge of the principles, accompanied by the skills, of providing patient and family education.

This chapter discusses the essentials of chemotherapy administration:

1. *Qualifications of the clinician administering chemotherapy*
2. *Assessment and education of the patient and family*
3. *Preparation and administration of chemotherapeutic agents*
4. *Routes of administration*
5. *Prevention and detection of extravasation*
6. *Chemotherapy delivery systems*

PROFESSIONAL QUALIFICATIONS

To ensure optimal quality of care and patient safety, the Oncology Nursing Society (ONS), the professional organization of oncology nurses, has recommended that only adequately prepared professional registered nurses who are proficient in chemotherapy administration assume the responsibility for actual drug delivery (ONS 1988b). The ONS has developed guidelines for the establishment of an educational program designed to train professional nurses in the administration of chemotherapy (ONS 1988a). These guidelines are divided into two major parts:

1. The *didactic component* includes the basic information on the science of oncology, the principles of cancer chemotherapy, the major principles governing the administration of chemotherapy, and the nursing management of the patient receiving chemotherapy.

2. The *clinical practicum* includes the clinical skills that the practitioner must demonstrate prior to being considered qualified to administer chemotherapy.

Chemotherapy administration training programs have been in existence since the late 1970s (Creaton et al 1991, Pilapil and Studva 1978, Welch-McCaffrey 1985). Knowledge about establishing continuing education programs in cancer nursing is now explicated in the literature (Belcher 1987, Fernsler 1987, Itano 1987, McMillan 1987, Volker 1987). Although the basic design of a chemotherapy education and training program to qualify registered nurses to administer chemotherapy will vary, depending on the resources of the particular institution or agency and the particular nurse practice act in the given state, the development of the Oncology Nursing Society guidelines greatly facilitates the establishment of a thorough educational program. Adherence to these guidelines, including both the didactic portion and the supervised clinical experience, will provide the practitioner with the necessary knowledge and skills to administer chemotherapy safely and expertly.

PREPARING THE PATIENT AND FAMILY: ASSESSMENT, EDUCATION, AND SUPPORT

Preparation of the patient and family is best accomplished through the collaborative efforts of the medical oncologist, the registered nurse, and the registered pharmacist. This preparation includes three main categories: (1) assessment of the patient's physical, psychological, social, and cognitive status; (2) education of the patient and family; and (3) the provision of support to the patient and family.

Assessment

Prior to the administration of chemotherapy, the nurse administering the chemotherapy should establish a pretreatment profile of the person and the disease status, including pertinent physical, psychological, and social parameters. Table 4.1 provides an outline/checklist for this assessment. This baseline assessment should be followed by ongoing assessments, all of which are essential to the decision of the treatment plan and to the design of interventions to assist the patient and family in optimal functioning.

TABLE 4.1. PRECHEMOTHERAPY ASSESSMENT

I. Physical
  A. Past medical history
    1. Cancer diagnosis and history
    2. Previous medical and surgical history
    3. Current medical and surgical problems
    4. Allergies
  B. Laboratory data
    1. Complete blood count, including granulocyte/neutrophil count
    2. Platelet count
    3. Other hematopoietic function, if indicated
    4. Liver function
    5. Renal function
  C. System review
    1. Cardiovascular function
    2. Dental and oral cavity status
    3. Dermatologic status
    4. Gastrointestinal function
    5. Neurologic function
    6. Respiratory function
    7. Sexual function
    8. Urologic function
  D. Prior cancer therapy toxicity
    1. Surgery
    2. Chemotherapy
    3. Radiation therapy
    4. Biological therapy
II. Psychologic and social assessment
  A. Life stage development
  B. Previous experience with chemotherapy
  C. Informed consent
  D. Fears
  E. Anxiety
  F. Depression
  G. Intrapersonal resources: coping
  H. Interpersonal resources: social support
III. Educational needs of patient and family
  A. Drug treatment protocol
  B. Potential side effects/adverse reactions
  C. Posttreatment care

Sources. Burke et al 1991, Holland 1990, ONS 1988a, Rowland 1990a,b.

The physical assessment should include review of the patient's most recent pertinent laboratory test results. The complete blood count (CBC) and platelet count are always included. The absolute granulocyte count (AGC) should be calculated if the white blood cell count (WBC) is low, that is, below 2500 cells/mm^3. The AGC is calculated by multiplying the percentages of neutrophils and segmented bands by the total WBC. When the AGC is less than

1500 cells/mm^3, chemotherapy may be withheld. Renal and liver function should also be assessed prior to the administration of chemotherapy, as related to the way in which the drugs are metabolized and eliminated. Dose reductions may be indicated if these indices are not in the normal range. A systemic assessment of the patient's physical status should also be done prior to the first administration of chemotherapy. In addition, assessment of the patient's performance status evaluates the ability of the individual to perform normal life activities. The Karnofsky and Zubrod scales provide a quantitative measure for subjective functional data (Brown and Hogan 1990).

The psychologic aspects that accompany the entire trajectory of the cancer experience play a significant role in how the patient will comply with and respond to his or her chemotherapy treatments. The patient's life stage, fears, anxieties, and coping skills should be included in the psychologic assessment.

The social support that is provided to the patient can also play a significant role in the success of the chemotherapeutic treatment. These interpersonal resources have not only been shown to diminish the psychic distress of cancer, but may also be important in modulating survival (Rowland 1990a). In assessing social support, the features that constitute support must be addressed (ie, type, source, availability, quality, and perceived use for), as should the characteristics of the provider and the recipient of that support (Rowland 1990a).

The patient's and family's cognitive abilities must also be included in the assessment. An important feature of this assessment is that regardless of the patient's and family's intellectual sophistication, the uniquely threatening nature of cancer and chemotherapy can alter cognitive abilities.

Education

Education of the patient and family is an ongoing process and must begin before chemotherapy is administered. This education must be individualized and must take into account the significant psychologic reactions that accompany the diagnosis of and treatment for cancer. It is normal for the patient and family to feel overwhelmed by the large amounts of information they must retain and use. Education of the patient and family must include both verbal and written avenues of delivery.

The importance of informed consent is emphasized by the fact that written or oral consent for chemotherapy treatment is now mandatory whether the patient is receiving standard or investigational treatment (see Chapter 7 for further discussion of this topic). Although the responsibility for obtaining informed consent is that of the physician, the professional nurse has the responsibility to develop, implement, and evaluate patient and family education programs (ONS 1989d).

Prior to the actual education of the patient and family, it is helpful to ascertain the knowledge base from which both the patient and family may be operating. It is frequently helpful for the practitioner, as well as therapeutic for the patient, to have the patient describe his or her cancer history. This is an excellent opportunity to identify the coping skills of the patient: as the patient relays the story from first symptom to diagnosis, the professional nurse can identify at least one way in which the patient deals with unexpected, unplanned stress. It is also helpful to have the patient and family describe their understanding of the information that the physician has communicated thus far, even if the nurse was present during this transaction. The nurse must also ascertain the patient's and family's perceptions of chemotherapy, to correct any misconceptions. Table 4.2 lists the questions to be used in this preparatory phase, as well as the topics to be included in the actual education of the patient and family.

TABLE 4.2. PATIENT AND FAMILY CHEMOTHERAPY EDUCATION

Preparatory Questions
1. What was your first symptom that something was wrong? What did you do about it?
2. What has your physician told you about your cancer and the chemotherapy treatments?
3. What does chemotherapy mean to you?

Topics to Be Included in Patient/Family Education
1. Names and actions of drugs to be given and taken
2. Schedule of drug administration
3. Length of treatment plan
4. Purpose of treatment plan (eg, cure or palliation)
5. Potential side effects and management of such
6. Self-care preventative management of side effects
7. Vascular access device care (if a vascular access device is to be used)
8. Procedure for contacting the nurse, physician, or clinic 24 hours a day, 7 days a week
9. Questions and concerns of patient and family

Support

The psychologic care of medical patients has become an important aspect of the total care of the patient. Patients with cancer experience unique psychologic needs, and appropriate interventions are necessary throughout the course of treatment. The health care professional involved in any aspect of the diagnosis and treatment of cancer should be cognizant of the psychologic demands placed on the patient and hence provide some element of emotional and psychologic support to the patient and family. Treatment with chemotherapy implies additional psychologic concerns for most patients. In addition to having a broad knowledge of chemotherapy, it is helpful for the clinician to possess the personal skills that encompass diplomacy, empathy, sensitivity, and personal integrity.

AMBULATORY AND HOME SETTINGS

In large part because of economic factors, the administration of chemotherapy is taking place in more varied settings. Formerly administered only in the hospital setting, chemotherapy is now frequently administered in a variety of ambulatory settings, such as outpatient clinics and physicians' private offices. Administration of chemotherapy in the patient's home has also increased. The majority of chemotherapeutic agents are now administered to patients who are well enough to commute to the ambulatory setting to receive the treatment and who are residing at home, not in the hospital.

PREPARATION AND ADMINISTRATION OF CHEMOTHERAPEUTIC AGENTS

Calculation of Chemotherapy Dosage

Most chemotherapy doses are computed on the basis of body surface area and are expressed in milligrams per square meter of body surface area (mg/m^2). Body surface area (BSA) is generally calculated from height and weight according to such equations as the classic Du Bois formula (Du Bois and Du Bois 1916). There are many published nomograms based on such equations, although some are inaccurate (Turcotte 1979). If the clinician is planning to calculate the BSA with a nomogram, it must be available at the time of calculation. An alternative to this approach is the use of a modification of an equation by Gehan and George (1970) reported by Mosteller (1987). This approach requires the use of a calculator with a square root key.

$$\text{BSA (m}^2\text{)} = \sqrt{\frac{\text{Ht (in.)} \times \text{Wt (lb)}}{3131}}$$

In metric:

$$\text{BSA (m}^2\text{)} = \sqrt{\frac{\text{Ht (cm)} \times \text{Wt (kg)}}{3600}}$$

Controversy surrounds the issue of whether to use the individual's actual (current) or ideal body weight. Usually, the lesser of actual or ideal weight is used in calculating body surface area to avoid overdosing obese patients or those with amputations. There are, however, many versions of ideal weight charts and the practice of using the lesser weight is by no means universal. On the basis of a retrospective study of 3732 patients entered on eight phase III combination chemotherapy protocols, Gelman and colleagues (1987) recommend that actual weight be used in setting initial chemotherapy doses in most phase III studies (excluding those using very high doses, such as bone marrow transplant studies) and in most patients (excluding those who are clinically obese, ie, 30% overweight). Until the controversy is resolved, the nurse, physician, and pharmacist should discuss dosage concerns related to obese patients or those with amputations on an individual patient basis.

Although body surface area is the preferred method of calculating the dosage, some drug doses are based on body weight alone, expressed as milligrams per kilogram (mg/kg). The body surface area method provides a better method of determining the individual's size than body weight because it minimizes the variation in similar-sized individuals resulting from weight and provides for dosage differences between adults and children (Brown and Hogan 1990, DeVita 1989).

Safe Handling of Cytotoxic Drugs

Safe handling of cytotoxic drugs has become an issue for health care providers, especially oncology nurses and pharmacists, because these drugs represent an occupational hazard. Chemotherapeutic agents are mutagens, carcinogens, and teratogens that can be absorbed, inhaled, or ingested by staff who handle them. Personnel can protect themselves from exposure to these agents by using appropriate protection (Occupational Safety and Health Administration 1986), and the use of such protection appears to be improving over time (Valanis et al 1991). Cancer chemotherapy for parenteral administration may be prepared by either a registered pharmacist or a registered nurse. In the majority of hospital settings, this responsibility is assumed by the staff pharmacist. A pharmaceutical company outside the hospital may also prepare the agent. In many physicians' offices, as well as in many home health care agencies, the registered nurse is responsible for preparation as well as administration of the drugs. In a few oncology units in hospital settings, the registered nurse is still preparing the drugs. In the vast majority of settings, however, the pharmacist has the responsibility for preparing cancer chemotherapy.

Regardless of where the chemotherapy is prepared, special equipment and procedures should be employed to ensure minimal exposure to and maximum protection from potentially dangerous agents (Gullo 1988). The Occupational Safety and Health Administration (OSHA) has prepared guidelines describing the hazards of cancer chemotherapy, identifying high-risk workers and recommending control work practice techniques that can be implemented to help prevent adverse health effects. The most recent of these guidelines was released January 29, 1986, and is entitled *Work Practice Guidelines for Personnel Dealing with Cytotoxic (Antineoplastic) Drugs,* OSHA Instructional Publication 8-1.1. Copies of these guidelines may be obtained from the local OSHA office or from the U.S. Department of Labor. The Oncology Nursing Society has also published *Safe Handling of Cytotoxic Drugs* (ONS 1989c), which articulates directions similar to those of OSHA. Table 4.3 summarizes the recommended guidelines from the ONS and OSHA for the safe handling and disposal of antineoplastic agents. The reader is urged to refer to the ONS publication for a detailed independent study module addressing safe handling of cytotoxic drugs.

ROUTES OF ADMINISTRATION

Chemotherapy is administered via multiple routes, although these routes can be divided into two fundamental methods of administration: *systemic* and *regional.* The goal of systemic chemotherapy is to attain a drug concentration sufficient to achieve a therapeutic cytotoxic effect in presumed or proven metastatic disease without causing excessive toxicity to normal tissues. Systemic chemotherapy may be given orally, intravenously, subcutaneously, intramuscularly, or intraosseously. Regional chemotherapy is directed toward the goal of delivering the drug(s) directly into the blood vessel supplying the tumor or the cavity in which the tumor is isolated. Frequently, regional chemotherapy permits higher doses of the drug to be delivered to the area of the tumor accompanied by less severe toxic effects, because a decreased amount of drug reaches the systemic circulation (Goodman 1991). Regional chemotherapy may be given through the routes of intrathecal, intraarterial, or intracavitary administration.

The route chosen is an important variable in optimal drug delivery. The most common routes used are oral and intravenous (Brown and Hogan 1990). Regardless of the route chosen, however, it is imperative that chemotherapeutic agents are administered safely and that this administration is accompanied by appropriate patient and family education. A chemotherapy administration checklist, such as that in Table 4.4, can facilitate the proper administration of chemotherapeutic agents.

Intravenous Drug Administration

The intravenous (IV) route of chemotherapy administration is the most commonly used route, with over 20 million hospitalized patients receiving intravenous medications or fluids each year (Von Hoff 1991). Although the benefits of administration of medications and fluids by the intravenous route are many, problems such as cellulitis, bacteremia, and venous thrombosis can occur.

Chemotherapy may be given intravenously by several methods: (1) IV push (direct push method, two-syringe technique); (2) IV sidearm (IV sideport, IV Y-site); (3) mini-infusion (IV piggyback); (4) IV infusion. The IV push method is the administration of the chemotherapeutic agent(s) directly into a vein through a single syringe (per antineoplastic agent), with the use of an additional syringe for flushing purposes. Administration of the drug(s) from a syringe through the sideport or a Y-site of a freely running IV line is referred to as IV sidearm. A mini-infusion, long called IV piggyback, is the administration of the chemotherapeutic agent diluted in a secondary IV bag, usually in 50 to 100 mL of diluent. The secondary line is usually attached to a needle and primary line or heparin lock and removed when not in use. IV infusion is the administration of the chemotherapy diluted in the main IV bag, usually in 250 to 1000 mL of IV solution.

TABLE 4.3. GUIDELINES FOR SAFE HANDLING AND DISPOSAL OF ANTINEOPLASTIC AGENTS

Drug Preparation
1. All antineoplastic drugs should be prepared by specially trained individuals in a centralized area to minimize interruptions and risk of contamination.
2. Drugs are prepared in a class II biologic safety cabinet (vertical laminar airflow hood) with vents to the outside, if possible. The blower is left on 24 hours a day, 7 days a week. The hood is serviced regularly according to the manufacturer's recommendations.
3. Eating, drinking, smoking, and applying cosmetics in the drug preparation area are prohibited.
4. The work surface is covered with a plastic absorbent pad to minimize contamination. This pad is changed immediately in the event of contamination and at the completion of drug preparation each day or shift.
5. The prescribed drug is prepared using aseptic technique according to the physician's orders, other pharmaceutic resources, or both.
6. Disposable surgical latex unpowdered gloves are used when handling the drugs. Gloves should be changed hourly or immediately if torn or punctured.
7. A disposable long-sleeved gown made of lint-free fabric with knitted cuffs and a closed front is worn during drug preparation.
8. A thermoplastic (Plexiglass) face shield or goggles and a powered air-purifying respirator should be used if a biologic safety cabinet is not available.
9. Because exposure can result when connnecting and disconnecting intravenous (IV) tubing, when injecting the drug into the IV line, when removing air from the syringe or infusion line, and when leakage occurs at the tubing, syringe, or stopcock connection, priming of all IV tubing is carried out under the protection of the hood.
10. Other measures to guard against drug leakage during drug preparation include venting the vial and using large-bore needles, luer-Lock fittings, and sterile gauze or sponge around the neck of the vial during needle withdrawal. Aerosolization may also be minimized by attaching an aerosol protection device (CytoGuard, Bristol-Myers) to the vial of drug before adding the diluent.
11. Once reconstituted, the drug is labeled according to institutional policies and procedures; the label should include the drug's vesicant properties and antineoplastic drug warning.
12. Antineoplastic drugs are transported in an impervious packing material and are marked with a distinctive warning label.
13. Personnel responsible for drug transport are knowledgeable of procedures to be followed in the event of drug spillage.

Drug Administration
1. Chemotherapeutic agents are administered by registered professional nurses who have been specially trained and designated as qualified according to specific institutional policies and procedures.
2. Before administering the drugs, the nurse ensures that informed consent has been given and clarifies any misconceptions the patient might have regarding the drugs and their side effects.
3. Appropriate laboratory results are evaluated and found to be within acceptable levels (eg, complete blood count, renal and liver function).
4. Measures to minimize side effects of the drugs are carried out before drug administration (eg, hydration, antiemetics and antianxiety agents, and patient comfort).
5. An appropriate route for drug administration is ensured according to the physician's order.
6. Personal protective equipment is worn, including disposable latex surgical gloves and a disposable gown made of a lint-free, low-permeability fabric with a closed front, long sleeves, and elastic or knit closed cuffs (optional).
7. The work surface is protected with a disposable absorbent pad.
8. The drug or drugs are administered according to established institutional policies and procedures.
9. Documentation of drug administration, including any adverse reaction, is made in the patient's medical record.
10. A mechanism for identification of patients receiving antineoplastic agents is established for the 48-hour period following drug dispensing.
11. Disposable surgical unpowdered latex gloves and a disposable gown are worn when handling body secretions such as blood, vomitus, or excreta from patients who received chemotherapy drugs within the previous 48 hours.
12. In the event of accidental exposure, contaminated gloves and gown should be removed immediately and discarded according to official procedures.
13. Wash the contaminated skin with soap and water.
14. An eye that is accidentally exposed to chemotherapy should be flooded with water or isotonic eye wash for at least 5 minutes.
15. A medical evaluation must be obtained as soon as possible after exposure and the incident documented according to institutional policies and procedures.

(continued)

TABLE 4.3. GUIDELINES FOR SAFE HANDLING AND DISPOSAL OF ANTINEOPLASTIC AGENTS (continued)

Drug Disposal

1. Regardless of the setting (hospital, ambulatory care, or home), all equipment and unused drugs are treated as hazardous and are disposed of according to the institution's policies and procedures.
2. All contaminated equipment, including needles, are disposed of intact to prevent aerosolization, leaks, and spills.
3. All contaminated materials used in drug preparation are disposed of in a leakproof, punctureproof container with a distinctive warning label and are placed in a sealable 4-mil polyethylene or 2-mil polypropylene bag with appropriate labeling.
4. Linen contaminated with bodily secretions of patients who have received chemotherapy within the previous 48 hours is placed in a specially marked laundry bag, which is then placed in an impervious bag that is marked with a distinctive warning label.
5. In the event of a spill, personnel should don double surgical latex unpowdered gloves; eye protection; and a disposable gown made of a lint-free, low-permeability fabric with a closed front, long sleeves, and elastic or knit closed cuffs.
6. Small amounts of liquids are cleaned up with gauze pads, whereas larger spills (more than 5 mL) are cleaned up with absorbent pads.
7. Small amounts of solids or spills involving powder are cleaned up with damp cloths or absorbent gauze pads.
8. The spill area is cleaned three times with a detergent followed by clean water.
9. Broken glassware and disposable contaminated materials are placed in a leakproof, punctureproof container and then placed in a sealable 4-mil polyethylene or 2-mil polypropylene bag and marked with a distinctive warning label.
10. Contaminated reusable items are washed by specially trained personnel wearing double surgical unpowdered latex gloves.
11. The spill should be documented according to established institutional policies and procedures.

From Goodman M. Delivery of cancer chemotherapy. In: Baird SB, McCorkle R, Grant M, eds. Cancer Nursing: A Comprehensive Textbook. Philadelphia: WB Saunders; 1991:291–320. Reprinted with permission.

The choice of an IV method is based on the following factors, which should be reflected in the institutional/agency policies and procedures (Goodman 1991):

1. Vesicant properties of the drug(s)
2. Potential vein irritation of the drug(s)
3. Potential for immediate or delayed complications of the drug(s), for example, anaphylaxis, hypertension, hypotension
4. The logistics of the specific treatment protocol

Most chemotherapy, including vesicants and nonvesicants, is administered by IV push. The main controversy over which intravenous method to employ usually concerns the administration of vesicants. Both the IV push and the IV sidearm methods are considered safe for the administration of vesicants; however, the IV push (two-syringe) method is preferable because venous pressure (resistance) and blood return are more readily assessed with this method, thereby permitting more precise and direct control of the fluid into the vein. A very important point is that all drugs, vesicant or nonvesicant, should be injected directly into a peripheral vein only after ample flushing with normal saline is performed to ascertain adequate blood flow and venous integrity (Goodman 1991).

Short-term infusions (30 minutes to 6 hours) are indicated when the chemotherapeutic agents produce complications or undesirable side effects when given via the IV push method. Long-term infusions (8 hours or longer), including continuous infusions, are increasing because of the accumulating knowledge of the advantages of this method. Continuous infusions have demonstrated advantages in (1) overcoming cytokinetic resistance and, thereby, minimizing toxic effects while enhancing tumor response; (2) maximizing the intracellular levels of the drugs by prolonging exposure to low extracellular concentrations of the drug(s); (3) enhancing the transport mechanisms of the cell membrane through the saturation process provided by continuous infusion therapy; and (4) avoiding peak plasma levels and, thereby, minimizing toxic effects (Goodman 1991).

Venipuncture. The intravenous administration of chemotherapeutic agents poses unique problems (eg, extravasation, frequency of venipuncture, physical condition of patient) as compared with many other types of medications. To provide a high standard of quality of care, intravenous chemotherapy should be administered only by health care providers knowledgeable, trained, and skilled in venipuncture and chemotherapy administration.

TABLE 4.4. CHEMOTHERAPY ADMINISTRATION CHECKLIST

1. Establish a professional relationship with the patient.
2. Conduct a pretreatment patient evaluation, which provides the following assessment data:
   a. Medical history relevant to chemotherapy
   b. Patient's/family's understanding of chemotherapy and previous experience with chemotherapy
   c. Patient/family knowledge base
   d. Patient/family emotional, psychologic, and cognitive levels
   e. Pertinent, current laboratory values
   f. Evidence that patient has given informed consent
   g. Patient's/family's ability to manage patient's postchemotherapy care
   h. Resources available to patient
3. Verify the name of drug(s) and dosage, route, rate, and timing of drug(s) administration with physician's order or protocol.
4. Have a working knowledge of the drug pharmacology: mechanism of action, usual dosage, route of administration, administrative precautions, immediate and delayed side effects, and route of excretion.
5. Discuss laboratory abnormalities with physician.
6. Calculate patient's body surface area if not done by physician or pharmacist; otherwise, recalculate patient's body surface area.
7. Recalculate drug dosage.
8. Verify physician's orders and body surface area and dosage calculations with another nurse.
9. Use proper procedure for identification of patient.
10. Develop and implement an individualized teaching plan for the patient and family, including the following:
    a. Chemotherapy procedure and schedule
    b. Potential side effects and their management
    c. Self-care preventative management of side effects
    d. Patient's/family's questions and concerns
11. Supplement verbal education with printed material and audiovisual aids, as needed.
12. Inform patient and family about causes and procedure for contacting the nurse, physician, or clinic 24 hours a day, 7 days a week.
13. Prepare antineoplastic agents according to manufacturers' suggestions, OSHA guidelines, and institution procedures. (This may be either a nursing or a pharmacy procedure.)
14. Administer any premedications (eg, antiemetics, sedatives) at least 20 to 30 minutes before chemotherapy starts. (Some antiemetics are begun the night prior to chemotherapy.)
15. Administer chemotherapy according to written institutional policies and procedures, based on ONS and OSHA guidelines.
16. Do not allow interruptions during the preparation or administration of chemotherapy.
17. Emergency drugs and an extravasation kit should be readily available at all times.
18. Incorporate the patient into the administration procedure, including vein selection and reactions to administration.
19. Dispose of all chemotherapy supplies according to OSHA guidelines and institutional policy.
20. Document drug administration according to institutional policy and procedures.

Sources. Burke et al 1991, ONS 1988b, Tenenbaum 1989.

Although starting a new intravenous line is preferable for the administration of most chemotherapeutic agents, a preexisting intravenous line may be used, but only under the following conditions: (1) The line has been in place less than 24 hours. (2) There are no signs or symptoms of phlebitis. (3) The blood return is quick and ample. A new line must be established if there is violation of any one of these conditions, for example, erythema, swelling, or sluggish or absent blood return. If a vesicant agent is to be given and the patient has a preexisting intravenous line, the same preceding criteria hold; however, it is preferable to consider a venous access device prior to the first administration of chemotherapy, especially if vesicant agents are part of the treatment plan. When using preexisting or newly started intravenous lines for chemotherapy, one dictum still rules: whenever any doubt exists about the integrity of the vein, a new intravenous line must be established prior to administering the chemotherapy (Burke et al 1991, Goodman 1991).

Venipuncture for the purpose of chemotherapy administration carries particular responsibilities. The clinician administering the antineoplastic agents should have special knowledge about venous selection, cannulation, and patency. The following 12 steps address this process.

1. *Assessment.* A thorough, systematic assessment of all available arm veins must be accomplished prior to venipuncture. Each entire arm must be fully visible, that is, free of jewelry and clothes, in good lighting, and on a firm surface (Goodman 1991).
2. *Location of vein.* Veins in a distal location (eg, the dorsum of the hand) should be chosen first, alternating proximal (closer to the heart) venipuncture sites with subsequent administrations. One exception to this is the administration of vesicant agents; the forearm is the preferred site for the administration of vesicant agents because this location has more underlying muscle and tissue to protect vital nerves and it provides extra tissue coverage if surgical management of an extravasation is necessary. For vesicant administration, if the forearm does not provide a usable vein, the dorsum of the hand is the next choice, followed by the wrist area. A large vein is always preferable to a small vein, even if the larger vein is on the dorsum of the hand and the smaller vein is in the forearm. Also, the antecubital fossa is avoided for vesicant drug administration because of the difficulty in detecting and treating extravasations in this area (Goodman 1991). For all chemotherapy administration, veins that are located in areas of decreased circulation, impaired lymphatic drainage, and in the legs and feet should be avoided.
3. *Type of vein.* Only veins that are smooth and pliable should be used for chemotherapy administration. Veins that are inflamed, sclerosed, bruised, or phlebitic should not be considered for venipuncture.
4. *Equipment.* All the necessary equipment for venipuncture, the anchoring of the needle and line, and the administration of chemotherapy should be assembled before venipuncture is attempted. This is also the time during which protective equipment should be donned by the individual administering the chemotherapy.
5. *Referrals.* If the health care professional preparing to do venipuncture cannot find a site for venipuncture, a colleague should be consulted. Also, if the health care professional cannot secure venous access after two unsuccessful attempts at venipuncture, another health care professional should attempt venipuncture. If a vascular access device has not been considered prior to this point, such assessment should definitely be accomplished at this time.
6. *Type of needle/cannula.* The choice of an angiocath or a butterfly needle is based on the following (Burke et al 1991, Knobf 1982):
   a. The individual patient
   b. The goal of the therapy
   c. The type of therapy to be given
   d. Length of time required for needle to be in place
   e. Risk of vein perforation
   A 25- or 23-gauge butterfly/scalp vein needle is preferable for short-term infusions (less than 60 minutes) and for direct push (two-syringe technique). An 18- to 21-gauge needle, such as a plastic thin-walled catheter, is appropriate for lengthy infusions, blood components, or hydration regimens that last 2 to 3 hours.
7. *Skin preparation.* The selected venipuncture site should be prepared by a 1-minute alcohol rub or a povidone–iodine and alcohol rub. To avoid contamination the area should not be repalpated after this cleansing.
8. *Venipuncture.* Venipuncture should be performed according to institutional policies and procedures. The scalp vein should enter the vein smoothly and directly and immediate blood return should be obvious. At this point the tourniquet should be released and a syringe of saline should be attached to the tubing. The needle should then be taped in place securely without obstructing the visualization of the entrance site. Air should be aspirated from the tubing and the catheter should be flushed with a minimum of 10 mL of saline. This tests the patency of the vein. During this time, the venipuncture site and proximal portion of the vein should be palpated and observed for any evidence of infiltration, including swelling, redness, and burning.
9. *Administration.* The chemotherapeutic agents may be injected only if the needle is resting securely in the vein and a brisk

blood return is observed, along with no evidence of infiltration. Blood return should be checked after every 2 mL of solution is administered. The vein must be flushed with a minimum of 5 mL of saline between agents and with 10 mL of saline before the needle is removed. If the chemotherapy is to be administered through the IV sidearm method, the venipuncture site must still be visualized, and any obstructive dressing removed. Blood return must be checked by aspirating the blood into the tubing or by lowering the infusion bag (Goodman 1991).

10. *Vesicant administration.* Infusing a vesicant agent into a peripheral vein places the patient at unnecessary risk for pain, anxiety, drug extravasation, and tissue damage. Given the ready availability of vascular access devices, the administration of vesicants through peripheral lines should become the exception rather than the rule. Vesicants should never be administered into a line that is infusing with the aid of an infusion pump. This could increase the potential for extravasation and could prevent the quick reversal of the direction of drug flow in the event of a possible extravasation. The vesicant agent should be administered first (after ample flushing and blood return check), before other chemotherapeutic agents, in anticipation of perivenous irritation or needle movement; however, a vesicant agent should never be injected distally to a previous puncture site. Additionally, vesicant agents should never be infused as a mini-infusion or continuous infusion into a peripheral vein. Vesicant agents always have the potential to cause tissue damage if infiltration occurs, regardless of the dilution (Goodman 1991).

11. *Order of administration.* Although the order of administration of drugs (vesicant first or last) is a controversial issue, it has not been shown to increase the risk of extravasation or decrease long-term venous integrity; however, other factors may also affect the order of administration. A drug known to be associated with rapid onset of nausea and vomiting (eg, high-dose cyclophosphamide or cisplatin) or with an aversive taste (eg, cyclophosphamide) is generally administered last. The important aspect in the order of the drug administration is the flushing of the line with saline before each drug, after each drug in a combination, and after the last drug at the end of treatment (Burke et al 1991, Goodman 1991).

12. *Vein observation during administration.* The entire course of the vein should be visible during venipuncture and infusion. The vein should be observed throughout the administration for any evidence of vein irritation. The patient should also be taught to play an active role by reporting any pain, burning, or itching during the administration (Goodman 1991).

Prevention and Detection of Extravasation. *Extravasation* is the leakage of caustic fluid from a vein into the surrounding subcutaneous tissues, causing tissue damage of varying degrees (Jameson and O'Donnell 1983). Chemotherapeutic agents are just one group of drugs that may cause tissue damage or extravasation. These drugs that have the potential to cause cellular damage or tissue destruction are referred to as *vesicants*. Injuries caused by the extravasation of vesicants can cause sloughing of tissue, severe prolonged pain, infection, and loss of mobility (Montrose 1987). Vesicants are contrasted with *irritants*, which are drugs that may produce pain and inflammation at the administration site or along the path of the vein through which they are administered, but do not cause tissue destruction. Table 4.5 lists the antineoplastic agents according to their vesicant or irritant properties.

The reported incidence of extravasation of antineoplastic agents ranges from 0.1% to 6% of all toxic reactions to chemotherapy (Goodman 1991, Ignoffo and Friedman 1980, Larson 1982, Montrose 1987). The majority of reported cases occurred with inexperienced personnel or with those lacking knowledge of the signs and symptoms of extravasation; however, even with a skilled practitioner, the incidence can be as great as 1% (Montrose 1987). Prevention, early detection, and prompt intervention are essential in dealing with the problem of extravasation. The treatment of extravasation is covered in Chapter 6; the remainder of this section will address prevention and detection.

Because of the severity of the tissue damage caused by extravasation, as well as the controversy regarding treatment of extravasation injuries, prevention of extravasation is essential. There are sev-

TABLE 4.5. VESICANT AND IRRITANT ANTINEOPLASTIC AGENTS

Vesicants

Amsacrine
Bisantrene (CL 216942, "orange crush," NSC-337766)
Dactinomycin
Daunorubicin
Doxorubicin
Epirubicin (Pharmorubicin®)
Maytansine (Maitansine)
Mechlorethamine
Mitomycin-c
Pyrazofurin (pyrazomycin)
Vinblastine
Vincristine
Vindesine

Irritants

Carmustine
Dacarbazine
Etoposide
Mitoguazone (Methyl-GAG)
Plicamycin
Streptozocin
Teniposide

---

eral factors that affect the risk of extravasation (Burke et al 1991, Goodman 1991). These risk factors are listed in Table 4.6.

Knowledge and Skill of the Practitioner. Chemotherapy should be administered only by registered nurses who are trained in chemotherapy administration. These practitioners should only attempt venipuncture twice, at which point a colleague should be consulted if the venipuncture is unsuccessful. These practitioners should also be knowledgeable about the signs and symptoms of extravasation. The institutional policies and procedures should be routinely reviewed and updated to reflect the changing standards and methods of practice; nursing practice should be based on these policies and procedures.

TABLE 4.6. RISK FACTORS FOR EXTRAVASATION

Knowledge and skill of the practitioner
Education and participation of patient
Condition of the vein
Location of the vein
Drug administration technique
Order of vesicant administration
Preexisting intravenous line

Sources. Burke et al 1991, Goodman 1991.

Education and Participation of the Patient. The patient can be an active participant in the prevention and detection of extravasation. By educating the patient about the signs and symptoms of extravasation (eg, burning, erythema) and the importance of prompt reporting of such, earlier detection is possible.

Location of the Vein. The large veins of the forearm (eg, the posterior basilic vein) are the optimal peripheral access sites for the administration of vesicant agents because there is normally sufficient tissue protecting nerves and tendons. If these veins are not usable, the metacarpal veins of the dorsum of the hand are the next choice; however, a large straight vein over the dorsum of the hand is preferable to a smaller, less accessible vein of the forearm. Any area in which extravasation would expose critical nerves and tendons should be avoided as injection sites, as extravasation in these areas can lead to permanent dysfunction. This includes veins over the wrist, the antecubital fossa, and the hands of thin, elderly patients. If the only apparent site of venipuncture is the antecubital fossa, the patient must receive a vascular access device. Chemotherapy should never be administered in areas of compromised circulation, such as the lower extremities, a mastectomy site, or areas with phlebitis, lymphedema, or hematomas (Brown and Hogan 1990, Goodman 1991, Montrose 1987).

The use of multiple puncture sites in the same vein should also be avoided, because of the possible resulting leakage into surrounding tissues once an intravenous line is established. If multiple venipuncture attempts are necessary, a different vein should be chosen each time. If venipuncture must be attempted more than once on the same vein, each subsequent puncture site must be proximal to the preceding site. If the multiple sites were selected in a distal progression, leakage would occur at the proximal puncture sites.

Preexisting Intravenous Lines. The clinician's skill at assessment is the critical factor in the determination of the use of a preexisting intravenous line. All dressings over the intravenous insertion site must be removed to allow full visualization of the vein during assessment and administration of the vesicant agent(s). Key components of the assessment that would necessitate a new venipuncture include the following:

68 CHEMOTHERAPY ADMINISTRATION AND NURSING CONSIDERATIONS

1. *Time of venipuncture.* The intravenous line was placed more than 6 hours earlier.
2. *Flow of fluid.* The intravenous fluid runs erratically and the intravenous line seems positional.
3. *Condition and location of the intravenous site.* The site is swollen, sore, or reddened, shows other evidence of infiltration, or is located over the wrist or in the antecubital fossa.
4. *Blood return.* The blood return is not brisk and consistent, but rather sluggish or absent.
5. *Patient participation.* The patient complains of burning or tingling at the venipuncture site or along the vein.

Drug Administration Technique. If vesicant agents are to be given peripherally, the two-syringe technique (IV push) and the use of the IV sidearm are the techniques of choice. These techniques are described in Table 4.7. Vesicant agents should never be administered into a peripheral vein as continuous infusions or through a controlled infusion pump. If a continuous infusion is necessary, the vesicant drug should be infused via an externally based central venous catheter. The incidence of vesicant drug extravasation from implanted ports used for continuous infusion presents a risk to be avoided (Goodman 1991). If the peripheral line is on a controlled infusion pump, the pump must be disconnected before the administration of chemotherapy.

Anaphylaxis. An anaphylactic reaction to chemotherapy, also referred to as an allergic or hypersensitivity reaction, can result from overstimulation of the immune system. There are four types of hypersensitivity reactions, with type I being the reaction most frequently seen in association with chemotherapy. This level of reaction is caused by the development of immunoglobulin E (IgE) antibodies as a result of exposure of the cell to a foreign substance or antigen. Sensitization then occurs, with subsequent exposures to the antigen resulting in allergic reactions. Symptoms associated with this level include agitation, urticaria, facial edema, rhinitis, dyspnea, and anaphylaxis. These symptoms can become progressively worse with each additional exposure to the antigen. Hypersensitivity reactions have been reported with intravenous use of the following drugs: L-asparaginase, bleomycin, cisplatin, cyclophosphamide, daunorubicin, doxorubicin, mechlorethamine, methotrexate, melphalan, teniposide, and zinostatin (Neocarzinostatin®) (Brown and Hogan 1990, Burke et al 1991). Table 4.8 describes the proce-

TABLE 4.7. ADMINISTRATION OF VESICANT AGENTS

Two-Syringe Technique
1. Select an appropriate vein.
2. Begin a new intravenous line using a scalp vein needle (25- or 23-gauge).
3. Access vein using a single approach.
4. Flush line with 8 to 10 mL of saline. Assess for brisk, full blood return and any evidence of infiltration. Check for swelling at the site, redness or pain, and lack of blood return.
5. Once access is ensured, switch to syringe of chemotherapy.
6. Dilute drugs according to the package insert.
7. Inject drugs slowly and with minimal resistance.
8. Assess for blood return every 1 to 2 mL of infusion.
9. Irrigate with 3 to 5 mL of saline between each drug and 8 to 10 mL at the completion of the infusion of the drug or drugs.

Sidearm Technique
1. Ensure proper venous access site. The intravenous fluid should be additive free.
2. The cannula used to access the vein should be at least a 20-gauge to ensure an adequate blood return and fluid flow.
3. Secure cannula but do not obstruct entrance site.
4. Pinch off tubing and assess for blood return.
5. Test the vein with 50 to 100 mL to ensure an adequate and swift drip of infusion.
6. With intravenous fluid continuing to drip, slowly inject vesicant into intravenous line.
7. Do not allow vesicant to flow backward.
8. Do not pinch off tubing except to assess for blood return.
9. Assess for blood return every 1 to 2 mL of injection.
10. Flush needle with saline at the completion of injection.

From Goodman M. Delivery of cancer chemotherapy. In: Baird SB, McCorkle R, Grant M, eds. *Cancer Nursing: A Comprehensive Textbook.* Philadelphia: WB Saunders; 1991:291–320. Reprinted with permission.

TABLE 4.8. MANAGEMENT OF ANAPHYLAXIS

1. Review the patient's allergy history and record baseline blood pressure, pulse, and respiration.
2. Consider prophylactic medication with hydrocortisone or an antihistamine in individuals with suspected hypersensitivity potential (this requires a physician's order).
3. Inform the patient of the potential for hypersensitivity reaction and the necessity to report any of the following symptoms immediately:
    a. Urticaria
    b. Localized/generalized itching
    c. Shortness of breath with or without wheezing
    d. Uneasiness or agitation
    e. Periorbital or facial edema
    f. Light-headedness/dizziness
    g. Tightness in the chest
    h. Abdominal cramping
    i. Chills
4. Ensure that emergency equipment (eg, oxygen, AMBU bag, intubation equipment) is readily available and that there is a patent IV line. Check the supply of the following drugs and be familiar with appropriate doses and routes:
    a. Epinephrine (Adrenaline® [Parke-Davis, Morris Plains, NJ])
    b. Diphenhydramine HCl (Benadryl® [Parke-Davis]) or other antihistamines
    c. Hydrocortisone sodium succinate (Solu Cortef® [The Upjohn Company, Kalamazoo, MI])
    d. Aminophylline
    e. Dopamine HCl (Intropin® [DuPont Pharmaceuticals, Wilmington, DE])
    f. Dexamethasone (Decadron® [Merck Sharp & Dohme, West Point, PA])
5. Before administering the initial dose of a drug with reports of increased incidence of hypersensitivity, a scratch test, intradermal skin test, or test dose may be performed first (all of these procedures require a physician's order):
    a. Observe the patient for at least 15 minutes after the test dose for a local positive reaction and/or a systemic reaction; if positive, notify the physician. A systemic reaction can occur up to an hour after the test dose.
    b. If no signs of hypersensitivity response occur, proceed with initial dosing.
    c. If administering drug by intravenous infusion, give slowly and observe patient closely for additional 25 minutes.
    d. If a hypersensitivity response is suspected, discontinue infusion of drug, maintain the intravenous line, administer emergency drugs if preordered, and notify the physician.
6. For a localized hypersensitivity response:
    a. Observe and evaluate symptoms: urticaria, wheals, localized erythema.
    b. Administer diphenhydramine and/or hydrocortisone, per physician's order.
    c. Monitor vital signs every 15 minutes for one hour.
    d. If patient is considered sensitized, avoid subsequent dosing. However, if drug is critical in treatment plan, premedication with antihistamines and corticosteroids may prevent a hypersensitivity response. A desensitization program may be indicated.
    e. If a "flare" reaction appears along the vein with doxorubicin or daunorubicin, stop the drug and flush the vein with saline:
        i. Assess for immediate manifestation of extravasation to determine if this is a flare reaction or extravasation.
        ii. If extravasation is not suspected, continue with saline flush and observe for resolution of flare reaction.
        iii. If resolution does not occur, administer hydrocortisone, 25–50 mg, and/or diphenhydramine, 25–50 mg, intravenously with a physician's order, followed by saline flush.
        iv. Once the flare reaction has resolved, resume infusion of the drug at a much slower rate.
        v. Monitor for repeated flare episodes. It may be preferable to change the intravenous site.
        vi. If the drug is to be readministered at a later date, consider premedication with antihistamines and glucocorticoids. Slower infusion rates and/or greater fluid volumes also may be helpful.
7. For a generalized hypersensitivity/anaphylactic response, suspect if any or all of the following signs/symptoms occur (usually within first 15 minutes from start of infusion/injection):
    a. Subjective signs/symptoms:
        i. Generalized itching
        ii. Chest tightness
        iii. Agitation
        iv. Dizziness
        v. Nausea
        vi. Cramps/abdominal pain
        vii. Anxiety

(continued)

TABLE 4.8. MANAGEMENT OF ANAPHYLAXIS (continued)

  viii. Chills
  ix. Burning/tingling sensations
  b. Objective signs/symptoms
      i. Localized or generalized urticaria
      ii. Flushed appearance (angioedema of face, neck, eyelids, hands, and feet)
      iii. Respiratory distress with or without wheezing
      iv. Hypotension
      v. Cyanosis
  c. Management
      i. Immediate action is imperative; many actions may need to be performed simultaneously.
      ii. Stop chemotherapy injection/infusion immediately.
      iii. Stay with patient; another staff member should notify physician.
      iv. Maintain intravenous line with normal saline or another appropriate solution to expand vascular space.
      v. Administer emergency drugs as per standing orders or physician's order: epinephrine, 0.1–0.5 mg (1:10,000 solution) intravenous push; repeat every 10 minutes as needed. Pediatric dosage is 0.01 mg/kg. Adult subcutaneous epinephrine (1:1000 solution) doses are 0.2–0.5 mg; pediatric patients can receive 0.01 mg/kg. Subcutaneous doses may be repeated every 10–15 minutes if needed.
      vi. Place patient in supine position.
      vii. Monitor vital signs every two minutes until stable, every five minutes for 30 minutes, then every 15 minutes until stable.
      viii. Maintain patient's airway, assessing for increasing edema of the respiratory passageway. Administer oxygen if needed. Anticipate the need for cardiopulmonary resuscitation.
      ix. Reassure patient and family.
      x. Administer other emergency drugs as needed:
          (1) Antihistamines such as diphenhydramine HCl (Benadryl) 25–50 mg intravenously to block further antigen-antibody reaction
          (2) Adrenal steroids such as Solu Medrol® (The Upjohn Company, Kalamazoo, MI) 30–60 mg IV or Solu Cortef 100–500 mg IV or dexamethasone (Decadron) 10–20 mg intravenously, to ease bronchoconstriction and cardiac dysfunction
          (3) Aminophylline 5 mg/kg over 30 minutes intravenously to produce bronchodilatation
          (4) Vasopressors such as dopamine (Intropin) 2–20 μm/kg/min to counter hypotension[55,56]
8. Document all treatment in patient's medical record.
9. Avoid using chemotherapy agent causing anaphylaxis/hypersensitivity in the future. If drug is necessary in treatment plan, however, health-care team should consider and discuss the following options:
  a. Physician-guided desensitization
  b. Premedication with antihistamines and/or corticosteroids
  c. Additional fluid for drug dilution
  d. Increased infusion time
  e. Substitution of a similar drug (eg, using *Erwinia* L-asparaginase instead of *E. coli*)

From Oncology Nursing Society. *Cancer Chemotherapy Guidelines: Recommendations for the Management of Vesicant Extravasation, Hypersensitivity and Anaphylaxis.* Pittsburgh, PA: Oncology Nursing Society; 1992. Reprinted with permission.

dures to be undertaken in the prevention and treatment of anaphylaxis.

Intraosseous Administration

Intraosseous administration is the administration of fluids into the marrow cavity. Intraosseous infusions were first reported in the early 1920s by Drinker et al (1922) and Doan (1922). Historically, this route has been used to resuscitate pediatric patients, but, until recently, has not been used for patients with prolonged illnesses who do not have ready vascular access (Von Hoff 1991).

Intraosseous infusion uses the rich vascular network of the long bones to transport fluids and medications into the systemic circulation (Miccolo 1990, Wheeler 1989). There are three aspects of a long bone: (1) diaphysis, or bone shaft; (2) epiphyses, or rounded, enlarged bone ends; and (3) metaphysis, the portion of bone between the diaphysis and the epiphysis (Manley et al 1988, Miccolo 1990, Wheeler 1989). The cavity at the center of the diaphysis, the medullary cavity, is filled with bone marrow which is rich with venous sinusoids that drain into a central venous sinus. This central venous sinus leaves the marrow via the nutrient veins and enters the systemic circulation. As a result, the marrow cavity serves as a virtually noncollapsible vein, because it is supported by the bony matrix (Miccolo 1990).

A new device called the Osteoport (U.S. Patent No. 4,772,261, D. Von Hoff, J. Kuhn, P. Leighton, H. Wakeman) has been designed to establish the potential usefulness of the intraosseous route of administration (Fig 4.1). This catheter is currently undergoing phase I clinical trials in humans. This device is described more fully under Chemotherapy Delivery Systems in this chapter.

Potential complications with intraosseous infusions are few and rarely occur. Von Hoff (1991) summarized the potential problems associated with intraosseous infusions. Those that were addressed include extravasation, osteomyelitis, fat emboli, ischemic necroses, and death. The reported extravasations occurred because the needle was not placed properly in the marrow cavity, the needle was forced through the opposite side of the bone, and, occasionally, there was leakage around the puncture site. The reported incidence of osteomyelitis is extremely low and was most often seen in patients in whom the needle had been left inserted for a long period or who had bacteremia prior to insertion of the needle. One patient was reported as developing ischemic necrosis of two toes, but this was from strapping the leg down too tightly during insertion of the device. One death was reported as a result of perforation of the pleural space by a sternal intraosseous infusion. Fat emboli have not been reported, although they are a potential complication of the procedure.

Von Hoff (1991) estimates approximately 50,000 to 200,000 intraosseous infusions could be used each year in the United States. This approach promises to be an exciting alternative route for the administration of chemotherapy.

Oral Drug Administration

The oral route is used for chemotherapeutic agents that are well absorbed and nonirritating to the gastrointestinal tract (Brown and Hogan 1990) (Table 4.9). Before the oral route is chosen, however, the following factors must be considered: (1) availability of the medication in oral form; (2) patency and functioning of the gastrointestinal tract; (3) presence of nausea, vomiting, or dysphagia; (4) patient's state of consciousness; (5) patient's ability and willingness to comply with the schedule (Burke et al 1991). To avoid an accidental overdose, only enough medication for a single course of treatment should be prescribed at a time. Because of the toxic nature of chemotherapeutic agents, accidental overdoses can be fatal.

Oral chemotherapy has been used in large part because of the conveniency of administration and the decrease in the cost and toxicity of the drug(s); however, as with all oral medication, the availability and concentration of oral antineoplastic agents can be incomplete and erratic for drugs that are poorly soluble, slowly absorbed, unstable, or extensively metabolized by the liver (Goodman 1991). The last is specifically a problem in patients with questionable liver or renal function.

The issue of compliance with oral chemotherapy is a critical area for future studies to determine the efficacy and the frequency of the oral route. Recent research into this area is demonstrating that noncompliance with oral therapy is a serious prob-

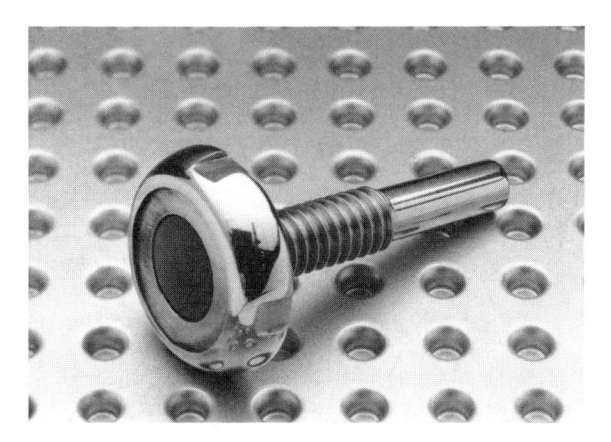

Figure 4.1. Osteoport.

TABLE 4.9. ORAL ANTINEOPLASTIC AGENTS

Altretamine (hexamethylmelamine, Hexalen)
Busulfan
Cyclophosphamide
Chlorambucil (Leukeran)
Etoposide (VP-16-213, VePesid)
Hydroxyurea
Lomustine
Melphalan
6-Mercaptopurine
Methotrexate
Procarbazine
Semustine (MeCCNU®) (not currently available)
6-Thioguanine

lem (Barofsky 1984; Levine et al 1987). Because of this, oral chemotherapy requires skillful assessment and education of the patient, including assessment of the patient's cognitive and emotional functioning, social support, physical abilities, and willingness to comply with the treatment plan. The education of the patient should include both verbal and written instructions. As with other chemotherapy, the patient should learn the names of the chemotherapeutic drugs he or she is taking and should keep a record of all other medications taken, prescription and over-the-counter, including the schedule and potential toxicity of each. Additionally, the patient should be instructed to check with the nurse or the physician before taking other medications.

Regional Drug Delivery

Systemic chemotherapy frequently fails to control disease because it is difficult to obtain the necessary, sufficient concentration of the drug at the tumor site without causing limiting toxic effects on the normal tissues. Regional administration of chemotherapy seeks to alleviate this problem by increasing the concentration of the drug at the tumor site and simultaneously lowering the systemic drug exposure, thereby improving the therapeutic index (Goodman 1991, Keizer and Pinedo 1985).

Regional administration of chemotherapy includes the following methods: (1) intrathecal or intraventricular; (2) intraarterial; (3) intracavitary, including intraperitoneal and intravesical (bladder). With the advent of a wide selection of access devices, including implantable pumps, ports, and catheters, regional chemotherapy is becoming more widely used.

Intrathecal and Intraventricular Administration.

The administration of chemotherapy intrathecally involves the insertion of a needle into the lumbar region and the injection of the drug through the dura and the arachnoid into the subarachnoid space, thereby allowing the drug to reach the central nervous system (Burke et al 1991, Goodman 1991). This technique is used to treat meningeal metastases, most commonly seen in breast cancer, gastrointestinal carcinoma, lung cancer, leukemia, and lymphoma. Tumor cells in the central nervous system are not affected by most systemically administered chemotherapy, because the drugs cannot cross the blood–brain barrier in sufficient concentrations to be therapeutic. Intrathecal or intraventricular chemotherapy administration allows for the delivery of drugs directly into the cerebrospinal fluid.

Intrathecal administration is accomplished by either lumbar puncture or the use of an indwelling subcutaneous cerebrospinal fluid reservoir, such as the Ommaya reservoir (Burke et al 1991). The lumbar puncture technique does not always ensure cisternal and ventricular distribution of the drug, regardless of the positioning. Additionally, the ascent of the drug to the ventricles following lumbar puncture is probably inhibited by the large production of cerebrospinal fluid from the ventricles and the pressure generated by the subsequent outflow (Goodman 1991). To counteract this problem, the Ommaya reservoir is more commonly used. The Ommaya reservoir is a small, mushroom-shaped, reusable, self-sealing, silicone port with an extension catheter. It is surgically implanted through the cranium into a lateral ventricle (Fig 4.2). The placement of the reservoir is verified by radiograph, and then the scalp-flap is sutured. Access to the reservoir is allowed after a waiting period of 24 to 48 hours (Goodman 1991). The reservoir is accessed by inserting a small-gauged butterfly needle with an attached three-way stopcock and syringe, directly into the dome. A volume of cerebrospinal fluid equal to that of the medication to be injected is removed. The medication is

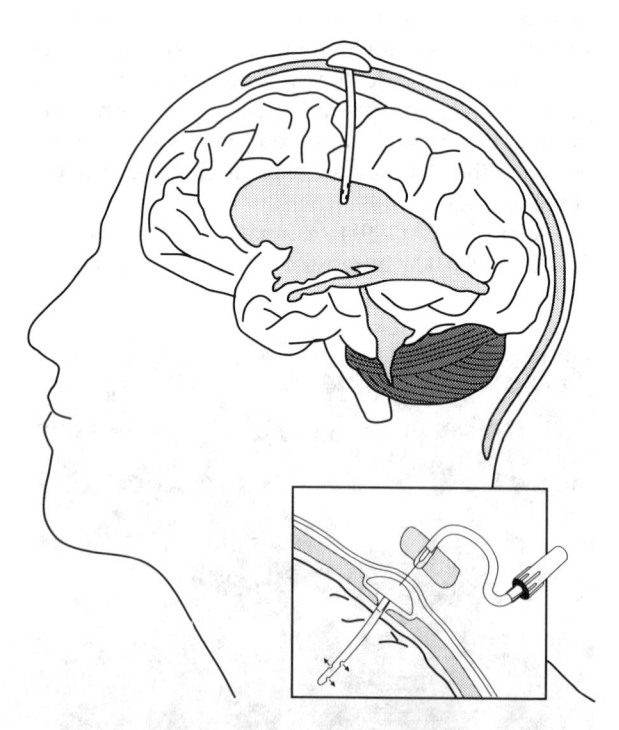

Figure 4.2. Ommaya reservoir. *(From Goodman M. Delivery of cancer chemotherapy. In: Baird SB, McCorkle R, Grant M, eds. Cancer Nursing: A Comprehensive Textbook. Philadelphia: WB Saunders; 1991:291–320. Reprinted with permission.)*

then injected into the reservoir over 5 to 10 minutes, the needle is removed, and the domed reservoir is manually compressed and released to mix the medication with the cerebrospinal fluid. The medication used for intrathecal therapy may be mixed with the patient's own cerebrospinal fluid or with a preservative-free saline (8–12 mL). The medication and the diluent should contain no preservatives. The patient is instructed to remain supine for 30 minutes following the procedure. Acute complications include nausea, vomiting, fever, headache, and rigidity of the neck, all of which usually subside within 72 hours.

Intraarterial Chemotherapy. Intraarterial administration of chemotherapy is most commonly used to treat an isolated organ. The intraarterial drugs are administered through a catheter inserted into an artery that supplies the tumor. This technique has been used to treat primary hepatoma, metastatic disease of the liver, bladder carcinoma, brain tumors, cervical carcinoma, head and neck carcinoma, melanoma, and osteogenic sarcoma (Burke et al 1991, Goodman 1991). The toxic effects associated with intraarterial chemotherapy relate to the region that is perfused. Rarely, minimal systemic toxic effects may also be present.

Intraperitoneal Chemotherapy. The administration of chemotherapy directly into the abdominal cavity is referred to as intraperitoneal chemotherapy and allows a higher drug concentration at the tumor site. The peritoneal cavity is the region bordered by the parietal layer of the peritoneum and contains all the abdominal organs exclusive of the kidneys. Ovarian carcinoma, gastrointestinal malignancies, and metastatic disease of the liver are the types of cancers that may benefit from intraperitoneal chemotherapy. Most chemotherapeutic agents are either metabolized or detoxified in the liver, which leads to numerous complications. Intraperitoneal administration of chemotherapy reduces these drug toxic effects, because the majority of abdominal cavity fluid is absorbed and detoxified in the portal circulation after passing through the liver just one time (Goodman 1991).

Intravesical Bladder Chemotherapy. The majority of patients with superficial transitional cell carcinoma of the bladder have recurrent disease following traditional therapy (Goodman 1991). In an effort to prevent recurrence of the cancer and the need for a cystectomy, intravesical bladder chemotherapy is used to destroy any viable cancer cells in the bladder. This technique allows a high concentration of the antineoplastic agent to come into contact with the urothelium over a relatively long period. Minimal systemic toxic effects are seen with this therapy and urinary and sexual function is preserved.

The chemotherapeutic agent is typically instilled into the bladder through a urinary catheter, and retained for about 1 to 3 hours. The patient must change positions at 15-minute intervals to ensure optimal bladder exposure. The most common side effects of intravesical bladder chemotherapy include bladder spasms, dysuria, hematuria, and polyuria. The drug should be kept in the bladder only for the specified period, as increased exposure can result in cystitis and excessive exfoliation of the bladder epithelium.

Documentation

Documentation of the administration of chemotherapy is a critical part of professional oncology nursing practice. As with any documentation, the purpose of chemotherapy administration documentation is to ensure continuity of quality patient care (Miaskowsky and Nielsen 1991).

There are many methods that result in competent documentation of chemotherapy administration. Documentation tools and flowsheets that are time-efficient, yet comprehensive, are the more desired form of documenting chemotherapy administration. There are several advantages to using documentation tools and flowsheets: time efficiency, provision of timely and consistent documentation, improvement of continuity of nursing care, provision of concise and comprehensive overview of chemotherapy administration and vascular access device care, provision of a database for quality assurance monitoring, and minimization of loss of revenue because of lack of documentation (Mikos and Finn 1990).

Two examples of general chemotherapy documentation tools are depicted in Figures 4.3 and 4.4. Figures 4.5 and 4.6 demonstrate tools that are specifically used for vascular access devices, including a flowsheet and a monitoring tool.

CHEMOTHERAPY DELIVERY SYSTEMS

The problem of difficult vascular access has long plagued clinicians who administer chemotherapy. In response to the need for safe, effective administration of chemotherapy, drug delivery systems are

CONFIDENTIAL INFORMATION

Date 10-14-91 R. Pickett, RN, MSN RN Signature

Check below any condition that may apply or list others that may influence the vasculature or venous access in extremity being used for chemotherapy.

	L	R		L	R
Mastectomy	X		Immobility		
Radiation to Arm			Severe Arthritis		
Radiation to Axilla			History of DVT		
Axillary Node Dissection	X		Previous Chemo Infiltration		
Radiation to Supraclavicular Area			Ecchymosis		
Surgery/Prior Limb Trauma			Other ______		
Peripheral Vascular Disease			Other ______		

Pre-chemotherapy Drugs Given:

	Dose	Route	Time
Compazine		/	
Decadron	10 mg	IV	1000
Benadryl			
Ativan			
Reglan			
Zofran	10mg	IV	10:05

Nurses Notes
(For any added comments regarding chemo)

Chemotherapy Drug(s)

#1 Adriamycin
Dose 90 mg
Route: IVP X Drip ____
Infusion Time: 1030 To 1040
Given via IV Saline: Yes X No __
Blood Return Present: (Yes) No

#2 Cytoxan
Dose 900 mg
Route: IVP X Drip ____
Infusion Time: 1041 To 1050
Given via IV Saline: Yes X No __
Blood Return Present: (Yes) No

#3 5 FU
Dose 900 mg
Route: IVP X Drip ____
Infusion Time: 1051 To 1058
Given via IV Saline: Yes X No __
Blood Return Present: (Yes) No

#4 ______
Dose ______
Route: IVP ____ Drip ____
Infusion Time: ____ To ____
Given via IV Saline: Yes __ No __
Blood Return Present: Yes No

#5 ______
Dose ______
Route: IVP ____ Drip ____
Infusion Time: ____ To ____
Given via IV Saline: Yes __ No __
Blood Return Present: Yes No

(For professional use only)

ST. MARY'S HOSPITAL
DECATUR, ILLINOIS 62521-3883

OUTPATIENT ONCOLOGY
CHEMOTHERAPY DOCUMENTATION

Orig. 11/90

Addressograph Purposes Only:

Figure 4.3. St. Mary's Hospital, Decatur, IL, outpatient oncology chemotherapy documentation. *(From Pickett RR. Outpatient oncology chemotherapy documentation tool. Oncol Nurs Forum. 1992;19(3):515–517. Reprinted with permission.)*

ADMINISTRATION OF CANCER CHEMOTHERAPY AGENTS 75

CONFIDENTIAL INFORMATION FOR MATION

Needle Type and Size (for periph IV's only)

Site No. 1	Site No. 2	Site No. 3
Intracath _____ gauge	Intracath _____ gauge	Intracath _____ gauge
Butterfly __23__ gauge	Butterfly _____ gauge	Butterfly _____ gauge
Other _____ gauge	Other _____ gauge	Other _____ gauge

Site No. 4	
Intracath _____ gauge	Time IV Started __1000__
Butterfly _____ gauge	Time IV D'cd __1100__
Other _____ gauge	Solution Used __250 ml NS__

Vein Condition

Number of IV attempts in extremity drug(s) given __1__

Soft, pliable __X__   Thready _____

Fragile, thin _____   Hard, knotty _____

Other _____

Reactions Observed During or Immediately After Chemotherapy

KEY A = Localized
     B = Follows path of vein
     C = Generalized, over entire limb
     D = Discontinued IV

Type	IV Site #	Yes	No	Key
Subjective Signs & Symptoms				
Burning	1		X	
Pruritis (Itching)	1		X	
Throbbing	1		X	
Pain	1		X	
Numbness	1		X	
Objective Signs & Symptoms				
Erythema	1		X	
Swelling	1		X	
Urticaria (hives)	1		X	
Rash	1		X	
Temp. change	1		X	

Drug Infusion Location (For periph. IVs only)
(Mark an "X" where IV inserted)

Ventral (Underside of Arm)   Dorsal (Top of Arm)

(Circle L or **R**)

Vascular Access Devices

Type: Port _____ Hickman _____ Groshong _____

Other _____

Site Appearance (Circle)

 Pre-chemo: Clear Red Edematous Ecchymotic
   Other: _____

 Post-chemo: Clear Red Edematous Ecchymotic
   Other: _____

Port Needle Size: _____ Gauge _____ Length

Port Accessed: With difficulty _____

              Without difficulty _____

Blood Return: Yes _____ No _____

After Chemotherapy:

 Saline Flush _____ cc's

 Heparin Flush _____ cc's

(For professional use only)

ST. MARY'S HOSPITAL
DECATUR, ILLINOIS 62521-3883
**OUTPATIENT ONCOLOGY
CHEMOTHERAPY DOCUMENTATION**

Orig. 11/90

Addressograph Purposes Only:

Figure 4.3. Continued.

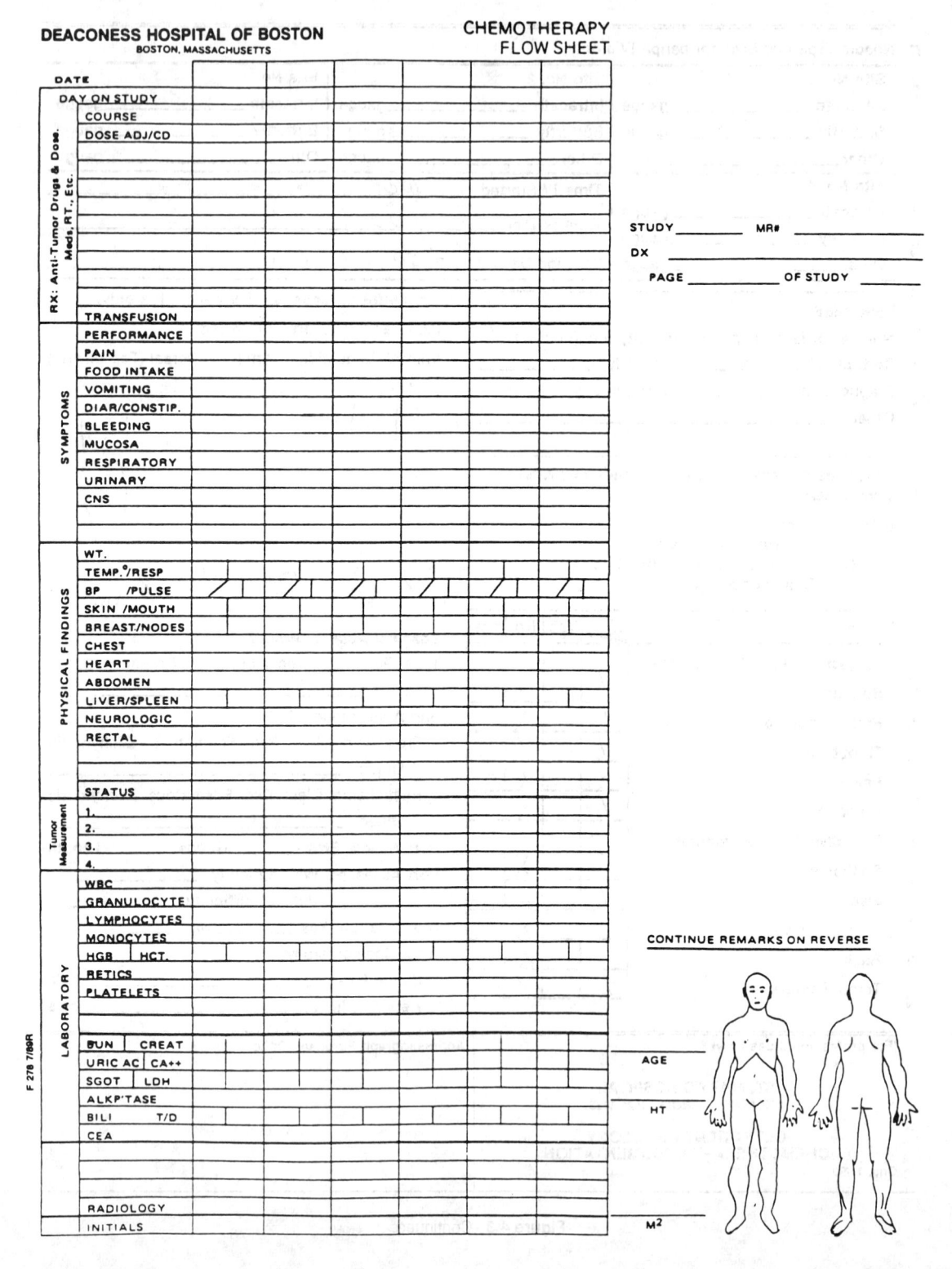

Figure 4.4. Deaconess Hospital of Boston Chemotherapy flowsheet. *(From Lynch M, Yanes L. Flowsheet documentation of chemotherapy administration and patient teaching. Oncol Nurs Forum. 1991;18(4):777–783. Reprinted with permission.)*

Administration	DATE:						
	IV Site						
	Needle Type & Size						
	Adverse Reactions						
Patient Teaching	Treatment Schedule: Drug & Method of Administration:						
	Instructions per NEDH Instruction Sheets for:						
	Self-Care Measures per NEDH Standards of Care for: Nausea/Vomiting Myelosuppression Mouth Care						
Nursing Observations/Assessments/Management	Acknowledgement of Initial Teaching (Signature of Patient)						
	Nurse:						
	I = Initial Teaching R = Reviewed W = Written Materials Given P = See Progress Note N/A = Not applicable S = Side effects verbalized or reported						
Key			RN		RN		RN
			RN		RN		RN

Figure 4.4. Continued.

VASCULAR ACCESS DEVICE FLOWSHEET

Allergies _____

Date Device Inserted _____

TYPE OF DEVICE	Date AM	Date PM	Date AM	Date PM	Date AM	Date PM	Date AM	Date PM	Date AM	Date PM
Subclavian										
Single/Double/Triple										
Site Assessment										
Dressing Change										
Cap(s) Changed										
Catheter Patency										
Hickman/Broviac										
Site Assessment										
Dressing Change										
Cap(s) Changed										
Catheter Patency										
Implantable Ports										
Model:										
Single/Double										
Site Assessment										
Needle Change										
Dressing Change										
Cap(s) Changed										
Catheter Patency										
Other Devices										
Type:										
Site Assessment										
Dressing Change										
Cap(s) Changed										
Catheter Patency										
Line 1 Heparinization (u)										
Line 2 Heparinization (u)										
Line 3 Heparinization (u)										
UROKINASE										
Complications — See Progress Notes										

Initials	Full Signature	Title	Initials	Full Signature	Title

Figure 4.5. Christ Hospital and Medical Center, Oaklawn, IL, vascular access device flowsheet. *(From Mikos KA, Finn TR. Quality assurance monitoring through use of a vascular access device flowsheet. Oncol Nurs Forum. 1990;17(3):427–432. Reprinted with permission.)*

Monitoring
Period ______________________

Unit ______________________

Documentation Code: Present +
Absent –
Not Applicable NA

							Dressing Changes				Clinical Observation + Present – Absent						Complications		
Medical Record #	Diagnosis	Type Of Device	Date Inserted	Date Removed	Catheter Patency (every shift)	Site Assessment (every shift)	Subclavians, Hickmans®, Broviacs®, Groshongs™, Perm-Caths® (every 72 hours)	Implantable Ports (every 5 days)	CAP(s) Change (every 72 Hours)	Needle Change – implantable ports ONLY (every 5 days)	Site Redness/ Swelling	Site Drainage	Tenderness	Warmth at Site/ Tunnel	Elevated Temperature	Elevated WBC Count	Infected Catheter	Clotted Catheter	Catheter Displacement

Figure 4.6. Monitoring tool: management of vascular access device. *(From Mikos KA, Finn TR. Quality assurance monitoring through use of a vascular access device flowsheet. Oncol Nurs Forum. 1990;17(3):427–432. Reprinted with permission.)*

being designed and marketed at an accelerated rate. These devices facilitate the administration of chemotherapy through a variety of routes: intravenous, intraosseous, intraarterial, and intracavitary. Table 4.10 outlines the classification of chemotherapy delivery systems. As the most common route of antineoplastic drug delivery is the intravenous one, the vascular access devices (VADs) that facilitate this type of administration are the most commonly used. The advent of VADs has greatly increased the ability of the patient to receive chemotherapy safely, with much less discomfort than with previous intravenous drug delivery. Additionally, VADs facilitate blood component therapy, blood sampling, continuous-infusion therapy of vesicant and nonvesicant drugs, and the concurrent administration of multiple drug and fluid therapies. The administration of chemotherapy in ambulatory and home settings has also increased in large part because of VADs (Garvey 1987).

Although the benefits of vascular access devices are many, they are not without risk. Indeed, all medications and fluids given intravenously, with or without VADs, pose some problems, as mentioned previously in this chapter. A significant body of literature exists that addresses the problems associated with central venous catheters and implanted ports (eg, Johnston-Anderson et al 1987, Prager and Hertzberg 1987, Reed et al 1985, Stellato et al 1985, Strum and McDermed 1985, Sznajder et al 1986). Table 4.11 summarizes the most commonly reported complications. A multidisciplinary approach to the management of VADs can significantly reduce complications, increase catheter life, enhance quality assurance, and improve the quality of patient care (Bosserman et al 1990).

The nurse is frequently the health care professional in the pivotal role of identifying the need for a VAD, as well as organizing the resources that enable the insertion of the VAD. The nurse must be cognizant of the factors to consider in determining the need for a VAD. Table 4.12 identifies basic criteria for the clinician to use in determining if a patient is a potential candidate for a VAD. The early placement of a vascular access device can greatly benefit a large proportion of individuals undergoing treatment with chemotherapeutic agents.

TABLE 4.10. CLASSIFICATION OF CHEMOTHERAPY DELIVERY SYSTEMS

I. Catheters
   A. Venous catheters
      1. Short-term, not tunneled
      2. Long-term, tunneled, percutaneously placed
      3. Long-term, peripherally placed
   B. Midline (longarm) catheters
   C. Arterial catheters
   D. Intraperitoneal catheters
      1. Percutaneously placed temporary flexible Silastic
      2. Surgically placed Tenckhoff
   E. Epidural catheters (analgesic use)
      1. Short-term
      2. Permanent indwelling
II. Implanted ports and reservoirs
   A. Vascular implanted ports
      1. Conventional ports
      2. Skin-parallel access ports
   B. Intraosseous implanted ports
   C. Intraperitoneal implanted ports
   D. Intraventricular implanted reservoirs
   E. Epidural implanted ports/reservoirs
III. Pump—infusion systems
   A. External infusion systems
   B. Internal implantable infusion systems

Sources. ONS 1989a–d, 1990, Tenenbaum 1989, Von Hoff 1991, Wickham 1987.

TABLE 4.11. POTENTIAL COMPLICATIONS AND PROBLEMS ASSOCIATED WITH CENTRAL VENOUS CATHETERS AND IMPLANTED PORTS

1. Infection (can lead to sepsis)
2. Formation of fibrin sheath
3. Clotting in the vein (thrombosis)
4. Clotting of the catheter (occlusion)
5. Pinching or kinking of the catheter
6. Pneumothorax (puncturing of lung during insertion of needle)
7. Hemothorax
8. Vessel erosion
9. Ruptured or sheared catheter
10. Tumor metastases developing in device implant sites
11. Malposition and/or migration of catheter with embolization to the right atrium
12. Acute thyroiditis
13. Difficulty in securing nontunneled catheters in adults and most catheters in children
14. Cost of operative procedure to place catheter or port
15. Cosmetic dissatisfaction (protruding catheter or bump over port)
16. Stress of home care (catheters)

Sources. Bosserman et al 1990, Lokich et al 1985, Stellato et al 1985, Von Hoff 1991.

Vascular Access Catheters

The central venous catheters used for the administration of chemotherapy are typically divided into

ADMINISTRATION OF CANCER CHEMOTHERAPY AGENTS 81

TABLE 4.12. FACTORS IN DETERMINING NEED FOR VASCULAR ACCESS DEVICES

Criterion	VAD Indicated	VAD Possibility
Venous integrity	Multiple (>2) venipunctures to secure venous access	Venous access with 2 or fewer venipunctures
	Venous access limited to one extremity	Both extremities available
	Prior tissue damage as a result of extravasation	
	Venous thrombosis/sclerosis as a result of previous IV therapy	No previous IV therapy
	Impaired venous or lymph flow secondary to surgical procedures, radiation therapy, or disease progression	
Frequency of venous access	Frequent venous access	Infrequent venous access
	Extensive or prolonged intravenous therapy (including antibiotics, blood products, chemotherapy, nutritional supplements)	
Length of treatment	3 or more months	<3 months
Mode of administration	Continuous-infusion chemotherapy	Intermittent single injections
	Home-infusion chemotherapy	
Type of drug	Vesicant/irritating drugs	Nonvesicant/nonirritating drugs
Patient preference	Patient prefers VAD	Patient does not prefer VAD
	Financially feasible for patient	

Sources. Burke et al 1991, Goodman 1991, Goodman and Wickham 1984, Simon 1987.

three groups: (1) indwelling, percutaneously placed, long-term Silastic right atrial catheters; (2) short-term central venous catheters; and (3) long-term peripherally inserted central venous catheters. Midline or longarm catheters constitute another category of catheters used for chemotherapy administration of chemotherapy. Catheters are also inserted into the arteries, peritoneum, and epidural space for the administration of chemotherapy and supportive drugs.

Central Venous Catheters

Indwelling Silastic Right Atrial Catheters. Indwelling, long-term Silastic right atrial catheters have become the frontrunners not only for the choice of venous access device, but also for the surgical technique of inserting such catheters (Burke et al 1991). This type of catheter is placed on the anterior chest and tunneled beneath the skin, resting in the cephalic vein, internal or external jugular vein, subclavian vein, or superior vena cava. The tip terminates in or near the right atrium (Goodman 1991, Tenenbaum 1989). Figure 4.7 demonstrates the anatomic location of a long-term Silastic right atrial catheter. An alternate placement site is the saphenous vein with the tip resting in the inferior vena cava; the exit site is either on the lower abdomen or in the groin. This site is associated with more difficulty in drawing blood but may be indicated in patients experiencing superior vena cava syndrome, subclavian vein thrombosis, severe radiation changes, or tumor invasion of the chest and underlying tissues (Goodman 1991).

The Broviac® Silastic catheter (Davol, Salt Lake City, UT) was originally reported in 1973 as a safe mechanism for infusing total parenteral nutrition (TPN) on a long-term basis (Broviac et al 1973). This first Silastic catheter was a small-bore, 18-gauge catheter. A larger version of the Broviac catheter, the 16-gauge Hickman catheter, was reported in 1979 to be safe for intravenous infusions including blood

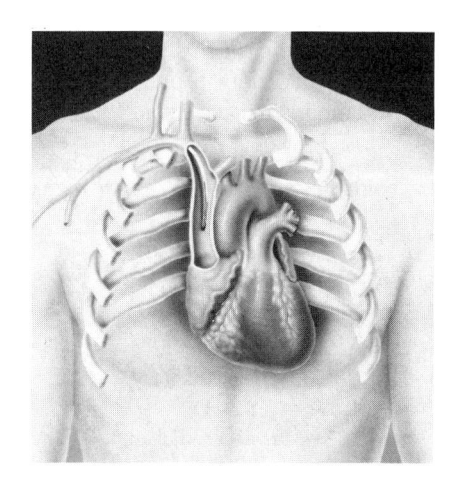

Figure 4.7. Right atrial catheter placement (Bard).

transfusions and blood sampling (Burke et al 1991, Hickman et al 1979, Simon 1987). The more flexible and nonirritating Silastic rubber, as well as the subcutaneous "tunneling" of these catheters, gave them a distinct advantage over the conventional central venous (subclavian) lines (Simon 1987). These improved catheters have reduced infection, the most undesirable complication in the long-term use of catheters (Raaf 1985).

There are distinct advantages to use of the indwelling central venous catheter: (1) the catheter passes through the subcutaneous tissue of the chest wall and exits to the right or left of the midline on the chest wall, and (2) a Dacron cuff forms a seal around the catheter. The cuff serves the dual functions of stabilizing the catheter and preventing retrograde migration of organisms. An infection-control device called a Vitacuff (Vitaphore Corp.) may be placed around the catheter at the time of insertion to further minimize the incidence of infection (Goodman 1991).

Numerous indwelling Silastic right atrial catheters are available on the market, including single-lumen, double-lumen, and triple-lumen (Figs 4.8 and 4.9) models. The number and size of the lumens vary, depending on the particular catheter. The unique medical care needs of the patient determine which catheter is most appropriate (Goodman 1991). The different lumens can be used for the infusion of blood products, intravenous medications/solutions, and total parenteral nutrition, as well as for the aspiration of blood for blood samples.

A tunneled right atrial catheter called the Groshong® catheter (Bard, Salt Lake City, UT) (Fig 4.10) is popular because of the unique three-way valve within its lumen (Fig 4.11) which eliminates the need for daily heparin flushes. This valve also minimizes blood backflow problems and reduces the risk of air embolism (Burke et al 1991).

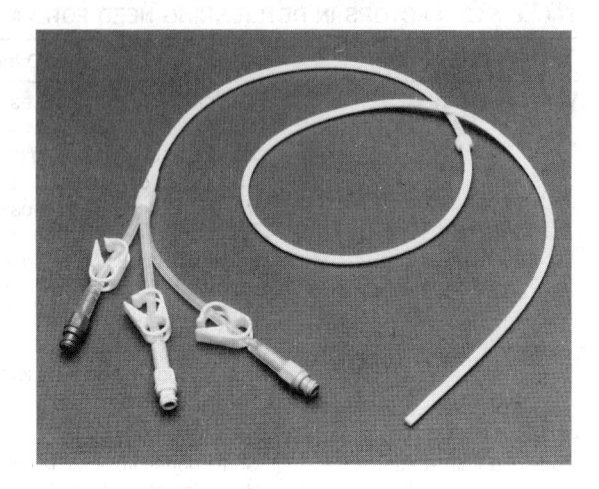

Figure 4.9. Triple-lumen right atrial catheter (Quinton Instrument Co., Seattle, WA).

Care of indwelling Silastic right atrial catheters involves irrigation and dressing and cap changes. The volume and dose of heparin solution as well as the frequency of flushing vary greatly across institutions and remain controversial issues. In general, these tunneled catheters (excluding the Groshong catheter) are irrigated every other day, three times a week, or weekly with 3 to 5 mL of heparinized saline solution (100 to 1000 units of heparin/mL). Weekly flushings are supported by a study of 82 patients with 89 catheter insertions over a 3-year period in which the overall infection rate was 0.15 per 100 catheter days (Kelly et al 1992), an acceptable rate. The Groshong catheter, because of its pressure-release valve that prevents blood from backing up into the catheter unless suction is exerted by a syringe to withdraw blood, does not need to be irri-

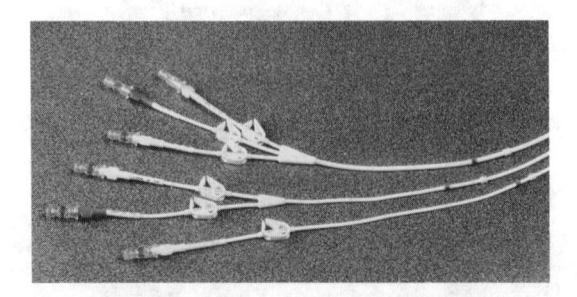

Figure 4.8. Hickman catheters: single, double, and triple lumens (Bard, Salt Lake City, UT).

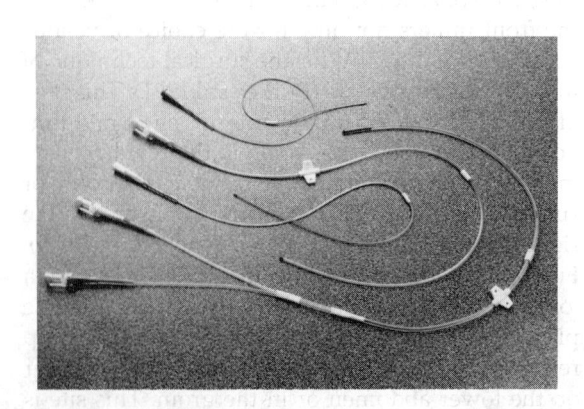

Figure 4.10. Groshong® catheters (Bard, Salt Lake City, UT).

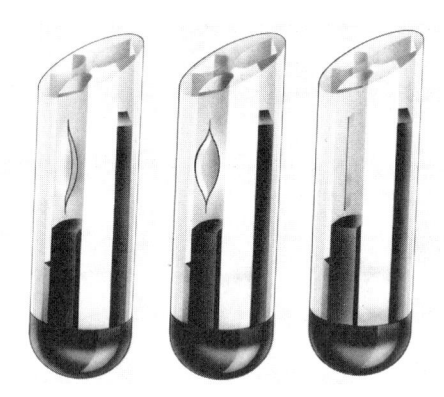

Figure 4.11. Groshong® three-position valve (Bard, Salt Lake City, UT).

gated with heparin. Additionally, a clamp is never indicated for use with a Groshong. This catheter is flushed once a week with 5 to 10 mL of saline when not being used and with 10 to 20 mL of saline after drawing blood. The caps of all indwelling catheters are changed weekly or monthly, depending on the frequency of use of the catheter. Immediately after placement of a tunneled catheter, an occlusive dressing is placed over the exit site and remains in place for up to 48 hours. After 7 to 14 days, a dressing is no longer required, provided the patient is not immunocompromised and practices good personal hygiene. Most patients, however, prefer to wear a light dressing (2 × 2 gauze and tape) or an adhesive bandage over the exit site to stabilize and secure the catheter in place. Whether or not a dressing is used, the catheter should always be taped to the patient to prevent the inadvertent removal of the catheter.

Short-term Central Venous Catheters. Central venous catheters may be used for short-term continuous or intermittent administration of medications, fluids, or blood components, as well as for drawing blood samples. The subclavian catheters that are placed percutaneously have been used in the acute care setting when vascular access was necessary and peripheral venous access was a problem (Simon 1987). These catheters terminate in the superior vena cava or the right atrium. Most are inserted by a physician, at the bedside or in the clinic, into the subclavian or jugular vein, and are usually 15- to 19-gauge in size for adults. Unlike surgically implanted long-term catheters, short-term catheters have no cuff and do not pass through a subcutaneous tunnel (Tenenbaum 1989). Because of these factors, the potential for infection and/or septicemia is increased. Strict aseptic technique is required for catheter site

skin care and dressing changes. When not in use these lines are maintained with a daily heparin flush (Slater et al 1985). One advantage of these catheters is the ability to remove and replace the old catheter with a new catheter at the same insertion site using a guidewire (Bottino et al 1979, Slater et al 1985). The usual duration of placement for short-term catheters is 30 to 60 days. Although somewhat common, but not desired, one of these catheters may be inserted for a short-term indication or a trial basis and then left in place for a longer period. This emphasizes the need for accurate assessment and education of the patient prior to the placement of a vascular access device. Even though the development of the silicone elastomer central venous catheter (Centrasil, Travenol) has enabled longer duration of placement and fewer complications than previously seen with Teflon and polyethylene catheters (Legha et al 1985), if the patient will need long-term vascular access, it is best not to involve a short-term central venous catheter.

Long-term Peripherally Inserted Central Venous Catheters. Peripherally inserted central venous catheters may be used for long-term indications. These catheters may be inserted by a specially trained nurse at the patient's bedside and are advantageous for patients with chest wall involvement by tumor or radiation fibrosis. These catheters are also indicated for patients needing a shorter duration of venous access, a trial of vesicant chemotherapeutic agents, or other chemotherapy necessitating central venous access.

The Per-Q-Cath® (Gesco International, San Antonio, TX) (Fig 4.12) is inserted into the vein much like a peripheral IV catheter, such as an angiocath. An introducer needle surrounded by a plastic catheter (Excalibur, Gesco International) (Fig 4.13) is first

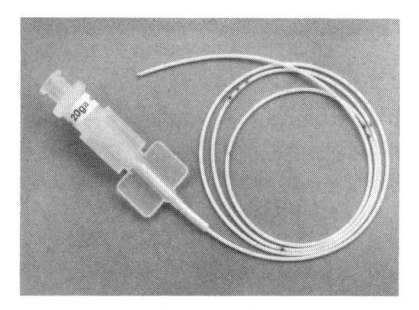

Figure 4.12. Per-Q-Cath® (Gesco International, San Antonio, TX), a peripherally placed central venous catheter.

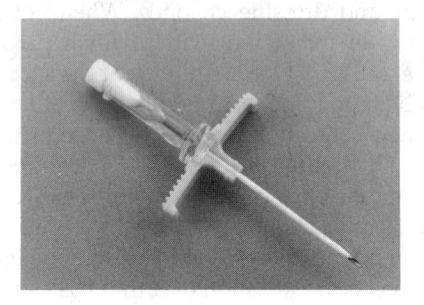

Figure 4.13. Excalibur® introducer needle (Gesco International, San Antonio, TX).

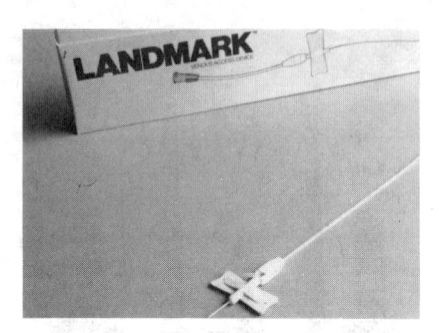

Figure 4.15. Landmark® midline venous catheter (Menlo Care, Inc., Menlo Park, CA).

inserted into the vein, then the metal stylet is removed. The soft silicon catheter (Per-Q-Cath) is inserted through the plastic cannula. After the Per-Q-Cath is in place, the plastic catheter is removed from the patient by breaking it into two pieces and slitting it apart. This leaves the Per-Q-Cath in the patient (Fig 4.14) without the need for sutures. The Per-Q-Cath as a single lumen comes in 2, 3, 4, or 5 French; it is also available as a 4- and 5-French double lumen.

The Intrasil® (Baxter, Deerfield, IL) is a 16- to 18-gauge central venous catheter that is inserted peripherally into the right or left basilic or cephalic vein in the antecubital fossa (Simon 1987, Tenenbaum 1989). This catheter, which has been in use for many years, is sutured through the eyelets in the catheter hub to stabilize it in place.

Long-term peripherally inserted central venous catheters require daily irrigation with heparin. Because they are nontunneled, strict sterile technique is necessary during dressing changes. A transparent dressing is placed over the exit site; an extension tubing should extend beyond the dressing for easy access. The incidence of infection is low and similar to that for the percutaneous tunneled catheter, if proper care and maintenance are practiced (Goodman 1991).

Midline Venous Catheters. Midline venous catheters provide an additional option for vascular access. A midline catheter is inserted peripherally, but rather than being inserted into the central venous system, the midline catheter is inserted through the veins of the antecubital area and advanced into the veins in the upper arm (Hadaway 1990). The medications and fluids infused via this route will be diluted by a larger amount of blood than those infused via venipuncture in the hand or forearm. This results in a significant reduction in the amount of irritation to the vein. The midline catheter can be used for intermediate-length therapies of 1 to 6 weeks (Fontaine 1991), and can be used in home, ambulatory, and acute care settings.

The Landmark® catheter (Menlo Care, Inc., Menlo Park, CA) (Fig 4.15) is constructed of a new bioconforming polymer called Aquavene® (Menlo Care, Inc.). When dry, Aquavene® is stiff and can therefore be advanced without the use of guidewires. Once the catheter is placed in the vein, the Aquavene® will absorb fluid from the blood and soften dramatically. It will also expand by two gauge sizes to provide an increased flow rate (Fontaine 1991, Hadaway 1990) (Fig 4.16). The Landmark® catheter, unlike other longarm devices, uses an over-the-needle method of introduction rather than a through-the-needle method. This prevents the damage that can occur to catheters when passed through an introducer needle. After venipuncture, the needle is retracted into a needle safety tube on the distal end of the catheter where it is permanently housed.

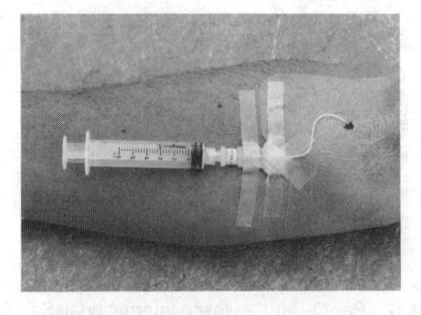

Figure 4.14. Inserted Per-Q-Cath® (Gesco International, San Antonio, TX).

Arterial Catheters. Intraarterial administration of chemotherapeutic agents is accomplished by the use

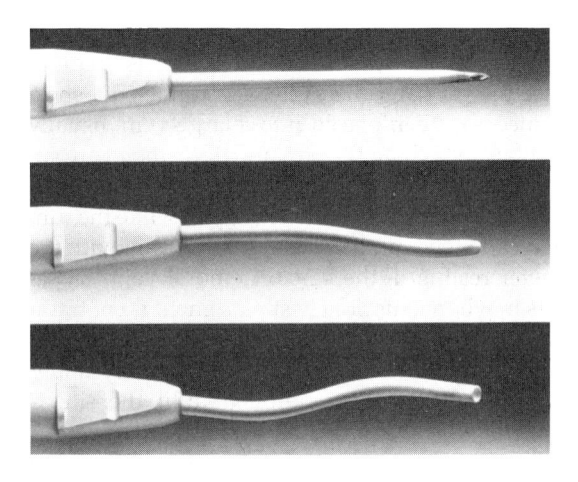

Figure 4.16. Landmark® midline catheter before and after Aquavene® material has been hydrated (Menlo Care, Inc., Menlo Park, CA).

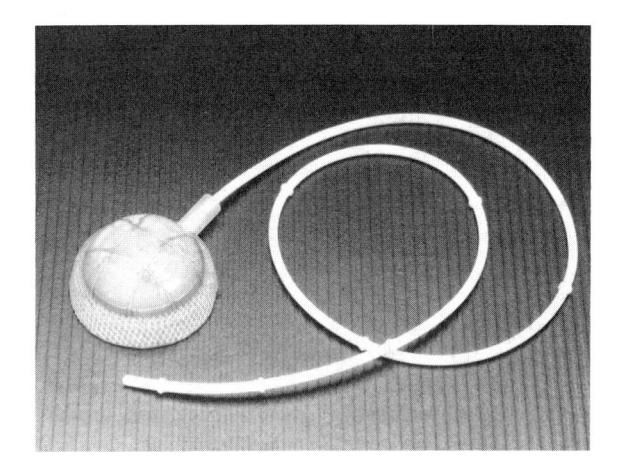

Figure 4.18. OmegaPort-AB® intraarterial port (Norfolk Medical, Skokie, IL).

of a catheter that is placed within the artery supplying the tumor. This arterial catheterization is accomplished by one of three methods: (1) arterial catheter, (2) arterial catheter connected to an implanted port, and (3) arterial catheter connected to an implanted pump. When catheterization without the addition of a port or pump is the method of choice, a stiff catheter is employed for arterial perfusion. The area of treatment is immobilized during treatment, which can last from several minutes to several hours, and the site is assessed frequently for bleeding. The catheter is removed after the treatment. When arterial catheterization is necessary for longer-term use, a flexible, silicone catheter is surgically placed into the artery and sutured to the skin, or connected to an implanted port. Daily irrigation is necessary to maintain patency for the external catheter; the implanted port is irrigated weekly with heparinized saline. An external infusion pump may be connected to either the catheter or the implanted port to allow for infusion chemotherapy (Goodman 1991). To provide constant infusion of the involved organ, a totally implanted infusion pump may be used.

Intraperitoneal Catheters. The most commonly used intraperitoneal catheter is the Tenckhoff catheter. One end of this indwelling, flexible, Silastic catheter lies in the abdominal cavity and the other end passes through the abdominal wall and extends externally to the skin (Hoff 1987) (Fig 4.17). There are also several implanted ports that are made to be connected to a Tenckhoff or similar catheter (see next section).

Implantable Vascular Access Ports

Implanted vascular access ports are used primarily for intravenous therapy but can be used to administer drugs into the arteries (Fig 4.18) and into the peritoneum (Fig 4.19) (Goodman 1991, Tenenbaum 1989). The arterial ports, such as the OmegaPort-AB (Norfolk Medical), provides chronic access to the hepatic artery for repeated drug delivery via bolus or protracted infusions. The intraperitoneal ports provide chronic access to the peritoneal cavity for repeated drug delivery via bolus or protracted infusions and for fluid withdrawal. Numerous types of implanted ports are currently available, including both front-entrance and side-entrance ports. Venous access ports are available as a single-port or a double-port system (Fig 4.20). Additionally, newer models, such as the OmegaPort® (Norfolk Medical,

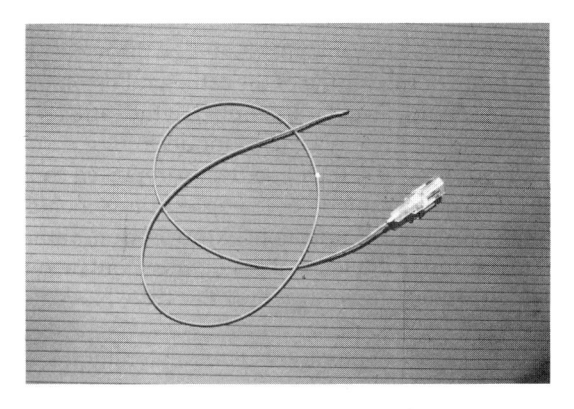

Figure 4.17. Tenckhoff intraperitoneal catheter (Bard, Salt Lake City, UT).

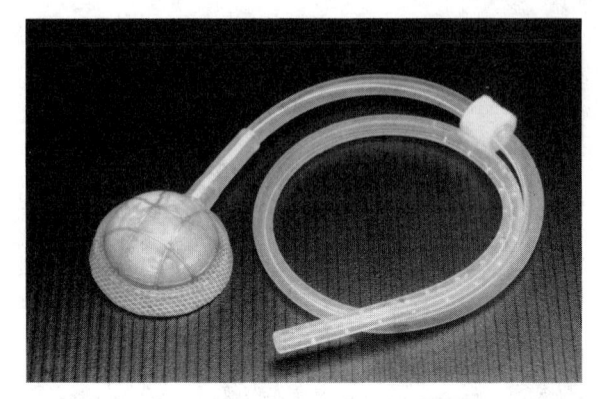

Figure 4.19. OmegaPort-PT® intraperitoneal port (Norfolk Medical, Skokie, IL).

Skokie, IL) (Fig 4.21), provide omnidirectional 360-degree directional accessibility with 160 degrees of entry angles.

The majority of implanted ports are constructed from titanium and silicone rubber and consist of two main features: (1) the port housing, made of titanium, plastic, or stainless steel, including a resealable silicone septum, and (2) the Silastic catheter, which either is preattached to the housing or may be attached during the insertion procedure (Fig 4.22). The port septum is made of a dense silicone that is capable of withstanding up to 2000 needle injections (Goodman 1991). The port is accessed by a needle puncture through the skin into the silicone septum. Only specially designed, deflected (Huber)-point needles are used to gain access to these ports; these needles also prevent damage to the septum with repeated injections.

The insertion procedure is similar to that for indwelling Silastic right atrial catheters. The optimal placement for implanted venous access ports is on the upper chest at the midclavicular line (Goodman 1991). Under local anesthesia, a pocket is made to house the port and the catheter is tunneled a short distance and then placed into a large vein, usually the subclavian. Both the port and the catheter are sutured into place, and the pocket containing the port is closed (Burke et al 1991). These ports, like the tunneled catheters, can be placed in the groin, with the catheter resting in the iliac or femoral vein for patients in whom anterior chest placement is contraindicated (Goodman 1991). Once the insertion is completed, the venous access port is completely under the skin. A dressing is applied until the site is healed, at which time no further dressing is needed. These ports can remain in place indefinitely and can be used to infuse blood products, total parenteral nutrition, and intravenous medications/solutions, as well as to draw blood. Vesicant drugs can be administered through venous access ports, but not as a long-term infusion on an outpatient basis. This is due to the risk of needle dislodgment and subsequent drug extravasation. If continuous infusion of a vesicant is necessary, the patient should be monitored throughout the infusion.

The port is accessed only by use of a Huber-point needle, which is inserted transdermally through the septum until it meets the back of the port. These needles are either straight or have a 90-degree angle. Long and Ovaska (1992) documented no infection with or without the use of sterile gloves in the accessing of venous access ports. The presence of blood return ensures the proper placement of the needle; however, blood return is frequently absent. If a blood return is not obtained, the port can be irrigated with 20 to 30 mL of saline to check for tissue swelling. If there is no tissue swelling, the needle is assumed to be placed properly (Burke et al 1991, Goodman 1991). The inability to irrigate or aspirate is usually caused by malpositioning of the needle in the septum or by clotting of the catheter. Forceful irrigation should never be attempted. If the catheter is clotted, urokinase may be used for declotting.

In addition to catheter occlusion, reported complications of implanted venous access ports include venous thrombosis, infection, extravasation, catheter migration, catheter embolus, and spontaneous fracture of the catheter (Moore et al 1986, Noyen et al 1987).

Implanted venous access ports are preferable to indwelling Silastic catheters in patients who are unable to care for a Silastic catheter or who choose the cosmetic appearance of a port over a catheter. The

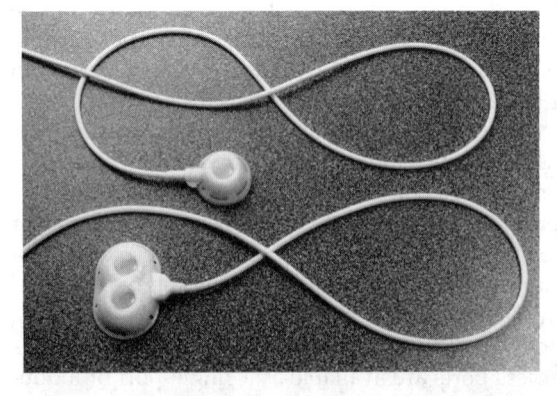

Figure 4.20. MRI single and double ports (Bard, Salt Lake City, UT).

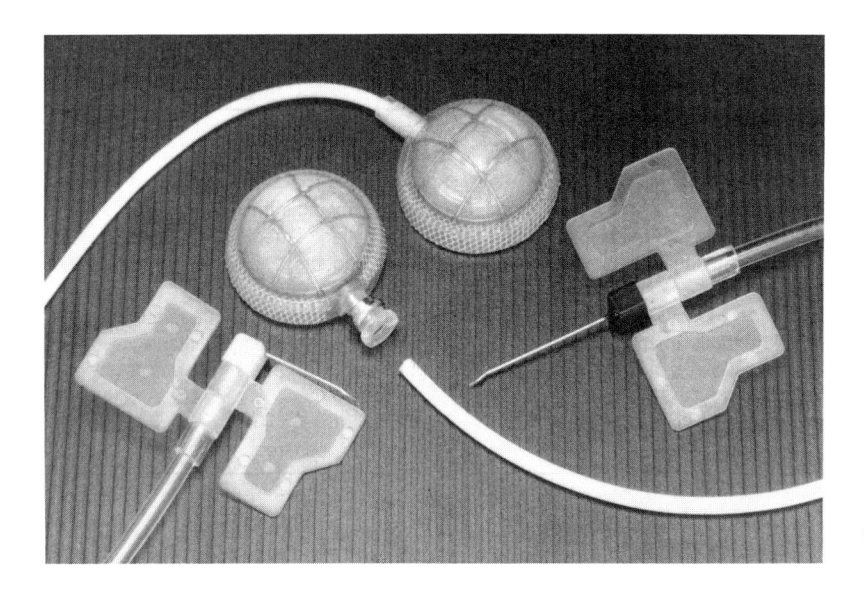

Figure 4.21. OmegaPort venous access port and Huber needles (Norfolk Medical, Skokie, IL).

care of these ports is minimal, consisting of heparin flushes after each use or every 3 to 4 weeks when not in use. Additionally, there are no restrictions on activities such as bathing and swimming.

Choosing Between a Catheter and an Implanted Port

Although there are several types of long-term vascular access devices in use today, both external and implantable, the choice for most patients is between an indwelling catheter and an implanted port. Although there are some similarities between these two types of devices, there are also important differences. These differences include the insertion procedure, the use of the device, activity restrictions, and home care (Conroy 1990, Wainstock 1987). These factors should be considered when the decision for a particular type of vascular access device is necessary. The patient's individual preference should be the primary factor considered in decision making (Brown and Hogan 1990), although the particular brand of access device used is often determined by the surgeon's experience and preference (Lokich et al 1985). To ensure the best results with a vascular access device, the patient and health care team together must make the decision based on the particular physical, emotional, intellectual, and supportive resources of the patient. Education of the patient and family about the advantages and disadvantages of each device is imperative. Table 4.13 lists the factors to be considered by the patient in contributing to this decision.

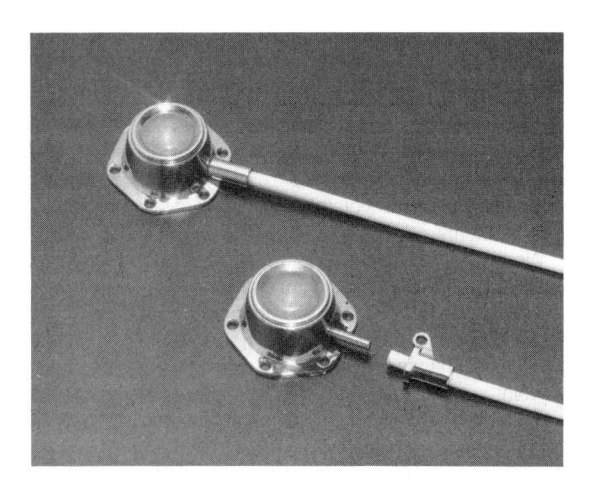

Figure 4.22. Q-Port with preattached and unattached catheters (Quinton Instrument Co., Seattle, WA).

Osteoport

The Osteoport (US Patent No. 4,772,261, D. Von Hoff, J. Kuhn, P. Leighton, H. Wakeman) has been designed to allow the intraosseous route of administration to serve as a useful access for chemotherapy, as well as many other medications and fluids. This port is actually an implantable needle with a Silastic self-sealing membrane or septum at the top of the needle (see Fig 4.1). The Osteoport is made of medical implant-grade titanium; the Silastic membrane is made of medical implant-grade Silastic, such as that commonly used in intravenous catheters and im-

TABLE 4.13. PATIENT CONSIDERATIONS FOR USE OF CATHETER VERSUS PORT

Factor	Catheter	Port
Activity restrictions	Avoid swimming and vigorous sports	No restrictions
Insertion procedure	Surgery	Surgery
Method of removal	Usually office procedure; sometimes surgery	Surgery
Use of the device	Drawing of blood samples	Drawing of blood samples
	Administration of medications, IV fluids, blood products, and some nutritional supplements	Administration of medications, IV fluids, blood products, and some nutritional supplements
Accessing the device	Painless	Possibly some pain when needle is inserted
Blood drawing	Usually easy for the nurse to draw blood	Blood drawing sometimes difficult
Cosmetic appearance	Sticks out of chest about 6 in.	Slight bump over area where port is implanted
Home care	Change bandage, change cap, flush catheter	No home care
Maintenance cost	Supplies and routine flushes	No supplies, less frequent flushing

Sources. Conroy 1990, Wainstock 1987.

planted ports. The implantable feature of the Osteoport prevents a direct conduit from outside the body into the bone marrow, thereby decreasing the rate of osteomyelitis and cellulitis. Threads were added to the needle to decrease the complications of insertion; this allows precise placing of the intraosseous needle within the marrow. To decrease leakage, a cone was added to provide a tight seal between the bone and the Osteoport (Miller 1990). The catheter is a 1.5-in. needle with threads along the upper third of the needle. The catheter may be implanted into several bones, for example, the iliac crest and the tibia. As with other implanted ports, it is concealed totally under the skin (Von Hoff 1991).

The device is implanted into the bone by the drilling of a pilot hole into which the self-tapping catheter is screwed. This is done through a small skin incision. The device is accessed similarly to other implanted ports: the skin is prepped and the needle on the end of the intravenous tubing is inserted through the skin into the catheter. The advantages of the Osteoport are listed in Table 4.14.

Internal Implantable Infusion Pumps

The first implantable pump was placed for the continuous infusion of heparin in 1975, and continuous chemotherapy infusions began in 1977 (Buchwald and Rohde 1984). The goals of implantable pumps are to maximize portability and to protect against infection (Hagle 1987). Currently, two pumps are commonly used: the Infusaid 400® (Pfizer Infusaid, Strato Medical, Beverly, MA, Fig 4.23) and the Medtronic® (Walpole, MA) pump. A newer pump is currently undergoing clinical trials: Therex 3000 (Therex, Fig 4.24). Table 4.15 compares the three pumps. These pumps can be filled with chemotherapy or saline and provide constant infusion, usually to the liver via the hepatic artery. The pumps are refilled by percutaneous injection. Tables 4.16 and 4.17 describe the procedures for filling the Infusaid 400 and Therex 3000 respectively.

The Infusaid 400 pump is made of titanium with two silicone rubber septums, a connected Silastic catheter, and a 50-mL reservoir. It consists of two chambers separated by a flexible metal bellows. The inner chamber contains the drug and the outer chamber contains a fluorocarbon liquid. When a liquid such as fluorocarbon is in equilibrium with its vapor phase at a given temperature, regardless of

TABLE 4.14. ADVANTAGES OF THE OSTEOPORT

1. No venous clotting problems (catheter is not in the vein) or phlebitis
2. No cosmetic problems
3. Possibly less infection (although osteomyelitis could be a problem)
4. No difficulty securing in children
5. Little chance for occlusion of catheter
6. No chance for migration of catheter
7. No chance for pneumothorax
8. Minimal chance for leakage of toxic drugs outside of the vein
9. No pulmonary embolism (although fat embolism is a theoretical problem)

From Von Hoff DD. Intraosseous infusions: An important but forgotten method of vascular access. Cancer Invest. 1991;9(5):521–528. Reprinted with permission.

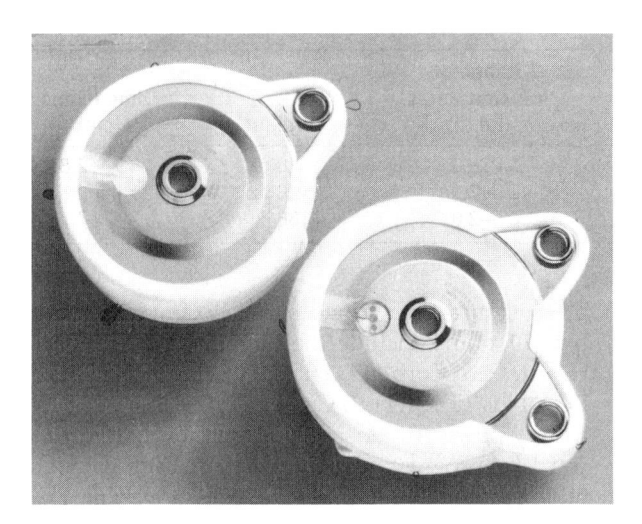

Figure 4.23. Infusaid 400 internal implanted pump.

the enclosing volume, a constant pressure is exerted. Therefore, because fluorocarbon is in a liquid and gaseous state at body temperature, a constant pressure on the inner chamber and its contents is exerted by the fluorocarbon as a result of the relatively constant temperature of the body (Hagle 1987). The pump is refilled by percutaneous injection through the septum. When the drug chamber is filled, the bellows are forced to expand and compress the outer chamber. This condenses the fluorocarbon vapor and subsequently recharges the power source. The drug is forced from the reservoir through the Silastic catheter into the artery or vein. Flow rate is determined by the preset length and diameter of the Silastic catheter, the pressure at the catheter exit site, arterial or venous placement, viscosity and concentration of the infusate, and the patient's body temperature (Burke et al 1991, Hagle 1987). Bolus injections can be accomplished by the use of a second septum, a Sideport, which directly accesses the catheter and bypasses the drug delivery system. The flow rate is preset between 1.0 and 6.0 mL/d.

The Medtronic pump, which is also made of titanium, houses a collapsible 20-mL reservoir and is powered by a lithium battery. This battery powers the peristaltic roller pump, the silicone rubber septum, the alarm mechanism, and the microprocessor circuit. The battery has an expected life of 2 years, and must be replaced by removal of the pump. Radio signals are used by a noninvasive programmer and handheld telemetry wand to relay information to the pump. The flow rate can be set from 2.0 to 200 mL/d via bolus, bolus delay, or continuous infusion (Hagle 1987).

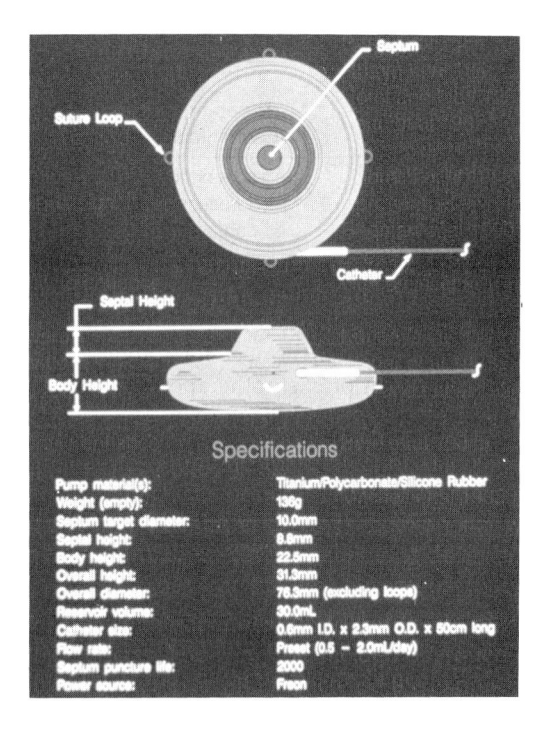

Figure 4.24. Therex 3000 internal implanted pump (Therex, Walpole, MA).

The Therex 3000, a titanium pump with an attached silicone rubber catheter, is currently under investigational use. This pump will deliver 30 mL of infusate at a preset flow rate and is refilled percutaneously using a Therex Huber-point noncoring needle and tubing set as supplied in the Therex Refill Kit. Bolus injections are performed percutaneously using the Therex Special Bolus Needle. The inside of the Therex Pump is divided into inner and outer chambers by an accordion-like bellows. The inner chamber contains the drug to be infused. The outer chamber contains a propellant permanently sealed inside. The temperature of the patient's body warms the propellant, which then exerts a constant pressure on the bellows, causing the drug to flow out of the inner chamber, through a filter and flow restrictor, and then slowly out the catheter. Refilling the pump with drug expands the bellows and starts the pump on the next cycle of drug infusion.

External (Ambulatory) Infusion Pumps

The shift from hospital care to home care and ambulatory care settings has greatly increased the need

TABLE 4.15. IMPLANTABLE PUMPS

Name	Pumping Mechanism	Reservoir (mL)	Range of Infusion Rates (mL/d)	Weight	Dimensions (cm)
Pfizer Infusaid 400	Self-contained	50	1.0–6.0	8 oz	8.7 × 2.8
Medtronic	Microprocessor	20	2.0–200	6 oz	7.0 × 2.8
Therex 3000	Self-contained	30	0.5–2.0	136 g	3.1 × 7.75

for alternative methods of drug delivery. Paramount among these is the need for ambulatory, continuous infusion of chemotherapeutic agents. The development of reliable microvolume infusion pumps and safe long-term vascular access has made this possible. There are now numerous ambulatory infusion pumps available, all of which fall into three general categories: (1) the battery-powered syringe or pulsatile pump, (2) the battery-powered peristaltic pump, and (3) the balloon pump. The battery-powered pulsatile pump moves fluid out of the syringe and into the catheter through the force of the plunger into the syringe barrel. Examples of this type of pump include the Auto Syringe® (Baxter Health Care Corp., Deerfield, IL) and the LifeCare PCA Plus II® (Abbott, Chicago, IL) (Fig 4.25). The battery-powered peristaltic pump moves fluid forward by progressively squeezing the intravenous tubing around a wheel or other pressure point. The CADD® pump (Deltec-Pharmacia, St. Paul, MN) and the Pancretec® pump (Pancretec Inc.) are examples of this type of pump. The balloon-powered pump moves fluid at a constant rate as the balloon deflates; thus, the distended elastomer balloon acts

TABLE 4.16. FILLING THE INFUSAID PUMP

Equipment

- 50-mL syringe (remove plunger)
- 50-mL syringe filled with chemotherapy or saline and heparin 50,000 U (total volume always equal to 50 mL)
- 1½-in. 22-gauge Huber-point needle (curved) with connecting tubing or 1½-in. 22-gauge straight needle with three-way stopcock
- Povidone–iodine swabs (3)
- Alcohol wipes (3)
- Adhesive bandage
- Sterile gloves

Procedure

1. Prepare a sterile field containing sterile equipment.
2. Palpate pump; attempt to locate septum.
3. Cleanse area over pump with alcohol and povidone–iodine swabs three times using a circular motion.
4. Don sterile gloves. Place Huber-point needle on a three-way stopcock and attach 50-mL syringe. Turn stopcock to off **or** attach needle to tubing and attach 50-mL syringe to the tubing. Clamp tubing. Relocate septum. Insert the needle perpendicular to the septum. The needle will puncture the septum and meet the needle stop. Open stopcock or clamp and observe fluid rising in the syringe as the pump empties.
5. Once fluid has stopped rising in the syringe, note amount and disconnect syringe from stopcock or tubing. The needle will be open to air, but air will not enter the pump because it is pressurized. Discard pump fluid properly as one would chemotherapy.
6. Connect the syringe filled with chemotherapy or saline to the stopcock or tubing. While maintaining the needle in the pump, inject contents of the syringe.
7. Check for correct placement (fluid will rise in syringe when pressure is released from plunger).
8. Once completed, remove the syringe and needle while stabilizing the pump. Apply an adhesive bandage.
9. Calculate the rate of flow by subtracting the amount left in the syringe at the time of emptying from 50 mL and divide by the total number of days since pump was filled. This will reveal the mL/d and ensure that the patient is receiving the appropriate dose of the drug as planned. Most pumps will infuse between 1.5 and 2.5 mL/d (consult individual manufacturer's insert). Temperature elevation and the use of less than 50,000 units of heparin in 50 mL of solution will increase the speed of the pump.

From Goodman M. Delivery of cancer chemotherapy. In: Baird SB, McCorkle R, Grant M, eds. Cancer Nursing: A Comprehensive Textbook. Philadelphia: WB Saunders; 1991:291–320. Reprinted with permission.

TABLE 4.17. FILLING THE THEREX 3000 PUMP

Equipment

A Therex Refill Kit containing the necessary materials (excluding gloves, drug, and syringe) should be used to accomplish a pump refill. The kit contains a helpful picture poster of the refill procedure and the refill data sticker. Only properly trained and qualified physicians, registered nurses, and medical personnel may perform and assist in the pump refill procedure.

Procedure

1. It is critical to the safe functioning of the pump that only a Therex needle be used to penetrate the septum.
2. Do not aspirate fluid from the pump. Aspiration will cause blood to be drawn into catheter and result in occlusion.
3. It is important to follow the pump refill instructions precisely to complete the pump refill procedure successfully. If the needle is not properly positioned, and verified as detailed in the Pump Refill Procedures, there is a possibility that a drug extravasation or a direct bolus of drug to the patient will occur.
4. Place patient in a supine position. Expose the pump pocket site. Palpate the pump site and locate the raised septum.
5. Fill a 30-mL syringe with appropriate refill solution and a 10-mL syringe with saline solution.
6. Using sterile technique, open refill kit and expose kit components.
7. Don sterile gloves. Use three iodine swabsticks to prep the pump site in a circular fashion, extending the prepped area beyond the periphery of the pump. Allow prepped area to dry. Place fenestrated drape over pump site.
8. Tighten all connections on the needle/tubing set/stopcock assembly. Ensure that the stopcock is in the **closed** position.
9. Repalpate the pump site and locate the raised septum.
10. Insert the noncoring needle **perpendicular** to the pump septum. Advance the needle until it is in contact with the needle stop.
11. Attach the empty syringe barrel to the stopcock. **Open stopcock** and allow the pump reservoir to empty. If no fluid returns during pump emptying or during the refill injection procedure, proceed as follows:
    a. Confirm needle position and that a Therex 22-gauge, noncoring Huber needle is being used. Check that the needle is **perpendicular** to the pump septum and is fully depressed and in contact with the needle stop. If no volume returns, proceed with steps b, c, and d.
    b. Attach a 10-mL syringe containing saline solution to the refill tubing set.
    c. Keep downward pressure on the needle and inject 5 mL of saline into the pump. Release pressure on the syringe plunger and allow the fluid to return to the syringe. If fluid returns, then the needle is in the proper position and indicates that the pump was empty at the start of the refill procedure. Replace the 10-mL syringe with the 30-mL syringe containing the pump refill solution and continue with the refill procedure (steps 17 and 18).
    d. If there is still no fluid return after injection of the 5 mL of saline, remove the needle and refill tubing set. Flush the refill set to confirm that the system is patent. Reinsert the needle perpendicular into the pump septum until it is in contact with the needle stop. Repeat step c.
    e. If there is still no fluid return after injection of the 5 mL of saline, contact Therex Corporation for assistance (1–800–322–1507 or 508–660–1122).
12. After emptying, approximately 1.5 mL of fluid from the previous refill will remain in the pump.
13. **Close stopcock.** Place the syringe cap in the open end of the syringe barrel. Disconnect the stopcock and syringe barrel, leaving the needle and refill set in place. Note the returned volume (mL) and record on refill data sticker provided. Discard syringe barrel and stopcock, leaving the needle and refill set in place.
14. Expel air from the 10-mL syringe of saline. Attach the syringe to the proximal end of the refill set and confirm that the needle is still in contact with the needle stop. Keep downward pressure on the needle and inject 5 mL of saline into the pump.
15. Release pressure on the plunger and allow the 5 mL injected to return to the syringe. This procedure reconfirms correct positioning of the needle. If no fluid returns, refer to steps a–e above. Disconnect the syringe from the refill set.
16. Expel air from the refill syringe. Attach the syringe to the proximal end of the refill set and confirm that the needle is still in contact with the needle stop.
17. Keep downward pressure on the needle and begin to inject refill solution into the pump. Release pressure on plunger at 5-mL increments and allow 1 mL of solution to return to syringe. This will verify that the needle is in the correct position and the pump reservoir is being filled. Continue to inject and check needle placement until the syringe is emptied.
18. If no fluid returns to the syringe on release of the plunger, **do not continue to inject refill solution until you have verified the needle placement.**
19. After injecting the entire 30 mL, keep pressure on the syringe plunger and pull the needle out of the pump septum. Remove drape and iodine. Apply adhesive bandage to access site.

Reprinted with permission of the Therex Corporation, 1991.

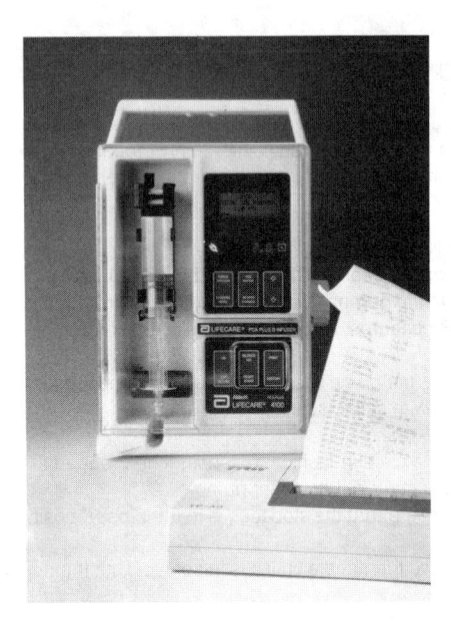

Figure 4.25. Lifecare PCA Plus II infusor (Abbott, Chicago, IL), an external ambulatory pump.

as the energy source. The Baxter 5- and 7-day infusor pumps are included in this category (Burke et al 1991, Mioduszewski and Zarbo 1987) (Fig 4.26).

Outpatient administration of chemotherapy using an ambulatory infusion pump can significantly reduce patient and hospital costs. This method of drug delivery also offers more autonomy to the patient.

SUMMARY

The methods for administration of chemotherapy have greatly improved over the past several decades. The responsibilities inherent in this complex group of procedures extend beyond that of the actual task of drug delivery; decisions regarding administrative techniques, methods of drug delivery, patient/family participation, and education of the patient and family are now considered part of the routine practice of the administration of antineoplastic agents. Additionally, there are numerous research opportunities for the health care team to address in the areas of drug delivery systems and management, safe handling of antineoplastics, extravasation management, and education techniques.

REFERENCES

Barofsky I. Therapeutic compliance and the cancer patient. *Health Educ.* 1984;**10**:43–56.

Belcher AE. Developing continuing education programs in cancer nursing: Defining content and methods. *Oncol Nurs Forum.* 1987;**14**(5):65–67.

Bosserman G, McGuire DB, McGuire WP, Nicholls D. Multidisciplinary management of vascular access devices. *Oncol Nurs Forum.* 1990;**17**(6):879–886.

Bottino J, McCredie KB, Groschel DHM, Lawson M. Long-term intravenous therapy with peripherally inserted silicone elastomer central venous catheters in patients with malignant diseases. *Cancer.* 1979;**43**:1937–1943.

Broviac JW, Cole JJ, Scribner GH. A silicone rubber atrial catheter for prolonged parenteral alimentation. *Surg Gynecol Obstet.* 1973;**136**:602–606.

Brown JK, Hogan CM. Chemotherapy. In: Groenwald SL, Frogge MH, Goodman M, Yarbro CH, eds. *Cancer Nursing: Principles and Practice.* 2nd ed. Boston: Jones and Bartlett; 1990:pp. 230–283.

Buchwald H, Rohde TD. Implantable infusion pumps. In: Shires GT, ed. *Advances in Surgery.* Chicago: Year Book; 1984;vol 18:177–221.

Burke MB, Wilkes GM, Berg D, Bean CK, Ingwersen K. Principles of chemotherapy administration and drug delivery systems. In: *Cancer Chemotherapy: A Nursing Process Approach.* Boston: Jones and Bartlett; 1991:375–423.

Conroy CS. Groshong catheter or implanted port: Which is better for you? *Oncol Nurs Forum.* 1990;**17**(5):745–749.

Creaton EM, Leonard FE, Day AL. A hospital-based chemotherapy education and training program. *Cancer Nurs.* 1991;**14**(2):79–90.

DeVita VT. Principles of chemotherapy. In: DeVita VT, Hellman S, Rosenberg SA, eds. *Cancer: Principles and Practice of Oncology.* 3rd ed. Philadelphia: Lippincott; 1989:276–300.

Doan CA. Circulation of bone marrow. *Contrib Embryol.* 1922;**14**:27.

Drinker CK, Drinker KR, Lund CC. Circulation in mam-

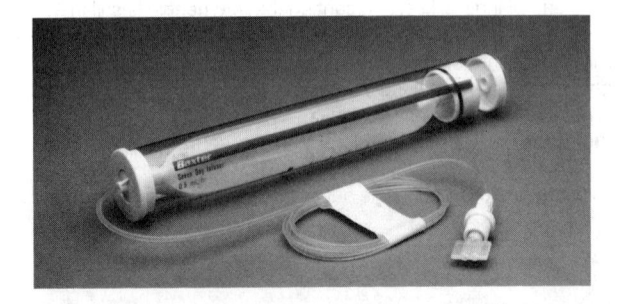

Figure 4.26. Baxter 7-day infusor (Baxter, Deerfield, IL), an external ambulatory pump.

malian bone marrows with special reference concerned in movement of red blood cells from bone marrows into circulating blood as disclosed by perfusion of tibia of dog and by injections of bone marrow in rabbit and cat. *Annu J Physiol.* 1922;**62**:1–92.

Du Bois D, Du Bois EF. A formula to estimate the approximate surface area if height and weight be known. *Arch Intern Med.* 1916;**17**:863–871.

Fernsler J. Developing continuing education programs in cancer nursing: An overview. *Oncol Nurs Forum.* 1987;**14**(5):59–60.

Fontaine PJ. Performance of a new softening expanding midline catheter in home intravenous therapy patients. *J Intravenous Nurs.* 1991;**14**(2):91–99.

Garvey EC. Current and future nursing issues in the home administration of chemotherapy. *Semin Oncol Nurs.* 1987;**3**:142–147.

Gehan EA, George SL. Estimation of human body surface area from height and weight. *Cancer Chemother Rep.* 1970;**54**:225–235.

Gelman RS, Tormey DC, Betensky R, et al. Actual versus ideal weight in the calculation of surface area: Effects on dose of 11 chemotherapy agents. *Cancer Treat Rep.* 1987;**71**:907–911.

Goodman M. Delivery of cancer chemotherapy. In: Baird SB, McCorkle R, Grant M, eds. *Cancer Nursing: A Comprehensive Textbook.* Philadelphia: WB Saunders; 1991:291–320.

Goodman MS, Wickham R. Venous access devices: An overview. *Oncol Nurs Forum.* 1984;**11**(5):16–23.

Gullo SM. Safe handling of antineoplastic drugs: Translating the recommendations into practice. *Oncol Nurs Forum.* 1988;**15**(5):595–601.

Hadaway LC. A midline alternative to central and peripheral venous access. *Caring.* 1990:45–50.

Hagle ME. Implantable devices for chemotherapy: Access and delivery. *Semin Oncol Nurs.* 1987;**3**(2):96–105.

Hickman RO, Buckner CD, Clift RA, Sanders JE, Stewart P, Thomas ED. A modified right atrial catheter for access to the venous system in marrow transplant recipients. *Surg Gynecol Obstet.* 1979;**148**:871–875.

Hilkemeyer R. A historical perspective in cancer nursing. *Oncol Nurs Forum.* 1982;**9**(2):47–56.

Hoff ST. Concepts in intraperitoneal chemotherapy. *Semin Oncol Nurs.* 1987;**3**(2):112–117.

Holland JC. Fears and abnormal reactions to cancer in physically healthy individuals. In: Holland JC, Rowland JH, eds. *Handbook of Psychooncology: Psychological Care of the Patient With Cancer.* New York: Oxford University Press; 1990:13–21.

Ignoffo RT, Friedman MA. Therapy of local toxicities caused by extravasation of cancer chemotherapeutic drugs. *Cancer Treat Rev.* 1980;**7**:17–27.

Itano J. Developing continuing education programs in cancer nursing: Developing educational objectives. *Oncol Nurs Forum.* 1987;**14**(5):62–65.

Jameson J, O'Donnell J. Guidelines for extravasation of intravenous drugs. *Infusion.* 1983;**7**:157–162.

Johnston-Anderson A, Krasnow SH, Boyer MW. Hickman catheter clots: A common occurrence despite daily heparin flushing. *Cancer Treat Rep.* 1987;**71**:651–653.

Keizer JH, Pinedo HJ. Cancer chemotherapy: Alternative routes of drug administration—A review. *Cancer Drug Delivery.* 1985;**2**:147–169.

Kelly C, Dumenko L, McGregor SE, McHutchion ME. A change in flushing protocols of central venous catheters. *Oncol Nurs Forum.* 1992;**19**(4):599–605.

Knobf T. Intravenous therapy guidelines for oncology practice. *Oncol Nurs Forum.* 1982;**9**(2):30–34.

Larson DL. Treatment of tissue extravasation of antitumor agents. *Cancer.* 1982;**49**:1796–1799.

Legha SS, Haq M, Rabinowits M, Lawson M, McCredie K. Evaluation of silicone elastomer catheters for long-term intravenous chemotherapy. *Arch Intern Med.* 1985;**145**:1208–1211.

Levine AM, Richardson JL, Marks G, et al. Compliance with oral drug therapy in patients with hematological malignancy. *J Clin Oncol.* 1987;**5**:1469–1476.

Lind J, Bush NJ. Nursing's role in chemotherapy and administration. *Semin Oncol Nurs.* 1987;**3**(2):83–86.

Lokich J, Bothe A, Benotti P. Complications and management of implanted venous access catheters. *J Clin Oncol.* 1985;**3**:710–717.

Long MC, Ovaska M. Comparative study of nursing protocols for venous access ports. *Cancer Nurs.* 1992;**15**(1):18–21.

Lynch M, Yanes L. Flowsheet documentation of chemotherapy administration and patient teaching. *Oncol Nurs Forum.* 1991;**18**(4):777–783.

Manley L, Haley K, Dick M. Intraosseous infusion: Rapid vascular access for critically ill or injured infants and children. *J Emergency Nurs.* 1988;**14**(2):63–69.

McMillan SC. Developing continuing education programs in cancer nursing: Program evaluation. *Oncol Nurs Forum.* 1987;**14**(5):67–70.

Miaskowsky C, Nielsen B. Documentation of the nursing process in cancer nursing. In: Baird S, McCorkle R, Grant M, eds. *Cancer Nursing: A Comprehensive Textbook.* Philadelphia: WB Saunders; 1991:1126–1138.

Miccolo MA. Intraosseous infusion. *Crit Care Nurse.* 1990;**10**(10):35–47.

Mikos KA, Finn TR. Quality assurance monitoring through use of a vascular access device flowsheet. *Oncol Nurs Forum.* 1990;**17**(3):427–432.

Miller LJ. *Intraosseous (IO) infusions: An enduring method of intravenous access.* Unpublished manuscript; 1990.

Mioduszewski J, Zarbo AG. Ambulatory infusion pumps: A practical view at an alternative approach. *Seminars in Oncology Nursing.* 1987;**3**(2):106–111.

Montrose PA. Extravasation management. *Semin Oncol Nurs.* 1987;**3**(2):128–132.

Moore CL, Erikson KA, Yanes LB, Franklin M, Gonsalves

L. Nursing care and management of venous access ports. *Oncol Nurs Forum.* 1986;**13**(3):35–39.

Mosteller RD. Simplified calculation of body-surface area. *N Engl J Med.* 1987;**317**(17):1098.

Noyen J, Hoorntje J, de Lange Z, Lemmslag J-W, Sleijfer D. Spontaneous fracture of the catheter of a totally implantable venous access port: Case report of a rare complication. *J Clin Oncol.* 1987;**5**(8):1295–1299.

Occupational Safety and Health Administration. *Work Practice Guidelines for Personnel Dealing With Cytotoxic (Antineoplastic) Drugs.* OSHA Instructional Publication 8-1.1. Washington, DC: Office of Occupational Medicine; 1986.

Oncology Nursing Society. *Cancer Chemotherapy Guidelines:* Module I. *Recommendations for Cancer Chemotherapy. Course Content and Clinical Practicum.* Pittsburgh, PA: Oncology Nursing Society; 1988a.

Oncology Nursing Society. *Cancer Chemotherapy Guidelines:* Module II. *Recommendations for Nursing Practice in the Acute Care Setting.* Pittsburgh, PA: Oncology Nursing Society; 1988b.

Oncology Nursing Society. *Cancer Chemotherapy Guidelines:* Module III. *Recommendations for Nursing Practice in the Outpatient Setting.* Pittsburgh, PA: Oncology Nursing Society; 1988c.

Oncology Nursing Society. *Cancer Chemotherapy Guidelines:* Module IV. *Recommendations for Nursing Practice in the Home Care Setting.* Pittsburgh, PA: Oncology Nursing Society; 1988d.

Oncology Nursing Society. *Cancer Chemotherapy Guidelines:* Module V. *Recommendations for the Management of Extravasation and Anaphylaxis.* Pittsburgh, PA: Oncology Nursing Society; 1988e.

Oncology Nursing Society. *Access Device Guidelines:* Module I. *Catheters. Recommendations for Nursing Education and Practice.* Pittsburgh, PA: Oncology Nursing Society; 1989a.

Oncology Nursing Society. *Access Device Guidelines:* Module II. *Implanted Ports and Reservoirs. Recommendations for Nursing Education and Practice.* Pittsburgh, PA: Oncology Nursing Society; 1989b.

Oncology Nursing Society. *Safe Handling of Cytotoxic Drugs: Independent Study Module.* Pittsburgh, PA: Oncology Nursing Society; 1989c.

Oncology Nursing Society. *Standard of Oncology Education: Patient/Family and Public.* Pittsburgh, PA: Oncology Nursing Society; 1989d.

Oncology Nursing Society. *Access Device Guidelines:* Module III. *Pumps (Infusion Systems). Recommendations for Nursing Education and Practice.* Pittsburgh, PA: Oncology Nursing Society; 1990.

Pickett RR. Outpatient oncology chemotherapy documentation tool. *Oncol Nurs Forum.* 1992;**19**(3):515–517.

Pilapil F, Studva KV. Cancer chemotherapy. *Cancer Nurs.* 1978;**1**(2):153–164.

Prager D, Hertzberg RW. Spontaneous intravenous catheter fracture and embolization from an implanted venous access port and analysis by scanning electron microscopy. *Cancer.* 1987;**60**:270–273.

Raaf JH. Results from use of 826 vascular access devices in cancer patients. *Cancer.* 1985;**55**:1312–1321.

Reed WP, Newman KA, Applefeld MM, Sutton FJ. Drug extravasations as a complication of venous access ports. *Ann Intern Med.* 1985;**102**:788–790.

Rogers B, Emmett EA. Handling antineoplastic agents: Urine mutagenicity in nurses. *Image: J Nurs Scholarship.* 1987;**19**(3):108–113.

Rowland JH. Interpersonal resources: Social support. In: Holland JC, Rowland JH, eds. *Handbook of Psychooncology: Psychological Care of the Patient With Cancer.* New York: Oxford University Press; 1990a:58–71.

Rowland JH. Intrapersonal resources: Coping. In: Holland JC, Rowland JH, eds. *Handbook of Psychooncology: Psychological Care of the Patient With Cancer.* New York: Oxford University Press; 1990b:44–57.

Simon RC. Small gauge central venous catheters and right atrial catheters. *Semin Oncol Nurs.* 1987;**3**(2):87–95.

Slater H, Goldfar IW, Jacob HE, Hill JB, Srodes CH. Experience with long-term outpatient venous access utilizing percutaneously placed silicone elastomer catheters. *Cancer.* 1985;**56**:2074–2077.

Stellato TA, Gauderer MWL, Kazura J. Tumor metastasis from multiple myeloma and Burkitt's lymphoma in Broviac catheter tracts. *Cancer.* 1985;**55**:2715–2717.

Strum SB, McDermed JE. Drug extravasation and the Port-a-Cath system. *Ann Intern Med.* 1985;**103**:472–473.

Sznajder JI, Zveibil FR, Bitterman H, Weiner P, Bursztein S. Central vein catheterization—Failure and complication rate by three percutaneous approaches. *Arch Intern Med.* 1986;**146**:259–261.

Tenenbaum L. *Cancer Chemotherapy: A Reference Guide.* Philadelphia: WB Saunders; 1989.

Turcotte G. Erroneous nomograms for body-surface area. *N Engl J Med.* 1979;**300**:1339.

Valanis B, McNeil V, Driscoll K. Staff members' compliance with their facility's antineoplastic drug handling policy. *Oncol Nurs Forum.* 1991;**18**(3):571–576.

Volker DL. Developing continuing education programs in cancer nursing: Learning needs assessment. *Oncol Nurs Forum.* 1987;**14**(5):60–62.

Von Hoff DD. Intraosseous infusions: An important but forgotten method of vascular access. *Cancer Invest.* 1991;**9**(5):521–528.

Wainstock JM. Making a choice: The vein access method you prefer. *Oncol Nurs Forum.* 1987;**14**(1):79–82.

Welch-McCaffrey D. Rationale, development, and evaluation of a chemotherapy certification course for nurses. *Cancer Nurs.* 1985;**8**(5):255–262.

Wheeler CA. Pediatric intraosseous infusion: An old technique in modern health care technology. *J Intravenous Nurs.* 1989;**12**(6):371–376.

Wickham R. Techniques for long-term venous access. *Proceedings from the Fifth National Conference on Cancer Nursing,* Atlanta: American Cancer Society; 1987.

Chapter 5

Alternative Routes of Chemotherapy Administration

James M. Koeller and Suzanne Fields

In an attempt to increase the antitumor activity of chemotherapeutic agents, researchers have explored alternative routes of drug administration. The major routes that have been used include intrathecal, intraperitoneal, and intrapleural drug administration. It is often difficult to obtain therapeutic drug concentrations in the central nervous system and the abdominal cavity following systemic drug administration due to the presence of membranous boundaries that act as diffusion barriers for the drug. Following intracavitary drug administration, however, these boundaries are beneficial in that they allow for slow diffusion of the drug out of the cavity resulting in increased exposure time of the tumor cell to drug. Furthermore, by delivering the chemotherapeutic drug locally to the area of the tumor one is able to obtain pharmacologic drug concentrations that may be therapeutically advantageous to the concentrations that can be obtained with systemic administration. Intracavitary drug administration may also minimize some of the systemic toxicities associated with the drug due to the lower plasma concentrations that are achieved.

INTRATHECAL CHEMOTHERAPY

As systemic chemotherapy for acute lymphocytic leukemia (ALL) continues to show prolonged remissions in children, the central nervous system (CNS) has emerged as the primary site of relapse (Nies et al 1965, Evans et al 1970, Price and Johnson 1973). Prior to therapy targeted at the CNS, relapse rates exceeding 50% had been reported (Hardisty and Norman 1967, Evans et al 1970). This is because the blood–brain barrier acts as "tumor sanctuary," not allowing penetration of many of the systematically administered chemotherapeutic agents. Drugs that demonstrate poor penetration into the CNS at more standard chemotherapeutic dosages are shown in Table 5.1. This lack of "drug penetration" causes problems not only for ALL patients but, in addition, for patients with other tumors that have a propensity to metastasize to the meninges. These tumors include breast cancer, small cell lung cancer, non-Hodgkin's lymphoma, and gastric, prostate, and pancreatic carcinoma. Because of the limitations of systemic chemotherapy, strategies involving the direct treatment of the CNS have evolved. With direct intrathecal administration of chemotherapeutic agents either alone or in combination with radiation therapy, the relapse rate in ALL has decreased to less than 10% (Aur et al 1971). Although this percentage may appear low, the latent mental impairment described by Poplack and Brouwers (1983) and the meningeal relapse that has a very poor prognosis are ample reasons for more effective therapy for CNS involvement.

Meningeal involvement is often revealed by signs of headache, vomiting, visual disturbances, or other symptoms of increased intracranial pressure. Cranial nerve involvement and focal extremity deficits are seen along with confusion, back pain, and seizures. Analysis of the CSF fluid will typically show a decreased glucose and an elevated protein.

Mellett (1977) described five criteria that would favor blood–brain barrier penetration of a drug

TABLE 5.1. DRUGS WITH POOR CENTRAL NERVOUS SYSTEM PENETRATION

L-Asparaginase	5-Fluorouracil
Cyclophosphamide	Methotrexate
Cytarabine	Procarbazine
Daunomycin	Teniposide
Daunorubicin	Vincristine

given systemically. Drugs that are un-ionized, have a high lipid/aqueous partitioning coefficient, low protein binding, and a small molecular size, and sustained drug levels of drug would have the best CNS penetration. The large molecular weight of most antineoplastic agents appears to be the major limiting factor for poor CNS penetration. For significant CNS concentrations of drug to be achieved, direct CNS administration is generally required.

INTRATHECAL DRUG THERAPY

The antimetabolites methotrexate and cytarabine and the alkylating agent thiotepa have had the most use with intrathecal administration and have demonstrated good clinical results, although data on the intrathecal administration of other agents such as 6-mercaptopurine, diaziquone, dacarbazine, interferon alfa, etoposide and various immunotoxins have also been reported. Of all these agents, methotrexate continues to be the most studied.

Methotrexate

(Also see Part III, Methotrexate, Special Applications.) Intrathecal methotrexate alone or in combination with cytarabine is the most common treatment and preventive regimen for meningeal leukemia. Weekly administration of intrathecal methotrexate (Duttera et al 1973) for 8 to 10 doses can produce responses in over 80% of patients treated. A prolongation in remission can be achieved with subsequent monthly injections. For CNS prevention, Bleyer and Poplack (1985) demonstrated that methotrexate administered during the induction phase and continued through maintenance provided the optimal treatment for patients with low-risk ALL.

Systemic chemotherapy is generally dosed on the basis of body weight or surface area. Bleyer (1977) showed that methotrexate CNS concentrations were highly variable following a 12 mg/m² dose and correlated better with patient age. Knowing that the cerebrospinal fluid (CSF) volume is relatively constant from age 3 through 40, a single methotrexate dose can be given. Bleyer and Dedrick (1977) established the pharmacokinetics of intrathecal methotrexate. The terminal half-life was 14 hours, and the peak serum concentration from a 12 mg/m² dose was 2×10^{-7} M seen 3 to 12 hours after the dose. These data were confirmed by Blasberg et al (1977), although Shapiro and colleagues (1975) also demonstrated that ventricular CSF concentrations are highly variable following intralumbar administration and are approximately 10% of simultaneously drawn lumbar levels. Because of this epidural and subdural leakage following what appears to be successful intrathecal methotrexate administration, Shapiro and co-workers also recommended the use of a Ommaya reservoir. Bleyer and Poplack (1978) went on to demonstrate the advantage of regional administration of methotrexate by achieving a CSF concentration 100 times greater than that of plasma. At the same time, they also showed that the CSF acts as a reservoir for the slow systemic release of methotrexate. Serum concentration of 0.01 µmol/L are maintained twice as long with intrathecal administration than with systemic administration.

Reports of toxicity as a result of intrathecal methotrexate administration are quite common (Bleyer 1981). Multiple factors have been implicated in methotrexate intrathecal toxicity (Poplack and Brouwers 1985). Increased toxicity has been noted in the presence of overt meningeal involvement versus that seen with prophylactic therapy. Increased age has also been associated with worsened toxicity. Sustained CSF drug levels have correlated with increased toxicity. Finally, the use of hyper- or hypotonic diluents or those with bacteriostatic ingredients (methyl and propyl parabens and benzyl alcohol) have been linked to increased toxicity than more physiologic solutions such as normal saline or Ringer's lactate injection, USP (all without preservatives) (Hahn et al 1983).

The most common toxic reaction reported is an acute chemical arachnoiditis that is characterized by headache, back pain, vomiting, fever, and nuchal rigidity (Kaplan and Wiernik 1982). Other toxic effects noted included leukoencephalopathy (Bleyer et al 1973; Shapiro et al 1973), paraplegia (Gagliano and Costanzi 1976), cerebral calcifications (Mueller et al 1976), and death as a result of drug or diluent hypersensitivity (Back 1969). The possible mechanisms for these various toxic effects include reduced cerebral glucose and protein metabolism, altered blood–brain barrier permeability, impaired neurotransmitter synthesis, and depletion of cerebral reduced folate (Phillips 1991).

Long-term follow-up of children with acute lymphocytic leukemia treated prophylactically or for meningeal involvement have revealed poor school performance, growth retardation, behavioral changes, hormonal imbalances, and abnormal CAT scan findings (cerebral atrophy, intracerebral calcifications). It is unclear how much of this can be related directly to the radiation therapy, although methotrexate alone can produce many of these symptoms (Poplack and Brouwers 1985).

Accidental overdose with intrathecal methotrexate has been reported (Addiego et al 1981). Doses under 100 mg without CSF drainage may produce acute chemical meningitis. Doses exceeding 500 mg can cause myelopathy and encephalopathy, which can be fatal. For accidental CNS methotrexate overdose, Jakobson et al (1992) recommend lumbar cerebrospinal fluid exchange.

Modulation of methotrexate neurotoxicity with the administration of systemic leucovorin has been reported by Winick et al (1992). Gregory et al (1991) have reported sustained systemic methotrexate levels following intrathecal administration in patients with renal dysfunction. They calculated half-lives exceeding 40 hours in some patients with renal dysfunction. A case report of acute systemic tumor lysis syndrome was reported by Simmons and Somberg (1991) following a single intrathecal dose of methotrexate. Sustained, low-level (10^{-8} M) methotrexate levels were implicated in the clinical picture of tumor lysis.

Cytarabine

(Also see Part III, Cytarabine, Special Applications.) Bromylee et al (1968) were the first to administer cytarabine intrathecally. Behind methotrexate, cytarabine is the second most commonly administered intrathecal agent for the prevention or treatment of meningeal leukemia. Numerous doses and dosing schedules have been used. Schedules ranging from weekly to monthly administration have been employed, whereas doses have ranged from 30 to 100 mg/m². All dose levels were generally well tolerated, with transient headaches and vomiting seen at doses exceeding 27 mg/m². More recently, a standardized dose of 100 mg of cytarabine has been given for prophylaxis or treatment in adults and children over 5 years of age.

Systemic cytarabine is rapidly metabolized to its inactive metabolite, uracil arabinoside, by the enzyme cytidine deaminase (Camiener and Smith 1965). Because of the lower levels of cytidine deaminase in the CNS, the conversion of cytarabine to uracil arabinoside is very slow. This is responsible for the prolonged CSF levels of cytarabine found in the CSF versus serum. For a 30-mg intrathecal dose of cytarabine, peak CSF concentrations exceed 2 µmol/L and remain above 1 µmol/L for greater than 24 hours (Zimm et al 1984). Serum samples from the same intrathecal dose show no detectable drug concentration.

The most frequent toxic effect noted with intrathecal cytarabine is chemical arachnoiditis (Phillips and Reinhard 1991), although reactions including paraparesis (Breuer et al 1977), fatal paralysis (Frederick 1991), and seizures (Eden et al 1978) have been reported. Others have described serious toxicity when cytarabine and methotrexate have been used together, establishing both agents as potentially neurotoxic (Saiki et al 1972), although the risk of serious neurologic toxicity is less with cytarabine than with methotrexate (Phillips and Reinhard 1991).

Thiophosphoramide

(Also see Part III, Thiophosphoramide, Special Applications.) Intrathecal thiophosphoramide has been evaluated for the treatment of meningeal leukemia and ependymoma (Gutin et al 1976). Thiophosphoramide was given twice weekly at a dose ranging from 1 to 10 mg/m². Mild toxicity was noted including transient paresthesias of the lower extremities. Recent pharmacokinetic data have limited the use of thiophosphoramide intrathecally (Strong et al 1986). Data indicate that thiophosphoramide distribution is limited in the CSF because of rapid diffusion out of the CNS. In addition, TEPA, the active metabolite, is not found in the CSF following intrathecal administration. In fact, after systemic administration of thiophosphoramide, CSF and plasma concentrations are almost equivalent as a result of the rapid passage across the blood–brain barrier. This would indicate that systemic administration may be the preferred route for intrathecal treatment.

Other Agents

Although 6-mercaptopurine has been used as standard maintenance therapy in acute lymphocytic leukemia for years, intrathecal administration had never been tried. Adamson and co-workers (1991) studied the effects of a 10-mg intrathecal dose of 6-mercaptopurine in leukemic children who had failed other forms of therapy. This dose was selected on the basis of Rhesus monkey data that indicated a 1 μM concentration of drug could be maintained longer than 12 hours. They administered this dose twice weekly for 4 weeks. Seven of nine patients responded. Mild headache and nausea were the only reported toxic effects.

Diaziquone is an alkylating agent that was designed to have enhanced CNS penetration (Ettinger et al 1990). Phase II trials have demonstrated activity against both leukemia and CNS malignancies (Ettinger et al 1990, Faletta et al 1990), although hematologic toxicity severely limits its usefulness by systemic administration. Even though diaziquone is cleared somewhat quickly from the CNS, lumbar levels were sevenfold greater when given by intrathecal administration than when given systematically (Zimm et al 1984). More recently, Berg and colleagues (1992) studied intrathecal diaziquone in refractory meningeal diseases. One- or two-milligram doses were given twice weekly for 4 weeks, or the $C \times T$ (concentration × time) administration method was used by giving 0.5 mg every 6 hours for three doses. The overall response rate was 62% (38% complete responses). No difference in dose or schedule was noted except for toxicity in which the 2 mg dose twice weekly produced more headache and nausea and vomiting.

Champagne and Silver (1992) reported two patients treated with intrathecal dacarbazine in doses ranging from 5 to 20 mg given twice weekly. Headache, neck stiffness, and hypertension were the reported toxic effects. The severe hypertension seen in one patient was noted with intraventricular, not intralumbar, administration.

Another brief report has described the intrathecal administration of etoposide to two patients (Gaast et al 1992). Intrathecal etoposide was administered as a 0.5-mg dose daily for 5 days, followed in 21 days by a second course of 0.5 mg twice daily for 5 days. No treatment-related side effects were noted in either patient. CSF concentrations of 5.2 µg/mL were achieved. Both patients showed evidence of response.

A single patient with metastatic melanoma was treated with intrathecal interferon alfa (Roferon-A®, Intron A®) (Dorval et al 1991). Three-times-weekly doses ranging from 3 to 10×10^6 units were administered intrathecally. Marked clinical improvement was seen and no side effects were noted.

Finally, there is an excellent review (Hall and Fodstad 1992) of the use of immunotoxins in meningeal disease.

INTRATHECAL INJECTION

Drug administration into the CSF is usually performed by lumbar puncture (between L_4 and L_5) or by intraventricular administration using a subcutaneous implanted reservoir (Ommaya). Rieselbach and colleagues (1962) were able to show that the volume administered, not the site of injection, was the critical determinant for adequate distribution. The optimal volume in monkeys appeared to be one-fourth the total CSF volume (equal to roughly 30 mL in humans). Although this is not practical in most human applications, Gutin et al (1976) found that 20 mL of thiophosphoramide was well tolerated. Today, the most common volumes administered range from 5 to 10 mL. These are generally well tolerated if CSF is removed first or used as the diluent.

The diluent used for intrathecal chemotherapy preparation also appears to be important when considering toxicity. Although none of the studies are conclusive, there tends to be more toxicity when nonphysiologic solutions and when solutions with preservatives are used (Duttera et al 1973). Most believe an unpreserved isotonic, buffered diluent should be used. Methotrexate is now available in an unpreserved lyophilized form for intrathecal use. If cytarabine is used, the diluent provided in the container should not be used (it is benzyl alcohol preserved). For intrathecal administration, either sodium chloride USP (unpreserved) or Ringer's injection USP (unpreserved) should be used as the diluent. These will offer a buffered vehicle that is roughly isotonic. To avoid contamination, it is suggested that strict aseptic technique be used in preparation.

INTRAPERITONEAL CHEMOTHERAPY

The primary goal of intraperitoneal chemotherapy administration is to expose intraabdominal tumors to increased drug concentrations for longer periods than would be possible following intravenous drug administration. Furthermore, it is hoped that the systemic toxicity of the drug may also be minimized because of the lower drug plasma concentrations compared with the intraperitoneal cavity.

The origin of intraperitoneal chemotherapy administration as a therapeutic treatment modality is twofold. In the early 1970s, Chabner and Young (1973) reported on the pharmacokinetic effects of methotrexate in patients with large-volume pleural effusions or peritoneal ascites. Following methotrexate administration patients with significant ascites experienced prolonged myelosuppression and sustained blood methotrexate concentrations as a result of third-spacing of the drug in the peritoneal cavity. The slow release of the methotrexate from the peritoneal cavity back into the plasma suggested that drugs could be administered directly into the peritoneal cavity and that the peritoneum would act as a diffusion barrier. The second impetus for intraperitoneal chemotherapy occurred several years later when Dedrick and his colleagues at the National Cancer Institute devised mathematical models that provided the pharmacokinetic rationale for peritoneal drug administration (Dedrick et al 1978).

Several pharmacokinetic principles determine the advantages of intraperitoneal drug delivery compared with intravenous administration. To obtain a concentration advantage, the total body clearance of the drug must be more rapid than the peritoneal clearance. Drugs administered directly into the peritoneum exit the cavity via three routes: (1) diffusion of the drug across the peritoneal surface, (2) absorption of the drug by the lymphatic system, and (3) uptake of the drug into the portal venous system (Wolf and Sugarbaker 1988, Markman 1986). All of these routes will influence the rate of peritoneal clearance; however, passive peritoneal diffusion and portal venous uptake of the drug appear to be most important in determining peritoneal clearance.

Passive diffusion of the drug across the peritoneum is influenced by several factors including molecular weight, lipid solubility, and ionization. Therefore, the ideal drug for intraperitoneal administration or the drug that would exhibit the slowest clearance rate from the peritoneal cavity would be a large molecule that is ionized and water soluble. Rapid clearance of the drug once it is absorbed into the systemic circulation is also necessary to maintain the concentration advantage of intraperitoneal administration. Because many antineoplastic agents are hydrophilic and have molecular weights between 100 and 1000, their peritoneal clearance is less than 30 mL/min (Surbone and Myers 1988). When compared with total body clearance for many drugs, this will result in clearance ratios (total body clearance/peritoneal clearance) as high as several thousand, illustrating the pharmacologic advantages of intraperitoneal drug administration.

The portal venous uptake of drugs from the peritoneal cavity is important for two reasons. First, for drugs that undergo primarily hepatic metabolism, the first pass of the drug through the liver from the peritoneal cavity would minimize the amount of active drug that reaches the systemic circulation (Markman 1985). As a result, the systemic toxic effects of the drug may be decreased or avoided, allowing the administration of higher drug dosages. Second, absorption of drugs by the portal venous system results in the delivery of high drug concentrations to the liver (Brenner 1986). In a study conducted by Speyer et al (1981) the portal vein concentrations of 5-fluorouracil following intraperitoneal drug administration were comparable to the concentrations achieved with intraarterial drug administration and 4 to 10 times higher than systemic plasma concentrations. The administration of drugs with high hepatic extraction ratios by the intraperitoneal route would provide high drug concentrations in the liver, which could benefit patients with hepatic metastases.

Following intravenous administration, chemotherapy drugs reach the tumor via the capillary vasculature. In contrast, following intraperitoneal administration the drug reaches the site of antitumor activity through direct tumor contact and diffusion. Because of this difference, treatment volume and tumor penetration are important considerations with intraperitoneal chemotherapy administration. To maximize drug contact with tumor, the solution containing the drug must distribute evenly throughout the peritoneal cavity. This may be difficult in patients with intraabdominal tumors secondary to large tumor masses, surgical scarring, and/or adhesion formation. A study conducted in monkeys by Rosenshein et al (1978) demonstrated that large fluid volumes result in uniform drug distribution in the peritoneum, whereas small fluid volumes do not flow freely and miss areas such as the surface of the diaphragm. These results have been confirmed in several trials in patients conducted using radioimaging techniques (Dunnick et al 1979, Howell et al 1982, Gyves et al 1984). As a result it is recommended that intraperitoneal chemotherapy be administered in 1.5 to 2 L of fluid to obtain abdominal distension and uniform drug distribution throughout the peritoneal cavity.

The ability of the drug to penetrate the tumor is also an important consideration with intraperitoneal drug administration. Unfortunately, little information is available about the penetration of antineoplastic agents following direct contact with solid tumor cell surfaces. Ozols and his colleagues determined that doxorubicin penetrates the outermost five to six cell layers of tumor following intraperitoneal administration in mice with ovarian teratomas (Ozols et al 1979). The tumor penetration of cisplatin following intraperitoneal administration is slightly better than that of doxorubicin as drug penetrates as deep as 3 mm into the tumor, which is equivalent to approximately 50 cell layers (McVie et al 1985). The depth of tumor drug penetration varies among the chemotherapeutic agents and may be influenced by many factors, including intracellular/extracellular drug ratios, surface area available for diffusion, duration of cell surface exposure, diffusion coefficient for the administered drug, rate of cellular uptake, and drug half-life in the extracellular fluid and in the tumor cell (Markman 1987). Animal studies have also demonstrated that larger molecules may penetrate deeper into tumor nodules than smaller molecules (Dedrick 1985). All of these factors should be considered when choosing a drug for intraperitoneal therapy. Furthermore, because of the limited depth of tumor penetration it appears that only patients with microscopic disease or smaller tumor nodules (≤0.5 cm) would potentially benefit from intraperitoneal chemotherapy administration. Long-term survivals have been compared in patients with minimal disease (<2 cm) and bulky disease (>2 cm) at the time of treatment with cisplatin-based intraperitoneal therapy (Howell et al 1987b). The patients with minimal disease survived a median of 49+ months compared with only 8 months in the patients with bulky disease. This further illustrates the significance of extent of disease at the time of treatment.

Another important consideration with intraperitoneal therapy is the method used for drug delivery. If the chemotherapy is administered infrequently (every few weeks) then the insertion of a percutaneous catheter at the time of each treatment might be feasible; however, many of these patients may have severe adhesions secondary to previous surgeries and the risk of bowel perforation is significant. As a result, the surgical implantation of two different semipermanent catheter types has been explored for intraperitoneal drug administration. Many researchers have used the Tenckhoff catheter system for intraperitoneal drug delivery because of its extensive use in patients undergoing chronic ambulatory peritoneal dialysis. Once the catheter is in place it can be used for drug delivery or ascites drainage with cytology determination. These catheters are associated with some problems, however. In a retrospective analysis conducted in three institutions, the following complications were associated with catheter placement in 143 patients: bowel perforation (3.5%), bleeding with transfusion requirements (12.5%), ileus development (4.8%), and leakage of fluid around the catheter (11.1%) (Piccart et al 1985). Approximately one half of the patients also experienced either partial outflow obstruction or a total inability to drain the catheter after placement. The infection rate associated with the Tenckhoff catheter was relatively low, as 6.2% of patients experienced an infection at the exit site and 5.5% developed peritonitis. One disadvantage of the Tenckhoff catheter is that it requires continuous maintenance which may lead to low patient acceptability.

As a result of these complications, Pfeifle and his colleagues (1984) have promoted the use of a totally implantable system (Port-A-Cath) for intraperitoneal access. When compared with the Tenckhoff catheter, the complications following Port-A-Cath implantation are much less (Piccart et al 1985). Bowel perforation and leakage of fluid around the catheter each occurred in less than 2% of patients, and no patients developed an ileus or bleeding requiring transfusions after catheter placement. None of the patients with Port-A-Caths experienced cutaneous infections, but the incidence of peritonitis was slightly higher than reported with the Tenckhoff catheter (8.0 versus 5.5%). Approximately one half of the patients experienced either partial outflow obstruction or a total inability to drain the catheter after a period of time. This is similar to the experience with the Tenckhoff catheter and is thought to result from development of a fibrous sheath and fibrin clots around the catheter tip (Pfeifle et al 1984, Piccart et al 1985). With both catheters the outflow problems were not associated with inflow problems and the system was still usable for drug administration. Potential disadvantages of the Port-A-Cath system include more time for drug instillation than the Tenckhoff catheter and surgical removal if any problems develop once it is implanted.

In addition to the complications and infections associated with the intraperitoneal catheters, there are also local and systemic toxic effects that occur with drug administration. Instillation of chemotherapy agents into the peritoneal cavity can cause a chemical irritation of the peritoneal lining (Markman 1987). In a phase I trial the development of chemical peritonitis was the dose-limiting toxicity with intraperitoneal doxorubicin (Ozols et al 1982). Chemical peritonitis may be associated with such symptoms as fever, inflammation, and abdominal pain and therefore may be mistaken for infectious peritonitis. Because of the seriousness of an abdominal infection, any patient with these symptoms should be empirically started on antibiotic therapy until culture results from the peritoneal fluid can be obtained. The most common bacteria causing infection in patients with intraperitoneal catheters are skin organisms including *Staphylococcus epidermidis* and *Staphylococcus aureus*. Antibiotics with adequate coverage of these organisms should be used. Patients may also experience pain during drug administration because of expansion of the peritoneal cavity and the presence of adhesions. Other potential local toxic effects that may occur with intraperitoneal therapy are adhesion formation and bowel obstruction (Markman et al 1986a). Because the chemotherapy agents are absorbed into the systemic circulation from the peritoneal cavity, patients may also experience the systemic toxic effects associated with intravenous drug administration such as nausea, vomiting, myelosuppression, mucositis, nephrotoxicity, and neurotoxicity. In many of the clinical trials these systemic toxic effects were the dose-limiting toxic effects of the chemotherapy regimens.

The pharmacologic advantages of intraperitoneal drug administration has clearly been established; however, whether or not the exposure of tumor cells to higher concentrations of antineoplastic agents will result in increased antitumor activity remains to be determined. Numerous phase I and II trials with single agents, combination regimens, and immunotherapy have been conducted. These trials have been primarily in patients with ovarian cancer, gastrointestinal malignancies, and peritoneal mesothelioma because these diseases are frequently limited to the peritoneal cavity. Some of the patients included in these trials had bulky intraabdominal disease at the time of treatment. Because of the minimal penetration depth of antineoplastic agents into tumor nodules, the use of intraperitoneal therapy may be most effective for minimal residual disease following surgery or as adjuvant therapy to prevent tumor recurrence or spread (Sugarbaker et al 1989, Ozols 1985, Vlasveld et al 1991). This remains to be established for any of the three tumor types.

5-Fluorouracil

Several phase I and II trials have been conducted with intraperitoneal 5-fluorouracil in patients with ovarian cancer and gastrointestinal malignancies (Ozols et al 1984, Gyves et al 1984, Ekberg et al 1988, Speyer et al 1980). The toxic effects encountered in these trials included peritonitis, myelosuppression, and mucositis. Objective responses to intraperitoneal 5-fluorouracil therapy were obtained in 4 of the 35 patients treated in these studies. Sugarbaker and his colleagues (1985) conducted a prospective, randomized trial of intravenous versus intraperitoneal 5-fluorouracil in patients with colon or rectal cancer. The patients receiving intraperitoneal therapy were able to receive higher doses of 5-fluorouracil and experienced less hematologic and hepatic toxicity than the patients treated by the intravenous route. The patients receiving intravenous drug also experienced more disease recurrence on peritoneal surfaces, but time to relapse and survival were not different between the two groups. Reichman and colleagues conducted a phase I trial of concurrent intraperitoneal and continuous intravenous infusion of 5-fluorouracil in an attempt to achieve maximal local-regional and systemic drug exposure. The regimen was well tolerated and one patient experienced a complete remission following therapy (Reichman et al 1988).

Cisplatin

Clinical trials have also been conducted with single-agent intraperitoneal cisplatin (Hacker et al 1987, tenBokkel Huinink et al 1985). Complete remissions were obtained in approximately 30% of patients, most of whom had minimal residual disease. In an attempt to decrease the systemic toxicity, Howell and co-workers (1982) administered systemic thiosulfate (an intravenous neutralizing agent) in combination with intraperitoneal cisplatin. The administration of thiosulfate allowed escalation of the cisplatin dose to 270 mg/m^2 without causing systemic toxicity. The patients that did not receive systemic thiosulfate were able to tolerate only 90 mg/m² intraperitoneal cisplatin before they experienced nephrotoxicity.

Doxorubicin/Mitoxantrone

Intraperitoneal doxorubicin administration has also been investigated in phase I trials (Ozols et al 1982, Demicheli et al 1985). As mentioned previously, the dose-limiting toxic effect in these trials was chemical peritonitis secondary to the doxorubicin. The peritonitis was dose dependent and was tolerable to doxorubicin concentrations below 36 µM. Furthermore, the drug demonstrated significant antitumor activity in patients with refractory ovarian cancer. Because of similar antitumor activity and lack of vesicant activity, mitoxantrone has also been administered by the intraperitoneal route (Alberts et al 1988, Blöchl-Daum et al 1988). The dose-limiting toxic effects in these studies were chemical peritonitis and leukopenia. No complete responses were reported, but several patients experienced partial remissions, a reduction or disappearance of ascites, and decreases in serum tumor markers.

Other Single Agents

A pharmacokinetic advantage for intraperitoneal drug administration has also been established for carboplatin, melphalan, bleomycin, methotrexate, and cytosine arabinoside (Elferink et al 1988, Howell et al 1981, 1987, Jones et al 1981, King et al 1984). The dose-limiting toxic effect for melphalan was myelosuppression and the investigators were able to give three times the maximally tolerated intravenous dose by the intraperitoneal route. Intraperitoneal bleomycin was associated with the development of abdominal pain in approximately half of the patients. Local dose-limiting toxic effects will probably not allow for dose escalation with bleomycin, which would limit its intraperitoneal utility. The administration of intraperitoneal methotrexate has also resulted in a concentration advantage compared with the systemic circulation. The addition of systemic leucovorin to the regimen also allowed dose escalation of the methotrexate while minimizing systemic toxicity. The dose-limiting toxic effect of the regimen was, however, myelosuppression. Cytosine arabinoside was predicted to be an ideal agent for intraperitoneal administration in a pharmacokinetic model. As a result, a small 10-patient trial was conducted in patients with ovarian carcinoma (King et al 1984). Two of the four patients treated experienced a complete response to therapy that was sustained for over a year.

Combination Regimens

Because of its activity as a single agent, cytosine arabinoside has been administered in combination with various other antineoplastic agents in an attempt to increase tumor response. In the first trial cytosine arabinoside was administered in combination with cisplatin and doxorubicin (Markman et al 1984). Approximately 30% of the patients demonstrated a clinical response to therapy, most of whom had minimal disease at the time of treatment. The primary side effect associated with the regimen was abdominal pain secondary to the doxorubicin administration. In a similar trial cisplatin, cytarabine, and bleomycin were administered in combination (Markman et al 1986b). Once again, complete responses were obtained in approximately one third of the patients who had minimal residual disease at the time of treatment; however, most patients experienced severe abdominal pain after bleomycin administration which limited the amount of drug that could be given. Piver and his colleagues conducted a trial in 31 patients with stage III and IV ovarian cancer with the same drug combination (Piver et al 1988). All of the patients in this trial had their disease evaluated surgically before and after treatment with intraperitoneal therapy. Twenty-six percent of the patients demonstrated a response (five complete, three partial) to therapy. All of these responders had stage III ovarian cancer with 1-cm or less minimal residual disease and had previously responded to cisplatin-based intravenous therapy.

In an attempt to decrease the toxicity of these combination regimens while maintaining the antitumor activity, Markman and co-workers (1985) conducted a trial with only cisplatin and cytarabine. The response rate with the two-drug regimen was similar to that obtained with the three-drug regimen (approximately 30%) and the toxic effects were significantly lessened because of the elimination of doxorubicin or bleomycin from the regimen. Based on the success of this trial, the investigators conducted another trial with cisplatin and cytarabine that used a multiple-day dosing regimen and surgical reevaluation of the disease following treatment (Markman et al 1991a). The dose-limiting toxic effect of this regimen was severe thrombocytopenia. Furthermore, in patients with less than 1 cm disease there was a 30% surgically defined complete response. No complete responses were reported in patients with bulky intraabdominal disease at the time of treatment.

Two clinical trials have been conducted with the combination of intraperitoneal cisplatin and etoposide in patients with ovarian cancer. In the first trial patients with refractory or recurrent ovarian cancer received cisplatin (100 mg/m^2) and etoposide (200 mg/m^2) monthly for 6 months (Reichman et al 1989). All of the patients had previously received intravenous cisplatin therapy. Of the 57 patients who were evaluable, 21% obtained a surgically defined complete response and 19% obtained a surgically defined partial response. In patients with refractory disease, the majority of responses were reported in patients with minimal residual disease less than 0.5 cm. With recurrent disease, patients with all categories of residual disease responded to therapy. Howell and his colleagues (1990) also conducted a trial with intraperitoneal cisplatin (100 mg/m^2) and etoposide (350 mg/m^2) on a monthly basis in patients with newly diagnosed stage III and IV ovarian cancer. Because of the high doses of cisplatin, systemic sodium thiosulfate was administered concomitantly to minimize nephrotoxicity. Fifty-six percent (13/56) of the patients obtained a complete clinical remission after six cycles of treatment. Seven of these thirteen patients underwent a second-look laparotomy which confirmed three pathologic complete remissions. The primary toxic effects reported with this regimen included nausea, vomiting, and myelosuppression.

Biologic Agents

Intraperitoneal therapy with the biologic agents has also been explored in an attempt to decrease some of the systemic toxic effects associated with these agents. The biologic agents that have been investigated to date include bacillus Calmette-Guérin; interferons alfa, beta, and gamma; and interleukin-2 (Falk et al 1976, Rambaldi et al 1985, Berek et al 1985, Chapman et al 1986, Lotze et al 1986). As with the antineoplastic agents, clinical responses have been reported in a few patients who have minimal residual disease at the time of treatment. The true utility of administering these new agents by the intraperitoneal route remains to be established in definitive clinical trials.

Investigational Drugs

Because of the activity of Taxol® against ovarian cancer in early clinical trials, Markman and his colleagues (1991b) have recently conducted a trial using intraperitoneal Taxol® administration. This drug possesses many pharmacologic properties that make it appropriate for intraperitoneal administration including a high molecular weight, bulky chemical structure, primarily hepatic metabolism, and activity in ovarian cancer. The dose-limiting toxic effect in this trial was severe abdominal pain; myelosuppression was also reported. Pharmacokinetic studies also demonstrated that Taxol® has an intraperitoneal/systemic area-under-the-curve ratio of 1000 after intraperitoneal drug administration. On the basis of these data, the Gynecologic Oncology Group is currently conducting a study exploring weekly intraperitoneal Taxol® administration in patients with measurable ovarian cancer.

INTRAPLEURAL CHEMOTHERAPY

The intrapleural administration of drugs such as talc, tetracycline, and bleomycin has been used for many years for sclerosing malignant pleural effusions caused by malignancies. Because of the pharmacokinetic advantages and antitumor activity obtained with intraperitoneal chemotherapy administration, researchers began to investigate intrapleural drug administration for the treatment of tumors that are confined to the pleural cavity, such as mesothelioma. It is hoped that the intrapleural administration of chemotherapy will treat the underlying malignancy and provide local control of the effusion. The primary difference between using a chemotherapy agent for sclerosis and for active tumor treatment is the fluid volume employed for drug administration (Markman 1987). When used as a sclerosing agent, the drug is administered as concentrated solution in a small volume of fluid. On the other hand, when the drug is being used as active treatment a larger fluid volume is used for drug administration to obtain uniform distribution throughout the cavity. Numerous trials establishing the activity of intrapleural chemotherapy administration have been conducted, but until recently the pharmacokinetics of intrapleural drug administration had not been delineated. Two separate clinical trials of intrapleural cisplatin or intrapleural cisplatin and mitomycin have confirmed that the pharmacokinetics of intrapleural drug administration are indeed similar to those of intraperitoneal chemotherapy administration (Bogliolo et al 1991, Rusch et al 1992). In both studies the pleural fluid concentrations were significantly higher than the plasma concentrations, resulting in a pleural fluid/plasma area-under-the-curve concentration advantage.

Single-Agent Therapy

Single-agent intrapleural therapy trials have been conducted with various chemotherapeutic and biologic agents including bleomycin, mitoxantrone, doxorubicin, mitomycin-C, cisplatin, etoposide, OK-432, bacillus Calmette-Guérin, and interferon gamma (Ruckdeschel et al 1991, Paladine et al 1976, Ostrowski 1986, Groth et al 1991, Masuno et al 1991, Ike et al 1991, Markman et al 1986c, Holoye et al 1990, Macchiarini et al 1991, Boutin et al 1991). Various methods have been used to determine treatment response including the presence of fluid reaccumulation or disappearance of fluid on serial chest x-rays, thoracoscopic examination, and computed tomography scanning. In general, the administration of intrapleural therapy prevented the recurrence of the pleural effusion in 40 to 80% of patients and the toxic effects associated with therapy were minimal.

Combination Regimen

The use of combination regimens for intrapleural administration is also being explored in clinical trials. The Lung Cancer Study Group evaluated intrapleural cisplatin in combination with cytarabine in patients with pleural effusions associated with malignant mesothelioma (Rusch et al 1991). The rationale for this study was based on the in vitro data suggesting synergy between these two drugs and the use of this regimen in intraperitoneal trials. Six of the thirty-seven evaluable patients had complete disappearance of their effusion at 3 weeks posttreatment (complete response) and 12 additional patients experienced a 75% or greater decrease in the amount of their effusion on serial chest x-rays (partial response). The median durations of response were 9 months in the complete responders and 5.1 months in the patients with a partial response. The primary toxic effects associated with the regimen were nausea and vomiting, myelosuppression, pain, and cardiopulmonary symptoms that were thought to result from fluid overload. Currently, the Lung Cancer Study Group is conducting another trial using this treatment regimen in combination with surgical debulking of pleural tumor in patients with malignant mesothelioma.

REFERENCES

Adamson PC, Balis FM, Arndt CA, et al. Intrathecal 6-mercaptopurine: Preclinical pharmacology, phase I/II trial and pharmacokinetic study. *Cancer Res.* 1991;**51**:6079–6083.

Addiego JE, Ridgway D, Bleyer WA. The acute management of intrathecal methotrexate overdose: Pharmacology rationale and guidelines. *J Pediatr.* 1981;**98**:825–831.

Alberts DS, Surwit EA, Peng YM, et al. Phase I clinical and pharmacokinetic study of mitoxantrone given to patients by intraperitoneal administration. *Cancer Res.* 1988;**48**:5874–5877.

Aur RJ, Simone JV, Hustu HO, et al. Central nervous system therapy and combination chemotherapy of childhood lymphocytic leukemia. *Blood.* 1971;**37**:272–281.

Back EH. Deaths after intrathecal methotrexate. *Lancet.* 1969;**11**:1005.

Band PR, Holland JF, Bernard J, et al. Treatment of central nervous system leukemia with intrathecal cytosine arabinosine. *Cancer.* 1973;**32**:744–748.

Berek JS, Hacker NF, Lichtenstein A, et al. Intraperitoneal recombinant alpha-interferon for "salvage" immunotherapy in stage III epithelial ovarian cancer: A Gynecologic Oncology Group study. *Cancer Res.* 1985;**45**:4447–4453.

Berg SL, Balis FM, Zimm S, et al. Phase I/II trial and pharmacokinetics of intrathecal diaziquone in refractory meningeal malignancies. *J Clin Oncol.* 1992;**10**:143–148.

Blasberg RG, Patlak CS, Shapiro WR. Distribution of methotrexate in the cerebrospinal fluid and brain after intraventricular administration. *Cancer Treat Rep.* 1977;**61**:633–641.

Bleyer WA. Clinical pharmacology of intrathecal methotrexate. II. An improved dosage regimen derived from age-related pharmacokinetics. *Cancer Treat Rep.* 1977;**61**:1419–1425.

Bleyer WA. Neurologic sequelae of methotrexate and ionizing radiation: A new classification. *Cancer Treat Rep.* 1981;**65**(suppl 1):89–98.

Bleyer WA, Dedrick RL. Clinical pharmacology of intrathecal methotrexate. I. Pharmacokinetics in nontoxic patients after lumbar injection. *Cancer Treat Rep.* 1977;**61**:703–708.

Bleyer WA, Drake JC, Chabner BA. Neurotoxicity and elevated cerebrospinal-fluid methotrexate concentration in meningeal leukemia. *N Engl J Med.* 1973;**289**:770–773.

Bleyer WA, Poplack DG. Clinical studies on the central nervous system pharmacology of methotrexate. In: Pinedo HM, ed. Clinical Pharmacology of Anti-neoplastic Drugs. Amsterdam: Elsevier/North-Holland Biomedical; 1978:115–131.

Bleyer WA, Poplack DG. Prophylaxis and treatment of leukemia in the central nervous system and other sanctuaries. *Semin Oncol.* 1985;**12**:131–148.

Blöchl-Daum B, Eichler HG, Rainer H, et al. Escalating dose regimen of intraperitoneal mitoxantrone: Phase I study—clinical and pharmacokinetic evaluation. *Eur J Cancer Clin Oncol.* 1988;**24**:1133–1138.

Bogliolo GV, Lerza R, Bottino GB, et al. Regional pharmacokinetic selectivity of intrapleural cisplatin. *Eur J Cancer.* 1991;**27**:839–842.

Boutin C, Viallat JR, Zadwijk NV, et al. Activity of intrapleural recombinant gamma interferon in malignant mesothelioma. *Cancer.* 1991;**67**:2033–2037.

Brenner DE. Intraperitoneal chemotherapy: A review. *J Clin Oncol.* 1986;**4**:1135–1147.

Breuer AC, Pitman WS, Dawson DM, et al. Paraparesis following intrathecal cytosine arabinoside. *Cancer.* 1977;**40**:2817–2822.

Bromylee RW, Scott PB, Talley RW, et al. Clinical experience with cytosine arabinoside administered intrathecally to thirteen patients with demonstrable cerebral metastases. *Proc Am Soc Clin Oncol.* 1968;**1**:9.

Camiener GN, Smith CG. Studies of the enzymatic deamination of cytosine arabinoside. I. Enzyme distribution and species specialty. *Biochem Pharmacol.* 1965;**14**:1405–1416.

Chabner BA, Young RC. Threshold methotrexate concentration for in vivo inhibition of DNA synthesis in normal and tumorous target tissues. *J Clin Invest.* 1973;**52**:1804–1811.

Champagne MA, Silver HK. Intrathecal dacarbazine treatment of leptomeningeal malignant melanoma. *J Natl Cancer Inst.* 1992;**84**:1203–1204.

Chapman PB, Hakes T, Gabrilove JL, et al. A phase I pilot study of intraperitoneal rIL-2 in ovarian cancer (abstract). *Proc Am Soc Clin Oncol.* 1986;**5**:23.

Dedrick RL. Theoretical and experimental bases of intraperitoneal chemotherapy. *Semin Oncol.* 1985;**3** (suppl 4):1–6.

Dedrick RL, Myers CE, Bungay PM, DeVita VT Jr. Pharmacokinetic rationale for peritoneal drug administration in the treatment of ovarian cancer. *Cancer Treat Rep.* 1978;**62**:1–11.

Demicheli R, Bonciarelli G, Jirillo A, et al. Pharmacologic data and technical feasibility of intraperitoneal doxorubicin administration. *Tumor.* 1985;**71**:63–68.

Dorval T, Beuzeboc P, Garcia-Giralt E, et al. Malignant melanoma: Treatment of metastatic meningitis with intrathecal interferon alpha-2b. *Eur J Cancer.* 1991;**28**:244–245.

Duffner PK, Cohen ME. The long-term effects of central nervous system therapy on children with brain tumors. *Neurol Clin.* 1991;**9**:479–486.

Dunnick NR, Jones RB, Doppman JL, et al. Intraperitoneal contrast infusion for assessment of intraperitoneal fluid dynamics. *AJR.* 1979;**133**:221–223.

Duttera MJ, Bleyer WA, Pomeroy TC, et al. Irradiation, methotrexate toxicity and the treatment of meningeal leukemia. *Lancet.* 1973;**2**:703–707.

Eden OB, Goldie W, Wood T. Seizures following intrathecal cytosine arabinoside in young children with acute lymphocytic leukemia. *Cancer.* 1978;**42**:53–58.

Ekberg H, Tranberg KG, Persson B, et al. Intraperitoneal infusion of 5-FU in liver metastases from colorectal cancer. *J Surg Oncol.* 1988;**37**:94–99.

Elferink F, van der Vijgh WJF, Klein I, ten Bokkel Huinink WW, Dubbelman R, McVie JG. Pharmacokinetics of carboplatin after intraperitoneal administration. *Cancer Chemother Pharmacol.* 1988;**21**:57–60.

Ettinger LJ, Ru N, Krailo MD. A phase II study of diaziquone in children with recurrent or progressive solid tumors: Report from the Children's Cancer Study Group. *Am J Pedia Hematol/Oncol.* 1990;**12**:301–305.

Evans AE, Gilbert ES, Zandstra R. The increasing incidence of central nervous system leukemia in children. *Cancer.* 1970;**26**:404–409.

Faletta J, Cushing B, Lauer S, et al. Phase I evaluation of diaziquone in childhood leukemia: A Pediatric Oncology Group study. *Invest New Drugs.* 1990;**8**:167–170.

Falk RE, MacGregor AB, Landi S, Ambus U, Langer B. Immunostimulation with intraperitoneally administered Bacille Calmette-Guérin for advanced malignant tumors of the gastrointestinal tract. *Surg Gynecol Obstet.* 1976;**142**:363–368.

Frederick E. Rare neurotoxicity related to intrathecal Cytosar. *Oncol Nurs Forum.* 1991;**18**:603–604.

Gaast AV, Sonneveld P, Mans DR, et al. Intrathecal administration of etoposide in the treatment of malignant meningitis: Feasibility and pharmacokinetic data. *Cancer Chemother Pharmacol.* 1992;**29**:335–337.

Gagliano RG, Costanzi JJ. Paraplegia following intrathecal methotrexate. *Cancer.* 1976;**37**:1663–1668.

Gregory RE, Pui CH, Crom WR. Raised plasma methotrexate concentrations following intrathecal administration in children with renal dysfunction. *Leukemia.* 1991;**5**:994–1003.

Groth G, Gatzemeier U, Häußingen K, et al. Intrapleural palliative treatment of malignant pleural effusions with mitoxantrone versus placebo (pleural tube alone). *Ann Oncol.* 1991;**2**:213–215.

Gutin PH, Weiss HD, Wiernik WA, et al. Intrathecal N, N', N", triethylenethiophosphoramide [thio-TEPA (NSC-6396)] in the treatment of malignant meningeal disease. *Cancer.* 1976;**38**:1529–1534.

Gyves JW, Ensminger WD, Stetson P. Constant intraperitoneal 5-fluorouracil infusion through a totally implanted system. *Clin Pharmacol Ther.* 1984;**35**:83–89.

Hacker NF, Berek JS, Pretorius G, Zuckerman J, Eisenkop S, Lagasse LD. Intraperitoneal cis-platinum as salvage therapy for refractory epithelial ovarian cancer. *Obstet Gynecol.* 1987;**70**:759–764.

Hahn AF, Feasby TE, Gilbert JJ. Paraparesis following intrathecal chemotherapy. *Neurology.* 1983;**33**:1032.

Hall WA, Fodstad O. Immunotoxins and central nervous system neoplasia. *J Neurosurg.* 1992;**76**:1–12.

Hardisty RM, Norman PM. Meningeal leukemia. *Arch Dis Child.* 1967;**42**:441–447.

Holoye PY, Jeffries DG, Dhingra HM, et al. Intrapleural etoposide for malignant effusion. *Cancer Chemother Pharmacol.* 1990;**26**:147–150.

Howell SB, Chu BCF, Wung WE, Metha BM, Mendelsohn J. Long-duration intracavitary infusion of methotrexate with systemic leucovorin protection in patients with malignant effusion. *J Clin Invest.* 1981;**67**:1161–1170.

Howell SB, Kirmani S, Lucas WE, et al. A phase II trial of intraperitoneal cisplatin and etoposide for primary treatment of ovarian epithelial cancer. *J Clin Oncol.* 1990;**8**:137–145.

Howell SB, Pfeifle CE, Olshen RA. Intraperitoneal chemotherapy with melphalan. *Ann Intern Med.* 1984;**101**:14–18.

Howell SB, Pfeifle CL, Wung WE, et al. Intraperitoneal cisplatin with systemic thiosulfate protection. *Ann Intern Med.* 1982;**97**:845–851.

Howell SB, Schiefer M, Andrews PA, Markman M, Abramson I. The pharmacology of intraperitoneally administered bleomycin. *J Clin Oncol.* 1987a;**5**:2009–2016.

Howell SB, Zimm S, Markman M, et al. Long-term survival of advanced refractory ovarian carcinoma patients with small-volume disease treated with intraperitoneal chemotherapy. *J Clin Oncol.* 1987b;**5**:1607–1612.

Ike O, Shimizu Y, Hitomi S, Wada R, Ikada Y. Treatment of malignant pleural effusions with doxorubicin hydrochloride-containing poly(L-lactic acid) microspheres. *Chest.* 1991;**99**:911–915.

Jakobson AM, Kreuger A, Mortimer O, et al. Cerebral-spinal fluid exchange after intrathecal methotrexate overdose. A report of two cases. *Acta Pediatr.* 1992;**81**:359–361.

Jones RB, Collins JM, Myers CE, et al. High-volume intraperitoneal chemotherapy with methotrexate in patients with cancer. *Cancer Res.* 1981;**41**:55–59.

Kaplan RS, Wiernik PH. Neurotoxicity of antineoplastic drugs. *Semin Oncol.* 1982;**9**:103–130.

King ME, Pfeifle CE, Howell SB. Intraperitoneal cytosine arabinoside therapy in ovarian carcinoma. *J Clin Oncol.* 1984;**2**:662–669.

Lotze MT, Custer MC, Rosenberg SA. Intraperitoneal administration of interleukin-2 in patients with cancer. *Arch Surg.* 1986;**121**:1373–1379.

Macchiarini P, Hardin M, Angeletti CA. Long-term evaluation of intrapleural Bacillus Calmette-Guerin with or without adjuvant chemotherapy in completely resected stages II and III non-small cell lung cancer. *Am J Clin Oncol.* 1991;**14**:291–297.

Markman M. Intracavitary chemotherapy for malignant disease confined to body cavities. *West J Med.* 1985;**142**:364–368.

Markman M. Intraperitoneal antineoplastic agents for tumors principally confined to the peritoneal cavity. *Cancer Treat Rev.* 1986;**13**:219–242.

Markman M. Intraperitoneal "belly-bath" chemotherapy. In: Lokich JJ, ed. *Cancer Chemotherapy by Infusion.* Chicago: Precept Press; 1987:502–524.

Markman M, Cleary S, Howell SB, Lucas WE. Complications of extensive adhesion formation after intraperitoneal chemotherapy. *Surg Gynecol Obstet.* 1986a;**162**:445–448.

Markman M, Cleary S, Lucas WE, Howell SB. Intraperitoneal chemotherapy with high-dose cisplatin and cytosine arabinoside for refractory ovarian carcinoma and other malignancies principally involving the peritoneal cavity. *J Clin Oncol.* 1985;**3**:925–931.

Markman M, Cleary S, Lucas W, Weiss R, Howell SB. Ip chemotherapy employing a regimen of cisplatin, cytarabine, and bleomycin. *Cancer Treat Rep.* 1986b;**70**:755–760.

Markman M, Cleary S, Pfeifle C, et al. Cisplatin administered by the intracavitary route as treatment for malignant mesothelioma. *Cancer.* 1986c;**58**:18–21.

Markman M, Hakes T, Reichman B, et al. Intraperitoneal cisplatin and cytarabine in the treatment of refractory or recurrent ovarian carcinoma. *J Clin Oncol.* 1991a;**9**:204–210.

Markman M, Howell SB, Lucas WE, Pfeifle CE, Green MR. Combination intraperitoneal chemotherapy with cisplatin, cytarabine, and doxorubicin for refractory ovarian carcinoma and other malignancies principally confined to the peritoneal cavity. *J Clin Oncol.* 1984;**2**:1321–1326.

Markman MM, Rowinsky E, Hakes T, et al. Phase I study of taxol administered by the intraperitoneal route (abstract). *Proc Am Soc Clin Oncol.* 1991b;**10**:601.

Masuno T, Kishimoto S, Ogura T, et al. A comparative trial of LC9018 plus doxorubicin and doxorubicin alone for the treatment of malignant pleural effusion secondary to lung cancer. *Cancer.* 1991;**68**:1495–1500.

McVie JG, Dikhoff T, van der Heide J, et al. Tissue concentration of platinum after intraperitoneal cisplatin administration in patients (abstract). *Proc Am Assoc Cancer Res.* 1985;**26**:162.

Mellett LB. Physiochemical considerations and pharmacokinetic behavior in delivery of drugs to the central nervous system. *Cancer Treat Rep.* 1977;**61**:527–531.

Mueller S, Bell W, Seibert J. Cerebral calcifications associated with intrathecal methotrexate therapy in acute lymphocytic leukemia. *Pediatrics.* 1976;**83**:650–653.

Nies BA, Thomas LB, Friereich EJ. Meningeal leukemia. *Cancer.* 1965;**18**:546–553.

Ostrowski MJ. An assessment of the long-term results of controlling the reaccumulation of malignant effusions using intracavitary bleomycin. *Cancer.* 1986;**57**:721–727.

Ozols R. Intraperitoneal chemotherapy in the management of ovarian cancer. *Semin Oncol.* 1985;**12**(suppl 4):75–80.

Ozols RF, Locker GY, Doroshow JH, Grotzinger KR, Myers CE, Young RC. Pharmacokinetics of Adriamycin and tissue penetration in murine ovarian carcinoma. *Cancer Res.* 1979;**39**:3209–3214.

Ozols RF, Speyer JL, Jenkins J, Myers CE. Phase II trial of 5-FU administered Ip to patients with refractory ovarian cancer. *Cancer Treat Rep.* 1984;**68**:1229–1232.

Ozols RF, Young RC, Speyer JL, et al. Phase I and pharmacological studies of Adriamycin administered intraperitoneally to patients with ovarian cancer. *Cancer Res.* 1982;**42**:4265–4269.

Paladine W, Cunningham TJ, Sponzo R, Donavan M, Olson K, Horton J. Intracavitary bleomycin in the management of malignant effusions. *Cancer.* 1976;**38**:1903–1908.

Pfeifle CE, Howell SB, Markman M, Lucas WE. Totally implantable system for peritoneal access. *J Clin Oncol.* 1984;**2**:1277–1280.

Phillips PC. Methotrexate neurotoxicity. In: Rottenberg DA, ed. *Neurological Complications of Cancer Treatment.* Boston: Butterworth-Heinemann; 1991:115–123.

Phillips PC, Reinhard CS. Antipyrimidine neurotoxicity: Cytosine arabinoside and 5-fluorouracil. In: Rottenberg DA, ed. *Neurological Complications of Cancer Treatment.* Boston: Butterworth-Geinemann; 1991:97–118.

Piccart MJ, Speyer JL, Markman M, et al. Intraperitoneal chemotherapy: Technical experience at five institutions. *Semin Oncol.* 1985;**12**(suppl 4):90–96.

Piver MS, Lele SB, Marchetti DL, Baker TR, Emrich LJ, Hartman AB. Surgically documented response to intraperitoneal cisplatin, cytarabine, and bleomycin after intravenous cisplatin-based chemotherapy in advanced ovarian adenocarcinoma. *J Clin Oncol.* 1988;**6**:1679–1684.

Poplack DG, Brouwers P. Adverse sequelae of central nervous system therapy. *Clin Oncol.* 1985;**4**:263–270.

Price RA, Johnson WW. The central nervous system in childhood leukemia. I. The arachnoid. *Cancer.* 1973;**31**:520–533.

Rambaldi A, Introna M, Colotta F, et al. Intraperitoneal administration of interferon-beta in ovarian cancer patients. *Cancer.* 1985;**56**:294–301.

Reichman B, Markman M, Hakes T, et al. Phase I trial of concurrent intraperitoneal and continuous intravenous infusion of fluorouracil in patients with refractory cancer. *J Clin Oncol.* 1988;**6**:158–162.

Reichman B, Markman M, Hakes T, et al. Intraperitoneal cisplatin and etoposide in the treatment of refractory/recurrent ovarian carcinoma. *J Clin Oncol.* 1989;**7**:1327–1332.

Rosenshein N, Blake D, McIntyre P, et al. The effect of volume on the distribution of substances instilled into the peritoneal cavity. *Gynecol Oncol.* 1978;**6**:106–110.

Ruckdeschel JC, Moores D, Lee JY, et al. Intrapleural therapy for malignant pleural effusions. A randomized comparison of bleomycin and tetracycline. *Chest.* 1991;**100**:1528–1535.

Rusch VW, Figlin R, Godwin D, Piantadosi S. Intrapleural cisplatin and cytarabine in the management of malignant pleural effusions: A Lung Cancer Study Group trial. *J Clin Oncol.* 1991;**9**:313–319.

Rusch VW, Niedzwiecki D, Tao Y, et al. Intrapleural cisplatin and mitomycin for malignant mesothelioma following pleurectomy: Pharmacokinetic studies. *J Clin Oncol.* 1992;**10**:1001–1006.

Saiki JH, Thompson S, Smith F, et al. Paraplegia following intrathecal chemotherapy. *Cancer.* 1972;**29**:370–374.

Shapiro WR, Chernik NL, Posner JB. Necrotizing encephalopathy following intraventricle instillation of methotrexate. *Arch Neurol.* 1973;**28**:96–100.

Shapiro WR, Young DF, Mehta BM. Methotrexate distribution in cerebrospinal fluid after intravenous ventricular and lumbar injections. *N Engl J Med.* 1975;**293**:161–166.

Simmons ED, Somberg DA. Acute tumor lysis syndrome after intrathecal methotrexate administration. *Cancer.* 1991;**67**:2062–2065.

Speyer JL, Collins JM, Dedrick RL, et al. Phase I and pharmacological studies of 5-fluorouracil administered intraperitoneally. *Cancer Res.* 1980;**40**:567–572.

Speyer JL, Sugarbaker PH, Collins JM, Dedrick RL, Klecker RW Jr, Myers CE. Portal levels and hepatic clearance of 5-fluorouracil after intraperitoneal administration in humans. *Cancer Res.* 1981;**41**:1916–1922.

Strong JM, Collins JM, Lester C, et al. Pharmacokinetics of intraventricular and intravenous N, N', N", triethylene-thio-phosphoramide (Thiotepa) in Rhesus monkeys and humans. *Cancer Res.* 1986;**46**:6101–6104.

Sugarbaker PH, Cunliffe WJ, Belliveau J, et al. Rationale for integrating early postoperative intraperitoneal chemotherapy into the surgical treatment of gastrointestinal cancer. *Semin Oncol.* 1989;**16**(suppl 6): 83–97.

Sugarbaker PH, Gianola FJ, Speyer JC, Wesley R, Barofsky I, Meyers CE. Prospective, randomized trial of intravenous versus intraperitoneal 5-fluorouracil in patients with advanced primary colon or rectal cancer. *Surgery.* 1985;**98**:414–421.

Surbone A, Myers CE. Principles and practice of intraperitoneal therapy. *Antibiot Chemother.* 1988;**40**:14–25.

ten Bokkel Huinink WW, Dubbelman R, Aartsen E, Franklin H, McVie JG. Experimental and clinical results with intraperitoneal cisplatin. *Semin Oncol.* 1985;**12**(suppl 4): 43–46.

Vlasveld LT, Gallee MPW, Rodenhuis S, Taal BG. Intraperitoneal chemotherapy for malignant peritoneal mesothelioma. *Eur J Cancer.* 1991;**27**:732–734.

Winick NJ, Bowman WP, Kamen BA, et al. Unexpected acute neurologic toxicity in the treatment of children with acute lymphoblastic leukemia. *J Natl Cancer Inst.* 1992;**84**:252–256.

Wolf BE, Sugarbaker PH. Intraperitoneal chemotherapy and immunotherapy. *Recent Results Cancer Res.* 1988;**110**:254–273.

Zimm S, Collins JM, Curt GA, et al. Cerebral spinal fluid pharmacokinetics of intraventricular and intravenous aziridinylbenzoquinone. *Cancer Res.* 1984;**44**:1696–1701.

Chapter 6

Pharmacologic Management of Vesicant Chemotherapy Extravasations

Robert T. Dorr

Most chemotherapy agents are not ulcerogenic (vesicants) if inadvertently extravasated or otherwise delivered outside the vascular compartment. Table 6.1 summarizes these nonvesicant agents, which include most of the antimetabolites, a few alkylating agents, all of the hormonal agents, and all of the protein-based agents. A separate category of anticancer agents can be classified as local irritants with the potential to cause soft tissue ulcers only if a large amount of concentrated drug solution is inadvertently extravasated (Table 6.2). These irritant agents include a variety of nonclassic alkylating agents and the DNA-binding drugs mitoxantrone and plicamycin. The final category of true vesicants includes the vinca alkaloids, several alkylating agents, and the DNA-intercalating anthracycline antibiotics (Table 6.3).

Procedures used to minimize the likelihood of extravasation include (1) the administration of vesicants only by personnel specifically trained and experienced in oncology practice; (2) continuous monitoring of intravenous infusions using serial blood return challenges and constant patient/site assessment during an infusion; (3) interruption of an infusion for such evaluations at the first sign of discomfort, altered infusion flow, or a local reaction; (4) the use of central vein vascular access devices; and (5) the rapid use of defined local antidotes for different vesicant drugs. Specific guidelines for chemotherapy administration are reviewed in Chapter 4 and this chapter focuses on the pharmacologic management of vesicant chemotherapy extravasations.

VASCULAR ACCESS DEVICES

The use of central venous access devices (CVADs), either subcutaneous implanted ports or peripherally inserted (central) catheters (PIC lines), clearly reduces but does not eliminate the risk of inadvertent drug extravasation. In one series of over 329 procedures in 300 patients, an extravasation incidence of 6.4% was described (Brothers et al 1988). Several cases of drug extravasation from CVADs were also described by Reed et al (1985). In this instance, necrosis occurred on the chest wall following the extravasation of fluoropyrimidine solutions. Central venous ports and catheters may leak as a result of (1) catheter separation from the port body, (2) a nick in the outflow catheter, (3) a rupture or tear in the port septum, (4) excessive backpressure around the needle due to a fibrin sheath at the catheter outflow tip (Gemlo et al 1988), and (5) incomplete or no penetration of the injection needle through the port septum. In addition, spontaneous retraction of the catheter tip from the subclavian vein has also been reported (Meranze et al 1988). Thus, CVADs should not be considered foolproof with respect to drug extravasation.

DNA-INTERCALATING AGENTS

The DNA-intercalating agents include some of the most commonly used anticancer agents such as doxorubicin, daunorubicin, dactinomycin, and mitoxantrone. These agents bind noncovalently to DNA and have relatively long plasma half-lives and even longer tissue half-lives.

Doxorubicin

Doxorubicin given by peripheral vein infusion has a reported extravasation incidence of 0.5% (Laughlin et al 1979) up to 6.5% (Barlock et al 1979). The drug can also cause local venous flare reactions in up to 3% of peripheral vein infusions (Etcubanas and Wilbur 1974, Souhami and Feld 1978, Vogelzang 1979). These common reactions are characterized by delayed venous erythema and itching from local histamine release and do not connote serious sequelae. In contrast, doxorubicin extravasations are characterized by severe pain and swelling. Symptoms are usually immediate in onset although extravasations

TABLE 6.1. NONVESICANT CHEMOTHERAPAY AGENTS

Class	Specific Agent
Antimetabolites	Cytarabine
	Methotrexate
	Pentostatin
Alkylating agents	Cyclophosphamide
	Thiophosphoramide
	Melphalan
Biologics	Granulocyte colony-stimulating factor[a]
	Granulocyte–macrophage colony-stimulating factor[a]
	Tumor necrosis factor[a]
	Interleukin-2[a]
	Interferons alpha, beta, and gamma
Miscellaneous	Bleomycin
	L-Asparaginase
Hormonal agents	Hydrocortisone
	Dexamethasone
	Methylprednisone
	Testosterone
	Leuprolide
	Goserelin

[a]Occasional local site irritation.

TABLE 6.2. OCCASIONAL LOCAL IRRITANT ANTICANCER AGENTS AND/OR AGENTS WITH A WEAK VESICANT POTENTIAL[a]

Class	Specific Agent	References
Antimetabolites	Fluorouracil	Teta and O'Connor 1984
		Reed et al 1985
		Seyfer and Solimando 1983
	Floxuridine	Reed et al 1985
DNA-intercalating antibiotics	Menogaril	McGovren et al 1984
		Sessa et al 1988
	Aclacinomycins	Preuss and Partoft 1987
	Mitoxantrone	Dorr et al 1986
		Von Hoff et al 1980
		Peters et al 1987
	Liposomal doxorubicin	Forssen and Tokes 1983
		Balazsovits et al 1989
Epipodophyllotoxins	Etoposide	Preuss and Partoft 1987
		Dorr and Alberts 1983b
	Teniposide	Dorr and Alberts 1983b
Alkylating or DNA-binding agents	Cisplatin	Buchanan et al 1985
		Dorr et al 1986
		Leyden and Sullivan 1986
		Lewis and Medina 1980
		Algarra et al 1986
	Dacarbazine	Dorr et al 1987
	Carmustine	DeVita et al 1965
		Dorr 1990
Miscellaneous	Bleomycin	Seyfer and Solimando 1983
		Preuss and Partoft 1987

[a]Soft tissue ulceration is rare unless doses near the MTD are extravasated in a concentrated solution.

TABLE 6.3. VESICANT ANTICANCER AGENTS

Class/Specific Agent	Clinical Comment	Reference
Alkylating Agents		
Mechlorethamine (nitrogen mustard)	Causes phlebitis and immediate pain if extravasated; lesions heal poorly	Chait and Dinner 1975 Goodman et al 1946
Mitomycin-C	Symptoms are sometimes delayed months; skin lesions rarely develop distal to injection site; lesions can expand over weeks	
DNA-intercalating antibiotics		
Doxorubicin	Usually immediate pain; lesions form slowly over weeks and expand locally over months	Rudolph et al 1976 Reilly et al 1977 Barlock et al 1979 Linder et al 1983
	Long tissue retention of unchanged drug	Sonneveld et al 1984 Garnick et al 1981 Dorr et al 1989
Daunorubicin	Same as doxorubicin	Dragon and Braine 1979
Dactinomycin	Same as doxorubicin	Moore et al 1958 Frei 1974
Vinca alkaloids		
Vincristine	Painful ulceration with slow healing and local paresthesia	James and George 1964
Vinblastine	Same as vincristine	Preuss and Partoft 1987 Larson 1982
Vindesine	Occasionally delayed onset of symptoms; otherwise like the other vinca alkaloids	Dorr and Jones 1979

into chest wall tissues can be much less noticeable (author's unpublished observations). Doxorubicin skin reactions can also "recall" or synergize with prior radiotherapy-induced skin toxicity and/or prior doxorubicin therapy. This synergy may involve (1) overlapping mechanisms of action involving oxygen free radical production and (2) the relatively long retention of doxorubicin in the DNA of affected cells. Thus, repeated doxorubicin injections can sometimes cause prior healed extravasation sites to react with pain, swelling, and rarely tissue necrosis even though the drug is unquestionably administered into a patent vein distal to the prior site. Fortunately, this occurrence is rare and idiosyncratic.

If a doxorubicin extravasation is suspected (poor blood return, local pain and swelling), the indwelling needle should be used to evacuate extravasated fluid, if possible, from the site. The needle can then be removed. Surgical follow-up of doxorubicin extravasations is indicated in patients with residual pain and swelling at the site 2 weeks after the event (Larson 1982). If surgery is required, a wide local excision of involved tissue is needed to facilitate engraftment and to remove entrapped drug. Pharmacologic studies have documented prolonged local retention of high concentrations of intact (unchanged) drug (Garnick et al 1981, Sonneveld et al 1984, Dorr et al 1989). Thus, surgery can act to remove drug from the site to halt further expansion of a necrotic lesion. For this reason, early surgical consultation is recommended if pain and swelling persist for several weeks after the extravasation. Clearly, the development of an open ulcer represents a very late stage in the evolution of any extravasation lesion and should not be used as the criterion for definitive reconstructive surgery.

Antidotes to Doxorubicin Extravasation

A variety of pharmacologic antidotes to doxorubicin extravasation have been experimentally evaluated (Dorr 1990). Unfortunately, the only agents that chemically inactivate this drug, the radical morpholinyl dimers of Koch and Averbuch, are not available for clinical use (Averbuch et al 1985, 1986, 1988). Glucocorticosteroids such as hydrocortisone have been used anecdotally (Rudolph et al 1976, Reilly et al 1977, Barlock et al 1979) but lack a clear pharmacologic rationale for use as doxorubicin antidotes (Luedke et al 1979, Petro et al 1979, Cohen 1979). Furthermore, glucocorticosteroids in high concentrations can be locally deleterious (Dorr et al 1980). Other ineffective local antidotes include sodium bicarbonate (Dorr et al 1980, Petro et al 1979, Upton et al 1986, Coleman et al 1983, Ignoffo et al 1981) and other agents including antihistamines, lidocaine, and N-acetylcysteine (Dorr et al 1981). Experimental antidotes that have not been clinically tested include β-adrenergics (Dorr and Alberts 1981), antioxidants such as butylated hydroxytoluene (BHT [Babich 1982, Daugherty and Khurana 1985]) and dimethylsulfoxide with vitamin E (Ludwig et al 1987).

Dimethylsulfoxide. In contrast, the antioxidant dimethylsulfoxide (DMSO) has been evaluated as a topical antidote in both experimental and clinical settings. Complete protection from experimental doxorubicin skin ulceration was described in studies in a pig model (Desai and Teres 1982) and a rat model (Svingen et al 1981), but not mice (Dorr and Alberts 1983a). Of note, one negative trial of topical DMSO in the pig model has also been described (Van Sloten-Harwood and Bachur, 1987). In contrast, several anecdotal clinical case reports have also described protection from doxorubicin ulceration with combination antidote regimens containing topical DMSO (Lawrence and Goodnight 1983, Olver and Schwarz 1983). A seminal prospective clinical trial also showed efficacy for 99% DMSO solution (1.5 mL) applied topically every 6 hours for 14 days (Olver et al 1988). In this trial, none of 20 patients experiencing an anthracycline (doxorubicin or daunorubicin) extravasation developed significant local toxicity. The DMSO treatments did not prevent some initial pain and swelling, and DMSO apparently caused a transient burning sensation with erythema and urticaria (Olver et al 1988).

Topical Cooling. Topical cooling has also been shown to be highly effective against experimental and clinical doxorubicin extravasation injuries. Cooling dramatically reduces experimental skin lesions in both mice (Dorr et al 1985a) and in pigs (Van Sloten-Harwood and Bachur 1987). Conversely, mild topical heating synergistically increases experimental doxorubicin skin lesions (Dorr et al 1985a), and heat increases doxorubicin tumor cell cytotoxicity in vitro (Ohnoshi et al 1985). Sunlight also appears to increase the severity of doxorubicin extravasation reactions. Cooling is also known to be effective at blocking doxorubicin-induced alopecia in patients with solid tumors (Dean et al 1979). Topical cooling does not reduce doxorubicin skin concentrations (Dorr et al 1985a), but rather may alter cell membrane fluidity to block doxorubicin cellular uptake and lethality (Lane et al 1987).

Other DNA Intercalators

The related anthracycline daunorubicin is also a vesicant but antidote studies are largely unavailable (Lippman et al 1972, Greene et al 1972, Dragon and Braine 1979). A single experimental antidote trial in a mouse model has suggested limited efficacy for topical DMSO (Soble et al 1987). The modified doxorubicin analogs epirubicin, esorubicin, and idarubicin appear to have substantially reduced clinical extravasation risks; however, all of these compounds are potent experimental vesicants and esorubicin is known to produce a high incidence of venous flare reaction (Leek et al 1987). The cyanomorpholinyl derivatives of doxorubicin have significantly increased vesicant potency along with enhanced antitumor potency (Johnston et al 1983). In contrast, liposomal encapsulated doxorubicin possesses much less vesicant potential (Forssen and Tokes 1983). The semisynthetic anthracycline antibiotic menogaril produces potent vesicant reactions in experimental animals (Averbuch et al 1988), but clinical extravasations have not produced necrosis (Dorr et al 1985b). More commonly, menogaril causes phlebitis and swelling along the vein used for infusion. These symptoms typically resolve after 1 to 2 weeks but a residual hard, palpable venous "cord" may remain over the affected vein. This reaction may increase if highly concentrated solutions greater than 1 mg/mL are used or if infusion times are prolonged (more than 2 hours).

Other DNA intercalating agents with vesicant potential include dactinomycin, amsacrine, and mitoxantrone. Extravasation necrosis from dactinomycin has been characterized in experimental animals (Barr et al 1981, Buchanan et al 1985, Soble et al 1987) and in patients (Moore et al 1958, Frei 1974). These lesions develop and expand slowly and, like doxorubicin lesions, can synergize or "recall" prior reactions with radiotherapy or earlier drug therapy. Unfortunately, experimental studies in rodents could not demonstrate efficacy for a large number of potential antidotes including DMSO, cold, thiosulfate, hyaluronidase, and β-adrenergic agents (Buchanan et al 1985, Soble et al 1987).

Amsacrine has similarly produced experimental extravasation necrosis in animal models (Henry et al 1980) and in at least one clinical case (Legha et al 1978). The drug also produces a high incidence of phlebitis (Louie and Issell 1985). Clinical antidotes are not known for amsacrine, although topical DMSO was active in a mouse model and should probably be evaluated in the clinic (Soble et al 1987).

Mitoxantrone is an anthracene-based DNA-intercalating agent with a very low propensity to cause extravasation necrosis in humans (Dorr 1990). In the mouse model, intradermal mitoxantrone was a nonvesicant (Dorr et al 1986). Soft tissue necrosis is described in only 3 of 13 (23%) cases of mitoxantrone extravasation (Dorr 1990). One of these lesions spontaneously resolved without any therapy (Khoury 1986). Typically, mitoxantrone extravasations produce only a blue discoloration of the skin, but in two cases, surgery was required to excise a 4 (x) 6-cm lesion in one patient (Peters et al 1987) and a residual flexion deformity of the elbow in another patient (Khoury 1986). Antidotes to mitoxantrone extravasation are not known.

ALKYLATING AGENTS

As summarized in Table 6.3, several DNA alkylating or binding agents are also consistent vesicants if extravasated. The prototype bifunctional alkylator mechlorethamine is a well-known vesicant which causes immediate severe pain and protracted necrosis if extravasated. These lesions can widen and not undergo healing for months if untreated (Chait and Dinner 1975). The preferred systemic antidote to mechlorethamine extravasations is sodium thiosulfate in a $\frac{1}{6}$ or 0.17 M (isotonic) concentration. This sulfur nucleophile provides an alternative target for alkylation by mechlorethamine to form nontoxic thioethers which can be excreted into the urine. Thiosulfate is effective as a systemic antidote (Bonadonna and Karnofsky 1965) or as an experimental local extravasation antidote (Dorr et al 1988). It has shown clinical efficacy in preventing soft tissue damage from an accidental intramuscular injection of mechlorethamine (Owen et al 1980). Studies in mice suggest that rapid use following mechlorethamine extravasation is vital for maximal efficacy (Dorr et al 1988). Also, a double-strength solution of 0.34 M was much more active in the mouse model (Dorr et al 1988). Neither heat nor cooling aided mechlorethamine-induced ulcer healing.

CISPLATIN

The platinum-containing agent cisplatin has rarely produced extravasation necrosis and only when large amounts of a highly concentrated solution are extravasated. Cisplatin-induced necrosis has been reported after leakage of up to 100 mL of 0.75 mg/mL solution into the dorsum of the hand (Leyden and Sullivan 1986). A large necrotic lesion subsequently developed over several weeks and required surgical debridement and skin grafts to effect healing. In another case an arterial extravasation of a 1 mg/mL solution led to a 3-cm black eschar after 1 month. This lesion developed in spite of the use of topical antibiotics and glucocorticosteroids (Leyden and Sullivan 1986). In contrast, cisplatin is only weakly ulcerogenic in mice (Dorr et al 1986). Fortunately, $\frac{1}{6}$ M sodium thiosulfate is an effective cisplatin antagonist (Howell and Taetle 1980) and would be useful in treating a large cisplatin extravasation; however, unless a large volume (> 20 mL) of concentrated solution (> 0.5 mg/mL) is extravasated, probably no therapy is needed.

MITOMYCIN-C

The natural product alkylator mitomycin-C is a potent vesicant which can cause unusually delayed symptoms in some patients. In one series, the average time to the onset of local tissue toxicity following mitomycin-C extravasation was about 3 months (Wood and Ellerhorst-Ryan 1984, Aizawa and Tagami 1987). There are also reports of reactions distal to the site of drug administration following uneventful venous injections (Johnston-Early and Cohen 1981). Mitomycin skin ulcers involve a crescendo of pain and can slowly enlarge over weeks (Argenta and Manders 1983). Sunlight is known to aggravate these lesions (Fuller et al 1981). Surgical debridement is necessary once lesions have developed, and the clinical use of corticosteroids does not prevent ulceration (Argenta and Manders 1983). Experimental studies in mice have confirmed that steroids are ineffective but some antidotal activity was noted with $\frac{1}{3}$ M sodium thiosulfate or the radical morpholinyl dimers (moderate protection). Surprisingly, topical DMSO provided complete protection in the mouse skin model (Dorr et al 1986). Ineffective mitomycin-C antidotes included hyaluronidase, hydrocortisone, vitamin E, N-acetylcysteine, and diphenydramine. Topical DMSO has also been shown to be effective in three clinical cases (Alberts and Dorr 1991). In this brief series a 99% (w/v) solution of DMSO was applied to the site every 6 hours for at least 14 consecutive days. This is the same DMSO schedule used with doxorubicin extravasations (Olver et al 1988). A single application of DMSO was not effective in one case report (Herrera and Burnham 1989). Confirmatory trials of DMSO using the commercial 50% (w/v) solution are clearly needed. Nonetheless, DMSO applied topically does not produce any significant toxicity and therefore might be useful in treating mitomycin-C extravasations until more definitive antidote information is available.

Other alkylators that cause occasional local toxicity include dacarbazine, the nitrosourea carmustine, ifosfamide, and carboplatin (Marnocha and Hutson, 1992). In experimental models neither DTIC nor BCNU produces extravasation necrosis. In the clinic both agents are known to cause phlebitis and local site irritation; however, neither drug is associated with extravasation necrosis and thus these drugs should be classified as irritant but not vesicant drugs.

VINCA ALKALOIDS AND EPIPODOPHYLLOTOXINS

Vinca alkaloids and epipodophyllotoxins constitute the final major category of vesicant and irritant anticancer drugs, respectively. The epipodophyllotoxins include etoposide and teniposide, which are potent inhibitors of DNA topoisomerase II enzymes. Neither drug is a true vesicant although both are associated with local venous reactions consisting of phlebitis, urticaria, and erythemia (Rozencweig et al 1977). Much of this toxicity is due to the lipophilic solvents used in the commercial drug formulations. Indeed in the mouse, intradermal injections of the teniposide solvent system alone produce small local ulcers which healed rapidly (Dorr and Alberts 1983b). The enzyme hyaluronidase injected proximally was found to completely prevent these lesions (Dorr and Alberts 1983b). This enzyme is available in a highly purified form derived from bovine testes. It acts to dissolve hyaluronic acid bonds in tissues to expand the interstitial space, thereby creating a larger surface area for drug absorption. For most epipodophyllotoxin extravasations, however, hyaluronidase is not necessary as these drugs are usually only mild irritants.

With the vinca alkaloids vincristine and vinblastine, serious soft tissue ulcers can result from even small extravasations. These reactions are usually noted by immediate pain and swelling but occasionally symptoms are delayed for several hours. This was noted with the vinblastine derivative vindesine (Dorr and Jones 1979). More commonly vinca alkaloid skin lesions form blisters after a few days and evolve slowly over weeks to necrotic ulcers. These are unlike doxorubicin lesions in that some healing may eventually occur even though neurologic sequelae may remain. These symptoms include tingling paresthesias and sensory deficits at the site which may be permanent. Although there are anecdotal reports on the use of corticosteroids to treat vinca extravasations (Choy 1979, Bellone 1981), hydrocortisone was found to significantly increase vinca skin ulceration in a quantitative mouse model (Dorr and Alberts 1985). Other purported vinca antidotes have included glutamic acid (Vaitkevicius et al 1962), sodium bicarbonate (Ignoffo et al 1981), and hyaluronidase (Johnson et al 1963). This last antidote was found to be highly effective at preventing ulcers in a mouse model wherein the enzyme was shown to promote very rapid dispersal of [^{3}H]-vinblastine from the local skin site (Dorr and Alberts 1985). Mild local warming was also effective, whereas cooling significantly increased vinca skin toxicity. Other ineffective antidotes in the mouse model included leucovorin, diphenhydramine, hydrocortisone, bicarbonate, and vitamin A.

CONCLUSIONS

Only a few antidotes have proven efficacy at reducing vesicant cancer drug extravasation injuries. These antidotes are summarized in Table 6.4 and should be readily available in the clinic as delayed treatment with most antidotes is ineffective. Confirmatory trials are needed to assess the efficacy of topical DMSO for anthracyclines and mitomycin-C. A particularly pertinent question is whether the commercially available 50% solution (Rimso 50^R) is as efficacious as the more concentrated solutions used in the experimental and early clinical trials. On the other hand, none of the recommended antidotes produce serious intrinsic toxicities. Thus, their use should not be impaired by concern over increased local tissue damage. It must also be remembered that not all vesicant drug extravasations will produce local necrosis. In Larson's series (1982), only

TABLE 6.4. RECOMMENDED EXTRAVASATION ANTIDOTES

Class/Specific Agents	Local Antidote Recommended	Specific Procedure

Alkylating agents
  Cisplatin[a]
  Mechlorethamine
	$\frac{1}{6}$ or $\frac{1}{3}$ M sodium thiosulfate	Mix 4–8 mL 10% sodium thiosulfate U.S.P. with 6 mL of sterile water for injection, U.S.P. for a $\frac{1}{6}$ or $\frac{1}{3}$ M solution. Inject 2 mL into site for each milligram of mechlorethamine or 100 mg of cisplatin extravasated.

Mitomycin-C	Dimethylsulfoxide 50–99% (w/v)	Apply 1.5 mL to the site every 6 hours for 14 days. Allow to air-dry; do not cover.
DNA intercalators Doxorubicin, daunorubicin, amsacrine	Cold compresses	Apply immediately for 30–60 minutes, then alternate off/on every 15 minutes for 1 day.
	Dimethylsulfoxide 50–99% (w/v) solution	Apply 1.5 mL to the site every 6 hours for 14 days. Allow to air-dry; do not cover.
Vinca alkaloids Vinblastine, vincristine	Warm compresses Hyaluronidase	Apply immediately for 30–60 minutes, then alternate off/on every 15 minutes for 1 day. Inject 150 U hyaluronidase (Wydase, others) into site.
Epipodophyllotoxins[a] Etoposide, teniposide	Warm compresses Hyaluronidase	Apply immediately for 30–60 minutes, then alternate off/on every 15 min for 1 day. Inject 150 U hyaluronidase (Wydase, others) into site.

[a]Treatment indicated only for large extravasations (eg, doses one half or more of the planned total dose for that course of therapy).

one third of all vesicant extravasations produced local tissue breakdown. Thus, it is easy to be misguided by anecdotal case reports of antidotal efficacy as 67% of patients may have a good outcome with only conservative therapy. Finally, early surgical referral for evolving lesions is of utmost importance to prevent further damage. With agents such as doxorubicin, surgical tissue excision can remove substantial drug quantities and thereby spare adjacent tissues.

A combined approach to vesicant drug extravasation is recommended: early detection to halt further drug delivery, rapid use of experimentally proven antidotes, and early surgical excision for evolving lesions.

REFERENCES

Aizawa H, Tagami H. Delayed tissue necrosis due to mitomycin-C. *Acta Dermato venereol* (Stock). 1987;**67**:364–366.

Alberts DS, Dorr RT. Case Report: Topical DMSO for mitomycin C-induced skin ulceration. *Oncol Nurs Forum* 1991;**19**:693–695.

Algarra SM, Dy C, Bilbao I, Aparicio LA. Cutaneous necrosis after intra-arterial treatment with cisplatin. *Cancer Treat Rep.* 1986;**70**:687–688.

Argenta LC, Manders EK. Mitomycin-C extravasation injuries. *Cancer.* 1983;**51**:1080–1082.

Averbuch SD, Boldt M, Gaudiano G, et al. Experimental chemotherapy-induced skin necrosis in swine: Mechanistic studies of anthracycline antibiotic toxicity and protection with a radical dimer compound. *J Clin Invest.* 1988;**81**:142–148.

Averbuch SD, Gaudiano G, Koch TH, Bachur NR. Radical dimer rescue of toxicity and improved therapeutic index of Adriamycin in tumor-bearing mice. *Cancer Res.* 1985;**45**:6200–6204.

Averbuch SD, Gaudiano G, Koch TH, Bachur NR. Doxorubicin-induced skin necrosis in the swine model: Protection with a novel radical dimer. *J Clin Oncol.* 1986;**4**(1):88–94.

Babich H. Butylated hydroxytoluene (BHT): A review. *Environ Res* 1982;**29**:1–21.

Barlock AL, Howser DM, Hubbard SM. Nursing management of Adriamycin extravasation. *Am J Nurs.* 1979;**137**:94–96.

Balazsovits JAE, Mayer LD, Bally MB, et al. Analysis of the effect of liposome encapsulation on the vesicant properties, acute and cardiac toxicities, and antitumor efficacy of doxorubicin. *Cancer Chemother Pharmacol* 1989;**23**:81–86.

Barr RD, Benton SG, Belbeck LW. Soft tissue necrosis induced by extravasated cancer chemotherapeutic agents. *J Natl Cancer Inst.* 1981;**66**:1129–1136.

Barr RD, Sertic J. Soft-tissue necrosis induced by extravasated cancer chemotherapeutic agents: A study of active intervention. *Br J Cancer.* 1981;**44**:267–269.

Bellone JD. Treatment of vincristine extravasation (letter). *JAMA.* 1981;**245**:343.

Bonadonna G, Karnofsky DA. Protection studies with sodium thiosulfate against methyl bis(β-chloroethyl) amine hydrochloride (HN$_2$) and its ethyleneimmonium derivative. *Clin Pharmacol Ther.* 1965; **6**(1):50–64.

Brothers TE, Niederhuber JE, Roberts JA, Ensminger WD. Experience with subcutaneous infusion ports in three hundred patients. *Surg Gynecol Obstet.* 1988;**166(4)**:295–301.

Buchanan GR, Buchsbaum HJ, O'Banion K, Gojer B. Extravasation of dactinomycin, vincristine, and cisplatin: Studies in an animal model. *Med Pediatr Oncol.* 1985;**13**:375–380.

Chait LA, Dinner MI. Ulceration caused by cytotoxic drugs. *South Afr Med J.* 1975;**49**:1935–1936.

Choy DS. Effective treatment of inadvertent intramuscular administration of vincristine (letter). *JAMA.* 1979; **241**:695.

Cohen MH. Amelioration of Adriamycin skin necrosis: An experimental study. *Cancer Treat Rep.* 1979;**63**(6):1003–1004.

Coleman JJ, Walker AP, Didolkar MS. Treatment of adriamycin-induced skin ulcers: A prospective controlled study. *J Surg Oncol* 1983;**22**:129–135.

Daugherty JP, Khurana A. Amelioration of doxorubicin-induced skin necrosis in mice by butylated hydroxytoluene. *Cancer Chemother Pharmacol.* 1985; **14**:243–246.

Dean JC, Salmon SE, Griffith KS. Prevention of doxorubicin-induced hair loss with scalp hypothermia. *N Engl J Med.* 1979;**301**(26):1427–1429.

Desai MH, Teres D. Prevention of doxorubicin-induced skin ulcers in the rat and pig with dimethyl sulfoxide (DMSO). *Cancer Treat Rep.* 1982;**66**(6):1371–1374.

DeVita VT, Carbone PP, Owens AH Jr, et al. Clinical trials with 1, 3-bis (2-chloroethyl)-1-nitrosourea, NSC-409962. *Cancer Res.* 1965;**25**:1876–1881.

Dorr RT. Antidotes to vesicant chemotherapy extravasations. *Blood Reviews* 1990;**4**:41–60.

Dorr RT, Alberts DS. Pharmacologic antidotes to experimental doxorubicin skin toxicity: A suggested role for beta-adrenergic compounds. *Cancer Treat Rep.* 1981; **65**(11/12):1001–1006.

Dorr RT, Alberts DS, Einspahr J, Mason-Liddil N, Soble MJ. Experimental dacarbazine antitumor activity and skin toxicity in relation to light exposure and pharmacologic antidotes. *Cancer Treat Rep* 1987;**71**:267–272.

Dorr RT, Alberts DS. Failure of DMSO and vitamin E to prevent doxorubicin skin ulceration in the mouse. *Cancer Treat Rep.* 1983a;**67**(5):499–501.

Dorr RT, Alberts DS. Skin ulceration potential without therapeutic anticancer activity for epipodophyllotoxin commercial diluents. *Invest New Drugs.* 1983b;**1**:151–159.

Dorr RT, Alberts DS. Vinca alkaloid skin toxicity: Antidote and drug disposition studies in the mouse. *J Natl Cancer Inst.* 1985;**74**:113–120.

Dorr RT, Alberts DS, Chen HSG. The limited role of corticosteroids in ameliorating experimental doxorubicin skin toxicity in the mouse. *Cancer Chemother Pharmacol.* 1980;**5**:17–20.

Dorr RT, Alberts DS, Stone A. Cold protection and heat enhancement of doxorubicin skin toxicity in the mouse. *Cancer Treat Rep.* 1985a;**69**(4):431–437.

Dorr RT, Dordal MS, Koenig LM, et al. High doxorubicin tissue levels in a patient experiencing extravasation during a four day infusion. *Cancer.* 1989;**64**(12):2462–2464.

Dorr RT, Jones SE. Inapparent infiltrations associated with vindesine administration. *Med Pediatr Oncol.* 1979;**6**:285–288.

Dorr RT, Soble M, Alberts DS. Efficacy of sodium thiosulfate as a local antidote to mechlorethamine skin toxicity in the mouse. *Cancer Chemother Pharmacol.* 1988;**22**:299–302.

Dorr RT, Soble M, Liddil JD, Keller JH. Mitomycin-C skin toxicity studies in mice: Reduced ulceration and altered pharmacokinetics with topical dimethyl sulfoxide. *J Clin Oncol.* 1986;**4**(9):1399–1404.

Dorr A Von Hoff D, Kuhn J, Kisner D. Phase I clinical trial of menogaril (abstract). *Proc Am Soc Clin Oncol.* 1985b;**4**:39.

Dragon LH, Braine HG. Necrosis of the hand after daunorubicin infusion distal to an arteriovenous fistula. *Ann Intern Med.* 1979;**91**:58–59.

Etcubanas E, Wilbur JR. Uncommon side effects of Adriamycin (NSC-123127). *Cancer Chemother Rep Pt 1.* 1974;**58**(6):757–758.

Forssen EA, Tokes ZA. Attenuation of dermal toxicity of doxorubicin by liposome encapsulation. *Cancer Treat Rep.* 1983;**67**(5):481–484.

Frei E. The clinical use of actinomycin. *Cancer Chemother Rep.* 1974;**58**(1):49–54.

Fuller B, Lind M, Bonomi P. Mitomycin-C extravasation exacerbated by sunlight. *Ann Intern Med.* 1981;**94**(4):542.

Garnick M, Israel M, Knetarpal IV, Luce J. Persistence of anthracycline levels following dermal and subcutaneous Adriamycin extravasation (abstract). *Proc Am Soc Clin Oncol.* 1981;**22**:173.

Gemlo BT, Rayner AA, Swanson RJ, et al. Extravasation: A serious complication of the split-sheath introducer technique for venous access. *Arch Surg* 1988;**123**:490–492.

Goodman LS, Wintrobe MM, Dameshek M. Nitrogen mustard therapy. *J Amer Med Assoc* 1946;**132**:126–132.

Greene W, Huffman D, Wiernik PH, et al. High dose daunorubicin therapy for acute nonlymphocytic leukemia: Correlation of response and toxicity with pharmacokinetics and intracellular daunorubicin reductase activity. *Cancer.* 1972;**30**:1419–1427.

Henry MC, Port CD, Levine BS. Preclinical toxicologic evaluation of 4'-(9-acridinylamino) methanesulfon-*m*-

anisidide (AMSA) in mice, dogs, and monkeys. *Cancer Treat Rep.* 1980;**64**(8/9):855–860.

Herrera D, Burnham D. DMSO and extravasation of mitomycin. *Oncol Nurs Forum.* 1989;**16**:155.

Howell SB, Taetle R. Effect of sodium thiosulfate on *cis*-dichlorodiammineplatinum (II) toxicity and antitumor activity in L1210 leukemia. *Cancer Treat Rep.* 1980;**64**(4/5):611–616.

Ignoffo RJ, Friedman MA. Therapy of local toxicities caused by extravasation of cancer chemotherapeutic drugs. *Cancer Treat Rev.* 1980;**7**:17–27.

Ignoffo RJ, Tomlin W, Rubinstein E, Friedman MA. A model for skin toxicity of antineoplastic drugs: Doxorubicin (DOX), mitomycin-C (MMC), and vincristine (VCR). *Clin Res.* 1981;**29**(2):437A.

James DH, George P. Vincristine in children with malignant solid tumors. *J Pediatr* 1964;**64**:534–541.

Johnson IS, Armstrong JG, Gorman M, Burnett JP Jr. The vinca alkaloids: A new class of oncolytic agents. *Cancer Res.* 1963;**23**:1390–1427.

Johnston-Early A, Cohen M. Mitomycin-C–induced skin ulceration remote from infusion site. *Cancer Treat Rep.* 1981;**65**:5–6.

Johnston JB, Habernicht B, Acton EM, Glazer RI. 3'-(3-cyano-4-morpholinyl)-3'-deamino adriamycin: A new anthracycline with intense potency. *Biochemical Pharmacol* 1983;**32**:3255–3258.

Khoury GG. Local tissue damage as a result of extravasation of mitozantrone. *Br Med J.* 1986;**292**:802.

Lane P, Vichi P, Bain DL, Tritton TR. Temperature dependence studies of Adriamycin uptake and cytotoxicity. *Cancer Res.* 1987;**47**:4038–4042.

Larson DL. Treatment of tissue extravasation by antitumor agents. *Cancer.* 1982;**49**:1796–1799.

Laughlin RA, Landeen JM, Habal MB. The management of inadvertent subcutaneous Adriamycin infiltration. *Am J Surg.* 1979;**137**:408–412.

Lawrence HJ, Goodnight SH Jr. Dimethyl sulfoxide and extravasation of anthracycline agents. *Ann Int Med.* 1983;**98**:1025.

Leek M, Dorr RT, Robertone A. High incidence of local venous reactions to esorubicin. *Invest New Drugs* 1987;**5**:43–47.

Legha SS, Gutterman JU, Hall SW. Phase I clinical investigation of 4'-(9-acridinylamino)methansulfon-*m*-anisidide (NSC 249992), a new acridine derivative. *Cancer Res.* 1978;**38**:3712–3716.

Lewis KP, Medina WD. Cellulitis and fibrosis due to *cis*-diamminedichloroplatinum(II) (platinol) infiltration. *Cancer Treat Rep.* 1980;**64**(10):1162–1163.

Leyden M, Sullivan J. Cutaneous necrosis after intra-arterial treatment with cisplatin. *Cancer Treat Rep.* 1986;**70**(5):687.

Linder RM, Upton J, Osteen R. Management of extensive doxorubicin hydrochloride extravasation injuries. *J Hand Surg.* 1983;**8**(1):32–38.

Lippman M, Zager R, Henderson ES. High dose daunorubicin (NSC-83142) in the treatment of advanced acute myelogenous leukemia. *Cancer Chemother Rep.* 1972;**56**(6):755–760.

Louie AC, Issell BF. Amsacrine (AMSA)—A clinical review. *J Clin Oncol.* 1985;**3**(3):562–590.

Ludwig CV, Stoll H, Obrist R. Prevention of cytotoxic drug-induced skin ulcers with dimethylsulfoxide (DMSO) and alpha-tocopherol. *Eur J Clin Oncol.* 1987;**23**:327–329.

Luedke DW, Kennedy PS, Rietschel RL. Histopathogenesis of skin and subcutaneous injury induced by Adriamycin. *Plast Reconstruct Surg.* 1979;**63**(4):463–465.

Marnocha RSM, Hutson PR. Intradermal carboplatin and ifosfamide extravasation in the mouse. *Cancer.* 1992;**70**:850–853.

McGovren JP, Nelson KG, Lassus M, et al. Menogaril: A new anthracycline agent entering clinical trials. *Invest New Drugs* 1984;**2**:359–367.

Meranze SG, Burke DR, Feurer ID, Mullen JL. Spontaneous retraction of indwelling catheters: Previously unreported complications. *J Parent Enteral Nutr* 1988;**12**(3):312–320.

Moore GE, DiPaolo JA, Kondo T. The chemotherapeutic effects and complications of actinomycin D in patients with advanced cancer. *Cancer.* 1958;**11**:1204–1214.

Nobbs P, Barr RD. Soft-tissue injury caused by antineoplastic drugs is inhibited by topical dimethyl sulphoxide and alpha tocopherol. *Br J Cancer.* 1983;**48**:873–876.

Ohnoshi T, Ohnuma T, Beranek JT, Holland JF. Combined cytotoxicity effect of hyperthermia and anthracycline antibiotics on human tumor cells. *J Natl Cancer Inst.* 1985;**74**(2):275–281.

Okano T, Ohnuma T, Efremidis A, Holland JF. Doxorubicin-induced skin ulcer in the piglet. *Cancer Treat Rep.* 1983;**67**(12):1075–1078.

Olver IN, Aisner J, Hament A, et al. A prospective study of topical dimethyl sulfoxide for treating anthracycline extravasation. *J Clin Oncol.* 1988;**6**(11):1732–1735.

Olver IN, Schwarz MA. Use of dimethylsulfoxide in limiting tissue damage caused by extravasation of doxorubicin. *Cancer Treat Rep* 1983;**67**:407–408.

Owen OE, Dellatorre DL, Van Scott EJ, Cohen MR. Accidental intramuscular injection of mechlorethamine. *Cancer.* 1980;**45**:2225–2226.

Peters FTM, Beijnen JH, ten Bokkel-Huinink WT. Nitoxantrone extravasation injury. *Cancer Treat Rep* 1987;**7**:992–993.

Petro JA, Graham WP, III, Miller SH, et al. Experimental and clinical studies of ulcers induced with Adriamycin. *Surg Forum.* 1979;**30**:535–537.

Preuss P, Partoft S. Cytostatic extravasations. *Ann Plast Surg.* 1987;**19**:323–329.

Reed WP, Newman KA, Applefeld MM, Sutton FJ. Drug extravasation as a complication of venous access ports. *Ann Intern Med.* 1985;**102**(6):788–790.

Reilly JJ, Neifeld JP, Rosenberg SA. Clinical course and management of accidental Adriamycin extravasation. *Cancer.* 1977;**40**(5):2053–2056.

Rozencweig M, Von Hoff DD, Henney JE, Muggia FM.

VM 26 and VP 16-213: A comparative analysis. *Cancer.* 1977;**40**:334–342.

Rudolph R, Stein RS, Pattillo RA. Skin ulcers due to Adriamycin. *Cancer.* 1976;**38**:1087–1094.

Sessa G, Gundersen S, ten Bokkel-Huinink W, Renard J, Cavalli F. Phase II study of intravenous menogaril in patients with advanced breast cancer. *J Natl Cancer Inst* 1988;**80**:1066–1069.

Seyfer AE, Solimando DA Jr. Toxic lesions of the hand associated with chemotherapy. *J Hand Surg.* 1983;**8**(1):39–42.

Soble MJ, Dorr RT, Plezia P, Breckenridge S. Dose-dependent skin ulcers in mice treated with DNA binding antitumor antibiotics. *Cancer Chemother Pharmacol.* 1987;**20**:33–36.

Sonneveld P, Wassenaar HA, Nooter K. Long persistence of doxorubicin in human skin after extravasation. *Cancer Treat Rep.* 1984;**68**(6):895–896.

Souhami L Jr, Feld R. Urticaria following intravenous doxorubicin administration. *JAMA.* 1978;**240**(15):1624–1626.

Svingen BA, Powis G, Appel PL, Scott M. Protection against Adriamycin-induced skin necrosis in the rat by dimethyl sulfoxide and α-tocopherol. *Cancer Res.* 1981;**41**:3395–3399.

Teta JB, O'Connor L. Local tissue damage from 5-fluorouracil extravasation. *Oncol Nurs Forum.* 1984;**11**(4):77.

Upton PG, Yamaguchi KT, Myers S, et al. Effects of antioxidants and hyperbaric oxygen in ameliorating experimental doxorubicin skin toxicity in the rat. *Cancer Treat Rep.* 1986;**70**(4):503–507.

Vaitkevicius VK, Talley RW, Tucker JL, Brennan MJ. Cytological and clinical observations during vincaleukoblastine therapy of disseminated cancer. *Cancer.* 1962;**15**:294–306.

Van Sloten-Harwood K, Bachur N. Evaluation of dimethyl sulfoxide and local cooling as antidotes for doxorubicin extravasation in a pig model. *Oncol Nurs Forum.* 1987;**14**(1):39–44.

Vogelzang NJ. "Adriamycin flare": A skin reaction resembling extravasation. *Cancer Treat Rep.* 1979;**63**(11/12):2067–2069.

Wood HA, Ellerhorst-Ryan JM. Delayed adverse skin reactions associated with mitomycin-C administration. *Oncol Nurs Forum.* 1984;**11**(4):14–18.

Chapter 7 ◻ ◻ ◻ ◻ ◻

Legal Implications for the Nurse Involved in the Administration of Cytotoxic Agents

Suzanne A. Miller

Prior to 1970, the intravenous administration of cytotoxic agents was primarily the responsibility of the physician. With the advent of combination chemotherapeutic regimens such as MOPP (mechlorethamine, vincristine, prednisone, and procarbazine) and the introduction of the exciting anthracycline antibiotic doxorubicin, it was felt that curative potential existed for a wide spectrum of disease activities. About that time, physicians turned to nurses for assistance in the delivery of these cytotoxic agents. Initially, nurses were enlisted to administer a few select drugs only, and gradually their responsibilities expanded to encompass the many areas that oncology nurses are involved in today. In light of these new demands, nurses found there was a need to be aware of their legal responsibilities when administering cancer chemotherapeutic agents.

This area of oncology nurse practice appears to be one of many areas in which nursing practice overlaps medical practice. Many of the statements herein reflect the laws of the author's state of California. Naturally, these will vary somewhat in individual states, and for that reason it is recommended that nurses become familiar with laws regarding nursing practice in their own state. Perhaps legal "gray zones" of overlapping responsibility will always exist in some form because nursing is a dynamic field in which the practice is continually evolving to include more sophisticated patient care activities. The California Nurse Practice Act states: "It is the legislative intent to recognize the existence of overlapping function between physicians and nurses and to permit additional sharing of functions within the organized health care systems which provide for collaboration between physicians and nurses" (Business and Professional Code 1975). This statement acknowledges areas of overlap and also encourages future developments in nursing that may extend this overlap. When nursing functions or acts represent an overlap of medical practice, then standards of care must be developed. Over the last decade nurses have made great strides in formulating standards of care for delivering nursing care to oncology patients while protecting their welfare and defining nurses' roles and responsibilities. This chapter discusses legal implications for the nurse related to the administration of cytotoxic agents.

INFORMED CONSENT

We live in a time when patients not only want to know what is happening to them medically, but the courts are insisting that they must be informed.

Thus, over the past few years, state supreme courts have shown a trend toward establishing legally imposed standards for informed consent. These legal standards set forth a minimum amount of information that must be available to the patient. Ultimately it is the physician's responsibility to provide that information, and any breach of this duty may constitute negligence.

In addition, many states are adopting variations of an ethical code known as the Patient's Bill of Rights. This bill was adopted by the American Hospital Association in 1973 and states that the patient should receive information about her or his medical care and that failure to ensure that the patient is adequately informed about his or her care places both professionals and hospitals in danger of liability. In California, this code states that the patient has a right to receive as much information about any proposed treatment or procedure as he or she may need to give informed consent or to refuse this course of treatment. In addition, patients must receive a copy of the Patient's Bill of Rights. Except in emergencies, this information should include a description of the procedure or treatment, the medically significant risks involved in the treatment, alternate courses of treatment or nontreatment, the risks involved in each, and the name of the person who will carry out the procedure or treatment.

It makes sense that this is the kind of information patients must receive to participate intelligently in decisions regarding treatment that can significantly affect their lives. Additionally, patients who are fully informed have better rapport with doctors and nurses. With adequate opportunity to have questions answered, they are less likely to consider litigation in the future.

Consent to treatment can be either written or oral. Written consent implies documentation of informed consent; oral consent, if mutually accepted, is equally as binding as written consent. Oral consent can often be difficult to prove, however, and for that reason many institutions and some states require that informed consent be evidenced by a signed, written statement. The consent should be specific enough so that the patient understands the nature of treatment. A written and signed consent, however, does not prove understanding, but merely serves as evidence of the patient's signature on a legal document. It does not limit the legal liability of those involved in the patient's care. Although it is not necessary to obtain written consent for standard therapies, it is recommended, and is standard practice in many treatment centers.

What exactly constitutes proper consent and adequate proof of informed consent is a complex matter. No agreement exists as to how complete written informed consent must be. Consent forms vary in scope and content. They range from general treatment consents with some additional information added to photocopies of drug package inserts. Some institutions feel that a general hospital consent is sufficient coverage for the administration of cytotoxic agents. Undoubtedly, most courts would find that such general authorization is insufficient because it does not designate the exact nature of the treatment. On the other hand, the manufacturer's package inserts for many drugs could needlessly alarm many patients. As patients vary in their ability to comprehend medical language, it becomes difficult to inform the patient adequately without either under- or overestimating the risks.

If consent has not been obtained, the hospital or institution could be held liable if treatment is administered. Failure to obtain a patient's consent may constitute battery. *Battery* is defined as any physical contact of a patient without his or her permission. Performed within the scope of employment, treatment without prior informed consent could constitute battery and the hospital and nurse would be liable (Springer 1970). It should be reemphasized that without consent, any "touching" (ie, treatment) of a patient is battery, whereas a failure to obtain informed consent constitutes negligence. Most hospital consents are designed to satisfy the former but not the latter.

If there is doubt that the patient has given an informed consent, then chemotherapy should not be administered until there is proof of consent. State laws vary, but most feel it is ultimately the physician's duty to reveal to the patient the nature of the illness, the type and goal of treatment, a description of the treatment plan, a review of the possible risks and toxic effects, the name of the responsible physician, an explanation of alternative treatments that may be available with the risks and benefits of each, and the implications of nontreatment. In most situations, nurses are not permitted to inform the patient initially. The Oncology Nursing Society has developed policies, outcomes, and procedures as a tool for guiding nurses regarding their role in the informed consent process (Oncology Nursing Society 1988b). A review of these guidelines provides nurses with a framework for integration of their facility's policies with those recommended by the Oncology Nursing Society. Although it is the physician's responsibility to inform the patient initially, it is beneficial for the nurse to be present during the initial discussion. This allows the nurse and patient to be comfortable with questions that may arise later. In addition, many physicians rely heavily on the nurse to teach patients about problems related to their chemotherapy, such as effective methods of controlling nausea, vomiting, and constipation; dietary modifications; mouth care; and hair loss.

Comprehension of the information conveyed in informed consent can be hampered by the high anxiety level frequently experienced by oncology patients. Therefore, many practitioners deliver patient education materials along with the informed consent form 24 to 48 hours prior to the signing of the informed consent to allow the patient and family adequate time to review the materials, express concerns, and ask questions about therapy. The nurse's role in patient education and the informed consent process should be clearly defined by the individual facility. One facility delivers written information to patients on the side effects of chemotherapy with suggestions to minimize these effects before patients sign that the material was received and reviewed. Their state Nursing Association and institution have deemed it the nurse's responsibility to provide patients with knowledge about medications, side effects, methods to minimize side effects, and what constitutes a medical emergency (Krohner 1987).

When clinical research trials involve experimentation on human subjects, federal regulations mandate that the patient be provided with a statement regarding the study, including an explanation of the purpose, duration of study, description of study procedures, and identification of those procedures that are experimental. Additional disclosure should include a description of risks and benefits inherent in the study or its treatment, alternatives to participation in the study, a statement of confidentiality and how it will be maintained, an explanation of any compensation associated with participation, directions for obtaining further information, and a statement of the subject's voluntary participation in the study. It is important that nurses reinforce the voluntary nature of the clinical research trial and explain that refusal of therapy (voluntary withdrawal from protocol) will not jeopardize future medical care. Occasionally, patients confide that they "just don't want anymore." They may be afraid of offending the physician or feel that they "owe something to medical science." It is the nurse's responsibility, as patient advocate, to communicate these concerns to the physician.

Consenting to the use of investigational drugs poses another problem. Because little is known about many new phase I and II drugs, it is difficult to obtain as informed a consent as is possible when commercially available drugs are involved. For instance, as more experience with a new drug is accrued, new adverse side effects may be discovered that were unsuspected at the outset. The physician and nurse share the responsibility of keeping the patient informed as new information is obtained about the drug. Because of strict federal requirements, there must be a written consent obtained for each new investigational protocol into which a patient is entered. The consent form signed by the patient should state that the safety and usefulness of the drug for the specific condition mentioned are being investigated and that its use is still unproved by medical experience. The patient should acknowledge that no guarantee of the efficacy of the drug has been made to him or her and that, with full knowledge of this, he or she voluntarily consents to treatment.

As patient advocates, nurses should view their role in the informed consent process as reinforcing, clarifying, and supplementing information delivered by the physician. Clearly, there is a need to incorporate patient education programs and materials into the informed consent process.

SUPERVISION OF ONCOLOGY NURSES

Should a suit be brought against a nurse working within an institution, usually the hospital, physician, or employing facility will also be held liable under the doctrine of "respondeat superior." Loosely translated, *respondeat superior* means "let the master answer." If the nurse is negligent while acting within the course and scope of employment duties, the doctrine of respondeat superior requires that the hospital, the physician, or the employer be held accountable for the nurse's negligence. Because the nurse is not absolved, it is advantageous to have clearly defined in writing who is responsible for supervision and what tasks and responsibilities will be included in the scope of the job. Some institutions have developed cytotoxic drug administration policies that prohibit nurses from being left alone in the clinic while chemotherapy is infusing. For example, some chemotherapy drugs can cause allergic or other adverse reactions. A nurse left alone in either situation is potentially liable.

A statement such as the following might protect the clinic or office nurse who works alone while the physician is in the hospital or out in the community. "The nurse . . . will not administer direct intravenous medications without another nurse or responsible physician in the immediate area." Some drug companies also feel that nurses should not be left unsupervised when administering their products. The package information for cisplatin states: "Platinol (cisplatin) should be administered under the supervision of a qualified physician experienced in the use of cancer chemotherapeutic agents." Obviously one must use some judgment in interpreting what is actually meant by the term *supervision* in these recommendations. It should not be implied that direct, physical supervision by the physician is required for the administration of this drug. There is, however, a responsibility placed on the nurse to administer the drug properly and in accordance with the physician's order and that the physician or her or his qualified designate be readily available when treatment is given.

Although not challenged yet in the courts, a gray area exists of overlapping functions for nurses who practice in expanded roles once thought to belong to the physician. Independent practitioners, research or protocol nurses, and those practicing with a degree of autonomy have accepted responsibilities once thought solely within the realm of physician practice. In an expanded role, nurses may have a certain degree of autonomy in practicing within the framework of their job descriptions. Indeed, this role may require the performance of duties such as ordering tests, making patient referrals to other health professionals, performing physical examinations, initiating therapeutic interventions, adjusting medications, or administering phase I and II investigational agents in the home or office setting. When nurses accept such duties, they should have in writing a statement of support from their employer.

In reality, routine nursing care can involve the performance of tasks that go far beyond nursing practice as defined by law or the American Nursing Association. During the course of the workday, nurses are often asked to perform tasks that do not lie within the realm of their written job descriptions. Thus, no one is assuming responsibility for supervision when these tasks are performed. Unfortunately, it will be difficult, perhaps impossible, to eliminate the risk that nurses might be held liable for when performing tasks not defined in their job descriptions. It is therefore important when considering the legal liability of nursing care that job descriptions be concise and unambiguous, with clear definitions of the lines of supervision.

EXPERT NURSING CARE

It is the responsibility of professional nurses to learn and be accountable for the skills necessary to perform their duties. There must be a definition of what is expected, what the standards of care are at the employing facility, what policies and procedures are in existence, what the scope of duties includes, and what "reasonable care" means in a particular area of practice. Duties must be performed with at least the same care and skill that an ordinary, responsible, and prudent nurse in the same or similar circumstances would use. Nurses are expected to observe and evaluate a patient's condition. In addition, they are personally responsible for all their wrongful or negligent acts.

Nurses are moving away from the traditional role of guardian of the patient through the assumption of duties requiring judgments that must be backed by a firm base of knowledge. The development of new therapeutic concepts is likely to make the administration of cytotoxic agents increasingly complex, thus requiring that nurses continue to expand their base of knowledge and refine their clinical skills. As new medical biotechnologic devices become available to improve the therapeutic index, decrease costs, reduce disease and treatment-related morbidity, and permit greater patient freedom outside of the medical environment, nurses find they are required to become expert in technical and mechanical areas previously not envisioned as encompassing nursing care roles. When nurses work with state-of-the-art ambulatory infusion pumps, implantable vascular access devices, indwelling atrial catheters, and other computerized devices that deliver cytotoxic agents, they must be adequately trained and supervised and express a degree of confidence in being able to survive in this highly sophisticated arena that encompasses "expert nursing care."

NURSE CERTIFICATION

In 1984 the Oncology Nursing Society addressed the issue of ensuring "expert" nursing care through the formation of the Oncology Nursing Certification

Corporation (ONCC), a nonprofit Pennsylvania corporation. This was, in part, the result of many years of discussion and research regarding the need to ensure that "expert" nursing care was being delivered to oncology patients. An independent, nonprofit corporation was engaged for test development, test administration, and education research. Certification is defined as the process by which a nongovernmental agency or association certifies that an individual licensed to practice a profession has met certain predetermined standards specified by that profession for specialty practice. Its purpose is to ensure various publics that an individual has mastered a body of knowledge and acquired skills in a particular specialty. Certification is viewed as a measure of documenting, to some extent, continued professional development (Steel 1985). Although certification is voluntary, oncology nurses are encouraged to become certified to improve consumer protection, to permit self-regulation rather than governmental regulation, and to enable a degree of recognition and enhancement of earning power to those certified.

Currently, the oncology nursing certification examination includes test questions based on the Oncology Nursing Core Curriculum. As such, the examination is aimed at testing the general knowledge base of the professional oncology nurse. At this time, separate oncology nursing subspecialty examinations, such as for chemotherapy, are not available, although chemotherapy-related test questions are included in the certification examination. The Oncology Nursing Society has developed a computer-assisted instruction (CAI) self-assessment program to assist the nurse in preparation for the examination. As of May 1993, 11,863 nurses were certified as Oncology Certified Nurses (OCNs).

INTRAVENOUS CHEMOTHERAPY

According to Creighton (1981) professional competence is the best protection for nurses. Yet, there are no guarantees that a nurse will not be named in a malpractice suit. Should nurses, therefore, receive special training to give chemotherapy? The law in many states gives nurses the right to administer intravenous infusions and the right to administer medications. The employing facility then has the responsibility to determine what the standard of care will be for the individual nurse in administering intravenous cytotoxic agents. Standards of care are important because it may become necessary in a litigation to determine what the standards of care have been. The California Medical Association, the California Hospital Association, and the California Nurses Association have issued a statement on the intravenous administration of fluids, including the addition of drugs by nurses licensed to practice in California. It should be emphasized that the statement is not law, but it is a recommendation by this committee. The criteria outlined are as follows:

1. The nurse has had special training in the technique.
2. The nurse performs the technique on the order of a licensed doctor of medicine.
3. The order is for a specific patient.
4. The technique is to be performed within the framework of designated practice established for the hospital or employing agency.... A committee composed of representatives from the medical staff, department of nursing, and administration shall compose a written framework of preparation and practice for the nurse to adhere to.

The committee shall:

1. Decide if the nurse may perform the technique.
2. Determine the special method of teaching to be required.
3. Establish in-service teaching of the technique.
4. Delineate the solutions that may be safely given and which types of fluids or medications the nurses may administer intravenously.
5. Determine whether the physician's orders should be written or oral. (California Medical Association 1976)

In attempting to promote further a high quality of care, the responsible institutional committee should have a policy statement (or standard of care) for nurses who administer intravenous medications. Standards of care do not guarantee that the nurse will perform to the highest degree of excellence, but they do provide a framework within which the nurse can learn. Such a standard of care optimally might include the following:

1. A request by a responsible physician for a particular nurse to learn how to administer chemotherapy.
2. Prior approval for nurses to administer each individual drug or drug classification.
3. Authorization for the individual nurse by the responsible committee prior to the administration of intravenous chemotherapy.
4. Initial venipuncture class for the nurse to demonstrate skill and proficiency in starting intravenous infusions.
5. Yearly cardiopulmonary resuscitation classes.
6. Orientation to the cytotoxic agents to include normal dose ranges, adverse effects, nursing intervention for adverse reactions, and expected physiologic effect.
7. A written examination at the completion of the orientation program.
8. A written, dated, and signed physician's order, which must be in the nurse's possession before intravenous chemotherapy is given, specifying the drug and dose for each individual patient.
9. A statement that the nurse will not administer intravenous chemotherapy without another nurse or responsible person being present.
10. A statement that the nurse will have a clinical practicum with a qualified preceptor with dates specified for reverification of clinical and didactic knowledge.

Also attached to this policy statement should be a list of the individual nurses who have been approved to administer intravenous chemotherapy and the drugs the nurse may administer.

Obviously, such a statement should be tailored to the nurse's area of practice and the responsibilities that the employing facility delegates. Such a policy will protect not only the patient but also the nurse who is asked to administer new investigational agents about which little is known. Thus, it may be desirable in some institutions to restrict the administration of new investigational agents to physicians until reasonable safety has been established. If, however, a facility elects to employ a nurse in an expanded role, this responsibility may be written into the job description.

Additional skills are necessary for the nurse who administers intravenous chemotherapy. This includes knowledge of the side effects and toxicities of individual drugs, not only because this has been stated in the hospital's written standards of care for the purposes of legal protection, but also because it is an essential part of patient education. Indeed, increasing consumer advocacy has promoted the patient's right to be actively involved in treatment decisions and self-care activities. Self-care cannot occur without prior knowledge, and the responsibility for this lies primarily with the oncology nurse. For example, doxorubicin can cause a pink- to reddish-tinged urine several hours after it has been administered; therefore, good nursing care includes informing the patient of this fact to allay fears. Likewise, the potential renal damage associated with cisplatin can be greatly minimized by adequately educating patients about the side effects and self-care management with this cytotoxic agent.

When nurses reconstitute, store, and administer drugs, they must accept responsibility for their actions. For example, if a drug is stored incorrectly and its potency and therefore its efficacy are decreased, or if a drug is not diluted correctly and causes vein irritation, the nurse could be held negligent. Specific training for these responsibilities should be provided to ensure that the nurse is capable of performing them accurately. In addition, when nurses assume responsibility for admixing cytotoxic agents, on-the-job training should include training with a skilled oncology pharmacist in drug handling safety techniques and precautions. Nurses who admix drugs report that initially the procedure of working in a biologic safety cabinet while wearing a gown and gloves is quite cumbersome, so adequate time should be permitted for the nurse to practice the procedure with normal saline. It is known that many cytotoxic agents are carcinogenic, mutagenic, and teratogenic in animals, and in humans pharmacologic doses of some cytotoxic agents are carcinogenic and teratogenic. What is not known at this time, however, is the risk, if any, of long-term, continuous exposure to small amounts of cytotoxic agents. Because of this unknown, it is essential to minimize exposure to these agents through good self-protective techniques. Miller (1987) lists drug handling safety recommendations for drug preparation and equipment disposal that can be adapted to policies and procedures for individual settings. Individual facilities have the responsibility of educating employees to avoid unnecessary exposure to potentially hazardous cytotoxic agents. It is hoped that informing employees of the potential hazards associated with these agents will prevent litigation.

A nurse's training should also include an understanding of normal dose ranges. If there is doubt about the physician's written order, the nurse has the responsibility of confirming the accuracy and intent of the order. A decimal point could be in the wrong place or missing, and an order could be written for 70 mg of vinblastine instead of a normal dose of 7.0 mg. Or the physician may mean to write 5-fluorouracil 200 mg, but instead writes an order for 2000 mg.

Nurses have a duty to stop the intravenous chemotherapy administration if the patient complains of pain or burning at the needle insertion site. If swelling, obvious infiltration, or local allergic reactions are noted, the nurse must know what steps to take. Individual facilities should develop standards of care or protocols for dealing with these situations, for example, whether the nurse should discontinue the infusion or keep it open with a maintenance solution. If the nurse notices that the intravenous chemotherapy infusion has infiltrated and does nothing, or does not act in accordance with established policies and procedures for drug extravasation, a charge of negligence could result. Many intravenous chemotherapy extravasations have led to prolonged, expensive, and psychologically traumatic hospitalizations for the patient. Skin grafting of the affected area may be necessary, and it is possible that a severely damaged limb may need amputation. Surely no nurse should assume the responsibility of administering intravenous chemotherapy without knowing the consequences and feeling personally responsible for becoming technically competent.

In 1984 the Oncology Nursing Society developed *Cancer Chemotherapy: Guidelines and Recommendations for Nursing Education and Practice.* Revised in modular format in 1986, they were designed to assist in the development of courses for a basic didactic component and a clinical practicum experience (Oncology Nursing Society 1988a). These excellent guidelines permit adaptation to a variety of practice settings. Additional modules are available for the acute care setting, home care setting, and outpatient area. Also in module format are recommendations for the management of vesicant extravasation, hypersensitivity, and anaphylaxis. The availability of such tools enables the instructor and the practitioner to meet the standards recommended by the professional organization that represents oncology nurses. Of equal importance is the need for nurses to be periodically evaluated for knowledge and skill in chemotherapy administration. Ongoing participation in continuing education programs is recommended to maintain a current knowledge base in the rapidly changing specialty of oncology nursing.

DOCUMENTATION

Nurses who practice in a variety of settings today are confronted with numerous challenges that impact their ability to adequately document the delivery of care. Increasingly complex multimodality treatment regimens, the nursing shortage, an increase in the number of visits to outpatient settings or alternative care settings, and the addition of expanded nursing responsibilities provide time challenges to the nurse when documenting nursing care. Yet it is important for medicolegal purposes that nurses be able to recall what their actions were at any given time. A sound practice is the consistent, timely notation on the patient's record of pertinent nursing interventions.

The following example emphasizes the importance of adequately documenting nursing care: A nurse is called into court 3 years after an apparent inadvertent extravasation of a cytotoxic agent and permitted to review the nursing note which read, "Intravenous Adriamycin appears to have extravasated. Dr. White notified." With such scanty charting, none of the particular circumstances regarding the event would readily be called to mind. If long and painful hospitalization and debridements, skin grafting, or possible amputation were the result of a cytotoxic agent extravasating into the tissues, the nurse must be able to prove that "reasonable, prudent, and safe" nursing interventions occurred. To prove this at a later date, it must be documented.

Increasingly, medical records are being presented as important evidence in legal proceedings, and if called on to recall events of a particular occurrence, nurses are permitted to review their nursing notes. Medical records are carefully scrutinized for completeness, consistency, and contradictory events. Late-entry notes (written several hours after the incident), crossed-out notes, and advance-written notes (written before the treatment) are viewed with suspicion (Schulmeister 1987).

The Oncology Nursing Society (1988b) provides guidelines for the documentation of chemotherapy administration. Essential elements felt necessary to include in chemotherapy documentation are date, time, needle size and type, insertion site, drug sequence, drug administration technique, drugs and dosages administered, amount and type of flushing solution, description of the site after treatment, adverse reactions, if noted, side effects discussed or experienced, reactions to treatment, and specific discharge instructions. Should extravasation occur, important additional information to include is the time of all events, the approximate amount of drug extravasated, nursing interventions and management of the possible infiltrate, photographic documentation if it is the institutional policy, patient's statements and complaints, appearance of the site, notification of the physician, follow-up measures, and the nurse's signature. In addition, if co-workers have witnessed the event, they should be referenced and all follow-up telephone calls and return visits should reflect that nursing followed the event closely.

Oncology nurses have exhibited creativity in developing chemotherapy forms to record pertinent information regarding drug administration and the occurrence of extravasation. Standardization of documentation ensures that important points are included, while saving time for nurses in charting. Appropriate institutional committees should review new documents prior to their utilization in the practice setting. Increasingly, computerized programs are being developed to document various aspects of medical and nursing care. One facility has successfully implemented computerized nursing documents for the administration of cytotoxic agents (Cross-Skinner 1989). They feel it is an accurate, reliable, and accessible tool for documenting cytotoxic drug administration. In addition, it can be useful for research activities, quality analysis, and verification for third-party payment. What remains as yet to be determined is the legality of computerized documentation when submitted in litigation proceedings. Obviously, safeguards must be ensured to protect confidentiality, prevent erasure of notes, and permit nursing entry of notes only by authorized nurses. Unfortunately, society's focus on litigation has emphasized the need for defensive documentation. Nurses must seek to satisfy the employing institution's need for documenting the care delivered while realizing that governmental bodies and third-party reimbursement agencies must be informed of nursing actions.

PROFESSIONAL LIABILITY INSURANCE

From the preceding discussion, it is clear that this is an era of nurse specialists. Indeed, the number of oncology nurse clinicians who administer cytotoxic agents is increasing. This is also a time when the number of lawsuits is increasing. Accordingly, many experts feel that the nurse should carry individual professional liability insurance. When professional services are provided, the professional may be held legally responsible for any harm the patient suffers as a result of negligence. Grace Barbee, formerly an attorney for the California Nurses Association, states: "It can be expensive to prove your innocence" (Creighton 1981). In obtaining professional liability insurance, protection is sought to reduce the risk of legal and financial loss through liability. As oncology nurses become increasingly entrepreneurial and creative in designing nontraditional nursing roles, they risk stepping out from under the protective umbrella previously provided by hospitals. An increasing trend reflects that specialty nurses are obtaining their own professional liability insurance to supplement the coverage provided by their employer. It is possible that a nurse could be sued individually as well as in a suit brought against the employer. In addition, when the employer is required to pay damages, the insurance company may seek restitution from the nurse (Schulmeister 1987). In general, malpractice insurance, whether provided by the employer or an individual insurance company, provides three major benefits to the policyholder:

1. In the event of the award of damages against the nurse, the insurance pays any sum within the specified limits of the policy.
2. The insurance pays the cost of the lawyer who defends the nurse.
3. The insurance pays for bond for a nurse in the event it is required in an appeal.

The decision to obtain professional liability insurance is a highly individual one. Some believe it is a necessity for nurses today, some believe it is an added security, and many believe it is too much of an individual matter to generalize. There are several points to consider when contemplating liability insurance:

1. The extent to which the nurse is covered by the employer's policy: The nurse should ask to see a copy of the policy and attempt to ascertain whether the insurance policy protects the employee's interests only to the extent it is necessary to do so in the course of protecting the hospital's interests.
2. Whether the nurse practices in a "high-risk" area: High-risk areas might include the type of nursing a particular nurse performs, the geographic area in which a nurse lives, and the inclination of patients in the area to sue nurses. Many feel that oncology nurses who administer cytotoxic agents fall within a "high-risk" group.
3. The cost of the policy: Group policies obtained through a national, state, or local professional organization may be less expensive. Cost alone should not be a deciding factor for nurses who feel they need individual coverage and practice in a "high-risk" area.

In response to the well-publicized professional liability insurance crisis of 1987, the American Nurses Association joined forces with an independent insurance company to establish the National Nurses' Claims Data Base. Its ultimate goal is to identify the extent of litigation occurring against nurses and to monitor professional liability claims and incidences for the entire profession. Secondary goals include serving as a source of information to nurses facing a lawsuit by providing them with information regarding how similar cases were decided in court, providing access for nurses to standards of care in their community, assisting nurses with what to expect throughout the process of litigation, assisting specialty nursing organizations with information to use in negotiation with insurance carriers, and providing information to assist in the development of nursing malpractice prevention programs. Although the program is strictly confidential, nurses may be hesitant to report litigious situations for fear of repercussion. Indeed, only approximately 70 cases have been self-reported in the first 2 years.

Currently, only the state of Missouri has mandatory reporting of all malpractice claims. By tapping into reported cases involving nurses, the National Nurses' Claims Data Base hopes to expand their knowledge base of the extent and outcome of litigation so that nurses will not be denied professional liability insurance nor be exposed to exorbitant and escalating insurance premiums.

CONCLUSIONS

The next decade will undoubtedly see many changes in the responsibilities of nurses who administer cytotoxic agents. As health care moves from the medical institution to the home, and as staffing shortages continue, nurses must be flexible yet aware of their legal responsibilities as defined by law, the government, and the employing facility. Educational tools must meet the needs of patients who will be empowered to assume a more active role in their care. Indeed, many patients, as prosumers, will attempt to convince medicine that they are capable of managing their care at home with limited assistance. Cost-containment efforts will undoubtedly support this shift in care.

Because nurses are held responsible for their professional judgments, they should have defined, in writing, what is their responsibility regarding informed consent, who their supervisors are, what constitutes acceptable institutional documentation, and what standards of care are before employment begins. Above all, nurses should express confidence in being able to manage the complexities associated with caring for the oncology patient today. Only after these issues have been addressed will the nurse be adequately prepared to deliver nursing care responsibly in and beyond the 1990s in this dynamic and rapidly evolving specialty.

REFERENCES

Business and Professional Code. Registered Nurses, Chapter 913, Assembly Bill No. 2725, 1975 Amendment, p. 9.

California Medical Association, California Hospital Association, California Nurses Association. *Joint Statement for Standardized Procedures: The Intravenous Administration of Fluids, Including the Addition of Drugs and the Start-*

ing and Administration of Blood by Nurses Licensed to Practice in California. January 30, 1976.

Creighton H. *Law Every Nurse Should Know.* 4th ed. Philadelphia: WB Saunders; 1981.

Cross-Skinner S. Computerized documentation of outpatient chemotherapy administration. In: *Out-Patient Chemotherapy.* New York: Burroughs Wellcome Co. 1989; vol 3(3):9–11.

Krohner K. Patient education tool serves as consent. *Oncol Nurs Forum.* 1987;**14**(4):91–92.

Miller SA. Issues in cytotoxic drug handling safety. *Semin Oncol Nurs.* 1987;**3**(2):133–141.

Oncology Nursing Society. *Cancer Chemotherapy Guidelines: Module I. Recommendations for Cancer Chemotherapy: Course Content and Clinical Practicum.* Pittsburgh, PA: Oncology Nursing Society; 1988a:2–7.

Oncology Nursing Society. Informed Consent to Administer Chemotherapy. *Cancer Chemotherapy Guidelines: Module III. Recommendations for Nursing Practice in the Outpatient Setting.* Pittsburgh, PA: Oncology Nursing Society; 1988b:3.

Oncology Nursing Society. *Cancer Chemotherapy Guidelines: Module V. Recommendations for the Management and Vesicant Extravasation, Hypersensitivity, and Anaphylaxsis.* Pittsburgh, PA: Oncology Nursing Society; 1992.

Oncology Nursing Society. *Oncology Nursing Review: A Computer-Assisted Instruction (CAI) Program.* Pittsburgh, PA: Oncology Nursing Society; 1993.

Schulmeister L. Litigation involving oncology nurses. *Oncol Nurs Forum.* 1987;**14**(2):25–28.

Steel JE. Getting our "C's" in order. *Oncol Nurs Forum.* 1985;**12**(3):88.

Springer EW. *Nursing and the Law.* Pittsburgh, PA: L.L.B. Health Law Center, Aspen Systems Corp; 1970.

Part III

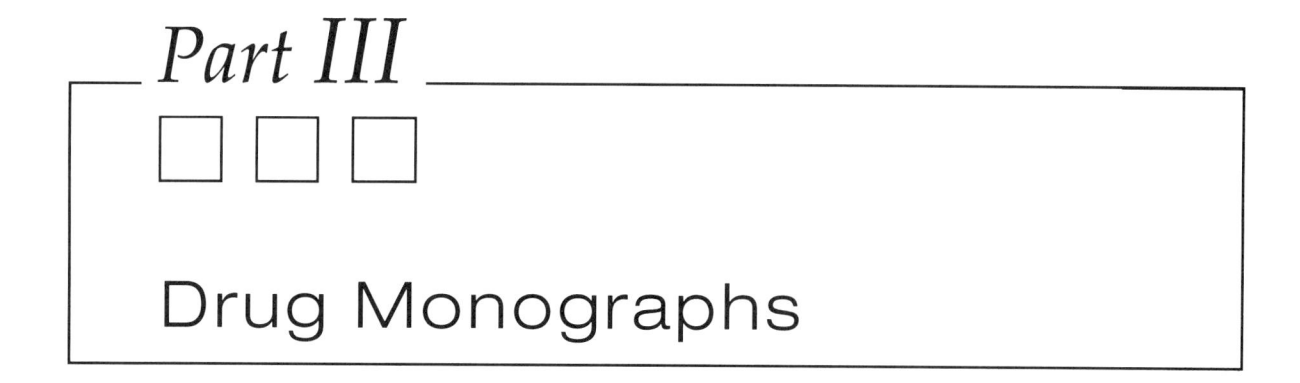

Drug Monographs

This section of the book was designed to provide an initial guide or quick reference for health professionals who deal directly with the preparation and administration of cancer chemotherapeutic agents. Specific information pertaining to each drug includes synonyms, chemical and physical properties, tumor activity, mechanism of action, preparation, stability, administration, toxicities, special precautions, drug interactions, availability, storage, pharmacokinetics, special applications, and selected references. This section is not intended to recommend drug therapy for specific patients or disease states nor to act as a sole source of cancer drug information. It is offered to provide useful guidelines for some of the practical aspects of cancer chemotherapy. Some of the procedures discussed with particular agents are investigational and may not have universal applicability. Also, many of these agents are available only to approved investigators through established protocols and are included in this text for reference only.

Many of the agents described in this section are undergoing early phase testing and thus, little clinical information was available at the time of publication. In some cases only animal data or limited Phase I dose-finding studies were available. Thus, extra caution should be used in reviewing the data for these agents, since drug tolerable doses and schedules for specific cancers may not be described. The same is true for important toxicities which often are not apparent until large-scale trials are performed. The authors strongly recommend that practitioners review the primary literature on these agents, particularly for current dosing guidelines and side-effect profiles.

Acivicin

■ Other Names

U-42126; AT-125; NSC-163501; L-(αS, 5S)-α-amino-3-chloro-4,5-dihydro-5-isoxazoleacetic acid.

■ Chemistry

Structure of acivicin

Acivicin is an L-erythro amino acid isolated from the fermentation broth of *Streptomyces sviceus* (Hanka and Dietz 1973, Martin et al 1973). It is an amino acid antimetabolite. The compound had excellent activity in a number of mouse cell lines and against human tumor xenografts growing in male mice (Hanka et al 1973), Houchens et al 1978). Good reviews of the clinical and preclinical aspects of acivicin have been published by O'Dwyer et al (1984) and by Earhart (1987).

■ Antitumor Activity

Acivicin is still an investigational agent; however, acivicin has had hints of antitumor activity against a number of tumor types including non-small cell lung cancer (Kramer et al 1986, Maroun et al 1984), colon cancer (Earhart et al 1983, 1987), and gastric cancer (Weiss et al 1982). The drug has been found to be inactive in patients with hepatocellular carcinoma (Falkson et al 1990), ovarian cancer (McGuire et al 1986, Earhart et al 1989), renal cell carcinoma (Elson et al 1988), acute leukemia (Powell et al 1988), colon cancer (Adolphson et al 1986, Eisenhauer et al 1987), mesothelioma (Falkson et al 1987), and breast cancer (Willson et al 1986, Booth et al 1986, Fleishman et al 1983). Most recently, Taylor et al (1991) have noted four objective responses (one complete and three partial) in 32 patients with recurrent gliobastana multiforme.

■ Mechanism of Action

Acivicin is an antagonist of L-glutamine. It inhibits a variety of enzymes that require glutamine as a cofactor. The in vitro inhibition of L1210 cell growth by acivicin is antagonized by L-glutamine (Jayaram et al 1975) or by a combination of cytosine and guanosine ribonucleosides or deoxyribonucleosides (Neil et al 1979). Cytidine triphosphate synthetase, a glutamine-dependent amidotransferase that is the primary target of 3-deazauridine activity, is strongly inhibited by acivicin. The cytotoxic effects of acivicin are probably largely due to inhibition of cytidine triphosphate synthetase (EC 6.3.4.2). Elevation of cellular UTP pools with concomitant decreases in CTP and GTP pools indicates that the cytotoxic effects of acivicin may be mediated by inhibition of CTP synthetase as well as of xanthosine monophosphate aminase, another glutamine-dependent enzyme (Neil et al 1979). Inhibitory effects of acivicin on several other enzymes involved in de novo purine and pyrimidine synthesis are probably of secondary importance (Jayaram et al 1975), as are effects on other glutamine-dependent enzymes.

The biochemical effects of acivicin, summarized in the preceding, would suggest its classification as an S-phase-specific agent. This is supported by cytokinetic and flow cytometry studies (Meck et al 1981). A variety of animal and clinical evidence suggests that such agents are best administered by continuous infusion over periods that are tolerated by the normal marrow stem cell pool (Valeriote and Edelstein 1977, Tannock 1978).

■ Availability and Storage

Acivicin is supplied by the National Cancer Institute in sterile lyophilized form in vials containing 25 mg of drug and 25 mg of mannitol. Unopened vials should be stored at room temperature.

■ Preparation for Use, Stability, and Admixture

Each vial is to be aseptically reconstituted with 2.0 mL of sterile water for injection (without preservative), yielding a drug concentration of 12.5 mg/mL. The appropriate daily dose of this solution should be infused by Harvard pump for 24 hours.

Acivicin is chemically stable for 14 days in solution at 28°C, but reconstituted solutions should be used within 24 hours in accordance with good pharmaceutical technique. Caution should be exercised in handling the powder and preparation of the solution; the use of gloves is recommended.

■ Administration

The optimal schedule for acivicin has not yet been determined. As described under Dosage, a variety of schedules have been explored. The 72-hour infusion schedule is currently being explored using Aminosyn® to protect against the neurotoxicity. When that trial is complete it is hoped an optimal schedule of administration can be arrived at.

■ Special Precautions

The drug causes severe central nervous system (CNS) toxicity and a trial using Aminosyn® to decrease or prevent this toxicity is currently ongoing.

■ Drug Interactions

None are known.

■ Dosage

A number of phase I studies have been performed with acivicin. They are outlined in the following table.

■ Pharmacokinetics

In all but one of the phase I studies (the daily × 5 schedule) noted in the table, central nervous system toxicity was the dose-limiting toxicity. Clearly, acivicin's CNS toxicity was not related to peak plasma drug levels. There was a rough correlation between CNS toxicity and area under (integral of) the concentration × time curve (AUC); however, the data also support the interpretation that CNS toxicity ensues only when plasma acivicin levels exceed 0.9 µg/mL for more than 16 hours.

The table on the opposite page summarizes the pharmacokinetics available. (These have all been obtained using a microbiological method.)

McGovren et al (1985) found that urinary excretion of intact acivicin ranged from 2 to 42% in the first 24 hours.

■ Side Effects and Toxicity

As noted earlier, the dose-limiting toxicity of acivicin involves central nervous system effects. When given by 72-hour continuous intravenous infusion, acivicin produces dose-limiting CNS toxicity (lethargy, somnolence, anxiety, hallucinations, and paranoid psychoses) at doses greater than 75 mg/m^2 per course (Earhart et al 1983). Myelosuppression, including both leukopenia and thrombocytopenia, was dose related as were emesis, diarrhea, malaise, and anorexia. A syndrome of diaphoresis followed by chills, without fever, and occasional ataxia and dizziness, was seen at 75 mg/m^2 per course. By 24-hour infusion (Weiss et al 1982), similar CNS toxicity was dose limiting at 160 mg/m^2 per course, whereas gastrointestinal and hematologic toxic effects were variable and not dose related. When acivicin was administered as a brief single infusion (Taylor et al 1984), CNS toxicity was also dose limiting at 150 mg/m^2 per course, with dose-related gastrointestinal toxicity, mild diarrhea, infrequent chills and fever, and occasional transient rises in serum glutamic oxaloacetic transaminase. Myelosuppression was absent. In contrast, five daily brief infusions (Sridhar et al 1983) produced dose-limiting myelosuppression with acute gastrointestinal toxicity and less common but qualitatively similar neurotoxicity.

The mechanism responsible for the CNS toxicity of acivicin is not known, although several hypotheses have been suggested (Earhart and Neil 1986). Acivicin crosses the blood–brain barrier in mice (McGovren et al 1981) and dogs and monkeys (McGovren et al 1982). In tumor cells in vitro, one study suggests that acivicin transport is mediated by the L-system common to large neutral amino acids (Allen and Yunis 1983). In another study with a different tumor line, transport was inhibited by L-glutamine (Jayaram et al 1985). Brain transport of large neutral amino acids is thought to be mediated by a carrier that is specific and saturable and that

PHASE I TRIALS OF ACIVICIN

Schedule	Dose Range Explored (mg/m^2)	Recommended Phase II Dose (mg/mL)	Dose-Limiting Toxic Effect	Reference
72-hour infusion	3–90	60	CNS effects	Earhart et al 1983
24-hour infusion	—	160 mg/m^2	CNS effects	Weiss et al 1982
Bolus	2.0–150	None	CNS effects	Taylor et al 1984
Daily × 5	0.7–20	12–15	Hemotologic and CNS effects	Sridhar et al 1983
14- to 21-day infusion	1–3.3 mg m^2/d × 14–21 days	—	Mucositis	Poplin et al 1991

PHARMACOKINETICS OF ACIVICIN

Schedule	Half-Life (h) α	Half-Life (h) β	Peak Plasma Level (μg/mL)	Volume of Distribution (L/m²)	Total Body Clearance (L/h/m²)	Reference
Daily × 5	0.32 ± 0.05	9.9 ± 3.9	2.05	21.79 ± 294	1.69 ± 0.48	McGovren et al 1985, 1988
72-hour infusion	0.2–1.1	0.5–1.1	0.09 1.10	—	—	Earhart et al 1983
24-hour continuous	—	6–9	4.66	—	—	Weiss et al 1982
Bolus	—	—	13.85	—	—	Taylor et al 1984

shows competitive effects between different substrates (James and Fisher 1981).

Toxicology studies at the Upjohn Company have demonstrated that adult cats treated with acivicin exhibit clinical signs of CNS toxicity, including ataxia, somnolence, vomiting, and mydriasis (McGovren and Williams 1986). This model has been used to test the hypothesis that uptake of acivicin across the blood–brain barrier might be selectively inhibited by elevated levels of amino acids and that such treatment might prevent the clinical toxic effects. Cats were given continuous intravenous infusions of Aminosyn® 10% or 0.9% Sodium Chloride for Injection, USP, for 22 hours at a rate of 21 mL/h. The Aminosyn® infusion represented an amino acid load equivalent to 18 g/kg/d in cats that averaged 2.8 kg in weight.

The commercial amino acid solution Aminosyn® clearly prevented some of the signs of acivicin intoxication in cats (sedation, ataxia) and lowered the incidence of vomiting, but had little effect on mydriasis (Williams et al 1990). This hypothesis is now being tested in an ongoing phase I clinical trial in San Antonio where acivicin is being given with ammolyn 10% for protection from CNS toxicity. That study is not yet complete.

Other toxic effects (in addition to CNS effects and myelosuppression) of acivicin include mucositis vomiting, diarrhea, and a blue-green discoloration at infusion sites.

■ Special Applications

None are known to date.

REFERENCES

Adolphson CC, Ajani JA, Stroehlein JR, et al. Phase II trial of acivicin in patients with advanced colorectal carcinoma. *Am J Clin Oncol.* 1986;**9**(3):189–191.

Allen LM, Yunis AA. Cellular transport of the glutamine analog acivicin does not require gamma-glutamyl transpeptidase. *ICRS Med Sci.* 1983;**11**:125–126.

Booth BW, Korzun AH, Weiss RB, et al. Phase II trial of acivicin in advanced breast carcinoma: A cancer and leukemia group B study. *Cancer Treat Rep.* 1986;**70**(10):1247–1248.

Earhart RH. Acivicin: A new antimetabolite. *Cancer Treat Res.* 1987;**36**:161–181.

Earhart RH, Khandekar JD, Farassi D, Schinella RA, Davis TE. Phase II trial of continuous drug infusions in advanced ovarian carcinoma: Acivicin versus vinblastine. *Invest New Drugs.* 1989;**7**(2–3):255–260.

Earhart RH, Koeller JM, Davis TE, et al. Phase I trial and pharmacokinetics of acivicin administered by 72-hour infusion. *Cancer Treat Rep.* 1983;**67**(7–8):683–692.

Earhart RH, Mussia FM, Falkson G, Benson AB III, Bennett JM, Schutt AJ. Activity of acivicin in colorectal carcinoma (meeting abstract). *Proc Annu Meet Am Assoc Cancer Res.* 1987;**28**:200.

Earhart RH, Neil GL. Acivicin in 1985. *Adv Enzyme Regul.* 1986;**24**:179–205.

Eisenhauer EA, Maroun JA, Fields AL, Walde PL. Phase II study of acivicin as a 72-hr continuous infusion in patients with untreated colorectal cancer. A National Cancer Institute of Canada Clinical Trials Group study. *Invest New Drugs.* 1987;**5**(4):375–378.

Elson PJ, Kvols LK, Vosl SE, et al. Phase II trials of 5-day vinblastine infusion (NSC-49842), L-alanosine (NSC-153353), acivicin (NSC-163501), and aminothiadiazole (NSC-4728) in patients with recurrent or metastatic renal cell carcinoma. *Invest New Drugs.* 1988;**6**(2):97–103.

Falkson G, Cnaan A, Simson IW, et al. A randomized phase II study of acivicin and 4'-deoxydoxorubicin in patients with hepatocellular carcinoma in an Eastern Cooperative Oncology Group study. *Am J Clin Oncol.* 1990;**13**(6):510–515.

Falkson G, Vorobiof DA, Simson IW, Borden EC. Phase II trial of acivicin in malignant mesothelioma. *Cancer Treat Rep.* 1987;**71**(5):545–546.

Fleishman G, Yap HY, Murphy WK, Bodey G. Phase II trial of acivicin in advanced metastatic breast cancer. *Cancer Treat Rep.* 1983;**67**(9):843–844.

Hanka LJ, Dietz A. U-42126, a new antimetabolite antibiotic: Production, biological activity, and taxonomy of the producing microorganism. *Antimicrob Agents Chemother.* 1973;**3**:425–431.

Hanka LJ, Martin DG, Neil GL. A new antimetabolite, (αS,5S)-α-amino-3-chloro-4,5-dihydro-5-isoxazoleacetic acid (NSC-163501): Antimicrobial reversal studies and preliminary evaluation against L1210 mouse leukemia in vivo. *Cancer Chemother Rep.* 1973;**57**:141–148.

Houchens D, Ovejera A, Johnson R, Bogden A, Neil GL. Therapy of mouse tumors and human tumor xenografts by the antitumor antibiotic AT-125 (NSC-163501). *Proc Am Assoc Cancer Res.* 1978;**19**:40.

James JH, Fischer JE. Transport of neutral amino acids at the blood–brain barrier. *Pharmacology.* 1981;**22**:1–17.

Jayaram HN, Ardalan B, Deas M, Johnson RK. Mechanism of resistance of a variant of P388 leukemia to L-(αS,5S)-α-amino-3-chloro-4,5-dihydro-5-isoxazoleacetic acid (acivicin). *Cancer Res.* 1985;**45**:207–212.

Jayaram HN, Cooney DA, Ryan JA, Neil GL, Dion RL, Bono VH. L-(αS,5S)-α-amino-3-chloro-4,5-isoxazoleacetic acid (NSC-163501). A new amino acid antibiotic with the properties of an antagonist of L-glutamine. *Cancer Chemother Rep.* 1975;**59**:481–491.

Kramer BS, Birch R, Greco A, Prestridge K, Johnson R. Phase II evaluation of acivicin in lung cancer: A Southwestern Cancer Study Group trial. *Cancer Treat Rep.* 1986;**70**(8):1031–1032.

Maroun J, Maksymiuk A, Eisenhauer E, Stewart D, Young V, Pater J. A phase II trial of acivicin (AT-125, NSC 163501) in metastatic nonsmall cell lung cancer (NSCLC). A Canadian National Cancer Institute Study. *Proc Am Soc Clin Oncol* 1984;**3**:218.

Martin DG, Duchamp DJ, Chidester CG. The isolation, structure, and absolute configuration of U-42126, a novel antitumor antibiotic. *Tetrahedron Lett.* 1973;**27**:2549–2552.

McGovren JP, Neil GL, Sern PCC, Stewart JC. Sex- and age-related mouse toxicity and disposition of the amino acid antitumor agent, acivicin. *J Pharmacol Exp Ther.* 1981;**216**:433–440.

McGovren JP, Pratt EA, Belt RJ, et al. Pharmacokinetic and biochemical studies on acivicin in phase I clinical trials. *Cancer Res.* 1985;**45**(9):4460–4463.

McGovren JP, Stewart JC, Elfring GL, et al. Plasma and cerebrospinal fluid pharmacokinetics of acivicin in Ommaya reservoir-bearing monkeys. *Cancer Treat Rep.* 1982;**66**:1333–1341.

McGovren JP, Williams JP. Prevention of acivicin-induced CNS toxicity by concomitant amino acid infusion. *Proc Am Assoc Cancer Res* 1986;**27**:421.

McGovren JP, Williams MG, Stewart JC. Interspecies comparison of acivicin pharmacokinetics. *Drug Metab Dispos.* 1988;**16**(1):18–22.

McGuire WP, Blessin JA, DiSaia PJ, Buchsbaum HJ. Phase II trial of acivicin in patients with advanced epithelial ovarian carcinoma. A Gynecologic Oncology Group study. *Invest New Drugs.* 1986;**4**(1):49–52.

Meck RA, Clubb KJ, Allen LM, Yunis AA. Inhibition of cell cycle progression of human pancreatic carcinoma cells in vitro by L-(αS,5S)-α-amino-3-chloro-4,5-dihydro-5-isoxazoleacetic acid, acivicin (NSC-163501). *Cancer Res.* 1981;**41**:4547–4553.

Neil GL, Berger AE, McPartland RP, Grindey GB, Bloch A. Biochemical and pharmacological effects of the fermentation-derived antitumor agent, (αS,5S)-α-amino-3-chloro-4,5-isoxazoleacetic acid (AT-125). *Cancer Res.* 1979;**39**:852–856.

O'Dwyer PJ, Alonso MT, Leyland-Jones B. Acivicin: A new glutamine antagonist in clinical trials. *J Clin Oncol.* 1984;**2**(9):1064–1071.

Poplin E, LoRusso P, Foster B. Acivicin by continuous low-dose infusion: A phase I trial. *Am Assoc Cancer Res.* 1991;**32**:202.

Powell BL, Crais JB, Capizzi RL, Richards F. Phase I–II trial of acivicin in adult acute leukemia. *Invest New Drugs.* 1988;**6**(1):41–44.

Sridhar KS, Ohnuma T, Chahinian AP, Holland JF. Phase I study of acivicin in patients with advanced cancer. *Cancer Treat Rep.* 1983;**67**(7–8):701–703.

Tannock I. Cell kinetics and chemotherapy: A critical review. *Cancer Treat Rep.* 1978;**62**:1117–1133.

Taylor S, Belt RJ, Joseph U, Haas CD, Hoogstraten B. Phase I evaluation of AT-125 single dose every three weeks. *Invest New Drugs.* 1984;**2**:311–314.

Taylor SA, Crowley J, Pollock TW, et al. Objective antitumor activity of acivicin in patients with recurrent CNS malignancies: A Southwest Oncology Group Trial. *J Clin Oncol.* 1991;**9**(8):1476–1479.

Valeriote FA, Edelstein MB. The role of cell kinetics in cancer chemotherapy. *Semin Oncol.* 1977;**4**:217–226.

Weiss GR, McGovren JP, Schade D, Kufe DW. Phase I and pharmacological study of acivicin by 24-hour continuous infusion. *Cancer Res.* 1982;**42**(9):3892–3895.

Williams MG, Earhart RH, Bailey H, McGovren JP. Prevention of central nervous system toxicity of the antitumor antibiotic acivicin by concomitant infusion of an amino acid mixture. *Cancer Res.* 1990;**50**(17):5475–5480.

Willson JK, Knuiman ME, Skeel RT, et al. Phase II clinical trial of acivicin in advanced breast cancer: An Eastern Cooperative Oncology Group study. *Cancer Treat Rep.* 1986;**70**(10):1237–1238.

Aclarubicin

Other Names

Aclacinomycin; aclacinomycin A; ACM; NSC-209834.

Chemistry

Structure of aclarubicin

Aclarubicin (ACM) is an anthracycline similar to doxorubicin possessing three modified sugars linked glycosidically at the C-7 position of the planar anthracycline chromophore. The three sugars, rhodosamine, 2-deoxyfucose, and cinerulose, are each linked via a glycosidic bond. The drug was originally isolated from *Streptomyces galilaeus* (Oki et al 1975). The complete chemical name is 2-ethyl-1,2,3,4,6,11-hexahydro-2,5,7-trihydroxy-6,11-dioxo-4-[[2,3,6-trideoxy-4-O-[2,6-dideoxy-4-O-[2R-*trans*-tetrahydro-6-methyl-5-oxo-2H-pyran-2-yl]-α-L-lyxo-hexopyranosyl]-3-(dimethylamino)-α-L-lyxo-hexopyranosyl]oxy]-1-naphthacenecarboxylic acid methyl ester. The molecular weight is 884.4 with a molecular formula of $C_{42}H_{53}NO_{15}$ HCl·$2H_2O$. Besides the different sugars, ACM has ethyl and acetyl substitutions at the C-1 and C-2 positions and a hydroxyl at the C-4 position. These each differ from doxorubicin (Egorin et al 1982). Aclarubicin has a pK_a of 7.3 and is more lipophilic than either doxorubicin (DOX) or daunorubicin (DAUNO) (Zenebergh et al 1982). Thus, the octanol/water coefficient of ACM is 21.8 compared with 3.3 and 0.5 for DAUNO and DOX, respectively.

Antitumor Activity

In preclinical studies ACM has shown activity in a variety of murine models including P-388 leukemia, CD8F mammary carcinoma, and colon-38 (Oki 1977). Early clinical trials in Europe and Japan have shown activity for ACM in leukemia (Mathe et al 1978; Suzuki et al 1979), in lymphoma (Mathe et al 1978, Ogawa et al 1979, Oka 1978), and in several solid tumors including cancers of the lung, breast, and stomach (Furue et al 1978, Kumashiro et al 1980, Ogawa et al 1979).

In phase II trials, ACM produced responses in myelogenous leukemia (Dabich et al 1986), advanced lymphomas (Case et al 1985), and rarely in multiple myeloma (Karanes et al 1990).

Aclarubicin is active in some acute non-lymphocytic leukemia patients who did not respond to other anthracyclines. Activity has also been observed in acute nonlymphocytic leukemia patients treated with ACM either alone (Pedersen-Bjergaard et al 1984) or in combination with etoposide (Rowe et al 1988). Some activity has also been observed in soft tissue sarcoma (Bertrand et al 1985) and rarely in breast cancer (Casper et al 1981). The table on page 136 summarizes these data. Overall, there is not a clear unique clinical indication for ACM and the drug is currently unavailable for further clinical trials in the United States.

Mechanism of Action

Aclarubicin produces potent inhibition of nucleic acid synthesis with an eightfold greater effect on RNA synthesis than DNA synthesis (Tone et al 1985). In L-1210 cells the 50% inhibitory ACM concentrations were 0.038 for RNA synthesis and 0.30 for DNA synthesis. Both RNA polymerase and DNA polymerase activities are also inhibited by the drug (Tone et al 1985). Aclacinomycin binds to DNA by an intercalative type of mechanism with one ACM binding site per 4 bp at saturating drug concentrations (Yamaki et al 1978, Katenkamp et al 1983).

With short-term drug exposures, sigmoidal cytotoxicity curves are produced in leukemia cells in vitro. Prolonging the drug exposure period to 24 hours changes the response to a simple, steep exponential curve, suggesting enhanced cytotoxicity for prolonged ACM exposures. Other in vitro studies in

PHASE II ANTITUMOR ACTIVITY OF ACLACINOMYCIN

Tumor Type	Partial Response Rate	Reference
Acute nonlymphocytic leukemia	2/20 (10%)	Dabich et al 1986
Acute lymphocytic leukemia	0/4	
Advanced lymphomas	5/53 (15%) (0 in anthracycline-refractory patients)	Case et al 1985
Multiple myeloma	1/43	Karanes et al 1990
	0/35	Gockerman et al 1987
Sarcoma	30%	Bertrand et al 1985
Breast cancer	Rare	Casper et al 1981
Head and neck cancer	None	Carugati et al 1986
Non-small cell lung cancer	None	Chiuten et al 1985
		Ettinger et al 1985
Advanced small cell lung cancer	None	Abeloff et al 1985

synchronized leukemia cells show that ACM blocks cell cycle progression at the G_1–S border and also in late S phase (Tanabe et al 1980).

The cellular pharmacology of ACM may differ from that of other anthracyclines in that distribution into cytosol may be greater than nuclear uptake as measured by fluorescence (Egorin et al 1979). Another study using high-performance liquid chromatographic drug measurements contradicts this, however, showing that 90% of ACM *is* concentrated in the nucleus of L-1210 cells after 5 hours of incubation (Zenebergh et al 1982). Seeber et al (1980) also showed major ACM uptake into the nucleus. One explanation for the prior finding of little ACM nuclear uptake may be the large amount of quenching of anthracycline fluorescence by DNA (Du Verney et al 1979).

Aclarubicin is also concentrated in lysosomes and appears to be taken up into cells more rapidly than is DOX (Zenebergh et al 1982). These features may relate to the greater ionization of ACM at physiologic pH and the greater degree of lipophilicity, respectively. Other mechanistic effects that distinguish ACM from DOX include (1) ACM antagonism of etoposide or AMSA-induced formation of a "cleavable complex" between DNA and topoisomerase II (Jensen et al 1990) and (2) the lack of mutagenic activity in vitro (Umezawa et al 1978). If given prior to other topoisomerase II inhibitory drugs, ACM may antagonize their effects instead of producing additive inhibition (see Drug Interactions); however, one preliminary study has reported that ACM produces DNA single-strand breaks in P-388 cells (Li et al 1990). Thus, ACM may cause DNA strand breaks by a mechanism not involving an alteration of topoisomerase II.

■ Availability and Storage

Aclacinomycin was available investigationally from the National Cancer Institute in 10-mL amber vials containing 10 mg lyophilized powdered drug and 100 mg lactose. The intact vials should be stored under refrigeration and are stable for at least 4 years after manufacture (U.S. Department of Health and Human Services [USDHHS] 1987).

■ Preparation for Use, Stability, and Admixture

Each vial is reconstituted with 5 mL of 0.9% Sodium Chloride for Injection, USP, resulting in a 4 mg/mL concentration at a pH of 4.5 to 6.5. Paraben-preserved diluents were not recommended because of possible precipitate formation (USDHHS 1987). Slow decomposition (4% over 72 hours) may occur in sunlight and overall stability is pH sensitive. Greater stability is observed at pH 6.2, with degradation noted at pH 3 or less (Poochikian et al 1981). The drug is stable for at least 24 hours at room temperature at a concentration of 128 µg/mL in the following intravenous infusion solutions: 5% dextrose in water (D5W), 0.9% sodium chloride (saline), lactated Ringer's injection, and Normosol-R, pH 7.4 (Poochikian et al 1981).

■ Administration

Aclarubicin is administered intravenously. Typical infusions involve drug dilution into 50 to 100 mL of

D5W or saline given over 20–30 minutes (Woolley et al 1982, Dabich et al 1986). The drug has also been administered as a continuous infusion over 24 hours (Chiuten et al 1985). See Special Applications for an investigational intraperitoneal ACM regimen and an arterial chemoembolization regimen.

■ Dose

The following table summarizes the recommended intravenous doses for different aclarubicin schedules. Note that significant dose reductions are recommended for poor-risk patients (extensive prior therapy and/or poor performance status).

■ Drug Interactions

Human small cell lung cancer cells exposed to noncytotoxic concentrations of ACM in vitro become almost completely insensitive to etoposide (Jensen et al 1990). If aclarubicin is given after etoposide, no interaction is seen. The mechanism for the sequence-dependent interaction may involve inhibition by ACM of cleavable complex formation between topoisomerase II enzymes and DNA. Both effects, etoposide inhibition and the lack of an effect on topoisomerase II, are different from the activities of other DNA intercalators such as doxorubicin (Tewey et al 1984). Despite this in vitro interaction, the clinical combination of etoposide and aclarubicin given sequentially is active in patients with acute myelogenous leukemias who are refractory to other anthracyclines (Rowe et al 1988).

■ Pharmacokinetics

Aclarubicin displays the typical triphasic plasma disappearance pattern common to other anthracyclines (see the table on page 138); however, the terminal elimination phase for ACM is much shorter at 2.7 hours than with other anthracyclines.

The plasma kinetics of the drug do not appear to be altered with increasing doses (Malspeis et al 1981). The drug appears to selectively concentrate in leukocytes (Ando et al 1986). Several metabolites of ACM with longer plasma half-lives have been identified (Egorin et al 1982). Some, containing intact rhodosamine, are active (Malspeis et al 1981). One more nonpolar inactive metabolite is a drug–drug aglycone dimer, bisanhydroaklavinone, formed by microsomal NADPH–cytochrome P450 reductase (Egorin et al 1982). Metabolites more polar than ACM have also been observed in humans. Metabolites form slowly over a 24-hour period following drug injection by two types of reactions: (1) enzymatic reduction of the terminal keto sugar to form stereoisomeric active glycosidic metabolites, and (2) enzymatic cleavage of the trisaccharide yielding the inactive aglycone, 7-deoxyaklavinone (Egorin et al 1982).

■ Side Effects and Toxicity

The dose-limiting toxic effect of ACM is myelosuppression, primarily thrombocytopenia. The platelet nadir occurs on about day 10 after dosing (Casper et al 1981). Granulocytopenia is more variable and is occasionally prolonged, without full recovery even after 21 days. Median nadirs are reported to occur between 16 and 20 days (Van Echo et al 1982). In some cases a transient "rebound" thrombocytosis is noted following the initial platelet depression. None of the myelosuppressive effects of ACM appear to be cumulative.

Nausea and vomiting of mild to moderate in-

ACLARUBICIN DOSES WITH DIFFERENT INTRAVENOUS SCHEDULES

Dose (mg/m^2)						
Good Risk	Poor Risk*	Days	Repeat Course (wk)	Infusion Method	Disease	Reference
100	60	1	4	Bolus	Solid tumors	Van Echo et al 1982
100	80	1	3	Bolus	Tumors	Casper et al 1981
85	85	1	Weekly × 4	Bolus	Solid tumors	Baker et al 1981
75[†]	75[†]	1–4[†]	3	Bolus	Leukemia	Dabich et al 1986
25	20	1–5	4	Bolus	Solid tumors	Woolley et al 1982
120	120	1	3–4	Continuous 24-hour	NSCLC[‡]	Chiuten et al 1985

*Heavily pretreated patients and/or those with poor performance status.
[†]Total dose of 300 mg/m^2 in refractory leukemics in highly myelosuppressive and is not indicated in solid tumor patients.
[‡]Non-small cell lung cancer.

Pharmacokinetic Parameter	Value
Half-life	
α (min)	2.5
β (min)	20
γ (h)	2.7
Volume of distribution (L/m^2)	
Central	60
γ Phase	938
Total body clearance (L/min/m^2)	4

tensity are common following ACM. Anorexia and malaise may also be seen, but mucositis and diarrhea are rare. Transient hepatic enzyme elevation is occasionally reported (Ogawa et al 1979, Van Echo et al 1982). Hyperbilirubinemia was also noted in early Japanese trials (Ogawa et al 1979). Typically, renal and hepatic toxic effects have not been reported (Woolley et al 1982, Casper et al 1981). Alopecia also appears to be minimal with ACM (Woolley et al 1982). The drug does not typically cause phlebitis although venous urticaria has been described rarely (Van Echo et al 1982). Aclarubicin may also cause a venous "flare" reaction characterized by erythema, pain, and swelling along the path of the vein used for infusion (Glass 1982). In animals, ACM is much less active as a vesicant (Dantchev et al 1978, Jenkins and Corden 1983), suggesting that extravasations may not produce the severe necrosis seen with DOX in humans.

Cardiotoxicity studies in animals demonstrate significantly less cardiotoxicity for ACM compared with either DOX or DAUNO (Tone et al 1985, Hori et al 1977, Oki 1977). Clinically insignificant transient electrocardiographic changes were noted in early trials of ACM (Ogawa et al 1979) whereas latter phase I studies occasionally reported premature atrial and ventricular beats with complete heart block described in a single case (Van Echo et al 1982). The acute cardiac toxic effects of ACM may be heralded by a flushed feeling with diaphoresis which is reported in up to 39% of patients receiving ACM (Van Echo et al 1982). Supraventricular tachycardia is reported in about 25% of patients (Chiuten et al 1985). These acute cardiovascular effects generally disappear within 1 to 5 hours of drug administration. Some late rhythm disturbances are also described (Dabich et al 1986). A prospective study of ACM cardiac toxicity showed minimal changes in left ventricular ejection fractions (LVEF) with cumulative ACM doses up to 700 mg/m^2 (Unverferth et al 1982); however, one patient at that dose level examined by endomyocardial biopsy did show slight dilation of tubular structures and mitochondria with some myofibrillar dropout. Another patient developed a 28% drop in LVEF after receiving 380 mg/m^2 DOX and 100 mg/m^2 ACM (Woolley et al 1982). Overall, ACM appears to be clinically less cardiotoxic than other anthracyclines but it does produce similar toxic effects and the cardiac damage is at least additive with that of other anthracyclines.

■ Special Applications

Intraperitoneal ACM has been tested in patients with various solid tumors: five ovarian, one breast, one colon, and one leiomyosarcoma (Kerr et al 1987). Each dose was diluted in 2 L of 1.5% Dianeal solution. Doses of 25 to 75 mg of ACM were instilled intraperitoneally via a Tenckhoff catheter and produced intraperitoneal levels of 7.7 to 24.8 μg/mL. No drug was detectable in the plasma at any dose or time point. The intraperitoneal concentration × time products were 7 to 3, 13 to 25, and 1300 to 6200 μg · min/mL for intraperitoneal doses of 25, 50, and 75 mg, respectively. Clearance from the intraperitoneal space ranged from 7 to 60 mL/min (median 12.7 mL/min). The major dose-limiting toxic effects were moderate to severe abdominal pain, as a result of chemical peritonitis, and mild nausea and vomiting (Kerr et al 1987). Two patients had a reduced amount of ascites from ovarian cancer following the intraperitoneal ACM treatments.

Arterial chemoembolization has also been performed with ACM to treat 62 patients with primary hepatocellular carcinoma (Ichihara et al 1989). Microspheres of polylactic acid (200 μm in diameter) containing 10% (w/w) aclarubicin were infused via the hepatic artery for one to eight courses. More than 80% of patients had reduced α-fetoprotein levels and tumor shrinkage with a cumulative survival rate at 1, 2, and 3 years of 54, 25, and 19%, respectively. Toxic effects consisted of nausea and vomiting (66%), abdominal pain and fever (40%), increased amylase levels (34%), and jaundice (8%). Myelosuppression was not observed and high hepatic drug levels (> 200 μg/g liver) were documented (Ichihara et al 1989).

REFERENCES

Abeloff MD, Finkelstein DM, Chang AY-C, et al. Phase II study of aclarubicin and diaziquone in the treatment of advanced small cell bronchogenic carcinoma (EST 4581): An Eastern Cooperative Oncology Group study. *Cancer Treat Rep.* 1985;**69**:451–452.

Ando S, Nakamura T, Kagawa D, et al. Pharmacokinetics of aclarubicin and its metabolites in humans and their disposition in blood cells. *Cancer Treat Rep.* 1986;**70**:835–841.

Baker L, Samson M, Young J, Franco L. Phase I evaluation of aclacinomycin A (NSC-208734) in a weekly I.V. schedule. *Am Soc Clin Oncol.* 1981;**21**:353.

Bertrand M, Multhauf P, Bartolucci A, et al. Phase II study of aclarubicin in previously untreated patients with advanced soft tissue sarcoma: A Southeastern Cancer Study Group trial. *Cancer Treat Rep.* 1985;**69**:725–726.

Carugati AA, Olivari AJ, Campos DM, et al. Phase II trial of aclarubicin in epidermoid carcinoma of the head and neck. *Cancer Treat Rep.* 1986;**70**:799–800.

Case DC Jr, Boyd MA, Hayes DM. Phase II study of aclarubicin in patients with lymphoma. *Cancer Treat Rep.* 1985;**69**:1315–1316.

Casper ES, Gralla RJ, Young CW. Clinical phase I study of aclacinomycin A by evaluation of an intermittent intravenous administration schedule. *Cancer Res.* 1981;**41**:2417–2420.

Chiuten DF, Umsawasdi T, Dhingra HM, et al. Aclarubicin given as continuous infusion in non-small cell bronchogenic carcinoma. *Cancer Treat Rep.* 1985;**69**:1327–1328.

Dabich L, Bull FE, Beltran G, et al. Phase II evaluation of aclarubicin in refractory adult acute leukemia: A Southwest Oncology Group study. *Cancer Treat Rep.* 1986;**70**:967–969.

Dantchev D, Slioussartchouk V, Paintrand M, et al. Electron microscopic studies of the heart and light microscopic studies of the skin after treatment of Golden hamsters with Adriamycin, detorubicin, AD-32, and aclacinomycin. *Cancer Treat Rep.* 1978;**63**:875–888.

Du Verney VH, Pachter JA, Crooke ST. Deoxyribonucleic acid binding studies on several new anthracycline antitumor antibiotics. Sequence preference and structure–activity relationships of marcellomycin and its analogues as compared to Adriamycin. *Biochemistry.* 1979;**18**:4024–4030.

Egorin MJ, Clawson RE, Ross LA. Cellular accumulation and disposition of aclacinomycin A. *Cancer Res.* 1979;**39**:4396–4401.

Egorin MJ, Van Echo D, Fox BM, et al. Plasma kinetics of aclacinomycin A and its major metabolites in man. *Cancer Chemother Pharmacol.* 1982;**8**:41–46.

Ettinger DS, Finkelstein DM, Haper GR, et al. Phase II study of mitoxantrone, aclarubicin, and diaziquone in the treatment of non-small cell lung carcinoma: An Eastern Cooperative Oncology Group study. *Cancer Treat Rep.* 1985;**69**:1033–1034.

Furue H, Komita T, Nakao I, et al. Clinical experiences with aclacinomycin-A. Recent results. *Cancer Res.* 1978;**63**:241–246.

Glass EC. Aclacinomycin A flare. *Cancer Treat Rep.* 1982;**66**:1683.

Gockerman JP, Silberman HH, Bartolucci AA. Phase II evaluation of aclarubicin in refractory multiple myeloma: A Southeastern Cancer Study Group trial. *Cancer Treat Rep.* 1987;**71**:773–774.

Hori S, Shirai M, Hirano S, et al. Antitumor activity of new anthracycline antibiotics, aclacinomycin-A and its analogs, and their toxicity. *Gann.* 1977;**68**:685–690.

Ichihara T, Sakamoto K, Mori K, Akagi M. Transcatheter arterial chemoembolization therapy for hepatocellular carcinoma using polylactic acid microspheres containing aclarubicin hydrochloride. *Cancer Res.* 1989;**49**:4357–4362.

Jenkins J, Corden BJ. Vesicant activity of chemotherapeutic agents. *Cancer Treat Rep.* 1983;**67**:409.

Jensen PB, Sorensen BS, Demant EJF, et al. Antagonistic effect of aclarubicin on the cytotoxicity of etoposide and 4'-(9-acridinylamino)methanesulfon-*m*-anisidide in human small cell lung cancer cell line and on topoisomerase II-mediated DNA cleavage. *Cancer Res.* 1990;**50**:3311–3316.

Karanes C, Crowley J, Sawkar L, et al. Aclacinomycin A in the treatment of multiple myeloma: A Southwest Oncology Group study. *Invest New Drugs.* 1990;**8**:101–104.

Katenkamp U, Stretter E, Petri I, et al. Interaction of anthracycline antibiotics with biopolymers. VII. Binding parameters of aclacinomycin A to DNA. *J Antibiot.* 1983;**36**:1222.

Kerr IG, Archer S, DeAngelis C, et al. Phase I and pharmacokinetic study of high volume intraperitoneal aclacinomycin-A (aclarubicin). *Invest New Drugs.* 1987;**5**:171–176.

Kumashiro R, Tamada R, Kanematsu T, Inokuchi K. A clinical study of intermittent high-dose administration of aclacinomycin-A in patients with advanced cancer. In: *Eleventh International Congress of Chemotherapy, Program and Abstracts.* Washington, DC: American Society of Microbiology, 1980: Abstract 386.

Li ZR, Yin MB, Rustum YM. Cytotoxicity and DNA damage induced by aclacinomycin A and B in Adriamycin-sensitive and -resistant P388 cells. *Am Assoc Cancer Res.* 1990;**31**:356.

Malspeis L, Neidhart J, Staubus A, et al. HPLC determination of aclacinomycin A (NSC-208734, ACM) in plasma and application to preliminary clinical pharmacokinetic studies. *Am Assoc Cancer Res.* 1981;**22**:242.

Mathe G, Baussas M, Gouveia J, et al. Preliminary results of a phase II trial of aclacinomycin in acute leukemia and lymphosarcoma. *Cancer Chemother Pharmacol.* 1978;**1**:259–262.

Ogawa M, Inagaki J, Horikoshi N, et al. Clinical study of aclacinomycin A. *Cancer Treat Rep.* 1979;**63**:931–934.

Oka S. A review of clinical studies on aclacinomycin A—Phase I and preliminary phase II evaluation of ACM. *Sci Rep Res Inst Tohoku Univ Ser C.* 1978;**25**:37–49.

Oki T. New anthracycline antibiotics. *Jpn J Antibiot.* 1977;**30**(suppl):70–84.

Oki T, Matsuzawa Y, Yoshimoto A, et al. New antitumor antibiotics, aclacinomycins A and B. *J Antibiot (Tokyo).* 1975;**28**:830–834.

Pedersen-Bjergaard J, Brincker H, Ellegaard J, et al. Aclarubicin in the treatment of acute nonlymphocytic leukemia refractory to treatment with daunomycin and cytarabine: A phase II trial. *Cancer Treat Rep.* 1984;**68**:1233–1238.

Poochikian GK, Cradock JC, Flora KF. Anthracycline antitumor agents: Stability in infusion fluids by high-performance liquid chromatography. *Am J Hosp Pharm.* 1981;**38**:483–486.

Rowe JM, Chang AYC, Bennett JM. Aclacinomycin A and etoposide (VP-16-213). An effective regimen in previously treated patients with refractory acute myelogenous leukemia. *Blood.* 1988;**71**:992–996.

Seeber S, Loth H, Crooke ST. Comparative nuclear and cellular incorporation of daunorubicin, doxorubicin, carminomycin, marcellomycin, aclacinomycin A and AD-32 in daunorubicin-sensitive and -resistant Ehrlich ascites in vitro. *J Cancer Res Clin Oncol.* 1980;**98**:109–118.

Suzuki H, Kawashima K, Yamada K. Aclacinomycin A, a new antileukemic agent. *Lancet.* 1979;**1**:870–871.

Tanabe M, Miyamoto T, Nakajima Y, Terashima T. Lethal effect of aclacinomycin A on cultured mouse L cells. *Gann.* 1980;**71**:699.

Tewey KM, Rowe TC, Yang L. Adriamycin-induced DNA damage mediated by mammalian DNA topoisomerase II. *Science.* 1984;**226**:466–468.

Tone H, Nishida H, Takeuchi T, Umezawa H. Experimental studies on aclacinomycin. *Drugs Exp Clin Res.* 1985;**11**:9–15.

Umezawa K, Sawamura M, Matsushima T, Sugimura T. Mutagenicity of aclacinomycin A and daunomycin derivatives. *Cancer Res.* 1978;**38**:1782.

Unverferth DV, Balcerzak SP, Neidhart JA. Cardiac evaluation of aclacinomycin (ACLAC) and dihydroxyanthracenedione (DHAD). *Am Assoc Cancer Res.* 1982; **23**:135.

U.S. Department of Health and Human Services. Aclarubicin hydrochloride (NSC-208734). In: *NCI Investigational Drugs—Pharmaceutical Data.* Washington, DC: U.S. Govt Printing Office, 1987:96–99.

Van Echo DA, Whitacre MY, Aisner J, et al. Phase I trial of aclacinomycin A. *Cancer Treat Rep.* 1982;**66**:1127–1132.

Woolley PV, Ayoob MJ, Levenson SM, Smith FP. A phase I clinical trial of aclacinomycin A administered on a five-consecutive-day schedule. *J Clin Pharmacol.* 1982;**22**:359–365.

Yamaki H, Suzuki H, Nishimura T, Tanaka N. Mechanism of action of aclacinomycin A1. The effect on macromolecular synthesis. *J Antibiot.* 1978;**31**:1149.

Zenebergh A, Baurain R, Trouet A. Cellular pharmacokinetics of aclacinomycin A in cultured L1210 cells. *Cancer Chemother Pharmacol.* 1982;**8**:243–249.

Acodazole

■ Other Names

N-methyl-*N*-[4-[(7-methyl-1*H*- imidazo [4,5-*f*]-quinoline-9-yl)amino]phenyl]acetamide, monohydride; acodazole hydrochloride; NSC-305884.

■ Chemistry

Structure of acodazole

Acodazole is a water-soluble imidazoquinolone derivative with a molecular weight of 381.86 and a molecular formula of $C_{20}H_{19}N_5O \cdot HCl$. The compound was originally synthesized by Snyder and colleagues (1977) as an antibacterial agent.

■ Antitumor Activity

This agent was investigated in phase I dose-finding studies only. No complete or partial responses were noted in those trials. Because of the major organ toxic effects noted in early trials, the agent has not been advanced to phase II efficacy studies.

■ Mechanism of Action

In vitro studies have suggested that acodazole probably works as an intercalating agent. Acodazole stabilizes DNA to thermal denaturation, produces protein-associated DNA single-strand breaks, and nonselectively blocks nucleic acid and protein synthesis. The compound was active against intraperitoneally implanted B-16 melanoma and P-388 leukemia. It was inactive against four sublines of P-388 leukemia resistant to unrelated DNA intercalators (amsacrine, doxorubicin, mitoxantrone, and ellipticine [Johnson 1981]).

■ Availability and Storage

This agent is not currently available for clinical trials. Acodazole was investigationally available from the National Cancer Institute as a sterile light yellow lyophilized powder. Each vial contains 200 mg of acodazole with 120 mg of mannitol. The intact vial should be stored under refrigeration (2–8°C).

■ Preparation for Use, Stability, and Admixture

To each 200-mg vial 3.6 mL of Sodium Chloride Injection, USP, is added. Each milliliter of the resulting solution will contain 50 mg of acodazole hydrochloride and 30 mg of mannitol at pH 3.0 to 5.0. At a concentration of 50 mg/mL in both distilled water and sodium chloride injection, acodazole exhibited no decomposition over 12 days at room temperature in normal laboratory light. Diluted to a concentration of 1 mg/mL in 5% Dextrose Injection, USP, or in 0.90% Sodium Chloride Injection, USP, less than 2% decomposition occurred in 12 days at room temperature under normal laboratory light. As the single-use vial contains no antibacterial preservatives, it is advised that the reconstituted product be discarded 8 hours after initial entry.

■ Administration

In phase I trials of acodazole, a variety of schedules of administration were tried, including the following:

Single IV dose from 48 to 480 mg/m² repeated monthly	Grever et al (1986)
Daily IV dose for 5 days ranging from 38 to 342 mg/m²/d	Grever et al (1986)
Continuous IV infusion for 5 days ranging from 38 to 304 mg/m²/d	Grever et al (1986)
1-hour infusion once weekly × 4	Trump et al (1987)
1-hour infusion every 21 days	Pazdur et al (1988)

Because of severe toxic effects in phase I studies no schedule for phase II studies of acodazole can be recommended. These toxic effects include cardiac toxicity on the weekly × 4 (Trump et al 1987) and 1-hour infusion every 21 days (Pazdur et al 1988) schedules, acute tubular necrosis on the single-dose schedule (Grever et al 1986), painful paresthesias on the daily × 5 days schedule (Grever et al 1986), and phlebitis on the continuous infusion schedule (Grever et al 1986).

■ Special Precautions

It is clear acodazole causes significant cardiac, renal, and vein toxic effects. Patients with preexisting cardiac or renal disease of any kind should be excluded from receiving this agent.

■ Drug Interactions

None have been described.

■ Dosage

The maximally tolerated dose (MTD) on each schedule is outlined in the table below.

■ Pharmacokinetics

Pharmacokinetic studies are summarized in the table on page 142.

The plasma profile exhibited a triexponential decay. The volumes of distribution were large, which is indicative of a very high degree of tissue binding of the drug. In dogs the compound was found in high levels in myocardium (53-fold higher than plasma), liver (102-fold higher than plasma), and kidney (114-fold higher than plasma) (Pazdur et al 1988). In humans, there was no apparent relationship between acodazole blood levels and prolongation of the QT interval on the electrocardiogram (Trump et al 1987).

■ Side Effects and Toxicity

On the weekly × 4 schedule the dose-limiting toxic effect was prolongation of the QT interval (Trump et al 1987). One patient developed a polymorphic ventricular tachycardia (torsades des pointes). Nausea and vomiting as well as burning at the site of infu-

PHASE I TRIAL OF ACODAZOLE

Schedule	MTD (mg/m²)	Reference
Single dose monthly	480	Grever et al 1986
Daily × 5	342 (per day)	Grever et al 1986
Continuous infusion × 5 days	304 (per day)	Grever et al 1986
1-Hour infusion every 21 days	1370	Pazdur et al 1988
Weekly × 4	1000	Trump et al 1987

PHARMACOKINETICS OF ACODAZOLE

Schedule (Reference)	Peak Plasma Concentration C_P (µg/mL)	AUC (mg·hL)	Half-life α (min)	Half-life β (h)	Half-life γ (h)	MRT* (h)	Total Body Clearance (mL/min/m²)	Volume of Distribution (L/m²) Central	Volume of Distribution (L/m²) Steady State	Volume of Distribution (L/m²) $V_{d_\gamma}^*$	Urinary Recovery (% dose)
Weekly × 4 (Trump et al 1987)	4.81–13.60	23.6–73.5	6.55	2.21	20.7	20.2	256 ± 73.5	21.9 ± 9.6	319 ± 42.5	454 ± 76.7	25.8 ± 8.1 (72 h)
Variable (Staubus et al 1985)	—	—	17.8	2.86	20.8	20.71	295 ± 75.9	61.1	377	555.9	—
1-Hour IV infusion (Pazdur et al 1988)	9.8–19.2	34.5–85.8	8.4	2.5	19.5	—	226	16.7 ± 2.1	238 ± 18	370 ± 34	29 ± 2 (48 h)

*V_{d_γ}, terminal phase volume of distribution; MRT, mean residence time.

sion were also noted. Pazdur et al (1988), using the 1-hour infusion every 21 days, also noted dose-limiting toxic effects consisting of multiple premature ventricular contractions, QT_c interval prolongation, and decreasing heart rate. Nausea and vomiting as well as local reactions at the intravenous site (requiring use of a central venous catheter) were reported. Grever and colleagues (1986) noted renal toxicity (acute tubular necrosis in one patient) on the single dose every month schedule. Mild (grade 1) renal toxicity was also noted on the daily × 5 schedule as were grade 2 nausea and vomiting, hypotension, and painful paresthesias. When they explored the 5-day continuous infusion there was reversible local tissue erythema and edema. No tissue necrosis was observed. Dilution of the daily dose in a total volume of 3 L/d did not ameliorate this local toxicity.

■ **Special Applications**

None are known at this time.

REFERENCES

Grever MR, Gochnour DC, Neidhart JA, Kraut EH, Balcerzak SP, Malspeis L. A phase I clinical investigation of acodazole. *Proc Am Soc Clin Oncol.* 1986;**5**:53.

Johnson RK. *Final Progress Report on Acodazole.* Arthur D. Little, Inc., Contract N01 CM8-7186. Washington, DC: National Cancer Institute, 1981.

Pazdur R, Chabot GG, Campbell CA, Lehmann MH, Kloner RA, Baker LH. Acodazole hydrochloride: Phase I trial, pharmacokinetics, and evaluation of cardiotoxicity in dogs. *Cancer Res.* 1988;**48**:4423–4426.

Snyder HR Jr, Spencer CF, Freedman R. Imidazo[4,5-f]quinolines. III. Antibacterial: 7-methyl-9-(substituted arylamino)imidazo[4,5-f] quinolines. *J Pharm Sci.* 1977;**66**:1204–1206.

Staubus AE, DeSouza JJV, Grever MR, Neidhart JA, Malspeis L. Clinical pharmacokinetics of acodazole hydrochloride (HSC305884). *Proc Am Assoc Cancer Res.* 1985;**26**:160.

Trump DL, Tutsch KD, Willson JKV, et al. Phase I clinical trial and pharmacokinetics evaluation of acodazole (HSC 305884), an imidazoquinoline derivative with electrophysiological effects on the heart. *Cancer Res.* 1987;**47**:3895–3900.

Acronycine

■ **Other Names**

NSC-403169.

■ **Chemistry**

Structure of acronycine

Acronycine is a natural alkaloid isolated from the bark of the scrub ash or yellowwood, *Acronychia baueri* Schott (Liska 1972). These trees are native to Australia and New Zealand (Svoboda et al 1966). The chemical name of the drug is 3,12-dihydro-6-methoxy-3,3,12-trimethyl-7H-pyrano-[2,3-C]acridin-7-one. The natural alkaloids are highly lipophilic (log P = 2.6 for acronycine) and have weak bases which are typically dissolved only in strong acids or in an alcoholic cosolvent system (Dorr and Liddil 1988). The molecular formula of acronycine is $C_{20}H_{19}O_3N_1$ with a molecular weight of approximately 321.

■ **Antitumor Activity**

Acronycine initially showed activity in a broad range of murine tumors studied at Eli Lilly and Company. These included AKR lymphoma; B-82, C-1498, and L-5178 lymphocytic leukemias; Ridgeway osteosarcoma; LPC-1 and X5563 myelomas; and S-91 melanoma (Svoboda et al 1966). The drug was not active in the four NCI mouse tumor models used for new agent selection at the time (P-388 and L-1210 leukemia, B-16 melanoma, and Lewis lung cancer [Suffness and Douros 1980]). An investigational aqueous parenteral formulation of acronycine also demonstrated significant antitumor activity in MOPC-315 murine plasmacytoma, in colon-38, and in nude mice bearing the human MCF-7 breast cancer (Dorr et al 1989). Unfortunately, acronycine was not consistently active against multidrug-resistant tumor lines expressing the P-glycoprotein (Dorr et al 1989); however, acronycine was active against a variety of fresh human tumors studied in a colony-forming assay in vitro. Sensitive human tumors included bladder cancer (50%), breast cancer (33%), uterine cancer (25–67%), and carcinomas of unknown primary (67%).

The difficulty in achieving an aqueous solution led to the testing of oral acronycine capsules in the initial clinical trials. In phase I and II clinical trials activity was noted in a number of patients with multiple myeloma (Gerzon 1983). A follow-up British trial also noted objective responses in 2 of 16 patients with multiple myeloma. Remissions were maintained in the two responding patients for 20 and 72 weeks (Scarffe et al 1983); however, because of the lack of an injectable formulation and its unimpressive activity in the NCI mouse tumor screen, interest was lost in this novel compound in the mid 1980s.

■ Mechanism of Action

Acronycine produces a number of unusual biochemical effects that do not relate to DNA synthesis. In L5178Y lymphoblasts, acronycine inhibits RNA synthesis (Gout et al 1971). This is apparently mediated by an interaction with cell surface components (Kessel 1977), leading to reduced intracellular pools of uridine and thymidine. The effect does not involve RNA polymerase inhibition, but is instead caused by inhibition of uptake of extracellular nucleosides and also formate (Dunn et al 1973). Acronycine causes swelling and destruction of cellular organelles, especially Golgi complexes and, less commonly, the mitochondria (Tan and Auersperg 1973). Cells exposed to acronycine show unique delayed effects including binucleation, altered melanosome translocation, reduced adhesion, and cessation of mitotic activity. The dose-dependent binucleating effect was believed to be caused by interference with cytokinesis and is mechanistically similar to effects of cytochalasin B (Low and Auersperg 1981).

■ Availability and Storage

Acronycine is no longer available investigationally. It was originally supplied by Eli Lilly and Company (Indianapolis, IN) as 200-mg capsules for oral ingestion (Scarffe et al 1983). An aqueous injectable formulation of the etoposide cosolvent system was also evaluated preclinically (Dorr and Liddil 1988).

■ Administration

Acronycine was administered orally in limited clinical trials.

■ Dose

In an unpublished phase I study performed in 28 patients at the National Cancer Institute, continuous oral doses of 100 to 675 mg/m^2/d for several months were evaluated. In the British myeloma trial dosing was begun at 200 mg/m^2/d and then escalated at 100 mg/m^2 increments to a maximum of 500 mg/m^2/d. These doses were administered daily for up to 90 weeks in responding patients (Scarffe et al 1983). Of note, antitumor responses were obtained only when a daily dose of 400 mg/m^2 was achieved (Scarffe et al 1983). This is probably the maximally tolerated oral dose as nausea and vomiting became quite prominent at doses of 300 mg/m^2/d and higher.

■ Pharmacokinetics

The drug's disposition has not been studied in humans. In mice, acronycine is rapidly eliminated from the plasma (see the table). The bioavailability of an aqueous solution of acronycine was only 50% in mice. It is therefore likely that the availability of acronycine powder from the capsules was much lower, as dissolution of the lipophilic drug in aqueous medium is difficult.

Major metabolites in rodents and humans have been identified in the urine and bile. They are mono- or dihydroxy derivatives of acronycine, with substitution occurring at the 9-, 10-, and 11-positions. Unlike guinea pigs, O-demethylation is not involved in acronycine metabolism in humans (Gerzon 1983). A large fraction of an acronycine dose is recovered as metabolites in the feces. After parenteral injection,

PHARMACOKINETICS OF ACRONYCINE IN MICE

Parameter	Oral Dosing	Intraperitoneal Dosing
K$_{absorp}$ (min^{-1})	17.2	2.3
T$_{max}$ (min)	45.2	10
C$_{max}$ (μg/mL)	1.04	3.0
Half-life (min)		
α	50.9	44.3
β	—	109
Volume of distribution (L/kg)	—	8.3
AUC (μg/ML · min)	5.3	10.58

90% of a radiolabeled acronycine dose was recovered in the feces after 48 hours. This fraction was reduced to 12.5% after oral dosing, reflecting the relatively poor oral bioavailability of acronycine powder in capsules (Gerzon 1983).

■ Side Effects and Toxicity

Preclinical studies showed that the oral LD_{50} in mice and rats were 350 to 680 g and 560 to 675 mg/kg, respectively (Gerzon 1983). In cats, a single dose of 100 mg/kg was tolerable. Most deaths were delayed and signs included hypoactivity, anorexia, and weakness. In chronic dosing studies, rats showed weight loss, anemia, leukopenia, and death. In mice, liver weight increased and anemia, leukopenia, and thymic atrophy occurred. Dogs additionally displayed elevations in liver enzymes, especially alkaline phosphatase and blood urea nitrogen, when high dose levels were tested.

When administered intraperitoneally in rodents the lethal doses were two- to threefold lower than oral doses. Repeated intraperitoneal injections led to peritoneal sarcomas and other local tumors in carcinogenesis studies performed at the NCI (Gerzon 1983). Male animals also showed osteosarcomas and mammary tumors were noted in female mice given chronic intraperitoneal injections of acronycine in polysorbate 80 (Tween 80®).

In clinical trials, nausea and vomiting were the most common side effects. These effects were universal at oral doses above 200 mg/m²/d for 14 weeks or longer in the unpublished NCI trial (Carcinogenicity Test Program, National Cancer Institute 1979). In the British trial in myeloma patients, anorexia was common but actual episodes of nausea and vomiting occurred in only 7 of 11 patients receiving doses of 300 mg/m²/d or higher. Treatment had to be stopped because of toxicity in only one of these patients (Scarffe et al 1983). One responding myeloma patient developed severe ataxia at a chronic (93-week) oral dose of 400 mg/m²/d. This disappeared within 8 weeks of stopping the drug. A rise in liver function enzymes was noted in one patient and mild myelosuppression in two patients. The latter two myeloma patients each had advancing disease in the bone marrow so it is unclear whether oral acronycine truly produces clinical myelosuppression.

Currently, acronycine is no longer available for clinical trials.

REFERENCES

Carcinogenicity Test Program, National Cancer Institute, Bethesda, MD. Bio-assay of acronycine for possible carcinogenicity, CAS No. 7008-42-6. Reported in *Chem Abstr*. 1979;**90**:-097501[h]; NIOSH Registry, Suspected Carcinogens, 2nd Edition, Cincinnati, OH 45226, Dec 1976, Code No. UQ03300.

Dorr RT, Liddil JD. Development of a parenteral formulation for the antitumour agent acronycine. *J Drug Dev*. 1988;**1**(1):31–39.

Dorr RT, Liddil JD, Von Hoff DD, Soble M, Osborne CK. Antitumor activity and murine pharmacokinetics of parenteral acronycine. *Cancer Res*. 1989;**49**:340–344.

Dunn BP, Gout PW, Beer CT. Effects of the antineoplastic alkaloid acronycine on nucleoside uptake and incorporation into nucleic acids by cultured L5178Y cells. *Cancer Res*. 1973;**33**:2310–2319.

Gerzon K. Acridone alkaloids: Experimental antitumor activity of acronycine. In: Gerzon K, Svoboda GH, eds. *The Alkaloids*, Vol. 21. New York: Academic Press; 1983;1–28.

Gout PW, Dunn BP, Beer CT. Effects of acronycine on nucleic acid synthesis and population growth in mammalian tumor cell cultures. *J Cell Physiol*. 1971;**78**:127–138.

Kessel D. Effects of acronycine on cell-surface properties of murine leukemia cells. *Biochem Pharmacol*. 1977;**26**:1077–1081.

Liska KJ. Preparation and antitumor properties of analogs of acronycine. *J Med Chem*. 1972;**15**(11):1177–1179.

Low RS, Auersperg N. Effects of acronycine and of cytochalasin B on the division of rat leukemia cells. *Exp Cell Res*. 1981;**131**:15–24.

Scarffe JH, Beaumont AR, Crowther D. Phase I–II evaluation of acronycine in patients with multiple myeloma. *Cancer Treat Rep*. 1983;**67**(1):93–94.

Suffness M, Douros J. Miscellaneous natural products with antitumor activity. In: Cassady JM, Douros JD, eds. *Anti-cancer Agents Based on Natural Product Models*. New York: Academic Press; 1980:470–477.

Svoboda GH, Poore GA, Simpson PJ, Boder GB. Alkaloids of *Acronychia baueri* Schott I. *J Pharm Sci*. 1966;**55**(8):758–768.

Tan P, Auersperg N. Effects of the antineoplastic alkaloid acronycine on the ultrastructure and growth patterns of cultured cells. *Cancer Res*. 1973;**33**:2320–2329.

Adozelesin

■ Other Names

U-73975 (Upjohn Company).

■ Chemistry

U-78, 057

Adozelesin

Carzelesin

Adozelesin is one of several compounds related to CC-1065, a cyclopropylpyrrolindole derivative originally isolated from broths of *Streptomyces zelensis*. These agents bind to DNA by a unique, site-specific mechanism. The molecular weight is 502.2 and the bulk drug powder is a beige color. Adozelesin is insoluble in water, slightly soluble in methanol or acetone, and soluble in dimethylformamide, dimethylsulfoxide, and dimethylacetamide. A newer analog of adozelesin, carzelesin, has even broader antitumor activity in preclinical models. The compound U-78, 057 was dropped from development due to delayed death syndrome.

■ Antitumor Activity

Adozelesin demonstrates significant antitumor activity in a variety of preclinical systems. Highly responsive tumors include murine L- 1210 leukemia, B-16 melanoma, M5076 sarcoma, Lewis lung cancer, and colon-38 adenocarcinoma. The relatively drug-resistant pancreas-02 carcinoma is also moderately sensitive to adozelesin (Li et al 1991). Human tumor xenografts of LX-1 lung tumor, clear cell carcinoma, CX-1 colon carcinoma, and ovarian 2780 carcinoma growing in nude mice are also sensitive to the agent (Li et al 1991).

In phase I clinical trials, sentinel responses were obtained in patients with gastric carcinoma, and melanoma. Phase II trials in patients with these tumors are currently underway.

■ Mechanism of Action

Like the original isolate CC-1065, adozelesin associates within the minor groove of DNA and alkylates N^3-adenines using the cyclopropyl group on the pyrroloindole moiety. Binding to DNA is complete within 2 hours and there is a specificity for adenine–thymine-rich sites in DNA (Swenson et al 1982). The effect of this group of agents on helical DNA occurs in two steps; a reversible binding or "fit" in the minor groove of DNA is followed by cyclopropyl ring opening and covalent bonding to the N^3 position on adenine (Swenson et al 1982). DNA polymerase activity and DNA synthesis are preferentially inhibited over RNA synthesis and there is little effect on protein synthesis (Li et al 1992). These drugs do not cause strand breaks and, in contrast, appear to stabilize the native B-form DNA helix.

Adozelesin induces a blockade in cell cycle progression in G_2 phase and slows cycle progression through S phase (Bhuyan et al 1992). Thus, tumor cells in late G_1 phase and early S phase are most sensitive to the drug, but overall, cell killing is not cell cycle phase specific.

■ Availability and Storage

Adozelesin is available as an investigational agent from the Upjohn Company (Kalamazoo, MI). It is supplied in glass ampules containing 1.2 mL of sterile solution (1.0 mg/mL adozelesin). The nonaqueous vehicle contains a 2:1 mixture of polyethylene glycol 400:ethanol with polysorbate 80 at a concentration of 10% (v/v). The ampules are stored frozen at −20°C prior to use and should be protected from light. The frozen drug is supplied with separate 10.5-mL ampules of sterile vehicle (as above) for subsequent dilution. The vehicle ampules may be stored at room temperature.

Preparation for Use, Stability, and Admixture

The concentrated 1 mg/mL adozelesin solution is diluted through a filter needle in 1/10 (v/v) proportions with the special diluent and injected into a sterile glass vial for mixing. The required diluted dose for injection is then removed from the vial. These solutions should be protected from light and should not be mixed with other drug solutions. Adozelesin solutions should be used within 2 hours of preparation.

Administration

Due to the high potency, adozelesin is administered by careful intravenous injection only. Initial studies with adozelesin are using syringe pumps to deliver low doses over a 10-minute period through tubing primed with an equivalent concentration of drug solution. These doses are given by constant intravenous infusion over 10 minutes through the side port of an intravenous solution containing 5% dextrose in water flowing at a rate of 1 mL/min.

Extravasation of adozelesin solutions should be avoided as the drug is a vesicant in animal models. Local dilution with 0.9% sodium chloride was an effective antidote procedure for adozelesin extravasations in mice.

Dosage

The maximally tolerated and/or effective clinical dose of adozelesin is not known but phase II studies are being initiated at 150 µg/m² IV as a 10-minute infusion every 4 weeks. The original starting dose for clinical trials was 10 µg/m², which is 1/30th the mouse equivalent lethal dose (MELD). For reference, a single dose of 200 µg/kg is lethal in the mouse, but 100 µg/kg doses are well tolerated and active in tumor-bearing mice (Li et al 1991). A lower dose of 25 to 50 µg/kg of adozelesin is used in mice on a day 1, 5, 9 schedule. These doses are well tolerated in the mouse. This contrasts with the delayed lethality seen with the original analog, CC-1065, following doses of 7 µg/kg × 1 or 0.14 µg/kg/d × 5 consecutive days (McGovren et al 1984).

Pharmacokinetics

Biologic assays in tumor-bearing mice suggest that adozelesin antitumor activity rapidly diminishes following intravenous injection (Li et al 1992). In those trials, adozelesin was administered intravenously at various times prior to intraperitoneal implantation of L-1210. The resulting survival effects demonstrated the residual antitumor activity present at the time of tumor implantation. With adozelesin, approximately 50% of antitumor activity was lost by 2 hours, and at 6 hours only minimal activity remained. Injections at 0.5 and 1 hour and were also slightly less effective than simultaneous drug/tumor injections (Li et al 1992). Based on these data, the crude biologic half-life of adozelesin antitumor activity in mice is approximately 1 to 2 hours. These experiments also demonstrated a significantly longer biologic half-life for the second-generation analog, carzelesin (Li et al 1992).

Radiolabeled drug studies in mice have demonstrated a plasma clearance of 2.57 L/h and a volume of distribution of 8.75 L/kg. A three-phase elimination pattern was evident, with the majority of drug in the bloodstream localized to the plasma compartment and with little binding to various blood cells. The terminal half-life of radiolabel in these studies was 47 hours. In tissues, the bulk of radioactivity is tightly associated with DNA.

Preliminary clinical studies using a high-performance liquid chromatographic assay suggest that peak plasma levels up to 10 ng/mL are achieved following intravenous doses of 70 µg/m² given as a 10-minute intravenous bolus. These levels fall to undetectable levels (< 1 ng/mL) within 30 minutes of injection.

Drug Interactions

There are no known drug interactions for adozelesin. Prior studies with the related analog CC-1065 in mice also could not show any effect from the addition of microsomal enzyme-inducing agents, phenobarbital, Aroclor 1254, or methylcholanthrene on delayed hepatic lethality (McGovren et al 1984). The sulfhydryl-containing compounds WR-2721 and N-acetylcysteine were similarly ineffective in this preclinical study (McGovren et al 1984).

Side Effects and Toxicity

Animal toxicology tests with the first analog, CC-1065, produced fatal hepatic necrosis 70 days after dosing (McGovren et al 1984). This delayed lethality has not been observed with either adozelesin or carzelesin (Li et al 1992). Otherwise, the major preclinical toxic effects of adozelesin are myelosuppression, acute gastrointestinal toxicity, and venous irritation. In addition, the compound produces severe local tissue reactions with ulcer formation following subcutaneous injection in experimental animals. The dose–response curve for adozelesin is steep and small increments in dose may produce substantial increases in toxicity.

For clinical trials, myelosuppression, primarily thrombocytopenia, is believed to be the primary dose-limiting toxic effect (Burris et al 1992). In one set of phase I trials, pulmonary toxicity was observed 3 months after a few patients received doses of 30 and 60 μg/m^2. Pulmonary effects included mostly patchy infiltrates which resolved without treatment. One case of severe diffuse bilateral infiltrate was described; however, no pulmonary complications were observed in animals. Thus, the relationship of adozelesin to pulmonary toxicity is unknown.

In phase I studies, doses of 100 μg/m^2 and greater have been associated with significant myelosuppression, primarily thrombocytopenia. Other effects include visual disturbances such as "spots" in the visual field, dizziness, headache, and muscle pains. Toxic effects seen with a 24-hour infusion have included emesis, abdominal cramping, chills, hypoxemia, and renal dysfunction. The latter complication was associated with hematuria, proteinuria, and elevated serum creatinine (Fleming et al 1992).

REFERENCES

Bhuyan BK, Smith KS, Adams EG, et al. Adozelesin, a potent new alkylating agent: Cell-killing kinetics and cell-cycle effects. *Cancer Chemother Pharmacol.* 1992;**30**:348–354.

Burris H, Earhart R, Kuhn J, et al. A phase I trial of adozelesin, a novel DNA sequence-specific alkylating agent. *Proc Am Assoc Cancer Res* 1992;**33**:520 (abstract 3106).

Fleming GF, Ratain MJ, O'Brien SM, Vogelzang NJ, Earhart RH. Phase I study of adozelesin by 24-hour infusion. *Proc Am Assoc Cancer Res* 1992;**33**:265 (abstract 1590).

Li LH, DeKoning TF, Kelly RC, et al. Cytotoxicity and antitumor activity of carzelesin, a prodrug cyclopropylpyrroloindole analogue. *Cancer Res.* 1992;**52**:4904–4913.

Li LH, Kelly RC, Warpehoski MA, et al. Adozelesin, a selected lead among cyclopropylpyrroloindole analogs of the DNA-binding antibiotic, CC-1065. *Invest New Drugs.* 1991;**9**:137–148.

McGovren JP, Clarke GL, Pratt EA, et al. Preliminary toxicity studies with the DNA-binding antibiotic, CC-1065. *J Antibiot.* 1984;**37**(1):63–70.

Swenson DH, Li LH, Hurley LH, et al. Mechanism of interaction of CC-1065 (NSC-298223) with DNA. *Cancer Res.* 1982;**42**:2821–2828.

Alanosine

■ Other Names

L-Alanosine; NSC-153353.

■ Chemistry

$$\text{HO}-\underset{\underset{N=O}{|}}{N}-CH_2-\underset{\underset{NH_2}{|}}{CH}-\overset{\overset{O}{\|}}{C}-OH$$

Structure of alanosine

Alanosine is an antibiotic produced by *Streptomyces alanosinicus* (Murthy et al 1966). The chemical name is L-2-amino-3-[(N-nitroso)hydroxylamino]propionic acid. The molecular weight is 149 and the molecular formula is $C_3H_7N_3O_4$ (Coronelli et al 1966). As the monosodium salt (NSC-153353), the molecular weight is 171.1.

■ Antitumor Activity

Preclinical studies have shown activity in murine tumors and in viral models (Murthy et al 1966). Antitumor activity has been seen in P-388 leukemia, L5178Y lymphocytic leukemia, B-16 melanoma, CD8F mammary carcinoma, colon-26 and -38, and intracerebrally injected ependymoblastoma.

In phase II clinical trials, alanosine was inactive in patients with malignant melanoma (Creagan et al 1984), colorectal cancer (Rubin et al 1983), head and neck cancer (Creagan et al 1983), and acute nonlymphocytic leukemia (Weick et al 1983). No activity was also reported in a more recent trial of alanosine in heavily pretreated patients with advanced breast cancer (Von Hoff et al 1991). The combination of alanosine with N-phosphonacetyl-L-aspartate in malignant melanoma produced only one partial response in 21 patients (Morton et al 1987). The lack of significant antitumor activity has led to the discontinuance of clinical trials with alanosine.

■ Mechanism of Action

Alanosine is an antimetabolite that inhibits de novo purine synthesis, primarily the formation of adenosine monophosphate (AMP). The specific site of inhibition is the enzyme adenylosuccinate synthetase (Graff and Plagemann 1976). This blocks the first reaction in the conversion of inosine monophosphate (IMP) to AMP: the condensation of IMP with as-

RECOMMENDED DOSES OF ALANOSINE BY DIFFERENT SCHEDULES

Dose (mg/m²)	Days	Repeat Course (wk)	IV Administration Method	Reference
160	1–5	4	Bolus	Rubin et al 1983
250	1–3	3	Bolus	Dosik et al 1982
125	1–5	3	Continuous infusion	Weick et al 1983

partic acid (Gale and Schmidt 1967). Intermediate metabolites of alanosine appear to mediate this inhibition (Gale and Smith 1968). Ultimately, there is inhibition of DNA, RNA, and protein synthesis leading to cell death (Graff and Plagemann 1976). Inhibition of DNA synthesis appears to be the primary effect of alanosine. Glutamine and aspartic acid do not reverse the effects of alanosine, indicating that cytotoxicity is not due to depletion of these specific nucleotide precursors. Alanosine also does not block ribonucleotide reductase.

■ Availability and Storage

Alanosine was investigationally available from the National Cancer Institute in 10-mL vials containing 100 mg of lyophilized powder. Sodium hydroxide is added to the vials to adjust pH to 6.5 to 8.0. The intact vials are stored at room temperature. This agent is no longer available for clinical trials.

■ Preparation for Use, Stability, and Admixture

Each 100-mg vial is reconstituted with 5 mL of Sodium Chloride for Injection, USP. This results in a clear solution containing 20 mg/mL alanosine at a pH of about 6 to 7.

■ Administration

Alanosine is administered intravenously, usually as a brief infusion in 50 to 100 mL of saline over 10 to 20 minutes. Continuous infusion over 5 days has also been described (Weick et al 1983).

■ Dosage

The phase I recommended doses of alanosine are given in the table. Not shown in the table is a single intravenous bolus schedule of 5 g/m² which was not tolerated in two patients treated at the Mayo Clinic because of severe renal toxicity among other toxic effects. The continuous infusion dose of 125 mg/m²/d was most highly recommended for phase II trials.

■ Pharmacokinetics

Alanosine is rapidly cleared from the plasma. The plasma pharmacokinetics can be described by a two-compartment model with an α half-life of 14 minutes and a β half-life of 99 minutes (Weick et al 1983). Metabolism is the major mechanism of clearance and less than 4% of a dose is excreted intact in the urine over 24 hours. One major metabolite has tentatively been identified as the condensation product of alanosine with aminoimidazole ribonucleotide. These pharmacokinetic features suggest that prolonged continuous infusion might provide optimal antitumor activity with possibly reduced toxicity.

■ Side Effects and Toxicity

The usual dose-limiting toxic effect of alanosine is mucositis, which can occur as early as day 3 or 4 of treatment (Goldsmith et al 1983). Leukopenia was also evident in about 33% of patients at doses of 80 mg/m²/d × 5 days or greater. Thrombocytopenia was much less common, affecting only 9% of patients. Potentially life-threatening hypotension has occurred in some studies (Goldsmith et al 1983, Von Hoff et al 1991).

Mild to moderate nausea and vomiting are seen in less than 5 to 10% of patients. Rare toxic effects include rash, somnolence, weight loss, leg cramps, uremia, hypertension, and pleurisy (Von Hoff et al 1991). Phlebitis and cellulitis are also reported infrequently (Rubin et al 1983). With a single large bolus dose of 5 g/m², extreme renal toxicity is also described. At lower dose levels, renal or hepatic toxicity is not encountered.

REFERENCES

Coronelli C, Pasqualucci CR, Tamoni G, et al. Isolation and structure of alanosine, a new antibiotic. *Farmaco.* 1966;4:269–277.

Creagan ET, Long HJ, Ahmann DL, Green SJ. Phase II

evaluation of L-alanosine (NSC-153353) for patients with disseminated malignant melanoma. *Am J Clin Oncol.* 1984;**7**:543–544.

Creagan ET, Schutt AJ, Ingle JN, O'Fallon JR. Phase II clinical trial of L-alanosine in advanced upper aerodigestive cancer. *Cancer Treat Rep.* 1983;**67**:1047.

Dosik GM, Stewart D, Valdivieso M, et al. Phase I study of L-alanosine using a daily × 3 schedule. *Cancer Treat Rep.* 1982;**66**:73–76.

Gale GR, Schmidt GB. Mode of action of alanosine. *Biochem Pharmacol.* 1967;**17**:363–368.

Gale GR, Smith AB. Alanosine and hadicidin. Comparative effects on adenylosuccinate synthetase. *Biochem Pharmacol.* 1968;**17**:2495–2498.

Goldsmith MA, Ohnuma T, Spigelman M, et al. Phase I study of L-alanosine (NSC-153353). *Cancer.* 1983;**51**:378–380.

Graff JC, Plagemann PGW. Alanosine toxicity in Novikoff rat hepatoma cells due to inhibition of the conversion of inosine monophosphate to adenosine monophosphate. *Cancer Res.* 1976;**36**:1428–1440.

Morton RF, Creagan ET, Cullinan SA, et al. Phase II studies of single-agent cimetidine and the combination N-phosphonacetyl-L-aspartate (NSC-224131) plus L-alanosine (NSC-153353) in advanced malignant melanoma. *J Clin Oncol.* 1987;**5**:1078–1082.

Murthy YKS, Thieman JE, Coronelli C, Sensi P. Alanosine, a new antiviral and antitumor agent isolated from a *Streptomyces*. *Nature.* 1966;**211**:1198–1199.

Rubin J, Schutt AJ, Hineman V, et al. A phase II study of alanosine in advanced large bowel carcinoma. *Am J Clin Oncol.* 1983;**6**:191–193.

Von Hoff DD, Green SJ, Neidhart JA, et al. Phase II study of L-alanosine (NSC-153353) in patients with advanced breast cancer. *Invest New Drugs.* 1991;**9**:87–88.

Weick JK, Tranum BL, Morrison FS. The treatment of acute leukemia with continuous infusion L-alanosine. *Invest New Drugs.* 1983;**1**:249–252.

Aldesleukin

Other Names

Interleukin-2 (IL-2); T-cell growth factor; Proleukin® (Cetus Oncology; Teceleukin® (Hoffman-La Roche).

Chemistry

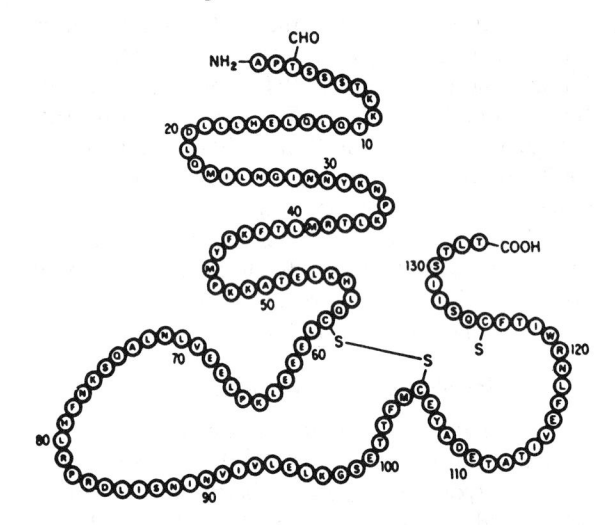

Structure of aldesleukin

Human interleukin-2 (IL-2) is produced in mature T lymphocytes from a precursor protein consisting of 153 amino acids. Following the removal of a 20-amino-acid signal sequence, the resultant "secreted" protein has 133 amino acids and a molecular weight of approximately 15,000 kD (Taniguchi et al 1983). There is one disulfide bond between amino acids 58 and 105 and denaturation of this bond produces a rapid loss of activity. The secreted molecule is normally glycosylated, although this is not known to affect antitumor activities (Robb and Smith 1981). Natural IL-2 is markedly hydrophobic and about 50% of the molecule has a helical structure.

Recombinant IL-2 produced by Cetus Oncology, Emeryville, California (Proleukin®), differs from the natural molecule in that (1) it is not glycosylated, (2) it lacks the N-terminal alanine, and (3) a serine is substituted for cysteine at amino acid position number 125. The Cetus-supplied material is produced in *Escherichia coli* into which a modified human IL-2 gene has been inserted. A recombinant IL-2 from Hoffman-La Roche is also produced in *E. coli* and is nonglycosylated, but conforms to natural human IL-2 in amino acid sequence with the exception of the additional N-terminal methionine residue. Another recombinant human IL-2 was produced by Ortho Pharmaceutical Corporation (Raritan, NJ) and has alanine substituted for cysteine at amino acid position number 125 and an N-terminal methionine residue (Schoof et al 1988).

Interleukin-2 Units. Interleukin-2 activity is now standardized in International Units (IU). This activity is based on stimulation of T-cell growth in vitro using standardized human cell lines (Gearing and Thorpe 1988). On this basis, 1 Cetus U = 6 IU and 1 Roche U = 3 IU.

■ Antitumor Activity

Interleukin-2 is poorly cytotoxic when used alone on tumor cells in vitro. Thus, most antitumor effects are probably mediated indirectly through lymphokine release and the generation of lymphokine-activated killer (LAK) cells. A particularly effective LAK cell is the tumor-infiltrating lymphocyte (TIL) derived from lymphocytes in individual tumors (Rosenberg et al 1988). Rosenberg originally described IL-2 antitumor activity for exogenously generated LAK cells in a variety of animal tumor models. This form of therapy has been termed *adoptive immunotherapy* and involves the in vitro generation of LAK cells which are then infused in large quantities to mediate tumor cell lysis. Animal tumors sensitive to this therapy include murine B-16 and M-3 melanomas, several sarcomas, colon-38, and 1660 bladder carcinoma (Rosenberg et al 1985).

Early trials in humans explored high-dose bolus IL-2 with aggressive infusion of in vitro LAK cells (Rosenberg et al 1986). Objective responses were noted in 11 of 25 (44%) patients including patients with malignant melanoma, colon cancer, renal cell cancer, and lung tumor. A subsequent report described objective clinical responses in 21% of 105 patients receiving LAK cells plus IL-2 and in 6 of 46 (13%) patients receiving high-dose IL-2 alone (Rosenberg et al 1987). Toxicity was severe but short-lived. Similarly, a large multicenter trial of the high-dose IL-2/LAK regimen showed slightly lower response rates and severe (rarely fatal) cardiopulmonary toxicity (Dutcher et al 1989, Margolin et al 1989) (see the table). A combined IL-2 bolus and infusion regimen with LAK cells has produced a 14% response rate in 50 patients with advanced malignant melanoma (Bar et al 1990).

Antitumor activity has been most consistently observed in metastatic renal cell cancer (Rosenberg et al 1985, 1987, Fisher et al 1987, West et al 1987, Sosman et al 1988a). Patients who are good candidates for responding to IL-2 or IL-2/LAK regimens have several common characteristics. These include (1) aggressive surgical excision of the primary tumor, (2) metastases limited primarily to the lung, (3) excellent performance status, and (4) no cardiovascular impairment. Within this framework, some patients have achieved prolonged unmaintained

COMPARISON OF IL-2/LAK CELL REGIMENS AND RESPONSE RATES IN PATIENTS WITH SOLID TUMORS*

Total Dose	Margolin et al (1989)	Rosenberg et al (1987)
LAK cells	7.6×10^{10}	7.6×10^{10}
IL-2 (IU × 10^6/kg)	6–8.4	7.8
Objective responses		
Renal cell, CR + PR[†]	5/35 (16%)	12/36 (33%)
No. CR/No. PR	2/3	4/8
Malignant melanoma		
CR + PR/Total	6/32 (19%)	6/26 (23%)
No. CR/No. PR	1/5	2/4
Colon cancer		
CR + PR/Total	5/22 (22%)	3/26 (12%)
No. CR/No. PR	1/4	1/2

*6×10^5 IU/kg IV over 15 minutes every 8 hours on days 1–5, before LAK cells, then on days 12–15 with LAK cell infusions (Proleukin®, Cetus Corporation).
[†]CR, complete response; PR, partial response.
Data from Margolin KA, Rayner AA, Hawkins MJ, Atkins MB, et al. Interleukin-2 and lymphokine-activated killer cell therapy of solid tumors: Analysis of toxicity and management guidelines. *J Clin Oncol.* 1989;7:486–498.

disease-free remissions of renal cell carcinoma following a few courses of aggressive IL-2/LAK cell therapy.

It is unclear what the optimal IL-2 dose is for antitumor efficacy and whether in vitro LAK cell or TIL generation is required. In this regard, preliminary clinical trials suggest that prolonged continuous IL-2 infusions with LAK cells (Paciucci et al 1989) or without LAK cells (Sosman et al 1988b) may be as efficacious as the more toxic high-dose IL-2 bolus/LAK cell reinfusion programs (Rosenberg et al 1985).

Responses to low-dose IL-2 therapy in outpatients have been noted in patients with malignant lymphoma or chronic lymphocytic leukemia. In one trial, 3 of 12 (25%) patients responded objectively with remission durations lasting 1 to 17 months (Allison et al 1989).

■ Mechanism of Action

Like all protein hormones, IL-2 affects only cells that express a specific cell surface receptor. Two classes of IL-2 receptors have been identified on activated T lymphocytes. Only about 10% or 500 to 5000 of the total number of cellular IL-2 receptors are high-affinity receptors that mediate the biologic activity of the compound (Robb et al 1984). The high-affinity receptor consists of two subunits that interact to change weak independent subunit binding of IL-2 into high-affinity binding. The IL-2–receptor complex is then internalized and subsequent signal transduction may involve tyrosine kinase activity (Bernard et al 1987).

Interleukin-2 was originally identified as a small molecule with the ability to maintain T-lymphocyte cell growth in vitro (Morgan et al 1976). The molecule performs a number of normal cell regulatory functions including the stimulation of activated T-cell growth and differentiation, proliferation and immunoglobulin production in B lymphocytes, macrophage cytotoxic activity, oligodendrocyte proliferation, and generation of LAK cell activity. This last effect, and especially the generation of TILs, is believed ultimately to mediate the antitumor effects of IL-2. In activated T cells, IL-2 stimulates cell entry into S phase and the simultaneous acquisition of cytotoxic activity.

Lymphokine-activated killer cells generated from IL-2 usually do not express either B- or T-cell markers and are now believed to be indistinct from natural killer (NK) lymphocytes (Herberman et al 1987). In addition to NK cell activation, IL-2 also stimulates the production of several other cytokines, notably interferons alfa and gamma and tumor necrosis factor (Herberman 1989).

Following IL-2 exposure, at least 48 hours is required for LAK cells to generate maximal cytotoxic efficacy (Grimm 1986). These cells can then display a broad range of specificity for tumor cell lysis, although high effector (LAK cell)-to-target (tumor) cell ratios are required in vitro. Thus, for LAK cells, effector:target ratios of 200:1 to 10:1 are needed, whereas with TILs, the effector:target ratios are much lower. This suggests that LAK cells generated *within* a particular tumor (TILs) are the ultimate mediators of IL-2 cytotoxicity.

It is also now clear that IL-2 cytotoxicity is probably mediated by as yet uncharacterized periplasmic cytolysins released from LAK cells interacting with a particular tumor cell. Activated LAK cells can be shown to develop cytoplasmic granules containing cytolytic proteins in the same time course as antitumor activity develops. The cytoplasmic granules are known to contain pore-forming proteins that literally produce holes in the plasma membrane of adjacent target tumor cells (Hook et al 1988).

■ Availability and Storage

Two recombinant forms of nonglycosylated IL-2 are available. Proleukin® is a modified IL-2 manufactured by Cetus Oncology (Emeryville, CA). It is commercially available in glass vials containing 1.2 mg of lyophilized powder (22×10^6 IU). The vials also contain sodium dodecyl sulfate and are adjusted to a pH of 7.2 to 7.8. An investigational formulation of this product is a combination of Proleukin® and polyethylene glycol. The polyethylene glycol is covalently linked to the modified IL-2 to decrease antigenicity and to extend the pharmacokinetic half-life by blocking the rapid clearance of the protein.

Recombinant IL-2 was also investigationally available as Teceleukin® from Hoffman-La Roche. It was supplied in vials containing 100 µg of IL-2, with 25 mg of human albumin/10^6 units and 5 mg of mannitol/10^6 units of IL-2 (Gustavson et al 1989).

All formulations of IL-2 require storage under refrigeration (4–8°C). Proleukin® is stable for 18 months from the date of manufacture and should be protected from exposure to heat and light.

Preparation for Use, Stability, and Admixture

Proleukin® vials are reconstituted with 1.2 mL of solution to contain 1.3 mg or 22×10^6 IU to yield 18×10^6 IU/mL. Hoffman-La Roche-supplied IL-2 is typically reconstituted with Sodium Chloride for Injection, USP. Dilutions of Proleukin® in polyvinylchloride infusion bags containing 5% Dextrose Injection, USP, and 2% human albumin are stable for 48 hours at room temperature. It is recommended that IL-2 solutions not be filtered because of possible adsorption of drug with a loss of biologic activity. In addition, Proleukin® may precipitate with preservatives such as benzyl alcohol and methyl/propyl paraben. Therefore, the drug should not be reconstituted with bacteriostatic solutions nor 0.9% sodium chloride.

Administration

Interleukin-2 has been administered by a variety of parenteral routes including intravenous, subcutaneous, and intramuscular routes. The drug is usually given intravenously. Intravenous "bolus" doses are usually diluted into 50 to 100 mL of 5% dextrose and administered over 15 to 30 minutes. Continuous prolonged infusions of IL-2 are usually administered in daily (24-hour) fractions in 250 to 500 mL of fluid (Thompson et al 1988, West et al 1987). Interleukin-2 doses for subcutaneous or intramuscular administration are usually administered without further dilution from the original vial (Thompson et al 1987); however, subcutaneous administration has led to a high incidence of IL-2 of nonneutralizing antibody induction in one study (Krigel et al 1988) but not to increased local site toxicity (Thompson et al 1987).

Special Precautions

Interleukin-2 can induce severe hypotension and life-threatening cardiovascular toxicity manifested by a hyperdynamic state when given at the maximally tolerated dose. Patients receiving high-dose IL-2 thus require close cardiac monitoring (Margolin et al 1989). This may prevent severe cardial toxicity or severe pulmonary edema caused by dose- and route-dependent decrements in peripheral vascular resistance with increased extravascular fluid accumulation. Facilities must be available to rapidly treat patients receiving high-dose IL-2 with vasopressor agents for any severe symptoms including low blood pressure, tachycardia, labored respiration, and occasionally delirium.

Dosage

The United States FDA-approved dose of aldesleukin (Proleukin®) for renal cell carcinoma is 600,000 IU/kg (0.037 mg/kg) per dose as a 15-minute intravenous infusion every 8 hours for 14 doses. Two such 14-dose courses are administered with a 9-day rest period inbetween. Doses used in the original IL-2/LAK cell regimen and in subsequent investigations are detailed in the table on page 154. This summary shows that there is a broad range of reported IL-2 dose levels. Studies with teceleukin suggest that administration by continuous infusion tends to substantially increase both the activity and toxicity of a given dose of IL-2 (Thompson et al 1988).

There is some evidence that continuous intravenous infusion of IL-2 for several days may allow the delivery of higher total doses, while simultaneously reducing the incidence of acute life-threatening toxic effects (Sosman et al 1988a). Indeed, recent animal studies suggest that prolongation of serum IL-2 levels by continuous infusion may lead to enhanced immunologic activity (Talmadge et al 1987). Furthermore, prolonged low-dose IL-2 regimens with LAK cell reinfusion have produced clinical responses with markedly reduced toxicity (Schoof et al 1988). Similarly, reducing the number of "priming" bolus IL-2 doses while extending a low-dose continuous IL-2 infusion during LAK cell administration also lowers toxicity while maintaining clinical activity in patients with solid tumors (Bar et al 1990).

Drug Interactions

Interleukin-2 has been shown to interact with a number of other agents (see table on page 155). Many of these interactions have documented clinical significance. Indomethacin has occasionally been added to IL-2 regimens to decrease some of the acute toxic effects of the drug. Although indomethacin does not alter IL-2-induced immune response parameters, there is some suggestion that renal dysfunction and the capillary leak syndrome may worsen with indomethacin (Sosman et al 1988b). In mice with experimental metastases of B-16 melanoma, indomethacin can increase IL-2 levels by blocking prostaglandin E_2 production in host monocytes (Parker and Lala 1987).

DOSES AND REQUISITE TREATMENT SETTINGS FOR DIFFERENT SCHEDULES OF INTERLEUKIN-2

Method of IV Administration	Schedule of Administration	Approximate Daily Dose* ($IU \times 10^6/m^2$)	Type of IL-2	Required Treatment Setting[†]	Author, Date
15-minute infusion every 8 hours	14 doses, 9 days rest, then 14 doses	600,000 IU/kg	Cetus	H	Cetus Oncology 1992
Bolus every 8 hours (with LAK cells)	Days 1–5 and 12–16	72[‡]	Cetus	ICU	Rosenberg et al 1985
Infusion over 24 hours	Days 1–5 and 12–16	18	Cetus	ICU	West et al 1987
Bolus	Daily × 5 days for 2 weeks	18	Cetus	OP	Cetus Oncology 1989
Bolus	Daily × 5 days every other week	18	Cetus	OP	Allison et al 1989
Bolus	Daily × 7 days	3	Roche	H	Kohler et al 1989
Bolus	Daily (every 8 hours) days 1–5 and 8–23 (23 doses)	~10	Ortho	H	Schoof et al 1988
Bolus	3 times weekly	36	Cetus	H	Cetus Oncology 1989
Infusion over 24 hours	Weekly × 6	54	Cetus	H	Richards et al 1988
Bolus	Weekly	30	Cetus	OP	Cetus Oncology 1989
2-hour infusion	Daily × 5, every other week × 4 weeks	1.8	Hoffman-La Roche	H	Thompson et al 1988
24-hour infusion		1.8			
2-hour infusion		18			
24-hour infusion		18			
Bolus every 8 hours		18			
24-hour infusion	Daily × 4 per week × 4 weeks	1 or 13	Hoffman-La Roche	OP	Sosman et al 1988b
24-hour infusion	Daily × 4	1	Hoffman-La Roche	H	Kohler et al 1989

*All doses were converted to International Units (IU) in this table (see Chemistry section for conversions). These listings should not be used for therapeutic dose calculations; check original citations for all clinical dose recommendations.
[†]ICU, hospital intensive care unit; H, hospital; OP, outpatient
[‡]Fixed dose.
From Cetus Corporation. Proleukin®—Recombinant Interleukin-2 (Human). Investigational brochure information for investigators. April 28, 1989:1–44. Adapted with permission.

Glucocorticosteroids have been shown to block the antitumor efficacy of IL-2 in mice (Papa et al 1986). Interestingly, cortisone acetate did not affect LAK cell generation in this same study. Hydrocortisone has also been observed to inhibit the binding of IL-2 to its receptors in murine spleen cells (Horst and Flad 1987) and to decrease LAK cell activity in human lymphocytes stimulated by IL-2 (Grimm et al 1985). This effect may be caused by the well-documented decrease in circulating lymphocytes in the peripheral blood of humans given corticosteroids (Fauci and Dale 1974). In patients receiving IL-2 and LAK cells, dexamethasone (4 mg IV every 6 hours) significantly reduced IL-2-induced toxic effects, including dyspnea, fever, pruritus, and high serum creatinine and bilirubin levels (Vetto et al 1987). Interestingly, hematologic side effects were not reduced; however, none of the 32 patients treated with IL-2/LAK and dexamethasone showed evidence of objective response compared with 9 of 27 persons in a matched (historical) control group (Vetto et al 1987). This suggests that corticosteroids should be avoided in patients receiving IL-2 unless to reverse side effects of IL-2.

Tumor necrosis factor has been shown to synergistically enhance the generation of LAK cells exposed to IL-2 (Chouaib et al 1988). Interferon gamma also synergized with IL-2 by enhancing the expression of IL-2 cell surface receptors (Herrmann et al 1985). This combination has been evaluated clinically and is active in patients with various advanced cancers (Redman et al 1990). In this trial, the

DRUG INTERACTIONS WITH INTERLEUKIN-2

Agent	Effect on IL-2	Reference
Nonsteroidal anti-inflammatories		
Indomethacin	Lessens clinical toxicity; may worsen renal function	Sosman et al 1988b
Glucocorticosteroids		
Dexamethasone	Blocks antitumor action	Papa et al 1986
Hydrocortisone	Decreases LAK activity	Grimm et al 1985
	Blocks IL-2 receptors	Horst and Flad 1987
	Reduces IL-2-induced clinical toxic effects	Vetto et al 1987
Other Biologics		
Tumor necrosis factor	Enhances LAK cell generation	Chouaib et al 1988
Interferon gamma	Increases IL-2 receptor expression	Herrmann et al 1985
	Is active clinically	Redman et al 1990
Interferon alfa	Is active clinically	Lee et al 1989
	Increases tumor antigenicity to enhance LAK cell recognition	Gracomini et al 1984
Interferons alfa and beta	Has antitumor synergy in vitro	Kuribayashi et al 1981
	Has antitumor synergy in vivo	Weber et al 1987, Brunda et al 1986
Cytotoxic agents		
Cyclophosphamide	Depletes T-cell suppressors to enhance LAK cell production	Berd et al 1984a
	Is active clinically	Mitchell et al 1988

maximally tolerated doses were 1×10^6 IU/m²/d IL-2 by continuous 5-day infusion and 0.5 mg/m²/d interferon gamma by intramuscular injection for 5 days. Dose-limiting toxicity involved pulmonary fluid accumulation, with responses noted in 5 of 26 patients including those with lymphomas and renal cell carcinoma.

Interleukin-2 has also been combined clinically with interferon alfa-2a in patients with metastatic cancer (Lee et al 1989). In this phase I trial, patients received daily continuous-infusion IL-2 along with daily intramuscular interferon alfa-2a. Both agents were administered for 4 days per week for 4 weeks, with treatment repeated after 2 to 4 weeks of therapy. The maximum tolerated daily IL-2 dose was 18 $\times 10^6$ IU/m² combined with 5 to 10×10^6 U/m² interferon alfa-2a. Importantly, there were 7 objective responses in 25 patients including 1 complete and 4 partial responses in 10 patients with malignant melanoma (Lee et al 1989). Toxic effects included fever, chills, hypotension, fluid retention, nausea/vomiting, erythrodermia, weight loss, elevated liver function tests, thrombocytopenia, and some central nervous system toxicity manifested by somnolence and confusion. Chronic fatigue appeared to be cumulative.

This trial suggests that IL-2 and interferon alfa may interact therapeutically through a number of biologic effects. These include the demonstrated capability of interferon alfa to increase the expression of tumor-associated antigens and class I major histocompatibility antigens (Gracomini et al 1984), a major determinant of responsiveness to IL-2 in mice (Weber et al 1987). In preclinical models, the combination of interferon alfa or beta with IL-2 produced antitumor synergy both in vitro (Kuribayashi et al 1981) and in vivo (Iigo et al 1988, Weber et al 1987, Brunda et al 1986). Second, interferons are known to augment NK cell activity, which is believed to be the final common mediator of antitumor effects from IL-2 (Herberman et al 1987). Although the combination of interferon alfa and IL-2 is active in vivo, it is still unclear whether truly synergistic antitumor effects are produced.

Mitchell et al (1988) have investigated the combination of IL-2 with cyclophosphamide in patients with metastatic malignant melanoma. This combination was based on the observation that low doses of cyclophosphamide could selectively deplete suppressor T cells in humans (Berd et al 1984a) and might thereby augment IL-2-induced LAK cell production. The depletion of suppressor cells by cyclophosphamide was manifested 3 to 6 days after dosing. This potentiated both humoral and cell-mediated immunity in humans (Berd et al 1984b). In the Mitchell et al study, cyclophosphamide (350 mg/m^2) was given intravenously 3 days before starting a 5-day IL-2 regimen (3.6×10^6 U/m^2/d IV). Responses were noted in 6 of 24 (25%) evaluable patients and toxic effects were not substantially different from those of regimens using IL-2 alone (Mitchell et al 1988).

Interleukin-2 also alters the disposition of dacarbazine in patients with malignant melanoma (Chabot et al 1990). Patients receiving IL-2 appear to have an increase in dacarbazine clearance from 6.7 to 9.3 L/h·m^2 and an increase in steady-state volume of distribution from 22.6 to 30.8 L/m^2 (Chabot et al 1990). The terminal dacarbazine half-life was unchanged at 2.8 hours and the area under the concentration × time curve (AUC) decreased by a mean of about 28%. There was also a similar change in the AUC of the primary dacarbazine metabolite, 5-aminoimidazole-4-carboxamide, when IL-2 was given before dacarbazine. These findings suggest that IL-2 may decrease the systemic exposure to dacarbazine, but the clinical significance of this pharmacokinetic effect is unknown.

■ Pharmacokinetics

Interleukin-2 is rapidly cleared from the bloodstream following parenteral administration (see table). The elimination of a partially purified IL-2 is reported to be biphasic in patients given an intravenous bolus injection (Lotze et al 1985). In one study, the plasma half-lives of Hoffman-La Roche brand IL-2 were 5 to 7 minutes (α), with a second β-phase half-life of 45 minutes (± 10 minutes) (Kohler et al 1989), and 30 to 120 minutes (Thompson et al 1987). For the Cetus Oncology IL-2 product, the α and β half-lives were 12.9 and 85 minutes, respectively (Konrad et al 1990). The total body clearances for Hoffman-La Roche IL-2 given by bolus intravenous injection were 26 and 47 mL/min/m^2 for a continuous infusion (Kohler et al 1989). Steady-state levels for the continuous infusion ranged from 25 to 40 U/mL and were achieved 2 to 4 hours after starting the 4-day infusion (Kohler et al 1989).

A β half-life of 60 minutes is reported for Cetus Oncology IL-2 (Mitchell et al 1988). Thirty minutes after injection, over 95% of the dose is cleared from the bloodstream. Infusions of 3×10^6 U of recombinant IL-2 (Hoffman-La Roche) are associated with blood levels of ≥ 223 or 16 U/mL for 1- and 24-hour infusions, respectively (Thompson et al 1987). Peak levels of 800 to 900 U/mL are described in patients given 18×10^6 IU of Cetus Oncology IL-2 as a 15-minute intravenous infusion (Mitchell et al 1988).

Following a subcutaneous injection of 18×10^6 IU (Cetus), IL-2 serum levels greater than 20 U/mL were maintained for over 9 hours. The apparent IL-2 half-lives following three different administration routes were 30 minutes for the 24-hour infusion, 70 minutes for the 2-hour infusion, and 4 hours for the subcutaneous injection. Of note, the apparent time to achieve peak plasma levels following the subcutaneous injection is approximately 5 hours (Thompson et al 1987). After an intramuscular injection of Cetus IL-2, only about 30% of IL-2 activity is recovered systemically (Konrad et al 1990).

The primary route of IL-2 elimination is believed to be renal, involving catabolism in the renal tubules. Hepatic metabolism is not believed to constitute a major route of drug elimination. Also, although IL-2 can produce neurotoxicity, the parent protein is not believed to penetrate into the central nervous system; however, the sodium dodecyl sulfate and mannitol in the Cetus preparation have been associated with a significant increase in cerebrovascular permeability in cats given both Proleukin® and the Proleukin® diluent containing sodium dodecyl sulfate (Ellison et al 1987). This effect was associated with endothelial lesions, expanded intracellular spaces, and disrupted neuronal and glial processes. The clinical significance of this observation is unknown.

■ Side Effects and Toxicity

Interleukin-2 produces a broad range of acute, noncumulative toxic effects (Kintzel and Calis 1991). The intensity of such toxic effects is clearly dose and duration dependent (Thompson et al 1987). It is also clear that most of the toxicity of the IL-2/LAK cell regimen is related to IL-2, as LAK cell infusions alone produce relatively minor side effects (Mazumder and Rosenberg 1984).

Flulike Syndrome. All patients receiving IL-2 experience a general malaise with fever and chills which are partially responsive to acetaminophen and indomethacin. Nausea, vomiting, and diarrhea are also common during the latter days of daily repetitive administration cycles (Rosenberg et al 1987). These symptoms are highly responsive to antiemetics and antidiarrheal agents. Peptic ulcers are uncommon when most patients are prophylactially treated with H$_2$ antagonists, usually ranitidine.

HUMAN SERUM PHARMACOKINETICS OF INTERLEUKIN-2

IL-2 Manufacturer	Route of Administration	Time to Peak (min)	Dose (10⁶/U/m²)	Peak Plasma Level (U/mL)	Half-life (minutes) α	Half-life (minutes) β	Volume of Distribution Steady State	Volume of Distribution Control	Total Body Clearance	AUC (U/mL)
Cetus Oncology*	IV bolus	0	6	400	12.9	85	7.9 L	4.3 L	120 mL/min	18,200
Cetus Oncology*	IM	150	0.24–4	1.3–160	—	—	—	—	—	0.37 (AUC IM/AUC IV)
Cetus Oncology*	SC	180	0.5–1.0	4.5–12	—	—	—	—	—	—
Cetus Oncology*	IP	—	1–10	8–34	—	4–11 h	—	—	—	28,900

Manufacturer	Route		Dose (10⁶/U/m²)	Peak Plasma Level (U/mL)	Half-life (h) α	Half-life (h) β	Volume of Distribution Area (L)	Control	Steady-State Clearance (L/h)	AUC (U/h/mL)
Hoffman-La Roche†	IV 2-hour infusion	—	0.3	19	—	0.7	13.7		8.3	—
		—	1.0	79	—	0.65	13.3		10.6	219
		—	3.0	434	—	1.05	7.39		4.48	1,340
		—	10	1150	—	1.46	10.1		4.26	3,680
		—	30	3680	—	1.74	8.7		3.3	6,130

Manufacturer	Route		Dose (10⁶/U/m²)	Level at Steady State	α	β	Area (L)	Control		AUC (U/h/mL)
Hoffman-La Roche†	IV 24-hour infusion	—	0.3	3.1	—	—	—	4.0		
		—	1.0	6.3	—	0.75	9.0	10		
		—	3.0	46	—	1.05	6.3	5.5		
		—	10	111	—	1.25	10.6	8.0		
		—	30	324	—	1.35	7.5	3.9		

Manufacturer	Route	Time To Peak (h)	Dose	Peak	α	β				AUC
Hoffman-La Roche†	SC	3.5	0.3	11	—	4.3	—	—		120
		3.9	1.0	25	—	4.6	—	—		177
		2.7	3.0	41	—	5.3	—	—		359

*Konrad et al (1990).
†Gustavson et al (1989).

There is also a consistent increase in serum bilirubin which returns to pretreatment levels within 4 days of stopping IL-2.

Capillary Leak Syndrome. The major dose-limiting side effect of IL-2 is pulmonary edema resulting from an increase in capillary permeability. This has been termed the *capillary leak syndrome* and begins with the first dose and increases in magnitude with each repetitive dose. Symptoms include hypotension, interstitial pulmonary edema, and a general decrease in peripheral vascular resistance (Rosenberg et al 1987). This often leads to substantial weight gain (>10% of body weight) as a result of fluid accumulation in peripheral tissues. The resultant contraction in intravascular volume reduces cardiac output, which can result in prerenal azotemia, oliguria, and sodium retention. Serious IL-2-induced hypotension requires vasopressor therapy with dopamine and cautious replacement of fluids, with attention to avoid aggravating peripheral fluid accumulations. For these reasons, high-dose-intensity IL-2 regimens may require treatment in intensive care units (see earlier table). Likewise, severe pulmonary edema from IL-2 typically correlates with the degree of general fluid retention and may necessitate intubation and respiratory therapy.

Renal Toxicity. Serum creatinine levels are often transiently increased. This toxic effect has been likened to endotoxemia with the development of respiratory alkalosis (pH 7.44, pCO_2 30) (Kozeny et al 1988). There is also an intracellular shift of phosphorus accompanied by increased renal phosphorus reabsorption, but such patients experience neither altered calcium or magnesium excretion nor glycosuria (Kozeny et al 1988). Detailed studies of renal function in IL-2-treated patients show that the degree of renal insufficiency is out of proportion to the decrease in renal perfusion (Shalmi et al 1990). Glomerular filtration rates fell a mean of 43% in 9 of 10 patients, and the filtration fraction decreased from 23 to 15% on day 4 of IL-2 therapy. This suggests that there may be an intrarenal component of IL-2-induced renal toxicity (Shalmi et al 1990). All of these effects resolve within 5 to 7 days of stopping IL-2, but they can be life-threatening in a significant subset of patients.

Hematologic Toxicity. There is some bone marrow suppression from IL-2 although most hematopoietic effects resolve rapidly with drug discontinuation. Some renal cell cancer patients given high-dose (bolus) IL-2 have experienced significant anemia requiring red cell transfusions (Rosenberg et al 1987). Thrombocytopenia (<100,000/mm^3) occurs in about 13% of courses and neutropenia (<500/mm^3) occurs in about 4% of high-dose bolus IL-2 trials. Significant eosinophilia (> 5%) is also quite common in patients receiving IL-2 (Lotze et al 1985). This also resolves rapidly after the drug is stopped.

Cardiac Toxicity. Myocardial infarctions (MIs) can be fatal in patients receiving IL-2/LAK cell therapy. In one trial 2 of 106 patients died of a MI related to the IL-2/LAK regimen (Rosenberg et al 1987). In a multicenter trial of this same therapy, nonfatal MIs occurred unexpectedly in 3 of 10 patients who did not have either a preexisting poor performance status or any specific cardiovascular risk factors (Nora et al 1989). Of note, two of these MIs were clinically silent.

Transient atrial arrhythmias have also been observed during IL-2 infusions (Rosenberg et al 1987), and most patients will develop a reflex tachycardia during therapy. This constellation of cardiac symptoms is believed to reflect a hyperdynamic state characterized by a significant increase in the cardiac index. Simultaneously, there are profound decreases in mean arterial pressure, systemic vascular resistance, and left ventricular stroke work index (Nora et al 1989). These effects appear to involve primarily increased permeability in vascular endothelia (Ettinghausen et al 1988) and not direct myocardial cell injury (Dorr and Shipp 1989).

Central Nervous System Toxicity. Interleukin-2 also produces neuropsychiatric effects, most often characterized by transient somnolence and rarely coma, delirium, or marked confusion (Rosenberg et al 1987). Again, these effects resolve rapidly following the cessation of IL-2 therapy.

Skin Toxicity. There are no reports of serious venous or local site irritation with IL-2. However subcutaneous IL-2 injections may cause local inflammation and induration (Thompson et al 1987). A number of patients develop purpuric skin rashes and urticaria with facial swelling and distal erythema (Lotze et al 1986); however, the drug does not produce a high incidence of anaphylactoid-type reactions. Two cases of life-threatening bullous eruptions of the arms, legs, and trunk have been reported (Staunton et al 1991). There are also isolated cases of erythema nodosum and pemphigus vulgaris associated with IL-2 therapy (Weinstein et al 1987, Ramseur et al 1989).

■ Special Applications

Interleukin-2 has been administered as a continuous perfusion of the urinary bladder (Huland and Huland 1989). The total IL-2 dose in this trial was 15×10^6 U (n-interleukin-2, Biotest Corporation, Frankfurt, West Germany), administered as a continuous 24-hour perfusion for 5 days (2 mL/min, 1000 U/mL concentration). Cycles were repeated at 4- to 12-week intervals and some local responses were noted in 1 of 5 patients with advanced bladder cancer. No local or systemic side effects were observed in this pilot study.

Interleukin-2 has also been administered intraperitoneally to patients with advanced ovarian cancer. A range of doses up to 10×10^6 IU/m² have been administered as a 30-minute instillation in 500 mL of fluid. There is a long apparent half-life of IL-2 monitored both in intraperitoneal fluid (median, 22 hours) and in the serum (median, 4 hours) (Konrad et al 1990). This suggests that IL-2 is transported very slowly from the intraperitoneal space to the blood leading to very high AUCs in the intraperitoneal compartment.

REFERENCES

Allison MAK, Jones SE, McGuffey P. Phase II trial of outpatient interleukin-2 in malignant lymphoma, chronic lymphocytic leukemia, and selected solid tumors. *J Clin Oncol.* 1989;**7**:75–80.

Bar MH, Sznol M, Atkins MB, et al. Metastatic malignant melanoma treated with combined bolus and continuous infusion interleukin-2 and lymphokine-activated killer cells. *J Clin Oncol.* 1990;**8**(7):1138–1147.

Berd D, Maguire HC Jr, Mastrangelo MJ. Impairment of concanavalin A-inducible suppressor activity following administration of cyclophosphamide to patients with advanced cancer. *Cancer Res.* 1984a;**44**:1275–1280.

Berd D, Maguire HC Jr, Mastrangelo MJ. Potentiation of human cell-mediated and humoral immunity by low-dose cyclophosphamide. *Cancer Res.* 1984b;**44**:5439–5443.

Bernard O, De St Groth F, Ullrich A, Green W, Schlessinger J. High affinity interleukin 2 binding by an oncogenic hybrid interleukin 2–epidermal growth factor receptor molecule. *Proc Natl Acad Sci USA.* 1987;**84**:2125–2129.

Brunda MJ, Tarnowski D, Davatelis V, et al. Effect of combinations of recombinant interferon alpha and interleukin-2 on tumor metastases and cytotoxic cell function. In: Lotzova E, Herberman RB, eds. *Natural Immunity, Cancer and Biological Response Modification.* Basel, Switzerland: Karger; 1986:235–241.

Cetus Corporation. *Proleukin®*—Recombinant Interleukin-2 (Human). Investigational Brochure Information for Investigators, April 28, 1989:1–44.

Chabot GG, Flaherty LE, Valdivieso M, Baker LH. Alteration of dacarbazine pharmacokinetics after interleukin-2 administration in melanoma patients. *Cancer Chemother Pharmacol.* 1990;**27**:157–160.

Chiron/Cetus Oncology Corporation. *Proleukin®: Aldesleukin for Injection.* Package insert. Emeryville, CA; 1992.

Chouaib S, Bertoglio J, Blay J-Y, et al. Generation of lymphokine-activated killer cells: Synergy between tumor necrosis factor and interleukin 2. *Proc Natl Acad Sci USA.* 1988;**85**:6875–6879.

Dorr RT, Shipp NG. Effect of interferon, interleukin-2 and tumor necrosis factor on myocardial cell viability and doxorubicin cardiotoxicity in vitro. *Immunopharmacology.* 1989;**18**:31–38.

Dutcher JP, Creekmore S, Weiss GR, et al. A phase II study of interleukin-2 and lymphokine-activated killer cells in patients with metastatic malignant melanoma. *J Clin Oncol.* 1989;**7**:477–485.

Ellison MD, Povlishock JT, Merchant RE. Blood–brain barrier dysfunction in cats following recombinant interleukin-2 infusion. *Cancer Res.* 1987;**47**:5765–5770.

Ettinghausen SE, Puri RK, Rosenberg SA. Increased vascular permeability in organs mediated by the systemic administration of lymphokine-activated killer cells and recombinant interleukin-2 in mice. *J Natl Cancer Inst.* 1988;**80**:177–188.

Fauci AS, Dale DC. The effect of in vivo hydrocortisone on subpopulations of human lymphocytes. *J Clin Invest.* 1974;**53**:240–246.

Fisher RI, et al. Phase II clinical trial of interleukin 2 plus lymphokine activated killer cells (IL-2/LAK) in metastatic renal cancer. *Proc Am Soc Clin Oncol.* 1987;**6**:244.

Gearing AJH, Thorpe R. The international standard for human interleukin-2. Calibration by international collaborative study. *J Immunol Methods.* 1988;**114**:3–9.

Gracomini P, Aguzzi A, Pestka PS, et al. Modulation by recombinant DNA leukocyte (alpha) and fibroblast (beta) interferons of the expression and shedding of HLA- and tumor-associated antigens by human melanoma cells. *J Immunol.* 1984;**133**:1649.

Grimm EA. Human lymphokine-activated killer cells (LAK cells) as a potential immunotherapeutic modality. *Biochim Biophys Acta.* 1986;**865**:267–279.

Grimm EA, Muul LM, Wilson DJ. The differential inhibitory effects exerted by cyclosporine and hydrocortisone on the activation of human cytotoxic lymphocytes by recombinant interleukin-2 versus allospecific CTL. *Transplantation.* 1985;**39**:537–540.

Gustavson LE, Nadeau RW, Oldfield NF. Pharmacokinetics of Teceleukin (recombinant human interleukin-2) after intravenous or subcutaneous administration to patients with cancer. *J Biol Respir Med.* 1989;**8**:440–449.

Herberman RB. Interleukin-2 therapy of human cancer: Potential benefits versus toxicity. *J Clin Oncol.* 1989;**7**:1–4.

Herberman RB, Balch C, Bolhuis R, et al. Lymphokine-activated killer cell activity: Characteristics of effector cells and their progenitors in blood and spleen. *Immunol Today.* 1987;**8**:178–181.

Herrmann F, Cannistra SA, Levine H, Griffin JN. Expression of interleukin 2 receptors and binding of interleukin 2 by γ- interferon-induced human leukemic and normal monocytic cells. *J Exp Med.* 1985;**162**:1111–1116.

Hook GR, Greenwood MA, Barba D, et al. Morphology of interleukin-2 stimulated human peripheral blood mononuclear effector cells killing glioma-derived tumor cells in vitro. *J Natl Cancer Inst.* 1988;**80**:171–177.

Horst H-J, Flad H-D. Corticosteroid–interleukin 2 interactions: Inhibition of binding of interleukin 2 to interleukin 2 receptors. *Clin Exp Immunol.* 1987;**68**:156–161.

Huland E, Huland H. Local continuous high dose interleukin 2: A new therapeutic model for the treatment of advanced bladder carcinoma. *Cancer Res.* 1989;**49**:5469–5474.

Iigo M, Sakurai M, Tamura T, et al. In vivo antitumor activity of multiple injections of recombinant interleukin-2 alone and in combination with three different types of recombinant interferon on various syngeneic murine tumors. *Cancer Res.* 1988;**48**:260–264.

Kintzel PE, Calis KA. Recombinant interleukin-2: A biological response modifier. *Clin Pharmacol.* 1991;**10**:110–128.

Kohler PC, Hank JA, Moore KH, et al. Phase I clinical trial of recombinant interleukin-2: A comparison of bolus and continuous intravenous infusion. *Cancer Invest.* 1989;**7**(3):213–223.

Konrad MW, Hemstreet G, Hersh EM, et al. Pharmacokinetics of recombinant interleukin 2 in humans. *Cancer Res.* 1990;**50**:2009–2017.

Kozeny GA, Nicolas JD, Creekmore S, et al. Effects of interleukin-2 immunotherapy on renal function. *J Clin Oncol.* 1988;**6**:1170–1176.

Krigel R, Padavic K, Comis R, Rudolph A. A phase I study of recombinant interleukin 2 (rIL-2) plus recombinant β interferon (IFN-β). *Cancer Res.* 1988;**48**:3875–3881.

Kuribayashi K, Gillis S, Kern DE, et al. Murine NK cell cultures: Effects of interleukin-2 and interferon on cell growth and cytotoxic reactivity. *J Immunol.* 1981;**126**:2321–2327.

Lee KH, Talpaz M. Rothberg JM, et al. Concomitant administration of recombinant human interleukin-2 and recombinant interferon α-2A in cancer patients: A phase I study. *J Clin Oncol.* 1989;**7**(11):1726–1732.

Lotze MT, Frana LW, Sharrow SO, et al. In vivo administration of purified human interleukin 2. I. Half-life and immunologic effects of the Jurkat cell line-derived interleukin 2. *J Immunol.* 1985;**134**(1):157–166.

Lotze MT, Matory YL, Rayner AA, et al. Clinical effects and toxicity of interleukin-2 in patients with cancer. *Cancer.* 1986;**58**:2764–2772.

Margolin KA, Rayner AA, Hawkins MJ, Atkins MB, et al. Interleukin-2 and lymphokine-activated killer cell therapy of solid tumors: Analysis of toxicity and management guidelines. *J Clin Oncol.* 1989;**7**:486–498.

Mazumder A, Rosenberg SA. Successful immunotherapy of natural killer resistant established pulmonary melanoma metastases by the intravenous adoptive transfer of syneneic lymphocytes activated in vitro by interleukin-2. *J Exp Med.* 1984;**159**:495–507.

Mitchell MS, Kempf RA, Harel W, et al. Effectiveness and tolerability of low-dose cyclophosphamide and low-dose intravenous interleukin-2 in disseminated melanoma. *J Clin Oncol.* 1988;**6**:409–424.

Morgan DA, Ruscetti FW, Gallo RC. Selective in vitro growth of T-lymphocytes from normal bone marrows. *Science.* 1976;**193**:1007–1008.

Nora R, Abrams JS, Tait NS, et al. Myocardial toxic effects during recombinant interleukin-2 therapy. *J Natl Cancer Inst.* 1989;**81**:59–63.

Paciucci PA, Holland JF, Glidewell O, Odchimar R. Recombinant interleukin-2 by continuous infusion and adoptive transfer of recombinant interleukin-2-activated cells in patients with advanced cancer. *J Clin Oncol.* 1989;**7**:869–878.

Papa MZ, Vetto JT, Ettinghausen E, et al. Effect of corticosteroid on the antitumor activity of lymphokine-activated killer cells and interleukin 2 in mice. *Cancer Res.* 1986;**46**:5618–5623.

Parker RS, Lala PK. Amelioration of B-16F10 melanoma lung metastases in mice by a combination therapy with indomethacin and interleukin-2. *J Exp Med.* 1987;**165**:14–28.

Ramseur WL, Richard F II, Duggan DB. A case of fatal pemphigus vulgaris in association with beta interferon and interleukin-2 therapy. *Cancer.* 1989;**63**:2005–2007.

Redman BG, Flaherty L, Chou T-H, et al. A phase I trial of recombinant interleukin-2 combined with recombinant interferon-gamma in patients with cancer. *J Clin Oncol.* 1990;**8**:1269–1276.

Richards JM, Barker E, Latta J, et al: Phase I study of weekly 24-hour infusions of recombinant human interleukin-2. *J Natl Cancer Inst.* 1988;**80**:1325–1328.

Robb RJ, Greene WC, Rusk CM. Low and high affinity cellular receptors for interleukin 2. *J Exp Med.* 1984;**160**:1126–1146.

Robb RJ, Smith KA. Heterogeneity of human T-cell growth factor(s) due to variable glycosylation. *Mol Immunol.* 1981;**18**:1087–1094.

Rosenberg SA, Lotze MT, Muul LM, et al. Observations on the systemic administration of autologous lymphokine-activated killer cells and recombinant interleukin-2 to patients with metastatic cancer. *N Engl J Med.* 1985;**313**(23):1485–1492.

Rosenberg SA, Lotze MT, Muul LM, et al. A progress report on the treatment of 157 patients with advanced cancer using lymphokine-activated killer cells and interleukin-2 or high-dose interleukin-2 alone. *N Engl J Med.* 1987;**316:**889–897.

Rosenberg SA, Packard BS, Aebersold PM, et al. Use of tumor-infiltrating lymphocytes in the immunotherapy of patients with metastatic melanoma. *N Engl J Med.* 1988;**319:**1676–1680.

Rosenberg SA, Spiess P, Lafreniere R. A new approach to the adoptive immunotherapy of cancer with tumor-infiltrating lymphocytes. *Science.* 1986;**233:**1318–1321.

Schoof DD, Gramolini BA, Davidson DL, Massaro AF, Wilson RE, Eberlein TJ. Adoptive immunotherapy of human cancer using low-dose recombinant interleukin 2 and lymphokine-activated killer cells. *Cancer Res.* 1988;**48:**5007–5010.

Shalmi CL, Dutcher JP, Feinfeld DA, et al. Acute renal dysfunction during interleukin-2 treatment: Suggestion of an intrinsic renal lesion. *J Clin Oncol.* 1990;**8:**1839–1846.

Sosman JA, Kohler PC, Hank J, et al. Repetitive weekly cycles of recombinant human interleukin-2: Responses of renal carcinoma with acceptable toxicity. *J Natl Cancer Inst.* 1988a;**80:**60–63.

Sosman JA, Kohler PC, Hank JA, et al. Repetitive weekly cycles of interleukin-2. II. Clinical and immunologic effects of dose, schedule, and addition of indomethacin. *J Natl Cancer Inst.* 1988b;**80:**1451–1461.

Staunton MR, Scully MC, Le Boit PE, Aronson FR. Life-threatening bullous skin eruptions during interleukin-2 therapy. *J Natl Cancer Inst.* 1991;**83:**56–57.

Talmadge JE, Phillips H, Shindler J, Tribble H, Pennington R. Systematic preclinical study on the therapeutic properties of recombinant human interleukin 2 for the treatment of metastatic disease. *Cancer Res.* 1987;**49:**415–422.

Taniguchi, et al. Structure and expression of a cloned cDNA for human interleukin 2. *Nature.* 1983;**302:**305–310.

Thompson JA, Lee DJ, Cox WW, et al. Recombinant interleukin 2 toxicity, pharmacokinetics, and immunomodulatory effects in a phase I trial. *Cancer Res.* 1987;**47:**4202–4207.

Thompson JA, Lee DJ, Lindgren CG, et al. Influence of dose and duration of infusion of interleukin-2 on toxicity and immunomodulation. *J Clin Oncol.* 1988;**6:**669–678.

Vetto JT, Papa MZ, Lotze MT, et al. Reduction of toxicity of interleukin-2 and lymphokine-activated killer cells in humans by the administration of corticosteroids. *J Clin Oncol.* 1987;**5**(3):496–503.

Weber JS, Jay G, Tanaka K, et al. Immunotherapy of a murine tumor with interleukin-2: Increased sensitivity after MHC class I gene transfection. *J Exp Med.* 1987;**166:**1716–1733.

Weinstein A, Bujak D, Mittelman A, et al. Erythema nodosum in a patient with renal cell carcinoma treated with interleukin 2 and lymphokine-activated killer cells (letter). *JAMA.* 1987;**258:**3120–3121.

West WH, Tauer KW, Yannelli JR, et al. Constant-infusion recombinant interleukin-2 in adoptive immunotherapy of advanced cancer. *N Engl J Med.* 1987;**316:**898–905.

Allopurinol Sodium

■ Other Names

Zyloprim (100- and 300-mg scored tablets, Burroughs Wellcome); allopurinol sodium (injection); NSC-1390 (Burroughs-Wellcome).

■ Chemistry

Structure of allopurinol

Chemically the drug is 1, 5-dihydro-4*H*-pyrazolo [3,4-*d*]pyrimidin-4-one and has a molecular weight of 136. Allopurinol is an acidic compound with a pK_a of $\simeq$ 9.4. An injectable monosodium salt is available as an investigational agent. It forms a solution in water (500 mg/25 mL) with a resultant pH of 10.5.

■ Antitumor Activity

In cancer patients allopurinol is used mainly to prevent acute hyperuricemia and acute urate nephropathy from tumor lysis syndrome caused by cytoreductive chemotherapy in highly proliferative tumors of massive burden (DeConti and Calabresi 1966, Krakoff and Meyer 1965).

Allopurinol does not have direct antitumor activity; however the drug can greatly increase the antitumor effects and toxicity of azathioprine (Imuran®), 6-mercaptopurine, and possibly, and to a lesser extent, cyclophosphamide. It may also alter the toxicity of other antimetabolites (see Drug Interactions). In addition there is also some evidence for activity as an antiparasitic agent in the treatment of leishmaniasis and trypanosomiasis (Marr et al 1978).

■ Mechanism of Action

Allopurinol is a structural analog of hypoxanthine and is a potent inhibitor of the enzyme xanthine oxidase. In humans, xanthine oxidase converts the water-soluble acids hypoxanthine and xanthine to the much less soluble end product, uric acid. Thus, allopurinol metabolically blocks uric acid production from its normal purine precursors. This activity is also shared by the major metabolite of allopurinol, oxipurinol. Both diminish de novo purine synthesis by creating an intracellular accumulation of inosinic, xanthylic, adenylic, and guanylic acids. A feedback inhibition produced by the latter two purines inhibits phosphoribosylpyrophosphate amidotransferase (PRPPase). The inhibition of PRPPase ultimately blocks de novo purine synthesis by inhibiting essential phosphoribosyl enzymes (McCollister et al 1977).

De novo pyrimidine synthesis is also inhibited by allopurinol. The effect is mediated primarily by an alteration of orotic acid metabolism. This occurs by the buildup of xanthylic acid and by ribonucleotide metabolites of allopurinol (Kelley and Beardmore 1970). The buildup of the ribonucleotide metabolites inhibits the enzyme orotidylic decarboxylase.

The onset of pharmacologic effects from allopurinol does not appear to be more rapid with intravenous dosing. Thus, intravenous allopurinol (which is investigational) should probably be reserved for those emergency situations in which a patient is unable to take oral medications (Kann et al 1968).

■ Availability and Storage

Allopurinol tablets are stored at room temperature. Intact vials may be stored at room temperature but stability is enhanced if stored under refrigeration. For parenteral use, allopurinol is supplied investigationally as lyophilized powder in 500-mg vials of monosodium allopurinol.

■ Preparation for Use, Stability, and Admixture

The investigational powder may be reconstituted with 25 mL of sterile water for injection. Ideally, it should be further diluted with D5W or normal saline to a final concentration not greater than 1.2 mg/mL. This acts to reduce the concentration of alkaline solution infused and thus may reduce the likelihood of thrombophlebitis. The reconstituted drug should be used within 24 hours of preparation and any remainder discarded because of the potential risk of inadvertent contamination; however, unbuffered drug is chemically stable for several weeks at room temperature (Gressel and Galleli 1968). On prolonged standing at room temperature, the major degradation product of the injectable formulation is the 3-amino-4-pyrazolocarboxamide which is inactive. Allopurinol sodium is physically incompatible with methotrexate and should, therefore, not be diluted or administered within the same intravenous fluids.

■ Administration

The required dose, diluted as described earlier, should be administered over a period of at least 1 hour. Twenty-four-hour infusions have also been used to deliver large daily doses. Single daily doses of 105 to 660 mg can be given in 25 to 50 mL of D5W over a 15- to 30-minute period (Brown et al 1970).

■ Dosage

The optimal dose of injectable allopurinol in cancer chemotherapy is not well established. Common doses range from 200 to 400 mg/m^2/d. Of note, a dose–response relationship is reported up to 1200 mg allopurinol per day (Rundles and Hitchings 1966). It should also be remembered that allopurinol dose reduction is required in patients with moderate to severe renal impairment to prevent significant drug accumulation from the 14-hour half-life of the active metabolite oxipurinol. This long half-life indicates that maximal steady-state responses to allopurinol would not be obtained until after 3 to 5 days of single daily dosing. Therefore, initially higher loading doses of up to 1.2 g/m^2/d may be required to achieve a rapid effect. Prolonged effects from allopurinol are obtained with single daily doses, and although multiple daily dosing has been studied it offers no practical advantages in general use (Rodnan et al 1975). As previously stated, the use of the intravenous preparation has not shown a significantly more rapid onset of effects than observed after equivalent oral doses and is recommended only for situations in which gastrointestinal absorption is impaired.

■ Drug Interactions

Because allopurinol blocks the metabolism of both 6-mercaptopurine and azathioprine, doses of either agent must be reduced to one-third or one-fourth the normal dose with concomitant allopurinol therapy (Coffey et al 1972). Allopurinol was reported to potentiate bone marrow suppression from other cytotoxic drugs, particularly cyclophosphamide (Boston Collaborative Drug Surveillance Program 1974). A preclinical study also reported that allopurinol increased cyclophosphamide antitumor activity but not myelosuppression (Alberts and van Daalen Wetters 1976). However, a follow-up clinical study did not show that allopurinol increased myelosuppression in lymphoma patients receiving three to six cycles of combination chemotherapy regimens that included cyclophosphamide (Stolbach et al 1982). Thus, a role for allopurinol in enhancing myelosuppression caused by cyclophosphamide is not firmly established.

Interactions with 5-Fluorouracil. Clinical reports have described allopurinol modulation of 5-fluorouracil (5-FU) toxicity, allowing high dose, continuously infused 5-FU to be administered (Fox et al 1979, 1981). The mechanism of this interaction was believed to involve oxipurinol-induced inhibition of the activation of 5-FU by orotate phosphoribosylpyrophosphatase and, to a lesser degree, reduced thymidylate synthetase inhibition by 5-FU (Fox et al 1981). When administered by continuous intravenous infusion, 5-FU doses can be increased approximately fourfold with concomitant allopurinol (Howell et al 1981). Dose-limiting mucositis is reached at 5-FU doses of 2 g/m^2/d × 5 consecutive days with allopurinol doses of 300 mg PO every 8 hours (Howell et al 1981).

With the administration of single bolus doses of 5-FU, allopurinol doses of 600 mg/d reduce the amount of myelosuppression, allowing 5-FU dose escalation to 1.8 g/m^2 every 4 weeks (Woolley et al 1985). 5-FU neurotoxicity was dose limiting and the allopurinol regimen was well tolerated. Nonetheless, allopurinol combined with high-dose 5-FU has not produced significantly higher response rates and neurotoxicity has been consistently problematic (Campbell et al 1982). Thus, both the therapeutic advantage and the biochemical rationale for this drug combination are unclear.

The allopurinol metabolite oxipurinol does not inhibit cytotoxicity from 5-FU in human breast, ovary, and colon tumor cells studied in colony-forming assays in vitro (Garewal et al 1983). In contrast, allopurinol can partially reverse the antitumor effects of methotrexate in vitro (Grindey and Moran 1975). This may be caused by an allopurinol-mediated increase in cellular concentrations of hypoxanthine and other xanthines that can act to overcome methotrexate's inhibition of thymidine synthesis.

Other reported interactions with allopurinol include severe neurotoxicity when combined with the antiviral agent vidarabine (adenine arabinoside, Ara-A, Vira-A®) (Friedman and Grasela 1981) and inhibition of theophylline metabolism by long-term allopurinol (Manfredi and Vesell 1981). In the case of vidarabine, the mechanism of interaction is believed to involve inhibition of hypoxanthine arabinoside metabolism, which is normally mediated by xanthine oxidase. The effect of allopurinol on theophylline results in a 27% increase in systemic theophylline exposure and a 25% increase in the half-life of theophylline (Manfredi and Vesell 1981). This contradicts prior studies that demonstrated no interaction for lower doses of allopurinol combined with theophylline (Grygiel et al 1979, Vozeh et al 1980).

Another reported potential drug interaction with allopurinol includes a prolongation in the half-lives of warfarin and oral antidiabetic drugs because of depressed hepatic microsomal metabolism by allopurinol. The clinical significance of these interactions in humans is not established. Epidemiologic studies, however, have demonstrated an increased incidence of rash when allopurinol was given with penicillin antibiotics, particularly ampicillin, and also with thiazide diuretics (Young et al 1974).

■ Pharmacokinetics

Allopurinol is rapidly cleared from the plasma by conversion to oxipurinol. The half-life of allopurinol is reported to range from 40 minutes in a specific assay (Hande et al 1978) to 2 hours in a nonspecific biochemical assay (Elion et al 1966). Oxipurinol, the major allopurinol metabolite, has a much longer half-life of approximately 14 hours in the plasma. The range of oxipurinol half-life ranged from 18 to 30 hours in the study by Elion et al (1968) and from 14 to 28 hours in other studies (Hande et al 1978, Appelbaum et al 1982). Oxipurinol has roughly one-fifth to one-tenth the enzymatic-inhibitory activity of allopurinol; however, because of the longer half-life, oxipurinol is probably most responsible for the antihyperuricemic effects of allopurinol. Neither allopurinol nor oxipurinol is protein bound (Elion et al 1966), and the volume of distribution is about twice that of total body water or about 1.6 L/kg (Appelbaum et al 1982). Both allopurinol and oxipurinol are ultimately excreted into the urine, although oxipurinol is reabsorbed in the proximal tubules. Thus, with severely impaired renal function, the half-life of oxipurinol is greatly increased, and the daily doses should be reduced (see Dosage).

The bulk of an administered allopurinol dose is excreted as oxipurinol, which is slowly eliminated. The renal clearance is 12 to 15 mL/min (Hande et al

1978, Appelbaum et al 1982). The inhibition of xanthine oxidase by allopurinol also does not slow the metabolic oxidation of allopurinol to oxipurinol. This suggests that allopurinol can be metabolized by alternate non-xanthine oxidase metabolic routes.

Adult patients receiving 300-mg oral doses develop mean allopurinol and oxipurinol levels of 3×10^{-5} and 9×10^{-5} M, respectively (Hande et al 1978), with peak allopurinol levels occurring 2 to 3 hours after the tablets are ingested. According to Elion et al (1966), about 80% of an oral dose is absorbed in 48 hours. A subsequent pharmacokinetic trial using a more specific gas chromatographic assay showed an absolute oral bioavailability of 67% in normal male subjects (Appelbaum et al 1982). Approximately 90% oral bioavailability was reported in another trial (Breithaupt and Tittel 1982).

■ Side Effects and Toxicity

Allopurinol is usually well tolerated; however, about 2 to 3% of patients may develop a pruritic maculopapular rash or, less commonly, exfoliative dermatitis. These reactions appear to be much more common in patients with renal insufficiency or those receiving concurrent ampicillin or thiazides. In patients with a history of gout, acute exacerbations may be precipitated on initiation of allopurinol therapy.

Severe hypersensitivity reactions to allopurinol have been rarely reported. Granulomatous hepatitis has also been described (Ohsawa and Ohtsubo 1985, Simmons et al 1972). Allopurinol hepatotoxicity is more common in patients receiving diuretics or in those with compromised renal function. It is also unclear whether glucocorticosteroids help in resolving the hepatitis (Al-kawas et al 1981). Ocular lesions, alopecia, slight bone marrow suppression, drowsiness, peripheral neuropathy, and gastrointestinal upset have also been reported (Young 1975).

Thrombophlebitis has been noted with the intravenous formulation and may relate to this formulation's high pH. Dilution with D5W may prevent phlebitis.

Serious reactions from allopurinol are very rare. They include aplastic agranulocytosis (Greenberg and Zambrano 1972), several cases of toxic epidermal necrolysis with some fatal outcomes (Kantor 1970, Ellman et al 1975), and severe systemic vasculitis (Jarzobski et al 1970, Bailey et al 1976). A single case of arteritis with atypical seizures has also been reported (Weiss et al 1978).

■ Special Applications

Allopurinol Suppositories. Allopurinol has been investigationally formulated into rectal suppositories using either cocoa butter or polyethylene glycol (Chang et al 1981, Appelbaum et al 1980). The bioavailability of a 300-mg suppository was poor, with absorption ranging from 0 to 5.89%. Absorption was slightly higher with cocoa butter than with polyethylene glycol; however, both bases facilitated poor overall allopurinol absorption.

Allopurinol Mouthwash. Allopurinol solutions (1 mg/mL) in 0.5% carboxymethylcellulose in cherry-flavored Kool-Aid® have been evaluated as a topical means of preventing 5-fluorouracil-induced stomatitis (Van der Vliet et al 1989). Ten to fifteen milliliters of the agent was given as an oral swish immediately after and 1, 2, and 3 hours following intravenous 5-fluorouracil. Although there was one positive report on the efficacy of this procedure (Clark and Slevin 1985), a follow-up trial demonstrated no benefit for the allopurinol mouthwash (Van der Vliet et al 1989). The preparation is stable at 4°C or at room temperature for at least 8 months (Loprinzi et al 1989).

REFERENCES

Alberts DS, van Daalen Wetters T. The effect of allopurinol in cyclophosphamide antitumor activity. *Cancer Res.* 1976;**36**:2790–2794.

Al-Kawas FH, Seeff LB, Berendson RA, et al. Allopurinol hepatotoxicity. *Ann Intern Med.* 1981;**95**:588–590.

Applebaum SJ, Mayersohn M, Dorr RT, Perrier D. Allopurinol kinetics and bioavailability: Intravenous, oral and rectal administration. *Cancer Chemother Pharmacol.* 1982;**8**:93–98.

Applebaum SJ, Mayersohn M, Perrier D, Dorr RT. Allopurinol absorption from rectal suppositories. *Drug Intell Clin Pharm.* 1980;**14**:789.

Bailey RR, Neale TJ, Lynn KL. Allopurinol-associated arteritis. *Lancet.* 1976;**2**:907.

Boston Collaborative Drug Surveillance Program. Allopurinol and cytotoxic drugs: Interaction in relation to bone marrow depression. *JAMA.* 1974;**227**(9):1036–1041.

Breithaupt H, Tittel M. Kinetics of allopurinol after single intravenous and oral doses: Noninteraction with benzbromarone and hydrochlorothiazide. *Eur J Clin Pharmacol.* 1982;**22**:77–84.

Brown CH III, Sashick E, Carbone P. Clinical efficacy and lack of toxicity of allopurinol (NSC-1390) given intravenously. *Cancer Chem Ther Rep, Part I.* 1970;**54**(2):125–129.

Campbell TN, Howell SB, Pfeifle C, House BA. High-dose allopurinol modulation of 5-FU toxicity: Phase I trial of an outpatient dose schedule. *Cancer Treat Rep.* 1982;**66**:1723–1727.

Chang S-L, Kramer WG, Feldman S, et al. Bioavailability of allopurinol oral and rectal dosage forms. *Am J Hosp Pharm.* 1981;**38**:365–368.

Clark PI, Slevin ML. Allopurinol mouthwashes and 5-fluorouracil induced oral toxicity. *Eur J Surg Oncol.* 1985;**11**:267–268.

Coffey JJ, White CA, Lesk AB, et al. Effect of allopurinol on the pharmacokinetics of 6-mercaptopurine in cancer patients. *Cancer Res.* 1972;**32**:1283–1289.

DeConti RC, Calabresi P. Use of allopurinol for prevention and control of hyperuricemia in patients with neoplastic disease. *N Engl J Med.* 1966;**274**:481–486.

Elion GB, Kovensky A, Hitchings GH, et al. Metabolic studies of allopurinol, an inhibitor of xanthine oxidase. *Biochem Pharmacol.* 1966;**15**:863–880.

Elion GB, Yu T-F, Gutman AB, et al. Renal clearance of oxipurinol: The chief metabolite of allopurinol. *Am J Med.* 1968;**45**:69–77.

Ellman MH, Fretzen DF, Olson W. Toxic epidermal necrolysis associated with allopurinol administration. *Arch Dermatol.* 1975;**111**:986–990.

Fox RM, Woods RL, Tattersall MHN. Allopurinol modulation of high-dose fluorouracil toxicity. *Lancet.* 1979;**1**:677.

Fox RM, Woods RL, Tattersall MHN, et al. Allopurinol modulation of fluorouracil toxicity. *Cancer Chemother Pharmacol.* 1981;**5**:151–155.

Friedman HM, Grasela T. Adenine arabinoside and allopurinol—Possible adverse drug interaction. *N Engl J Med.* 1981;**304**:423.

Garewal HS, Ahmann FR, Alberts DS. Lack of inhibition by oxypurinol of 5-FU toxicity against human tumor cell lines. *Cancer Treat Rep.* 1983;**67**:495–498.

Greenberg MS, Zambrano SS. Aplastic agranulocytosis after allopurinol therapy. *Arthritis Rheum.* 1972;**15**:415–416.

Gressel PD, Galleli JF. Quantitative analysis and alkaline stability studies of allopurinol. *J Pharm Sci.* 1968;**57**(2):335–338.

Grindey G, Moran R. Effects of allopurinol on the therapeutic efficacy of methotrexate. *Cancer Res.* 1975;**35**:1702–1705.

Grygiel JJ, Wing LMH, Farka J. Effects of allopurinol on theophylline metabolism and clearance. *Clin Pharmacol Ther.* 1979;**26**:660–667.

Hande K, Reed E, Chabner O. Allopurinol kinetics. *Clin Pharmacol Ther.* 1978;**23**(5):598–605.

Howell SB, Wung WE, Taetle R, et al. Modulation of 5-fluorouracil toxicity by allopurinol in man. *Cancer.* 1981;**48**:1281–1289.

Jarzobski J, Ferry J, Womboldt D, et al. Vasculitis with allopurinol therapy. *Am J Heart.* 1970;**79**:116–121.

Kann HE Jr, Wells JH, Gallelli JF, et al. The development and use of an intravenous preparation of allopurinol. *Am J Sci.* 1968;**256**:53–63.

Kantor CL. Toxic epidermal necrolysis, azotemia and death after allopurinol therapy. *JAMA.* 1970;**212**:478–479.

Kelley W, Beardmore T. Allopurinol: Alteration in pyrimidine metabolism in man. *Science.* 1970;**169**:388–390.

Krakoff LH, Meyer R. Prevention of hyperuricemia in leukemia and lymphoma: Use of allopurinol. *JAMA.* 1965;**193**:1–12.

Loprinzi CL, Burnham NL, O'Connell MJ, et al. Allopurinol mouthwash kinetic and stability information based on normal volunteers. *Hosp Pharm.* 1989;**24**:353–373.

Manfredi RL, Vesell ES. Inhibition of theophylline metabolism by long term allopurinol administration. *Clin Pharmacol Ther.* 1981;**29**:224–229.

Marr JJ, Berens RL, Nelson DJ. Antitrypanosomal effect of allopurinol: Conversion in vivo to aminopyrazolopyrimidine nucleotides by *Trypanosoma cruzi*. *Science.* 1978;**201**:1918–1920.

McCollister RH, Gilbert WR, Ashton DM, Wyngaarden JB. Pseudo-feedback inhibition of purine synthesis by 6-mercaptopurine ribonucleotide and other purine analogues. *J Biol Chem.* 1977;**239**:1560–1563.

Ohsawa T, Ohtsubo M. Hepatitis associated with allopurinol. *Drug Intell Clin Pharm.* 1985;**19**:431–432.

Rodnan GP, Robin JA, Tolchin SF, Elion GB. Allopurinol and gouty hyperuricemia—Efficacy of a single daily dose. *JAMA.* 1975;**231**:1143–1147.

Rundles RW, Hitchings B. Allopurinol in the treatment of gout. *Ann Intern Med.* 1966;**64**:229–258.

Schwartz PM, Handschumacher RE. Selective antagonism of 5-fluorouracil cytotoxicity by 4-hydroxypyrazolopyrimidine (allopurinol) in vitro. *Cancer Res.* 1979;**39**:3095–3101.

Simmons F, Feldman B, Gerenty D. Granulomatous hepatitis in a patient receiving allopurinol. *Gastroenterology.* 1972;**62**:101–104.

Stolbach L, Begg C, Bennett JM, et al. Evaluation of bone marrow toxic reaction in patients treated with allopurinol. *JAMA.* 1982;**247**(3):334–336.

Van der Vliet W, Erlichman C, Elhakim T. Allopurinol mouthwash for prevention of fluorouracil-induced stomatitis. *Clin Pharm.* 1989;**8**:655–658.

Vozeh S, Powell JR, Cupit GC, et al. Influence of allopurinol on theophylline disposition in adults. *Clin Pharmacol Ther.* 1980;**27**:194–197.

Weiss EB, Forman P, Rosenthal IM. Allopurinol-induced arteritis in partial HGPRTase deficiency. *Arch Intern Med.* 1978;**138**:1743–1744.

Woolley PV, Ayoob MJ, Smith FP, et al. A controlled trial of the effect of 4-hydroxypyrazolopyrimidine (allopurinol) on the toxicity of a single bolus dose of 5-fluorouracil. *J Clin Oncol.* 1985;**3**(1):103–109.

Young JL, Bosewll RB, Nies AS. Severe allopurinol hypersensitivity: Association with thiazides and prior renal compromise. *Arch Intern Med.* 1974;**134**:533–558.

Young L. Gout and hyperuricemia. In: Koda-Kimble MA, Young LY (eds). Applied Therapeutics for Clinical Pharmacists. San Francisco: Applied Therapeutics; Inc; 1992;74:1–15.

Altretamine

Other Names

Hexamethylmelamine; NSC-13875; HXM; HMM; Hexalen® (U.S. Bioscience, Inc).

Chemistry

Structure of altretamine

Altretamine (hexamethylmelamine) is one of the synthetic, substituted melamines derived from cyanuric chloride. It is structurally similar to the ethylenimonium alkylating agent triethylenemelamine (TEM). It has the empiric formula of $C_9H_{18}N_6$, with a molecular weight of 210.3 and a melting point of 172°C. The chemical name is N, N, N', N', N'', N''-hexamethyl-1,3,5-triazine-2,4,6-triamine. It is soluble at a concentration of 0.92 mg/mL in water, 47 mg/mL in ethyl ether, and 220 mg/mL in chloroform. The drug is more water soluble at acid pH (< 3.0).

Antitumor Activity

In experimental animal systems altretamine demonstrated significant antitumor effects in Walker 256 carcinosarcoma but was interestingly inactive in the prior NCI mouse tumor screen (L-1210 and P-388 leukemia, Lewis lung cancer, and B-16 melanoma) (Venditti 1975).

In clinical studies, the drug demonstrated usefulness in combination or as a single-agent therapy for a variety of solid tumors (Bergevin et al 1973, Blum et al 1973). It has shown activity in bronchogenic carcinoma (Takita and Didolkar 1974), ovarian carcinoma (Wampler et al 1972), cervical cancer (Stolinsky and Bateman 1973), breast cancer (Wilson et al 1970, Wampler et al 1972), and lymphomas (Wilson et al 1970). Some activity was also described in childhood leukemias and solid tumors (Dyment et al 1973). In a phase II trial, however, Leite (1978) was unable to detect any clinical effectiveness for altretamine in refractory breast cancer patients given high doses of the drug. Similarly, Lawson et al (1979) and Denefrio and Vogel (1978) have recently confirmed the relative inactivity of the drug for use in heavily pretreated patients with advanced breast cancer. In this combination drug study, it represented no improvement over mitomycin-C alone. Altretamine is active in non-Hodgkin's lymphomas with a 28% response rate (Legha et al 1976) and in cervical cancer (19% response rate [Stolinsky and Bateman 1973]). In the combination chemotherapy of lung cancer, altretamine has demonstrated antitumor efficacy in small cell lung cancer alone (De La Garza et al 1968) or in combination either with etoposide and/or procarbazine or with doxorubicin, cyclophosphamide, and vincristine (Ettinger et al 1987). Activity was also noted in both advanced small cell and non-small cell, epidermoid, and anaplastic lung cancer in combination with doxorubicin (Schultz et al 1979), and in advanced non-small cell lung cancer with mitomycin, platinum, and lomustine (Chaninian et al 1979). Clinical studies have shown altretamine to be active in some alkylator-resistant tumors (Stolinksy et al 1972, Takita and Didolkar 1974, Wampler et al 1972) including ovarian cancer (Johnson et al 1978).

The most positive clinical trials with altretamine are in the chemotherapy of ovarian carcinoma (Rosen et al 1987, Hainsworth et al 1990). Young et al (1978) have reported a 76% response rate with the "Hexa-CAF" regimen. Alberts et al (1979) also reported a 48% overall response rate in ovarian cancer when altretamine was combined with 5-fluorouracil and cisplatin. The "CHAP" or "CHAD" regimens are also widely reported as effective therapy for advanced ovarian carcinoma. These regimens consist of altretamine combined with doxorubicin, cisplatin, and cyclophosphamide (CHAD: Vogl et al 1979, CHAP: Kane et al 1979). Despite its major activity as part of a combination regimen, altretamine is currently FDA-approved as a second-line single agent for refractory ovarian cancer (Rosen et al 1987, Manetta et al 1990). In this setting 5/52 patients responded to altretamine therapy with a median survival of at least 41 months (Manetta et al 1990). A slightly higher partial response rate of 25% was reported by Hainsworth et al (1987) in patients receiving altretamine after relapsing on cisplatin-based regimens.

Mechanism of Action

Structurally, altretamine is similar to triethylenemelamine, an alkylating agent. The seemingly small structural differences between the two compounds nevertheless produce significant differences in activity and probably in mechanism of action. The exact cytotoxic mechanism of action of altretamine, however, is not known. While it does not act as an alkylating agent in vitro (Worzalla et al 1974), but it is possible that it is activated to an alkylating agent in the body. Metabolism of altretamine to *N*-hydroxymethylpentamethylmelamine (also called *N*-methylolpentamethylmelamine) by microsomal enzymes is dependent on NADPH and oxygen. This carbinolamine intermediate has been shown to bind covalently to microsomal proteins and to DNA, perhaps explaining some of the antitumor activity of the compound (Ames et al 1983, Gescher et al 1980). The breakdown of the *N*-methylolmelamines to formaldehyde may also mediate some of the cytotoxicity of this agent (Rutty and Abel 1980). As previously discussed, several clinical studies have demonstrated that altretamine is active in alkylating agent-resistant tumors (Stolinksy et al 1973, Takita and Didolkar 1974, Wampler et al 1973). Altretamine also inhibits incorporation of nucleotides into DNA and RNA. The mechanism of this inhibition is unknown (Heere and Donnelly 1971).

Availability and Storage

Altretamine is commercially available as 50-mg hard gelatin capsules (U.S. Bioscience). The capsules also contain lactose and calcium sterate as excipients. They should be stored at room temperature (22°C) in a tightly sealed bottle containing a desiccant. The intact capsules are stable for at least 2 years.

An investigational parenteral formulation has used 10% Intralipid® (intravenous fat emulsion) as the vehicle for drug dissolution (Ames and Kovach 1982). Powdered drug (500 mg) was initially dissolved in 27.5 mL of 0.1 N HCl and filtered through a 0.22-µm filter. A volume of 10% Intralipid® was added to achieve a concentration of 5.1 mg/mL to which sterile sodium bicarbonate (1 mEq/mL) was added (0.1 mL/20 mg drug). This final solution contained about 4 mg/mL of drug at a pH of 5.5 to 6.0 (Ames et al 1990). This formulation is not yet available for multicenter investigational trials.

Administration

Altretamine is administered orally. Dose-limiting gastrointestinal toxic effects may be partially relieved if the doses are given after meals and/or after prophylactic antiemetics. Effects of food on the oral bioavailability of altretamine are unknown.

The investigational parenteral formulation of altretamine in 10% Intralipid® was administered as an intravenous infusion at a rate of 2 or 8 mg/min (Ames et al 1990). Fifty milliliters of normal saline was given at the completion of the infusion.

Dosage

Several different dosing schedules of altretamine have been used. The usual dose as a single agent ranges from 4 to 12 mg/kg/d. Most investigators now give the total daily dose in four divided increments, after meals and at bedtime. The approved dose for single-agent therapy of advanced ovarian cancer is 260 mg/m^2/d administered in four divided daily doses for 14 to 21 days of a 28-day treatment cycle. When combined with other myelosuppressive agents the daily dose is typically 150 mg/m^2 for 14 consecutive days of a 28-day cycle. Altretamine dose intensification has been possible in some drug combinations in patients with advanced ovarian cancer (Bruckner et al 1989). The maximally tolerated dose of the investigational parenteral formulation ranged from 850 mg/m^2 for 1 day to 630 mg/m^2/d for 5 days (Ames et al 1990).

Drug Interactions

Because of marked altretamine metabolism by cytochrome P450 enzymes, several drug interactions are possible. Pretreatment of rats with phenobarbital to induce P450 enzymes led to greater covalent binding by the drug (Ames et al 1981). Conversely, the administration of SKF-525A, to block microsomal enzymes, or glutathione, which could bind active altretamine metabolites, led to a reduction in the covalent binding of the drug to hepatic proteins in vivo (Ames et al 1981). Similarly, the H$_2$ antagonist cimetidine has been shown to increase the lethality of altretamine in rats (Hande et al 1986). This was due to inhibition of microsomal metabolism, leading to a dose-related extension of the drug's half-live in vivo (Hande et al 1986).

It was believed that concurrent administration of pyridoxine (vitamin B$_6$) might decrease the incidence and severity of the neurologic complications. Leite (1978), however, was unable to detect any benefit for concurrent pyridoxine therapy in a phase II breast cancer study.

■ Pharmacokinetics

Altretamine is rapidly metabolized by N-demethylation through hepatic microsomes (Louis et al 1967). Eight and possibly nine demethylated metabolites are known. The main metabolites of altretamine are water soluble and include pentamethylmelamine and tetramethylmelamine. The triazine ring of altretamine does not appear to be metabolically cleaved. Following prolonged daily administration, approximately 60% of a dose is excreted into the urine as demethylated metabolites by 24 hours; more than 90% is excreted after 72 hours (Bryan et al 1968). Less than 1% of the drug is excreted intact in the urine. A small amount of the drug appears to be excreted by the lungs and trace amounts appear in the gut. The table below summarizes the pharmacokinetics of altretamine.

D'Incalci et al (1978) have recently described highly variable oral absorption of altretamine (120–300 mg/m^2) in humans. Using a specific gas chromatographic method, they documented peak plasma levels from 0.2 to 20.8 µg/mL achieved between 0.5 and 3 hours after dosing. The total area under the curve (reflecting the completeness of drug absorption) ranged from 70 to over 3000 µg/mL · min, with a terminal drug half-life range of 4.66 to 10.2 hours (average, 6.9 hours). Thus, there was considerable variation in altretamine bioavailability and pharmacokinetics after oral dosing (D'Incalci et al 1978); however, there is no dose dependence for absorption in an individual patient. Even with the variable absorption, no drug accumulation in plasma was detected during the daily treatment for up to 2 to 3 weeks. The drug is highly bound to plasma proteins with free fractions of 6, 25, and 50% for altretamine, pentamethylmelamine, and tetramethylmelamine, respectively. In the report by D'Incalci et al (1979) there were no differences in these parameters for patients with ascites, except that it took about 4 hours for ascitic fluid, drug, and metabolite levels to equilibrate with plasma levels. After 12 hours the levels of parent drug and pentamethylmelamine were equal to those in plasma. There is also some evidence of saturable N-demethylation in patients given high doses of the parenteral formulation (Ames et al 1990).

Ames (1979) described preliminary drug metabolism in animals and found extensive hepatic microsomal drug metabolism. These animal data confirm that the demethylated derivatives of altretamine predominate. In murine studies, Morimoto et al (1979) were unable to detect intact drug in the liver, brain, or small intestine 1 hour after ingestion. Unexpectedly, the major difference between altretamine and pentamethylmelamine in this study was a threefold greater brain concentration of the more water-soluble metabolite, pentamethylmelamine.

■ Side Effects and Toxicity

Three main types of altretamine toxicity have been noted. Gastrointestinal toxicity is usually dose limiting and manifests as anorexia, nausea, vomiting, diarrhea, and abdominal cramps (Wilson et al 1970). It is often severe in patients receiving doses of 12

ALTRETAMINE PHARMACOKINETICS

	Mean Pharmacokinetic Parameters						
Formulation	Peak Plasma Level [µg/mL (Dose)]	Time to Peak	Half-life (min) α	β	γ	Total Body Clearance (L/min/m^2)	Volume of Distribution (L/m^2)
IV*	10 (540 mg/m^2)	0–5 min	11	109	622	0.72	460
Caps†	15 (12 mg/kg) 6 (9 mg/kg) ≅ 5 (6 mg/kg)	2–3 h	—	~480	—	—	—
Caps‡	0.2–20.8 (120–200 mg/m^2) 0.13–2.66 (pentamethylmelamine)	0.5–4 h (1–4 h)	—	180–600	—	—	—

*Ames et al 1990.
†Bryan et al 1968.
‡D'Incalci et al 1979.

mg/kg/d, but it occurs less frequently at a dose of 8 mg/kg/d. Some tolerance to this effect has been noted. Neurotoxicity with altretamine involves various peripheral neuropathies which are predominantly sensory and characterized by loss of deep tendon reflexes, ataxia, and paresthesia. Central nervous system effects include agitation, confusion, hallucinations, depression, and parkinsonian-like symptoms. Petit mal-type seizures have rarely been described. The neurologic symptoms are usually reversible with discontinuation of therapy and are more common with continuous daily dosing for longer than 3 months compared with intermittent pulse-dosing regimens. Of interest, neurotoxicity was not observed in patients treated with the parenteral formulation (Ames et al 1990).

Hematologic toxicity is generally mild and may be related to cumulative dose and/or duration of on therapy. It consists of leukopenia and thrombocytopenia with typical respective nadirs of 3 to 4 weeks after a 14-day regimen. Recovery is usually rapid, occurring within 1 week after drug discontinuation.

There have been rare reports of alopecia, cystitis, and an eczematous condition. A drug-related skin rash with or without pruritus is also reported. There are also rare elevations in alkaline phosphatase, blood urea nitrogen, and/or serum creatinine (Manetta et al 1990).

REFERENCES

Alberts DS, Hilgers RD, Moon TE, et al. Combination chemotherapy for alkylator-resistant ovarian carcinoma: A preliminary report of a Southwest Oncology Group trial. *Cancer Treat Rep.* 1979;**63**(7):151–155.

Ames MW. Pharmacologic studies of pentamethylmelamine and hexamethylmelamine. *Proc Am Assoc Cancer Res ASCO.* 1979;**20**(abstract 636):158.

Ames MM, Kovach JS. Parenteral formulation of hexamethylmelamine potentially suitable for use in man. *Cancer Treat Rep.* 1982;**66**:1579–1581.

Ames MM, Richardson RL, Kovach JS, et al. Phase I and clinical pharmacological evaluation of a parenteral hexamethylmelamine formulation. *Cancer Res.* 1990;**50**:206–210.

Ames MM, Sanders ME, Tiede WS. Metabolic activation of hexamethylmelamine and pentamethylmelamine by liver microsomal preparations. *Life Sci.* 1981;**29**:1591–1598.

Ames MM, Sanders ME, Tiede WS. Role of N-methylolpentamethylmelamine in the metabolic activation of hexamethylmelamine. *Cancer Res.* 1983;**43**:500–504.

Bergevin PR, Tormey DC, Blom J. Clinical evaluation of hexamethylmelamine (NSC-13875). *Cancer Chemother Rep.* 1973;**57**:51–58.

Blum RH, Livingston RB, Carter SK. Hexamethylmelamine—A new drug with activity in solid tumors. *Eur J Cancer.* 1973;**9**:195–200.

Bruckner HW, Cohen CJ, Feuer E, Holland JF. Modulation and intensification of a cyclophosphamide, hexamethylmelamine, doxorubicin, and cisplatin ovarian cancer regimen. *Obstet Gynecol* 1989;**73**:349–356.

Bryan GT, Worzalla JF, Gorski AL, Ramirez G. Plasma levels and urinary excretion of hexamethylmelamine following oral administration to human subjects with cancer. *Clin Pharmacol Ther.* 1968;**9**:777–782.

Chaninian A, Chamberlain KB, Holland JF. A new four drug combination in advanced lung cancer (LC). *Proc Am Assoc Cancer Res ASCO.* 1979;**20**(abstract C-607):437.

De La Garza JG, Carr DT, Bisel HF. Hexamethylmelamine (NSC-13875) in the treatment of primary cancer of the lung with metastasis. *Cancer.* 1968;**22**:571–575.

Denefrio JM, Vogel CL. Phase II study of hexamethylmelamine in women with advanced breast cancer refractory to standard cytotoxic therapy. *Cancer Treat Rep.* 1978;**62**(1):173–175.

D'Incalci MD, Bolis G, Mangioni C, et al. Variable oral absorption of hexamethylmelamine in man. *Cancer Treat Rep.* 1978;**62**(12):2117–2119.

D'Incalci MD, Sessa C, Belloni C, et al. Hexamethylmelamine (HMM) and pentamethylmelamine (PMM) levels in plasma and ascites after oral administration to ovarian cancer patients. *Proc Am Assoc Cancer Res ASCO.* 1979;**20**(abstract 185):46.

Dyment PG, Fernback DJ, Sutow WW. Hexamethylmelamine (NSC-18375) for acute leukemia and solid tumors in children. *J Clin Pharmacol.* 1973;**15**:111–113.

Ettinger DS, Mehta CR, Abeloff MD. et al. Maintenance chemotherapy versus no maintenance chemotherapy in complete responders following induction chemotherapy in extensive disease smallcell lung cancer. *Proc Amer Soc Clin Oncol.* 1987;**6**:175.

Gescher A, D'Incalci M, Fanelli R, Farina P. N-Hydroxymethylpentamethylmelamine, a major in vitro metabolite of hexamethylmelamine. *Life Sci.* 1980;**26**:147–154.

Gordon IL, Kar R, Opfell RW, Wile AG. Pharmacokinetics of hexamethylmelamine in intralipid following hepatic regional administration in rabbits. *Cancer Res.* 1988;**48**:5070–5073.

Hainsworth JD, Jones HW, Burnett LS, Johnson DH, Greco FA. The role of hexamethylmelamine in the combination chemotherapy of advanced ovarian cancer: A comparison of hexamethylmelamine, cyclophosphamide, doxorubicin and cisplatin (H-CAP) versus cyclophosphamide, doxorubicin and cisplatin (CAP). *Am J Clin Oncol.* 1990;**13**:410–415.

Hande K, Combs G, Swingle R, et al. Effect of cimetidine and ranitidine on the metabolism and toxicity of hexamethylmelamine. *Cancer Treat Rep.* 1986;**70**:1443–1445.

Heere LJ, Donnelly ST. Antitumor activity of hexamethylmelamine and imidazole carboxamide. *Proc Am Assoc Cancer Res.* 1971;**12**:101.

Johnson BL, Fisher RI, Bender RA, et al. Hexamethylmelamine in alkylating agent-resistant ovarian carcinoma. *Cancer.* 1978;**42**:2157–2161.

Kane R, Andrews T, Bernath A, et al. Phase II trial of cyclophosphamide, hexamethylmelamine, Adriamycin and *cis*-platinum therapy (CHAP) in advanced ovarian carcinoma. *Proc Am Assoc Cancer Res ASCO.* 1979;**20**(abstract C-53):329.

Lawson DH, Moore MR, Smalley RV. An evaluation of hexamethylmelamine, *cis*-dichloroplatinum and mitomycin-C in advanced breast cancer. *Proc Am Assoc Cancer Res ASCO.* 1979;**20**(abstract C-322):369.

Legha SS, Slavik M, Carter SK. Hexamethylmelamine—An evaluation of its role in the therapy of cancer. *Cancer.* 1976;**38**(1):27–35.

Leite C. Hexamethylmelamine (HEX) with or without pyridoxine (PYR) in refractory breast cancer. *Proc Am Assoc Cancer Res ASCO.* 1978;**19**(abstract C-341):392.

Louis J, Louis NB, Linman JW, et al. The clinical pharmacology of hexamethylmelamine—Phase I study. *Clin Pharmacol Ther.* 1967;**8**:55–64.

Manetta A, MacNeill C, Lyter JA, et al. Hexamethylmelamine as a single second-line agent in ovarian cancer. *Gynecol. Oncol.* 1990;**36**:93–96.

Morimoto M, Schein PS, Engle R. Comparative pharmacology of pentamethylmelamine (PMM) and hexamethylmelamine (HMM) in mice. *Proc Am Assoc Cancer Res ASCO.* 1979;**20**(abstract 980):220.

Rosen GF, Lurain JR, Newton M. Hexamethylmelamine in ovarian cancer after failure of cisplatin-based multiple agent chemotherapy. *Gynecol Oncol.* 1987;**27**:173–179.

Rutty CJ, Abel G. In vitro cytotoxicity of the methylmelamines. *Chem–Biol Interact.* 1980;**29**:235–246.

Schultz MJ, Armentrout SA, Slater LM, Bateman JR. Adriamycin/hexamethylmelamine (ArmA) vs. CCNU, vincristine, cytoxan, bleomycin (ArmB) in advanced oat cell, epidermoid and anaplastic (NOS) lung cancer. *Proc Am Assoc Cancer Res ASCO.* 1979;**20**(abstract C-565):427.

Stolinsky DC, Bateman JR. Further experience with hexamethylmelamine (NSC-13875) in the treatment of carcinoma of the cervix. *Cancer Chemother Rep.* 1973;**57**:497–499.

Stolinsky DC, Bogdon DL, Solomon J, Bateman JR. Hexamethylmelamine (NSC-13875) alone and in combination with 5-(3,3-dimethyl-triazeno)imidazole-4-carboxamide (NSC-45388) in the treatment of advanced cancer. *Cancer.* 1972;**30**:654–659.

Takita H, Didolkar MS. Effects of hexamethylmelamine (NSC-13875) on small cell carcinoma of the lung (phase II study). *Cancer Chemother Rep.* 1974;**58**:371–374.

Venditti JM. Relevance of transplantable animal tumor systems to the selection of new agents for clinical trial. In: Goldin A, Venditti JM (eds). *Pharmacological Basis of Cancer Chemotherapy.* Baltimore: Williams & Wilkins; 1975:245–270.

Vogl SE, Berenzweig M, Kaplan BH, et al. The CHAD and HAD regimens in advanced ovarian cancer combination chemotherapy including cyclophosphamide, hexamethylmetamine, Adriamycin and *cis*-dichlorodiammineplatinum(II). *Cancer Treat Rep.* 1979;**63**:311–317.

Wampler GL, Mallette SJ, Kumperming M, Regelson W. Hexamethylmelamine (NSC-13875) in the treatment of advanced cancer. *Cancer Chemother Rep.* 1972;**56**:505–514.

Wilson WL, Bisel HF, Cole D, et al. Prolonged low-dosage administration of hexamethylmelamine (NSC-13875). *Cancer.* 1970;**25**:568–570.

Worzalla JE, Kaiman BD, Johnson BM, et al. Metabolism of hexamethylmelamine-ring-^{14}C in rats and man. *Cancer Res.* 1974;**34**:2669–2674.

Young RC, Chabner BC, Hubbard SP, et al. Advanced ovarian adenocarcinoma: A prospective clinical trial of melphalan (L-PAM) vs. combination chemotherapy. *N Engl J Med.* 1978;**299**(23):1261–1266.

Aminoglutethimide

■ Other Names

Cytadren; Elipten; BA-16038 (Ciba-Geigy); Orimeten.

■ Chemistry

Structure of aminoglutethimide

Aminoglutethimide (AG) is a nonsteroidal inhibitor of corticosteroid biosynthesis. The complete chemical name is 3-(4-aminophenyl)-3-ethyl-2,6-piperidinedione. It is a simple chemical derivative of the sedative glutethimide (Doriden®, Doriden-Sed,® Elrodorm®). The commercial product is supplied as the racemic mixture of D- and L-stereoisomers which have different pharmacologic potencies (Brodie and Santen 1986). The D-isomer is 30 times more potent at inhibiting aromatase activity, whereas the L-isomer is more potent at inhibiting cholesterol side-chain cleavage (see Mechanism of Action). The molecular weight of AG is 232.28, and the melting point, 149 to 150°C. It is soluble in most organic solvents but is only slightly soluble in water. Thus, AG is lipophilic with a log P value of −0.23, indicating preferential partitioning into lipid over water.

Antitumor Activity

Aminoglutethimide is an antihormonal agent that metabolically blocks corticosteroid production. When combined with hydrocortisone, AG produces a "medical adrenalectomy." It is therefore used to provide symptomatic palliation in Cushing's disease, in hormonally responsive breast cancer (Lipton and Santen 1974), and in prostate carcinoma (Sanford et al 1976). Newsome et al (1977) observed a 50% response rate in 18 postmenopausal patients with metastatic breast cancer. Similarly, Santen et al (1977a) observed a 38% response rate in 50 patients with widely metastatic disease. Smith et al (1978) reported a similar response rate of 37.5% in postmenopausal patients with advanced metastatic breast cancer. Responses to AG are usually greatest in breast cancer patients who have previously responded to other hormonal manipulations, particularly in patients who are estrogen receptor positive (Horsley et al 1982, Santen et al 1982) in which response rates of up to 50% have occurred (Santen 1981, Santen et al 1982). Importantly, responses are observed in both soft tissue (47%) and in bone (35%), with durations of 30 and 14 months for complete and partial responders, respectively (Santen et al 1982). Local breast cancer recurrence is also significantly reduced by AG (Coombes et al 1987). Responses are less frequently observed in visceral metastases including those in lung (11%) and liver (7%) (Asbury et al 1981). A low response rate of 16% is reported in patients failing all conventional therapies (Crivellari et al 1989).

Low-dose AG without steroid replacement is less effective and potentially hazardous in breast cancer patients (Murray and Pitt 1985). Similarly, the addition of AG to tamoxifen does not increase response rates (Milsted et al 1985). Conversely, AG appears to be as active as high-dose medroxyprogesterone acetate (Amen,® Depo-Provera,® Provera®) in advanced breast cancer (Canney et al 1988). Aminoglutethimide is also active in up to 63% of patients relapsing after initially responding to tamoxifen (Santen 1981).

In prostate cancer, AG plus hydrocortisone has been combined with cytotoxic chemotherapy to produce high initial objective response rates of about 35% (Manni et al 1988); however, median response durations are relatively short at 10 months and there is only a minimal impact on survival in prostate cancer. One explanation for the limited efficacy of AG in prostate cancer is that adrenal steroid levels are not completely suppressed and may actually rise in up to one third of orchiectomized patients given AG plus hydrocortisone (Ahmann et al 1987). Nonetheless, subjective improvements, primarily in bone pain, may be observed in up to 48% of prostate patients failing other treatments (Ponder et al 1984).

Mechanism of Action

Aminoglutethimide was originally introduced as an anticonvulsant but it was found to cause adrenal insufficiency (Hughes and Burley 1970). This serendipitous finding stimulated research into its use to block adrenal steroidogenesis. Aminoglutethimide binds to cytochrome P450 enzymes, interfering with the conversion of cholesterol to Δ^5-pregnenolone by inhibiting aromatase enzymes in adrenal mitochondria and in peripheral (nonhormonal) tissues. This ultimately blocks the biosynthesis of all corticosteroid hormones (glucocorticosteroids, estrogens, and androgens). Aminoglutethimide also interferes with cytochrome P450-mediated hydroxylation in the adrenal gland. This includes reactions mediated by 21-hydroxylase, 11β-hydroxylase, and 18-hydroxylase activities (Harris et al 1983). Aminoglutethimide additionally blocks the conversion of androgens to estrogens (Camacho et al 1967). In essence, AG causes a reversible chemical adrenalectomy (Santen et al 1974).

The failure of the adrenals to biosynthesize 11-hydroxycorticosteroids following AG causes a large release of adrenocorticotropin from the pituitary. This can overcome the steroidal blockade unless a pituitary-suppressive glucocorticoid is concurrently administered. Hydrocortisone or dexamethasone has been used for this purpose; however, because aminoglutethimide increases the metabolic clearance of dexamethasone, adrenal escape may occur after 3 to 7 days (Santen et al 1974). In contrast, hydrocortisone metabolism is unaffected by AG. The hydrocortisone–aminoglutethimide regimen is therefore preferred (Santen et al 1977a, b). Typical hydrocortisone doses range from 20 to 50 mg/d.

During AG treatment in women, plasma estrone and estradiol levels fall to 45 and 62% of basal levels, respectively. Pituitary gonadotropin levels do not change but thyroid-stimulating hormone levels may double as a result of inhibition of thyroxine synthesis by AG. Aldosterone biosynthesis is also reduced by AG but mineralocorticoid replacement is not always necessary. In premenopausal women, AG does not lower estrogen levels, which indicates that ovarian aromatase enzymes are insensitive to AG (Santen et al 1980). In orchiectomized men, steroidogenesis is variably reduced by AG–hydrocortisone combinations. Consequently, dehydroepiandrostenedione sulfate, androstenedione, and testosterone levels are reduced by 87, 52, and 49%, respectively (Ahmann et al 1987, Plowman et al 1987). Testosterone levels may, however, rise in some patients following AG, thereby limiting clinical efficacy of the drug in prostate cancer (see Antitumor Activity).

■ Availability and Storage

Aminoglutethimide is investigationally available in 250-mg tablets that may be stored at room temperature.

■ Administration

The tablets may be administered orally. Nausea and vomiting are usually not problematic with this drug. Most doses are given in divided fractions, two to three times per day.

■ Special Precautions

More than 60% of patients treated with aminoglutethimide will initially manifest an allergic response, usually a rash. This typically resolves with dosage reduction and does not generally require drug discontinuance. Also, about 20 to 50% of patients treated with aminoglutethimide will require mineralocorticoid replacement. This may be managed with fludrocortisone (Florinef®) 0.1 mg daily or three times per week.

■ Dosage

In adults, the dose range for adrenal suppression is 750 to 1500 mg/d given in divided oral doses. The upper dosing limit according to the manufacturer is 2.0 g/d; however, Griffiths et al (1973) reported using daily doses up to 2.5 g. Dexamethasone (2–5 mg/d) or hydrocortisone (20–40 mg/d) is also required to produce effective adrenal suppression (eg, in the treatment of metastatic breast cancer). Santen et al (1977a, b) have documented that a daily regimen of 1000 mg aminoglutethimide and 40 to 60 mg hydrocortisone produces greater hormone suppression compared with the equivalent doses of aminoglutethimide combined with dexamethasone.

Low-dose AG (250 mg/d) without hydrocortisone is ineffective in women with advanced breast cancer (Murray and Pitt 1985); however, the combination of 500 mg AG plus 50 mg hydrocortisone has been demonstrated to possess activity in patients with metastatic breast cancer (Crivellari et al 1989).

■ Drug Interactions

Aminoglutethimide can alter the metabolism of a number of other drugs. It is known to induce its own metabolism and that of some glucocorticosteroids, including dexamethasone and medroxyprogesterone acetate (Van Deijk et al 1985). Hydrocortisone is unaffected. Other highly metabolized drugs may also be effected by AG, resulting in increased clearance rates (see table below). These include warfarin (Lonning et al 1986), antipyrine, theophylline, and digitoxin (Lonning et al 1984).

The mechanism by which AG stimulates the metabolism of other drugs is unclear, as AG is known to bind selectively to the cytochrome P450 enzymes involved in oxidative drug metabolism. For the corticosteroids, steady-state plasma levels can decrease by 50% after treatment with AG is initiated (Van Deijk et al 1985). Aminoglutethimide also reduces the steady-state plasma levels of tamoxifen and its primary active metabolites, including N-desmethyltamoxifen (Lien et al 1990). The clearance rate of tamoxifen clearance was increased over threefold, from 189 to 608 mL/min. Conversely, tamoxifen did not alter the pharmacokinetics of AG (Lien et al 1990). AG also suppresses plasma prostaglandin $F_{1\alpha}$ and $F_{2\alpha}$ levels in breast cancer patients (Harris et al 1983).

■ Pharmacokinetics

Aminoglutethimide exhibits a mono- or biphasic elimination pattern. The mean elimination half-life was reported to be 13.3 hours using a spectrophotometric assay (Murray et al 1979) and 15.5 hours using a radioimmunoassay (Lonning et al 1985). These half-lives decrease by 40 to 50% to 7 to 9 hours during chronic AG dosing for several months. This suggests that AG induces its own metabolism; however, AG clearance was only slightly increased during chronic therapy in another trial.

DRUGS WHOSE CLEARANCE IS INCREASED BY AMINOGLUTETHIMIDE

Class	Individual Drug	Reference
Corticosteroids	Medroxyprogesterone	Van Deijk et al 1985
	Dexamethasone	Santen et al 1977a
Antiestrogens	Tamoxifen	Lien et al 1990
Miscellaneous	Warfarin	Lonning et al 1986
	Theophylline	Lonning et al 1984
	Digitoxin	

CLINICAL PHARMACOKINETICS OF AMINOGLUTETHIMIDE AND ITS PRIMARY METABOLITE

	Volume of Distribution (L)	Total Body Clearance (L/h)	Half-life (h)	% Urinary Excretion
Aminoglutethimide				
Initial therapy	76	3.49	15.5	40–50%
Chronic therapy	53	4.42	8.9	
N-Acetylaminoglutethimide				
Initial therapy	NR*	NR	15.3	20–50%
Chronic therapy	NR	NR	9.6	

*Not reported.
Data from Lonning PE, Schanche JS, Kvinnsland S, Ueland PM. Single-dose and steady-state pharmacokinetics of aminoglutethimide. Clin Pharmacokinet. 1985;10:353–364.

This was due to a simultaneous and proportional decrease in the volume of distribution from 76 to 53 L (Lonning et al 1985). Plasma protein binding of AG is minimal at 21 to 25% and is not dose dependent (Thompson et al 1981). The drug is concentrated about 1.4 to 1.7 times in cells compared with plasma. Two 250-mg tablets taken orally produce peak plasma concentrations of 5.6 to 6.3 µg/mL with 0.7 to 1.5 hours after ingestion. This dose produced a mean AUC_{0-} of 97 ± 7 µg·h/mL (Thompson et al 1981). A dose of 1 g/d yields plasma levels of 9 µg/mL on day 7 and 6 to 7 µg/mL after 1 month of therapy (Miller et al 1987). Biphasic drug elimination with an apparent α half-life of about 2 to 3 hours and a β half-life of about 13 hours was observed (Thompson et al 1981). The half-lives are similar to those described in breast cancer patients by Miller et al (1987). Clearance averaged 5.5 L/h in this trial but plasma levels of aminoglutethimide did not correlate with clinical response (Miller et al 1987). (See the table above.)

There is some suggestion of dose-dependent renal elimination of AG with increased urinary recovery observed after a 500-mg dose (54%) compared with a 250-mg dose (39%) (Douglas and Nichols 1965). Actual renal clearance rates in two subjects given 500 mg of drug orally were 30 and 38 mL/min (Thompson et al 1981).

Aminoglutethimide undergoes significant metabolism to N-acetylaminoglutethimide (NAG) (Douglas and Nichols 1972). Up to 50% of a dose may be excreted as NAG which has only 20% of the hormone inhibitory activity of AG (Brodie and Santen 1986). Patients with a rapid acetylator phenotype will form larger amounts of NAG and therefore probably require higher AG doses than patients who slowly acetylate the drug (Adam et al 1984). Of interest, NAG formation decreased with chronic dosing in one study (Jarman et al 1983). The half-life of NAG apparently is the same as for aminoglutethimide, about 7 to 10 hours (Miller et al 1987). Other AG metabolites recovered from the urine include N-formylaminoglutethimide and nitroglutethimide (Baker et al 1981) and hydroxylaminoglutethimide (Jarman et al 1983). Minor urinary metabolites include p-amino-5-hydroxyglutethimide, p-amino-1'-hydroxyglutethimide, and lactone from p-amino-2'-hydroxyglutethimide (Foster et al 1984). All of the urinary metabolites except NAG are inactive.

A preclinical study with AG in rats shows that the drug readily penetrates the blood–brain barrier (Unger et al 1986). Following intravenous drug injection of AG dissolved in olive oil, the cerebrospinal fluid/blood levels were 0.53 at 10 minutes and 0.26 at 60 minutes. Thus, AG achieves nearly equal distribution into central nervous system tissues as into the plasma. This clearly results from the drug's low molecular weight, high lipophilicity, and low degree of protein binding.

■ Side Effects and Toxicity

About 50% of the patients treated with aminoglutethimide will experience an adverse reaction. Skin reactions are most common and are typified by a morbilliform maculopapular rash, which is usually observed within the first week of treatment in about one third of patients. It is usually self-limiting and disappears after 5 to 8 days. If the rash does not clear within this period, the drug should be discontinued. Santen (1981) also recommend an initial hydrocortisone dose of 100 mg/d for 2 weeks to help control acute dermatologic reactions. The second most common acute toxic effect, however, is lethargy which is usually transient but may be quite severe in individual patients (Wells et al 1978). Smith et al (1978) reported that somnolence was initially severe and was greatest in elderly patients, many of whom also described visual blurring and dizziness as well as a feeling of "walking on air."

Hematologic reactions including leukopenia and agranulocytosis are rare. Lawrence et al (1978) have additionally reported a single nonfatal case of aminoglutethimide-induced pancytopenia complicated by gram-negative septicemia and bleeding. An immunologic mechanism was felt to be responsible for the reaction. There was rapid resolution of the pancytopenia following drug discontinuance. Thrombocytopenia is reported in only 0.37% of patients and leukopenia in less than 1% of patients (Young et al 1984). Pancytopenia has been rarely described in 0.37% of 1345 patients as reviewed by Young et al (1984); however, deaths from agranulocytosis are described with AG (Coombes et al 1987).

Thyroid complications, including hypothyroidism with the development of a goiter, have been reported in several children treated with AG for seizure disorders (Rallison et al 1967) and in some breast cancer patients. Other hormonal alterations include a consistent decrease in aldosterone secretion, leading to postural hypotension and hyponatremia, and a drug-induced addisonian condition (Fishman et al 1968). Virilization, probably as a result of malfunctions in peripheral aromatization, has also been seen (Cash et al 1969). Other drug-induced effects include mild nausea, vomiting, and anorexia. Facial flushing and periorbital edema have also been observed. Neurologic side effects include mild vertigo, nystagmus, and ataxia. These effects generally abate with slight dosage reduction (Lipton and Santen 1974).

REFERENCES

Adam AM, Rogers MJ, Smiel SA, et al. The effect of acetylator phenotype on the disposition of aminoglutethimide. *Br J Clin Pharmacol.* 1984;**18**:495–505.

Ahmann FR, Crawford ED, Kreis W, et al. Adrenal steroid levels in castrated men with prostatic carcinoma treated with aminoglutethimide plus hydrocortisone. *Cancer Res.* 1987;**47**:4736–4739.

Asbury RF, Bakemeier RF, Folsch E, et al. Treatment of metastatic breast cancer with aminoglutethimide. *Cancer.* 1981;**47**:1954–1958.

Baker MH, Foster AB, Harland SJ, et al. Metabolism of aminoglutethimide in humans: Formation of N-formylaminoglutethimide and nitroglutethimide. *Br J Pharmacol.* 1981;**74**:243P–244P.

Brodie AM, Santen RJ. Aromatase in breast cancer and the role of aminoglutethimide and other aromatase inhibitors. *CRC Crit Rev Hematol Oncol.* 1986;**5**:361–396.

Camacho AM, Cash R, Brough AJ, Wilroy RS. Inhibition of adrenal steroidogenesis by amino-glutethimide and the mechanism of action. *JAMA.* 1967;**202**:20.

Canney PA, Priestman TJ, Griffiths T, et al. Randomized trial comparing aminoglutethimide with high-dose medroxyprogesterone acetate in therapy for advanced breast carcinoma. *J Natl Cancer Inst.* 1988;**80**:1147–1151.

Cash R, Petrini MA, Brough AJ. Ovarian dysfunction associated with an anticonvulsant drug. *JAMA.* 1969;**208**:1149.

Coombes RC, Powles TJ, Easton D, et al. Adjuvant aminoglutethimide therapy for postmenopausal patients with primary breast cancer. *Cancer Res.* 1987;**47**:2496–2499.

Crivellari D, Galligioni E, Frustaci S, et al. Low-dose aminoglutethimide plus steroid replacement in advanced breast cancer patients resistant to conventional therapies. *Cancer Invest.* 1989;**7**(2):113–116.

Douglas JS, Nichols PJ. The urinary excretion of aminoglutethimide in man. *J Pharm Pharmacol.* 1965;**17**(suppl):115S–117S.

Douglas JS, Nichols PJ. The partial fate of aminoglutethimide in man. *J Pharm Pharmacol.* 1972;**17**:150P.

Fishman LM, Liddle GW, Island DP, et al. Effects of amino-glutethimide on adrenal function in man. *J Clin Endocrinol Metab.* 1968;**27**:481–490.

Foster AB, Griggs LJ, Howe I, et al. Metabolism of aminoglutethimide in humans. Identification of four new urinary metabolites. *Drug Metab Dispos.* 1984;**12**:511–516.

Griffiths CT, Hall TC, Saba Z, et al. Preliminary trial of aminoglutethimide in breast cancer. *Cancer.* 1973;**32**(1):31–37.

Harris AL, Mitchell MD, Smith IE, Powles TJ. Suppression of plasma 6-keto-prostaglandin $F_{1\alpha}$ and 13,14-dihydro-15-keto-prostaglandin $F_{2\alpha}$ by aminoglutethimide in advanced breast cancer. *Br J Cancer.* 1983;**48**:595–598.

Horsley JS III, Newsome HH, Brown PW, et al. Medical adrenalectomy in patients with advanced breast cancer. *Cancer.* 1982;**49**:1145–1149.

Hughes SW, Burley DM. Amino-glutethimide: A "side-effect" turned to therapeutic advantage. *Postgrad Med J.* 1970;**46**:409–416.

Jarman M, Foster AB, Goss PE, et al. Metabolism of aminoglutethimide in humans: Identification of hydroxyglutethimide as an induced metabolite. *Biomed Mass Spectrom.* 1983;**10**:620–625.

Lawrence B, Santen RJ, Lipton A, et al. Pancytopenia induced by aminoglutethimide in the treatment of breast cancer. *Cancer Treat Rep.* 1978;**62**:1581–1583.

Lien EA, Anker G, Lonning PE, et al. Decreased serum concentrations of tamoxifen and its metabolites induced by aminoglutethimide. *Cancer Res.* 1990;**50**:5851–5857.

Lipton A, Santen RJ. Medical adrenalectomy using aminoglutethimide and dexamethasone in advanced breast cancer. *Cancer*. 1974;**33**:503–512.

Lonning PE, Kvinnsland S, Bakke OM. Effect of aminoglutethimide on antipyrine, theophylline, and digitoxin disposition in breast cancer. *Clin Pharmacol Ther*. 1984;**36**:796–802.

Lonning PE, Schanche JS, Kvinnsland S, Ueland PM. Single-dose and steady-state pharmacokinetics of aminoglutethimide. *Clin Pharmacokinet*. 1985;**10**:353–364.

Lonning PE, Ueland PM, Kvinnsland S. The influence of a graded dose schedule of aminoglutethimide on the disposition of the optical enantiomers of warfarin in patients with breast cancer. *Cancer Chemother Pharmacol*. 1986;**17**:177–181.

Manni A, Bartholomew M, Caplan R, et al. Androgen priming and chemotherapy in advanced prostate cancer: Evaluation of determinants of clinical outcome. *J Clin Oncol*. 1988;**6**:1456–1466.

Miller AA, Miller BE, Hoffken K, Schmidt CG. Clinical pharmacology of aminoglutethimide in patients with metastatic breast cancer. *Cancer Chemother Pharmacol*. 1987;**20**:337–341.

Milsted R, Habeshaw T, Kaye S, et al. A randomised trial of tamoxifen versus tamoxifen with aminoglutethimide in post-menopausal women with advanced breast cancer. *Cancer Chemother Pharmacol*. 1985;**14**:272–273.

Murray FT, Santner S, Samojlik E, Santer RJ. Serum aminoglutethimide levels: Studies of serum half-life clearance and patient compliance. *J Clin Pharmacol*. 1979;**19**:704–711.

Murray R, Pitt P. Low-dose aminoglutethimide without steroid replacement in the treatment of postmenopausal women with advanced breast cancer. *Eur J Cancer Clin Oncol*. 1985;**21**(1):19–22.

Newsome HH, Brown PW, Terz JJ, Lawrence W. Medical and surgical adrenalectomy in patients with advanced breast carcinoma. *Cancer*. 1977;**39**:542–546.

Plowman PN, Perry LA, Chard T. Androgen suppression by hydrocortisone without aminoglutethimide in orchiectomised men with prostatic cancer. *Br J Urol*. 1987;**59**:255–257.

Ponder BAJ, Shearer RJ, Pocock RD, et al. Response to aminoglutethimide and cortisone acetate in advanced prostatic cancer. *Br J Cancer*. 1984;**50**:757–763.

Rallison ML, Kumagae LF, Tyler FH. Goitrous hypothyroidism induced by amino-glutethimide, anti-convulsant drug. *J Clin Endocrinol Metab*. 1967;**27**:265–269.

Sanford EJ, Drago JR, Rohner TJ, et al. Amino-glutethimide medical adrenalectomy for advanced prostatic carcinoma. *J Urol*. 1976;**115**:170–174.

Santen RJ. Suppression of estrogens with aminoglutethimide and hydrocortisone (medical adrenalectomy) as treatment of advanced breast carcinoma: A review. *Breast Cancer Res Treat*. 1981;**1**:183–202.

Santen RJ, Lipton A, Kendall J. Successful medical adrenalectomy with aminoglutethimide. Role of altered drug metabolism. *JAMA*. 1974;**230**:1661–1665.

Santen RJ, Samojlik E, Lipton E, et al. Kinetic, hormonal and clinical studies with aminoglutethimide in breast cancer. *Cancer*. 1977a;**39**(6 suppl):2948–2958.

Santen RJ, Samojlik E, Wells SA. Resistance of the ovary to blockade of aromatization with aminoglutethimide. *J Clin Endocrinol Metab*. 1980;**51**:473–477.

Santen RJ, Wells SA, Runic S, et al. Adrenal suppression with aminoglutethimide. I. Differential effects of aminoglutethimide on glucocorticoid metabolism as a rationale for use of hydrocortisone. *J Clin Endocrinol Metab*. 1977b;**45**:469–479.

Santen RJ, Worgul TJ, Lipton A, et al. Aminoglutethimide as treatment of postmenopausal women with advanced breast carcnoma. *Ann Intern Med*. 1982;**96**:94–101.

Smith IE, Fitzharris BM, McKinna JA, Fahmy DR, Nash AG, Neville AM, et al. Aminoglutethimide in treatment of metastatic breast carcinoma. *Lancet* 1978;**2**:646–649.

Thompson TA, Vermeulen JD, Wagner WE Jr, Le Sher AR. Aminoglutethimide bioavailability, pharmacokinetics, and binding to blood constituents. *J Pharm Sci*. 1981;**70**(9):1040–1043.

Unger C, Eibl H, von Heyden H-W, et al. Aminoglutethimide. Penetration of the blood brain barrier. *Invest New Drugs*. 1986;**4**:237–240.

Van Deijk WA, Blijham GH, Mellink WAM, et al. Influence of aminoglutethimide on plasma levels of medroxyprogesterone acetate: Its correlation with serum cortisol. *Cancer Treat Rep*. 1985;**69**:85–90.

Wells SA, Santen RJ, Lipton A, et al. Medical adrenalectomy with aminoglutethimide. *Ann Surg*. 1978;**187**(3):475–484.

Young JA, Newcomer LN, Keller AM. Aminoglutethimide-induce bone marrow injury: Report of a case and review of the literature. *Cancer*. 1984;**54**:1731–1733.

Amonafide

■ Other Names

Nafidamide; NSC-308847; 5-amino-2-[2-(dimethylamine)ethyl]-1H-benz[de-]isoquinoline-1,3-(2*H*)-dione.

■ Chemistry

Structure of amonafide

Amonafide is a synthetic organic compound that possesses both potent antiviral and cytotoxic activity (Brana et al 1978, 1980, 1981, Gancedo et al 1982). The drug has the formula $C_{16}H_{17}N_3O_2$ and a molecular weight of 283.33.

■ Antitumor Activity

In phase I trials of amonafide, responses were noted in patients with non-small cell lung cancer and prostate cancer (Saez et al, 1989).

The drug has been found to have some antitumor activity in patients with hormone-refractory prostate cancer (Craig and Crawford 1989). The drug has not had activity in other prostate cancer studies (Shevrin et al 1991) and is inactive in patients with sarcoma (Perez et al 1992).

Amonafide has had a response rate of 23% in women with no previous chemotherapy for metastatic breast cancer (Costanza et al 1990). In phase II studies of amonafide in women who have failed one or two regimens for breast cancer, a daily dose for 5 days of 300 mg/m² every 21 days induced a response in 3 of 10 patients with no prior doxorubicin and 0 of 12 patients with prior doxorubicin (Allen et al 1991b). Similar results have been reported by Scheithauer et al (1991).

No responses have been noted in patients with previously untreated extensive small cell lung cancer (Evans et al 1990).

Amonafide has been found to be inactive in patients with previously untreated pancreatic cancer (Linke et al 1991) and in patients with previously untreated non-small cell lung cancer (Kreis et al 1989), malignant melanoma (Slavik et al 1991), and renal cell carcinoma (Higano et al 1989).

■ Mechanism of Action

Amonafide has been identified as an intercalating agent (Waring et al 1979) as well as an inhibitor of topoisomerase II (Andersson et al 1987).

■ Availability and Storage

Amonafide is supplied as an investigational agent by the National Cancer Institute as a sterile 100-mg (prepared as a yellow to orange or red-orange) lyophilized powder with hydrochloric acid to adjust pH in 5-mL vials.

The intact vials should be stored under refrigeration (2–8°C).

■ Preparation for Use, Stability, and Admixture

The 100-mg vial is reconstituted with 4 mL of Sterile Water for Injection, USP, or 0.9% Sodium Chloride Injection, USP, which results in a solution containing 25 mg/mL amonafide with hydrochloric acid to adjust to pH 5 to 7. The reconstituted solution may vary in color from yellow to red-orange or red.

Shelf-life surveillance of the intact vials is ongoing. Amonafide is stable in aqueous phosphate-buffered solutions over the pH range 5.4 to 9.4, exhibiting little or no decomposition over 8 hours at 90°C. At lower pH values, however, increased rates of decomposition occur.

When reconstituted as directed with Sterile Water for Injection, USP, or 0.9% Sodium Chloride Injection, USP, amonafide solutions exhibit no decomposition over 14 days at room temperature or under refrigeration. Further dilution to a concentration of 0.25 mg/mL in 0.9% Sodium Chloride Injection, USP, results in a solution that exhibits no decomposition over 14 days of storage at room temperature or under refrigeration.

Amonafide is very unstable in dextrose-containing solutions. Approximately 25 to 35% decomposition occurs over 24 hours at room temperature in 5% Dextrose Injection, USP, 5% Dextrose in 0.9% Sodium Chloride Injection, USP, and 5% Dextrose in 0.45% Sodium Chloride Injection, USP. The dextrose content may be catalyzing the degradation.

CAUTION: The single-dose lyophilized dosage form contains no antibacterial preservatives. Therefore, it is advised that the reconstituted product be discarded 8 hours after initial entry.

■ Administration

The optimal dose and schedule for administration of amonafide have not yet been determined. The Dosage section outlines the dosage and schedule studied in phase I trials. One of the most common schedules being used in phase II trials is 300 to 400 mg/m² daily × 5 given as a 60-minute infusion.

■ Special Precautions

Rapid infusions (over < 1 hour) are associated with dizziness, tinnitus, headaches, diaphoresis, and flushing.

■ Drug Interactions

None have been reported to date.

Dosage

The following phase I trials (see table below) have been performed to obtain the optimal dose and schedule.

Pharmacokinetics

The table on page 178 summarizes the pharmacokinetic parameters of amonafide.

As noted in the table plasma levels decline in a biexponential manner (Saez et al 1989). Less than 5% of the total dose of amonafide is excreted in the urine (Saez et al 1989). Other investigators have reported that up to 23% is excreted in the urine (Felder et al 1987).

N-Acetylamonafide is major metabolite of amonafide in plasma and urine (Felder et al 1988). There is some evidence that amonafide is metabolized via acetylation and that there may be many genetic variations of the acetylating enzyme responsible for the predominant metabolism of amonafide (Kreis et al 1991).

N-Acetylation phenotypes (using sulfapyridine) can be used to predict the ability of a patient to N-acetylate amonafide (Grever et al 1990). The toxicity of amonafide is correlated with acetylator phenotype, with a rapid acetylator being at greater risk for severe toxicity (myelosuppression) (Ratain et al 1990, 1991). Felder et al (1987) have described up to eight urinary metabolites of amonafide. Some are cytotoxic.

Ratain et al (1988) have developed a limiting sampling model approach (two timed plasma concentrations) to facilitate population pharmacodynamic studies in ongoing phase II studies with amonafide.

Side Effects and Toxicity

The usual dose-limiting toxic effect of amonafide has been granulocytopenia (Saez et al 1989, Hochster et al 1990, Allen et al 1991a).

Other toxic effects have included infusion-rate related diaphoresis, flushing, dizziness, tinnitus, and headache (Legha et al 1987, Saez et al 1989, Hochster et al 1990) and mild nausea and vomiting (Legha et al 1987). Irritation at the infection site has also been reported (Scheithauer et al 1991, Allen et al 1991).

In a phase I study in patients with leukemia, dose-limiting toxic effects included mucositis and a painful skin erythema (O'Brian et al 1991). A transient orange discoloration of the skin was also noted in that study.

Correlations between decreases in leukemia blasts induced by amonafide and increases in levels of polyamines have been noted by Benvenuto and Nishioka (1991).

Special Applications

None have been reported to date.

PHASE I STUDIES OF AMONAFIDE

Schedule	Dose Range (mg/m^2)	Dose-Limiting Toxic Effect	Recommended Phase II Dose (mg/m^2)	Reference
Once every 28 days over 30–120 minutes	18–1104	Granulocytopenia	918	Saez et al 1989
Weekly × 4 over 1 hour, rest 1 week, every 35 days	200–540	Granulocytopenia	—	Hochster et al 1990
Daily × 2 every 21 days over 1–2 hours	300–800	Myelosuppression	800	Allen et al 1991a
Daily × 2 every 21 days over 1 hour	300–900	Not reached	—	Puccio et al 1991
Daily × 5 over 2–4 hours	600–1800	Mucositis + painful skin erythema	1100–1400	O'Brian et al 1991*
Daily × 5 over 30–60 minutes	10–625	Myelosuppression	400 good risk 300–320 poor risk	Legha et al 1987
Bolus	18.4–1125	Leukopemia	—	Leiby et al 1988
Daily × 5	7.6–288.1	Leukopemia	220	
24-hour continuous IV infusion every 4 weeks	6.1–720	Not reached	—	Richardson et al 1987

*Leukemia patients.

PHARMACOKINETICS OF AMONAFIDE

Schedule	Peak Plasma Level	Half-life (h) α	Half-life (h) β	AUC (μg · h/mL)	Total Body Clearance (L/h/m^2)	Volume of Distribution (L/m^2) Central	Volume of Distribution (L/m^2) Steady State	Reference
Once every 28 days over 30–120 minutes	0.5–4.40	0.66 ± 0.8	5.5 ± 3.9	0.29–16.67	84.5 ± 30.5	231.2 ± 60.8	531.5 ± 268.9	Saez et al 1989
Daily × 5 over 2.4 hours	—	—	4.6	—	—	—	—	O'Brian et al 1991
Daily × 5 30-minute infusion	—	—	3.5	—	—	—	—	Felder et al 1987

REFERENCES

Allen SL, Fusco D, Budman D, et al. Phase I trial of amonafide (AM) given IV daily × 2. *Proc Am Soc Clin Oncol.* 1991a;**10**:110.

Allen SL, Ratain M, Korzun AH, et al. Phase II study of amonafide in previously treated metastatic breast cancer (CALGB 8841). *Proc Am Assoc Cancer Res.* 1991b;**32**:183.

Andersson BS, Beran M, Bakic M, Silberman LE, Newman RA, Zwelling LA. In vitro toxicity and DNA cleaving capacity of benzisoquinolinedine (nafidimide; NSC-308847) in human leukemia. *Cancer Res.* 1987;**47**(4):1040–1044.

Benvenuto JA, Nishioka K. The correlation of response with plasma pharmacokinetics and polyamines in patients with AML receiving amonafide (AMF). *Proc Am Assoc Cancer Res.* 1991;**32**:177.

Brana MF, Castellano JM, Jimeniz A, et al. Synthesis, cytostatic activity and mode of action of a new series of imide derivatives of 3-nitro-1,8, naphthalic acid. *Curr Chemother* (Proc 10th Int Congr Chemother 1977). 1978;**2**:1216–1217.

Brana MF, Castellano JM, Roldan CM, Santos A, Vazquez D, Jimenez A. Synthesis and mode(s) of action of a new series of imide derivatives of 3-nitro-1,8-naphthalic acid. *Cancer Chemother Pharmacol.* 1980;**4**:61–66.

Brana MF, Sanz AM, Castellano JM, Roldan CM, Roldan C. Synthesis and cytostatic activity of benz(de)-isoquinolin-1,3, diones. Structure–activity relationships. *Eur J Med Chem–Chim Ther.* 1981;**16**:207–212.

Costanza ME, Korzun AH, Henderson IC, Rice MA, Wood WC, Norton L. Amonafide: An active agent in metastatic breast cancer (CALGB 8642) (meeting abstract). *Proc Am Soc Clin Oncol.* 1990;**9**:31.

Craig J, Crawford E. Phase II trial of amonafide in advanced prostate cancer: A Southwest Oncology Group study (meeting abstract). *Proc Am Soc Clin Oncol.* 1989;**8**:147.

Evans WK, Eisenhauer EA, Cormier Y, et al. Phase II study of amonafide: Results of treatment and lessons learned from the study of an investigational agent in previously untreated patients with extensive small-cell lung cancer (comment). *J Clin Oncol.* 1990;**8**(3):374–377.

Felder TB, Benvenuto JA, Andersson BS, Newman RA. Disposition of amonafide in adults with acute leukemia (meeting abstract). *Proc Am Assoc Cancer Res.* 1988;**29**:278.

Felder TB, McLean MA, Vestal ML, et al. Pharmacokinetics and metabolism of the antitumor drug amonafide (NSC-308847) in humans. *Drug Metab Dispos.* 1987;**15**(6):773–778.

Gancedo AG, Gil-Fernandez C, Vilas P, et al. Imide derivatives of 3-nitro-1,8-naphthalic acid: Their inhibitory activity against DNA viruses. *Arch Virol.* 1982;**74**:157–165.

Grever MR, Staubus AE, Malspeis L. Correlation of N-acetylation phenotype with plasma levels of the N-acetyl metabolite of amonafide (NSC-308847). *Proc Am Assoc Cancer Res.* 1990;**31**:178.

Higano CB, Craig J, Goodman P, Blumenstein B, Wettlaufer J, Crawford E. A phase I trial of amonafide in advanced renal cell carcinoma (meeting abstract). *Proc Am Soc Clin Oncol.* 1989;**8**:147.

Hochster H, Oratz R, Wernz J, et al. Weekly amonafide: Phase I study of a novel schedule. *Proc Am Soc Clin Oncol.* 1990;**9**:69.

Kreis W, Budman DR, Lesser M, et al. Acetylation-phenotype in 43 patients treated with continuous 1 hr IV infusion of amonafide. *Proc Am Assoc Cancer Res.* 1991;**32**:179.

Kris MG, Gralla RJ, Berger MZ, et al. Phase II trial of amonafide in patients with advanced non-small cell lung cancer (meeting abstract). *Proc Am Assoc Cancer Res.* 1989;**30**:270.

Legha SS, Ring S, Raber M, Felder TB, Newman RA, Krakoff IH. Phase I clinical investigation of benzisoquinolinedine. *Cancer Treat Rep.* 1987;**71**(12):1165–1169.

Leiby JM, Malspeis L, Straubus AE, Kraut EH, Grever MR. Amonafide (NSC-308847): A clinical phase I study of two schedules of administration (meeting abstract). *Proc Am Assoc Cancer Res.* 1988;**29**:278.

Linke K, Pazdur R, Ajani J, et al. Phase II trial of amonafide in advanced pancreatic carcinoma. *Proc Am Soc Oncol.* 1991;**10**:146.

O'Brian S, Benvenuto JA, Estey E, Beran M, Felder TB, Keating M. Phase I clinical investigation of benzisoquinolinedione (amonafide) in adults with refractory or relapsed acute leukemia. *Cancer Res.* 1991;**51**(3):935–938.

Perez RP, Nash SL, Ozols RF, et al. Phase II study of amonafide in advanced and recurrent sarcoma patients. *Invest New Drugs.* 1992;**10**:99–101.

Puccio C, Mittelman A, Ahmed T, et al. Phase I trial and pharmacokinetics of amonafide. *Proc Am Soc Clin Oncol.* 1991;**10**:112.

Ratain MJ, Mick R, Berezin F, et al. Prospective correlation of acetylator phenotype with amonafide toxicity. *Proc Am Soc Clin Oncol.* 1991;**10**:101.

Ratain MJ, Propert K, Costanza M, et al. Population pharmacodynamic study of amonafide: CALGB 8862. *Proc Am Assoc Cancer Res.* 1990;**31**:181.

Ratain MJ, Staubus AE, Schilsky RL, Malspeis L. Limited sampling models for amonafide (NSC-308847) pharmacokinetics. *Cancer Res.* 1988;**48**(14):4127–4130.

Richardson RL, Schutt AJ, O'Connell MJ, Creagan ET, Loprinzi CL, Powis G. Phase I study of amonafide (A) (NSC-308847) given by 24 hour continuous intravenous infusion (24H-CIV) every 4 weeks (meeting abstract). *Proc Am Soc Clin Oncol.* 1987;**6**:35.

Saez R, Craig JB, Kuhn JG, et al. Phase I clinical investigation of amonafide. *J Clin Oncol.* 1989;**7**(9):1351–1358.

Scheithauer W, Dittrich C, Kornek G, Linkesch W, Haider K, Depisch D. A phase II trial of amonafide in metastatic breast cancer. *Proc Am Soc Clin Oncol.* 1991;**10**:66.

Shevrin D, Khandekar J, Kilton L, et al. Amonafide in advanced hormone-resistant prostate cancer (HRPC): An Illinois Cancer Council phase II study. *Proc Am Soc Clin Oncol.* 1991;**10**:180.

Slavik M, Kopecky K, Craig J, Sondak V, Samson M. Evaluation of amonafide in disseminated malignant melanoma. *Proc Am Soc Clin Oncol.* 1991;**10**:292.

Waring MJ, Gonzalez A, Jimenez A, Vazquez D. Intercalative binding of DNA of antitumor drugs derived from 3-nitro-1,8-naphthalic acid. *Nucleic Acids Res.* 1979; **7**:217–230.

Ampligen

■ Other Names

Mismatched double-stranded RNA; $rI_n \cdot r(C_{12}, U)_n$.

■ Chemistry

Ampligen belongs to a unique category of agents, the double-stranded (ds) RNAs. In Ampligen, uridine is substituted at intervals of one uridine for every 12 cytidines in the polycytidylic acid chain. This modification makes the dsRNA more susceptible to degradation by hydrolytic enzymes (Levy 1987, Strayer et al 1981). The first dsRNAs, polyinosinic–polycytidylic acid (poly I, C) and poly (I, CL), a complex between poly-L-lysine and poly(I, C), which were developed as antiviral/antitumor agents, had substantial toxic effects, including fever, severe allergic reactions, liver dysfunction, antibody formation, bone marrow suppression, and hypotension (Robinson et al 1976, Freeman et al 1977, Krown et al 1983, Levy and Riley 1984). Ampligen, designated $rI_n \cdot r(C_{12}, U)_n$, is a mismatched dsRNA that purportedly retains its ability to induce interferon while being less toxic is preclinical systems (Carter et al 1985a, 1976). The compound is prepared by a method detailed by Carter et al in 1972. The compound was designed to work as an interferon inducer. To provide for less toxicity, it was felt that if alterations were made in the normal double-helix structure of RNA, there would be more rapid clearance of the drug (Carter et al 1985b).

■ Antitumor and Antihuman Immunodeficiency Activity

There are no reports of formal phase II studies with this agent. In phase I and phase I–II trials an occasional response has been noted, including complete responses in patients with renal cell cancer (Brodsky et al 1985) and adenocarcinoma of the lung and melanoma (Strayer et al 1986a, 1987b). Some minor activity in a patient with multiple myeloma has also been reported (Strayer et al 1981); however, on the basis of available evidence there is as yet no indication that the agent is useful in patients with cancer.

Montefiori and Mitchell (1987) found that Ampligen protected cells from human immunodeficiency (HIV) infection but had no effect on cell division, RNA and protein synthesis, or viral replication. Carter and colleagues (1987a) have reported on 10 HIV-positive patients with acquired immunodeficiency syndrome (AIDS), AIDS-related complex (ARC), or lymphadenopathy syndrome (LAS) who were given 200 to 250 mg of Ampligen twice a week without side effects. The patients had a decrease in HIV level, an augmentation of delayed-type hypersensitivity skin reactions, and a rise in titer of neutralizing antibodies against HIV. Of note, one patient cleared a chronic oral candida infection. This experience was updated 1 year later. Of 25 patients treated with 100 to 200 mg of Ampligen, 83% showed an improvement in delayed-type hypersensitivity. Mean p24 levels decreased by 28% in the patients. Patients reported improvement in diarrhea, night sweats, and fatigue. Patients also had a decrease in lymphadenopathy. No Ampligen-related lymphadenopathy was noted.

With the aforementioned activity it is likely ampligen will continue to be tested in patients with HIV infections. Of additional interest is the finding that Ampligen is synergistic with zidovudine (azidothymine [AZT]) in in vitro HIV systems (Mitchell et al 1987).

In preclinical systems, the compound has been found active against human tumor colony-forming units growing in vitro (particularly gliomas, renal cell carcinomas, and carcinoids), as well as human tumor cell lines (Carter et al 1985a, b, Hubbell et al 1984, Strayer et al 1986b, 1987a) and renal cell carcinomas and bladder cancer growing in nude mice (Carter et al 1985a, b, Hubbell et al 1985). It has been found more active than $rI_n \cdot rC_n$ against a small cell lung cancer line growing in vitro (Carter et al 1985a).

Finally, Ampligen has been found to be synergistic with some types of interferon beta as well as interferon alfa in in vitro preclinical systems (Carter et al 1985a, Hubbell 1985, Rosenblum and Gutterman 1985, Strayer et al 1985).

Mechanism of Action

In general, dsRNAs are thought to be inducers of interferons and lymphokines and stimulators of immune surveillance and also to possess a direct inhibitory effect on tumor cell growth (Carter and DeClerq 1974). Several lines of evidence suggest Ampligen may work through mechanism(s) in addition to induction of interferon (Carter et al 1985a). In patients receiving Ampligen there are significant increases in natural killer lymphocyte activity as well as 2', 5'-oligoadenylate synthetase, an antiviral protein that produces polyadenylate strands from ATP (Brodsky et al 1985).

Availability and Storage

This agent is available from HEM Pharmaceutical Corporation, Rockville, Maryland. It is supplied in vials as a frozen solution containing 200, 400, or 700 mg.

Preparation for Use, Stability, and Admixture

No published information is available.

Administration

The schedule used in published studies is a twice weekly intravenous dose ranging from 10 to 300 mg (Carter et al 1987, Brodsky et al 1985).

Special Precautions

None have been reported at this time.

Drug Interactions

None have been reported at this time.

Dosage

As noted under Administration, doses of Ampligen range from 10 to 300 mg intravenously twice per week. A recommended dose for patients has not yet been consistently reported. HIV patients have received 200 to 250 mg twice per week. This appears to be the most commonly used dose (Carter et al 1987).

Pharmacokinetics

Only limited data are available on the pharmacokinetics of Ampligen. Krueger and colleagues (1985) have used a modification of the Quickblot® technique of nucleic acid immobilization and hybridization to determine serum levels of the agent. In their limited report (an abstract), they reported detectable Ampligen at least 2 hours after drug infusion with an estimated half-life of 15 to 90 minutes. A second report estimated the half-life at 53 minutes (Krueger et al 1986). No specific data were given on serum levels.

Side Effects and Toxicity

Brodsky and colleagues (1985) have summarized the clinical studies with ampligen in patients with malignancies. The doses have ranged from 10 to 300 mg twice weekly (Strayer et al 1986). Low-grade transient fever (< 100.5°F) as well as occasional fatigue and flulike symptoms (Strayer et al 1981) were noted. No Ampligen-induced changes in hematologic, hepatic, or renal function parameters have been reported. No antibody formation has been reported in patients receiving up to 14 months of Ampligen, with cumulative doses ranging over 4 g. On the basis of these data, it is unclear whether the doses of the agent have been pushed high enough.

Special Applications

See preceding sections for use of Ampligen in patients with HIV infections.

REFERENCES

Brodsky I, Strayer DR, Krueger LJ, Carter WA. Clinical studies with ampligen (mismatched double-stranded RNA). *J Biol Resp Mod.* 1985;**4**:669–675.

Carter WA, Brodsky I, Pellegrino MG, et al. Clinical immunological and virological effects of ampligen, a mismatched double-stranded RNA, in patients with AIDS or AIDs-related complex. *Lancet.* 1987;**1**:1286–1292.

Carter WA, DeClerq E. Viral infection—Host defense. *Science.* 1974;**186**:1172–1178.

Carter WA, Hubbell HR, Krueger LJ, Strayer DR. Comparative studies of ampligen (mismatched double-stranded RNA) and interferons. *J Biol Resp Mod.* 1985a;**4**:613–620.

Carter WA, O'Malley J, Beeson M, et al. An integrated and comparative study of the antiviral effects and other biological properties of the $rI_n \cdot rC_n$ duplex and its mismatched analogs. III. Chronic effects, immunologic features. *Mol Pharmacol.* 1976;**12**:440–453.

Carter WA, Pitha PM, Marshall LW, Tazawa I, Tazwa S, Ts'o P. Structural requirements of the $rI_n \cdot rC_n$ complex for induction of human interferon. *J Mol Biol.* 1972b;**70**:567–587.

Carter WA, Strayer DR, Hubbell HR, Brodsky I. Preclinical studies with ampligen (mismatched double-stranded RNA). *J Biol Resp Mod.* 1985b;**4**:495–502.

Freeman AI, Al-Bussam N, O'Malley J, Stutzman L, Bjornsjon S, Carter WA. Pharmacologic effects of poly I·C in man. *J Med Virol.* 1977;**1**:79–93.

Hubbell HR. Synergistic antiproliferative effect of human interferons in combination with mismatched double-stranded RNA (ampligen) on human tumor cell. *Proc Am Assoc Cancer Res.* 1985;**26**:277.

Hubbell HR, Kualines-Krick K, Carter WA, Strayer DR. Antiproliferative and immunomodulatory actions of interferon β and double-stranded RNA, individually and in combination, in human bladder tumor xenografts in nude mice. *Cancer Res.* 1985;**45**:2481–2486.

Hubbell HR, Lui R-S, Maxwell BL. Independent sensitivity of human tumor cell lines to interferon and double stranded RNA. *Cancer Res.* 1984;**44**:3252–3257.

Krown SE, Fruden BG, Khonsur T, Davies ME, Oettgen HF, Field AK. Phase I trial with the interferon induces poly I:C/poly-L-lysine (poly ICL). *J Interferon Res.* 1983;**3**:281–290.

Krueger LJ, Andryuk PJ, Burigin MJ. Nucleic and hybridization in plasma: Method for quantitation of poly(I). Poly(C_{12}, U) in plasma of cancer patients. *J Biol Resp Mod.* 1986;**5**:539–547.

Krueger LJ, Strayer DS, Andryuk PJ, Kieffer GL, Carter WA. Pharmacokinetic analysis of dsRNA therapy in cancer: Measurement of ampligen levels. *Proc Am Soc Clin Oncol.* 1985;**4**:221.

Levy HB. Clinical studies with polynucleotides. The interferon system. A current review to 1987. In: Baron S, et al, eds. *The University of Texas Medical Branch Series in Biomedical Science.* Austin: University of Texas Press; 1987;469–475.

Levy HB, Riley FL. Utilization of stabilized forms of polynucleotides. In: Came PE, Carter WA, eds. *Handbook of Experimental Pharmacology.* Berlin: Springer-Verlag, 1984:515–533.

Mitchell WM, Montefiori DC, Robinson WE, Strayer DR, Carter WA. Mismatched double-stranded RNA (ampligen) reduces concentrations of zidovudine (azidothymidine) required for in vitro inhibition of human immunodeficiency virus. *Lancet.* 1987;**1**:890–892.

Montefiori DC, Mitchell WM. Antiviral activity of mismatched double-stranded RNA against human immunodeficiency virus in vitro. *Proc Natl Acad Sci USA.* 1987;**84**:2985–2989.

Robinson RA, Devita VT, Levy HB, Baron S, Hubbard SP, Levine AS. A phase I–II trial of multiple-dose polyriboinosinic–polyribocytidylic acid in patients with leukemia or solid tumors. *J Natl Cancer Inst.* 1976;**57**:599–602.

Rosenblum M, Gutterman J. Human leukocyte interferon (IFN) and mismatched double-stranded RNA (dsRNA): Synergistic antiproliferative activity in vitro. *Proc Am Assoc Cancer Res.* 1985;**26**:280.

Strayer DR, Carter WA, Brodsky I, Gillespie DH, Greene JT, Ts'o P. Clinical studies with mismatched double-stranded RNA. *Tex Rep Biol Med.* 1981;**41**:663–671.

Strayer DR, Carter WA, Crilley P, Novak S, Brodsky I. Complete clinical responses in solid tumor patients without side effects or toxicity using mismatched double-stranded RNA (ampligen). *Proc Am Soc Clin Oncol.* 1987b;**6**:240.

Strayer DR, Carter WA, Crilley P, Pologruto DG, Brodsky I. Phase I study of mismatched double-stranded RNA (ampligen). *Proc Am Assoc Cancer Res.* 1986a;**27**:209.

Strayer DR, Watson P, Carter WA, Brodsky I. Antiproliferative effect of mismatched double-stranded RNA on fresh human tumor cells analyzed in a clonogenic assay. *J Interferon Res.* 1986b;**6**:373–379.

Strayer DR, Watson P, Weisbaud J, Carter WA. Synergistic antitumor effects of interferon α and mismatched double-stranded RNA (ampligen) in human renal cell carcinoma. *Proc Am Assoc Cancer Res.* 1985;**26**:367.

Strayer DR, Weisbaud J, Carter WA, Black P, Nidzgorski F, Cook A. Growth of astrocytomas in the human tumor clonogenic assay and sensitivity to mismatched dsRNA and interferons. *Am J Clin Oncol.* 1987a;**4**:281–284.

Amsacrine

■ Other Names

Acridinylanisidide. AMSA; *m*-AMSA; Amsidine® (Parke-Davis); NSC-141549; NSC-249992.

■ Chemistry

Structure of amsacrine

Amsacrine is a derivative of the acridine dye class. Its chemical name is *N*-[4-(9-acridinylamino)-3-methoxyphenyl]methanesulfonamide. It is one of a number of acridine derivatives with antitumor activity that were synthesized by Cain and colleagues in 1974 (Cain and Atwell 1974, Cain et al 1974). The compound has three coplanar rings and is structurally similar to the tricyclic antidepressant drug imipramine. It has an empiric formula of $C_{21}H_{19}N_3O_3S$ with a molecular weight of 394 for the base, 429.9 for the hydrochloride salt, and 466.0 for the hydrated ($2H_2O$) hydrochloride salt. The melting point of the bright yellow crystals is 189 to 200°C, and the molecule is more soluble in organic solvents than in water (0.3 mg/mL). Solubility in ethanol is 2.3 mg/mL; in dimethylformamide, 29 mg/mL; and in dimethylsulfoxide, 60 mg/mL. The bulk powder is very stable, with no decomposition noted after 30 days at 60°C.

■ Antitumor Activity

Amsacrine has been noted to have significant antitumor activity in a wide range of transplantable animal tumor systems: Lewis lung, mouse mammary, and colon cancers; L-1210 leukemia; B-16 melanoma; P-388 leukemia (Cain et al 1974). Most notably, clinical responses have been observed in refractory acute nonlymphocytic leukemia (ANLL), advanced ovarian carcinoma, and lymphomas (see table).

The drug is active in a variety of pediatric malignancies including ANLL and acute lymphocytic leukemias (ALL) (Hutter and Meyskens 1982, Goldman and Malpas 1982). The drug is also occasionally active in neuroblastoma (Civin et al 1982), but it has been inactive in various pediatric sarcomas (Goldman and Malpas 1982). In adults, major activity has been seen in refractory ANLL with response rates up to 23% (Legha et al 1982). When combined with high-dose cytarabine in refractory ANLL patients, significantly greater toxicity was observed without enhanced antitumor activity. These studies have called into question the role of amsacrine, if any, in refractory acute leukemia.

Response rates of 25 to 42% have been described in refractory ALL (Arlin et al 1980, Weil et al 1982). Occasional responses are noted in chronic myelogenous leukemia in blast crisis (Omura et al 1983). Common drug combinations that have demonstrated activity in leukemia include amsacrine

CLINICAL ANTITUMOR ACTIVITY OF AMSACRINE*

Tumor Type	Overall Response Rate (CR + PR %)	Other Drugs	Reference
Adult leukemias			
Acute myeloblastic leukemia	17	None	Louie and Issell 1985
	70	Cytarabine	Hines et al 1983
	50	Azacytidine	Kahn et al 1983
	25	Cytarabine, vincristine, prednisone	McCredie et al 1981
Acute lymphocytic leukemia	17	None	Louie and Issell 1985
	46	Cytarabine	Weil et al 1982
	11	Cytarabine, vincristine, prednisone	McCredie et al 1981
Pediatric leukemias			
ALL	15	None	Louie and Issell 1985
ANLL	35	None	Louie and Issell 1985
Adult lymphomas			
Hodgkin's	20		
Non-Hodgkin's	35		
Adult solid tumors			
Lung cancer (SCLC, NSCLC)*	<10	None	Louie and Issell 1985
Breast cancer	<10	None	Louie and Issell 1985
Melanoma	<10	None	Louie and Issell 1985
Colon, pancreas, gastric	< 5	None	Louie and Issell 1985
Ovary, cervix, endometrial	15–25	None	Louie and Issell 1985
Head and neck cancer		None	Louie and Issell 1985
Pediatric solid tumors			
Neuroblastoma	< 5		Goldman and Malpas 1982
Soft tissue sarcomas			Civin et al 1982
Osteogenic sarcoma			

*SCLC and NSCLC, small cell and non-small cell lung cancer.

plus either cytarabine (Hines et al 1983), azacitidine (Kahn et al 1983), or cytarabine, vincristine, and prednisone (McCredie et al 1981). Amsacrine is also active in about 20% of adults with Hodgkin's or non-Hodgkin's lymphomas (Weick et al 1983).

Very low (<15%) response rates have been reported in adult solid tumors including breast cancer (Legha et al 1979); large cell and small cell lung cancer; melanoma; colorectal, pancreatic, and gastric cancer; and various gynecologic neoplasms including ovarian, cervical, and endometrial carcinoma (reviewed in Louie and Issell 1985). From experimental models, amsacrine also possesses antiviral (Byrd 1977) and immunosuppressive activities (Baguley et al 1974).

■ Mechanism of Action

In 1933 Mellanby noted that acridine and similar dye derivatives had slight antibacterial and antiviral properties (Mellanby 1933). Later, Ledochowski and Cain evaluated several synthetic derivatives of acridine, of which amsacrine appeared most active (Cain et al 1974).

Amsacrine is known to intercalate between DNA base pairs, resulting in the inhibition of DNA synthesis (Waring 1976). The binding to DNA is tight, and the anilino side chain is believed to provide additional electrostatic bonding in the minor groove of DNA (Denny et al 1983). The primary binding is, however, intercalative with complex dissociation kinetics (Denny and Wakelin 1986).

As with other DNA intercalators, amsacrine induces protein-linked DNA strand breaks (Zwelling et al 1981). This activity is believed to result from the stabilization of a cleavable complex between subunits of the enzyme topoisomerase II and the 5' terminus of a broken DNA strand (Nelson et al 1984). Amsacrine produces a higher incidence of DNA single-strand breaks than does doxorubicin and this activity is dependent on topoisomerase II levels in the G_2 phase of the cell cycle. Cytotoxicity is tenfold greater in cycling versus noncycling human tumor cells, and the drug may cause cell cycle arrest in G_2 phase (Drewinko et al 1982). Of interest, the O-amsacrine isomer is inactive as an anticancer agent although it does intercalate into DNA (Zwelling et al 1981).

■ Availability and Storage

Amsacrine is investigationally available from the National Cancer Institute. It is supplied in a Duopack®, containing two sterile liquids that are aseptically mixed before use: (1) 1.5 mL of 50 mg/mL drug in anhydrous N,N-dimethylacetamide (in a 2-mL glass ampule) and (2) 13.5 mL of 0.0353 M L-lactic acid diluent in a 20-mL amber vial. Both vials should be stored under refrigeration (National Cancer Institute 1978) and are stable for at least 1 year.

Two other investigational formulations were previously available: 1) AMSA-gluconate (Warner-Lambert, Morris Plains, NJ) and 2) AMSA-lactate alone, without N,N-dimethylacetamide (Bristol-Myers Oncology Division, Evansville, IN) (Louie and Issell 1985). The latter preparation was available in 50- and 100-mg vials, which were reconstituted to a concentration of 2 mg/mL with 25 to 50 mL of Sterile Water for Injection, USP, or 5% dextrose. Saline cannot be used for dilution of amsacrine formulations; the drug can even precipitate when in contact with saline-washed glassware or administration sets (Engelking et al 1984).

■ Preparation for Use, Stability, and Admixture

The solution for injection is prepared by aseptically adding the drug solution to the lactic acid diluent. This results in a 10% (v/v) combined solution (5 mg/ml amsacrine in 0.0318 M L-lactic acid). The concentrated solvent N,N-dimethylacetamide can degrade certain plastic components and the use of glass syringes for reconstitution is recommended (National Cancer Institute 1978). It is stable at room temperature and under normal light conditions for at least 48 hours; however, use of this solution within 8 hours of mixing is recommended as no bacteriostatic agent is included.

The combined solution (amsacrine plus N,N-dimethylacetamide solvent) is not stable with any chloride-containing solutions because of the poor aqueous solubility of hydrochloride salt. Careful flushing of tubing should be used to remove any saline prior to amsacrine administration (Kuehnle and Moore 1979). Admixtures in 5% dextrose, however, are chemically stable for at least 48 hours at room temperature and light conditions. Caution is urged to prevent direct exposure of skin or mucous membranes to amsacrine powder or solution.

■ Administration

Amsacrine should be administered as a slow intravenous infusion over several hours. For phase I–II trials, the dose has been diluted into 500 mL of 5% dextrose and cautiously infused over several hours. Close monitoring of the infusion is required and venous patency should be ensured before administration.

Amsacrine has been given orally to mice (Cysyk et al 1978) and to humans in investigational studies (DeJager et al 1979, 1980); however, the oral route is not indicated because of incomplete and variable bioavailability.

■ Special Precautions

Acute ventricular arrhythmias have been reported in adults and children receiving amsacrine. The propensity for life-threatening ventricular arrhythmias is believed to be enhanced by rapid infusion of highly concentrated solutions and by administration to hypokalemic patients (Riela et al 1981). Serum potassium levels should be checked and corrected if low (<2.5 mEq/mL) prior to drug administration (Steinherz et al 1982). A minimal infusion volume of 500 mL is also recommended to reduce phlebitis (Von Hoff et al 1978).

■ Dosage

Preliminary phase I trials in patients with leukemia and solid tumors have confirmed that the maximally tolerated dose is 120 mg/m^2 injected as a single dose over 120 minutes or 40 mg/m^2/d as a 60 to 120-minute infusion for 3 consecutive days repeated at 4-week intervals (Legha et al 1978). Although leukopenia may be severe at doses above 70 mg/m^2, dose escalation up to 160 mg/m^2 was accomplished in selected patients. Phase I studies in leukemia have suggested a need for doses up to 75 to 90 mg/m^2/d for 5 consecutive days (Goldsmith et al 1980). Generally, maximal antileukemic effects are usually not observed until a total (cumulative) dose of 500 mg/m^2 is administered (Legha et al 1982).

For poor-risk patients a single dose of 50 mg/m^2 every 14 days for three doses or 90 mg/m^2 every 3 weeks was recommended in a phase I clinical trial in patients with solid tumors and Hodgkin's disease (Van Echo et al 1979). For good-risk patients, a dose of 70 mg/m^2 every 14 days or 120 mg/m^2 every 3 weeks was recommended.

Dose Adjustment in Hepatic/Renal Dysfunction. Patients with impaired liver function may experience increased myelosuppression and therefore their doses should be reduced (Legha et al 1978). It is known that patients with hepatic and/or renal dysfunction who received full doses of amsacrine have experienced severe myelosuppression and stomatitis (Mahla et al 1981, Hall et al 1983). In patients with hepatobiliary dysfunction manifested by a serum bilirubin above 2 mg/dL, a 25% amsacrine dose reduction is recommended (Mahla et al 1981). A 30 to 40% dose reduction is recommended for patients with renal and/or hepatic dysfunction manifested by a serum blood urea nitrogen greater than 20 mg/dL or serum creatinine greater than 1.5 mg/dL (Hall et al 1983).

■ Drug Interactions

Heating tumor cells prior to amsacrine exposure reduces experimental drug-induced DNA damage and is not recommended (Kampinga et al 1989). Conversely, amsacrine blocks the cytotoxicity of the antibiotic novobiocin, presumably by altering the activity of DNA topoisomerase II (Utsumi et al 1990). The polyamine synthesis inhibitor eflornithine (α-DFMO) significantly enhances DNA strand scission by amsacrine (Zwelling et al 1985).

Experimental metabolic interactions include a decrease in amsacrine clearance by cimetidine or L-buthionine sulfoximine and an increase by phenobarbital in the rabbit (Paxton et al 1986). Doxorubicin, nafcillin, and warfarin also appear to increase the biliary excretion of amsacrine in experimental rat models (Mitchell et al 1982).

■ Pharmacokinetics

Pharmacokinetic studies using 9-^{14}C-radiolabeled amsacrine have reported a mean terminal half-life (of radiolabel) of 46 hours in cancer patients with metastatic malignancies (Hall et al 1983). The plasma half-life of unchanged amsacrine was 7.4 and 17.2 hours in patients with normal and reduced renal function, respectively. Cumulative 72-hour urinary excretion of radiolabel averaged 35% of a dose (12% intact drug) in patients with normal hepatorenal function, and 49% of a dose (20% intact drug) in patients with hepatic dysfunction. Patients with renal insufficiency excreted only 2 to 16% of a dose, with only 2% of the dose excreted unchanged in the urine.

In a pharmacokinetic study using fluorescent drug detection, a biphasic disposition pattern was detected. The initial (distributive) half-life was 10 to 15 minutes with a second, terminal disposition half-life of 8 to 9 hours for total fluorescent species and

3 hours for unchanged amsacrine (Van Echo et al 1979). A similar biphasic disposition pattern was observed in leukemic patients monitored using a specific high-performance liquid chromatographic assay procedure (Paul et al 1987). In this trial the terminal half-life was 6.3 to 7.1 hours with a mean volume of distribution of about 100 L/m². Clearance averaged about 12 L/m²/h with an AUC of 6-10 µg/mL·h following a dose of 75 mg/m²/d × 7 days (Paul et al 1987).

Drug disposition and metabolism studies after intravenous and oral dosing have been done with ^{14}C-labeled amsacrine in animals. Cysyk et al (1977) demonstrated drug localization in the liver, mainly as metabolites. There also appeared to be rapid drug elimination into the bile: more than 50% by 2 hours. With therapeutic doses, however, the biliary transport system appeared saturable (Shoemaker et al 1980).

The major metabolites produced were alkyl-thiol derivatives of acridine. Nonenzymatic attack at the number 9 carbon by endogenous thiols appears to account for 90 to 95% of drug metabolism. The main metabolic product can then be eliminated in urine and bile. The small fraction interacting with protein-thiols facilitates prolonged retention of the acridine moiety. Amsacrine does not significantly penetrate into the central nervous system (Hall et al 1983). Amsacrine levels in the cerebrospinal fluid were only 2% of the simultaneous plasma level. The primary biliary metabolite appears to be a glutathione conjugate with amsacrine at the 5'-position in the anilino ring (Shoemaker et al 1980, 1982).

Importantly, microsomal activation of the drug results in enhanced formation of protein-linked DNA lesions (Gorsky and Morin 1990). This means that amsacrine metabolites may contribute significantly to the inhibitory effects on topoisomerase II. These metabolites may thereby contribute to antitumor cytotoxic effects.

■ Side Effects and Toxicity

Hematologic toxicity appears to be the dose-limiting effect of amsacrine (Von Hoff et al 1978). Significant leukopenia is common with doses over 70 mg/m², the nadir occurring within 10 days and recovery by day 25. Amsacrine appears to be relatively platelet sparing, and thrombocytopenia below 100,000/mm³ is unusual.

Phlebitis is common and dilution in 500 mL D5W is recommended although this may not entirely prevent vein irritation. Serum alkaline phosphatase levels are commonly elevated by the drug, and the urine will characteristically appear orange after drug administration. Increased serum bilirubin has also been observed and appears to be the result of cholestasis rather than direct hepatocellular toxicity. Drug extravasation into subcutaneous tissues is anticipated to produce severe soft tissue ulcers based on animal skin toxicity studies (Henry et al 1976).

Other less common adverse effects of amsacrine include nausea and vomiting which occur in about 16% of patients (Legha et al 1978). Skin rashes are also occasionally described but typically resolve rapidly after treatment is discontinued (Henry et al 1976).

Cardiac arrest has also been reported during amsacrine infusions (Steinherz et al 1982). One event was fatal, and a diluent-related toxic effect was suspected but not confirmed. Acute lethality may occur in 12% of patients who develop arrhythmias while receiving amsacrine (Grillo-Lopez and Hess 1983). Acute ventricular fibrillation is associated with hypokalemia (Riela et al 1981) but may also occur in normokalemic patients (Steinherz et al 1982). These life-threatening reactions have also been more common in patients who have received prior anthracycline therapy (> 400 mg/m²) and those who received the drug as a brief infusion (Von Hoff et al 1980). Nonetheless, most patients who manifest cardiac effects in response to amsacrine have a history of anthracycline exposure and were hypokalemic at the time of amsacrine therapy.

Congestive heart failure has been observed in children receiving amsacrine (Miller et al 1983). Radionuclide cardiac ejection fraction tests may be useful to screen for serious amsacrine heart toxicity (Vorobiof et al 1983). Other reviews have suggested that amsacrine heart toxicity is not additive with anthracyclines in the production of drug-induced cumulative congestive heart failure (Fanucchi and Arlin 1982).

Amsacrine-related neurotoxicity is uncommon. These effects include peripheral neuropathy, headache, dizziness, central nervous system and depression (Louie and Issell 1985). Grand mal seizures have been described in a few patients who also had other central nervous system predisposing signs and especially hypokalemia (Mittelman and Arlin 1982). Peripheral neuropathy is rare (< 2% of patients) but may present as Guillain–Barré syndrome in children (Goldman and Malpas 1982). Headaches are also described in pediatric patients (Hutter and Meyskens 1982) and rarely in adults (Legha et al 1978).

Gastrointestinal toxic effects are common with amsacrine and include nausea, vomiting, and diarrhea. The incidence of nausea and vomiting ranges from 0 to 3%, with diarrhea described in only 13% of patients (Legha et al 1982). Anorexia is described in one third of patients (DeJager et al 1983). Mucositis is also quite common and is both dose and duration dependent. Up to 80% of patients may experience mucositis in dose-intensive amsacrine regimens (Louie and Issell 1985).

Hair loss also occurs in amsacrine-treated patients. Allergic reactions are rare but include anaphylaxis (Land et al 1981), localized (venous) allergic reactions (Ettinger et al 1983), arm edema (Brenner et al 1982), and acute hypersensitivity skin reactions (Weil et al 1982, Rosenfelt et al 1982). These reactions manifest as a burning sensation at the injection site and sometimes as a local urticarial rash (DeLena et al 1982). Generalized allergic reactions have also been reported (Welt et al 1981).

Other side effects of amsacrine include malaise (Casper et al 1980) and a transient loss of fertility (DaCunha et al 1982). Allergic reactions have rarely been reported in pharmacy personnel mixing the drug (Reynolds et al 1982). In a mouse model, amsacrine induces severe extravasation necrosis which is reduced by topical dimethylsulfoxide treatment (Soble et al 1987).

REFERENCES

Arlin ZA, Sklaroff RB, Gee TS, et al. Phase I and II trial of 4'-(9-acridinylamino)-methanesulfon-*m*-anisidide in patients with acute leukemia. *Cancer Res.* 1980;**40**:3304–3306.

Baguley BC, Falkenhaug EM, Rastrick JM, Marbrook J. An assessment of the immunosuppressive activity of the antitumor compound 4'-[(9 acridinyl)-amino]methane-sulfon-*m*-anisidide (*m*-AMSA). *Eur J Cancer.* 1974; **10**:169–176.

Brenner D, Barbino C, Kasdorf H, et al. A phase II trial of *m*-AMSA in the treatment of advanced gynecologic malignancies. *Am J Clin Oncol.* 1982;**5**:291–295.

Byrd DM. Antiviral activities of 4'-(9-acridinylamino)-methanesulfon-*m*-anisidide (SN11841). *Ann NY Acad Sci.* 1977;**284**:463–471.

Cain BF, Atwell GJ. The experimental antitumor properties of three cogeners of the acridinylmethane-sulphonanilide (AMSA) series. *Eur J Cancer.* 1974; **10**:539–549.

Cain BF, Seelye RN, Atwell GJ. Potential antitumor agents. XIV. Acridinylmethanesulfonanilides. *J Med Chem.* 1974;**17**:922–930.

Casper ES, Gralla RJ, Kelsen DP, et al. Phase II evaluation of 4'-(9-acridinylamino)-methanesulfon-*m*-anisidide (AMSA) in patients with non-small cell lung cancer. *Cancer Treat Rep.* 1980;**64**:345–347.

Civin CI, Land VJ, Nitschke R, et al. *m*-AMSA (methanesulfon-*m*-anisidine, 4'-(9-acridinylamino) (NSC-249992) activity in pediatric solid tumors (abstract). *Proc Am Soc Clin Oncol.* 1982;**1**:178.

Cysyk RL, Shoemaker D, Adamson RH. The pharmacologic disposition of 4'-(9-acridinylamino)methanesulfon *m*-anisidide in mice and rats. *Drug Metab Dispos.* 1977;**5**(6):579–590.

Cysyk RL, Shoemaker DD, Ayers OC, Adamson RH. Oral absorption and selective tissue localization of 4'-(9-acridinylamino)-methanesulfon-*m*-anisidide. *Pharmacology (Basel).* 1978;**16**:206–216.

DaCunha MF, Meistrich ML, Haq MM, et al. Temporary effects of AMSA (4'-(9-acridinylamino)-methanesulfon-*m*-anisidide) chemotherapy on spermatogenesis. *Cancer.* 1982;**49**:2459–2462.

DeJager R, Body JJ, Dupont D, et al. Phase I study of oral 4'-(9-acridinylamino)-methanesulfon-*m*-anisidide (*m*-AMSA, NSC 249992) (abstract). *Proc Am Soc Clin Oncol.* 1979;**20**:429.

DeJager R, Dupont D, Body JJ. Phase II study of oral 4'-(9-acridinylamino)-methanesulfon-*m*-anisidide (*m*-AMSA, NSC 24992) (abstract). *Proc Am Assoc Cancer Res.* 1980;**21**:146.

DeJager R, Siegenthaler P, Cavalli F, et al. Phase II study of amsacrine in solid tumors. Report of the EORTC early clinical trial group. *Eur J Cancer Clin Oncol.* 1983;**19**:289–293.

DeLena M, Rossi A, Bonadonna G. Phase II trial of AMSA in refractory breast cancer. *Cancer Treat Rep.* 1982; **66**:403–404.

Denny WA, Baguley BC, Cain BF, Waring MJ. Antitumor acridines. In: Neidle S, Waring MJ, eds. *Molecular Aspects of Anticancer Drug Action.* New York: MacMillan; 1983:1–34.

Denny WA, Wakelin LPG. Kinetic and equilibrium studies of the interaction of amsacrine and anilino ring-substituted analogues with DNA. *Cancer Res.* 1986;**46**:1717–1721.

Drewinko B, Yang LY, Barlogie B. Lethal activity and kinetic response of cultured human cells to 4'-(9-acridinylamino)-methanesulfon-*m*-anisidide. *Cancer Res.* 1982;**42**:107–111.

Engelking C, Sullivan P, Agoliati G, Arlin ZA. Amsacrine administration: A precautionary note. *Cancer Chemother Pharmacol.* 1984;**13**:150.

Ettinger DS, Day R, Ferraro JA, et al. A randomized phase II study of *m*-AMSA (NSC 249992) and neocarzinostatin (NSC 157365) in non-small cell bronchogenic carcinoma. *Am J Clin Oncol.* 1983;**6**:167–170.

Fanucchi MP, Arlin ZA. Successful treatment of a patient with acute nonlymphoblastic leukemia (ANLL) and anthracycline cardiomyopathy with 4'-(9-acridinylamino)-methanesulfon-*m*-anisidide (AMSA). *Cancer Chemother Pharmacol.* 1982;**10**:27–28.

Goldman A, Malpas JS. Phase I and II study of AMSA in childhood tumours. *Cancer Chemother Pharmacol.* 1982;**9**:53–56.

Goldsmith MA, Bhardwaj S, Ohnuma T, et al. Phase I study of *m*-AMSA in patients with solid tumors and leukemias. *Cancer Clin Trials.* 1980;**3**:197–202.

Gorsky LD, Morin MJ. Microsomal activation and increased production of 4'-(9-acridinylamino)-3-methanesulfon-*m*-anisidide (*m*-AMSA)-dependent, topoisomerase-associated DNA lesions in nuclei from human HL-60 leukemia cells. *Biochem Pharmacol.* 1990;**39**(9):1481–1484.

Grillo-Lopez AJ, Hess F. Carditoxicity associated with amsacrine (abstract C-712). *Proc Am Soc Clin Oncol.* 1983;**2**:183.

Hall SW, Friedman J, Legha SS, et al. Human pharmacokinetics of a new acridine derivative, 4'-(9-acridinylamino)methanesulfon-*m*-anisidide (NSC-249992). *Cancer Res.* 1983;**43**:3422–3426.

Henry MC, Port CD, Guarino AM, et al. *Preclinical Toxicologic Evaluation of 4'-(9-Acridinylamino)-Methanesulphon-m-Anisidide Monochloride in Mice, Dogs and Monkeys.* Report 11TRI-TOX 249992-76-2. Washington, DC: National Cancer Institute, National Institutes of Health; 1976.

Hines JD, Oken MM, Mazza J, et al. High dose cytosine arabinoside (Ara-C) and *m*-AMSA in relapsed acute non-lymphocytic leukemia (ANLL). *Proc Am Soc Clin Oncol.* 1983;**2**:173.

Hutter JJ, Meyskens FL. AMSA therapy for children with lymphoblastic malignancy. *Cancer Treat Rep.* 1982;**66**:593–594.

Kahn SB, Sklaroff R, Lebedda J, et al. 4'-(9-Acridinylamino)-methanesulfon-*m*-anisidide (*m*-AMSA) and 4-azacytidine (AZA) in the treatment of relapsed adult acute leukemia. *Am J Clin Oncol.* 1983;**6**:493–502.

Kampinga HH, Kruk G.v.d., Konings WT. Reduced DNA break formation and cytotoxicity of the topoisomerase II drug 4'-(9'-acridinylamino)methomesulfon-*m*-anisidide when combined with hyperthermia in human and rodent cell lines. *Cancer Res.* 1989;**49**:1712–1717.

Kuehnle C, Moore TD. Sodium chloride residue provides potential for drug incompatibilities. *Am J Hosp Pharm.* 1979;**36**:881.

Land VJ, Civin CI, Ragab AH, et al. Efficacy and toxicity of methanesulfon-*m*-anisidine,4'-(9-acridinylamino) (NSC-249992) (*m*-AMSA) in advanced childhood leukemia (abstract). *Proc Am Assoc Cancer Res.* 1981;**22**:403.

Legha SS, Blumenschein GR, Buzdar AU, et al. Phase II study of 4'-(9-acridinylamino)-methanesulfon-*m*-anisidide (AMSA) in metastatic breast cancer. *Cancer Treat Rep.* 1979;**63**:1961–1964.

Legha SS, Gutterman JU, Hall SW, et al. Phase I clinical investigation of 4'-(9-acridinylamino) methanesulfon-*m*-anisidide (NSC 249992), a new acridine derivative. *Cancer Res.* 1978;**38**:3712–3716.

Legha SS, Keating MJ, McCredie KB, et al. Evaluation of AMSA in previously treated patients with acute leukemia: Results of therapy in 109 adults. *Blood.* 1982;**60**:484–490.

Louie AC, Issell BF. Amsacrine (AMA)—A clinical review. *J Clin Oncol.* 1985;**3**(4):562–590.

Mahla PS, Legha SS, Valdivieso M, et al. AMSA toxicity in patients with abnormal liver function. *Eur J Cancer.* 1981;**17**:1343–1348.

McCredie KB, Keating MJ, Estey EH, et al. Use of 4'-(9-acridinylamino)-methanesulfon-*m*-anisidide (AMSA), cytosine arabinoside (ara-C), vincristine, prednisone combination (AMSA-OAP) in poor risk patients in acute leukemia (abstract). *Proc Am Soc Clin Oncol.* 1981;**22**:479.

Mellanby A. *British Empire Cancer Campaign, 10th Annual Report.* 1933.

Miller L, Miller D, Meyers P, et al. Combination chemotherapy with amsacrine (AMSA) and cyclocytidine in refractory leukemia: Preliminary observations of a phase II study. *Cancer Treat Rep.* 1983;**67**:439–443.

Mitchell E, Rahman A. Gutierrez P, et al. The pharmacologic interaction of *m*-AMSA with other drugs. *Proc Am Assoc Cancer Res.* 1982;**23**:205.

Mittelman A, Arlin ZA. AMSA-induced seizures in patients with hypokalemia. *Cancer Treat Rep.* 1982;**67**(1):102–103.

National Cancer Institute, Division of Cancer Treatment. *Investigational Drug–Pharmaceutical Data Sheet: Acridinyl Anisidide (AMSA).* Washington, DC: Pharmaceutical Resources Branch; January 1978.

Nelson EM, Tewey KM, Liu LF. Mechanism of antitumor drug action: Poisoning of mammalian DNA topoisomerase II on DNA by 4'-(9-acridinylamino)-methanesulfon-*m*-anisidide. *Proc Natl Acad Sci USA* 1984;**81**:1361–1365.

Omura GA, Winton EF, Vogler WR, et al. Phase II study of amsacrine gluconate in refractory leukemia. *Cancer Treat Rep.* 1983;**67**:1131–1132.

Paul CY, Liliemark JO, Farmen RH, et al. Comparison of the pharmacokinetics of AMSA and AMSA-lactate in patients with acute nonlymphoblastic leukemia. *Ther Drug Monitor.* 1987;**9**(3):263–271.

Paxton JW, Foote SE, Singh RM. The effect of buthionine sulphoximine, cimetidine and phenobarbitone on the disposition of amsacrine in the rabbit. *Cancer Chemother Pharmacol.* 1986;**18**:208–212.

Reynolds RD, Ignoffo R, Lawrence J, et al. Adverse reactions to AMSA in medical personnel. *Cancer Treat Rep.* 1982;**66**:1885.

Riela AR, Kimball JC, Pattersen RB, et al. Cardiac arrhythmia associated with AMSA in a child: A Southwest Oncology Group study. *Cancer Treat Rep.* 1981;**65**:1121–1123.

Rosenfelt FP, Rosenbloom BE, Weinstein IM. Allergic reaction following administration of AMSA. *Cancer Treat Rep.* 1982;**66**:594–595.

Shoemaker DD, Cysyk RL, Padmanabhan S, et al. Identification of the principal biliary metabolite of 4'-(9-acridinylamino)methanesulfon-*m*-anisidide in rats. *Am Soc Pharmacol Exp Ther.* 1982;**10**(1):35–39.

Shoemaker DD, Gormley PE, Cysyk RL. Biliary excretion of 4'-(9-acridinylamino)methanesulfon-*m*-anisidide (AMSA) in rats. *Drug Metab Dispos.* 1980;**8**:467–468.

Soble MJ, Dorr RT, Plezia P et al. Dose-dependent skin ulcers in mice treated with DNA binding antitumor antibiotics. *Cancer Chemother Pharmacol.* 1987;**20**:33–36.

Steinherz LJ, Steinhertz PG, Mangiacasale D, et la. Cardiac abnormalities after AMSA administration. *Cancer Treat Rep.* 1982;**66**:483–488.

Utsumi H, Shibuya ML, Kosaka T, et al. Abrogation by novobiocin of cytotoxicity due to the topoisomerase II inhibitor amsacrine in Chinese hamster cells. *Cancer Res.* 1990;**50**:2577–2581.

Van Echo DA, Chiuten DF, Gormley PE, et al. Phase I clinical and pharmacological study of 4'-(9-acridinylamino)-methanesulfon-*m*-anisidide using an intermittent biweekly schedule. *Cancer Res.* 1979;**39**:3881–3884.

Von Hoff DD, Elson D, Polk G, et al. Acute ventricular fibrillation and death during infusion of 4'-(9-acridinylamino)-methanesulfon-*m*-anisidide (AMSA). *Cancer Treat Rep.* 1980;**64**:356–357.

Von Hoff DD, Howser D, Gormley P, et al. Phase I study of 4'-(9-acridinylamino)methanesulfon-*m*-anisidide (NSC-24992, *m*-AMSA) using a single dose schedule. *Cancer Treat Rep.* 1978;**62**:1421–1426.

Vorobiof DA, Iturralde M, Falkson G. Amsacrine cardiotoxicity: Assessment of ventricular function by radionuclide angiography. *Cancer Treat Rep.* 1983;**67**:1115–1117.

Waring MJ. DNA-binding characteristics of acridinylmethanesulphonanilide drugs: Comparison with antitumor properties. *Eur J Cancer.* 1976;**12**:995–1001.

Weick JK, Jones SE, Ryan DH. Phase II study of amsacrine (*m*-AMSDA) in advanced lymphomas: A Southwest Oncology Group study. *Cancer Treat Rep.* 1983;**67**:489–492.

Weil M, Auclerc MF, Schaison G, et al. Activite clinique de la *m*-AMSA et de l'association de *m*-AMSA et de cytosine arabinoside. *Nouv Presse Med.* 1982;**11**:2911–2914.

Welt S, Dellaquila C, Arlin ZA. Allergic reaction following administration of AMSA. *Cancer Treat Rep.* 1981;**65**:919.

Zwelling LA, Kerrigan D, Marton LJ. Effect of difluoromethylornithine, an inhibitor of polyamine biosynthesis, on the topoisomerase II-mediated DNA scission produced by 4'-(9-acridinylamino)methanesulfon-*m*-anisidide in L1210 murine leukemia cells. *Cancer Res.* 1985;**45**:1122–1126.

Zwelling LA, Michaels S, Erickson C, et al. Protein-associated deoxyribonucleic acid strand breaks in L1210 cells treated with the deoxyribonucleic acid intercalating agents 4'-(9-acridinylamino)methanesulfon-*m*-anisidide and Adriamycin. *Biochemistry.* 1981;**20**:6553–6563.

Androgens

■ Chemistry

Structures of five androgens

Androgens are steroidal derivatives of the natural hormone testosterone. The synthetic preparations useful in cancer appear to have somewhat selective structure–activity relationships. Two basic chemical classes include 17-alkyl derivatives (Segaloff et al 1964) and various testosterone esters. The 17-methylated compounds are associated with a greater incidence of cholestatic jaundice, but are also thought to be less virilizing than natural testosterone. The 17β-hydroxy compounds, particularly dromostanolone and nandrolone, have a greater proportional anabolic/androgenic activity ratio. Concerning antitumor activity, Segaloff (1957) showed that for most of the available androgens, loss of virilizing activity was commensurate with loss of antitumor efficacy. Further work with the more recent (and purportedly more specific) synthetic agent calusterone (Methosarb®) has shown that it also has significant androgenic potential (Brodkin and Cooper 1978). In 1957, Kennedy noted equivalent antitumor and androgenic action comparing the halogenated testosterone derivative fluoxymesterone and testosterone propionate. Similar results were subsequently obtained by Blackburn and Childs (1959) and Thomas et al (1962) with 2α-methylandrostan-17-β-ol-3-one (2α-methyldihydrotestosterone) propionate and by Segaloff et al (1962) with Δ¹-testolactone. In summary, few androgens surpass testosterone propionate in antitumor efficacy and virilization, and most other androgenic side effects appear to be roughly comparable.

■ Antitumor Activity

Androgens offer some palliation in about 20% of postmenopausal, hormonally sensitive advanced breast cancers (Cooperative Breast Cancer Group 1964, Segaloff 1958, Goldenberg 1964), but rarely in renal carcinomas. The antitumor effects are not well elucidated but are limited to advanced postmenopausal/postcastration breast cancer patients (Brodsky 1973). Occasionally, metastatic hypernephroma patients may also benefit. In breast cancer, the impeded androgens calusterone and danazol appear to have significantly less virilizing activity than other androgens. Testolactone also possesses little virilizing activity and, like calusterone, is active in advanced breast cancer (Goldenberg 1969). Stanozolol is also active in advanced breast cancer (Daniel et al 1991) as is fluoxymesterone (Kennedy 1958). The newer impeded androgen danazol is also active in nonmalignant cystic disease of the breast (Madanes and Farber 1982) and in advanced breast cancer, with response rates ranging from 6 to 17% (Brodovsky et al 1987, Coombes et al 1980). It is also active in postmenopausal breast cancer patients when combined with other hormonal agents (tamoxifen and aminoglutethimide) (Powles 1984). Unfortunately, androgens have not been useful in refractory epithelial ovarian cancer (Kavanagh et al 1987).

Androgens have also been used historically to stimulate prostate cancer cells before treatment with phosphorus-32 (Donati et al 1966, Edland 1974). The objective of this therapy is to stimulate tumor growth, thereby potentiating the cytotoxic effects of radiophosphorus on bony metastases. Numerous other studies have shown that although exogenous testosterone stimulates most prostatic cancers (Prout and Brewer 1967), it has no real role in combination with cytotoxic chemotherapy (Fowler and Whitemore 1982). Androgens were also used historically to stimulate erythropoiesis and thrombopoiesis in various disorders characterized by bone marrow failure (Sahidi 1973). In severe aplastic anemia, however, androgens are associated with negligible activity and appear to offer no advantage over bone marrow transplantation (Camitta et al 1979).

■ Mechanism of Action

Androgens have diverse biologic effects. It is known that the androgens are not always pure reciprocal antagonists to estrogens, although this may constitute their main mechanism of antitumor action. In fact, a few effects are complementary. Androgens also may impair tumor growth by suppressing pituitary function. The presence of specific cell hormone receptor proteins has been described by some as essential for effect.

Danazol is a weak androgen which also appears to have additional antigonadotropin activity in animal models and in the hypergonadotropic states that follow castration or menopause in humans (Madanes and Farber 1982). Thus, danazol reduces the levels of follicle-stimulating hormone (FSH) and luteinizing hormone (LH), especially in response to exogenous gonadotropin-releasing hormone (Fraser and Thornburn 1978). Danazol reduces testosterone levels in males and blocks ovulation in females as a result of the lack of the normal midcycle surge of LH and FSH. Danazol also binds to estrogen and progesterone receptors, which results in a blockade of estradiol binding (Chamness et al 1980) and a mild progestational effect (Wentz et al 1976). Danazol also blocks the enzymatic synthesis of androgens and estrogens in the ovary. This activity involves the inhibition of 17α-hydroxylase, 17, 20-lyase, 3β-hydroxysteroid dehydrogenase, and various mitochondrial enzymes involved in sex steroid biotransformation (Barbieri et al 1977). Fortunately, glucocorticosteroid synthesis is unaffected by danazol (Wentz et al 1975).

Other general activities of all androgens include a significant protein anabolic effect with retention of nitrogen, potassium, calcium, and phosphorus; a mild stimulatory effect or erythropoiesis; and augmentation of immune responses and stimulation of the fibrinolytic system (Rigberg and Brodsky 1975).

Costlow et al (1976) and Quadri et al (1974) have additionally suggested that the antitumor activity of androgens is due to reduction or competitive inhibition of prolactin receptors.

Other popular theories concerning the antitumor mechanism include inhibition of estrogen synthesis from adrenal steroid precursors (McGuire 1977), competitive inhibition at the estrogen receptor (Zava and McGuire 1977), and estrogen production in vivo via peripheral conversion of androgenic substances (McGuire 1977). Overall, androgen-induced estrogen depletion appears to be most highly favored. This has been metabolically documented by Fishman and Hellman (1976), at least for calusterone. Thus, the antitumor effects of androgens may relate more to antigonadotropic effects than to direct tumor tissue receptor interactions.

■ Availability and Storage

For availability, see the table on page 192. Follow manufacturers' guidelines for storage.

■ Preparation for Use, Stability, and Admixture

All intramuscular injections should be observed for clarity and shaken to obtain a good suspension. Most compounds are extremely stable; however, the specific manufacturers' recommendations should be followed. Admixture of injectable testosterone preparations with other medications is not recommended.

■ Administration

Intramuscular injections should be administered with extreme caution to avoid inadvertent intravenous or subcutaneous administration. This can result in considerable pain and discomfort and the possibility of a serious oil embolism. Some patients may also become sensitized to the oil carriers in the depot testosterone preparations. Overall, oral administration may be preferred for convenience although occasionally oral absorption is erratic.

■ Dosage

Generally, relatively large pharmacologic doses of androgens must be employed in hormonally sensitive tumors. Because prolonged hormonal suppression is usually required to inhibit tumor growth, therapy dosing should continue for at least 2 to 3 months before therapeutic failure is clearly documented. Dosage reductions are required in patients with liver function abnormalities, especially if a 17-methyl derivative is used. Thus, liver function tests including serum bilirubin should be routinely followed while a patient is on androgen therapy. For specific dosage recommendations, see the table.

■ Pharmacokinetics

Testosterone is generally well absorbed orally. Radiolabeled testosterone precursors are rapidly cleared in humans: 90% in the urine and 6% in the feces after 2 days (Brotherton 1976). Extensive and rapid biotransformation occurs in the liver. Most androgens are primarily glucuronidated and are excreted in the urine (Dorfman and Ungar 1965). Some natural androgens are metabolized to estrogenic substances and etiocholanolone, a potent pyrogen. Free (unbound) testosterone has a half-life of approximately 15 minutes, and at physiologic levels of approximately 500 ng/dL, greater than 95% of the drug is bound to proteins (Nisula and Dunn 1979). These proteins include testosterone–estradiol-binding globulin and albumin. Testosterone can be converted back to androstenedione via the reversible 17-keto reductase step. Alternatively, the drug is normally "activated" by 5α-methylase reduction of the double bond at position 5 to form dihydrotestosterone. A third route of metabolic clearance involves reduction of the keto group at the 3-position, producing an alcohol. These latter products which are weakly androgenic include 5α-androsterone and the 5β-isomer of etiocholanolone. Both metabolites are excreted in the urine as sulfate or glucuronide conjugates.

Synthetic androgens such as danazol are also metabolized in the liver. To date, several methylestrione metabolites have been identified. About 11% of a dose is excreted as metabolites, largely as 2-hydroxymethylethisterone. This metabolite appears in the plasma at levels that are 10-fold greater than those of the parent drug (80–293 ng/mL), but the metabolite lacks antigonadotropic activity (Potts 1977). A danazol dose of 200 mg twice daily leads to steady-state levels of 511 mg/mL. Steady-state levels are achieved at 7 days with a daily dose of 200 mg and at 14 days with a daily dose of 400 mg (Williams et al 1978). The plasma half-life of danazol is 23.8 hours with an absorption half-time of approximately 10 minutes (Potts et al 1980). Peak plasma concentrations are dose dependent and range from 90 to 214 ng/mL for doses of 50 to 400 mg. Concentrations × time products (AUC) for these dose levels range from 571 to 1683 ng/mL·h (Potts et al 1980).

Injectable androgens are formulated as poorly soluble oil-based esters and possess slow-release characteristics and prolonged biologic effects in vivo.

■ Side Effects and Toxicity

The androgens are generally well tolerated and possess a wide margin of safety. Acute side effects include dose-related nausea and vomiting. Hyper-

ANDROGEN AVAILABILITY, DOSES, AND CLINICAL APPLICATIONS

Drug	Available Preparations	Uses	Usual Dose	Chemical Name
Oral preparations				
Danazol (Danocrine®)	Capsules: 50, 100, 200 mg	Fibrocystic breast disease, endometriosis, advanced breast cancer	100–400 mg/d (in two daily fractions)	17α-Pregna-2,4-diene-20-yno[2,3-*d*] isoxazol-17-ol
Fluoxymesterone (Halotestin®)	Tablets: 2, 5, 10 mg	Advanced breast cancer	10–30 mg/d (0.5–1 mg/kg/d) orally	9α-Fluoro-11β,17β-dihydroxy-17α-methyl-4-androsten-3-one
Methandrosteneolone (Dianabol®)	Tablets: 2.5, 5 mg	Protein anabolism	5–10 mg/day (0.25–3 mg/kg/d) orally	17α-Methyl-17β-hydroxy-2-androsta-1,4-dien-3-one
Methyltestosterone [Oreton® (M)]	Tablets: 2, 5, 10, 25mg Buccal TABS: 5 mg, 10 mg CAPS: 10 mg	Breast cancer Protein anabolism	25–100 mg/d (0.5–2 mg/kg/d) sublingually, orally = 50–200 mg/d	17α-Methyltestosterone
Calusterone (Methosarb®)	Currently out of production	Advanced breast cancer	40 mg QID orally	7β, 17α-Dimethyltestosterone
Oxymethalone (Anadrol-50®, Anapolon®, Adroyd®, OraTestryl®)	Tablets: 50 mg	Refractory anemia, anabolic effects	1–5 mg/kg/d (0.25–4 mg/kg/d)	17α-Methyl-17β-hydroxy-2-hydroxymethylene-5α-androstan-3-one
Stanozolol (Winstrol®)	Tablets: 2 mg	Breast cancer (not approved)	5–10 mg/d	17-Methyl-2′*H*-5α-androst-2-eno[3,2-*c*]pyrazol-17β-ol
Testolactone (Teslac®)	Tablets: 50 mg	Advanced breast cancer, refractory anemia	250 mg QID orally	D-Homo-17α-oxa-androstra-1,4-diene-3,17-dione
Injections				
Testosterone propionate (Oreton®)	Injection in oil 25, 50, 100 mg/mL	Advanced breast cancer	50–100 mg IM three times weekly	Testosterone propionate
Testosterone enanthate (Deletestry)®	Injection in oil 100, 200 mg/mL	Advanced breast cancer	200–400 mg IM every 24 weeks	Testosterone heptanoate
Testosterone cypionate (Depo-Testosterone®)	Injection in oil 50, 100, 200 mg/mL	Advanced breast cancer, refractory anemia	600–1200 mg IM weekly 200–400 mg IM every 2–4 weeks	Testosterone cyclopentyl propionate
Dormastonalone propionate (Drolban®)	Injection in oil 50 mg/mL	Advanced breast cancer, protein anabolism, refractory anemia	4–7 mg/kg/wk IM	17β-Hydroxy-2α-methyl-5α-androstan-3-one propionate
Nandrolone phenylpropionate (Durabolin®)	Injection in oil 25, 50 mg/mL	Protein anabolism, refractory anemia, breast cancer	100 mg IM three times weekly 25–50 mg IM three times 50–100 mg IM weekly	19-Nortestosterone phenylpropionate
Nandrolone decanoate (Deca-Durabolin®)	Injection in oil 50, 100 mg/mL	Refractory anemia	1–1.5 mg/kg/wk IM	19-Nortestosterone decanoate
Testolactone (Teslac®)	Injection: aqueous suspension, 100 mg/mL	Advanced breast cancer	100 mg IM three times weekly	17α-Oxaandrostra-1,4-diene-3,17-dione

calcemia may also occur on initiation of therapy, especially in immobilized patients with bony disease. As a result of the anabolic retention of nitrogen, potassium, calcium, and phosphorus, androgens should be administered with extreme caution in patients with serious renal diseases. Edema may also be encountered and is the result of a small degree of sodium retention. Androgens should therefore be used with some caution in patients with compromised cardiovascular or renal function.

With synthetic androgens such as danazol and calusterone, there is less of the usual androgenic and antiestrogenic effects. Patients may experience muscle cramps, which can be associated with elevated serum creatinine phosphokinase; however, frank creatinuria is most common with the 17α-methyl compounds (Wilkins and Fleischmann 1945). Fatigue, somnolence, headache, and skin rashes are also described.

Prolonged, high-dose therapy with methylated androgens such as fluoxymesterone, methandrostenolone, testosterone, and methyltestosterone has been associated with intrahepatic biliary stasis often producing clinical jaundice (Werner et al 1950). Other liver function abnormalities noted with the methyl derivatives are usually not dose limiting. Hepatic adenocarcinomas have also been associated with chronic use of any 17-alkyl androgen (Bernstein et al 1971, Henderson et al 1973).

Virilization in females is commonly observed and is characterized by the growth of facial hair, acne, clitoral hypertrophy, and increased libido. Voice deepening is also seen, along with a patchy type of alopecia. These effects are androgenic, not toxic; however, patients should be warned well in advance about these potentially unwelcome androgenic effects. Typical antiestrogenic effects include decreased breast size, vasomotor flushing, irregular vaginal bleeding, and decreased libido.

Dosage adjustment is required in the presence of severe liver disease. The stimulatory effect of erythropoiesis may cause a slightly increased red cell mass but this is rarely of any clinical consequence (Sahidi 1973). Fever has been noted with some androgens, especially calusterone (Gordon et al 1970). Calusterone curiously lacks erythropoietic activity, but retains platelet and leukocyte stimulatory activity (Brodkin and Cooper 1978).

REFERENCES

Barbieri RL, Canick JA, Makris A, et al. Danazol inhibits steroidogenesis. *Fertil Steril.* 1977;**28**:809–813.

Bernstein MS, Hunter RL, Hachnin S. Hepatoma and peliosis hepatitis in Franconi's anemia. *N Engl J Med.* 1971;**284**:1135–1136.

Blackburn CM, Childs DS Jr. Use of a 2-α-methyl-androstan-17-β-91-3-one (2α-methyl-dihydrotestosterone) in the treatment of advanced cancer of the breast. *Proc Mayo Clin.* 1959;**34**:113–126.

Brodkin RA, Cooper MR. Calusterone. *Ann Intern Med.* 1978;**89**:945–948.

Brodovsky HS, Holroyde CP, Laucius JF, et al. Danazol in the treatment of women with metastatic breast cancer. *Cancer Treat Rep.* 1987;**71**:875–876.

Brodsky I. The role of androgens and anabolic steroids in the treatment of cancer. *Semin Drug Treat.* 1973;**3**:15–25.

Brotherton J. *Sex Hormone Pharmacology.* London: Academic Press; 1976.

Camitta BM, Thomas D, Nathan DG, et al. A prospective study of androgens and bone marrow transplantation for treatment of severe aplastic anemia. *Blood.* 1979;**53**(3):504–514.

Chamness GC, Asch RH, Pauerstein CJ. Danazol binding and translocation of steroid receptors. *Am J Obstet Gynecol.* 1980;**136**:426–429.

Coombes RC, Dearnaley D, Humphreys J, et al. Danazol treatment of advanced breast cancer. *Cancer Treat Rep.* 1980;**64**:1073–1076.

Cooperative Breast Cancer Group. Testosterone propionate therapy in breast cancer—a cooperative study. *JAMA.* 1964;**188**:1069–1077.

Costlow ME, Buschow RA, McGuire WL. Prolactin receptors and androgen-induced regression of 7,12-dimethylbenz(a)anthracene-induced mammary carcinoma. Cancer Res. 1976;**36**:3324–3329.

Daniel F, Rao DG, Tyrrell CJ. A pilot study of stanozolol for advanced breast carcinoma. *Cancer.* 1991;**36**:2966–2968.

Donati RM, Ellis H. Gallagher NI. Testosterone potentiated P-32 therapy in prostatic carcinoma. *Cancer.* 1966;**19**:1088–1090.

Dorfman RI, Ungar F. *Metabolism of Steroid Hormones.* New York: Academic Press; 1965.

Edland RW. Testosterone potentiated radiophosphorus therapy of osseous metastases in prostatic cancer. *Am J Roentgenol Radiat Ther Nucl Med.* 1974;**120**:678–683.

Fishman J, Hellman L. 7β,17α-Dimethyltestosterone (calusterone)-induced changes in the metabolism, production rate, and excretion of estrogens in women with breast cancer: A possible mechanism of action. *J Clin Endocrinol Metab.* 1976;**42**:365–369.

Fowler JE Jr, Whitmore WF Jr. Considerations for the use of testosterone with systemic chemotherapy in prostatic cancer. *Cancer.* 1982;**49**:1373–1377.

Fraser IS, Thornburn GD. Effects of danazol on pituitary gonadotrophins in post-menopausal women. *Aust NZ J Obstet Gynecol.* 1978;**18**:247–249.

Goldenberg IS. Testosterone propionate therapy in breast cancer—A cooperative study. *JAMA.* 1964;**183**:1069.

Goldenberg IS. Clinical trial of testolactone (NSC-23759),

medroxyprogesterone acetate (NSC-26386) and oxylone acetate (NSC-47438) in advanced female mammary cancer. *Cancer.* 1969;**23**:109–112.

Gordan GS, Halden A. Walter RM. Antitumor efficacy of 7β,17α-dimethyltestosterone (calusterone) in advanced female breast cancer. *Calif Med.* 1970;**113**:1.

Henderson JT, Richmond J, Sumerling MD. Androgenic-anabolic steroid therapy and hepatocellular carcinoma. *Lancet.* 1973;**1**:934.

Kavanagh JJ, Wharton JT, Roberts WS. Androgen therapy in the treatment of refractory epithelial ovarian cancer. *Cancer Treat Rep.* 1987;**71**(5):537–538.

Kennedy BJ. Fluoxymesterone in the treatment of advanced breast cancer. *Cancer.* 1957;**10**:813–818.

Kennedy BJ. Fluoxymesterone therapy in advanced breast cancer. *N Engl J Med.* 1958;**259**:673–675.

Madanes AE, Farber M. Danazol. *Ann Intern Med.* 1982;**96**:625–630.

McGuire WL. *Breast Cancer.* New York: Plenum; 1977;240–245.

Nisula BC, Dunn JF. Measurement of the testosterone binding parameters for both testosterone–estradiol binding globulin and albumin in individual serum samples. *Steroids.* 1979;**34**:771–791.

Potts GO. Pharmacology of danazol. *J Int Med Res.* 1977;**5**:1–14.

Potts GO, Schane HP, Edelson J. Pharmacology and pharmacokinetics of danazol. *Drugs.* 1980;**19**:321–330.

Powles TJ. The role of aromatase inhibitors in breast cancer. *Semin Oncol.* 1984;**10**:20–24.

Prout GR, Brewer WR. Response of men with advanced prostatic carcinoma to exogenous administration of testosterone. *Cancer.* 1967;**20**:1871–1878.

Quadri SK, Kledzik GS, Meites J. Counteraction by prolactin of androgen-induced inhibition of mammary tumor growth in rats. *J Natl Cancer Inst.* 1974;**52**:875–878.

Rigberg SV, Brodsky I. Potential roles of androgens and the anabolic steroids in the treatment of cancer—A review. *J Med.* 1975;**6**(3,4):271–290.

Sahidi NT. Androgens and erythropoiesis. *N Engl J Med.* 1973;**289**:72–80.

Segaloff A. Testosterone and miscellaneous steroids in the treatment of advanced mammary cancer. *Cancer.* 1957;**10**:808–812.

Segaloff A. The therapy of advanced breast cancer with androgens. In: *Breast Cancer* (2nd Biennial Louisiana Cancer Conference), St. Louis MO: CV Mosby; 1958:203.

Segaloff A, Weeth JB, Cunningham M, Meyer KK. Hormonal therapy in cancer of the breast. XXIII. Effect of 17α-methyl-19-nortestosterone acetate (17α-methyl-estr-4-en-3-one, 17β-ol acetate) or testosterone propionate on a clinical course and hormonal excretion. *Cancer.* 1964;**17**:1248.

Segaloff A, Weeth JB, Rongone EL, et al. Hormonal therapy in cancer of the breast. XVI. The effect of Δ¹-tes-tololactone on clinical course and hormonal excretion. *Cancer.* 1962;**15**:633–635.

Thomas AN, Gordan GS, Goldman L, Lowe R. Antitumor efficacy of 2α-methyl dihydrotestosterone propionate in advanced breast cancer. *Cancer.* 1962;**15**:176–178.

Wentz AC, Jones GS, Andrews MC, et al. Adrenal function during chronic danazol administration. *Fertil Steril.* 1975;**26**:1113–1115.

Wentz AC, Jones GS, Saap KC, et al. Progestational activity of danazol in the human female subject. *Am J Obstet Gynecol.* 1976;**126**:378–384.

Werner SC, Hanger FM, Kritzler R. Jaundice during methyl testosterone therapy. *Am J Med.* 1950;**8**:325.

Wilkins L. Fleischmann W. Studies on the creatinuria due to methylated steroids. *J Clin Invest.* 1945;**24**:21–32.

Williams TA, Edelson J, Ross RW. A radioimmunoassay for danazol. *Steroids.* 1978;**31**:205–217.

Zava DT, McGuire WL. Estrogen receptors in androgen-induced breast tumor regression. *Cancer Res.* 1977;**37**(6):1608–1610.

Anguidine

■ Other Names

Diacetoxyscirpenol, NSC-141537.

■ Chemistry

Structure of anguidine

Anguidine has a complex structure with an empiric formula of $C_{19}H_{24}O_7$ and a molecular weight of 366.4. It is one of a series of derivatives of a parasitic plant fungus, *Fusarium equiseti*, that were originally noted to produce severe scorching and death when sprayed on plants (Brian et al 1961). Anguidine has a water and 5% dextrose solubility of 2 mg/mL.

Antitumor Activity

Anguidine has demonstrated antitumor effects in animal systems including various leukemias and a colon cancer model. Synergism with 5-fluorouracil was noted in the latter system (Corbett and Griswold 1977). Phase II testing of the agent in patients with colorectal cancer (DeSimone et al 1986) and a variety of other malignancies has not clearly demonstrated any antitumor activity in humans (Adler et al 1984). Adler et al (1984) reported that one patient with gastric cancer had a partial response lasting 80 weeks and one with prostate cancer had a 12-week partial response. Based on their study, they felt the drug was inactive in previously treated patients with colon cancer, non-small cell lung cancer, renal cell carcinoma, head and neck cancer, melanoma, and breast cancer. Of some interest is the 14% response rate noted in patients with gliomas who were refractory to other standard treatment (Goodwin et al 1983).

Mechanism of Action

Anguidine appears to act in a manner unrelated to existing chemotherapeutic agents. The primary site of attack appears to be polyribosomes, causing disaggregation and interruption of protein synthesis (Uneo et al 1973). DNA but not RNA synthesis has also been shown to be affected. Cell cycle phase specificity and the exact cytotoxic mechanism are not known. The main action of the drug, however, appears to involve an irreversible blockade of protein synthesis (Liao et al 1976).

Availability and Storage

Anguidine was investigationally available from the Investigational Drug Branch of the National Cancer Institute in 5-mL vials also containing 100 mg of mannitol. Intact vials may be stored at room temperature up to 2 years from the date of manufacture.

Preparation for Use, Stability, and Admixture

Vials are reconstituted with 9.8 mL of Sterile Water for Injection, USP. This yields a solution of pH 6.0 to 8.0 containing 0.5 mg/mL anguidine and 10 mg/mL mannitol which is chemically stable for at least 7 days at room temperature; however, solutions should optimally be freshly prepared before administration and used within 8 hours as no bacteriostatic preservative is included. It is recommended that the preceding initial reconstitution be further diluted into 50 to 500 mL of D5W or normal saline for infusion. This final dilution is reportedly chemically stable for at least 24 hours.

Administration

Freshly prepared solutions of anguidine were initially recommended to be given as a 4- to 6-hour infusion in at least 500 mL of D5W. Shorter infusion times are thought to increase the incidence and severity of somnolence, erythema, nausea, and vomiting; however, Murphy et al (1978) have recently recommended dilution of the daily doses in 50 to 100 mL of 5% dextrose solution for administration over 30 to 60 minutes.

Special Precautions

Because of the irritating nature of the drug, extravasation must be avoided. A flush of 5 to 10 mL of saline or dextrose before and after administration is recommended. Close supervision of the infusion is necessary. Murphy et al (1978) have recommended a substantially reduced dosage in patients with liver dysfunction to decrease the diffuse erythema and burning sensation seen in these patients. Also, because of potential hypotensive effects, similarly reduced doses are recommended for patients with cardiovascular instability.

Drug Interactions

None are known.

Dosage

The optimal therapeutic dose of anguidine remains to be defined. In phase I studies of the daily ($\times$ 5) schedule, doses of 0.2 to 7.5 mg/m^2 were investigated. In patients with impaired liver function and/or prior nitrosourea therapy, a starting dose of 3.0 mg/m^2 for phase-II trials was recommended by Haas et al (1977). Murphy et al (1978) have recommended a 5 mg/m^2 daily dose for 5 consecutive days. For patients with liver enzyme elevation ($\geq$ 50%) or mild increase in bilirubin (< 2.5 mg/100 mL), these authors similarly recommend initial doses of 3.0 mg/m^2/d $\times$ 5. Phase II studies have used doses of 5 mg/m^2/d $\times$ 4 days (by continuous infusion) repeated every 32 days (Adler et al 1984), 5 mg/m^2 as a 4-hour infusion given weekly (Goodwin et al., 1983), and 5 mg/m^2 daily $\times$ 5 every 3 weeks.

Pharmacokinetics

No pharmacokinetic studies have been performed with this agent.

Side Effects and Toxicity

With short infusions (30 minutes to 1-2 hours), dose–limiting acute gastrointestinal and central nervous system toxic effects may be greater. These include nausea and vomiting, which may lead to dehydration and somnolence, and also local erythemia (Haas et al 1977). Fever and chills, myelosuppression, headache, and malaise may also be noted. Evidence of cerebral dysfunction has been observed by electroencephalographic analysis during periods of somnolence and disorientation. With a longer infusion time (4–6 hours), the preceding effects may be diminished in severity, and myelosuppression becomes the dose-limiting toxic effects (Haas et al 1977). Maximal myelosuppression is noted 12 days after initiation of therapy (Murphy et al 1978). Thrombocytopenia with a 28-day nadir appears to characterize the myelosuppression; however, milder degrees of leukopenia are also observed. There is additionally some evidence that cumulative myelotoxicity is possible with repeated courses of anguidine. Renal dysfunction (blood urea nitrogen elevation), hypotension (often severe), hyperuricemia, and elevations in liver function tests (serum glutamic–oxalacetic transaminase and alkaline phosphatase) are also seen. Patients with hepatic metastases have experienced unusual and severe nonhematologic toxic effects. These have included diffuse erythema and a burning sensation. Infrequently, marked motor weakness, skin desquamation, and diarrhea are observed.

Special Applications

Anguidine can potentiate the activity of cisplatin in a variety of cisplatin-resistant tumors in vitro and in vivo (Hromas and Yung 1986, Hormas et al 1983, 1984, 1985). This finding has not yet been studied in humans.

REFERENCES

Adler SS, Lowenbraun S, Birch B, et al. Anguidine: A broad phase II study of the Southeastern Cancer Study Group. *Cancer Treat Rep.* 1984;**68**:423–425.

Brian PW, Dawkens AW, Grove JF, et al. Phytotoxic compounds produced by *Fusarium equiseti*. *J Exp Bot.* 1961;**12**:1–12.

Corbett TH, Griswold DP. Treatment of colon adenocarcinomas in mice with anguidine (NSC-141537) and anguidine + 5FU (NSC-19893). *Proc Am Assoc Cancer Res.* 1977;**18**:115.

DeSimone AP, Greco FA, Lersner HF, et al. Phase II evaluation of anguidine (NSC-141537) in 5-day courses in colorectal adenocarcinoma. A Southeastern Cancer Study Group trial. *Am J Clin Oncol.* 1986;**9**:187–188.

Goodwin W, Bottomly R, Vaughn C, et al. Anguidine (diacetoxyscirpenol) in central nervous system tumors. A Southwest Oncology Group study. *Proc Am Soc Clin Oncol.* 1983;**2**:230.

Haas C, Goodwin W, Leite C, et al. Phase I study of anguidine (diacetoxyscirpenol, NSC-141537). *Proc Am Soc Clin Oncol.* 1977;**18**:296.

Hromas RA, Barlogie B, Meyn RE, et al. Diverse mechanisms and methods of overcoming cis-platinum resistance in L1210 leukemia cells. *Proc Am Assoc Cancer Res.* 1985;**26**:261.

Hromas R, Barlogie B, Swartzendruber D, et al. Potentiation of DNA-reactive antineoplastic agents and protection against S-phase-specific agents by anguidine in Chinese hamster ovary cells. *Cancer Res.* 1983;**43**:3070–3073.

Hromas R, Meyn R, Jenkins S, et al. Anguidine enhances cis-platinum-induced DNA crosslinks in Chinese hamster ovary cells. *Proc Am Assoc Cancer Res.* 1984;**25**:370.

Hromas RA, Yung WK. Anguidine potentiates cis-platinum in human brain tumor cells. *J Neurooncol.* 1986;**3**:343–348.

Liao LL, Grollman AP, Horwitz SB. Mechanism of action of the 12,13-epoxytrichothecene, anguidine: An inhibitor of protein synthesis. *Biochim Biophys Acta.* 1976;**454**:273–284.

Murphy WK, Burgess AM, Valdivieso M, et al. Phase I clinical evaluation of anguidine. *Cancer Treat Rep.* 1978;**62**(10):1497–1502.

Uneo Y, Nakajima M, Saki K, et al. Comparative toxicology or trichothec mycotoxins: Inhibition of protein synthesis in animal cells. *J Biochem.* 1973;**74**:285–296.

Aphidicolin Glycinate

Other Names

NSC-234714.

Chemistry

Structure of aphidicolin glycinate

Aphidicolin is a tetracyclic diterpene tetraol antibiotic isolated from the fungi *Cephalosporium aphidicol* (Bucknall et al 1973) and *Nigrospora sphaerica* (Starratt and Loschiavo 1974). The structure resembles that of a steroid but contains unusual terpenoid rings. The molecular formula of aphidicolin is $C_{20}H_{33}O_4$ and its molecular weight 337 (excluding the glycinate of the injectable formulation). Aphidicolin is soluble in dimethylsulfoxide, methanol, and ethanol but has very limited solubility in water. The commercial preparation for parenteral use is an ester of glycinate–hydrochloride at the 17-position.

Antitumor Activity

Aphidicolin is a mycotoxin that is highly effective at blocking cell growth. This is due to inhibition of DNA synthesis (Ikegami et al 1978). Growth inhibition has been noted in human HeLa tumor cells (Pedrali-Noy and Spadari 1979), in human melanoma cells (Lonn and Lonn 1983), and in L-1210 mouse leukemia cells (Sessa et al 1991). In the latter model, L-1210 tumor colony formation was inhibited in vitro by about 90% (1 log) after exposure to a concentration of 30 µg/mL for 6 hours. After exposure to a concentration of 3 µg/mL for 24 hours, a cell kill of over 3 logs (99.9%) was achieved. A number of rodent tumors are also sensitive to aphidicolin administered in vivo (Lobbezoo et al 1987). In addition, several human tumor cell lines were similarly inhibited by aphidicolin glycinate in vitro. Typically, long exposures are required for cytotoxicity in vitro. Sensitive tumors included 7 of 8 breast, 15 of 17 colon, 12 of 14 kidney, 14 of 17 lung, 7 of 11 ovarian, 4 of 6 melanoma, 2 of 2 mesothelioma, and 1 of 1 sarcoma specimens (Lobbezoo et al 1987).

Aphidicolin also blocks the repair of cisplatin-induced DNA damage in human ovarian cancer cell lines in vitro (Masuda et al 1988). When used alone in the ovarian cancer cells, aphidicolin produced a maximal 63% growth inhibition at a concentration of 4 µg/mL for 6 hours (Masuda et al 1988).

In an initial phase I clinical trial, no objective responses were observed in 41 adult patients with a variety of solid tumors (Sessa et al 1991). Similarly, no responses were observed in another European trial of 17 patients pretreated with other chemotherapy (Zucchetti et al 1990).

Mechanism of Action

Aphidicolin produces a reversible inhibition of DNA polymerase α and, to some extent, DNA polymerase Σ (Ikegami et al 1978). This results in near-total blockade of DNA synthesis. The drug appears to interact with an accessory subunit of DNA polymerase α and not with the catalytic subunit (Plevani et al 1980). The other DNA polymerases are not affected by aphidicolin (Ikegami et al 1978). The inhibition of DNA synthesis is competitive with respect to deoxycytidine triphosphates; however, aphidicolin inhibition of DNA is uncompetitive with other individual deoxynucleotide triphosphates (dNTPs) (Oguro et al 1979). Nonetheless, when aphidicolin is added with all four dNTPs (including deoxycytidine triphosphate), competitive enzyme inhibition is observed (Oguro et al 1980).

Aphidicolin binds only to DNA polymerase molecules which themselves have not yet bound dNTP. Notwithstanding this, the drug does not appear to directly bind to the dNTP binding sites on DNA polymerase α. This suggests that aphidicolin binds primarily to the DNA/polymerase complex and not to the free polymerase (Huberman 1981). Such aphidicolin binding sites are found in virtually all eukaryotic cells. They can also be found in the α-like DNA polymerases of some plants (Sala et al 1980) and in the DNA polymerases encoded by the vaccinia and herpes viruses (Pedrali-Noy and

Spadari 1979). Aphidicolin-resistant mammalian cell mutants are known to express increased amounts of DNA polymerase α (Nishimura et al 1979, Sugino and Nakayama 1980).

Aphidicolin reversibly blocks cell cycle traverse in early S phase. Thus, cells are able to progress through the G_1/S boundary but are then halted in early S phase. If the drug is then removed, DNA synthesis can proceed in a population of synchronized cells (Cordeiro-Stone and Kaufman 1985). In contrast, cells in G_2, M, and G_1 phases during aphidicolin exposure continue to progress through the cell cycle (Pedrali-Noy et al 1980).

■ Availability and Storage

Aphidicolin glycinate is investigationally available in vials containing 250 mg of lyophilized powder (ICI Pharmaceuticals, Alderly-Park, Chesire, UK).

■ Preparation for Use, Stability, and Admixture

Aphidicolin is initially reconstituted in 2.5 mL of Sterile Water for Injection, USP, yielding a clear solution that contains 100 mg/mL. This solution is then added to 0.9% sodium chloride to a final concentration of 1 mg/mL for intravenous bolus administration and 0.5 mg/mL for prolonged intravenous infusions.

■ Dosage

In a phase I clinical trial, a maximally tolerated dose of 4500 mg/m² was reported for a 24-hour continuous infusion (Zucchetti et al 1990). The recommended dose was 2250 mg/m²/d for 5 consecutive days (Sessa et al 1991). For planned phase I studies of aphidicolin used to prevent repair of cisplatin DNA damage, an aphidicolin dose of ≥ 3000 mg/m²/24-h infusion was recommended (Sessa et al 1991).

■ Pharmacokinetics

A gas chromatographic assay has been used to study aphidicolin's pharmacokinetic behavior in cancer patients (Rotondo et al 1989). Aphidicolin is rapidly eliminated from the plasma with a terminal half-life of approximately 2 hours.

Pharmacokinetics are not dose related and a two-compartment model appears to adequately describe the disposition of this drug in plasma (Sessa et al 1991; see tables on pages 198 and 199). There is

MEAN PHARMACOKINETICS OF APHIDICOLIN GLYCINATE

Pharmacokinetic Parameter	Mean	SE
Half-life (h)	2	0.2
Clearance (L/m²/h)	59	6
Volume of distribution (L/m²)	160	20
Urinary elimination (% of dose)	<0.1	

*One-hour drug infusion.
Data from Sessa C, Zucchetti M, Davoli E, et al. Phase I and clinical pharmacological evaluation of aphidicolin glycinate. J Natl Cancer Inst. 1991;83(16):1160–1164. Reprinted with permission.

also a proportional increase in the systemic exposure (AUC) with the dose administered, which appears to be independent of the infusion time. The volume of distribution for aphidicolin ranges from 50 ± 5 L/m²/h for a 24-hour infusion to 59 ± 6 L/m²/h for a 1-hour infusion.

Interestingly, the AUC in mice given the LD_{10} (100 mg/kg) was 40.1 μg/mL·h (Zucchetti et al 1990) which is similar to AUCs achieved at a dose of 2000 mg/m² given over 1 or 24 hours.

Other studies have shown that 3-keto-aphidicolin is a major metabolite in humans (Zucchetti et al 1990). Indeed, about half of the renally excreted drug is accounted for as the 3-keto-aphidicolin glucuronide and half as the aphidicolin glucuronide. Overall, less than 0.1% of the intact drug is excreted renally in humans. These findings suggest that biliary secretion of glucuronide conjugates may constitute the major route of aphidicolin elimination in humans.

■ Side Effects and Toxicity

The major dose-limiting toxic effect of 24-hour aphidicolin infusions are local erythema and pain (Sessa et al 1991). These effects are prominent within hours of drug administration and subside after 24 to 48 hours. Fortunately, the local toxic effects did not lead to long-term complications after the 24-hour infusions; however, with the five daily 1-hour infusions, local venous toxicity again predominated. Pain and erythema along the skin overlying the vein were both dose related and dose limiting.

Other effects included dose-related leukopenia which was both mild and reversible. Elevations in liver function enzymes, particularly alkaline phosphatase and serum glutamic–oxalacetic transaminase, were also observed. These effects were reversible and did not appear to be cumulative. One

MEAN APHIDICOLIN PLASMA LEVELS FOR DIFFERENT DOSES AND SCHEDULES

Dose (mg/m^2)	Infusion Time (h)	Number of Patients	Peak or Steady-State Level (μg/mL)	AUC (μg/mL · h)
290	1	3	4.6	4.36
435	1	3	6.1	7.28
435	24	2	0.11–0.4	4.2
650	1	3	5.6	8.87
650	24	2	0.3–0.74	10.64
1000	1	3	7.3	10.3
1000	24	3	0.2–0.9	15.2
1500	1	1	9.9	12.2
2000	24	3	0.9–1.6	32.0
2250	1	3	30.8	62.5
3000	24	3	1.32–3.3	56.2
4500	24	3	4.25–8.0	157.5

Data from Sessa C, Zucchetti M, Davoli E, et al. Phase I and clinical pharmacological evaluation of aphidicolin glycinate. *J Natl Cancer Inst.* 1991;83(16):1160–1164.

patient receiving a first dose of 2250 mg/m^2 as a 1-hour infusion also experienced asymptomatic bradycardia. This worsened on administration of the second dose whereupon dizziness occurred. It was eliminated entirely by switching to a 3-hour infusion in this patient. Of interest, this patient achieved a very high peak plasma level of 63.7 μg/mL after the first dose.

REFERENCES

Bucknall RA, Moores H, Simms R, Hesp B. Antiviral effects of aphidicolin, a new antibiotic produced by *Cephalosporium aphidicol. Antimicrob Agents Chemother.* 1973;4:294–298.

Cordeiro-Stone M, Kaufman DG. Kinetics of DNA replication in C3H 10T1/2 cells synchronized by aphidicolin. *Biochemistry.* 1985;24:4815–4822.

Huberman JA. New views of the biochemistry of eucaryotic DNA replication revealed by aphidicolin, an unusual inhibitor of DNA polymerase α. *Cell.* 1981;23:647–648.

Ikegami S, Taguchi T, Ohashi M, et al. Aphidicolin prevents mitotic cell division by interfering with the activity of DNA polymerase-α. *Nature.* 1978;275:458–460.

Lobbezoo MW, Winograd B, Pinedo HM, Malspeis L, et al. Preclinical drug profile of aphidicolin glycinate (NSC-303812). *Proc Am Assoc Cancer Res.* 1987;28:311 (abstract 1232).

Lonn U, Lonn S. Aphidicolin inhibits the synthesis and joining of short DNA fragments but not the union of 10-kilobase DNA replication intermediates. *Proc Natl Acad Sci USA.* 1983;80:3996–3999.

Masuda H, Ozols RF, Lai GM, et al. Increased DNA repair as a mechanism of acquired resistance to cisdiamminedichloroplatinum(II) in human ovarian cancer cell lines. *Cancer Res.* 1988;48:5713–5716.

Nishimura M, Yasuda H, Ikegami S, et al. Aphidicolin resistant mutant of which DNA polymerase alpha is induced by this drug. *Biochem Biophys Res Commun.* 1979;91:939–945.

Oguro M, Shioda M, Nagano H, Mano Y. The mode of action of aphidicolin on DNA synthesis in isolated nuclei. *Biochem Biophys Res Comm.* 1980;92(1):13–19.

Oguro M, Suzuki-Hori C, Nagano H, et al. The mode of inhibitory action by aphidicolin on eukaryotic DNA polymerase α. *Eur J Biochem.* 1979;97:603–607.

Pedrali-Noy G, Spadari S. Effect of aphidicolon on viral and human DNA polymerases. *Biochem Biophys Res Comm.* 1979;88(4):1194–1202.

Pedrali-Noy G, Spadari S, Miller-Faures A, et al. Synchronization of HeLa cell cultures by inhibition of DNA polymerase α with aphidicolin. *Nucleic Acids Res.* 1980;8(2):377–387.

Plevani P, Badaracco G, Ginelli E, Sora S. Effect and mechanism of action of aphidicolon on yeast deoxyribonucleic acid polymerases. *Antimicrob Agents Chemother.* 1980;18:50–57.

Rotondo S, Zucchetti M, Sessa C, et al. A gas chromatographic mass spectrometric assay for the determination of aphidicolin in plasma of cancer patients. *J Pharm Sci.* 1989;78(5):399–401.

Sala F, Parisi B, Burroni D, et al. Specific and reversible inhibition by aphidicolin of the α-like DNA polymerase of plant cells. *FEBS Lett.* 1980;117(1):93–98.

Sessa C, Zucchetti M, Davoli E, et al. Phase I and clinical pharmacological evaluation of aphidicolin glycinate. *J Natl Cancer Inst.* 1991;83(16):1160–1164.

Starratt AN, Loschiavo SR. The production of aphidicolin by *Nigrospora sphaerica. Can J Microbiol.* 1974;**20**:416–417.

Sugino A, Nakayama K. DNA polymerase alpha mutants from a *Drosophila melanogaster* cell line. *Proc Natl Acad Sci USA.* 1980;**77**:7049–7053.

Zucchetti M, Davoli E, Sulkes A, et al. Pharmacokinetics of aphidicolin (AP) given as a 24-hr continuous infusion (CI). *Proc Am Assoc Cancer Res.* 1990;**31**:180(abstract 1968).

Asaley

■ Other Names

NSC-167780; acetyl-sarcolysin L-leucine.

■ Chemistry

Structure of asaley

The complete chemical name is L-leucine,*N*-[*N*-acetyl-4(bis(2-chloroethyl)amino-DL-phenylalanyl]ethyl ester. Asaley is the leucine amino acid derivative of acetylated melphalan developed in the Soviet Union. The compound has a molecular weight of 488.16 and an empiric formula of $C_{23}H_{35}Cl_2N_3O_4$.

■ Antitumor Activity

Initially, asaley showed activity in animal sarcoma tumor models. It also produced a rough doubling of survival in murine P-388 and L-1210 leukemia models (Zubrod et al 1977). In addition, preclinical activity was observed in sarcoma 180, Walker's carcinosarcoma, and Harding–Passie melanoma. In the Soviet Union, asaley has been evaluated in patients with acute leukemia and solid tumors (Larionov et al 1965). Clinical "response rates" in these trials were 25% in ovarian cancer, 31% in breast cancer, 36% in multiple myeloma, and 43% in "lymphogranulomatosis." No activity was detected in carcinoma of the lung, esophagus, rectum, or stomach. Leukemia trials in the United States showed little activity for asaley. In phase II trials of patients with solid tumors in the United States, partial responses were observed in only 2 of 24 patients with malignant melanoma (Bodey et al 1977). Minimal activity (less than a partial response) was noted in colon cancer, myeloma, breast cancer, and thyroid cancer (Bodey et al 1977). The drug is currently not under active study.

■ Mechanism of Action

Asaley, as a derivative of melphalan, acts by alkylation of DNA, ultimately forming DNA–DNA crosslinks that block cell division. It is a non-cell cycle phase-specific agent and possesses greater activity in cycling cells versus plateau phase tumor cells.

■ Administration and Dose

Asaley was supplied as 250-mg capsules given orally at doses of 600 to 800 mg/m^2/d × 4 (Bodey et al 1977) or 250 to 330 mg/m^2 every other or every day for 18 to 27 days (Zaytseva et al 1971).

■ Side Effects and Toxicity

Toxic effects have included dose-related leukopenia and thrombocytopenia occurring in 80 and 40% of patients, respectively. Gastrointestinal toxicity and central nervous system disturbances were also noted. Central nervous system symptoms included lethargy, mental confusion, and transient focal neurologic signs. In animals the drug was shown to cross the blood–brain barrier and this may explain the central nervous system activity of the drug.

REFERENCES

Bodey GP, Gottlieb JA, Burgess A. Clinical evaluation of asaley. *Med Pediatr Oncol.* 1977;**3**(4):365–371.

Larionov LF, Bukharova JK, Shanayeva YM. Experimental studies of the toxicity and antineoplastic activity of the ethyl ester of acetyl-sarcolysin L-leucine (asaley). *Vopr Onkol (Leningr).* 1965;**11**:78–80.

Zaytseva LA, Borodkina RP, Lapatin PV, Syrkin AB. Antineoplastic effect of asalin and asalay with course-wise and single internal, intramuscular and rectal administration. *Pharmikol Toksikol.* 1971;**4**:460–463.

Zubrod CG, Schepartz SA, Carter SK. The linear array. In: Saunders JF, Carter SK, eds. *Methods of Development of New Anticancer Drugs.* NCI Monograph 45. Washington, DC: Department of Health and Human Services, 1977:13–35.

Asparaginase

■ Other Names

Elspar® (Merck, Sharpe & Dohme Laboratories, Inc); L-asparaginase, EC 3.5.1.1; colaspase; L-ASP; Crasnitin®; L-asnase; L-asparaginase amidohydrolase; NSC-109229 (*Escherichia coli*); *Erwinia* asparaginase (Porton-Down Ltd) (NSC-106997 [*Erwinia*]).

■ Chemistry

Asparaginase is an enzyme (EC 3.5.1.1) isolated from a number of natural sources: *Escherichia coli, Serratia marcescens, Erwinia caratovora,* and guinea pig serum. Clinically useful antitumor enzymes are obtained from the gram-negative bacteria *E. coli* and from the plant parasite *E. caratovora*. Preparations from these sources have a specific activity of 300 to 600 IU/mg protein (Ho et al 1969). The active enzyme has a molecular weight of 144,000 to 141,000 (Maita and Matsuda 1980). The isoelectric point is 4.9 to 5.6 for the *E. coli* enzyme, and numerous aspartic acid residues are present. The active structure has four subunits each with one active site per molecule (Jackson et al 1969). Each subunit has a molecular weight of approximately 34,080 (*E. coli*) or 32,000 (*E. carotovora*). The international L-asparaginase unit denotes enzyme activity sufficient to release 1 μmol of ammonia in 1 minute under the sodium borate buffer test conditions.

An investigational formulation of L-asparaginase covalently conjugated to polyethylene glycol (PEG-LA, Enzon, Inc, South Plainfield, NJ) has also been evaluated (Muss et al 1990).

■ Antitumor Activity

Asparaginase is officially indicated for the induction treatment of acute lymphocytic leukemia, and is conventionally used in combination with other cytotoxic drugs (Jones et al 1977). Occasional responses have also been noted in malignant melanoma (Oettgen et al 1968), chronic myelocytic leukemia, acute myelocytic leukemia (Ohnuma et al 1970), and some non-Hodgkin's lymphomas (Haskell et al 1969). The polyethylene glycol conjugate of L-asparaginase is also active in non-Hodgkin's lymphoma (Muss et al 1990). Antitumor activity has also been observed with asparaginase in central nervous system leukemia in a murine system (Burchenal et al 1970) and clinically in humans (Tallal et al 1970).

L-Asparaginase has specifically been found to lack activity in pancreatic carcinoma (Lessner et al 1980). Interestingly, L-asparaginase may increase the therapeutic activity of methotrexate in breast

```
                          10                            20                            30
Leu-Pro-Asn-Ile-Thr-Ile-Leu-Ala-Thr-Gly-Gly-Thr-Ile-Ala-Gly-Gly-Gly-Asp-Ser-Ala-Thr-Lys-Ser-Asn-Tyr-Thr-Ala-Gly-Lys-Val-
                          40                            50                            60
Gly-Val-Glu-Asn-Leu-Val-Asn-Ala-Val-Pro-Gln-Leu-Lys-Asp-Ile-Ala-Asn-Val-Lys-Gly-Glu-Gln-Val-Val-Asn-Ile-Gly-Ser-Gln-Asp-
                          70                            80                            90
Met-Asn-Asp-Asp-Val-Trp-Leu-Thr-Leu-Ala-Lys-Lys-Ile-Asn-Thr-Asp-Cys-Asp-Lys-Thr-Asp-Gly-Phe-Val-Ile-Thr-His-Gly-Thr-Asp-
                          100                           110                           120
Thr-Met-Glu-Glu-Thr-Ala-Tyr-Phe-Leu-Asp-Leu-Thr-Val-Lys-Cys-Asp-Lys-Pro-Val-Met-Val-Gly-Ala-Met-Arg-Pro-Ser-Thr-Ser-Met-
                          130                           140                           150
Ser-Ala-Asp-Gly-Pro-Phe-Asn-Leu-Tyr-Asn-Ala-Val-Thr-Ala-Ala-Asp-Lys-Ala-Ser-Ala-Asn-Arg-Gly-Val-Leu-Val-Met-Asn-Asp-Thr-
                          160                           170                           180
Val-Leu-Asp-Gly-Arg-Asp-Val-Thr-Lys-Thr-Asn-Thr-Thr-Asp-Val-Ala-Thr-Phe-Lys-Ser-Val-Asn-Tyr-Gly-Pro-Leu-Gly-Tyr-Ile-His-
                          190                           200                           210
Asp-Gly-Lys-Ile-Asp-Tyr-Gln-Arg-Thy-Pro-Ala-Arg-Lys-His-Thr-Ser-Asp-Thr-Pro-Phe-Asp-Val-Ser-Lys-Leu-Asn-Glu-Leu-Pro-Lys-
                          220                           230                           240
Val-Gly-Ile-Val-Tyr-Asn-Tyr-Ala-Asn-Ala-Ser-Asp-Leu-Pro-Ala-Lys-Ala-Leu-Val-Asp-Ala-Gly-Tyr-Asp-Gly-Ile-Val-Ser-Ala-Gly-
                          250                           260                           270
Val-Gly-Asp-Gly-Asn-Leu-Tyr-Lys-Thr-Val-Phe-Asp-Thr-Leu-Ala-Thr-Ala-Ala-Lys-Asp-Gly-Thr-Ala-Val-Arg-Ser-Ser-Arg-Val-Pro-
                          280                           290                           300
Thr-Gly-Ala-Thr-Thr-Gln-Asp-Ala-Glu-Val-Asp-Asp-Ala-Lys-Tyr-Gly-Phe-Val-Ala-Ser-Gly-Thr-Leu-Asn-Pro-Gln-Lys-Ala-Arg-Val-
                          310                           320
Leu-Leu-Gln-Ala-Leu-Thr-Gln-Thr-Lys-Asp-Pro-Gln-Gln-Ile-Gln-Gln-Ile-Phe-Asn-Gln-Tyr
```

Amino acid sequence of asparaginase

cancer by reducing methotrexate-induced myelotoxicity (Yap et al 1979) (see Drug Interactions also).

■ Mechanism of Action

Asparaginase is an enzyme that acts indirectly to inhibit protein synthesis in certain tumor cells dependent on exogenous asparagine, a nonessential amino acid in humans. Although normal cells generally possess the ability to synthesize most amino acids including asparagine (Capizzi et al 1971), some tumors such as most acute lymphoblastic leukemia do not have this capacity and, therefore, require exogenous asparagine. Asparaginase hydrolyzes asparagine in the bloodstream to aspartic acid and ammonia, thereby depriving the tumor cells of a required amino acid. Circulating glutamine levels are also reduced (Miller et al 1969, Capizzi et al 1971). The binding constant (k_M) for asparaginase is about 1×10^{-5} M for *E. coli* asparaginase (Jackson and Handschumacher 1970). The D-isomer has 10% or less of the activity of the L-isomer in this capacity. Enzymatic activity results in liberation of a free amine from asparagine during the formation of an enzyme–aspartyl intermediate (Liu and Chabner 1982). This is followed by hydrolytic cleavage to free L-aspartate and active enzyme. Asparagine-dependent protein synthesis is thereby interrupted, which inhibits tumor cell proliferation. Protein synthesis is rapidly halted with delayed inhibition of DNA and RNA synthesis. The inhibitory activity is maximal in the postmitotic (G_1) phase of the cell cycle. In sensitive cells, cell death occurs rapidly.

Tumor cell resistance to L-asparaginase involves an increase in L-asparagine synthetase activity (Haskell and Canellos 1969, Horowitz et al 1968). Likewise, cells resistant to L-asparaginase have high intrinsic asparagine synthetase activity (Haskell and Canellos 1969).

■ Availability and Storage

Asparaginase is provided in 10,000-IU vials as lyophilized caked materials from two natural sources, *E. coli* (commercial preparation) and *Erwinia* (investigational preparation). It should be stored between 0 and 5°C, if possible, or under refrigeration. Commercial asparaginase is obtained from the active EC-2 enzyme derived from *E. coli*. Enzymes derived from *E. caratovora* are available investigationally for patients with allergic reactions to *E. coli* asparaginase. The commercial product (10,000 IU) also contains 80 mg mannitol per vial and possesses a specific activity of at least 225 IU/mg (Product Information, Elspar, Merck, Sharpe & Dohme, 1978).

Erwinia asparaginase obtained from *E. carotovora* is investigationally available from the National Cancer Institute in 10,000-IU 2-mL vials containing 0.6 mg sodium chloride and 20 mg dextrose with a specific activity of 700 to 850 IU/mg of protein.

■ Preparation for Use, Stability, and Admixture

The contents of each vial should be diluted with approximately 2 to 5 mL of nonpreserved normal saline or sterile water. For intramuscular injections a maximum volume of 2 mL should be used for individual injections at separate sites. Vigorous agitation of the reconstituted vials can result in a significant loss of potency, up to 20% after 1 hour of mechanical shaking (Department of Health and Human Services 1970). In common practice, however, this amount of agitation would be highly unlikely. After reconstitution, no loss in potency has been noted after storage for 1 week at room temperature. The reconstituted drug may appear as either a clear or a slightly cloudy solution; however, care must be taken to ascertain that gross precipitation, noted occasionally with D5W or saline, has not occurred. Further dilutions in physiologic saline or dextrose are relatively stable at room temperature (Trissel 1977).

The Porton (*Erwinia*) product is stable for 4 years under refrigeration and 2 years at room temperature. Once reconstituted at concentrations up to 35 IU/mL, it is stable for 20 days under refrigeration or at room temperature.

The manufacturer of the commercial product, however, recommends storage for only 8 hours after reconstitution, as a bacteriostatic preservative is not present. Additionally, asparaginase should not be infused through a final filter because of potential physicochemical binding to the filter material.

■ Administration

The reconstituted drug may be given intramuscularly or by infusion. For intravenous applications a slow push over at least 30 minutes is recommended. Because the drug is derived from a gram-negative bacteria it can contain foreign, potentially antigenic proteins. Various types of allergic reactions have been reported, including life-threatening, anaphylactic-type reactions. This type of reaction can occur in up to 20% of patients treated with asparaginase;

therefore, facilities should be available for resuscitation and support.

Several series have noted that the severe, anaphylactoid reactions are less common when asparaginase is administered intramuscularly (Nesbit et al 1979). In one report severe reactions were noted in 6 of 15 children following intravenous injection versus 0 of 9 children following intramuscular injections (Lobel et al 1979). An alternative explanation for this phenomenon is that absorption after intramuscular injection is slower, resulting in a delayed onset of symptomatology and less severe acute reactions. Therefore, prolonged monitoring has been recommended after intramuscular asparaginase (Spiegel et al 1980). A maximal 2-mL volume is recommended for intramuscular injections. When severe hypersensitivity reactions occur, it is recommended that the *Erwinia* preparation be used along with the prophylactic administration of antihistamines and/or subcutaneous epinephrine in oil.

■ Special Precautions

Reactive antibodies can be detected in the absence of plasma asparaginase activity; however, skin test reactivity does not predict hypersensitivity reactions in all individuals. Antibodies apparently occur more frequently in adults than in children (28–79% versus 16–25%, respectively) (Killander et al 1976). Hypersensitivity reactions also appear to be more common when plasma asparaginase activity is decreasing. Dialysis with extracorporeal perfusion with asparaginase has also been used, but this is a highly technical experimental remedy to prevent systemic exposure to the drug and subsequent anaphylaxis (Pralle and Loffler 1977).

Skin testing before asparaginase administration is recommended by the manufacturer. The intradermal skin test (a 0.1-mL solution containing 2.0 IU in normal saline) is given at least a week after the last asparaginase dose, and the patient is observed for wheal or flare formation for at least 1 hour. Hypersensitivity reactions may, however, still occur despite a negative skin test (Ohnuma et al 1970). Test doses of 50 IU are also common (Evans et al 1982).

The intradermal test solution is prepared by performing a 1:100 dilution of a stock 10,000-IU vial diluted with 5 mL of unpreserved saline (0.1 mL of stock solution added to 9.9 mL of saline diluent). Of interest, Ohnuma et al (1970) have incidentally observed that a noticeable fall in plasma asparagine levels occurs after similar test doses of 0.2 IU/kg.

Desensitization is rarely used currently. One desensitization regimen calls for administering an initial intravenous unit and then double the dose at 10-minute intervals as long as no toxicity occurs. This escalation continues until the desired total daily dose has been given (Clarkson et al 1970).

The crossover anaphylactoid reaction rate (*E. caratovora*) in children is about 25% and a few will react to the first dose of *Erwinia* asparaginase (Evans et al 1982). Importantly, only a few "sensitive" patients reacted to the intravenous 50-IU test dose, but all reactions ensued within 30 minutes of administration. Fortunately, fatal reactions are rare if careful monitoring and rapid treatment are performed. Limited the duration of L-asparginase therapy to 10 days may also lessen the incidence of anaphylactic reactions (Rausen et al 1979).

■ Dosage

Asparaginase is not indicated for use as a sole induction agent in leukemia. When given alone, doses of 200 IU/d for 28 days have produced very short remissions (Clarkson et al 1970, Haskell et al 1969, Zubrod 1970). Thus, it is incorporated into various combination drug regimens. In pediatric acute lymphocytic leukemia, asparaginase 1000 IU/kg/d IV × 10 days is typically started on day 22 after prednisone and vincristine. Another scheme calls for 6000 IU/m^2/d IM for nine injections every third day, starting the fourth day after cytotoxic therapy (Ortega et al 1977).

High-dose intramuscular regimens have been associated with high response rates in previously treated children with ALL. Doses of 12,000 IU/m^2 three times weekly resulted in a 63% response rate in one trial (Ertel et al 1979). The addition of 6-mercaptopurine (75 mg/m^2 PO) was felt to significantly reduce hypersensitivity reactions which occurred in only 6.5% of patients.

Sutow et al (1976) found that different dosing schedules, such as a continuous daily regimen (for 5 days) or intermittent 5-day pulses, produced comparable response rates in childhood leukemia. The three doses used in this study were 6000, 2000, and 500 IU/m^2. Pratt et al (1970) found that 20,000 IU/m^2 given intravenously as a single dose per week produced less toxicity and equivalent therapeutic effects than a schedule consisting of 4000 IU IV daily for 14 doses. In this study, treatment with asparaginase for longer than 2 weeks was not beneficial.

Peg-Asparaginase. The dose of the polyethylene glycol–L-asparaginase preparation used in studies to date was 2000 U/m² given by intramuscular injection every 2 weeks (Muss et al 1990 [see Special Applications]).

■ Drug Interactions

Asparaginase significantly affects cellular protein synthesis, resulting in a number of drug interactions (see table). In experimental murine systems, asparaginase with methotrexate has shown both therapeutic antagonism (Connors and Jones 1970, Capizzi et al 1970a, b) and synergism (Capizzi et al 1972). The result of the interaction is apparently schedule dependent (Vadlamudi et al 1973). Specifically, separating the administration of methotrexate and that of asparaginase by 9 to 10 days (the duration of asparaginase-induced depressed protein synthesis) has a sound theoretical basis. The report by Lobel et al (1979) confirms such schedule-dependent therapeutic synergy. These investigators additionally suggest that asparaginase, through protein inhibition, may attenuate methotrexate's toxicity without ameliorating its antileukemic activity. This has also been noted by others (Capizzi et al 1970b, 1975, Yap et al 1979). The mechanism for this observation involves inhibition of protein synthesis which may reduce the polyglutamation of methotrexate needed for drug retention intracellularly (Jolivet et al 1985).

Antitumor synergism was shown to be dependent on concomitant therapy in the cytarabine–asparaginase combination regimen used in a murine leukemia model by Avery and Roberts (1973). Additive neurotoxicity can be produced with concomitant vincristine. Administration of L-aspariginase after vincristine VCR may lessen this effect. Similarly, enhanced hyperglycemia may occur with concomitant prednisone therapy. In this regard it is important to note that L-asparaginase transiently inhibits insulin synthesis. This could contribute to hyperglycemia from clinical drug regimens involving prednisone. Insulin therapy may be needed in these situations. Hemostatic complications can result from the decrease in coagulation factors by L-asparaginase combined with the thrombocytopenic effects of cytotoxic agents (Pui et al 1983).

■ Pharmacokinetics

After intravenous administration there is minimal distribution of asparaginase out of the vascular compartment. This probably relates to its large molecular size and highly ionized state at physiologic conditions. Studies in dogs have shown the following pattern of minimal distribution to other tissues (expressed as a percentage of simultaneous intravenous levels): 25% in thoracic lymph fluid, 6% in bile fluid, and 1% in cerebrospinal fluid (Ho et al 1971). Thus, the apparent volume of distribution is only slightly larger than plasma volume. Also, an immunologic response (with production of binding antibody) may account for the apparent wide spectrum of individual responses and pharmacokinetics seen with the enzyme. Additionally, Ohnuma et al (1970) showed that rapid plasma clearance of enzyme occurred with the development of an immunologic reaction.

After intravenous injection, initial drug levels appear to be dose related. Peak intramuscular asparaginase levels have been found to be approximately half those of equivalent intravenous doses (Schwartz et al 1970). Ho et al (1971) found that only minimal urinary and biliary excretion occurs.

In an earlier study, Ho et al (1970) reported that individual asparaginase half-lives varied from 8 to 30 hours, and daily dosing produced cumulative plasma level increases. Within an individual, however, the half-life remained constant. There is apparently no correlation of asparaginase disposition kinetics with drug level, age, sex, body mass, or renal or hepatic function. Haskell et al (1969) described a biphasic elimination: the initial half-life was 4 to 9 hours, whereas the terminal half-life was 1.4 to 1.8

CLINICAL DRUG INTERACTIONS WITH L-ASPARAGINASE

Agent	L-Asparaginase Schedule	Effect
Cytarabine	Concomitant	Synergistic antitumor activity
Methotrexate	9–10 days before or just after methotrexate	Reduced toxicity
Prednisone	Concomitant	Augmented hyperglycemia
6-Mercaptopurine and/or prednisone	Concomitant	Reduced hypersensitivity to L-asparaginase
Vincristine	Before or concomitant with methotrexate	Additive or enhanced neurotoxicity

days. Rapid binding of enzyme to peri- and intravascular binding sites was also noted in this study. Thus, the enzyme appears to be very slowly and unpredictably cleared from the plasma, with exceptionally poor extravascular tissue penetration. In the blood, however, levels of active enzyme are detectable 13 to 22 days after intravenous dosing in humans (Ohnuma et al 1970). There is also some suggestion that hepatic sequestration of drug by the reticuloendothelial system may be a major means of elimination (Cooney and Handschumacher 1970).

■ Side Effects and Toxicity

Hypersensitivity reactions are common with asparaginase. They occur in 20 to 35% of patients. They can be life threatening but are usually mild, producing only urticarial eruptions. The latter are sometimes controlled with antihistamines (Capizzi et al 1970a). Anaphylactoid symptoms from asparaginase reactions include laryngeal constriction, hypotension, diaphoresis, edema, asthma, and loss of consciousness. Because anaphylactoid reactions are common, medical personnel and life-support equipment should be readily available whenever the drug is given. Other symptoms include fever, aches, and chills. It should be remembered that the incidence of anaphylactoid reactions increases with each subsequent drug administration. Bivalent antibodies to the enzyme are commonly produced during therapy (Killander et al 1976), but there is only a general correlation of antibody presence to anaphylaxis. Both, however, occur more commonly after repeated doses and in older populations. Likewise, intradermal skin testing offers only a general but not completely reliable method for predicting severe immunologic reactions (Ohnuma et al 1970).

The incidences of hypersensitivity reactions are equivalent for *E. coli*- and *E. caratovora*-derived enzyme (Dellinger and Miale 1976). Zubrod (1970) noted two deaths from the *E. coli* preparation in 300 patients treated. Although antibodies to the enzyme are commonly found, they do not predict toxic reactions. Most serious hypersensitivity reactions tend to occur after several doses have been administered; however, anaphylactic reactions have also been noted with the first dose (Mathe et al 1970). Again, the two enzyme preparations are usually not cross-reactive and thus may be substituted for one another when hypersensitivity to one product develops (Dellinger and Miale 1976).

Other effects include the potential for a slight degree of immunosuppression as detected by in vitro measurements (Capizzi et al 1970a). Bone marrow suppression is not usually significant with asparaginase. Thus, even though a slight anemia may occur, serious leukopenia or thrombocytopenia is rare (Haskell et al 1969).

Gastrointestinal complaints include malaise, anorexia, and generally mild nausea and vomiting. Some weight loss may also occur possibly as a result of asparaginase-induced hepatic toxicity. Hepatic complications are common with asparaginase. Several liver function tests may be abnormally elevated beginning within the first 2 weeks of treatment, including bromsulphalein retention, serum glutamic–oxalacetic transaminase, bilirubin, and alkaline phosphatase (Oettgen et al 1970). Liver biopsies performed during these periods characteristically demonstrate fatty hepatocellular metamorphosis (Pratt and Johnson 1971). Hepatic protein synthesis is also generally depressed and hypoalbuminemia may occasionally be severe. This may rarely produce massive anasarca (Capizzi et al 1970a). Similarly-depressed proteins include cholesterol-carrying proteins (which may lead to hypercholesterolemia) and the hepatically derived clotting factors: prothrombin, fibrinogen, and factors V, VII, VIII, and IX (Ramsay et al 1977). Antithrombin III levels are also depressed by asparaginase (Liebman et al 1982). Severe bleeding, however, is uncommon with asparaginase (Whitecar et al 1970, Ramsay et al 1977). Fortunately, disseminated intravascular coagulation is also rare with L-asparaginase and fibrinogen survival times are typically normal. Furthermore, fibrinogen, which is synthesized in the presence of L-asparaginase, does not have an abnormal rate of catabolism (Alving et al 1984).

Renal complications are rare and usually associated with other serious toxic effects; however, frank oliguric renal failure has been observed (Haskell et al 1969).

Pancreatic lesions have been observed, including manifestations of endocrine and exocrine dysfunction, and may reflect a drug-induced acute pancreatitis. In children, a latent onset of pancreatitis may be noted (Weetman and Baehener 1974); however, because of protein synthesis depression, amylase and lipase may be normal (Haskell et al 1969). Insulin is usually effective in controlling hyperosmotic, nonketotic hyperglycemia (Capizzi et al 1970a, Falletta et al 1972). Diabetic ketoacidosis has been noted in children and at least one fatality has been reported (Land et al 1972). Of note, hyperamylasemia can result from an elevation in salivary amylase (Adams et al 1985). Thus, not all L-asparaginase-induced hyperamylasemia is due to pancreatitis.

Central nervous system toxicity has occurred principally in adults treated with asparaginase. Lethargy and somnolence are the most common symptoms of central nervous system toxicity; however, frank coma is not a rare occurrence (Haskell et al 1969). Electroencephalographic changes are characteristically noted during toxic periods (Moure et al 1970). Ohnuma et al (1970) found a high incidence of mild to moderate brain dysfunction, often delayed in onset for up to 1 week and lasting up to 1 month. Disorientation, confabulation, easy suggestability, and loss of recent memory were noted in this study.

Although asparaginase does not appear to cross into the central nervous system, cerebrospinal fluid levels of both asparagine and glutamine have been noted to decrease after intravenous dosing (Capizzi et al 1970a). This is probably due to the creation of a central nervous system–blood asparagine concentration gradient.

"Asparagine rescue" infusions have been successfully used to reverse serious drug-induced acute brain dysfunction syndromes (Ohnuma et al 1970). Doses of asparagine used were 1 to 2 mmol/kg/24 h given by continuous infusion for 5 days.

Fatalities from asparaginase have been reported as a result of severe pancreatitis and hepatic complications (Land et al 1972) and hypersensitivity reactions (Mathe et al 1970, Zubrod 1970).

Teratogenic effects have also been noted in pregnant rabbits treated with asparaginase (Adamson 1968), but confirmatory human data are lacking.

■ Special Applications

Intrathecal asparaginase has been administered to patients with acute lymphoblastic leukemia and central nervous system involvement (Tan and Oettgen 1969, Tallal et al 1970). The first study used doses of 100 to 5000 IU daily which were generally well tolerated. Intraventricular administration has also been used to produce higher cerebrospinal fluid asparaginase levels in the central nervous system. Once in the central nervous system, asparaginase is rapidly transported to the plasma and, after 24 hours, cerebrospinal fluid drug activity is negligible (Schwartz et al 1970). Intrathecal asparaginase, however, has not demonstrated clinical superiority over conventional central nervous system radiotherapy and chemotherapy regimens.

Modified L-Asparaginase Products. L-Asparaginase has been chemically modified to eliminate glutaminase activity present in some *E. coli* preparations and to reduce the immunogenicity of the preparation. The latter effect has been achieved by adding multiple poly DL-alanine side-chain polymers (n = 14–334) to the enzyme. This does not significantly change the enzymatic activity of the drug, but increases the half-life sevenfold and renders the molecule resistant to tryptic degradation (Uren and Ragin 1979). Conjugation of the enzyme to dextran or polyethylene glycol (PEG) similarly reduces the immunogenicity of the complex (Abuchowski et al 1979). This results in prolonged stability and enhanced antitumor efficacy at least for the polyethylene glycol preparation (Abuchowski et al 1984). A copolymer of L-asparaginase with albumin is also markedly less antigenic in experimental settings (Yasura et al 1981).

The PEG–L-asparaginase preparation (Enzon Inc) has shown activity in non-Hodgkin's lymphoma (Muss et al 1990). In preclinical systems this modified L-asparaginase has an extended plasma half-life of 2 to 3 weeks and exhibits minimal immunogenicity (Bendich et al 1982, Abuchowski et al 1979). This preparation produces typical side effects but gastrointestinal toxic effects may be more severe. These consist of protracted nausea and vomiting, diarrhea, and abdominal pain (Muss et al 1990). An increased partial thromboplastin time and a 50% or greater decrease in fibrinogen without bleeding have also been observed. In addition, central nervous system toxicity (confusion, somnolence) has been reported. Fatigue and weakness have been observed in one third of patients. A moderate degree of leukopenia occurred but only a few patients had transient elevations in hepatic transaminase enzyme levels. In adult patients with lymphoma, tumor lysis has also occurred.

Other novel applications include conjugation of L-asparaginase to fixed matrices such as hollow-fiber dialysis tubing (Mazzola and Vecchio 1980) and to acrylamide microspheres (Edman et al 1987).

Intraarterial L-asparaginase has been investigationally administered via the hepatic artery at a dose of 20,000 IU/d for 7 to 10 days in adults with insulinomas.

REFERENCES

Abuchowski A, Kago G, Verhoest C, et al. Cancer therapy with chemically modified properties of polyethylene glycolasparaginase conjugates. *Cancer Biochem Biophys.* 1984;**7**:175–186.

Abuchowski A, Van Es T, Palczuk NC, et al. Treatment of L5178Y tumor-bearing BDF mice with a nonimmunogenic L-glutaminase L-asparaginase. *Cancer Treat Rep.* 1979;**63**:1127–1132.

Adams LJ, Antonow DR, Ash R, McClain CJ. Salivary hyperamylasemia after L-asparaginase therapy. *Cancer Treat Rep.* 1985;**69**(12):1437–1438.

Adamson RH. Antitumor activity and other biological properties of L-asparaginase: A review. *Cancer Chemother Rep.* 1968;**52**:617.

Alving BM, Barr CF, Tang DB. L-Asparaginase: Acute effects on protein synthesis in rabbits with normal and increased fibrinogen production. *Blood.* 1984;**63**(4):823–827.

Avery T, Roberts D. Combination chemotherapy with cytosine arabinoside L-asparaginase and 6-azuridine for transplantable murine leukemias. *Cancer Res.* 1973;**33**:791–799.

Bendich A, Kafkewitz D, Abuchowski A, Davis FF. Immunological effects of native and polyethylene glycol-modified asparaginases from *Vibrio succinogenes* and *Escherichia coli* in normal and tumor-bearing mice. *Clin Exp Immunol.* 1982;**48**:273–278.

Burchenal JH, Bevenisti D, Dollinger M. Experimental studies with L-asparaginase in mouse leukemias. *Recent Results Cancer Res.* 1970;**33**:102.

Capizzi RL. Improvement in the therapeutic index of methotrexate (NSC-740) by L-asparaginase NSC-10922. *Cancer Chemother Rep.* 1975;**6**:37–41.

Capizzi RL, Bertino JR, Handschumacher RE. L-Asparaginase. *Annu Rev Med.* 1970a;**21**:2433–2444.

Capizzi RL, Bertino JR, Steel RT, et al. L-Asparaginase: Clinical biochemical, pharmacological and immunological studies. *Ann Intern Med.* 1971;**24**:893–901.

Capizzi RL, Nichols R, Millis J. Long-term survival of leukemic mice by therapeutic synergism between asparaginase (A'Ase) and methotrexate (MTX). *Fed Proc.* 1972;**31**:553.

Capizzi RL, Summers WP, Bertino JR. Antagonism of the antineoplastic effect of methotrexate (MTX) by L-asparaginase or L-asparagine deprivation. *Proc Am Assoc Cancer Res.* 1970b;**11**:14.

Clarkson B, Krakoff I, Burchenol J, et al. Clinical results of treatment with *E. coli* L-asparaginase in adults with leukemia, lymphoma and solid tumors. *Cancer.* 1970;**25**:279–305.

Connors TA, Jones M. Antagonism of the anti-tumor effects of asparaginase by methotrexate. *Biochem Pharmacol.* 1970;**19**:2927–2929.

Cooney DA, Handschumacher RE. L-Asparaginase metabolism. *Annu Rev Pharmacol.* 1970;**10**:421–440.

Dellinger Ct, Miale TD. Comparison of anaphylactic reactions to asparaginase derived from *Escherichia coli* and from *Erwinia* cultures. *Cancer.* 1976;**38**:1843–1846.

Department of Health and Human Services. *Investigational Drug Pharmaceutical Data Sheet: L-Asparaginase, NSC-109220, and NSC-106977.* Washington, DC: Pharmaceutical Resources Branch, Division of Cancer Treatment, National Cancer Institute.

Edman P, Artursson P, Bjork E, et al. Immobilized L-asparaginase–L-glutaminase from *Acinetobacter glutaminasificans* in microspheres: Some properties in vivo and in an extracorporeal system. *Int J Pharm.* 1987;**34**:225–230.

Ertel IJ, Nesbit ME, Hammond D, et al. Effective dose of L-asparaginase for induction of remission in previously treated children with acute lymphocytic leukemia: A report from Childrens Cancer Study Group. *Cancer Res.* 1979;**39**:3893–3896.

Evans WE, Tsiatis A, Rivera G, et al. Anaphylactoid reactions to *Escherichia coli* and *Erwinia* asparaginase in children with leukemia and lymphoma. Cancer. 1982;**49**:1378–1383.

Falletta JM, Steuba CP, Hayes JW, et al. Nonketotic hyperglycemia due to prednisone (NSC-10023) following ketotic hyperglycemia due to L-asparaginase (NSC-109229) plus prednisone. *Cancer Chemother Rep.* 1972;**56**:781–782.

Haskell CM, Canellos GP. L-Asparaginase resistance in human leukemia—Asparagine synthetase. *Biochem Pharmacol.* 1969;**18**:2578–2580.

Haskell CM, Canellos GP, Leventhal BG, et al. L-Asparaginase: Therapeutic and toxic effects in patients with neoplastic disease. *N Engl J Med.* 1969;**281**:1028–1034.

Ho DHW, Carter CJK, Therford B, Frei E III. Distribution and mechanism of clearance of L-asparaginase (NSC 109299). *Cancer Chemother Rep Part I.* 1971;**55**(5):539–545.

Ho PPK, Frank BH, Burck PJ. Crystalline L-asparaginase from *Escherichia coli* B. *Science* 1969;**165**:510–511.

Ho DHW, Therford B, Carter CJK, et al. Clinical pharmacologic studies of L-asparaginase. *Clin Pharmacol Ther.* 1970;**11**:408–417.

Horowitz B, Madras BK, Meister A, et al. Asparagine synthetase activity of mouse leukemia. *Science.* 1968;**160**:533–555.

Jackson RC, Cooney DA, Handschumacher RE. Studies of the catalytic center in L-asparaginase. *Fed Proc.* 1969;**28**:601.

Jackson RC, Handschumacher RE. *Eschericia coli* L-asparaginase. Catalytic activity and subunit nature. *Biochemistry.* 1970;**9**:3585–3590.

Jolivet J, Cole DE, Holcenberg JS, Poplack DG. Prevention of methotrexate cytotoxicity by asparaginase inhibition of methotrexate polyglutamate formation. *Cancer Res.* 1985;**45**:217–220.

Jones B, Holland JF, Glidewell O, et al. Optimal use of L-asparaginase (NSC-109229) in acute lymphocytic leukemia. *Med Pediatr Oncol.* 1977;**3**:387–400.

Killander D, Dohlwitz A, Engstedt L, et al. Hypersensitivity reactions and antibody formation during L-asparaginase treatment of children and adults with acute leukemia. *Cancer.* 1976;**37**:220–228.

Land VJ, Sutow WW, Fernbach DJ, et al. Toxicity of L-asparaginase in children with advanced leukemia. *Cancer.* 1972;**30**:339–347.

Lessner HE, Valenstein S, Kaplan R, et al. Phase II study of L-asparaginase in the treatment of pancreatic carcinoma. *Cancer Treat Rep.* 1980;**64**:1359–1361.

Liebman HA, Wada JK, Patch MJ, McGehee W. Depression of functional and antigenic plasma antithrombin III (AT-III) due to therapy with L-asparaginase. *Cancer.* 1982;**50**:451–456.

Liu YP, Chabner BA. Enzyme therapy: L-Asparaginase. In: Chabner B, ed. *Pharmacologic Principles of Cancer Treatment.* Philadelphia: WB Saunders; 1982:435–443.

Lobel JS, O'Brien RT, McIntosh S, et al. Methotrexate and asparaginase combination chemotherapy in refractory acute lymphoblastic leukemia of childhood. *Cancer.* 1979;**43**:1089–1094.

Maita T, Matsuda G. The primary structure of L-asparaginase from *Escherichia coli. Hoppe Seyler's Z Physiol Chem.* 1980;**361**:105–117.

Mathe G, Amiel JL, Clarysse A, et al. The place of L-asparaginase in the treatment of acute leukemias. Recent results. *Cancer Res.* 1970;**33**:279–287.

Mazzola G, Vecchio G. Immobilization and characterization of L-asparaginase on hollow fibers. *Int J Artif Organs.* 1980;**3**:120–127.

Miller HK, Slaser JS, Balis ME. Amino acid levels following L-asparagine aminohydrolase (EC.3.5.1.1) therapy. *Cancer Res.* 1969;**29**:183–187.

Moure JMB, Whitecar JP, Bodey GP. Electroencephalogram changes secondary to asparaginase. *Arch Neurol.* 1970;**23**:365–368.

Muss HB, Spell N, Scudiery D, et al. A phase II trial of peg-L-asparaginase in the treatment of non-Hodgkin's lymphoma. *Invest New Drugs.* 1990;**8**:125–130.

Nesbit M, Karon M, Chard R, Hammond GD, et al. Evaluation of intramuscular versus intravenous administration of L-asparaginase in childhood leukemia. *Am J Pediatr Hematol Oncol.* 1979;**1**(1):9–13.

Oettgen HF, Old LJ, Boyse EA, Schwartz MK. Therapeutic effects of L-asparaginase on asparagine-dependent neoplasms: Laboratory and clinical studies. *J Clin Invest.* 1968;**47**:74a.

Oettgen HF, Stephenson PA, Schwartz MK, et al. Toxicity of *E. coli* L-asparaginase in man. *Cancer.* 1970;**25**:253–278.

Ohnuma, T, Holland JF, Freeman A, et al. Biochemical and pharmacological studies with asparaginase in man. *Cancer Res.* 1970;**30**:2297–2305.

Ortega JA, Nesbitt ME, Donaldson MH. L-Asparaginase, vincristine and prednisone for induction of first remission in acute lymphocytic leukemia. *Cancer Res.* 1977;**37**:535–540.

Pralle H, Loffler H. Extrakorporal asparaginase therapie bei allergie und toxischen nebenwirkungen. *Blut.* 1977;**35**:179–186.

Pratt CB, Johnson WW. Duration and severity of fatty metamorphosis of the liver following L-asparaginase therapy. *Cancer.* 1971;**28**:361–364.

Pratt CB, Simone JV, Zee P, et al. Comparison of daily versus weekly L-asparaginase for the treatment of childhood acute leukemia. *J Pediatr.* 1970;**77**(3):474–483.

Pui C-H, Jackson CW, Chesney C, et al. Sequential changes in platelet function and coagulation in leukemic children treated with L-asparaginase, prednisone, and vincristine. *J Clin Oncol.* 1983;**1**(6):380–385.

Ramsay NKC, Coccia PF, Krivit W, et al. The effect of L-asparaginase on plasma coagulation factors in acute lymphoblastic leukemia. *Cancer.* 1977;**40**:1398–1401.

Rausen AR, Cuttner J, Glidewell O, et al. Superiority of L-asparaginase combination chemotherapy in advanced acute lymphocytic leukemia of childhood. Randomized comparative trial of combination verus solo therapy. *Cancer Clin Trials.* 1979;**2**:137–144.

Schwartz MK, Lash ED, Oettgen HF, Tomao FA. L-Asparaginase activity in plasma and other biological fluids. *Cancer.* 1970;**25**:244–252.

Spiegel RJ, Echelberger CK, Poplack DG. Delayed allergic reactions following intramuscular L-asparaginase. *Med Pediatr Oncol.* 1980;**8**:123–125.

Sutow WW, George S, Lowman JT, et al. Evaluation of dose and schedule of L-asparaginase in multidrug therapy of childhood leukemia. *Med Pediatr Oncol.* 1976;**2**:387–395.

Tallal L, Tan C, Oettgen H, et al. *E. Coli* asparaginase in the treatment of leukemia and solid tumors in 131 children. *Cancer.* 1970;**25**:306–320.

Tan C, Oettgen H. Clinical experience with L-asparaginase administered intrathecally. *Proc Am Assoc Cancer Res.* 1969;**10**:92.

Trissell LA. *Handbook on Injectable Drugs.* Washington, DC: American Society of Hospital Pharmacists; 1977:408.

Uren JR, Ragin RC. Improvement in the therapeutic, immunological, and clearance properties of *E. coli* and *Erwinia carotovora* L-asparaginase by attachment of poly-DL-alanyl peptides. *Cancer Res.* 1979;**39**:1927–1933.

Vadlamudi S, Krishna B, Redd B, Goldin A. Schedule-dependent therapeutic synergism for L-asparaginase and methotrexate in leukemic (L51784) mice. *Cancer Res.* 1973;**33**:2014–2019.

Weetman RM, Baehener RL. Latent onset of clinical pancreatitis in children receiving L-asparaginase therapy. *Cancer.* 1974;**34**:780–785.

Whitecar JP Jr, Bodey GP, Harris JE, et al. L-Asparaginase. *N Engl J Med.* 1970;**282**:732–734.

Yap H-Y, Benjamin RS, Blumenschein GR, et al. Phase II study with sequential L-asparaginase and methotrexate in advanced refractory breast cancer. *Cancer Treat Rep.* 1979;**63**(1):77–83.

Yasura T, Kamisaki Y, Wada H, et al. Immunological studies on modified enzymes. I. Soluble L-asparaginase/mouse albumin copolymer with enzyme activity and substantial loss of immunosensitivity. *Int Arch Allergy Appl Immunol.* 1981;**64**:11–18.

Zubrod CG. The clinical toxicities of L-asparaginase in treatment of leukemia and lymphoma. *Pediatrics.* 1970;**45**:555–559.

5-Azacytidine

■ Other Names

NSC-102816; 5-AC; 4-amino-1-β-D-ribofuranosyl-1,3,5-triazine-2(1*H*)-one; Mylosar®.

■ Chemistry

Structure of 5-azacytidine

5-Azacytidine has an empiric formula of $C_8H_{12}N_4O_5$ and a molecular weight of 244. Structurally, 5-azacytidine is a ring analog of the natural pyrimidine nucleoside cytidine, differing only by a nitrogen instead of the number 5 carbon (Bergy and Herr 1966).

■ Antitumor Activity

In humans, significant activity has generally been limited to acute myelogenous leukemia (Karon et al 1973, McCredie et al 1973, Von Hoff et al 1976), with lesser activity observed in acute lymphocytic leukemia. A comprehensive review of 5-azacytidine has been published by Glover et al (1987).

No significant activity has been noted in patients with a variety of human solid tumors, including breast, lung, and colorectal tumors (Moertel et al 1972). It similarly lacked substantial activity in chronic myelogenous leukemia (McCredie et al 1973), multiple myeloma, and melanoma.

Saiki et al (1978) have demonstrated significant activity in patients with acute leukemia only when administered intravenously over a 5-day period. With every-8-hour dosing, the response rate was 24% as a single agent. Bolus dosing was ineffective, and the drug appeared to lack any activity in acute lymphoblastic leukemias.

More recently 5-azacytidine has continued to demonstrate single-agent activity as well as activity when used in combination with other agents (eg etoposide) in relapsed leukemic patients (Gaynon and Baum 1983, Kalwinsky et al 1983, 1986). Of particular note is the combination of 5-azacytidine and mitoxantrone, which has demonstrated significant activity in patients with chronic myelogenous leukemia in accelerated phase and blast crisis (6 complete responses and 2 partial responses in 40 patients) (Dutcher et al 1989).

■ Mechanism of Action

As a pyrimidine ring analog (antimetabolite) 5-azacytidine probably acts by interfering with nucleic acid metabolism. Its primary mechanism of action is not well established. Several mechanisms have been proposed with documentation supporting each. 5-Azacytidine is incorporated into both RNA and DNA (Zadrazil et al 1965) and thereby interferes with protein synthesis (Paces et al 1968). 5-Azacytidine and its phosphorylated metabolite have shown activity in blocking the production of cytidine and uridine (Vadlamudi et al 1970). It competes for incorporation into nucleic acids where it acts as a false pyrimidine. Both messenger RNA and transfer RNA containing 5-azacytidine are structurally and functionally inhibited, and therefore do not allow normal protein synthesis to occur. Additionally, DNA formed in the presence of 5-azacytidine is less stable and more susceptible to breakage (Zadrazil et al 1965). Although 5-azacytidine appears to have some activity in all phases of the cell cycle, its activity seems to be maximal in S phase (Li et al 1970).

A unique feature of 5-azacytidine activity is reduced methylation of DNA, which can induce the expression of otherwise repressed genes. This may relate to the inability of incorporated 5-azacytidine to be methylated because of inhibition of methyltransferase enzymes (Friedman 1981). This effect has been experimentally used to induce the expression of fetal hemoglobin and other normally repressed embryonic or fetal gene products (Jones et al 1983).

■ Availability and Storage

5-Azacytidine is supplied as a white lyophilized powder in 30-mL vials containing 100 mg of drug with an equal amount of mannitol. The undiluted drug is stable for at least 2 years if stored under refrigeration, preferably between 4 and 10°C. Storage at room temperature (22–25°C) for 2 years has not altered the chemical potency; however, degradation rapidly ensues at higher temperatures.

■ Preparation for Use, Stability, and Admixture

Vials are reconstituted with 19.9 mL sterile water for injection, resulting in a clear solution of pH 6.0 to 7.5 containing 5 mg of drug and 5 mg mannitol per milliliter. The aqueous stability of 5-azacytidine is relatively short (decomposition half-life at 40°C = 4.4 hours; therefore the initial dilution should be used within 30 minutes by further dilution into Ringer's lactate solution. At room temperature this provides for optimal pH (about 6.2–6.5) and temperature conditions, and 90% potency is thus maintained for 14 to 15 hours (decomposition half-life [20°C] = 94–100 hours [Israili et al 1976]).

Dilution in nonbuffered media or admixture with highly acidic or basic drugs would greatly accelerate degradation and is contraindicated. It is therefore recommended that dilution be done in Ringer's lactate only and that a new solution be prepared every 8 hours for continuous-infusion regimens. A chemical degradation scheme is reported by Notari and De Young (1975).

■ Administration

5-Azacytidine has been given by intravenous push, subcutaneously, and by intravenous infusion. Pharmacokinetic behavior and toxicity tend to favor more frequent administration. Drug levels are not drastically different after subcutaneous administration, and the drug is relatively nonirritating. Optimally, all doses should be prepared immediately before use and discarded after 8 hours. Any convenient volume of lactated Ringer's solution may be used as a vehicle to deliver the dose. For subcutaneous doses, a dilution of 3 mL/50 to 100 mg of drug has been successfully used (Bellet et al 1974).

For intravenous dosing, continuous infusion is preferred. Both Vogler et al (1975) and Lomen et al (1975) have noted much less gastrointestinal toxicity with continuous dosing. Intravenous push administration as used by McCredie et al (1973) is not currently recommended; however, subcutaneous dosing offers a reasonable alternative when vein access is a serious problem.

■ Special Precautions

See stability data given earlier.

■ Drug Interactions

Neil et al (1974) have shown a schedule-dependent synergism for azacitidine given 10 hours after cytarabine in experimental mouse L-1210 leukemia. Human data have additionally demonstrated a lack of cross-resistance for the two similar drugs (McCredie et al 1973). Experimentally, 5-azacytidine is also synergistic with emetine in L-1210 leukemia.

■ Dosage

In acute myelogenous leukemia, doses of 100 to 250 mg/m^2 biweekly, 150 to 400 mg/m^2/d × 5 days IV and continuous 5- to 10-day infusions have demonstrated approximately equivalent remission rates (Von Hoff et al 1976). Subcutaneous doses of 275 to 850 mg/m^2 (total) given over 10 days are recommended for patients with solid tumors (Bellet et al 1974). McCredie et al (1973) used 400 mg/m^2 given as a 15- to 30-minute intravenous push in 50 to 200 mL of D5W (note that this was before the instability of the drug in D5W was noted). Maintenance subcutaneous doses ranged from 35 to 90 mg/m^2/wk in the study of Bellet et al (1974).

Saiki et al (1978) have evaluated three different regimens of 5-azacytidine administration in acute leukemia. In that study, clinical responses were noted only after administration of 300 mg/m^2 daily doses either as a divided fraction every 8 hours or as a continuous infusion, both given for 5 consecutive days. No responses were noted when a single 750 mg/m^2 bolus injection was given every 2 to 3 weeks. Of great interest would be an attempt at greater dose escalations with the currently available new antiemetic and bone marrow support regimens.

■ Pharmacokinetics

Troetel et al (1972) studied the pharmacokinetics of radiolabeled 5-azacytidine after both subcutaneous and intravenous administration. Subcutaneous doses gave peak levels at 0.5 hour, equilibrated with the initially higher intravenous levels by 2 hours, and thereafter remained equal. Thus, subcutaneous drug is absorbed rapidly and fairly efficiently. Subcutaneously administered drug showed less urinary drug recovery with a plasma half-life of 3.5 hours. This was comparable to a plasma half-life after intravenous dosing of 4.2 hours. Higher tumor and normal tissue drug levels were also produced with intravenous doses, and traces of radioactivity were still present 6 days after dosing.

Israili et al (1974, 1976) noted a multiphasic plasma decline, a volume of distribution less than that of body water, and 24-hour urinary recovery of more than 90% of the administered dose. A cerebrospinal fluid/plasma ratio less than 0.1 was noted, although drug binding to albumin was not observed. Fecal excretion appears to be negligible.

■ Side Effects and Toxicity

Hematologic toxicity is most often dose limiting and dose related, occurring significantly in about a third of the patients treated. With a daily schedule in solid tumors, the nadir for leukopenia is about 25 days (Moertel et al 1972). It is slightly longer with 10-day continuous infusions, also seen with subcutaneous regimens. Occasionally, prolonged leukopenia may be seen in patients with leukemia (Von Hoff et al 1976).

Thrombocytopenia, also dose dependent, is more unusual, occurring in less than 20% of those treated, with a nadir and duration comparable to those of leukopenia; however, Bellet et al (1974) reported two deaths from thrombocytopenia. Severe anemia has generally not been a problem.

Gastrointestinal toxicity (nausea, vomiting, and diarrhea) may be very severe with most 5-azacytidine regimens. Both Vogler et al (1975) and Lomen et al (1975) showed substantially reduced toxicity for continuous infusions over intravenous or subcutaneous pulse dosing. Nonetheless, a high incidence is manifest. Symptoms generally ensue 1 to 3 hours after injection, clear in 3 to 4 hours, and recur with subsequent doses. Bellet et al (1974) achieved some control with moderate doses of antiemetics administered prophylactically and also noted that tolerance to the nausea and vomiting developed rapidly; by day 10 patients required no prophylaxis. The use of more recently developed antiemetics (eg metoclopramide or andansetron) has not been explored.

Hepatic toxicity thought to be caused by the drug is a rare but serious complication. Bellet et al (1974) noted that 5 of 22 patients developed deterioration in liver function studies. In three of those patients frank hepatic coma and death ensued. These patients were older and had received extensive prior chemotherapy and had a significant hepatic tumor burden. Based on these data, the administration of 5-azacytidine has been contraindicated in patients with hepatic metastases and/or serum albumin values below 3 g 100 mL and/or serum glutamic–oxalacetic transaminase above 120 IU/mL (Bellet et al 1973).

Neurologic complications, although rare (2.7%), also appear to be dose dependent and are characterized by a slow onset of generalized muscle pain, weakness, and lethargy (Levi and Wiernik 1975).

Other toxic effects include a transient fever during and up to 24 hours after drug administration. Hypotension, a pruritic drug rash, and stomatitis have also been noted.

Rhabdomyolysis (Koeffler and Haskell 1978) and profound symptomatic hypophosphatemia (Ho et al 1976) may also occur with 5-azacytidine. Both syndromes are characterized by severe muscle pain and tenderness. The exact mechanism of these effects is not known. In the latter syndrome, excess phosphate elimination did not occur and serum phosphate levels returned to normal without the need for replacement therapy.

■ Special Applications

5-Azacytidine has been used to treat patients with sickle cell anemia. Early uncontrolled trials of 5-azacytidine seem to indicate that treated patients have increased levels of fetal hemoglobin along with decreased anemia and fewer vaso-occlusive sickle cell crises (Dover and Charache, 1987a, b).

REFERENCES

Bellet RE, Mastrangelo MJ, Engstrom PF, Custer RP. Hepatotoxicity of 5-azacytidine (NSC-102816) (a clinical and pathologic study). *Neoplasma (Bratisl.)* 1973;**20**:303–309.

Bellet RE, Mastrangelo MJ, Engstrom PF, Strawitz JG, Weiss AJ, Yarbro JW. Clinical trial with subcutaneously administered 5-azacytidine (NSC-102816). *Cancer Chemother Rep.* 1974;**58**:217–222.

Bergy ME, Herr RR. Microbiological production of 5-azacytidine. II. Isolation and chemical structure. *Antimicrob Agents Chemother.* 1966;**6**:624–630.

Dover GJ, Charache S. Increasing fetal hemoglobin production in sickle cell disease: Results of clinical trials. *Prog Clin Biol Res.* 1987a;**251**:455–466.

Dover GJ, Charache S. The effect of increased fetal hemoglobin production on the frequency of vaso-occlusive crisis in sickle cell disease. *Prog Clin Biol Res.* 1987b;**240**:277–285.

Dutcher JP, Wiernik PH, Arlin Z, et al. Mitoxantrone and 5-azacytidine for patients with accelerated or blast crisis PH1 + chronic myeloid leukemia (meeting abstract). *Proc Ann Meet Am Soc Clin Oncol.* 1989;**8**:205.

Friedman S. The inhibition of DNA (cytosine-5)methylases by 5-azacytidine. The effect of azacytosine-containing DNA. *Mol Pharmacol.* 1981;**19**:314–320.

Gaynon PS, Baum ES. Continuous infusion of 5-azacytidine as induction for acute nonlymphocytic leukemia in patients with previous exposure to 5-azacytidine. *Oncology.* 1983;**40**(3):92–94.

Glover AB, Leyland-Jones BR, Chun HG, Davies B, Hoth DF. Azacitidine: 10 years later. *Cancer Treat Rep.* 1987;**71**(7–8):737–746.

Ho M, Bear RA, Garvey MB. Symptomatic hypophosphatemia secondary to 5-azacytidine therapy of acute nonlymphocytic leukemia. *Cancer Treat Rep* 1976;**60**:1400–1402.

Israili ZH, Vogler WR, Mingioli ES, Pirkle JL, Smithwick RW, Goldstein JH. Studies of the disposition of 5-azacytidine-^{14}C in man. *Pharmacologist.* 1974;**16**:231.

Israili ZH, Vogler WR, Mingioli ES, Pirkle JL, Smithwick RW, Goldstein JH. The disposition and pharmacokinetics in humans of 5-azacytidine administered intravenously as a bolus or by continuous infusion. *Cancer Res.* 1976;**36**:1453–1461.

Jones PA, Taylor SM, Wilson SV. DNA modification, differentiation and transformation. *J Exp Zool.* 1983;**228**:287–295.

Kalwinsky D, Dahl G, Look T, Mirro J, Simone J. AML-80: An intensive therapy regimen for childhood acute myeloid leukemia (AML). *Proc Am Soc Clin Oncol* 1983;**2**:C664.

Kalwinsky DK, Dahl BF, Mirro J, Jackson CW, Look AT. Induction failures in childhood acute nonlymphocytic leukemia: Etoposide/5-azacytidine for cases refractory to daunorubicin/cytarabine. *Med Pediatr Oncol.* 1986;**14**(5):245–250.

Karon M, Sieger L, Leimbrock S, Finklestein J, Nesbit M, Swaney J. 5-Azacytidine: A new active agent for the treatment of acute leukemia. *Blood.* 1973;**42**:359–365.

Koeffler HP, Haskell CM. Rhabdomyolysis is a complication of 5-azacytidine (letter). *Cancer Treat Rep.* 1978;**62**(4):573–574.

Levi JA, Wiernik PH. A comparative study of 5-azacytidine and guanazole in previously treated adult acute non-lymphocytic leukemia. *Cancer Chemother Rep.* 1975;**59**:1043–1045.

Li LH, Olin EJ, Fraser TJ, Bhuylan BK. Phase specificity of 5-azacytidine against mammalian cells in tissue culture. *Cancer Res.* 1970;**30**:2770–2775.

Lomen, Pave L, Baker LH, Neil GL, Samson MK. Phase I study of 5-azacytidine (NSC-102816) using 24-hour continuous infusion for 5 days. *Cancer Chemother Rep Part 1.* 1975;**59**:1123–1126.

McCredie KB, Bodey GP, Burgess MA, et al. Treatment of acute leukemia with 5-azacytidine (NSC-102816). *Cancer Chemother Rep.* 1973;**57**:319–323.

Moertel CG, Schutt AJ, Reitemeier RJ, Hahn RG. Phase II study of 5-azacytidine (NSC-102816) in the treatment of advanced gastrointestinal cancer. *Cancer Chemother Rep.* 1972;**56**:649–652.

Neil GL, Gray LG, Berger AE. Combination chemotherapy of L1210 leukemia with cytarabine and 5-azacytidine-temporal aspects (abstract). *Pharmacologist.* 1974;**16**:209.

Notari RE, De Young JL. Kinetics and mechanisms of degradation of anti-leukemic agent 5-azacytidine in aqueous solutions. *J Pharm Sci.* 1975;**64**:1148–1156.

Paces V, Doskocil J, Sorm F. Incorporation of 5-azacytidine into nucleic acids of *Escherichia coli. Biochim Biophys Acta.* 1968;**161**:352–360.

Saiki JH, McCredie KB, Vietti RJ, et al. 5-Azacytidine in acute leukemia. *Cancer.* 1978;**42**:2111–2114.

Troetel WM, Weiss AJ, Stambaugh JE. Absorption, distribution, and excretion of 5-azacytidine (NSC-102816) in man. *Cancer Chemother Rep.* 1972;**56**:405–411.

Vadlamudi S, Choudry JN, Waravdekar VS, Kline I, Goldin A. Effect of combination treatment with 5-azacytidine and cytidine on the life span and spleen and bone marrow cells of leukemic (L1210) and non-leukemic mice. *Cancer Res.* 1970;**30**:362–369.

Vogler WR, Miller D, Keller JW. Remission induction in refractory myeloblastic leukemia with continuous infusion of 5-azacytidine (abstract). *Proc Am Assoc Cancer Res.* 1975;**16**:155.

Von Hoff D, Slavik M, Muggia F. 5-Azacytidine—a new anticancer drug with effectiveness in acute myelogenous leukemia. *Ann Intern Med.* 1976;**85**(2):237–245.

Zadrazil S, Fucik V, Bartl P, Sormova Z, Sorm F. The structure of DNA from *Escherichia coli* cultured in the presence of 5-azacytidine. *Biochim Biophys Acta.* 1965;**108**:701–703.

Azathioprine

■ Other Names

Imuran®; BW-57-322 (Burroughs Wellcome).

■ Chemistry

Structure of azathioprine

Azathioprine is the 1-methyl-4-nitro-5-imidazolyl derivative of 6-mercaptopurine. It has a molecular weight of 277.29 and an empiric formula of

$C_9H_7N_7O_2S$. The complete chemical name is 6-[(1-methyl-4-nitro-1H-imidazol-5-yl)thio]-1H-purine.

■ Antitumor Activity

Azathioprine is officially indicated in the prevention of renal transplant graft rejection. It is also used as an immunosuppressant in a variety of "autoimmune" diseases, including regional and ulcerative colitis, chronic active hepatitis and biliary cirrhosis, rheumatoid arthritis, systemic lupus erythematosus, glomerulonephritis and nephrotic syndrome, and certain skin lesions (Rosman and Bertino 1973).

In human malignancies, azathioprine has shown limited utility in the treatment of multiple myeloma (Woodruff 1981) and has demonstrated activity in patients with acute leukemia (Rundles et al 1961). Other tumors may also occasionally respond to azathioprine (Elion et al 1961).

■ Mechanism of Action

Azathioprine was originally synthesized by Hitchings and Elion in 1961 to block the rapid oxidation and methylation of 6-mercaptopurine. The primary cytotoxic mechanism of action involves the substitution of active metabolites into biosynthetic reactions which block de novo purine synthesis. This ultimately halts DNA synthesis and RNA synthesis. Cytotoxicity is afforded by close chemical similarity of the main metabolite of azathioprine (mercaptopurine) to physiologic purine bases. The agent can thus act as a "false" purine or an antimetabolite. With azathioprine there is an initial reduction of the sulfur linkage to the nitroimidazole moiety. This liberates 6-mercaptopurine. The process can be mediated nonenzymatically by sulfhydryl compounds including glutathione. There is subsequent activation of the metabolite to the ribonucleotide form which can substitute in RNA or DNA for the normal RNA or DNA bases guanine, adenine, and hypoxanthine (Hitchings and Elion 1972). Purine biosynthesis is thereby halted, and resultant DNA and RNA synthesis is impaired.

The activity of azathioprine probably is greatest in S phase of the cell cycle.

■ Availability and Storage

The drug is available commercially (Burroughs Wellcome, Research Triangle Park, NC) as an oral 50-mg tablet and investigationally as the sodium salt injection containing 100 mg of lyophilized drug in a 20-mL vial. Both may be stored at room temperature.

Oral. The oral formulation of azathioprine is available as a light-sensitive yellow powder that is insoluble in water and alcohol. The molecule is stable under neutral or acidic conditions; however, the imidazolyl group can be cleaved under alkaline conditions to yield free 6-mercaptopurine.

Injectable. The investigational injectable formulation is supplied as the sodium salt with a resultant water solubility sufficient to allow a 1.0% solution. On prolonged storage at room temperature for 72 weeks, free mercaptopurine is produced. Free 6-mercaptopurine can also be produced by exposure of the parent compound to sulfhydryl-containing compounds such as glutathione, cysteine, and hydrogen sulfide.

■ Preparation for Use, Stability, and Admixture

The investigational injection is prepared by the addition of 10 mL of sterile water for injection to each vial. The vials are then gently swirled to obtain a clear solution. This solution has a pH of 9.6 and 2-week stability at room temperature; however, the manufacturer recommends use within 24 hours of reconstitution.

For infusion, the stock solution may be further diluted in normal saline or D5W. Data on stability and compatibility with other diluents or drugs are not available; however, the infusion is stable for at least 24 hours at room temperature and light conditions. Addition of the drug to an alkaline medium could allow hydrolysis of azathioprine to the active metabolite mercaptopurine. Admixture to any solution with an alkaline pH should therefore be avoided.

■ Administration

Intravenous doses may be given by slow intravenous push or by continuous infusion. Vein patency should be ensured with a 5- to 10-mL flush of normal saline or D5W before or after administration.

■ Special Precautions

The dose should be reduced to one third to one fourth of the usual dose if allopurinol is concomitantly administered. There is also a general recommendation to reduce doses in patients with liver dysfunction (Kaplan and Calabresi 1973). Azathioprine is also reported to inhibit its own hepatic metabolism in vivo (Kaplowitz and Kuhlenkamp 1978). In addition, dose reduction in patients with renal dysfunction is recommended since a large fraction of a dose is excreted intact in the urine as 6-mercaptopurine (see Dosage). There is one report of decreased elimination of azathioprine metabolites in a patient with severe renal insufficiency (Bach and Dardenne 1971).

■ Dosage

In a single multiple myeloma study, daily doses of 300 mg orally were given each morning before breakfast.

Azathioprine, however, is generally not used as an anticancer agent. For immunosuppression, initial doses recommended by the manufacturer range from 3 to 5 mg/kg/d both orally and intravenously. Subsequently 1 to 2 mg/kg/d is recommended as a maintenance dose. Repeat dosing should be based on hematologic status and renal function. With anuria the plasma half-life increases from 3 to as long as 50 hours, thereby necessitating dosage reduction commensurate with the degree of renal impairment. One source has suggested that when creatinine clearance reaches the range 10 to 50 mL/h, the dosing interval be increased to 24 to 36 hours. At a creatinine clearance of 7 to 10 mL/h the dosing interval should be increased to 24 to 48 hours (Clarysse and Mathe 1976).

■ Drug Interactions

With concurrent allopurinol administration, the dose of azathioprine must be reduced to one fourth or one third of the usual dose. Patients with renal failure frequently have hyperuricemia and receive allopurinol so that extra care must be taken with these patients when administering azathioprine.

Azathioprine can inhibit cyclic AMP phosphodiesterase and may thereby alter the effects of adrenergic or other agents on neuromuscular transmission (Dretchen et al 1976). The neuromuscular blockade produced by nondepolarizing blockers (eg, curariform agents) is inhibited by azathioprine. In contrast the neuromuscular blockade produced by succinylcholine may be enhanced.

■ Pharmacokinetics

The oral formulation of azathioprine is reported to be well absorbed; however, only 50% of a radiolabeled oral dose appears in the urine 24 hours after dosing. A peak level of 1 to 2 µg/mL was achieved 2 hours after oral dosing in one patient. After intravenous injection, the drug is rapidly cleared from the plasma. Little intact drug is excreted in the urine, and hepatic metabolism is significant for both formulations.

The major metabolite of azathioprine is 6-mercaptopurine, formed from cleavage of the imidazolyl group by sulfhydryl compounds. Less than 10% of a dose is metabolized to an inactive sulfur derivative. A very small fraction of a dose may also be converted to an 8-hydroxy derivative by aldehyde oxidase (Chalmers 1975). With normal renal function, the half-life of the drug is reported to be 3 hours; with anuria, a half-life of up to 50 hours is described. Approximately 30% of a dose is protein bound; however, both free drug and metabolites can be effectively hemodialyzed.

For a more in-depth discussion of the primary metabolite of azathioprine, see 6-Mercaptopurine.

■ Side Effects and Toxicity

Hematologic suppression is the usual dose-limiting toxic effect. This manifests as leukopenia, thrombocytopenia, and anemia (Rundles et al 1961). The anemia seen with long-term dosing appears to be dose related and has been associated with macrocytosis and megaloblastic changes (McGrath et al 1975). These effects may occur independently of and precede neutropenia. The bone marrow suppressive effects of azathioprine can persist days or weeks after the drug is discontinued.

Gastrointestinal effects are not common at low doses. Vomiting and diarrhea are common at higher doses. Oral ulceration and, rarely, rashes, fever, and serum sickness are also reported.

Pulmonary complications with long-term therapy are also reported. Rubin et al (1972) described a single case of acute restrictive lung disease in a young patient taking 100 mg/d. After drug cessation, there was steady resolution of respiratory function to normal.

Hepatic toxicity with jaundice has also been noted including both hepatocellular and cholestatic types. Zarday et al (1972) reported a case of irreversible liver damage in a young female renal transplant patient on chronic azathioprine (3 mg/kg/d). Therefore, liver function tests should be periodically performed while a patient is on the drug.

Pancreatitis is also an occasional complication of azathioprine when combined with prednisone (Herskowitz et al 1979) or with azathioprine alone (Paloyan et al 1977). This has usually required immediate drug discontinuance. Acute renal failure is also described following azathioprine although it was felt to be due to a hypersensitivity reaction (Sloth and Thomsen 1971).

Other toxic effects include alopecia, retinopathy, and arthalgia.

Carcinogenic and teratogenic changes are well documented with long-term, continuous administration of azathioprine. In animal models, azathioprine is a well-documented carcinogen (Cohen et al 1983). Thus, the incidence of malignancy, especially lymphoma, is much higher in transplant patients receiving the drug (Penn and Starzl 1972). The incidence of cerebral lymphoma and acute myeloid leukemia appears to be markedly enhanced.

Azathioprine is also known to damage chromosomes (Van Went 1979). Nonetheless, several successful pregnancies have been reported after continuous azathioprine therapy throughout the pregnancy (Erkman and Blythe 1972). There are also anecdotal reports of successful impregnation by azathioprine-treated males. Chromosomal aberrations, however, as a result of the drug are documented and should be kept in mind in this discussion (Jensen 1970).

Infectious complications of therapy include disseminated viral diseases, such as measles, cytomegalovirus, and chicken pox, and diffuse bacterial, fungal, or protozoal diseases (eg, *Pneumocystic carinii*). Thus, opportunistic infection is highly likely while on azathioprine. *Pseudomonas aeruginosa* infection is one such documented complication (Steinberg et al 1972).

REFERENCES

Bach JF, Dardenne M. Metabolism of azathioprine in renal failure. *Transplant.* 1971;**12**(4):253–259.

Chalmers AH. A spectrophotometric method for the estimation of urinary azathioprine, 6-mercaptopurine and 6-thiouric acid. *Biochem Med.* 1975;**12**:234.

Clarysse A, Mathe G. Malignant diseases. In: Avery GS, ed. *Drug Treatment*. Boston: Publishing Sciences Group, Inc; 1976:973.

Cohen SM, Erturk E, Skibba JL, Bryan GT. Azathioprine induction of lymphomas and squamous cell carcinomas in rats. *Cancer Res.* 1983;**43**:2768–2772.

Dretchen KL, Morgenroth VH III, Standaert FG, et al. Azathioprine: Effects on neuromuscular transmission. *Anesthesiology.* 1976;**45**:604.

Elion G, Callahan S, Bieber S, et al. A summary of investigations with 6-(1-methyl-4-nitro-γ-imidazolyl)thio purine (BW 57-322). *Cancer Chemother Rep.* 1961;**14**:93–98.

Erkman J, Blythe JG. Azathioprine therapy complicated by pregnancy. *Obstet Gynecol.* 1972;**40**(5):708–710.

Herskowitz LJ, Olansky S, Lang PG. Acute pancreatitis associated with long-term azathioprine therapy. *Arch Dermatol.* 1979;**115**:179.

Hitchings GH, Elion GB. Purine analogues. In: Brodsky L. Moyer JH, Kahn SB, eds. *Cancer Chemotherapy II, Twenty-Second Hahneman Symposium*. New York: Grune and Stratton; 1972:23–32.

Jensen MK. Effect of azathioprine on the chromosome complement of human bone marrow cells. *Int J Cancer.* 1970;**5**:147–151.

Kaplan SR, Calabresi P. Immunosuppressive agents. *N Engl J Med.* 1973;**289**:1234.

Kaplowitz N, Kuhlenkamp J. Inhibition of hepatic metabolism of azathioprine in vivo. *Gastroenterology.* 1978;**74**:90.

McGrath BP, Ibels IS, Raik E, et al. Erythroid toxicity of azathioprine. *Q J Med.* 1975;**44**(173):57–63.

Paloyan D, Levin B, Simonowitz D. Azathioprine-associated acute pancreatitis. *Am J Dig Dis.* 1977;**22**(9):839–840.

Penn I, Starzl TE. A summary of the status of de novo cancer in transplant patients. *Transplant Proc.* 1972;**4**:719–732.

Rosman M, Bertino JR. Azathioprine. *Ann Intern Med.* 1973;**79**:694–700.

Rubin G, Baume P, Vandenberg R. Azathioprine and acute restrictive lung disease. *Aust NZ J Med.* 1972;**2**:272–274.

Rundles RW, Laszlo J, Hoge T, et al. Clinical and hematological study of 6-[(1-methyl-4-nitro-5-imidazolyl)thio]-purine (B.W. 57-322) and related compounds. *Cancer Chemother Rep.* 1961;**14**:99–115.

Sloth K, Thomsen AC. Acute renal insufficiency during treatment with azathioprine. *Acta Med Scand.* 1971;**189**:145–148.

Steinberg AD, Plotz PH, Wolff SM, et al. Cytotoxic drugs in the treatment of nonmalignant diseases. *Ann Intern Med.* 1972;**76**:619–642.

Van Went GF. Investigations into the mutagenic activity of azathioprine (Imuran) in different test systems. *Mutat Res.* 1979;**68**:153.

Woodruff R. Treatment of multiple myeloma. *Cancer Treat Rev.* 1981;**8**:225–270.

Zarday Z, Vlith FJ, Getlman ML, et al. Irreversible liver damage after azathioprine. *JAMA* 1972;**222**:690–691.

Bacillus Calmette–Guérin (BCG)

■ Other Names

BCG live (intravesical), TheraCys® (NSC-116341) (Connaught Laboratories); Tice® BCG (NSC-116327) (Organon Inc).

■ Chemistry

Connaught BCG is a freeze-dried suspension of an attenuated strain of *Mycobacterium bovis* (bacillus Calmette-Guérin) that has been grown on a potato and glycerin based medium. Tice® BCG is an attenuated live culture preparation of the BCG strain of *M. bovis*. The Tice strain was developed at the University of Illinois. The strain originated at the Pasteur Institute.

■ Antitumor Activity

Both TheraCys® and Tice® BCG are approved for intravesical treatment of carcinoma in situ of the urinary bladder (Morales et al 1981, Zinche et al 1983, Mori et al 1986, Martinez-Pireiro et al 1990, Badalament et al 1987). TheraCys® is approved for carcinoma in situ with or without associated papillary tumors but is not indicated for the treatment of papillary tumors alone. It is not approved as an immunizing agent to prevent tuberculosis.

In a randomized controlled trial of TheraCys® versus intravesical doxorubicin, TheraCys® was superior to doxorubicin in percentage of complete response (74% versus 42%) and in progressive disease (13% versus 42%). Median time to treatment failure was 48.2 months for the TheraCys® arm and 5.9 months for the doxorubicin arm; however, there was no survival benefit for patients receiving TheraCys.®

Tice® BCG is also indicated for intravesical instillation to treat carcinoma in situ of the bladder (Melekos 1990, Khanna et al 1988, 1990, DeJager et al 1990). Tice® BCG had significantly reduced the need for cystectomies (DeJager et al 1990). Of interest is that the recurrence rate for smokers is greater in patients receiving BCG than it is in non-smokers (Garvin et al 1990). The agent is also indicated for percutaneous use for immunization against tuberculosis. This monograph does not present any of the data for that indication.

In the late 1960s and early 1970s, a flurry of publications indicated that BCG might prevent relapse in patients with leukemia (Mathe et al 1969, Zuhrie et al 1980, Powles 1973, Crowther et al 1973). However, use of BCG for that purpose has not been widely adapted (Vogler et al 1984, Omura et al 1982, Whittaker et al 1980).

Bacillus Calmette–Guérin has been found not to have a salutary effect for patients with ovarian cancer (Alberts et al 1989a, b, Creasman et al 1990), ocular melanoma (Melekos 1990, McLean et al 1990), breast cancer (Crowe et al 1990), non-small cell lung cancer (Millar et al 1982, Roeslin et al 1989), colorectal cancer (Abdi et al 1989, Panettiere et al 1988, Wolmark et al 1988) malignant melanoma (Costanzi et al 1982, Veronesi et al 1982), and malignant lymphoma (Jones et al 1985). A salutary effect of BCG in patients with large cell lymphomas (improved survival) was reported by Jones et al (1983) for the Southwest Oncology Group. Ravaud et al (1990) have demonstrated (in a small trial) that BCG given by scarification may improve survival for patients with clinical stage I and II intermediate and high-grade non-Hodgkin's lymphoma. Slightly improved survival was noted in patients with prostate cancer treated with BCG (Guinan et al 1982).

For the preceding indications, BCG has been given by dermal scarification, intradermal or subcutaneous injection, intrapleural or intraperitoneal injection, and oral or aerosol routes. These routes of administration are not in general use today and will not be covered in this monograph. The reader who is interested in these modes of administration is referred to the first edition of this book.

■ Mechanism of Action

Intravesical BCG promotes an inflammatory reaction in the bladder that is associated with a reduction of carcinoma in situ lesions in the bladder (Morales et al 1981, Zinche et al 1983, Mori et al 1986). The precise mechanism of action is, however, unknown (Mikkelson and Ratliff 1989). Numerous other specific mechanisms have been suggested. These include (1) a "broad-spectrum" nonspecific anamnestic or "recall" immune response to a variety of antigens; (2) a nonspecific inflammatory reaction at injected local tumor sites, facilitating lymphocyte– and macrophage–tumor cell interactions; (3) cross-reactivity of BCG antigens to tumor-associated antigens; (4) augmentation of the phagocytic ability of macrophages; (5) stimulation of simple lymphocytosis; and (6) possible augmentation of a humoral, tumor-cytotoxic system.

■ Availability and Storage

TheraCys® contains 27 mg (dry weight) of BCG per vial ($3.4 \pm 3.0 \times 10^8$ CFU/vial) and 5% monosodium glutamate. There are no preservatives in the vial. The accompanying diluent (1.0 mL) contains 0.85% sodium chloride, 0.025% polysorbate 80, and 0.06% (w/v) sodium dihydrogen phosphate. The diluent also contains no preservatives. The BCG and the diluent must be stored continuously at 2 to 8°C (35 to 46°F) until use. Neither the unentered vial nor the reconstituted solution should be exposed to sunlight. Exposure to artificial light should also be kept to a minimum.

The Tice® BCG is freeze-dried BCG in glass-sealed ampules each of which contains 1 to 8×10^8 CFU of the Tice® BCG equivalent to approximately 50 mg wet weight. No preservatives have been added. Tice® BCG is supplied by Organon in a box of one 2-mL ampule. The intact ampule must be stored at 2 to 8°C and protected from light.

■ Preparation for Use, Stability, and Admixture

Each vial of TheraCys® is reconstituted with the accompanying 1.0 mL of diluent. To prepare for intravesical use, one dose, which consists of three pooled vials of reconstituted material, is further diluted in preservative-free sterile saline. The diluted product should be used immediately after it is reconstituted. The final dose (three reconstituted vials) is further diluted in an additional 50 mL of preservative-free sterile saline for a total of 53 mL. The drug should always be handled as an infectious agent. All persons who handle the drug should wear masks and gloves. (Please see the package insert for other important details in the preparation of the dose.)

Tice® BCG is prepared with gloves, mask, and gown. One milliliter of preservative-free saline (0.9% Sodium Chloride Injection, USP) at 4 to 25°C should be drawn up in a small (3-mL) syringe and added to 1 ampule of Tice® BCG. To make a suspension, the mixture should be carefully barbotaged to ensure mixing. The BCG suspension should be added to 49 mL of saline in a catheter-tip syringe to make a total volume of 50 mL. The suspended material should be used immediately. It should be discarded after 2 hours.

■ Administration

The initial clinical trials with TheraCys® included percutaneous administration of 0.5 mL of BCG (live) solution which was reconstituted in the diluent and further diluted with 50 mL sterile preservative-free saline. This was given along with each intravesical dose. The utility of this additional subcutaneous dose is not certain.

TheraCys® is usually given 7 to 14 days after the biopsy diagnosis of carcinoma in situ. The usual dose is three vials of TheraCys® intravesically under aseptic conditions once a week for 6 weeks. The drug is given through a urethral catheter after the bladder is drained by instilling the 53-mL solution slowly by gravity. After the catheter is withdrawn, the patient should lie on each side, prone, and supine for 15 minutes each. The suspension should be retained for another 60 minutes (a total of 2 hours). The patient can then be allowed to void (in a seated position) and maintain hydration after that. After the usual 6 weeks of induction therapy, a single treatment can be given again at 3, 6, 12, 18, and 24 months after the initial therapy.

Voided urine (up to 6 hours postinstillation) should be disinfected with an equal volume of 5% undiluted household bleach (5% hypochloride) and allowed to work for 15 minutes before flushing.

The techniques for administration of the Tice® BCG are similar to that for TheraCys® (see package insert for details).

In a trial of oral BCG versus intravesical administration, the intravesical route was more effective (D'Ancona et al 1991, Lamm et al 1990).

■ Special Precautions

If the urethral catheterization is felt to be traumatic, the BCG should not be administered for at least 1 week. Also, intravesical BCG should not be given any sooner than 1 week following transurethral resection. After administration, all equipment and material should be treated as biohazards.

Immunocompromised hosts should not be given BCG because of the risk of sepsis from the mycobacterium. This is particularly true for patients who are positive for the human immunodeficiency virus or who are receiving steroids. It should also not be given to patients with a fever or with a urinary tract infection.

Of additional importance is that intravesical administration of BCG can cause conversion of a negative to a positive tuberculosis skin test.

There has been some concern that BCG might promote the formation of second primary tumors (Kendrick and Comstock 1981). These concerns have been disproven by recent studies (Bilik et al 1989).

■ Drug Interactions

Concomitant administration of immunosuppressive agents may block the response to intravesical BCG.

■ Dosage

Please see Administration.

■ Pharmacokinetics

No pharmacokinetic studies have been performed with BCG.

■ Side Effects and Toxicity

Intravesical administration of BCG has been associated with hematuria, urinary frequency, dysuria, and bacterial urinary tract infections. These symptoms may last 1 to 3 days after instillation. Systemic BCG infections with death have also occurred. Disseminated BCG infections may be heralded by a cough. Granulomatous hepatitis has also been observed.

■ Special Applications

There are none besides those already outlined.

REFERENCES

Abdi EA, Hanson J, Harbora DE, Young DG, McPherson TA. Adjuvant chemoimmuno- and immunotherapy in Dukes' stage B2 and C colorectal carcinoma: A 7-year follow-up analysis. *Br J Haematol.* 1989;71(1):161–162.

Alberts DS, Mason-Liddil N, O'Toole RV, et al. Randomized phase III trial of chemoimmunotherapy in patients with previously untreated stages III and IV suboptimal disease ovarian cancer: A Southwest Oncology Group study. *Gynecol Oncol.* 1989a;32(1):8–15.

Alberts DS, Mason-Liddil N, O'Toole RV, et al. Randomized phase II trial of chemoimmunotherapy in patients with previously untreated stage III optimal disease ovarian cancer: A Southwest Oncology Group study. *Gynecol Oncol.* 1989b;32(1):16–21.

Badalament RA, Herr HW, Wong GY, et al. A prospective randomized trial of maintenance versus nonmaintenance intravesical bacillus Calmette–Guérin therapy of superficial bladder cancer. *J Clin Oncol.* 1987;5(3):441–449.

Bilik J, Sosnowski JT, Lamm DL, et al. Comparison of second primaries in bladder tumor patients treated with BCG or doxorubicin: A Southwest Oncology Group study (meeting abstract). *J Urol.* 1989;141(4, p2):333A.

Costanzi JJ, Al-Sarraf M, Groppe C, et al. Combination chemotherapy plus BCG in the treatment of disseminated malignant melanoma: A Southwest Oncology Group study. *Med Pediatr Oncol.* 1982;10(3):251–258.

Creasman WT, Omura GA, Brady MF, Yordan E, DiSaia PJ, Beecham J. A randomized trial of cyclophosphamide, doxorubicin, and cisplatin with or without bacillus Calmette–Guérin in patients with suboptimal stage II and IV ovarian cancer: A Gynecologic Oncology Group study. *Gynecol Oncol.* 1990;39(3):239–243.

Crowe JP Jr, Gordon NH, Shenk RR, et al. Short term tamoxifen plus chemotherapy: Superior results in node-positive breast cancer. *Surgery.* 1990;108(4):281–282.

Crowther D, Powles RL, Bateman CJT, et al. Management of adult acute myelogenous leukemia. *Br Med J.* 1973;1:131–137.

D'Ancona CA, Netto NR Jr, Claro JA, Ikari O. Oral or intravesical bacillus Calmette–Guérin immunoprophylaxis in bladder carcinoma. *J Urol.* 1991;145(3):498–501.

DeJager R, Guinan P, Lamm D, et al. Long-term complete remission in bladder carcinoma *in situ* (CIS) with intravesical Tice bacillus Calmette–Guérin (BCG). *Proc Am Soc Clin Oncol.* 1990;9:135.

Garvin TJ, Fuan JJJ, Ratliff TL, Catalona WJ. The effect of cigarette smoking on bladder cancer response to intravesical bacillus Calmette–Guérin (BCG). *Proc Am Assoc Cancer Res.* 1990;31:187.

Guinan P, Toronchi E, Shaw M, Crispin R, Sharifi R. Bacillus Calmette–Guérin (BCG) adjuvant therapy in stage D prostate cancer. *Urology.* 1982;20(4):401–403.

Jones SE, Grozea PN, Metz EN, et al. Improved complete remission rates and survival for patients with large cell lymphoma treated with chemoimmunotherapy. A Southwest Oncology Group study. *Cancer.* 1983;51(6):1083–1090.

Jones SE, Grozea PN, Miller TP, et al. Chemotherapy with cyclophosphamide, doxorubicin, vincristine, and prednisone alone or with levamisole or with levamisole plus BCG for malignant lymphoma: A Southwest Oncology Group study. *J Clin Oncol.* 1985;3(10):1318–1324.

Kendrick MA, Comstock GW. BCG vaccination and the subsequent development of cancer in humans. *J Natl Cancer Inst.* 1981;66(3):431–437.

Khanna OP, Son DL, Mazer H, et al. Superficial bladder cancer treated with intravesical bacillus Calmette–Guérin or Adriamycin: Follow-up report. *Urology.* 1988;31(4):287–293.

Khanna OP, Son DL, Mazer H, et al. Multicenter study of superficial bladder cancer treated with intravesical bacillus Calmette–Guérin or Adriamycin. *J Clin Oncol.* 1990;8(4):608–614.

Lamm DL, DeHaven JI, Shriver J, Crispen R, Grau D, Sarosdy MF. A randomized prospective comparison of oral versus intravesical and percutaneous bacillus

Calmette–Guérin for superficial bladder cancer. *J Urol.* 1990;**144**(1):65–67.

Martinez-Pireiro JA, Jimenez Leon J, Martinez-Pineiro L Jr, et al. Bacillus Calmette–Guérin versus doxorubicin versus thiotepa: A randomized prospective study in 202 patients with superficial bladder cancer. *J Urol.* 1990;**143**(3):502–506.

Mathe G, Ameil JL, Schwarzenberg L, et al. Active immunotherapy for acute lymphoblastic leukemia. *Lancet.* 1969;**1**:697–699.

McLean IW, Bred D, Mastrangelo MJ, et al. A randomized study of methanol-extraction residue of bacillus Calmette–Guérin as postsurgical adjuvant therapy of uveal melanoma. *Am J Ophthalmol.* 1990;**110**:522–526.

Melekos MD. Intravesical bacillus Calmette–Guérin prophylactic treatment for superficial bladder tumors: Results of a controlled prospective study. *Urol Int.* 1990;**45**(3):137–141.

Mikkelson DJ, Ratliff TL. Mechanisms of action of intravesical bacillus Calmette–Guérin for bladder cancer. *Cancer Treat Res.* 1989;**46**:195–211.

Millar JW, Roscoe P, Pearce SJ, Ludgate S, Horne NW. Five year results of a controlled study of BCG immunotherapy after surgical resection in bronchogenic carcinoma. *Thorax.* 1982;**37**(1):57–60.

Morales A, Ottenhof P, Emerson L. Treatment of residual non-infiltrating bladder cancer with bacillus Calmette–Guérin. *J Urol.* 1981;**125**:649.

Mori K, Lamm DL, Crawford ED. A trial of bacillus Calmette–Guérin versus Adriamycin in superficial bladder cancer: A Southwest Oncology Group study. *Urol Int.* 1986;**41**:254–259.

Omura GA, Vogler WR, Lefante J, et al. Treatment of acute myelogenous leukemia: Influence of three induction regimens and maintenance with chemotherapy or BCG immunotherapy. *Cancer.* 1982;**49**(8):1530–1536.

Panettiere FJ, Goodman PJ, Costanzi JJ, et al. Adjuvant therapy in large bowel adenocarcinoma: Long-term results of a Southwest Oncology Group study. *J Clin Oncol.* 1988;**6**(6):947–954.

Powles R. Immunotherapy of acute myelogenous leukemia in man. *Natl Cancer Inst Monogr.* 1973;**39**:243–246.

Ravaud A, Eghbali H, Trojani M, Hoerni-Simon G, Soubeyran P, Hoerni B. Adjuvant bacillus Calmette–Guérin therapy in non-Hodgkin's malignant lymphomas: Long-term results of a randomized trial in a single institution. *J Clin Oncol.* 1990;**8**(4):608–614.

Roeslin N, Dumont P, Morand G, Wihlm JM, Witz JP. Immunotherapy as an adjuvant to surgery in carcinoma of bronchus. Results in three randomized trials. *Eur J Cardiothorac Surg.* 1989;**3**(5):430–435.

Veronesi U, Adamus J, Aubert C, et al. A randomized trial of adjuvant chemotherapy and immunotherapy in cutaneous melanoma. *N Engl J Med.* 1982;**307**(15):913–916.

Vogler WR, Winton EF, Gordon DS, Raney MR, Go B, Meyer L. A randomized comparison of postremission therapy in acute myelogenous leukemia: A Southeastern Cancer Group trial. *Blood.* 1984;**63**(5):1039–1045.

Whittaker JA, Bailey-Wood R, Hutchins S. Active immunotherapy for the treatment of acute myelogenous leukaemia: Report of two controlled trials. *Br J Haematol.* 1980;**45**(3):389–400.

Wolmark N, Fisher B, Rockette H, et al. Postoperative adjuvant chemotherapy or BCG for colon cancer: Results from NSABP protocol C-01. *J Natl Cancer Inst.* 1988;**80**(1):30–36.

Zinche H, Utz DC, Taylor WF, Myers RP, Leary FJ. Influence of thiotepa and doxorubicin instillation at time of transurethral surgical treatment of bladder cancer on tumor recurrence: A prospective, randomized, double-blind, controlled trial. *J Urol.* 1983;**129**:505–509.

Zuhrie SR, Harris R, Freeman CB, et al. Immunotherapy alone vs no maintenance treatment in acute myelogenous leukaemia. *Br J Cancer.* 1980;**41**(3):372–377.

Baker's Antifol (Soluble)

■ Other Names

NSC-139105; ethanesulfonic acid compound; BAF; triazinate; TZT.

■ Chemistry

Structure of Baker's antifol (soluble)

Baker's antifol (BAF) compound has a molecular weight of 539 and is soluble to the extent of 25 mg/mL in both water and alcohol. The complete chemical is a compound of ethanesulfonic acid with α-[2-chloro-4-(4,6-diamino-2,2-dimethyl-s-triazin-1-(2H)-yl)phenoxy]-N,N-dimethyl-m-toluamid (1:1). It was synthesized by the late Dr. B. R. Baker as a dihydro-s-triazine, active-site-directed inhibitor of dihydrofolate reductase (Baker 1971).

■ Antitumor Activity

In animal studies, BAF was highly effective against ascites carcinoma (Skeel et al 1973), whereas in vitro studies with human cells noted activity similar to that of methotrexate in acute lymphocytic and myelogenous leukemia, melanoma, and breast cancer (Skeel et al 1974). Phase I clinical studies by Rodriguez et al (1976) noted activity in adenocarcinomas of the lung, colon, and breast and in transitional bladder carcinoma. A follow-up phase II study in 138 patients (Rodriguez et al 1977) confirmed slight objective antitumor activity in lung (31 patients) colorectal (25 patients), and renal cell carcinoma (6 patients). Another study of BAF in combination treatment of colorectal cancer detected no advantage over 5-fluorouracil alone. BAF is similarly inactive in acute lymphocytic leukemia in children (Nitschke et al 1978), in recurrent or inoperable head and neck cancer (Krasnow et al 1986), in resistant osteogenic sarcoma in children (Nitschke et al 1981), and in pancreatic cancer (Gastrointestinal Tumor Study Group 1987).

Baker's antifol was active in advanced gastric cancer, producing a 17% response rate among 23 evaluable patients (Bruckner et al 1982). The drug was also active in primary brain cancer when combined with carmustine. Dose-dependent response rates of 20 to 57% were produced in this trial (Eagan et al 1984). The drug also elicited a 6% partial response rate in patients with advanced breast cancer refractory to other agents (Cummings et al 1981).

■ Mechanism of Action

Baker's antifol is a "nonclassic" folic acid antagonist as opposed to "classic" antifolates such as methotrexate. Although both types of antifols have the common target enzyme, dihydrofolic acid reductase, the drugs differ in their transport mechanisms. Methotrexate penetrates cell membranes by active transport using the same transport system used for reduced folic acid metabolites. It was originally thought that BAF also entered cells by passive diffusion. It is currently thought to be taken up by active transport but through a different system than methotrexate. Thus, these drugs may possess different tumor specificity because of different selective transport mechanisms. Baker's antifol is a cell cycle phase-specific agent that acts in S phase. It inhibits DNA synthesis through reversible inhibition of dihydrofolate reductase with a subsequent blockade of thymidylate synthetase.

■ Availability and Storage

The lyophilized powder was investigationally available from the National Cancer Institute in 100 mg/10 mL and 250 mg/mL vials. The intact vials are stable for at least 2 years at room temperature. It is no longer available.

■ Preparation for Use, Stability, and Admixture

When the 100-mg vial is diluted with 5 mL of Sterile Water for Injection, USP, each milliliter contains 20 mg of soluble Baker's antifol and has a pH of 5.0 to 7.0. When the 250-mg vial is diluted with 10 mL of Sterile Water for Injection, USP, each milliliter contains 25 mg of soluble Baker's antifol and has a pH of 6.0 to 7.0.

After reconstitution, the drug is stable for at least 96 hours at room temperature or under refrigeration. The stability is not affected by ultraviolet light or further dilution in D5W or normal saline. As no preservative has been added, it is recommended that the solution be discarded 24 hours after initial reconstitution.

■ Administration

Baker's antifol should be given by intravenous infusion over at least 30 minutes. More rapid infusions have been noted to cause visual disturbances, convulsions, and severe respiratory depression. Thus, the initial reconstitution is usually further diluted in either D5W or normal saline prior to administration. Rodriguez et al (1977) diluted the dose into 100 to 200 mL of D5W and infused the solution over 1 to 2 hours.

■ Dosage

Courses of 100 to 250 mg/m^2 have been administered every day for 3 to 5 consecutive days with repetition at 2- to 3-week intervals (Rodriguez et al 1977). The standard starting dose has been 250 mg/m^2/d for 3 consecutive days with dosage adjustment by response. It is recommended that patients with abnormal liver function receive a decreased dose because of depressed drug elimination, but specific dosing guidelines are not available (Benjamin et al 1975). Single doses of 300 to 600 mg/m^2 infused over 0.5 to 3 hours in adults have caused marked but transient neurologic and respiratory impairment.

■ Special Precautions

Patients with poor renal and liver function or with preexisting dermatologic disease are more likely to develop severe skin toxicity and should receive appropriately reduced doses: 150 mg/m^2/d × 3 (Rodriguez et al 1977).

Pharmacokinetics

Baker's antifol is poorly absorbed orally and produces only 10% of the levels of equivalent intravenous doses. After intravenous administration, the half-life has been reported to be 1.2 to 6 hours. Urinary excretion reported in the first 12 hours varies from 15 to 60%; thus the drug is excreted primarily by the liver. Cerebrospinal fluid levels appear to be 2 to 5% of serum levels; however, a brain tissue analysis in several patients revealed a 1000-fold excess of drug over the serum levels at the same time.

Animal studies demonstrate a biphasic plasma clearance. The drug is concentrated in the liver, kidney, brain, and spleen of experimental animals (Cashmore et al 1975).

In humans, intravenous administration of 300 mg/m^2 produces serum levels of 10^{-5} M or higher for 8 hours. In this study, Skeel et al (1976) showed that urinary excretion of the drug ranged from 12 to 72% of the administered dose at 24 hours. The average amount excreted in the urine was 43% of a dose. Benjamin et al (1975) have described the half-life in normal persons as 5.3 hours, whereas in patients with markedly abnormal liver function the terminal half-life increased to 8.3 hours and the area under the plasma × time curve was fourfold greater.

Side Effects and Toxicity

Gastrointestinal reactions include stomatitis, varying degrees of nausea, vomiting, and diarrhea. The nausea and vomiting are generally mild with Baker's antifol, although occasionally severe diarrhea may occur.

A skin rash occurs in 40% of patients. The rash may progress to exfoliative dermatitis and can be fatal. The rash may develop any time during drug therapy but most commonly appears 1 week after drug administration. Skin rashes are probably the typical dose-limiting toxic effect. A radiation recall skin rash has also been reported. Stomatitis is uncommon with BAF except in patients with liver dysfunction. Symptoms include redness, soreness, and angular stomatitis, but no significant ulceration (Skeel et al 1976). In the pediatric leukemia study of Nitschke et al (1978) skin lesions were the predominant toxic effect. Oral lesions in this study appeared within 5 days and lasted 2 to 8 days.

Neurologic side effects have been reported following high-dose short infusions. Signs and symptoms included respiratory depression, headache, dizziness, somnolence, blurred vision, and weakness (Skeel et al 1976). These symptoms usually disappear rapidly after the dose is administered.

Mild to moderate myelosuppression has been reported. Thrombocytopenia and leukopenia with a nadir on or about the ninth day are typical. Rodriguez et al (1977) noted myelosuppression in 30% of patients treated. Both thrombocytopenia and leukopenia were well tolerated and generally resolved within 5 days in most patients.

All observed side effects and toxic effects are much more common in patients with compromised liver function.

REFERENCES

Baker BR. Active-site directed irreversible inhibitors of dihydrofolate reductase. *Ann NY Acad Sci.* 1971;**186**:214–226.

Benjamin RS, Loo TL, Friedman J, et al. Liver disease and clinical pharmacology of Baker's antifolate BAF, NSC-139105. *Pharmacologist.* 1975;**17**:265.

Bruckner HW, Lokich JJ, Stablein DM. Studies of Baker's antifol, methotrexate, and razoxane in advanced gastric cancer: A Gastrointestinal Tumor Study Group report. *Cancer Treat Rep.* 1982;**66**:1713–1717.

Cashmore AR, Skell RT, Makulu DR. Pharmacology of a new triazine antifolate in mice, rats, dogs and monkeys. *Cancer Res.* 1975;**35**(1):17–22.

Cummings FJ, Gelman R, Skeel RT, et al. Phase II trials of Baker's antifol, bleomycin, CCNU, streptozotocin, tilorone, and 5-fluorodeoxyuridine plus arabinosyl cytosine in metastatic breast cancer. *Cancer.* 1981;**48**:681–685.

Eagan RT, Dinapoli RP, Herman RC Jr, et al. Carmustine and Baker's antifol combination chemotherapy for primary brain tumors progressive after irradiation and chemotherapy. *Cancer Treat Rep.* 1984;**68**(2):431–433.

Gastrointestinal Tumor Study Group. Phase II trials of the single agents Baker's antifol, diaziquone, and epirubicin in advanced pancreatic cancer. *Cancer Treat Rep.* 1987;**71**(9):865–867.

Krasnow S, Green M, Perry DJ, et al. Phase II trial of Baker's antifol in patients with recurrent or inoperable head and neck cancer. *Cancer Treat Rep.* 1986;**70**(8):1039–1040.

Nitschke R, Morgan Sk, Land VJ. Baker's antifol in children with therapy-resistant solid tumors: A Southwest Oncology Group study. *Cancer Treat Rep.* 1981;**65**(7/8):725–727.

Nitschke R, Vietti T, Ragab A, Dyment P. Baker's antifol in children with late-stage acute lymphocytic leukemia. *Cancer Treat Rep.* 1978;**62**(1):2109–2110.

Rodriguez V, Gottlieb J, Burgess MA, et al. Phase I studies with Baker's antifol (BAF) (NSC-139105). *Cancer.* 1976;**38**:690–694.

Rodriguez V, Richman SP, Benjamin RS, et al. Phase 2 study with Baker's antifol in solid tumors. *Cancer Res.* 1977;**37**:980–983.

Skeel RT, Cashmore AR, Sawicki WL. Clinical and pharmacologic evaluation of triazinate in humans. *Cancer Res.* 1976;**36**:48–54.

Skeel R, Rodriguez V, Freireich EJ, Bertino J. Clinical and pharmacological studies of the folate antagonist, triazinate (Baker's antifol TXT). *Proc Am Assoc Cancer Res.* 1974;**15**:77.

Skeel R, Sawicki WL, Cashmore AR, Bertino JR. The basis for the disparate sensitivity of L1210 leukemia and Walker 256 carcinoma to a new triazine folate antagonist. *Cancer Res.* 1973;**33**:2972–2976.

Beta-2'-Deoxythioguanosine

■ Other Names

βTGdr; NSC-71261.

■ Chemistry

Structure of beta-2'-deoxythioguanosine

Beta-2'-doxythioguanosine (βTGdr) is a purine nucleoside analog of 6-thioguanine. Chemically, the drug behaves similarly to thioguanine (6-TG) except for relative acid instability caused by a glycosyl bond (Iwamoto et al 1963). The active pharmacologic form is the β anomer. βTGdr can be easily dissolved in sodium hydroxide but unlike thioguanine is unstable in acid media.

■ Antitumor Activity

Beta-2'-deoxythioguanosine was investigated in a variety of solid tumors and in acute leukemia. In an initial study by Bodey et al (1976) βTGdr demonstrated some activity in leukemia but not in several solid tumors. Others noted slight activity in colorectal carcinoma when combined with semustine (methyl-CCNU) (Brooks et al 1976, Douglass et al 1976). In pancreatic cancer, only 2 of 32 (6%) patients responded to βTGdr (Gastrointestinal Tumor Study Group 1985).

In combination regimens, βTGdr has not added significant antitumor efficacy to standard treatments. The combination of azacitidine followed by βTGdr in adult acute leukemia patients produced a 24% response rate, similar to that of azacitidine alone (Omura et al 1979). Cytarabine also does not improve the response rate to βTGdr in acute leukemia (Bodey et al 1976). Likewise, the combination of βTGdr with mitomycin-C in colorectal cancer produced a 20% response rate compared with 30% for mitomycin-C plus semustine (Gagliano et al 1981).

■ Mechanism of Action

Beta-2'-deoxythioguanosine is an antimetabolite similar to thioguanine that is incorporated into DNA, ultimately producing cell death (Peery and Le Page 1969). In murine tumors, four mechanisms of resistance to thioguanine have been well described (Le Page et al 1964). βTGdr is phosphorylated to a nucleotide form which can theoretically bypass the metabolic blocks involved in thioguanine resistance; however, the agent has been shown to lack activity in thioguanine-resistant tumors (Nelson et al 1975). DNA synthesis is affected by βTGdr but lethality may correlate better with drug-induced mutations in DNA replication. A delay in cell cycle progression has not been noted but cell cycle phase specificity has been observed, with optimal cytotoxic effects occurring in the early and midportions of S phase of the cell cycle (Barranco and Humphrey 1971).

■ Availability and Storage

Beta-2'-deoxythioguanosine was available investigationally from the National Cancer Institute as a lyophilized powder in 200-mg vials that required refrigerated storage. They were chemically stable for only 24 hours at room temperature. It is no longer experimentally available.

■ Preparation for Use, Stability, and Admixture

Vials may be diluted in 50 to 150 mL of D5W or normal saline. Extremely acidic infusion solutions should be avoided. In addition, the recommended admixtures are stable only for 2 hours after mixing (room temperature).

■ Administration

Beta-2'-deoxythioguanosine has been given as either a rapid or a short intravenous infusion. A 30- to 60-minute infusion time is recommended.

■ Dosage

The most efficacious dosage scheme for βTGdr in human cancers is not known. As a single agent in phase II clinical trials, doses of 200 to 500 mg/m^2/d × 5 days repeated at 2-week intervals produced severe marrow toxicity (Omura 1975). In combination with other cytotoxic anticancer agents, doses of 60 to 120 mg/m^2 concurrently or 100 to 200 mg/m^2 6 days after other chemotherapy drugs, repeated at 2- to 3-week intervals, were more safely used (Bodey et al 1976). Myelotoxicity becomes much more pronounced after doses greater than 125 mg/m^2/d.

■ Drug Interactions

Animal data originally suggested that βTGdr is synergistic with cytarabine (Rao et al 1974). This, however, has not been borne out in human trials (Bodey et al 1976). Similarly, although synthesized as a non-cross-resistant replacement for thioguanine, it apparently lacks activity in two experimental tumors resistant to 6-thioguanine (Nelson et al 1975).

Concurrent allopurinol administration (270 mg/m^2) with βTGdr increased only the percentage of methylxanthine with a proportionate decrease in the methylthioguanine fraction (Loo and Lu 1974). The relative distribution of other βTGdr metabolites remains unchanged. This would tend to support the use of both βTGdr and allopurinol concurrently without dosage reduction of βTGdr (similar to thioguanine, but opposite to mercaptopurine).

■ Pharmacokinetics

After an injection of 80 to 100 mg/kg IV in dogs, a plasma half-life of 4.5 hours is described (Loo et al 1970). In this study the apparent volume of distribution exceeded total body water, and βTGdr appeared to be extensively metabolized. Cumulative urinary excretion accounted for 35 to 40% of a dose (radioactively labeled drug) by 5 hours; less than 20% of the drug is excreted unchanged in the urine. The predominant initial metabolite is thioguanine, but 6-thiouric acid predominates by 3 hours after injection.

Intravenous injection of 200 mg/m^2 radioactively labeled drug in humans revealed an initial half-life of about 1 hour and a prolonged terminal half-life of about 24 hours (Loo and Lu 1974). Again, the drug appeared to undergo significant liver metabolism. One hour after injection urinary metabolites consist primarily of thioguanine (35%), βTGdr (27%), thioxanthine (22%), and thiouric acid (11%), with only trace amounts of methylthioxanthine and methylthioguanine. By 13 hours after injection, distribution of metabolites shifts considerably to favor the more highly metabolized drug derivatives: thiouric acid (28%), methylthioguanine (21%), and thioxanthine (15%), with only 6% as thioguanine and 5% as intact βTGdr. Cumulative 24-hour urine excretion accounts for 65% of βTGdr in humans (Lu et al 1982).

■ Side Effects and Toxicity

With high doses (300–500 mg/m^2/d × 5 every 2 to 3 weeks), severe, often life-threatening granulocytopenia may occur which is a dose-limiting effect (Omura 1975); however, there has been no evidence to date of cumulative myelotoxicity. Both leukopenia and thrombocytopenia are characteristic.

Both granulocytes and platelets are depressed with a typical nadir of about 2 weeks (Bodey et al 1976).

Minor toxic effects include alopecia, nausea and vomiting, and mild anemia (Omura 1975). Dermal reactions have also been reported including photosensitivity and hyperpigmentation (Le Page and Gottlieb 1973). A few patients have developed transient abnormalities in liver function characterized by elevated serum glutamic–oxalacetic transaminase and serum bilirubin values. Patients with preexisting liver disease have also had worsening of liver function while receiving the drug (Bodey et al 1976). Only one patient in these studies reported stomatitis while on the drug.

REFERENCES

Barranco SC, Humphrey RM. The effects of β-2'-deoxythioguanosine on survival and progression in mammalian cells. *Cancer Res.* 1971;**31**:583.

Bodey GP, McCredie KB, Whitecar JP, et al. Clinical studies of beta-thioguanine deoxyriboside alone and in combination with arabinosylcytosine. *Med Pediatr Oncol.* 1976;**2**:199–205.

Brooks JC, Douglass HO Jr, Reyes J, et al. Treatment of advanced solid tumors with combination of methyl-CCNU and β-2'-deoxythioguanosine. *Proc Am Soc Clin Oncol.* 1976;**17**:306.

Douglass HR Jr, Moertel C. Chemotherapy of previously treated colorectal adenocarcinoma with methyl-CCNU or β-2'-deoxythioguanosine (βTGdr), a phase II–III study of ECOG. *Proc Am Soc Clin Oncol.* 1976;**17**:306.

Gagliano RG, Stuckey WJ, Panettiere FJ, et al. Evaluation of beta-2'-deoxythioguanosine combined with methyl-CCNU or mitomycin in advanced colorectal cancer. A Southwest Oncology Group study. *Cancer Clin Trials.* 1981;**4**:401–405.

Gastrointestinal Tumor Study Group. Phase II trials of hexamethylmelamine, dianhydrogalactitol, Razoxane, and β-2'-deoxythioguanosine as single agents against advanced measurable tumors of the pancreas. *Cancer Treat Rep.* 1985;**69**:713–716.

Iwamoto RH, Acton EM, Goodman L. β-2'-Deoxythioguanosine and related nucleotides. *J Med Chem.* 1963;**6**:684.

Le Page GA, Gottlieb JA. Deoxythioguanosine and thioguanine. *Clin Pharmacol Ther.* 1973;**14**:966.

Le Page GA, Junga IG, Bowman B. Biochemical and carcinostatic effects of β-2'-deoxythioguanosine. *Cancer Res.* 1964;**24**:835.

Loo TL, Lu K. Pharmacologic disposition of thioguanine (TG) and β-deoxythioguanosine (β-TGdr) in man. *Proc Am Assoc Cancer Res.* 1974;**15**:139.

Loo TL, Lu K, Richards MT, et al. Pharmacologic disposition of arabinosyl-6-mercaptopurine and β-2'-deoxythioguanosine. *Pharmacologist.* 1970;**12**:555.

Lu K, Benvenuto JA, Bodey GP, Gottlieb JA. Pharmacokinetics of metabolism of β-2'-deoxythioguanosine and 6-thioguanine in man. *Cancer Chemother Pharmacol.* 1982;**8**:119–123.

Nelson JA, Kuhns JN, Carpenter JW. Lack of activity of β-2'-deoxythioguanosine against two tumors resistant to 6-thioguanine. *Cancer Res.* 1975;**35**:1372.

Omura GA. Phase II trial of β-deoxythioguanosine (β-TGdr, NSC-71261) in refractory adult acute leukemia. *Proc Am Assoc Cancer Res.* 1975;**16**:140.

Omura GA, Vogler WR, Bartolucci A, et al. Treatment of refractory adult acute leukemia with 5-azacytidine plus β-2'-deoxythioguanosine. *Cancer Treat Rep.* 1979;**63**(2): 209–210.

Peery A, Le Page GA. Nucleotide formation from alpha and β-2'-deoxythioguanosine in extracts of murine and human tissues. *Cancer Res.* 1969;**29**:617.

Rao RN, Freireich EJ, Bodey GP, et al. In vitro evaluation of 1-β-D-arabinofuranosyl cytosine-β-2'-deoxythioguanosine combination chemotherapy. *Cancer Res.* 1974; **34**:2539–2543.

Bisantrene HCl

■ Other Names

CL-216942; NSC-337766.

■ Chemistry

Structure of bisantrene HCl

Bisantrene is a modified anthracene with the chemical name, 9,10-anthracenedicarboxaldehyde bis[(4,5-dihydro-1*H*-imidazol-2-yl)hydrazone]dihydrochloride. The molecular formula is $C_{22}H_{22}N_8 \cdot 2HCl$ and the molecular weight, 471.4. The akyl-imidazol side chains are very basic and, at physiologic pH, are positively charged. This is believed to facilitate electrostatic attractions to negatively charged ribose phosphate groups in DNA.

■ Antitumor Activity

Bisantrene showed excellent antitumor activity in murine tumor models including P-388 leukemia and B-16 melanoma (Citarella et al 1980). Human tumor cells that were sensitive to bisantrene as assessed by in vitro colony-forming assays include breast cancer, ovarian cancer, renal cancer, small cell and non-small cell lung cancer, lymphoma, acute myelogenous leukemia, melanoma, gastric cancer, adrenal cancer, and head and neck cancer (Von Hoff et al 1981a). In phase I clinical trials bisantrene showed activity in hepatocellular cancer and hypernephroma (one patient each, Von Hoff et al 1981b) and in lymphoma, myeloma, melanoma, renal cancer, and tumors of the bladder and lung (Alberts et al 1982). Phase I activity was also observed in two other hypernephroma patients (Spiegel et al 1982). Bisantrene was inactive in human colon cancer tested in vitro or in vivo (Perry et al 1982, Von Hoff et al 1981a,b). It was also inactive in refractory malignant melanoma (Alberts et al 1987).

In phase II clinical trials, bisantrene was particularly active in patients with metastatic breast cancer (Yap et al 1983, Osborne et al 1984). Partial response rates of 20% were observed in heavily pretreated patients with advanced breast cancer. Despite this demonstrated clinical activity, bisantrene studies were terminated by the drug's sponsor, Lederle Laboratories. Presumably this was done because of the excessive local toxicity with bisantrene and the availability of better analogs such as mitoxantrone which has superior antitumor activity.

■ Mechanism of Action

Bisantrene has been shown to induce altered DNA supercoiling indicative of DNA intercalation (Bowden et al 1985). In L-1210 leukemia cells bisantrene was also shown to induce protein-associated DNA strand breaks typical of drug-induced inhibition of DNA topoisomerase II enzymes (Bowden et al 1985). Both cytotoxicity and the DNA strand breaks appear to be reduced in hypoxic conditions (Ludwig et al 1984). The noncovalent binding of bisantrene to DNA appears to comprise two types of interactions: (1) intercalation of the planar anthracene moiety between DNA base pairs, and (2) electrostatic binding between negatively charged ribose phosphates of DNA and positively charged basic nitrogens on the alkyl side chains of the drug. This is reflected in the biphasic DNA dissociation curves for bisantrene in calf thymus DNA in vitro (Foye et al 1986).

■ Availability and Storage

Bisantrene was investigationally available from Lederle Laboratories, Pearl River, New Jersey, as a lyophilized orange powder in vials containing 50 or 250 mg of the free base. It was recommended that the vials be stored at room temperature.

■ Preparation for Use, Stability, and Admixture

Bisantrene vials were reconstituted with 2 to 5 mL of Sterile Water for Injection, USP, and then diluted to approximately 0.1 to 0.5 mg/mL in D5W. Bisantrene is incompatible with saline and unstable in light (Powis et al 1982). The final bisantrene solutions in dextrose are stable for 2 hours at room temperature and should be protected from light.

■ Administration

Because of severe local venous toxicity, bisantrene doses were usually infused via central venous access devices over 1 hour (Von Hoff et al 1981b). Bisantrene was infused through peripheral veins over 2 hours. It was often "piggybacked" into a running dextrose infusion in an attempt to lessen delayed swelling in the arm used for infusion.

■ Special Precautions

To reduce venous irritation, hyperpigmentation, drug extravasation, and anaphylactoid reactions, patients were often given hydrocortisone (50 mg IV) and the antihistamine diphenhydramine (50 mg IM) immediately prior to bisantrene (Alberts et al 1982). Bisantrene is known to stain the skin orange, and as with all anticancer drugs, direct contact with the drug should be avoided.

■ Dosage

The maximally tolerated doses for different bisantrene phase I schedules are described in the table.

■ Drug Interactions

Bisantrene is physically incompatible with sodium chloride solutions, forming a precipitate. It is also chemically inactivated by high-pH solutions such as sodium bicarbonate (1 mEq/mL, pH 10) (Dorr et al 1984). Bisantrene is reported to produce additive cytotoxic effects in tumor cells when combined with radiation (Hernandez and Rosenshein 1985). The clinical significance of this interaction, if any, is unknown.

BISANTRENE PHASE I MAXIMALLY TOLERATED DOSING SCHEDULES

Dose (mg/m^2)	Schedule	Reference
200 (150)*	Weekly × 3	Alberts et al 1982
150	Weekly × 3 (repeat every 4–5 wk)	Yap et al 1982
260 (240)*	Monthly (every 3–4 wk)	Von Hoff et al 1981b
80	Daily × 5 (repeat every 4 wk)	Spiegel et al 1982

*Lower dose for patients with poor bone marrow reserve (eg, those who have received radiotherapy or extensive chemotherapy regimens).

Pharmacokinetics

More than 95% of bisantrene is bound to plasma proteins and the drug has a long terminal plasma half-life. There appears to be three phases of elimination: an initial distributive phase of 6 minutes, a beta phase of approximately 1.5 hours, and a final gamma elimination phase of 23 to 54 hours (Alberts et al 1983). Typical areas under the plasma concentration × time curve are 4.4 to 5.7 mg · h/mL following intravenous doses of 260 to 340 mg/m^2, respectively (Alberts et al 1983). Less than 7% of a bisantrene dose is excreted in the urine and the majority of the drug is eliminated by the hepatobiliary route. The drug may be metabolized to some extent in vivo. In vitro bisantrene is a substrate for hepatic microsomal enzymes but specific metabolites have not been identified. Preclinical drug distribution studies showed that the tissues with the highest concentration (in descending order) are kidney, liver, gallbladder, spleen, lung, and heart. Brain levels were extremely low although the drug did distribute to lymph nodes and bone marrow (Wu and Nicolau 1982).

Side Effects and Toxicity

The major dose-limiting toxic effect of bisantrene is leukopenia (Von Hoff et al 1981b, Alberts et al 1982, Spiegel et al 1982, Yap et al 1982). On a schedule of every 3 to 4 weeks, the nadir for myelosuppression was 9 days with recovery by 19 days (Von Hoff et al 1981b). Thrombocytopenia was mild although bisantrene can also inhibit platelet aggregation (Rybak et al 1986). Anemia and cumulative myelosuppressive toxic effects were not encountered with this drug.

In addition to myelosuppression, bisantrene produced severe phlebitis along peripheral veins used for drug infusion (Von Hoff et al 1981b, Alberts et al 1982). This may have been caused by drug precipitation in veins which has been documented in experimental models (Powis and Kovach 1983). The drug is a potent vesicant and produces severe local tissue necrosis if inadvertently extravasated (Von Hoff et al 1981b). Oftentimes severe arm swelling, hyperpigmented veins, and punctate perivenous orange discolorations appeared following bisantrene infusions given through peripheral veins. The arm swelling appeared to be the result of a localized capillary leak syndrome in the arm used for infusion. In an experimental mouse skin model, extravasation necrosis was blocked with a local injection of sodium bicarbonate which physically decomposes bisantrene (Dorr et al 1984).

Up to 10% of patients experienced anaphylactoid reactions following a bisantrene infusion (Myers et al 1983). Symptoms included chills, chest pain, shortness of breath, flushing, and pruritis. These effects may be caused by drug-induced histamine release. Hypotension is also reported with bisantrene, and prolongation of the infusion was recommended to reduce this complication (Von Hoff et al 1981b). In addition, a few patients experienced diaphoresis and palpitations, usually near the end of a bisantrene infusion (Von Hoff et al 1981b). The drug was not cardiotoxic in animals and its potential to cause cumulative dose-related cardiotoxicity in humans is unknown. No patients experienced electrocardiographic changes while receiving the drug.

Of note, bisantrene produces very little nausea and vomiting. Alopecia is also less intense with bisantrene compared with doxorubicin (Cowan et al 1991); however, bisantrene can produce a mild fever in some patients and malaise may be particularly common. This was reported by up to one half of patients studied (Yap et al 1982).

Although bisantrene was clearly active, the range and severity of toxic effects, particularly the troublesome local venous and anaphylactoid reactions, probably precluded further clinical development of this agent.

REFERENCES

Alberts DS, Mackel C, Pocelinko R, Salmon SE. Phase I clinical investigation of 9,10-anthracenedicarboxaldehyde bis[(4,5-dihydro-1*H*-imidazol-2-yl)hydrazone] dihydrochloride with correlative in vitro human tumor clonogenic assay. *Cancer Res.* 1982;**42**:1170–1175.

Alberts DS, Mason-Liddil N, Green SJ, Cowan JD. Phase II evaluation of bisantrene hydrochloride in refractory malignant melanoma. *Invest New Drugs.* 1987;**5**:289–292.

Alberts DS, Peng Y-M, Leigh S, Davis TP, Woodward DL. Pharmacokinetics of bisantrene in cancer patients. In: Coltman C, ed. *Proceedings, 13th International Congress on Chemotherapy.* Vienna: Verlag H. Egermann, 1983.

Bowden GT, Roberts R, Alberts DS, Peng Y-M, Garcia D. Comparative molecular pharmacology in leukemic L1210 cells of the anthracene anticancer drugs mitoxantrone and bisantrene. *Cancer Res.* 1985;**45**:4915–4920.

Citarella RV, Wallace RE, Murdock KC, Angier RB, Durr FE. Anti-tumor activity of CL-216942: 9,10-Anthracenedicarboxaldehyde bis[(4,5-dihydro-1*H*-imidazol-2-yl)-hydrazone)]dihydrochloride (Abstract #23). In: *Abstracts of the 20th Interscience Conference on Antimicrobial Agents and Chemotherapy*, Bethesda, MD: American Society for Microbiology. September 1980.

Cowan JD, Neidhart J, McClure S, et al. Randomized trial of doxorubicin, bisantrene, and mitoxantrone in advanced breast cancer: A Southwest Oncology Group study. *J Natl Cancer Inst.* 1991;**83**:1077–1084.

Dorr RT, Peng Y-M, Alberts DS. Bisantrene solubility and skin toxicity studies: Efficacy of sodium bicarbonate as a local ulceration antidote. *Invest New Drugs.* 1984;**2**:351–357.

Foye WO, Karnik PS, Sengupta SK. DNA-binding abilities of bisguanylhydrazones of anthracene-9,10-dicarboxaldehyde. *Anti-Cancer Drug Design.* 1986;**1**:65–71.

Hernandez E, Rosenshein NB. Interaction between bisantrene and radiation. *Int J Radiat Oncol Biol Phys.* 1985;**11**:1395–1399.

Ludwig CU, Bowden GT, Roberts RA, Alberts DS. Reduced bisantrene-induced cytotoxicity and protein-associated DNA strand breaks under hypoxic condition. *Cancer Treat Rep.* 1984;**68**:367–372.

Myers JW, Von Hoff DD, Kuhn JG, Osborne CK, Sanbach JF, Pocelinko R. Anaphylactoid reactions associated with bisantrene infusions. *Invest New Drugs.* 1983;**1**:85–88.

Osborne CK, Von Hoff DD, Cowan JD, Sandbach J. Bisantrene, an active drug in patients with advanced breast cancer. *Cancer Treat Rep.* 1984;**68**:357–360.

Perry MC, Forastiere AA, Richards F II, Weiss RB, Anbar D. Phase II trial of bisantrene in advanced colorectal cancer: A cancer and leukemia group B study. *Cancer Treat Rep.* 1982;**66**(11):1997–1998.

Powis G, Kovach JS. Disposition of bisantrene in humans and rabbits: Evidence for intravascular deposition of drug as a cause of phlebitis. *Cancer Res.* 1983;**43**:925–929.

Powis G, Kvols LK, Rubin J, Kovach JS. Pharmacokinetic study of ADAH in humans and sensitivity of ADAH to light (abstract #C-74). *ASCO Proc.* 1982;**1**:19.

Rybak ME, Badstubner B, Griffin T. The effects of bisantrene on human platelets. *Invest New Drugs.* 1986;**4**:119–125.

Spiegel RJ, Blum RH, Levin M, et al. Phase I clinical trial of 9,10-anthracene dicarboxaldehyde (bisantrene) administered in a five-day schedule. *Cancer Res.* 1982;**42**:354–358.

Von Hoff DD, Coltman CA Jr, Forseth B. Activity of 9,10-anthracenedicarboxaldehyde bis[(4,5-dihydro-1*H*-imidazol-2-yl)hydrazone]dihydrochloride (CL216,942) in a human tumor cloning system. *Cancer Chemother Pharmacol.* 1981a;**6**:141–144.

Von Hoff DD, Myers JW, Kuhn J, et al. Phase I clinical investigation of 9,10-anthracenedicarboxaldehyde bis[(4,5-dihydro-1*H*-imidazol-2-yl)hydrazone]dihydrochloride (CL216, 942). *Cancer Res.* 1981b;**41**:3118–3121.

Wu WH, Nicolau G. Disposition and metabolic profile of a new antitumor agent: CL 216,942 (bisantrene) in laboratory animals. *Cancer Treat Rep.* 1982;**66**(5):1173–1185.

Yap B-S, Yap H-Y, Blumenschein GR, Bedikian AY, Pocelinko R, Bodey GP. Phase I clinical evaluation of 9,10-anthracenedicarboxaldehyde[bis(4,5-dihydro-1*H*-imidazol-2-yl)hydrazone]dihydrochloride (bisantrene). *Cancer Treat Rep.* 1982;**66**:1517–1520.

Yap H-Y, Yap B-S, Blumenschein GR, Barnes BC, Schell FC, Bodey GP. Bisantrene, an active new drug in the treatment of metastatic breast cancer. *Cancer Res.* 1983;**43**:1402–1404.

Bleomycin Sulfate

■ Other Names

NSC-125066; Blenoxane® (Bristol-Myers Oncology Division); BLM[2]; "Bleo."

■ Chemistry

Structure of bleomycin sulfate

The bleomycins are antineoplastic antibiotics produced by fermentation from *Streptomyces verticillus*, a strain of *Actinomyces* (Umezawa 1974). Thirteen identifiable glycopeptide fractions have been isolated and are designated A_1 to A_6, A_2, and B_1 to B_6 (Tomoshisa et al 1972). The main component is bleomycin A_2 (approximate molecular weight 1400), which constitutes at least 50% of the bleomycin species in the commercial formulation. Bleomycins are sulfur-containing polypeptides, soluble in water and methanol but not in other organic solvents. The potency varies between 1.2 and 1.7 U/mg; however, with current nomenclature redefined, 1 mg of bleomycin is equal to 1 U of inhibitory activity against *Mycobacterium smegmatis* in vitro (Crooke and Bradner 1976). The commercial product contains at least 65% A fraction and less than 0.1% copper by weight. The bleomycin A_2 and B_2 fractions represent 55 to 70% and 25 to 32% of the total weight, respectively. Thus, bleomycin A_2 is the predominant active component. The active conformation of bleomycin juxtaposes six distinct nitrogens in a "ring" which can bind metals such as Fe, Cu^{2+}, and Zn(II). The functional groups contributing to this binding include two nitrogens from L-β-aminoalaninecarboxamide, one nitrogen from pyrimidinylmethyl, two nitrogens from the L-erythro(β)-hydroxyhistidine group, and one oxygen from the carbonyl group of the 3-O-carbamoyl-α-D-mannopyranoside unit. The bleomycin–iron complex is believed to be the active form; bleomycin–copper complexes are inactive.

Antitumor Activity

Bleomycin has demonstrated significant activity in a number of human malignancies including squamous cell carcinomas of the head and neck, cervix, vulvovaginal area, skin, penis, and rectum (as reviewed by Blum et al 1973); Hodgkin's and non-Hodgkin's lymphomas (Blum et al 1973); mycosis fungoides (Spigel and Coltman 1973); testicular tumors (Samuels et al 1975); and lung cancer (Livingston et al 1975a, b). Bleomycin is usually given in full doses with other effective agents. This is possible because of the lack of additional myelotoxicity from bleomycin. Examples of active combinations include MOPP–BLEO in Hodgkin's disease (Frei et al 1973); BACOP in non-Hodgkin's lymphoma (Schein et al 1976); MOB in uterine cervix cancer (Baker et al 1976); platinum–vinblastine(velban)–BLEO in testicular carcinoma (Einhorn and Donohue 1977); and BACON or COMB in lung cancer (Livingston et al 1975b and a, respectively).

Mechanism of Action

Bleomycin causes scission of both single- and double-stranded DNA (Crooke and Bradner 1976). Single-strand breaks appear to predominate. Several low-molecular-weight fragments of DNA are observed after bleomycin interacts with cells (Haidle et al 1972). These effects are mediated by oxygen free radicals generated in a stepwise process from a bleomycin–iron–oxygen complex. The initial step involves bleomycin binding to DNA, a process mediated by the amino-terminal tripeptide and by partial intercalation of the bithiazole rings between G–C base pairs (Kasai et al 1978).

The binding constant for the bleomycin–DNA complex is around 10^{-5} M, and at saturating drug concentrations there is one bleomycin bound per 4 to 5 bp (Chien et al 1977). Some specificity for strand damage is observed at linker DNA regions and at sites of active DNA transcription (Mirabelli et al 1983). Bleomycin strand damage results from oxygen free radicals such as superoxide and hydroxyl which are generated by the bleomycin–Fe(II)–oxygen complex. The complex is thereafter oxidized to an inactive state and any further activity requires enzymatic reduction of the iron.

Three-dimensional analysis of the active bleomycin–iron complex shows a rigid square-pyramidal structure with oxygen bound directly to the iron.

Single-strand breaks occur primarily at the C-4' to C-3' bond in deoxyribose, leaving a broken strand and free base propenals of all four DNA bases. DNA synthesis and, to a lesser degree, RNA and protein synthesis are inhibited by the drug. Experimentally, the cytotoxic reaction is enhanced in the presence of intercalating agents (dactinomycin) and is inhibited by nonferrous divalent cations.

Bleomycin is cell cycle phase specific, producing its major cytotoxic effect in the G_2 and M phases. In decreasing order of sensitivity are early S phase, late S phase, and G_1. Aside from the cytotoxic effects, bleomycin appears to inhibit cell progression out of G_2 phase (Tobey 1972). Some have used this effect to "synchronize" cells kinetically before subsequent drug therapy (Barranco et al 1973, Livingston et al 1973).

Other pharmacologic effects of bleomycin that are experimentally documented in animals appear to be histaminergic in nature. These include contraction of mouse intestines, which is blocked by atropine and diphenhydramine; transient blood pressure decrease in all species; increased capillary permeability; and mast cell degeneration noted in rat mesenteries (Crooke and Bradner 1976).

Resistance. The cytosolic enzyme bleomycin hydrolase removes an amino group from the molecule. The enzyme is a cysteine protease that converts bleomycin to the inactive desamido form (Sebti et al 1987, 1989). In rabbits this enzyme is an acidic hydrophobic pentamer containing five identical 50,000-dalton subunits (total molecular weight, 250,000). An uneven distribution of the enzyme may explain the relative resistance to bleomycin in sarcoma tissues which have high levels of the hydrolase. In contrast, sensitive carcinomatous tissues have low hydrolase levels (Umezawa et al 1972). Lung tissues also contain little hydrolase activity and have a high relative oxygen tension. This may explain the unique sensitivity of pulmonary tissues to bleomycin toxicity as drug inactivation is negligible and oxygen is plentiful for free radical generation (Lazo et al 1990).

Septi et al (1991) have also shown that bleomycin resistance in human tumor xenografts is associated with rapid drug metabolism and decreased accumulation.

■ Availability and Storage

Bleomycin is commercially available as Blenoxane® (Bristol-Myers Oncology Division, Princeton, NJ) in ampules as a white or yellowish lyophilized powder containing 15 mg of drug (equivalent to 15 U). The more recent designation is units of activity because the older designation of milligrams varied by the composition of bleomycin subfractions. Intact ampules of bleomycin have been shown to be chemically stable for 2 years when stored at 1 to 35°C.

■ Preparation for Use, Stability, and Admixture

Bleomycin should be dissolved in 1 to 5 mL of sterile water, D5W, or normal saline for injection. The diluent may contain a bacteriostatic agent if prolonged storage is anticipated. After dilution as described, the resulting solution is stable for 90 days frozen, 14 days if refrigerated, and 96 hours at room temperature; however, long-term storage of unpreserved solutions at room temperature is not recommended because of the possibility of bacterial or other contamination. Admixture compatibility with heparin is undetermined; however, bleomycin does chelate various divalent and trivalent cations (Umezawa 1974). Therefore the drug should not be admixed with solutions containing these ions, especially copper.

The table reviews the compatibility of bleomycin with several other medications. Bleomycin is compatible with filters, and although one study described slight absorption to polyvinyl chloride infusion bags (Benvenuto et al 1981), this has not been seen in other studies. Thus, bleomycin appears to be stable and is not appreciably bound to either glass or plastic infusion containers (Dorr et al 1982).

■ Administration

Bleomycin may be given by the intramuscular, intravenous, intraarterial, intratumoral, subcutaneous, or intracavitary route. Adverse reactions do not appear to be concentration or route dependent. Therefore, any convenient volume may be used to administer an individual dose. Specific recommendations for unusual drug administration routes (intrapleural, others) are described under Special Applications. Most brief infusions of bleomycin are delivered in 50 to 100 mL of solution. Intramuscular doses are equivalent to intravenous doses and both are active in patients with advanced lymphomas (Durkin et al 1976).

In some tumors there may be an enhanced therapeutic effect produced by prolonged administration of drug as a continuous intravenous infusion (Krakoff et al 1977, Baker et al 1978). There is also experimental evidence that continuous infusions of bleomycin produces less serious pulmonary toxicity while maintaining or increasing therapeutic activity. This has been observed in rats (Sikic et al 1978) and in humans (Cooper and Hong 1981). Continuous 24-hour infusion doses are usually delivered in 1 L of D5W or saline for 4 to 5 days.

■ Special Precautions

Historically, a few patients with lymphomas may be at risk of severe hyperpyrexic responses to bleomycin. To detect sensitive individuals it has been recommended that patients be tested first with 1 or 2 U bleomycin IM. If no acute reaction occurs after 2 to 4 hours, then regular dosing may commence. This maneuver is not generally recom-

BLEOMYCIN COMPATIBILITY AND STABILITY

Compatible Drugs (>24 h at Room Temperature and Light)	Incompatible Drugs
Amikacin	Aminophylline
Cephapirin	Ascorbic acid
Cisplatin	Carbenicillin
Cyclophosphamide	Cefazolin
Dexamethasone sodium phosphate	Cephalothin
Diphenhydramine	Diazepam
Doxorubicin	Hydrocortisone sodium succinate
Droperidol	
5-Fluorouracil	Methotrexate
Gentamicin	Mitomycin-C
Heparin	Nafcillin
Hydrocortisone sodium phosphate	Penicillin
Leucovorin	Terbutaline
Metoclopramide	
Ondansetron (4 h)†	
Streptomycin	
Tobramycin	
Vinblastine	
Vincristine	

*Dorr et al 1982, Cohen et al 1985.
†Trissel et al 1990.

mended as the incidence of severe acute reactions to bleomycin is very low.

Cumulative (lifetime) bleomycin doses greater than 400 U by any route should be given with great caution if at all. The incidence of pulmonary toxicity rises sharply with increasing total doses (> 400 U) and with increasing age (>70 years). Therefore, total doses should be limited to 400 units and the drug should not be administered to elderly patients with any degree of pulmonary insufficiency. Bleomycin must also be used with extreme caution in patients with significant pulmonary or renal disease and in patients receiving hyperbaric oxygen exposure, as from anesthetic gas delivery during surgery (see Dosage).

■ Dosage

The standard dosage for bleomycin as a single agent is 10 to 20 U/m² given one or two times per week (0.25–0.5 mg/kg IV or IM). Several "low-dose" schedules (3–4 units/m²) are also employed in combination regimens (eg, MOPP + low-dose BLEO). Equivalent continuous intravenous or intraarterial infusion doses may also be given. As a continuous intravenous infusion, 15 mg/m² over 24 hours daily for 4 days has been used. A multiple-dose subcutaneous bleomycin regimen was also developed to simulate continuous infusions (Alberts and Peng 1979). In this preliminary study, steady-state bleomycin levels of 0.1, 0.05, and 0.01 mU/mL could be sustained with subcutaneous bleomycin doses of 6.1, 3.1, and 0.6 U/m² given every 8 hours for 4 days (Alberts and Peng 1979).

Doses of up to 60 U/d have been given intraarterially to local tumor sites to provide increased local concentrations. These doses may be given daily but should not surpass the 400-U total dose for patients with normal renal function. This dose limit is reduced further for elderly patients and for those with significant chronic renal dysfunction. Severe cutaneous toxicity, hypertension, confusion, and urinary burning have resulted from single biweekly intravenous doses of more than 25 mg/m² (Chabner et al 1977), although in some series doses of 30 U/d × 4 to 5 days have been used without undue toxicity.

Significant dosage reduction is recommended in patients with renal failure. Nonetheless, bleomycin has been active and safe in regimens using reduced doses given once per week, even in patients with complete renal failure. In this regard it is important to note that the drug is not effectively hemodialyzed (Crooke et al 1977). Generally, dosage adjustment is not required until the patient's creatinine clearance falls below 40 mL/min (see table). The Blenoxane® package insert suggests that for moderate degrees of renal failure (serum creatinine 1.5–2.0), doses be reduced by 50%. For more severe degrees of renal failure, the table below presents a generalized schedule for dose reduction; however, this nomogram has not been evaluated in a prospective or retrospective clinical trial. Caution is also recommended for use in patients over age 70 wherein reduced cumulative dosing is recommended.

■ Drug Interactions

Bleomycin has been shown to be therapeutically synergistic with other anticancer drugs in a number of experimental tumor systems (reviewed by Crooke and Bradner 1976). Bleomycin induces partial synchrony of susceptible cells in G_2 phase and has demonstrated schedule-dependent synergy when followed in about 6 to 12 hours by a vinca alkaloid such as vincristine (Barranco et al 1973); however, corroborative clinical studies have not been performed.

Drugs such as L-buthionine sulfoximine that deplete cellular glutathione can increase the antitumor activity of bleomycin (Russo et al 1984). In animal models phenothiazines such as chlorpromazine (Thorazine®) may also enhance bleomycin cytotoxicity without enhancing pulmonary toxicity (Hait et al 1988). Of interest, tumor cells that were inherently resistant to bleomycin were quite sensitive to bleomycin–anticalmodulin drug combinations (Lazo et al 1985).

BLEOMYCIN PHARMACOKINETICS AND DOSE REDUCTIONS IN PATIENTS WITH COMPROMISED RENAL FUNCTION

Patient's Creatinine Clearance (mL/min)	Terminal Elimination Half-Life* (h)	% of Normal Dose Suggested[†]
>35	2–3	100
30	NL[‡]	55
25	NL	53
20	5.7	50
15	11	48
10	21	45
5	21	40

*From Crooke et al 1977.
[†]General formula of Anderson et al 1976, using a fractional urinary bleomycin excretion of 45% of a dose.
[‡]NL, Not listed in original citation.

The use of other nephrotoxic drugs such as cisplatin can alter bleomycin elimination and increase toxicity (see Pharmacokinetics). Also, hyperoxia and concomitant radiation therapy can significantly increase bleomycin pulmonary toxicity (see Side Effects and Toxicity).

■ Pharmacokinetics

The peak blood level of bleomycin after intramuscular injection is obtained in about 30 to 60 minutes and is about one-third that of a similar dose given intravenously. Pharmacokinetic studies indicate a volume of distribution of 20 L, approximating intra- and extracellular fluid volumes. After intravenous administration, the drug has a rapid initial distribution half-life of 10 to 20 minutes, followed by an elimination half-life of about 2 to 3 hours (Hall et al 1977, Alberts et al 1978) (see the table below). Even though there is significant biotransformation of the drug, about 50% of a dose can be recovered in the urine at 24 hours. Only 20 to 40% of drug recovered in urine is active drug. Tissue inactivation of bleomycin is apparently rapid, especially by the liver and kidney (Ohnuma et al 1974). Enzymatic inactivation is notably reduced in skin and lung (Chabner et al 1977).

Bleomycin pharmacokinetics has been studied in a few patients with renal failure (Crooke et al 1977). These studies show that renal failure significantly prolongs the plasma half-life and reduces the magnitude of drug excreted into the urine. The clearance of bleomycin correlates fairly well with creatinine clearance in individual patients (see Dosage for recommendations). Furthermore, the prior use of nephrotoxic drugs such as cisplatin can reduce bleomycin clearance with a resultant increase in the plasma half-life and clinical toxicity of bleomycin (Yee et al 1983). In one case, total plasma clearance decreased from 39 to 18 mL/min/m² with an increase in the half-life to 6 hours.

Bleomycin's binding to plasma proteins is less than 10%. The drug is also well-absorbed following intramuscular injection, with mean peak serum concentrations of 0.13, 0.33, and 0.59 mU/mL obtained 1 hour after intramuscular doses of 2, 5, and 10 U/m², respectively (Oken et al 1981). Urinary excretion over the 24 hours after intramuscular dosing averaged 61% of an intramuscular dose (Oken et al 1981).

Bleomycin apparently can also selectively localize in a number of tumor tissues. This has facilitated its use as a radionuclide tumor-scanning agent with limited success. Isotopes include indium (^{111}In)-labeled bleomycin and cobalt (^{57}Co)-labeled bleomycin (Lilien et al 1975).

Alberts and Peng (1979) have also reported roughly equivalent blood levels for continuous intravenous infusion of 30 U/d × 4 compared to subcutaneous doses of 10 U Q 8 hours × 4 days (see Dosage for steady-state levels obtained with subcutaneous dosing every 8 hours). The study by Ginsberg et al (1979) also suggests that effective steady-state levels of 6 to 10 μU/mL may be obtained by low-dose continuous infusion, in this case as part of the "CHOP–BLEO" regimen (2 U/24 hours × 5 days, repeated every 21 days).

■ Side Effects and Toxicity

Anaphylactoid reactions can occur following the administration of bleomycin. Furthermore, a high incidence of fever with or without chills may occur after each dose. Approximately 50% of all patients experience some degree of fever with bleomycin. In lymphoma patients the fever may be followed by excessive sweating and dehydration with resultant hypotension. Severe fever and hypotension leading to death or renal failure have been rarely reported. This syndrome may occur several hours after a dose of bleomycin. The incidence of chills and fever may

BLEOMYCIN PHARMACOKINETICS IN PATIENTS WITH NORMAL RENAL FUNCTION

Route	Dose (U/m²)	Half-life α (min)	Half-life β (hr)	Concentration × Time (mU · min/mL)	Clearance (mL/min/m²)	Volume of Distribution	Reference
Intravenous bolus	15	24	4	300	51	17.5 L/m²	Alberts et al 1978
10-min infusion	7–10	22	2	NL*	128	0.35 L/kg	Kramer et al 1978
4- to 5-day infusion	15–30/d	5	3	NL	119	0.45 L/kg	Kramer et al 1978
Intramuscular	2–10	NL	2.6	30–207	NL	NL	Oken et al 1981
Intraperitoneal	15	NL	5.5	904	NL	NL	Alberts et al 1979
Intrapleural	15	NL	3.6	548			

*NL, Not listed in original citation.

decrease with subsequent doses, especially if antipyretics are administered prophylactically. The drug appears to produce fever by liberating endogenous pyrogens from white cells (Dinarello et al 1973). Pretreatment with glucocorticosteroids but not antihistamines is effective at preventing this in animal models (Oken and Loch 1979).

Because bleomycin concentrates in the skin, cutaneous reactions are the most common type of toxicity encountered (Cohen et al 1973). "Staining" or hyperpigmentation of the skin may occur after subcutaneous dosing (Alberts and Peng 1979). Mild stomatitis is frequently observed and numerous other cutaneous manifestations may also occur. These include generalized hyperpigmentation, edema, and erythema of the skin and thickening of nail beds (Shetty 1977). Bleomycin skin toxicity correlates with the total drug dose but not with the route of administration or the specific schedule used. In some instances, skin toxicity may become dose limiting.

Mild to moderate dose-related alopecia begins several weeks after therapy. Typically there is regrowth of hair several months later. Other uncommon adverse reactions include headache, pruritis, and pain at the tumor site. Nausea, vomiting, and anorexia are reported but are usually self-limited and mild.

Late effects occur and by far the most serious toxic effect is lung damage. The pulmonary toxicity of bleomycin presents as pneumonitis with dry cough, dyspnea, rales, and infiltrates. It can progress steadily over weeks to radiographically documented fibrosis (Rudders and Hensley 1973, Perez-Guerra et al 1972). Histologically, there is a shift of type I to type II pneumonocytes in the lung. Pulmonary function studies taken during this process will variably show arterial hypoxemia, decreased carbon monoxide diffusing capacity, and restrictive ventilatory changes. Carbon monoxide diffusing capacity has been demonstrated by some to be a sensitive indicator of pulmonary toxicity (Van Barneveld et al 1987, Comis et al 1979, Sorenson et al 1985); however, several groups have recently reported that carbon monoxide diffusing capacity is not a reliable test to predict the development of clinically significant bleomycin lung damage (Lewis and Izbicki 1980, McKeage et al 1990). Clinical respiratory symptoms and auscultatory signs and serial chest x-rays can also be used to follow bleomycin-treated patients. One recommended hallmark for halting therapy is the finding of end-inspiratory crackles.

Neither pleural effusions nor hilar disease has been reported with bleomycin. It is reported that pulmonary toxicity is more common in patients over 70 years, in those receiving prior pulmonary radiation (Samuels et al 1976), and when total doses greater than 400 U are used. Acute pulmonary reactions are unpredictable, however, and have occurred at much lower total doses (Blum et al 1973). At total doses below 150 mg, life-threatening pulmonary toxicity is rare, but nonetheless can occur. At doses above 283 mg/m^2 pulmonary toxicity has reportedly occurred in 55% of patients and in 66% of those receiving 359 mg/m^2 or higher doses (Sostman et al 1977). Bleomycin pulmonary toxicity is significantly potentiated by thoracic radiation (Samuels et al 1976, Catane et al 1979) and by hyperoxia used during surgical anesthesia (Goldiner et al 1978, Ingrassia et al 1991).

A distinct low-dose hypersensitivity pneumonitis may occur at low total bleomycin doses. Fortunately, this reaction is responsive to corticosteroids (Holoye et al 1978). Because serious pulmonary toxicity is definitely related to the total dose administered, dosing should be halted and appropriate cultures taken to rule out intercurrent infection at the first signs or symptoms of toxicity. Even with rapid drug discontinuance respiratory fatalities may still occur and corticosteroids may be beneficial (Sostman et al 1977).

There are clinical data showing that bleomycin pulmonary toxicity is probably a continual process and that classic signs and symptoms are merely recognized relatively late in the clinical progression of the disease (Pascual et al 1973). Patients with compromised renal function may be more prone to bleomycin toxicity but elevations in serum creatinine or blood urea nitrogen seen in some patients have not correlated with the significant decrease in bleomycin elimination and increase in toxicity (Yee et al 1983).

In the review by Crooke and Bradner (1976), significant bleomycin toxicity occurred in about 11% of patients. From their review of 14 studies involving about 2000 patients, deaths from pulmonary toxicity from bleomycin occurred in 0 to 6% of cases. Others have reported a relatively low incidence of serious pulmonary fibrosis. For example, this was noted in about 2 to 3% of cases whereas fatal toxic effects occurred in only 1 to 2% of cases (Yagoda et al 1972).

Bleomycin appears to produce insignificant myelosuppressive effects. This allows for its incorporation into numerous combination chemotherapy regimens without adding significantly to bone marrow depression.

■ Special Applications

Malignant Effusions. Intracavitary bleomycin, in doses ranging from 15 to 240 U, has been used for control of malignant effusions. The most commonly used doses range from 60 to 120 U. For malignant pleural effusions, the drug is diluted into 100 mL of normal saline which is instilled into the pleural cavity via a thoracostomy tube that is clamped for 24 hours. Excessive fluid is drained for 2 to 3 days thereafter, and the tube removed. This has controlled malignant effusions in 60 to 80% of cases (Paladine et al 1976, Cunningham et al 1972).

Responses to intrapleural bleomycin are obtained in patients previously treated with tetracycline. Several prospective randomized trials have shown superiority in remission duration obtained with bleomycin compared with tetracycline (Johnson and Curzon 1985). Chest pain and fever are reported in only 10.5% of these patients and myelosuppression is not a problem (Ostrowski 1989). About 45% of an intrapleural dose is systemically absorbed and the terminal plasma half-life is 3.6 hours (similar to that following intravenous dosing [Alberts et al 1979]). The mean concentration × time product for a 60-U dose was 548 mU·min/mL and about 17% of the intrapleural dose was excreted in the urine.

Intraperitoneal instillation of bleomycin has been used to manage malignant ascites (Ostrowski and Halsall 1982, Bitran et al 1981). After peritoneal drainage for 12 to 24 hours, intraperitoneal bleomycin doses of 60 to 150 mg were instilled in 100 mL of saline and then the catheter was removed. Bleomycin doses of 60 mg appeared to produce the maximal response rates of 47% (Ostrowski and Halsall 1982) to 60% reported (Bitran et al 1981). Side effects include pain and fever in 21% of patients, nausea and vomiting in 6%, and rarely, erythema and dyspnea. The plasma half-life of bleomycin following intraperitoneal dosing was 5.5 hours, which is slightly longer than that following intravenous doses (about 4 hours [Alberts et al 1979]). This suggests a slow release of drug from the intraperitoneal space into the systemic circulation. About 25% of an intraperitoneal dose is recovered in the urine and the concentration × time product for a 60-U dose is 904 mU·min/mL, representing about 50% systemic bioavailability (Alberts et al 1979).

Bladder Instillation. Bleomycin has also been used with limited success by intravesicular administration for superficial bladder tumors. Doses of 30 to 120 U in 60 to 30 mL of water, respectively, have been instilled by urinary catheter and retained by the patient for 2 hours. Systemic absorption as assessed by bleomycin blood levels is minimal and is less than the therapeutic or toxic levels obtained with this route of administration (Bracken et al 1977).

Intratumoral Injection. Bleomycin has also been injected into malignant cutaneous lesions with some success. For this purpose small bleomycin doses are diluted in a minimal volume of normal saline and combined with lidocaine without obvious precipitation. Systemic drug absorption from this route of administration has been observed in subcutaneous dosing studies in mice (Crooke and Bradner 1976); however, a Japanese study reported no detectable systemic absorption following intratumoral bleomycin (as reviewed by Crooke and Bradner 1976). Local skin and soft tissue toxicity may be severe and this method of administration is not generally recommended.

Intraarterial Administration. Bleomycin in relatively large doses has been administered by continuous intraarterial infusion in squamous cell carcinomas of the uterine cervix (Huntington et al 1973), in head and neck cancer (Bilder and Hornova 1974), and in hepatic malignant melanoma (Kondi et al 1974). Intraarterial bleomycin serum concentration peaks were reported to be three times higher than levels from comparable intravenous doses (Crooke and Bradner 1976). See Dosage for specific doses reported in these studies.

Topical Application. In Japan, topical bleomycin has been used to treat a variety of cutaneous malignant lesions. The lyophilized powdered drug is reportedly quite stable in petrolatum (7% loss of activity after 2 years) but is unstable in Dermabase® or benzoin tincture (Crooke and Bradner 1976). Pharmacokinetic studies in mice have shown that only about 1% of topically applied bleomycin is absorbed systemically through intact skin. About 10% was absorbed through abraded tissue. In human studies, a 1% ointment is applied followed by an occlusive dressing. This was reported to be effective in condyloma acuminatum, actinic keratosis, and various types of warts (Crooke and Bradner 1976). Much lower response rates were reported in basal cell or squamous cell carcinomas of the skin.

Oral Administration. Bleomycin has also been used as a topical oral solution dissolved in dimethylsulfoxide. This formulation was used to treat localized lesions of leukoplakia (Wong et al 1989). A cotton wool pledget soaked in the solution was applied daily for 5 minutes each day for 2 weeks. A 0.5% solution reduced ulcer size but did not eliminate lesions. The use of a 1.0% solution caused complete ulcer resolution in three patients (Wong et al 1989).

REFERENCES

Alberts DS, Chen HSG, Liv R, et al. Bleomycin pharmacokinetics in man. *Cancer Chemother Pharmacol.* 1978;**1**:1–5.

Alberts DS, Chen HSG, Mayersohn M, et al. Bleomycin pharmacokinetics in man. II. Intracavitary administration. *Cancer Chemother Pharmacol.* 1979;**2**:127–132.

Alberts DS, Peng YM. Effective simulation of the minimum cytotoxic concentrations of continuous infusion (CI) bleomycin (BLEO) with multiple subcutaneous injections (MSC) in cancer patients. *Proc Am Assoc Cancer Res ASCO.* 1979;**20**:432.

Anderson EE, Gambertoglio JG, Schrier RW. *Clinical Use of Drugs in Renal Failure*, pp 15–17. Springfield, IL: Charles C. Thomas Publishers, 1976.

Baker L, Opipari M, Izbick R. Phase II study of mitomycin-C, vincristine, and bleomycin in advanced squamous cell carcinoma of the uterine cervix. *Cancer.* 1976;**38**:2222–2224.

Baker LH, Opipari MI, Wilson H, et al. Mitomycin-C, vincristine, and belomycin therapy for advanced cervical cancer. *Obstet Gynecol.* 1978;**52**(2):146–150.

Barranco SC, Kue JK, Romsdahl MM, Humphrey RM. Bleomycin as a possible synchronizing agent for human tumor cells in vivo. *Cancer Res.* 1973;**33**:882–887.

Benvenuto JA, Anderson RW, Kerkof K, et al. Stability and compatibility of antitumor agents in glass or plastic containers. *Am J Hosp Pharm.* 1981;**38**:1914–1918.

Bilder J, Hornova T. Synchronized combination bleomycin–methotrexate in regional chemotherapy of orofacial carcinomas. *Neoplasma (Bratisl.).* 1974;**21**:335–342.

Bitran JD, Brown C, Desser RK, et al. Intracavitary bleomycin for the control of malignant effusions. *J Surg Oncol.* 1981;**16**:273–277.

Blum RH, Carter SK, Agre K. A clinical review of bleomycin—a new, antineoplastic agent. *Cancer.* 1973;**31**:903–914.

Bracken RB, Johnson DE, Rodriquez L, et al. Treatment of multiple superficial tumors of the bladder with intravesical bleomycin. *Urology.* 1977;**9**(2):161–163.

Catane R, Schwade JG, Turrisi AT III, et al. Pulmonary toxicity after radiation and bleomycin: A Review. *Int J Radiat Oncol Biol Phys.* 1979;**5**:1513–1518.

Chabner BA, Myers CE, Oliverio VT. Clinical pharmacology of anticancer drugs. *Semin Oncol.* 1977;**4**:165–191.

Chien M, Grollman AP, Horwitz SB. Bleomycin–DNA interactions: Fluorescence and proton magnetic resonance studies. *Biochemistry.* 1977;**16**:3641.

Cohen MH, Johnston-Early A, Hood MA, et al. Drug precipitation within IV tubing: A potential hazard of chemotherapy administration. *Cancer Treat Rep.* 1985;**69**:1325–1326.

Cohen IS, Mosher MB, O'Keefe EJ, et al. Cutaneous toxicity of bleomycin therapy. *Arch Dermatol.* 1973;**107**:553–555.

Comis RL, Kuppinger MS, Ginsberg SJ, et al. Role of single-breath carbon monoxide-diffusing capacity in monitoring the pulmonary effects of bleomycin in germ cell tumor patients. *Cancer Res.* 1979;**39**:5046–5050.

Cooper KR, Hong WK. Prospective study of the pulmonary toxicity of continuously infused bleomycin. *Cancer Treat Rep.* 1981;**65**:419–425.

Crooke ST, Bradner WT. Bleomycin: A review. *J Med.* 1976;**7**:333–428.

Crooke ST, Friedrich L, Broughton A, et al. Bleomycin serum pharmacokinetics as determined by a radio-immunoassay and a microbiologic assay in a patient with compromised renal function. *Cancer.* 1977;**39**:1430–1434.

Cunningham TJ, Olson KB, Horton J, et al. A clinical trial of intravenous and intracavitary bleomycin. *Cancer.* 1972;**29**:1413–1419.

Dinarello CA, et al. Pyrogenic properties of bleomycin (NSC-125066). *Cancer Chemother Rep Part 1.* 1973;**57**:393–398.

Dorr RT, Peng YM, Alberts DS. Bleomycin compatibility with selected intravenous medications. *J Med.* 1982;**13**:121–130.

Durkin W, Pugh R, Solomon J, et al. Intravenous versus intramuscular bleomycin in far-advanced lymphomatous malignancy. Prospective randomized study (abstract #C-53). *Proc Am Soc Clin Oncol AACR.* 1976;**17**:250.

Einhorn LH, Donohue J. cis-Diamminedichloroplatinum, vinblastine, and bleomycin combination chemotherapy in disseminated testicular cancer. *Ann Intern Med.* 1977;**87**:293–298.

Frei E, Luce J, Gamble J, et al. Combination chemotherapy in advanced Hodgkin's disease—Induction and maintenance of remission. *Ann Intern Med.* 1973;**79**:376–382.

Ginsberg SJ, Gottlieb AJ, Bloomfield CD, et al. Combination chemotherapy with continuous infusion, low dose bleomycin in lymphoma. *Proc Am Assoc Cancer Res ASCO.* 1979;**20**:322.

Goldiner PL, Carlon GC, Cvitkovic E, et al. Factors influencing postoperative morbidity and mortality in patients treated with bleomycin. *Br Med J.* 1978;**1**:1664–1667.

Haidle CW, Weiss KK, Klo MT. Release of freebases from deoxyribonucleic acid after reaction with bleomycin. *Mol Pharmacol.* 1972;**8**:531–537.

Hait WN, Lazo JS, Chen DL, et al. Antitumor and toxic effects of combination chemotherapy with bleomycin and a phenothiazine anticalmodulin agent. *J Natl Cancer Inst.* 1988;**80**:246–250.

Hall SW, Broughton A, Strong JE, Benjamin RS. Clinical pharmacology of bleomycin by radioimmunoassay. *Clin Res.* 1977;**25**:407A.

Holoye PY, Luna M, MacKay B, Bedrossian CWM. Bleomycin hypersensitivity pneumonitis. *Ann Intern Med.* 1978;**88**:47–49.

Huntington MC, Dupriest RW, Fletcher WC. Intra-arterial bleomycin therapy in inoperable squamous cell carcinomas. *Cancer.* 1973;**31**:153–158.

Ingrassia TS, Ryu JH, Trastek VF, Rosenow EC III. Oxygen-exacerbated bleomycin pulmonary toxicity. *Mayo Clin Proc.* 1991;**66**:173–178.

Johnson CE, Curzon PGD. Comparison of intrapleural bleomycin and tetracycline in the treatment of malignant pleural effusions. *Thorax.* 1985;**40**:210.

Kasai H, Naganawa H, Takita T, et al. Chemistry of bleomycin. XXII. Interaction of bleomycin with nucleic acids, preferential binding to guanine base and electrostatic effect of the terminal amine. *J Antibiot (Tokyo).* 1978;**31**:1316.

Kondi ES, Gallitano AL, Eviy JT, Barnard DE. Prolonged survival in a patient with hepatic malignant melanoma treated by intra-arterial bleomycin and oral hydroxyurea. *Am J Surg.* 1974;**128**:85–87.

Kramer WG, Feldman S, Broughton A, et al. The pharmacokinetics of bleomycin in man. *J Clin Pharmacol.* 1978;**18**:346–352.

Krakoff IH, Cvitkovic E, Currie V, et al. Clinical pharmacologic and therapeutic studies of bleomycin given by continuous infusion. *Cancer.* 1977;**40**:2027–2037.

Lazo JS, Hait WN, Kennedy KA, et al. Enhanced bleomycin-induced DNA damage and cytotoxicity with calmodulin antagonists. *Mol Pharmacol.* 1985;**27**:387–393.

Lazo JS, Hoyt DG, Sebti SM, Pitt BR. Bleomycin: A pharmacologic tool in the study of the pathogenesis of interstitial pulmonary fibrosis. *Pharmacol Ther.* 1990;**47**:347–358.

Lewis BM, Izbicki R. Routine pulmonary function tests during bleomycin therapy. Tests may be ineffective and potentially misleading. *JAMA.* 1980;**243**:347–351.

Lilien DL, Jones SE, O'Mara RE. A clinical evaluation of indium-III bleomycin as a tumor-imaging agent. *Cancer.* 1975;**35**:1036–1049.

Livingston R, et al. Kinetic scheduling of vincristine and bleomycin in patients with lung cancer and other malignant tumors. *Cancer Chemother Rep.* 1973;**57**:219–224.

Livingston RB, Einhorn LH, Bodey GP, Burgess MA, et al. COMB (cyclophosphamide, oncovin, methyl-CCNU and bleomycin): A four drug combination in solid tumors. *Cancer.* 1975a;**36**:327–332.

Livingston RB, Einhorn LH, Burgess MA, et al. Combination chemotherapy with bleomycin (NSC-125066), Adriamycin (NSC-123127), CCNU (NSC-79037), vincristine (NSC-67574) and mechlorethamine (NSC-762) (BACON) in squamous cell lung cancer: Experience with 50 patients. *Cancer Chemother Rep Part 3.* 1975b;**6**:361–367.

McKeage MJ, Evans BD, Atkinson C, et al. Carbon monoxide diffusing capacity is a poor predictor of clinically significant bleomycin lung. *J Clin Oncol.* 1990;**8**:779–783.

Mirabelli CK, Haung CH, Crooke ST. Role of deoxyribonucleic acid topology in altering the site/sequence specificity of cleavage of deoxyribonucleic acid by bleomycin and talisomysin. *Biochemistry.* 1983;**22**:300–306.

Ohnuma T, Holand JF, Masuda H, et al. Microbiological assay of bleomycin: Inactivation, tissue distribution and clearance. *Cancer.* 1974;**33**:1230–1238.

Oken MM, Crooke ST, Elson MK, et al. Pharmacokinetics of bleomycin after IM administration in man. *Cancer Treat Rep.* 1981;**65**:485–489.

Oken MM, Loch J. Corticosteroid and antihistamine modification of bleomycin-induced fever. *Proc Soc Exp Biol Med.* 1979;**161**:594–596.

Ostrowski MJ. Intracavitary therapy with bleomycin for the treatment of malignant pleural effusions. *J Surg Oncol (Suppl).* 1989;**1**:7–13.

Ostrowski MJ, Halsall GM. Intracavitary bleomycin in the management of malignant effusions: A multicenter study. *Cancer Treat Rep.* 1982;**66**:1903–1907.

Paladine W, Cunningham TJ, Sponzo R. Intracavity bleomycin in the management of malignant effusions. *Cancer.* 1976;**38**:1903–1908.

Pascual RS, Mosher MB, Sikand RS, et al. Effects of bleomycin on pulmonary function in man. *Am Rev Respir Dis.* 1973;**108**:211–220.

Perez-Guerra K, Harkleroad LE, Walsh RE, et al. Acute bleomycin lung. *Am Rev Respir Dis.* 1972;**106**:909–913.

Rudders RA, Hensley GT. Bleomycin pulmonary toxicity. *Chest.* 1973;**63**:626–628.

Russo A, Mitchell JB, McPherson S, Friedman N. Alteration of bleomycin cytotoxicity by glutathione depletion or elevation. *Int J Radiat Oncol Biol Phys.* 1984;**10**:1675–1678.

Samuels ML, Holoye PY, Johnson DE. Bleomycin combination chemotherapy in the management of testicular neoplasia. *Cancer.* 1975;**36**:318–326.

Samuels ML, Johnson DE, Holoye PY, et al. Large-dose bleomycin therapy and pulmonary toxicity. A possible role of prior radiotherapy. *JAMA.* 1976;**35**:1117–1120.

Schein PS, DeVita VT, Hubbard S, et al. Bleomycin, Adriamycin, cyclophosphamide, vincristine, and prednisone (BACOP) combination chemotherapy in the treatment of advanced diffuse histiocytic lymphoma. *Ann Intern Med.* 1976;**85**:417–422.

Sebti SM, DeLeon JC, Lazo JS. Purification, characterization, and amino acid composition of rabbit pulmonary bleomycin hydrolase. *Biochemistry.* 1987;**26**:4213–4219.

Sebti SM, Mignano JE, Jani JP, et al. Bleomycin hydrolase: Molecular cloning, sequencing and biochemical studies reveal membership in the cysteine proteinase family. *Biochemistry.* 1989;**28**:6544–6548.

Sebti SM, Jani JP, Mistry JS, et al. Metabolic inactivation: A mechanism of human tumor resistance to bleomycin. *Cancer Res.* 1991;**51**:227–232.

Shetty MR. Case of pigmented banding of the nail caused by bleomycin. *Cancer Treat Rep.* 1977;**61**:501–502.

Sikic BI, Collins JM, Minnaugh EG, Gram TE. Improved therapeutic index of bleomycin when administered by continuous infusion in mice. *Cancer Treat Rep.* 1978;**62**:2011–2017.

Sorenson PG, Rossing N, Rorth M. Carbon-monoxide diffusing capacity: A reliable indicator of bleomycin-induced pulmonary toxicity. *Eur J Respir Dis.* 1985;**66**:333–340.

Sostman HD, Matthay RA, Putnam CE. Cytotoxic-induced lung disease. *Am J Med.* 1977;**62**:608–615.

Spigel SC, Coltman CA Jr. Therapy of mycosis fungoides with bleomycin. *Cancer.* 1973;**32**:767.

Tobey RA. Arrest of Chinese hamster cells in G_2 following treatment with the antitumor drug bleomycin. *J Cell Physiol.* 1972;**79**:259–266.

Tomoshisa J, et al. The chemistry of bleomycin. IX. The structures of bleomycin and phleomycin. *J Antibiot (Tokyo).* 1972;**25**:755–757.

Trissel LA, Fulton B, Tramonte SM. Visual compatibility of ondansetron with chemotherapeutic agents, antibiotics, and other selected drugs during simulated Y-site injection (abstract #P-468R). In: 25th Annual ASHP Midyear Clinical Meetings and Exhibit, Las Vegas, Nevada.

Umezawa H. Chemistry and mechanism of action of bleomycin. *Fed Proc.* 1974;**33**:2296–2302.

Umezawa H, Takeuchi T, Hori S, et al. Studies on the mechanism of antitumor effect of bleomycin on squamous cell carcinoma. *J Antibiot (Tokyo).* 1972;**20**:15–24.

Van Barneveld PWC, Sleijfer DT, Van Der Mark TW, et al. Natural course of bleomycin-induced pneumonitis. *Am Rev Respir Dis.* 1987;**135**:48–51.

Wong F, Epstein J, Millner A. Treatment of oral leukoplakia with topical bleomycin. A pilot study. *Cancer.* 1989;**64**:361–365.

Yagoda A, Mukherji B, Young C, et al. Bleomycin, an antitumor antibiotic. Clinical experience in 274 patients. *Ann Intern Med.* 1972;**77**:861–870.

Yee GC, Crom WR, Champion JE, et al. Cisplatin-induced changes in bleomycin elimination. *Cancer Treat Rep.* 1983;**67**:587–589.

Busulfan

■ Other Names

Myleran® (Burroughs Wellcome); BSF; NSC-750; busulphan.

■ Chemistry

$$CH_3-\underset{O}{\overset{O}{\underset{\|}{\overset{\|}{S}}}}-O-CH_2CH_2CH_2CH_2-O-\underset{O}{\overset{O}{\underset{\|}{\overset{\|}{S}}}}-CH_3$$

Structure of busulfan

Chemically, busulfan is 1,4-butanediol dimethanesulfonate. It is poorly water soluble and has a molecular weight of 246.32. It was synthesized by Timnis as a disulfonic ester molecule with a four-carbon chain in an attempt to find a less toxic analog of nitrogen mustard. A related seven-carbon analog, hepsulfam, is currently in early clinical trials and appears to have enhanced cytotoxic potency over busulfan in vitro (Pacheco et al 1989).

■ Antitumor Activity

Busulfan was first noted to have activity against murine ascites carcinoma. Although it has lacked significant clinical activity in acute and chronic lymphocytic leukemias, Galton and colleagues were the first to report significant antitumor effects in chronic myelogenous leukemia (Galton 1953, Galton et al 1958). It is for this indication that busulfan has been almost exclusively employed when used in standard doses (Hyman and Gelhorn 1956, Korbitz and Reiquam 1969). Busulfan at standard doses lacks activity in most solid tumors (Arduino and Mellinger 1967). High doses of both busulfan and cyclophosphamide are useful as a preparative regimen for bone marrow transplantation (BMT) in refractory leukemias (Santos et al 1984), in lymphomas (Lu et al 1984), and in several advanced pediatric solid tumors (Hartmann et al 1986) (see Special Applications).

See also Special Applications section at end of monograph for High Dose Applications with Bone Marrow Transplantation.

Mechanism of Action

Busulfan is the only commercially available methanesulfonate-type alkylating agent currently in use. The drug has purported cytotoxic selectivity for the granulocytic white blood cells. This is clinically seen at low doses with relative sparing of platelets and lymphocytes. At higher doses, all nucleated bone marrow cell lines are affected. Busulfan acts as a polyfunctional alkylating agent and thus shares many of the diverse cytotoxic effects of the nitrogen mustard-type alkylating agents. Warwick (1963), however, has shown that unlike other polyfunctional alkylators, busulfan appears to interact with cellular thiol groups as well as with nucleic acids. Busulfan produces a small amount of DNA–DNA (interstrand) crosslinking and a large amount of DNA–protein crosslinking. Both lesions form slowly in vitro, peaking 12 hours after drug exposure in L-1210 cells (Pacheco et al 1989). Busulfan is known to undergo SN_2-type alkylations of DNA with binding to the N-7 position of guanine (Brookes and Lawley 1961). Nonetheless, very little DNA–DNA crosslinking can be detected (Michell and Walker 1972). Warwick further postulated that endocrine gland suppression may explain a portion of busulfan's antitumor activity. This hypothesis has not been firmly substantiated. The antitumor activity of busulfan is not cell cycle phase specific.

Availability and Storage

Busulfan is available commercially from Burroughs Wellcome, Research Triangle Park, North Carolina. It is supplied as 2-mg scored tablets which have good stability if kept dry at room temperature.

Administration

Busulfan in common doses is generally well tolerated orally and may be taken any time during the day. (See Special Applications for high-dose busulfan in bone marrow transplantation.)

Dosage

This particular alkylating agent is most commonly used in an intermittent schedule in the management of the nonacute phase of chronic myelocytic leukemia. Initially, doses of 4 to 12 mg/d are given for several weeks. The higher doses in this range require close hematologic control and rapid tapering as the leukocyte count falls to avoid serious bone marrow aplasia. Subsequent dosing is based on the degree of symptomatic and hematologic control (eg, white blood cell [WBC] count) desired and on any evident toxicity. When used, maintenance doses have ranged from 1 to 3 mg/d; however, continuous dosing is generally not required in chronic myelogenous leukemia since long unmaintained remissions are characteristic and relapsing patients generally respond to additional busulfan therapy. In chronic myelocytic leukemia, busulfan therapy is usually stopped at a WBC count of 2500 or greater because the count will continue to fall for 2 to 3 weeks without further busulfan therapy. Because cumulative myelotoxicity can occur with this drug, chronic daily administration can involve considerable risk and is therefore not recommended. (See Special Applications for high-dose busulfan therapy in bone marrow transplantation.) In children receiving high-dose preparative therapy for BMT treatment, dosing on a mg/m^2 basis is suggested (Grochow et al 1990).

Pharmacokinetics

Busulfan is reportedly well absorbed orally. In adults, the oral absorption of busulfan from the tablets displays zero-order kinetics, with a mean lag time of 0.6 hour and a duration of 2 hours to the end of absorption (Ehrsson et al 1983). The elimination half-life in this trial was 2.51 hours and was not dose dependent. Mean plasma concentration × time (AUC) values were dose dependent, with peak levels of 24 to 130 ng/mL for doses of 2 to 6 mg. On hydrolysis, busulfan undergoes nucleophilic attack to yield 4-methanesulfonyloxybutanol. This metabolite breaks down further to yield the final decomposition products, tetrahydrofuran and methanesulfonic acid (Hassan and Ehrsson 1987). Busulfan also forms a sulfonium ion metabolite in the presence of glutathione transferases (Hassan and Ehrsson 1987).

The table on page 238 summarizes the clinical pharmacokinetic parameters of oral busulfan, particularly from reports of high-dose preparative therapy for BMT. These results show that busulfan clearance is more rapid in children, suggesting that busulfan doses could be increased in children (Grochow et al 1990). There is also evidence from one trial that the terminal half-life decreases after multiple dosing, suggesting an induced clearance (Hassan et al 1989b). The drug also readily distributes in spinal fluid with a cerebrospinal fluid: plasma ratio of 1.3:1.0 (range, 0.9–1.7) (Hassan et al 1989a). The half-life of busul-

CLINICAL PHARMACOKINETICS OF HIGH-DOSE ORAL BUSULFAN

Dose (mg/kg)	Patients	Volume of Distribution (L/kg)	Half-Life (h)	Clearance (mL/min/m^2)	AUC (μmol·min/L)	Peak (μmol/L)	Reference
1–2	Children	1.42	1.5	197	715 (1 mg)	1.4–2	Grochow et al 1990
1–2	Adults	0.60	2.3	95	2180 (1 mg)	4.25	Grochow et al 1990
1 every 6 h × 4 d	Adults	—	2.3	—	7590*	1.7[†]	Hassan et al 1989b
2[‡]			2.6		125*	28[†]	
4[‡]	Adults	—	2.1		290*	65[†]	Ehrsson et al 1983
6[‡]			2.5		366*	83[†]	

*AUC values in ng·h/mL.
[†]Peak plasma levels in ng/mL.
[‡]Fixed dose (not mg/kg).

fan in the cerebrospinal fluid (2.8 hours) is similar to the plasma half-life (Vassal et al 1990). Distribution into saliva is also equivalent to that into plasma (Hassan et al 1989b). The drug achieves transplacental uptake into the fetus and can cause teratogenic malformations (Diamond et al 1960).

Busulfan binding to plasma proteins was only 7.4%. Unique urinary metabolites identified in this trial include sulfoxane, 3-hydroxysulfoxane and tetrahydrothiophene-1-oxide (Hassan et al 1989b).

The pharmacologic action of the drug appears to be terminated by extensive metabolism to inactive compounds that are excreted renally. The majority of an oral dose is excreted in the urine as methanesulfonic acid. The remaining metabolites and excretion patterns are not well elucidated; however, little intact drug is found in the urine (Warwick 1963). Only 1% of unchanged busulfan was collected in the urine in one trial.

■ Side Effects and Toxicity

At low doses busulfan is purported to have somewhat selective activity on granulocytic cell lines, with relative sparing of platelets and lymphoid elements (Louis et al 1956). At high doses, all hematopoietic cell lines may be affected and busulfan-induced aplastic anemia is reported (Williams et al 1973). Compared with other alkylating agents, the nadir for myelosuppression with busulfan may be uncharacteristically long. Neutropenic nadirs may range from 11 to 30 days. Recovery is also prolonged, requiring more than to 24 to 54 days off therapy. This may explain the delayed and refractory pancytopenias reported for busulfan (Stuart et al 1976). In the one reported case of busulfan-induced aplastic bone marrow reactions, matched donor transfusion therapy was used. In these life-threatening reactions, bone marrow transplantation has also been used with a good outcome depending on the degree of HLA match with the donor marrow. According to Williams et al (1973) corticosteroids are not indicated. Lethality is reported in 20 to 90% of busulfan pancytopenias. Therefore, close hematologic monitoring with early drug discontinuance is strongly recommended to prevent this catastrophic complication.

Interstitial pulmonary fibrosis with cellular dysplasia within a year of starting therapy was first noted by Oliner et al (1961). It apparently is a rare complication usually occurring after long-term therapy (Burns et al 1970). Symptomatology may be delayed for up to 10 years in onset (average 4 years) and has generally been fatal within 6 months of diagnosis (Heard and Cooke 1968). Symptoms of the process include anorexia, cough, dyspnea, and fever. There is usually rapid progression to diffuse fibrosis and death (Leake et al 1963). Occasionally, patients have benefited from the prompt institution of high-dose corticosteroids (Oliner et al 1961).

Hormonal effects from busulfan include occasional gynecomastia and addisonian symptoms, with adrenal insufficiency and decreased adrenocorticotropin stores noted in the pituitary (Korbitz and Reiquam 1969). Drug discontinuance usually reverses this effect. There are also individual reports of testicular atrophy, impotence, and amenorrhea following busulfan. Surprisingly, there are at least nine case reports of successful pregnancies in women receiving the drug, some for the entire duration of the pregnancy (Korbitz and Reiquam 1969, Dugdale and Fort 1967); however, the drug is a known teratogen in humans, producing fetal malformation and cytomegaly (Diamond et al 1960).

Generally, nausea and vomiting are not problems with standard-dose busulfan but are quite prominent with high-dose therapy. There are, however, a few reports of unusual gastrointestinal complications such as severe diarrhea. Minor hepatotoxicity has also been reported, usually transient elevations of various hepatic enzymes. Other gastrointestinal symptoms have included cheilosis, glossitis, and anhydrosis.

Dermatologic hyperpigmentation is a frequent complication of busulfan therapy (Feingold and Koss 1969). It is thought to be the result of increased melanin synthesis and/or dispersion in the skin. It is most often noted at skin creases, particularly in the hands and nail beds, although total body hyperpigmentation is also described. Kyle (1961) has postulated that busulfan interacts with specific groups of glutathione in tissues. This process could potentially dethiolate sulfhydryl groups in the skin and thereby remove an inhibitor of melanin synthesis.

Cytologic dysplasia of cells of various organs is a common finding with busulfan (Bishop and Wassom 1986). Busulfan-induced chromosomal alterations have also been observed in Philadelphia chromosome-positive chronic myelocytic leukemia cells and in normal bone marrow (Becher and Prescher 1988). Cytogenetic aberrations included sister chromatid exchanges. Other affected epithelial cells include pulmonary alveoli, renal tubules, cervix and uterus, pancreas, thyroid and parathyroid, as well as arteriole and nerve trunk tissues (Gureli et al 1963, Koss et al 1965, Min and Gyorkey 1968).

■ Special Applications

High Doses with BMT. High-dose busulfan has been combined with cyclophosphamide and autologous or allogeneic BMT in the experimental treatment of a variety of refractory cancers. These include acute and chronic leukemias or malignant lymphomas treated with a total busulfan dose of 16 mg/kg plus cyclophosphamide 200 mg/kg (Geller et al 1989, Santos 1984, Lu et al 1984) or amsacrine 200 mg/m^2/d × 3 days in acute myeloid leukemia (Huijgens et al 1987), and for a variety of advanced pediatric solid tumors (Hartmann et al 1986). In children under 5 years, Hassan et al (1990) have shown that half-lives are shorter and AUCs lower than in older children and adults. There was also a 24-hour cyclic variation in busulfan plasma levels, with higher levels occurring at night. Thus, sampling times and drug doses may require modification in specific patient populations.

Response rates to high-dose busulfan/cyclophosphamide and BMT in relapsed and/or refractory acute and chronic leukemias and lymphoma are high and typically involve a high percentage of complete responders (Lu et al 1984, Santos et al 1984); however, relapses with 3 months of therapy may occur in over half of the responders (Lu et al 1984, Hartmann et al 1986). In relapsed acute myelogenous leukemia, patients treated in complete remission following initial induction therapy have the most profound benefit in terms of increased survival (Geller et al 1989). As a single agent, high-dose busulfan (16–20 mg/kg) produced partial responses in two of five patients with malignant melanoma but with relatively short durations of only 2 to 3 months (Peters et al 1987).

A total busulfan dose of 16 mg/kg is typically administered orally at a dose rate of 4 mg/kg/d for 4 consecutive days, followed by intravenous cyclophosphamide 50 mg/kg/d × 4 (Lu et al 1984). Pharmacokinetic studies with high-dose busulfan were summarized in the earlier table. Typical doses of 16 mg/kg given over a 4-day period produce steady-state plasma levels between 2 and 10 μM (Peters et al 1987). Mutagenic material can be recovered in the patient's urine for up to 48 hours after the last dose is administered.

As anticipated, severe myelosuppression is produced with high-dose busulfan therapy. Mean recovery of neutrophils starts on day 19 and platelets starting to increase on day 30. There is relative sparing of lymphocytic elements (Peters et al 1987); however, the typical dose-limiting toxic effects are mucositis, anorexia, and hepatic toxicity. Treatment deaths may occur in up to 20% of patients and are usually due to massive opportunistic infections (Lu et al 1984) or graft-versus-host disease (unless cyclosporine and/or methylprednisolone are added) (Geller et al 1989). *Candida albicans* infections may be particularly common (Peters et al 1987). Skin reactions typically involve mild desquamation with marked melanoderma (Hartmann et al 1986). Interstitial pneumonitis is also described, but the relative contributions of busulfan and cyclophosphamide to this common toxic effect is unknown. Moderate to severe nausea, vomiting, and diarrhea are common but are amenable to vigorous prophylaxis. Severe stomatitis, often as a result of herpes simplex, is described in about 70% of patients.

Other toxic effects attributed to busulfan include fatal hepatoveno-occlusive disease (VOD) in 10% of patients and transient elevations of liver enzymes and serum bilirubin. Hepatic VOD is also associated with unusually high systemic exposures obtained with fixed-dose schedules of busulfan in some patients (Grochow et al 1989). In this trial in which patients received 4 mg/kg/d × 4 days, AUCs greater than 3000 µmol·min/L were found in a patient who developed VOD. This compares with a mean of 2012 µmol·min/L for nonhepatotoxic patients. Unexplained hyperbilirubinemia with levels in excess of 5 mg/dL is also encountered frequently.

Generalized seizures are also observed and typically occur on days 3 to 4 of high-dose busulfan therapy (Marcus and Goldman 1984, Hartmann et al 1986, Sureda et al 1989). In children seizures usually occur 2 to 4 hours after dosing (Vassal et al 1990). The events involve classic tonic–clonic seizures without focal neurologic findings. Phenytoin is apparently an effective prophylaxis when used in a loading dose regimen of 18 mg/kg prior to busulfan, with a 300-mg phenytoin maintenance dose given on busulfan therapy days thereafter (Grigg et al 1989). Clonazepam prophylaxis (0.1 mg/kg/d by continuous intravenous infusion during busulfan therapy) may also be used to protect against seizures in pediatric patients (Vassal et al 1990). Another trial has shown that busulfan neurotoxicity in children is dose dependent (Vassal et al 1990). Only 1 of 57 children given a total dose of 16 mg/kg developed seizures compared with 6 of 39 children receiving 600 mg/m^2 (16–28 mg/kg). A slightly higher cerebrospinal fluid: plasma ratio of 1.4:1.0 was obtained in the high-dose patients compared with the low-dose ratio of 1.02 (Vassal et al 1990).

Unexplained pain at tumor sites is also described in a few patients, along with transient autoimmune disorders including rash and severe seronegative arthritis, development of antigranulocyte and antiplatelet antibodies, and chronic active hepatitis (Peters et al 1987).

REFERENCES

Arduino LJ, Mellinger GT. Clinical trial of busulfan (NSC-750) in advanced carcinoma of prostate. *Chemother Rep.* 1967;**51**:295–303.

Becher R, Prescher G. Induction of sister chromatid exchanges and chromosomal aberrations by busulfan in Philadelphia chromosome-positive chronic myeloid leukemia and normal bone marrow. *Cancer Res.* 1988;**48**:3435–3439.

Bishop JB, Wassom JS. Toxicological review of busulfan (Myleran). *Mutat Res.* 1986;**168**:15–45.

Brookes P, Lawley PD. The alkylation of guanosine and guanylic acid. *Biochem J.* 1961;**80**:486.

Burns WA, McFarland W, Matthews MJ. Busulphan induced pulmonary disease: Report of a case and review of the literature. *Am Rev Respir Dis.* 1970;**101**:408–413.

Diamond I, Anderson MM, McCreadie SR. Transplacental transmission of busulfan (myleran) in a mother with leukemia. Production of fetal malformation and cytomegaly. *Pediatrics.* 1960;**25**:85–90.

Dugdale M, Fort AT. Busulfan treatment of leukemia during pregnancy. *JAMA.* 1967;**199**:167–169.

Ehrsson H, Hassan M, Ehrnebo M, Beran M. Busulfan kinetics. *Clin Pharmacol Ther.* 1983;**34**(1):86–89.

Feingold ML, Koss LG. Effects of long term administration of busulfan. *Arch Intern Med.* 1969;**124**:66–71.

Galton DAG. Myleran in chronic myeloid leukaemia. *Lancet.* 1953;**1**:208–213.

Galton DAG, Till M, Wiltshaw E. Busulfan: Summary of clinical results. *Ann NY Acad Sci.* 1958;**68**:967–973.

Geller RB, Saral R, Piantadosi S, et al. Allogeneic bone marrow transplantation after high-dose busulfan and cyclophosphamide in patients with acute non-lymphocytic leukemia. *Blood.* 1989;**73**(8):2209–2218.

Grigg AP, Shepherd JD, Phillips GL. Busulphan and phenytoin. *Ann Intern Med.* 1989;**111**(12):1049–1050.

Grochow LB, Jones RJ, Brundrett RB, et al. Pharmacokinetics of busulfan: Correlation with veno-occlusive disease in patients undergoing bone marrow transplantation. *Cancer Chemother Pharmacol.* 1989;**25**:55–61.

Grochow LB, Krivit W, Whitley CB, Blazar B. Busulfan disposition in children. *Blood.* 1990;**75**(8):1723–1727.

Gureli N, Denham SW, Root SW. Cytologic dysplasia related to busulfan (Myleran) therapy. Report of a case. *Obstet Gynecol.* 1963;**21**:466–470.

Hartmann O, Benhamou E, Beaujean F, et al. High-dose busulfan and cyclophosphamide with autologous bone marrow transplantation support in advanced malignancies in children: A phase II study. *J Clin Oncol.* 1986;**4**:1804–1810.

Hassan M, Ehrsson H. Metabolism of ^{14}C-busulfan in isolated perfused rat liver. *Eur J Drug Metab Pharmacokinet.* 1987;**13**:301–305.

Hassan M, Ehrsson H, Smedmyr B, et al. Cerebrospinal fluid and plasma concentrations of busulfan during high-dose therapy. *Bone Marrow Transplant.* 1989a;**4**:113–114.

Hassan M, Oberg G, Bekassy A, et al. Pharmacokinetics of busulfan during high-dose therapy in relation to age and chronopharmacology. *J Cancer Res Clin Oncol.* 1990;**116**(suppl):580.

Hassan M, Oberg G, Ehrsson H, et al. Pharmacokinetic

and metabolic studies of high-dose busulphan in adults. *Eur J Clin Pharmacol.* 1986b;**36**:525–530.
Heard BE, Cooke RA. Busulfan lung. *Thorax.* 1968;**23**:187–193.
Huijgens PC, Ossenkoppele GJ, van der Weide M, et al. High-dose busulfan and amsacrine with autologous bone marrow rescue in patients with acute myeloid leukemia in first remission. *Cancer Treat Rep.* 1987;**71**(5):552–553.
Hyman GA, Gelhorn A. Myleran therapy in malignant neoplastic disease: Use of 1,4-dimethanesulfonoxybutane with emphasis on chronic granulocytic leukemia. *JAMA.* 1956;**161**:944–947.
Korbitz BC, Reiquam CW. Busulfan in chronic granulocytic leukemia, a spectrum of clinical considerations. *Clin Med.* 1969;**76**:16–22.
Koss LG, Melamed MR, Mayer K. The effect of busulfan in human epithelia. *Am J Clin Pathol.* 1965;**44**:385–394.
Kyle RA. A syndrome resembling adrenocortical insufficiency associated with long-term busulfan (Myleran) therapy. *Blood.* 1961;**18**:497–510.
Leake E, Smith WG, Woodliff HJ. Diffuse interstitial pulmonary fibrosis after busulphan therapy. *Lancet.* 1963;**2**:432–434.
Louis J, Limarzi LR, Best W. Treatment of chronic granulocytic leukemia with Myleran. *Arch Intern Med.* 1956;**97**:299–308.
Lu C, Braine HG, Kaizer H, et al. Preliminary results of high-dose busulfan and cyclophosphamide with syngeneic or autologous bone marrow rescue. *Cancer Treat Rep.* 1984;**68**(5):711–717.
Marcus RE, Goldman M. Convulsions due to high-dose busulphan. *Lancet.* 1984;**2**:1463.
Michell MP, Walker IG. Studies on the cytotoxicity of Myleran and dimethylMyleran. *Can J Biochem.* 1972;**50**:1074–1078.
Min KW, Gyorkey F. Interstitial pulmonary fibrous, atypical epithelial changes and bronchiolar cell carcinoma following busulfan therapy. *Cancer.* 1968;**22**:1027–1032.
Oliner H, Schwartz R, Rubio F, Dameshek W. Interstitial pulmonary fibrosis following busulfan therapy. *Am J Med.* 1961;**31**:134–139.
Pacheco DY, Stratton NK, Gibson NW. Comparison of the mechanism of action of busulfan with hepsulfam, a new antileukemic agent, in the L1210 cell line. *Cancer Res.* 1989;**49**:5108–5110.
Peters WP, Henner WD, Grochow LB, et al. Clinical and pharmacologic effects of high dose single agent busulfan with autologous bone marrow support in the treatment of solid tumors. *Cancer Res.* 1987;**47**:6402–6406.
Santos GW, Tutschka PJ, Brookmeyer R, et al. Marrow transplantation for acute non-lymphocytic leukemia after treatment with busulfan and cyclophosphamide. *N Engl J Med.* 1984;**309**:1347–1352.
Stuart JJ, Crocker DL, Roberts HR. Treatment of busulfan-induced pancytopenia. *Arch Intern Med.* 1976;**136**:1181–1183.
Sureda A, Oteyza JP, Larana JG, Odriozola J. High-dose busulfan and seizures. *Ann Intern Med.* 1989;**111**(6):543–544.
Vassal G, Deroussent A, Hartmann O, et al. Dose-dependent neurotoxicity of high-dose busulfan in children: A clinical and pharmacological study. *Cancer Res.* 1990;**50**:6203–6207.
Warwick GP. The mechanism of action of alkylating agents. *Cancer Res.* 1963;**23**:1315–1333.
Williams DM, Lynch RE, Cartwright GE. Drug induced aplastic anemia. *Semin Hematol.* 1973;**10**:195–223.

Buthionine Sulfoximine

■ Other Names

BSO; NSC-326231.

■ Chemistry

Structure of buthionine sulfoximine

DL-Buthionine-SR-sulfoximine is a structural analog of the amino acid L-methionine. The complete chemical name is 2-amino-4-(S-butylsulfonimidoyl)-2S-butanoic acid. It has a molecular formula of $C_8H_{18}N_2O_3S$ and a molecular weight of 222.3. The water solubility of buthionine sulfoximine is approximately 11.2 g/100 mL or 0.5 M. The L-isomer is the active form of the molecule which is commercially supplied as a racemic DL product.

■ Antitumor Activity

Buthionine sulfoximine (BSO) is primarily a modulator of glutathione synthesis (Meister 1978) which may block the inactivation of several types of antitumor agents, particularly alkylating agents (Arrick and Nathan 1984). In some tumor cell lines, BSO has been shown to produce direct inhibition of colony formation when glutathione (GSH) levels are chronically depressed to 10% or less of control (Dorr et al 1986). This was observed most prominently in 8226 multiple myeloma (B-lymphocyte) cell lines.

In combination with other antitumor agents,

L-BSO has been shown to sensitize tumor cells to the cytotoxic effects of the alkylating agent melphalan (Green et al 1984, Somfai-Relle et al 1984, Suzukake et al 1982), to the DNA intercalating agent doxorubicin (Russo and Mitchell 1985), to cisplatin in ovarian cancer cells (Andrews et al 1988), to bleomycin in Chinese hamster ovary cells (Russo et al 1984), and to mitomycin-C in EMT6/SF mouse fibrosarcoma cells. The cytotoxic activity of cisplatin and carboplatin in vitro are increased following exposure to L-BSO (Lee et al 1992). Interestingly, the activity of oxaliplatin was not enhanced by L-BSO (Boughattas et al 1992). Not all studies, however, demonstrate an augmentation of cytotoxicity by BSO in vitro. Doxorubicin, mitomycin-C, vinblastine, cytarabine, and carmustine did not produce greater cytotoxic effects in murine P-815 fibrosarcoma cells when incubated with BSO (Arrick et al 1983). Similarly, with anticancer agents such as neocarzinostatin (DeGraff et al 1985) and Taxol® (Liebmann et al 1992), BSO can decrease drug cytotoxicity in these instances (see Drug Interactions).

Buthionine sulfoximine also sensitizes cells to the cytotoxic effects of other antitumor modalities. These include radiation therapy (Durand 1984, Biaglow and Varnes 1983, Biaglow et al 1986, Bertsche and Schorn 1986), hyperthermia (Mitchell and Russo 1983, Freeman et al 1985), and a diverse number of radiosensitizing oxidants such as misonidazole (Yu and Brown 1984), sesquiterpene lactones (Arrick et al 1983), and hydrogen peroxide (Arrick et al 1982).

In tumor cell lines, BSO can reverse drug resistance to agents such as melphalan (Kramer et al 1987) and cisplatin (Hamilton et al 1985, 1986, Andrews et al 1988). When BSO is combined with resistance modulators such as verapamil, additional cytotoxicity may be expressed in multidrug-resistant cells that possess the 180,000-molecular-weight P-glycoprotein (Kramer et al 1988); however, a more recent in vitro study has not confirmed this finding in human colon carcinoma cell lines (Lutzky et al 1992).

In mice bearing MOPC-315 plasmacytomas, BSO slightly enhanced the antitumor effects of low doses of doxorubicin, melphalan, carmustine, and cyclophosphamide (Soble and Dorr 1987). At high doses of the antitumor agents, acute lethality was enhanced by the addition of L-BSO. In nude mice bearing human ovarian cancer cells, BSO combined with melphalan significantly increased antitumor effects (Hamilton et al 1985, 1986, Ozols et al 1987). In mice bearing melphalan-resistant L-1210 leukemia tumors, however, survival was not significantly enhanced by BSO in two other trials (Kramer et al 1987, Somfai-Relle et al 1984).

Overall, these results suggest that BSO can modulate intracellular GSH levels and alter experimental tumor cell responses to alkylating agents and anthracyclines. The degree of enhancement is highly dependent on the BSO dose and on the timing of the two treatments (BSO prior to the cytotoxic modality). Of note, not all studies show enhanced antitumor efficacy for BSO combined with sulfhydryl-dependent antitumor agents (Soble and Dorr 1988).

In early clinical trials, one partial response was achieved with intravenous BSO plus intravenous melphalan in a patient with locally extensive ovarian cancer (LaCreta et al 1991). Other clinical trials are still exploring phase I dose escalations of L-BSO and have not described antitumor effects (Bailey et al 1992).

■ Mechanism of Action

Buthionine sulfoximine blocks the formation of the tripeptide glutathione by irreversibly inhibiting the rate-limiting enzyme, γ-glutamyl-cysteine synthetase (see figure on opposite page) (Griffith 1982). Thus, BSO acts as suicide substrate inhibitor to block the conjugation of cysteine and glutamate (Meister 1978). This directly blocks replenishment of the cytosolic pool of reduced glutathione which is lost principally by oxidation to the dimer GSSG as a result of normal metabolic reactions. The smaller pool of mitochondrial GSH is not affected by BSO treatments (Meister and Griffith 1983) and this pool may provide sufficient GSH for continued cell growth in the face of continued treatment with BSO (Gaetjens et al 1984).

Kinetic studies of enzyme inactivation by DL-BSO show that the initial binding constant is less than 100 μM with a pseudo-first-order rate constant for inactivation of 3.7 min^{-1} (half-life for inhibition of about 11 seconds) (Griffith 1982). Binding and enzyme inactivation are normally irreversible if magnesium and ATP are available. Unlike the lower homologs methionine sulfoximine and prothionine sulfoximine, BSO has little or none of the inhibitory activity for the α-glutamyl cycle which led to convulsions and other central nervous system toxic effects in mice (Griffith and Meister 1979). The larger chemical homologs of BSO, hexathionine sulfoximine and heptathionine sulfoximine, produced potent lethality and were similarly abandoned for clinical trial consideration (Griffith 1982).

Following the administration of BSO to rodents, glutathione levels are slowly depleted in sev-

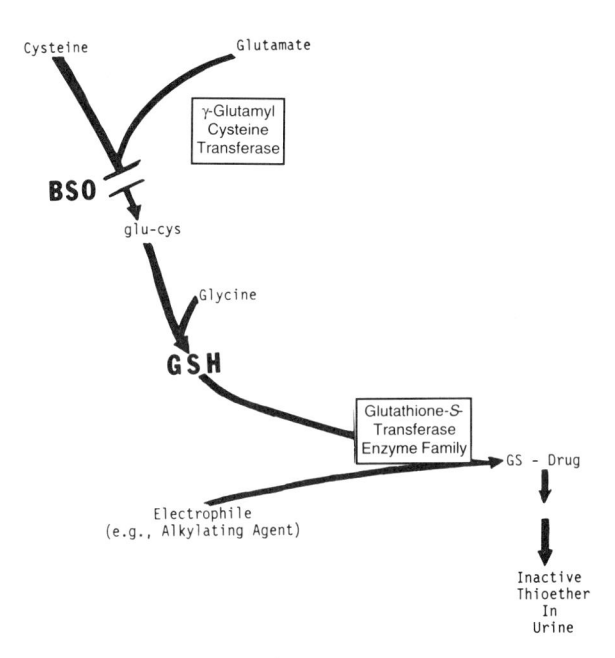

Inhibition of glutathione (GSH) synthesis by buthionine sulfoximine (BSO)

REDUCED GLUTATHIONE (GSH) LEVELS IN PERIPHERAL BLOOD MONONUCLEAR CELLS (PBMCS) FOLLOWING ADMINISTRATION OF L-BUTHIONINE SULFOXIMINE (L-BSO) IN HUMANS

L-BSO (mg/m² IV)	% Control*	% Control†	% Control, BSO + Melphalan
1500	90	72	54
3000	30	50	39
4500	15–20	—	—
4800	—	42	47

*La Creta et al 1991.
†Baily et al 1991 (GSH in lymphocytes measured 72 hours after dosing).

eral normal tissues as well as in tumor cells. In mice maximal GSH depletion is achieved after 2 to 4 hours in the plasma, 5 hours in the liver, 3 hours in the kidney, and 5 to 10 hours in anaplastic and fibrosarcoma tumors, respectively (Minchinton et al 1984, Soble and Dorr 1987). Intracellular GSH depletion may not, however, explain cell growth inhibition following exposure to L-BSO (Kang 1992). Rather, BSO may be inhibiting extracellular amino acid uptake, particularly cysteine (Kang 1992). Thus, BSO-induced cytostasis in vitro can be overcome by supplying exogenous GSH *or* L-cysteine (Kang 1992).

Buthionine sulfoximine also decreases the activity of DNA polymerases α, β, and γ (Ali-Osman and Rairkar 1992). The maximal decrease was 45% for DNA polymerase α and was obtained 48 hours after a 24-hour BSO exposure. This may explain an inhibitory effect of L-BSO on DNA repair which is postulated to enhance tumor cell sensitivity to alkylating agents, including platinum-containing compounds.

Pharmacodynamic studies of GSH depletion by BSO in humans are outlined in the table. These studies have shown that GSH depletion in peripheral blood lymphocytes (PBLs) is non-dose dependent, with maximum depletion of 60 to 70% of GSH content (200–300 ng/10⁶ cells). This depletion was achieved at 72 hours after dosing (Bailey et al 1992). On a 12-hour oral dosing interval, GSH levels have returned to normal prior to the next dose. Importantly, the patterns of GSH depletion in PBLs were similar to that in ascites tumor cells in one patient (Bailey et al 1992). On the basis of rodent data, it may be possible to sequentially administer an anticancer agent after BSO to take advantage of the more rapid GSH replenishment in normal organs compared with solid tumors (Minchinton et al 1984; Russo et al 1986a).

■ Availability and Storage

Buthionine sulfoximine has been available commercially as a laboratory reagent from Chemical Dynamics Corporation, Plainfield, New Jersey. It is supplied as a nonsterile powder of approximately 90% purity that has been used for laboratory research. An investigational sterile injection is available from the National Cancer Institute. The product is supplied as a 10% sterile solution containing 100 mg/mL in 10-mL vials (1 g/vial). The pH of the solution is adjusted to 7 to 8 with sodium hydroxide. The intact vials are recommended to be stored at room temperature.

■ Preparation for Use, Stability, and Admixture

The sterile 10% solution can be diluted to a final concentration of 0.1 mg/mL in 5% Dextrose for Injection, USP, or into 0.9% Sodium Chloride for Injection, USP. The drug is also compatible in either glass or polyvinyl chloride plastic infusate containers for a 14-day period at room temperature (20°C). The drug is unstable at acid pH values, but is stable for at least 48 hours at pH between 6 and 9.9 at 90°C (Department of Health and Human Services 1987).

Administration

Buthionine sulfoximine is intravenously administered as either a brief injection or a more prolonged infusion. The drug has also been administered orally in experimental animals, although bioavailability may be as low as 2% (in the mouse). In phase I studies, BSO has been infused intravenously over 30 minutes in 100 to 250 mL of saline or dextrose (LaCreta et al 1991).

Special Precautions

In high doses in animals, BSO has produced severe central nervous system toxicity characterized by convulsions and death. Patients with preexisting central nervous system disorders are currently ineligible for phase I studies with L-BSO because of these concerns. It is also clear that some cytotoxic drugs may produce severe toxicity when combined with BSO. This has been noted for the combination of cyclophosphamide with BSO (Friedman et al 1990) (see Drug Interactions) and may also occur with other as yet untested drug combinations. Thus, extreme caution should be exercised when considering a combination of BSO with any drug that itself is inactivated even partially by reduced thiols.

Dosage

In experimental animals, tolerable doses have ranged from 1600 mg/kg/per dose (every 4 hours × 6 doses) in the mouse and 100 mg/kg/per dose (every 8 hours for 15 doses) in the beagle dog. Single intravenous doses of 3.2 g/kg or 10 oral doses of 800 mg/kg given every 8 hours have been lethal in the dog (Department of Health and Human Services 1987). In initial phase I trials in humans, BSO has been given at a dose of 1500 mg/m^2 to 10.08 g/m^2 over 30 minutes intravenously every 12 hours for six doses (Bailey et al 1991, 1992, LaCreta et al 1991). The dose of melphalan has been fixed at 15 mg/m^2 IV (Hamilton et al 1990, Bailey et al 1992).

Drug Interactions

Buthionine sulfoximine significantly lowers the lethal dose of cyclophosphamide in experimental rodent models (Soble and Dorr 1988, Friedman et al 1990). The latter study clearly shows that cyclophosphamide cardiotoxicity is significantly enhanced by concomitant BSO. In the rabbit, BSO has also been shown to significantly reduce the clearance of the DNA intercalator amsacrine (Paxton et al 1986). This could potentially increase the severity of amsacrine-induced myelotoxicity. Kramer et al (1985) have also described synergistic nephrotoxicity for the combination of BSO with the nitrosourea semustine in B44 rats. Besides potentiating nephrotoxicity, the combination produced hepatotoxicity that was not seen with either agent alone. Grade 4 hepatotoxicity was observed in one patient receiving BSO + melphalan and a quinolone antibiotic. The BSO therapy may have enhanced the toxicity of the antibiotic in this single case (LaCreta et al 1991).

Conversely, L-BSO reduces the experimental cytotoxic activity of neocarzinostatin (DeGraff et al 1985) and Taxol® in vitro (Liebmann et al 1992). The latter effect may relate to altered tubulin formation induced by GSH depletion.

Pharmacokinetics

The pharmacokinetics of BSO has been studied in CD2F1 mice and in beagle dogs given intravenous doses of up to 2.4 g/m^2. There appears to be a biphasic and rapid elimination of the drug (see table). The low volume of distribution suggests that the drug is not highly bound to tissues or plasma proteins and is distributed predominantly into total body water. Of interest, plasma drug clearance was similar in both species (see table). Metabolic studies in rats given radiolabeled L-BSO have shown that only about 3% of a dose is recovered as carbon dioxide, implying that little metabolism occurs (Griffith 1982). About 60% of the administered radiolabel is recovered as the intact molecule and 90% of the remainder was thought to be N-acetylated L-buthionine-SR-sulfoximine. The compound appears to be readily excreted in the urine, and in rats nearly all the drug can be recovered in the urine within 24 hours of administration (Griffith 1982).

Initial oral bioavailability studies in mice given

PHARMACOKINETICS OF INTRAVENOUS BUTHIONINE SULFOXIMINE IN MICE AND DOGS GIVEN 2.4 g/m^2

Parameter	CD2F1 Mouse	Beagle Dog
Clearance (mL/min/m^2)	84	104
Half-life (min)		
α	5	8
β	37	36
Volume of distribution at steady state (mL/kg)	280	233
AUC (g/mL · min)	28.5	23.8

PHARMACODYNAMICS OF GLUTATHIONE DEPLETION FOLLOWING ADMINISTRATION OF BUTHIONINE SULFOXIMINE (BSO) IN MICE

Dose (mg/kg Orally)	GSH Depletion (Time After BSO Administration)			
	Plasma	Liver	Kidney	Lung
100 × 15	61–72% (4 h)		41% (4 h)	39% (4 h)
400 × 15	61–72% (4 h)	35% (4 h)	82% (4 h)	48% (4 h)
800 × 15	61–72% (4 h)	35% (4 h)	89% (4 h)	60% (4 h)
1200 × 1	70% (8 h)	88% (4 h)*	NM†	NM
	37% (24 h)	73% (8 h)		
1600 × 1	70% (8 h)	88% (4 h)*	NM	NM
	53% (24 h)	73% (8 h)		
		0% (24 h)		

*Intravenous doses.
†NM, not measured.

BSO in the drinking water showed that only about 2% of the drug was absorbed intact from the gastrointestinal tract. Despite this finding, GSH suppression was equivalent after oral or intravenous doses of 2.4 g/m².

The pharmacodynamics of BSO-induced suppression of GSH levels in different tissues is shown in the above table. These results show that there is not always a good correlation between the dose and the level of GSH reduction in a specific tissue. This was especially true in the liver, where all doses produced significant GSH depletion 4 hours after drug administration (See Mechanism of Action also). Although the plasma GSH levels were significantly depressed in both mice and dogs, the extent of GSH depletion was dependent on both the dose and the duration of treatment only in the dog. In mice, plasma GSH was depleted in a non-dose-dependent fashion.

In humans, GSH levels fall to 20% or less of control in peripheral blood mononuclear cells examined 48 hours after the sixth dose of 1500 mg/m² BSO given intravenously every 12 hours (Hamilton et al 1990). There is a dose-dependent reduction in GSH levels in peripheral blood mononuclear cells (PBMCs) (see the above table). The pharmacokinetics of the drug in humans do not show stereoselectivity except for the smaller volume of distribution at steady state for the R-BSO isomer (see the table below). These studies show that the drug is rapidly eliminated with a distribution volume approximating total body water (LaCreta et al 1991). A reduction in PBMC GSH levels to about 20 to 48% of control is achieved at BSO doses of 4500 to 4800 mg/m², respectively (LaCreta et al 1991 and Bailey et al 1991, respectively). The nadir in GSH levels is achieved 72 hours after dosing, with recovery at 120 hours (LaCreta et al 1991). There is also evidence of slightly enhanced GSH depletion with BSO combined with melphalan (Bailey et al 1991) (see the above table). Glutathione depletion to 20% or less of control was also observed in ascites tumor cells in five of eight ovarian cancer patients treated in a phase I trial (LaCreta et al 1991).

■ Side Effects and Toxicity

Preclinical Studies. Buthionine sulfoximine produces only a transient 67% decrease in peripheral white blood cells in mice. A slight (10%) degree of weight loss occurred in female mice given the highest dose of intravenous BSO (1600 mg/kg every 4 hours for six doses). No gross or microscopic lesions were observed at this dose level. Mice given this dose of BSO followed by melphalan (5 mg/kg IV) experienced atrophy of bone marrow, splenic my-

CLINICAL PHARMACOKINETICS OF L-BUTHIONINE SULFOXIMINE (L-BSO) STEREOISOMERS IN HUMANS

Pharmacokinetic Parameters at Dose of 1.5 g/m² (n = 3)	L-BSO Stereoisomer	
	R (53%)	S (47%)
Half-life		
α (min)	19.4	17.9
β (h)	3.5	3.4
Clearance (mL/min/kg)	2.45	2.22
Volume of distribution (L/kg)		
Central	0.13	0.14
Steady state	0.36	.56

Data from LaCreta F, Brennan J, Padavic K, et al. Phase I clinical, biochemical and pharmacokinetic study of buthionine sulfoximine (BSO) in combination with melphalan (L-PAM). Proc Am Soc Clin Oncol. 1991;10:104.

eloid tissues, and mesenteric lymph nodes with the new appearance of renal nephrosis and a significant increase in blood urea nitrogen levels (Page et al 1987).

In contrast, a single intravenous dose of 3.2 g/kg in the dog produced tonic–clonic convulsions and hematuria which were lethal (Smith et al 1987). There was also damage to the exocrine pancreas and attendant changes in the serum chemistries of these animals, including significant elevations in liver enzymes (serum glutamic–oxalacetic transaminase [SGOT], serum glutamic–pyruvic transaminase [SGPT], and alkaline phosphatase), hyperglycemia, and serum chloride concentrations. With a multiple-dose schedule of 800 mg/kg every 8 hours BSO produced nonlethal emesis, diarrhea, hyperactivity, and convulsions after 9 to 10 doses were administered. The lower dose levels of 100 and 400 mg/kg produced diarrhea and emesis. Increased alkaline phosphatase and liver transaminase activities (SGOT, SGPT) were also observed with the 400 and 800 mg/kg multiple dose schedules; however, no microscopic lesions were noted in either of these lower-dose groups.

As noted earlier, BSO does not appear to significantly increase myelotoxicity from some antitumor agents in mice. This effect has been observed for combinations with cyclophosphamide (Soble and Dorr, 1987), carmustine (Soble and Dorr 1987), and doxorubicin (Soble and Dorr 1987). With melphalan, there are conflicting reports that describe either little myelotoxic synergy (Russo et al 1986b, Kramer et al 1986, Soble and Dorr 1987) or significantly enhanced myelotoxicity for L-BSO + melphalan over melphalan alone (Liao et al 1989). The combination of cyclophosphamide and BSO has, however, led to acute lethality 2 to 4 hours after administration of otherwise nonlethal cyclophosphamide doses in the mouse (Soble and Dorr 1987). Friedman et al (1990) have studied this phenomenon in rats and have described acute elevations in serum potassium, blood urea nitrogen, and creatinine phosphokinase levels with resultant renal failure. Skeletal muscle biopsies showed distortions of type 2 myofibrils with a loss of sarcomere definition and mitochondrial clustering. In the heart, the combination produced mitochondrial swelling but no other changes; however, rats dying after combined BSO and cyclophosphamide all exhibited acute myocardial ischemia, hypotension, and finally complete heart block and ventricular fibrillation (Friedman et al 1990). These findings suggest that BSO may be a poor candidate to consider in combination with oxazophosphorine alkylating agents such as cyclophosphamide and ifosfamide.

Buthionine sulfoximine combined with the nitrosourea semustine (CCNU) produces synergistic nephrotoxicity in rats (Kramer et al 1985). This combination also produced severe hepatotoxicity which did not occur with semustine alone (Kramer et al 1985). This finding suggests that combinations of BSO with nitrosoureas should be avoided to prevent nitrosourea-induced hepatotoxicity and nephrotoxicity, as seen after high-dose therapy in the absence of BSO (Weiss et al 1983).

Clinical Toxicity. Little if any toxicity has been associated with BSO alone in phase I studies (Bailey et al 1991, LaCreta et al 1991). When BSO is combined with intravenous melphalan (15 mg/m^2), grade 3 myelosuppression and moderate nausea and vomiting are observed. These are the standard anticipated side effects of melphalan. Myelosuppression from the fixed melphalan dose appears to be increased by BSO in a dose-dependent fashion (LaCreta et al 1991). Neutropenia is the predominant effect although thrombocytopenia is also observed (LaCreta et al 1991, Bailey et al 1991). In a preliminary phase I clinical report, the addition of BSO increased melphalan myelotoxicity, reflected by grade 4 neutropenia and thrombocytopenia in three of three and two of three patients, respectively (Hamilton et al 1990).

REFERENCES

Ali-Osman, Rairkar A. Alterations in DNA polymerases α, β and γ in human brain tumor cells after glutathione (GSH) depletion. *Proc Am Assoc Cancer Res.* 1992;**33**:497.

Andrews PA, Schiefer MA, Murphy MP, Howell SB. Enhanced potentiation of cisplatin cytotoxicity in human ovarian carcinoma cells by prolonged glutathione depletion. *Chem–Biol Interact.* 1988;**65**:51–58.

Arrick BA, Nathan CF. Glutathione metabolism as a determinant of therapeutic efficacy: A review. *Cancer Res.* 1984;**44**:4224–4232.

Arrick BA, Nathan CF, Cohn ZA. Inhibition of glutathione synthesis augments lysis of murine tumor cells by sulfhydryl-reactive antineoplastics. *J Clin Invest.* 1983;**71**: 258–267.

Arrick BA, Nathan CF, Griffith OW, Cohn ZA. Glutathione depletion sensitizes tumor cells to oxidative cytolysis. *J Biol Chem.* 1982;**257**:1231–1237.

Bailey H, Mulcahy RT, Tutsch K, et al. Phase I trial of intravenous L-buthionine sulfoximine (BSO) and melphalan (L-PAM): An attempt at modulation of glutathione

(GSH) chemoprotection. *Proc Am Soc Clin Oncol.* 1991; **10:**100.

Bailey H, Mulcahy RT, Tutsch KD, et al. Glutathione levels and γ-glutamylcysteine synthetase activity in patients undergoing phase I treatment with L-buthionine sulfoximine and melphalan. *Proc Am Assoc Cancer Res.* 1992;**33:**479.

Bertsche U, Schorn H. Glutathione depletion by DL-buthionine-*SR*-sulfoximine (BSO) potentiates X-ray-induced chromosome lesions after liquid holding recovery. *Radiat Res.* 1986;**105:**351–369.

Biaglow JE, Varnes ME. Symposium: Thiols—The role of thiols in cellular response to radiation and drugs. *Radiat Res.* 1983;**95:**437–455.

Biaglow JE, Varnes ME, Tuttle SW, et al. (1986) The effect of L-buthionine sulfoximine on the aerobic radiation response of A549 human lung carcinoma cells. *Int J Radiat Oncol Biol Phys.* 1986;**12:**1139–1142.

Boughattas NA, Filipski J, Lemaigre G, et al. Buthionine sulfoximine (BSO) affects circadian rhythms (CR) in toxicity of cisplatin (CDDP) and oxaliplatin (1-OHP) in mice. *Proc Am Assoc Cancer Res.* 1992;**33:**540.

DeGraff WG, Russo A, Mitchell JB. Glutathione depletion greatly reduces neocarzinostatin cytotoxicity in Chinese hamster V79 cells. *J Biol Chem.* 1985;**260:**8312–8315.

Department of Health and Human Services. *Buthionine Sulfoximine Investigators Brochure.* Washington, DC: National Cancer Institute, Division of Cancer Treatment; 1989.

Dorr RT, Liddil JD, Soble MJ. Cytotoxic effects of glutathione synthesis inhibition by L-buthionine-(*SR*)-sulfoximine on human and murine tumor cells. *Invest New Drugs.* 1986;**4:**305–313.

Durand RE. Roles of thiols in cellular radiosensitivity. *Int J Radiat Oncol Biol Phys.* 1984;**10:**1235–1238.

Freeman ML, Malcolm AW, Meredith MJ. Decreased intracellular glutathione concentration and increased hyperthermic cytotoxicity in an acid environment. *Cancer Res.* 1985;**45:**504–508.

Friedman HS, Colvin OM, Aisaka K, et al. Glutathione protects cardiac and skeletal muscle from cyclophosphamide-induced toxicity. *Cancer Res.* 1990;**50:** 2455–2462.

Gaetjens EC, Chen P, Broome JD. L1210(A) mouse lymphoma cells depleted of glutathione with L-buthionine-*SR*-sulfoximine proliferate in tissue culture. *Biochem Biophys Res Commun.* 1984;**123:**626–632.

Green JA, Vistica DT, Young RC, Hamilton TC, Rogan AM, Ozols RF. Potentiation of melphalan cytotoxicity in human ovarian cancer cell lines by glutathione depletion. *Cancer Res.* 1984;**44:**5427–5431.

Griffith OW. Mechanism of action, metabolism, and toxicity of buthionine sulfoximine and its higher homologs, potent inhibitors of glutathione synthesis. *J Biol Chem.* 1982;**257:**13704–13712.

Griffith OW, Meister A. Potent and specific inhibition of glutathione synthesis by buthionine sulfoximine (*S-n*-butyl homocysteine sulfoximine). *J Biol Chem.* 1979;**254:** 7558–7560.

Hamilton T, O'Dwyer P, Young R, et al. Phase I trial of buthionine sulfoximine (BSO) plus melphalan (L-PAM) in patients with advanced cancer (abstract #281). *Proc Am Soc Clin Oncol.* 1990;**9:**73.

Hamilton TC, Winker MA, Louie KG, et al. Augmentation of Adriamycin, melphalan, and cisplatin cytotoxicity in drug-resistant and -sensitive human ovarian carcinoma cell lines by buthionine sulfoximine mediated glutathione depletion. *Biochem Pharmacol.* 1985;**34:**2583–2586.

Hamilton TC, Young RC, Masuda H, Grozzinger KR, McKoy W, Ozols RF. Effect of buthionine sulfoximine (BSO) on the activity of anticancer drugs in vitro and in vivo in human ovarian cancer (HOC) (abstract #1562). *Proc Am Assoc Cancer Res.* 1986;**27:**393.

Kang YJ. Effect of exogenous glutathione on buthionine sulfoximine induced homeostasis. *Proc Am Assoc Cancer Res* 1992;**33:**497.

Kramer RA, Ahmad S, Vistica D. Toxicologic considerations in chemosensitization of melphalan (L-PAM) by buthionine sulfoximine (BSO) in mice (abstract #1665). *Proc Am Assoc Cancer Res.* 1986;**27:**419.

Kramer RA, Greene K, Ahmad S, et al. Chemosensitization of L-phenylalanine mustard by the thiol-modulating agent buthionine sulfoximine. *Cancer Res.* 1987;**47:**1593–1597.

Kramer RA, Schuller HM, Smith AC. Effects of buthionine sulfoximine on the nephrotoxicity of 1-(2-chloroethyl)-3-(*trans*-4-methylcyclohexyl)-1-nitrosourea (MeCCNU). *J Pharmacol Exp Ther.* 1985;**234:**498–506.

Kramer RA, Zakher J, Kim G. Role of the glutathione redox cycle in acquired and de novo multidrug resistance. *Science.* 1988;**241:**694–697.

LaCreta F, Brennan J, Padavic K, et al. Phase I clinical, biochemical and pharmacokinetic study of buthionine sulfoximine (BSO) in combination with melphalan (L-PAM). *Proc Am Soc Clin Oncol.* 1991;**10:**104.

Lee FYF, Allalunis-Turner MJ, Siemann DW. Depletion of tumour versus normal tissue glutathione by buthionine sulfoximine. *Br J Cancer.* 1987;**56:**33–38.

Lee KS, Kim H-K, Kang JH. Effects on cellular thiol and cytotoxicities of cisplatin and carboplatin by buthionine sulfoximine (BSO) in human stomach cancer cell lines (SNO-1 and cisplatin resistant SNU-1®). *Proc Am Assoc Cancer Res.* 1992;**33:**496.

Liao JT, Merriman TN, Collins WT, Gieshaber CK, Smith AC. The intravenous toxicity of L-buthionine sulfoximine (NSC-326231) and its effect on melphalan (NSC-8806) induced toxicity in mice (abstract #2492). *Proc Am Assoc Cancer Res.* 1989;**30:**626.

Liebmann JE, Hahn SM, Mitchell JB, et al. Glutathione depletion by buthionine sulfoximine antagonizes Taxol® cytotoxicity. *Proc Am Assoc Cancer Res.* 1992;**33:**423.

Lutzky J, Canada AL, Yamanishi DT, et al. Effect of verapamil and buthionine sulfoximine (BSO) on daunorubicin (DNR) cytotoxicity and multidrug-resistant human melanoma cell lines overexpressing P-glycoprotein and glutathione-*S*-transferases. *Proc Am Assoc Cancer Res.* 1992;**33**:554.

Meister A. Inhibition of glutamine synthesis and γ-glutamylcysteine synthetase by methionine sulfoximine and related compounds. In: Seiler P, Jung MJ, Koch Weser J, eds. *Enzyme-Activated Irreversible Inhibitors.* Amsterdam: Elsevier/North-Holland Biomedical Press; 1978;187–210.

Meister A, Griffith OW. Effect of buthionine sulfoximine and related compounds on mitochondrial glutathione levels (abstract #2642). *Fed Proc.* 1983;**42**:2210.

Minchinton AI, Rojas A, Smith A, et al. Glutathione depletion in tissues after administration of buthionine sulphoximine. *Int J Radiat Oncol Biol Phys.* 1984;**10**:1261–1264.

Mitchell JB, Russo A. Thiols, thiol depletion, and thermosensitivity. *Radiat Res.* 1983;**95**:471–485.

Ozols RF, Louie KG, Plowman J, et al. Enhanced melphalan cytotoxicity in human ovarian cancer in vitro and in tumor-bearing nude mice by buthionine sulfoximine depletion of glutathione. *Biochem Pharmacol.* 1987;**36**:147–153.

Page JG, Carlton BD, Smith AC, Kastello MD, Grieshaber CK. Preclinical toxicology and pharmacokinetic studies of buthionine sulfoximine (BSO, NSC-326231) in CD2F1 mice (abstract #1745). *Proc Am Assoc Cancer Res.* 1987;**28**:440.

Paxton JW, Foote SF, Singh RM. The effect of buthionine sulphoximine, cimetidine and phenobarbitone on the disposition of amsacrine in the rabbit. *Cancer Chemother Pharmacol.* 1986;**18**:208–212.

Russo A, Degraff W, Friedman N, et al. Selective modulation of glutathione levels in human normal versus tumor cells and subsequent differential response to chemotherapy drugs. *Cancer Res.* 1986a;**46**:2845–2848.

Russo A, Mitchell JB. Potentiation and protection of doxorubicin cytotoxicity by cellular glutathione modulation. *Cancer Treat Rep* 1985;**69**:1293–1296.

Russo A, Mitchell JB, McPheson S, Friedman N. Alteration of bleomycin cytotoxicity by glutathione depletion or elevation. *Int J Radiat Oncol Biol Phys.* 1984;**10**:1675–1678.

Russo A, Tochner Z, Phillips T, et al. In vivo modulation of glutathione by buthionine sulfoximine: Effect on marrow response to melphalan. *Int J Radiat Oncol Biol Phys.* 1986b;**12**:1187–1189.

Smith AC, Page JG, Carlton BD, Kastello MD, Grieshaber CK. Preclinical toxicology and pharmacokinetic studies of buthionine sulfoximine (BSO, NSC-326231) in beagle dogs (abstract #1746). *Proc Am Assoc Cancer Res.* 1987;**28**:440.

Soble MJ, Dorr RT. Lack of enhanced myelotoxicity with buthionine sulfoximine and sulfhydryl-dependent anticancer agents in mice. *Res Commun Chem Pathol Pharmacol.* 1987;**55**:161–180.

Soble MJ, Dorr RT. Lack of enhanced antitumor efficacy for L-buthionine sulfoximine in combination with carmustine, cyclophosphamide, doxorubicin or melphalan in mice. *Anticancer Res.* 1988;**8**:17–22.

Somfai-Relle S, Suzukake K, Vistica BP, et al. Reduction in cellular glutathione by buthionine sulfoximine and sensitization of murine tumor cells resistant to L-phenylalanine mustard. *Biochem Pharmacol.* 1984;**33**:485–490.

Suzukake K, Petro BJ, Vistica DT. Reduction in glutathione content of L-PAM resistant L-1210 cells confers drug sensitivity. *Biochem Pharmacol.* 1982;**31**:121–124.

Weiss RB, Posada JG Jr, Kramer RA, Boyd MR. Nephrotoxicity of semustine. *Cancer Treat Rep.* 1983;**67**(12):1105–1112.

Yu NY, Brown JM. Depletion of glutathione in vivo as a method of improving the therapeutic ratio of misonidazole and Sr 2508. *Int J Radiat Oncol Biol Phys.* 1984;**10**:1265–1269.

BWA 773U82

■ Other Names

Arylmethylaminopropanediol; BW 773; AMAP 773.

■ Chemistry

Structure of BWA 773U82

The complete chemical name is 2-[(1-fluoranthenylmethyl)amino]-2-methyl-1,3-propanediol. This compound is one of four arylmethylaminopropanediols being evaluated in phase I and II clinical trials. The other compounds are crisnatol (BWA 770U), BW 502A 502U83·HCl, and BW 7U85 discussed elsewhere in this book. These compounds have a common methylaminopropanediol side chain linked to different carbocyclic rings (Bair et al 1986). BWA 773U82 has a fluoranthene ring. The drug is a yellow crystalline powder, with molecular weights of 355.98 as the hydrochloride salt and 319.4 as the free base. The empiric formulas of the hydrochloride and mesylate salts are $C_{21}H_{21}NO_2 \cdot HCl$ and CH_3SO_3H, respectively.

The solubility of the hydrochloride formulation is 4 mg/mL compared with 12 mg/mL for the mesylate formulation. The latter (current) formulation was used for clinical trials. The log P(–log octanol/water) partition coefficient is 0.2 (slightly lipophilic). The pH of a 1.16×10^{-6} M solution BWA 773U82 mesylate is 5.2. At 25°C this formulation has a solubility (w/v) of 23.3 mg/mL in distilled water, 21.9 mg/mL in 5% dextrose, and 0.38 mg/mL in 0.9% Sodium Chloride for Injection, USP.

■ Antitumor Activity

No clinical antitumor activity has been established in humans. In animals, the compound has activity against P-388 mouse leukemia, L-1210 mouse lymphoid leukemia, B-16 melanoma, and Lewis lung carcinoma. The compound did not have activity against the MX-1 mammary carcinoma (Knick et al 1986).

■ Mechanism of Action

BWA 773U82 blocks the macromolecular synthesis of both RNA and DNA. This activity does not involve the uptake, phosphorylation, or retention of nucleotide precursors (Carter et al 1991). The agent intercalates into DNA but also inhibits DNA topoisomerase II enzymes (Bellamy et al 1989). BWA 773U82 produced concentration-dependent single strand breaks and DNA–protein crosslinks in DNA. DNA double strand breaks were produced in higher frequency as would be anticipated for a drug interacting with topoisomerase II enzymes to stabilize the "cleavable complex" between a homodimeric subunit of the enzyme and a host double-stranded fragment of DNA. In vitro tumor studies suggest that prolonged exposure times may significantly enhance cytotoxicity. Some cross-resistance with other intercalating agents was observed in preclinical in vitro and in vivo test systems (Bair et al 1986, Knick et al 1986). The cytotoxic effects are not cell cycle (phase) specific but may be maximal in S/G_2-phase cells.

■ Availability and Storage

BWA 773U82 is investigationally supplied by the Burroughs Wellcome, Research Triangle Park, North Carolina, in a sterile, amber 10-mL vial containing 50 mg of the free base as the hydrochloride salt in 10 mL sterile water for injection as a 5 mg/mL solution. The mesylate formulation is available in amber vials containing 360 mg of the free base. The intact vials should be stored at room temperature (59–77°F). They should remain in individual cartons as further protection from direct light. Early studies used a hydrochloride salt formulation, whereas later batches used the more water soluble mesylate salt formulation.

■ Preparation for Use, Stability, and Admixture

BWA 773U82 solution should be passed through a 0.22-μm filter as it is diluted for infusion with 5% Dextrose Injection, USP, in polyvinyl chloride intravenous bags. Solutions containing up to 1 mg/mL BWA 773U82 prepared by diluting solutions in 5% Dextrose Injection, USP, in polyvinyl chloride bags remained chemically stable at refrigeration temperature for 24 hours. Solutions containing up to 1 mg/mL BWA 773U82 diluted with 5% dextrose should be used within 8 hours if stored at room temperature. Solutions of the mesylate 1 mg/mL in D5W are chemically stable for 48 hours at 4 or 25°C. The drug is compatible with glass or polyvinyl chloride plastic infusion containers.

■ Administration

All doses should be filtered through a 0.45-μm filter. The only reported phase I dose schedule with this agent has been the single dose given as a 1-, 2-, 4-, or 6-hour infusion every 28 days. Fifty-eight courses at doses of 15 to 980 mg/m^2 have been administered to 36 patients. Neurologic toxicity with blurred vision was noted at 720 mg/m^2. On this schedule a drug-induced hemolysis was the dose-limiting toxic effect (Havlin et al 1989a,b, 1991). Other administration schedules are currently being evaluated in phase I trials. It is currently believed that the hemolysis is most likely due to the concentration of drug infused in the vein, as in vitro studies have shown that high concentrations of the drug can cause hemolysis.

■ Special Precautions

The diluted drug should be administered through a fresh, free-flowing intravenous line and should not be injected directly into a vein. The drug should never be administered undiluted.

Because of the proposed mechanism of action of BWA 773U82, care should be taken to prevent contact of the drug with the skin and procedures should be followed to reduce or to prevent inhalation of aerosolized particles of drug.

Drug Interactions

In P-388 mouse leukemia, BWA 773U82 shows additive or supraadditive antitumor effects with a variety of other clinically used antitumor agents. Additive effects were observed with etoposide, 5-fluorouracil, methotrexate, cyclophosphamide, and melphalan. Supraadditive antitumor effects were observed with doxorubicin, carmustine, and cisplatin. Less than additive effects were noted with vincristine and dacarbazine (Knick et al 1988).

Dosage

Based on phase I trials to date with this agent, no phase I dose has yet been established. Because of the hemolysis noted with the 1- to 6-hour infusion of the agent, that schedule cannot be recommended (Havlin et al 1989a,b, 1991). Doses up to 980 mg/m^2 have been administered by this schedule with some episodes of acute hemolytic toxicity seen at 700 mg/m^2 or higher doses. With 24- to 48-hour intravenous infusions, doses up to 4000 mg/m^2 have been administered. Grade 3 and 4 leukopenia occurred at the highest dose of 4 g/m^2/48 h (Arbuck et al 1990). One phase I trial has recommended a daily dose of 800 mg/m^2 given intravenously over 4 hours for 3 consecutive days, repeated at 3- to 4-week intervals.

Pharmacokinetics

In the earlier mentioned phase I study, BWA 773U82 plasma concentrations were determined by a high-pressure liquid chromatography method. After infusion, a biexponential decline in plasma concentrations was seen with an average terminal half-life of 4 hours. The mean peak plasma level at 840 mg/m^2 was 3.04 µg/mL. Total body clearance was 74.7 L/h/m^2 with an apparent volume of distribution at steady state of 297 L/m^2 (Havlin et al 1989a,b, 1991).

Side Effects and Toxicity

As noted earlier, when BWA 773U82 was given as a 1-hour infusion, blurred vision and generalized weakness occurred at 720 mg/m^2. With prolongation of the infusion to 6 hours, neurologic symptoms were not observed, but gross hemolysis was noted in plasma samples from patients given 980 mg/m^2. This hemolysis was the dose-limiting toxic effect. It was felt that prolonging the infusion to 24 hours may decrease the concentration and thereby avoid hemolysis. In addition to the hemolysis noted on the 1- to 6-hour infusion schedule, moderate phlebitis was also evident (Havlin et al 1989a,b).

With prolonged infusions of higher doses (> 350 mg/m^2) myelosuppression is common, but not clearly dose dependent. Fortunately, hemolysis is largely absent. Leukopenia is typically dose limiting (Arbuck et al 1990). Thrombocytopenia and anemia are rarely observed. Cardiovascular side effects are sporadic but are known to involve supraventricular arrhythmias and premature ventricular contractions. Mild hypertension is also noted in some patients.

Nausea and vomiting are dose related and especially prominent at doses above 600 mg/m^2. Antiemetics greatly lessen or eliminate this toxic effect. Central nervous system effects can be common but are not clearly dose dependent. Symptoms include lightheadedness, dizziness, tremors, drowsiness, insomnia, confusion, and transient visual problems such as amblyopia and diplopia. Importantly, only one seizure was described in a patient known to have cerebral metastases.

Special Applications

There are none.

REFERENCES

Arbuck S, Creaven P, Solomon J, et al. A phase I trial of 773U-HCl administered by 24 or 48 hours continuous infusion, every 28 days. *Proc Am Assoc Cancer Res.* 1990;**31**:1075.

Bair KW, Andres WC, Tuttle RL, Knick VC, McKee DD, Cory M. Biophysical studies and murine antitumor activity of arylmethylaminopropanediol (AMAP), a new class of DNA binding drugs. *Proc Am Assoc Cancer Res.* 1986;**27**:424.

Bellamy W, Dorr R, Bair K, et al. Cytotoxicity and mechanism of action of 3 arylmethylaminopropanediols (AMAPs). *Proc Am Assoc Cancer Res.* 1989;**30**:2236.

Carter CA, Bair KW. Effects of isomeric 2-(arylmethylamino)-1,3-propanediols (AMAPs) and clinically established agents on macromolecular synthesis in P388 and MCF-7 cells. *Invest New Drugs.* 1991;**9**:125–136.

Havlin K, Kuhn J, Craig J, et al. Clinical trials with the new arylmethylaminopropanediols (AMAPs). In: *Proceedings, Sixth Annual NCI–EORTC Meeting, The Netherlands, March 7–10,* 1989a.

Havlin K, Kuhn J, Craig J, et al. Phase I clinical and pharmacokinetic study of BW A773U, an arylmethylaminopropanediol. *Proc Am Soc Clin Oncol.* 1989b;**8**:79(Abstract 306).

Havlin K, Kuhn J, Craig J, et al. Phase I evaluation of 773 U820-HCL, a member of a new class of DNA intercalators. *Anti-Cancer Drugs* 1991;**2**:357–363.

Knick V, Tuttle R, Bair K. Murine chemotherapy studies of

three arylmethylaminopropanediols (AMAPs) combined with clinical active drugs. *Proc Am Assoc Cancer Res.* 1988;**29**:479.

Knick VC, Tuttle RL, Bair KW, Von Hoff DD. Murine and human tumor stem cell activity of three candidate arylmethylaminopropanediols (AMAPs). *Proc Am Assoc Cancer Res.* 1986;**27**:424.

BW 502U83·HCl

■ Other Names

Arylmethylaminopropanediol; BW A502U; AMAP-A.

■ Chemistry

Structure of BW 502A 502U83·HCl

The complete chemical name is 2-[(10-(2-hydroxyethoxy)-anthracen-9-ylmethyl)amino]-2-methyl-1,3-propanediol. This compound is one of four arylmethylaminopropanediols currently being evaluated in phase I and II clinical trials. The other compounds are crisnatol (BWA 770U), BWA 773U82, and BW 7U8J discussed elsewhere in this book. These compounds have a common methylaminopropanediol side chain linked to different carbocyclic rings (Bair et al 1986). BW 502U83·HCl has an anthracene ring and molecular weights of 391.89 and 355.43 for the hydrochloride salt and free base, respectively.

■ Antitumor Activity

No antitumor activity has been established in humans because the compound is only now undergoing phase I studies. In animals the compound has activity against P-388 mouse leukemia, L-1210 mouse lymphoid leukemia, B-16 melanoma, and Lewis lung carcinoma. The compound did not have activity against the MX-1 mammary carcinoma (Knick et al 1986).

■ Mechanism of Action

The mode of action of BW 502U83·HCl is currently unknown. The agent presumably works through intercalation with DNA. This assumption is based on its structure, DNA binding experiments, and cross-resistance patterns with some intercalating agents in preclinical in vitro and in vivo test systems (Bair et al 1986, Knick et al 1986).

■ Availability and Storage

BW 502U83·HCl is supplied by the Burroughs Wellcome, Research Triangle Park, North Carolina, as a sterile, lyophilized powder in an amber 10-mL vial containing BW 502U83·HCl equivalent to 100 mg of BW 502U83·HCl free base. The intact vials should be stored at room temperature (15–30°C). They should remain in individual cartons as further protection from light.

■ Preparation for Use, Stability, and Admixture

Vials of BW 502U83·HCl sterile powder should be reconstituted with 10 mL Water for Injection, USP, to produce a solution containing 10 mg/mL. Reconstituted BW 502U83·HCl can be further diluted with either 5% Dextrose Injection, USP, or 0.9% NaCl injection, USP.

The diluted solutions can be stored in polyvinyl chloride bags and should be administered within 8 hours if stored at room temperature or within 24 hours if refrigerated (5°C).

■ Administration

The only reported phase I dose schedule with this agent has been the single dose given over 1 hour every 28 days. In 48 courses given to 31 patients with refractory solid tumors, prolongation of the PR, QRS, and QT intervals on electrocardiograms was noted. This prolongation was dose related and dose limiting (Havlin et al 1989, Von Hoff et al 1990). Other administration schedules are currently being evaluated (Schilsky et al 1989).

Diluted drug should be administered through a fresh, free-flowing intravenous line; it should never be injected directly into a vein.

■ Special Precautions

With what is now known about BW 502U83·HCl (eg, the prolongation of the QT interval), it would not be advisable to administer BW 502U83·HCl to patients with hypokalemia or hypomagnesemia, both of which cause prolongation of the QT interval. Also, care will have to be exercised in patients who are receiving other agents known to prolong the QT interval (eg, antiarrhythmics such as quinidine, procainamide, and diisopyramide; phenothiazines; and tricyclic antidepressants). All of the preceding interactions are only theoretical and not based on clinical experience with the interactions.

Because of the proposed mechanism of action of BW 502U83·HCl, care should be taken to prevent contact of the drug with the skin and procedures should be followed to reduce or prevent inhalation of aerosolized particles of drug.

■ Drug Interactions

See Special Precautions.

■ Dosage

Based on phase I trials to date with this agent, no phase II dose has yet been established. Because of prolongation of the cardiac conduction intervals, the 1- to 4-hour infusion schedule cannot be recommended (Havlin et al 1989, Von Hoff et al 1990).

■ Pharmacokinetics

In the earlier mentioned phase I study, BW 502U83·HCl plasma concentrations were determined by a high-pressure liquid chromatography method. After infusion, the plasma concentrations declined in a triexponential manner with a terminal half-life of 11.44 hours. The mean apparent volume of distribution at steady state and the total body clearance were 182 L/m^2 and 43 L/h/m^2, respectively, indicative of extensive tissue distribution and probably rapid hepatic clearance (Von Hoff et al 1990). At the maximum dose given, 2000 mg/m^2, the concentration × time product was 43 to 45 µg/L/h and the peak concentration was 12 to 23 µg/mL.

■ Side Effects and Toxicity

As noted earlier, dose-related prolongation of the PR, QRS, and QT intervals on the electrocardiogram has been the dose-limiting toxic effect noted with the 1- to 4-hour infusion of the drug. These prolongations were totally reversible in 24 hours. No episodes of prolongation of these intervals have resulted in any rhythm disturbances. (Von Hoff et al 1990). Other toxic effects include sporadic, mild to moderate nausea and vomiting. No hematologic toxicity has been observed.

With the 24-hour continuous infusion schedule, no cardiac interval prolongation was observed. One patient with a malar rash and facial swelling lasting 24 hours has been described (Schilsky et al 1989).

■ Special Applications

BW 502U83·HCl was administered intraarterially to three patients with hepatocellular carcinoma (Van der Graaf et al 1992). Doses of 3 to 7.5 g/m^2 produced little systemic toxicity except for a rise in serum lactate dehydrogenase levels. One patient obtained a partial response.

REFERENCES

Bair KW, Andrews CW, Tuttle RL, Knick VC, McKee DD, Cory M. Biophysical studies and murine antitumor activity of arylmethylaminopropanediol (AMAP), a new class of DNA binding drugs. *Proc Am Assoc Cancer Res.* 1986;**27**:424.

Havlin K, Craig J, Turner J, et al. Phase I clinical and pharmacokinetic study of BWA 502U, an arylmethylaminopropanediol. *Proc Am Assoc Cancer Res.* 1989;**30**:286.

Knick VC, Tuttle RL, Bair KW, Von Hoff DD. Murine and human tumor stem cell activity of three candidate arylmethylaminopropanediols (AMAP). *Proc Am Assoc Cancer Res.* 1986;**27**:424.

Schilsky RL, Ratain M, Grayhock J, et al. Phase I clinical and pharmacologic study of BWA 502U HCl administered by 24 hour continuous intravenous infusion. *Proc Am Soc Clin Oncol.* 1989;**8**:75.

Van der Graaf WTA, Zijlstra JG, de Jong S, et al. In vitro activity of BWA 502U, an arylmethylaminopropanediol, and clinical activity after intra-arterial infusion. *Proc Am Assoc Cancer Res.* 1992;**33**:519.

Von Hoff DD, Kuhn JG, Havlin KA, et al. Phase I and clinical pharmacology trial of BWA 502U using a monthly single dose schedule. *Cancer Res.* 1990;**50**:7496–7500.

BW 7U85 Mesylate

Other Names

7U85 mesylate.

Chemistry

Structure of BW 7U85 mesylate

BW 7U85 mesylate is an arylmethylaminopropanediol (AMAP). Other AMAPs include crisnatol (BWA 770U), BWA 773U82, and BW 502U83·HCl, discussed elsewhere in this book. This compound differs from the other AMAPs by the presence of the heteroatom nitrogen in the benzo(C)carbazole ring system.

Antitumor Activity

BW 7U85 is similar in activity to the other AMAPs in a variety of preclinical tumor systems (Knick et al 1986). The agent has activity in those systems when administered by the intravenous, intraperitoneal, and oral routes.

BW 7U85 is an investigational agent currently undergoing phase I clinical trials. No antitumor activity has yet been established for patients with cancer (Hendricks et al 1992).

Mechanism of Action

BW 7U85 has been shown to intercalate DNA and inhibit topoisomerase II (Bair et al 1986). This agent also blocks macromolecular synthesis, affecting the synthesis of DNA, RNA, and, to a lesser degree, protein (Carter and Bair 1991). The IC_{50} values in P-388 cells were 8.3, 5.9, and 11.6 μM for these three macromolecules, respectively. Unlike other AMAPs, BW 7U85 also decreased the specific activity of cellular thymidine pools by approximately 30% (Carter and Bair 1991).

Availability and Storage

BW 7U85 is investigationally supplied by the Burroughs Wellcome, Research Triangle Park, North Carolina, as a sterile amber 30-mL vial containing BW 7U85 mesylate equivalent to 450 mg of BW 7U85 free base in 30 mL sterile water for injection as a 15 mg/mL solution. All doses and labeling are expressed as the free base, not the mesylate salt (eg, a 50-mg dose is equivalent to 64 mg of BW 7U85 mesylate).

Vials should be stored at room temperature (59–77°F). They should remain in individual cartons as further protection from light.

Preparation for Use, Stability, and Admixture

The appropriate daily dose of BW 7U85 should be drawn from the vial(s), passed through a 0.22-μm filter, and diluted in 250 mL of D5W for administration over 2 hours. Alternatively, the final solution may be filtered at the time of administration. BW 7U85 *cannot* be diluted in normal saline as precipitation may occur. The concentration and rate at which BW 7U85 is administered should not exceed 1.0 mg/mL and 2.08 mg/min, respectively. The observation of clinical toxicity or continued dose escalation may require the administration of larger fluid volumes or an adjustment in the duration of the infusion.

The preceding recommendations are a result of preclinical data regarding rate-related pharmacologic effects and in vitro hemolysis and flocculation studies. These recommendations may be modified as clinical data are obtained.

Solutions containing 5 mg/mL BW 7U85 mesylate, prepared by dilution in D5W, remain chemically and physically stable when stored for up to 72 hours at room temperature or refrigerated (41°F, 5°C), protected or unprotected from light, in polyvinylchloride bags. If stored at room temperature, the diluted solutions should be administered within 8 hours of initial dilution to minimize the potential for inadvertent microbiologic contamination.

Administration

BW 7U85 may cause irritation at the injection site. Diluted drug should be administered through a fresh, free-flowing intravenous line; it should not be injected directly into a vein. The access site should be checked frequently during the infusion to ensure proper intravenous administration. Drug should only be given using a controlled infusion pump. The company guidelines stated are based on preclinical data and may be modified as clinical experience evolves.

The phase I trials with the agent are ongoing and no best schedule of administration has been determined. Initial trials have used a 2-hour intravenous infusion given daily for 5 days (Hendricks et al 1992).

■ Special Precautions

None are known at this time.

■ Drug Interactions

None are known to date.

■ Dosage

This drug is just undergoing phase I trials with the single bolus dose and the daily ×5 schedules. Ongoing phase I studies suggest that the maximum tolerated dose for the latter schedule will be about 54 to 80 mg/m^2/d × 5 days, repeated every 28 days (Hendricks et al 1992).

■ Pharmacokinetics

Pharmacokinetic studies on dogs have noted half-lives of 3 to 4 hours with extensive metabolism (Patel et al 1991). The clinical pharmacokinetic studies are ongoing at the time of this writing. At an 80 mg/m^2 dose, the peak plasma concentration was 2016 ng/mL and the terminal half-life was 15.3 hours (Hendricks et al 1992).

In dogs, about 83% of a radiolabeled drug dose is excreted via the feces (Patel et al 1991). There was significant first-pass clearance after oral dosing and mean half-lives varied between 3.99 and 3.1 hours for oral and intravenous therapy, respectively. Several possible metabolites were identified but not characterized (Patel et al 1991).

■ Side Effects and Toxicity

The dose-limiting toxic effect of BW 7U85 is neutropenia with a lesser degree of thrombocytopenia (Hendricks et al 1992). Nonhematologic toxic effects include nausea and vomiting (16%), mucositis (6.5%) and rash and hypertension (1 patient each). Phlebitis occurred in 13% of patients and appeared to be dose related (Hendricks et al 1992). The lack of dose-limiting central nervous system toxicity with BW 7U85 may be due to the heteroatom in the carbocyclic ring system (Hendricks et al 1992).

■ Special Applications

None are known at this time.

REFERENCES

Bair KW, Andrews CW, Tuttle RL, et al. Biophysical studies and murine antitumor activity of arylmethylaminopropanediol (AMAP), a new class of DNA binding drugs. *Proc Am Assoc Cancer Res.* 1986;**27**:424.

Carter CA, Bair KW. Effects of isomeric 2-(arylmethylamino)-1,3-propanediols (AMAPs) and clinically established agents on macromolecular synthesis in P388 and MCF-7 cells. *Invest New Drugs.* 1991;**9**:125–136.

Hendricks C, Von Hoff D, Rowinsky E, et al. Phase I and pharmacokinetic (PK) study of 7U85 mesylate. *Proc Am Soc Clin Oncol.* 1992;**11**:115.

Knick VC, Tuttle RL, Bair KW, et al. Murine and human tumor stem cell activity of three candidate arylmethylaminopropanediols (AMAPs). *Proc Am Assoc Cancer Res.* 1986;**27**:424.

Patel DK, Lewis RP, Schroeder DH, et al. Disposition of the new antitumor agent 7U85, a heterocyclic arylmethylaminopropanediol (AMAP), in dogs. *Proc Am Assoc Cancer Res.* 1991;**32**:346.

Caracemide

■ Other Names

NSC-253272.

■ Chemistry

Structure of caracemide

Caracemide is a methylurea compound with the complete chemical name *N*-[(methylamino) carbonyl]-*N*-[[(methylamino)-carbonyl]oxy]acetamide. It has a molecular weight of 189.2 and a molecular formula of $C_6H_{11}N_3O_4$. The compound was developed by Dow Chemical as a derivative of *N'*-methyl-*N*-acetyl-*N*-hydroxyurea *N*-methyl-*N'*-acetyl-isohydroxyurea (Moore and Loo 1984). It is synthesized from acetohydroxamic acid and methyl isocyanate (Newman et al 1986).

Antitumor Activity

In preclinical models, caracemide was active in P-388 murine leukemia and in several human tumors xenografted into athymic nude mice. These include MX-1 mammary carcinoma and CX-1 colon carcinoma. In contrast, a large number of tumors were insensitive to caracemide including the mouse tumors B-16 melanoma, L-1210 leukemia, and Lewis lung cancer. Human LX-1 lung cancer in nude mice was similarly insensitive to caracemide (Raber et al 1987). Of interest, caracemide is not cross-resistant to Chinese hamster ovary cells selected for resistance to hydroxyurea (Newman et al 1986).

Although not designed to detect activity, caracemide produced no objective responses in phase I studies of 20 patients with various advanced carcinomas (Pazdur et al 1987) or 42 patients with other advanced malignancies (Raber et al 1987). One patient in the latter study had a transient minor response (< 50% tumor shrinkage) (Raber et al 1985, 1987).

Mechanism of Action

Caracemide inhibits macromolecular synthesis in P-388 leukemia cells in vitro. In these studies, the inhibition of DNA synthesis was more sensitive than was inhibition of either protein synthesis or RNA synthesis (Newman et al 1986). At high drug concentrations of 100 μM or greater, caracemide also induces DNA strand breaks. Lower drug concentrations did not induce DNA strand breaks and their relationship to the cytotoxic mechanism is therefore not established.

Like hydroxyurea, caracemide also inhibits ribonucleotide reductase. This inhibitory activity is noted by a blockade in the reduction of cytidine diphosphate to deoxycytidine diphosphate. In this regard, it is about one ninth as potent as hydroxyurea on crude or partially purified enzyme (Moore and Loo 1984). Unfortunately, the inhibition constant (K_i) for the enzymatic activation of ribonucleotide reductase could not be calculated; however, the 50% inhibitory concentration of caracemide appears to range from 0.5 to 1.1 mM (95–208 μg/mL) in vitro using reductase enzymes from rat Novikoff tumor (Moore and Loo 1984). For comparison, 0.21 mM hydroxyurea was approximately equipotent to 1.8 mM caracemide (Moore and Loo 1984).

The lack of cross-resistance in hydroxyurea-resistant Chinese hamster ovary cells suggests that the mechanism of action for caracemide is different from that of hydroxyurea. Therefore, caracemide may produce hybrid actions in tumor cells involving DNA strand breakage, DNA synthesis inhibition, and inhibition of ribonucleotide reductase. In contrast to the actions of hydroxyurea which are cell cycle (phase) specific for S phase, caracemide cytotoxicity is not cell cycle specific (Newman et al 1986).

Availability and Storage

Caracemide is investigationally available in 250 mg/10 mL glass vials. The drug is supplied from Dow Chemical to the National Cancer Institute as a white lyophilized powder containing a sodium phosphate/sodium hydroxide buffer. The intact vials are stable for at least 5 years at room temperature (Department of Health and Human Services 1990). The vials are unstable at 50°C and higher temperatures.

Preparation for Use, Stability, and Admixture

Each 250-mg vial can be reconstituted with 4.7 mL of Sterile Water for Injection, USP, or 0.9% Sodium Chloride for Injection, USP. This yields a clear solution containing 50 mg/mL caracemide in 0.1 M buffer. The final pH is between 4.5 and 5.5 (Department of Health and Human Services 1990). At a pH above 7.0, extensive and rapid inactivation occurs. At room temperature there is 3% or less decomposition of caracemide (50 mg/mL) at 8 hours and 5 to 6% decomposition at 24 hours (Department of Health and Human Services 1990). When diluted to 0.5 to 1.0 mg/mL in 5% dextrose or normal saline, however, there is about 8 to 15% decomposition in 4 hours at room temperature (Department of Health and Human Services 1990). In human plasma at 37°C, there is 55% degradation of caracemide after 30 minutes and 75% after 1 hour (Newman et al 1986).

Dosage

The recommended dose for Phase II studies was 525 mg/m^2 as an intravenous bolus for 5 consecutive days (Raber et al 1987). The recommended dose for continuous 5-day infusions was 650 mg/m^2/d in this same trial. As a 4-hour infusion, the maximally tolerated dose was 795 mg/m^2 (Pazdur et al 1987).

Pharmacokinetics

In dogs, the pharmacokinetics of caracemide have demonstrated biphasic half-lives of 5 minutes and 3.1 hours (Lu et al 1985). Total body clearance was 37 mL/kg/min and 16% of a dose was excreted in the urine (Lu et al 1985); less than 1% of this was excreted intact. The disposition of drug into various organs showed that the liver contained the highest proportion of a dose (7.7%), followed by the small intestine at 1.7%, the kidney and lung at 0.4% each, the stomach and large intestine at 0.3% each, the spleen and brain at 0.2% each, and the pancreas at 0.1% (Lu et al 1985).

In humans, the terminal plasma half-life of caracemide is about 2.5 minutes, with a volume of distribution of 39 L/m^2 and a total body clearance of 11.5 L/min/m^2 (Pazdur et al 1987). The distribution volume of the drug approximates the extracellular fluid compartment. Doses of 425 mg/m^2 produced caracemide levels of 0.74 to 2.31 µg/mL during a half-hour infusion and 0.15 to 0.18 µg/mL with a 4-hour infusion. With a 4-hour infusion of 595 mg/m^2, blood levels of 0.33 µg/mL were achieved (Pazdur et al 1987).

Side Effects and Toxicity

Caracemide produces a dose-limiting burning pain during infusion. This can begin within 15 minutes to 3 hours of starting an infusion. The pain can involve the perioral mucosa and typically spreads to the neck, chest, and abdomen (Pazdur et al 1987). Excessive lacrimation is also observed. One other patient developed an allergic reaction manifested by hives and wheezing. This abated with corticosteroids and discontinuance of caracemide (Pazdur et al 1987).

With a bolus infusion over 30 minutes, pain at the infusion site was dose limiting. Frank phlebitis did not develop in these patients (Raber et al 1987). Nonetheless, local venous reactions necessitated placement of central venous catheters in some patients. A burning perioral pain was again common in patients receiving doses above 525 mg/m^2. This was associated with nasal stuffiness and flushing and was ameliorated with prolonging infusions to 4 hours or longer. Thrombocytopenia was noted in two of seven patients given 650 mg/m^2. With continuous infusions, no hematologic changes were observed. Mild nausea and vomiting were also observed in most patients at these dose levels (Raber et al 1987).

Manifestations of caracemide-induced central nervous system toxicity include lethargy, disorientation, confusion, and cognitive dysfunction. A combative agitated type of behavior may be noted. Electroencephalographs obtained in affected patients receiving high doses showed diffuse slowing with occasional irritative activity in the temporal lobes (Raber et al 1987). Once evident, caracemide-induced dementia slowly resolves with drug discontinuance and may not completely remit if high doses have been administered (> 1200 mg/m^2). The most sensitive cognitive alterations involve short-term memory loss and visual spatial disorientation (Adams et al 1985). The pathophysiology of the disorder may involve cholinergic overdrive with compensatory noradrenergic responses (Adams et al 1985).

The severe toxic effects noted in these early trials do not support continued broad testing of caracemide. Furthermore, it is unclear if ribonucleotide reductase inhibitory concentrations can be achieved in vivo.

REFERENCES

Adams F, Kavanagh J, Raber M, et al. Neuropsychiatric manifestations of caracemide toxicity in a phase I trial (abstract #C-191). *Proc Am Soc Clin Oncol.* 1985;**4**:50.

Department of Health and Human Services. *Caracemide—NSC-253272.* NIH Publication No. 91-2141. Washington, DC: Investigational Drug Branch, National Cancer Institute: 1990:27–28.

Lu K, Savaraj N, Feun LG, et al. Pharmacokinetics of caracemide (CAR, NSC-253272) in dogs (abstract #1418). *Proc Am Assoc Cancer Res.* 1985;**26**:359.

Moore EC, Loo TL. Inhibition of ribonucleotide reductase by caracemide. *Cancer Treat Rep.* 1984;**68**(10):1293–1294.

Newman RA, Farquhar D, Lu K, et al. Biochemical pharmacology of N-acetyl-N-(methylcarbamoyloxy)-N'-methylurea (caracemide; NSC-253272). *Biochem Pharmacol.* 1986;**35**(16):2781–2787.

Pazdur R, Chabot GG, Baker LH. Phase I study and pharmacokinetics of caracemide (NSC-253272) administered as a short infusion. *Invest New Drugs.* 1987;**5**:365–371.

Raber MN, Adams F, Kavanagh J, et al. Phase I trial of caracemide using bolus and infusion schedules. *Cancer Treat Rep.* 1987;**71**(4):349–352.

Raber MN, Dimery LI, Kavanagh J, et al. Phase I study of caracemide (abstract #C-174). *Proc Am Soc Clin Oncol.* 1985;**4**:46.

Carbetimer

Other Names

Carbethimer; N-137; NED-137; carboxyimamidate; polima.

Chemistry

Molecular structure of carbetimer

Carbetimer is a synthetic low-molecular-weight (1600) imide/amide derivative of a precursor copolymer of ethylene and maleic anhydride polyelectrolyte. A comprises 14 to 25% of the total A + B units. Carbetimer has had antitumor activity in a variety of tumor models (Fields et al 1982, Rees et al 1982, Kisner et al 1984, Fromm et al 1985).

Antitumor Activity

Carbetimer has been carefully studied in phase I and in limited phase II studies. In phase I trials a partial response was noted in one patient with melanoma (Dodion et al 1986). In phase II studies to date, no antitumor activity has been noted in patients with non-small cell lung cancer (Keaton et al 1990) and in patients with previously untreated metastatic colorectal carcinoma (Audeh et al 1990).

Mechanism of Action

The mechanism of action of carbetimer has not been well defined. Preliminary evidence for an immunomodulatory effect has been reported. In rodents, augmentation of B-cell differentiation has been reported (Teodorcyk-Injeyan et al 1982, 1983). Carbetimer increases IgM production in T-cell-depleted rats after exposure to cellular antigens (Rotstein et al 1980). When compared with other immunologic adjuvants in murine tumor models, carbetimer led to a superior prolongation of survival (Falk et al 1980). In addition to its effects on the immune system, carbetimer has also been reported to inhibit uptake and incorporation of radiolabeled pyrimidine nucleosides into sensitive melanoma cells in vitro and in vivo and to inhibit the enzyme cyclic nucleotide phosphodiesterase (Ardalan and Paget 1986, Hrishikeshavan et al 1986). The compound has also been reported to be a differentiating agent (Hepburn et al 1988) and an antimetastatic agent (Ardalan et al 1988).

Availability and Storage

Carbetimer is available as an investigational agent through G. D. Searle. It is supplied as sterile lyophilized material in 1-g vials. The vials are stored at 4°C.

Preparation for Use, Stability, and Admixture

The appropriate dose of carbetimer is further diluted to a total volume of 250 to 500 mL in D5W. Reconstituted material must be used within 8 hours.

Administration

The solution of carbetimer in D5W is infused over 1 to 2 hours through a free-flowing peripheral intravenous line. At doses greater than 4000 mg/m^2 several patients in one study complained of pain at the infusion site. Therefore, administration over 2 hours was required. In addition, at very high doses (16,690 mg/m^2) a central venous catheter had to be used with a concomitant decrease in infusion time to 1 hour (Fromm et al 1989).

Special Precautions

See Drug Interactions.

Drug Interactions

None have been described to date; however, because carbetimer has been reported to prolong prothrombin and partial thromboplastin times concomitant use of anticoagulants should be avoided.

Dosage

The most appropriate dose and schedule for carbetimer are not clear. The table on page 258 describes phase I trials that have been conducted.

Pharmacokinetics

Unfortunately a satisfactory assay for the compound has not yet been developed. Therefore, no clinical pharmacology data are available on the compound.

CARBETIMER DOSE RECOMMENDATIONS FROM PHASE I CLINICAL TRIALS

Schedule	Dose Range (mg/m^2)	Dose-Limiting Toxic Effect	Recommended Phase II Dose (mg/m^2)	Reference
Single dose every 28 days	180–8500	Hypercalcemia	6500	Hanauske et al 1988
Single dose every 28 days	180–16,690	Visual disturbance	—	Fromm et al 1989
Daily × 5	1080–11,000	Hypercalcemia	—	Dodion et al 1989
Daily × 5	100–11,000	Hypercalcemia	8500	Grunberg et al 1990
Continuous infusion for 21 days	200–?	Not reached	—	Ardalan et al 1989

■ Side Effects and Toxicity

Two different dose-limiting toxic effects have been described for carbetimer. These include hypercalcemia (Hanauske et al 1988) and visual disturbances (flashing lights and seeing stars) (Fromm et al 1989). The hypercalcemia is reversible. Calcium balance studies have revealed an increase in urinary cyclic AMP and phosphate excretion accompanied by a mild elevation in serum parathyroid hormone (Hanauske et al 1988). In a detailed short-term study, Bodey et al (1989) noted an initial fall in plasma ionized calcium followed by an increase in plasma parathyroid hormone. These changes were best explained by a carbetimerinduced chelation of calcium.

The visual disturbances were felt to be the result of retinal ischemia caused by high concentrations of carbetimer in the retinal vessels (Fromm et al 1989).

Other toxic effects have included nausea and vomiting, mild proteinuria (non-dose dependent), reversible prolongation of partial thromboplastin times and prothrombin times, and pain at the infusion site (see Administration) (Hanauske et al 1988, Keaton et al 1990, Fromm et al 1989, Audeh et al 1990, Dodion et al 1989, Grunberg et al 1990).

■ Special Applications

Immunologic studies in patients receiving carbetimer have revealed increases in the percentage of peripheral helper T cells. An increase in the T helper/suppressor cell ratio was also observed (Hanauske et al 1988).

REFERENCES

Ardalan B, Hepburn M, Shanahan W, Shield M. Carbetimer, a new antineoplastic agent with antimetastatic properties (meeting abstract). *Proc Am Assoc Cancer Res.* 1988;**29**:501.

Ardalan B, Hussein A, Shanahan W, et al. Phase I continuous intravenous (IV) infusion of carbetimer (CBT) in refractory malignancies (meeting abstract). *Proc Am Assoc Cancer Res.* 1989; **30**(283):1125.

Ardalan B, Paget GE. Mechanism of action of a new antitumor agent, carbetimer. *Cancer Res.* 1986;**46**(11):5473–5476.

Audeh MW, Jacobs CD, Davis TE, Carlson RW. A phase II trial of carbetimer for the treatment of colorectal cancer. A trial of the Northern California Oncology Group. *Am J Clin Oncol.* 1990;**13**(4):324–326.

Bodey JJ, Magritte A, Cleeren A, Borkowski A, Dodion P. Short-term effects of carbetimer on calcium and bone metabolism in man. *Eur J Cancer Clin Oncol.* 1989;**25**(12):1831–1835.

Dodion P, Abrams J, Crespeigne N, et al. Phase I trial with carbetimer given on a 5 day schedule. *Proc Am Soc Clin Oncol.* 1986;**5**:30.

Dodion P, de Valeriola D, Body JJ, Phase I clinical trial with carbetimer. *Eur J Cancer Clin Oncol.* 1989;**25**:(2):279–286.

Falk RE, Makowka L, Nossal NA, Rotstein LE, Falk JA. Comparison of the antitumor effects of a synthetic biopolymer and standard adjuvants. *Surgery.* 1980;**88**:126–136.

Fields JE, Asculai SS, Johnson JH, Johnson RK. Carboxyimamidate, a low-molecular-weight polyelectrolyte with antitumor properties and low toxicity. *J Med Chem.* 1982;**25**:1060–1064.

Fromm M, Berdel WE, Schick HD, et al. Experience with the polyelectrolyte carbetimer in early clinical trials. *Contrib Oncol.* 1989;**37**:12–19.

Fromm M, Schick HD, Scheiber H, et al. Assay-dependent toxicity of the low-molecular-weight polyelectrolyte carbetimer in cells from human tumors and leukemias *in vitro* and report on a clinical phase I trial. *Proc Am Soc Clin Oncol.* 1985;**4**:29.

Grunberg SM, Ehler E, Francis RB Jr, Mitchell MS. Phase I trial of a 5-day course of carbetimer. *Invest New Drugs.* 1990;**8**(1):S41–S49.

Hanauske A-R, Melink TJ, Harman GS. Phase I clinical trial of carbetimer. *Cancer Res.* 1988;**48**:5353–5357.

Hepburn M, Ardalan B, Shanahan W, Shield M, Richman

S. Differentiating properties of carbetimer, a new antineoplastic agent (meeting abstract). *Proc Am Assoc Cancer Res.* 1988;**29**:514.

Hrishikeshaven HJ, Ardalan B, Paget E. Inhibition of cyclic nucleotide phosphodiesterase by carbetimer in a human melanoma. *Proc Am Assoc Cancer Res.* 1986;**27**:280.

Keaton M, Brown T, Craig J, et al. Phase II study of carbetimer in non-small cell lung cancer. *Invest New Drugs.* 1990;**8**(4):385–386.

Kisner D, Mehta P, Paget GE, Von Hoff D. Activity of carbetimer in a human tumor cloning system. *Invest New Drugs.* 1984;**2**:55–58.

Rees RC, Potter CW, Clegg A, Hall JM. Studies on the antitumor effects of NED-137. *Chemotherapy.* 1982;**28**:283–290.

Rotstein LE, Makowka L, Falk RE, Kirby TJ, Nossal N, Falk JA. Selective immune stimulation during induction of allograft tolerance in the rat by radical immunosuppression. *Transplantation.* 1980;**30**:417–420.

Teodorcyk-Injeyan JA, Filion L, Falk J, Falk R, Makowka L. Mechanisms of enhanced humoral response in rodents to a synthetic polymer. *J Immunopharmacol.* 1983;**5**:147–172.

Carboplatin

■ Other Names

Paraplatin® (Bristol-Myers Oncology Division); CBDCA; JM-8; NSC-241240.

■ Chemistry

Structure of carboplatin

Carboplatin has a molecular formula of $C_6H_{12}N_2O_7Pt$ with a formula weight of 371.25. The chemical name is diammine [1,1-cyclobutanedicarboxylato(2-)-*O, O'*]-platinum (II), (SP-4-2). The drug is soluble in water and very slightly soluble in ethanol, acetone, and dimethylacetamide. Of note, the water solubility of carboplatin (14 mg/mL) is approximately ten times that of cisplatin. The carboxylato bonds in carboplatin are slowly hydrolyzed to yield transient aquated intermediates. These activated platinum species are believed to lead directly to irreversible adducts to DNA or protein. Overall, the rate of hydrolysis of carboplatin is significantly slower than that of cisplatin, leading to much slower reactivity with DNA (Gaver et al 1987).

■ Antitumor Activity

Carboplatin is officially marketed in the United States for the treatment of patients with advanced ovarian cancer. When used as a single agent in patients previously treated with cisplatin, response rates to carboplatin range from 14% (Pohl et al 1986) to 32% (Ogawa et al 1987). Typically, the complete response rate is low in this group of patients, ranging from 0% (Colombo et al 1986) to 13% (Ozols et al 1987). Response rates increase dramatically when single-agent carboplatin is used as first-line therapy in ovarian cancer. In this setting, overall response rates of up to 85% (62% complete) are described for high-dose regimens (George et al 1988). Overall response rates of 50% (Ogawa et al 1987) and 68% are reported for standard-dose regimens (Calvert et al 1984). Importantly, complete response rates in ovarian cancer are maintained for prolonged periods with first-line carboplatin therapy. Rates up to 29% are consistently described (Wiltshaw et al 1986, Calvert et al 1984).

Carboplatin demonstrates equivalent or slightly superior activity when compared directly with cisplatin in randomized phase III trials in ovarian cancer (Alberts et al 1990). The median duration of response in these different studies averages about 16 months (Wiltshaw et al 1985). Unfortunately, when carboplatin is combined with other cytotoxic agents in first-line treatment of ovarian cancer, overall response rates are not significantly improved. This includes combinations of carboplatin with chlorambucil (57% response rate [Evans et al 1988]), cyclophosphamide (57% response rate [Meerpohl 1988]), cisplatin (43% response rate [Lund et al 1988]), and doxorubicin, cyclophosphamide, and hexamethylmelamine (48% response rate [ten Bokkel Huinink et al 1985]). A similar result was described in a phase III trial comparing carboplatin combinations with the same-named drugs combined with cisplatin. The response rates, 45% versus 56% respectively, were not significantly different (ten Bokkel Huinink et al 1988).

It is important to note that carboplatin is usually not active in ovarian tumors that have acquired resistance to cisplatin in vitro (Behrens et al 1987) or in vivo (Alberts et al 1990). This argues that carboplatin will be most active when used early in the management of ovarian cancer before generic platinum resistance is produced.

Carboplatin is active in a number of other solid tumors including non-small cell lung cancer (Bunn 1990), head and neck cancer (Eisenberger et al 1989), and testicular cancer (Williams et al 1989). Single-agent carboplatin response rates in small cell lung cancer range from 14 to 28%, with a complete response rate of about 10% (Bunn 1989). Response rates are lower in head and neck cancer: 26% overall with a 7% complete rate (Eisenberger et al 1989). Another trial in 40 patients with recurrent and metastatic squamous cell carcinoma of the head and neck showed that carboplatin was equal to methotrexate, with each drug producing responses in 5 of 20 patients (Eisenberger et al 1989). In one trial of heavily pretreated patients with nonseminomatous testicular cancer, the combination of high-dose carboplatin + etoposide produced a 44% overall response with 25% complete response rates (Nichols et al 1989); however, conventional-dose carboplatin was ineffective as a single agent in a larger group of heavily pretreated patients (Motzer et al 1987, Horwich et al 1989). In metastatic seminoma, a single-agent monthly carboplatin regimen produced an actuarial 2-year survival rate of 94% in 34 patients (Horwich et al 1989). This therapy was therefore recommended as the treatment of choice for advanced-stage malignant seminoma.

There is also some activity for carboplatin in relapsed and refractory acute leukemia. A 28.5% overall response rate including two complete responses is described in 28 patients receiving a 5-day high-dose continuous-infusion regimen (Meyers et al 1989). Low but consistent response rates are also reported for carboplatin in bladder cancer. Response rates of 9% (Ogawa et al 1987) to 28% (Mechl et al 1987) are described in this tumor type. Other solid tumors that have responded to carboplatin in 20% or more patients include endometrial cancer (28% response rate [Long et al 1988]) and recurrent brain tumors in children, particularly medulloblastomas in which a 43% response rate is described (Allen et al 1987). Carboplatin appears to be inferior to cisplatin in advanced carcinoma of the uterine cervix with a response rate of only 15% (McGuire et al 1989).

■ Mechanism of Action

The precise molecular mechanism(s) of platinum antitumor effects is not known although DNA appears to constitute the predominant intracellular target. Like cisplatin, carboplatin must first undergo sequential losses of the non-amine-chelated ligands. Although this process proceeds readily with the loss of the chlorides in cisplatin (Horacek and Drobnik 1971), the rate of leaving or "opening" of the carboxylato moieties in carboplatin is much slower.

After a 2-hour drug exposure in L-1210 cells, carboplatin produced concentration-dependent DNA–DNA interstrand crosslinks as well as DNA–protein crosslinks (Micetich et al 1985). The molar potency of carboplatin in creating these DNA lesions and cytotoxicity was observed to be roughly one-fiftieth that of cisplatin in vitro (Micetich et al 1985) and up to one-third to one-fourth that of cisplatin in vivo (DeNeve et al 1990). A more striking difference is the markedly delayed onset of peak crosslinking for carboplatin compared with cisplatin. With carboplatin, maximal DNA crosslinking occurs 18 hours after exposure, compared with 6 to 12 hours for cisplatin (Micetich et al 1985). In addition, carboplatin-induced DNA crosslinks appear to have a slower rate of removal than do cisplatin-induced crosslinks. This slower onset and repair of carboplatin crosslinking are believed to be a direct result of a slow rate of monofunctional adduct formation and/or a slower rate of conversion of monoadducts to crosslinks. In another trial, however, no difference was noted in the rate of crosslink formation for both drugs tested in AKR tumor cells implanted in mice (DeNeve et al 1990). In this study, 13-fold higher carboplatin doses were required for equivalent antitumor effects, even though DNA crosslinks were equal with only 3- to 4-fold greater doses of carboplatin. This suggests that there may be a discrepancy between DNA crosslinking and antitumor activity for carboplatin in vivo.

Harrap (1985) has described nuclear protein phosphorylation in a variety of rat tissues following treatment with both cisplatin and carboplatin. These events appear to correlate to cell killing (Wilkinson et al 1978). Of interest, carboplatin appeared to produce selective phosphorylation of nuclear proteins in tumor cells over normal kidney or liver cells (Harrap 1985).

It is also possible that carboplatin may form intrastrand DNA crosslinks as has been noted with cisplatin (Zwelling and Kohn 1979). These lesions involve a bifunctional platinum adduct to a single strand of DNA. This could lead to transcriptional miscoding and inhibition of DNA synthesis. Carboplatin-induced cytotoxicity, like that induced by cisplatin, is not cell cycle phase specific but can nonetheless be maximized if exposed to cells in S phase. Carboplatin's antitumor activity may also be somewhat schedule dependent in that maximal cytotoxicity in human ovarian cancer cells treated in vitro is greatest when drug exposure is increased from 1 to 24 hours (Curt et al 1983).

■ Availability and Storage

Carboplatin (Paraplatin®, Bristol-Myers Oncology Division, Princeton, New Jersey) is supplied in glass vials containing 50, 150, and 450 mg of sterile, lyophilized powder. Each vial contains an equivalent amount of mannitol. The vials can be stored at room temperature (15 to 30°C or 59 to 86°F) and should be protected from light. The vials generally have a shelf-life of 3 years after manufacture; however, the user is cautioned to observed the stated expiration date printed on each vial.

■ Preparation for Use, Stability, and Admixture

Carboplatin vials can be reconstituted with Sterile Water for Injection, USP, 5% Dextrose in Water, USP, or Sodium Chloride Injection, USP. The recommended amounts of diluent are 5, 15, and 45 mL for 50-, 150-, and 450-mg vials, respectively, yielding a 10 mg/mL concentration. The pH of this solution is 5 to 7 and it is chemically stable for at least 24 hours (Cheung et al 1987). Nonetheless, the manufacturer recommends use within 8 hours of reconstitution because no antibacterial agent is included in the commercial formulation.

Aluminum can react with carboplatin to yield an inactive complex and a resultant loss of antitumor potency. Thus, as for cisplatin, aluminum-containing needles and infusion sets should not be used to prepare or administer carboplatin solutions.

Carboplatin solutions can be diluted to 0.5 mg/mL for administration to patients. At 5 mg/mL, carboplatin is physically stable for 4 hours with a 1 mg/mL solution of ondansetron 1 mg/mL (Trissel et al 1990).

■ Administration

Carboplatin is usually administered as a brief infusion over 15 minutes or longer in either 0.9% sodium chloride or D5W. Typically the drug is diluted into 500 mL of fluid and infused intravenously over 15 to 30 minutes without further hydration (McGuire et al 1989) or over 1 hour (Calvert et al 1982, Horwich et al 1989). Carboplatin has also been administered as a continuous 24-hour intravenous infusion for 1 day (Curt et al 1983), for 4 days (Shea et al 1989), for 5 days (Meyers et al 1989) or as a continuous intravenous infusion for 21 days (Smit et al 1991).

■ Dosage

The official dose recommendation for single-agent carboplatin in ovarian cancer patients with good bone marrow reserve is 360 mg/m² IV every 4 weeks. A wide variety of other dosing schedules have also been evaluated in phase I clinical trials. The table lists the recommended doses for phase II carboplatin trials. This summary shows a wide variation in maximally tolerated doses for different schedules of carboplatin administration.

Dose Adjustment. Because of the potential for severe and sometimes fatal myelosuppression from carboplatin, several dose adjustment guidelines have been promulgated. These patient-specific recommendations are usually based on renal function (Calvert et al 1989) or renal function and the effect of prior therapy on the platelet count (Egorin et al 1984). The latter method distinguishes between previously treated and previously untreated patients to

CARBOPLATIN DOSE RECOMMENDATIONS FROM PHASE I CLINICAL TRIALS

Intravenous Dosing Schedule	Frequency (wk)	Total Dose (mg/m²)	Reference
Bolus × 1	4	400–500	Calvert et al 1982
Bolus × 5	5–6	100	Van Echo et al 1984 Rozencweig et al 1983
Weekly × 4	6	150	Woolley et al 1984
(high-dose 24-hour continuous infusion)	4	320	Curt et al 1983
Continuous infusion over 5 days (high-dose leukemia induction therapy)	3	1000–1500	Meyers et al 1989
Continuous infusion over 4 days (required autologous bone marrow transplantation)	—	2000	Shea et al 1989
21-Day continuous IV infusion	—	30/d	Smit et al 1991

take into account the loss of bone marrow reserve, particularly platelet-regenerating capacity:

For Previously Untreated Patients

Dose (mg/m^2) = 317
[(pretreatment platelet count
− platelet nadir desired/pretreatment platelet count) 100 − 82.1]
× (body surface area/creatinine clearance) + 447

For Previously Treated Patients

Dose (mg/m^2) = 317
[(pretreatment platelet count
− platelet nadir desired/pretreatment platelet count) 100 − 92.4]
× (body surface area/creatinine clearance) + 447

In the simpler Calvert formula dose adjustments are based on creatinine clearance or glomerular filtration rate (GFR) and a desired serum concentration × time product (AUC) for carboplatin antitumor activity, dose (mg) = target AUC × (GFR + 25), with desired target AUCs of 4 to 6 mg/mL · min for previously treated patients and 6 to 8 mg/mL · min for previously untreated patients (Calvert et al 1989). Note that doses in the Calvert method are total mg *not* mg/m^2 and that the GFR determinations were based on actual ethylenediaminetetraacetic acid clearance rather than estimated from serum creatinine.

Both methods have been prospectively evaluated and offer the potential to adjust carboplatin doses in patients with impaired renal function. This will avoid severe toxicity and maintain the therapeutic efficacy of the drug. Because of its simplicity, the Calvert method may be easier to apply in diverse clinical settings. Although the use of measured creatinine clearance is recommended by Calvert et al, creatinine clearance values calculated from serum creatinine using the Cockroft and Gault (1976) method or the Jeliffe method (Jelliffe and Jelliffe 1972) may also be applicable. The relationship between increasing carboplatin AUCs and response in ovarian cancer has been discussed in a recent preliminary study. Unfortunately, the data showed that increasing the AUC above 5 to 7 mg/mL · min does not increase response rates but does increase myelotoxicity, primarily thrombocytopenia (Egorin et al 1991). Clearly, other studies will be needed to confirm these findings.

■ Drug Interactions

The combination of carboplatin and thymidine has produced enhanced cytotoxicity in human T-cell leukemia in vitro (Cohen et al 1989). In addition, carboplatin plus hyperthermia similarly produces enhanced antitumor cytotoxicity (Cohen and Robins 1987). The hyperthermic synergizing effect can also be increased further with thymidine in an experimental setting (Cohen et al 1989).

■ Pharmacokinetics

The pharmacokinetics of carboplatin differ significantly from that of cisplatin. As the table below shows, the plasma clearance of carboplatin is biphasic and slower than that of cisplatin, with a much higher percentage of drug excreted in the urine. Unlike cisplatin, relatively little carboplatin is bound to plasma proteins; however, about 30% of the platinum degraded from carboplatin can be irreversibly bound with a half-life of elimination of 5 days. Free platinum released from carboplatin has a plasma half-life of about 90 minutes (Newell et al 1987, Harland et al 1984). The major route of elimination of carboplatin is glomerular filtration and tubular secretion. There is little if any true metabolism of the drug. In an anephric patient, the half-life of carboplatin was 36 hours with peritoneal dialysis and 4 hours with hemodialysis (Weitzman et al 1991). Kinetic studies indicate that hemodialysis can remove drug at a rate 25% that of the kidney. Peritoneal dialysis is ineffective as a means of eliminating carboplatin. Therefore, in anephric patients, dose adjustments should correspond to the method and length of dialysis.

Because up to 65% of a carboplatin dose is excreted in the urine, significant dose adjustments are recommended for patients with creatinine clearance values less than 60 mL/min (see Dose Adjustment). The table on the opposite page lists the different

CARBOPLATIN PHARMACOKINETICS

Cumulative 24-hour urinary excretion	65% (if creatinine clearance > 60 mL/min)
Plasma half-life	
α (free drug)	90 min
β (free drug)	180 min
β [free Pt (II)]	90 min
Protein-bound drug	> 5 d
Volume of distribution	16–20 L
Protein binding	30% (slow equilibration)

AUCs for various carboplatin regimens. This analysis shows that a wide range of systemic carboplatin exposures can be achieved in patients. Importantly, these pharmacokinetic data can be used to adjust dosing to achieve a target exposure in an individual patient (Calvert et al 1989). With a continuous (21-day) infusion, mean steady-state levels of ultrafilterable drug were 160 ± 10 μg/L (Smit et al 1991). Approximately 21% of the drug was present as the free (ultrafilterable) fraction at 21 days with an AUC of 4921 ± 302 mg · min/L. Total body clearance of ultrafilterable drug in this study was 0.248 mL/min, or twice the maximal glomerular filtration rate. Plasma level decay was triexponential, with half-lives of 44, 111, and 1387 minutes for the α, β and γ phases, respectively (Smit et al 1991).

Carboplatin is also widely distributed in body fluids (Van Echo et al 1984) and achieves good penetration into pleural effusions and ascites fluid (Shea et al 1989). Carboplatin also distributes into cerebrospinal fluid (CSF) of children with brain tumors (Riccardi et al 1992). The mean AUCs for free (unbound) carboplatin in CSF and plasma were 2.3 and 8.2 mg/mL/min following intravenous doses of 600 mg/m^2. There was greater variability in CSF levels and the ratio of CSF:plasma concentration ranged from 0.17 to 0.46 (mean 0.28). Thus, about 30% of the systemic exposure is achieved in the central nervous system following intravenous carboplatin dosing. Of interest, this correlated with objective antitumor responses in patients with medulloblastoma (Riccardi et al 1992).

The pharmacokinetics of high-dose carboplatin in pediatric patients is similar to that in adults. The mean terminal half-life was 3.6 hours (range, 2.1–14.2 hours) and the mean clearance 45.8 mL/min/m^2 (range, 25.5–65.3 mL/min/m^2) (Madden et al 1992). Clearance correlated to body surface area (55 × body surface area in m^2). Clearance of carboplatin was significantly lower in patients receiving prior cumulative cisplatin doses of 960 mg/m^2 or greater (Madden et al 1992). Finally, pharmacokinetic studies in patients receiving continuous carboplatin infusions show that although total platinum levels increase over the course of the infusion, free or active platinum levels can decrease from 78% on day 1 to 38% on day 4 of a 4-day infusion.

■ Side Effects and Toxicity

Carboplatin toxicity differs significantly from that of cisplatin. The usual dose-limiting toxic effect of carboplatin is bone marrow suppression, particularly thrombocytopenia (Calvert et al 1982). Leukopenia and anemia also occur but are less severe. Nonetheless, transfusions may need to be given to about one fifth of all patients receiving carboplatin (Canetta et al 1985). They may not be necessary unless the patient has received heavy prior myelosuppressive therapy.

The platelet nadir is achieved 3 weeks following an intravenous bolus injection and recovery is generally complete 4 to 5 weeks after dosing; however, patients with poor bone marrow reserve from previous chemo- or radiotherapy can have more profound thrombocytopenia and leukopenia with carboplatin. This can sometimes persist several weeks after dosing (see Dose Adjustment for guidelines in this regard).

Nausea and vomiting induced by carboplatin are much less severe than with cisplatin and rarely last beyond 24 hours. Emesis can usually be blocked entirely with aggressive therapy using antiemetic drug combinations (Plezia et al 1984). Diarrhea has

AREA UNDER THE (PLASMA CONCENTRATION) CURVE (AUC) FOR DIFFERENT CARBOPLATIN DOSES

	AUC	Reference
Dose (mg/m^2)		
77–99 (bolus)	145–709 μg/mL/min	Van Echo et al 1984
400–600 (bolus)*	6–8 mg/mL · min	Calvert et al 1989
1600 (bolus)	10.800–25.4 mg/mL/min	Newell et al 1987
Infusion × 4 days		
500	262 μmol/L · h	
1200	893 μmol/L · h	Shea et al 1989
1600	1035 μmol/L · h	
2400	1545 μmol/L · h	

*Assuming normal creatinine clearance in previously untreated patients.

been reported in only 6% and constipation in 3% of carboplatin-treated patients (Canetta et al 1985).

Nephrotoxicity has been reported with carboplatin, but it is much less common and less severe than with cisplatin. In a large review series, transient elevations in serum creatinine and blood urea nitrogen were described in 7 and 16% of patients (Canetta et al 1985). Measured creatinine clearances dropped in 25% of patients and a slight increase in uric acid was described in the same percentage of patients. There can, however, be a significant loss of serum electrolytes including potassium (16% of patients) and especially magnesium (37% of patients). Serum calcium is only rarely decreased following carboplatin (Canetta et al 1985).

A few cases of carboplatin-induced hematuria have been described: in one leukemic adult who had previously experienced cyclophosphamide-induced hemorrhagic cystitis and in another pediatric patient who had no significant past history or previous thrombocytopenia from the drug. Both patients recovered uneventfully. There is also a single case of hepatic veno-occlusive disease in postmortem specimens from a patient who received high-dose carboplatin and etoposide during an autologous bone marrow transplantation regimen. Another possible carboplatin fatality was reported in a patient who developed marked encephalopathy and coma in association with thrombotic microangiopathic hemolytic anemia (Walker et al 1989). Severe microvascular thrombosis was observed in the heart, kidney and brain of this 62-year-old patient who had been cured of recurrent medulloblastoma after receiving 175 mg/m^2 of carboplatin weekly × 4, every 7 weeks for nine courses.

Hepatic enzyme elevations occasionally occur with carboplatin (Canetta et al 1985). Alkaline phosphatase was transiently increased in 36% of patients and serum glutamic–oxalacetic and glutamic-pyruvic transaminases in about 15% of patients. Serum bilirubin levels are also only rarely elevated (4% of over 250 patients) (Canetta et al 1985).

Similarly, neurotoxicity is very uncommon following carboplatin and was described in only 25 of 428 (6%) of patients treated on a variety of schedules for different tumor types (Canetta et al 1985). Mild paresthesias have been reported in a few patients receiving cumulative carboplatin doses above 1.6 g/m^2 (Calvert et al 1982). Unlike cisplatin, these peripheral nerve toxic effects rarely produce any disabling symptoms. Indeed, in most series, no neurotoxicity is described from the drug (Wiltshaw et al 1985). The relative lack of significant neurotoxicity from carboplatin has helped to propel the drug forward for routine use as first-line therapy of ovarian cancer (Alberts et al 1990).

Ototoxicity also does not appear to be problematic with carboplatin and only 8 of 710 (1.1%) patients have described clinical hearing deficits, mainly tinnitus (Canetta et al 1985); however, if pretreatment and serial audiometric tests are performed, up to 15% of patients may be found to have experienced some decrease in audio acuity. Fortunately, ototoxicity from carboplatin can sometimes improve once therapy is halted. And, as with cisplatin, greater ototoxicity from carboplatin can be expected in patients with preexisting hearing loss and/or in those given other ototoxic drugs such as aminoglycosides concurrently.

Other rare carboplatin toxic effects include alopecia (2%), mucositis (2%), skin rash (1.7%), injection site irritation without extravasation necrosis (0.4%), and a flulike syndrome (1.3%) (Canetta et al 1985). Alterations in taste sensation are also described. Skin disorders with carboplatin may appear as an erythematous rash in exposed areas (Calvert et al 1982) and do not occur in all patients who had developed similar rashes on cisplatin. In a mouse model, highly concentrated carboplatin solutions were toxic following intradermal injection (Marnocha and Hutson 1992). However, the drug has not been associated with necrosis following inadvertent extravasations in humans.

With the high doses of carboplatin used in autologous bone marrow transplantation programs other toxic effects may ensue. These include hepatotoxicity (both hepatitis and cholestasis) and severe renal dysfunction (Shea et al 1989). Nausea, vomiting, and electrolyte wasting are also more profound with high-dose carboplatin treatments. In addition, other unusual toxic effects may occur. These include hemorrhagic colitis, optic neuritis, and interstitial pneumonitis.

■ Special Applications

Intraperitoneal Administration in Ovarian Cancer. Patients with advanced ovarian cancer have been treated with intraperitoneal carboplatin in doses of 200 to 400 mg/m^2/mo (Columbo et al 1987) and up to 650 mg/m^2 (ten Bokkel Huinink et al 1987a). Doses are typically diluted into 2 L of saline, which is instilled for 2 to 4 hours, then drained by gravity. A response rate of 10% was described in one trial involving 27 patients (ten Bokkel Huinink et al 1987a) and a 50% response rate was reported in a smaller series of 14 patients with minimal residual disease. These patients were treated with carboplatin following surgery and systemic cisplatin therapy (Columbo et al 1987). No chemical peritonitis or renal toxicity has been encountered, although some myelotoxicity is characteristically seen. A 53% response rate was reported in another trial involving 17 patients treated with 400 mg/m^2. Of note, patients in this latter trial all had bulky disease which had recurred following other treatments including cisplatin therapy (Kopecny et al 1987).

Another recent trial has also reported favorable results for intraperitoneal carboplatin in women with minimal residual disease after cisplatin therapy (Speyer et al 1990). Doses were escalated from 200 mg/m^2 to a median of 525 mg/m^2 with caution if the creatinine clearance was 60 mL/min or less. Each dose was diluted into 2 L of 1.5% dextrose and given intraperitoneally with a 4-hour dwell time every 6 weeks. Complete pathologic responses were observed in 6 of 23 (26%) evaluable patients, with ongoing response durations ranging from 3 to 40 months (median for all patients, 14 months). The dose-limiting side effect was thrombocytopenia which was more severe in patients with compromised renal function. Again, no local toxic effects were described, and overall, the treatments were well tolerated.

REFERENCES

Alberts DS, Canetta R, Mason-Liddil N. Carboplatin in the first-line chemotherapy of ovarian cancer. *Semin Oncol.* 1990;**17**(1):54–60.

Allen JC, Walker R, Luks E, et al. Carboplatin and recurrent childhood brain tumors. *J Clin Oncol.* 1987;**5**:459–463.

Behrens BC, Hamilton TC, Masuda H. Characterization of cis-diamminedichloroplatinum (II) resistant human ovarian cancer cell line and its use in evaluation of platinum analogues. *Cancer Res.* 1987;**47**:414–419.

Bunn PA Jr. Review of therapeutic trials of carboplatin in lung cancer. *Semin Oncol* 1989; **16**(2)(suppl 5):27–34.

Calvert AH, Baker JW, Dalley VM, et al. Phase II trial of *cis*-diammine-1, 1-cyclobutane dicarboxylate platinum II (CBDCA, JM8) in patients with carcinoma of the ovary not previously treated with cisplatin (abstract). In: Hacker MP, Double EB, Krakoff IH, eds. *Platinum Coordination Complexes in Cancer Chemotherapy.* Boston: Martinus Nijhoff; 1984:353.

Calvert AH, Harland SJ, Newell DR, et al. Early clinical studies with *cis*-diammine-1,1-cyclobutane dicarboxylate platinum II. *Cancer Chemother Pharmacol.* 1982;**9**:140–147.

Calvert AH, Newell DR, Gumbrell LA, et al. Carboplatin dosage: Prospective evaluation of a simple formula based on renal function. *J Clin Oncol.* 1989;**7**(11):1748–1756.

Canetta R, Rozencweig M, Carter SK. Carboplatin: The clinical spectrum to date. *Cancer Treat Rev.* 1985;**12**(suppl A):125–136.

Cheung Y-W, Cradock JC, Vishnuvajjala BR, et al. Stability of cisplatin, iproplatin, carboplatin, and tetraplatin in commonly used intravenous solutions. *Am J Hosp Pharm.* 1987;**44**:124–130.

Cockcroft DW, Gault MH. Prediction of creatinine clearance from serum creatinine. *Nephron.* 1976;**16**:31–41.

Cohen JD, Robins HI. Hyperthermic enhancement of *cis*-diammine-1, 1-cyclobutane dicarboxylate platinum (II) cytotoxicity in human leukemia cells in vitro. *Caner Res.* 1987;**47**:4335–4337.

Cohen JD, Robins HI, Schmitt CL, et al. Interactions of thymidine, hyperthermia, and *cis*-diammine-1, 1-cyclobutane dicarboxylate platinum(II) in human T-cell leukemia. *Cancer Res.* 1989;**49**:5805–5809.

Colombo N, Speyer JL, Green MD, et al. Carboplatin (CBDCA) as salvage in ovarian cancer (OC): Unpredictable myelotoxicity (abstract). *Proc Am Soc Clin Oncol.* 1986;**5**:123.

Colombo N, Speyer J, Wernz J, et al. Phase I–II study of intraperitoneal CBDCA in patients (pts) with advanced ovarian cancer (oc). *Proc Am Soc Clin Oncol.* 1987;**6**:113.

Curt GA, Grygiel JJ, Corden BJ, et al. A phase I and pharmacokinetic study of diamminecyclobutanedicarboxylatoplatinum (NSC-241240). *Cancer Res.* 1983;**43**:4470–4473.

DeNeve W, Valeriote F, Tapazoglou E, et al. Discrepancy between cytotoxicity and DNA interstrand crosslinking of carboplatin and cisplatin in vivo. *Invest New Drugs.* 1990;**8**:17–24.

Egorin M, Jodrell D, Canetta R, et al. Tumor response & toxicity in ovarian cancer correlates with carboplatin (CBDCA) area under the curve (AUC) (abstract). *Proc Am Soc Clin Oncol.* 1991;**10**:184.

Egorin MJ, Van Echo DA, Tiping SJ, et al. Pharmacokinetics and dosage reduction of carboplatin in patients with impaired renal function. *Cancer Res.*1984;**44**:5432–5438.

Eisenberger M, Krasnow S, Ellenberg S, et al. A comparison of carboplatin plus methotrexate versus methotrexate alone in patients with recurrent and metastatic head and neck cancer. *J Clin Oncol.* 1989;**7**:1341–1345.

Evans BD, Chapman P, Dady P, et al. A phase II study of carboplatin (JM8) and chlorambucil in previously untreated patients with advanced ovarian cancer (abstract). *Proc Am Soc Clin Oncol.* 1988;**7**:139.

Gaver RC, George AM, Deeb G. In vitro stability, plasma protein binding and blood cell partitioning of ^{14}C-carboplatin. *Cancer Chemother Pharmacol.* 1987;**20**:271–276.

George M, Kerbrat P, Herron JF, et al. Phase I–II study of

high-dose carboplatin (HDC) as first line chemotherapy (CT) of extensive epithelial ovarian cancer (OC) (abstract). *Proc Am Soc Clin Oncol.* 1988;**7**:140.

Harland SJ, Newell DR, Siddik ZH, et al. Pharmacokinetics of *cis*-diammine-1, 1-cyclobutane dicarboxylate platinum (II) in patients with normal and impaired renal function. *Cancer Res.* 1984;**44**:1693–1697.

Harrap KR. Preclinical studies identifying carboplatin as a viable cisplatin alternative. *Cancer Treat Rev.* 1985;**12**(suppl A):21–33.

Horacek P, Drobnik J. Interaction of *cis*-dichlorodiammineplatinum(II) with DNA. *Biochim Biophys Acta.* 1971;**254**:341–347.

Horwich A, Dearnaley DP, Duchesne GM, et al. Simple nontoxic treatment of advanced metastatic seminoma with carboplatin. *J Clin Oncol.* 1989;**7**(8):1150–1156.

Jelliffe RW, Jelliffe SM. A computer program for estimation of creatinine clearance from unstable serum creatinine levels, age, sex, and weight. *Math Biosci.* 1972;**14**:17–24.

Kopecny J, Nechl Z, Kiss F, et al. Clinical study of intraperitoneal carboplatin in ovarian cancer therapy (abstract). *Proc ECCO.* 1987;**4**:217.

Long HJ, Pfeifle DM, Wieand HS, et al. Phase II evaluation of carboplatin in advanced endometrial carcinoma. *J Natl Cancer Inst.* 1988;**80**:276–278.

Lund B, Hansen M, Hansen OP, et al. Combined high-dose carbo- and cisplatin in ovarian cancer patients (abstract). *Proc Am Soc Clin Oncol.* 1988;**7**:148.

Madden T, Sunderland M, Santana VM, et al. The pharmacokinetics of high-dose carboplatin in pediatric patients with cancer. *Clin Pharmacol Ther.* 1992;**51**:701–707.

Marnocha RSM, Hutson PR: Intradermal carboplatin and ifosfamide extravasation in the mouse. *Cancer* 1992;**70**:850–855.

McGuire WP III, Arseneau J, Blessing JA, et al. A randomized comparative trial of carboplatin and iproplatin in advanced squamous carcinoma of the uterine cervix: A Gynecologic Oncology Group study. *J Clin Oncol.* 1989;**7**(10):1462–1468.

Mechl Z, Sopkova B, Nekulova M, et al. Phase II trial of carboplatin in advanced bladder cancer. *Proc ECCO.* 1987;**4**:237.

Meerpohl HG, Carboplatin (CBDCA) in patients with advanced ovarian cancer: Results of two phase II studies (abstract). *J Cancer Res Clin Oncol.* 1988;**114**(suppl):S60.

Meyers FJ, Welborn J, Lewis JP, et al. Infusion carboplatin treatment of relapsed and refractory acute leukemia: Evidence of efficacy with minimal extramedullary toxicity at intermediate doses. *J Clin Oncol.* 1989;**7**(2):173–178.

Micetich KC, Barnes D, Erickson LC. A comparative study of the cytotoxicity and DNA-damaging effects of *cis*-(diammino)(1,1-cyclobutanedicarboxylato)-platinum(II) and *cis*-diamminedichloroplatinum(II) on L1210 cells. *Cancer Res.* 1985;**45**:4043–4047.

Motzer RJ, Bosl GJ, Taver K, et al. Phase II trial of carboplatin in patients with advanced germ cell tumors refractory to cisplatin. *Cancer Treat Rep.* 1987;**71**:197–198.

Newell DR, Siddik ZH, Gumbrell LA, Boxall FE, Gore ME et al. Plasma free platinum pharmacokinetics in patients treated with high dose carboplatin. *Europ J Cancer Clin Oncol.* 1987; **23**:1399–1405.

Nichols CR, Tricot G, Williams SD. Dose-intensive chemotherapy in refractory germ cell cancer—A phase I/II trial of high-dose carboplatin and etoposide with autologous bone marrow transplantation. *J Clin Oncol.* 1989;**7**(7):932–939.

Ogawa M, Inuyama Y, Kato T, et al. Phase II study of carboplatin (abstract). *Proc Am Soc Clin Oncol.* 1987;**6**:20.

Ozols RF, Ostchega Y, Curt G, et al. High-dose carboplatin in refractory ovarian cancer patients. *J Clin Oncol.* 1987;**5**:197–201.

Plezia PM, Alberts DS, Kessler J, et al. Immediate termination of intractable vomiting induced by cisplatin combination chemotherapy using an intensive five-drug antiemetic regimen. *Cancer Treat Rep.* 1984;**68**(12):1493–1495.

Pohl J, Meerpohl HG, Pfleiderer A. A phase II clinical trial of carboplatin in advanced ovarian cancer (abstract). In: *Fifth NCI–EORTC Symposium on New Drugs in Cancer Therapy.* Brussels: European Organization for Research and Treatment of Cancer; 1986.

Riccardi R, Riccardi A, De Rocco C, et al. Cerebrospinal fluid pharmacokinetics of carboplatin in children with brain tumors. *Cancer Chemother Pharmacol.* 1992;**30**:21–24.

Rozencweig M, Nicaise C, Beer M, et al. Phase I study of carboplatin given on a five-day intravenous schedule. *J Clin Oncol.* 1983;**1**(10):621–626.

Shea TC, Flaherty M, Elias A, et al. A phase I clinical and pharmacokinetic study of carboplatin and autologous bone marrow support. *J Clin Oncol.* 1989;**7**(5):651–661.

Smit EF, Willomse PHB, Sleijfer DTh, et al. Continuous infusion carboplatin on a 21-day schedule: A phase I and pharmacokinetic study. *J Clin Oncol.* 1991;**9**:100–110.

Speyer JL, Beller U, Colombo N, et al. Intraperitoneal carboplatin: Favorable results in women with minimal residual ovarian cancer after cisplatin therapy. *J Clin Oncol.* 1990;**8**:1335–1341.

Ten Bokkel Huinink WW, Heintz AP, Dubbelman R, et al. Intraperitoneal carboplatin and refractory ovarian cancer: A phase I study. *Proc ECCO.* 1987a;**4**:826.

Ten Bokkel Huinink WW, van der Berg MEL, van Oosterom AT, et al. A pilot study of CHAC-1. *Cancer Treat Rev.* 1985;**23**(suppl A):77–82.

Ten Bokkel Huinink WW, van der Berg MEL, van Oosterom AT, et al. Carboplatin in combination chemotherapy for ovarian cancer. *Cancer Treat Rev.* 1988;**15**(suppl B):9–15.

Ten Bokkel Huinink, Wanders J, Dubbelman A, et al. High dose carboplatin in refractory ovarian cancer: A phase II trial assessing the protective role against myelosuppression by diethyldithiocarbamate (DDTC). *Proc ECCO.* 1987b;**4**:214.

Trissel LA, Fulton B, Tramonte SM. Visual compatibility of ondansetron with chemotherapeutic agents, antibiotics, and other selected drugs during simulated Y-site injection (abstract #P-468R). In: *25th Annual ASHP Midyear Clinical Meetings and Exhibit, Las Vegas, Nevada*, Las Vegas: American Society of Hospital Pharmacists, 1990.

Van Echo DA, Egorin MJ, Whitacre MY, et al. Phase I clinical and pharmacologic trial of carboplatin daily for 5 days. *Cancer Treat Rep.* 1984;**68**:1103–1114.

Walker RW, Rosenblum MK, Kempin SJ, et al. Carboplatin-associated thrombotic microangiopathic hemolytic anemia. *Cancer.* 1989;**64**:1017–1020.

Weitzman S, Klein J, Koren G. Pharmacokinetics of carboplatinum in an anephric child with recurrent Wilms' tumor. *Proc Am Soc Clin Oncol.* 1991;**10**:116.

Wilkinson R, Cox PJ, Jones M, et al. Selection of potential second generation platinum compounds. *Biochimistry.* 1978;**60**:851–857.

Williams SD, Nichols CR, Jansen J. Use of carboplatin in the treatment of testicular cancer. *Semin Oncol.* 1989;**16**(2)(suppl 5):42–45.

Wiltshaw E. Ovarian trials at the Royal Marsden. *Cancer Treat Rev.* 1985;**12**(suppl A):67–71.

Wiltshaw E, Evans BD, Jones AC, et al. JM8, successor to cisplatin in advanced ovarian carcinoma. *Lancet.* 1985;**1**:587.

Wiltshaw E, Smales E, Gallagher CJ, et al. Carboplatin (paraplatin) in ovarian cancer. In: Lapis, Eckhardt, eds. *Lectures and Symposia, 14th International Cancer Congress, Budapest, 1986.* Basel: S. Karger; 1987; 9:3–8.

Woolley PV, Priego VM, Luc PV, et al. Clinical pharmacokinetics of diammine [1,1-cyclobutanedicarboxylato (2-)]-O, O'-platinum (CBDCA). *Dev Oncol.* 1984;**17**:82–89.

Zwelling LA, Kohn KW. Mechanism of action of *cis*-dichlorodiammineplatinum(II). *Cancer Treat Rep.* 1979;**63**:1439–1444.

Carmustine

■ Other Names

NSC-409962; BCNU; bischloronitrosourea; BiCNU® (Bristol-Myers Oncology Division).

■ Chemistry

$$ClCH_2CH_2\underset{NO}{\overset{\overset{O}{\|}}{N}}CNH-CH_2CH_2Cl$$

Structure of carmustine

Chemically, carmustine is 1,3-bis(2-chloroethyl)-1-nitrosourea. One gram is soluble in about 250 mL of normal saline or 80 mL of propylene glycol. It is a highly lipid soluble, un-ionized drug of low molecular weight (214.06). It is also soluble in water, 5 mg/mL, and absolute alcohol, 100 mg/mL (Zackheim et al 1977). The drug has a melting point of 27°C (80.6°F). The octanol/water coefficient (log *P*) value is 1.54, indicating significant lipophilicity.

■ Antitumor Activity

Carmustine was originally developed on the basis of the antileukemic activity observed with the related compound methylnitrosoguanidine (MNNG). Carmustine originally demonstrated activity in central nervous system tumors in mice (Schabel et al 1963) and in humans with a variety of advanced cancers (Rall et al 1963, DeVita et al 1965, Walker 1973). In brain cancers, an overall response rate of 48% was described. Fifty-three percent of patients with glioblastoma responded (Fewer et al 1972). It has activity in multiple myeloma, generally as part of first-line drug combinations (Salmon 1976, Cohen et al 1976). It also has activity in advanced, refractory Hodgkin's disease (Anderson et al 1976, Young et al 1971, Rege and Owens 1974) and in non-Hodgkin's lymphoma (Bennet et al 1976). A topical solution has been investigationally successful in controlling dermal disease in the cutaneous T-cell lymphoma mycosis fungoides (Zackheim and Epstein 1975). In combination with other cytotoxic agents, intravenous carmustine also has some activity in malignant melanoma (Moon 1970).

See Special Applications for high-dose applications with bone marrow transplantation.

■ Mechanism of Action

Carmustine acts primarily as an alkylating agent through metabolites containing chloroethyl moieties (Wheeler and Chumley 1967). The drug inhibits a number of key enzymatic reactions involved with DNA synthesis. Because carmustine possesses two functional chloroethyl groups, DNA crosslinking is possible. With carmustine the formation of DNA–DNA interstrand crosslinks is relatively slow, whereas DNA–protein crosslinks form rapidly (Kohn et al 1981). This creates a relatively long duration of inhibition of DNA synthesis (Wheeler and Alexander 1976). Of interest, cells that rapidly remove monoadducts from DNA by the enzyme O^6-alkyltransferase (MER + cells) have increased resistance to carmustine (Erickson et al 1980). It has also been shown that transcriptionally active regions of chromatin are preferentially attacked by carmustine in HeLa cells (Tew 1981).

Kann et al (1974a) noted inhibition of DNA repair and carbamoylation of cellular proteins at the ε-amino group of lysine caused by the isocyanate protein of the drug. Although carbamoylation does not correlate with antitumor activity, the 2-chloroethylisocyanate does inactivate red blood cell glutathione reductase (Frischer and Ahmad 1977). Of more importance, carbamoylation by isocyanate appears to be solely responsible for the inhibition of DNA repair caused by carmustine (Kann 1981). Conversely, the repair of carmustine-induced damage appears to involve ADP-ribosylation (Smulson et al 1981). A later study additionally showed that carmustine interferes with the synthesis of RNA and proteins (Wheeler and Bowden 1965, Kann et al 1974b) as well as DNA synthesis (Wheeler and Alexander 1974). The drug also blocks the uptake of nucleic acid bases into cells (Ludlum et al 1975). Wheeler and Chumley (1967) noted interruption of DNA polymerase activity. Thus, the cytotoxic activity of the drug is thought to be mediated through the action of metabolites that can alkylate DNA and interfere with several other DNA enzymatic processes. Unfortunately, cross-resistance to classic alkylating agents is usually noted with carmustine. Nonetheless, clinical responses to carmustine have occasionally been obtained in patients with tumors resistant to classic alkylating agents. Carmustine does not appear to be cell cycle phase specific although a G_2 arrest has been observed (Tobey and Crissman 1975). In addition, Bhuyan et al (1972) and Barranco and Humphrey (1971) have observed maximal cytotoxicity from nitrosoureas in late G_1 phase or early S phase.

■ Availability and Storage

Carmustine is commercially available from Bristol-Myers Oncology Division, Princeton, New Jersey. It is supplied as a 100-mg lyophilized powder in 30-mL amber vials along with a separate 3.5-mL vial of absolute alcohol diluent. Unopened, dry vials can be stored under refrigeration (2–8°C) for up to 3 years. Storage of the intact vials at room temperature results in a slow decomposition (approximately 3% over 36 days) (Montgomery et al 1967). Because of the low melting point, exposure to temperatures in excess of 27°C (80.6°F) will cause the drug to liquefy and appear as an oil film in the bottom of the vial. This is evidence of decomposition; if present, the vial should be discarded (Kleinman et al 1976).

■ Preparation for Use, Stability, and Admixture

Carmustine should be initially diluted with 3 mL of the absolute alcohol diluent. After this, 27.0 mL of Sterile Water for Injection, USP, should be aseptically added. This results in a clear, colorless solution of pH 5.6 to 6.0 with a 10% ethanol concentration containing 3.3 mg of drug per milliliter. For stability under various conditions refer to the table on the opposite page. The lyophilized drug vials do not contain a preservative and therefore should not be used as a multidose container.

Carmustine solutions are light sensitive with stability times at 25°C of 6 hours without light and 3.5 to 0.6 hours dependent on light energy (Fredriksson et al 1986). Maximum stability was observed at pH 3.3 to 4.8. Significant adsorption of carmustine to plastics has been documented. This is especially important with polyvinyl chloride-based infusion containers (Benvenuto et al 1981, Fredriksson et al 1986). The degree of adsorption can be minimized by using tubing with internal polyethylene linings and by administering the drug at high solution flow rates above 250 mL/h. Carmustine stability is also temperature dependent, with enhanced stability at 4°C (Laskar and Ayres 1977).

In 5% dextrose at room temperature, carmustine is stable for only 0.5 hour in plastic containers and 7.7 hours in glass containers (Benvenuto et al 1981). The drug is stable for 4 hours in 5% dextrose containing 1 mg/mL ondansetron (Trissel et al 1990). The drug is also incompatible with sodium bicarbonate solutions, noted by 10% degradation in 15 minutes and 27% loss in 90 minutes (Colvin et al 1980).

■ Administration

Rapid intravenous infusion of carmustine is not recommended as it is associated with severe burning along the vein and generalized flushing. A longer infusion period of 1 to 2 hours can alleviate this side effect. In general, a 15- to 45-minute infusion in 100 to 250 mL D5W is preferred, with constant monitoring of the patient for arm or venous pain. Because of the pain and vein irritation, it is advisable to administer carmustine last if several drugs are to be given in sequence through a single site. Additionally, a 5- to 10-mL flush (D5W or normal saline) is recom-

CARMUSTINE STABILITY WITH VARIOUS PREPARATIONS

Carmustine Concentration	Final Alcohol Concentration	Temperature/Light	Stability	Reference
Unopened vials	—	4°C (refrigeration) 20°C (room temperature)	2 y 3% loss in potency in 36 d	Manufacturer
Concentrated solution	95%	0–5°C	10% degradation by 78 d 3 mo	Laskar and Ayres 1977 Chan and Zackheim 1973
3.3 mg/mL (0.33%) (recommended initial)	10% (alcohol/water mixture)	4°C 20°C in light (room temperature)	2 h—no decomposition* 24 h—4.1% decomposition* 1 h—0.9% decomposition* 2 h—2.7% decomposition 6 h—8.0% decomposition 21 h—19.2% decomposition	
Above diluted into 500 mL normal saline or D5W	—	4°C (refrigeration), protected from light	Stable 48 h	Manufacturer's product brochure
0.5–0.6 mg/mL (aqueous topical solution)	<1% in distilled H_2O	0–5°C	Half-life 19.0 d	Chan and Zackheim 1973

mended both before and after drug administration to ensure vein patency and flush any remaining drug from the tubing.

■ Dosage

Two basic dosing schedules for carmustine have been used: up to 75 to 100 mg/m² IV daily for 2 consecutive days or up to 200 mg/m² IV in a single injection for primary brain cancer. Because of delayed toxic effects, successive treatments with the drug are usually given no more frequently than every 6 to 8 weeks (Salmon 1976). (See Special Applications for high-dose regimens used with bone marrow transplantation.)

■ Drug Interactions

Cohen (1972) demonstrated experimental antitumor enhancement with carmustine in vitro when vitamin A and caffeine were present. Theophylline and carmustine are synergistic against tumors in vivo (DeWys and Bathina 1980). In a clinical study, Present et al (1976, 1980) have additionally shown an increased therapeutic ratio for the combination of carmustine with amphotericin B (Fungizone®). In these situations, amphotericin is believed to enhance cellular uptake of the nitrosourea by disrupting tumor cell membrane function.

The H_2 antihistamine cimetidine (Tagamet®) has been shown to potentiate carmustine toxicity in preclinical systems (Dorr and Soble 1989) and in cancer patients (Volkin et al 1982, Selker et al 1978). Conversely, hepatic microsomal enzyme inducers such as phenobarbital block experimental carmustine toxic effects in animals (Klubes et al 1979, Levin et al 1979). In contrast, phenytoin, dexamethasone, and methylprednisolone had no such effect in the mouse model (Levin et al 1979). Because of these effects, the use of microsomal enzyme inducers of inhibitors is not recommended with carmustine.

■ Pharmacokinetics

Biotransformation of carmustine is considerable and rapid. The biologic half-life of the drug in vivo is short (DeVita et al 1967, Chirigos et al 1965). The table on page 270 summarizes the clinical pharmacokinetics of the drug using specific assays for carmustine. Note that there is no difference in the disposition of high doses used in bone marrow transplantation programs and standard doses. With hepatic arterial administration, mean hepatic vein drug levels of 4.3 μg/mL are 2.5-fold higher than portal vein levels of 1.8 μg/mL following a 200 mg/m² intraarterial dose (Ensminger et al 1978). This differential is lost rapidly once the 2-hour hepatic artery infusion ends. Nonetheless, a 2.3-fold higher AUC is achieved in the liver with the intraarterial infusion (Ensminger et al 1978). The ex-

CLINICAL PHARMACOKINETICS OF INTRAVENOUS CARMUSTINE

Half-life	
α	6.1 min
β	21.5 min
Volume of distribution at steady state	3.25 L/kg
Total plasma clearance	56 mL/min/kg

Information taken from Levin VA, Hoffman W, Weinkam RJ. Pharmacokinetics of BCNU in man: A preliminary study of 20 patients. Cancer Treat Rep. 1978;62:1305–1312.

cretion of carmustine metabolites in the urine accounts for only 30% of drug elimination after 24 hours. Liver metabolism by microsomal enzymes appears to partially metabolize the drug to active species. The resultant metabolic breakdown products show prolonged plasma levels; however, only 60 to 70% of a dose is recovered in the urine as the metabolites within 96 hours.

The prolonged plasma metabolite levels also demonstrate biphasic peaks. These early and late peaks may be caused by enterohepatic circulation (documented in mice) or uptake and ultimate release from lipid storage depots (this agent is quite soluble in body fat stores). The blood–brain barrier is readily crossed by the drug and/or its metabolites and levels are usually more than 50% of those measured simultaneously in the plasma (DeVita et al 1967).

■ Side Effects and Toxicity

Overall, delayed hematopoietic toxicity has been the dose-limiting toxic effect of carmustine (DeVita et al 1965). Leukopenia and sometimes severe thrombocytopenia peak by 3 to 5 weeks after administration, and may occasionally persist for 1 to 3 weeks longer (Oliverio 1973). Thus, the nadir for white blood cell count suppression by carmustine occurs at 3 to 4 weeks and resolves more slowly than with other alkylating agents.

Immediate adverse reactions to carmustine consist of a burning sensation in the extremity used for infusion or pain at the intravenous site (although true thrombophlebitis is rare). Marked facial flushing may also occur, particularly after rapid intravenous infusions. According to Marsh et al (1971), severe nausea and vomiting commonly begin 2 hours after an intravenous dose and last 4 to 6 hours. Pretreatment with antiemetics is highly recommended. Of interest, Marsh et al (1971) observed diminished pain when the infusion rate and the final concentration of alcohol were reduced.

Other rare toxic effects of carmustine include liver and renal dysfunction. These too seem to occur at higher dosage ranges. Abnormal elevations of serum glutamic-oxalacetic transaminase, alkaline phosphatase, and serum bilirubin have occurred at widely differing and prolonged intervals after treatment (Lokich et al 1974). Jaundice without hepatic pain and hepatic coma have been reported. Biopsy findings in affected patients demonstrate subacute hepatitis with an intense inflammatory response. Renal toxicity, as evidenced by an unexplained elevation in the blood urea nitrogen, occurs in 10% of patients and bears no relationship to the time, dose, or schedule of the drug. These toxic effects are generally reversible.

With long-term therapy pulmonary fibrosis has also been reported (Holoye et al 1976). The associated mortality rate is high. Pulmonary fibrosis does not appear to be dose related and presents either as an insidious cough and dyspnea or a sudden onset of respiratory failure. Chest x-rays show interstitial infiltrates and pulmonary function tests reveal hypoxia associated with diffusion and restrictive defects. It is suggested that this reaction may be more common when carmustine is given in conjunction with cyclophosphamide. Treatment with prednisone does not appear to be of benefit (Durant et al 1979). Topical reactions are also possible with this agent. Thus, extra care should be taken to avoid contact of the solution with the skin or eyes. Pain and a brown staining of exposed tissues may also occur in these instances.

Other unusual toxic effects recently reported with carmustine include optic neuroretinitis (in association with procarbazine therapy) (McLennan and Taylor 1978) and gynecomastia (Schorer et al 1978). In both situations the precise etiologic mechanism is not known; however, the toxic effect appears to resolve once carmustine therapy stops.

■ Special Applications

High-Dose Carmustine with Autologous Bone Marrow Transplantation

Antitumor Activity. Carmustine has been used in a large number of high-dose drug combinations for treating refractory solid tumors. Malignancies responsive to high-dose carmustine-containing combinations include cancer of the breast (Eder et al 1986, Peters et al 1988), neuroblastoma (Hartmann et al 1987), gliomas (Johnson et al 1987, Phillips et al 1986), melanoma and sarcoma (Peters et al 1986, Slease et al 1988), and malignant lymphomas including Hodgkin's disease (Jagannath et al 1989, Phillips et al 1989, Taylor et al 1989, Korbling et al 1990) and non-Hodgkin's lymphomas (Wheeler et al 1990, Petersen et al 1990).

Administration. High-dose carmustine is usually given with several other agents. It is typically administered as a short intravenous infusion at a rate not greater than 3 mg/m^2/min to avoid excessive flushing, agitation, and hypotension (Peters et al 1986). The drug dose is usually diluted into at least 500 mL of 5% dextrose to lessen phlebitis, and infusions usually run for at least 2 hours. Alternatively, the total carmustine dose can be divided into two even fractions and administered at 12-hour intervals (Henner et al 1986). When carmustine is used as a single agent in the treatment of gliomas, mannitol infusions or short-term dexamethasone is administered to prevent cerebral edema (Phillips et al 1986). Other cytotoxic agents are administered concomitantly with high-dose carmustine (in separate infusions).

Dose. In combination with other cytotoxic agents and autologous bone marrow transplantation (ABMT), carmustine doses of 450 to 600 mg/m^2 are typical (Wheeler et al 1990, Peters et al 1986). A higher carmustine dose of 900 mg/m^2 was used with cyclophosphamide (160 mg/kg) in patients with various refractory solid tumors (Slease et al 1988). In Hodgkin's disease lower carmustine doses of 300 mg/m^2 have been combined with high doses of cyclophosphamide and etoposide (Jagannath et al 1989). As a single agent in malignant gliomas, carmustine has been used at doses of 1050 to 1350 mg/m^2 (Phillips et al 1986, Johnson et al 1987). Herzig et al (1981) explored doses up to 2850 mg/m^2 as a single agent and found fatal necrosis at doses above 2 g/m^2. A "safe" upper high dose of carmustine was felt to be 1200 mg/m^2 for a single course. [*Note:* All of the doses here above would be fatal without the subsequent administration of autologous bone marrow.]

Drug Disposition. The pharmacokinetics of high-dose carmustine (300–750 mg/m^2) has been studied using high-performance liquid chromatography and ultraviolet detection (Henner et al 1986). The table summarizes the pharmacokinetics of ultrafilterable (unbound or free) carmustine in ten patients. The results show rapid clearance of drug, with about 23% of a dose free (unbound) in the plasma. Importantly, there was no evidence for dose-dependent pharmacokinetics at these higher doses of carmustine. As with lower doses, carmustine elimination is monophasic but clearances again may vary tenfold between different individuals. Finally, carmustine AUCs are much higher in breast cancer patients experiencing pulmonary injury following high-dose therapy with cisplatin, cyclophosphamide, and carmustine (Jones et al 1992). The mean carmustine AUC in patients developing pulmonary injury was 1266 µg·min/mL, compared with 676 µg·min/mL in the unaffected patients. This suggests that pulmonary toxicity may be associated with increased systemic exposure following high-dose carmustine regimen.

Toxicity. Besides the anticipated bone marrow aplasia, several other toxic effects are caused by high-dose carmustine therapy. These include severe nausea and vomiting, encephalopathy, hepatotoxicity, and pulmonary toxicity (Takvorian et al 1983). The latter two effects may be dose limiting and have been fatal in 15 to 20% of patients in some series. Nausea is apparent in 80% of patients but less than 40% may experience emesis (Johnson et al 1987). Hepatic toxicity usually involves transient elevations in liver enzymes to twice normal values within a week of treatment in 90% of patients (Peters et al 1986). These enzyme levels usually return to normal over the ensuing week; however, veno-occlusive disease (VOD) of the liver has been observed in about 5 to 20% of patients (Ayash et al 1990, Peters et al 1988) and can be fatal (McIntyre et al 1981). Hepatic veno-occlusive disease is thought to be more common in patients with preexisting metastatic cancer in the liver and in those receiving a single high-dose carmustine infusion versus a fractionated schedule (Ayash et al 1990). Signs and symptoms include right upper quadrant tenderness, hepatomegaly, jaundice, and ascites with or without en-

CLINICAL PHARMACOKINETICS OF HIGH-DOSE CARMUSTINE

AUC	0.322 mM · min*
Peak concentration	4.7 µM*
Half-life	22.2 min
Volume of distribution	5.1 L/kg
Clearance	
Free drug	326 mL/min/kg
Total	77.6 mL/min/kg
Unbound	23.3%

*Adjusted to a "standard" dose of 600 mg/m^2 for patients receiving 300 to 750 mg/m^2.
Data from Henner WD, Peters WP, Eder JP, et al. Pharmacokinetics and immediate effects of high-dose carmustine in man. *Cancer Treat Rep.* 1986;70:877–880.

cephalopathy and hyperbilirubinemia (Ayash et al 1990). Pathologically, livers show severe centrilobular and midzonal hemorrhagic necrosis without inflammation or thrombosis of large vessels but with evidence of biliary stasis (McIntyre et al 1981).

Pulmonary complications of high-dose carmustine include severe interstitial pneumonitis (Phillips et al 1986) and frequent supervening infections particularly by opportunistic pathogens such as cytomegalovirus (Peters et al 1986). Glucocorticosteroids are helpful for treating interstitial pneumonitis associated with high-dose carmustine. Many patients also experience a chronic loss of lung capacity manifested as a drop in carbon monoxide diffusing capacity with signs of mild to moderate obstructive disease. Indeed, some patients manifest progressive respiratory insufficiency with hypoxemia up to 2 months following high-dose therapy (Slease et al 1988).

Central nervous system toxic effects in patients with brain tumors have included encephalopathy seizures (Burger et al 1981), hyperprolactinemia and hypothyroidism (Constine et al 1987). Late neurologic deterioration has been observed in a number of trials and may lead to dementia (Phillips et al 1986). Endocrine dysfunction following high-dose carmustine and brain irradiation has been observed in about 50% of patients (Constine et al 1987). Decreased thyroxin (T_4) is noted in 21% but elevated thyroid-stimulating hormone is rare. Carmustine also appears to enhance radiation-induced hyperprolactinemia, which may lead to reduced libido in males and irregular menses and anovulatory cycles in females (Constine et al 1987).

Topical Solution. Carmustine in concentrations of 0.5 to 3.0 mg/mL in a 30% alcohol/aqueous solution has been used topically in the treatment of mycosis fungoides (a particular type of T-lymphocyte lymphoma of the skin) (Zackheim and Epstein 1975). For this purpose, 60 mL (usually adequate to cover the entire body) is painted on the entire body daily after a shower for up to 14 days. Side effects include a primary irritant dermatitis occurring in about half of the patients. This is usually responsive to a reduction in the concentration. Telangiectasias and temporary bone marrow suppression have been observed in a few patients treated in this fashion.

A follow-up study noted that the net percutaneous absorption of carmustine ranged from 5 to 28% in the first 48 hours (Zackheim et al 1977). Also, patients with more severe cutaneous disease predictably absorbed larger amounts of drug (76–90%).

Carmustine topical solutions should be refrigerated and protected from light. It should be clearly labeled for topical use only and applied with protective rubber gloves. The eyes should be protected from splashes of the solution. Carmustine stored at 5°C, away from light, has a half-life of 19 days diluted in distilled water and 3 months diluted in either 95 or 100% ethanol (see stability table on page 269).

Intraarterial Carmustine. Ensminger et al (1978) have studied carmustine 200 mg/m^2 administered via the hepatic artery in patients with liver tumors. With a 60-minute infusion, steady-state blood levels were attained after 50 minutes. Levels of nitrosourea were 2.5-fold higher in the hepatic vein than in a simultaneously measured peripheral vein. Interestingly, no significant drug-related hepatotoxicity was observed. Only one of three patients studied developed myelotoxicity, which consisted of profound but reversible leukopenia and thrombocytopenia.

Response rates to hepatic artery carmustine may be improved by concomitant administration of degradable starch microspheres to transiently occlude the vascular bed in the liver (Dakhil et al 1982). A dose of 10 mL of microspheres (9×10^6/mL) reduced hepatic blood flow by 80 to 100%. This similarly reduced the systemic exposure to carmustine by 50% following a 50 mg/m^2 dose. Toxicity included acute pain and a transient 1.5 to 2-fold increase in hepatic enzyme levels. Myelosuppression was not observed.

The drug has also been administered intraarterially via the carotid or vertebral artery to patients with lung carcinoma metastatic to the brain (Yamada et al 1979). Objective responses were observed in four of nine patients. Acute complications included pain in the eye, the orbit, and occipital area with focal seizures in seven patients and mild disorientation or nausea in two patients. In contrast to metastatic lung cancer, no patients with brain metastases from malignant melanoma responded to intraarterial carmustine at a dose of 100 mg/m^2 given every 4 weeks (Madajewicz et al 1981).

REFERENCES

Anderson T, DeVita VT, Young RC. BCNU (NSC-409963) in the treatment of advanced Hodgkin's disease: Its role in remission introduction and maintenance. *Cancer Treat Rep.* 1976;**60**(6):761–767.

Ayash LJ, Hunt M, Antman K. Hepatic occlusive disease

in autologous bone marrow transplantation of solid tumor and lymphomas. *J Clin Oncol.* 1990;**8**:1699–1706.

Barranco SC, Humphrey RM. The effects of 1,3-bis(2-chloroethyl)-1-nitrosuorea on survival and cell progression in Chinese hamster cells. *Cancer Res.* 1971; **31**:191–195.

Bennet NJ, Bakemier RF, Carme PP. Clinical trials with BCNU (NSC-409962) in malignant lymphomas by the Eastern Cooperative Oncology Group. *Cancer Treat Rep.* 1976;**60**(6):739–745.

Benvenuto JA, Anderson RW, Kerkof K, et al. Stability and compatibility of antitumor agents in glass and plastic containers. *Am J Hosp Pharm.* 1981;**38**:1914–1918.

Bhuyan BK, Scheidt LG, Fraser TJ. Cell cycle phase specificity of antitumor agents. *Cancer Res.* 1972;**32**:398–407.

Burger PC, Kamenar E, Schold SC, et al. Encephalomyelopathy following high-dose BCNU therapy. *Cancer.* 1981;**48**:1318–1327.

Chan KK, Zackheim HS. Stability of nitrosourea solutions (letter). *Arch Dermatol.* 1973;**107**:298.

Chirigos MA, Humphreys SP, Goldin A. Duration of effective levels of three antitumor drugs in mice with leukemia L1210 implanted intracerebrally and subcutaneously. *Cancer Chemother Rep.* 1965;**49**:15–19.

Cohen HJ, Abramson N, Bartolucci A, et al. BCNU cyclophosphamide and prednisone (BCP) vs. melphalan and prednisone (MP) in myeloma. *Proc Am Assoc Cancer Res.* 1976;**17**:280.

Cohen MH. Enhancement of the antitumor effect of 1,3-bis(2-chloroethyl)-1-nitrosourea by vitamin A and caffeine. *J Natl Cancer Inst.* 1972;**48**:927–932.

Colvin M, Hartner J, Summerfield M. Stability of carmustine in the presence of sodium bicarbonate. *Am J Hosp Pharm.* 1980;**37**:677–678.

Constine LS, Rubin P, Woolf PD, et al. Hyperprolactinemia and hypothyroidism following cytotoxic therapy for central nervous system malignancies. *J Clin Oncol.* 1987;**5**(11):1841–1851.

Dakhil S, Ensminger W, Cho K, et al. Improved regional selectivity of hepatic arterial BCNU with degradable microspheres. *Cancer.* 1982;**50**:631–635.

DeVita VT, Carbone PP, Owens AB, et al. Clinical trials with 1,3-bis(2-chloroethyl)-1-nitrosourea, NSC-409962. *Cancer Res.* 1965;**25**:1876–1881.

DeVita VT, Denham C, Davidson J, et al. The physiological disposition of carcinostatic 1,3-bis(2-chloroethyl)-1-nitrosourea (BCNU) in man and animals. *Clin Pharmacol Ther.* 1967;**8**:566–577.

DeWys WD, Bathina SH. Synergistic antileukemic effect of theophylline and 1,3-bis(2-chloroethyl)-1-nitrosourea. *Cancer Res.* 1980;**40**:2202–2208.

Dorr RT, Soble MJ. H_2-Antagonists and carmustine. *J Cancer Res Clin Oncol.* 1989;**115**:41–46.

Durant JR, Norgard MJ, Murad TM, Bartolucci AA. Pulmonary toxicity associated with bis-chloroethyl nitrosourea (BCNU). *Ann Intern Med.* 1979;**90**:191–194.

Eder JP, Antman K, Peters W, et al. High-dose combination alkylating agent chemotherapy with autologous bone marrow support for metastatic breast cancer. *J Clin Oncol.* 1986;**4**:1592–1597.

Ensminger WD, Thompson M, Come S. Hepatic arterial BCNU: A pilot pharmacologic study in patients with liver tumors. *Cancer Treat Rep.* 1978;**62**(10):1509–1512.

Erickson LC, Laurent G, Sharkey N, et al. DNA crosslinking and monoadduct repair in nitrosourea-treated human tumour cells. *Nature.* 1980;**288**:727–729.

Fewer D, Wilson CB, Boldrey EB, et al. The chemotherapy of brain tumors. Clinical experience with carmustine (BCNU) and vincristine. *J Am A.* 1972;**222**(5):549–552.

Fredriksson K, Lundgren P, Landersjo L. Stability of carmustine—Kinetics and compatibility during administration. *Acta Pharm Suec.* 1986;**23**:115–124.

Frischer H, Ahmad T. Severe generalized glutathione reductase deficiency after antitumor chemotherapy with BCNU [1,3-bis(chloroethyl)-1-nitrosourea]. *J Lab Clin Med.* 1977;**89**(5):1080–1091.

Hartmann O, Benhamou E, Beaujean F, et al. Repeated high-dose chemotherapy followed by purged autologous bone marrow transplantation as consolidation therapy in metastatic neuroblastoma. *J Clin Oncol.* 1987;**5**:1205–1211.

Henner WD, Peters WP, Eder JP, et al. Pharmacokinetics and immediate effects of high-dose carmustine in man. *Cancer Treat Rep.* 1986;**70**:877–880.

Herzig GP, Phillips GL, Herzig RH, et al. High-dose nitrosourea (BCNU) and autologous bone marrow transplantation: A phase I study. In: Prestayko AW, Crooke ST, Baker LH, et al, eds. *Nitrosoureas: Current Status and New Developments.* New York: Academic Press; 1981:337–341.

Holoye PY, Jenkins DE, Greenberg SD. Pulmonary toxicity in long-term administration of BCNU. *Cancer Treat Rep.* 1976;**60**:1691–1693.

Jagannath S, Armitage JO, Dicke KA, et al. Prognostic factors for response and survival after high dose cyclophosphamide, carmustine and etoposide with autologous bone marrow transplantation for relapsed Hodgkin's disease. *J Clin Oncol.* 1989;**7**:179–185.

Johnson DB, Thompson JM, Carwin JA, et al. Prolongation of survival for high-grade malignant gliomas with adjuvant high-dose BCNU and autologous bone marrow transplantation. *J Clin Oncol.* 1987;**5**:783–789.

Jones RB, Matthes S, Shpall EJ, et al. BCNU plasma exposure (AUC) correlates with the risk of non-infectious pulmonary injury (P) following cyclophosphamide, cisplatin, and BCNU (CPA/cDDP/BCNU) with autologous bone marrow support (ABMS). *Proc Am Soc Clin Oncol.* 1992;**11**:132.

Kann HE Jr. Carbamoylating activity of nitrosoureas. In: Prestayko AW, Crooke ST, Baker LH, et al, eds. *Nitrosoureas: Current Status and New Developments.* New York: Academic Press; 1981:95–105.

Kann HE Jr, Kohn KW, Lyles TM. Inhibition of DNA repair by the 1,3-bis(2-chloroethyl)-1-nitrosoureas breakdown product, 2-chloroethyl isocyanate. *Cancer Res.* 1974a;**34**:398–402.

Kann HE Jr, Kohn KW, Widerlite L. Effects of 1,3-bits(2-chloroethyl)-1-nitrosourea and related compounds on nuclear RNA metabolism. *Cancer Res.* 1974b;**34**:1982–1988.

Kleinman LM, Davingnon JP, Cradock JC, et al. Investigational drugs. *Drug Intell Clin Pharm.* 1976;**10**(1):48–50.

Klubes P, Miller HG, Cerna I, Trevithick J. Alterations in the toxicity and antitumor activity of methyl-CCNU in mice following pretreatment with either phenobarbital or SKF 525A. *Cancer Treat Rep.* 1979;**63**:1901–1907.

Kohn KW, Erickson LC, Laurent G, et al. DNA crosslinking and the origin of sensitivity to chloroethylnitrosoureas. In: Prestayko AW, Crooke ST, Baker LH, et al, eds. *Nitrosoureas: Current Status and New Developments.* New York: Academic Press; 1981:69–83.

Korbling M, Holle R, Haas R, et al. Autologous blood stem-cell transplantation in patients with advanced Hodgkin's disease and prior radiation to the pelvic site. *J Clin Oncol.* 1990;**8**:978–985.

Laskar PA, Ayres JW. Degradation of carmustine in aqueous media. *J Pharm Sci.* 1977;**66**(8):1073–1078.

Levin VA, Hoffman W, Weinkam RJ. Pharmacokinetics of BCNU in man: A preliminary study of 20 patients. *Cancer Treat Rep.* 1978;**62**:1305–1312.

Levin VA, Stearns J, Byrd A, et al. The effect of phenobarbital pretreatment on the antitumor activity of 1,3-bis(2-chloroethyl)-1-nitrosourea (BCNU), 1-(2-chloroethyl)-3-cyclohexyl-1-nitrosourea (CCNU) and 1-(2-chloroethyl)-3-(2,6-dioxo)-3-piperidyl-1-nitrosourea (PCNU), and on the plasma pharmacokinetics and biotransformation of BCNU. *J Pharmacol Exp Ther.* 1979;**208**:1–6.

Lokich JJ, Drum DW, Kaplan W. Hepatic toxicity of nitrosourea analogues. *Clin Pharmacol Ther.* 1974;**16**:363–367.

Ludlum DB, Kramer BS, Wang J, et al. Reaction of 1,3-bis(2-chloroethyl)-1-nitrosourea with synthetic polynucleotides. *Biochemistry.* 1975;**14**:5480–5485.

Madajewicz S, West CR, Park HC, et al. Phase II study—Intra-arterial BCNU therapy for metastatic brain tumors. *Cancer.* 1981;**47**:653–657.

Marsh JC, DeConth RC, Hubbard SP. Treatment of Hodgkin's disease and other cancers with 1,3-bis(2-chloroethyl)-1-nitrosourea (BCNU-NSC-409962). *Cancer Chemother Rep.* 1971;**55**:599.

McIntyre RE, Magidson JG, Austin GE, Gale RP. Fatal veno-occlusive disease of the liver following high-dose 1,3-bis(2-chloroethyl)-1-nitrosourea (BCNU) and autologous bone marrow transplantation. *Am J Clin Pathol.* 1981;**74**(4):614–617.

McLennan R, Taylor HR. Optic neutroretinitis in association with BCNU and procarbazine. *Med Pediatr Oncol.* 1978;**4**:43–48.

Montgomery JA, James R, McCaleb GS, et al. The modes of decomposition of 1,3-bis(2-chloroethyl)-1-nitrosourea and related compounds. *J Med Chem.* 1967;**10**:668–674.

Moon JH. Combination chemotherapy in malignant melanoma. *Cancer.* 1970;**25**:468.

Oliverio VT. Toxicology and pharmacology of the nitrosoureas. *Cancer Chemother Rep Part 3.* 1973;**4**:13–20.

Peters WP, Eder JP, Henner WD, et al. High-dose combination alkylating agents with autologous bone marrow support: A phase I trial. *J Clin Oncol.* 1986;**4**:646–654.

Peters WP, Shpall EJ, Jones RB, et al. High-dose combination alkylating agents with bone marrow support as initial treatment for metastatic breast cancer. *J Clin Oncol.* 1988;**6**:1368–1376.

Petersen FB, Appelbaum FR, Hill R, et al. Autologous marrow transplantation for malignant lymphoma: A report of 101 cases from Seattle. *J Clin Oncol.* 1990;**8**:638–647.

Phillips GL, Reece DE, Barnett MJ, et al. Allogeneic marrow transplantation for refractory Hodgkin's disease. *J Clin Oncol.* 1989;**7**:1039–1045.

Phillips GL, Wolff SN, Fay JW, et al. Intensive 1,3-bis(2-chloroethyl)-1-nitrosourea (BCNU) monochemotherapy and autologous marrow transplantation for malignant glioma. *J Clin Oncol.* 1986;**4**:639–645.

Presant CA, Hillinger S, Klahr C. Phase II study of 1,3-bis(2-chloroethyl)-1-nitrosourea (BCNU, NSC-409962) with amphotericin B in bronchogenic carcinoma. *Cancer.* 1980;**45**:6–10.

Present GA, Klahr C, Olander J, Gatewood D. Amphotericin B plus 1,3-bis(2-chloroethyl)-1-nitrosourea (BCNU-NSC-409962) in advanced cancer. *Cancer.* 1976;**38**:1917–1921.

Rall DP, Ben M, McCarthy DM. 1,3-Bis-β-chloroethyl-1-nitrosourea (BCNU) toxicity and initial clinical trial. *Proc Am Assoc Cancer Res.* 1963;**4**:55.

Rege VB, Owens AH. BCNU (NSC-409962) in the treatment of advanced Hodgkin's disease, lymphosarcoma and reticulum cell sarcoma. *Cancer Chemother Rep.* 1974;**58**:383–393.

Salmon SE. Nitrosoureas in multiple myeloma. *Cancer Treat Rep.* 1976;**60**(6):789–794.

Schabel FM Jr, et al. Experimental evaluation of potential anticancer agents. VIII. Effects of certain nitrosoureas on intracerebral L1210. *Cancer Res.* 1963;**23**:725.

Schorer AE, et al. Gynecomastia with nitrosourea therapy. *Cancer Treat Rep.* 1978;**62**(4):574–576.

Selker RG, Moore P, LoDolce D. Bone-marrow depression with cimetidine plus carmustine. *N Engl J Med.* 1978;**299**(15):834.

Slease RB, Benear JB, Selby GB, et al. High-dose combination alkylating agent therapy with autologous bone marrow rescue for refractory solid tumors. *J Clin Oncol.* 1988;**6**:1314–1320.

Smulson M, Butt T, Sudhakar W, et al. ADP-ribosylation and DNA repair as induced by nitrosoureas. In: Prestayko AW, Crooke ST, Baker LH, et al, eds. *Nitrosoureas: Current Status and New Developments.* New York: Academic Press; 1981:123–142.

Takvorian T, Parker LM, Hochberg FH, Canellos GP. Autologous bone-marrow transplantation: Host effects of high-dose BCNU. *J Clin Oncol.* 1983;**1**(10):610–620.

Taylor KM, Jagannath S, Spitzer G, et al. Recombinant

human granulocyte colony-stimulating factor hastens granulocyte recovery after high-dose chemotherapy and autologous bone marrow transplantation in Hodgkin's disease. *J Clin Oncol.* 1989;**7**:1791–1799.

Tew KD. Chromatin and associated nuclear components as potential drug targets. In: Prestayko AW, Crooke ST, Baker LH, et al, eds. *Current Status and New Developments.* New York: Academic Press; 1981:101–120.

Tobey RA, Crissman HA. Comparative effects of three nitrosourea derivatives on mammalian cell cycle progression. *Cancer Res.* 1975;**35**:460–470.

Trissel LA, Fulton B, Framonte SM. Visual compatibility of ondansetron with chemotherapeutic agents, antibiotics, and other selected drugs during simulated Y-site injection (abstract P-468R). In: *25th Annual ASHP Midyear Clinical Meeting and Exhibit, Las Vegas, Nevada, December 1990.* Bethesda, MD: American Society of Hospital Pharmacists; 1990.

Volkin RL, Shadduck RK, Winkelstein A, et al. Potentiation of carmustine–cranial irradiation-induced myelosuppression by cimetidine. *Arch Intern Med.* 1982;**142**:243–245.

Walker MD. Nitrosoureas in central nervous system tumors. *Cancer Chemother Rep.* 1973;**4**:21–26.

Wheeler C, Antin JH, Churchill WH, et al. Cyclophosphamide, carmustine, and etoposide with autologous bone marrow transplantation in refractory Hodgkin's disease and non-Hodgkin's lymphoma: A dose-finding study. *J Clin Oncol.* 1990;**8**:648–656.

Wheeler GP, Alexander JA. Duration of inhibition of synthesis of DNA in tumors and host tissues after single doses of nitrosoureas. *Cancer Res.* 1974;**34**:1957–1964.

Wheeler GP, Alexander JA. Duration of inhibition of synthesis of DNA in tumors and host tissues after single doses of nitrosoureas. *Cancer Res.* 1976;**36**:1470–1474.

Wheeler GP, Bowdon BJ. Some effects of BCNU on the synthesis of protein and nucleic acids. *Cancer Res.* 1965;**25**:1770–1778.

Wheeler GP, Chumley S. Alkylating activity of 1,3-bis(2-chloroethyl)-1-nitrosourea and selected compounds. *J Med Chem.* 1967;**10**:259–265.

Yamada K, Bremer AM, West CR, et al. Intra-arterial BCNU therapy in the treatment of metastatic brain tumor from lung carcinoma. A preliminary report. *Cancer.* 1979;**44**:2000–2007.

Young RC, DeVita VT, Serpick AA, et al. Treatment of advanced Hodgkin's disease with 1,3-bis(2-chloroethyl)-1-nitrosourea BCNU. *N Engl J Med.*1971;**285**:475–479.

Zackheim HS, Epstein EH. Treatment of mycosis fungoides with topical nitrosourea compounds. *Arch Dermatol.* 1975;**111**:1564–1570.

Zackheim HS, Feldman RJ, Lindsay C, Maibach HI. Percutaneous absorption of 1,3-bis(2-chloroethyl)-1-nitrosourea (BCNU, carmustine) in mycosis fungoides. *Br J Dermatol.* 1977;**97**:65–67.

Chlorambucil

■ Other Names

NSC-3088; B-1348; Leukeran® (Burroughs Wellcome).

■ Chemistry

Structure of chlorambucil

Chlorambucil is a more stable derivative of nitrogen mustard. Chemically, it is 4-[bis(2-chlorethyl)amino]benzenebutyric acid. Chlorambucil has pK_a values of 1.3 and 5.8 and a molecular weight of 304.21.

■ Antitumor Activity

Chlorambucil has shown activity in a variety of human malignancies (Livingston and Carter 1970, Miller et al 1959). These include chronic lymphocytic leukemia (CLL) (Galton et al 1955, Han et al 1973, Knopse et al 1974), Hodgkin's and non-Hodgkin's lymphoma (Ezdinli and Stutzman 1965), choriocarcinoma and ovarian carcinoma (Williams et al 1985), and breast carcinoma (Freckman et al 1964). Moore et al (1968) found a response rate of 19% in 52 advanced breast cancer patients. In ovarian cancer a response rate of 26% was associated with a minor impact on survival of about 11 months (Williams et al 1985). Higher response rates of up to 50% were described in some earlier trials, but again, the impact on long-term survival in ovarian cancer was only moderate (Katz et al 1981). Chlorambucil has often been employed in the long-term maintenance management of chronic lymphocytic leukemia (CLL). A study by the Cancer and Acute Leukemia Group B has found that in CLL, response rates were slightly higher (47%) with intermittent monthly chlorambucil and prednisone rather than with a conventional daily dosing regimen (Sawitsky et al 1977). Response durations with chlorambucil average 2.5 to 3 years in this disease. Complete responses to chlorambucil in CLL occur in a small fraction of patients, about 10% (Huguley 1977); however, up to 70% of patients achieve significant objective responses with reduction of splenomegaly, leukocyte counts, and lymphadenopathy (Huguley 1977).

Chlorambucil alone or combined with prednisone is also used in Waldenström's macroglobinemia to reduce severe symptoms of increased plasma viscosity (McCallister et al 1967). In addition, chlorambucil has activity in choriocarcinoma when used in combination with methotrexate and dactinomycin in patients with poor prognosis metastatic disease (Surwit and Hammond 1980).

Several nonmalignant myeloproliferative disorders are responsive to chlorambucil including polycythemia vera and essential thrombocythemia (Case 1984). This use is questionable, however, because of the drug's established potential to cause acute myeloid leukemia after years of chronic low-dose therapy (Berk et al 1981).

■ Mechanism of Action

Chlorambucil is a classic alkylating agent of the nitrogen mustard type. It is considered cell cycle phase nonspecific. The drug produces DNA interstrand crosslinks via activation of the two chloroethyl side chains to yield unstable ethyleneimine intermediates and electrophilic carbonium ions. The rate of chloride leaving (activation) determines the rate of alkylation. This is nonenzymatic and relatively slow compared to nitrogen mustard. At the usual doses, chlorambucil has the slowest onset of activity, which may explain the low acute toxicity of this compound.

■ Availability and Storage

Chlorambucil (Leukeran®, Burroughs Wellcome, Research Triangle Park, North Carolina) is available as a 2-mg sugar-coated tablet. The tablets are stored at room temperature.

■ Administration

Chlorambucil is administered orally.

■ Dosage

The usual oral dose of chlorambucil in chronic lymphocytic leukemia is 0.1 to 0.2 mg/kg (4–10 mg total) daily for 3 to 6 weeks as required for remission induction. This is followed by a maintenance schedule of 2 to 4 mg daily. In advanced breast cancer, Moore et al (1968) used a continuous daily dose of 0.1 to 0.2 mg/kg.

In CLL the drug may optimally be administered on an intermittent basis in doses of 0.4 mg/kg every 4 weeks (Sawitsky et al 1977). Both the intermittent and continuous regimens commonly include prednisone. On the intermittent schedule, monthly pulse doses as high as 1.5 to 2.0 mg/kg were well tolerated in most patients and did not produce undue marrow toxicity. An effective biweekly dosing schedule with lessened hematologic toxicity is also reported: 0.4 mg/kg every 2 weeks, increasing by 0.1 mg/kg increments to toxicity or remission (Knopse et al 1974). The median maximum dose achieved in this trial was 0.9 mg/kg (range, 0.4–1.83 mg/kg); however, most patients required dose reductions at some point in their therapy (Knopse et al 1974).

Short pulses of high-dose chlorambucil have been evaluated in patients with advanced solid tumor malignancies. The recommended dose for phase II trials was 108 mg/m^2 given in six 6-hourly doses (Blumenreich et al 1988).

■ Drug Interactions

The toxicity of chlorambucil is reportedly increased when the drug is administered to patients previously treated with barbiturates. The mechanism for this increased toxicity is postulated to involve the induction of hepatic enzymes responsible for the activation of chlorambucil. In vitro chemical studies have also shown that the alkylation of certain DNA nucleotides by chlorambucil can be prevented by coincubation with dimethylsulfoxide or sodium thiosulfate (Wickstrom 1980).

■ Pharmacokinetics

According to the manufacturer, chlorambucil is well absorbed orally. In one clinical trial, the absolute oral bioavailability averaged 75.5% if taken with food. The range in bioavailability was 56 to 105% (Adair et al 1986). Peak plasma levels were significantly reduced to about 50% of those achieved when the drug was taken without a meal. Two patients in another trial were also given oral and intravenous chlorambucil and the oral bioavailability was 0.72 and 1.02, indicating relatively good absorption of this drug (Newell et al 1983). The hepatic extraction ratio for chlorambucil is low at 0.22 (Alberts et al 1980).

In rats, radioactive drug appears to be cleared from the blood rapidly, and at 1 hour the highest tissue concentration is found in the liver; however, fairly homogeneous tissue distribution was noted. The drug has also been shown to distribute well into ascitic fluid after subcutaneous administration. Sixty percent of drug radioactivity was excreted into the urine by 24 hours, with the majority of the remainder existing as tissue-bound drug (Hill and Riches 1975). Significant (99%) drug binding to plasma proteins has been observed in vitro. The majority of this binding is to albumin, although gamma globulins also bind the drug. Apparently little chlorambucil is excreted in the feces. Because a portion of the drug molecule has lipophilic properties, some fat storage of chlorambucil may occur. This creates a drug depot, facilitating delayed elimination of the drug, which could explain the prolonged myelosuppressive effects of chlorambucil occasionally observed in humans.

Pharmacokinetic data in humans have been obtained by Alberts et al (1979, 1980) using a gas chromatographic–mass spectrophotometric technique (see the table). These data indicate a terminal half-life of intact drug of about 2 hours. In this study 1% of unchanged drug was recovered in the urine over 24 hours. Thus, there appears to be extensive metabolic degradation of the drug and production of a major metabolite, aminophenylacetic acid. This metabolite appears to have some antineoplastic activity (McClean 1979) and a half-life of about 2.5 hours in humans. Other metabolites of chlorambucil have yet to be defined, although some have been suggested by thin-layer chromatography studies of radiolabeled drug (McClean 1979).

Renal function or at least glomerular filtration does not appear to be a major factor in the clearance of intact drug from the plasma (Adair et al 1986). Up to 60% of radiolabel is obtained in the urine of patients given labeled chlorambucil, but very little (< 1%) is intact chlorambucil or the phenylacetic acid metabolite (McClean 1979).

Chlorambucil is relatively stable in the plasma, compared with other alkylating agents such as melphalan (Alberts et al 1980). The hydrolysis rate for chlorambucil to mono- or dihydroxy derivatives in plasma at 37°C is approximately 1.4×10^{-3} min^{-1} yielding a half-life of about 8 hours.

■ Side Effects and Toxicity

In general, chlorambucil is one of the best tolerated oral alkylating agents. Bone marrow depression is the dose-limiting toxic effect and includes neutropenia and thrombocytopenia. Lymphocytopenia may also occur with prolonged use, and irreversible bone marrow damage has been reported.

Central nervous system stimulation has occurred with chlorambucil but is uncommon unless large doses are used. Seizures and coma were also noted at the highest dose tested (144 mg/m^2) (Blumenreich et al 1988), and myoclonic seizures were described following a chlorambucil overdose (Byrne et al 1981). Seizures may be more common in children being treated for nephrotic syndrome (Williams et al 1978).

Gastrointestinal distress with large chlorambucil doses can occur but it is usually not serious. In high-dose studies, chlorambucil has produced severe nausea and vomiting which were prevented by metoclopramide therapy (Blumenreich et al 1988). Hepatitis and disturbances of liver function have been rarely reported.

Drug fever and skin rash are also described in a few patients. Dermatologic effects include urticarial-like plaques on the face and scalp (Peterman and Braunstein 1986, Knisley et al 1971) and severe periorbital edema and rash (Millard and Rajah 1977). One case of toxic epidermal necrolysis has also been reported (Barone et al 1990).

Inadvertent toxic ingestions in children of 1.5 to 5 mg/kg have occurred without fatalities but with moderate toxicity. This is characterized by vomiting, agitation, irritability, and hyperactivity. These acute symptoms are followed by lethargy and eventual pancytopenia (Green and Naiman 1968, Wolfson and Olney 1957). An adult patient had inadvertently taken 250 mg chlorambucil (acute overdose) which produced two grand mal seizures and transient renal failure. Both effects resolved without se-

HUMAN PHARMACOKINETICS OF CHLORAMBUCIL IN TWO PATIENTS*

	Tissue Concentration (μg · min/mL)	Peak Level (μg/mL)	Half-Life (min^{-1}) β	24-Hour Urinary Excretion
Chlorambucil	168	1.4	86	0.5%
Phenylacetic acid mustard	210	0.77	162	0.29%

*Chlorambucil dose was 0.6 to 1.21 mg/kg.
Data from Alberts DS, Chang SY, Chen H-SG, et al. Comparative pharmacokinetics of chlorambucil and melphalan in man. *Recent Results Cancer Res.* 1980;74:124–131.

quelae (Blank et al 1983). Another patient who took a total dose of 8.2 mg/kg (30 mg/m² every 2 weeks) developed prolonged but eventually reversible bone marrow toxicity (Enck and Burnett 1977).

Chromosomal damage is well documented for chlorambucil although the exact mechanism is not well described (Reeves 1975). Lerner (1978) has described a high incidence of secondary acute myelogenous leukemia in breast cancer patients receiving continuous chlorambucil for 4 years or longer. A similar finding is reported for patients with polycythemia vera given a continuous regimen of 10 mg chlorambucil daily for 6 weeks with 30-day rest periods between cycles (Berk et al 1981).

Similar to some other alkylating agents, chlorambucil has also been reported to cause alveolar dysplasia and pulmonary fibrosis with long-term use. Cole et al (1978) reported a patient with lung toxicity who showed good clinical response to drug discontinuance and corticosteroids. However, fatal interstitial pneumonitis is described following high dose therapy (Lane et al 1981). Spermatogenesis is depressed during chlorambucil therapy (Richter et al 1970), and the drug is known to produce teratogenic effects. It should not be administered during pregnancy or to women of childbearing potential (Shotton and Monie 1963).

REFERENCES

Adair CG, Bridges JM, Desai ZR. Can food affect the bioavailability of chlorambucil in patients with haematological malignancies? *Cancer Chemother Pharmacol.* 1986;**17**:99–102.

Alberts DS, Chang SY, Chen H-SG. Pharmacokinetics and metabolism of chlorambucil in man: A preliminary report. *Cancer Treat Rev.* 1979;**6**(suppl):9.

Alberts DS, Chang SY, Chen H-SG, et al. Comparative pharmacokinetics of chlorambucil and melphalan in man. *Recent Results Cancer Res.* 1980;**74**:124–131.

Barone C, Cassano A, Astone A. Toxic epidermal necrolysis during chlorambucil therapy in chronic lymphocytic leukaemia. *Eur J Cancer.* 1990;**26**:1261.

Berk PD, Goldberg JD, Silverstein MN, et al. Increased incidence of acute leukemia in polycythemia vera associated with chlorambucil therapy. *N Engl J Med.* 1981;**304**:441–447.

Blank DW, Nanji AA, Schreiber DH, et al. Acute renal failure and seizures associated with chlorambucil overdose. *J Toxicol Clin Toxicol.* 1983;**20**:361–365.

Blumenreich MS, Woodcock TM, Sherrill EJ, et al. A phase I trial of chlorambucil administered in short pulses in patients with advanced malignancies. *Cancer Invest.* 1988;**6**(4):371–375.

Byrne TN Jr, Moseley TAE III, Finer MA. Myoclonic seizures following chlorambucil overdose. *Ann Neurol.* 1981;**9**:191–194.

Case DC Jr. Therapy of essential thrombocythemia with thiotepa and chlorambucil. *Blood.* 1984;**63**:51–54.

Cole SR, Myers JJ, Klatsky AU. Pulmonary disease with chlorambucil therapy. *Cancer.* 1978;**41**:455–459.

Enck RE, Burnett JM. Inadvertent chlorambucil overdose in the adult. *NY State J Med.* 1977;**77**:1480–1481.

Ezdinli EZ, Stutzman L. Chlorambucil therapy for lymphomas and chronic lymphocytic leukemia. *JAMA.* 1965;**191**:444–450.

Freckman HA, Fry HL, Mendez FL, et al. Chlorambucil–prednisone therapy for disseminated breast carcinoma. *JAMA.* 1964;**189**:23–26.

Galton DAG, Israels LG, Nabarro JBN, et al. Clinical trials of *p*-(di-2-chloroethylamino)-phenylbutyric acid (CB 1348) in malignant lymphoma. *Br Med J.* 1955;**2**:1172–1176.

Green AA, Naiman JL. Chlorambucil poisoning. *Am J Dis Child.* 1968;**116**:190–191.

Han T, Ezdinli EZ, Shimaoka K, Desai DV. Chlorambucil vs. combined chlorambucil-corticosteroid therapy in chronic lymphocytic leukemia. *Cancer.* 1973;**31**:502–512.

Hill BT, Riches PG. The absorption distribution and excretion of chlorambucil in rats bearing the Yoshida ascites sarcoma. *Eur J Cancer.* 1975;**11**:9–16.

Huguley CM Jr. Treatment of chronic lymphocytic leukemia. *Cancer Treat Rev.* 1977;**4**:261–273.

Katz ME, Schwartz PE, Kapp DS, et al. Epithelial carcinoma of the ovary—Current strategies. *Ann Intern Med.* 1981;**95**:98–111.

Knisley RE, Settipane GA, Albala MM. Unusual reaction to chlorambucil in a patient with chronic lymphocytic leukemia. *Arch Dermatol.* 1971;**104**:77–79.

Knopse WH, Loeb V Jr, Huguley CM Jr. Bi-weekly chlorambucil treatment of chronic lymphocytic leukemia. *Cancer.* 1974;**33**:555–561.

Lane SD, Besa EC, Justh G, et al. Fatal interstitial pneumonitis following high-dose intermittent chlorambucil therapy for chronic lymphocytic leukemia. *Cancer.* 1981;**47**:32–36.

Lerner HJ. Acute myelogenous leukemia in patients receiving chlorambucil as long-term adjuvant chemotherapy for stage II breast cancer. *Cancer Treat Rep.* 1978;**62**(8):1135–1138.

Livingston RB, Carter SK. *Single Agents in Cancer Chemotherapy.* New York: Plenum; 1970.

McCallister BD, Bayrd ED, Harrison EG Jr, et al. Primary macroglobulinemia—Review with a report on thirty-one cases and notes on the value of continuous cholorambucil therapy. *Am J Med.* 1967;**43**:394.

McLean A. Pharmacokinetics and metabolism of chlorambucil in patients with malignant disease. *Cancer Treat Rev.* 1979;**6**(suppl):33–42.

Millard LG, Rajah SM. Cutaneous reaction to chlorambucil. *Arch Dermatol.* 1977;**113**:1298.

Miller DG, Diamond HD, Craver LF. The clinical use of

chlorambucil: A critical study. *N Engl J Med.* 1959;**261**:525–528.

Moore G, Bross IDJ, Ausman R, et al. Effects of chlorambucil (NSC-3088) in 374 patients with advanced cancer. *Cancer Chemother Rep.* 1968;**52**:661–666.

Newell DR, Clavert AH, Harrap KR. Studies on the pharmacokinetics of chlorambucil and prednimustine in man. *Br J Clin Pharmacol.* 1983;**15**:253–258.

Peterman A, Braunstein B. Cutaneous reaction to chlorambucil therapy. *Arch Dermatol.* 1986;**122**:1358–1360.

Reeves BR. Chlorambucil and chromosomal damage. *Br Med J.* 1975;**4**:22–23.

Richter P, Calamera JC, Morganfeld MC, et al. Effect of chlorambucil on spermatogenesis in the human with malignant lymphoma. *Cancer.* 1970;**25**:1026–1030.

Sawitsky A, Rai KR, Glidewell O, et al (Cancer and Leukemia Group B). Comparison of daily versus intermittent chlorambucil and prednisone therapy in the treatment of patients with chronic lymphocytic leukemia. *Blood.* 1977;**50**(6):1049–1059.

Shotton D, Monie IW. Possible teratogenic effect of chlorambucil on a human fetus. *JAMA.* 1963;**186**:74–75.

Surwit EA, Hammond CB. Treatment of metastatic trophoblastic disease with poor prognosis. *Obstet Gynecol.* 1980;**55**:565–570.

Wickstrom E. Chlorambucil inhibition by dimethyl sulfoxide and thiosulfate: Implications for chlorambucil chemotherapy. *Med Hypoth.* 1980;**6**:1035–1041.

Williams SA, Makker SP, Grupe WE. Seizures—A significant side effect of chlorambucil therapy in children. *J Pediatr.* 1978;**93**:516–518.

Williams CJ, Mead GM, Macbeth FR, et al. Cisplatin combination chemotherapy versus chlorambucil in advanced ovarian carcinoma: Mature results of a randomized trial. *J Clin Oncol.* 1985;**3**:1455–1462.

Wolfson S, Olney MB. Accidental ingestion of a toxic dose of chlorambucil: Report of a case in a child. *JAMA.* 1957;**165**:239–240.

Chloroquinoxaline Sulfonamide

■ Other Names

NSC-339004; chlorsulfaquinoxaline; CQS.

■ Chemistry

Structure of chloroquinoxaline sulfonamide

Chloroquinoxaline sulfonamide (CQS) is a heterocyclic sulfonamide with a molecular weight of 334.8 and a formula of $C_{14}H_{11}ClN_4O_2S$. The complete chemical name is 4-amino-*N*-[5-chloro-2-quinoxalinyl]benzenesulfonamide. It was selected for clinical trials based on its in vitro activity in a human tumor cloning assay (Shoemaker 1986).

■ Antitumor Activity

Chloroquinoxaline sulfonamide is just now undergoing dose-finding phase I trials. In these ongoing trials there have been hints of antitumor activity in patients with colon cancer and non-small cell lung cancer.

■ Mechanism of Action

The mechanism of action of CQS is unknown (Branda et al 1987). Although it has structural similarity with sulfaquinoxaline, CQS does not block folic acid metabolism. In addition, leucovorin does not reverse CQS toxicities.

■ Availability and Storage

Chloroquinoxaline sulfonamide is available as an investigational agent from the Division of Cancer Treatment, National Cancer Institute. It is supplied for injection, 500 mg, prepared as a yellow lyophilized powder with 750 mg of meglumine (*n*-methylglucamine). The intact vial should be stored under refrigeration (2–8°C).

■ Preparation for Use, Stability, and Admixture

When the 500-mg vial is reconstituted with 9.2 mL of Sterile Water for Injection, USP, each milliliter of the resulting solution contains 50 mg of chlorsulfaquinoxaline and 75 mg of meglumine at pH 9.5 to 10.5.

Shelf-life stability studies of the intact vials are ongoing. When the vial contents are reconstituted, the solution is physically and chemically stable for at least 14 days at 0 and 25°C.

Further dilution to a concentration of 1 mg/mL in 5% Dextrose Injection, USP, or 0.9% Sodium Chloride Injection, USP, in both glass and polyvinyl chloride containers also results in stable solutions for 14 days at 0 and 25°C.

The single-use lyophilized dose form has no antibacterial preservatives and therefore the reconstituted vial should be discarded 8 hours after initial entry.

Caution: The addition of dilute acid to CQS solutions results in the formation of a precipitate.

■ Administration

At this time no recommendations regarding administration can be made. Phase I trials with the agent using a single dose ranging from 18 to 216 mg/m² are ongoing (Rigas et al 1990).

■ Special Precautions

Glucose monitoring is required with this agent and diabetic patients may be poor candidates to receive CQS.

■ Drug Interactions

None are known at this time.

■ Dosage

Phase I trials with the agent are ongoing. Therefore, no firm dosage recommendations can yet be made (Rigas et al 1990, Melink et al 1992). In a preliminary study, the maximally tolerated dose was 4,060 mg/m² as a 1 hr IV infusion every 28 days. The recommended dose for phase II trials was 4000 mg/m² on the same schedule (Rigas et al 1990, 1992).

■ Pharmacokinetics

In ongoing phase I trial, the pharmacokinetics best fit a three-compartment model with half-lives of (α) 1.9 hours (range, 1.3–3.4 hours) (β) 53 hours (range 27–74 hours), and (γ) 450 hours (range 230–820 hours). The steady-state volume of distribution was 37 L/m² (range, 48–116 L/m²) and total body clearance was 87 mL/min/m² (range, 45–132 mL/min/m²) (Rigas et al 1990). Plasma levels of >100 µg/mL were seen in all patients given doses of 72350 mg/m² (Rigas et al 1992).

■ Side Effects and Toxicity

In preliminary phase I studies, the dose-limiting toxicity at 4,870 mg/m² has been hypoglycemia (Rigas et al 1992). A few patients with prior cardiac disease have also experienced supraventricular tachyarrhythmias. Vomiting is rare and only slight myelosuppression is noted at maximally tolerated doses. There are also rare descriptions of alopecia perioral numbness, diarrhea, and hives at the injection site.

■ Special Applications

None are known to date.

REFERENCES

Branda RF, McCormack JJ, Perlmutter C. Cellular pharmacology of chloroquinoxaline sulfonamide (CQS) and a related compound (meeting abstract). *Proc Am Assoc Cancer Res.* 1987;**28**:303.

Melink T, Conley BA, Sorim MJ, et al. Phase I and pharmacokinetic (PK) trial of chloroquinoxaline sulfonamide (CQS) inpatients (Pts) with solid tumors. *Proc Am Soc Clin Oncol* 1992;**11**:114.

Rigas JR, Warrell RP Jr, Tong W, et al. Phase I clinical/pharmacologic study of chloroquinoxaline sulfonamide. *Proc Am Assoc Cancer Res.* 1990;**31**:177.

Rigas JR, Kris MG, Ton W, et al. Phase I trial of chloroquinoxaline sulfonamide (CQS): A unique agent selected for study based on activity in an in vitro stem cell assay. *Proc Am Assoc Cancer Res.* 1992;**33**:529.

Shoemaker RH. New approaches to antitumor drug screening: The human tumor colony-forming assay. *Cancer Treat Rep.* 1986;**70**(1):9–12.

Chlorozotocin

■ Other Names

DCNU; NSC-178248.

■ Chemistry

Structure of chlorozotocin

Chemically, chlorozotocin is 2-[[[(2-chloroethyl)-nitrosoamino]carbonyl]amino]-2-deoxy-D-glucose. Chlorozotocin is a water-soluble chlorethyl derivative of streptozotocin, with the cytotoxic group attached to the C-2 position of glucose. Previous studies have demonstrated that reduced myelotoxicity is afforded by this type of structure. It has a molecular weight of 313.7 and an empiric formula of $C_9H_{16}ClN_3O$.

■ Antitumor Activity

In animal leukemia models, chlorozotocin has demonstrated good antitumor activity and appears to share the lack of myelosuppressive toxicity seen with the other glucose-containing nitrosourea analog, streptozotocin (Anderson et al 1975). In phase I studies, clinical antitumor activity was shown in patients with melanoma, non-small cell carcinoma of the lung, and lymphoma (Hoth et al 1978).

Chlorozotocin has had extensive phase II testing over the last 15 years. Although responses have been seen in patients with islet cell tumors, melanoma, non-Hodgkins lymphoma, pancreatic cancer, breast cancer, colon cancer, small cell and non-small cell lung cancer, and sarcoma, the clinical response rates have not been high enough to pursue further testing (Houghton et al 1981, Ahmann et al 1980, Silver et al 1982, Van Amburg et al 1982, Amato et al 1985, Hoth et al 1980, Creagan et al 1979, Presant and Bartolucci 1984, Veronesi et al 1983, Von Hoff et al 1984, Haas et al 1983, 1984, Gralla and Yagoda 1979, Douglass et al 1988, Schutt et al 1984, Bukowski et al 1983, Ungerleider 1980, Gastrointestinal Tumor Study Group 1985, Creech et al 1982, Lawton et al 1981, Bleiberg et al 1981, Talley et al 1981).

■ Mechanism of Action

At equimolar doses, chlorozotocin has approximately twice the in vitro alkylating activity of carmustine (Schein et al 1973). Thus the cytotoxic effect appears to involve alkylation probably via 2-chloroethylamine, inhibiting the synthesis of DNA and RNA. Also, if similar to carmustine, chlorozotocin may prolong the S phase in treated cells before death although the cytotoxic mechanism is thought to be cell cycle (phase) nonspecific. Characteristically, the nitrosourea compounds are not cross-resistant to conventional alkylating agents, which appear to act in different phases of the cell cycle and to have less activity in the L-1210 leukemia model. The addition of glucose as the nitrosourea carrier group (similar to streptozotocin) appears to similarly afford a greatly reduced myelotoxic potential to the molecule (Schein et al 1978). Also, unlike the other nitrosoureas, chlorozotocin has essentially no carbamoylating activity. Byrne et al (1984) have later shown that although lomustine binds preferentially to transcriptionally active regions of chromatin, chlorozotocin alkylates predominantly the transcriptionally inactive regions. They postulated this would result in less myelosuppression.

■ Availability and Storage

Chlorozotocin is available as an investigational agent from the National Cancer Institute as a lyophilized powder in 50-mg vials also containing citric acid and sodium hydroxide to adjust pH to 3.8 to 4.2. These should be refrigerated and, as such, are stable at least 18 months.

■ Preparation for Use, Stability, and Admixture

Fifty-milligram vials are reconstituted with 5 mL Sterile Water for Injection, USP, or Sodium Chloride Injection, USP, to produce a 20 mg/mL solution of pH 3.8 to 4.2. At room temperature this solution is reportedly stable for 3 hours; under refrigeration it is stable 24 hours. Admixture information is not currently available. Under simulated physiologic conditions (phosphate buffer pH 7.4 or plasma in vitro), the nitrosoureas decompose to yield chlorethyl carbonium ions (Montgomery et al 1975). Thus, the chemical half-lives of chlorozotocin were 48 and 40 min, respectively (Panasci et al 1977).

■ Administration

In phase I studies the drug has been well tolerated when given by rapid intravenous injection; however, a 5- to 10-mL flush of either D5W or normal saline is recommended before and after drug administration, respectively, to test vein patency and to flush any remaining drug from the tubing. Alternatively, injection into the tubing of a free-flowing intravenous solution may be used.

■ Special Precautions

Pulmonary toxicity has been ascribed to chlorozotocin in about 1% of patients receiving the drug (Ahlgren et al 1981, Weiss et al 1981).

■ Drug Interactions

None are known.

Dosage

In the phase I study by Hoth et al (1978) doses of from 5 to 175 mg/m² every 6 weeks were explored. Dose-dependent thrombocytopenia occurred 4 weeks after doses significantly greater than 120 mg/m². Thus, the recommended dose for phase II studies from that report was 120 mg/m² IV every 6 weeks. Kovach et al (1979) explored a single dose and a daily × 5 schedule with doses ranging from 12.5 to 200 mg/m². On either schedule, dose-limiting toxic effects were leukopenia and thrombocytopenia at total doses of 150 to 200 mg/m².

Gralla and colleagues (1979) have explored the daily × 5 schedule and found dose-limiting thrombocytopenia and leukopenia at 150 mg/m² and higher doses.

Taylor et al (1980) used a schedule of a single dose every 6 weeks and revealed a maximally tolerated dose of 250 mg/m². A starting dose of 200 to 225 mg/m² was recommended for phase II studies.

In a weekly × 4 schedule, Moriconi et al (1985) recommended a dose of 40 mg/m²/wk × 4 every 8 weeks.

Pharmacokinetics

After rapid injection, Hoth et al (1978) noted three short phases of elimination of intact drug including an initial phase of 3 to 4.5 minutes, a secondary phase of 6 to 12 minutes, and a third phase of 18 to 30 minutes. This produced plasma concentrations greater than 10^{-5} M for at least 30 minutes. Seven days after bolus administration, 2% peak plasma concentrations (10^{-4} M) were detectable. These are very similar to the pharmacokinetic pattern for carmustine (De Vita et al 1967). From a radioisotope study about 50 to 60% of the dose of chlorozotocin appears to be excreted in the urine, primarily in highly metabolized forms. Therefore, a prolonged excretion phase of metabolites, many probably active, is possible as has been described for the other chloroethylnitrosoureas. Chlorozotocin, probably because of its water solubility, does not achieve significant levels in the cerebrospinal fluid. This is profoundly different from the other available nitrosourea compounds (eg, carmustine, lomustine, and methyl-CCNU).

Kovach and colleagues (1979) noted plasma half-lives for the intact N-nitroso groups of 9.5 minutes after doses up to 40 mg/m² and 12.5 minutes after doses of 150 or 200 mg/m². There was no evidence of drug accumulation on the daily × 5 schedule.

Side Effects and Toxicity

Phase I studies have shown that hematologic toxicity, especially thrombocytopenia, is dose limiting (Hoth et al 1978, Taylor et al 1980, Kovach et al 1979, Gralla et al 1975). The nadir was relatively late, occurring 4 weeks after administration.

Hepatic toxicity consisting of transient elevations in serum glutamic–oxalacetic and glutamic–pyruvic transaminases has been noted, without evidence of cumulative effects (Taylor et al 1980). Belt et al (1980) have described a cholestatic jaundice in those patients treated with intermittent high-dose chlorozotocin.

Gastrointestinal toxicity was common but mild. It consisted only of nausea and vomiting, which occurred within 1 to 2 hours, usually abated by 4 to 6 hours, and was effectively controlled with antiemetics.

Other toxic effects are significantly absent with this chloroethylnitrosourea. These include local vein irritation, diarrhea, stomatitis, and renal dysfunction (Houghton et al 1981, Ahmann et al 1980, Silver et al 1982, Van Amburg et al 1982, Creagen et al 1979).

Chlorozotocin pulmonary toxicity has been described by several investigators (Sordillo et al 1981, Weiss et al 1981, Ahlgren et al 1981). Lung biopsies have shown interstitial inflammation and early fibrosis (Ahlgren et al 1981).

A chemotherapy-induced pneumonitis in a patient receiving chlorozotocin and mitomycin-C has also been reported, suggesting additive or synergistic toxicity with that combination (Goedert et al 1983).

REFERENCES

Ahlgren JD, Smith FP, Kerwin DM, Sikic BI, Weiner JH, Schein PS. Pulmonary disease as a complication of chlorozotocin chemotherapy. *Cancer Treat Rep.* 1981; 65(3/4):223–229.

Ahmann DL, Frytak S, Kvois LK, et al. Phase II study of maytansine and chlorozotocin in patients with disseminated malignant melanoma. *Cancer Treat Rep.* 1980;**64**:721–723.

Amato DA, Borden EC, Hiraki M, et al. Evaluation of bleomycin, chlorozotocin, MGBG, and bruceantin in patients with advanced soft tissue sarcoma, bone sarcoma, or mesothelioma. *Invest New Drugs.* 1985;**3**(4):397–401.

Anderson T, McMenamin MG, Schein PS. Chlorozotocin 2-[3-(2-chloro ethyl)-3-nitrosoureidol]-D-glucopyranose, an antitumor agent with modified bone marrow toxicity. *Cancer Res.* 1975;**35**:761–765.

Belt RJ, McGregor D, Haas CD, Bhatia PS. Cholestatic jaundice associated with chlorozotocin. *Cancer Treat Rep.* 1980;**64**(12):1235–1239.

Bleiberg H, Rozencweig M, Michel J. Phase II trial with chlorozotocin in advanced colorectal cancer. *Eur J Cancer Clin Oncol.* 1981;**17**(8):863–866.

Bukowski RM, McCraken JD, Balcerzak SP, Fabian CJ. Phase II study of chlorozotocin in islet cell carcinoma. A Southwest Oncology Group study. *Cancer Chemother Pharmacol.* 1983;**11**(1):48–50.

Byrne P, Tew K, Jemionek J, MacVittie T, Erickson L, Schein P. Cellular and molecular mechanisms of the bone marrow sparing effects of glucose chloroethylnitrosourea chlorozotocin. *Blood.* 1984;**63**:759–767.

Creagen ET, Eagan RT, Fleming TR, Frytak S, Kvols LK, Ingle JN. Phase II evaluation of chlorozotocin in advanced bronchogenic carcinoma. *Cancer Treat Rep.* 1979;**63**(11/12):2105–2106.

Creech RH, Stanley K, Vogl SE, Ettinger DS, Bonomi PD, Salazar O. Phase II study of cisplatin, maytansine and chlorozotocin in small cell lung carcinoma. *Cancer Treat Rep.* 1982;**66**(6):1417–1419.

De Vita VT, Denham C, Davidson JD, Oliverio VT. The physiologic disposition of the carcinostatic 1,3-bis-(2-chloro ethyl)-1-nitrosourea (BCNU) in man and animals. *Clin Pharmacol Ther.* 1967;**8**:566–577.

Douglass HO Jr, Lefkopoulou M, Davis HL, et al. ECOG phase II trials of MGBG, chlorozotocin, COM multidrug therapy in advanced measurable colorectal cancer. *Am J Clin Oncol.* 1988;**11**(6):646–649.

Gastrointestinal Tumor Study Group. Phase II trials of maytansine, low-dose chlorozotocin, and high-dose chlorozotocin as single agents against advanced measurable adenocarcinoma of the pancreas. *Cancer Treat Rep.* 1985;**69**(4):417–420.

Goedert JJ, Smith FP, Tsou E, Weiss RB. Combination chemotherapy pneumonitis: A case report of possible synergistic toxicity. *Med Pediatr Oncol.* 1983;**11**(2):116–118.

Gralla RJ, Tan CTC, Young CW. Phase I trial of chlorozotocin. *Cancer Treat Rep.* 1979;**63**(1):17–20.

Gralla RJ, Yagoda A. Phase II evaluation of chlorozotocin in patients with renal cell carcinoma. *Cancer Treat Rep.* 1979;**63**(6):1007–1008.

Haas CD, McCracken JD, Vaughn CB, Stephens RL, Bukowski RM, Eyre HJ. Chlorozotocin: Results in colorectal carcinoma treated with high and low doses. A Southwest Oncology Group study. *Invest New Drugs.* 1984;**2**(4):401–404.

Haas CD, Stephens RL, Bukowski RM, et al. High-dose chlorozotocin in lung cancer: A Southwest Oncology Group phase II study. *Cancer Treat Rep.* 1983;**67**:705–707.

Hoth DF, Schein PS, Winokur S, A phase II study of chlorozotocin in metastatic malignant melanoma. *Cancer.* 1980;**46**:1544–1547.

Hoth D, Wooley P, Green D, et al. Phase I studies on chlorozotocin. *Clin Pharmacol Ther.* 1978;**23**(6):712–722.

Houghton AN, Camacho FJ, Gralla RJ, Wittes R. Phase II evaluation of chlorozotocin in patients with malignant melanoma. *Cancer Treat Rep.* 1981;**65**(7/8):705–706.

Kovach JS, Moertel CG, Schutt AJ, et al. A Phase I study of chlorozotocin (NSC-178248). *Cancer.* 1979;**43**:2189–2196.

Lawton JO, Giles GR, Hall J, et al. Phase II study of chlorozotocin in the treatment of advanced colorectal cancer. *Cancer Treat Rep.* 1981;**65**(1/2):13–15.

Montgomery JA, James R, McCaleb GS, Kirk MC, Johnston JP. Decomposition of N-2-(2-chloroethyl)-N-nitrosoureas in aqueous media. *J Med Chem.* 1975;**18**:568–570.

Moriconi WJ, Taylor S, Slavik M, Belt RJ, Haas CD, Hoogstraten B. Phase I evaluation of chlorozotocin (NSC-178248): Weekly schedule. *Invest New Drugs.* 1985;**3**(1):57–62.

Panasci LC, Green D, Nagourney R, Fox P, Schein PS. A structure activity analysis of chemical and biological parameters of chlorethylnitrosoureas in mice. *Cancer Res.* 1977;**37**:2615–2618.

Presant CA, Bartolucci AA. Phase II evaluation of chlorozotocin in metastatic sarcomas. *Med Pediatr Oncol.* 1984;**12**(1):25–27.

Schein PS, Bull JM, Doukas D, Hoth D. Sensitivity of human and murine hematopoietic precursor cells to chlorozotocin and BCNU. *Cancer Res.* 1978;**38**:257–260.

Schein PS, McMenamin M, Anderson T. 3-(Tetraacetyl glucopyranose-2-yl)-1-(2-chloroethyl)-1-nitrosourea, an antitumor agent with modified bone marrow toxicity. *Cancer Res.* 1973;**33**:2005–2009.

Schutt AJ, Hoth D, Moertel CG, Schein PS, Rubin J, O'Connell MJ. A phase II study of chlorozotocin in advanced large bowel carcinoma. A cooperative study between two institutions. *Am J Clin Oncol.* 1984;**7**(5):507–511.

Silver BA, Barlock AL, Lippman ME, Anderson T, Fisher RI. Phase II trial of chlorozotocin in malignant melanoma, breast cancer, and other solid tumors. *Cancer Treat Rep.* 1982;**66**(5):1229–1230.

Sordillo EM, Sordillo PP, Stover D, Magill GB. Chlorozotocin (DCNU)-induced pulmonary toxicity. *Cancer Clin Trials.* 1981;**4**(4):397–399.

Talley RW, Samson MK, Brownlee RW, Samhouri AM, Fraile RJ, Baker LH. Phase II evaluation of chlorozotocin (NSC-178248) in advanced human cancer. *Eur J Cancer.* 1981;**17**(3):337–343.

Taylor S, Belt RJ, Haas CD, Stephens RL, Hoogstraten B. Phase I evaluation of chlorozotocin: Single dose every six weeks. *Cancer.* 1980;**46**:2365–2368.

Ungerleider RS. Antitumor activity of chlorozotocin (NSC-178748). *Cancer Treat Rev.* 1980;**7**:191–195.

Van Amburg AL III, Presant CA, Burns D. Phase II study of chlorozotocin in malignant melanoma: A Southeastern Cancer Study Group report. *Cancer Treat Rep.* 1982;**66**(6):1431–1433.

Veronesi A, Magri MD, Tirelli U, et al. Chlorozotocin treatment of advanced gastrointestinal cancer. *Med Pediatr Oncol.* 1983;**11**:365–366.

Von Hoff DD, Amato DA, Kaufman JH, Falkson G, Cunningham TJ. Randomized trial of chlorozotocin, neocarzinostatin or methyl-CCNU in patients with malignant melanoma. *Am J Clin Oncol.* 1984;**7**(2):135–139.

Weiss RB, Poster DS, Penta JS. The nitrosoureas and pulmonary toxicity. *Cancer Treat Rev.* 1981;**8**(2):111–125.

Chromomycin A$_3$

■ Other Names

Toyomycin; NSC-58514.

■ Chemistry

Structure of chromomycin A$_3$

Chromomycin A$_3$ was isolated by Tatsuoka and colleagues in 1958. The complete chemical name is 6-[[2,6-dideoxy-4-O-(2,6-dideoxy-4-O-methyl-α-D-*lyxo*-hexopyranosyl)-β-D-*lyxo*-hexopyranosyl]oxy]-2-[O-2,6-dideoxy-3C-methyl-α-L-*arabino*-hexopyranosyl-(1→3)-O-2,6-dideoxy-β-D-*arabino*-hexopyranosyl-(1→3)-2,6-dideoxy-D-*arabino*-hexopyranosyl)oxy]-3-(3,4-dihydroxy-1-methoxy-2-oxopentyl)-3,4-dihydro-8,9-dihydroxy-7-methyl-1(2H)-anthracenone diacetate. Chemically, chromomycin A$_3$ closely resembles mithramycin. It is an antibiotic isolate from *Streptomyces griseus* with a high molecular weight (1182) and large complex glycosidic structure. It has the empiric formula $C_{57}H_{82}O_{26}$. The structure consists of a polycyclic chromophobic group linked with two chains of two and three sugars.

■ Antitumor Activity

Chromomycin A$_3$ is no longer used clinically in the United States but is still used in Japan. Chromomycin A$_3$ was being investigationally evaluated in humans following positive animal tumor results in sarcomas, hepatomas, and certain leukemias (Kaziwara et al 1961, Kuru 1961). In humans its clinical results in phase I solid tumor studies were not particularly encouraging (Reynolds et al 1976, Kovach et al 1973); however, a few objective responses were noted by Reynolds et al in 4 of 43 patients (1 each with Hodgkin's disease, melanoma, lung cancer, and rhabdomyosarcoma). The results of Samal et al (1978) demonstrated little drug activity in patients with advanced breast cancer. Similarly, Moertel et al (1975) were unable to confirm clinically significant drug activity in patients with colorectal carcinoma. In a broad phase II trial in children with various malignancies, no antitumor activity was noted except in patients with Hodgkin's disease (Krivit et al 1976).

■ Mechanism of Action

Chromomycin A$_3$ probably acts similarly to mithramycin and dactinomycin. This mechanism is similar to intercalation and involves anchoring of the drug into or around the DNA helix (Kamiyama 1968). Chromomycin A$_3$ binds to the purine region of DNA, specifically guanine, and acts to inhibit DNA-dependent RNA polymerase and thereby block DNA replication and RNA transcription (Kaziro and Kamiyama 1967). The bivalent cation Mg^{2+} appears to be necessary for this activity in vitro. This mechanism is probably cell cycle phase nonspecific.

■ Availability and Storage

Chromomycin A$_3$ was investigationally available from the National Cancer Institute in 0.5-mg vials as a lyophilized yellow powder. These vials could be stored at room temperature but should be protected from light. Each vial also contained 50 mg of sodium salicylate and 90 mg of sodium chloride. The intact vials remained stable for 2 years at room temperature and carried an imprinted expiration date. No preservative was included.

■ Preparation for Use, Stability, and Admixture

The addition of 10.0 mL of sterile water for injection resulted in an isotonic yellow solution of pH 5.0 to

5.5. Five percent dextrose could also be used as a diluent. The solution reconstituted as described was stable for up to 1 month if protected from light. Exposure to light resulted in from 10 to 30% loss in potency after 1 week. Increasing the dilution of the drug appeared to enhance light sensitivity, and minimal volumes were therefore recommended. For use within 24 hours of preparation, no special light precautions needed to be taken; however, as there was no preservative, the use of a dose within 8 hours of reconstitution was recommended.

■ Administration

The drug was usually given as a short infusion over 15 to 30 minutes or, in the minimal dilution described earlier, as a bolus injection through a well-established intravenous infusion. The infusion dose could be further diluted into 100 mL of D5W. Intravenous push doses were kept at the minimal total volume. In either case the patency of the intravenous infusion must be ensured. A 5- to 10-mL flush was recommended both before and after the dose was administered. Lengthy infusions or use of existing intravenous or blood administration sites was discouraged.

■ Special Precautions

Extreme local tissue damage can result from an extravasation (Falkson et al 1964). Therefore, the patient should be continuously monitored during the injection for any changes in sensation. This may herald an extravasation before any physical signs. The drug should never be administered by the intramuscular or subcutaneous route.

■ Drug Interactions

None are known.

■ Dosage

The dosage range in one phase I study varied from 0.5 to 1.1 mg/m^2/d for up to 5 days. A maximum total daily dose of 2.0 mg and a total course dose of 7.0 mg have also been recommended. These courses rarely have been condensed to a single one-time dose or expanded up to 14 days; however, subsequent courses by any schedule should not be repeated until toxicity, generally nephrotoxicity, has resolved, usually taking 4 weeks. The maximal tolerated dose in an advanced breast cancer study was 0.75 mg/m^2/d × 5 (Samal et al 1978).

There is also evidence that dosing every other day for five doses per course affords the use of slightly higher total doses (1.3 mg/m^2) without a significant increase in toxicity (Reynolds et al 1976).

■ Pharmacokinetics

An intravenous dose of chromomycin is cleared from the plasma in 3 hours. Both urinary excretion and biliary excretion are involved in total body clearance of the drug. Excretion of drug into the bile appears to predominate. In mice the highest concentration is found in the liver, kidneys, and intestine (Fujita 1971).

■ Side Effects and Toxicity

In Japan, most studies have reported mild leukopenia and hepatic dysfunction, rare hepatic necrosis, and frequent thrombophlebitis. Pain and eventual dermal necrosis have often occurred after extravasation. Nausea occurred when more than 1.0 mg of drug was given as a single bolus dose. Serious extravasations have required skin grafting (Samal et 1978).

In U.S. studies, renal function impairment has generally been the dose-limiting toxic effect. Elevation of the serum creatinine and blood urea nitrogen, proteinuria, and loss of concentrating ability were noted. This impairment usually showed improvement after 3 weeks and was more frequent at higher dosage ranges of 1.0 mg/m^2/d and upward (Kovach et al 1973, Krivit et al 1976, Moertel et al 1975). Renal tubular necrosis was evident on biopsy.

Other toxic effects include hypocalcemia, nausea, vomiting, and phlebitis. Leukopenia, thrombocytopenia, anemia, and coagulation problems were not significant. Rarely, stupor and semicoma may occur. The structural similarity to mithramycin may explain the hypocalcemia noted in some studies (Samal et al 1978).

■ Special Applications

The compound has been used clinically as a radiosensitizer (Falkson et al 1966). Chromomycin is also being used to label chromosomes to perform karyotyping using flow cytometry (Trask et al 1990).

REFERENCES

Falkson G, Sandison AG, Falkson HC, Fichardt T. Chemotherapy in advanced cancer. A clinical trial with chromomycin A$_3$. *Med Proc (South Africa)*. 1964;**10**:264–268.

Falkson G, Sandison AG, Falkson HC. Chromomycin A$_3$ (toyomycin) and radiotherapy in the treatment of advanced malignancy. *S Afr J Radiol.* 1966;**4**:38–39.

Fujita M. Comparative studies on the blood level, tissue distribution, excretion, and inactivation of anticancer drugs. *Jpn J Clin Oncol.* 1971;**1**:151–162.

Kamiyama M. Mechanism of action of chromomycin A$_3$. III. On binding of chromomycin A$_3$ with DNA and physico-chemical properties of the complex. *J Biochem (Tokyo).* 1968;**63**:566–572.

Kaziro Y, Kamiyama M. Mechanism of action of chromomycin A$_3$. II. Inhibition of RNA polymerase reaction. *J Biochem (Tokyo).* 1967;**62**:424–429.

Kaziwara K, Watanabe J, Komeda T, Usui T. Further observations on the inhibiting effects of chromomycin A$_3$ on transplantable tumors. *Cancer Chemother Rep.* 1961;**13**:99–106.

Kovach JS, Moertel CG, Ahmann DL, Hahn RG, Schutt AJ, Donadio JV Jr. Phase I study of chromomycin A$_3$ (NSC-58514). *Cancer Chemother Rep.* 1973;**57**:341–347.

Krivit W, Sonley M, Smith WB, Higgins G, Weiner T, Hammond D. Chromomycin A$_3$: A phase II study in childhood malignancies. *Proc Am Soc Clin Oncol ASCO.* 1976;**17**:176.

Kuru M. Clinical experience with a new antitumor agent chromomycin. *Cancer Chem Rep.* 1961;**13**:91–97.

Moertel CG, Schutt AJ, Hahn RG, Marciniak JA, Reitemer RJ. Phase II study of chromomycin A$_3$ (NSC-58514) in advanced colorectal carcinoma. *Cancer Chemother Rep.* 1975;**59**:577–579.

Reynolds RD, Fisher JI, Jensen PA, Pajak TF, Bateman JR. Phase I alternate-day dose study of chromomycin A$_3$. *Cancer Treat Rep.* 1976;**60**:1251–1255.

Samal B, Jones S, Brownlee RW, et al. Chromomycin A$_3$ for advanced breast cancer: A Southwest Oncology Group study. *Cancer Treat Rep.* 1978;**62**(1):19–22.

Tatsuoka S, Nakazawa K, Miyake A, et al. Isolation, anticancer activity and pharmacology of a new antibiotic chromomycin A$_3$. *Gann.* 1958;**49**(suppl):23.

Trask B, Van den Engh G, Nussbaum R, Suhwarts C, Gray J. Quantification of the DNA content of structurally abnormal Y chromosomes and X chromosome aneuploidy using high resolution bivariate flow karyotyping. *Cytometry.* 1990;**11**:184–195.

Cisplatin

Other Names

Platinol® (Bristol-Myers Oncology Division); NSC-119875; DDP; platinum; CACP.

Chemistry

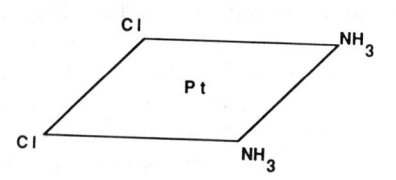

Structure of cisplatin

Cisplatin, or *cis*-diamminedichloroplatinum(II), has the empiric formula $N_2Cl_2PtH_6$. It is a planar inorganic compound with a molecular weight of 300. It is soluble in water at a concentration of 1 mg/mL. The "(II)" nomenclature denotes the (active) valence state of the platinum. The interatomic distance of the chlorides is 3.3 Å, which is different from the interatomic distance of the classic alkylating agents (5–7 Å). Only the *cis*-isomer is therapeutically active.

Antitumor Activity

Cisplatin has a wide spectrum of antitumor activity (Rozencweig et al 1977). Platinum activity was originally discovered serendipitously when it was noted that platinum electrodes immersed in a culture medium produced a bacteriostatic effect (Rosenberg et al 1965). In initial human trials the compound showed the greatest activity in germinal cell neoplasias of the testis, notably in combination with bleomycin and vinblastine (Einhorn and Donohue 1977), and in germ cell carcinoma of the ovary (Williams et al 1991). It also has shown clinical activity in patients with lymphoma (Rossoff et al 1972), ovarian carcinoma (Wiltshaw and Kroner 1976, Wiltshaw and Carr 1974), and squamous cell carcinoma of the head and neck (Hill et al 1975, Higby et al 1974, Jacobs et al 1978). More recent investigations have greatly expanded the use of cisplatin.

Non-Small Cell Lung Cancer. There is increasing evidence that cisplatin (with or without other agents) is effective for patients with non-small cell lung cancer (Ruckdeschel et al 1985). However, none of the platinum containing agents has clear superiority (Hainsworth et al 1989). Other investigators have found no place for cisplatin-containing combinations in patients with non-small cell lung cancer (Hainsworth et al 1989). Of great interest is a randomized trial result reported by Dillman et al (1986), who found that cisplatin + vinblastine + radiation therapy was superior to radiation therapy alone for treatment of patients with stage III non-small cell lung cancer. Chemotherapy was given in a neoadjuvant fashion prior to radiation therapy in this positive pilot study.

Small Cell Lung Cancer. Cisplatin combined with etoposide has been shown to be synergistic in animal models and produces objective response rates of up to 70% in patients with refractory small cell lung cancer (Sierocki et al 1979). A similar response rate is reported for cisplatin, etoposide, and doxorubicin (CAV) (Klastersky et al 1982). Despite these high response rates, survival has not been significantly improved in these settings.

Bladder Cancer. Loehrer et al (1990) have demonstrated that the cisplatin-containing combination MVAC is superior (in terms of response and survival) to cisplatin alone. Hillcoat and colleagues (1989) could not demonstrate a survival advantage for the use of cisplatin + methotrexate versus methotrexate alone. Troner et al (1982) and Khandekar et al (1985) also could not demonstrate an advantage for cisplatin + doxorubicin + cyclophosphamide versus cisplatin alone.

Breast Cancer. Cisplatin is just beginning to be explored at high doses and in combination for treatment of patients with advanced breast cancer (Cox et al 1989). At this time no treatment regimens can be recommended.

Penile Cancer. Cisplatin has been documented to have marginal activity (15%) in patients with carcinoma of the penis when given at doses of 50 mg/m^2 on days 1 and 8 (Gagliano et al 1989).

Osteosarcoma. Cisplatin has been placed in a number of adjuvant treatment programs for patients with osteogenic sarcoma (Winkler et al 1983).

Head and Neck Cancer. The use of cisplatin + 5-fluorouracil to treat patients with squamous cell head and neck cancer has become common (Al-Kourainy et al 1987). There is, however, controversy as to whether the combination is superior (in terms of survival) to treatment with cisplatin alone (Coninx et al 1988, Campbell et al 1987).

The combination of cisplatin + methotrexate has not been found superior to cisplatin alone for treatment of patients with advanced disease (Jacobs et al 1983).

Colorectal Carcinoma. Loehrer et al (1985) and O'Connell et al (1986) had reported in a pilot study that cisplatin + 5-fluorouracil appears to be an active combination for patients with advanced colorectal cancer. This finding has not been confirmed in controlled randomized clinical trials of cisplatin + 5-fluorouracil (Loehrer et al 1987).

Gastric Cancer. A response rate of 33% has been reported in patients with advanced gastric cancer (Leichman et al 1984). Combination studies are underway.

Pediatric Brain Tumors. Pediatric brain tumors have also been found to be responsive to cisplatin (Sexauer et al 1984).

Ovarian Cancer. Wiltshaw et al (1985) reported that *cis*-platinum and carboplatin are both effective agents for treatment of ovarian cancer patients (20% non-cross-resistance for both agents); however, carboplatin is clearly less toxic. Mangioni et al (1989) have compared cisplatin and carboplatin in patients with advanced ovarian cancer. Although it is less toxic, they could not conclude that the carboplatin was more active than cisplatin. Unfortunately, there is usually cross-resistance between cisplatin and carboplatin. Thus, carboplatin is not highly useful in patients refractory to cisplatin.

Alberts et al (1989) in the Southwest Oncology Group have compared carboplatin + cyclophosphamide with cisplatin + cyclophosphamide. They reported greatly reduced toxicity in the carboplatin + cyclophosphamide arm; however, no survival data were reported.

■ Mechanism of Action

It is very likely that cisplatin's interaction with DNA is its primary mode of action. The antitumor effect of cisplatin has been correlated with binding to DNA, production of intrastrand crosslinks, and formation of DNA adducts (Roberts and Pascoe 1972, Rosenberg 1975, Zwelling et al 1979, 1981, Fitchinger-Schepman et al 1987, Reed et al 1986). Intrastrand cisplatin adducts can cause changes in DNA conformation that may affect DNA replication (Rive et al 1988). This differs significantly from classic alkylating agents. Cisplatin also forms DNA–protein crosslinks but these do not correlate with antitumor activity. Of great interest has been the measurement of platinum–DNA adduct levels in patients' leukocytes and their correlation with clinical response (Fitchinger-Schepman et al 1987, Reed et al 1986, 1987).

Recently, more attention has been focused on the interaction of cisplatin with other components of the cell (eg, glutathione). The interested reader is referred to an excellent review of that subject by Andrews and Howell (1990).

■ Availability and Storage

Cisplatin is available from Bristol-Myers Oncology Division, Princeton, New Jersey, in amber vials containing either 10 or 50 mg of *cis*-platinum. Unopened vials of the powder should be stored at room temperature. The drug is also available as an aqueous solution (Platinol AQ).

■ Preparation for Use, Stability, and Admixture

The 10- and 50-mg vials should be reconstituted with 10 or 50 mL of sterile water for injection, respectively. Each vial will then contain 1 mg/mL *cis*-platinum. The solution should be clear and colorless. The unopened vial is stable for the lot life indicated on the package (if kept at room temperature). The reconstituted solution is stable for 20 hours at room temperature. It is important that the solution not be placed in the refrigerator as a precipitate may form. At concentrations greater than 0.6 mg/mL cisplatin solutions in normal saline under refrigeration for 24 hours can precipitate. Thus, more concentrated dilutions should be avoided if refrigerated storage is anticipated.

Cisplatin apparently degrades by aquation and the aquated platinum complex appears to be toxic (Cleare and Hoeschele 1973). The drug is also known to undergo photoaquation in aqueous solution, facilitating removal of the chloride ligands. Greene et al (1979) thus recommend light protection of cisplatin solutions.

When admixed with dextrose-containing solutions, by chromatographic analysis the drug appeared to be relatively unstable, with decomposition evident by 2 hours (Earhart 1978). It is clear that the sodium content does prevent the chlorides from leaving; thus, in normal saline or half-normal saline, less than 5% cisplatin solution at 25°C is lost after 48 hours (Le Roy 1979). Recent evidence indicates cisplatin should be mixed in solutions containing 0.9% NaCl because drug stability is inversely related to the concentration of chloride ions (Bohart and Ogawa 1979, Cheung et al 1987, Earhart et al 1978, Repta et al 1979, Le Roy 1979, Hincal et al 1979). Platinum can also form significant, colored complexes if directly admixed with mannitol and stored for 2 to 3 days (Eshaque et al 1976). Short-term (< 24 hours) admixtures, however, have been used successfully. Platinum may also react with aluminum, a metal found in many syringe needles. The interaction is apparently rapid and may result in a black plating on the metal surface and a loss of cisplatin potency (Prestayko et al 1979). Cisplatin (1–1.5 mg/mL) is physically compatible with ondansetron (1 mg/mL) in D5W (Trissel et al 1990). Admixtures of cisplatin (10 mg/50 mL saline) and etoposide (20 mg) in 50 mL of 0.9% sodium chloride in a polyvinyl chloride plastic bag are chemically stable for 7 days at room temperature (Lokich et al 1989).

■ Administration

Cisplatin is administered intravenously. Initially, the drug was administered by the intravenous push technique. It has been demonstrated that the nephrotoxicity of cisplatin may be greatly reduced or completely eliminated if a high urine flow is maintained (Hill et al 1975). Several methods of accomplishing this have been recommended. The patient should be well hydrated before therapy to ensure good urine flow. A convenient method to ensure good urine flow is to infuse the cisplatin with mannitol in the same solution (Hayes et al 1976). As a recommended regimen, pretreatment hydration with 1 to 2 L of fluid prior to cisplatin is recommended. The drug can be diluted in 2 L of 5% dextrose in normal saline containing 37.5 g of mannitol and infused over 6 to 8 hours. Adequate hydration and urinary output should be maintained during the next 24 hours.

A safe outpatient procedure using concurrent mannitol infusion appears to prevent serious nephrotoxicity. The desired dose of cisplatin plus 50 g mannitol is diluted to 1 L with D5W and 0.45% Sodium Chloride, USP (Rainey and Alberts 1978). This solution may then be infused at a rate no greater than 1 mg/min. For patients with known cardiac disease (congestive heart failure), the dose may be placed in 200 mL of a 10% mannitol solution and infused at a rate no greater than 1 mg/min. This is then followed by 200 mL of additional 10% mannitol. In an alternative regimen the drug is added to 400 mL of 10% mannitol which is then brought up to a 1 L volume with normal saline containing 3 g of magnesium sulfate and administered intravenously over 1 hour (Brock and Alberts 1986).

There are, additionally, a number of reports describing continuous intravenous infusion regimens with cisplatin. Jacobs et al (1978) used a continuous 24-hour infusion of cisplatin in patients with head and neck cancer. With the 80 mg/m^2 dose, responses equivalent to those to bolus injection were noted, and the authors felt that toxicity was reduced. Nonetheless, vomiting occurred in 76% of patients but may have been less severe than otherwise. Salem et al (1978), however, found greatly reduced nausea and vomiting in patients with a variety of tumors given 20 mg/m^2 cisplatin by continuous infusion daily for 5 days. Renal damage (21%) and ototoxicity (10%) were comparable to those after rapid infusion.

■ Special Precautions

This agent should be given (if at all) with great caution to patients with impaired renal function, impaired hearing, a preexisting peripheral neuropathy, or a past history of allergies to platinum.

■ Drug Interactions

Because cisplatin can reduce renal function, interactions with other renally eliminated drugs are possible. Thus, clinical studies have documented reduced drug clearance and increased half-lives following cisplatin therapy for several drugs including high-dose methotrexate (Crom et al 1984) and standard-dose bleomycin (Yee et al 1983). The toxicity of other renally eliminated drugs may also be enhanced by concomitant cisplatin therapy. This has been observed for hematologic suppression from ifosfamide (Lund et al 1990) or etoposide (Lokich et al 1989). Methotrexate-induced irreversible nephrotoxicity has similarly been enhanced in patients given concomitant cisplatin and high-dose methotrexate (Goren et al 1986). Dose reductions of these agents, using the patient's current creatinine clearance value as an index, are recommended in these settings.

The elimination of cisplatin via renal tubular secretion can be reduced by concomitant probenecid therapy (Jacobs et al 1984). In an experimental model, probenecid significantly enhanced cisplatin-induced nephrotoxicity (Daley-Yates and McBrien 1984). Cimetidine similarly enhances cisplatin lethality in mice (Dorr and Soble 1988). The antiplatelet agent dipyridamole also enhances cisplatin cytotoxicity in vitro (Howell et al 1987a). This is believed to be mediated by enhanced cisplatin uptake, possibly as a result of the effects of dipyridamole as a membrane nucleoside transport inhibitor. Whether this interaction is clinically significant or therapeutically useful is unknown.

Cytotoxic synergy has been described for cisplatin and etoposide in experimental animal tumor systems (Schabel et al 1979). This combination is also known to be highly effective in patients with lymphomas, non-small cell lung cancer, and testicular cancer (Loehrer and Einhorn 1984). Nonetheless, careful in vitro studies have not always noted true cytotoxic synergy for this combination (Tsai et al 1989). Sodium thiosulfate and mesna directly inactivate cisplatin and if given systemically together, decreased antitumor efficacy is noted in animals (Dorr and Lagel 1989). Clinical evidence exists for enhanced antitumor efficacy for cisplatin combined with tamoxifen in patients with malignant melanoma (McClay et al 1989). The mechanism for this beneficial interaction is not known.

■ Dosage

Livingston (1989) has recently reviewed the effect of dose and schedule of cisplatin administration. In general, he concluded that higher doses of cisplatin have more efficacy. The effect of schedule (eg, a continuous infusion) on efficacy was less clear (Livingston 1989, Gandara et al 1989). Typical dosage regimens include 20 mg/m^2 daily for 5 days repeated every 3 weeks (Einhorn and Donohue 1977), 100 to 120 mg/m^2 IV every 3 to 4 weeks (Bonomi et al 1985), and 100 mg/m^2 on days 1 and 8 repeated every 20 days (Gandara et al 1989).

The question of whether more cisplatin is better is still being addressed. Bonomi et al (1985) examined three regimens in patients with advanced squamous cell carcinoma of the cervix including 50 mg/m^2 every 21 days, 100 mg/m^2 every 21 days, and 20 mg/m^2 daily × 5 every 21 days. The response rate was highest in the 100 mg/m^2 arm, but there was no difference in complete response rate or survival.

High-Dose Cisplatin. Holleran and DeGregorio (1988) performed a review of high-dose (200 mg/m^2 per course) cisplatin. New dose-limiting toxic effects with the higher-dose regimens include severe neurotoxicity and myelosuppression. Responses have been seen, however, in patients refractory to conventional-dose cisplatin regimens (Bajorin et al 1987). Ozols and Young (1985) and Ozols et al (1984) have reported a complete response rate of 60% in patients with untreated ovarian cancer treated with high-dose cisplatin.

■ Pharmacokinetics

The table on page 290 details the pharmacokinetic parameters of cisplatin. In general, cisplatin demonstrates a triphasic disappearance curve with an α half-life of 20 minutes, β half-life of 48 to 70 minutes, and a γ half-life of 24 hours (Smith and Taylor 1974, DeConti et al 1973). The first two phases of disappearance represent clearance of free drug from the plasma; the third phase is probably removal of drug from the plasma proteins (> 90% bound Gormley et al 1979, DeConti et al 1973, Jacobs et al 1980). Ninety percent of the drug is removed by renal mechanisms (glomerular filtration and tubular secretion), whereas less than 10% is removed by biliary excretion (Casper et al 1979, Jacobs et al 1980).

Corden et al (1985) found that the mean half-life of ultrafilterable platinum was 50% longer for patients receiving high-dose cisplatin than for patients receiving conventional doses. Total systemic exposure was three times higher for the high-dose groups. Bajorin et al (1986) did not agree with those findings. No radiolabeled platinum has been detected in a single fecal sample (Smith and Taylor 1974). Stewart and colleagues (1989) noted that extracerebral and intracerebral tumor platinum concentrations were comparable.

■ Side Effects and Toxicity

Allergic Reactions. Anaphylactic hypersensitivity reactions consisting of tachycardia, wheezing, hypotension, and facial edema, within a few minutes of intravenous administration, have occasionally occurred after a dose of cisplatin in previously treated patients (Khan et al 1975, Von Hoff et al 1976). These hypersensitivity reactions have been controlled with corticosteroids, epinephrine, or antihistamines.

Wiesenfeld et al (1979) reported successful retreatment with cisplatin after apparent allergic reactions in two patients. In that report, in vivo and in vitro tests in one patient could not demonstrate an immunologic basis for the initial reaction. Both patients were successfully rechallenged with cisplatin after only diphenhydramine pretreatment. This

PHARMACOKINETICS OF CISPLATIN

Dose (mg/m^2)	Method	Number of Patients	Half-life (h) α	Half-life (h) β	Half-life (h) γ	Daily AUC (μg · min/mL)	Daily Total Body Clearance (mL/min/m^2)	% of Dose Excreted in Urine	Reference
70 over 1 h	FAAS*	8	23[†] 0.15[‡]	67[†] 0.72[‡]	—	—	—	23 ± 39% in 24 h	Gormley et al 1979
10 over 2–5 min	Isotopic	10	0.41–0.82	58–73	—	—	—	27–45% in 5 d	DeConti et al 1973
100 over 15 min without mannitol	FAAS	4	—	0.80	—	—	—	40% in 24 h	Belt et al 1979
+ Mannitol		4	—	0.98	—	—	—	16% in 24 h	
100 over 6 h without mannitol		4	—	0.43	—	—	—	75% in 24 h	
+Mannitol		3	—	0.43	—	—	—	20% in 24 h	
50–100 over 3–5 min	FAAS and HPLC	24		≥24[ξ] 0.32–0.50[″] 0.33–0.50[#]	—	—	—	—	Himmelstein et al 1981
40 daily × 5 over 30 min	FAAS	7	—	0.51	—	—	—	—	Corden et al 1985
20 daily × 5 over 30 min		4	—	0.31	—	—	—	—	
20 daily × 5		3	—	0.45	—	43	321	—	Bajorin et al 1986
20 daily × 5		3	—	0.55	—	37	345	—	
40 daily × 5		3	—	0.48	—	66	359	—	
100 days 1 and 8		5	—	—	—	0.573[**] 14.5	—	—	Gandara et al 1986

* FAAS, flameless atomic absorption spectrometry; HPLC, high-performance liquid chromatography. [†]Protein-bound platinum. [‡]Non-protein-bound plasma platinum. [ξ]Total platinum ["]Total filterable platinum. [#]Cisplatin. [**]Ultrafiltrate platinum.

suggests a nonallergic etiology for the acute hypersensitivity reactions occasionally seen with platinum.

Emesis. Acute and delayed nausea and vomiting occur in most patients. This reaction may be severe and usually starts within the first hour of treatment and may persist 24 to 48 hours (Higby et al 1974, Yagoda et al 1976). There has been considerable recent success in controlling these side effects. There are many effective antiemetic regimens to prevent cisplatininduced nausea and vomiting, including prochlorperazine + dexamethasone + lorazepam; metoclopramide + dexamethasone + lorazepam (Carr et al 1989); metoclopramide + dexamethasone (Kris et al 1989); metoclopramide + methylprednisolone (Roila et al 1987); and metoclopramide + lorazepam (Ziccarelli et al 1985).

Cisplatin emesis is well controlled with the new HT-3 receptor antagonist ondansetron. Specific regimens typically involve three intravenous ondansetron doses of 0.15 to 0.18 mg/kg given 15 minutes before dosing and again at 4 and 8 hours or 6 and 12 hours after cisplatin (Einhorn et al 1990). The response rate to 0.15 mg/kg ondansetron at 0, 4, and 8 hours was 79% (Cubeddu et al 1990), the response rate to 0.16 mg/kg at 0, 6, and 12 hours was 87% (Einhorn et al 1990), and the response rate to 0.18 mg/kg at 0, 6, and 12 hours was 83% (Hesketh et al 1989a).

Granisetron, another serotonin type 3 receptor antagonist, has also demonstrated major efficacy in preventing cisplatin-induced emesis (Hesketh et al 1989b). With time it is likely this agent will be incorporated into many anticancer regimens. Pollera and Giannarelli (1989) reported that regardless of the antiemetic regimen employed, patient characteristics such as sex, performance status, and age significantly affect cisplatin-related emesis.

Nephrotoxicity. Dose-related nephrotoxicity has been the major dose-limiting toxic effect of cisplatin (Leonard et al 1971). It manifests as renal tubular damage, resulting in an elevation of the blood urea nitrogen or serum creatinine (Hardaker et al 1974). The peak detrimental effect on renal function usually occurs between the 10th and 20th days after treatment. The renal damage is usually reversible. Patients concomitantly receiving gentamicin and cephalothin have been shown to be at greater risk of developing acute renal failure (Gonzalez-Vitale et al 1978).

Dentino et al (1978) serially observed 15 male patients receiving the 5-day 20 mg/m^2 cisplatin testicular regimen of Einhorn and Donohue (1977). After 6 months of therapy the mean creatinine clearance for the group had halved and significant elevations in plasma blood urea nitrogen were also present. These toxic effects were greater in patients receiving other potentially nephrotoxic drugs, especially aminoglycosides; however, neither proteinuria nor functional tubular defects could be discerned in this study. Madias and Harrington (1978) have characterized the renal damage of cisplatin as similar to that of mercury nephrotoxicity. Pathologically, renal tubular necrosis, degeneration, and interstitial edema without glomerular changes are noted. Thus, although clinically overt renal toxicity may be common there is usually resolution. Long-term damage is, however, quite probable. The renal-protective effect of hydration and mannitol is now well described both in animal models and in humans (Frick et al 1979, Rainey and Alberts 1978, Einhorn and Donohue 1977).

Ototoxicity. Ototoxicity secondary to cisplatin manifests as high-frequency hearing loss above the frequency of normal speech and may be seen in up to 30% of patients treated (Piehl et al 1974). This effect may be dose related and can be apparent unilaterally or bilaterally. Occasional tinnitus and, rarely, vestibular dysfunction have also been noted. The ototoxicity and nephrotoxicity may be prevented completely or partially by adequate hydration and the use of mannitol diuresis. Fleming and colleagues (1985) demonstrated that patients with lower-than-average threshold prior to chemotherapy with cisplatin were more likely to experience greater threshold shifts. Recent evidence also suggests that there is increased ototoxicity with cisplatin given after radiotherapy in pediatric patients with brain tumors (Kovnar et al 1991).

Cardiotoxicity. Possible cardiotoxicity (ST-T wave abnormalities and bundle branch block) has been reported but is probably quite rare (Wiltshaw and Carr 1974). Atrial fibrillation and supraventricular tachycardia have also been reported (Menard et al 1990; Hashima et al 1984).

Neurotoxicity. Peripheral neuropathy is becoming a more significant toxic effect with long-term administration of cisplatin. Kedar et al (1978) noted a patient with a "glove-and-stocking" type neuropathy while receiving cisplatin as a single agent. Numbness, tingling, and a sensory loss occurred distally in both arms and legs. Others have also documented this troublesome toxic effect (Von Hoff et al 1979, Ashraf et al 1983, Thompson et al 1984, Mollman et al 1988, Roelofs et al 1984, Marin and Rierson 1979).

Recently Gerritsen and colleagues (1989, 1990) reported that the adrenocorticotropin analog ORG 2766 significantly reduces the subclinical and clinical neuropathy induced by cisplatin. These findings await confirmation.

Focal encephalopathy with cortical blindness, seizures, and aphasia has been reported (Gorman et al 1989, Merd et al 1982, Berman and Mann 1980, Hitchins and Thomson 1988, Ostrow et al 1978, Lindeman et al 1990). In most patients it is reversible. Retinal toxicity has also been reported (Wilding et al 1985).

Hypomagnesemia. Symptomatic hypomagnesemia is frequently seen with cisplatin (Schilsky and Anderson 1979). In a study to determine the effects of magnesium supplementation on cisplatin-induced hypomagnesemia the administration of magnesium (oral + intravenous) with cisplatin resulted in less renal tubular damage and no compromise in efficacy compared with a group not supplemented with magnesium (Willox et al 1986).

Myelosuppression. Myelosuppression is infrequently seen with low doses of the agent but is more pronounced with the high-dose (≥ 200 mg/m^2) regimens (Talley et al 1973, Ozols et al 1984). Anemia, including a Coombs-positive hemolytic anemia, can be seen with cisplatin. Cisplatin-induced anemia has been shown to respond to recombinant erythropoietin (Henry et al 1990).

Hepatic Toxicity. Cavalli et al (1978) described a single case of liver toxicity associated, at least temporarily, with cisplatin administration. Signs and symptoms included transiently elevated serum bilirubin, alkaline phosphatase, and serum glutamic–oxalacetic transaminase values. Morphologically, steatosis, cholestasis, and periportal edema were noted. Complete recovery occurred in this case.

Local Toxicity. Extravasation of cisplatin has rarely been associated with cellulitis and fibrosis of the local tissue (Fields et al 1990, Lewis and Medina 1980). In animal models, cisplatin is weakly toxic to skin although it can be antagonized locally by 1/6 M sodium thiosulfate (Dorr 1990).

■ Drug Interactions

At least three sulfhydryl-containing agents have been introduced to decrease the toxic effects of cisplatin-induced renal or ototoxicity: sodium thiosulfate, diethyldithiocarbamate, and WR 2721. Howell and colleagues (1982) have demonstrated that use of systemic thiosulfate could protect patients from the side effects of intraperitoneally administered cisplatin. Kramer et al (1988) have examined the effects of diethyldithiocarbamate (DDTC) on response, toxicity, and pharmacology of cisplatin in patients with head and neck cancer. They found that DDTC does not alter the toxicity, pharmacokinetics, or clinical response to cisplatin.

WR 2721 has been reported to protect patients from nephrotoxicity and ototoxicity (Glover et al 1984, 1986, 1987). Confirmatory trials of these initial studies are ongoing. Each of these agents is believed to bind platinum to an activated sulfur in the antagonist. The resultant thioplatinum complex is inactive and can be more readily excreted in the urine. Selenium has also been reported to protect against experimental cisplatin nephrotoxicity (Baldew et al 1989) without reducing antitumor efficacy (Ohkawa et al 1988). This potential interaction has not been tested clinically.

■ Special Applications

Intraarterial Use. Cisplatin has been used by an intraarterial route. Investigators are now using doses of 120 mg/m^2 infused over longer periods of time ranging up to 45 hours. For these applications, the dose is diluted into normal saline, and from 15,000 to 25,000 U of heparin is added to maintain catheter patency and reduce thromboembolic complications. The drug has been used intraarterially for patients with head and neck cancer, glioma, bladder cancer, and melanoma. As yet there is no definitive evidence for the advantage of this route of administration (Gouyette et al 1986, Frost et al 1985, Stewart et al 1987).

Of note is that the incidence of severe encephalopathy encountered with the intraarterial administration of cisplatin for patients with glioma is 1.8% (Green et al 1989a).

Intravesical Use. Intravesical cisplatin has been used with limited success in the treatment of superficial bladder cancer (Horn et al 1985, Llopis et al 1985, Mobley et al 1986).

Intraperitoneal Use. As mentioned earlier, Howell et al (1982, 1987b) used intraperitoneal cisplatin to treat patients with peritoneum-predominant ovarian cancer. Doses ranged from 90 to 270 mg/m^2, usually given in 2 L of normal saline. Other cisplatin-containing combinations have also been used intraperitoneally (Doroshow et al 1986, Reichman et al 1988).

Use with Hyperthermia. The use of cisplatin at doses of 40 to 60 mg/m² given over 60 minutes with hyperthermia (up to 42°C) has been reported (Green et al 1989b).

Use as a Radiosensitizer. Choo et al (1986) reported a randomized trial of cisplatin + radiation therapy versus radiation therapy alone in patients with stage II and III cervical cancer. The complete response rate was 55% for the combination versus 20% for radiation therapy alone. Al-Sarraf et al (1985) documented that radiation therapy + cisplatin can be given with acceptable toxicity and a high degree of local control.

REFERENCES

Al-Kourainy K, Kish J, Ensley J, et al. Achievement of superior survival for histologically negative versus histologically positive clinical complete responders to cisplatin combination in patients with locally advanced head and neck cancer. *Cancer.* 1987;**59**(2):233–238.

Al-Sarraf M, Marcial V, Mowry P, et al. Superior local control with combination of high dose *cis*-platinum and radiotherapy. An RTOG study (abstract). *Proc Am Assoc Cancer Res.* 1985;**26**:169.

Alberts D, Green S, Hannigan E, et al. Improved efficacy of carboplatin (carbo D)/cyclophosphamide (CPA) vs cisplatin (CISP/CPA): Preliminary report of a phase III, randomized trial in stage III–IV suboptimal ovarian cancer (OV, CA). *Proc Am Soc Clin Oncol.* 1989;**8**:151.

Andrews PA, Howell SB. Cellular pharmacology of cisplatin: Perspectives on mechanisms of acquired resistance. *Cancer Cells.* 1990;**2**(2):35–43.

Ashraf M, Scotchel PL, Krall JM, Fink EB. *cis*-Platinum-induced hypomagnesemia and peripheral neuropathy. *Gynecol Oncol.* 1983;**16**:309–318.

Bajorin JF, Bosl GJ, Alcock NW, et al. Pharmacokinetics of *cis*-diamminedichloroplatinum(II) after administration in hypertonic saline. *Cancer Res.* 1986;**46**:5969–5972.

Bajorin D, Bosl GJ, Fein R. Phase I trial of escalating doses of cisplatin in hypertonic saline. *J Clin Oncol.* 1987;**5**(10):1589–1593.

Baldew GS, van den Hamer CJA, Los G, et al. Selenium-induced protection against *cis*-diamminedichloroplatinum(II) nephrotoxicity in mice and rats. *Cancer Res.* 1989;**49**:3020–3023.

Belt RJ, Himmelstein KJ, Patton TF, et al. Pharmacokinetics of non-protein-bound platinum species following administration of *cis*-dichlorodiammine-platinum(II). *Cancer Treat Rep.* 1979;**63**:1515–1521.

Berman IJ, Mann MP. Seizures and transient cortical blindness associated with *cis*-platinum(II) diamminedichloride (PPD) therapy in a thirty-year-old man. *Cancer.* 1980;**45**:764–766.

Bohart R, Ogawa G. An observation on the stability of *cis*-dichlorodiammineplatinum(II): A caution regarding its administration. *Cancer Treat Rep.* 1979;**63**:2117–2119.

Bonomi P, Blessing JA, Stehman FB, et al. Randomized trial of three cisplatin dose schedules in squamous-cell carcinoma of the cervix: A Gynecologic Oncology Group study. *J Clin Oncol.* 1985;**3**(8):1079–1085.

Brock J, Alberts DS. Safe, rapid administration of cisplatin in the outpatient clinic. *Cancer Treat Rep.* 1986;**70**:1409–1414.

Campbell JB, Dorman EB, McCormick M, et al. A randomized phase III trial of cisplatinum, methotrexate, cisplatinum + methotrexate, and cisplatinum + 5-fluorouracil in end-stage head and neck cancer. *Acta Otolaryngol (Stockh).* 1987;**103**(5/6):519–528.

Carr BI, Doroshow JH, Morgan RJ, et al. Combination antiemetic therapy based on high doses of either prochlorperazine or metoclopramide give complete protection against platinum-induced emesis (abstract). *Proc Am Soc Clin Oncol.* 1989;**8**:325.

Casper ES, Kelsen DP, Alcock NW, Young CW. Platinum concentrations in bile and plasma following rapid and six hour infusions of *cis*-dichlorodiammineplatinum(II). *Cancer Treat Rep.* 1979;**63**:2023–2025.

Cavalli F, Tschopp L, Sonntag RW, Zimmerman A. A case of liver toxicity following *cis*-diamminedichloroplatinum(II) treatment (letter). *Cancer Treat Rep.* 1978;**62**(12):2125–2126.

Cheung Y, Cradock JC, Vishnuvajjala BR, Flora KP. Stability of cisplatin, iproplatin, carboplatin, and tetraplatin in commonly used intravenous solutions. *Am J Hosp Pharm.* 1987;**44**:124–130.

Choo YC, Choy TK, Wong LC, Ma HK. Potentiation of radiotherapy by *cis*-dichlorodiammine platinum(II) in advanced cervical carcinoma. *Gynecol Oncol.* 1986;**23**(1):94–100.

Cleare MJ, Hoeschele JD. Studies on the antitumor activity of group 8 transition metal complexes. I. Platinum(II) complexes. *Bioinorg Chem.* 1973;**2**:187–210.

Coninx P, Nasca S, Lebrun D, et al. Sequential trial of initial chemotherapy for advanced cancer of the head and neck. DDP versus DDP + 5-fluorouracil. *Cancer.* 1988;**62**(9):1888–1892.

Corden BJ, Fine RL, Ozols RF, Collins JM. Clinical pharmacology of high dose cisplatin. *Cancer Chemother Pharmacol.* 1985;**14**:38–41.

Cox EB, Burton GV, Olsen GA, Vugrin D. Cisplatin and etoposide: An effective treatment for refractory breast carcinoma. *Am J Clin Oncol.* 1989;**12**(1):53–56.

Crom WR, Pratt CB, Green AA, et al. The effect of prior cisplatin therapy on the pharmacokinetics of high-dose methotrexate. *J Clin Oncol.* 1984;**2**(6):655–661.

Cubeddu LX, Hoffman IS, Fuenmayor NT, Finn AL. Efficacy of ondansetron (GR38032F) and the role of serotonin in cisplatin-induced nausea and vomiting. *N Engl J Med.* 1990;**322**:810–816.

Daley-Yates PT, McBrien DCH. Enhancement of cisplatin nephrotoxicity by probenecid. *Cancer Treat Rep.* 1984;**68**(2):445–446.

De Conti RC, Toftness BR, Lange RC, Creasey WA. Clinical and pharmacological studies with *cis*-diamminedichloroplatinum(II). *Cancer Res.* 1973;**33**:1310–1315.

Dentino M, Luft FC, Yum MN, et al. Long term effect of *cis*-diamminedichloride platinum (CDDP) on renal function and structure in man. *Cancer.* 1978;**41**:1274–1281.

Dillman RO, Seagren SL, Propert K, et al. Complete responses in regional stage III non-small cell lung cancer (NSCLC) with vinblastine (VLB) and cisplatinum (CDDP) (abstract). *Proc Am Soc Clin Oncol.* 1986;**5**:180.

Doroshow J, Braly P, Hoff S, et al. Intraperitoneal (IP) chemotherapy with cisplatin (P) and 5-fluorouracil (FU): An active regimen for refractory ovarian cancer (OC). *Proc Am Soc Clin Oncol.* 1986;**5**:117.

Dorr RT. Antidotes to vesicant chemotherapy extravasation. *Blood Rev.* 1990;**4**:31–60.

Dorr RT, Soble MJ. Cimetidine enhances cisplatin toxicity in mice. *J Cancer Res Clin Oncol.* 1988;**114**:1–2.

Dorr RT, Lagel K. Interaction between cisplatin and mesna in mice. *J Cancer Res Clin Oncol.* 1989;**115**:604–605.

Earhart RH. Instability of *cis*-dichlorodiammineplatinum in dextrose solution. *Cancer Treat Rep.* 1978;**62**(7):1105–1106.

Einhorn LH, Donohue J. *cis*-Diamminedichloroplatinum, vinblastine and bleomycin. Combination chemotherapy in disseminated testicular cancer. *Ann Intern Med.* 1977;**87**:293–298.

Einhorn LH, Nagy C, Werner K, Finn AL. Ondansetron: A neoantiemetic for patients receiving cisplatin chemotherapy. *J Clin Oncol.* 1990;**8**(4):731–735.

Eshaque M, McKay MJ, Theophande T. *p*-Mannitol platinum complexes. *Wadley Med Bull.* 1976;**7**(1):338–358.

Fields S, Loeller J, Topper RL, et al. Local soft tissue toxicity following cisplatin extravasation. *J Natl Cancer Inst.* 1990;**82**:1649–1659.

Fitchinger-Schepman AMJ, von Oosteram AT, Lohman PMH, Berends F. *cis*-Diamminedichloroplatinum(II) induced DNA adducts in peripheral leukocytes from seven cancer patients: Quantitative immunochemical detection of the adduct induction and removal after a single dose of *cis*-diamminedichloroplatinum(II). *Cancer Res.* 1987;**476**:3000–3004.

Fleming S, Peppard S, Ratanatharathorn V, et al. Ototoxicity from *cis*-platinum in patients with stages III and IV previously untreated squamous cell cancer of the head and neck. *Am J Clin Oncol.* 1985;**8**(4):302–306.

Frick GA, Ballentine R, Driever CW, Kramer WG. Renal excretion kinetics of high-dose *cis*-dichlorodiammineplatinum(II) administered with hydration and mannitol diuresis. *Cancer Treat Rep.* 1979;**63**(1):13–16.

Frost DB, Patt YZ, Mavligit G, et al. Arterial infusion of dacarbazine and cisplatin for recurrent regionally confined melanoma. *Arch Surg.* 1985;**120**:478–480.

Gagliano RG, Blumenstein BA, Crawford ED, et al. *cis*-diamminedichloroplatinum in the treatment of advanced epidermoid carcinoma of the penis: A Southwest Oncology Group study. *J Urol.* 1989;**141**(1):166–167.

Gandara DR, DeGregorio MW, Wold H, et al. High-dose cisplatin in hypertonic saline: Reduced toxicity of a modified dose schedule and correlation with plasma pharmacokinetics. A Northern California Oncology Group pilot study on non-small cell lung cancer. *J Clin Oncol.* 1986;**4**:1787–1793.

Gandara DR, Wold H, Perez EA, et al. Cisplatin dose intensity in non-small cell lung cancer: Phase II results of a day 1 and day 8 high-dose regimen. *J Natl Cancer Inst.* 1989;**81**:790–794.

Gerritsen van der Hoop R, Vecht C, Elderson A, et al. ORG 2766, an ACTH(4–9) analog, prevents cisplatin-induced neuropathy in ovarian cancer patients (abstract). *Proc Am Soc Clin Oncol.* 1989;**8**:150.

Gerritsen von der Hays P, Vecht CJ, van der Burg MFL, et al. Prevention of cisplatin neurotoxicity with an AITIL(4–9) analogue in patients with ovarian cancer. *N Engl J Med.* 1990;**322**:89–94.

Glover D, Glick JH, Weiler C, et al. Phase I trials of WR2721 and cisplatin. *Int J Radiat Oncol Biol Phys.* 1984;**10**:1781–1784.

Glover D, Glick J, Weiler C, et al. Phase I–II trials of WR2721 and cisplatin. *Int J Radiat Oncol Biol Phys.* 1986;**12**:1509–1512.

Glover D, Glick JH, Weiler C, et al. WR2721 and high-dose cisplatin: An active combination in the treatment of metastatic melanoma. *J Clin Oncol.* 1987;**5**:574–578.

Gonzalez-Vitale JC, Hayes DM, Civitkovic E, Sternberg SS. Acute renal failure after *cis*-dichlorodiammineplatinum(II) and gentamicin cephalothin therapies. *Cancer Treat Rep.* 1978;**62**(5):693–698.

Goren MP, Wright RK, Horowitz ME, Meyer WH. Enhancement of methotrexate nephrotoxicity after cisplatin therapy. *Cancer.* 1986;**58**:2617–2621.

Gorman DJ, Kefford R, Stuart-Harris R. Focal encephalopathy after cisplatin therapy. *Med J Aust.* 1989;**150**:339–401.

Gormley PE, Bull JM, LeRoy AF, Cysyk R. Kinetics of *cis*-dichlorodiammineplatinum. *Clin Pharmacol Ther.* 1979;**25**:351–357.

Gouyette A, Apchin A, Foka M, Richards JM. Pharmacokinetics of intraarterial and intravenous cisplatin in head and neck cancer patients. *Eur J Cancer Clin Oncol.* 1986;**22**:257–263.

Green BB, Shapiro WR, Burger PC, et al. Randomized comparison of intraarterial (IA) cisplatin and intravenous (IV) PCNU for the treatment of primary brain tumors (BTCG Study B420A) (abstract). *Proc Am Soc Clin Oncol.* 1989a;**8**:86.

Green DM, Burton GV, Cox EB, et al. A phase I/II study of combined cisplatin and hyperthermia treatment for refractory malignancy. *Int J Hyperthermia.* 1989b;**5**(1):13–21.

Greene RF, Chatterji AC, Hiranaka PK, Gallelli JF. Stability of cisplatin in aqueous solution. *Am J Hosp Pharm.* 1979;**36**:38–43.

Hainsworth JD, Johnson DH, Hande KR, Greco FA. Chemotherapy of advanced non-small-cell lung cancer: A randomized trial of three cisplatin-based chemotherapy regimens. *Am J Clin Oncol.* 1989;**12**(4):345–359.

Hardaker WT, Stone RA, McCoy R. Platinum nephrotoxicity. *Cancer.* 1974;**34**:1030–1032.

Hashima LA, Khalyl MF, Salem PA. Supraventricular tachycardia. A probable complication of platinum treatment. *Oncology.* 1984;**41**:174–175.

Hayes D, Civitkovic E, Golbey R, et al. Amelioration of renal toxicity of high dose *cis*-platinum diammine dichloride (CPDD) by mannitol induced diuresis (abstract). *Proc Am Assoc Cancer Res.* 1976;**17**:169.

Henry D, Keller A, Kugler J, et al. Treatment of anemia in cancer patients on cisplatin chemotherapy with recombinant human erythropoietin (RHUEPO). *Proc Am Soc Clin Oncol.* 1990;**9**:182.

Hesketh PJ, Kasimis BS, Schall S, et al. An open label dose comparison of intravenous GR 38032F in the prevention of emesis induced by high dose cisplatin (DDP). *Proc Am Soc Clin Oncol.* 1989a;**8**:333.

Hesketh PJ, Murphy WK, Lester EP, et al. GR 38032F (GR-C507/75): A novel compound effective in the prevention of acute cisplatin-induced emesis. *J Clin Oncol.* 1989b;**7**(6):700–705.

Higby DJ, Wallace HJ, Albert DJ, Holland JF. Diamminodichloroplatinum: A phase I study showing responses in testicular and other tumors. *Cancer.* 1974;**33**:1219–1225.

Hill JM, Loeb E, MacLellan A, et al. Clinical studies of platinum coordination compounds in the treatment of various malignant diseases. *Cancer Chemother Rep.* 1975;**59**:647–659.

Hillcoat BL, Raghavan D, Matthews J, et al. A randomized trial of cisplatin versus cisplatin plus methotrexate in advanced cancer of the urothelial tract. *J Clin Oncol.* 1989;**7**(6):706–709.

Himmelstein KT, Patton TE, Belt RJ, et al. Clinical kinetics of intact cisplatin and some related species. *Clin Pharmacol Ther.* 1981;**29**:658–664.

Hincal AA, Long DJ, Repta AJ. Cisplatin stability in aqueous parenteral vehicles. *J Parenteral Drug Assoc.* 1979;**33**:107–116.

Hitchins RN, Thomson DB. Encephalopathy following cisplatin, bleomycin and vinblastine therapy for nonseminomatous germ cell tumour of testis. *Aust NZ J Med.* 1988;**18**:67–68.

Holleran WM, DeGregorio MW. Evolution of high-dose cisplatin. *Invest New Drugs.* 1988;**6**(2):135–142.

Horn Y, Eidelman A, Walach N, et al. Intravesical chemotherapy of superficial bladder tumors in a controlled trial with *cis*-platinum versus *cis*-platinum plus hyaluronidase. *J Surg Oncol.* 1985;**28**(4):304–307.

Howell SB, Vick J, Andrews PA, et al. Biochemical modulation of cisplatin by dipyridimole. *Proc Am Assoc Cancer Res.* 1987a;**28**:313.

Howell SB, Zimm S, Markman M, et al. Long term survival of advanced refractory ovarian carcinoma patients with small volume disease treated with intraperitoneal chemotherapy. *J Clin Oncol.* 1987b;**5**:1607–1612.

Howell SR, Pferfle CE, Wung W, et al. Intraperitoneal cisplatin with systemic thiosulfate protection. *Ann Intern Med.* 1982;**97**:845–951.

Jacobs C, Bertino JR, Goffinet DR, et al. 24 Hour infusion of *cis*-platinum in head and neck cancers. *Cancer.* 1978;**42**:2135–2140.

Jacobs C, Coleman CN, Rich L, et al. Inhibition of *cis*-diamminedichloroplatinum secretion by the human kidney with probenecid. *Cancer Res.* 1984;**44**:3632–3635.

Jacobs C, Kalman SM, Tretton M, Weiner MW. Renal handling of *cis*-diamminedichloroplatinum(II). *Cancer Treat Rep.* 1980;**64**:1223–1226.

Jacobs C, Meyers F, Hendrickson C, et al. A randomized phase III study of cisplatin with or without methotrexate for recurrent squamous cell carcinoma of the head and neck. A Northern California Oncology Group study. *Cancer.* 1983;**52**(9):1563–1569.

Kedar A, Cohen ME, Freeman AL. Peripheral neuropathy as a complication of *cis*-dichlorodiammineplatinum(II) treatment: A case report. *Cancer Treat Rep.* 1978;**62**(5):819–821.

Khan A, Hill JM, Grater W, et al. Atopic hypersensitivity to *cis*-dichlorodiammineplatinum(II) and other platinum complexes. *Cancer Res.* 1975;**35**:2766–2770.

Khandekar JD, Elson PJ, DeWys WD, et al. Comparative activity and toxicity of *cis*-diamminedichloroplatinum (DDP) and a combination of doxorubicin, cyclophosphamide, and DDP in disseminated transitional cell carcinoma of the urinary tract. *J Clin Oncol.* 1985;**3**(4):539–545.

Klastersky J, Nicaise C, Longeval E, Stryckmans P. Cisplatin, Adriamycin and etoposide (CAV) for remission induction of small cell bronchogenic carcinoma. *Cancer.* 1982;**50**:652–658.

Kovnar E, McHaney V, Ayers D, et al. Effects of treatment sequence on ototoxicity due to cisplatin and radiation in pediatric brain tumor patients. *Proc Am Soc Clin Oncol.* 1991;**10**:311.

Kramer A, Paredes J, Dimery I, et al. The effect of diethyldithiocarbamate (DDTC) on responses, toxicity and pharmacology of cisplatin in patients with recurrent squamous cell carcinoma of the head and neck. *Dev Oncol.* 1988;**54**:484–490.

Kris MG, Gralia RJ, Tyson LB, et al. Controlling delayed vomiting: Double-blind, randomized trial comparing placebo, dexamethasone alone, and metoclopramide plus dexamethasone in patients receiving cisplatin. *J Clin Oncol.* 1989;**7**(1):108–114.

Leichman L, McDonald B, Dindogru A, et al. Cisplatin. An active drug in the treatment of disseminated gastric cancer. *Cancer.* 1984;**53**(1):18–22.

Leonard BJ, Eccleston E, Jones D, et al. Antileukemic and nephrotoxic properties of platinum compounds. *Nature (Lond).* 1971;**234**:43–45.

Le Roy AF. Some quantitative data on *cis*-dichlorodiammineplatinum(II) species in solution. *Cancer Treat Rep.* 1979;**63**:231–233.

Lewis KP, Medina WD. Cellulitis and fibrosis due to *cis*-diamminedichloroplatinum(II) (platinol) infiltration. *Cancer Treat Rep.* 1980;**64**:1162–1163.

Lindeman G, Kefford R, Stuart-Harris R. Cisplatin neurotoxicity (letter). *N Engl J Med.* 1990;**323**:64–65.

Livingston RB. Cisplatin in the treatment of solid tumors: Effect of dose and schedule (editorial). *J Natl Cancer Inst.* 1989;**81**:724–725.

Llopis B, Gallego J, Momp'o JA, et al. Thiotepa versus Adriamycin versus cisplatinum in the intravesical prophylaxis of superficial bladder tumors. *Eur Urol.* 1985;**11**:73–78.

Loehrer PJ, Einhorn LH. Cisplatin. *Ann Intern Med.* 1984;**100**:704–713.

Loehrer PJ, Elson P, Kuebler JP, et al. Advanced bladder cancer: A prospective intergroup trial comparing single agent (COOP) versus M-VAC combination therapy (INT 0078). *Proc Am Soc Clin Oncol.* 1990;**9**:132.

Loehrer PJ, Turner S, Kubitis P, et al. A prospective randomized study of 5-fluorouracil (5FU) alone or with cisplatin (P) in the treatment of metastatic colorectal cancer: A Hoosier Oncology Group trial. *Proc Am Soc Clin Oncol.* 1987;**6**:76.

Loehrer PJ, Einhorn LH, Williams SD, Hui SL, Estes NC, Penningtonk. Cisplatin plus 5-Fu for the treatment of adenocarcinoma of the colon. *Cancer Treat Rep.* 1985;**69**:1359–1363.

Lokich J, Anderson N, Bern M, et al. Etoposide admixed with cisplatin. Phase I clinical investigation of 72-hour infusion. *Cancer.* 1989;**63**:818–821.

Lund B, Hansen M, Hansen OP, Hansen HH. Combined high-dose carboplatin and cisplatin, and ifosfamide in previously untreated ovarian cancer patients with residual disease. *J Clin Oncol.* 1990;**8**(7):1226–1230.

Madias NE, Harrington JT. Platinum nephrotoxicity. *Am J Med.* 1978;**65**:307–314.

Mainsworth JD, Johnson DH, Hande KR, Greco FA. Chemotherapy of advanced non-small-cell lung cancer: A randomized trial of three cisplatin-based chemotherapy regimens. *Am J Clin Oncol.* 1989;**12**(4):345–349.

Mangioni C, Bolis G, Pecorelli S, et al. Randomized trial in advanced ovarian cancer comparing cisplatin and carboplatin. *J Natl Cancer Inst.* 1989;**81**(19):1464–1471.

Marin AC, Rierson B. Peripheral neuropathy secondary to *cis*-dichlorodiammino-platinum(II) (platinol): Treatment for advanced ovarian cancer. *Ariz Med.* 1979;**36**:898–899.

McClay EF, Mastrangelo MJ, Sprandio JD, et al. The importance of tamoxifen to a cisplatin-containing regimen in the treatment of metastatic melanoma. *Cancer* 1989;**63**:1292–1295.

Menard O, Martinet Y, Lamy P. Cisplatin-induced atrial fibrillation. *J Clin Oncol.* 1990;**8**:192–193.

Merd GM, Arnold AM, Green JA, et al. Epileptic seizure associated with cisplatin administration. *Cancer Treat Rep.* 1982;**66**:1719–1722.

Mobley WC, Loening SA, Narayana AS, Culp DA. Use of intravesical cisplatin and mitomycin-C for recurrent transitional cell carcinoma of bladder refractory to thiotepa. *Urology.* 1986;**27**:335–339.

Mollman JE, Hogan WM, Glover DJ, McCluskey LF. Unusual presentation of *cis*-platinum neuropathy. *Neurology.* 1988;**38**:488–490.

O'Connell MJ, Moertel CG, Kvols LK, et al. Clinical trial of cisplatin and intensive course 5-fluorouracil for the treatment of advanced colorectal cancer. *Am J Clin Oncol.* 1986;**9**(3):192–195.

Ohkawa K, Tsukada Y, Dohzono H, et al. The effects of co-administration of selenium and cis-platin (CDDP) on CDDP-induced toxicity and antitumor activity. *Br J Cancer.* 1988;**58**:38–41.

Ostrow S, Hahn D, Wiernik PH, Richard RD. Ophthalmologic toxicity after *cis*-dichlorodiammineplatinum(II) therapy. *Cancer Treat Rep.* 1978;**62**(10):1591–1594.

Ozols RF, Corden BF, Jacob J, et al. High dose cisplatin in hypertonic saline. *Ann Intern Med.* 1984;**100**:19–24.

Ozols RF, Young RC. High-dose cisplatin therapy in ovarian cancer. *Semin Oncol.* 1985;**12**(4S):21–30.

Piehl IJ, Meyer D, Perlia CP, Wolfe VI. Effects of *cis*-diamminedichloroplatinum (NSC-119875) on hearing function in man. *Cancer Chemother Rep.* 1974;**58**:871–875.

Pollera CF, Giannarelli D. Prognostic factors influencing cisplatin-induced emesis. Definition and validation of a predictive logistic model. *Cancer.* 1989;**64**(5):1117–1122.

Prestayko AW, Cadiz M, Crooke ST. Incompatibility of aluminum-containing IV administration equipment with *cis*-dichlorodiammineplatinum(II) administration. *Cancer Treat Rep.* 1979;**63**:2118–2119.

Rainey JM, Alberts DS. Rapid administration schedule for cisplatinum–mannitol. *Med Pediatr Oncol.* 1978;**4**:371–375.

Reed FF, Behrens BL, Yuspa SH, et al. Differences in cisplatin DNA adduct formation in sensitive and resistant sublines of human ovarian cancer cells. *Proc Am Assoc Cancer Res.* 1986;**27**:285.

Reed FF, Ozols RF, Torme R, et al. Platinum–DNA adducts in leukocyte DNA correlate with decreased response in ovarian cancer patients receiving platinum based chemotherapy. *Proc Natl Acad Sci USA.* 1987;**84**:5024–5028.

Reichman B, Markman M, Hakes T, et al. Phase II trial of intraperitoneal cisplatin and etoposide in recurrent refractory ovarian cancer (abstract). *Proc Am Soc Clin Oncol.* 1988;**7**:135.

Repta AJ, Long DF, Hincal AA. *cis*-Dichlorodiammineplatinum(II) stability in aqueous vehicles: An alternative view. *Cancer Treat Rep.* 1979;**63**:229–230.

Rive JA, Cruthers DM, Pinto AL, Lippard SJ. The major adduct of the antitumor drug cis-diamminedichloroplatinum(II) with DNA bends the diplex by 40° toward the major genome. *Proc Natl Acad Sci USA.* 1988;**85**:4158–4161.

Roberts JJ, Pascoe JM. Cross-linking of complementary strands of DNA in mammalian cells by antitumor platinum compounds. *Nature (Lond).* 1972;**235**:282–284.

Roelofs RI, Hrushesky W, Rogin J, Rosenberg L. Peripheral sensory neuropathy and cisplatin chemotherapy. *Neurology.* 1984;**34**:934–938.

Roila F, Tonato M, Basurto C, et al. Antiemetic activity of high doses of metoclopramide combined with methylprednisolone versus metoclopramide alone in cisplatin-treated cancer patients: A randomized double-blind trial of the Italian Oncology Group for Clinical Research. *J Clin Oncol.* 1987;**5**(1):141–149.

Rosenberg B. Possible mechanisms for the antitumor activity of platinum coordination complexes. *Cancer Chemother Rep.* 1975;**59**:589–598.

Rosenberg B, Van Camp L, Krigas T. Inhibition of cell division in *Escherichia coli* by electrolysis products from a platinum electrode. *Nature (Lond).* 1965;**205**:698–699.

Rossoff AH, Slayton RE, Perlia CP. Preliminary clinical experience with cis-diamminedichloroplatinum(II) (NSC119875, CACP). *Cancer.* 1972;**30**(6):1451–1456.

Rozencweig M, Von Hoff D, Slavik M, Muggia FM. Cis-diamminedichloroplatinum (II): A new anti-cancer drug. *Ann Intern Med.* 1977;**86**:803–812.

Ruckdeschel JC, Finkelstein DM, Mason BA, Creech RH. Chemotherapy for metastatic non-small-cell bronchogenic carcinoma: EST 2575, Generation V—A randomized comparison of four cisplatin-containing regimens. *J Clin Oncol.* 1985;**3**(1):72–79.

Salem P, Hall SW, Benjamin RS, et al. Clinical phase I–II study of cis-dichlorodiammineplatinum(II) given by continuous IV infusion. *Cancer Treat Rep.* 1978;**62**(10):1553–1555.

Schabel FM, Trader MW, Laster WR, Corbett TH, Griswold DP. Cis-dichlorodiammineplatinum(II): Combination chemotherapy and cross-resistance studies with tumors of mice. *Cancer Treat Rep.* 1979;**63**:1459–1473.

Schilsky RL, Anderson T. Hypomagnesemia and renal magnesium wasting in patients receiving cisplatin. *Ann Intern Med.* 1979;**90**:929–931.

Sexauer C, Khan A, Burger P, et al. Cisplatinum in recurrent pediatric brain tumors: A POG phase II study (abstract). *Proc Am Soc Clin Oncol.* 1984;**3**:84.

Sierocki JS, Hilaris BS, Hopfan S, et al. Dichlorodiammineplatinum(II) and VP-16-213: An active induction regimen for small-cell carcinoma of the lung. *Cancer Treat Rep.* 1979;**63**:1593–1597.

Smith PHS, Taylor DM. Distribution and retention of the antitumor agent ^{195m}Pt-cis-diamminedichloroplatinum(II) in man. *J Nucl Med.* 1974;**15**:349–351.

Stewart DJ, Eapen L, Hirte WE, et al. Intra-arterial cisplatin for bladder cancer. *J Urol.* 1987;**138**:302–305.

Stewart DJ, Molepo M, Hungerholtz H, et al. Concentrations of platinum in intracerebral vs extracerebral human tumors following intravenous cisplatin. *J Neurol Oncol.* 1989;**71**:527.

Talley RW, O'Bryan RM, Gutterman JU. Clinical evaluation of toxic effects of cis-diamminedichloroplatinum (NSC-119875): Phase I clinical study. *Cancer Chemother Rep.* 1973;**57**:465–471.

Thompson SW, Davis LE, Kornfeld M, et al. Cisplatin neuropathy: Clinical, electrophysiologic, morphologic, and toxicologic studies. *Cancer.* 1984;**54**:1269–1275.

Trissel LA, Fulton B, Tramonte SM. Visual compatibility of ondansetron with chemotherapeutic agents, antibiotics, and other selected drugs during simulated Y-site injection (abstract #P-468R). In: *25th Annual ASHP Midyear Clinical Meetings and Exhibit, Las Vegas, Nevada, December 1990.* Bethesda, MD: American Society of Hospital Pharmacists; 1990.

Troner M, Birch R, Omura GA, Williams S. Phase III comparison of cisplatin alone versus cisplatin, doxorubicin and cyclophosphamide in the treatment of bladder (urothelial) cancer: A Southeastern Cancer Study Group trial. *J Urol.* 1987;**137**(4):660–662.

Tsai C-M, Gazdar AF, Venzon DJ, et al. Lack of in vitro synergy between etoposide and cis-diamminedichloroplatinum(II). *Cancer Res.* 1989;**49**:2390–2397.

Von Hoff DD, Reichert CM, Cunco R, et al. Demyelination of peripheral nerves associated with cis-diamminedichloroplatinum(II) (DDP) therapy. *Proc Am Assoc Cancer Res.* 1979;**20**:91.

Von Hoff DD, Slavik M, Muggia FM. Allergic reactions to cis-platinum (letter). *Lancet.* 1976;**1**:90.

Wiesenfeld M, Reinders E, Corder M, et al. Successful retreatment with cis-dichlorodiammineplatinum(II) after allergic reactions. *Cancer Treat Rep.* 1979;**63**(2):219–221.

Wilding G, Caruso R, Lawrence TS, et al. Retinal toxicity after high-dose cisplatin therapy. *J Clin Oncol.* 1985;**3**:1683–1689.

Willox JC, McAllister EJ, Sangster G, Kaye SB. Effects of magnesium supplementation in testicular cancer patients receiving cisplatin: A randomized trial. *Br J Cancer.* 1986;**54**(1):19–23.

Wiltshaw E, Carr B. cis-Platinum(II) diamminedichloride. Clinical experience of the Royal Marsden Hospital and Institute of Cancer Research, London. *Recent Results Cancer Res.* 1974;**48**:178–182.

Wiltshaw E, Evans B, Harland S. Phase III randomized trial cisplatin versus JM8 (carboplatin) in 112 ovarian cancer patients, stages III and IV (abstract). *Proc Am Soc Clin Oncol.* 1985;**4**:121.

Wiltshaw E, Kroner T. Phase II study of cis-dichlorodiammineplatinum (NSC-119875) in advanced adenocarcinoma of the ovary. *Cancer Treat Rep.* 1976;**60**:55–60.

Winkler K, Beron G, Kotz R, et al. Adjuvant chemotherapy

in osteosarcoma—Effects of cisplatinum, BCD, and fibroblast interferon in sequential combination with HD-MTX and Adriamycin. Preliminary results of the Coss BO study. *J Cancer Res Clin Oncol.* 1983;**106S**:1–7.

Yagoda A, Watson RC, Gonzales-Vitale JC, et al. cis-Dichlorodiammineplatinum(II) in advanced bladder cancer. *Cancer Treat Rep.* 1976;**60**:917–923.

Yee GC, Crom WR, Champion JE, et al. Cisplatin-induced changes in bleomycin elimination. *Cancer Treat Rep.* 1983;**67**:587–589.

Ziccarelli A, Pazdur R, Al-Sarraf M, et al. Metoclopramide and lorazepam vs metoclopramide alone for prevention of cisplatin induced nausea and vomiting (abstract). *Proc Am Soc Clin Oncol.* 1985;**4**:262.

Zwelling LA, Anderson T, Koln KW. DNA–protein and DNA interstrand crosslinking by *cis-* and *trans-*platinum(II) diamminedichloride in L1210 mouse leukemia cells and its relation to cytotoxicity. *Cancer Res.* 1979;**39**:365–369.

Zwelling LA, Michaels S, Schwartz H, et al. DNA crosslinking as an indicator of sensitivity and resistance of mouse L1210 leukemia to *cis*-diamminedichloroplatinum(II) and L-phenylalanine mustard. *Cancer Res.* 1981;**41**:640–649.

Cladribine

■ Other Names

2-CdA; Leustatin® (Ortho Biotech); NSC-105014-F, 2-chlorodeoxyadenosine.

■ Chemistry

Structure of cladribine

The complete chemical name is 2-chloro-2′-deoxy-β-D-adenosine (CdA). This agent is an adenosine deaminase-resistant purine deoxynucleoside antimetabolite. Resistance to adenosine deaminase is afforded by the substitution of chlorine for hydrogen in the 2-position of the purine ring (Carson et al 1984). The drug is structurally related to fludarabine and pentostatin, but has a different mechanism of action. The molecular weight is 285.7.

■ Antitumor Activity

Cladribine has antitumor activity in a variety of lymphoid malignancies. It is currently approved by the U.S. Food and Drug Administration for first- and second-line therapy for hairy cell leukemia (see the table). A unique feature of this activity is the extremely high percentage of complete responses obtained even in pretreated patients (Tallman et al 1992). The median times for recovery of normal platelet counts and for correction of anemia are 2 and 6 weeks, respectively, from the start of therapy. Patients with active infections at the time of therapy recover their platelet and red blood cell counts at 5 and 13 weeks, respectively (Juliusson and Liliemark 1992).

Cladribine has some activity in heavily pretreated patients with non-Hodgkin's lymphoma. A 20% complete response rate is described in 40 patients with low-grade lymphocytic lymphoma treated with one to six courses of cladribine (Kay et al 1992). The median duration of response in this study was 6 months. Similarly, a 20% complete response rate is reported among 10 patients with cutaneous T-cell lymphomas (Saven et al 1989). The median duration of response was 19 months. A 33% overall response rate was reported among 12 patients with mycosis fungoides (Kuzel et al 1992).

Acute and chronic myelogenous leukemias are also sensitive to cladribine. A 100% complete response rate is reported in five patients with chronic myelogenous leukemia (Saven et al 1992a). A 47% complete response rate is described in relapsed acute myelogenous leukemia (Santana et al 1992). In contrast, acute and chronic lymphocytic leukemias are much less responsive to cladribine (Saven et al 1991, Piro et al 1988, Santana et al 1992); however, Tallman et al (1992) have recently described a 62% partial response rate in patients with refractory chronic lymphocytic leukemia.

In nonhematologic malignancies, a 29% partial response rate is reported in patients with astrocytomas (Saven et al 1992b).

In vitro cytotoxicity studies using human colony-forming tumor cells suggest that cladribine is

ANTITUMOR ACTIVITY OF CLADRIBINE IN HAIRY CELL LEUKEMIA

Number of Evaluable Patients	% Previously Treated*	Objective Response Overall (%)	Complete (%)	Median Duration (mo)	Reference
147	35	98	85	>14	Piro et al 1990, 1992
46	39	89	78	>7.8	Estey et al 1992
16	69	NL	75	>12	Juliusson and Liliemark 1992
16	87	100	75	NL	Lauria et al 1992
15	30	100	60	NL	Hoffman et al 1992

*Interferon alfa and/or pentostatin (2-deoxycoformycin).

much less active against solid tumors (Hutton and Von Hoff 1986). Relatively insensitive tumors (< 10% sensitive) included those derived from patients with breast, colorectal, kidney, and stomach cancer. A few solid tumors that were sensitive to cladribine at either 1.0 or 10 µg/mL include those derived from patients with lung cancer, breast cancer, and malignant melanoma (Hutton and Von Hoff 1986).

■ Mechanism of Action

For antitumor activity, cladribine must be phosphorylated intracellularly to its triphosphate form (CdATP), which is believed to be the active metabolite (Carson et al 1980). Unlike pentostatin, cladribine is not an inhibitor of adenosine deaminase. The phosphorylation of cladribine to 2-CdATP is mediated by deoxycytidine kinase (EC 2.7.1.74). Excess deoxycytidine can inhibit this required activation step. The triphosphate metabolite, 2-CdATP, accumulates in cells rich in kinase activity and poor in deoxynucleotidases. The drug is also incorporated into DNA (Carson et al 1983) and leads to the accumulation of DNA strand breaks (Seto et al 1985). The strand breaks probably result from drug-induced inhibition of several enzymes necessary for DNA repair. These include DNA polymerase, DNA ligase, and ribonucleotide reductase. RNA synthesis is also impaired by cladribine.

Importantly, nicotine adenine dinucleotide (NAD) levels fall progressively in lymphocytes treated with cladribine (Seto et al 1985). This depletion of NAD may be triggered by an increase in the repair-related poly-ADP-ribose formation following cladribine. Thus, in resting lymphocytes, NAD depletion followed by ATP depletion may constitute the principal mechanism of cytotoxicity (Seto et al 1985).

Other studies suggest that the final common pathway for cladribine-induced cytotoxicity involves apoptosis, or programmed cell death (Carrera et al 1991, Robertson et al 1991). This has been shown to occur in both normal and malignant lymphocytes treated with cladribine in vitro (Carrera et al 1991). This process may also explain the DNA strand breaks observed in other mechanistic studies of cladribine. Because these effects occur in both dividing and nondividing lymphocytes, cladribine is not believed to be cell cycle phase specific for S phase (Carrera et al 1992b). In contrast, cladribine does cause cells to accumulate at the G_1/S phase junction, suggesting that cytotoxicity is associated with events crucial to cell entry into S phase (Huang et al 1986).

■ Availability and Storage

Cladribine is commercially available from Ortho Biotech, Raritan, New Jersey. The drug is supplied as a 1 mg/mL sterile solution in 0.9% Sodium Chloride for Injection, USP. The intact vials should be stored under refrigeration (2–8°C). No preservative is present in the vial.

■ Preparation for Use, Stability, and Admixture

The desired dose is aseptically removed from the vial and added to 500 to 1000 mL of normal saline for infusion over 24 hours. These solutions are chemically stable for 72 hours but contain no preservative. The drug is stable with PVC plastic infusion containers for 24 hours at room temperature and light, and for 7 days in Pharmacia Deltec medication cassettes. Individual vials must *not* be used in a multidose fashion and should be discarded after a single use. The drug is also compatible with dextrose solutions containing saline, and with Bacteriostatic Sodium Chloride, USP (containing 0.9% benzyl alcohol) (Santana et al 1991).

Reconstitution in 5% dextrose is not recommended. The incompatibility with dextrose produces an immediate 13% loss on admixture. It is recommended that all solutions be filtered through a 0.22 µm filter prior to use. Freezing of vials is not recommended as precipitates may form. For the 7-day infusion dose, the drug should be reconstituted in bacteriostatic sodium chloride containing 0.9% benzyl alcohol.

■ Dosage

In hairy cell leukemia, the most commonly used dose is 0.1 mg/kg/d × 7 days, given as a continuous intravenous infusion (Piro et al 1990, 1992, Juliusson and Liliemark 1992). The same dose is used in the treatment of non-Hodgkin's lymphomas (Kay et al 1992) and in myelogenous leukemias (Saven et al 1992a, Santana et al 1992). The FDA-approved dose for hairy cell leukemia is 0.09 mg/kg/d as a continuous infusion for 7 consecutive days. On a body surface area basis, this dose is approximately 4 mg/m^2/d (Estey et al 1992). The recommended dose for further studies in acute leukemia in children is 8.9 mg/m^2/d × 5 days as a continuous intravenous infusion (Santana et al 1991).

■ Administration

Cladribine is administered intravenously as a continuous infusion for 5 to 7 days. A final volume of at least 100 mL and up to 500 mL is recommended. Investigational regimens using experimental enteric coated oral capsules and subcutaneous injections have also been evaluated in patients with chronic lymphocytic leukemia (Liliemark et al 1992).

■ Drug Interactions

In vitro studies suggest that there may be cross-resistance between cladribine and mechlorethamine (Nagourney et al 1992).

■ Pharmacokinetics

During the first few days of infusion (0.2 mg/kg/d), plasma cladribine levels were approximately 10 nM (Carson et al 1984). A 24-hour infusion of 0.14 mg/kg provided steady state plasma levels of 22.5 nM in another trial (Liliemark and Juliusson 1991). The drug appeared to be completely cleared from the plasma over a period of 1 to 3 days after stopping the infusion (Carson et al 1984).

By use of a high performance liquid chromatography technique, half-lives of 35 min (α) and 6.7 h (β) were reported (Lilliemark and Juliusson 1991). The volume of distribution was 9.2 +/− 5.4 L/kg. The mean area under the plasma concentration × time curve (AUC) was 763 nM · h and 724 nM · h for intravenous and subcutaneous doses of 0.14 mg/kg/d (Liliemark et al 1992). This represents 97% bioavailability for the subcutaneous dose. The AUC after an oral capsule dose of 0.28 mg/kg ranged from 210 to 480 nM · h (Liliemark et al 1992). This increased to 295 to 580 nM · h with an oral solution in saline. These investigational studies suggest that the oral bioavailability of cladribine is approximately 50% (Liliemark et al 1992).

■ Side Effects and Toxicity

Neutrophil counts decrease temporarily in approximately 60% of patients receiving cladribine. The decrease is maximal in the first 1 to 2 weeks after starting therapy and typically resolves by week 4 (Estey et al 1992). Most patients also experience significant decrements in the number of circulating CD-4 (helper) and CD-8 (suppressor) T cells. This may last for 26 to 34 weeks posttherapy (Estey et al 1992). Febrile episodes are common (46%) in hairy cell leukemia patients, but are not a direct side effect of the drug. Rather, the fevers appear to correspond to the time of maximal lysis of the malignant cells and may occur as a result of the release of endogenous pyrogen(s).

Infections are common in patients receiving cladribine. Typical sites of infection include the lungs and sites of venous access. The incidence of opportunistic infection is less than 30% in most series. Septicemia is also reported with cladribine therapy, but the etiologic agent is typically not identified; however, fungal infections have been documented in about 20 to 30% of cases. Hairy cell leukemia patients with pancytopenia and especially lymphopenia prior to cladribine appear to be at increased risk of developing a serious infection (Juliusson and Liliemark 1992).

A rash may occur in 50% of patients with hairy cell leukemia (Estey et al 1992). In contrast, most patients do not experience nausea and vomiting, hair loss, or abnormalities in liver or kidney function following cladribine therapy (Piro et al 1990).

REFERENCES

Carrera CJ, Cottam HB, Wasson DB, et al. Stability and oral activity of 2-chloro-2′-ara-fluoro-2′-deoxyadenosine (CAFdA) in a SCID mouse model of chronic lymphocytic leukemia (CLL). *Proc Am Soc Clin Oncol.* 1992a;**11**:112.

Carrera CJ, Piro LD, Saven A, et al. Chlorodeoxyadenosine toxicity in hairy cell leukemia. Effects of phorbol ester and polyamine synthesis inhibitors on apoptosis. *Proc Am Assoc Cancer Res.* 1992b;**33**:150.

Carrera CJ, Terai C, Piro L, et al. 2CdA chemotherapy triggers programmed cell death in normal and malignant lymphocytes. *Int J Purine Pyrimidine Res.* 1991;**2**(suppl 1):38.

Carson DA, Wasson DB, Beutler E. Antileukemic and immunosuppressive activity of 2-chloro-2′-deoxyadenosine. *Proc Natl Acad Sci USA.* 1984;**81**:2232–2236.

Carson DA, Wasson DB, Kaye J, et al. Deoxycytidine kinase-mediated toxicity of deoxyadenosine analogs toward malignant human lymphoblasts *in vitro* and toward murine L-1210 leukemia in vivo. *Proc Natl Acad Sci USA.* 1980;**77**:6865–6869.

Carson DA, Wasson DB, Taetle R, et al. Specific toxicity of 2-chlorodeoxyadenosine toward resting and proliferating human lymphocytes. *Blood.* 1983;**62**(4):737–743.

Estey EH, Kurzrock R, Kantarjian HM, et al. Treatment of hairy cell leukemia with 2-chlorodeoxyadenosine (2-CdA). *Blood.* 1992;**79**(4):882–887.

Hoffman M, Rai KR, Janson D, et al. Comparison of complete remission (CR) rates among previously treated or untreated hairy cell leukemia (HCL) patients (PTS) with 2-chlorodeoxyadenosine (CdA). *Proc Am Soc Clin Oncol.* 1992;**11**:271.

Huang M-C, Ashmun RA, Avery TL, et al. Effects of cytotoxicity of 2-chloro-2′-deoxyadenosine and 2-bromo-2′-deoxyadenosine on cell growth, clonogenicity, DNA synthesis, and cell cycle kinetics. *Cancer Res.* 1986;**46**:2362–2368.

Hutton JJ, Von Hoff DD. Cytotoxicity of 2-chlorodeoxyadenosine in a human tumor colony-forming assay. *Cancer Drug Delivery.* 1986;**3**(2):115–122.

Juliusson G, Liliemark J. Rapid recovery from cytopenia in hairy cell leukemia after treatment with 2-chloro-2′-deoxyadenosine (CdA): Relation to opportunistic infections. *Blood.* 1992;**79**(4):888–894.

Kay AC, Saven A, Carrera DA, et al. 2-Chlorodeoxyadenosine: Treatment of low grade lymphomas. *J Clin Oncol.* 1992;**10**:371–377.

Kuzel T, Samuelson E, Roenigk H, et al. Phase II trial of 2-chlorodeoxyadenosine (2-CdA) for the treatment of mycosis fungoides or the Sézary syndrome (MF/SS). *Proc Am Soc Clin Oncol.* 1992;**11**:321.

Lauria F, Benfenati D, Zinzani PL, et al. High complete remission rate in patients with hairy cell leukemia treated with 2-chlorodeoxyadenosine (abstract). *Ann Oncol.* 1992;**3**(suppl 1):139.

Liliemark J, Juliusson G. On the pharmacokinetics of 2-chloro-2′-deoxyadenosine in humans. *Cancer Res.* 1991;**51**:5570–5572.

Liliemark J, Albertioni F, Pettersson B, et al. Bioavailability of oral and subcutaneous 2-chloro-2′-deoxyadenosine (CdA). *Proc Am Soc Clin Oncol.* 1992;**11**:112.

Nagourney RA, Evans S, Su YZ, et al. 2-Chlorodeoxyadenosine cross-resistance patterns in human hematologic tumors. *Proc Am Assoc Cancer Res.* 1992;**33**:510.

Piro LD, Carrera CJ, Beutler E, et al. 2-Chlorodeoxyadenosine: An effective new agent for the treatment of chronic lymphocytic leukemia. *Blood.* 1988;**72**(3):1069–1073.

Piro LD, Carrera CJ, Carson DA, et al. Lasting remissions in hairy cell leukemia induced by a single infusion of 2-chlorodeoxyadenosine. *N Engl J Med.* 1990;**322**:1117–1121.

Piro LD, Saven A, Ellison D, et al. Prolonged complete remissions following 2-chlorodeoxyadenosine (2-CdA) in hairy cell leukemia (HCL). *Proc Am Soc Clin Oncol.* 1992;**11**:259.

Robertson L, Chubb S, Story M, et al. Induction of DNA cleavage in chronic lymphocytic leukemia cells by chlorodeoxyadenosine and fludarabine. *Proc Am Assoc Cancer Res.* 1991;**32**:415.

Santana VM, Mirro J Jr, Harwood FC, et al. A phase I clinical trial of 2-chlorodeoxyadenosine in pediatric patients with acute leukemia. *J Clin Oncol.* 1991;**9**(3):416–422.

Santana VM, Mirro JM, Kearns C, et al. 2-Chlorodeoxyadenosine produces a high rate of complete hematologic remission in relapsed acute myeloid leukemia. *J Clin Oncol.* 1992;**10**:364–370.

Saven A, Carrera CJ, Carson DA, et al. 2-Chlorodeoxyadenosine: An active agent in the treatment of cutaneous T-cell lymphomas (abstract). *Blood.* 1989;**74**(suppl 1):239A.

Saven A, Carrera CJ, Carson DA. 2-Chlorodeoxyadenosine treatment of refractory chronic lymphocytic leukemia. *Leuk Lymph.* 1991;**5**(suppl):133–138.

Saven A, Figueroa ML, Piro LD, et al. Complete hematological remissions in chronic myelogenous leukemia (CML) following 2-chlorodeoxyadenosine (2-CdA). *Proc Am Soc Clin Oncol.* 1992a;**11**:261.

Saven A, Waltz T, Carrera CJ, et al. Phase I study of 2-chlorodeoxyadenosine (2-CdA) in non-hematologic malignancies. *Proc Am Soc Clin Oncol.* 1992b;**11**:119.

Seto S, Carrera CJ, Kubota M, et al. Mechanism of deoxyadenosine and 2-chlorodeoxyadenosine toxicity to nondividing human lymphocytes. *J Clin Invest.* 1985;**75**:377–383.

Tallman M, Hakimian D, Variakojis D. A single cycle of 2-chlorodeoxyadenosine results in complete remissions in the majority of patients with hairy cell leukemia. *Blood* 1992;**80**:2203–2209.

Corticosteroids

■ Chemistry

Corticosteroids comprise the synthetic steroidal congeners of the natural adrenal hormone hydrocortisone (cortisol). They are also called *glucocorticoids*. The major derivatives include prednisone, methylprednisolone, triamcinolone, and dexamethasone. Pharmaceutical formulations include well-absorbed oral forms, injectable water-soluble esters, and repository forms, usually as the acetates.

Various structure–activity relationships have allowed the modification of these compounds to decrease mineralocorticoid activity (salt retention) to enhance potency and to extend the duration of action (see the table on the opposite page).

■ Antitumor Activity

Corticosteroids are most often employed for lympholytic effects in acute and chronic lymphocytic leukemias (Ezdinli et al 1969), in Hodgkin's and non-Hodgkin's lymphomas (Hall et al 1967), and in multiple myeloma (Alexanian et al 1986). Corticosteroids are also active in breast cancer (Lemon 1959), as in the "Cooper regimen" (CMF-VP) for estrogenic hormone-resistant disease (Cooper 1969).

Corticosteroids are also used in cancer patients for their anti-inflammatory effects (eg, the edema from cranial metastases); antihypercalcemic effects (by enhanced excretion of calcium and impaired calcium absorption); (3) effects as a mild euphoriant and appetite stimulant; suppression of tumor-related fever (eg, lymphomas or hypernephromas) or antiallergic effects (in the control of drug reactions, etc); and ability to block cortical pathways involved in emetic drug reactions to cancer chemotherapy (Plezia and Alberts 1985, Aapro et al 1981).

■ Mechanism of Action

The corticosteroids produce diverse physiologic effects. These include metabolic effects on glucose: increased blood glucose, increased gluconeogenesis and glycogenolysis, and decreased peripheral uptake of glucose. There are also effects on protein metabolism, mainly increased degradation and decreased synthesis; lipids are mobilized into the circulation as free fatty acids broken down from triglycerides. Circulatory effects of corticosteroids lead to increased cardiac output, sodium retention, and sensitivity to catecholamines. There is an increase in short-term musculoskeletal work capacity, but with chronic therapy muscular atrophy can ensue. Finally, corticosteroids are widely used for immunomodulation noted by reduced antibody formation, stabilization of mast cell and lysosomes, decreased leukocyte chemotaxis and phagocytosis, decreased Fc receptor expression, reduced blastogenic response to T-cell mitogens, and impaired delayed hypersensitivity.

The corticosteroids consistently alter the trafficking of peripheral blood leukocytes (Udkow 1978). Following single doses of either 100 to 200 mg hydrocortisone or 40 mg of prednisone, the total granulocyte pool is increased by about 4000/mm³. The peak occurs 4 to 6 hours after the dose and counts return to normal 24 hours after a dose. The increase in granulocytes is dually caused by increased bone marrow release and inhibition of white cell egress from the bloodstream. A slight shift of cells from the marginating (endothelial-adherent) fraction to the bloodstream also occurs;

FORMULATIONS AND DOSES OF GLUCOCORTICOSTEROIDS

Generic Drug Name (Exemplary Trade Name)	Preparations Available	Salt-Retaining Activity	Equivalent Dose* (mg)
Hydrocortisone sodium succinate (Solu-Cortef®)	Tablets: 5, 10, 20 mg Injection (aqueous): 100, 250, 500, 1000-mg vials (10-mL vial)	+	20
Hydrocortisone sodium phosphate (Hydrocortone®)	Injection: 50 mg/mL		20
Prednisone (Deltasone®, Meticorten®, many generics)	Tablets: 1, 2.5, 5, 20, 50 mg	+	5
Prednisolone sodium succinate (Delta-Cortef®, Meticortelone®)	Tablets: 1, 2.5, 5 mg	+	5
Methylprednisolone (Medrol®) Sodium succinate (Solu-Medrol®) Acetate (Depo-Medrol®)	Tablets: 2, 4, 16 mg Capsules: 2, 4 mg Injection: 40, 125, 500, 1000 mg Injection: 40 mg/mL	−	4
Triamcinolone (Aristocort®, Kenacort®)	Tablets: 1, 2, 4, 8 and 16 mg Syrup: 2 and 4 mg/5 mL	−	2
Dexamethasone phosphate (Decadron®)	Tablets: 0.25, 0.5, 0.75, 1.5, 4 mg Elixir: 500 µg/5 mL Injection: 4, 24 mg/mL	−	0.75

*Dose equivalent to 20 mg of hydrocortisone (eg, 20 mg hydrocortisone = 5 mg prednisone, etc).

however, diapedesis of cells out of the vascular compartment is impaired following administration of corticosteroids. An important implication of this in cancer patients is that delayed hypersensitivity skin test responses may be significantly "blunted" by most corticosteroids. A notable exception is dexamethasone, which actually enhances granulocyte egress and therefore accumulation at inflammatory sites (Peters et al 1972). Lymphocytes, particularly T cells, are also affected, as is the monocyte fraction. Both lymphocytes and monocytes are inhibited in movement out of the blood to inflammatory sites. Eosinophils are consistently depressed too.

Selective binding of cortisol to lymphoid cells has been observed and probably explains the apparent specificity of corticosteroid antitumor effects to lymph-derived tumors (Baxter et al 1971). Corticosteroid–protein binding to "receptors" in acute myeloblastic leukemia cells has also been noted (Lippman et al 1975).

A report by Lippman et al (1978) further delineated the role of glucocorticoid receptors in human leukemias. Although normal lymphoblasts contain relatively small numbers of receptors (< 2500 per cell), leukemic lymphoblasts possess significantly larger numbers of glucocorticoid receptors (2500–6000 per cell). Furthermore, they found that high receptor numbers correlated with complete remission duration following corticosteroid induction therapy. Interestingly, this correlation was independent of patient age, white blood cell count, or leukemic cell type. Thus, glucocorticoid receptors appear to have clinical significance in leukemia and may allow for more specific tailoring of corticosteroid therapy in this disease.

The exact cellular mechanisms for antitumor effects are not well known but probably relate to steroid-induced inhibition of glucose transport or phosphorylation reactions. This could induce intracellular deficits in the energy available for cellular division. Alternatively, glucocorticoids may be cytotoxic to immature lymphocytes by a process of programmed cell death or apoptosis (Duke et al 1983). This "cell suicide" process involves a sequential series of steps culminating in DNA fragmentation and has been well demonstrated in the destruction of immature normal thymocytes (Roholl et al 1983). Following glucocorticoid binding there is an increase in cytosolic Ca^{2+} followed by the synthesis of new mRNA and the activation of endonucleases that fragment DNA and produces cell killing. Some studies have suggested that DNA fragmentation may result from activation of topoisomerase II enzymes.

When corticosteroids are used as antiemetics, the mechanism of action involves blockade of cerebral cortical innervation of the emetic center. This is believed to be mediated by blocked release of arachidonic acid from phospholipids thereby inhibiting prostaglandin synthesis in the central nervous system (Gryglewski et al 1975, Hong and Levine 1976).

■ Availability and Storage

See the earlier table for availability. Follow manufacturer's recommendations for storage.

■ Preparation for Use, Stability, and Admixture

Because of the availability of numerous formulations of corticosteroids, individual manufacturers' recommendations should be followed. Several admixture incompatibilities are noted for the corticosteroids and other anticancer agents (see the table below). A more detailed review of compatibility and stability information is also available (Trissel 1988).

■ Administration

The water-soluble esters of the corticosteroids may generally be given by slow intravenous push or by intramuscular administration in minimal volumes for dilution. Intramuscular injection is required for the respository forms, which are usually acetate salts. Caution must be used with these preparations to avoid inadvertent intravenous administration of the poorly soluble intramuscular compounds. Although a transient burning sensation is often noted with both intramuscular and intravenous routes, serious hypersensitivity reactions are extremely rare.

■ Dosage

Specific corticosteroid doses for different oncologic indications are listed in the table on the opposite page. For alternate-day dosing, a single morning administration of a short-acting compound is employed. Doses of the different agents may be interconverted with the relative milligram equivalencies listed in the earlier table and with consideration of the relative duration of activity and the salt-retaining [mineralocorticoid] activity of the two compounds. Overall, intermittent administration regimens are probably preferable and can reduce the incidence of long-term steroid complications (Cushing's disease, serious infection, osteoporosis, and diabetes). In the treatment of adrenal carcinoma, corticosteroid replacement therapy (also required with mitotane or aminoglutethimide adrenal

COMPATIBILITY OF VARIOUS GLUCOCORTICOIDS WITH OTHER SELECTED AGENTS

Glucocorticoid	Compatible (at Least 24-h Stability)	Incompatible
Hydrocortisone sodium phosphate	Bleomycin Dacarbazine Heparin Ondansetron	
Hydrocortisone sodium succinate	Cytarabine (dextrose) Daunorubicin Metoclopramide Dexamethasone Fluorouracil Morphine Cytarabine with Methotrexate in Elliott's B solution or normal saline or D5W Ondansetron	Bleomycin Cytarabine (Ringer's lactate) Doxorubicin Diazepam
Dexamethasone	Bleomycin Metoclopramide Heparin Ondansetron	Daunorubicin Doxorubicin
Methylprednisolone	Cytarabine (in dextrose or normal saline) Heparin Metoclopramide	Cytarabine (in Ringer's injection)

From Trissel LA. Hydrocortisone sodium phosphate. In: ASHP Handbook on Injectable Drugs. 5th ed. New York: American Society of Hospital Pharmacists; 1988;356–368.

ablation) must be accomplished with small daily morning doses of 20 to 25 mg hydrocortisone. In addition, these doses must be increased as needed for trauma, infection, and stress. High-dose single-agent intermittent therapy is occasionally used in multiple myeloma (Alexanian et al 1986). A 40-mg oral dose of dexamethasone was administered every day for 4 days beginning on days 1, 9, and 17 of each cycle. The standard dose in the Hodgkin's lymphoma MOPP regimen is 40 mg/m^2 prednisone orally on days 1 to 14 of each cycle. In the non-Hodgkin's CHOP regimen a fixed 100-mg oral prednisone dose is given daily on days 1 to 5 of each treatment cycle. In breast cancer, oral prednisone 20 mg/m^2 is given on days 1 to 7 or 0.75 mg/kg is given on days 1 to 10 of each treatment cycle. In myeloma, a standard prednisone dose of 1 mg/kg is given three times a week with oral melphalan. Daily prednisone doses are generally limited to a maximum of 100 mg and are tapered after 4 weeks of therapy (Sporn and McIntyre 1986). In the VAD regimen for myeloma, dexamethasone is given in a dose of 40 mg orally each morning for 4 days of each cycle of therapy (Barlogie et al 1984).

In antiemetic regimens very high doses are used for a short duration before and after chemotherapy is administered. Total doses of up to 100 mg of dexamethasone and 2000 mg of methylprednisolone have been used (Plezia and Alberts 1985) (see the table). A typical antiemetic regimen called for 4 mg of dexamethasone orally every 4 to 6 hours plus 10 mg IV prior to chemotherapy. High-dose dexamethasone is also used for managing cerebral metastases from a variety of different primary tumors. Typical doses range from 16 to 24 mg/d in divided doses (Weinstein et al 1972).

■ Drug Interactions

A number of drug-drug interactions are possible with the corticosteroids. Phenytoin (Dilantin®) has been shown to enhance the metabolism of dexamethasone, perhaps as a result of enzyme induction (Choi et al 1971, Hague et al 1972), whereas aspirin appears to decrease steroid excretion rates (Elliot 1962). The anticancer drug mitotane (Lysodren®) is directly adrenocorticotoxic and also blocks the peripheral metabolism of endogenous corticosteroids (see *Mitotane*). Similarly, aminoglutethimide causes inhibition of proper steroidogenesis. Thus, replacement corticosteroids are indicated with both drug therapies.

Corticosteroids may enhance the expression of metallothionein, an enzyme associated with resistance to heavy metals including cisplatin (Kelley et al 1988); however, dexamethasone has been shown to have no effect on cisplatin antitumor activity in vitro or in vivo (Aapro et al 1983). Short-term responses have been reported in lung cancer patients receiving long- or short-term glucocorticosteroids (Thatcher et al 1982). It is unclear whether this is due to a drug interaction or stimulation of tumor growth

Indication	Usual Dosage Range*	Duration of Activity[†]	Reference
Hydrocortisone			
Postadrenalectomy	25–30 mg/d	Very short, < 8–12 h	
Prednisone			
Leukemia remission induction:	40–50 mg/m^2 · d	Short, < 24 h	
Hodgkin's disease	20–30 mg/d		
resistant patients—high dose	40–100 mg/m^2 · d		
Breast cancer	15–20 mg/d		
Intracranial metastases			
Initially	60–80 mg/d		
Reduce to	20–30 mg/d		
Hypercalcemia	60–80 mg/d (adults)		
Methylprednisolone			
Antiemetic use	250–500 mg for 2–4 doses over 24–48 h	Short, < 1.5 d	Plezia and Alberts 1985 Schallier et al 1985
Dexamethasone			
Antiemetic use	10–20 mg IV or PO for 2–4 doses in 24–48 h	Extended, > 3 d	Plezia and Alberts 1985 Allan et al 1984

*Doses for different treatment programs (MOPP, CMF-P, etc) vary widely, and individual regimens should be reviewed carefully before use.
[†]Based on hypothalamic–pituitary suppression (tissue effects, not plasma half-lives which are much shorter).

as observed in certain animal models (Sloman and Murphy 1984).

Methylprednisolone has been shown to partially synchronize C3H/HeJ cells in S phase in vitro, which results in greater cytotoxicity from subsequent treatment with cyclophosphamide and doxorubicin (Braunschweiger and Schiffer 1979). No such effects have been observed in vivo.

■ Pharmacokinetics

As a class, the corticosteroids are relatively well absorbed orally. For prednisolone, oral bioavailability ranges from 80 to 100% (Rose et al 1981). Hydrocortisone products peak blood levels within 2 hours and levels fall slowly over the next 8 to 12 hours (see the table). Hydrocortisone is significantly protein bound (> 90% for low doses) in the plasma, specifically to the globulin transcortin and secondarily, in a nonspecific fashion, to albumin. The synthetic congeners demonstrate important deviations in both binding affinity and metabolism. Thus, the relative potencies of these compounds are generally greater than that of hydrocortisone. There is also some evidence for nonlinear or dose-dependent pharmacokinetics of prednisone and prednisolone (Rose et al 1981). Longer half-lives are observed with higher doses, even though systemic clearance also increases with the dose (see the table).

All steroidal compounds are extensively metabolized in the liver (Berliner and Dougherty 1961). Additionally, prednisone requires reduction at the 2-keto position to produce a pharmacologically active steroid (prednisolone). Despite this, marked liver dysfunction has not been shown to significantly alter the metabolism or excretion (hence pharmacologic effects) of the corticosteroids. There is also marked interconversion between prednisone and prednisolone in vivo (Rose et al 1981, Jenkins and Sampson 1967). Corticosteroids are excreted predominantly in the urine as hepatic conjugates of sulfate esters and glucuronides.

■ Side Effects and Toxicity

Most of the "side effects" of the corticosteroids relate to simple extensions of characteristic pharmacologic effects from the large doses required in cancer therapy (Marmont and Fusco 1960). Generally, these untoward effects may be lessened by the use of intermittent dosing or alternate-day dosing. Patients at special risk for side effects include those with chronic granulomatous infections (eg, tuberculosis), hypertension and cardiovascular diseases (eg, heart failure), peptic ulcers, diabetes, and preexisting osteoporosis and psychologic disturbances; however, some acute corticosteroid side effects can often be beneficial, such as the mild euphoria and appetite stimulation occasionally noted in cancer patients receiving high-dose therapy.

A serious risk in any steroid treatment regimen is that of complete suppression of the adrenal–pituitary axis (adrenal atrophy). Thus, gradual tapering of doses after long-term administration should be employed and a regimen is reported (Byny 1976). Nonetheless, most regimens carry the certainty that some degree of cushingoid symptomatology will develop, noted by moon facies, truncal obesity,

GLUCOCORTICOSTEROID PHARMACOKINETICS IN HUMANS

Corticosteroid	Dose (mg)	Route	Plasma Half-life (h)	Volume of Distribution	Systemic Plasma Clearance	Reference
Prednisone	5–40	PO	3.4–3.5	—	572–2271 mL/min/1.73 m^2 (dose dependent)	Rose et al 1981
Prednisolone	5–40	IV	2.7–3.5	24–52 L/1.73 m^2 at steady state	111–194 mL/min/1.73 m^2	Rose et al 1981
Dexamethasone	6.66	IV	6.5–7.2	41–63 L (females, males, respectively)	245 mL/min	Tsuei et al 1979
Methylprednisolone sodium succinate	30 mg/kg	IV	3.5	—	—	Upjohn Company
Hydrocortisone	37	IV	2	—	—	Lima and Jusko 1980

striae, particularly of skin folds and pressure points, bruises, osteoporosis, and muscle weakness. Depression is often encountered especially when high-dose long-term therapy is discontinued. The signs and symptoms of this toxic syndrome include fatigue, psychosomatic complaints, crying spells, insomnia, and loss of drive or self-image. Fortunately, the depression is usually brief.

Spiegel et al (1979) studied adrenal function in cancer patients receiving short-term high-dose courses of prednisone. After 5 days of high-dose prednisone (40–100 mg/m^2) therapy most patients required 2 to 4 days to recover adrenal function, and, in a few, full recovery had not occurred by 7 days. In this population neither the dose nor the duration of therapy correlated with adrenal suppression.

Metabolic effects may also be noted. These include an electrolyte depletion syndrome (calcium and potassium) but with mild sodium retention for some compounds (prednisone and hydrocortisone, see table).

Another occasionally devastating effect results from steroidal suppression of cellular immunity. This can cause the development of serious systemic infection in the immunocompromised host. Very often, "opportunistic" organisms or unusual pathogens are encountered. Patients with positive tuberculin skin tests and/or a history of granulomatous disease should thus be considered for chemotherapeutic prophylaxis while on steroids (eg, INH for tuberculosis).

Diabetes is another potential consequence of steroidal effects on carbohydrate metabolism. It may become clinically significant in patients with a predisposition for overt diabetes. With high-dose regimens, steroid-induced hyperglycemia can be a common troubling side effect.

Peptic ulceration or gastric bleeding from ulcers has been presumptively linked to the use of steroids, possibly because of acid and pepsin stimulation and/or the impairment of wound healing; however, well-controlled epidemiology studies have failed to confirm this (Conn and Blitzer 1976). Prophylactic antacid therapy with H$_2$ antihistamines such as ranitidine (150 mg PO twice daily) may therefore be of benefit in patients who must receive corticosteroids and who develop symptoms of gastrointestinal upset.

Ocular side effects of high-dose corticosteroids have also been documented. These include increased ocular pressure and posterior subcapsular cataracts (Williamson et al 1969). Cataracts are also described following intermittent high-dose dexamethasone when used as a chemotherapy antiemetic (Bluming and Zeegen 1986).

Intradermal corticosteroids can cause epidermal thinning and other local complications (Gottlieb and Riskin 1980). Therefore, high-dose intradermal injections should be avoided.

Acute rectal itching may occur after injection of hydrocortisone sodium phosphate but not after injection of the sodium succinate salt (Novak et al 1976). In children and infants, long-term, high-dose corticosteroid use will retard growth. In adults, particularly postmenopausal women and those with limitations on physical activity, chronic steroids may also induce or aggravate osteoporosis.

REFERENCES

Aapro MS, Alberts DS. High-dose dexamethasone for prevention of cisplatin-induced vomiting. *Cancer Chemother Pharmacol.* 1981;**7**:11–14.

Aapro MS, Alberts DS, Serokman R. Lack of dexamethasone effect on the antitumor activity of cisplatin. *Cancer Treat Rep.* 1983;**67**:1013–1017.

Alexanian R, Barlogie B, Dixon D. High-dose glucocorticoid treatment of resistant myeloma. *Ann Intern Med.* 1986;**105**:8–11.

Allan SG, Cornbleet MA, Warrington PS, et al. Dexamethasone and high dose metoclopramide: Efficacy in controlling cisplatin induced nausea and vomiting. *Br Med J.* 1984;**289**:878–879.

Barlogie B, Smith L, Alexanian R. Effective treatment of advanced multiple myeloma refractory to alkylating agents. *N Engl J Med.* 1984;**310**:1353–1356.

Baxter JD, Harris AW, Tomkins GM, Cohn M. Glucocorticoid receptors in lymphoma cells in culture: Relationship to glucocorticoid killing activity. *Science.* 1971;**171**:189.

Berliner DL, Dougherty TF. Hepatic and extrahepatic regulation of corticosteroids. *Pharmacol Rev.* 1961;**13**:239.

Bluming AZ, Zeegen P. Cataracts induced by intermittent decadron used as an antiemetic. *J Clin Oncol.* 1986;**4**(2):221–223.

Braunschweiger PG, Schiffer LM. Effect of methylprednisolone on the cell kinetic response of C3H/HeJ mammary tumors to cyclophosphamide and Adriamycin. *Cancer Res.* 1979;**39**:3812–3815.

Byny RL. Withdrawal from glucocorticoid therapy. *N Engl J Med.* 1976;**295**(1):30–32.

Choi Y, Thrasher K, Werk EE, et al. Effect of diphenylhydantoin on cortisol kinetics in humans. *J Pharmacol Exp Ther.* 1971;**176**:27–34.

Conn HO, Blitzer BL. Nonassociation of adrenocorticosteroid therapy and peptic ulcer. *N Engl J Med.* 1976;**294**(9):473–479.

Cooper RJ. Combination chemotherapy in hormone resistant breast cancer. *Proc Am Assoc Cancer Res.* 1969;**10**:15.

Duke RC, Chervenak R, Cohen JJ. Endogenous endonuclease-induced DNA fragmentation: An early event in cell-mediated cytolysis. *Proc Natl Acad Sci USA.* 1983;**80**:6361–6365.

Elliot HC. Reduced adrenocortical steroid excretion rates in man following aspirin administration. *Metab Clin Exp.* 1962;**11**:1018–1025.

Ernst P, Killmann S. Perturbation of generation of human leukemic blast cells by cytostatic therapy in vivo: Effect of corticosteroids. *Blood.* 1970;**36**:689.

Ezdinli EZ, Stutzman L, Aungst WC, Firat D. Corticosteroid therapy for lymphomas and chronic lymphocytic leukemia. *Cancer J Clin.* 1969;**23**:900.

Gottlieb NL, Riskin WG. Complications of local corticosteroid infections. *JAMA* 1980;**243**(15):1547–1548.

Gryglewski RJ, Panczenko B, Korbut R, et al. Corticosteroids inhibit prostaglandin release from perfused mesenteric blood vessels of rabbit and prefused lungs of sensitized guinea pigs. *Prostaglandins.* 1975;**10**:343–355.

Hague N, Thrasher K, Werk EE, et al. Studies on dexamethasone metabolism in man: Effect of diphenylhydantoin. *J Clin Endocrinol Metab.* 1972;**34**:44–50.

Hall TC, Choi OS, Abadi A, Krant MJ. High-dose corticoid therapy in Hodgkin's disease and other lymphomas. *Ann Intern Med.* 1967;**66**:1144.

Hong SL, Levine L. Inhibition of arachidonic acid release from cells as the biochemical action of anti-inflammatory corticosteroids. *Proc Natl Acad Sci USA.* 1976;**73**:1730–1734.

Jenkins JS, Sampson PA. Conversion of cortisone to cortisol and prednisone to prednisolone. *Br Med J.* 1967;**2**:205–207.

Juleiz W, Meikle AW, Levison RA, et al. Effect of diphenylhydantoin on the metabolism of dexamethasone. *N Engl J Med.* 1970;**283**:11–14.

Kelley SL, Basu A, Teicher BA, et al. Overexpression of metallothionein confers resistance to anticancer drugs. *Science.* 1988;**241**:1813–1815.

Lemon HM. Prednisone therapy of advanced mammary cancer. *Cancer.* 1959;**12**:93.

Lima JJ, Jusko WJ. Bioavailability of hydrocortisone retention enemas in relation to absorption kinetics. *Clin Pharmacol Ther.* 1980;**28**(2):262–269.

Lippman ME, Perry S, Thompson EB. Glucocorticoid binding proteins in myeloblasts of acute myelogenous leukemia. *Am J Med.* 1975;**59**:224–227.

Lippman ME, Yarbro GK, Keventhal BG. Clinical implications of glucocorticoid receptors in human leukemia. *Cancer Res.* 1978;**38**:4251–4256.

Marmont A, Fusco FA. Massive doses of predni-steroids in the treatment of acute leukemia: Clinical experience and therapeutic considerations. *Minerva Med.* 1960;**51**:3437–3450.

McConkey DJ, Nicotera P, Hartzell P, et al. Glucocorticoids activate a suicide process in thymocytes through an elevation of cytosolic Ca^{2+} concentration. *Arch Biochem Biophys.* 1989;**269**:365–370.

McConkey DJ, Orrenlus S, Jondal M. Cellular signalling in programmed cell death (apoptosis). *Immunol Today.* 1990;**11**(4):120–121.

Meickel RP, Miller FP, Brodie BB. Interaction of non-steroidal anti-inflammatory agents with corticosteroids. *Pharmacologist.* 1966;**7**:182.

Munck A. Glucocorticoid inhibition of glucose uptake by peripheral tissues: Old and new evidence, molecular mechanisms, and physiological significance. *Perspect Biol Med.* 1971;**14**:265.

Novak E, Gilbertson TJ, Seckman CE, et al. Anorectal pruritus after intravenous hydrocortisone sodium succinate and sodium phosphate. *Clin Pharmacol Ther.* 1976;**20**(1): 109–112.

Peters WP, Holland JF, Senn H, et al. Corticosteroid administration and localized leukocyte mobilization in man. *N Engl J Med.* 1972;**282**:342–345.

Plezia PM, Alberts DS. Nausea and vomiting: Mechanisms and management. *Clin Oncol.* 1985;**4**(3):357–386.

Plezia PM, Alberts DS, Kessler J, et al. Immediate termination of intractable vomiting induced by cisplatin combination chemotherapy using an intensive five-drug antiemetic regimen. *Cancer Treat Rep.* 1984;**68**:1493–1495.

Roholl PJM, Al B, Hoeben K, Leene W. T-cell differentiation in the rabbit. II. Con A and PHA response of thymus, spleen and lymph node cells and of thymus subpopulations: influence of dexamethasone treatment. *Thymus.* 1983;**5**:167–178.

Rose JQ, Yurchak AM, Jusko WJ. Dose dependent pharmacokinetics of prednisone and prednisolone in man. *J Pharmacokinet Biopharm.* 1981;**9**(4):389–417.

Rosen F. Inhibition of glucose uptake in lymphosarcoma 1798 by cortisol and its relationship to the biosynthesis of deoxyribonucleic acid. *J Biol Chem.* 1970;**245**:2074.

Schallier D, Van Belle S, De Greve J, Willekens A. Methylprednisolone as an antiemetic drug. A randomized double blind study. *Cancer Chemother Pharmacol.* 1985;**14**: 235–237.

Spiegel RJ, Oliff AL, Bruton J, et al. Adrenal suppression after short-term corticosteroid therapy. *Lancet.* 1979;**1**:630–633.

Sporn JR, McIntyre OR. Chemotherapy of previously untreated multiple myeloma patients: An analysis of recent treatment results. *Semin Oncol.* 1986;**13**(3):318–325.

Trissel LA. Hydrocortisone sodium phosphate. In: *ASHP Handbook on Injectable Drugs.* 5th ed. Bethesda, MD: American Society of Hospital Pharmacists; 1988:356–368.

Trissel LA, Fulton B, Tramonte SM. Visual compatibility of ondansetron with chemotherapeutic agents, antibiotics, and other selected drugs during simulated Y-site injection (abstract P-468). In: *25th Annual ASHP Midyear Clinical Meeting, Las Vegas, Nevada, December,* Bethesda, MD: American Society Hospital Pharmacists; 1990.

Tsuei SE, Moore RG, Ashley JJ, McBride WG. Disposition of synthetic glucocorticoids. I. Pharmacokinetics of dexamethasone in healthy adults. *J Pharmacokinet Biopharm.* 1979;**7**(3):249–264.

Udkow G. Steroid effects on leukocyte counts. *Drug Ther.* 1978;**8**(1):172–177.

Weinstein JD, Toy FJ, Jaffe ME, Goldberg HI. The effect of dexamethasone on brain edema in patients with metastatic brain tumors. *Neurology.* 1972;**23**:121–129.

Williamson J, Paterson RWW, McGavin DDM, et al. Posterior subcapsular cataracts and glaucoma associated with long-term oral corticosteroid therapy. *Br J Ophthalmol.* 1969;**53**:361–371.

Corynebacterium parvum

■ Other Names

C. parvum; coparvax; NSC-197213 (Merieux Product); NSC-220537 (Burroughs Wellcome).

■ Chemistry

Corynebacterium parvum is a microbiologic preparation consisting of a suspension of whole killed gram-positive anaerobic bacilli. Certain strains of *C. parvum* are probably synonymous with *Propionibacterium acnes.* The preparation is usually a formalin-fixed suspension in thimerosal preservative. It is often derived from horse serum culture. There are French (Pasteur and Merieux [MER]), English (National Collection of Type Cultures), and various American (Burroughs Wellcome, HEW [National Institute of Allergy and Infectious Disease], Temple University, and Virginia Polytechnic) strains. All are reported as "*C. parvum*" in the literature. Activities vary from strain to strain (Wrba 1975).

■ Antitumor Activity

Antitumor effects in humans are probably mediated through immunopotentiation and have been noted in a variety of advanced neoplasms (Castro and Sadler 1975, Fisher et al 1975). These effects were first demonstrated by Halpern (1974) and Israel et al (1975). Tumors that have occasionally responded to *C. parvum* include small cell lung carcinoma, various sarcomas, metastatic breast cancer, and malignant melanoma (Band et al 1975, Carter and Slavik 1975, Cheng et al 1976, Fisher et al 1976a, Scott 1974). The agent has most often been combined with chemotherapy in the treatment of a variety of solid tumors (Gutterman et al 1976). In malignant melanoma, an advantage in disease-free survival was observed in a subgroup of patients with melanomas greater than 3 mm in thickness (Balch et al 1982). *C. parvum* has been used as adjuvant therapy following surgical resection of primary disease (Balch et al 1982). Thus, *C. parvum* does not appear to be efficacious in all stage I malignant melanoma patients (Murray et al 1983) but may be effective in selected subsets. Two separate clinical trials have compared *C. parvum* with bacillus Calmette–Guérin as adjuvant immunotherapy in stage II malignant melanoma. Both studies reported activity for *C. parvum* with either improved disease-free survival (Lipton et al 1983) or enhanced median survival (Balch et al 1984). A more recent survival analysis of these trials shows significantly enhanced disease-free survival and overall survival, particularly in patients younger than 60 years (Lipton et al 1991). In lung cancer *C. parvum* increased survival of patients with non-small cell disease when combined with cytotoxic chemotherapy; however, there was no increase in overall response rates nor in survival for other types of lung cancer (Chahinian et al 1982). Antitumor effects in acute leukemia have also been noted (Sexauer et al 1976b). A later trial showed that *C. parvum* did not prolong remission durations in acute myelocytic leukemia following cytotoxic combination induction regimens (Eppinger-Helft et al 1980). More recent studies in most solid tumors except melanoma have been similarly negative. Thus, *C. parvum* has not increased the activity of cytotoxic chemotherapy in lung cancer (treated with intrapleural *C. parvum* [Ludwig Cancer Study Group 1982]), in breast cancer (Pinsky et al 1977, Mayr et al 1978), in colorectal cancer (Souter et al 1982), in cervical cancer (DiSaia et al 1982), in head and neck cancer (Chen et al 1982), and finally in ovarian cancer (Wanebo et al 1977). There is, however, one positive trial of *C. parvum* with chemotherapy in advanced ovarian cancer (Gall et al 1982).

■ Mechanism of Action

In mice the intravenous or intraperitoneal administration of *C. parvum* causes an intense nonspecific stimulation of the immune system (Amiel et al 1969). Hyperplasia of the reticuloendothelial system results from *C. parvum* administration in animals. There is also documented augmentation of immunologic activity of macrophages and B lymphocytes; however, a temporary depression of T lymphocytes generally occurs (Adlam and Scott 1973). Animal studies have shown that the intense nonspecific stimulation produced by *C. parvum* can cause tumor regression or delay tumor growth. The mechanism of this tumor inhibition is thought to involve primarily activation of the macrophages with a slight but necessary boost from T lymphocytes (Scott 1972). Like bacillus Calmette–Guérin, *C. parvum* can increase macrophage responsiveness and possibly enhance the synthesis and release of tumor necrosis factor. *C. parvum* is known to increase macrophage precursors in the bone marrow (Wolmark and Fisher 1974) and activates circulating macrophages which may play an important role in immune surveillance against tumor cells (Christie and Bomford 1975, Bomford and Christie 1975).

Overall, the precise mechanism is not known and *C. parvum* may thus be termed a nonspecific immunopotentiator (Oettgen et al 1976). A protective effect of *C. parvum* (ie, experimental tumor prophylaxis) appears to develop rapidly in animals (Megirian et al 1980) and thus may not require specific tumor–antigen–antibody reaction for initiation (Baum and Breese 1976). In humans, delayed hypersensitivity reactions to recall antigens has increased after intravenous *C. parvum* administration (but not after subcutaneous administration in one study). It has changed unpredictably in other studies.

■ Availability and Storage

Corynebacterium parvum was investigationally available (Burroughs Wellcome, U.K.) as 7-mg (dry wt), 5-mL, and 20-mL sterile vials. The suspension is a washed, formalin-treated, thimerosal-preserved preparation of killed whole bacteria suspended in normal saline. This suspension is stored under refrigeration and should probably not be vigorously agitated nor warmed before use. The suspension must also be protected from heat and light. These off-white saline vials require refrigerated storage and are stable at least 18 months.

C. parvum is also available investigationally as a 2 mg/mL suspension of heat-killed bacilli in 2-mL ampules (Merieux). These also contain formalin (≤ 200 µg/mol) in normal saline at a pH of 7.13 (Institute Merieux: *C. parvum* strain 1M1585 of Institute Pasteur).

■ Preparation for Use, Stability, and Admixture

C. parvum is usually given by intravenous infusion. Initially, the vial should be gently shaken to ensure adequate resuspension of the mixture. Next, the desired dose is withdrawn aseptically from the vial and added to 100 to 500 mL of normal saline. This admixture is probably stable for several hours under refrigeration and protected from light.

Intraperitoneal, intratumoral, intramuscular, and subcutaneous doses do not need further dilution.

■ Administration

As an adjuvant to surgery in melanoma or lung cancer *C. parvum* has typically been administered subcutaneously, with the dose divided for injection among the four extremities (Balch et al 1982, Chahinian et al 1982). The drug has also been administered subcutaneously in combination with intravenous chemotherapy for acute leukemia (Eppinger-Helft et al 1980).

Intravenous doses are usually infused over 30 to 60 minutes or up to 4 hours. In England, infusions have been continued for up to 12 to 24 hours. Generally, brief infusions (< 30 minutes) are not advised as the preparation is of bacterial origin and therefore antigenic. Also, individual patients may not tolerate the cardiovascular challenge from the rapid saline infusion. Therefore, most North American investigators have used 2-hour infusion times. Inasmuch as the preparation is a suspension, the dose should not be run through a final or other type of in-line filter.

C. parvum has also been given intratumorally in malignant melanoma (Cunningham-Rundles et al 1975), intraperitoneally in cancer with malignant ascites, and only rarely by intramuscular routes (Woodruff et al 1975). Pain, local inflammation, and abscesses sometimes complicate the use of these routes. This has frequently and perhaps unnecessarily mandated dosage reduction. In mice, oral administration has also been shown to be ineffective (Sadler and Castro 1975).

■ Special Precautions

C. parvum should be given cautiously to patients with a documented hypersensitivity to either mercury or horse serum. De novo hypersensitivity to *C. parvum* may also occur and is more common after an initial (sensitizing) dose or regimen. Almost all patients develop chills and fever, which may be severe. Therefore most patients must be closely observed both during and after C. parvum infusion for signs of an exaggerated immunologic reaction or anaphylaxis. Emergency resuscitation equipment and personnel should be readily available to treat this condition.

■ Dosage

Intravenous infusion doses have ranged from 2 to 7.5 mg/m^2, generally given from once per week to once every other week, although daily infusions of similar doses for up to 3 weeks have been used (Israel et al 1975). The most common subcutaneous dose in adjuvant studies has been 3.5 to 4 mg/m^2 weekly for 3 months (Balch et al 1982). Fixed subcutaneous single doses of 2 to 15 mg/m^2 were given weekly in one trial (Reed et al 1975). The manufacturer recommends that individual intravenous doses not exceed 20 mg. Also, the maximally therapeutic safe dose of C. parvum has not yet been established. Maximum tolerated single doses have ranged from 2.5 to 50 mg (total doses 4–224 mg). The high doses are generally reached by daily escalations with careful constant monitoring for toxicity.

In malignant melanoma, doses of 4 to 8 mg/d for 5 days/wk of intratumorally administered C. parvum have elicited good responses. In one study an intraperitoneal dose of 4 mg/d showed limited success in controlling malignant ascites (Oettgen et al 1976).

■ Drug Interactions

A theoretical contraindication exists in the concurrent use of drugs requiring extensive hepatic metabolism: anesthetic drugs (Farquhar et al 1975, Mosedale and Smith 1975), phenothiazines, barbiturates, and others. Animal studies have documented anesthetic deaths in cases where otherwise normal doses of barbiturates were used to induce anesthesia in conjunction with relatively high doses of C. parvum (15 mg/kg). These effects were not seen with lower doses of C. parvum. Similar drug interactions may also be possible with anticancer drugs that are either hepatically activated (eg, cyclophosphamide [Fisher et al 1976b]) or hepatically detoxified (eg, doxorubicin [Harris 1976]).

■ Side Effects and Toxicity

Fever and chills almost invariably occur on intravenous administration but in only about 10% of subcutaneously administered doses (Hamilton 1975). Pain and swelling at the site of injection are also common with subcutaneous or intratumoral doses. Nausea and vomiting occur much less frequently. Both hypo- and hypertension have been reported. Two serious hypertensive reactions have also been reported. These were characterized by peripheral blanching, acrocyanosis, and chilling with dyspnea. Concurrent aberrations in cardiovascular and renal function were noted in these cases.

In general, most adverse reactions to C. parvum are evident within 2 hours and usually resolve by 48 hours. Malaise and drowsiness are also commonly reported but are usually clinically insignificant. In addition, leukopenia, hepatic dysfunction (noted by transient elevations in liver enzymes), and thrombocytopenia have been reported. One case of a severe but reversible intravascular coagulation syndrome has been seen.

If an autoimmune predisposition exists in a particular patient, C. parvum may be contraindicated. Also, patients with depressed hepatic and cardiovascular function will probably not tolerate the endotoxin type of C. parvum hypersensitivity reaction and are therefore poor candidates for C. parvum therapy.

Fever has typically been the dose-limiting toxic reaction with intravenous administration of C. parvum. In contrast, severe local inflammatory responses after subcutaneous administration have typically necessitated dose reduction in 30% of patients (Scott and Warner 1976).

A typical symptomatic reaction to the initial intravenous C. parvum injection consists of vigorous chills for 20 to 40 minutes, concurrent peripheral vasoconstriction (mild cyanosis or blanching), and a slight increase in blood pressure. Patients may feel nauseated and apprehensive; occasionally, they develop a mild headache. This is followed by high fever (up to 105°F) lasting 2 to 4 hours and then by gradual defervescence over the next 48 to 72 hours. During the latter period, patients may sweat profusely and thus often become slightly hypotensive (Oettgen et al 1976, Sexauer et al 1976a).

Reactions to subsequent doses are generally less intense. Thus, first doses are probably best managed in a hospital setting. An atypical low-grade fever may occasionally be noted after C. parvum therapy.

Adverse reactions to C. parvum appear to be dose related, become less severe with repeat doses, and do not decrease a patient's tolerance to concomitant chemotherapy or radiotherapy.

In one phase I study, investigators found that *C. parvum* reactions can be ameliorated by keeping patients warm, giving a mild tranquilizer at the start of a 1.5-hour infusion, giving a hot drink to patients at the onset of chills, keeping patients recumbent to decrease nausea (antiemetics were not beneficial), and giving antipyretics (1.2–1.8 g of aspirin) for fever.

■ Special Applications

Patt et al (1978) described the intraarterial use of *C. parvum* in patients with malignant lesions confined to the liver. The *C. parvum* (10 mg/m^2/d × 5) was infused continuously by infusion pump. To avoid physical incompatibility the daily dose was given in four aliquots diluted into 50 mL of Normal Saline, USP, with 1500 to 4000 U of heparin added, each given over a 6-hour period. Of the 63 infusion regimens conducted there were two serious *Staphylococcus* infections and four instances of arterial occlusion. Drug toxicity in the study consisted of fever, chills, an enlarged tender liver, and slight thrombocytopenia (perhaps secondary to the concurrent heparin). There was typically an initial and transient hepatic toxicity. Three patients, however, developed delayed and more severe hepatotoxicity. A few objective responses were noted in breast cancer and hepatocellular carcinoma metastatic to the liver. Significant benefits appeared to be limited to colon carcinoma metastatic to the liver.

REFERENCES

Adlam C, Scott MT. Lympho-reticular stimulatory properties of *Corynebacterium parvum* and related bacteria. *J Med Microbiol*. 1973;**6**:261–274.

Amiel JL, Litwin J, Beraudet M. Attempts at active nonspecific immunotherapy using formolized *Corynebacterium parvum*. *Rev Fr Etud Clin Biol*. 1969;**14**:909–915.

Balch CM, Murray DM, Presant C, et al. A randomized prospective comparison of BCG versus *C. parvum* adjuvant immunotherapy in melanoma patients with resected metastatic lymph nodes (abstract C-1031). *Am Soc Clin Oncol*. 1984;**3**:263.

Balch CM, Smalley RV, Bartolucci AA, et al. A randomized prospective clinical trial of adjuvant *C. parvum* immunotherapy in 260 patients with clinically localized melanoma (stage I). Prognostic factors, analysis and preliminary results of immunotherapy. *Cancer*. 1982;**49**:1079–1084.

Band PR, Jao-King C, Urtasun RC, Haraphongse M. Phase I study of *Corynebacterium parvum* in patients with solid tumors. *Cancer Chemother Rep*. 1975;**59**:1139–1145.

Baum M, Breese M. Antitumor effect of *Corynebacterium parvum*: Possible mode of action. *Br J Cancer*. 1976;**33**(4):468–473.

Bomford R, Christie GH. Mechanisms of macrophage activation by *Corynebacterium parvum*. II. In vitro experiments. *Cell Immunol*. 1975;**17**:150–155.

Carter SK, Slavik M. A chemotherapeutic perspective on clinical trials with *Corynebacterium parvum*. In: Halpern B, ed. *Corynebacterium parvum. Applications in Experimental and Clinical Oncology*. New York: Plenum; 1975:329–340.

Castro JE, Sadler TE. An analysis of the antitumor effects of *Corynebacterium parvum*. In: Halpern B, ed. *Corynebacterium parvum. Applications in Experimental and Clinical Oncology*. New York: Plenum; 1975:252–263.

Chahinian AP, Goldberg J, Holland JF, et al. Chemotherapy versus chemoimmunotherapy with levamisole or *Corynebacterium parvum* in advanced lung cancer. *Cancer Treat Rep*. 1982;**66**(6):1291–1297.

Chen VST, Suit HD, Wan CC, et al. Clinical trial of *Corynebacterium parvum* and radiotherapy in the treatment of head and neck carcinoma. In: Terry WD, Rosenberg SA, eds. *Immunotherapy of Human Cancer*. New York: Elsevier/North-Holland;1982:361.

Cheng VST, Suit HD, Wang CC, Cummings C. Nonspecific immunotherapy by *Corynebacterium parvum*: Phase I toxicity study in 12 patients with advanced cancer. *Cancer*. 1976;**37**(4):1687–1695.

Christie GH, Bomford R. Mechanisms of macrophage activation by *Corynebacterium parvum*. I. In vitro experiments. *Cell Immunol*. 1975;**17**:150–155.

Cunningham-Rundles WF, Hirshaut X, Pinsky CM, et al. Phase I trial of intralesional *Corynebacterium parvum* (abstract). *Clin Res*. 1975;**23**(3):337A.

DiSaia PJ, Gall S, Levy D, et al. Preliminary report on the treatment of women with cervical cancer, stage IIB, IIIB and IVA (confined to the pelvis and/or periaortic nodes), with radiotherapy alone versus radiotherapy plus immunotherapy with intravenous *Corynebacterium parvum*, phase III. In: Terry WD, Rosenberg SA, eds. *Immunotherapy of Human Cancer*. New York: Elsevier/North-Holland;1982:331.

Eppinger-Helft M, Pavlovsky S, Hidalgo G, et al. Chemoimmunotherapy with *Corynebacterium parvum* in acute myelocytic leukemia. *Cancer*. 1980;**45**:280–284.

Farquhar D, Loo TL, Reed R, Luna M. *Corynebacterium parvum* and anaesthetics (letter). *Lancet*. 1975;**1**:914.

Fisher B, Rubin H, Sartiano G, et al. Observations following *Corynebacterium parvum* administration to patients with advanced malignancy: A phase I study. *Cancer*. 1976a;**38**:119–130.

Fisher B, Wolmark N, Rubin H. Further observations on the inhibition of tumor growth by *Corynebacterium parvum* with cyclophosphamide. III. Effect of *C. parvum* on cyclophosphamide metabolism. *J Natl Cancer Inst*. 1976b;**57**:225–226.

Fisher B, Wolmark N, Saffer E, Fisher ER. Inhibitory effect of prolonged *Corynebacterium parvum* and cyclophosphamide administration on the growth of established tumors. *Cancer.* 1975;**35**:134–143.

Gall SA, Creasman WT, Blessing JA, et al. Chemoimmunotherapy in primary stage III ovarian epithelial cancer. In: Terry WD, Rosenberg SA, eds. *Immunotherapy of Human Cancer.* New York: Elsevier/North-Holland; 1982:337.

Gutterman JU, Mavligit GM, Hersh EM. Chemoimmunotherapy of human solid tumors. *Med Clin North Am.* 1976;**60**(3):441–462.

Halpern B. *Corynebacterium parvum:* An immunomodulator. In: Mathe G, Werner R, eds. *Recent Results in Cancer Research: Investigations and Stimulation of Immunity in Cancer Patients.* New York: Springer-Verlag; 1974:262.

Hamilton DNH. Side effects of intravenous *Corynebacterium parvum* (letter). *Lancet.* 1975;**2**:1263.

Harris PA. Phenobarbitol and *C. parvum* effects on Adriamycin elimination (abstract). *Proc Am Assoc Cancer Res.* 1976;**17**:131A.

Israel L, Edelstein R, Depierre A, Dimitrov N. Daily intravenous infusions with *Corynebacterium parvum* in twenty patients with disseminated cancer: A preliminary report of clinical and biologic findings. *J Natl Cancer Inst.* 1975;**55**:29–33.

Lipton A, Harvey HA, Balch CM, et al. *Corynebacterium parvum* versus bacille Calmette–Guérin adjuvant immunotherapy of stage II malignant melanoma. *J Clin Oncol.* 1991;**9**(7):1151–1156.

Lipton A, Harvey HA, Lawrence B, et al. *Corynebacterium parvum* versus BCG adjuvant immunotherapy in human malignant melanoma. *Cancer.* 1983;**51**:57–60.

Ludwig Cancer Study Group. Intrapleural *Corynebacterium parvum* as adjuvant therapy in operable bronchogenic non-small cell carcinoma: Preliminary report. In: Terry WD, Rosenberg SA, eds. *Immunotherapy of Human Cancer.* New York: Elsevier/North-Holland; 1982:111.

Mayr AC, Senn HJ, Gallmeier WM, et al. Randomized trial in advanced breast cancer using combination chemotherapy with or without *C. parvum:* Preliminary results. *Dev Biol Stand.* 1978;**38**:553.

Megirian R, Astry CL, Spoor RP, Loose L. Enhancement of the antitumor activity of *Corynebacterium parvum* by appropriate adjustment of dosage schedules. *Cancer Treat Rep.* 1980;**64**(8/9):915–920.

Mosedale B, Smith MA. *Corynebacterium parvum* and anesthetics. *Lancet.* 1975;**1**:168–170.

Murray JL, Ishmael DR, Bottomley RH, et al. Inefficacy of SC *Corynebacterium parvum* in stage I malignant melanoma: Preliminary results of a single-institution pilot study. *Cancer Treat Rep.* 1983;**67**(2):191–192.

Oettgen HE, Pinsky CM, Delmonte L. Treatment of cancer with immunomodulators *Corynebacterium parvum* and levamisole. *Med Clin North Am.* 1976;**60**(3):511–537.

Patt YZ, Wallace S, Hersh E, et al. Hepatic arterial infusion of *Corynebacterium parvum* and chemotherapy. *Surg Gynecol Oncol.* 1978;**147**:897–902.

Pinsky C, DeJaeger R, Wittes R, et al. *Corynebacterium parvum* as adjuvant to combination chemotherapy in patients with advanced breast cancer. In: Crispen RG, ed. *Neoplasm Immunity: Solid Tumor Therapy.* Philadelphia: Franklin Institute Press; 1977:145.

Reed RC, Gutterman JC, Mavligit GM, et al. Phase I trial of intravenous and subcutaneous *Corynebacterium parvum. Proc Am Soc Clin Oncol.* 1975;**16**:228.

Sadler TE, Castro JE. Lack of immunological and antitumor effects of orally administered *Corynebacterium parvum* in mice. *Br J Cancer.* 1975;**31**(3):359–363.

Scott MT. Biological effects of the adjuvant *Corynebacterium parvum.* II. Evidence for macrophage–T cell interaction. *Cell Immunol.* 1972;**5**:459–468.

Scott MT. *Corynebacterium parvum* as an immunotherapeutic anticancer agent. *Semin Oncol.* 1974;**1**:367.

Scott MT, Warner SL. The accumulated effects of repeated systemic or local injections of low doses of *Corynebacterium parvum. Cancer Res.* 1976;**36**:1335–1338.

Sexauer CL, Nitschke R, Humphrey GB. *Corynebacterium parvum* toxicity (letter). *Lancet.* 1976a;**2**:199.

Sexauer CL, Wells JR, Oleinick S, et al. Non-specific immunostimulation with *Corynebacterium parvum* in children with acute leukemia (abstract). *Clin Res.* 1976b;**24**(1):75A.

Sloman JC, Murphy MJ Jr. Dexamethasone-induced increase in in vitro clonogenicity of human neoplasms. *J Clin Oncol.* 1984;**2**(8):944–947.

Souter RG, Gill PG, Morris PJ. Adjuvant immunotherapy with *Corynebacterium parvum* in colorectal cancer. In: Terry WD, Rosenberg SA, eds. *Immunotherapy of Human Cancer.* New York: Elsevier/North-Holland; 1982:221.

Thatcher N, Wagstaff J, Wilkinson D, et al. Intermittent high dose cyclophosphamide with and without prednisolone: A study of the relationships between toxicity response and survival in metastatic lung cancer. *Cancer.* 1982;**50**(6):1051–1056.

Wanebo HJ, Ochoa M, Gunther U, et al. Randomized chemoimmunotherapy trial of CAF and intravenous *C. parvum* for residual ovarian cancer—Preliminary results (abstract). *Proc Am Assoc Cancer Res.* 1977;**18**:225.

Wolmark N, Fisher B. The effect of a single and repeated administration of *Corynebacterium parvum* on bone marrow macrophage colony production in syngeneic tumor bearing mice. *Cancer Res.* 1974;**34**:2869–2872.

Woodruff MFA, Clunie GJA, McBride WH, et al. The effect of intravenous and intramuscular injection of *Corynebacterium parvum.* In: Halpern B, ed. *Corynebacterium parvum. Applications in Experimental and Clinical Oncology.* New York: Plenum; 1975:383–388.

Wrba H. Comparative effects of various strains of *Corynebacterium parvum* and other prophylactic agents on tumor development in animals. In: Halpern B, ed. *Corynebacterium parvum. Applications in Experimental and Clinical Oncology.* New York: Plenum; 1975:314–318.

CPT-11

■ Other Names

Camptothecin-11; irinotecan.

■ Chemistry

Structure of CPT-11

The chemical name of CPT-11 is 7-ethyl-10-[4-(1-piperidino)-1-piperidino]barbonyloxycamptothecin. CPT-11 is a unique, water-soluble, semisynthetic analog of the alkaloid camptothecin, derived from the *Camptotheca acuminata* tree. CPT-11 has demonstrated excellent antitumor activity in a number of implantable animal tumor systems (Bissery et al 1991).

■ Antitumor Activity

CPT-11 is now undergoing phase I trials in the United States; however, the agent has already undergone phase I and early phase II clinical trials in Japan. In these trials the agent was reported to have a 46% response rate in patients with advanced colon cancer, including untreated and previously treated patients (Shimada et al 1991). The agent also was reported to have a 32% response rate in patients with non-small cell lung cancer (Fukuoka et al 1992). The median duration of response in patients showing a partial response was only 15 weeks. Equal responses were obtained in non-small cell lung cancer patients with adenocarcinoma and squamous cell carcinoma and in previously treated patients with advanced-stage disease (Fukuoka et al 1992). In small cell lung cancer an overall response rate of 33% is reported (Negoro et al 1991). Some responses have also been noted in patients with cervical cancer and ovarian cancer (Takeuchi et al 1991).

■ Mechanism of Action

CPT-11 is an inhibitor of topoisomerase I. Topoisomerase I is an enzyme with swivellike enzymatic activity which may be required for the elongation phase of DNA replication and RNA transcription (Stewart et al 1990). CPT-11 induces protein-linked DNA single-strand breaks that are dependent on topoisomerase I content in the cell (Hsiang et al 1985). Indeed, the protein linked to the DNA strand appears to be topoisomerase I (Hsiang and Liu et al 1988). Thus, like camptothecin, CPT-11 may cause the accumulation of an otherwise transient "cleavable complex" between DNA and topoisomerase I. This ultimately blocks both DNA synthesis and RNA synthesis in dividing cells (Hsiang et al 1985). The cytotoxic activity is cell cycle (phase) specific (Nagata 1987) and prevents cells from entering mitosis (Tobey 1972). The inhibition of topoisomerase I activity results in DNA damage which leads to cell death.

■ Availability and Storage

The drug is supplied by Yakult Honsha Company, Ltd, Tokyo, Japan, and Daicchi Pharmaceutical Company, Ltd, Tokyo, Japan, as a solution in 2- or 5-mL vials at a concentration of 20 mg/mL. The vials should be stored in a dry place at room temperature and protected from light.

■ Preparation for Use, Stability, and Admixture

CPT-11 is usually prepared by dilution and mixing in 500 mL of 5% glucose solution and administered over 90 minutes by drop infusion. Other solutions should not be used for dilution because the drug will not be stable.

■ Administration

CPT-11 is still undergoing phase I and early phase II studies. The optimal dose and schedule for drug administration are not known. The current dosages and schedules under investigation are outlined under Dosage.

■ Special Precautions

In preclinical studies it was noted that CPT-11 could be antigenic. Therefore, in early clinical trials a skin test (prick test) has been included in the prestudy testing. The prick test is performed by placing a small drop of CPT-11 (20 mg/mL) and a control solution (preservative-free normal saline) on the volar surface of the forearm. A disposable hypodermic needle (25–26 gauge) is placed through the drop and inserted into the skin surface at a low angle (bevel up). The needle tip is lifted up to elevate the upper dermis. The needle is then withdrawn and solution wiped away. Fifteen minutes after withdrawal of the needle the size of the reaction is measured. A positive test is a 4-mm or larger diameter of wheal formation or 15 mm or more of erythema which is twice as large as control. To date, however, no hypersensitivity has been noted in clinical trials, and the value of the skin test procedure is questionable.

■ Dosage

The recommended dose and schedule for administration of CPT-11 are still under investigation. Commonly used doses and schedules in early phase I and II clinical trials conducted in Japan include 100 mg/m² by 90-minute infusion every week (Fukuoka et al 1992) and 150 mg/m² given in a 5-day continuous infusion (Ohe et al 1991). In U.S. trial, a 90-minute infusion given four times weekly with a 2-week rest period as well as a bolus every 3 weeks dose regimen has been studied (Rowinsky et al 1992, Rothenberg et al 1992).

■ Pharmacokinetics

The pharmacokinetic studies performed with CPT-11 are very limited. Preclinically it is thought that the agent might be converted to an active form, SN-38, which is 100-fold more potent in vitro (Ohe et al 1991, Kawato et al 1991). Ohe et al (1991) found that after a 150 mg/m² dose given in a 120-hour continuous infusion in six patients, the AUC of CPT-11 was 20.6±6.2 µg/mL·h, whereas the AUC of SN-38 was 0.97±0.55 µg/mL·h. Chabot et al (1991) found that after a dose of 100 mg/m² given in a 30-minute infusion, peak plasma levels were 2566±531 ng/mL. Plasma elimination was triphasic with α, β, and γ half-lives of 0.07±0.01, 2.2±0.3, and 18.2±3 hours, respectively. The mean plasma AUC for parent CPT-11 in that study was 7562 ng/mL/h and clearance was 20.5 L/h/m². In contrast, peak levels of the active metabolite, SN-38, were much lower at 43 ng/mL, with a total AUC for SN-38 of only 236 ng/mL/h.

■ Side Effects and Toxicity

Dose-limiting toxic effects of CPT-11 include leukopenia in 50 to 60% of patients on the single-dose schedule (Fukuoka et al 1992) and diarrhea with the 5-day continuous infusion schedule (Ohe et al 1991) or with the four times weekly, 2-week rest schedule (Rothenberg et al 1992). Anemia was observed in 15% of non-small cell lung cancer patients and eosinophilia in 30% of patients (Fukuoka et al 1992). Other toxic effects have included moderate to severe nausea and vomiting in 35 to 60%, diarrhea in 60%, and alopecia in 33 to 40% of patients (Negoro et al 1991, Takeuchi et al 1991, Shimada et al 1991). One patient developed fatal interstitial pneumonitis in the non-small cell lung cancer trial (Fukuoka et al 1992). Six other patients (8%) developed diffuse interstitial infiltrates with fever and dyspnea, with an onset of 42 to 175 days. Glucocorticosteroids seemed to be beneficial in these patients. Transient elevations in hepatic enzymes occurred in a few patients without any sequelae.

■ Special Applications

None are known to date.

REFERENCES

Bissery MC, Mathieu-Boue A, Lavelle F. Preclinical evolution of CPT-11, a camptothecin derivative. *Proc Am Assoc Cancer Res.* 1991;**32**:402.

Chabot GG, Barilero I, Armand JP, et al Pharmacokinetics of the camptothecin analog CPT-11 and its active metabolite SN-38 in cancer patients. *Proc Am Assoc Cancer Res.* 1991;**32**:175.

Fukuoka M, Nitani H, Suzuki A, et al. A phase II study of CPT-11, a new derivative of camptothecin, for previously untreated non-small-cell lung cancer. *J Clin Oncol.* 1992;**10**(1):16–20.

Hsiang Y-H, Hertzberg R, Hecht S, Liu LF. Camptothecin induces protein-linked DNA breaks via mammalian DNA topoisomerase I. *J Biol Chem.* 1985;**260**(27):14873–14878.

Hsiang Y-H, Liu LF. Identification of mammalian DNA topoisomerase I as an intracellular target of the anticancer drug camptothecin. *Cancer Res.* 1988;**48**:1722–1726.

Kawato Y, Aohuma M, Hirota Y, et al. Intracellular roles of SN-38, a metabolite of the camptothecin derivative CPT-11, in the antitumor effect of CPT-11. *Cancer Res.* 1991;**51**:4187–4191.

Nagata H. Flow cytometric analysis of the effect of an antitumor alkaloid, camptothecin, on cell cycle progression of KB cell. *J Aichi Med Univ Assoc.* 1987;**15**:683–699.

Negoro S, Fukuoka M, Masuda N, et al. Phase I study of weekly intravenous infusions of CPT-11, a new derivative of camptothecin, in the treatment of advanced non-small-cell lung cancer. *J Natl Cancer Inst.* 1991;**83**(16):1164–1168.

Negoro S, Fukuoka M, Niitani H, Taguchi T. Phase II study of CPT-11, new camptothecin derivative, in small lung cancer (SCLC). *Proc Am Soc Clin Oncol.* 1991;**10**:241.

Ohe Y, Sasaki Y, Shinkai T, et al. Pharmacokinetics with a 5 day continuous infusion of a camptothecin derivative. *Proc Am Soc Clin Oncol.* 1991;**10**:117.

Rothenberg ML, Kuhn J, Burris HA, et al. A phase I and pharmacokinetic trial of CPT-II in patients with refractory solid tumors. *Proc Am Soc Clin Oncol.* 1992;**11**:113 (abstract #273).

Rowinsky E, Grochow L, Ettinger D, et al. Phase I and pharmacologic study of CPT-II, a semisynthetic topoisomerase I targeting agent, on a singe dose schedule. *Proc Am Soc Clin Oncol* 1992;**11**:115 (abstract #281).

Shimada Y, Yoshino M, Wakui A, et al. Phase II study of CPT-11, new camptothecin derivative, in the patients with metastatic colorectal cancer. *Proc Am Soc Clin Oncol.* 1991;**10**:135.

Stewart AF, Herrera RE, Nordheim A. Rapid induction of c-fos transcription reveals quantitative linkage of RNA polymerase II and DNA topoisomerase I enzyme activities. *Cell.* 1990;**60**:141–149.

Takeuchi S, Takamizawa H, Takeda T, et al. Clinical study of CPT-11, camptothecin derivative, for a gynecological malignancy. *Proc Am Soc Clin Oncol.* 1991;**10**:189.

Tobey RA. Effects of cytosine arabinoside, daunomycin, mithramycin, azacytidine, Adriamycin, and compt-tothecin on mammalian cell cycle transverse. *Cancer Res.* 1972;**32**:2720–2725.

Crisnatol

■ Other Names

BWA 770U mesylate.

■ Chemistry

Structure of crisnatol

The chemical name of crisnatol is 2[(6-chrysenylmethyl)amino]-2-methyl-1,3-propanediol. This compound is one of four arylmethylamino propanediols being evaluated in phase I and II trials. The other compounds are BWA 773U82, BW 7U85, and BW 502U83·HCl, discussed elsewhere in this book. These compounds have a common methylaminopropanediol side chain lined to different carbocyclic rings (Bair et al 1986). Crisnatol is a chrysene-based molecule. Crisnatol has molecular weights of 441.54 as the mesylate and 345.44 as the free base.

■ Antitumor Activity

In animals crisnatol has activity against P-388 mouse leukemia, L-1210 mouse lymphoid leukemia, B-16 melanoma, M-5076 sarcoma, Lewis lung carcinoma, and reticulum cell sarcoma (Bair et al 1986). The drug has borderline activity against colon-38 and was inactive against the MX-1 mammary xenograft (Knick et al 1986). Crisnatol has variable activity against the DNA intercalator-resistant P-388 subline.

Early phase II clinical trials have reported no activity in patients with malignant melanoma (Panella et al 1991). However there have been some intriguing responses observed in patients with gliomas (New et al 1992). There were 2 complete responders of 22 patients in this trial with remission durations of 23 and 35 months (New et al 1992). One other patient had disease stabilization for over 1 year. No responses were reported in 14 previously treated patients with ovarian cancer (Smalley et al 1992); however, higher concentrations might be active and intraperitoneal administration is being evaluated.

■ Mechanism of Action

The mode of action of crisnatol is currently unknown. The agent presumably acts through intercalation with DNA (Bair et al 1986). DNA binding experiments and cross-resistance patterns also show some correlations with other intercalating agents in preclinical in vitro and in vivo test systems (Bair et al 1986, Knick et al 1986). Crisnatol inhibition of topoisomerase II leading to protein-associated DNA double-strand breaks has been observed. In human tumor cells in vitro, crisnatol blocks macromolecular synthesis with IC_{50} values of 5 to 18 μM for DNA and RNA inhibition, respectively (Carter and Bair 1991). Inhibition of protein synthesis required higher concentrations and, overall, DNA synthesis inhibition may constitute the major cytotoxic lesion. In these experiments crisnatol did not alter nucleotide precursor uptake, phosphorylation, or retention. The cell killing by crisnatol is maximal on log-phase cells but is not cell cycle phase specific.

■ Availability and Storage

Crisnatol is investigationally supplied by Burroughs Wellcome, Research Triangle Park, North Carolina, as a sterile powder in amber vials containing 50 mg of BWA 770U as the free base. The intact vials should be stored under refrigeration (2–8°C) and should remain in individual cartons as further protection from direct light.

■ Preparation for Use, Stability, and Admixture

Vials of crisnatol should be reconstituted with 10 mL of Bacteriostatic Water for Injection, USP, only to produce a solution containing 5.0 mg/mL. The reconstituted solution should be passed through a 0.22-μm filter as it is further diluted with 5% Dextrose Injection, USP. The total volume of D5W is 1500 mL for doses of 292 mg and higher (Harman et al 1988).

Solutions containing 5 mg/mL crisnatol prepared by reconstituting the contents of one vial with 10 mL of bacteriostatic water remain chemically stable when stored under refrigeration or at room temperature for 48 hours. Solutions that are further diluted by D5W remain chemically stable under refrigeration or at room temperature for 48 hours. Studies have also shown that exposure to light will cause some degradation and solutions should be protected from light.

■ Administration

The drug is administered through a free-flowing intravenous line, using an infusion pump, over 6 hours as a single dose repeated every 28 days. Additional phase I trials using different schedules are now underway. It is hoped these alternate schedules will alleviate the neurotoxicity now seen with the drug (Harman et al 1988).

■ Special Precautions

Because of the proposed mechanism of action for crisnatol, care should be exercised to prevent contact of the drug with the skin and procedures should be followed to reduce or prevent inhalation of aerosolized particles of drug.

■ Drug Interactions

None have been described.

■ Dosage

The recommended phase II dose for the 6-hour infusion given every 28 days is 388 mg/m^2 (Harman et al 1988). With a prolonged infusion over 72 hours the maximally tolerated crisnatol dose is 2700 mg/m^2 (Poplin et al 1991). Lower doses would be indicated in patients with liver disease or poor performance status.

■ Pharmacokinetics

After infusion, plasma concentrations decline biexponentially with a terminal half-life of 2.85 hours. In a two-compartment model, the mean apparent volume of distribution at steady state was 58.8 and total body clearance was 18.3 L/h/m^2. These parameters include extensive tissue distribution and rapid hepatic clearance. Peak plasma levels at the end of unfusion averaged 5.48 ± 0.50 μg/mL at 388 mg/m^2 and correlated with the onset of neurologic toxicity (Harman et al 1988). With a prolonged infusion over 72 hours mean steady-state crisnatol levels were 2.7 and 3.8 μg/mL for doses of 2700 and 3400 mg/m^2, respectively (Poplin et al 1991). The mean terminal plasma half-life in this study was 3.3 hours with a total body clearance of 22.8 L/h/m^2 and a volume of distribution of 53 L/m^2 (Poplin et al 1991).

■ Side Effects and Toxicity

The dose-limiting toxic effect noted with the 6-hour infusion of crisnatol is reversible neurologic toxicity. This toxicity manifests as somnolence, dizziness, blurred vision, unsteady gait, and presence of gamma waves on the electroencephalogram. Other toxic effects have included severe phlebitis (alleviated somewhat with the 1500-mL volume of administration), mild to moderate nausea and vomiting, reversible sinus node arrest in one patient, and reversible mild hypertension (Harman et al 1988).

■ Special Applications

Because of the excellent dose–response effects noted with crisnatol in the human tumor cloning system (Knick et al 1986), intraarterial application of the agent is currently being considered.

REFERENCES

Bair KW, Andrews CW, Tuttle RL, Knick VC, McKee DD, Cory M. Biophysical studies and murine antitumor activity of Arylmethylaminopropanediol (AMAP), a new class of DNA binding drugs. *Proc Am Assoc Cancer Res.* 1986;**27**:424.

Carter CA, Bair KW. Effects of isomeric 2-(arylmethylamino)-1,3-propanediols (AMAPs) and clinically established agents on macromolecular synthesis in P388 and MCF-7 cells. *Invest New Drugs.* 1991;**9**:125–126.

Harman GS, Craig JB, Kuhn JG, et al. Phase I and clinical pharmacology trial of crisnatol (BWA 770U mesylate) using a monthly single-dose schedule. *Cancer Res.* 1988;**48**:4706–4710.

Knick VC, Tuttle RL, Bair KW, Von Hoff DD. Murine and human tumor stem cell activity of three candidate arylmethylaminopropanediols (AMAP). *Proc Am Assoc Cancer Res.* 1986;**27**:424.

New P, Vokes E, Rogers L, et al. Crisnatol mesylate in the treatment of progressive malignant glioma: A phase II study. *Proc Am Soc Clin Oncol.* 1992;**11**:154.

Panella TJ, Bell B, Lucas S, Wargin W, Clendeninn N,

Huang AT. Activity of crisnatol mesylate in metastatic melanoma: A phase II trial. *Proc Am Soc Clin Oncol.* 1991;**10**:296.

Poplin EA, Chabot GG, Tuttle RL, Lucas S, Wargin WA, Baker LH. Crisnatol mesylate: Phase I dose escalation by extending infusion duration. *Invest New Drugs.* 1991;**9**:41–47.

Smalley RV, Goldstein D, Bulkowski D, et al. A phase II study of crisnatol mesylate in patients with ovarian carcinoma. *Invest New Drugs.* 1992;**10**:107–112.

Cyclocytidine

■ Other Names

NSC-145668; Cyclo-C; ancitabine; 2,2′-O-cyclocytidine hydrochloride; O$^{2,2'}$-cyclocytidine.

■ Chemistry

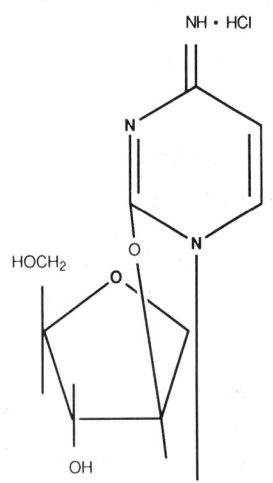

Structure of cyclocytidine

Cyclocytidine is an anhydride analog of cytarabine (Hoshi et al 1971). The complete chemical name is 2,3,3a,9a-tetrahydro-3-hydroxy-6-imino-6H-furo[2′,3′:4,5]oxazolo[3,2-a]pyrimidine-2-methanol. It has a molecular weight of 261.5. In solution it is slowly hydrolyzed to cytarabine.

■ Antitumor Activity

Cyclocytidine showed preclinical antitumor activity in L-1210 leukemia and sarcoma (Nakahara and Tokuzen 1972) and neuroblastoma (Finklestein et al 1973).

Cyclocytidine was evaluated for use primarily in acute leukemias, and was anticipated to have a spectrum of activity similar to that of its chemical analog cytarabine; however, in a phase II trial in childhood leukemia, there was only one response in 32 patients with acute lymphocytic leukemia. Furthermore, cyclocytidine was inactive in childhood myelogenous leukemia and in several pediatric sarcomas (Finklestein et al 1979). The drug was also inactive in adults with malignant melanoma (McKelvey et al 1978).

A definitive study has been carried out by the Children's Cancer Study Group in children with relapsed acute nonlymphocytic leukemia in which they were randomized to receive either daunomycin + cytosine arabinoside given intravenously every 12 hours or daunomycin + cyclocytidine (given once per day subcutaneously). The remission rates of the two regimens were not significantly different; however, the single subcutaneous dose of cyclocytidine was a more convenient way to treat patients with relapsed acute nonlymphocytic leukemia in an outpatient setting (Movassaghi et al 1984).

■ Mechanism of Action

Cyclocytidine is an analog of cytarabine which is not rapidly inactivated by the enzyme cytidine deaminase and other metabolic enzymes. Thus, cyclocytidine is not subject to in vivo deamination. Instead, it slowly releases cytarabine in the plasma (Ho 1974). Cyclocytidine may therefore be thought of as a "depot" or slow-release form of cytarabine.

Cyclocytidine is a cell cycle-specific, S-phase-dependent pyrimidine-based antimetabolite.

■ Availability and Storage

This agent is no longer supplied by the National Cancer Institute and was originally provided by the Kohgin Company in Tokyo, Japan. The compound was available in 100- and 500-mg vials which are stable at room temperature.

■ Preparation for Use, Stability, and Admixture

The contents of either vial may be reconstituted with sterile water for injection, normal saline solution, or 5% dextrose solution. The minimum recommended volume for either dosage form is 5 mL. The resultant pH of a 10% solution is between 5 and 6. The reconstituted solution may be further diluted with saline or dextrose solutions for administration by infusion.

The intact vials are stable at 60°C over 2

months. The reconstituted solutions are stable for at least 12 hours when stored at room temperature. Stability data on the infusion solutions have not been reported.

The dosage forms of cyclocytidine hydrochloride do not contain preservatives; therefore, the reconstituted solutions should be used within 8 hours of preparation.

■ Administration

Cyclocytidine can be diluted and injected intravenously, intramuscularly, or subcutaneously. Doses used range from 200 to 300 mg/m^2/d for 7 to 10 days, repeated at 2- to 4-week intervals.

■ Special Precautions

None are known.

■ Drug Interactions

None are known.

■ Dosage

The usual dose is 200 to 300 mg/m^2/d for 7 to 10 days, repeated every 2 to 4 weeks.

■ Pharmacokinetics

Using radiolabeled compound, Ho et al (1975) found that the plasma half-life of cytarabine following cyclocytidine administration is about 8 hours. Eighty percent is excreted in 24 hours with 70% as cyclocytidine, and 5% as cytarabine and 1-β-D-arabinofuranosyl uracil (ara-U). When cyclocytidine is given intramuscularly and subcutaneously the excretion ratios and plasma levels are not significantly different from those seen with the intravenous route of administration. The drug has poor oral bioavailability.

■ Side Effects and Toxicity

Side effects include hypotension, jaw pain, and mild gastrointestinal upset. Mylosuppression, however, is the usual dose-limiting toxic effect (Chawla et al 1974).

■ Special Applications

None are known.

REFERENCES

Chawla PL, Lokich JJ, Jaffe W, Frei E III. Phase I study of cyclocytidine. *Proc Am Assoc Cancer Res.* 1974;**15**:188.

Finklestein JZ, Arima E, Byfield PE, et al. Murine neuroblastoma: A model of human disease. *Cancer Chemother Rep.* 1973;**57**:405–412.

Finklestein JZ, Higgins G, Krivit W, Hammond D. Evaluation of cyclocytidine in children with advanced acute leukemia and solid tumors. *Cancer Treat Rep.* 1979;**63**:1331–1333.

Ho DHW. Biochemical studies of a new antitumor agent $O^{2,2'}$-cyclocytidine. *Biochem Pharmacol.* 1974;**23**:1235–1244.

Ho DHW, Rodriguez V, Loo TL, Bodes GP, Frereich FT. Clinical pharmacology of $O^{2,2'}$-cyclocytidine. *Clin Pharmacol.* 1975;**17**:69–72.

Hoshi A, Kanzawa F, Kuretami K, Saneyoshi M, Arai Y. 2,2′-*O*-cyclocytidine, an antitumor cytidine analog resistant to cytidine deaminase. *Gann.* 1971;**62**:145.

McKelvey EM, Hewlett JS, Thigpen T, Whitecar J. Cyclocytidine chemotherapy for malignant melanoma. *Cancer Treat Rep.* 1978;**62**:469–471.

Movassaghi N, Higgins G, Pyesmany A, et al. Evaluation of cyclocytidine in reinduction and maintenance of children with acute nonlymphocytic leukemia previously treated with cytosine arabinoside: A report from Children's Cancer Study Group. *Med Pediatr Oncol.* 1984;**12**:352–356.

Nakahara W, Tokuzen R. Effect of 2,2′-*O*-cyclocytidine on transplanted lymphocytic sarcoma and reticulum cell sarcoma in mice. *Gann.* 1972;**63**:379–381.

Cyclophosphamide

■ Other Names

NSC-26271; Cytoxan® (Bristol-Myers Oncology Division); CTX; CPM; Endoxan® (Asta-Werke AG-Chemische Fabrik); Neosar® (Adria Laboratories).

■ Chemistry

Structure of cyclophosphamide

Cyclophosphamide is 2-[bis(2-chloroethyl)amino] tetrahydro-2H-1,3,2-oxazaphosphorine 2-oxide monohydrate. It is a cyclic phosphamide ester of mechlorethamine and functions as an alkylating agent. The monohydrate (molecular weight 261.08) is unionized and lipid soluble. In normal saline or water it is soluble to a maximum of 4% at room temperature. It is also very soluble in ethanol, dichloromethane, and acetone and is readily soluble in chloroform. The anhydrous form is much less water soluble and less stable. The melting point range of cyclophosphamide is 48 to 53°C.

■ Antitumor Activity

Cyclophosphamide is useful in a wide spectrum of clinical indications. It is often included in combination regimens as in the induction therapy of non-Hodgkin's lymphomas (eg, BACOP [Skarin et al 1977] or COP [Luce et al 1971] and adult acute leukemia (eg, COAP [Whitecar et al 1972]) and can replace mechlorethamine in MOPP therapy of Hodgkin's disease (DeVita et al 1970). In this application, it has equal efficacy but is less sclerotic to veins and produces less emesis. It is also active in Burkitt's lymphoma (Ziegler et al 1970). Cyclophosphamide is frequently used in conjunction with doxorubicin in the primary and adjuvant management of breast cancer (Jones et al 1975) and endometrial carcinomas (Muggia et al 1977). It is also useful in combination therapy of small cell (oat cell) carcinoma of the lung (Livingston et al 1978) and has been useful in combination regimens in multiple myeloma (eg, MCP, VCAP, or VMCP) (Alexanian et al 1977). It also has activity in various sarcomas (Mullins and Colvin 1975, Wilbur et al 1975).

Cyclophosphamide is a potent immunosuppressive agent and is useful in a variety of nonmalignant disease processes, including nephrotic syndrome, Wegener's granulomatosis (Fauci and Wolff 1973), rheumatoid arthritis, and other autoimmune disease, and in the prevention of the graft versus host reaction in organ transplantations (Gershwin et al 1974). Conversely, low-dose cyclophosphamide (300 mg/m^2) can augment certain immune responses by selectively reducing suppressor T lymphocytes (Berd and Mastrangelo 1988, Hoon et al 1990).

See also Special Applications at the end of this monograph for high-dose applications with bone marrow transplantation.

■ Mechanism of Action

Cyclophosphamide is activated by hepatic microsomal (P450 mixed-function oxidase), enzymes forming two major intermediates (aldophosphamide and 4-hydroxycyclophosphamide) and ultimately forming at least two powerful intracellular alkylating metabolites, acrolein and phosphoramide mustard (Colvin et al 1973). Inasmuch as some of the enzymes necessary for activation of cyclophosphamide were thought to be relatively more prevalent in malignant cells (phosphamidases) and lymphocytes (phosphatases), some degree of selective cytotoxicity was believed possible (Arnold and Bourseaux 1958). This has subsequently been disproven experimentally.

As an alkylating agent, cyclophosphamide prevents cell division primarily by crosslinking DNA strands ("Proceedings" 1976). Because the cell continues to synthesize other cell constituents, such as RNA and protein, an imbalance occurs and the cell dies. A recent study has shown that DNA–DNA crosslinks form slowly but are rapidly removed from K562 cells following exposure to hepatocyte-activated cyclophosphamide (Crook et al 1986). Also, concentration- and time-dependent DNA–protein crosslinks and single-strand breaks formed after exposure to activated drug. The latter lesions were felt to be due to phosphoramide mustard, suggesting that some DNA damage and antitumor efficacy are not caused by acrolein (Crook et al 1986). There is controversy over whether 4-hydroxycyclophosphamide is the major transport form of the drug in vivo (Domeyer and Sladek 1980) or whether phosphoramide mustard constitutes the transport and cytotoxic moiety (Hipkens et al 1981) (see Pharmacokinetics for metabolic activation of cyclophosphamide). Cyclophosphamide is considered noncell cycle phase specific, with major activity against rapidly proliferating cells.

■ Availability and Storage

Cyclophosphamide is available in both oral and parenteral formulations from Bristol-Myers Oncology Division, Princeton, New Jersey (lyophilized Cytoxan®), and in a nonlyophilized injection from Adria Laboratories Division of Erbamont Inc, Dublin, Ohio (Neosar®), and from other generic manufacturers. The oral formulation is supplied in 25- and 50-mg tablets. The tablets (total weight about 240 mg with 50 mg cyclophosphamide) are coated but do dissolve in gastric juice at a rate not less than

75% after 45 minutes per USP basket test method. The parenteral formulation is available as white crystals with sodium chloride added as an excipient. The 100-mg dose is provided in a 10-mL vial, the 200-mg dose in a 20-mL vial, and the 500-mg dose in a 30-mL vial. For high-dose intravenous therapy, 1.0- and 2.0-g vials of lyophilized powder are available from Bristol-Myers. These vials are reconstituted with 50 and 100 mL Sterile Water for Injection, USP, for the 1- and 2-g vials, respectively. This yields a clear solution containing 20 mg/mL. All preparations, both tablets and injectable forms (before dilution), are stable at room temperature. Temperatures for extended storage of nonreconstituted products should not exceed 90°F.

■ Preparation for Use, Stability, and Admixture

Five milliliters of Sterile Water for Injection, USP, is added to the 100-mg vial, 10 mL to the 200-mg vial, and 25 mL to the 500-mg vial. Cyclophosphamide crystals in nonlyophilized preparations may be difficult to dissolve, and vigorous shaking with slight warming may be necessary to completely dissolve the drug. Only completely dissolved solutions should be used. Careful inspection for any remaining crystals is necessary before administration or further dilution. When the crystals are diluted in the preceding manner, the final concentration is 20 mg/mL. This solution has an approximate pH of 6.9 but this is highly dependent on the pH of the infusion fluid. The solutions as reconstituted in water will contain 3.54 mg sodium ion and 5.46 mg chloride ion from the cyclophosphamide formulation, yielding a tonicity of 378 mOsm/L. A 2% solution has a pH of 4 to 6. Bacteriostatic Water for Injection, USP (paraben-preserved only), may be used as the diluent; however, there is evidence that solutions prepared with benzyl alcohol-preserved diluents have a much higher rate of decomposition. Therefore, benzyl alcohol-preserved diluents should be avoided (Brooke et al 1973). It is recommended that unless a preserved diluent is used, the remaining portion of the vial should be discarded after 24 hours even if refrigerated. Aggressive heating of vials to obtain complete dissolution is not recommended. Even though 15 minutes of heating a 21 mg/mL solution of 50 or 60°C produces negligible decomposition, similarly heating to 70 and 80°C for the same period produces 10 and 23% decomposition, respectively (Brooke et al 1975).

Solutions reconstituted as described with either sterile water or paraben-preserved bacteriostatic water have 24-hour stability at room temperature (1.5% decomposition or less after 8 hours) and under refrigeration are stable for 6 days (Gallelli 1967). Cyclophosphamide diluted in D5W to a concentration of 1 mg/mL is physically stable for 4 hours with the antiemetic ondansetron at concentrations of 0.016 to 0.16 mg/mL (Trissel et al 1990).

According to the manufacturer, extemporaneous liquid preparations of cyclophosphamide intended for oral use may be prepared by dissolving Cytoxan® for injection into Aromatic Elixir, USP. Such preparations should be stored under refrigeration and used within 14 days.

■ Administration

Cyclophosphamide may be administered orally or intravenously. The drug may be given by intravenous push in the concentration described earlier or may be further diluted in a convenient volume of D5W or normal saline and administered by rapid or slow intravenous infusion. Intratumoral, intraperitoneal, and intrapleural routes have also been used but are not recommended as the drug is relatively inert until activated by hepatic microsomal enzymes.

The total oral drug dose may be administered all at once or divided depending on patient preference. Usually, doses of 400 mg given orally are divided into several smaller doses.

Adequate hydration of the patient both before and for 72 hours after high-dose intravenous cyclophosphamide therapy is recommended to reduce the incidence of cyclophosphamide-induced hemorrhagic cystitis. Enough fluids should be given either orally or intravenously to produce a copious urine output.

Drug interactions with cyclophosphamide and other drugs that stimulate liver metabolic enzymes (ie, barbiturates) may be significant. Other drugs that are not proven to interact significantly with cyclophosphamide include corticosteroids, succinylcholine, and allopurinol (see Drug Interactions).

See also Special Applications for high-dose administration with bone marrow transplantation.

■ Dosage

Cyclophosphamide is useful in treating many cancer types. The dosing schemes are numerous and depend on disease, individual response, and other therapy with either drugs or radiation. Two general schedules of treatment are used. In one schedule, a relatively large dose is given as a single dose once or in several divided doses over a short period (2–4 days) (Finklestein et al 1969). This approach typically includes other myelotoxic drugs, and additive effects must be considered in the dosing and frequency of cyclophosphamide administration. The other major type of dosing schedule involves relatively small doses given daily on a continuous basis.

Cyclophosphamide is usually given as a single dose ranging from 500 to 1500 mg/m^2 of body surface area (30–40 mg/kg) per treatment course. These courses can be repeated at approximately 2- to 4-week intervals. Such doses are usually administered intravenously and are not well tolerated orally.

When the continuous daily dosing method is employed, doses must be individualized to the patient. Doses of 60 to 120 mg/m^2 of body surface area or 1 to 2.5 mg/kg/d are commonly used. The dose must be titrated to the individual patient's tolerance. This involves frequent, careful assessment of the degree of myelosuppression.

See Special Applications for high-dose cyclophosphamide with bone marrow transplantation.

■ Special Precautions

It is important to keep the patient well hydrated during therapy (see Administration) to reduce the potential for hemorrhagic cystitis (see Drug Reactions).

■ Drug Interactions

A number of potential drug interactions are described with cyclophosphamide. These are summarized in the table. Only a few have been evaluated clinically; thus, clinical relevance is unknown in many of these "interactions" (see the table).

Allopurinol may possibly increase the incidence and degree of bone marrow suppression with cyclophosphamide by prolonging the half-life of cyclophosphamide (Bagley et al 1973). The total amount of alkylating metabolites, however, appears to remain unchanged. An interaction showing increased myelosuppression with cyclophosphamide and concurrent allopurinol has also been suggested by an epidemiologic review (Boston Collaborative Drug Surveillance Program 1974). However, a follow-up study could show no increase in myelosuppression from the combination of cyclophosphamide and allopurinol in 143 patients with malignant lymphoma (Stolbach et al 1982). Thus, the clinical significance of this interaction is not established.

Barbiturates and other inducers of hepatic microsomal enzymes such as phenytoin and chloral hydrate may increase the rate of hepatic conversion of cyclophosphamide to its toxic metabolites. Similarly, cyclophosphamide may block the metabolism of barbiturates, causing increased sedative effects (Bus et al 1973, Alberts and Van Daalen Wetters 1976). Although the clinical significance of these reactions is not clear, cyclophosphamide toxicity may be increased; however, even though pretreatment with phenobarbital decreases the half-life of cyclophosphamide from 4 to 1.6 hours, the total amount of alkylating metabolites produced apparently remains the same (Jao et al 1972). Thus, allopurinol and barbiturates appear to affect only the rates of activation, not the amount of active metabolites

DRUG INTERACTIONS WITH CYCLOPHOSPHAMIDE

Agent	Cyclophosphamide Potential Interaction	System
N-Acetylcysteine	Inactivation of acrolein without affecting antitumor activity	Rodents, humans
Allopurinol	Increased myelotoxicity in some studies; clinical significance not established	Humans, mice
Barbiturates	Enhanced clearance as a result of microsomal enzyme induction	Mice
Buthionine sulfoximine	Enhanced cardiotoxicity by glutathione depletion	Mice
Carbon tetrachloride	Enhanced toxicity as a result of delayed hepatic clearance	Mice
Cimetidine	Enhanced myelotoxicity enzyme inhibition	Mice
Corticosteroids	Blocked enzyme activation of cyclophosphamide	In vitro
Interferon	Enhanced antitumor effects; enhanced myelotoxicity of cyclophosphamide	Mice
Mesna	Binding (inactivation) of acrolein without affecting antitumor activity	In vitro, mice, humans
Ranitidine	Lack of interaction	Mice, humans
Succinylcholine	Blocked metabolism of succinylcholine	Rodents

produced. Nonetheless, the use of those interacting drugs before and during cyclophosphamide therapy should be avoided if possible.

Microsomal enzyme blockers such as SKF-525A and Lilly 18947 (2,4-dichloro-6-phenylphenoxyethyldiethylamine) reduce the lethality of cyclophosphamide without altering the antitumor activity (Hart and Adamson 1969). The blocker SKF-525A has also been shown to increase the amount of alkylating metabolites of cyclophosphamide in mice (Field et al 1972). Similarly, the H_2 antihistamine cimetidine has been shown to enhance cyclophosphamide's antitumor effects as a result of an increase in alkylating metabolites in mice (Dorr and Alberts 1982). Of interest, the related H_2 antagonist ranitidine did not alter cyclophosphamide activity in mice (Dorr et al 1986) nor in human cancer patients (Alberts et al 1991). A similar interaction involving enhanced cyclophosphamide toxicity may occur with interferon alfa combined with cyclophosphamide. Borden et al (1988) have described schedule-dependent inhibition of cyclophosphamide efficacy when combined with interferons alfa and beta. Other preclinical studies have also reported positive results for interferon combined with cyclophosphamide (Balkwill and Moodie 1984). In myeloma patients, interferon alfa doses greater than 3×10^6 U increased the myelosuppressive effects of cyclophosphamide (Durie et al 1986).

Corticosteroids may inhibit microsomal enzyme metabolism of cyclophosphamide and thereby reduce its effect (Hayakawa et al 1969, Faber and Mouridsen 1974). If a patient who is maintained on cyclophosphamide and corticosteroids has a sudden reduction in steroid dose, attention should be given to the possibility of increased toxicity of cyclophosphamide; however, this has not been clinically verified.

The enzyme pseudocholinesterase, which metabolizes succinylcholine, may be decreased during cyclophosphamide therapy. Therefore, prolonged apnea may occur after the coadministration of standard doses of succinylcholine with cyclophosphamide.

It has been reported that the general anesthetics halothane and nitrous oxide may cause increased mortality in patients receiving cyclophosphamide. This was based on animal studies and has not been reported in clinical situations. Carbon tetrachloride has also been reported to increase cyclophosphamide's antitumor effects because of delayed clearance of cyclophosphamide, ostensibly as a result of liver damage (Harris et al 1984).

A more serious interaction involves the depletion of glutathione by L-buthionine sulfoximine with cyclophosphamide (see Buthionine Sulfoximine). Pretreatment of mice with L-buthionine sulfoximine leads to a marked increase in the lethality of cyclophosphamide (Soble and Dorr 1987) without enhanced antitumor efficacy (Soble and Dorr 1988). The mechanism appears to involve enhanced myocardial muscle cell damage as a result of glutathione depletion therein (Friedman et al 1990).

Cyclophosphamide may also enhance the activity of immunopotentiating agents such as tumor vaccines by its selective inhibition of suppressor (CD8+) T lymphocytes (Berd et al 1984). This indirectly increases the percentage of helper T lymphocytes and can thereby increase patient response to melanoma vaccines as monitored by lymphocyte reactivity to lectins in vitro (Hoon et al 1990).

Finally, several sulfhydryl-containing agents are known to block cyclophosphamide-induced bladder damage. These agents bind acrolein in the urinary bladder. They include *N*-acetylcysteine (Primack 1971, Harrison et al 1983) and mesna (see Mesna).

■ Pharmacokinetics

Cyclophosphamide is probably well absorbed orally; however, studies with labeled cyclophosphamide have shown that only 31 to 66% of the total radioactivity (17–31% as unchanged drug) is present in the stools after oral administration (Bagley et al 1973). Wagner and Fenneberg (1984) have described 90% bioavailability of oral, unmetabolized cyclophosphamide with a first-pass effect of only 8%. Of interest, Struck et al (1986) have observed higher levels of alkylating metabolites following intravenous cyclophosphamide administration in contrast to an earlier study by Juma et al (1979).

The drug must be metabolized to be active (Sladek 1972). Although some cyclophosphamide may be activated by phosphatases and phosphamidases peripherally, the majority of the drug is metabolized by microsomal enzymes in the liver (Connors et al 1974, Jardine et al 1976). In rat hepatic tissue, the major forms of P450 involved in cyclophosphamide metabolism are the PB-1 and PB-4 isoenzymes (Clarke and Waxman 1989). Aldehyde dehydrogenase appears to play a minor role in cyclophosphamide metabolism (Hipkens et al 1981) and is not usually altered in cyclophosphamide-resistant cells (Lin and Lindahl 1987). There are also data suggesting that 4-hydroxycyclophosphamide serves as the transport form of the drug in the plasma following microsomal metabolism in the liver (Domeyer and Sladek 1980).

Cyclophosphamide is oxidatively metabolized to 4-hydroxycyclophosphamide by microsomal enzymes using NADPH as a cofactor. This relatively, stable active transport form can then break down via soluble enzymes or by spontaneous processes to the inactive metabolite 4-keto-cyclophosphamide. Conversely, 4-hydroxycyclophosphamide can be metabolized microsomally to aldophosphamide which will spontaneously yield another inactive metabolite, carboxyphosphamide, or the active alkylating species phosphoramide mustard

$$HO-\overset{\overset{O}{|}}{\underset{\underset{NH_2}{|}}{P}}-N-(CH_2-CH_2-Cl)_2$$

and acrolein ($H_2C{=}CHCH{=}O$). Phosphoramide mustard mediates the antitumor cytotoxic effect and may also constitute the transport form (Donelli et al 1976, Hipkens et al 1981). Conversely, acrolein binds avidly to proteins. Acrolein does not contribute to the antitumor effects of cyclophosphamide, but does produce hemorrhagic cystitis in the urinary bladder. Gurtoo et al (1981) have shown that glutathione and other sulfhydryl-containing compounds can protect against cyclophosphamide toxicity resulting from acrolein without inhibiting cyclophosphamide's antitumor activity. The sulfhydryl compound mesna similarly provides excellent site-selective inactivation of acrolein as a result of the breakdown of dimesna to active monomers in the renal tubules and bladder (see Mesna). Because active and toxic metabolites result from the activity of these enzymes on cyclophosphamide, many potential drug interactions may exist.

The pharmacokinetics of cyclophosphamide are reviewed in the table. Approximately 15% of the drug is excreted unchanged in the urine. Numerous inactive metabolites are also excreted in the urine (Jardine et al 1976). The plasma half-life after doses of 6 to 80 mg/kg appears to range from 4 to 6.5 hours (Bagley et al 1973). Cyclophosphamide is minimally bound to plasma proteins (Bagley et al 1973, Jardine et al 1978). In one patient, 24% of unmetabolized cyclophosphamide was bound in the plasma compared with 67% for phosphoramide mustard. The disposition of cyclophosphamide is biexponential, consisting of a rapid initial distribution phase and a slower phase associated with hepatic activation. Thus, over 24 hours, renal excretion accounts for 10% of the dose as a parent drug and 50% as metabolites.

Although cyclophosphamide is exclusively excreted by the kidney, because of the un-ionized nature of the intact drug molecule, tubular reabsorption is avid. Thus, a large fraction of the cyclophosphamide dose is eliminated by hepatic metabolism (Mouridsen et al 1974). The mean renal clearance of intact drug is approximately 11 mL/min, or 15% of creatinine clearance, whereas renal elimination remains the major route of disposition of the more polar, less lipid-soluble metabolites (Cohen et al 1971). In most patients, a low level of alkylating activity from the unbound metabolites is maintained in the plasma for a minimum of 24 hours. There may be significantly prolonged retention of active (alkylating) metabolites in patients with severe renal failure; however, Grochow and Colvin (1983) were unable to correlate cyclophosphamide-induced myelosuppression and the severity of renal failure in a retrospective review of 120

CLINICAL PHARMACOKINETICS OF CYCLOPHOSPHAMIDE AND SELECTED METABOLITES

Agent	Route	Half-life (h)	Volume of Distribution (L/kg)	Clearance (mL/min) Renal	Clearance (mL/min) Total Body	% Urinary Excretion	Reference
Cyclophosphamide	PO	1.3–6.8	0.48	—	—	—	Juma et al 1979, 1980
	IV	6–12.4	0.34	5.3	73	6.3	Juma et al 1979, 1980
Alkylating species	PO	9.9	—	—	—	—	Juma et al 1979, 1980
	IV	7.7	—	—	—	—	Juma et al 1979, 1980
Cyclophosphamide	IV	4.1–16	0.51–1.2	3.5–16.5	43–160	—	Edwards et al 1980

myeloma patients receiving doses of 60 mg/kg. Juma et al (1981) similarly recommended no dose adjustments in patients unless severe renal insufficiency (creatinine clearance < 20 mL/min) is present. In addition, Saul et al (1979) could find no association between the renal excretion of cyclophosphamide alkylating metabolites and the presence of only one functioning kidney.

In contrast, body weight may effect the elimination of the parent cyclophosphamide molecule. In women with a high body weight, cyclophosphamide clearance was low at about 20 mL/min/m^2. The plasma half-life was correspondingly long at more than 8 hours. Conversely, women with lower body weight had more rapid cyclophosphamide clearance values of 40 to 100 mL/min with plasma half-lives shorter than 8 hours (Powis et al 1987). There was no correlation for either parameter with response, the degree of myelosuppression, or the volume of distribution, which averaged 36 L (range, 19–62 L).

Distribution studies in humans have also detected that only minute quantities of drug and metabolites are excreted into expired air and into saliva, sweat, cerebrospinal fluid, and synovial fluid (Duncan et al 1973); however, in more recent studies cyclophosphamide has consistently been detected in breast milk using mass spectrometry techniques (Amato and Niblett 1977, Duradola 1979). Only 3.5% of cyclophosphamide can be recovered unchanged in the bile, although low levels of alkylating metabolites are detected up to 25 hours after dosing (Dooley et al 1982). It has not been possible to detect the drug in the central nervous system, but it appears in cerebrospinal fluid (Egorin et al 1982). Approximately 25% of plasma levels are achieved in amniotic fluid (D'Incalci et al 1982). Salivary secretion of cyclophosphamide has also been reported, with a plasma-to-saliva ratio of 1.61 (Ritschel et al 1981).

■ Side Effects and Toxicity

Myelosuppression consisting primarily of leukopenia is cyclophosphamide's principal dose-limiting toxic effect. The leukocyte nadir and time of recovery are rapid at 8 to 14 and 18 to 25 days, respectively. Although this drug is relatively "platelet sparing," significant thrombocytopenia has also occurred, especially after high doses. There is also a recent experimental case of recovery from chloramphenicol-induced aplastic anemia after treatment with cyclophosphamide (Baran et al 1977). A curious "priming" phenomenon with low-dose cyclophosphamide has recently been explained by Carmichael et al (1986). Low-dose cyclophosphamide given before other myelosuppressive drugs is known to reduce bone marrow toxicity. The mechanism appears to involve a cyclophosphamide-mediated initial depression and rebound elevation in the levels of glutathione and glutathione transferases in nucleated bone marrow cells. This renders the cell less susceptible to subsequent drug damage, especially from other alkylating agents which are detoxified by glutathione-based systems.

Acute sterile hemorrhagic cystitis is a severe toxic manifestation of cyclophosphamide and is associated with large single doses or with chronic low-dose therapy (Berkson et al 1973, Hutter et al 1969, Pearlman 1966). Commonly, this may constitute the dose-limiting toxic effect of cyclophosphamide. It is more common in poorly hydrated or renally compromised patients. The onset of this complication may be delayed from 24 hours to several weeks. It initially manifests as either gross hematuria or a microscopic hematuria of fewer than 20 erythrocytes/high-power field. The bleeding may persist but is generally transient. Prior to the use of prophylactic mesna, less severe presentations were treated with 5 to 10% formalin instillations to control bleeding. Primack (1971) also used acetylcysteine irrigation in severe presentations. Prophylactic hydration with intake of at least 3 L/d may also lessen cyclophosphamide-induced bladder damage. With continued cyclophosphamide therapy, patients may characteristically develop a fibrotic "small bladder," and urinary frequency may become a permanent problem (Johnson and Meadows 1971). Current regimens using mesna appear to provide more effective prevention of cyclophosphamide-induced bladder damage. Mesna should be considered for all high-dose cyclophosphamide regimens (see Mesna or Special Applications in this monograph).

The syndrome of inappropriate antidiuretic hormone (SIADH), or "water intoxication," has been reported after cyclophosphamide (Steele et al 1973). This is more common with intravenous doses greater than 50 mg/kg and is both a limitation to and consequence of fluid loading which should be kept in mind (DeFronzo et al 1973).

Bladder carcinomas and cellular dysplasias have all been reported after cyclophosphamide therapy (Wall and Clausen 1975). This is most common after chronic closing in patients with immunologic diseases.

Alopecia is severe in at least half of all patients treated. It should be expected to some degree in all patients. Resolution may ensue even with continuing treatment.

Gastrointestinal toxicity is more common with high-oral-dose therapy and comprises anorexia, nausea, and vomiting. Antiemetics are usually helpful. Dose-related hepatotoxicity manifests as a transient elevation in serum aminotransferase levels (Honjo et al 1988). The incidence was 33% at doses below 400 mg/m^2 and 77% at higher doses. The toxic effects were also associated with reduced formation of the acrolein conjugate 3-hydroxypropylmercapturic acid in patients receiving the higher doses of cyclophosphamide. Hepatotoxicity has also been reported in a patient with systemic lupus erythematosus. In animals, transient hypercholesterolemia and hypertriglyceridemia have been reported (Loudet et al 1984).

Extravasation of the drug does not produce necrosis as with other alkylating agents; however, a sterile phlebitis at the injection site has been reported.

In addition, a rare pulmonary toxic effect that is characterized by pneumonitis and is similar to "busulfan lung" has been reported (Rodin et al 1970). The typical picture is that of an interstitial pneumonitis usually occurring after long-term and continuous low-dose therapy (Topelow et al 1973). The onset of symptoms is insidious. Pathologically, there can be alveolitis with eventual fibrosis and atypical type II pneumocytes. Of seven reported cases, three patients died with respiratory failure and four survived with minimal residual deficit. Glucocorticosteroids may be beneficial in this syndrome (Topelow et al 1973).

Other toxic effects include testicular atrophy (Fairley et al 1972, Hyman and Gilbert 1972), sometimes with reversible oligospermia and azoospermia (Buchanan et al 1975), and amenorrhea with ovarian failure (Kumar et al 1972, Warne et al 1963). As with all alkylating agents, drug-induced congenital abnormalities including toe and cardiac defects have been associated with cyclophosphamide therapy (Greenberg and Tanaka 1964, Toledo et al 1971). Cyclophosphamide can also have carcinogenic effects, especially when low daily doses are administered for prolonged periods as in rheumatoid arthritis. Urinary bladder cancers and skin cancers tend to predominate in this setting (Baker et al 1987). Similarly, urinary bladder cancer has been described in lymphoma patients treated with cyclophosphamide. The cumulative risk was 3.5% 8 years after the start of therapy and 10.7% 12 years after the start of therapy (Pederson-Bjergaard et al 1988). Another study reports a ninefold increased risk of bladder cancer following cyclophosphamide (Fairchild et al 1979).

Other unusual toxic effects include a fleeting oropharyngeal sensation with bolus injection (Arena 1972) and urticaria, which resolved when cyclophosphamide was replaced by chlorambucil (Krutchik et al 1978). Karchmer and Hansen (1977) describe a similar case with a "tongue-burning" sensation, urticaria, and hypotension during a bolus injection. Transient blurring of vision is also reported (Kende et al 1979).

Cyclophosphamide allergic reactions have also occurred in mechlorethamine-sensitive patients (Ross and Chabner 1977). Conversely, a patient allergic to cyclophosphamide was successfully treated with mechlorethamine and ifosfamide without cross-sensitivity (Legha and Hall 1977). With high-dose therapy, cyclophosphamide-associated cardiac toxicity has been reported (Buckner et al 1972) (see Special Applications).

■ Special Applications

High Doses with BMT. Cyclophosphamide is one of several antineoplastic agents used in high doses, either alone or in combination with bone marrow transplantation (BMT). The drug has been used with autologous BMT in the treatment of acute lymphoblastic leukemia (Thomas et al 1979a, b), for recurrent acute myelogenous leukemias, and for severe aplastic anemia (Camitta et al 1976). In solid tumors, high-dose cyclophosphamide is usually combined with other agents such as carmustine and cisplatin for metastatic breast cancer (Eder et al 1986); with only carmustine for solid tumors such as melanoma, sarcoma, colon cancer, and breast carcinoma (Slease et al 1988), and with carmustine and etoposide for refractory Hodgkin's disease (Phillips et al 1989). Hematopoietic colony-stimulating factors such as GM-CSF have been evaluated in combination with these regimens to enhance and hasten bone marrow engraftment (Taylor et al 1989).

The table on the opposite page summarizes the various cyclophosphamide doses in these regimens. The maximal cyclophosphamide dose that can be administered as a single agent without BMT is 7 g/m^2, or 190 mg/kg (Buckner et al 1972, 1974, Smith et al 1983). This results in severe myelosuppression with hematologic recovery after about 3 weeks. Objective response rates in refractory lymphoma or

CYCLOPHOSPHAMIDE IN HIGH DOSE REGIMENS

CTX Dose	Other Agents (dose, mg/m^2)	Autologous Bone Marrow Transplantation	Indication	Reference
7 g/m^2 (190 mg/kg)	None	No	Ovarian cancer	Piver et al 1975
				Buckner et al 1974
	None	No	Small cell lung cancer	Souhami et al 1985
60–120 mg/kg	None	No	Various (ovary, testis, colon)	Buckner et al 1972
7 g/m^2	GM-CSF (5.5 μg/kg/d)	No	Breast, lymphoma	Gianni et al 1990
120 mg/kg	None	No	Lymphomas, solid tumor	Collins et al 1989
5.625 g/m^2	Cisplatin (165) Carmustine (600)	Yes	Breast	Eder et al 1986
160 mg/kg	Carmustine (900)	Yes	Solid tumors	Slease et al 1988
1.8 g/m^2	Carmustine (600) Etoposide (2400)	Yes	Hodgkin's disease	Phillips et al 1989
7.2 g/m^2	Carmustine (450) Etoposide (2000)	Yes	Lymphomas	Wheeler et al 1990

solid tumor malignancies can be as high as 60%; the majority of patients achieve a partial response and 10 to 15% complete remissions are described (Collins et al 1989). Unfortunately, remission durations tend to be short, 1 to 5 months, although there are usually a few long-term survivors. In metastatic breast cancer a median survival of 8 months is reported following high-dose combination chemotherapy including cyclophosphamide (Eder et al 1986). In other solid tumors, the median duration of response was even shorter, 4 months (Slease et al 1988). Much longer response durations are reported in Hodgkin's disease (Phillips et al 1989) and in non-Hodgkin's lymphomas (Wheeler et al 1990).

The pharmacokinetics of high-dose cyclophosphamide do not differ from that at low doses (see table on page 328). Even at doses of 5 g/m^2, there is no evidence that enzymes responsible for cyclophosphamide biotransformation and detoxification are saturated (Wilkinson et al 1983, Milsted and Jarman 1982). The average steady-state plasma level following a dose of 180 mg/kg given over 13 hours was 140 μg/mL in one trial, and the addition of high-dose etoposide did not alter cyclophosphamide disposition (Cunningham et al 1988). One group has reported that the half-life of cyclophosphamide sequentially decreased from 7.1 to 4.3 hours over the course of four daily administrations of 50 mg/kg/d (Schuler et al 1987). In the same period, systemic exposure to activated, unbound metabolites increased from 10.5 to 26.0 nmol·h/mL.

Thus, cyclophosphamide may rapidly induce activating enzymes or there may be transient saturation of protein binding sites with daily high-dose regimens. In another pharmacokinetic trial of high-dose cyclophosphamide, the pharmacokinetics of 4-hydroxycyclophosphamide was found to be relatively constant despite marked variations in the half-life of the parent compound (Sladek et al 1984). The half-life of the 4-hydroxy metabolite ranged between 2 and 3 hours with a systemic AUC of 5 mM·min in this trial. Similarly, the half-life and AUC of the active alkylating species, phosphoramide mustard, were relatively constant at 50 to 300 min and 15 mM·min, respec- tively (Sladek et al 1984).

Besides myelosuppression, the other usual toxic effects of cyclophosphamide are similarly increased following high-dose therapy. Nausea and vomiting develop between 6 and 12 hours after the start of a 1-hour cyclophosphamide infusion (Fetting et al 1982). The symptoms usually peak at 12 hours and have typically subsided after 24 hours, although nausea may persist for longer periods. Hemorrhagic cystitis also occurs at a very high incidence in high-dose therapy regimens.

Cardiotoxicity is uniquely associated with high-dose cyclophosphamide (Buckner et al 1972) and is believed to involve endothelial injury producing hemorrhagic necrosis (Gottdiener et al 1981). This can result in massive cardiac necrosis. Left ventricular systolic function has been observed to de-

PHARMACOKINETICS OF HIGH-DOSE CYCLOPHOSPHAMIDE

Dose (mg/kg)	Clearance (L/h)	Half-life (h)	Volume of Distribution (L)	AUC (mM · min)	24-h Urinary Excretion (% Dose)	Reference
180	6.5–7.2	1.9–2.6	18–20	—	3.7–16.9	Cunningham et al 1988
50–60	—	1–8	—	10–188		Sladek et al 1984

cline serially following a 4-day high-dose cyclophosphamide regimen (Gottdiener et al 1981). Pericardial effusions were noted in 33% of patients and electrocardiographic voltage decreased 5 to 14 days after cyclophosphamide was started. This led to congestive heart failure in 28% of patients without 3 weeks. Mortality was 19% in this study (Gottdiener et al 1981).

Unique histologic findings include fibrin microthrombi in cardiac capillaries with fibrin strands in muscle cells and interstitium (Appelbaum et al 1976). These findings are not limited to adults but are related to the cyclophosphamide dose, particularly when calculated on weight instead of body surface area (Goldberg et al 1986). This group recommended limiting the cyclophosphamide dose to 1.55 g/m^2/d × 4 days as preparative treatment for BMT in patients with a variety of dysfunctional bone marrow diseases (Goldberg et al 1986). The overall incidence of cyclophosphamide cardiotoxicity from several series is 22%, with a mortality rate of 11% (Steinherz et al 1981, Gottdiener et al 1981). Two fatalities have also been reported at relatively low cyclophosphamide doses of 144 and 168 mg/kg (Mills and Roberts 1979). There may also be synergy with prior anthracycline exposure (> 100 mg/m^2 daunorubicin or doxorubicin) (Steinherz et al 1981). It has also been suggested that large single infusions over short periods may enhance the likelihood of developing cyclophosphamide cardiomyopathy. Thus, twice daily infusions of high-dose cyclophosphamide have been shown to allow greater total dose delivery with reduced cardiotoxic risks in a prospective clinical study (Braverman et al 1991).

The mechanism of cardiac injury is not known; however, it may involve cellular thiols (Friedman et al 1990). Cyclophosphamide is known to deplete endomyocardial glutathione levels in patients (Peters et al 1988) and there is a known toxic synergy with the glutathione-depleting agent buthionine sulfoximine (Soble and Dorr 1987, Friedman et al 1990).

REFERENCES

Alberts DS, Mason-Liddil NM, Plezia P. Lack of ranitidine effects on cyclophosphamide bone marrow toxicity or metabolism: A placebo controlled clinical trial. *J Natl Cancer Inst.* 1991;**83**(23):1739–1743.

Alberts DS, Van Daalen Wetters T. The effect of phenobarbital on cyclophosphamide anti-tumor activity. *Cancer Res.* 1976;**36**:2785–2789.

Alexanian R, Salmon S, Bonnet J, et al. Combination therapy for multiple myeloma. *Cancer.* 1977;**40**:2765–2771.

Amato D, Niblett JS. Neutropenia from cyclophosphamide in breast milk. *Med J Aust.* 1977;**1**:383–384.

Appelbaum FR, Strauchen JA, Graw RG Jr, et al. Acute lethal carditis caused by high-dose combination chemotherapy. A unique clinical and pathological entity. *Lancet.* 1976;**1**:58–62.

Arena PJ. Oropharyngeal sensation associated with rapid intravenous administration of cyclophosphamide (NSC-26271). *Cancer Chemother Rep Part I.* 1972;**56**(6):779–780.

Arnold H, Bourseaux F. Sythese und Abbau cytostatisch wirksame cydischer N-phosphamidester des bis-(β-chlorathyl)-amis. *Agnew Chem (Engl).* 1958;**70**:539–544.

Bagley CM. Boslick FW, DeVita VT. Clinical pharmacology of cyclophosphamide. *Cancer Res.* 1973;**33**:226–233.

Baker GL, Kahl LE, Zee BC, et al. Malignancy following treatment of rheumatoid arthritis with cyclophosphamide. Long-term case-control follow-up study. *Am J Med.* 1987;**83**:1–9.

Balkwill FR, Moodie EM. Positive interactions between human interferon and cyclophosphamide or Adriamycin in a human tumor model system. *Cancer Res.* 1984;**44**:904–908.

Baran DT, Griner PF, Klemperer MR. Recovery from aplastic anemia after treatment with cyclophosphamide. *N Engl J Med.* 1977;**295**(27):1522–1523.

Berd D, Maguire HC Jr, Mastrangelo MJ. Immunopotentiation by cyclophosphamide and other cytotoxic agents. In: RL Fenichel, MA Chirigos, eds. *Immune Modulation Agents and Their Mechanisms.* New York: Marcel Dekker; 1984:39–61.

Berd D, Mastrangelo MJ. Effect of low dose cyclophosphamide on the immune system of cancer patients: Depletion of CD4$^+$,2H4$^+$ suppressor-inducer T-cells. *Cancer Res.* 1988;**48**:1671–1675.

Berkson GM, Lome LG, Shapiro I. Severe cystitis induced by cyclophosphamide. *JAMA*. 1973;**225:**605–606.

Borden EC, Sidky YA, Hatcher JF, Bryan GT. Schedule-dependent variations in the response of murine P388 leukemia to cyclophosphamide in combination with interferons-α/β. *Cancer Res*. 1988;**48:**2329–2334.

Boston Collaborative Drug Surveillance Program. Allopurinol and cytotoxic drugs. *JAMA*. 1974;**227**(9):1036–1040.

Braverman AC, Antin JH, Plappert MT, et al. Cyclophosphamide cardiotoxicity in bone marrow transplantation: A prospective evaluation of new dosing regimens. *J Clin Oncol*. 1991;**9**(7):1215–1223.

Brooke D, Bequette RJ, Davis RE. Chemical stability of cyclophosphamide in parenteral solutions. *Am J Hosp Pharm*. 1973;**30:**134–171.

Brooke D, Scott JA, Bequette RJ. Effect of briefly heating cyclophosphamide solutions. *Am J Hosp Pharm*. 1975;**32:**44–45.

Buchanan JD, Fairley KF, Barrie JU. Return of spermatogenesis after stopping cyclophosphamide therapy. *Lancet*. 1975;**2:**156–157.

Buckner CD, Briggs R, Clift RA, et al. Intermittent high-dose cyclophosphamide (NSC-26271) treatment of stage III ovarian carcinoma. *Cancer Chemother Rep*. 1974;**58:**697–703.

Buckner CD, Rudolph RH, Fefer A, et al. High-dose cyclophosphamide therapy for malignant disease. Toxicity, tumor response, and the effects of stored autologous marrow. *Cancer*. 1972;**29:**357–365.

Bus J, Short R, Gibson J. Effect of phenobarbital and SKF525A on the toxicity, elimination and metabolism of cyclophosphamide in newborn mice. *J Pharmacol Exp Ther*. 1973;**184**(3):749–756.

Camitta BM, Thomas ED, Nathan DG, et al. Severe aplastic anemia: A prospective study of the effect of early marrow transplantation on acute mortality. *Blood*. 1976;**48:**63–70.

Carmichael J, Adams DJ, Ansell J, et al. Glutathione and glutathione transferase levels in mouse granulocytes following cyclophosphamide administration. *Cancer Res*. 1986;**46:**735–739.

Clarke L, Waxman DJ. Oxidative metabolism of cyclophosphamide: Identification of the hepatic monooxygenase catalysts of drug activation. *Cancer Res*. 1989;**49:**2344–2350.

Cohen JL, Jao JY, Jusko WJ. Pharmacokinetics of cyclophosphamide in man. *Br J Pharmacol*. 1971;**43:**667–680.

Collins C, Mortimer J, Livingston RB. High-dose cyclophosphamide in the treatment of refractory lymphomas and solid tumor malignancies. *Cancer*. 1989;**63:**228–232.

Colvin M, Padgett CA, Fenselau C. A biologically active metabolite of cyclophosphamide. *Cancer Res*. 1973;**33:**915–918.

Connors TA, Cox PJ, Farmer PB, et al. Some studies of the active metabolites formed in the microsomal metabolism of cyclophosphamide and isophosphamide. *Biochem Pharmacol*. 1974;**23:**115–129.

Crook TR, Souhami RL, McLean AEM. Cytotoxicity, DNA cross-linking, and single strand breaks induced by activated cyclophosphamide and acrolein in human leukemia cells. *Cancer Res*. 1986;**46:**5029–5034.

Cunningham D, Cummings J, Blackie RB, et al. The pharmacokinetics of high dose cyclophosphamide and high dose etoposide. *Med Oncol Tumor Pharmacother*. 1988;**5**(2):117–123.

DeFronzo RA, Braine H, Colvin OM, et al. Water intoxication in man after cyclophosphamide therapy. Time course and relation to drug activation. *Ann Intern Med*. 1973;**78:**861–869.

DeVita VT, Serpick AA, Carbone PP. Combination chemotherapy in the treatment of advanced Hodgkin's disease. *Ann Intern Med*. 1970;**73**(6):881–895.

D'Incalci M, Sessa C, Columbo N, et al. Transplacental passage of cyclophosphamide. *Cancer Treat Rep*. 1982;**66:**1681–1682.

Domeyer BE, Sladek NE. Kinetics of cyclophosphamide biotransformation in vivo. *Cancer Res*. 1980;**40:**174–180.

Donelli MG, Bartosek I, Guaitani A. Importance of pharmacokinetic studies on cyclophosphamide (NSC-26271) in understanding its cytotoxic effect. *Cancer Treat Rep*. 1976;**60**(4):395–401.

Dooley JS, James CA, Rogers HJ, Stuart-Harris R. Biliary elimination of cyclophosphamide in man. *Cancer Chemother Pharmacol*. 1982;**9:**26–29.

Dorr RT, Alberts DS. Cimetidine enhancement of cyclophosphamide antitumor activity. *Br J Cancer*. 1982;**45:**35–43.

Dorr RT, Soble MJ, Alberts DS. Interaction of cimetidine but not ranitidine with cyclophosphamide in mice. *Cancer Res*. 1986;**46:**1795–1799.

Duncan JH, Colvin MO, Fenselau C. Mass spectrophotometric study of the distribution of cyclophosphamide in humans. *Toxicol Appl Pharmacol*. 1973;**24:**317–323.

Duradola JI. Administration of cyclophosphamide during late pregnancy and early lactation: A case report. *J Natl Med Assoc*. 1979;**71**(2):165–166.

Durie BGM, Clouse L, Braich T, et al. Interferon alfa-2b–cyclophosphamide combination studies: In vitro and phase I–II clinical results. *Semin Oncol*. 1986;**13**(suppl 2):84–88.

Eder JP, Antman K, Peters W, et al. High-dose combination alkylating agent chemotherapy with autologous bone marrow support for metastatic breast cancer. *J Clin Oncol*. 1986;**4:**1592–1597.

Edwards G, Calvert RT, Crowther D, et al. Repeated investigations of cyclophosphamide disposition in myeloma patients receiving intermittent chemotherapy. *Br J Clin Pharmacol*. 1980;**10:**281–285.

Egorin M, Kaplan RS, Salcman M, et al. Cyclophosphamide plasma and cerebrospinal fluid kinetics with and without dimethyl sulfoxide. *Clin Pharmacol Ther*. 1982;**32:**122–128.

Faber OK, Mouridsen HT. Cyclophosphamide activation and corticosteroids. *N Engl J Med.* 1974;**291**:211.

Fairchild WV, Spence CR, Solomon HD, Gangai MP. The incidence of bladder cancer after cyclophosphamide therapy. *J Urol.* 1979;**122**:163–164.

Fairley KF, Barrie JU, Johnson W. Sterility and testicular atrophy related to cyclophosphamide therapy. *Lancet.* 1972;**1**:568–569.

Fauci AS, Wolff SM. Wegener's granulomatosis: Studies in eighteen patients and a review of the literature. *Medicine (Baltimore).* 1973;**52**:533–561.

Fetting JH, Grochow LB, Folstein MF, et al. The course of nausea and vomiting after high dose cyclophosphamide. *Cancer Treat Rep.* 1982;**66**:1487–1493.

Field RB, Gang M, Kline I, et al. The effect of phenobarbital or 2-diethylaminoethyl 2,2-diphenylvalerate on the activation of cyclophosphamide in vivo. *J Pharmacol Exp Ther.* 1972;**180**:475–483.

Finklestein JZ, Hittle RF, Hammond GD. Evaluation of a high dose cyclophosphamide regimen in children. *Cancer Chemother Rep.* 1969;**54**:35–39.

Friedman HS, Colvin OM, Aisaka K, et al. Glutathione protects cardiac and skeletal muscle from cyclophosphamide-induced toxicity. *Cancer Res.* 1990;**50**:2455–2462.

Gallelli JF. Stability studies of drugs used in intravenous solutions. Part 1. *Am J Hosp Pharm.* 1967;**24**:425–433.

Gershwin ME, Goetel EJ, Steinberg AD. Cyclophosphamide: Use in practice. *Ann Intern Med.* 1974;**80**:531–540.

Gianni AM, Bregni M, Siena S, et al. Recombinant human granulocyte–macrophage colony-stimulating factor reduces hematologic toxicity and widens clinical applicability of high-dose cyclophosphamide treatment in breast cancer and non-Hodgkin's lymphoma. *J Clin Oncol.* 1990;**8**:768–778.

Goldberg MA, Antin JH, Guinan EC, Rappeport JM. Cyclophosphamide cardiotoxicity: An analysis of dosing as a risk factor. *Blood.* 1986;**68**(5):1114–1118.

Gottdiener JS, Appelbaum FR, Ferrans VJ, et al. Cardiotoxicity associated with high-dose cyclophosphamide therapy. *Arch Intern Med.* 1981;**141**:758–763.

Greenberg LH, Tanaka KR. Congenital anomalies probably induced by cyclophosphamide. *JAMA.* 1964;**188**:423–426.

Grochow LB, Colvin M. Clinical pharmacokinetics of cyclophosphamide. *Clin Pharmacokinet.* 1983;**4**:380–394.

Gurtoo HL, Marinello AJ, Struck RF. Studies on the mechanism of denaturation of cytochrome P-450 by cyclophosphamide and its metabolites. *J Biol Chem.* 1981;**256**:11691–11701.

Harris RN, Basseches PJ, Appel PL, et al. Carbon tetrachloride-induced increase in the antitumor activity of cyclophosphamide in mice: A pharmacokinetic study. *Cancer Chemother Pharmacol.* 1984;**12**:167–172.

Harrison EF, Fuquay ME, Hunter HL. Effect of N-acetylcysteine on the antitumor activity of cyclophosphamide against Walker-256 carcinosarcoma in rats. *Semin Oncol.* 1983;**10**(1):25–28.

Hart LG, Adamson RH. Effect of microsomal enzyme modifiers on toxicity and therapeutic activity of cyclophosphamide in mice. *Arch Int Pharmacodyn.* 1969;**180**(2):391–401.

Hayakawa T, Kanai N, Yamada R, et al. Effect of steroid hormone on activation of Endoxan (cyclophosphamide). *Biochem Pharmacol.* 1969;**18**:129–135.

Hipkens JH, Struck RF, Gurtoo HL. Role of aldehyde dehydrogenase in the metabolism-dependent biological activity of cyclophosphamide. *Cancer Res.* 1981;**41**:5371–5383.

Honjo I, Suou T, Hirayama C. Hepatotoxicity of cyclophosphamide in man: Pharmacokinetic analysis. *Res Commun Chem Pathol Pharmacol.* 1988;**61**(2):149–165.

Hoon DSB, Foshag LJ, Nizze AS, et al. Suppressor cell activity in a randomized trial of patients receiving active specific immunotherapy with melanoma cell vaccine and low dosages of cyclophosphamide. *Cancer Res.* 1990;**50**:5358–5364.

Hutter AM, Bauman AW, Frank IN. Cyclophosphamide and severe hemorrhagic cystitis. *NY State J Med.* 1969;**69**:305–309.

Hyman LR, Gilbert EF. Testicular atrophy in a prepubescent male after cyclophosphamide therapy. *Lancet.* 1972;**2**:426–427.

Jao JY, Jusko WJ, Cohen JL. Phenobarbital effects on cyclophosphamide pharmacokinetics in man. *Cancer Res.* 1972;**32**:2761–2764.

Jardine I, Brundett R, Colvin M, et al. Approaches to the pharmacokinetics of cyclophosphamide (NSC-26271): Quantitation of metabolites. *Cancer Treat Rep.* 1976;**60**:403–408.

Jardine I, Fenselau C, Appler M, et al. Quantitation by gas chromatography of cyclophosphamide, phosphoramide mustard and nornitrogen mustard in the plasma and urine of patients receiving cyclophosphamide therapy. *Cancer Res.* 1978;**38**:408–415.

Johnson WW, Meadows EC. Urinary-bladder fibrosis and telangiectasia associated with long-term cyclophosphamide therapy. *N Engl J Med.* 1971;**284**:290–294.

Jones SE, Durie BGM, Salmon SE. Combination chemotherapy with Adriamycin and cyclophosphamide for advanced breast carcinoma. *Cancer.* 1975;**36**:90–97.

Juma FD, Rogers HJ, Trounce JR. Pharmacokinetics of cyclophosphamide and alkylating activity in man after intravenous and oral administration. *Br J Clin Pharmacol.* 1979;**8**:209–217.

Juma FD, Rogers HJ, Trounce JR. The pharmacokinetics of cyclophosphamide, phosphoramide mustard and NOR-nitrogen mustard studied by gas chromatography in patients receiving cyclophosphamide therapy. *Br J Clin Pharmacol.* 1980;**10**:327–335.

Juma FD, Rogers HJ, Trounce JR. Effect of renal insufficiency on the pharmacokinetics of cyclophosphamide and some of its metabolites. *Eur J Clin Pharmacol.* 1981;**19**:443–451.

Karchmer RK, Hansen VL. Possible anaphylactic reaction to intravenous cyclophosphamide. *JAMA.* 1977;**237**(5):475.

Kende G, Sirkin SR, Thomas PRM, Freeman AI. Blurring of vision. A previously undescribed complication of cyclophosphamide therapy. *Cancer.* 1979;**44**:69–71.

Krutchik AN, Buzdar AU, Tashima CK. Cyclophosphamide-induced urticaria. *Arch Intern Med.* 1978;**138**:1725.

Kumar R, McEvoy J, Biggart JD, et al. Cyclophosphamide and reproductive function. *Lancet.* 1972;**1**:1212–1214.

Legha SS, Hall S. Acute cyclophosphamide hypersensitivity reaction: Possible lack of cross-sensitivity to mechlorethamine and isophosphoramide. *Cancer Treat Rep.* 1977;**62**:180–181.

Lin K-H, Lindahl R. Role of aldehyde dehydrogenase activity in cyclophosphamide metabolism in rat hepatoma cell lines. *Biochem Pharmacol.* 1987;**36**(19):3305–3307.

Livingston RB, Moore TW, Heilbrum L, et al. Small cell carcinoma of the lung: Combined chemotherapy and radiation. *Ann Intern Med.* 1978;**88**:194–199.

Loudet A-M, Dousset N, Carton M, Douste-Blazy L. Effects of an antimitotic agent (cyclophosphamide) on plasma lipoproteins. *Biochem Pharmacol.* 1984;**33**(19):2961–2965.

Luce JK, Gamble JF, Wilson HE, et al. Combined cyclophosphamide, vincristine and prednisone therapy of malignant lymphoma. *Cancer.* 1971;**28**:306–317.

Mills BA, Roberts RW. Cyclophosphamide-induced cardiomyopathy. A report of two cases and review of the English literature. *Cancer.* 1979;**43**:2223–2226.

Milsted RAV, Jarman M. Metabolism of high doses of cyclophosphamide. *Cancer Chemother Pharmacol.* 1982;**8**:311–313.

Mouridsen HT, Faber O, Skvosted L. The biotransformation of cyclophosphamide in man: Analysis of the variation in normal subjects. *Acta Pharmacol Toxicol.* 1974;**35**:98–106.

Muggia FM, Chia G, Reed LJ, Romney SL. Doxorubicin–cyclophosphamide. Effective chemotherapy for advanced endometrial adenocarcinoma. *J Obstet Gynecol.* 1977;**128**:314–319.

Mullins GM, Colvin M. Intensive cyclophosphamide (NSC-26271) therapy for solid tumors. *Cancer Chemother Rep.* 1975;**59**:411–419.

Pearlman CK. Cystitis due to cytoxan: Case report. *J Urol.* 1966;**95**:713–715.

Pedersen-Bjergaard J, Ersboll J, Hansen VL, et al. Carcinoma of the urinary bladder after treatment with cyclophosphamide for non-Hodgkin's lymphoma. *N Engl J Med.* 1988;**318**:1028–1032.

Peters WP, Rodeheaver DP, Menzel DB, et al. Effect of high dose alkylating agents on endomyocardial glutathione levels and cardiac performance in man. *Proc Am Assoc Cancer Res.* 1988;**29**:268.

Phillips GL, Reece DE, Barnett MJ, et al. Allogeneic marrow transplantation for refractory Hodgkin's disease. *J Clin Oncol.* 1989;**7**:1039–1045.

Piver MS, Barlow JJ, Chung WS. High-dose cyclophosphamide (NSC-26271) for recurrent or progressive ovarian adenocarcinoma. *Cancer Chemother Rep.* 1975;**59**:1157–1158.

Powis G, Reece P, Ahmann DL, Ingle JN. Effect of body weight on the pharmacokinetics of cyclophosphamide in breast cancer patients. *Cancer Chemother Pharmacol.* 1987;**20**:219–222.

Primack A. Amelioration of cyclophosphamide induced cystitis. *J Natl Cancer Inst.* 1971;**47**:223–227.

Proceedings of the symposium on the metabolism and mechanism of action of cyclophosphamide. 1976;**60**:299–525.

Ritschel WA, Bykadi G, Norman EJ, et al. Salivary elimination of cyclophosphamide in man. *J Clin Pharmacol.* 1981;**21**:461–465.

Rodin AE, Haggard ME, Travis LB. Lung changes and chemotherapeutic agents in childhood: Report of a case associated with cyclophosphamide therapy. *Am J Dis Child.* 1970;**120**:337–340.

Ross WE, Chabner BE. Allergic reaction to cyclophosphamide in a mechlorethamine-sensitive patient. *Cancer Treat Rep.* 1977;**61**(3):495–496.

Saul G, Matthias M, Rose H, et al. Excretion patterns of alkylating metabolites in urine following cyclophosphamide treatment of tumor patients: Influence of application route, dosage, liver and kidney function. *J Cancer Res Clin Oncol.* 1979;**94**:277–286.

Schuler U, Ehninger G, Wagner T. Repeated high-dose cyclophosphamide administration in bone marrow transplantation: Exposure to activated metabolites. *Cancer Chemother Pharmacol.* 1987;**20**:248–252.

Skarin AT, Rosenthal DS, Moloney WC, Frei E III. Combination chemotherapy of advanced non-Hodgkin's lymphoma with bleomycin, Adriamycin, cyclophosphamide, vincristine, and prednisone (BACOP). *Blood.* 1977;**49**(5):759–770.

Sladek NE. Therapeutic efficacy of cyclophosphamide as a function of its metabolism. *Cancer Res.* 1972;**32**:535–542.

Sladek NE, Doeden D, Powers JF, Krivit W. Plasma concentrations of 4-hydroxycyclophosphamide and phosphoramide mustard in patients repeatedly given high doses of cyclophosphamide in preparation for bone marrow transplantation. *Cancer Treat Rep.* 1984;**68**:1247–1254.

Slease RB, Benear JB, Selby GB, et al. High-dose combination alkylating agent therapy with autologous bone marrow rescue for refractory solid tumors. *J Clin Oncol.* 1988;**6**:1314–1320.

Smith IE, Evans BD, Harland SJ, Millar JL. Autologous bone marrow rescue is unnecessary after very high-dose cyclophosphamide. *Lancet.* 1983;**1**:76–77.

Soble MJ, Dorr RT. Lack of enhanced myelotoxicity with buthionine sulfoximine and sulhydryl-dependent anticancer agents in mice. *Res Commun Chem Pathol Pharmacol.* 1987;**55**(2):161–180.

Soble MJ, Dorr RT. Lack of enhanced antitumor efficacy for L-buthionine sulfoximine in combination with carmustine, cyclophosphamide, doxorubicin or melphalan in mice. *Anticancer Res.* 1988;**8**:17–22.

Souhami RL, Finn G, Gregory WM, et al. High-dose cyclophosphamide in small-cell carcinoma of the lung. *J Clin Oncol.* 1985;**3**:958–962.

Steele TH, Serpick AA, Block JB. Antidiuretic response to cyclophosphamide in man. *J Pharmacol Exp Ther.* 1973;**185**:245–253.

Steinherz LJ, Steinherz PG, Mangiacasale D, et al. Cardiac changes with cyclophosphamide. *Med Pediatr Oncol.* 1981;**9**:417–422.

Stolbach L, Begg C, Bennett JM, et al. Evaluation of bone marrow toxic reaction in patients treated with allopurinol. *JAMA.* 1982;**247**:334–336.

Struck RF, Horne K, Phillips JG, et al. Plasma levels and AUC data for the antitumor-active metabolites of cyclophosphamide (CPA) in cancer patients treated intravenously (i.v.) or orally (p.o.) with cyclophosphamide (abstract 663). *Proc Am Assoc Cancer Res.* 1986;**27**:167.

Taylor K, Jagannath S, Spitzer G, et al. Recombinant human granulocyte colony-stimulating factor hastens granulocyte recovery after high-dose chemotherapy and autologous bone marrow transplantations in Hodgkin's disease. *J Clin Oncol.* 1989;**7**:1791–1799.

Thomas ED, Buckner CD, Clift RA, et al. Marrow transplantation for acute non lymphoblastic leukemia in first remission. *N Engl J Med.* 1979a;**301**:597–599.

Thomas ED, Sanders JE, Flournoy N, et al. Marrow transplantation for patients with acute lymphoblastic leukemia in remission. *Blood.* 1979b;**54**:468–476.

Toledo TM, Harper RC, Moser RH. Fetal effects during cyclophosphamide and irradiation therapy. *Ann Intern Med.* 1971;**74**:87–91.

Topelow AA, Rothenberg SP, Cottrell TS. Interstitial pneumonia after prolonged treatment with cyclophosphamide. *Am Rev Respir Dis.* 1973;**108**:114–117.

Trissel LA, Fulton B, Tramonte SM. Visual compatibility of ondansetron with chemotherapeutic agents, antibiotics, and other selected drugs during simulated Y-site injection (abstract P-468R). In: 25th Annual ASHP Midyear Clinical Meeting and Exhibit, Las Vegas, Nevada, 1990.

Wagner T, Fenneberg K. Pharmacokinetics and bioavailability of cyclophosphamide from oral formulations. *Arzneim-Forsch.* 1984;**34**:313–316.

Wall RL, Clausen KP. Carcinoma of the urinary bladder in patients receiving cyclophosphamide. *N Engl J Med.* 1975;**293**:271–275.

Warne GL, Fairley KF, Hobbs JB, Martin FIR. Cyclophosphamide-induced ovarian failure. *N Engl J Med.* 1963;**289**:1159–1162.

Wheeler C, Antin JH, Hallowell W, et al. Cyclophosphamide, carmustine, and etoposide with autologous bone marrow transplantation in refractory Hodgkin's disease and non-Hodgkin's lymphoma: A dose-finding study. *J Clin Oncol.* 1990;**8**:648–656.

Whitecar JP, Bodey GP, Freireich EJ, et al. Cyclophosphamide, vincristine, cytosine arabinoside and prednisone (COAP) combination chemotherapy for acute leukemia in adults. *Cancer Chemother Rep.* 1972;**56**:543–550.

Wilbur JR, Sutow WW, Sullivan MP, Gottlieb JA. Chemotherapy of sarcomas. *Cancer.* 1975;**36**:765–769.

Wilkinson PM, O'Neill PA, Thatcher N, Lucas SB. Pharmacokinetics of high-dose cyclophosphamide in patients with metastatic bronchogenic carcinoma. *Cancer Chemother Pharmacol.* 1983;**11**:196–199.

Ziegler JL, Morrow RH, Fass L, et al. Treatment of Burkitt's tumor with cyclophosphamide. *Cancer.* 1970;**26**:474–484.

Cytarabine

■ Other Names

Ara-C; cytosine arabinoside; Cytosar-U® (Upjohn); NSC-63878.

■ Chemistry

Structure of cytarabine

Chemically, cytarabine, or 4-amino-1-β-D-arabinofuranosyl-2(1*H*)-pyrimidinone, is a congener of the nucleosides cytidine and deoxycytidine differing in the presence of an altered sugar (arabinose) instead of ribose or deoxyribose, respectively. The molecular weight is 243.22 and the formula is $C_9H_{13}N_3O_5$.

■ Antitumor Activity

Cytarabine is most useful clinically in hematologic malignancies usually in combination with other cytotoxic agents. It is used most commonly in the remission induction and consolidation therapy of acute myelogenous leukemia in adults (Bodey et al 1976).

Patients with advanced refractory myeloid leukemia can be treated with high-dose cytarabine without producing excess toxicity (Rudnick et al 1979). In an initial trial, high-dose cytarabine produced objective responses in two of four patients with acute myelogenous leukemia (AML), three of five patients with acute lymphocytic leukemia, and one patient with chronic myelogenous leukemia (Rudnick et al 1979). When combined with intercalating agents such as amsacrine, high-dose cytarabine regimens can produce remission induction rates of up to 70% in patients with relapsing acute nonlymphocytic leukemia (ANLL) (Hines et al 1984). A similar induction regimen with daunorubicin is highly effective as consolidation therapy for ANLL (Wolff et al 1985). High-dose cytarabine alone also has significant activity in patients with secondary ANLL from prior alkylator therapy (Preisler et al 1983). Intrathecal cytarabine is highly effective in both the prophylaxis and primary treatment of central nervous system leukemia (Band et al 1973).

■ Mechanism of Action

In vivo, cytarabine is metabolized by deoxycytidine kinases to ultimately form the triphosphorylated nucleotide, 1-β-D-arabinofuranosylcytosine-5'-triphosphatase (Ara-CTP) (Momparler 1972). This metabolite acts as a competitive inhibitor of DNA polymerase after incorporation into a DNA chain (Furth and Cohen 1968). Chain elongation is thereafter profoundly halted (Ross et al 1990).

The crucial step for cytotoxicity appears to comprise the phosphorylation of the parent drug to the triphosphate by sequential kinase activity. This activity is also upregulated in most forms of cellular resistance to cytarabine (Coleman et al 1975). Because cytarabine competes for enzymes involved in the conversion of the natural base cytidine to deoxycytidine nucleotides, deoxycytidine levels are depleted at the expense of producing the Ara-CTP nucleotide. Both processes block further polymerization of DNA as noted by the production of short DNA strands following exposure to cytarabine (Fram and Kufe 1982).

Cytarabine has no effect on nonproliferating cells, and minimal actions on proliferating cells treated in any phases other than S phase. In this capacity, it is a classic example of a cell cycle phase-specific antineoplastic drug (Skipper et al 1967).

■ Availability and Storage

Cytarabine is commercially available from the Upjohn Company, Kalamazoo, Michigan, (Cytosar-U®), and from several generic manufacturers (eg, Cetus Corporation, Emeryville, California). It is supplied in 100-mg, 500-mg, 1-g, and 2-g glass vials. The freeze-dried powder is recommended to be stored under refrigeration. A commercial diluent, containing 0.9% benzyl alcohol in water, provides for a bacteriostatic solution when added to the drug powder. The final commercial formulation may also contain small amounts of either hydrochloric acid, sodium hydroxide, or both to adjust the pH. At 22°C the drug is stable for at least 2 years (Notari et al 1972).

■ Preparation for Use, Stability, and Admixture

The manufacturer recommends that for the 100-mg vial, 5 mL of diluent be added, and for the 500-mg vial, 10 mL of diluent be added, to yield solutions of 20 and 50 mg/mL, respectively. For the 1- and 2-g vials, 10 and 20 mL of diluent are added, respectively, to yield a 100 mg/mL colorless solution. The pH of this solution is about 5, although some generic cytarabine formulations may have lower pH values in solution. Occasionally, this has caused precipitation of drugs combined for intrathecal use: hydrocortisone, methotrexate, and cytarabine. Cytarabine solutions should be stored at room temperature and optimally used within 48 hours of reconstitution. Any solution that is hazy or cloudy should not be used.

This solution is chemically stable for 1 week. Other aqueous diluents may also be used to reconstitute cytarabine (eg, sterile water for injection, normal saline, or D5W). The dry powder also does not require the volumes recommended by the manufacturer for dissolution, and minimal volumes of diluent (1 to 2 mL) may be used (particularly for subcutaneous injections) (up to 100 mg/mL). For infusions, the drug reconstituted variously as described may be added to any convenient volume of D5W or normal saline. In controlled tests with ultraviolet assay, infusion solutions containing cytarabine at 0.5 mg/mL in water, D5W, or normal saline retained chemical stability at room temperature for 7 days (package insert, Cytosar®, 1976).

The following are the results of spectrophotometric analysis of cytarabine mixed with different agents (McCrae and King 1976). Compatible admixtures with cytarabine (no change in spectrum of either drug, no physical alterations noted) include prednisolone sodium phosphate, sodium cephalothin, and vincristine. Use with caution (1) 5-fluorouracil (change in the spectrum of the 5-fluorouracil only, when admixed with cytarabine) and (2) methotrexate (very slight change noted in the spectrum of methotrexate). Cytarabine (50 mg/mL in water) is also physically stable with ondansetron for 4 hours (Trissel et al 1990).

Studies performed at Upjohn Laboratories show that cytarabine is also incompatible with carbenicillin, nafcillin, and gentamicin, the last in a highly concentrated solution containing 240 mg gentamicin and 300 mg cytarabine in 100 mL of D5W. In contrast, a mixture of 80 mg gentamicin and 100 mg cytarabine is physically compatible for 24 hours. Further studies showed that cytarabine was compatible for 4 to 8 hours with vancomycin (1–3 g) and for 24 hours with penicillin G sodium (1 million units with 100 mg cytarabine in 500 mL of D5W).

Cytarabine has also been found to be compatible with corticotropin, potassium chloride, and sodium bicarbonate (Trissel 1988). It was incompatible with heparin (haze formation) and insulin (immediate fine precipitate) (Trissel 1988).

■ Administration

Cytarabine can be administered by a variety of parenteral routes: subcutaneously, intramuscularly, or intravenously either as a bolus "push" or as a continuous infusion. In remission induction therapy for adult leukemia, the use of 5- to 10-day continuous intravenous infusions may be optimal for antitumor cytotoxicity because of an S-phase-specific mechanism of action (Bodey et al 1976, Wang and Pratt 1970). Small reconstitution volumes using isotonic diluents are preferred for subcutaneous or intramuscular administration. The drug is generally well tolerated and does not produce excessive pain or irritation at injection sites. Subcutaneous doses can be applied in a rotating site fashion to areas of body fat: thighs, abdomen, and flank regions. Repeated administration to a single site or region may be harmful and should be avoided.

For the intramuscular injection of cytarabine rotation of sites is again recommended.

Intravenous cytarabine is often administered as a continuous infusion over 24 hours for several consecutive days. Generally, both the infusion and the intravenous push administration are well tolerated, although thrombophlebitis has been rarely reported at the site. Intravenous push doses may be given rapidly. Injection volume is not an important determinant. Extravasations of the drug usually do not produce severe consequences; however, every effort should be made to ensure vein patency before administration and throughout the infusion.

■ Dosage

Single large doses of up to 3.0 g have been administered without serious hematologic toxicity; however, maintenance of low continuous blood levels for more than 5 days results in greater hematologic depression in leukemia therapy. Thus, significantly higher remission durations are noted for low-dose cytarabine infusions compared with equivalent bolus doses (Frei et al 1969). For leukemia, doses of 100 to 150 mg/m^2 have been used for 5 to 10 days, given either as a continuous 24-hour infusion or in daily divided doses (every 6–12 hours) (Bodey et al 1976). Alternately, 3 mg/kg/d has been recommended in the same setting. Again, marked bone marrow depression or hypoplasia necessitates dosage reduction or a reduction in the number of days of administration.

After each treatment, a period of no treatment is often introduced to facilitate bone marrow recovery (usually 5–9 days). Subcutaneous doses of up to 1 mg/kg once or twice weekly are recommended by the manufacturer, although doses of 70 to 100 mg/m^2 in divided doses for 5 days are often used in actual practice.

Cytarabine is unusual in that very high doses can be tolerated without the need for bone marrow transplantation. Typical high-dose regimens use 3 g/m^2 as a 1-hour infusion every 12 hours for 8 to 12 doses (Rudnick et al 1979, Early et al 1982). Individual doses up to 7.5 g/m^2 have also been tested but are not more efficacious than the 3 g/m^2 dose. The 3 g/m^2 doses can successfully be combined with DNA intercalators such as amsacrine (100 mg/m^2 × 3 [Hines et al 1984]) or daunorubicin (30 mg/m^2 × 2 or 3 doses [Wolff et al 1985]).

■ Drug Interactions

Cytarabine has been reported to decrease the cellular uptake of methotrexate and thereby reduce its effectiveness. Methotrexate, on the other hand, may decrease the intracellular activation of cytarabine (Tattersall and Harrap 1973). These antagonistic effects still require further clinical investigation but should be considered when using these drugs concurrently. Avery and Roberts (1972) have in fact shown synergism for methotrexate–cytarabine in a murine model. Therapeutic synergism for the combination was also noted by Edelstein et al (1975) and Hoovis and Chu (1973).

Thymidine has been shown experimentally to enhance the metabolic conversion of cytarabine to its triphosphate form in rats (Danhauser and Rustum 1985). This translated to a slight enhancement in antitumor effects in rats bearing a chemically induced colon carcinoma (Danhauser and Rustum 1980). Bromodeoxyuridine may similarly enhance cytarabine activation in vitro (Ross et al 1988).

Conversely, King et al (1984) have demonstrated that dipyridamole can block cytarabine toxicity in tumor cells by inhibiting drug uptake. This appears to follow the general ability of dipyridamole to bind to plasma membranes and inhibit nucleoside transport (Patterson et al 1980).

Hydroxyurea is reported to enhance cytarabine cytotoxicity in vitro by decreasing deoxycytidine triphosphate levels intracellularly (Streifel and Howell 1981). This can overcome cytarabine resistance presumably by increasing the phosphorylation of cytarabine to the active triphosphate form. Although this combination is highly active in leukemic mice (Schabel et al 1971), it was ineffective at reversing cytarabine resistance in 22 patients with refractory lymphoma or leukemia (Pfeifle and Howell 1983).

The hematopoietic colony-stimulating factor rhGM-CSF (Schering Corporation) increases the incorporation of cytarabine into human acute myelocytic leukemia marrow cells in vitro (Karp et al 1990). Cellular proliferation was also enhanced by rhGM-CSF, suggesting that this factor might enhance cytarabine cytotoxicity in vivo.

Pharmacokinetics

Cytarabine is not orally effective because of extensive and rapid deamination within the gut lumen, allowing for only 20% absorption of intact drug (Finklestein et al 1970). Cytidine deaminase, the inactivating enzyme, is a widely distributed enzyme in the body, but is concentrated in the liver. Intravenous doses of cytarabine appear to exhibit biphasic elimination (Ho and Frei 1971). There is an initial half-life of about 15 minutes wherein a major fraction of a dose is hepatically metabolized by cytidine deaminase to uracil arabinoside, which is inactive. The secondary elimination half-life is longer, about 2 hours. Other authors have described much shorter terminal half-lives: 8 to 19 minutes (Van Prooijen et al 1977), 3 to 14 minutes (Baguley and Falkenhaug 1975), and 15 minutes (Momparler 1972). Because the ratio of the active triphosphate to the uracil metabolite appears to be dose dependent, the use of larger doses may favor greater cytotoxicity by shifting the equilibrium toward formation of cytarabine triphosphate.

At 24 hours, 90% of a given dose has been eliminated, mostly in the urine (renal clearance, 90 mL/min) (Dedrick et al 1973). Some is eliminated into the bile (Finklestein et al 1970). Ninety percent of the excreted products are uracil arabinoside, which is inactive. Cerebrospinal fluid levels are about 40 to 50% of the simultaneous plasma level reached with continuous intravenous infusions; thus the cerebrospinal fluid-to-plasma ratio is 0.4 (Ho and Frei 1971). The high cerebrospinal fluid levels presumably result from a lack of cytidine deaminase activity in the cerebrospinal fluid. Intrathecally administered doses are therefore eliminated very slowly with a cerebrospinal fluid half-life that may range from 2 to 11 hours (Chabner et al 1977).

Finally, according to Wan et al (1974), plasma levels of 0.01 to 0.15 µg/mL are necessary to achieve cytotoxic effects and are achievable with the use of continuous or sequential bolus regimens of 100 to 200 mg/m^2.

The pharmacokinetics of high-dose cytarabine has been studied in patients with ANLL. Following 2-hour infusion of 1.8 to 3 g/m^2, steady-state plasma levels were 32 to 97 µM (8–24 µg/mL) and declined with half-lives of 7.8 to 12.6 minutes (Breithaupt et al 1982). The total clearance of cytarabine varied between 1.7 and 2.9 L/kg · h, and the volume of distribution ranged from 0.44 to 0.86 L/kg; however, cerebrospinal fluid levels of cytarabine were only 10 to 15% of the steady-state plasma concentrations. In another trial, the cytarabine β half-life was 12 to 98 minutes and there was some evidence for a γ half-life of 130 to 340 minutes (Pommier et al 1983). Peak cerebrospinal fluid concentrations were 13% of simultaneous plasma levels. Of interest, no relationship between high cytarabine levels and plasma cytidine deaminase activity was detected in individual patients. Significant cytarabine distribution into tear fluid is also documented; drug levels of 22 to 33 µM in tears (6–8 µg/mL) are produced following intravenous cytarabine doses of 3 g/m² (Hande et al 1981). In another trial, plasma levels of cytarabine following a 1-hour infusion of 2 to 3 g/m² were 18 and 30 µg/mL, respectively (Early et al 1982). In contrast, steady-state cytarabine levels of about 20 µM (5 µg/mL) are achieved during infusions of 250 mg/m²/h (total dose, 3–9 g/m²) (Spriggs et al 1985).

■ Side Effects and Toxicity

The acute dose-limiting toxic effects for cytarabine are generally those of hematopoietic depression. High cumulative doses can also lead to permanent central nervous system damage.

Cytarabine-induced bone marrow damage typically presents as peripheral leukopenia and thrombocytopenia of brief duration. Although clinically significant, anemia occurs rarely; megaloblastosis of erythroid precursors in the bone marrow is quite common. These hematologic toxic effects are more prominent after higher doses and especially if continuous infusions are used.

Other toxic effects involve rapidly proliferating tissues such as the gastrointestinal tract. Nausea and vomiting are quite common and may be more pronounced with the rapid intravenous push administration of divided doses than with the infusion method. Diarrhea may also be common. Stomatitis, anorexia, and gastrointestinal hemorrhage may sometimes occur, whereas mild oral ulceration is fairly common.

A flulike syndrome has been reported to occasionally follow cytarabine and consists of fevers, arthralgias, and sometimes rashes on the palms, soles, neck, and chest. Rashes are also commonly described but may be related to the concomitant use of other drugs such as allopurinol. Acral erythema has also been observed on the hands of patients receiving cytarabine (Burgdorf et al 1982). The erythema develops on the palms and soles. It is rarely followed by bulla formation, desquamation, and then healing (Levine et al 1985).

Hepatic dysfunction has occurred rarely (< 7% in one series) and may be evidenced by transient enzyme elevations. The drug may be hepatotoxic but this is unproven to date and must be rare. Several cases of acute pancreatitis following cytarabine have also been reported (Altman et al 1982).

Congenital limb abnormalities have been described in leukemic mothers treated with cytarabine and thioguanine (Schafer 1981) or with cytarabine alone (Wagner et al 1980). Thus, cytarabine is a teratogenic agent that must be avoided in pregnant females.

High-Dose Toxicities. Doses of cytarabine greater than 200 mg/m² produce greater myelosuppression which is readily reversible in leukemic patients. Central nervous system toxicity is seen in about 10% of patients and may be related to total (cumulative) doses, reduced renal function, or age above 50 (Rudnick et al 1979). Conjunctivitis is also seen and can be ameliorated with the prophylactic use of corticosteroid eye drops. A typical regimen calls for instillation of 1 or 2 drops of 0.1% dexamethasone ophthalmic solution into each eye every 4 to 6 hours, while awake, for 7 days following high-dose cytarabine.

Ocular toxicity from cytarabine is noted by excessive tearing, photophobia, pain, and blurred vision (Ritch et al 1983). Ophthalmologic findings include conjunctival injection, central punctate cornal opacities with subepithelial deposits, and decreased visual acuity. The symptoms usually resolve in a few days, but visual acuity problems may take weeks to resolve fully. This toxic effect appears to result from a drug-induced blockade of corneal epithelial DNA synthesis (Kaufman et al 1964).

Cerebellar dysfunction is the dose-limiting toxic effect of short infusions of high-dose cytarabine. The onset occurs about 6 to 8 days after the first dose and the effect lasts about 3 to 7 days in one study (Lazarus et al 1981). Cerebellar dysfunction is characterized by nystagmus, dysarthria, disdiadochokinesia, ataxia, and slurring of speech (Rudnick et al 1979). A cumulative dose phenomenon has been suggested by Lazarus et al (see table), and some patients develop irreversible toxic reactions even at relatively low cumulative doses (Barnett et al 1985). An extremely high local incidence of cerebellar dysfunction with low doses was associated with a generic cytarabine formulation that is no longer available (Jolson et al 1992).

Postmortem examinations of the brains of patients with severe cytarabine central nervous system toxic effects reveal a loss of Purkinje cells, a Bergmann-type gliosis, and a loss of nerve cells in the dentate nucleus with spongifor changes (Barnett et al 1985). There does not appear to be an association between central nervous system toxicity and the particular induction schedule or the disease state, but patients over 50 years of age may have a 6- to 10-fold greater risk of developing a toxic reaction

DOSE RELATIONSHIP FOR HIGH-DOSE CYTARABINE CENTRAL NERVOUS SYSTEM TOXICITY

Cumulative Dose Level (g/m^2)	Number of Patients Toxic/Total Patients	%
24	0/12	0
36	3/19	16
48	1/12	8
54	4/6*	67

*Two patients (50% of those affected) had irreversible central nervous system toxicity.

Data from Lazarus HM, Herzig RH, Herzig GP, et al. Central nervous system toxicity of high-dose systemic cytosine arabinoside. Cancer. 1981;48:2577–2582.

(Herzig et al 1985, 1987). Another retrospective analysis also suggested age greater than 50 years as a risk factor for central nervous system toxicity (Graves and Hooks 1989). One author suggests that toxic reactions can occur at relatively low dose levels of 30 g/m^2 (Dworkin et al 1985). The cause of this toxicity is unknown but recent experimental evidence suggests that cytarabine can be directly cytotoxic to postmitotic neurons by depleting 2'-deoxycytidine or by noncompetitively blocking nerve growth factor activity (Wallace and Johnson 1989). Recently, renal insufficiency and not age or dose has been associated with high-dose cytarabine neurotoxicity (Damon et al 1989, Jolson et al 1992). In the former study, 76% of patients with estimated creatinine clearances below 60 mL/min developed neurotoxicity. In contrast only 8% of patients with good renal function (estimated creatinine clearances > 60 mL/min) developed central nervous system toxicity. These authors recommended dose reductions for patients receiving high-dose cytarabine during renal insufficiency (Damon et al 1989). The use of longer infusions up to 3 hours may also reduce cytarabine central nervous system toxicity (Capizzi, et al 1984). One explanation for the role of the kidney is an accumulation of the deaminated metabolite, uracil arabinoside, which is a direct neurotoxin when injected into the cerebrospinal fluid of primates (Lopez and Agarwal 1984). Another study lists the following risk factors for neurotoxicity from high-dose cytarabine: (1) creatinine >1.2 mg/dL, (2) age ≥ 40 years, and (3) alkaline phosphatase level greater or equal to three times normal (Rubin et al 1992). Any two of these factors appeared to place patients at increased risk of developing neurotoxicity.

Noncardiogenic pulmonary edema has also been reported in patients receiving cytarabine doses of 16 mg/kg/d for 1 to 3 days (Haupt et al 1981). Respiratory failure was the major feature with an onset between 22 and 27 days after cessation of therapy. Clinical features included tachypnea and hypoxemia, with diffuse pulmonary infiltrates noted on x-ray examination. Histologic examinations from postmortem lung specimens show the presence of a highly proteinaceous intraalveolar infiltrate with no evidence of an inflammatory reaction (Andersson et al 1990). Treatments involve fluid restriction, diuretic therapy, and mechanical ventilation which can be helpful in some patients. An incidence of 13% was reported in one series of 103 patients, and in 9 of 13 affected, the complication was fatal (Andersson et al 1990). There does appear to be some relationship to high-dose regimens (Andersson et al 1985), but not to other factors such as cardiogenic and infectious episodes (Jehn et al 1988) or age and prior chemotherapy (Andersson et al 1990). There is also a single case of pericarditis with tamponade in a leukemic patient given high-dose cytarabine (Vaickus and Letendre 1984). The patient improved immediately after pericardiocentesis and there was no evidence of malignant cells in the pericardial fluid.

■ Special Applications

Intrathecal Use

Mechanism. Cytarabine has been shown to be an effective prophylactic antineoplastic when injected intrathecally to prevent central nervous system relapses (Spiers and Firth 1972). It should be remembered that the central nervous system is generally a drug sanctuary because most parenteral drugs do not easily cross the blood–brain barrier. In this capacity cytarabine has been used both singly and in combination with hydrocortisone and/or methotrexate. Naturally, it is also an effective treatment of overt central nervous system disease. Any cytarabine diffusing back to the blood is rapidly deaminated; thus, systemic toxicity is unusual after intrathecal administration.

Dosage. Intrathecal doses have ranged from 5 to 70 mg/m^2 for up to 3 days per week (Wang and Pratt 1970).

Another reported series used single doses from 4.5 to 73 mg/m^2. The median dose used in this study was 45 mg/m^2. Transient headaches and vomiting were seen more frequently at 27 mg/m^2; however, no hematologic toxicity or other severe reactions were noted at any of the doses used (Band et al 1973). Thus, an effective, simple, and generally well-tolerated (no undue complications) dose in ongoing adult studies has been 100 mg/m². Wolff et al (1979) reported a case of paraplegia following the fifth intrathecal dose of 170 mg (100 mg/m² × 5) in a young male patient. Symptoms in this case developed within a week and lasted over 8 weeks. They concluded that administration of the same dose might be safe only if divided with 3- to 5-day intervals between consecutive doses.

Preparation. Intrathecal cytarabine should be reconstituted in Elliott's B solution if available (to approximate normal cerebrospinal fluid), other physiologic buffered diluents such as Ringer's lactate, or the patient's own cerebrospinal fluid. *Note:* The bacteriostatic diluent provided is not physiologic and contains 0.9% (w/v) benzyl alcohol, which has been associated with a higher incidence of neurologic toxicity (Band et al 1973). It therefore should be avoided for intrathecal applications.

Generally, the volume to be given is in the range of 5 to 10 mL and should correspond to an equivalent amount of cerebrospinal fluid removed. Intrathecal volumes as high as 20 mL (14% of average adult cerebrospinal fluid volume) in adults have been well tolerated for drug administrations. Again, strict aseptic techniques must be used in administering the drug, and the use of mask, gloves, and laminar flow conditions for reconstitution is also recommended (see Pharmacokinetics for intrathecal cytarabine elimination pattern).

Adverse Reactions. Systemic toxicity from intrathecal cytarabine is not usually expected. Meningismus, paresthesias, paraplegias (Saiki et al 1972), and rare seizures in leukemic children (Eden et al 1978) have all been amply documented. Other, more common but less serious toxic effects include pleocytosis (increased number of cells in the cerebrospinal fluid), transient headaches, vomiting, and fever. A single case of cardiac arrest after intrathecal drug administration has been reported, as has development of spastic paraparesis (Breur et al 1977).

Intraperitoneal Administration. Cytarabine has been investigationally administered by the intraperitoneal route (Pfeifle and Howell 1983, Markman et al 1984). In one study, patients with advanced ovarian cancer received 2 L of dialysate containing 10, 100, and 1000 µM cytarabine. Intraperitoneal dwell times were 6 hours and produced peak plasma levels of 0.1 to 0.3 for the 100 µM dialysate and 0.8 to 2.2 µM for the 1000 µM dialysate. The intraperitoneal half-life of the drug ranged between 90 and 210 minutes and produced a 2 to 3 log increase in the intraperitoneal concentration gradient over plasma levels (King et al 1984). In a clinical trial, 2 of 10 patients with advanced ovarian cancer responded to a regimen of five daily 6-hour exchanges of 30 mg cytarabine in 2 L of fluid (62 µM) (King et al 1984). Toxicity included mild leukopenia and thrombocytopenia, one case of hypersensitivity, and nine episodes of bacterial peritonitis, but no chemical peritonitis.

Intraperitoneal cytarabine (2 g) has also been combined with high-dose intraperitoneal cisplatin (100–200 mg) both in 2 L of dialysate (Markman et al 1984). Sodium thiosulfate (4 /m² bolus, then 2 g/m² infusion) was administered intravenously to reduce cisplatin nephrotoxicity. This regimen produced objective responses in 9 of 18 patients and toxicity was mild (Markman et al 1984).

Isolated Limb Perfusion. Sondak et al (1989) have combined high-dose cytarabine (200, 400, 600, or 2000 mg) with cisplatin (200 mg) in eight patients with malignant melanoma. Thiosulfate was given intravenously along with furosemide and heparin to achieve systemic anticoagulation. The anticancer drugs were administered by regional limb perfusion in a normothermic perfusate flowing at a rate between 300 and 600 mL/min. There were four partial responses and one complete response. Toxicity was absent in five patients but was severe in the one patient given 2000 mg of cytarabine. This consisted of local pain and severe swelling (compartment syndrome), which were relieved by an intravenous injection of 1 g methylprednisolone (Sondak et al 1989).

REFERENCES

Altman AJ, Dinndorf P, Quinn JJ. Acute pancreatitis in association with cytosine arabinoside therapy. *Cancer.* 1982;**49**:1384–1386.

Andersson BS, Cogan BM, Keating MJ, et al. Subacute pulmonary failure complicating therapy with high-dose Ara-C in acute leukemia. *Cancer.* 1985;**56**:2181–2184.

Andersson BS, Luna MA, Yee C, et al. Fatal pulmonary failure complicating high-dose cytosine arabinoside therapy in acute leukemia. *Cancer.* 1990;**65**:1079–1084.

Avery T, Roberts D. Dose-related synergism of cytosine arabinoside and methotrexate against murine leukemia L1210. *Eur J Cancer.* 1972;**10**:425–429.

Baguley BC, Falkenhaug E-M. Plasma half-life of cytosine arabinoside in patients with leukemia—The effect of uridine. *Eur J Cancer.* 1975;**11**:43–49.

Band PR, Holland JF, Bernard J, et al. Treatment of central nervous system leukemia with intrathecal cytosine arabinoside. *Cancer.* 1973;**32**:744–748.

Barnett MJ, Richards MA, Ganesan TS, et al. Central ner-

vous system toxicity of high-dose cytosine arabinoside. *Semin Oncol.* 1985;**2**(3):227–232.
Bodey GP, Coltman CA, Hewlett JS, Freireich EJ. Progress in the treatment of adults with acute leukemia. *Arch Intern Med.* 1976;**136**:1383–1388.
Breithaupt H, Pralle H, Eckhardt T, et al. Clinical results and pharmacokinetics of high-dose cytosine arabinoside (HD ARA-C). *Cancer.* 1982;**50**:1248–1257.
Breuer AC, Pitman SW, Danson DM, Schoene WC. Paraparesis following intrathecal cytosine arabinoside. *Cancer.* 1977;**40**:2817–2822.
Burgdorf WHC, Gilmore WA, Ganick RG. Peculiar acral erythema secondary to high-dose chemotherapy for acute myelogenous leukemia. *Ann Intern Med.* 1982;**97**(1):61–62.
Capizzi RL, Poole M, Cooper MR, et al. Treatment of poor risk acute leukemia with sequential high-dose ARA-C and asparaginase. *Blood.* 1984;**63**:694–700.
Chabner BA, Myers CE, Oliverio VT. Clinical pharmacology of anticancer drugs. *Semin Oncol.* 1977;**4**(2):165–191.
Coleman CN, Johns DG, Chabner BA. Studies on mechanisms of resistance to cytosine arabinoside: Problems in the determination of related enzyme activities in leukemic cells. *Ann NY Acad Sci.* 1975;**255**:247–251.
Damon LE, Mass R, Linker CA. The association between high-dose cytarabine neurotoxicity and renal insufficiency. *J Clin Oncol.* 1989;**7**(10):1563–1568.
Danhauser LL, Rustum YM. Effect of thymidine on the toxicity, antitumor activity, and metabolism of 1-β-D-arabinofuranosylcytosine in rats bearing a chemically induced colon carcinoma. *Cancer Res.* 1980;**40**:1274–1280.
Danhauser LL, Rustum YM. Potential for selective enhancement of the in vivo metabolism of 1-β-D-arabinofuranosylcytosine in rats by thymidine pretreatment. *Cancer Res.* 1985;**45**:2002–2007.
Dedrick RL, Forrester DD, Cannon JN, et al. Pharmacokinetics of 1-β-D-arabinofuranosylcytosine (ARA-C) deamination in several species. *Biochem Pharmacol.* 1973;**22**:2405–2417.
Dworkin LA, Goldman RD, Zivin LS, et al. Cerebellar toxicity following high-dose cytosine arabinoside. *J Clin Oncol.* 1985;**3**(5):613–616.
Early AP, Preisler HD, Slocum H, et al. A pilot study of high-dose 1-β-D-arabinofuranosylcytosine for acute leukemia and refractory lymphoma: Clinical response and pharmacology. *Cancer Res.* 1982;**42**:1587–1594.
Edelstein M, Vietti J, Valeriote F. The enhanced cytotoxicity of combinations of 1-β-D-arabinofuranosylcytosine and methotrexate. *Cancer Res.* 1975;**35**:1555–1558.
Eden OB, Goldie W, Wood T, Etucubanas E. Seizures following intrathecal cytosine arabinoside in young children with acute lymphoblastic leukemia. *Cancer.* 1978;**42**:53–58.
Finklestein JZ, Scher J, Karen M. Pharmacologic studies of titrated cytosine arabinoside (NSC-63878) in children. *Cancer Chemother Rep.* 1970;**54**:35–39.
Fram RJ, Kufe DW. DNA strand breaks caused by inhibitors of DNA synthesis: 1-β-D-Arabinofuranosylcytosine and aphidicolin. *Cancer Res.* 1982;**42**:4050–4053.

Frei E III, Bickers JN, Hewlett JS, et al. Dose schedule and antitumor studies of arabinosylcytosine (NSC-63878). *Cancer Res.* 1969;**29**:1325–1332.
Furth JJ, Cohen SS. Inhibition of mammalian DNA polymerase by the 5′-triphosphate of 1-β-D-arabinofuranosylcytosine and the 5′-triphosphate of 9-β-D-arabinofuranosyladenine. *Cancer Res.* 1968;**28**:2061.
Graves T, Hooks MA. Drug-induced toxicities associated with high-dose cytosine arabinoside infusions. *Pharmacotherapy.* 1989;**9**(1):23–28.
Hande KR, Stein RS, McDonough DA, et al. Pharmacokinetics of high-dose cytosine arabinoside (Ara-C). *Clin Res.* 1981;**29**:436A.
Haupt HM, Hutchins GM, Moore GW. Ara-C lung: Noncardiogenic pulmonary edema complicating cytosine arabinoside therapy of leukemia. *Am J Med.* 1981;**70**:256–261.
Herzig RH, Hines JD, Herzig GP, et al. Cerebellar toxicity with high-dose cytosine arabinoside. *J Clin Oncol.* 1987;**5**(6):927–932.
Herzig RH, Lazarus HM, Herzig GP, et al. Central nervous system toxicity with high-dose cytosine arabinoside. *Semin Oncol.* 1985;**12**(2):233–236.
Hines JD, Oken MM, Mazza JJ, et al. High-dose cytosine arabinoside and m-AMSA is effective therapy in relapsed acute nonlymphocytic leukemia. *J Clin Oncol.* 1984;**2**(6):545–549.
Ho DHW, Frei E III. Clinical pharmacology of 1-β-D-arabinofuranosyl cytosine. *Clin Pharmacol.* 1971;**12**:944–954.
Hoovis ML, Chu MY. Enhancement of the natiproliferative action of 1-β-D-arabinosylcytosine by methotrexate in murine leukemic cells (L517BY). *Cancer Res.* 1973;**33**:521–525.
Jehn U, Goldel N, Rienmuller R, et al. Non-cardiogenic pulmonary edema complicating intermediate and high-dose Ara C treatment for relapsed acute leukemia. *Med Oncol Tumor Pharmacother.* 1988;**5**(1):41–47.
Jolson HM, Bosco L, Bufton MG, et al. Clustering of adverse drug events: Analysis of risk factors for cerebellar toxicity with high-dose cytarabine. *J Natl Cancer Inst.* 1992;**84**:500–505.
Karp JE, Burke PJ, Donehower RC. Effects of rhGM-CSF on intracellular Ara-C pharmacology in vitro in acute myelocytic leukemia: Comparability with drug-induced humoral stimulatory activity. *Leukemia.* 1990;**4**:553–556.
Kaufman HE, Capella JA, Maloney ED, et al. Corneal toxicity of cytosine arabinoside. *Arch Ophthalmol.* 1964;**72**:535–540.
King ME, Naporn A, Young B, et al. Modulation of cytarabine uptake and toxicity by dipyridamole. *Cancer Treat Rep.* 1984;**68**:361–366.
King ME, Pfeifle CE, Howell SB. Intraperitoneal cytosine arabinoside therapy in ovarian carcinoma. *J Clin Oncol.* 1984;**2**:662–669.
Lazarus HM, Herzig RH, Herzig GP, et al. Central nervous system toxicity of high-dose systemic cytosine arabinoside. *Cancer.* 1981;**48**:2577–2582.
Levine LE, Medenica MM, Lorinez AL, et al. Distinctive

acral erythema occurring during therapy for severe myelogenous leukemia. *Arch Dermatol.* 1985;**121**:102–104.

Lopez JA, Agarwal RP. Acute cerebellar toxicity after high-dose cytarabine associated with CNS accumulation of its metabolite, uracil arabinoside. *Cancer Treat Rep.* 1984;**68**(10):1309–1310.

Markman M, Howell SB, Pfeifle CE, et al. Intraperitoneal (IP) chemotherapy with high dose cisplatin (DDP) and cytarabine (Ara-C) in patients with refractory ovarian carcinoma and other malignancies confined to the abdominal cavity (abstract C-643). *Proc Am Soc Clin Oncol.* 1984;**3**:165.

McRae MP, King JC. Compatibility of antineoplastic, antibiotic and corticosteroid drugs in intravenous admixtures. *Am J Hosp Pharm.* 1976;**33**:1010–1013.

Momparler RL. Kinetic and template studies with 1-β-D-arabinofuranosylcytosine-5′-triphosphatase and mammalian deoxyribonucleic acid polymerase. *Mol Pharmacol.* 1972;**8**:362–370.

Notari RE, Chin ML, Wittebort R. Arabinosylcytosine stability in aqueous solutions: pH profile and shelf-life predictions. *J Pharm Sci.* 1972;**61**:1189–1196.

Patterson ARP, Lau EY, Dahlig E, et al. A common basis for inhibition of nucleoside transport by dipyridamole and nitrobenzylthioinosine. *Mol Pharmacol.* 1980;**18**:40–44.

Pfeifle CE, Howell SB. Phase I trial of cytarabine and hydroxyurea. *Cancer Treat Rep.* 1983;**67**(12):1127–1129.

Pommier Y, Pochat L, Marie J-P, et al. High-dose cytarabine in acute leukemia: Toxicity and pharmacokinetics. *Cancer Treat Rep.* 1983;**67**(4):371–372.

Preisler HD, Early AP, Raza A, et al. Therapy of secondary acute nonlymphocytic leukemia with cytarabine. *N Engl J Med.* 1983;**308**(1):21–23.

Ritch PS, Hansen RM, Heuer DK. Ocular toxicity from high-dose cytosine arabinoside. *Cancer.* 1983;**51**:430–432.

Ross DD, Chen S-RS, Cuddy DP. Effects of 1-β-D-arabinofuranosylcytosine on DNA replication intermediates monitored by pH-step alkaline elution. *Cancer Res.* 1990;**50**:2658–2666.

Ross DD, Joneckis CC, Song TH, et al. Bromodeoxyuridine enhancement of 1-β-D-arabinofuranosylcytosine metabolic activation and toxicity in HL-60 leukemic cells. *Cancer Res.* 1988;**48**:517–521.

Rubin EH, Andersen JW, Berg DT. Risk factors for high-dose cytarabine neurotoxicity: An analysis of a cancer and leukemia Group B trial in patients with acute myeloid leukemia. *J Clin Oncol.* 1992;**10**:948–953.

Rudnick SA, Cadman EC, Capizzi RL, et al. High dose cytosine arabinoside (HDARAC) in refractory acute leukemia. *Cancer.* 1979;**44**:1189–1193.

Saiki JH, Thompson S, Smith F, Atkinson R. Paraplegia following intrathecal chemotherapy. *Cancer.* 1972;**29**:370–374.

Schabel FM Jr, Laster WR Jr, Trader MW. Specific DNA inhibitors vs leukemia L1210. Development of resistance to Ara-C and ribonucleotide reductase inhibitors. *Proc Am Assoc Cancer Res ASCO.* 1971;**12**:67.

Schafer AI. Teratogenic effects of antileukemic chemotherapy. *Arch Intern Med.* 1981;**141**:514–515.

Skipper HE, Schabel FM, Wilcox WS. Experimental evaluation of potential anticancer agents. XXI. Scheduling of arabinosyl cytosine to take advantage of its S-phase specificity against leukemic cells. *Cancer Chemother Rep.* 1967;**51**:125–141.

Sondak VK, Wong J, Lazar GS, et al. Cytosine arabinoside and cisplatin isolation perfusion for the treatment of malignant melanoma: Clinical validation of an in vitro observation. *Reg Cancer Treat.* 1989;**2**:125–130.

Spiers ASD, Firth JL. Treating the nervous system in acute leukemia. *Lancet.* 1972;**2**:1433.

Spriggs DR, Robbins G, Takvorian T, et al. Continuous infusion of high-dose 1-β-D-arabinofuranosylcytosine: A phase I and pharmacological study. *Cancer Res.* 1985;**45**:3932–3936.

Streifel JA, Howell SB. Synergistic interaction between 1-β-D-arabinofuranosylcytosine, thymidine, and hydroxyurea against human B cells and leukemic blasts in vitro. *Proc Natl Acad Sci USA.* 1981;**78**:5132–5136.

Tattersall MHN, Harrap KR. Combination chemotherapy: The antagonism of methotrexate and cytosine arabinoside. *Eur J Cancer.* 1973;**9**:229–232.

Trissel LA. *ASHP Handbook on Injectable Drugs.* 5th ed. Bethesda, MD: American Society of Hospital Pharmacists; 1988:217–220.

Trissel LA, Fulton B, Tramonte SM. Visual compatibility of ondansetron with chemotherapeutic agents, antibiotics, and other selected drugs during simulated Y-site injection (abstract P-468R). In: *25th Annual ASHP Midyear Clinical Meetings and Exhibit, Las Vegas, Nevada, December 1990.* Bethesda, MD: American Society of Hospital Pharmacists; 1990.

Vaickus L, Letendre L. Pericarditis induced by high-dose cytarabine therapy. *Arch Intern Med.* 1984;**144**:1868–1869.

Van Prooijen, Rix, Kleijn EVD, Haanen C. Pharmacokinetics of cytosine arabinoside in acute myeloid leukemia. *Clin Pharmacol Ther.* 1977;**21**(6):744–750.

Wagner VM, Hill JS, Weaver D, Baehner RL. Congenital abnormalities in baby born to cytarabine treated mother. *Lancet.* 1980;**2**:98–99.

Wallace TL, Johnson EM Jr. Cytosine arabinoside kills postmitotic neurons: Evidence that deoxycytidine may have a role in neuronal survival that is independent of DNA synthesis. *J Neurosci.* 1989;**9**(1):115–124.

Wan SH, Huffman DH, Azarnoff DL, et al. Pharmacokinetics of 1-β-D-arabinofuranosylcytosine in humans. *Cancer Res.* 1974;**34**:392–397.

Wang JJ, Pratt CB. Intrathecal arabinosyl cytosine in meningeal leukemia. *Cancer.* 1970;**25**:531–534.

Wolff SN, Marion J, Stein RS, et al. High-dose cytosine arabinoside and daunorubicin as consolidation therapy for acute nonlymphocytic leukemia in first remissions: A pilot study. *Blood.* 1985;**65**(6):1407–1411.

Wolff L, Zighelboim J, Gale RP. Paraplegia following intrathecal cytosine arabinoside. *Cancer.* 1979;**43**:83–85.

Cytembena

Other Names

MBBA; NSC-104801; sodium bromebrate.

Chemistry

Structure of cytembena

Cytembena is a crotonolactone derivative with the empiric formula of $C_{11}H_8O_4BrNa$ and a molecular weight of 307.

Antitumor Activity

Phase II trials with cytembena have been limited because of the "autonomic storm" noted as the dose-limiting side effect of the compound. In European studies the compound induced objective response rates in 10 to 19% of patients with cervical cancer (Dvorak and Bauer 1971), 38% of patients with endometrial cancer, and about 50% of patients with ovarian cancer (Dvorak 1971). The only phase II trial in the United States was in patients with colorectal cancer in whom the drug was found to be inactive (Moertel et al 1975). Of note is that one patient with pancreatic cancer in the phase I study of cytembena had a complete response (Frytak et al 1975). That lead was never followed up. An overall review of the European and U.S. trials has been done by Von Hoff et al (1977).

Mechanism of Action

Cytembena is an antineoplastic agent with an unidentified mechanism of action. In the lab it has demonstrated inhibitory effects on purine synthesis, tetrahydrofolate formylase, incorporation or utilization of amino acids, oxidative phosphorylation, succinic acid dehydrogenase, and DNA biosynthesis. Cell cycle phase specificity is not known.

Availability and Storage

Cytembena was available from the National Cancer Institute in a lyophilized form with 200 mg per vial. The unopened vial should be stored at room temperature.

Preparation for Use, Stability, and Admixture

When reconstituted with 3.9 mL of Sterile Water for Injection, USP, each milliliter contains 50 mg of cytembena. If desired, the solutions may be further diluted in 5% Dextrose in Water, USP, or Sodium Chloride Injection, USP. The initial vials are stable at room temperature for at least 5 years. Reconstituted solutions are chemically stable for 48 hours at room temperature.

Administration

See Dosage.

Special Precautions

See Side Effects and Toxicity.

Drug Interactions

None are known.

Dosage

The usual dosages are 400 mg/m²/d × 5 days, repeated every 5 weeks, and 300 mg/m²/d × 20 days. Some European studies used a peanut oil suspension intramuscularly; a few studies used intracavitary injections with or without a local anesthetic. Use of 10% topical ointment and solution is also reported (Von Hoff et al 1977).

Pharmacokinetics

The agent is assayed by a chromatographic method. The half-life of the agent is 13.5 to 15 hours. It is likely the drug is excreted via a nonrenal mechanism. Only 8% of the drug was found in the urine. The agent has a large volume of distribution (30 L) (Grafnetterova et al 1971).

Side Effects and Toxicity

The unusual dose-limiting toxic effect of cytembena is an "autonomic storm" characterized by facial flushing and paresthesias, hypermotility, hypertension, anxiousness, and chest pain (with electrocardiographic changes). Nausea, vomiting, and diarrhea also occurred along with extreme pain at the injection site. Hematologic and hepatic toxic effects were not significant.

Special Applications

Cytembena has significant immunosuppressive activity and has also been used as an antiarthritic agent in Czechoslovakia.

REFERENCES

Dvorak O. Cytembena treatment of advanced gynecological carcinomas. *Neoplasma.* 1971;**13**:461–464.

Dvorak O, Bauer J. Cytembena treatment of advanced and relapsing uterine cervix carcinoma. *Neoplasma.* 1971;**18**:465–466.

Frytak S, Moertel CG, Schutz AS, Ahmann DL, Donadio JV, Weinshilbourn PM. A phase I study of cytembena. *Proc Am Assoc Cancer Res.* 1975;**16**:36.

Grafnetterova J, Schuck S, Mabel O. Pharmacokinetics of cytembena in man. *Neuroplasma.* 1971;**18**:447–454.

Moertel CG, Schutt AJ, Hahn RG, Marciniak TA, Reitemeir RJ. Phase II study of cytembena (NSC-104801) in advanced colorectal carcinoma. *Cancer Chemother Rep.* 1975;**59**:581–583.

Von Hoff DD, Rozencweig M, Muggia FM. Cytembena: A new anticancer compound with a unique structure. *Biomedicine.* 1977;**26**:388–392.

Dabis Maleate

■ Other Names

CBH; NSC-57198.

■ Chemistry

Structure of dabis maleate

Dabis maleate is a quaternary ammonium salt first described in 1969 (Fessler et al). The chemical name is 1,4-bis(2′-chloroethyl)-1,4-diazabicyclo[2.2.1]heptane diperchlorate. The compound has a molecular formula of $C_{17}H_{24}C_{12}N_2O_8$ and a molecular weight of 455. It is soluble in water. Pettit et al (1979, 1981) have suggested that the active component of the drug is formed through production of a very reactive carbon–carbon or carbon–nitrogen bond in vivo.

■ Antitumor Activity

The compound is close to undergoing phase I trials in humans. The drug has demonstrated excellent antitumor activity in a number of animal tumor systems (Goldin et al 1981) including L-1210, B-16, MX-1 mammary, P-388, and colon-26 and -38. Clinical trials will likely begin at the Rotterdam Cancer Institute in the near future.

■ Mechanism of Action

The precise mechanism of action of dabis maleate is unknown. It most likely is an alkylating agent (Traganos et al 1984). The drug has limited in vitro activity (may require in vivo activation).

■ Availability and Storage

The drug has just been formulated for clinical use and no data on these parameters is available.

■ Preparation for Use, Stability, and Admixture

The drug has just been formulated for clinical use and no data on these parameters is available.

■ Administration

In phase I trials, the drug has been diluted in 5% dextrose and administered either as a 5-to-15-minute (van der Burg et al 1992) or a 15-to-360-minute (Verweij et al 1992) intravenous infusion.

■ Special Precautions

None are known to date.

■ Drug Interactions

None have been described in preclinical testing.

■ Dosage

In a phase I trial, van der Burg et al (1991) administered dabis maleate in doses of 50 to 1400 mg/m^2 once every three weeks. In another phase I trial, Verweij et al (1992) administered dabis maleate either as a bolus injection in doses of 250 mg/m^2/d for 3 days every 3 weeks or 500 to 750 mg/m^2/week or as a 6-hour infusion weekly in doses of 500 to 750 mg/m^2. Neurotoxicity was the close-limiting toxicity in both trials. Doses recommended for phase II studies include 750 mg/m^2 once every three weeks as a 15-minute infusion and 500 mg/m^2/week as a 6-hour infusion for 6 weeks, followed by a 3-week rest period.

Pharmacokinetics

The pharmacokinetics of dabis maleate has not yet been determined.

Side Effects and Toxicity

Neurotoxicity, characterized by paresthesias and ataxia, is the dose-limiting toxicity associated with dabis maleate occurring routinely at doses of 750 mg/m^2 or higher. Symptoms usually last from 1 to 48 hours (van der Burg et al 1991, Verweij et al 1992), although severe paresthesias lasted for more than 28 days at doses of 900 to 1400 mg/m^2. Other observed toxic effects included nausea and vomiting, as well as brief hypotension (van der Burg et al 1991).

Effects will be determined in phase I clinical trials.

Special Applications

None are known.

REFERENCES

Fessler DC, Pettit GR, Settepani JA. Antineoplastic agents. XXV. 1,4-Diazabicyclo[2.2.1]heptanes. *J Med Chem.* 1969; **12**:542–543.

Goldin A, Venditti JM, Macdonald JS, Muggia FM, Henney JE, Devita VT. Current results of the screening program at the Division of Cancer Treatment, National Cancer Institute. *Eur J Cancer.* 1981;**17**:129–142.

Pettit GR, Gieschen DP, Pettit WE. Antineoplastic agents. LXIV. 1,4-Bis(2'-chloroethyl)-1,4-diazabicyclo[2.2.1]heptane dihydrogen dimaleate. *J Pharm Sci.* 1979;**68**:1539–1542.

Pettit GR, Gieschen DP, Pettit WE. Stability of the 1,4-bis(2'-haloethyl)-1,4-diazabicyclo[2.2.1]heptane dication. *Can J Chem.* 1981;**59**:212–221.

Traganos F, Darzynkiewicz Z, Bueti C, Melamed MR. Effects of a prospective antitumor agent, 1,4-bis(2'-chloroethyl)-1,4-diazabicyclo[2.2.1]heptane diperchlorate, on cultured mammalian cells. *Cancer Invest.* 1984;**2**(1):1–13.

van der Burg MEL, Planting AS, Stoter G, McDaniel C, Vecht CJ, Verweij J. Phase I study of dabis maleate given once every 3 weeks. *Eur J Cancer.* 1991;**27**:1635–1637.

Verweij J, Planting ASTh, de Boer M, van der Burg MEL, Stoter G. Frequent administration of dabis maleate, a phase I study. *Ann Oncol.* 1992;**3**:241–242.

Dacarbazine

Other Names

DIC; DTIC-Dome® (Miles Pharmaceutical Division); dimethyl-triazeno-imidazole-carboxamide; NSC-45388.

Chemistry

Structure of dacarbazine

The complete chemical name of dacarbazine is 5-(3,3-dimethyl-1-triazenyl)-1*H*-imidazole-4-carboxamide. It has a molecular weight of 182 and a melting point of about 199°C. It occurs physically as colorless to ivory-colored crystals and is extremely light sensitive. Solubility for the pure powder is markedly enhanced in 10% citric acid (60 mg/mL) compared with water (1 mg/mL). Thus, the commercial preparation includes citric acid to enhance aqueous solubility.

Antitumor Activity

Dacarbazine appears to have its greatest activity in advanced malignant melanoma (Carter and Friedman 1972, Luce 1975). When used singly or in various combinations, it produces objective responses in about 20% of patients. Approximately 5 to 6% of these responses are complete with a median duration of about 5 to 6 months (Comis 1976, Gottlieb et al 1976). It has been combined with other cytotoxic agents such as carmustine and vincristine (Luce et al 1970b, Cohen et al 1972) or with carmustine and hydroxyurea in the "BHD" regimen (Costanzi et al 1975). It has additionally been used in some soft tissue sarcomas (Wilbur et al 1975) and is commonly used in treating Hodgkin's disease in the ABVD regimen (Adriamycin, bleomycin, vinblastine, and dacarbazine) (Bonadonna et al 1974).

Mechanism of Action

The exact cytotoxic mechanism(s) for dacarbazine has not been established but there is some evidence for activity via three mechanisms: (1) monoalkylation by methyldiazonium ions (Loo et al 1976), (2) antimetabolite activity as a purine precursor, and (3) interaction with sulfhydryl (SH) groups in proteins (Loo et al 1968). The drug clearly inhibits synthesis of protein, RNA, and especially DNA. Methylation of nucleic acids has been documented in both rats and humans following dacarbazine (Skibba and Bryan 1971). Interestingly, the inhibition of DNA synthesis is enhanced following light exposure which may activate the molecule (Loo et al 1976) (see the figure below). Alkylation through a methyldiazonium ion metabolite is the most likely mechanism involved in dacarbazine antitumor activity. This monoalkylation does not lead to DNA–DNA strand crosslinking. Although dacarbazine is a structural analog of 5-aminoimidazole-4-carboxamide (AIC), a precursor of purine bases, it apparently does not function in this fashion in vivo and the AIC portion of the molecule is not required for activity (Schmid and Hutchison 1974). Bioactivation of the drug can be mediated by hepatic microsomal oxidases, yielding active hydroxylated and N-demethylated species (Skibba et al 1970). Light-induced conversion of dacarbazine to 5-diazoimidazole-4-carboxamide and subsequent cyclization to 2-azahypoxanthine is alternatively postulated to explain some of the drug's activity and/or toxicity (Montgomery 1976). Dacarbazine appears to be more active on cells in late G_2 phase, but has activity throughout the cell cycle and probably is not particularly cell cycle phase specific.

Availability and Storage

Dacarbazine is commercially available from Miles Pharmaceutical Division, West Haven, Connecticut (DTIC-Dome®) in amber glass vials containing either 100, 200, or 500 mg of lyophilized drug (without preservatives added). The intact vial is stable for 4 years from the date of manufacture when refrigerated; however, storage of vials at room temperature for several months does not adversely affect stability. The vials also contain anhydrous citric acid and mannitol to buffer the pH and add bulk, respectively. Protection from light is required during storage.

Preparation for Use, Stability, and Admixture

Sterile water, normal saline, or D5W may be used to reconstitute dacarbazine vials. A minimum of 2 mL of diluent must be used. The recommended reconstitution volumes of 9.9, 19.7, and 49.5 mL of sterile water are more commonly used for the 100-, 200- and 500-mg vials, respectively. This results in a

Activated dacarbazine molecule following light exposure

clear, colorless to pale yellow solution of 10 mg/mL dacarbazine with a pH of 3.0 to 4.0. This solution is chemically stable for only 8 hours at room temperature (20°C) and 72 hours under refrigeration (4°C). A change in the color of the solution from pale yellow to pink denotes decomposition of the drug (Kleinman et al 1976).

Further dilution of the initial admixture into D5W or normal saline (200–500 mL) provides a solution reportedly stable for 24 hours with only 5% loss of activity if protected from light, and 50% loss of activity after only 4 hours if exposed to light at room temperatures. Intravenous push doses should probably be reconstituted with D5W or normal saline rather than sterile water to ensure isotonicity. Baird and Willoughby (1978) additionally suggest that the breakdown products from photodegradation of dacarbazine in solution (5-diazoimidazole carboxamide and 2-azahypoxanthine) may be responsible for the acute local toxicity (burning and vein pain) as well as some systemic complications of the drug (including nausea, vomiting, and hepatotoxicity). Although more work is necessary to characterize this reaction, it is probably prudent to protect dacarbazine solutions from light exposure.

Dacarbazine forms an immediate precipitate with hydrocortisone sodium succinate (Solu-Cortef®). This change was not noted on admixture with the sodium phosphate salt of hydrocortisone (Hydrocortone®) nor with lidocaine 1 to 2%. Einhorn et al (1973) reported no compatibility problems when dacarbazine was admixed with 2000 U heparin in 500 mL D5W. Bottles were changed every 8 hours because of the light sensitivity consideration. The drug also appears to be physically compatible with doxorubicin, dactinomycin, cyclophosphamide, methotrexate, 5-fluorouracil, cytarabine, and carmustine (Horton and Stevens 1979) and for at least 4 hours with ondansetron (Trissel et al 1990).

■ Administration

Both the intravenous push and infusion methods have been used with dacarbazine. Oral absorption is erratic and therefore dacarbazine should not be administered orally. For intravenous push doses, administration in any convenient volume (5–10 mL) of D5W or normal saline over at least 1 minute is recommended (although this may be painful). Optimally, the patency of the vein should be tested first with a 5- to 10-mL flush of D5W or normal saline and with the same solutions after infusion to flush any remaining drug from the tubing.

Extravasation of dacarbazine solutions is likely to be associated with pain but not necrosis (Dorr et al 1987). Most commonly, DTIC is administered as a brief infusion over 15 to 30 minutes in 250 to 500 mL of fluid. In addition, there are reports that light-protected dacarbazine solutions may produce less vein irritation and pain (Koriech and Shukla 1980). Thus, light protection of prolonged infusion solutions may be warranted to prevent photodegradation (Baird and Willoughby 1978). This latter form of administration does not seem to cause pain along the injection site as with more rapid intravenous push techniques.

■ Dosage

There are two basic treatment schemes for dacarbazine: (1) a consecutive daily schedule for 10 or 5 days (Costanzi et al 1975), and (2) a single-dose regimen. Both schedules are repeated at 34-week intervals. For the 10-day course, doses of from 2 to 4.5 mg/kg/d IV are given for 10 consecutive days. Up to 250 mg/m² for 5 consecutive days interspersed with bacillus Calmette–Guérin immunotherapy has also been given (Gutterman et al 1976).

Treatments can be repeated when myelosupression has resolved: generally 4 weeks after a 10-day drug course and 3 weeks after a 5-day drug course. Doses should also be reduced in the presence of severely impaired renal function (especially tubular secreting function).

Dacarbazine may be given as a single dose of up to 850 mg/m² on day 1 of therapy, with doses repeated at 3- to 4-week intervals (Gardere et al 1972). This dose has also been combined with single doses of cyclophosphamide and vincristine on day 1 without excess toxicity (Pritchard et al 1980). As a single agent Cowan and Bersagel (1971) used single doses of from 650 to 1450 mg/m² repeated at 4- to 6-week intervals and Buesa et al (1984) used single doses of 850 to 1980 mg/m². These doses produced dose-limiting hypotension and flulike toxic reactions. High dacarbazine doses of 350 mg/m² to 2.5 g/m² given by 24-hour infusion have also been combined with hemibody radiation in patients with malignant melanoma (Thatcher et al 1986). These high-dose courses were repeated every 3 weeks.

■ Drug Interactions

The metabolism of dacarbazine may be induced by drugs such as phenytoin (Dilantin®) and phenobarbital. Experimentally, the enzyme xanthine oxidase is inhibited by dacarbazine, producing additive ef-

DACARBAZINE PHARMACOKINETICS

Administration Method	Reference	Dose	Half-life (min) α	Half-life (min) β	Volume of Distribution	Clearance (mL/kg/min) Total Body	Clearance (mL/kg/min) Renal	Urinary Recovery (% Dose)
Intravenous bolus	Breithaupt et al 1982	2.7–6.9 mg/kg	2.9	41	0.2	15.4	3–5	46–52
Hepatic perfusion in dogs	Breithaupt et al 1983	50–250 mg	—	66.4	—	18.4	—	—

fects with allopurinol and potentially increased toxicity if given concomitantly with azathioprine or 6-mercaptopurine.

The cytokine interleukin-2 significantly alters dacarbazine pharmacokinetics in melanoma patients (Chabot et al 1990). With interleukin-2, dacarbazine areas under the plasma concentration × time curve are lowered by 20%, the volume of distribution is increased by 36%, and clearance is increased by 38%. The dacarbazine half-life was unchanged at approximately 3 hours. The immune adjuvant *Corynebacterium parvum* may also depress hepatic N-demethylation and thereby impair dacarbazine elimination (Lipton et al 1978). Interestingly, the addition of dactinomycin reverses the effect of *C. parvum* on dacarbazine elimination.

■ Pharmacokinetics

Loo et al (1968) showed erratic and incomplete oral absorption of dacarbazine. Injected dacarbazine initially disappears rapidly from the plasma probably as a result of hepatic metabolism (Householder and Loo 1971). The terminal plasma half-life of intact drug is reported to be approximately 35 minutes (see first table). The pharmacokinetics of the inactive 5-amino-4-imidazole carboxamide metabolite (AIC) are similar to that of dacarbazine, although much less AIC is excreted in the urine (see second table). Of interest, the half-life of dacarbazine, measured by high-performance liquid chromatography (HPLC) in this study, was approximately 40 minutes. This is much shorter than the half-life of several hours reported by Chabot et al (1990) using the HPLC method and shorter than the half-life described by Loo et al (1976) using a nonspecific colorimetric assay. Loo et al (1976) did observe prolonged elimination of dacarbazine in patients with renal and hepatic dysfunction. In either case there could be 44% increase in the half-life. As dacarbazine can be hepatotoxic, dose reductions in patients with renal or hepatic dysfunction are probably indicated.

There is relatively little distribution of the drug into the cerebrospinal fluid. This relates to the poor lipid solubility of dacarbazine. Urinary excretion accounts for approximately 30 to 45% of a dose and this is maximal after about 5 hours. Fifty percent of the 6-hour excretion fraction can be found as intact drug and 50% as the N-demethylated metabolite AIC. The pattern of metabolism suggests that induction of microsomal liver enzyme systems by drugs like phenobarbital and phenytoin might enhance the conversion of dacarbazine to AIC and other metabolites.

Within standard dose ranges, only about 5% of administered drug is protein bound. It also appears that renal tubular secretion rather than glomerular filtration facilitates urinary elimination of drug and metabolite(s).

■ Side Effects and Toxicity

The usual dose-limiting toxic effect of dacarbazine is a moderate degree of myelosuppression. The typical nadir of leukopenia and thrombocytopenia ranges

---

PHARMACOKINETICS OF THE PRIMARY DACARBAZINE METABOLITE 5-AMINOIMIDAZOLE-4-CARBOXAMIDE

Administration method	Intravenous bolus
Dose	6.5 mg/kg
Half-life (mean)	43–116 min (76 min)
Clearance	26 mL/kg/min
Urinary recovery (mean)	9–18% dose (13% dose)

From Breithaupt H, Dammann A, Aigner K. Pharmacokinetics of dacarbazine (DTIC) and its metabolite 5-aminoimidazole-4-carboxamide (AIC) following different dose schedules. Cancer Chemother Pharmacol. 1982;9:103–109. Reprinted with permission.

from 21 to 25 days after drug administration (Comis 1976). Anemia is also sometimes noted but is rarely severe.

The most common acute toxic effect of dacarbazine is severe nausea and vomiting. Over 90% of patients experience this side effect, which characteristically lessens with each subsequent dose. Emetic episodes following dacarbazine may last 1 to 12 hours and aggressive antiemetic prophylaxis is suggested.

Hepatic toxicity is well described with dacarbazine (Ceci et al 1988). Effects range from delayed hepatic failure (Frosch et al 1979) to acute dystrophy with fatal thrombosis (Feaux de Lacroix 1983). Allergic vasculitis has been forwarded to explain this toxicity (McClay et al 1987, Cznaretzki and Macher 1981).

A flulike syndrome has been consistently reported in patients receiving large doses of dacarbazine (Buesa et al 1984). This syndrome manifests as fever, myalgia, and malaise with an onset of 7 days. It may last 1 to 3 weeks. Another acute effect of high-dose therapy is hypotension, possibly related to calcium chelation by the citric acid present in the commercial formulation (Buesa et al 1984). Infusion of calcium gluconate was suggested to alleviate this reaction. Other high-dose toxic effects include a severe reaction to sunlight with intense burning and pain on the head and hands if sun exposed. No erythema or edema was noted although blurred vision occurred in two patients given high-dose therapy. Photosensitivity is well described with dacarbazine (Beck et al 1980). Other rare toxic effects include alopecia, facial flushing, and facial paresthesias (Luce et al 1970). A giant urticarial reaction emanating from the injection site has also been described. Fortunately, extravasations do not lead to necrosis in patients (Buesa et al 1984) and the drug had very weak vesicant potential in an animal model (Dorr et al 1987). In rodent models, metabolites of dacarbazine have been demonstrated to be potent carcinogens (Skibba et al 1970).

■ Special Applications

Intraarterial Administration. Dacarbazine has been used intraarterially via hepatic artery cannulation of the femoral or brachial arteries (Banzet et al 1975, Joray et al 1977). In this experimental application, dacarbazine doses of 200 mg/m^2/d as a 24-hour infusion in 1000 mL of D5W for 5 days have been used to treat hepatic metastases from various solid tumors. Einhorn et al (1973) used a regimen of 250 mg/m^2/d for 5 consecutive days followed by 16 days off. In this trial the drug was diluted into 500 mL of D5W and new solutions were freshly prepared every 8 hours. The overall response rate in malignant melanoma was 41% and systemic toxicity was less than that from equivalent intravenous injections.

In a dog model, intraarterially administered dacarbazine rapidly forms the AIC metabolite and is cleared at a mean rate of 18 mL/min (Breithaupt et al 1982).

Intrathecal or Intraventricular Administration. Intrathecal or intraventricular administration of dacarbazine has been used in three patients with leptomeningeal malignant melanoma (Yamasaki et al 1989, Champagne and Silver 1992). Individual dacarbazine doses ranged from 5 to 20 mg in one series (Champagne and Silver 1992) and up to 30 mg in another single case (Yamasaki et al 1989). One group reported specific mixing procedures for the intrathecal doses: (1) for a 5 mg dose, reconstitute 5 mg dacarbazine in 0.5 mL of normal saline; (2) add 0.2 mL of 8.4% sodium bicarbonate solution (1 mEq/mL); (3) mix with 4 mL of the patient's cerebrospinal fluid (for a final volume of approximately 4.7 mL). The volumes of dacarbazine solution and sodium bicarbonate, but not cerebrospinal fluid, are then doubled for the 10-mg dose, and for the 20-mg dose, the drug mixture in saline (20 mg/2.0 mL) is combined with 0.8 mL of 8.4% sodium bicarbonate and 4 to 5 mL of the patient's cerebrospinal fluid (Champagne and Silver, 1992). Sodium bicarbonate is added to neutralize the 1% citric acid present in commercial dacarbazine formulations (DTIC-Dome®).

Intrathecal and intraventricular dacarbazine doses have been administered twice weekly (Champagne and Silver 1992) or intrathecally every third day for 1 month (Yamasaki et al 1989). The total (cumulative) dacarbazine dose given intrathecally in the latter study was 210 mg. These intrathecal treatments have reduced two patients' disease symptoms (Champagne and Silver 1992) and delayed tumor growth in one patient (Yamasaki et al 1989); however, there is no objective evidence of local tumor shrinkage following intrathecal or inventricular therapy with dacarbazine. Symptoms have ranged from transient headache and nuchal rigidity to a hypertensive episode with flushing and fecal incontinence but not loss of consciousness or seizure activity (Champagne and Silver 1992). This reaction occurred after an intraventricular dose, the patient's sixth dacarbazine treatment. In another patient given intrathecal dacarbazine, no symptoms were reported following multiple treatments (Yamasaki et al 1989).

The pharmacokinetics of intrathecal dacarbazine were studied in one patient using a reverse-phase HPLC assay. The elimination of parent dacarbazine from the cerebrospinal fluid was biphasic with half-lives of 30 minutes (α) and 5 hours (β) (Yamasaki et al 1989). The level of AIC was unchanged at 0.3 µg/mL over the sampling period.

REFERENCES

Baird GM, Willoughby MLN. Photodegradation of dacarbazine (letter). *Lancet.* 1978;**2**:681.

Banzet P, et al. Treatment of malignant melanomas. Trial of DTIC by intraarterial infusion (English abstract). *Nouv Presse Med.* 1975;**4**(20):1477–1480.

Beck TM, Hart NE, Smith CE. Photosensitivity reaction following DTIC administration: Report of two cases. *Cancer Treat Rep.* 1980;**64**(4/5):725–726.

Bonadonna G, Zucali R, Monfardini S, et al. Combination chemotherapy of Hodgkin's disease with adriamycin, bleomycin, vinblastine and imidazole carboxamide versus MOPP. *Cancer* 1975;**36**:252–259.

Breithaupt H, Aigner K, Hechtel R. Kinetics of methotrexate, dacarbazine and 5-fluorouracil during isolated liver perfusion. *Cancer Res.* 1983;**86**:116–121.

Breithaupt H, Dammann A, Aigner K. Pharmacokinetics of dacarbazine (DTIC) and its metabolite 5-aminoimidazole-4-carboxamide (AIC) following different dose schedules. *Cancer Chemother Pharmacol.* 1982;**9**:103–109.

Buesa JM, Gracia M, Valle M, et al. Phase I trial of intermittent high-dose dacarbazine. *Cancer Treat Rep.* 1984;**68**(3):499–504.

Carter SK, Friedman MA. 5-(3,3-Dimethyl-1-triazeno)-imidazole-4-carboxamide (DTIC, DIC, NSC-45388)—A new antitumor agent with activity against malignant melanoma. *Eur J Cancer.* 1972;**8**:85–92.

Ceci G, Bella M, Melissari M, et al. Fatal hepatic vascular toxicity of DTIC. Is it really a rare event? *Cancer.* 1988;**61**:1988–1991.

Chabot GG, Flaherty LE, Valdivieso M, Baker LH. Alteration of dacarbazine pharmacokinetics after interleukin-2 administration in melanoma patients. *Cancer Chemother Pharmacol.* 1990;**27**:157–160.

Champagne MA, Silver HKB. Intrathecal dacarbazine treatment of leptomeningeal malignant melanoma. *J Natl Cancer Inst.* 1992;**84**:1203–1204.

Cohen SM, Greenspan EM, Weiner MJ, et al. Triple combination chemotherapy of disseminated melanoma. *Cancer.* 1972;**29**:1489–1495.

Comis RL. DTIC (NSC-45388) in malignant melanoma: A perspective. *Cancer Treat Rep.* 1976;**60**:165–176.

Costanzi JJ, Vaitkevicius UK, Quagliana JM, et al. Combination chemotherapy for disseminated malignant melanoma. *Cancer.* 1975;**35**:342–346.

Cowan DH, Bersagel DE. Intermittent treatment of metastatic malignant melanoma with high dose 5-(3,3-dimethyl-1-triazeno)imidazole-4-carboxamide (NSC-45388). *Cancer Chemother Rep.* 1971;**55**:175–181.

Cznaretzki BM, Macher E. DTIC (dacarbazine)-induced hepatic damage: Possible pathogenesis and prevention. *Arch Dermatol Res.* 1981;**270**:375–376.

Dorr RT, Alberts DS, Einspahr J, et al. Experimental dacarbazine antitumor activity and skin toxicity in relation to light exposure and pharmacologic antidotes. *Cancer Treat Rep.* 1987;**71**:267–272.

Einhorn LH, McBride CM, Luce JK, et al. Intraarterial infusion therapy with 5-(3,3-dimethyl-1-triazeno)imidazole-4-carboxamide (NSC-45388) for malignant melanoma. *Cancer.* 1973;**32**(4):749–755.

Feaux de Lacroix W, Runne W, Hauk U, et al. Acute liver dystrophy with thrombosis of hepatic veins: A fatal complication of dacarbazine treatment. *Cancer Treat Rep.* 1983;**67**:779–784.

Frosch PJ, Czarnetzki BM, Macher E, et al. Hepatic failure in a patient treated with dacarbazine (DTIC) for malignant melanoma. *J Cancer Res Clin Oncol.* 1979;**95**:281–286.

Gardere S, Hussain S, Cowan DH. Treatment of metastatic malignant melanoma with a combination of 5-(3,3-dimethyl-1-triazeno)-imidazole-4-carboxamide (NSC-45388), cyclo-phosphamide (NSC-26271), and vincristine (NSC-67574). *Cancer Chemother Rep.* **56**:357–361.

Gottlieb J, Benjamin RS, Baker LH, et al. Role of DTIC (NSC-45388) in the chemotherapy of sarcomas. *Cancer Treat Rep.* 1976;**60**(2):199–203.

Gutterman JV, Mavligit GM, Hersh EM. Chemoimmunotherapy of human solid tumors. *Med Clin North Am.* 1976;**60**(3):441–462.

Horton JK, Stevens MFG. Search for drug interactions between the antitumor agent DTIC and other cytotoxic agents. *J Pharm Pharmacol.* 1979;**31**(suppl):64P.

Householder GE, Loo TL. Disposition of 5-(3,3-dimethyl-1-triazeno)imidazole-4-carboxamide—A new antitumor agent. *J Pharmacol Exp Ther.* 1971;**179**:386–395.

Joray AM, et al. Regional chemotherapy of maxillo facial malignant melanoma with intracarotid artery infusion of DTIC. *Tumori.* 1977;**63**(3):299–302.

Kleinman, LM, Davignon JP, Cradock JC, et al. Investigational drug information: Dacarbazine. *Drug Intell Clin Pharm.* 1976;**10**:48–49.

Koriech O, Shukla V. Reduced toxicity of DTIC with administration in the dark (abstract 672). *Proc Am Assoc Cancer Res ASCO.* 1980;**21**:168.

Lipton A, Hepner GW, White DS, et al. Decreased hepatic drug demethylation in patients receiving chemoimmunotherapy. *Cancer.* 1978;**41**:1680.

Loo TL, Householder CE, Gerulath AH, et al. Mechanism of action and pharmacology studies with DTIC (NSC-45399). *Cancer Treat Rep.* 1976;**60**:149–152.

Loo TL, Luce JK, Jardine JH, et al. Pharmacologic studies of the antitumor agent 5-(dimethyl-triazeno)-imidazole-4-carboxamide. *Cancer Res.* 1968;**28**:2448–2453.

Luce JK. Chemotherapy of melanoma. *Semin Oncol.* 1975;**2**(2):179–185.

Luce JK, Thurman WG, Isaacs BL, et al. Clinical trials with the antitumor agent 5-(3,3-dimethyl-1-triazeno)-imidazole-4-carboxamide (NSC-45388). *Cancer Chemother Rep.* 1970a;**54**:119–124.

Luce JK, Torn LB, Price H. Combination dimethyl triazeno imidazole carboxamide (NSC-45388: DIC), vincristine (NSC-67574), and 1,3-bis(2-chloroethyl)-1-nitrosourea (NSC-409962: BCNU) chemotherapy of disseminated malignant melanoma. *Proc Am Assoc Cancer Res.* 1970b;**11**:50.

McClay E, Lusch CJ, Mastrangelo MJ. Allergy-induced hepatic toxicity associated with dacarbazine. *Cancer Treat Rep.* 1987;**71**(2):219–220.

Montgomery JA. Experimental studies at Southern Research Institute with DTIC (NSC-45388). *Cancer Treat Rep.* 1976;**60**:125.

Pritchard KI, Quirt IC, Cowan DH, et al. DTIC therapy in metastatic malignant melanoma: A simplified dose schedule. *Cancer Treat Rep.* 1980;**64**(10/11):1123–1126.

Schmid FA, Hutchison DJ. Chemotherapeutic, carcinogenic, and cell-regulatory effects of triazenes. *Cancer Res.* 1974;**34**:1671.

Skibba JL, Bryan GT. Methylation of nucleic acids and urinary excretion of ^{14}C-labelled 2-methylguanine by rats and man after administration of 4(5)-(3,3-dimethyl-1-triazeno)imidazole-5(4)-carboxamide. *Toxicol Appl Pharmacol.* 1971;**18**:707.

Skibba JL, Erturik E, Bryan GT. Induction of thymic lymphosarcoma and mammary adenocarcinomas in rats by oral administration of the antitumor agent 4(5)-(3,3-dimethyl-1-triazeno)imidazole-5(4)-carboxamide. *Cancer.* 1970;**26**:1000–1005.

Thatcher N, Anderson H, James R, et al. Treatment of metastatic melanoma by 24-hour DTIC infusions and hemibody irradiation. *Cancer.* 1986;**57**:2103–2107.

Trissel LA, Fulton B, Tramonte SM. Visual compatibility of ondansetron with chemotherapeutic agents, antibiotics, and other selected drugs during simulated Y-site injection (abstract P-468R). In: *25th Annual ASHP Midyear Clinical Meetings and Exhibit, Las Vegas, Nevada, December 1990.* Bethesda, MD: American Society of Hospital Pharmacists, 1990.

Wilbur JR, Sutow WW, Sullivan MP, Gottlieb JA. Chemotherapy of sarcomas. *Cancer.* 1975;**36**:765–769.

Yamasaki T, Kikuchi H, Yamashita J, et al. Primary spinal intramedullary malignant melanoma: Case report. *Neurosurgery.* 1989;**25**:117–121.

Dactinomycin

■ Other Names

Actinomycin D; ACT-D; DACT; actinomycin C_1; Cosmegen® (Merck & Company, Inc); NSC-3053.

■ Chemistry

Structure of dactinomycin

Dactinomycin has a molecular weight of 1255. The drug is a phenoxazine pentapeptide containing antibiotic isolated from *Streptomyces parvullus*. The molecular structure includes two peptide loops linked to a three-ring chromophoric phenoxazone ring system (actinocin) (Woodruff and Waksman 1960). The two pentapeptide loops are identical and consist of, in order, L-threonine, D-valine, L-proline, sarcosine, and L-methylvaline (Brockmann 1974). The drug is highly soluble in water, forming an amber- to gold-colored solution.

■ Antitumor Activity

Dactinomycin has activity in a number of experimental tumor systems (Goldin and Johnson 1974) and in a variety of human solid tumors (see table on page 350) (Frei 1974). Alone or in combination with methotrexate, it is potentially curative in 50 to 70% of patients with gestational choriocarcinoma (Lewis

1972). When it is combined with surgery and radiotherapy, cure rates of 80% have been obtained in Wilms' tumor (Farber 1966). It is also active with or without vincristine in nonepidemic (African) forms of Kaposi's sarcoma. Other dactinomycin-sensitive solid tumors include Ewing's sarcoma (Hustu et al 1972), rhabdomyosarcoma (Frei 1974), and melanoma (Samson et al 1978). It also has activity in embryonal carcinoma of the testis as well as other testicular tumors (Ansfield et al 1969).

Dactinomycin appears to lack significant activity in carcinomas of the gastrointestinal tract, lung, kidney, and head and neck (Frei 1974). Minor activity has additionally been observed in breast cancer (Grimm et al 1980) and in childhood acute lymphocytic leukemia in responding patients had not received prior anthracyclines (Green et al 1978). Dactinomycin also has antibacterial properties, but on a molar basis it is one of the most potent antineoplastic agents available. In addition, the drug can inhibit osteoclast growth and thus has hypocalcemic activity similar to plicamycin (Reyes and Talley 1965).

■ Mechanism of Action

Dactinomycin becomes noncovalently bound between purine–pyrimidine base pairs in DNA by intercalation. The synthesis of DNA-dependent ribosomal RNA and new messenger RNA is selectively inhibited. The peptide loops appear to facilitate tighter binding to DNA, as the intercalating actinocin (phenoxazone) moiety alone is inactive (Reich 1963). Intercalative binding is due to pi–pi bonding or "stacking forces" between the chromophore moiety and guanine. This can occur adjacent to any guanine–cytosine pair in DNA. Binding at a given site distorts the DNA double helix and thereby disfavors binding by another dactinomycin closer than 6 bp away (Muller and Crothers 1968).

The DNA helix distortion caused by dactinomycin appears to be caused by hydrogen bonds formed between deoxyribose ring oxygens and –CONH– groups on the chromophore. Bound dactinomycin molecules dissociate very slowly from DNA as a result of electrostatic interactions of the cyclic peptide rings with each strand of the DNA double helix (Muller and Crothers 1968). This process, which stabilizes the intercalative interaction, appears to be crucial for cytotoxicity. There is also some evidence for the formation of an anionic free radical of dactinomycin which can be produced after reduction of the molecule with cytochrome P450 reductase and NADPH (Nakazawa et al 1981).

Although maximal cytotoxicity is noted in G_1 phase (Baserga et al 1965), the cytotoxic action is thought to be primarily cell cycle nonspecific. As anticipated, actively proliferating cells have generally been more sensitive than quiescent cells to the cytotoxic effects of the drug (Schwartz 1974, Valeriote et al 1973).

■ Availability and Storage

Dactinomycin is commercially available from Merck & Company, Inc, West Point, Pennsylvania, as a lyophilized, amorphous, yellow powder in vials containing 0.5 mg (500 µg) of drug with 20 mg of mannitol. The intact vials are stored at room temperature.

ANTITUMOR ACTIVITY OF DACTINOMYCIN IN HUMAN CANCER

Tumor Type	Regimen	Response Rate (%)
Wilms' tumor	Combined with surgery and radiotherapy	40–80
Embryonal rhabdomyosarcoma	Combined with surgery and radiotherapy	30
Trophoblastic carcinoma (choriocarcinoma)	Combined with methotrexate and other agents	50–70 (cure rate)
Malignant melanoma	Single and combination	35
Testicular tumors	Combined with other agents	20–60
Hodgkin's and non-Hodgkin's lymphomas	Single agent	40–50
African Kaposi's sarcoma	Combined with vincristine	70
Breast and colon cancer		<10
Head and neck, lung, kidney, and pancreatic cancer	Single agents	None

Data from Frei E III. The clinical use of actinomycin. Cancer Chemother Rep. 1974;58:49–54.

■ Preparation for Use, Stability, and Admixture

Initially, 1.1 mL of preservative-free Sterile Water for Injection, USP, is added to yield a final concentration of 0.5 mg/mL. The manufacturer states that the use of a preserved diluent may cause precipitation and should be avoided. The solution is gold colored and has been shown to be chemically stable for 2 to 5 months after reconstitution at room temperature. Any unused portion of the solution should be discarded after 24 hours to minimize possible bacterial growth. Rusmin et al (1977) have additionally shown that significant binding of drug occurs with micrometer nitrocellulose filter materials. Thus, filtration of dactinomycin solutions using standard filters should be avoided. Instead, stainless-steel filters may be used.

When dactinomycin is mixed with dacarbazine, no change in the ultraviolet spectrum of dactinomycin is noted. This implies compatibility (Horton and Stevens 1979). Dactinomycin at a 4 mg/mL concentration is also physically stable with ondansetron (1 mg/mL) for at least 4 hours (Trissel et al 1990).

■ Administration

Dactinomycin is administered intravenously by slow intravenous push, preferably into the tubing of a freely running intravenous solution. A 5- to 10-mL flush of D5W or normal saline is recommended both before and after dactinomycin administration to ensure venous patency and to flush any remaining drug from the tubing and proximal vein.

■ Special Precautions

Avoid extravasation. Dactinomycin is extremely damaging to soft tissue and will cause a severe local reaction if extravasation occurs (Frei 1974).

Dactinomycin is typically dosed in micrograms per kilogram or per square meter. Doses must be calculated and prepared carefully to prevent inadvertent overdosage of this drug. No specific antidote to overdosage is known, although hematopoietic colony-stimulating factors might be useful.

■ Dosage

Dactinomycin is commonly given in short "pulse" doses of 500 µg daily for up to 5 days in adults with solid tumors. Another common dosing regimen involves a single weekly 2-mg dose given for 3 consecutive weeks. In children with sarcoma, 15 µg/kg or 450 µg/m^2/d is given (up to a maximum of 500 µg). This is administered for up to 5 days and can be repeated every 3 to 8 weeks. Alternatively, 2.4 mg/m^2 in divided doses may be given over a 1-week period (Frei 1974). If necessary, such courses may be repeated at 2-week intervals provided toxic effects have resolved.

Benjamin et al (1976) have recommended a single dose of 2 mg/m^2 IV every 3 to 4 weeks for adult solid tumor therapy. This was based on experimental data demonstrating a relatively long biologic half-life for dactinomycin activity in animals (Galbraith and Mellett 1975). Similar prolonged effects following a short drug exposure have been observed in leukemic cells (Valeriote et al 1973). Indeed, several clinical studies have clearly documented equal efficacy and toxicity for single-dose regimens compared with 5-day dosing schedules (Blatt et al 1981, Petrilli and Morrow 1980, Petrilli et al 1987). In nonmetastatic gestational trophoblastic cancer, a single intravenous dose of 1.25 mg/m^2 every 14 days produced a 99% remission rate after four courses of therapy (Petrilli et al 1987). Compared with five divided doses of 0.5 mg/d, the single-dose method produced slightly greater total toxicity, primarily mild to moderate hematologic toxicity; however, severe myelosuppression was similar in both groups (Petrilli and Morrow 1980). When combined with dacarbazine (650 (mg/m^2) in melanoma, dactinomycin doses of 1 mg/m^2 every 3 to 4 weeks were active and well tolerated (Samson et al 1978).

In pediatric solid tumor patients, single-dose regimens of 60 µg/kg have occasionally been associated with severe hepato-veno-occlusive disease (Bjork et al 1975, Green et al 1990), and the National Wilms' Tumor Study group therefore recommends limiting single dactinomycin doses to 45 µg/kg (Green et al 1988).

■ Drug/Therapeutic Interactions

Dactinomycin has potent immunosuppressant activity and can inhibit the effectiveness of vaccinations given following drug administration. The drug also produces radiation "recall" damage to skin and soft tissues when given after ionizing radiation (see Side Effects and Toxicity). Additive hepatotoxicity may be produced when general anesthetics such as enflurane and halothane are administered after high-dose dactinomycin (Green et al 1990).

Dactinomycin produces complex interactions in vitro with heat. There is synergistic cytotoxicity when cancer cells are heated to 43°C and simultaneously exposed to dactinomycin (Donaldson et al 1978). In contrast, the application of heat *before* or *after* dactinomycin actually protects cells from cytotoxicity.

■ Pharmacokinetics

Tattersall et al (1975) have studied the pharmacokinetics of radiolabeled (^{3}H) dactinomycin in patients with malignant melanoma. In this study the drug appeared to be only minimally metabolized and was concentrated in nucleated cells. Thus, there was a greater distribution of drug into bone marrow compared with plasma. Drug penetration into the central nervous system was not observed. Urinary and fecal recovery of dactinomycin totaled only 15% each after 1 week and there was significant drug retention in lymphocytes and granulocytes. This may explain the prolonged terminal plasma half-life of 36 hours observed after single dactinomycin doses (Tattersall et al 1975). Pharmacodynamic studies in normal and leukemic cells show that cytotoxic effects in mice are maintained for at least 24 hours following a short drug exposure (Vietti and Valeriote 1971).

Animal studies have noted some hepatic metabolism and biliary excretion of dactinomycin (Weissbach et al 1966). In humans, however, there appears to be little metabolism as about 90% of the small fraction of drug excreted in the urine is collected as the intact molecule (Tattersall et al 1975). Some monolactone forms of dactinomycin are recovered in the urine. These phenoxazone cleavage products are inactive and can also be produced by incubating the drug with rat liver cells in vitro.

By use of a more specific radioimmunoassay, a much shorter dactinomycin half-life is described in both dogs (34 minutes) and humans (α = 0.78 minutes, β = 3.5 hours) (Brothman et al 1982). The reason for the discrepancy between these findings and those of Tattersall et al may relate to the different assays used. With the radiolabeling technique there is no discrimination between intact drug and radioactive metabolites which may be inactive.

■ Side Effects and Toxicity

Myelosuppression is the dose-limiting toxic effect of dactinomycin. The onset is usually within 7 to 10 days of dosing. All formed blood elements appear to be affected but the platelets and leukocytes are primarily depressed. There can be a relatively delayed nadir of about 3 weeks and the bone marrow typically appears hypocellular by 3 to 4 days. There is also some evidence of normal hematopoietic stem cell damage with this drug (Vietti and Valeriote 1971). Immunosuppression is another well-known effect of dactinomycin, and the drug has historically been used as an immunosuppressant in organ transplantations. Because of this effect, patients should not receive the drug before live virus vaccinations (such as vaccinia) or during an active viral infection because of the risk of developing more severe disease.

Severe gastrointestinal effects such as vomiting can occasionally constitute the acute dose-limiting toxic effect of the drug. Vomiting can last 4 to 20 hours but is well controlled by combination antiemetic regimens (Frei 1974). Mucositis with dactinomycin can also be severe. It is characterized by severe oral ulcerations and diarrhea in 30% of patients.

Reversible alopecia may occur with dactinomycin. A variety of other skin manifestations have been reported including acneiform changes, erythema, and hyperpigmentation (Moore et al 1958). Green et al (1978) noted the temporal concurrence of a maculopapular skin rash with the thrombocytopenic nadir of the drug.

Dactinomycin is similar to the anthracyclines in that it can interact with radiation skin damage to produce delayed radiation "recall" skin reactions (D'Angio et al 1959). Thus, previously irradiated or even irritated skin may become reddened and inflamed following drug administration. Frank necrosis has occasionally been reported. Oral ulcers may also develop following radiotherapy. These reactions may occur months after radiation therapy. Experimentally, radiotherapy given *after* dactinomycin does not produce this effect.

Extravasation of the drug can produce immediate pain and swelling and the drug is locally ulcerogenic in animal models (Henry and Marlow 1973). With clinical extravasations, indolent poor healing of necrotic ulcers characteristically occurs. Thus, every effort should be made to ensure venous patency during dactinomycin administration. In a rat paw model, dactinomycin produced dose-related inflammatory changes that could be partially blocked by indomethacin but not by aspirin or hydrocortisone (Giri et al 1975). Extravasation antidote studies in mice have demonstrated antidotal effects for topical cooling following dactinomycin extravasation (Buchanan et al 1985, Soble et al 1987). The efficacy of local antidotes has not been tested in well-controlled trials in humans.

Unexpected hepatotoxicity was described in children with Wilms' tumor (D'Angio 1987). Hepato-veno-occlusive toxicity manifested as elevated serum glutamic–oxalacetic transaminase (900–19,000 U/mL) and bilirubin (0.9–20.2 mg/dL) levels. In addition, ascites and liver enlargement also occurred with an onset within days of drug administration (Green et al 1990). A retrospective analysis from the National Wilms' Tumor Study Group has shown a significant dose- and schedule-dependent incidence of severe hepatotoxicity. The incidence was 14.3% with 60 µg/kg, 3.7% with 45 µg/kg, and 2.8% with five 15 µg/kg (Green et al 1990); however, other schedules also elicited a low incidence of severe hepatotoxicity (0.4%), which is higher than that observed in prior studies. Multiple factors were associated with these severe toxic reactions: (1) the administration of other hepatotoxic agents, especially halogenated inhalation anesthetics such as enflurane and halothane; (2) the use of the single-dose dactinomycin regimen over five daily doses; and (3) the administration of dactinomycin at 60 µg/kg (Green et al 1990). Similar hepatic toxic effects have also been seen with standard 5-day dactinomycin regimens in other trials with Wilms' tumor patients (Bjork et al 1985).

An inadvertent overdose of 3.3 mg/m^2 in a 17-year-old man produced a generalized convulsion, hyponatremia, hypokalemia, hypocalcemia, and hypomagnesemia (Choonara et al 1988). The patient subsequently developed generalized limb edema, intense erythema with desquamation and bullae, gastrointestinal ulceration with profuse diarrhea, mucositis, and febrile neutropenia. Fortunately, there was complete resolution of these effects within 3 weeks.

■ Special Applications

Dactinomycin has been investigationally administered by the isolated limb arterial perfusion technique (Creech et al 1959). The perfusion dose (up to 35–50 µg/kg) may be increased over those commonly given by the systemic route. Isolated perfusions of the upper extremities have usually been limited to a dose of 35 µg/kg. Greater dilution of the drug in 150–500 mL of physiologic solutions is required if this investigational route of administration is used. In dogs, dactinomycin given via the renal artery has been combined with simultaneous injection of degradable starch microspheres to transiently occlude an artery and enhance local drug disposition (Tuma et al 1982). In this study, arterial dactinomycin increased renal drug levels 6.4-fold over intravenous drug administration without starch and by 13- to 15-fold with the starch microspheres.

REFERENCES

Ansfield FJ, Korbitz BC, Davis HL Jr, et al. Triple drug therapy in testicular tumors. *Cancer.* 1969;**24**:442–446.

Baserga R, Estensen RD, Petersen RO. Inhibition of DNA synthesis in Ehrlich ascites cells by actinomycin D. II. The presynthetic block in the cell cycle. *Proc Natl Acad Sci USA.* 1965;**54**:1141–1148.

Benjamin RS, Hall SW, Burgess MA, et al. A pharmacokinetically based phase I–II study of single dose actinomycin D (NSC-3053). *Cancer Treat Rep.* 1976;**60**:289–291.

Bjork O, Eklof O, Willi U, Ahstrom L. Veno-occlusive disease and peliosis of the liver complicating the course of Wilms' tumor. *Acta Radiol Diagn.* 1985;**26**:589–597.

Blatt J, Trigg ME, Pizzo PA, Glaubiger D. Tolerance to single-dose dactinomycin in combination chemotherapy for solid tumors. *Cancer Treat Rep.* 1981;**65**:145–147.

Brockmann H. History and chemistry: Modification of the actinomycin molecule. *Cancer Chemother Rep Part 1.* 1974;**58**(1):9.

Brothman AR, Davis TP, Duffy JJ, Lindell TJ. Development of an antibody to actinomycin D and its application for the detection of serum levels by radioimmunoassay. *Cancer Res.* 1982;**42**:1184–1187.

Buchanan GR, Buchsbaum HR, O'Banion K, Gojer B. Extravasation of dactinomycin, vincristine, and cisplatin: Studies in an animal model. *Med Pediatr Oncol.* 1985;**3**:375–380.

Choonara IA, Kendall-Smith S, Bailey CC. Accidental actinomycin D overdosage in man, a case report. *Cancer Chemother Pharmacol.* 1988;**21**:173–174.

Creech O Jr, Krementz ET, Ryan RF, Reemtsma K, Elliot JL. Perfusion treatment of patients with cancer. *JAMA.* 1959;**171**:2069–2075.

D'Angio GJ. Unexpected toxicity encountered in the national Wilms' tumor study. *Cancer Treat Rep.* 1987;**71**(10):993.

D'Angio GJ, Farber S, Maddock CL. Potentiation of x-ray effects by actinomycin D. *Radiology.* 1959;**73**:175–177.

Donaldson SS, Gordon LF, Hahn GM. Protective effect of hyperthermia against the cytotoxicity of actinomycin D on Chinese hamster cells. *Cancer Treat Rep.* 1978;**62**:1489–1495.

Farber S. Chemotherapy in the treatment of leukemia and Wilm's tumor. *JAMA.* 1966;**198**:826–836.

Frei E III. The clinical use of actinomycin. *Cancer Chemother Rep.* 1974;**58**:49–54.

Galbraith WM, Mellett LB. Tissue disposition of ^{3}H-actinomycin D (NSC-3053) in the rat, monkey, and dog. *Cancer Chemother Rep.* 1975;**59**:1061–1069.

Giri SN, Rice S, Bacchetti P. Characteristic features of actinomycin D-induced paw inflammation of the rat. *Exp Mol Pathol.* 1975;**23**:367–378.

Goldin A, Johnson RK. Evaluation of actinomycins in experimental systems. *Cancer Chemother Rep Part I.* 1974;**58**(1):63–77.

Green DM, Finklestein JZ, Norkool P, D'Angio GJ. Severe hepatic toxicity after treatment with single-dose dactinomycin and vincristine. *Cancer.* 1988;**62**:270–273.

Green DM, Norkool P, Breslow NE, et al. Severe hepatic toxicity after treatment with vincristine and dactinomycin using single-dose or divided-dose schedules: A report from the National Wilms' Tumor Study. *J Clin Oncol.* 1990;**8**:1525–1530.

Green DM, Sallan SE, Krishan A. Actinomycin D in childhood acute lymphocytic leukemia. *Cancer Treat Rep.* 1978;**62**:829–831.

Grimm RA, Muss HB, White DR et al. Actinomycin D in the treatment of advanced breast cancer. *Cancer Chemother Pharmacol.* 1980;**4**:195–197.

Henry MC, Marlow M. Preclinical toxicologic study of actinomycin D (NSC-3053). *Cancer Chemother Rep Part 4.* 1973;(pt 3, No. 1):77–84.

Horton JK, Stevens MFG. Search for drug interactions between the antitumor agent DTIC and other cytotoxic drugs. *J Pharm Pharmacol.* 1979;**31**(suppl):64P.

Hustu HO, Pinkel D, Pratt CB. Treatment of clinically localized Ewing's sarcoma with radiotherapy and combination chemotherapy. *Cancer.* 1972;**30**:1522–1527.

Lewis JL Jr. Chemotherapy of gestational choriocarcinoma. *Cancer.* 1972;**30**:1517–1521.

Moore GE, DiPaolo JA, Kondo T. The chemotherapeutic effects and complications of actinomycin D in patients with advanced cancer. *Cancer.* 1958;**11**(6):1204–1214.

Muller W, Crothers DM. Studies of the binding of actinomycin and related compounds to DNA. *J Molec Biol.* 1968;**35**:251–290.

Nakazawa H, Chou F-TE, Andrews PA, Bachur NR. Chemical reduction of actinomycin D and phenoxazone analogues to free radicals. *J Organ Chem.* 1981;**46**(7):1493–1496.

Petrilli ES, Morrow CP. Actinomycin D toxicity in the treatment of trophoblastic disease. *Gynecol Oncol.* 1980;**9**:18–22.

Petrilli ES, Twiggs LB, Blessing JA, Teng NNH, Curry S. Single-dose actinomycin-D treatment for nonmetastatic gestational trophoblastic disease: A prospective phase II trial of the Gynecologic Oncology Group. *Cancer.* 1987;**60**:2173–2176.

Philips RS, Schwartz HS, Sternberg SS, Tan CTC. The toxicity of actinomycin D. *Ann NY Acad Sci.* 1970;**89**:348–360.

Reich E. Biochemistry of actinomycin. *Cancer Res.* 1963;**28**:1428.

Reyes EL, Talley RW. The hypocalcemic effects of actinomycin D and mithramycin. *Henry Ford Hosp Med J.* 1965;**62**:43–49.

Rusmin S, Welton S, DeLuca P, DeLuca PP. Effect of inline filtration on the potency of drugs administered intravenously. *Am J Hosp Pharm.* 1977;**34**:1071–1074.

Samson MK, Baker LH, Talley RW, Fraile RJ, McDonald B. Phase I–II study of intermittent bolus administraton of DTIC and actinomycin D in metastatic malignant melanoma. *Cancer Treat Rep.* 1978;**62**(8):1223–1225.

Schwartz HS. Some determinants of the therapeutic efficacy of actinomycin D (NSC-3053), Adriamycin (NSC-123127) and daunorubicin (NSC-83142). *Cancer Chemother Rep.* 1974;**58**:55–62.

Soble MJ, Dorr RT, Plezia P, Breckenridge S. Dose-dependent skin ulcers in mice treated with DNA binding antitumor antibiotics. *Cancer Chemother Pharmacol.* 1987;**20**:33–36.

Tattersall MHN, Sodegren JE, Sergupta SK, Trites DH, Modest EJ, Frei E. Pharmacokinetics of actinomycin D in patients with malignant melanoma. *Clin Pharmacol Ther.* 1975;**17**:701–708.

Trissell LA, Fulton B, Tramonte SM. Visual compatibility of ondansetron with chemotherapeutic agents, antibiotics, and other selected drugs during simulated Y-site injection (abstract #P-468R). In: *25th Annual ASHP Midyear Clinical Meetings and Exhibit, Las Vegas, Nevada.*

Tuma RF, Forsberg JO, Agerup B. Enhanced uptake of actinomycin D in the dog kidney by simultaneous injection of degradable starch microspheres into the renal artery. *Cancer.* 1982;**50**:1–5.

Valeriote F, Vietti T, Tolen S. Kinetics of the lethal effect of actinomycin D on normal and leukemic cells. *Cancer Res.* 1973;**33**:2658–2661.

Vietti T, Valeriote F. Actinomycin D: Kinetics of its lethal action on a transplantable leukemia. *J Natl Cancer Inst.* 1971;**46**:1177–1181.

Weissbach H, Redfield B, O'Connor T, Chirigos MA. Studies on the disposition of actinomycin D 3H in virus-infected and tumor-bearing mice. *Cancer Res.* 1966;**26**:1832–1838.

Woodruff HB, Waksman SA. The actinomycins—Historical background. *Ann NY Acad Sci.* 1960;**89**:287–298.

Daunorubicin HCl

■ Other Names

Daunomycin HCl; rubidomycin HCl; NSC-83142; Cerubidine® (Wyeth-Ayerst Laboratories).

■ Chemistry

Structure of daunorubicin HCl

Daunorubicin is an anthracycline analog of doxorubicin differing in the lack of a hydroxyl at the acetyl side chain of the 9-position on the D-ring in the aglycone (daunomycinone) portion of the molecule. Both molecules contain the same amino sugar, daunosamine, linked glycosidically to the number 7 carbon on the D-ring. Daunorubicin was originally isolated from *Streptomyces caeruleorubidus* by Rhone-Poulenc chemists in 1962. It was then known as rubidomycin. It was later isolated from cultures of *Streptomyces peucetius* by Farmitalin chemists and called daunomycin (Grein et al 1963). The complete chemical name is 7-(3-amino-2,3,6-trideoxy-L-lyxohexosyloxy)-9-acetyl-7,8,9,10-tetrahydro-6,9,11-trihydroxy-4-methoxy-5,12-naphthacenequinone hydrochloride. The molecular weight is 563.99 and the molecular formula $C_{27}H_{29}NO_{10}HCl$. The commercial hydrochloride salt of daunorubicin is hygroscopic and is soluble in water and slightly soluble in alcohol. The pK_a of the nitrogen on the amino group in daunosamine is 10.3. The glycosidic bond is unstable in solutions with a pH value above 8. Decomposition is noted by a color change from the normal red/orange to purple (Trissell 1988) (see Preparation for Use, Stability, and Admixture).

■ Antitumor Activity

Daunorubicin originally produced significant antitumor activity in a variety of experimental models including L-1210 leukemia and Walker 256 carcinosarcoma in vivo and in Hela cells in vitro (DiMarco et al 1964). In human cancer, the drug is approved in the United States for the treatment of acute non-lymphocytic leukemia (ANLL) in adults (Lippman et al 1972). It is typically combined with other cytotoxic agents such cytarabine, prednisone, and a thiopurine (eg, 6-mercaptopurine and 6-thioguanine) (Gale 1979, Bloomfield 1980). Complete remission rates of 50 to 80% are common with such regimens, although more than one induction course may be needed in up to 33% of patients (Wiernik et al 1976, Glucksberg et al 1975). The drug is similar to doxorubicin at inducing complete remissions in ANLL when both anthracyclines are used in combination with cytarabine infusions (Yates et al 1982). Daunorubicin is active in several subtypes of ANLL. For example, it is active in erythroleukemia, and in combination with other agents, response rates up to 78% have have reported (Bloomfield et al 1974). Unfortunately, the drug is not active in nor does it prevent meningeal leukemia (Jones et al 1971). This is probably due to poor penetration into the CNS central nervous system (see Pharmacokinetics).

Acute lymphocytic leukemia in adults and children will also respond to combination regimens containing daunorubicin (Matthews and Colebatch 1972, Sallan et al 1978, Jones et al 1971, Holton et al 1969). Daunorubicin is highly indicated for patients who relapse after induction with a vincristine/prednisone combination or have poor prognostic features on initial presentation (Reaman et al 1980).

Daunorubicin has also shown limited activity in adult and pediatric solid tumors as reviewed by Von Hoff (1984) (see respective tables on page 356). In solid tumors such as soft tissue sarcoma, lymphoma, and small cell lung cancer, response rates to daunorubicin are lower than those obtained with doxorubicin (Von Hoff 1984). Furthermore, daunorubicin was not active in several diseases known to be sensitive to doxorubicin. These include Kaposi's sarcoma, ovarian cancer, and, most notably, breast cancer (see table on top of page 356). Similar low response rates are observed in pediatric solid tumors wherein Ewing's sarcoma and rhabdomyosarcoma were the only malignancies sensitive to single-agent daunorubicin.

■ Mechanism of Action

As do the other anthracyclines, daunorubicin produces a number of cellular lesions which may con-

SENSITIVITY OF ADULT SOLID TUMORS TO SINGLE-AGENT DAUNORUBICIN*

Responsive Tumors (Number of Patients)	% Response	Nonresponsive Tumors <15% Response Rate (Number of Patients Evaluated)
Soft tissue sarcomas (54)	20	Non-small cell lung cancer (10)
Hodgkin's lymphoma (64)	20	Colon cancer (66)
Small cell lung cancer (4)	25	Melanoma (9)
Bladder cancer (intravesical) (4)	50	Testicular cancer (9)
Multiple myeloma (2)	50	Renal cell carcinoma (8)
Prostate (2)	50	Head and neck cancer (intraarterial) (7)
Choriocarcinoma (1)	100	Breast cancer (4)
Neuroblastoma (1)	100	Mesothelioma (2)
		Kaposi's sarcoma (2)
		Ovary (2)
		Stomach (2)
		Wilms' tumor (1)
		Hepatoma (1)
		Ewing's sarcoma (1)

*Responsive = complete response + partial response rate ≥ 15% of evaluable patients.
Data from Von Hoff D. Use of daunorubicin in patients with solid tumors. Semin Oncol. 1984;11(4,suppl 3):23–27.

tribute to the antitumor effects of the drug. Most of these effects relate to DNA-based damage from both direct and indirect mechanisms. Perhaps best studied is the capability of the agent to intercalate the planar aglycone between stacked DNA base pairs. This noncovalent association uses pi electrons in the tetracyclic daunomycinone moiety to form pi–pi-type bonds with DNA bases above and below the plane of the intercalated anthracycline (Kersten et al 1966, Pigram et al 1972). In addition, the amino sugar provides an electrostatic type of bond to DNA (Calendi et al 1965). Three-dimensional DNA modeling suggests that the C-3 portion of the amino sugar moiety rests in the minor groove of DNA. This enables the ionized amino group to interact with a negatively charged phosphate proximal to the intercalation site (Pigram et al 1972). This electrostatic type of bond may thereby help to "stabilize" the intercalated chromophore in DNA.

Daunomycin inhibits synthesis of both DNA and RNA (Dimarco 1975, Dano et al 1972, Meriwether and Bachur 1972). In Ehrlich ascites cells RNA synthesis was slightly more sensitive than DNA to the inhibiting effect of daunomycin. Similar effects have been observed in tumor cells treated in vivo (Theologides et al 1968, Hartmann et al 1964). In addition, daunomycin has been observed to directly inhibit both DNA-dependent RNA polymerase and DNA polymerase (Ward et al 1965).

Cellular DNA may also be indirectly damaged by daunomycin-induced interference with the ligase activity of DNA topoisomerase II (Tewey et al 1984). This enzyme normally binds covalently to

SENSITIVITY OF PEDIATRIC SOLID TUMORS TO SINGLE-AGENT DAUNORUBICIN*

Responsive Tumors (Number Evaluable)	% Response	Nonresponsive Tumors (Number Evaluable)
Rhabdomyosarcoma (24)	21	Neuroblastoma (119)
Letterer–Siwe disease (1)	100	Osteogenic sarcoma (8)
Testicular cancer (1)	100	Wilms' tumor (8)
Ewing's sarcoma (16)	19	Teratoma (1)
		Medulloblastoma (1)
		Lymphomas
		Hodgkin's (3)
		Non-Hodgkins (8)
		Unspecified (3)

*Responsive = complete response + partial response rate ≥ 15% of evaluable patients.
Data from Von Hoff D. Use of daunorubicin in patients with solid tumors. Semin Oncol. 1984;11(4,suppl 3):23–27.

DNA and induces double-strand breaks to facilitate strand passage (knotting or unknotting of supercoiled DNA). The enzyme then reseals the breaks. This is followed by detachment of the enzyme from DNA (Lock and Ross 1987). Drugs such as daunomycin interfere with the latter operations of topoisomerase II, leading to stabilization of the "cleavable complex" between the enzyme and DNA. This can be noted experimentally by the production of protein-associated DNA double strand breaks under denaturing (alkaline) conditions. Overall, however, the cytotoxic effect of daunomycin is maximal but not exclusively limited to S phase (Cheng and Zee-Cheng 1972, Kim et al 1968). Thus, daunomycin is a cell cycle nonspecific agent (Stryckmans et al 1973).

Another toxic effect of daunomycin involves the generation of oxygen free radicals. This is believed to result from redox cycling of the quinone moiety on the C-ring of the aglycone (Bender et al 1978). This activity appears to be dependent on the availability of molecular oxygen, a suitable reducing environment or enzyme (like cytochrome P450 reductase), and certain divalent metals, especially iron. The oxygen free radical cascade postulated from such a reduction of the quinone to the semiquinone is believed to produce superoxide and hydroxyl radicals, which can act to peroxide lipids and produce diverse damage to cellular membranes. Thus, daunomycin has been shown to increase red blood cell membrane fragility (Schioppocassi and Schwartz 1977). This effect could be blocked by the divalent chelator ethylenediaminetetraacetic acid (EDTA) (Schioppocassi and Schwartz 1977) and by the related intracellular chelating compounds razoxane (ICRF-159) and ICRF-187. It is believed that divalent metals can bind with anthracyclines to form complexes capable of redox cycling which is otherwise unfavored. This type of damage may also explain anthracycline cardiotoxicity, as heart cells are relatively deficient in antioxidant defenses such as reduced thiols (glutathione) as well as the free radical scavenging enzymes superoxide dismutase (SOD) and catalase (Doroshow et al 1980). The ability of free radical scavengers and antioxidants such as vitamin E and exogenous thiols to block daunomycin-induced membrane damage and experimental cardiac damage lends support to this hypothesis. In the heart, anthracyclines may also block the uptake of adenine, amino acids, and glucose (Reese et al 1987) and selectively interrupt the formation of high-energy phosphates such as ATP (Gosalvez et al 1979). Digoxin has been reported to reverse this inhibition in vitro (Burns and Dow 1980).

In addition to these direct cytotoxic effects toward tumor cells, daunorubicin also has antibacterial activity and immunosuppressive effects. It is also both carcinogenic and teratogenic in experimental animal models (Bender et al 1978).

■ Availability and Storage

Daunorubicin (Cerubidine®) is commercially available from Wyeth-Ayerst Laboratories, Philadelphia, Pennsylvania, in butyl rubber-stoppered glass vials which contain 20 mg of base daunomycin activity (21.4 mg of the hydrochloride salt form) and 100 mg of mannitol. These vials may be stored at room temperature but should be protected from light.

■ Preparation for Use, Stability, and Admixture

Each 20-mg vial can be reconstituted with 4 mL of Sterile Water for Injection, USP, to yield a 5 mg/mL red solution. According to Wyeth-Ayerst Laboratories this solution is reportedly stable for at least 24 hours at room temperature and 48 hours under refrigeration. Stability is highly dependent on the pH of the solution, with decomposition observed at pH values above 8. There is progressively enhanced stability at lower pH values from 7.4 to 4.5 (Poochikian et al 1981). Daunorubicin should be protected from fluorescent light to decrease photoinactivation noted after storage in solution for several days. It is especially significant with irradiation at 366 nm (Williams and Tritton 1981). At very low concentrations ($< 5 \times 10^{-8}$ M), daunorubicin may also self-associate to form dimers and possibly "n"-mers at higher concentrations (Barthelemy-Clavey et al 1974). The clinical significance of this finding is unclear.

Daunorubicin is physically compatible with 5% Dextrose, Normosol-R®, lactated Ringer's injection, and 0.9% sodium chloride; stability times (< 10% decomposition) at room temperature range from at least 24 hours (Poochikian et al 1981) to 4 weeks if stored in the dark (Beijnen et al 1985). The table on page 358 summarizes the physical compatibility of daunorubicin with other drug admixtures and with different infusion system components.

■ Administration

For most applications, daunorubicin should be administered as a short intravenous "push" infusion over 1 to 5 minutes into a recently established, unquestionably patent intravenous site. This can be ac-

PHYSICAL COMPATIBILITY OF DAUNORUBICIN ADMIXTURES WITH OTHER DRUGS AND INTRAVENOUS ADMINISTRATION DEVICES

Compatible (Reference)	Incompatible (Reference)
Cytarabine*	Aluminum needles cause solution darkening (Ogawa et al 1985)
Hydrocortisone*	Dexamethasone phosphate (Dorr 1979)
Sodium succinate (Trissel 1988)	Heparin sodium (Trissel 1988)
Ondansetron (Trissel 1988)	
Polyvinyl chloride plastic (no adsorption)*	
Nitrocellulose filters (no adsorption)*	

*Author's unpublished observations using high-performance liquid chromatography assay for daunorubicin (1 mg/mL over 24 hours in saline or dextrose).

complished by injection into the tubing of a free-flowing intravenous infusion (one not previously used for blood or other drug administration). The drug has also been given as a short intravenous infusion in 100 mL normal saline or D5W over 15 to 30 minutes. Because the drug can cause severe deep tissue damage if extravasated, a constantly attended slow intravenous injection over 2 to 3 minutes is generally recommended. During this procedure, the patient should be instructed to report immediately any change in sensation, such as stinging, which may be a symptom of drug extravasation. In any case, a 5- to 10-mL flush of intravenous solution is recommended both before and after drug administration to test vein patency and flush any remaining drug from the tubing and the local site.

■ Dosage

For adult ANLL remission induction therapy the daunorubicin dose is 45 to 60 mg/m^2/d × 3 consecutive days when used in combination with other agents such as prednisone, vincristine, and cytarabine. For remission induction therapy in pediatric acute lymphocytic leukemia, the dose of daunorubicin is 25 mg/m^2 on day 1 every week in combination with oral prednisone and vincristine intravenous. The manufacturer also recommends that in children under 2 years or smaller than 0.5 m^2 in body surface area, daunorubicin doses should be based on weight (mg/kg).

Doses used in solid tumor therapy have ranged from 15 to 30 mg/m^2/d × 5. Of interest, in one randomized clinical trial of childhood solid tumors there was no significant difference between these two doses (15 and 30 mg/m^2/d × 5) (Evans et al 1974). As a single intravenous bolus in solid tumors, doses of 80 to 120 mg/m^2 have also been administered (Alberts et al 1971). In contrast, leukemic patients, given a single intravenous bolus dose of 180 mg/m^2 experienced significant mortality (42%) during induction therapy (Greene et al 1972). This high dose is clearly contraindicated, and overall, the consecutive day dosing schedules are recommended over a single large intravenous bolus dose.

In patients with elevated serum bilirubin or reduced renal function, dose reductions are recommended (see next table). These dose reductions have not been prospectively evaluated.

■ Drug Interactions

Daunorubicin is physically incompatible with heparin sodium and with dexamethasone phosphate when directly admixed (see physical compatibility table).

In animal models, daunorubicin has decreased the effectiveness of methotrexate by decreasing the cellular uptake of methotrexate when given just before or concurrently (Zager et al 1973). Huffman et al (1972), though, have stated that because of a large degree of cytoplasmic metabolism, drug interactions with microsomal enzymes should not be as significant with daunorubicin as with doxorubicin (see *Doxorubicin* for specific examples).

Because daunorubicin is affected by the multidrug resistance (MDR) phenomenon (Dano 1973) it has been evaluated with a variety of drugs used to reverse tumor cell resistance. These agents are believed to alter the function of the 180,000-molecular-weight membrane protein also known as the P-glycoprotein. This protein acts as an active (energy-dependent) efflux pump for diverse natural product-based antitumor agents. Drugs that have been shown to modulate experimental daunorubicin MDR include amphotericin B (Riggs 1984), verapamil (Willingham et al 1987, Slater et al 1982, Yanovich and Preston 1984, Kessel and Wilberding 1985a), tiapamil (Kessel and Wilberding 1985b), and perhexilene maleate (Kessel and Wilberding 1985a). Clinical trials with some of these modulators are currently in progress.

DAUNORUBICIN DOSE ADJUSTMENTS BASED ON BILIRUBIN OR SERUM CREATININE

Serum Bilirubin (mg/dL)	Serum Creatinine (mg/dL)	Fraction of Recommended Dose to Administer
1.2–3.0	<3.0	3/4
>3.0	<3.0	1/2
<1.2	>3.0	1/2

Data from Cerubidine® Package Insert, Wyeth-Ayerst Laboratories, 1980.

Besides interactions with MDR-positive tumor cells, some modulators may also alter daunorubicin toxicity in normal host tissues. For example, one study has described slower elimination of daunorubicin from the plasma when verapamil is administered to rats (Nooter et al 1987). There was also two- to three-fold greater daunorubicin accumulation in the heart, liver, and lungs following verapamil therapy. Whether verapamil similarly enhances daunorubicin toxicity in humans is unknown.

There is experimental evidence that iron chelating agents like ICRF-159 and ICRF-187 can block some of the cardiotoxic effects of anthracyclines such as daunorubicin (Wang et al 1981, Giuliani et al 1981). This has already been clinically confirmed with doxorubicin in women with advanced breast cancer (Speyer et al 1988). This interaction appears to be the result of decomplexation of Fe(II)–anthracycline complexes which are believed to mediate myocyte damage via the generation of oxygen free radicals (Herman and Ferrans 1987). Studies have shown that anthracycline heart toxicity is selectively reduced and antitumor efficacy is maintained both experimentally (Woodman et al 1975) and clinically (Speyer et al 1988).

■ Pharmacokinetics

Daunorubicin has pharmacokinetic patterns similar to those of doxorubicin. Both drugs have long terminal plasma half-lives because of extensive tissue binding. Hepatobiliary secretion into feces is the predominant route of elimination of both parent drug and hydroxylated metabolites. The table on page 360 summarizes the pharmacokinetic parameters for daunorubicin disposition in adult cancer patients. These findings show that the majority of plasma anthracycline exposure is not to the parent drug but to the 13-hydroxylated metabolite, daunorubicinol. This metabolite is formed by a ubiquitous cytosolic aldo/keto reductase enzyme (Bachur 1971). Daunorubicinol has about one tenth of the cytotoxic activity of the parent in human ovarian cancer cells (Ozols et al 1980) and in human bone marrow stem cells (Dessypris et al 1986). It also has some in vitro activity against human leukemic cells in vitro (Beran et al 1979, Yesair et al 1980); however, clinical studies in human cancer patients showed little evidence of significant or improved antitumor activity for daunorubicinol compared with the parent molecule (Chauvergne et al 1976).

Both daunorubicin and daunorubicinol are excreted into the urine in small amounts. This averages about 13 to 15% of a dose for daunorubicin (Alberts et al 1971) and about 3% of a dose for daunorubicinol (Takanashi and Bachur 1975). About 2% of a dose is excreted in the urine as conjugates to sulfate and glucuronide (Takanashi and Bachur 1975). Other metabolites that can be recovered in the urine in small amounts include the 7-deoxy daunorubicin and daunorubicinol aglycones, and demethyldeoxyaglycone, and conjugates of each of these with sulfate or glucuronide.

Microsomal cytochrome P450 reductase metabolism of daunorubicin is involved in the glycosidase reactions that form the various aglycones. Some unspeciated glycosidic metabolites are also formed by another reaction pathway. Both reactions use NADPH as a cofactor (Bachur and Cradock 1971). These reactions are highly dependent on molecular oxygen but are only weakly blocked by classic microsomal enzyme inhibitors such as SKF-525A and carbon monoxide (Bachur and Gee 1976).

There are some clinical data to suggest that the rate of formation of daunorubicinol in leukemic myeloblasts correlates with responses in ANLL. In this regard, patients with elevated daunorubicin reductase activity in blast cells compared with normal cells had a greater likelihood of obtaining a remission (Huffman et al 1972, Greene et al 1972); however, the higher enzyme ratios in responders in the latter high-dose study may have involved a statistical artifact due to a high mortality rate of 43% in the patients with low ratios of tumor/normal cell re-

PHARMACOKINETICS OF DAUNORUBICIN IN ADULT CANCER PATIENTS

Anthracycline Species	Daunorubicin Dose (mg/m²)	Elimination Half-Life (h)	AUC (μM · h)
Daunorubicin	75*	20.6	1.97
Total fluorescent species	—	29.3	15.95
Daunorubicinol	—	27.9	6.07
Metabolite D5†	—	23.1	2.23
Total fluorescence	80	—	9.2
Total fluorescence	120	—	13.9
Total fluorescence	180	—	38.4
Daunorubicin	—	19.8	9.3
Daunorubicinol	—	39.7	21.8

*Daunorubicin combined with cytarabine, 6-thioguanine, and pyrimethamine (Wiernik et al 1976); all other doses used single-agent daunorubicin.
†D5 is a daunorubicin aglycone identified by Huffman et al 1972.
Data from Riggs CE Jr. Clinical pharmacology of daunorubicin in patients with actue leukemia. Semin Oncol. 1984;11(4,suppl 3):2–11.

ductase activity (Greene et al 1972). Daunorubicinol is also the only discernible metabolite observed in human myeloblasts of leukemic or normal bone marrow origin. Both cell types convert about 5 to 10% of intracellular daunorubicin to daunorubicinol over a 24-hour incubation period (DeGregorio et al 1982). There does not appear to be a correlation between daunorubicin concentrations in the plasma and bone marrow (Kokenberg et al 1988). There was a positive correlation between drug concentrations in the white blood cells and in nucleated bone marrow cells and an inverse correlation between drug levels in white blood cells and the number of peripheral blast cells at diagnosis. This suggests that the achievement of effective drug levels in peripheral leukemic cells is a function of total tumor cell burden (Kokenberg et al 1988).

Drug distribution studies from autopsy tissues taken 24 hours after drug injection showed that the liver contains about 25% of the total dose as both daunorubicin and metabolites (Alberts et al 1971); however, the highest concentrations of drug per gram of tissue were found in the kidneys. In another high-dose study, the heart was found to contain the highest concentration of aglycone metabolites (Greene et al 1972).

One anomaly with high doses of 180 mg/m² given as a single agent was that plasma anthracycline fluorescence appeared to increase 4 to 12 hours after injection (Greene et al 1972). This could be the result of enterohepatic recirculation. The levels then began to fall with the typical elimination half-life of 20 to 30 hours. Of interest, a similar early plasma accumulation phase is also noted with a lower 75 mg/m² daunorubicin dose given in combination with 6-thioguanine, pyrimethamine, and cytosine arabinoside (Wiernik et al 1976). This produced an AUC for daunorubicin greater than that obtained from a higher daunorubicin dose of 120 mg/m² given as a single agent (Riggs 1984). One possible explanation for the effect of other drugs on daunomycin disposition may involve altered hepatic biotransformation of the agent.

■ Side Effects and Toxicity

Myelosuppression. Hematologic suppression is the major toxic effect of daunorubicin. Leukocyte and platelet nadirs occur 10 to 14 days following drug administration (Jones et al 1971, Boiron et al 1969). Full recovery is usually achieved within 3 weeks of administration. The myelotoxic effects are enhanced when other myelosuppressive drugs are given and/or in patients with preexisting poor bone marrow reserve. In leukemic patients, daunorubicin is routinely associated with septic fever and chills as a result of myelosuppression, 5 to 10 days after administration; however, the drug has also rarely produced transient fever and chills during or shortly after infusion (Jones et al 1971; Greene et al 1972, Wiernik and Serpick 1972). One case of fulminant hyperpyrexia has also been described (Ma and Isbister 1980). Also, because of potential transient hyperuricemia, as a result of massive cell lysis, all leukemic patients should receive prophylactic allopurinol to prevent acute urate nephropathy.

Gastrointestinal Effects. Gastrointestinal effects include stomatitis, which is typically mild with initial courses. Subsequent remission induction courses or the use of prolonged daunorubicin infusions may increase the duration and severity of the mucositis. The typical onset of mucositis involves initial erythema and burning of the oral mucosa followed by ulceration in 2 to 3 days.

Nausea and vomiting with daunorubicin are usually of only mild to moderate intensity and are well managed with prophylactic antiemetics. These effects rarely persist beyond 24 to 48 hours. Diarrhea is occasionally noted but is rarely, if ever, dose limiting (Boiron et al 1969).

Dermatologic Effects. Daunorubicin causes a significant degree of alopecia in most patients. This involves all body hair areas including the scalp, pubic, and axillary sites. The drug has also caused hyperpigmented bands in the nail beds in some patients (Demarinis et al 1978). Other rare dermatologic side effects include contact dermatitis (Reich and Bachur 1975), a generalized rash, and urticaria (Freeman 1970). The last complication can be associated with local allergic reactions caused by histamine release from mast cells along the vein used for infusion. As do the other anthracyclines, daunorubicin can reactivate skin damage from prior radiotherapy. This radiation recall effect is temporally dependent on the sequence of drug following radiotherapy by 2 to 6 weeks.

Hepatorenal Toxicity. Daunorubicin usually does not produce specific toxic effects in the kidney or liver; however, transient elevations in serum bilirubin are common following daunorubicin induction therapy in leukemia (Katz and Cassileth 1977). Other hepatic enzymes that may be concomitantly elevated include serum glutamic–oxalacetic transaminase and alkaline phosphatase (Menard et al 1980, Weil et al 1973). Drug elimination is impaired in patients with hepatobiliary dysfunction and doses therein must be reduced significantly to prevent severe, life-threatening toxicity (see Dosage). Daunorubicin also imparts a red color to the urine as a result of urinary excretion of up to 15% of a dose. This does not represent toxicity and should be explained to patients.

Extravasation. Extravasation of daunorubicin can lead to painful soft tissue ulcers which heal poorly if at all (Wiernik and Serpick 1972; Bender et al 1978). Surgical excision of evolving necrotic lesions is recommended to prevent progressive ulceration into adjacent tissues. A variety of potential local antidotes have also been evaluated to treat daunorubicin extravasations. Ineffective antidotes include heparin, hydrocortisone, sodium bicarbonate, hyaluronidase, and saline. Topical demethyl-sulfoxide (DMSO) was partially effective in an animal model (Soble et al 1987) and has shown clinical utility with extravasations of the close congener, doxorubicin (Olver et al 1988). The recommended investigational regimen calls for 1.5 mL of DMSO to the site every 6 hours for 14 days. The DMSO should be allowed to air-dry and should never be injected into the site (see Chapter 6).

Cardiotoxicity. Cardiotoxicity is a major risk with daunorubicin. It manifests as a total dose-dependent congestive heart failure characterized by fatigue, dyspnea on exertion, and various arrhythmias. Electrocardiographic findings indicate that there are two types of cardiac effects: early transient arrhythmias and electrocardiographic changes and subsequent total-dose-related changes. Early cardiac effects may occur during or immediately after infusion. These effects include ST-T wave changes, a low-voltage QRS complex, and flattened T waves (Halazun et al 1974). Several types of anthracycline arrhythmias have also been described including sinus tachycaria, heart block, and premature ventricular contractions (Bristow et al 1978a). Most of these arrhythmias are transient, non-dose related, and relatively nonserious; however, a few cases of an early pericarditis–myocarditis syndrome have been noted in a few patients (Bristow et al 1978b).

The incidence of a congestive cardiomyopathy from daunomycin is dose related (see table on page 362). Thus, it is seen rarely after only a few doses are given (Starkebaum and Durack 1975, Ipoliti et al 1976). With increasing doses, the incidence rises proportionately (Von Hoff et al 1977). There is also evidence that children and infants may be more susceptible to daunorubicin-induced congestive heart failure (Von Hoff et al 1977, Mosijczuk et al 1979). Recently, late cardiac effects from anthracycline therapy have been described in survivors of childhood leukemia (Lipshultz et al 1991). The official (package insert) total dose limitation calls for halting therapy after 550 mg/m^2 has been administered. This dose correlates to a 1 to 2% incidence of congestive heart failure (Von Hoff et al 1977); however, higher total doses have occasionally been administered without cardiotoxicity. This may be facilitated by the administration of daunorubicin as a continuous infusion over 3 to 4 days but confirmatory clinical data are not yet available.

The cardiomyopathy from daunorubicin is treatable by salt restriction, diuretics, and digitalis; however, the condition is usually permanent and has been noted to have a very long latency period in

INCIDENCE OF DAUNORUBICIN-INDUCED CONGESTIVE HEART FAILURE (CHF) ACCORDING TO TOTAL CUMULATIVE DOSES

Total Dose (mg/m^2)	% Incidence (Approx) CHF Development
550	1–2
800	5
950	10
1100	20
1200	30
1400	≥60

*Retrospective analysis of 110 cases (includes adults and children). Data from Von Hoff DD, Rozencweig M, Layard M, et al. Daunomycin-induced cardiotoxicity in children and adults. Am J Med. 1977;62:200–208.

some pediatric patients (Gilladoga et al 1976). If prior radiotherapy ports have involved the heart, total daunorubicin doses should be 400 to 450 mg/m^2 (Bristow et al 1978a). Similarly, patients with preexisting heart disease or prior anthracycline therapy are at increased risk of cardiotoxic effects and total doses should be lowered accordingly. Prospective monitoring should include radionuclide measures of left ventricular ejection fractions, with therapy halted after a 10 to 20% decrement from baseline is registered. Endomyocardial biopsies may provide a more definitive histopathologic endpoint for dosing patients at higher cumulative dose limits.

REFERENCES

Alberts DS, Bachur NR, Holtzman JL. The pharmacokinetics of daunomycin in man. *Clin Pharmacol Ther.* 1971;**12**:96–104.

Bachur NR. Daunorubicinol, a major metabolite of daunorubicin: Isolation from human urine and enzymatic reactions. *J Pharmacol Exp Ther.* 1971;**177**:573–578.

Bachur NR, Cradock JC. Daunomycin metabolism in rat tissue slices. *J Pharmacol Exp Ther.* 1971;**175**:331–337.

Bachur NR, Gee M. Microsomal reductive glycosidase. *J Pharmacol Exp Ther.* 1976;**197**:681–686.

Barthelemy-Clavey V, Maurizot J-C, Dimicoli J-L, Sicard P. Self-association of daunorubicin. *FEBS Lett.* 1974;**46**(1):5–10.

Beijnen JH, Rosing H, deVries PA, et al. Stability of anthracycline antitumor agents in infusion fluids. *J Parenter Sci Technol.* 1985;**39**(Nov–Dec):220–222.

Bender RA, Zwelling LA, Doroshow JH, et al. Antineoplastic drugs: Clinical pharmacology and therapeutic use. *Drugs.* 1978;**16**:46–87.

Beran M, Andersson B, Eksborg S, Ehrsson H. Comparative studies on the in vitro killing of human normal and leukemic clonogenic cells (CFUC) by daunorubicin, daunorubicinol and daunorubicin–DNA complex. *Cancer Chemother Pharmacol.* 1979;**2**:19–24.

Bloomfield CD. Treatment of adult acute nonlymphocytic leukemia (editorial). *Ann Intern Med.* 1980;**93**(I):133–135.

Bloomfield CD, Brunning RD, Kennedy BJ. Daunorubicin–prednisone treatment of erythroleukemia. *Ann Intern Med.* 1974;**81**:746–750.

Boiron M, Jacquillat C, Weil M, et al. Daunorubicin in the treatment of acute myelocytic leukemia. *Lancet.* 1969;**1**:330–333.

Bristow MR, Mason JW, Billingham ME, et al. Doxorubicin cardiomyopathy: Evaluation by phonocardiography, endomyocardial biopsy, and cardiac catheterization. *Ann Intern Med.* 1978a;**88**:168–175.

Bristow MR, Thompson PD, Martin PR, et al. Early anthracycline cardiotoxicity. *Am J Med.* 1978b;**65**:823–832.

Burns JH, Dow JW. Daunorubicin-induced myocardial failure: Reversal by digoxin of an inability to use ATP for contraction. *J Mol Cell Cardiol.* **12**:95–108.

Calendi E, DiMarco A, Reggiani M, et al. On physicochemical interactions between daunomycin and nucleic acids. *Biochim Biophys Acta.* 1965;**103**:25–49.

Chauvergne J, Carton M, Berlie J, et al. Essau de chimotherapie anticancereuse par la duborimycine. Analyse de 151 observations. *Bull Cancer.* 1976;**63**:41–58.

Cheng CC, Zee-Cheng KY. Some antineoplastic antibiotics. *J Pharm Sci.* 1972;**61**:485–501.

Dano K. Active outward transport of daunomycin in resistant Ehrlich ascites tumor cells. *Biochim Biophys Acta.* 1973;**323**:466–483.

Dano K, Frederiksen S, Hellung-Larsen P. Inhibition of DNA and RNA synthesis by daunorubicin in sensitive and resistant Ehrlich ascites tumor cells in vitro. *Cancer Res.* 1972;**32**:1307–1314.

DeGregorio MW, Carrera CJ, Klock JC. Uptake of free and DNA-bound daunorubicin and doxorubicin into human leukemic cells. *Cancer Chemother Pharmacol.* 1982;**10**:29–32.

Demarinis M, Hendricks A, Stoltzner G. Nail pigmentation with daunorubicin therapy. *Ann Intern Med.* 1978;**89**:516–517.

Dessypris EN, Brenner DE, Hande KR. Toxicity of doxorubicin metabolites to human marrow erythroid and myeloid progenitors in vitro. *Cancer Treat Rep.* 1986;**70**:487–490.

DiMarco A. Adriamycin (NSC-123127): Mode and mechanism of action. *Cancer Chemother Rep.* 1975;**6**:91–106.

DiMarco A, Gaetani M, Davigotti L, et al. Daunomycin: A new antibiotic with antitumor activity. *Cancer Chemother Rep.* 1964;**38**:31–38.

Doroshow JH, Locker GY, Myers CE, et al. Enzymatic defenses of the mouse heart against reactive oxygen metabolites: Alterations produced by doxorubicin. *J Clin Invest.* 1980;**65**:128–135.

Dorr RT. Incompatibilities with parenteral anticancer drugs. *Am J IV Ther.* 1979;6(Feb–Mar):42, 45, 46, 52.

Evans AE, Baehner RL, Chard RL Jr, et al. Comparison of daunorubicin (NSC-83142) with Adriamycin (NSC-123127) in the treatment of late stage childhood solid tumors. *Cancer Chemother Rep.* 1974;58:671–676.

Freeman AI. Allergic reaction to daunomycin (NSC-82151). *Cancer Chemother Rep.* 1970;54:475–476.

Gale RP. Advances in the treatment of acute myelogenous leukemia. *N Engl J Med.* 1979;300:1189–1199.

Gilladoga AC, Manuel C, Tan CTC, et al. The cardiotoxicity of Adriamycin and daunomycin in children. *Cancer.* 1976;37(suppl):1070–1078.

Giuliani F, Casazza AM, Di Marco A, Savi G. Studies in mice treated with ICRF-159 combined with daunorubicin or doxorubicin. *Cancer Treat Rep.* 1981;65:267–276.

Glucksberg H, Buckner CD, Fefer A, et al. Combination chemotherapy for acute nonlymphoblastic leukemia in adults. *Cancer Chemother Rep.* 1975;59(6):1131–1137.

Gosalvez M, van Rossum GD, Blanco MF, et al. Inhibition of sodium–potassium-activated adenosine 5′-triphosphatase and ion transport by Adriamycin. *Cancer Res.* 1979;39:257–261.

Greene W, Huffman D, Wiernik PH, et al. High-dose daunorubicin therapy for acute nonlymphocytic leukemia. *Cancer.* 1972;30:1419–1427.

Grein A, Spalla C, DiMarco A. Decrizione e classificanzone di un attinomycete (*Streptomyces peucetius* sp. Nova) Produttore di una sostavia ad affivita antitumorale: La dawnomicina. *G. Microbiol.* 1963;11:19–115.

Halazun JF, Wagner HR, Gaeta JF, et al. Daunorubicin cardiac toxicity in children with acute lymphocytic leukemia. *Cancer.* 1974;33:545–554.

Hartmann G, Goller G, Koschel K, et al. Hemmung der DNA-abhangigen RNA-und DNA-synthese durch antiobiotica. *Biochem Zeitschrift.* 1964;341:126–128.

Herman EH, Ferrans VJ. Amelioration of chronic anthracycline cardiotoxicity by ICRF-187 and other compounds. *Cancer Treat Rev.* 1987;14:225–229.

Holton CP, Vietti TJ, Nora AH, et al. Clinical study of daunomycin and prednisone for induction of remission in children with advanced leukemia. *N Engl J Med.* 1969;280:171–174.

Huffman DH, Benjamin RS, Bachur NR. Daunorubicin metabolism in acute nonlymphocytic leukemia. *Clin Pharmacol Ther.* 1972;13:895–905.

Ipoliti G, Cassirola G, Marini G, et al. Daunorubicin cardiotoxicity. *Lancet.* 1976;1:430–431.

Jones B, Holland JF, Morrison AR, et al. Daunorubicin (NSC-82151) in the treatment of advanced childhood lymphoblastic leukemia. *Cancer Res.* 1971;31:84–90.

Katz ME, Cassileth PA. Hyperbilirubinemia during induction therapy of acute granulocytic leukemia. *Cancer.* 1977;40:1390–1392.

Kersten W, Kersten H, Szybalski E, et al. Physiochemical properties of complexes between deoxyribonucleic acid and antibiotics which affect ribonucleic acid synthesis (actinomycin, daunomycin, cinerubin, nogalomycin, chromomycin, mithramycin and olivomycin). *Biochemistry.* 1966;5:236–241.

Kessel D, Wilberding C. Anthracycline resistance in P388 murine leukemia and its circumvention by calcium antagonists. *Cancer Res.* 1985a;45:1687–1691.

Kessel D, Wilberding C. Promotion of daunorubicin uptake and toxicity by the calcium antagonist tiapamil and its analogs. *Cancer Treat Rep.* 1985b;69(6):673–676.

Kim JH, Gelbard AS, Djordjevic B, et al. Action of daunomycin on the nucleic acid metabolism and viability of HeLa cells. *Cancer Res.* 1968;28:2437–2442.

Kokenberg E, Sonneveld P, Sizoo W, et al. Cellular pharmacokinetics of daunorubicin: Relationships with the response to treatment in patients with acute myeloid leukemia. *J Clin Oncol.* 1988;6(5):802–812.

Lippman M, Zager R, Henderson ES. High dose daunorubicin (NSC-83142) in the treatment of advanced acute myelogenous leukemia. *Cancer Chemother Rep.* 1972;56:755–760.

Lipshultz SE, Colan SD, Gelber RD, et al. Late cardiac effects of doxorubicin therapy for acute lymphoblastic leukemia in childhood. *N Engl J Med.* 1991;324:808–815.

Lock RB, Ross WE. DNA topoisomerases in cancer therapy. *Anti-Cancer Drug Design.* 1987;2:151–164.

Ma DDF, Isbister JP. Cytotoxic-induced fulminant hyperpyrexia. *Cancer.* 45:2249–2251.

Matthews RN, Colebatch JH. Daunorubicin: Results in childhood leukemia. *Arch Dis Child.* 1972;47:272–277.

Menard DB, Gisselbrecht C, Marty M, et al. Antineoplastic agents and the liver. *Gastroenterology.* 1980;78:142–164.

Meriwether VD, Bachur NR. Inhibition of DNA and RNA metabolism by daunorubicin and Adriamycin in L1210 mouse leukemia. *Cancer Res.* 1972;32:1137–1142.

Mosijczuk AD, Ruymann FB, Mease AD, et al. Anthracycline cardiomyopathy in children—Report of two cases. *Cancer.* 1979;44:1582–1587.

Nooter K, Oostrum R, Deurloo J. Effects of verapamil on the pharmacokinetics of daunomycin in the rat. *Cancer Chemother Pharmacol.* 1987;20:176–178.

Ogawa GS, Young R, Munar M. Dispensing-pin problems. *Am J Hosp Pharm.* 1985;42:1042, 1045.

Olver IN, Aisner J, Hament A, et al. A prospective study of topical dimethyl sulfoxide for treating anthracycline extravasation. *J Clin Oncol.* 1988;6:1732–1735.

Ozols RF, Wilson JKV, Weltz MD, et al. Inhibition of human ovarian cancer colony formation by Adriamycin and its major metabolites. *Cancer Res.* 1980;40:4109–4117.

Pigram WJ, Fuller W, Hamilton LD, et al. Stereochemistry of intercalation: Interaction of daunomycin with DNA. *Nature New Biol.* 1972;235:17–19.

Poochikian GK, Cradock JC, Flora KP. Stability of anthracycline antitumor agents in four infusion fluids. *Am J Hosp Pharm.* 1981;38(Apr):483–486.

Reaman GH, Ladisch S, Echelberger C, et al. Improved

treatment results in the management of single and multiple relapses of acute lymphoblastic leukemia. *Cancer.* 1980;**45**:3090–3094.

Reese JB, Shirhatti V, Singh Y, et al. Daunomycin inhibits the uptake of adenine, amino acids and glucose into cardiac myocytes. *Toxicol Appl Pharmacol.* 1987;**88**:105–112.

Reich SD, Bachur NR. Contact dermatitis associated with Adriamycin (NSC-123127) and daunorubicin (NSC-82151) (letter). *Cancer Chemother Rep.* 1975;**59**:677–678.

Riggs CE Jr. Clinical pharmacology of daunorubicin in patients with acute leukemia. *Semin Oncol.* 1984;**11**(4, suppl 3):2–11.

Sallan SE, Camitta B, Cassady JR, et al. Intermittent combination chemotherapy with Adriamycin for childhood acute lymphoblastic leukemia: Clinical results. *Blood.* 1978;**51**(3):425–433.

Schioppocassi G, Schwartz HS. Membrane actions of daunorubicin in mammalian erythrocytes. *Res Commun Chem Pathol Pharmacol.* 1977;**18**:519–531.

Slater LM, Murray SL, Wetzel MW, et al. Verapamil restoration of daunorubicin responsiveness in daunomycin-resistant Ehrlich ascites carcinoma. *J Clin Invest.* 1982;**70**:1131–1134.

Soble MJ, Dorr RT, Pezia P, Breckenridge S. Dose-dependent skin ulcers in mice treated with DNA binding antitumor antibiotics. *Cancer Chemother Pharmacol.* 1987;**20**:33–36.

Speyer JL, Green MD, Kramer E, et al. Protective effect of the bispiperazinedione ICRF-187 against doxorubicin-induced cardiac toxicity in women with advanced breast cancer. *N Engl J Med.* 1988;**319**:745–752.

Starkebaum GA, Durack DT. Early onset of daunorubicin (daunomycin) cardiotoxicity (letter). *Lancet.* 1975;**2**:711–712.

Stryckmans PA, Manaster J, Lachapelle F, et al. Mode of action of chemotherapy in vivo on human acute leukemia. I. Daunomycin. *J Clin Invest.* 1973;**52**:126–133.

Takanashi S, Bachur NR. Daunorubicin metabolites in human urine. *J Pharmacol Exp Ther.* 1975;**195**(1):41–49.

Tewey KM, Chen GL, Nelson EM, et al. Intercalative drugs interfere with the breakage–reunion reaction of mammalian DNA topoisomerase II. *J Biol Chem.* 1984;**259**:9182–9187.

Theologides A, Yarbro JW, Kennedy BJ. Daunomycin inhibition of DNA and RNA synthesis. *Cancer.* 1968;**21**:16–21.

Trissel LA. *Handbook on Injectable Drugs.* Bethesda, MD: American Society of Hospital Pharmacists; 1988:222–223.

Von Hoff D. Use of daunorubicin in patients with solid tumors. *Semin Oncol.* 1984;**11**(4, suppl 3):23–27.

Von Hoff DD, Rozencweig M, Layard M, et al. Daunomycin-induced cardiotoxicity in children and adults. *Am J Med.* 1977;**62**:200–208.

Wang G, Finch MD, Trevan D, Hellmann K. Reduction of daunomycin toxicity by razoxane. *Br J Cancer.* 1981;**43**:871–877.

Ward DC, Reich E, Goldberg IH. Base specificity in the interaction of polynucleotides with antibiotic drugs. *Science.* 1965;**149**:1259–1263.

Weil M, Glidewell OJ, Jacquillat C, et al. Daunorubicin in the therapy of acute granulocytic leukemia. *Cancer Res.* 1973;**33**:921–928.

Wiernik PH, Schimpff SC, Schiffer CA, et al. Randomized clinical comparison of daunorubicin (NSC-82151) alone with a combination of daunorubicin, cytosine arabinoside (NSC-63878), 6-thioguanine (NSC-752), and pyrimethamine (NSC-3061) for the treatment of acute nonlymphocytic leukemia. *Cancer Treat Rep.* 1976;**60**:41–53.

Wiernik PH, Serpick AA. A randomized clinical trial of daunorubicin and a combination of prednisone, vincristine, 6-mercaptopurine and methotrexate in adult acute nonlymphocytic leukemia. *Cancer Res.* 1972;**32**:2023–2026.

Williams BA, Tritton T. Photoinactivation of anthracyclines. *Photochem Photobiol.* 1981;**34**:131–134.

Willingham MC, Cornwell MM, Cardarelli CO, et al. Single cell analysis of daunomycin uptake and efflux in multidrug-resistant and -sensitive KB cells: Effects of verapamil and other drugs. *Cancer Res.* 1987;**47**:5941–5946.

Woodman RJ, Cysyk RL, Kline I, et al. Enhancement of the effectiveness of daunorubicin (NSC-82151) or Adriamycin (NSC-123127) against early mouse L1210 leukemia with ICRF-159 (NSC-129943). *Cancer Chemother Rep.* 1975;**59**:689–695.

Yanovich S, Preston L. Effects of verapamil on daunomycin cellular retention and cytotoxicity in P388 leukemic cells. *Cancer Res.* 1984;**44**:1743–1747.

Yates J, Glidewell O, Wiernik P, et al. Cytosine arabinoside with daunorubicin or Adriamycin for therapy of acute myelocytic leukemia: A CALGB study. *Blood.* 1982;**60**(2):454–462.

Yesair M, Thayer PS, McNitt S, Teague K. Comparative uptake, metabolism and retention of anthracyclines by tumors growing in vitro. *Germ J Cancer.* 1980;**16**:901–907.

Zager R, Frisby S. Oliverio VT, et al. The effect of antibiotics and cancer chemotherapeutic agents in the cellular transport and antitumor activity of methotrexate in L-1210 murine leukemia. *Cancer Res.* 1973;**33**:1670–1676.

Deazauridine

Other Names

3-Deazauridine; DAU; NSC-126849.

Chemistry

Structure of deazauridine

The complete chemical name is 1-β-D-ribofuranosyl-2,4(1H,3H)-pyridinedione. Deazauridine has a molecular weight of 243 and the empiric formula $C_{10}H_{13}NO_6$. It is a pyridine analog of the naturally occurring pyrimidine nucleoside uridine. The pK_a for deazauridine is 6.5.

Antitumor Activity

Deazauridine showed antitumor activity in a number of preclinical models, including L-1210 leukemia and a leukemic cell line resistant to cytarabine (Brockman et al 1975). No responses were observed in a phase I trial of 44 adults with a variety of solid tumors including melanoma (9 patients), lymphoma (4 patients), lung cancer (7 patients), and a few other tumors (Stewart et al 1980). In adults with acute leukemia, 3 of 36 patients showed hematologic improvement but with no complete or partial responses reported (Yap et al 1981). Similarly, no objective responses to deazauridine were observed in 15 patients with advanced colorectal adenocarcinoma (Bruno et al 1982).

Mechanism of Action

Deazauridine is metabolized to the 5'-triphosphate nucleotide form. This metabolite inhibits the enzyme that synthesizes cytidine triphosphate (CTP) (McPartland et al 1974). Cellular pools of cytidine triphosphate are thereby significantly lowered by the drug (Barlogie et al 1981). Deazauridine is also a substrate for the enzyme uridine–cytidine kinase (EC 2.7.1.48). This enzyme may be low in cells that develop resistance to the drug (Ahmed et al 1980). Deazauridine in the undissociated form is transported across cell membranes by the nucleoside transporter protein for uridine (Dahlig-Harley et al 1984). At pH below 6.5, uptake of deazauridine is enhanced as the drug is primarily in the unionized form.

Deazauridine in the 5'-diphosphate form also inhibits the conversion of cytidine diphosphate to cytidine triphosphate, a process mediated by ribonucleotide reductase (Brockman et al 1975). Other metabolic effects of deazauridine include feedback inhibition of (1) thymidine kinase by a buildup of thymidine (Ives et al 1963) and (2) deoxycytidine monophosphate deaminase mediated by deazauridine and its 5'-monophosphate nucleotide metabolite (Maley and Maley 1962).

Deazauridine is cell cycle phase specific for S phase (Barlogie et al 1981).

Availability and Storage

Deazauridine was investigationally available from the National Cancer Institute. It was supplied in 20-mL, 500-mg vials (containing about 2 mEq/mL sodium as sodium hydroxide to adjust the pH) (National Cancer Institute, 1987). A 2.0-gm, 30-mL vial was also available (containing 7 mEq sodium per vial). The intact vials, stored under refrigeration, are stable for at least 2 years after manufacture and for 6 months at room temperature.

Preparation for Use, Stability, and Admixture

For the 500-mg vials, 9.8 mL of Sodium Chloride for Injection, USP, or Sterile Water for Injection, USP, is added. This yields a solution containing 50 mg/mL. The addition of 4.7 or 2.2 mL to the 500-mg vials yields a solution containing 100 or 200 mg/mL, respectively (National Cancer Institute 1987). The 2.0-g vials are reconstituted with 18.8 mL to yield a solution containing 100 mg/mL at a pH of 6.0 to 8.0. These solutions are chemically stable for at least 1 week at room temperature, but use within 8 hours is recommended as no antibacterial agent is present.

These initial solutions may be further diluted into 500 mL of 5% dextrose or 0.9% sodium chloride.

Administration

Deazauridine is administered intravenously, usually as a continuous infusion. This takes maximal advantage of the cell cycle phase specificity of the drug. Shorter 1-hour intravenous infusions have also been used (Creaven et al 1982, Bruno et al 1982).

Dosage

For solid tumor patients without extensive prior therapy, the recommended dose is 1000 mg/m^2/d as a 5-day continuous intravenous infusion (Stewart et al 1980). A slightly higher dose of 1200 mg/m^2/d × 5 as a 1-hour infusion recommended by Creaven et al (1982) was administered to patients with colorectal carcinoma (Bruno et al 1982). In leukemia, a dose of 2500 mg/m^2/d was recommended using a 5-day continuous intravenous infusion schedule (Yap et al 1981).

Drug Interactions

Deazauridine has shown enhanced, schedule-dependent cytotoxic effects in vitro when administered after cytarabine (Barlogie et al 1981). Deazauridine also synergistically potentiates the cytotoxicity of thymidine in tumor cells in vitro (Lockshin et al 1984).

Pharmacokinetics

Pharmacokinetic studies in cancer patients have demonstrated a biphasic elimination pattern for deazauridine (Benvenuto et al 1979, Creaven et al 1982). The mean terminal half-life of deazauridine following rapid infusion varies from 4.4 to 6.9 hours with an estimated volume of distribution of 0.57 L/kg. The half-life may increase up to 21.3 hours at the end of a 5-day continuous infusion regimen (Benvenuto et al 1979). Only about 8% of a deazauridine dose is excreted into the urine. High levels of deazauridine and its triphosphorylated metabolite have been recovered from a variety of tissues including brain, lung, and liver (Benvenuto et al 1979). Penetration into the central nervous system is particularly good, with 22.1% of the plasma concentration achieved in the central nervous system. Up to 50% central nervous system penetration was reported in two patients receiving a 5-day continuous infusion (Stewart et al 1979). Penetration into intracerebral tumor was equal to that in adjacent normal brain tissues, and in a tumor specimen high levels of deazauridine triphosphate were recovered. Two hours after the end of a 1.5 g/m^2 infusion over 30 minutes, the cerebrospinal fluid level of deazauridine was 3.1 µg/mL, and at 16 hours the level was only reduced to 1.9 µg/mL (Stewart et al 1979). Drug levels in subcutaneous breast cancer metastases have been measured at 0.4 µg/g 68 minutes after infusion (Creaven et al 1982).

The clearance of deazauridine was 3.7 L/h following the rapid infusion and 56.5 L/h after the continuous infusion (Benvenuto et al 1979). The majority of metabolites of deazauridine are excreted in the urine but they have not been identified (Creaven et al 1982).

Side Effects and Toxicity

The major dose-limiting toxic effects of deazauridine are leukopenia and thrombocytopenia. Granulocytopenia is the predominant effect and recovery is typically complete within 7 days of the nadir (Creaven et al 1982). Patients previously treated with nitrosoureas or radiation have more profound thrombocytopenia (Stewart et al 1980). A small percentage of patients experience nausea and vomiting. In contrast, mucositis may be severe, especially with the 5-day infusion regimens (Stewart et al 1980). Severe swelling of the tongue was described in one trial. Other toxic effects included rash, headache, chest pain, and blurred vision.

One patient with mild to moderate renal insufficiency (serum creatinine of 1.7 µg/dL) developed severe skin toxicity (Stevens–Johnson syndrome) and oral ulcerations (Creaven et al 1982). Thus, dose reductions in patients with renal insufficiency may be required, but specific guidelines have not yet been established.

REFERENCES

Ahmed NK, Germain GS, Welch AD, et al. Phosphorylation of nucleosides catalyzed by a mammalian enzyme other than uridine–cytidine kinase. *Biochem Biophys Res Commun.* 1980;**95**:440–445.

Barlogie B, Plunkett W, Raber M, et al. In vivo cellular kinetic and pharmacological studies of 1-β-D-arabinofuranosylcytosine and 3-deazauridine chemotherapy for relapsing acute leukemia. *Cancer Res.* 1981;**41**:1227–1235.

Benvenuto JA, Hall SW, Farquhar D, et al. Pharmacokinet-

ics and disposition of 3-deazauridine in humans. *Cancer Res.* 1979;**39**:349–352.
Brockman RW, Shaddix SC, Williams M, et al. The mechanism of action of 3-deazauridine in tumor cells sensitive and resistant to arabinosylcytosine. *Ann NY Acad Sci.* 1975;**255**:501–521.
Bruno S, Poster D, Creaven PJ, et al. Phase II study of 3-deazauridine in advanced colorectal adenocarcinoma. *Am J Clin Oncol.* 1982;**5**:69–71.
Creaven PJ, Priore RL, Mittelman A, et al. Phase I trial and pharmacokinetics of a daily × 5 schedule of 3-deazauridine. *Cancer Treat Rep.* 1982;**66**:81–84.
Dahlig-Harley E, Paterson ARP, Robins MJ, Cass CE. Transport of uridine and 3-deazauridine in cultured human lymphoblastoid cells. *Cancer Res.* 1984;**44**:161–165.
Ives DH, Morse PA Jr, Potter VR. Feedback inhibition of thymidine kinase by thymidine triphosphate. *J Biol Chem.* 1963;**238**:1467–1474.
Lockshin A, Mendoza JT, Giovanella BC, Stehlin JS Jr. Cytotoxic and biochemical effects of thymidine and 3-deazauridine on human tumor cells. *Cancer Res.* 1984;**44**:2534–2539.
Maley F, Maley GF. On the nature of a sparing effect by thymidine on the utilization of deoxycytidine. *Biochemistry.* 1962;**1**:847–851.
McPartland RP, Wang MC, Bloch A, Weinfeld H. Cytidine 5′-triphosphate synthetase as a target for inhibition by the antitumor agent 3-deazauridine. *Cancer Res.* 1974;**34**:3107–3111.
National Cancer Institute. NCI Investigational Drugs: *Pharmacological Data*. NIH Publication No. 88-2141. Washington, DC: U.S. Department of Health and Human Services, 1987:70–72.
Stewart DJ, Benvenuto JA, Leavens M, et al. Penetration of 3-deazauridine into human brain, intracerebral tumor, and cerebrospinal fluid. *Cancer Res.* 1979;**39**:4119–4122.
Stewart DJ, McCredie KD, Barlogie B, et al. Phase I study of 3-deazauridine in the treatment of adults with solid tumors. *Cancer Treat Rep.* 1980;**64**:1295–1299.
Yap B-S, McCredie KB, Keating MJ, et al. Phase I–II study of 3-deazauridine in adults with acute leukemia. *Cancer Treat Rep.* 1981;**65**:521–524.

Dexrazoxane

■ Other Names

ICRF-187; ADR-529; Zinecard® (Adria Laboratories); Cardioxane® (EuroCetus); NSC-169780.

■ Chemistry

Structure of dexrazoxane

The complete chemical name of dexrazoxane is 4,4′-(1-methyl-1,2-ethanediyl)-bis(2,6-piperazinedione). Dexrazoxane is the water-soluble (+) enantiomer of the racemic drug razoxane (ICRF-159). These agents are nonpolar derivatives of ethylenediaminetetraacetic acid (EDTA). Chemically it is a bisdioxopiperazine. Because of the lack of solubility of the racemic mixture, ICRF-159 could not be formulated for intravenous administration, and so dexrazoxane was developed (Repta et al 1976). Dexrazoxane has a molecular weight of 268.8 and an empiric formula of $C_{11}H_{16}N_4O_4$.

■ Antitumor Activity

Dexrazoxane had marginal antitumor activity in patients with non-Hodgkin's lymphoma, Kaposi's sarcoma, and colorectal carcinoma (Flannery et al 1978, Bellet et al 1976, Olweny et al 1976). There is experimental evidence that dexrazoxane can enhance the antitumor activity of several types of cytotoxic agents, including daunorubicin (Woodman et al 1975); however, dexrazoxane has not yet been demonstrated to have any substantial antitumor activity in phase II studies in patients with non-small cell lung cancer, renal cell carcinoma, and head and neck cancer (Natale et al 1983, Brubaker et al 1986, Wheeler et al 1984). Similarly, no responses were noted in 66 children with acute leukemia, Ewing's sarcoma, neuroblastoma, lymphomas, and several other solid tumors (Vats et al 1991).

The most interesting investigational use for dexrazoxane is in the area of protection from the cardiotoxic effects of doxorubicin. This effect was based on preclinical work by number of investigators in several animal cardiotoxicity models (Herman and Ferrans 1981, Herman et al 1979). Speyer et al (1988) conducted an elegant randomized trial of dexrazoxane at a dose of 1000 mg/m^2 prior to doxorubicin therapy in patients receiving 5-fluorouracil + doxorubicin + cyclophosphamide for their breast cancer. One half of the patients received the dexrazoxane. The patients receiving the dexrazoxane had a substantial decrease in the cardiotoxicity without a compromise in antitumor activity. This important finding is being retested in ongoing randomized phase III trials. For example, in small cell lung cancer, dexrazoxane lowers the cardiac toxicity of the CAV regimen (cyclophosphamide, doxorubicin, vincristine) from 29 to 12% without altering the overall objective response rate of about 67% (Feldmann et al 1992). The mechanism of this protection could be related to intracellular iron chelation seen in vitro (Hasinoff 1989) followed by an increased urinary excretion of iron noted with the agent in humans (Von Hoff et al 1981).

■ Mechanism of Action

The mode of action of dexrazoxane as an antitumor agent has not been fully elucidated. It is likely that dexrazoxane works as a metal chelator much like razoxane (ICRF-159), which is active in early mitosis (G$_2$/M phase) and inhibits DNA synthesis (Creighton et al 1969, Hellman and Field 1970, Sharp et al 1970). Although early studies suggested that these compounds might alkylate DNA, this has not been conclusively proven.

More recent evidence suggests that bisdioxopiperazine compounds like dexrazoxane inhibit topoisomerase II activity in a fashion distinct from that of epipodophyllotoxins such as etoposide (Ishida et al 1991, Tanabe et al 1991). Topoisomerase I activity was not inhibited. In contrast to drugs like etoposide, the bisdioxopiperazines do not stimulate cleavable complex formation and can even inhibit etoposide-induced strand breakage by topoisomerase (Tanabe et al 1991). Thus, these agents appear to block topoisomerase II activity prior to the formation of the cleavable complex between the enzyme and DNA double strands. Because cells are arrested in G$_2$/M phase, they typically possess a tetraploid DNA content (Ishida et al 1991).

As a cardioprotective agent, dexrazoxane is known to undergo intracellular hydrolysis of the piperazinyl rings to the double-ring-opened form capable of divalent metal chelation (Hasinoff 1989).

In this form, the drug can readily remove Fe^{2+} and Cu^{2+} from their complexes with doxorubicin (Hasinoff 1989). The reaction proceeds to 99% completion and is first order in both Fe^{2+} and doxorubicin. This thereby yields a second-order rate consistent with removal of iron from doxorubicin, 123 M^{-1} min^{-1}. The loss of iron and possibly also copper from doxorubicin protects against many oxidative biologic effects of the drug–metal complex. These include loss of cytochrome c oxidase activity (Hasinoff 1989) and, importantly, the generation of oxygen free radicals which are thought to mediate the cardiotoxic lipid peroxidative effects of the drug–metal complex (Butteridge 1984, Myers et al 1986).

Two recent pharmacokinetic studies have shown no influence of dexrazoxane on doxorubicin clearance in cancer patients. These results indicate that the cardioprotective mechanism does not involve enhanced elimination of doxorubicin (Narang et al 1992, Koning et al 1992).

It is of note that ICRF-159 can prevent metastases in experimental animal tumor systems, perhaps by an effect on tumor angiogenesis (Salsburg et al 1970, LeServe et al 1972).

■ Availability and Storage

Dexrazoxane is investigationally available from Adria Laboratories, Columbus, Ohio, in 30-mL vials each containing 250 mg of lyophilized dexrazoxane (+). The intact vials should be stored at room temperature and are stable for several months.

■ Preparation for Use, Stability, and Admixture

To each 30-mL vial, 25 mL of Sodium Chloride Injection, USP, is added. The resulting solution contains 10 mg/mL with a pH of 5.0 to 6.5 The solution is stable (5% degradation) for 8 hours at 22 to 25°C. Because the lyophilized solution contains no antibacterial preservatives, unused portions should be discarded 8 hours after initial reconstitution, although the drug is chemically stable in solution for up to 24 hours at room temperature. Solutions may be further diluted with saline or D5W.

■ Administration

Dexrazoxane has been given by several intravenous schedules including weekly × 4 weeks (followed by 2 weeks of rest), 1500 mg/m^2/d for 3 consecutive days, or 1000 mg/m^2 as a 48-hour infusion. Most schedules have used a repeat of the course every 3 weeks. For each of these schedules, the drug was diluted in D5W and run in over 30 to 60 minutes (except for the 48-hour continuous infusion schedule) (Natale et al 1983, Wheeler et al 1984, Brubaker et al 1986). For cardioprotection from doxorubicin, dexrazoxane is administered intravenously over 15 minutes, 30 minutes before doxorubicin (Speyer et al 1988).

■ Special Precautions

Although data are scarce, there is some indication that members of the ICRF family (ICRF-159 and dexrazoxane) may be leukemogenic in some patients (Joshi et al 1981). In addition, cases of basal cell and skin cancer have been reported in patients receiving ICRF-159 in colon adjuvant trials. These reports are not surprising, as the ICRFs are felt to be alkylating agents; however, the few case reports are *by no means* definitive.

■ Drug Interactions

Divalent metal chelation by dexrazoxane may mediate a number of interactions with other chemotherapy agents. Antitumor potentiation has been observed with anthracyclines (Monti and Sinha 1990, Wadler et al 1986, 1987) as reviewed by Koning et al (1991). The drug may also synergize with hyperthermia by blocking host toxicity to normal tissues (Baba et al 1991). A number of anthracycline antitumor agents produce less cardiotoxicity when combined with dexrazoxane (Alderton et al 1992). Less of a cardioprotective effect from dexrazoxane is observed with mitoxantrone (Alderton et al 1992, Shipp and Dorr 1993). These cardioprotective effects are mediated by intracellular iron chelation from the double-ring-opened hydrolysis product of dexrazoxane termed *ICRF-529* (Hasinoff et al 1991). By chelation of intracellular iron, the cardiotoxic generation of oxygen free radicals from iron–drug complexes was prevented (Gutteridge 1984; Hasinoff 1989). Dexrazoxane does facilitate the administration of larger cumulative doxorubicin doses (Speyer et al 1988) wherein increased myelotoxicity is described.

In contrast, dexrazoxane does not block pulmonary toxicity from the iron-dependent antitumor antibiotic bleomycin in a hamster model (Tryka 1989). Instead, dexrazoxane enhances pulmonary injury by an unknown mechanism. Dexrazonane does not alter doxorubicin's distribution metabolism or excretion (Hochster et al 1992).

■ Dosage

Usual dosages of dexrazoxane include 2.6 g/m^2/wk, 1250 to 1500 mg/m^2/d for 3 consecutive days, 1000 mg/m^2 as a 48-hour infusion, and 800 to 1250 mg/m^2/d × 5 (Liesmann et al 1981, Koeller et al 1981, Brubaker et al 1986, Von Hoff et al 1981). In a pediatric population, the maximally tolerated dose was considerably higher (3500 mg/m^2/d × 3) (Holcenbergh et al 1986). In adult patients with solid tumors, the recommended phase II doses for antitumor studies were 3.8 g/m^2/wk × 4 for heavily pretreated patients and 7.42 g/m^2/wk × 4 for good-risk patients (Vogel et al 1987). The dose shown to be cardioprotective against doxorubicin cardiotoxicity in breast cancer patients was 1000 mg/m^2 (Speyer et al 1988). More recently, a lower dexrazoxane dose of 500 mg/m^2 has been shown to block doxorubicin cardiotoxicity in breast cancer patients (Rosenfeld et al 1992). In children the maximally tolerated dose was 3.5 g/m^2, with a recommended dose of 3.0 g/m^2 IV every 3 weeks for studies of antitumor activity (Vats et al 1991). For blocking the cardiotoxicity of epirubicin, a dexrazoxane:epirubicin dose ratio of 9:1 (mg/m^2) was found to be safe and active (Basser et al 1992).

■ Pharmacokinetics

Earhart et al (1982), have carefully studied the kinetics of dexrazoxane in patients receiving the drug as 30-minute, 8-hour, or 48-hour infusions. Holcenbergh et al (1986) studied the 2-hour infusion daily × 3 schedule in pediatric patients. The table on page 370 summarizes the data from the two studies.

As can be seen from these data, the drug fits a two-compartment model. Children had a larger volume of distribution and a more rapid total body clearance than adults. Similar pharmacokinetic patterns are described by Hochster et al (1992). Urinary recovery averaged 37% in this trial and a mean AUC of 57,865 µg·h/L was reported following intravenous doses of 500 mg/m^2 (Hochster et al 1992).

■ Side Effects and Toxicity

The usual dose-limiting toxic effects for dexrazoxane are leukopenia and thrombocytopenia. Anemia is also noted at most dose levels above 1 g/m^2 (Vogel et al 1987). The nadir for neutropenia and thrombocytopenia ranges between 7 and 10 days with recovery by days 18 to 21 following a 3-day course of therapy. The anemia was not associated with hemolysis but a moderate degree of reticulocytosis was common at high doses (Vogel et

PHARMACOKINETIC PARAMETERS OF ICRF-187

Patients (Reference)	Half-life (min) α	Half-life (min) β	Volumes of Distribution (L/kg)* V_c	Volumes of Distribution (L/kg)* V_b	Clearance mL/min/kg	Clearance mL/min/m²	MRT (min)	Volume of Distribution at Steady State (L/kg)
Adults (Earhart et al 1982)	11.6	146	0.177	0.66	3.32	124	140	0.451
Children (9–12 y) (Holcenbergh et al 1986)	16	113	0.376	0.96	6.01	185	25	0.757
Adults (Hochster et al 1992)	28	250	NL†	NL	111#		NL	NL

*V_c = volume of central compartment, V_b = volume in postdistributive phase.
†Not listed.
#mL/m²/min.

From Holcenbergh JS, Tutsch KD, Earhart RH, et al. Phase I study of IRCF-187 in pediatric cancer patients and comparison of its pharmacokinetics in children and adults. Cancer Treat Rep. 1986;70:703–709. Adapted with permission.

al 1987). When dexrazoxane was combined with doxorubicin, slightly enhanced myelosuppression was consistently observed by Speyer et al (1988); however, this observation was not seen in another trial wherein none of the noncardiac toxic effects of doxorubicin were altered by concurrent dexrazoxane therapy (Curran et al 1992). Other toxic effects include nausea and rare vomiting, alopecia, transient elevation in liver function tests, low-grade fever, pain at the injection site, malaise, alopecia, and increased urinary clearance of iron and zinc (Von Hoff et al 1981). Hepatotoxicity is typically noted at all dose levels but is usually not dose limiting. Manifestations include elevated serum glutamic-oxalacetic transaminase with elevation of bilirubin or alkaline phosphatase. High doses have also produced fatigue. No necrosis was noted on inadvertent extravasation in one patient (Vogel et al 1987). Phlebitis is described in about 2% of patients.

■ Special Applications

As noted earlier, in one clinical study, dexrazoxane was found to protect against the cardiotoxicity of doxorubicin (Speyer et al 1988). This potentially important protective effect is being studied in ongoing confirmatory phase III studies.

REFERENCES

Alderton PM, Gross J, Green MD. Comparative study of doxorubicin, mitoxantrone, and epirubicin in combination with ICRF-187 (ADR-529) in a chronic cardiotoxicity animal model. *Cancer Res.* 1992;**52**:194–201.

Baba H, Stephens LC, Strebel FR, et al. Protective effect of ICRF-187 against normal tissue injury induced by Adriamycin in combination with whole body hyperthermia. *Cancer Res.* 1991;**51**:3568–3577.

Basser R, Duggan G, Rosenthal M, et al. Optimal dose ratio of ADR-529 (ICRF-187) and epirubicin. *Proc Am Soc Clin Oncol.* 1992;**11**:123.

Bellet RE, Engstrom PF, Catalano RB, Creech RH, Mastrangelo MJ. Phase II study of ICRF-159 in patients with metastatic colorectal carcinoma previously exposed to systemic chemotherapy. *Cancer Treat Rep.* 1976;**60**:1395–1397.

Brubaker LH, Vogel CL, Einhorn LH, Birch R. Treatment of advanced adenocarcinoma of the kidney with ICRF-187: A Southwestern Cancer Study Group trial. *Cancer Treat Rep.* 1986;**70**:915–916.

Butteridge JMC. Lipid peroxidation and possible hydroxyl radical formation stimulated by the self-reduction of doxorubicin–iron(III) complex. *Biochem Pharmacol.* 1984;**33**:1725–1728.

Creighton AM, Hellmann K, Whitecross S. Antitumor activity in a series of bisdeketopiperazines. *Nature.* 1969;**222**:382–383.

Curran C, Greenberg BR, Hochster H, et al. Minimal modification of non-cardiac doxorubicin (DOX) toxicities by dexrazoxane (DEXR), a cardioprotectant. *Proc Am Soc Clin Oncol.* 1992;**11**:140.

Earhart RH, Tutsch KD, Koeller JM et al. Pharmacokinetics of (+)-1, 2-di(3,5-dioxopiperazin-1-yl) Propane intravenous infusions in adult cancer patients. *Cancer Res.* 1982;**42**:5255–5261.

Feldmann JE, Jones SE, Weisberg SR, et al. Advanced small cell lung cancer treated with CAV (cyclophosphamide + Adriamycin® + vincristine) chemotherapy and the cardioprotective agent dexrazoxane (ADR-529, ICRF-187, Zinecard®). *Proc Am Soc Clin Oncol.* 1992;**11**:296.

Flannery EP, Corder MP, Sheehan WW, Papak TF, Bateman JR. Phase II study of ICRF-159 in non-Hodgkin's lymphomas. *Cancer Treat Rep.* 1978;**62**:465–467.

Hasinoff BB, Reinders FX, Clark V. The enzymatic hydrolysis-activation of the Adriamycin cardioprotective agent (+)-1,2-bis(3,5-dioxopiperazinyl-1-yl)propane. *Drug Metab Dispos.* 1991;**19**(1):74–80.

Hassinoff BB. The interaction of the cardioprotective agent ICRF-187; its hydrolysis product (ICRF-198) and other chelating agents with Fe (III) and CU (II) complexes of adriamycin. *Agents Actions.* 1989;**26**:378–385.

Hellmann K, Field EO. Effect of ICRF-159 on the mammalian cell cycle: Significance for its use in cancer chemotherapy. *J Natl Cancer Inst.* 1970;**44**:539–543.

Herman E, Ardalan B, Bier C, Waravdekar V, Krop S. Reduction of daunorubicin lethality and myocardial cellular alterations by pretreatment with ICRF-187 in Syrian Golden Hamsters. *Cancer Treat Rep.* 1979;**63**:89–92.

Herman EH, Ferrans VJ. Reduction of chronic doxorubicin cardiotoxicity in dogs by treatment with (+)-1,2-bis(3,5-dioxopiperazinyl-1-yl(propane (ICRP-187). *Cancer Res.* 1981;**41**:3436–3440.

Hochster H, Narang PK, Lewis RC, et al. Pharmacokinetics of cardioprotectant dexrazoxane (DZR) in advanced cancer patients. *Proc Am Soc Clin Oncol.* 1992;**11**:125.

Hochster H, Liebe SL, Wadler S et al. Pharmacokinetics of the cardioprotector ADR-529 (ICRF-187) in escalating doses combined with fixed dose doxorubicin. *J Natl Cancer Inst.* 1992;**84**:1725–1730.

Holcenbergh JS, Tutsch KD, Earhart RH, et al. Phase I study of ICRF-187 in pediatric cancer patients and comparison of its pharmacokinetics in children and adults. *Cancer Treat Rep.* 1986;**70**:703–709.

Ishida R, Miki T, Narita T, et al. Inhibition of intracellular topoisomerase II by antitumor bis(2,6-dioxopiperazine) derivatives: Mode of cell growth inhibition distinct from that of cleavable complex-forming type inhibitors. *Cancer Res.* 1991;**51**:4909–4916.

Joshi R, Smith B, Phillps RH, Barrett AJ. Acute myelomonocytic leukemia after rozoxane therapy. *Lancet.* 1981;**2**:1343.

Koeller JM, Earhart RH, Davis HL. Phase I trial of ICRP187 by 48 hour continuous infusion. *Cancer Treat Rep.* 1981;**65**:459–463.

Koning J, Beijnen JH, Ten Bokkel Huinink WW, et al. Pharmacokinetics (PK) of ICRF-187 and doxorubicin (DX) in patients receiving 5-FU, DX and cyclophosphamide (FAC). *Proc Am Assoc Cancer Res.* 1992;**33**:528.

Koning J, Palmer P, Franks CR, et al. Cardioxane—ICRF-187. Towards anticancer drug specificity through selective toxicity reduction. *Cancer Treat Rev.* 1991;**18**:1–19.

LeServe A, Hellmann K. Metastases and the normalization of tumor blood vessels with ICRF-159: A new type of drug action. *Br Med J.* 1972;**1**:597–601.

Liesmann T, Belt R, Haas C, Hoogstraten B. Phase I evaluation of ICRF-187 (NSC-169780) in patients with advanced malignancy. *Cancer.* 1981;**47**:1959–1962.

Monti E, Sinha BK. Potentiation of doxorubicin cytotoxicity by (+)-1,2-bis-(3,5-dioxopiperazin-1-yl)propane ICRF-187 in human leukemia HL-60 cells. *Cancer Commun.* 1990;**2**:145–149.

Myers CE, Gianni L, Zweier J, et al. The role of iron in Adriamycin biochemistry. *Fed Proc.* 1986;**45**:2792–2797.

Narang PK, Hochster H, Reynolds RD, et al. Does the cardioprotectant dexrazoxane (DZR) affect doxorubicin (DOX) kinetics/dynamics? *Proc Am Soc Clin Oncol.* 1992;**11**:126.

Natale RB, Wheller RH, Liepman MK, Sauder A, Bricker L. Phase II trial of ICRF-187 in non-small cell lung cancer. *Cancer Treat Rep.* 1983;**67**:311–313.

Olweny CLM, Masara JP, Sikyewunda W, Toya T. Treatment of Kaposi's sarcoma with ICRF-159 (NCS-129943). *Cancer Treat Rep.* 1976;**60**:111–113.

Repta AJ, Balfezor MJ, Bansal PC. Utilization of an enamtiomer as a solution to a pharmaceutical problem: Application to solubilization of 1,2-di(4-piperazine-2,6-dione)propane. *J Pharm Sci.* 1976;**65**:238–242.

Rosenfeld CS, Weisberg SR, York RM, et al. Prevention of Adriamycin® cardiomyopathy with dexrazoxane (ADR-529, ICRF-187). *Proc Am Soc Clin Oncol.* 1992;**11**:62.

Salsburg AJ, Burrage K, Hellmann K. Inhibition of metastatic spread by ICRF-159: Selective deletion of a malignant characteristic. *Br Med J.* 1970;**4**:344–346.

Sharp HBA, Field EO, Hellman K. Mode of action of the cytotoxic agent ICRF-159. *Nature.* 1970;**226**:524–526.

Shipp NG, Dorr RT, Alberts DS et al. Characterization of experimental mitoxantrone cardiotoxicity and its partial inhibition by ICRF-187 in cultured neonatal rat heart cells. *Cancer Res.* 1993;**53**:550–556.

Speyer JL, Green MD, Kramer E, et al. Protective effect of the bispiperazinedione ICRF-187 against doxorubicin induced cardiac toxicity in women with advanced breast cancer. *N Engl J Med.* 1988;**319**:745–752.

Tanabe K, Ikegami Y, Ishida R, et al. Inhibition of topoisomerase II by antitumor agents; Bis(2,6-dioxopiperazine) derivatives. *Cancer Res.* 1991;**51**:4903–4908.

Tryka AF. ICRF 187 and polyhydroxyphenyl derivatives fail to protect against bleomycin induced lung injury. *Toxicology.* 1989;**59**:127–138.

Vats T, Kamen B, Krischer JP. Phase II trial of ICRF-187 in children with solid tumors and acute leukemia. *Invest New Drugs.* 1991;**9**:333–337.

Vogel CL, Gorowski E, Davila E, et al. Phase I clinical trial and pharmacokinetics of weekly ICRF-187 (NSC-169780) infusion in patients with solid tumors. *Invest New Drugs.* 1987;**5**:187–198.

Von Hoff DD, Howser D, Lewis BJ, Holcenberg J, Weiss RB, Young RC. Phase I study of ICRF-187 using a daily for 3 days schedule. *Cancer Treat Res.* 1981;**65**:249–252.

Wadler S, Green MD, Basch R, et al. Lethal and sublethal effects of the combination of doxorubicin and the bisdioxopiperazine,(+)-1,2,-bis(3,5-deoxopiperazinyl-1-yl)propane (ICRF-187), on murine sarcoma S180 in vitro. *Biochem Pharmacol.* 1987;**36**:1495–1501.

Wadler S, Green MD, Muggia FM. Synergistic activity of doxorubicin and the bisdioxopiperazine (+)-1,2-bis(3,5-

dioxopiperazinyl-1-yl)propane (ICRF-187) against the murine sarcoma S180 cell line. *Cancer Res.* 1986;**46**:1176–1181.

Wheeler RH, Bricker LJ, Natale RB, Baker SR. Phase II trial of ICRF-187 in squamous cell carcinoma of the head and neck. *Cancer Treat Rep.* 1984;**68**:427–428.

Woodman RJ, Cysyk RL, Kline I, et al. Enhancement of the effectiveness of daunorubicin (NSC-82151) or Adriamycin (NSC-123127) against early mouse L1210 leukemia with ICRF-159 (NSC-129943). *Cancer Chemother Rep.* 1975;**59**(4):689–695.

Dianhydrogalactitol

■ Other Names

NSC-132313; DAG; galactitol.

■ Chemistry

Structure of dianhydrogalactitol

Galactitol is 1,2:5,6-dianhydrogalactitol. It is highly water soluble and has a molecular weight of 146. Chemically, it is the alkali conversion product of dibromodulcitol.

■ Antitumor Activity

Dianhydrogalactitol (DAG) showed preclinical antitumor activity in a wide range of animal leukemias and solid tumors including sarcomas, melanomas, and intracranial malignancies (Nemeth et al 1972). In humans, objective responses of 44% have also been observed in brain cancers treated with DAG (Chiuten et al 1981). In patients with malignant astrocytoma median survival was 31 weeks in one trial (Espana et al 1978) and 67 weeks in another trial (Eagan et al 1981a). Radiotherapy was combined with DAG in both trials. In contrast, DAG was inactive in children with primary brain tumors (Wienblatt et al 1981). As a single agent, DAG is inactive in a number of solid tumors including colon cancer (Perry et al 1976), breast cancer (Ahmann et al 1977, Hoogstratten et al 1978), malignant melanoma (Thigpen et al 1979), and sarcoma (Thigpen and Samson 1979). Some activity for DAG was reported in a pilot trial in renal cell carcinoma in which two of five patients responded (Eagan et al 1976); however, this was not confirmed in two larger cooperative group trials (Hahn et al 1979, Ratanatharathorn et al 1982).

In lung cancer DAG produced 2 (18%) responses in 11 large cell undifferentiated cancer cases and 4 (16%) responses in 25 epidermoid cancer cases. There were no responses in adenocarcinoma of the lung in one trial (Chiuten et al 1981) and 3 of 33 responders in another trial (Haus et al 1981). Small cell and squamous cell carcinomas were unresponsive. The drug possesses low activity in squamous cell carcinoma of the cervix, with response rates of 19% in one trial (Stehman et al 1983) and 11% in a larger follow-up study (Stehman et al 1984). A 15% objective response rate was also reported in ovarian cancer (Stehman et al 1983). The drug was inactive when combined with etoposide in colon cancer (Perry et al 1976) and when used as a single agent in endometrial adenocarcinoma (Stehman et al 1983), childhood acute leukemia (Vats et al 1981), and several solid tumors of childhood (Finklestein et al 1985). It is also inactive in pancreatic cancer (Gastrointestinal Tumor Study Group 1985) and in advanced head and neck cancer (Edmonson et al 1979), although one partial response is documented in a patient with anaplastic thyroid carcinoma (Haas et al 1983).

Dianhydrogalactitol has been combined with other anticancer agents including cisplatin and etoposide (Creagan et al 1981). In patients with recurrent brain tumors after radiotherapy, DAG + etoposide and DAG + etoposide + triazinate produced responses in 40 and 33% of patients, respectively (Eagan et al 1981a). When DAG was combined with carmustine, responses were observed in 47% of a similar patient population (Eagan et al 1982b). DAG was also active in advanced squamous cell lung cancer when combined with doxorubicin and cisplatin (Eagan et al 1981b). The overall response rate was 20/37 (54%) in this study.

Dianhydrogalactitol + cisplatin was inactive in uterine cancer (Vogl et al 1982). Finally, a three-drug combination of DAG with doxorubicin and cisplatin produced a 54% response rate in patients with advanced squamous cell carcinoma of the lung (Eagan et al 1981b).

Leukemia cells developed for resistance to DAG in vivo exhibit cross-resistance to other alkylating agents and partial cross-resistance to nitrosoureas (Bence et al 1986). In neural tumors, however, DAG was active in vitro against cells resistant to cyclophosphamide (Helson et al 1980). Antimetabolites and vinca alkaloids are active against the DAG-resistant cells that demonstrate a chromosomal deletion, as well as a submetacentric marker chromosome.

■ Mechanism of Action

Dianhydrogalactitol is a bifunctional alkylating agent that produces crosslinking of DNA strands (Kellner and Nemeth 1967, Horvath and Institoris 1967). In this regard, there is marked cross-resistance between DAG and the classic bischloroethylamine-based alkylating agents (eg, cyclophosphamide, melphalan). The epoxide-type moieties in DAG are more reactive than the halide-substituted alcohol sugar precursors in dibromodulcitol and dibromomannitol (Elson et al 1968). This probably explains the greater antitumor potency of DAG over the related dihalohexitols (Chiuten et al 1981).

As a consequence of alkylation, synthesis of DNA, RNA, and protein is inhibited by the drug. This activity is not believed to be cell cycle phase specific; however, in rat 9L brain tumor cells DAG does induce specific alterations in cell cycle progression noted by a prolongation of S phase, temporary accumulation in G_2 phase, and blocked progression past the $S-G_2$ boundary (Nomura et al 1978). Other in vitro studies in Chinese hamster ovary cells have shown that nondividing cells are almost twice as sensitive to DAG as are dividing cells (Barranco and Flournoy 1977).

■ Availability and Storage

Injectable DAG was investigationally available from the National Cancer Institute in 50 mg/10 mL vials which were stable for at least 2 years when stored under refrigeration (2–10°C). This formulation is no longer available. Oral preparations of DAG (Chinoin Pharmaceutical and Chemical Works, Ltd, Budapest, Hungary) have been evaluated in Europe.

■ Preparation for Use, Stability, and Admixture

The 50-mg vials are reconstituted with 5 mL of Sterile Water for Injection, USP. This forms a solution containing 10 mg/mL with a pH of 5.5 to 6.5. The solution is chemically stable at room temperature for 24 hours. Further dilution into 500 mL of Sodium Chloride for Injection, USP, or 5% Dextrose for Injection, USP, yields a solution that is stable for up to 8 hours.

■ Dosage

Phase I studies established a tolerable intravenous dose of 30 mg/m^2/d × 5 days (Haas et al 1976, Eagan et al 1976). In patients who received prior treatment with nitrosoureas or had abnormal hepatic function, the recommended dose was 25 mg/m^2/d × 5 days. A further reduction to 15 mg/m^2/d × 5 days was recommended in patients with impaired renal function (Haas et al 1983). In children with solid tumors, an intravenous dose of 50 mg/m^2 twice weekly for 2 consecutive weeks was given every 6 weeks (Finklestein et al 1985). In gynecologic cancer in adults, a weekly intravenous bolus dose of 60 to 75 mg/m^2 was tolerated for 4 to 12 consecutive weeks (Stehman et al 1984). A tolerable split-dosing regimen was 80 mg/m^2 given twice on day 1 only every 3 to 4 weeks for a total dose of 160 mg/m^2 (Eagan et al 1982a).

The recommended doses of oral DAG were 130 mg/m^2/d once monthly (Blum and Skarin 1976), 55 to 70 mg/m^2 weekly (Vogel et al 1976), 30 to 50 mg/m^2/d × 5 days (Haas et al 1976, Higgins et al 1976), and 10 mg/m^2/d × 10 days (Haas et al 1976). These doses were repeated at 3- to 4-week intervals.

When combined with other myelosuppressive drugs (such as etoposide), intravenous DAG doses have typically been reduced to 15 to 20 mg/m^2/d × 5 days (Eagan et al 1981b). Alternatively, a single monthly DAG dose of 60 mg/m^2 was found to be tolerable in combination with cisplatin (20 mg/m^2/d × 3) and etoposide (60 mg/m^2/d × 3) (Creagan et al 1981). When combined with carmustine (90 mg/m^2 IV), the DAG dose was 70 mg/m^2. Both were given once every 5 to 7 weeks (Eagan et al 1982b).

■ Pharmacokinetics

In humans, intravenously administered DAG doses of 50 mg/m^2 given as a 1-hour infusion produced peak plasma concentrations of 1.9 to 5.6 µg/mL (Eagan et al 1982a). The elimination of DAG was biphasic with an α half-life of 3.9 minutes and a β half-life of 31.3 minutes (Eagan et al 1982a). In one patient, urinary DAG elimination accounted for only 4.4% of the dose and disposition was otherwise normal in a few patients with abnormal liver or renal function. Overall, the primary route of DAG elimination is metabolism to a series of very polar metabolites which are excreted in the urine.

Pharmacokinetic studies with radiolabeled DAG demonstrated similar β half-lives of 40 minutes following intravenous injection and 80 minutes following oral administration (Horvath et al 1986). Interindividual absorption of oral DAG varies substantially as evidenced by the fractional absorption of 41 to 97% of the oral dose. The apparent volume of distribution ranged from 12 to 30 L, and about 20 to 30% of the drug is bound to plasma proteins. DAG appears to cross the blood–brain barrier into the cerebrospinal fluid. It also penetrates into malignant effusions but the extent of uptake has not been quantitated. Uptake into cerebrospinal fluid amounted to about 40% of the simultaneous plasma level (Horvath et al 1986). The half-life of DAG elimination from the cerebrospinal fluid was prolonged and averaged 20 hours (range, 3–24 hours) (Eckkardt et al 1977).

■ Side Effects and Toxicity

The dose-limiting toxic effect of DAG is myelosuppression, and thrombocytopenia is usually considered to be more severe than leukopenia (Haas et al 1976). Platelet function is depressed by DAG using in vitro aggregation assays (Kubisz et al 1981). In some trials there was an indication of cumulative myelosuppression (Perry et al 1976). Gastrointestinal toxicity consisting of mild to moderate nausea and vomiting is uncommon (Chiuten et al 1981).

Phlebitis and necrosis on extravasation have also been reported with intravenous DAG infusions (Vogel et al 1976). Other rare toxic effects include alopecia (Ahmann et al 1976), stomatitis, blurred vision, and/or paresthesias (Vogel et al 1976). Renal and hepatic toxic effects have not been reported with DAG.

REFERENCES

Ahmann DL, Bisel HF, Edmonson JH, et al. Phase II study of VP-16-213 versus dianhydrogalactitol in patients with metastatic malignant melanoma. *Cancer Treat Rep.* 1976;**60**:1681–1682.

Ahmann DL, O'Connell MJ, Bisel HF et al. Phase II study of dianhydrogalactitol and ICRF-159 in patients with advanced breast cancer previously exposed to cytotoxic chemotherapy. *Cancer Treat Rep.* 1977;**61**:81–82.

Barranco SC, Flournoy DR. Cell killing, kinetics, and recovery responses induced by 1,2:5,6-dianhydrogalactitol in dividing and nondividing cells in vitro. *J Natl Cancer Inst.* 1977;**58**:657–663.

Bence J, Somfai-Relle S Gati E. Development and some characteristics of a P388 leukemia strain resistant to 1,2:5,6-dianhydrogalactitol. *Eur J Cancer Clin Oncol.* 1986;**22**:773–780.

Blum RH, Skarin AT. Galactitol (G). Phase I–II study. *Proc Am Assoc Cancer Res Am Soc Clin Oncol.* 1976;**17**:272.

Chiuten DF, Rozencweig M, Von Hoff DD, Muggia FM. Clinical trials with the hexitol derivatives in the U.S. *Cancer.* 1981;**47**:442–451.

Creagan ET, Eagan RT, Kvols LK. Preliminary study of the combination, dianhydrogalactitol, *cis*-diamminedichloroplatinum(II), and VP-16-213 in patients with advanced cancer. *Oncology.* 1981;**38**:260–261.

Eagan RT, Ames MM, Powis G, Kovach JS. Clinical and pharmacologic evaluation of split-dose intermittent therapy with dianhydrogalactitol. *Cancer Treat Rep.* 1982a;**66**:283–287.

Eagan RT, Creagan ET, Bisel HF, et al. Phase II studies of dianhydrogalactitol-based combination chemotherapy for recurrent brain tumors. *Oncology.* 1981a;**38**:4–6.

Eagan RT, Dinapoli RP, Hermann RC Jr. et al. Combination carmustine (BCNU) and dianhydrogalactitol in the treatment of primary brain tumors recurring after irradiation. *Cancer Treat Rep.* 1982b;**66**:1647–1649.

Eagan RT, Frytak S, Nichols WC, et al. Phase II study of the combination of dianhydrogalactitol, doxorubicin, and cisplatin (DAP) in patients with advanced squamous cell lung cancer. *Cancer Treat Rep.* 1981b;**65**:517–519.

Eagan R, Moertel C, Hahn R, et al. Phase I study of a five day intermittent schedule for 1,2:5,6-dianhydrogalactitol (NSC-132313). *J Natl Cancer Inst.* 1976;**56**:179–181.

Eckhardt S, Csetenyi J, Horvath IP, et al. Uptake of labeled dianhydrogalactitol into human gliomas and nervous tissue. *Cancer Treat Rep.* 1977;**61**:841–847.

Edmonson JH, Frytak S, Letendre L, et al. Phase II evaluation of dianhydrogalactitol in advanced head and neck carcinomas. *Cancer Treat Rep.* 1979;**63**:2081–2083.

Elson LA, Jarman M, Ross WCJ. Toxicity, haematological effects and antitumour activity of epoxides derived from disubstituted hexitols. Mode of action of mannitol Myleran and dibromomannitol. *Eur J Cancer.* 1968;**4**:617–625.

Espana P, Wiernik PH, Walker MD. Phase II study of dianhydrogalactitol in malignant glioma. *Cancer Treat Rep.* 1978;**62**:1199–1200.

Finklestein JZ, Shore N, Krivit W, et al. Phase II trial of dianhydrogalactitol in the treatment of children with refractory childhood malignancies: A report from the Children's Cancer Study Group. *Cancer Treat Rep.* 1985;**69**:1331–1333.

Gastrointestinal Tumor Study Group. Phase II trials of hexamethylmelamine, dianhydrogalactitol, razoxane, and β-2'-deoxythioguanosine as single agents against advanced measurable tumors of the pancreas. *Cancer Treat Rep.* 1985;**69**:713–716.

Haas CD, Baker L, Thigpen T. Phase II evaluation of

dianhydrogalactitol in lung cancer: A Southwest Oncology Group study. *Cancer Treat Rep.* 1981;**65**:115–117.

Haas CD, Lehane D, Bottomley R. Phase II evaluation of galactitol in head and neck cancer: A Southwest Oncology Group study. *Med Pediatr Oncol.* 1983;**11**:281–283.

Haas CD, Stephens RL, Hollister M, Hoogstraten B. Phase I evaluation of dianhydrogalactitol (NSC-132313). *Cancer Treat Rep.* 1976;**60**:611–614.

Hahn RG, Bauer M, Wolter J, et al. Phase II study of single-agent therapy with megestrol acetate, VP-16-213, cyclophosphamide, and dianhydrogalactitol in advanced renal cell cancer. *Cancer Treat Rep.* 1979;**63**:513–515.

Helson L, Rozsa P, Hajdu E, Helson J-L. Dianhydrogalactitol and neural tumors: An in vitro, in vivo preclinical evaluation. *Cancer Treat Rep.* 1980;**64**:1287–1294.

Higgins GR, Shore NA, Etcubanas E, et al. Dianhydrogalactitol: Phase I clinical and pharmacological studies in childhood cancer. *Proc Am Assoc Cancer Res Am Soc Clin Oncol.* 1976;**17**:165.

Hoogstratten B, O'Bryan R, Jones S. 1,2:5,6-Dianhydrogalactitol in advanced breast cancer. *Cancer Treat Rep.* 1978;**62**:841–842.

Horvath IP, Csetenyi J, Kerpel-Fronius S, et al. Pharmacokinetics and metabolism of dianhydrogalactitol (DAG) in patients: A comparison with the human disposition of dibromodulcitol (DBD). *Eur J Cancer Clin Oncol.* 1986;**22**:163–171.

Horvath IP, Institoris L. Influence of the chemical structure on the biological tendency of cytostatic compounds related to dibromomannitol. II. Mechanism of action. *Arzneimittelforschung.* 1967;**17**:145–149.

Kellner B, Nemeth L. 1,6-Dibromo-1,6-dideoxy-dulcitol: A new antitumoral agent. *Nature.* 1967;**213**:402–403.

Kubisz P, Seghier F, Klener P, Cronberg S. Influence of dianhydrogalactitol on some platelet functions in vitro. *Acta Haematol.* 1981;**66**:27–30.

Nemeth L, Istitoris L, Somfai S, et al. Pharmacologic and antitumor effects of 1,2:5,6-dianhydrogalactitol (NSC-132313). *Cancer Chemother Rep.* 1972;**56**:593–602.

Nomura K, Hoshino T, Deen DF, Knebel KD. Perturbed cell kinetics of 9L rat brain tumor cells following dianhydrogalactitol. *Cancer Treat Rep.* 1978;**62**:2055–2061.

Perry MC, Moertel CG, Schutt AJ, et al. Phase II studies of dianhydrogalactitol and VP-16-213 in colorectal cancer. *Cancer Treat Rep.* 1976;**60**:1247–1250.

Ratanatharathorn V, Baker LH, Balducci L, et al. Phase II trial of dianhydrogalactitol in advanced renal cell carcinoma: A Southwest Oncology Group study. *Cancer Treat Rep.* 1982;**66**:1231–1232.

Stehman FB, Blessing JA, Delgado G, Louka M. Phase II evaluation of dianhydrogalactitol in the treatment of advanced endometrial adenocarcinoma: A Gynecologic Oncology Group study. *Cancer Treat Rep.* 1983;**67**:737.

Stehman FB, Blessing JA, Homesley HD, et al. Phase II evaluation of dianhydrogalactitol in the treatment of advanced non-squamous cervical carcinoma. *Invest New Drugs.* 1984;**2**:331–333.

Stehman FB, Blom J, Blessing JA, et al. Phase II trial of galactitol 1,2:5,6-dianhydro (NSC-132313) in the treatment of advanced gynecologic malignancies: A Gynecologic Oncology Group study. *Gynecol Oncol.* 1983;**15**:381–390.

Thigpen JT, Al-Sarraf M, Hewlett JS. Phase II trial of dianhydrogalactitol in metastatic malignant melanoma: A Southwest Oncology Group study. *Cancer Treat Rep.* 1979;**63**:525–528.

Thigpen JT, Samson MK. Phase II trial of dianhydrogalactitol in advanced soft tissue and bony sarcomas: A Southwest Oncology Group study. *Cancer Treat Rep.* 1979;**63**:553–555.

Vats TS, Lui V, Trueworthy R, van Eys J. Phase II clinical trial of dianhydrogalactitol for remission induction in children with acute leukemia: A Southwest Oncology Group study. *Cancer Treat Rep.* 1981;**65**:121–122.

Vogel CL, Winton EF, Moore MR, Sohner S. Phase I trial of dianhydrogalactitol administered i.v. in a weekly schedule. *Cancer Treat Rep.* 1976;**60**:895–901.

Vogl SE, Seltzer V, Camacho F, Calanog A. Dianhydrogalactitol and cisplatin in combination for advanced cancer of the uterine cervix. *Cancer Treat Rep.* 1982;**66**:1809–1812.

Wienblat ME, Ortega JA, Higgins GR, Siegel SE. Dianhydrogalactitol in the treatment of children with primary brain tumors. *Cancer Treat Rep.* 1981;**65**:923–924.

Diaziquone

■ Other Names

AZQ; NSC-182986; aziridinyl benzoquinone; carbamic acid.

■ Chemistry

Structure of diaziquone

The chemical name of diaziquone is 1,4-cyclohexyldiene-1,4-dicarbamic acid, 2,5-bis(1-aziridinyl)-3,6-dioxo-,diethyl ester. The molecular weight is 364.4 and the molecular formula $C_{16}H_{20}N_4O_6$. The drug is highly lipophilic and solubility in water is only 0.5 mg/mL. The compound is largely un-ionized at physiologic pH (Driscoll et al 1979).

■ Antitumor Activity

Diaziquone is active in a variety of preclinical tumor models including P-388 and L-1210 leukemia, B-16 melanoma, Lewis lung carcinoma, colon-26 carcinoma, and human breast and ovarian tumor xenografts in nude mice (Bender et al 1983). The compound is also active in intracerebral tumors because of its relatively high lipid solubility and low ionization (Driscoll et al 1979).

In human clinical trials, diaziquone has produced partial response rates of 20% in patients with primary brain cancer (Bender et al 1983, Curt et al 1983). In combination with carmustine, diaziquone has produced partial response rates of 22 and 30% in patients with glioblastoma and anaplastic astrocytoma, respectively (Schold et al 1987). And, in combination with procarbazine, diaziquone produced partial responses in 12 and 47% of patients with glioblastoma and anaplastic astrocytoma, respectively (Schold et al 1987). As a single agent the compound has not demonstrated activity in lung cancer (including small cell cancer), leukemia, breast cancer, colorectal cancer, renal cancer, melanoma, and lymphoma (Bender et al 1983).

Diaziquone has also produced objective responses in pediatric patients with several types of advanced malignancies. Objective regressions were noted in 3/5 patients with brain tumors and in 3/45 patients with acute lymphocytic leukemia (Falletta et al 1990).

■ Mechanism of Action

The two aziridinyl groups on the molecule are believed to produce covalent DNA crosslinks following enzymatic activation (Akhtar et al 1975). By the use of alkaline elution techniques, diaziquone has been shown to produce DNA–protein crosslinks and a small number of DNA strand breaks which are repaired over time (King et al 1984). The strand-breaking activity of the drug appears to involve the transfer of an electron from a reduced diaziquone molecule to molecular oxygen (Szmigiero and Kohn 1984, Szmigiero et al 1984). It has also been suggested that diaziquone forms a free radical anion intermediate which may augment the cytotoxic effect of the drug (Gutierrez et al 1982).

Studies on the cellular pharmacology of the drug in human leukemic cells indicate that concentrations of 0.05 nmol/mL or greater are required for growth inhibition (Egorin et al 1985). In addition, DNA synthesis is more sensitive to diaziquone than is RNA synthesis. Protein synthesis is unaffected by the drug (Egorin et al 1985). The metabolism of diaziquone to an active alkylator can be mediated by hepatic microsomal enzymes and is observed in sensitive tumor cell lines. Cell killing by diaziquone is not cell cycle phase specific but is maximal in Chinese hamster ovary cells treated in late S to early G_2 phase (Barranco et al 1983). Of further interest, nondividing Chinese hamster ovary cells were still sensitive to diaziquone (Barranco et al 1983).

■ Availability and Storage

Diaziquone is investigationally available from the Warner Lambert Company to the National Cancer Institute. It is supplied in a three-component package containing (1) a 10-mL vial of 10 mg diaziquone powder, (2) a 0.5-mL ampule of sterile anhydrous N,N-dimethylacetamide, and (3) a 10-mL ampule containing 9.5 mL of sterile 0.01 M, pH 6.5 phosphate buffer (8.02 mg sodium phosphate dibasic heptahydrate and 9.04 mg sodium phosphate monobasic monohydrate in Sterile Water for Injection, USP). The unreconstituted powder and the reconstituted solution may be stored at room temperature (< 86°F) (Bender et al 1983).

■ Preparation for Use, Stability, and Admixture

The 10 mg diaziquone powder is first dissolved into the 0.5 mL N, N-dimethylacetamide solution. This is then further diluted into the 9.5 mL buffer solution. This solution contains 1 mg/mL diaziquone and 5% (v/v) dimethylacetamide at pH 6.5. It is particularly important to completely dissolve all the diaziquone in the dimethylacetamide. Solid crystals of diaziquone dissolve very slowly in the second buffer solution (National Cancer Institute 1987). It is also recommended that the use of plastic filters and syringes be avoided when reconstituting the drug.

Diaziquone solutions are most stable at a pH around 7.0 (17- to 19-day half-life). At a pH of 3, the half-life is only 1 hour and at a pH of 5.0 the half-life is 3.5 days. Thus, a final diaziquone 1 mg/mL solution is stable (> 90% activity) for 84 hours at room temperature (Poochikian and Cradock 1981).

If diluted further, diaziquone (0.02 mg/mL) is stable for 36, 44, and 60 hours in 5% Dextrose Injection, USP, 0.9% Sodium Chloride Injection, USP, and Lactated Ringers Injection, USP, respectively (Poochikian and Cradock 1981). Because of short stability, dilution in 5% dextrose injection is not recommended (Bender et al 1983).

High concentrations of diaziquone (1 mg/mL) in whole blood can produce substantial hemolysis (Bender et al 1983). Some of this effect is believed to be caused by the pharmaceutical vehicle and can be prevented by lowering the infusion rate to achieve a 1:16(v:v) ratio of 1 mg/mL drug solution: blood.

■ Administration

Diaziquone is typically administered as a 5- to 15-minute intravenous infusion in 150 mL of 0.9% sodium chloride (Curt et al 1983). An alternate method was designed to provide for prolonged diaziquone plasma levels above the cytotoxic threshold defined in vitro by Egorin et al (1985): 0.05 nmol/mL. To accomplish this, one third of the dose is administered as an infusion over 20 minutes and the remaining two thirds is given as a continuous intravenous infusion over 4 to 6 hours (Bjornsson et al 1985, Schold et al 1987). Diaziquone has also been administered as a continuous intravenous infusion for 5 days (Bender et al 1983). Slow infusion of more dilute solutions may also help prevent incompatible ratios of drug to blood (see Preparation for Use, Stability, and Admixture).

In childhood cancer, weekly doses were administered as a 4-hour infusion (Falletta et al 1990).

■ Special Precautions

Diaziquone has produced anaphylactoid reactions in a number of patients (Budman et al 1982). Emergency resuscitation supplies and equipment should be available when administering this agent. Also, careful attention must be paid to completely dissolving the drug in the dimethylacetamide solution.

■ Dosage

In solid tumor therapy, diaziquone is most often administered every 3 to 4 weeks at doses of 40 to 50 mg/m^2; however, studies done at the Mayo Clinic suggest that the maximally tolerated dose ranges from 22.5 to 27.5 mg/m^2 every 4 to 5 weeks (Frytak et al 1984). In one trial, 20 mg/m^2 was administered on days 1 and 8 of a 28-day cycle (Curt et al 1983). Daily doses range from 8 to 12 mg/m^2/d for 5 consecutive days (Bender et al 1983). Doses have usually been lowered by 25% in heavily pretreated patients.

In childhood cancer, recommended weekly doses were 18 mg/m^2 for patients with solid tumors and 30 mg/m^2 for patients with leukemia. Doses were given weekly for 4 consecutive weeks (Falletta et al 1990).

■ Drug Interactions

Diaziquone is rapidly inactivated in solutions with a low pH such as 5% Dextrose Injection, USP. The H$_2$ antihistamine cimetidine has been shown to significantly alter the disposition of diaziquone in cancer patients (Loo et al 1983). The effect is presumed to involve inhibition of microsomal metabolism by cimetidine. Patients receiving diaziquone and cimetidine had diaziquone clearance reduced from 200 to 100 mL/kg/h with a commensurate increase in the terminal elimination half-life from 46 to 125 hours. The volume of distribution increased from 14 to 17 L/kg with cimetidine in this study (Loo et al 1983). These results suggest that excess toxicity could result from the combination of cimetidine and diaziquone.

■ Pharmacokinetics

Diaziquone is rapidly distributed and eliminated following intravenous administration. When administered as a 15-minute infusion, the drug was found to have an initial distribution half-life of 2.8 minutes and an elimination half-life of 33 minutes (Schilsky et al 1982). A similar half-life was reported for prolonged infusions of diaziquone (Curt et al 1983). Peak levels obtained after doses of 23 to 28 mg/m^2 ranged from 2 to 8 µg/mL (Frytak et al 1984). The mean total body clearance of the drug was 517 mL/min and the volume of distribution was 15.8 L in adult patients. Cerebrospinal fluid levels of diaziquone ranged from 60 to 90 ng/mL in samples taken 60 to 90 minutes after an intravenous dose of 15 to 20 mg/m^2 (Schilsky et al 1982). This represented fractional cerebrospinal fluid/plasma concentration ratios of 0.21 to 1.4, confirming the high degree of central nervous system uptake originally demonstrated in animals.

Brain tumor levels of radiolabeled diaziquone tend to be between 48 and 85% of concurrent plasma levels following intravenous infusions over 15 minutes (Savaraj et al 1983), however, only 18 to 45% of the total radioactivity in the brain tumor and 30 to 56% in the plasma were unchanged drug, suggesting that metabolism is extensive. The highest drug levels in this study were found in liver, followed by kidney. Normal brain tissue drug levels were equivalent to those in the tumor. These levels ranged from 22 to 31 ng/g, respectively (Savaraj et al 1983). Other pharmacokinetic studies have confirmed that high concentrations of drug are achieved in glioblastoma tumor specimens removed from patients 1 to 2 hours after drug administration (Curt et al 1983). These levels ranged from 27 to 624 ng/g of brain tumor tissue.

Other authors have reported shorter plasma elimination half-lives for diaziquone. Griffin et al (1982) describe an 18-minute half-life. Similarly, Schilcher et al (1983) reported a β half-life of only 17 minutes. The reason for the discrepancy with the data of Schilsky et al is unknown, but clearly, the drug is rapidly eliminated.

Very little drug is excreted in the urine. This ranges from 0.1% to 0.2% of a dose (Schilcher et al 1983, Schilsky et al 1982). A large fraction of diaziquone is protein bound; from 75 to 90% of drug in the blood (Curt et al 1983).

When administered intraventricularly to rhesus monkeys, diaziquone was eliminated with half-lives of 32 and 39 minutes in ventricular and lumbar spaces, respectively. This rapid clearance rate was fivefold greater than would be expected for cerebrospinal fluid bulk flow, indicating transcapillary drug passage or metabolism within the cerebrospinal fluid (Zimm et al 1984). In a single patient given 0.5 mg intraventricularly, peak diaziquone levels of 56 μM were achieved. The half-life of drug in the ventricular cerebrospinal fluid of this patient was 1.65 hours (Zimm et al 1984) (see Special Applications).

■ Side Effects and Toxicity

The dose-limiting toxic effect of diaziquone is myelosuppression, although thrombocytopenia is also prominent. The nadir for white blood cell or platelet suppression is 15 to 20 days following a single 15-minute intravenous infusion (Schilsky et al 1982). Recovery is generally complete by day 28 in most patients, although one study reported cumulative myelosuppression following diaziquone (Frytak et al 1984). This cumulative toxicity occasionally necessitated an 8-week delay in retreatment. Anemia was also described in 25% of patients receiving a dose of 20 mg/m² in this trial. At doses above 25 mg/m², anemia was noted in all patients. In some studies, a cumulative increase in the degree of myelosuppression has been noted after several cycles (Curt et al 1983); however, most authors have described noncumulative myelotoxicity with diaziquone.

Other toxic effects include mild to moderate nausea and vomiting in 30 to 40% of patients; most patients require little or no antiemetic therapy (Schold et al 1987). Alopecia and diarrhea were quite rare at doses below 25 mg/m² (Schilsky et al 1982). Pulmonary, renal, and cardiac toxicity has not been described with diaziquone. Liver function test elevation and stomatitis are only rarely reported (Bender et al 1983).

Anaphylactoid reactions to diaziquone have been described in several patients (Budman et al 1982). These typically manifest as hypotension, itching, sneezing, erythema, and bronchospasm. An incidence of 0 to 1.5% has been suggested for this reaction. There is also one report of acute myelogenous leukemia in a patient treated with diaziquone for a recurrent brain tumor.

■ Special Applications

Intraventricular Administration. Diaziquone has been administered intraventricularly to a single patient with refractory meningeal leukemia. The diaziquone dose of 0.5 mg was diluted into Elliott's B solution and administered via an Ommaya reservoir. The AUC for intraventricular diaziquone was 35-fold higher than levels obtained after standard intravenous doses are administered (Bachur et al 1982). Pharmacokinetic studies of intraventricular diaziquone show a biphasic elimination pattern with mean half-lives of 18.2 and 78.6 minutes (see the table below). These findings also show that a high AUC is achievable in the cerebrospinal fluid following a 1- to 2-mg intraventricular dose of diaziquone in adults (Berg et al 1992). The table summarizes these results. Neurotoxicity has not been produced in either rhesus monkeys or humans given intraventricular diaziquone (Zimm et al 1984, Berg et al 1992). In the one patient described by

PHARMACOKINETICS OF INTRAVENTRICULAR DIAZIQUONE IN PATIENTS WITH REFRACTORY MENINGEAL CANCER

Dose/Schedule	AUC (μmol/L/min)	Peak Ventricular Level	Clearance (mL/min)	Half-life (min) α	Half-life (min) β
2 mg twice weekly	5917–54,975	38–237	0.1	8–16	50–150
1 mg twice weekly	8061–12,344	64–105	0.22–0.37	18–42	45–83

RESPONSE TO INTRATHECAL DIAZIQUONE FOR REFRACTORY MENINGEAL CANCER

Dose/Schedule	Total Courses	Response Rate*/Number of Assessable Patients	
		CR	PR
2 mg twice weekly	6	1/3	1/3
1 mg twice weekly	9	3/8	4/8
0.5 mg every 6 h × 3, weekly	18	7/15	4/15

*CR, complete response; PR, partial response.

Zimm et al, intraventricular diaziquone produced a greater than 90% decrease in cerebrospinal fluid leukemic blast cells (Zimm et al 1984).

Intrathecal Administration. Two schedules of intrathecal diaziquone have been evaluated in patients with refractory meningeal malignancies. Diaziquone was administered either twice weekly at a dose of 1 or 2 mg, or weekly every 6 hours for three doses at a dose of 0.5 mg for each injection (Berg et al 1992). The dose-limiting toxic effect with the twice-weekly schedule was headache (three of six patients) and nausea or vomiting (two of six patients) at the 2 mg dose. The incidence of toxicity was halved at the 1-mg dose. The every-6-hour, 0.5-mg dosing schedule produced the same general pattern of toxicity as the 2-mg twice-weekly dose. In patients with assessable tumors, complete plus partial response rates were relatively high even though all patients were previously irradiated (see the table above). There were no significant differences in response rates between the twice-weekly and every-6-hour regimens. For all patients, the mean duration of complete response was 3.2 months (range, 0.5–9 months). Importantly, no chronic toxic effects were observed in this trial.

For the intrathecal trials, 10 mg diaziquone was dissolved in 0.5 mL of N,N-dimethylacetamide and then diluted with 9.5 mL sterile phosphate buffer, pH 6.5. This 1 mg/mL solution was then further diluted with Elliott's B solution to a final concentration not greater than 0.5 mg/mL. The intrathecal injections were isovolumetric in that an equal amount of cerebrospinal fluid was removed immediately prior to drug injection.

REFERENCES

Akhtar MH, Begleiter A, Johnson D, Lown JW, McLaughlin L, Sim S-K. Studies related to antitumor antibiotics. Part VI. Correlation of covalent cross-linking of DNA by bifunctional aziridinoquinones with their antineoplastic activity. *Cancer J Chem*. 1975;53:2891–2905.

Bachur NR, Collins JM, Kelley JA, et al. Diaziquone, 2,5-diaziridinyl-3,6-bis-carboethoxyamino-1,4-benzoquinone, plasma and cerebrospinal fluid kinetics. *Clin Pharmacol Ther*. 1982;31:650–655.

Barranco SC, Schechter GA, Boerwinkle WR, Howell KA, Rubin NH. Survival and cell cycle kinetics responses of Chinese hamster ovary cells, and clones of human adenocarcinoma of the stomach and astrocytoma to diaziquone (AZQ) in vitro. *Invest New Drugs*. 1983;1:11–20.

Bender JF, Grillo-Lopez AJ, Posada JG Jr. Diaziquone (AZQ). *Invest New Drugs*. 1983;1:71–84.

Berg SL, Balis FM, Zimm S, et al. Phase I/II trial and pharmacokinetics of intrathecal diaziquone in refractory meningeal malignancies. *J Clin Oncol*. 1992;10(1):143–148.

Bjornsson TD, Schold SC, Friedman HS, Schneider D, Falletta JM. Pharmacokinetics of diaziquone after three different dosage regimens. *Cancer Treat Rep*. 1985;69(12):1383–1385.

Budman DR, Schulman P, Vinciguerra V, Weiselberg L, Degnan TJ. Anaphylactoid reaction due to AZQ. *Cancer Chemother Pharmacol*. 1982;8:317.

Curt GA, Kelley JA, Kufta CV, et al. Phase II and pharmacokinetic study of aziridinylbenzoquinone [2,5-diaziridinyl-3,6-bis(carboethoxyamino)-1,4-benzoquinone, diaziquone, NSC-182986] in high-grade gliomas. *Cancer Res*. 1983;43:6102–6105.

Driscoll JS, Dudeck L, Congleton G, Geran RI. Potential CNS antitumor agents. VI. Aziridinylbenzoquinones III. *J Pharm Sci*. 1979;68:185–188.

Egorin MJ, Fox BM, Spiegel JF, Gutierrez PL, Friedman RD, Bachur NR. Cellular pharmacology in murine and human leukemic cell lines of diaqiquone (NSC-182986). *Cancer Res*. 1985;45:992–999.

Falletta JM, Cushing B, Lauer S, et al. Phase I evaluation of diaziquone in childhood cancer. A Pediatric Oncology Group study. *Invest New Drugs*. 1990;8:167–170.

Frytak S, Eagan RT, Ames MM, et al. Phase I study of diaziquone. *Cancer Treat Rep*. 1984;68(7/8):975–978.

Griffin JP, Newman RA, McCormack JJ, Krakoff IH. Clinical and clinical pharmacologic studies of aziridinylbenzoquinone. *Cancer Treat Rep*. 1982;66:1321–1325.

Gutierrez PL, Friedman RD, Bachur NR. Biochemical activation of AZQ [3,6-diaziridinyl-2,5-bis(carboethoxyamino)-1,4-benzoquinone] to its free radical species. *Cancer Treat Rep.* 1982;**66**:339–342.

King CL, Hittelman WN, Loo TL. Induction of DNA strand breaks and cross links by 2,5-diaziridinyl-3,6-bis(carboethoxyamino)-1,4-benzoquinone in Chinese hamster ovary cells. *Cancer Res.* 1984;**44**:5634–5637.

Loo TL, Yap BS, Lu K, Savaraj N. Effects of cimetidine on the clinical pharmacokinetics of 2,5-diaziridinyl-3,6-bis(carboethoxyamino)-1,4-benzoquinone (AZQ, NSC-182986). *Clin Pharmacol Ther.* 1983;**31**(2):245.

National Cancer Institute. *NCI Investigational Drugs: Pharmaceutical Data.* NIH Publication No. 88-241. Washington, DC: U.S. Department of Health and Human Services; 1987:90–93.

Poochikian GK and Cradock JC. 2,5-Diaziridinyl-3,6-bis(carboethoxyamino)-1,4-benzoquinone. I. Kinetics in aqueous solutions by high-performance liquid chromatography. *J Pharm Sci.* 1981;**70**(2):159–162.

Savaraj N, Lu K, Feun LG, et al. Intracerebral penetration and tissue distribution of 2,5-diaziridinyl 3,6-bis(carboethoxyamino)-1,4-benzoquinone(AZQ, NSC-182986). *J Neuro-Oncol.* 1983;**1**:15–19.

Schilcher RB, Young JD, Leichman LP, Haas CD, Baker LH. Phase I evaluation and pharmacokinetics of aziridinylbenzoquinone using a weekly intravenous schedule. *Cancer Res.* 1983;**43**:3907–3911.

Schilsky RL, Kelley JA, Ihde DC, Howser DM, Cordes RS, Young RC. Phase I trial and pharmacokinetics of aziridinylbenzoquinone (NSC-182986) in humans. *Cancer Res.* 1982;**42**:1582–1586.

Schold SC Jr, Mahaley MS Jr, Vick NA, et al. Phase II diaziquone-based chemotherapy trials in patients with anaplastic supratentorial astrocytic neoplasms. *J Clin Oncol.* 1987;**5**:464–471.

Szmigiero L, Erickson LC, Ewig RA, Kohn KW. DNA strand scission and cross-linking by diaziridinylbenzoquinone (diaziquone) in human cells and relation to cell killing. *Cancer Res.* 1984;**44**:4447–4452.

Szmigiero L, Kohn KW. Mechanisms of DNA strand breakage and interstrand cross-linking by diaziridinylbenzoquinone (diaziquone) in isolated nuclei from human cells. *Cancer Res.* 1984;**44**:4453–4457.

Zimm S, Collins JM, Curt GA, et al. Cerebrospinal fluid pharmacokinetics of intraventricular and intravenous aziridinylbenzoquinone. *Cancer Res.* 1984;**44**:1698–1701.

Dibromodulcitol

■ Other Names

NSC-104800; CAS Registry No. 10318-26-0; DBD; mitolactol; Mitolac® (Bristol-Myers); Elobromol® (Chinoin).

■ Chemistry

$$\begin{array}{c} CH_2-Br \\ | \\ H-C-OH \\ | \\ HO-C-H \\ | \\ HO-C-H \\ | \\ H-C-OH \\ | \\ CH_2-Br \end{array}$$

Structure of dibromodulcitol

Dibromodulcitol (DBD) is an omega-substituted hexitol with the molecular formula $C_6H_{12}Br_2O_4$ and a molecular weight of 308.0. It is described chemically as 1,6-dibromo-1,6-dideoxy-galactitol and has a melting point of 186 to 190°C. It is soluble in dimethylacetamide (6000 mg/100 mL) and water (30–40 mg/100 mL) and is poorly soluble in 10% ethanol or normal saline (5 mg/100 mL). Structurally, dibromodulcitol is similar to dianhydrogalactitol, mannitol Myleran, and dibromomannitol (Horvath and Institoris 1967). Chiuten et al (1981) have published a review comparing the hexitol derivatives dibromomannitol, dibromodulcitol, and dianhydrogalactitol.

■ Antitumor Activity

Dibromodulcitol is still an investigational antitumor agent in the United States. In early clinical trials the drug had hints of activity in patients with melanoma (Bellet et al 1978), breast cancer (Andrews et al 1971), Hodgkin's and non-Hodgkin's lymphoma (Andrews et al 1974), and colorectal carcinoma and in maintenance regimens for patients with acute lymphoblastic or undifferentiated leukemia. Of note is that patients maintained with the drug had lower incidence of central nervous system leukemia (Sitarz et al 1975).

Although DBD has been used in combination regimens for the treatment of patients with breast cancer, the contribution of the drug to the activity of the regimens against breast cancer is not clear (Skeel et al 1989, Falkson et al 1982). Single-agent activity against breast cancer is limited (Creech et al 1984).

More recently, Stehman et al (1989) have documented that DBD gave a 2% complete and a 27% partial response rate in patients with squamous cell carcinoma of the cervix.

A 10% response rate has been seen in patients with non-small cell lung cancer (Sorensen et al 1988, Brubaker et al 1986, Eagen et al 1981). Response rates of 9 to 24% in patients with metastatic melanoma have been reported by a number of investigators (Amato et al 1987, Simmonds et al 1985, Malden et al 1984). The response rate has not been as high in other studies (Medina and Kirkwood 1982, Hopkins et al 1984, Murray et al 1985).

Some activity of DBD has been seen in patients with squamous cell carcinoma of the bladder in Egypt (Gad-el-Maula et al 1989). Of interest is the finding that DBD is active in the treatment of metastatic hemangiopericytoma (Conroy et al 1982). The drug has not been found to be active in patients with other types of sarcomas (Borden et al 1982). The drug appears inactive in patients with squamous cell carcinoma of the head and neck (McHale et al 1986, Issell et al 1982). The drug also appears inactive in patients with colorectal and kidney cancer (Mischler et al 1981, Locker et al 1984). DBD has begun to be used in bone marrow transplantation regimens (Ratanatharathorn et al 1987).

Dibromodulcitol has been used in combination regimens for patients with brain tumors (adults and children). The contribution of DBD to the efficacy of those regimens is unclear (Elliot et al 1986, Afra et al 1983). The drug has had a 50% response rate in patients with medulloblastoma (Levin et al 1984). In combination with radiation therapy, DBD is as effective as radiation therapy + carmustine for control of high-grade astrocytomas (Elliott et al 1986).

■ Mechanism of Action

Dibromodulcitol is a halogenated sugar alcohol that appears to act primarily as an alkylating agent (Csanyi and Halasz 1967). In isolated systems Hidvegi et al (1967) described the metabolic effect of brominated hexitols as inhibition of DNA, RNA, and protein synthesis (in descending order of inhibition). Apparently, however, not all the drug's actions are explained on the basis of alkylation because (1) in vitro, nitrogen mustard has substantially greater alkylating activity; (2) aklyl group transfer is not absolutely required for drug activity; and (3) the chemical (alkylation) bonds formed are uncharacteristically more stable than with classic alkylating drugs (Institoris et al 1967). Dibromodulcitol only weakly and probably indirectly affects protein synthesis. After in vitro drug exposure, cytoplasmic alterations appear to precede nuclear aberrations (Palyi 1967); however, inhibition of nucleic acid synthesis or of an intermediate metabolic step in this process probably constitutes the major area for drug effects.

One recent finding is that tumor cells in hypoxic and slightly acidic conditions are more susceptible to dibromodulcitol (Jeney et al 1990).

■ Availability and Storage

Dibromodulcitol is an investigational agent available from the National Cancer Institute in 25-mg tablets. These also contain avicel and talc as excipients. The tablets are stable at least 2 years and may be stored at room temperature.

■ Preparation for Use, Stability, and Admixture

No preparation of the tablets is necessary. The tablets are stable for 2 years.

■ Administration

Dibromodulcitol is taken orally. Some investigators (Bellet et al 1978) have found that administration of the drug at bedtime may alleviate any gastrointestinal side effects.

■ Special Precautions

A number of authors have found that DBD is associated with an increased incidence of myelodysplastic syndrome or acute nonlymphocytic leukemia (Falkson et al 1989, 1990). Not all investigators have agreed with these findings (Bellet 1990, Szuts and Virag-Szasz 1990).

■ Drug Interactions

Antitumor therapeutic synergism has been described for dibromodulcitol combined with cyclophosphamide, doxorubicin and 5-fluorouracil in experimental animal tumor systems (Mischler et al 1979).

■ Dosage

Andrews et al (1971), in a phase I study, explored doses ranging from 0.25 to 5.0 mg/kg/d for 14 to 60 days. They recommended a dose for future studies of 3.5 mg/kg/d × 42 days. Sellei et al (1969) had earlier reported effective and well-tolerated doses of 5 mg/kg/d given until leukopenia occurred. Keyes et al (1971) found a daily dose of 200 mg/m² to be excessively myelotoxic, whereas at 100 mg/m² myelosuppression could not consistently be produced. They therefore recommended 130 mg/m²/d, an intermediate dose producing mild to moderate myelosuppression in four of five patients studied at that level.

As remission maintenance therapy in acute leukemia, Sitarz et al (1975) compared continuous dibromodulcitol with cyclophosphamide, both drugs given at 3 mg/kg/d until relapse. In a more recent phase II investigation, Bellet et al (1978) used DBD in patients with refractory metastatic melanoma. They treated them with 100 mg/m²/d until hematologic toxicity occurred.

Dosage adjustment is usually based on hematologic toxicity parameters. In this regard Bellet et al (1978) have successfully applied a 50% reduction for a white blood cell count between 2000 and 4000 cells/mm³ (100% of dose for white blood cell count ≥ 4000). Below a white blood cell count of 2000 or thrombocytopenia less than 50,000, the drug was not given. Thus an established dosage range for dibromodulcitol would appear to be 3 to 3.5 mg/kg/d or 130 mg/m²/d administered continuously until mild hematologic suppression.

Most recently, Kelley et al (1986) performed a single-dose repeated monthly trial of DBD. The recommended dose was 1500 to 1800 mg/m². The most commonly used dose in the phase II trial is 100 mg/m²/d orally × 35 days. Dose escalations are used if minimal hematologic toxic effects are noted (Simmonds et al 1985, Hopkins et al 1984).

■ Pharmacokinetics

Bellej et al (1972) studied the pharmacokinetics of ^{14}C-labeled dibromodulcitol. After oral administration of 15 mg/kg, systemic blood levels were observed in 15 minutes, denoting rapid absorption. Maximum blood levels of 15 to 20/µg/ml were obtained 1 hour after ingestion and were maintained for up to 3 hours; however, the parent molecule is rapidly hydrolyzed in plasma to various epoxies and debrominated derivatives including monobromodulcitol. Thus, the half-life of intact dibromodulcitol is short, although the radiolabeled metabolites decay more slowly with a plasma half-life of 8 hours. By 48 hours all of the radiolabel has been eliminated. At least three of the metabolites are stable epoxies capable of significant alkylation.

Bellej et al also found that the labeled metabolites appeared to penetrate biologic membranes well, producing concentrations roughly 50% of the simultaneous plasma concentration in cerebrospinal, ascitic, and pleural fluids, 5 hours after administration. Similar findings using neutron activation analyses were also noted by Sziklai et al (1990). The metabolites also appear to distribute well throughout most body tissues, including tumor tissues. Although protein binding is insignificant, the red blood cell appears to bind the drug firmly, producing red blood cell/plasma ratios of 0.43 at 1 hour and 0.95 at 24 hours.

Renal excretion appears to provide the predominant route of elimination for dibromodulcitol and its metabolites. Thus, within 48 hours of administration 70 to 80% of administered radioactivity may be recovered in the urine. The largest fractional urinary elimination rate occurs 3 to 6 hours after oral administration. This constitutes an early excretion rate of 5% per hour. Covalently bound bromide elimination initially parallels this rate. After the first 4-hour period though, urinary covalent bromide elimination slows considerably. Approximately 4 to 6% of drug bromide is excreted as free bromide over 48 hours.

More recently Kelley et al (1986) noted that the kinetics of DBD followed a one-compartment model with first-order absorption and elimination. The mean half-life of DBD in plasma was 158 minutes. The elimination constant was 0.005 ± 0.002 minute. The apparent volume of distribution was 1.03 ± 0.4 L/kg. The peak level was 47.1 ± 16.8 µmol/L. Elimination was reduced in patients with abnormal hepatic function. The half-life in the Kelley et al study was much shorter than the half-life of 4 to 8 hours of total radioactivity in plasma noted by Horvath et al (1982).

■ Side Effects and Toxicity

Hematologic depression, particularly thrombocytopenia, is the usual dose-limiting toxic effect of dibromodulcitol (Andrews et al 1971, 1974, Bellet et al 1978). It is most often noted with a nadir by day 35 (Bellet et al 1978).

Leukopenia, severe granulocytopenia, and anemia are also side effects of the drug (Kelley et al 1986). Other toxic effects noted include nausea and vomiting (<20% of patients), transient liver enzyme elevations in 7% of patients, pruritus and vertigo, skin pigmentation, and, rarely, elevation of the blood urea nitrogen.

As noted under Special Precautions, DBD appears to be leukemogenic (Falkson et al 1989).

■ Special Applications

None have been noted to date.

REFERENCES

Afra D, Kocsis B, Dobay J, Eckhardt S. Combined radiotherapy and chemotherapy with dibromodulcitol and CCNU in the postoperative treatment of malignant gliomas. *J Neurosurg.* 1983;**59**(1):106–110.

Amato DA, Bruckner H, Guerry D IV, et al. Phase II evaluation of dibromodulcitol and actinomycin D, hydroxyurea, and cyclophosphamide in previously untreated patients with malignant melanoma. *Invest New Drugs.* 1987;**5**(3):293–297.

Andrews NC, Weiss AJ, Ansfield FJ, Rochlin DB, Mason JH. Phase I study of dibromodulcitol (NSC-104800). *Cancer Chemother Rep.* 1971;**55**:61–65.

Andrews NC, Weiss AJ, Wilson W, Nealon T. Phase II study of dibromodulcitol (NSC-104800). *Cancer Chemother Rep.* 1974;**58**:653–660.

Bellej MA, Troetel WM, Weiss AJ, Strambaugh JE, Manthei RW. The absorption and metabolism of dibromodulcitol in patients with advanced cancer. *Clin Pharmacol Ther.* 1972;**13**:563–572.

Bellet RE. Bone marrow stem cell disorders and mitolactol (letter). *J Clin Oncol.* 1990;**8**(4):751.

Bellet RE, Catalano RB, Mastrangelo MJ, Berd D. Positive phase II trial of dibromodulcitol in patients with metastatic melanoma refractory to DTIC and nitrosourea. *Cancer Treat Rep.* 1978;**62**(12):2095–2099.

Borden EC, Ash A, Enterline HT, et al. Phase II evaluation of dibromodulcitol, ICRF-159, and maytansine for sarcomas. *Am J Clin Oncol.* 1982;**5**(4):417–420.

Brubaker LH, Nelson MO Jr, Birch R, Williams S. Treatment of advanced adenocarcinoma of the kidney with mitolactol: A Southwestern Cancer Study Group trial. *Cancer Treat Rep.* 1986;**70**(2):305–306.

Chiuten DF, Rozencweig M, Von Hoff DD, Muggia FM. Clinical trials with the hexitol derivatives in the U.S. *Cancer.* 1981;**47**:442–451.

Conroy JF, Roda PI, Prasasvinichal S. Dibromodulcitol in the treatment of metastatic hemangiopericytoma. *Am J Clin Oncol.* 1982;**5**(4):453–456.

Creech RH, Catalano RB, Dierks KM, Shah MK. Phase II study of mitolactol in chemotherapy-refractory metastatic breast cancer. *Cancer Treat Rep.* 1984;**68**(12):1499–1501.

Csanyi E, Halasz M. Cross-resistance studies on 1,6-dibromodideoxy-D-mannitol (DBM)-resistant Yoshida SC sarcoma. *Br J Cancer.* 1967;**21**:353–357.

Eagen RT, Frytak S, Nichols WC, et al. Evaluation of an intermittent schedule of mitolactol in advanced non-small cell lung cancer. *Cancer Treat Rep.* 1981;**65**(11/12):1099–1101.

Elliott T, Dinapoli R, O'Fallon J, et al. Randomized trial of radiation therapy (RT) plus dibromodulcitol (DBD) vs RT plus BCNU in high grade astrocytoma (meeting abstract). *Proc Annu Meet Am Soc Clin Oncol.* 1986;**5**:130.

Falkson G, Gelman RS, Dreicer R, et al. Myelodysplastic syndrome and acute nonlymphocytic leukemia secondary to mitolactol treatment in patients with breast cancer. *J Clin Oncol.* 1989;**7**(9):1252–1259.

Falkson G, Gelman RS, Tormey DC, Bennett JM. Reply (letter). *J Clin Oncol* 1990;**8**(4):751–753.

Falkson G, Pretorius L, Falkson HC. Dibromodulcitol in the treatment of breast cancer. *Cancer Treat Rev.* 1982;**9**(4):261–266.

Gad-el-Maula N, Hamza MR, Zikri ZK, et al. Chemotherapy in invasive carcinoma of the bladder. A review of phase II trials in Egypt. *Acta Oncol.* 1989;**28**(1):73–76.

Hidvegi EJ, Lonai P, Holland J, Antoni F, Institoris L, Horvath IP. The effect of mannitolmyleran and two new dibromohexitols on the metabolic activities on nucleic acids and proteins, I. *Biochem Pharmacol.* 1967;**16**:2143–2153.

Hopkins J, Richards F, Case D. et al. A phase II study of dibromodulcitol (DBD) in stage IV melanoma. *Am J Clin Oncol.* 1984;**7**:555–556.

Horvath IP, Csetenyl J, Hindy I, et al. Metabolism and pharmacokinetics of dibromodulcitol (DBD, NSC-104800) in man. II. Pharmacokinetics of DBD. *Eur J Cancer Clin Oncol.* 1982;**18**(11):1211–1219.

Horvath IP, Institoris L. Influence of the chemical structure on the biological tendency of cytostatic compounds related to dibromomannitol. I. Structure–activity correlations. *Arzneim Forsch.* 1967;**17**:145–149.

Institoris L, Horvath IP, Pethes G. Some characteristic features of the biotransport of the cytostatic agent 1,6-dibromo-1,6-di-deoxy-dulcitol. *Int J Cancer.* 1967;**2**:21–25.

Issell BF, Borsos G, D'Aoust JB, Banhidy F, Crooke ST, Eckhardt S. Dibromodulcitol plus bleomycin compared with bleomycin alone in head and neck cancer. *Cancer Chemother Pharmacol.* 1982;**8**(2):171–173.

Jeney A, Lapis K, Papay J, Nagy-Olahne II. Further studies on the mode of action of dibromodulcitol. *Am Assoc Cancer Res.* 1990;**31**:2360.

Kelley SL, Peters WP, Anderson J, Furlog EA, Frei E III, Henner WD. Pharmacokinetics of dibromodulcitol in humans: A phase I study. *J Clin Oncol.* 1986;**4**(5):753–761.

Keyes JW, Selawry OS, Hansen HH. Initial clinical trials of dibromodulcitol (NSC-104800) in patients with advanced cancer. *Cancer Chemother Rep.* 1971;**55**:583–589.

Levin VA, Edwards MS, Gutin PH, et al. Phase II evaluation of dibromodulcitol in the treatment of recurrent medulloblastoma, ependymoma, and malignant astrocytoma. *J Neurosurg.* 1984;**61**(6):1063–1068.

Locker GY, Lanzotti V, Sweet D, et al. Phase II trial of mitolactol in previously treated and untreated patients with advanced colorectal cancer: An Illinois Cancer Council trial. *Cancer Treat Rep.* 1984;**68**(10):1303–1304.

Malden LT, Coates AS, Milton GW, et al. Mitolactol chemotherapy for malignant melanoma: A phase II study. *Cancer Treat Rep.* 1984;**68**(7/8):1045–1046.

McHale MS, Velez-Garcia E, Nelson O, Williams SD, Maddox W, Birch R. Phase II evaluation of mitolactol in squamous cell carcinoma of the head and neck: A Southwestern Cancer Study Group trial. *Cancer Treat Rep.* 1986;**70**(7):925–926.

Medina W, Kirkwood JM. Phase II trials of mitolactol in patients with metastatic melanoma. *Cancer Treat Rep.* 1982;**66**(1):195–196.

Mischler NE, Earhart RH, Carr B, Tormey DC. Dibromodulcitol. *Cancer Treat Rev.* 1979;**6**:191–204.

Mischler NE, Tormey DC, Klotz J, et al. Phase II study of dibromodulcitol in colorectal, kidney, and other carcinomas. *Cancer Clin Trials.* 1981;**4**(4):407–410.

Murray N, Silver H, Shah A, Wilson K. Phase II study of mitolactol in advanced malignant melanoma. *Cancer Treat Rep.* 1985;**69**(6):723–724.

Palyi I. Effect of antitumor agents: Degranol, mannitol Myeleran, dibromomannitol and dibromodulcitol on cell morphology in tissue cultures. *Neoplasma (Bratis).* 1967;**14**:159–166.

Ratanatharathorn V, Karanes C, Lewkow L, et al. High-dose L-Pam and dibromodulcitol (DBD) followed by autologous bone marrow transplant in patients with metastatic malignant melanoma. A phase I–II study (meeting abstract). *Proc Annu Meet Am Assoc Cancer Res.* 1987;**28**:217.

Sellei C, Eckhardt S, Horvath IP, Kralovansky J, Istitoris L. Clinical and pharmacologic experience with dibromodulcitol (NSC-104800), a new antitumor agent. *Cancer Chemother Rep.* 1969;**53**:377–383.

Simmonds MA, Lipton A, Harvey HA, Ellison N, White DS. Phase II study of mitolactol in metastatic malignant melanoma. *Cancer Treat Rep.* 1985;**69**(1):65–67.

Sitarz AL, Albo V, Movassaghi N, et al. Dibromodulcitol (NSC-104800) compared with cyclophosphamide (NSC-26271) as remission maintenance therapy in previously treated children with acute lymphoblastic leukemia or acute undifferentiated leukemia: Possible effectiveness in reducing the incidence of central nervous system leukemia. *Cancer Chemother Rep Part I.* 1975;**59**(5):989–994.

Skeel RT, Anderson JW, Tormey DC, Benson AB III, Asbury RF, Falkson G. Combination chemotherapy of advanced breast cancer. Comparison of dibromodulcitol, doxorubicin, vincristine, and fluoxymesterone and thiotepa, doxorubicin, vinblastine, and fluoxymesterone: An Eastern Cooperative Oncology Group study. *Cancer.* 1989;**64**(7):1393–1399.

Sorensen JB, Clerici M, Hensen HH. Single-agent chemotherapy for advanced adenocarcinoma of the lung: A review. *Cancer Chemother Pharmacol.* 1988;**21**(2):89–102.

Stehman FB, Blessing JA, McGehee R, Barrett RJ. A phase II evaluation of mitolactol in patients with advanced squamous cell carcinoma of the cervix: A Gynecologic Oncology Group study. *J Clin Oncol.* 1989;**7**(12):1892–1895.

Sziklai IL, Afra D, Ordogh M, Institoris L, Kerpel-Fronius S, Szabo E. The distribution of bromine content of dibromodulcitol in the central nervous system of patients with malignant gliomas. *Eur J Cancer.* 1990;**26**(2):79–82.

Szuts T, Virag-Szasz Z. Mitolactol: Further considerations (letter). *J Clin Oncol.* 1990;**8**(4):751.

Didemnin B

■ Other Names

NSC-325319.

■ Chemistry

Structure of didemnin B

Didemnin B is a potent depsipeptide isolated by Rinehart and co-workers (1981a, b) from the marine tunicate *Trididemnum*. The complete chemical name is *N*-(1-(*N*-(4-((3-hydroxy-*r*-((*N*-(1-(2-hydroxy-1-oxopropyl)-L-prolyl)-*N*-methyl-L-leucyl)-L-threonyl)-5-methyl-1-oxoheptyl)oxy)-2,5-dimethyl-1,3-dioxohexyl)-L-leucyl)-L-proly)-*N*,*O*-dimethyl-L-tyrosine, phi-lactone (9CI). The active compounds isolated from the tunicate include didemnins A, B, and C. All extracts inhibit in vitro growth of both DNA and RNA tumor viruses as well as L-1210 leukemia cells

(Rinehart et al 1981c,1983). Didemnin B (a derivative of didemnin A) is the most potent derivative in terms of inhibition of viral replication and also has the greatest *in vivo* antitumor activity. On the basis of these observations, didemnin B was chosen for further development as a new antineoplastic agent. In addition the didemnins represent a novel structure with novel ring peptide structures containing hydroxyisovalerylpropionate and a new stereoisomer of the highly unusual amino acid statine (Hamada et al, 1989, Hassain et al 1988). Didemnin B has a molecular weight of 1112 and the empiric formula $C_{57}H_{89}N_7O_{15}$. An excellent review article on the preclinical development of didemnin B has been published by Chun et al (1986).

■ Antitumor Activity

Didemnin B has been tested in a human tumor cloning system (Jiang et al 1983, Rossof et al 1983). There is a relationship between concentration and amount of *in vitro* activity. Continuous drug exposure produced greater cytotoxicity than short-term exposure. The spectrum of activity was rather wide, including leukemic cells and a variety of solid tumors such as breast, ovary, kidney, sarcoma, and mesothelioma (Jiang et al 1983). These data also indicate that for significant antitumor activity to be noted in the clinic, peak plasma concentrations need to range from 0.1 to 1.0 µg/mL.

At present, didemnin B is still undergoing phase I and II clinical trials. It remains an investigational agent. In phase II trials there has been some activity in patients with glioblastoma multiforme (one complete response) (Razis et al 1991). That finding is being followed up.

The drug has not had any antitumor activity in patients with renal cell carcinoma (Taylor et al 1989), colorectal cancer (Rossof et al 1989, Abbruzzese et al 1988), and non-small cell lung cancer (Murphy et al 1989). It was similarly inactive in patients with metastatic breast cancer (Benvenuto et al 1992).

■ Mechanism of Action

The mode of action of the didemnins in inhibiting L-1210 and viral growth is uncertain. By utilization of radiolabel incorporation techniques, both DNA and protein synthesis inhibition have been noted on treatment of L-1210 cells with didemnin A or B. There seems to be evidence that inhibition of DNA and protein synthesis is an important mechanism of action for didemnin B (Crampton et al 1984).

■ Availability and Storage

Didemnin B is supplied by the Division of Cancer Treatment, National Cancer Institute. The intact ampule should be stored under refrigeration (2–8°C).

■ Preparation for Use, Stability, and Admixture

Didemnin B is supplied as a sterile 1-mL ampule containing 1 mg didemnin B, ethanol 5% (v/v), Cremophor EL® 5% (v/v), and normal saline to make a total volume of 1 mL. The dose is diluted in 150 mL of normal saline and administered through a well-flowing intravenous line over 30 minutes.

No decomposition has been detected at room temperature or with refrigeration storage after 2 months. These studies continue. *Caution:* The single-use vial contains no antibacterial preservatives. Therefore it is advised that the reconstituted product be discarded 8 hours after initial entry.

■ Administration

The drug is diluted in 150 mL of normal saline and administered intravenously over 30 minutes.

■ Dosage

The recommended dose of didemnin B for phase II trials is not yet established. Dorr and colleagues (1988) noted dose-limiting nausea and vomiting when administering 4.51 mg/m^2 as a 30-minute infusion every 28 days with phenothiazine antiemetics. This toxicity could possibly have been ameliorated with the use of more effective antiemetic regimens such as serotonin antagonists. Other toxic effects in the trial included an allergic reaction characterized by chills, hypotension, dizziness, and flushing (an anaphylactic reaction) and mild elevations in liver transaminases.

Maroun et al (1989) have studied a weekly × 4 every-6-week schedule of the compound. Doses ranged from 0.4 to 1.2 mg/m^2. They noted dose-limiting nausea and vomiting. Other toxic effects include phlebitis and local skin reactions, anorexia, diarrhea, and asthenia. Hypersensitivity reactions, presumably caused by the drug vehicle Cremophor EL®, were also noted. Cremophor EL® is known to cause histamine release, which can cause vein swelling and acute hypersensitivity characterized by bronchoconstriction, hypotension, and dyspnea. Slow infusions of dilute solutions may reduce these reactions. Maroun et al determined that the maximum tolerated dose of didemnin B in patients not receiving antiemetics was 1.0 mg/m^2/wk.

Stewart and colleagues (1986) have studied a daily X 5 schedule of the agent with doses up to 0.67 mg/m^2/d; however no maximal tolerated dose has been reported to date.

Most recently, Shin and colleagues (1991) have aggressively escalated the dose of didemnin B using multiple antiemetics and methylprednisolone. Doses ranged from 3.47 to 9.1 mg/m^2. They also noted severe, dose-limiting neuromuscular toxicity at doses of 6.3 mg/m^2 and greater. This was accompanied by massive elevations in serum creatine kinase and aldolase levels in some patients. They also noted allergic reactions. They have recommended a dose of 6.3 mg/m^2 for phase II trials along with careful neurologic evaluations including electromyograms and muscle biopsies.

■ Special Precautions

Anaphylaxis and anaphylactoid reactions have been noted with didemnin B. It is presumed these reactions are secondary to the Cremophor EL® vehicle. Taylor et al (1989) felt didemnin B was associated with an exacerbation of coronary artery disease in two patients as well as with the onset of insulin-dependent diabetes in one patient.

■ Pharmacokinetics

The pharmacokinetics of didemnin B has been studied in only one patient, using a radioimmunoassay with an antibody raised in a rabbit. The half-life of the compound appeared to be very rapid (Dorr et al 1988). A competitive inhibition enzyme immunoassay determined that didemnin produced a biphasic elimination pattern in breast cancer patients (Benvenuto et al 1992). The initial (α) half-life was 0.12 hour and the terminal (β) half-life was 4.8 hours. Clearance averaged 29.7 L/h/m^2 with a mean volume of distribution of 57.6 L/m^2. The mean area under the plasma concentration × time curve was 233 ng·h/mL (range, 134–462) for intravenous doses of 5.6 to 7.6 mg/m^2 (Benvenuto et al 1992).

Using tritium-labeled didemnin B for in vitro incubation with whole blood specimens, Phillips and colleagues (1989) noted that only 55% of the agent remained in the plasma. The rest was found concentrated in red blood cells and in lymphocytes. No specific association with a lymphocyte subset was detected. Didemnin B does not appear to bind to plasma proteins (Benvenuto et al 1992).

■ Side Effects and Toxicity

The primary toxic effects of didemnin B include moderate nausea and vomiting seen in all patients and leukopenia of short duration in about 25% of patients (Benvenuto et al 1992). Occasionally, moderate to severe myalgias may be dose limiting (Shin et al 1991). Electromyography examinations are normal in these patients. Hypersensitivity reactions have also been noted and are characterized by flushing, hypotension, shortness of breath, and bronchospasm. Some life-threatening anaphylactic reactions have been reported. Severe cardiotoxicity has also been reported in patients with a history of other cardiac problems. Cardiac effects include supraventricular tachycardia, ischemia, and four cases of myocardial infarction within 30 days of receiving didemnin B. Some patients experience symptoms of congestive heart failure prior to infarction. The mechanism of these cardiac effects and their causal relationship to didemnin B are unknown.

Phase II clinical trials report mild to moderate renal toxicity and some myelosuppression. Abnormal liver function tests are occasionally described.

See also Administration and Special Applications for a list of side effects and toxicity by different routes.

■ Special Applications

Didemnin B is immunosuppressive in vitro. Montgomery and colleagues (Montgomery and Zukowski 1983, Montgomery et al 1987) demonstrated inhibition of protein synthesis in murine lymphocytes at micromolar levels of didemnin B. This has also been demonstrated in in vivo systems. Of note is that the structure of didemnin B is similar to the structure of cyclosporin A. The use of didemnin B as an immunosuppressive agent in a transplant situation is being explored in animal model systems.

REFERENCES

Abbruzzese J, Ajani J, Blackburn R, Faintuch J, Patt Y, Levin B. Phase II study of didemnin-B in advanced colorectal cancer. *Proc Ann Meet Am Assoc Cancer Res.* 1988;**29**:A805.

Benvenuto JA, Newman RA, Bignami GS, et al. Phase II clinical and pharmacological study of didemnin B in patients with metastatic breast cancer. *Invest New Drugs.* 1992;**10**:113–117.

Chun HB, Davies B, Hoth D. Didemnin B. The first marine compound entering clinical trials as an antineoplastic agent. *Invest New Drugs.* 1986;**4**(3):279–284.

Crampton SL, Adams EG, Kuentzel SL, Li LH, Badinez G, Bhuyon BK. Biochemical and cellular effects of didemnins A and B. *Cancer Res.* 1984;**44**:1796–1801.

Dorr FA, Kuhn JG, Phillips J, Von Hoff DD. Phase I clinical and pharmacokinetic investigation of didemnin B, a cyclic depsipeptide. *Eur J Cancer Clin Oncol.* 1988;**24**(11):1699–1706.

Hamada Y, Kondo Y, Shibata M, et al. Efficient total synthesis of didemnins A and B. *J Am Chem Soc.* 1989;**111**:669–673.

Hassain MB, vander Helm D, Antel J, et al. Crystal and molecular structure of didemnin B, an antiviral and cytotoxic depsipeptide. *Proc Natl Acad Sci USA.* 1988;**85**:4118–4123.

Jiang TL, Lin RH, Salmon JE. Antitumor activity of didemnin B in the human tumor stem cell assay. *Cancer Chemother Pharmacol.* 1983;**11**:1–4.

Maroun JA, Stewart DJ, Verma S, Eisenhaur E. Phase I study of didemnin B given in a weekly schedule. *Proc Annu Meet Am Assoc Cancer Res.* 1989;**30**:284.

Montgomery DW, Celniker A, Zukoski CF. Didemnin B—An immunosuppressive cyclic peptide that stimulates murine hemagglutinating antibody response and induces leukocytosis in vivo. *Transplantation.* 1987;**43**:133–138.

Montgomery DW, Zukowski CF. Inhibition of lymphocyte nitogenesis by sub-nanomolar concentrations of the depsipeptide, didemnin B. *Fed Proc.* 1983;**42**:374.

Murphy WV Holoye, PY Raber MN, Jeffries DG. Phase I study of didemnin B in non-small cell bronchogenic carcinoma. *Proc Am Assoc Cancer Res.* 1989;**30**:271.

Phillips JL, Schwartz R, Von Hoff DD. In vitro distribution of diacetyl didemnin B in human blood cells and plasma. *Cancer Invest.* 1989;**7**(2):123–128.

Razis E, Mittleman A, Puccio M, et al. Phase II clinical trial of didemnin B in patients with glioblastoma multiforme. *Proc Am Soc Clin Oncol.* 1991;**10**:126.

Rinehart KL, Jr, Gloer JB, Cook JC Jr. Structure of the didemnins, antiviral and cytotoxic depsipeptides from a Caribbean tunicate. *J Am Chem Soc.* 1981a;**103**:1857–1859.

Rinehart KL, Jr, Gloer JB, Hughes RG, Jr, Didemnins: Antiviral and antitumor depsipeptides from a Caribbean tunicate. *Science.* 1981b;**212**:933–935.

Rinehart KL, Jr, Gloer JB, Wilson GR, et al. Antiviral and antitumor compounds from tunicates. *Fed Proc.* 1983;**42**:87–90.

Rinehart KL, Jr, Shaw PD, Shield LS, et al. Marine natural products as sources of antiviral, antimicrobial, and antineoplastic agents. *Pure Appl Chem.* 1981c;**53**:795–817.

Rossof AH, Johnson PA, Kimmell BD, Graham JE, Roseman DL. In vitro phase II study of didemnin B in human cancer. *Proc Am Assoc Cancer Res.* 1983;**24**:315.

Rossof AH, Rowland K, Khandekar J, et al. Phase II trial of didemnin-B in previously untreated patients with measurable metastatic colorectal carcinoma: An Illinois Cancer Council Study. *Proc Am Soc Clin Oncol.* 1989;**8**:113.

Shin DM, Holoye PY, Murphy WK, et al. Phase I clinical trial of didemnin B (NSC-325319: DN-B) in non-small cell lung cancer (NSCLC): Neuromuscular toxicity (NMT) is dose-limiting. *Proc Am Soc Clin Oncol.* 1991;**10**:95.

Stewart JA, Tong WP, Hartshorn JN, McCormack JJ. Phase I evaluation of didemnin B (NSC-325319). *Proc Am Soc Clin Oncol.* 1986;**5**:33.

Taylor S, Pistone B, Stephens RL, Crawford ED. Phase II trial of didemnin B (DID-B) in advanced adenocarcinoma of the kidney: A Southwest Oncology Group study. *Proc Am Soc Clin Oncol.* 1989;**8**:145.

Diethyldithiocarbamate

■ Other Names

DTC; DDTC; Imuthiol® (Institute Merieux, Inc).

■ Chemistry

Structure of diethyldithiocarbamate

Two diethyldithiocarbamate molecules are formed in the chemical reduction of disulfiram (tetraethylthiuram disulfide, Antabuse®). The molecule is supplied as the monosodium salt which has a molecular weight of 171. The molecular formula is $C_5H_{10}N_1S_2$. The drug is very soluble in water and polar solvents (ethanol, dimethylsulfoxide, and pyridine). Many actions of diethyldithiocarbamate (DDTC) are mediated by the two sulfur molecules which can chelate certain heavy metals. There are two forms of DDTC depending on the pH of the solution. In a strongly acidic environment the nitrogen is protonated and one sulfur exists as the sulfhydryl, but the molecule is rapidly denatured to yield $(C_2H_5)_2N^+H_2$ and carbon disulfide. At a neutral or slightly alkaline pH, drug stability is enhanced. The aqueous solution has an absorption maximum of 283 nm.

■ Antitumor Activity

Diethyldithiocarbamate does not produce significant antitumor effects when used alone. Rather, it appears to modulate the toxicity of DNA binding agents, particularly the platinum-containing drugs cisplatin and carboplatin as well as alkylating agents such as cyclophosphamide. Importantly, these protective effects do not compromise the antitumor efficacy of either agent (Borch et al 1980, Gale et al 1982, Qazi et al 1988). In mice, DDTC has also been shown to block the hematopoietic toxicity of doxorubicin and cyclophosphamide (Pannacciulli et al 1989).

In a recent phase I clinical trial of DDTC with cisplatin, Qazi et al (1988) noted no nephrotoxicity and a possible reduction in nausea and vomiting; however, a standard mannitol/diuresis regimen was also used in this trial. High DDTC plasma levels were obtained (see Pharmacokinetics) and an appropriate dosing interval was used (a DDTC infusion starting 45 minutes *after* cisplatin). Toxicity at a DDTC dose of 150 mg/kg, however, precluded cisplatin dose escalations above 120 mg/m². No significant hematologic toxic effects were observed in this trial and 4 of 10 solid tumor patients achieved partial remissions with the cisplatin–DDTC combination. In contrast, Berry et al (1990) found that a 1-hour infusion of DDTC at 4 g/m² begun 45 minutes after cisplatin allowed for cisplatin dose escalation to 160 mg/m² without excessive nephrotoxicity. Cisplatin-induced ototoxicity was dose limiting in this study. Lower doses of DDTC (200 mg/m²) are uniformly inactive at modulating cisplatin therapy (Paredes et al 1988).

A similar trial has been performed with high-dose carboplatin (800 mg/m²) followed in 3 hours by DDTC (4 g/m²) (Rothenberg et al 1988). Unfortunately, significant hematologic toxicity occurred in this trial, including three treatment-related septic deaths. And, there was a trend toward more severe white blood cell and platelet nadirs with carboplatin, which persisted for shorter periods with DDTC treatment (Rothenberg et al 1988). Objective partial responses were again observed in 4 of 21 women with relapsed ovarian cancer. Thus, in contrast to the animal data (Dibble et al 1987), these two clinical studies do not establish a clear role for DDTC as a means of escalating the dose of platinum-containing antitumor agents.

Diethyldithiocarbamate also has activity as an immunorestorative adjuvant. Immunologic effects of DDTC in normal volunteers and cancer patients include an increase in T_4 (helper) lymphocytes with an enhanced T_4/T_8 ratio and augmented cytotoxic activity in natural killer (NK) lymphocytes.

■ Mechanism of Action

Diethyldithiocarbamate is known to have several effects on cells. It is an immunomodulator of T-lymphocyte function (Renoux and Renoux 1984) and is a metal chelator that has been used to treat metal intoxication from nickel (Sunderman 1981), cadmium (Gale et al 1981), and copper in Wilson's disease (Sunderman 1964). Metal chelation probably explains the inhibition by DDTC of a diverse number of metal-containing enzymes, including the following metalloenzymes: copper-containing dopamine β-hydroxylase (Goldstein et al 1964), the zinc-containing superoxide dismutase (Heikkila et al 1976), zinc-containing glutathione peroxidase (Goldstein et al 1979), iron-containing cytochrome oxidase complex (Frank et al 1978), and iron-containing ribonucleotide reductase. The effect on ribonucleotide reductase may explain DDTC-induced inhibition of DNA synthesis in rat thymocytes (Spath and Tempel 1987). There is also a suggestion that DNA polymerase α is inhibited by the drug.

The immunologic effects of DDTC are primarily restorative and not immunostimulatory in nature. In other words, DDTC may restore normal immunologic reactivity but it does not increase immune reactivity above a normal baseline. In animals, DDTC causes T-cell differentiation from null cells, T-lymphocyte proliferation in response to mitogens, and increased expression of T-cell markers (Renoux and Renoux 1979). There is also speculative evidence that DDTC can cause the liver to produce a thymic hormone-like activity (haptosin) that is dependent on the left neocortex of the brain (Renoux 1984).

The primary use of DDTC in cancer patients has been as a modifier of the renal and hematologic toxicity from various DNA binding agents including the platinum-containing drugs cisplatin (Gale et al 1982, Evans et al 1984) and carboplatin (Rothenberg et al 1988) and classic alkylating agents such as cyclophosphamide (Hacket el al 1982). With the platinum-containing agents, DDTC may block platinum binding to sulfhydryl-containing renal tubular enzymes such as Na$^+$, K-ATPase to prevent nephrotoxicity. A similar mechanism may explain DDTC-induced protection from platinum nephrotoxicity. DDTC may maintain renal enzyme levels which are reduced following platinum exposure. These include γ-glutamyl transpeptidase and glutathione peroxidase, as well as renal glutathione levels (Leyland-Jones et al 1983).

With isolated plasma proteins, DDTC has been observed to completely prevent cisplatin-induced crosslinking (Gonias et al 1984). Furthermore, DDTC can also reverse preformed crosslinks, indicating an affinity for cisplatin binding greater than that of DNA or protein. With carboplatin, DDTC's protection of the bone marrow appears to involve stimulation of DNA synthesis and proliferation following a drug-induced injury (Schmalbach and Borch 1989).

■ Availability and Storage

Diethyldithiocarbamate is available investigationally from Institute Merrieux, Paris, France. It is supplied as an injectable white hydrophilic powder in 500-mg clear glass, 20-mL vials (Imuthiol®, Institute Merieux, Inc). A special buffered diluent vial of 125 mL is also supplied by the manufacturer. In addition, investigational capsules of DDTC (125 mg) are available. All dosage forms and diluents may be stored at room temperature.

■ Preparation for Use, Stability, and Admixture

Injectable DDTC powder is reconstituted using the special alkaline-buffered diluent to achieve a final concentration of 4 mg/mL. These solutions are stable for at least 24 hours at room temperature and do not require protection from light. Further dilutions into 250 mL of 5% dextrose solution have also been used (Rothenberg et al 1988). The pH should be maintained above 6.5 for maximum stability.

■ Administration

Parenteral DDTC doses are typically administered intravenously as a brief infusion over 30 minutes (Qazi et al 1988) or 90 minutes (Rothenberg et al 1988).

■ Dosage

The maximally tolerated DDTC dose when combined with 120 mg/m^2 cisplatin is 150 mg/kg (Qazi et al 1988). DDTC doses of 4 g/m^2 have been used with carboplatin (Berry et al 1990). It is recommended that DDTC follow either cisplatin or carboplatin by at least 1 to 3 hours to allow for maximal platinum-induced antitumor activity and still provide protection from toxicity (Leyland-Jones 1988).

■ Drug Interactions

Diethyldithiocarbamate has some disulfiram-like activity because of the inhibition of aldehyde dehydrogenase activity. Therefore, alcohol should be avoided while taking DDTC. DDTC also has produced sulfhydryl-dependent interactions with other anticancer agents in experimental models, including inhibition of the immunosuppressive effect of azathioprine (Renoux et al 1983) and cytotoxic synergy with bleomycin (Lin et al 1980). The clinical significance of these interactions is unknown.

■ Pharmacokinetics

Diethyldithiocarbamate is rapidly metabolized and eliminated primarily by glomerular filtration into the urine. In humans, the plasma half-life is approximately 11 to 13 minutes. Peak blood levels are dose dependent (see table on page 390).

With oral DDTC, bioavailability is both incomplete and variable. When DDTC is used as a modulator of cisplatin toxicity, tolerable oral doses of the DDTC precursor disulfiram (2 g/m^2) produced very low peak plasma DDTC levels of 1 to 2 μM (Stewart et al 1987). These levels, which were far too low to provide protection from cisplatin toxicity, nonetheless produced dose-limiting central nervous system toxicity (Stewart et al 1987).

Diethyldithiocarbamate is extensively metabolized to a methyl diester derivative. In dogs, this metabolite has a much slower elimination with a plasma half-life of 49 minutes, compared with 4 minutes for the parent compound (Cobby et al 1978). About 27% of a DDTC dose is S-methylated. The biologic activity (if any) of the methylated DDTC metabolite is unknown.

PHARMACOKINETICS OF DIETHYLDITHIOCARBAMATE IN CANCER PATIENTS

Intravenous Dose	Half-life (min)	Peak Plasma Level (μM)	AUC (mg/mL · min)	Volume of Distribution (mL/kg)	Plasma Clearance (mL/min/kg)
75 mg/kg*	13.4	400	20.8	290	14.7
150 mg/kg*	13.1	1000	55	275	13.0
4 g/m²†	NL‡	442–446	NL	NL	NL

*Qazi et al 1988
†DeGregorio et al 1989
‡Not listed.

■ Side Effects and Toxicity

When DDTC was infused at the maximal intravenous dose of 150 mg/kg, severe acute toxic effects were occasionally encountered. These acute effects include numbness or local burning in the arm used for infusion with concomitant facial flushing and general agitation (Qazi et al 1988). These symptoms were often accompanied by severe diaphoresis, chest discomfort, and hypertension. A transient increase in systolic blood pressure, 20 to 40 mm Hg, typically resolved without treatment. Acute neurotoxic effects of DDTC are also seen with oral disulfiram. This condition has been described as mixed autonomic hyperactivity with anxiety and hypertension followed by hypotension, flushed skin, and conjunctival injection. Heavy sedation with benzodiazepines and barbiturates may exacerbate the depressive second phase of this reaction (Rothenberg et al 1988).

Diethyldithiocarbamate is not teratogenic in rodents but did show some teratogenic effects in rabbits. The compound was also nonmutagenic in vitro in both the Ames assay and the micronucleus test.

REFERENCES

Berry JM, Jacobs C, Sikic B, et al. Modification of cisplatin toxicity with diethyldithiocarbamate. *J Clin Oncol.* 1990;**8**:1585–1590.

Borch RF, Katz JC, Lieder PH, Pleasants ME. Effect of diethyldithiocarbamate rescue on tumor response to cis-platinum in a rat model. *Proc Natl Acad Sci USA.* 77:5441–5444.

Cobby J, Mayersohn M, Selliah S. Disposition kinetics in dogs of diethyldithiocarbamate, a metabolite of disulfiram. *J Pharmacokinet Biopharma.* 1978;**6**:369–387.

DeGregorio MW, Gandara DR, Holleran WM, et al. High-dose cisplatin with diethyldithiocarbamate (DDTC) rescue therapy: Preliminary pharmacologic observations. *Cancer Chemother Pharmacol.* 1989;**23**:276–278.

Dibble SE, Siddik ZH, Boxhall FE. The effect of diethyldithiocarbamate on the hematologic toxicity and antitumor activity of carboplatin. *Eur J Cancer Clin Oncol.* 1987;**23**:813–818.

Evans RG, Wheatley C, Engel C, et al. Modification of the bone marrow toxicity of cis-diamminedichloroplatinum(II) in mice by diethyldithiocarbamate. *Cancer Res.* 1984;**44**:3686–3690.

Frank L, Wood DL, Roberts RJ. Effect of diethyldithiocarbamate on oxygen toxicity and lung enzymes activity in immature and adult rats. *Biochem Pharmacol.* 1978;**27**:251–254.

Gale GR, Atkins LM. Cisplatin and diethyldithiocarbamate in treatment of L1210 leukemia. *J Clin Hematol Oncol.* 1981;**11**:41–45.

Gale GR, Atkins LM, Walker EM Jr. Further evaluation of diethyldithiocarbamate as an antagonist of cisplatin toxicity. *Ann Clin Lab Sci.* 1982;**12**:345–355.

Gale GR, Smith AB, Walker EM Jr. Diethyldithiocarbamate in the treatment of acute cadmium poisoning. *Ann Clin Lab Sci.* 1981;**11**:476–483.

Goldstein BD, Anagnoste B, Lauber E, McKereghan MR. Inhibition of dopamine β-hydroxylase by disulfiram. *Life Sci.* 1964;**3**:763–767.

Goldstein BD, Rozen MG, Quintavilla JC, Amaruso MA. Decrease in mouse lung and liver glutathione peroxidase activity and potentiation of the lethal effect of ozone and paraquat by the superoxide dismutase inhibitor diethyldithiocarbamate. *Biochem Pharmacol.* 1979;**28**:27–30.

Gonias SL, Oakley AC, Walther PJ, Pizzo SV. Effects of diethyldithiocarbamate and nine other nucleophiles on the intersubunit protein cross-linking and inactivation of purified human $α_2$-macroglobulin by cis-diamminedichloroplatinum(II). *Cancer Res.* 1984;**44**:5764–5770.

Hack MP, Ershler WB, Newman RA, Gamelli RL. Effect of disulfiram (tetraethylthiuram disulfide) and diethyldithiocarbamate on the bladder toxicity and antitumor activity of cyclophosphamide in mice. *Cancer Res.* 1982;**42**:4490–4494.

Heikkila RE, Cabbat FS, Cohen G. In vivo inhibition of superoxide dismutase in mice by diethyldithiocarbamate. *J Biol Chem.* 1976;**251**:2182–2185.

Leyland-Jones B. Whither the modulation of platinum? *J Natl Cancer Inst.* 1988;**80**:1432–1433.

Leyland-Jones B, Marrow C, Tate S, et al. cis-Diamminedichloroplatinum(II) nephrotoxicity and its relationship to renal gamma-glutamyl transpeptidase and glutathione. *Cancer Res.* 1983;**43**:6072–6076.

Lin PS, Kwock LK, Goodchild NT. Copper chelator enhancement by bleomycin cytotoxicity. *Cancer.* 1980;**46**:2360.

Pannacciulli IM, Lerza RA, Bogliolo GV, et al. Effect of diethyldithiocarbamate on toxicity of doxorubicin, cyclophosphamide and *cis*-diamminedichloroplatinum (II) on mice haemopoietic progenitor cells. *Br J Cancer.* 1989;**59**:371–374.

Paredes J, Hong WK, Felder TB, et al. Prospective randomized trial of high dose cisplatin and flurouracil infusion with or without sodium diethyldithiocarbamate in recurrent and/or metastatic squamous cell carcinoma of the head and neck. *J. Clin Oncol.* 1988;**6**:955–992.

Qazi R, Chang AYC, Borch RF, et al. Phase I clinical and pharmacokinetic study of diethyldithiocarbamate as a chemoprotector from toxic effects of cisplatin. *J Natl Cancer Inst.* 1988;**80**:1486–1488.

Renoux G. The mode of action of Imuthiol (sodium diethyldithiocarbamate): A new role for the brain neocortex and the endocrine liver in the regulation of the T-cell linage. In: Fenichel RL, Chirigos MA, eds. *Immune Modulation Agents and Their Mechanisms.* New York/Basel: Marcel Dekker; 1984;607–623.

Renoux G, Renoux M. Immunopotentiation and anabolism induced by sodium diethyldithiocarbamate. *Int J Immunopharmacol.* 1979;**1**:247.

Renoux G, Renoux M. Diethyldithiocarbamate (DTC): A biological augmenting agent specific for T cells. In: Fenichel RL, Chirigos MA, eds. *Immune Modulation Agents and Their Mechanisms.* New York/Basel: Marcel Dekker; 1984:7–20.

Renoux G, Renoux M, Lemaire E, Sodium diethyldithiocarbamate (Imuthiol) and cancer. In: Klein T, ed. *Biological Response Modifiers in Human Oncology and Immunology.* New York: Plenum; 1983:223–239.

Rothenberg ML, Ostchega Y, Steinberg SM, et al. High-dose carboplatin with diethyldithiocarbamate chemoprotection in treatment of women with relapsed ovarian cancer. *J Natl Cancer Inst.* 1988;**80**:1488–1492.

Schmalbach TK, Borch RF. Diethyldithiocarbamate modulation of murine bone marrow toxicity induced by *cis*-diammine(cyclobutanedicarboxylato)platinum(II). *Cancer Res.* 1989;**49**:6629–6633.

Spath A, Tempel K. Diethyldithiocarbamate inhibits scheduled and unscheduled DNA synthesis of rat thymocytes in vitro and in vivo—Dose–effect relationships and mechanisms of action. *Chem–Biol Interact.* 1987;**64**:151–166.

Stewart DJ, Verma S, Maroun JA. Phase I study of the combination of disulfiram with cisplatin. *Am J Clin Oncol.* 1987;**10**:517–519.

Sunderman FW Sr. Nickel and copper mobilization by sodium diethyldithiocarbamate. *J New Drugs.* 1964;**4**:154–161.

Sunderman FW Sr. Chelation therapy in nickel poisoning. *Ann Clin Lab Sci.* 1981;**11**:1–8.

Diglycoaldehyde

■ Other Names

NSC-118994; inosine dialdehyde; Inox; Wy-5321.

■ Chemistry

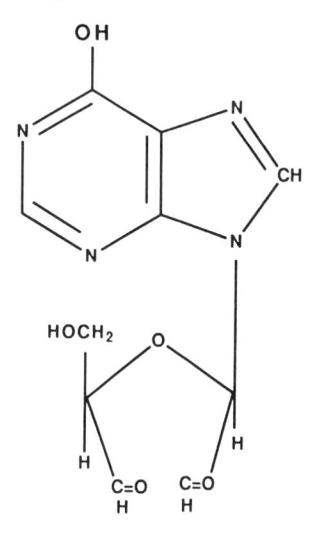

Structure of diglycoaldehyde

The complete chemical name of diglycoaldehyde is α-(hydroxymethyl)-α'-hydroxy-9H-purine-9-yl diglycoaldehyde.

■ Antitumor Activity

Although hints of antitumor activity were noted in early clinical trials (seminoma, non-small cell lung cancer, melanoma, acute leukemia), the agent did not prove to be useful in further phase II testing (Chiuten et al 1981, Vosika et al 1981, Higgins et al 1980, Shaw et al 1980). Because of lack of efficacy and because of excessive toxic effects this agent is no longer being developed.

■ Mechanism of Action

The exact biochemical mechanism of action of diglycoaldehyde is unknown; however, some inferences may be drawn from work with similar compounds (Dvonch et al 1966). These periodate oxidation compounds (including diglycoaldehyde) possess highly reactive aldehyde groups which may form Schiff bases with a variety of cellular proteins. Crosslinking of macromolecules by these aldehyde groups has also been proposed. Diglycoaldehyde is not incorporated into nucleic acids and does not interact with purine synthesis enzymes or with xanthine oxidase.

■ Availability and Storage

Diglycoaldehyde is available investigationally as a lyophilized powder in 1.0-gram (20-mL) vials which may be stored at room temperature (22°C) for at least 6 months.

■ Preparation for Use, Stability, and Admixture

The 1-g vials may be reconstituted with 9.0 mL of sterile water for injection to obtain a solution containing 100 mg diglycoaldehyde per milliliter. This acidic solution (pH 3.0–4.0) is chemically stable for at least 48 hours at room temperature (22°C) under either light or dark conditions. Without the use of a bacteriostatic preservative, it is recommended that solutions be used within 8 hours.

To reduce the irritation reported from the acidic initial reconstitution, diglycoaldehyde should be further diluted to 500 to 1000 mL of either D5W or normal saline. Buffering to a pH of about 7.5 with sodium bicarbonate (about 500 mg/1.0 g of diglycoaldehyde) is recommended to achieve the pH of 7.5 to 8.0 required for maximum stability; however, sodium bicarbonate is not recommended as the initial diluent.

The final buffered drug solution is reported to be chemically stable 48 hours at room temperature but optimally should be used within 24 hours.

■ Administration

Diglycoaldehyde is usually diluted in 1 L of buffered D5W or normal saline and is generally given as a 6-hour infusion. Shorter infusion times, a more concentrated solution, or use of unbuffered diluents may predispose patients to increased local vein irritation and skin reactions.

■ Special Precautions

Diglycoaldehyde should be used with extreme caution in patients with compromised renal function (serum creatinine > 1.5, BUN ≥ 20 mg 100 mL, or evidence of proteinuria).

■ Drug Interactions

None have been reported.

■ Dosage

In phase I studies (Kaufman and Mittelman 1975) doses of 1.5 to 2.0 $g/m^2/d \times 5$ days every 10 days and 3 $g/m^2 \times 5$ days have been used. Early hematologic and renal dose-limiting toxic effects were seen with these regimens. Recommendations for phase II investigations were $1.5/g/m^2/d \times 5$ days and 2 $g/m^2/d \times 5$ days given every 3 to 4 weeks to allow for complete resolution of toxicity.

■ Pharmacokinetics

Pharmacokinetic studies in dogs reveal a biphasic elimination curve after bolus dosing with a high peak and a very slow terminal elimination phase (Cysyk 1975). The drug is probably excreted quantitatively unchanged in the urine. No pharmacokinetic studies have been reported in humans.

■ Side Effects and Toxicity

The dose-limiting toxic effect of diglycoaldehyde given on the daily × 5 schedule is renal tubular damage manifested as proteinuria. It begins during the infusion period (day 4) and is generally resolved by day 14. Other toxic effects noted with a 2 $g/m^2/d \times 5$ course include mild leukopenia and thrombocytopenia (nadir at 10 days, recovery by 3–4 weeks), a Coombs-positive hemolytic anemia (Coombs' test remained positive for 2 months after treatment), and a prolonged partial thromboplastin time.

Additional toxic effects have included hypocalcemia (seems to be an effect on osseous disease sites rather than on calcium excretion), mild to moderate nausea and vomiting, and severe venous thrombosis with extravasation necrosis (which can be avoided if the drug is infused in buffered solution as described earlier).

■ Special Applications

None have been reported, although the compound may be looked at again for treatment of hypercalcemia in patients.

REFERENCES

Chiuten DF, Vosika GJ, Gisselbrecht C, et al. Clinical trials with diglycoaldehyde (NSC-118994): Review and reasons for withdrawals from clinical trial. *Anticancer Res.* 1981;**1**:121–124.

Cysyk R. Chemical assay for the antitumor agent inosine

dialdehyde (NSC-118994) in biologic fluids. *Cancer Treat Rep.* 1975;**59:**(4):685–687.

Dvonch W, Fletcher H III, Gregory FJ, Healey EH, Warren GH, Alburn HE. Antitumor activity of periodate-oxidation products of carbohydrates and their derivatives. *Cancer Res.* 1966;**26**:2386–2389.

Higgins GR, Finklestein J, Krivit W, Hammond D. Phase II evaluation of diglycoaldehyde (INOX) in children with acute leukemia. A Children's Cancer Study Group report. *Cancer Treat Rep.* 1980;**64**:625–628.

Kaufman J, Mittelman A. Clinical phase I trial of inosine dialdehyde (NSC-118994). *Cancer Treat Rep Part 1.* 1975;**59**(5):1007–1014.

Shaw MT, Morrison FS, Stuckey WJ, Trowbridge AA. Treatment of advanced adult leukemia with diglycoaldehyde: A Southwest Oncology Group study. *Cancer Treat Rep.* 1980;**64**:985–986.

Vosika GJ, Briscoe K, Carey RW, et al. Phase II study of diglycoaldehyde in malignant melanomas and soft tissue sarcomas. *Cancer Treat Rep.* 1981;**65**:823–825.

Dihydro-5-Azacytidine

■ Other Names

NSC-264880; 5,6-dihydro-5-azacytidine; DHAC.

■ Chemistry

The complete chemical name is 4-amino-3,6-dihydro-1-β-D-ribofuranosyl-1,3,5-triazin-2(1*H*)-ine monohydrochloride. It has a molecular weight of 282.7 and the formula $C_8H_{14}N_4O_5 \cdot HCl$.

Structure of 5,6-dihydro-5-azacytidine

Dihydro-5-azacytidine (DHAC) was developed as an alternative to 5-azacytidine (azacitidine), which possesses antitumor activity in patients with acute leukemia. 5-Azacytidine was unstable in aqueous solution. Therefore, Beisler et al (1976, 1977) synthesized DHAC which was stable for long periods (weeks) at room temperature over a broad range of pH in aqueous solutions.

■ Antitumor Activity

In phase I studies DHAC demonstrated some antitumor activity in patients with refractory lymphoma and in patients with mesothelioma (Curt et al 1985).

Because dihydro-5-azacytidine produces pleurisy some investigators examined the activity of DHAC in patients with mesothelioma (Harmon et al 1991). In a phase II trial conducted by Cancer and Acute Leukemia Group B, objective responses were noted in 17% of patients (Harmon et al 1991); however, other investigators have not been able to replicate these results in mesothelioma (Dhingra et al 1991).

Unfortunately, the drug has not produced significant activity in patients with non-small cell lung cancer (Carr et al 1987; Holoye et al 1987) or breast cancer (Nevinny et al 1989).

■ Mechanism of Action

Dihydro-5-azacytidine is incorporated into nuclear RNA. It inhibits methylation of ribosomal and transfer RNA. It also inhibits transcription of ribosomal RNA and nuclear RNA. The overall effect is a decrease in the synthesis of methylated bases into RNA and a decrease in protein synthesis (Glazer et al 1980, Lin and Glazer 1981). DHAC can substantially reduce DNA methylation levels (Avramis et al 1989, Antonsson et al 1987). Cytidine deaminase will inactivate DHAC (Voytek et al 1977). DHAC is a cell cycle-specific agent (Traganos et al 1981).

■ Availability and Storage

Dihydro-5-azacytidine is available as a 500-mg investigational vial of white lyophilized powder from the National Cancer Institute, Bethesda, Maryland. The intact 20-mL vials are stable for at least 4 years at room temperature or at 4°C.

■ Preparation for Use, Stability, and Admixture

Each 500-mg vial is reconstituted with 9.6 mL of Sterile Water for Injection, USP. This results in a clear solution containing 50 mg of DHAC and 30 mg of mannitol at a pH of 3 to 5. The drug can be diluted in multiple types of intravenous infusion solutions. The reconstituted solutions are stable for at least 48 hours at room temperature. DHAC is also stable for

PHARMACOKINETICS OF DIHYDRO-5-AZACYTIDINE

Schedule	Dose Range (mg/m^2)	Maximally Tolerated Dose (mg/m^2)	Dose-Limiting Toxic Effect	Recommended Phase II Dose (mg/m^2)
Daily × 5 bolus	30–3500	2500	Pleurisy Diarrhea Nausea and vomiting	—
Daily × 5 bolus	30–2500	1650	Pleurisy Vomiting	1650
Daily × 5 continuous infusion*	210–2500	2500	—	2500
24-h continuous infusion	1000–7000	7000	Pleurisy	5000–7000

*The daily × 5 continuous infusion (120 hours) is the schedule most often used.

48 hours when diluted into 5% dextrose, 0.9% sodium chloride, and Lactated Ringer's Injection, USP (data from the National Cancer Institute 1990).

■ Administration

The drug is most often given at a dose of 1500 mg/m^2 by a 120-hour continuous infusion repeated every 21 days.

■ Special Precautions

The patient should be watched carefully for any clinical signs of supraventricular tachycardia.

■ Drug Interactions

None have been reported.

■ Dosage

Daily × 5 bolus and infusions and 24-hour infusions have been explored in phase I studies of DHAC (see table above).

■ Pharmacokinetics

Pharmacokinetic studies performed in nine patients receiving a 24-hour infusion of DHAC showed that steady-state plasma levels were achieved within 8 hours. The β half-life was 90 ± 22 minutes and the mean total body clearance was 311 ± 76 mL/min/m^2. Of the administered dose, 8 to 20.5% was recovered unchanged in the urine. Like cytarabine, this agent appears to be extensively metabolized by cytidine deaminase in human plasma (Curt et al 1985). (See table above.)

■ Side Effects and Toxicity

The dose-limiting toxic effect of DHAC has been pleurisy, sometimes severe enough to require morphine (Harmon et al 1991, Curt et al 1985, Carr et al 1987).

Other toxic effects noted with the agent have included supraventricular tachycardia, pericardial effusions, mucositis, and nausea and vomiting (Harmon et al 1991, Curt et al 1985, Carr et al 1987). Hematologic, renal, and hepatic toxic effects have not been noted with DHAC. Carr et al (1987) reported on four patients who developed positive antinuclear antibodies while on treatment.

■ Special Applications

Carr et al (1987) noted that DHAC-treated patients had significant increases in fetal hemoglobin levels. That finding raises the possibility of using DHAC for the treatment of patients with sickle cell anemia.

REFERENCES

Antonsson BE, Avramis VI, Nyce J, Holcengerg JS. Effect of 5-azacytidine and congeners on DNA methylation and expression of deoxycytidine kinase in the human lymphoid cell lines CCF/CEM/O and CCRF/CEM/dCk(-). *Cancer Res.* 1987;**47**:3672–3678.

Avramis VI, Powell WC, Mecum RA. Cellular metabolism of 5,6-dihydro-5-azacytidine and its incorporation into DNA and RNA of human lymphoid cells CEM/O and CEM/dCk(-). *Cancer Chemother Pharmacol.* 1989;**24**:155–160.

Beisler JA, Abbasi MM, Driscoll JS. Dihydro-5-azacytidine hydrochloride, a biologically active and chemically stable analog of 5-azacytidine. *Cancer Treat Rep.* 1976;**60**:1671–1674.

Beisler JA, Abbasi MM, Kelley JA, Driscoll JS. Synthesis and antitumor activity of dihydro-5-azacytidine, a hydrolytically stable analogue of 5-azacytidine. *J Med Chem* 1977;**20**:806–812.

Carr BI, Rahbar S, Doroshow JH, et al. Fetal hemoglobin gene activation in a phase II study of 5,6-dihydro-5-azacytidine for bronchogenic carcinoma. *Cancer Res.* 1987;**47**(5):4199–4201.

Curt GA, Kelley JA, Fine RL, et al. A phase I and pharmacokinetic study of dihydro-5-azacytidine (NSC-2684880). *Cancer Res.* 1985;**45**:3359–3363.

Dhingra HM, Murphy WK, Winn RJ, Rabar MN, Hong WK. Phase II trial of 5,6-dihydro-5-azacytidine in pleural malignant mesothelioma. *Invest New Drugs.* 1991;**9**(1):69–72.

Glazer RI, Peale AL, Beisler JA, Abbasi MM. The effect of 5-azacytidine and dihydro-5-azacytidine on nuclear ribosomal RNA and poly(A) RNA synthesis in L1210 cells in vitro. *Mol Pharmacol.* 1980;**17**:111–117.

Harmon D, Vogelzang N, Roboz J, et al. Dihydro-5-azacytidine (DHAC) in malignant mesothelioma (MISO) using serum hyaluronic acid (SHA) as a tumor marker: A phase II trial of the CALGB (abstract #1248). *Am Soc Clin Oncol.* 1991;**10**:351.

Holoye PY, Dhingra HM, Umsawasdi T, Murphy WK, Carr DT, Lee JS. Phase II study of 5,6-dihydro-5-azacytidine in extensive, untreated non-small cell lung cancer. *Cancer Treat Rep.* 1987;**71**(9):859–860.

Lin HL, Glazer RI. Comparative effects of 5-azacytidine and dihydro-5-azacytidine on polysomal RNA in Ehrlich ascites cells in vitro. *Mol Pharmacol.* 1981;**20**:644–648.

National Cancer Institute. *NCI Investigational Drugs: Pharmaceutical Data.* Washington, DC: Department of Health and Human Services; 1990.

Nevinny H, Kilton L, Wade I, Braud E, Blough R, Weidner L. Phase II trial of 5,6-dihydro-5-azacytidine (DHAC) in metastatic adenocarcinoma of breast: An Illinois Cancer Council study (meeting abstract). *Proc Am Soc Clin Oncol.* 1989;**8**:40.

Traganos F, Staiano-Corco L, Darzynikiewicz Z, Melamed MR. Effect of dihydro-5-azacytidine on cell survival and cell cycle progression of cultured mammalian cells. *Cancer Res.* 1981;**41**:780–789.

Voytek P, Beisler JA, Abbasi MM, Wolpert-Defillippes MK. Comparative studies of the cytostatic action and metabolism of 5-azacytidine and 5,6-dihydro-5-azacytidine. *Cancer Res.* 1977;**37**:1956–1961.

Doxorubicin

■ Other Names

Adriamycin® (Adria Laboratories); Rubex® (Immunex Corporation); doxorubicin HCl (Cetus Corporation and Astra Pharmaceutical Products); NSC-123127; Adria; hydroxyl daunorubicin; DOX.

■ Chemistry

Structure of doxorubicin

Doxorubicin (molecular weight 580) is an anthracycline antibiotic obtained from *Streptomyces peucetius var caesius.* It is the hydroxylated congener of daunorubicin. The doxorubicin (DOX) structure includes a water-soluble basic amino sugar, daunosamine. This is linked glycosidically to carbon 7 on the D-ring of the water-insoluble chromophore, adriamycinone. This four-ringed aglycone is actually a substituted naphthacene quinone with a methoxy group at the 4-position of the A-ring and two substitutions at the D-ring: a hydroxyl moiety and a hydroxyacetyl group at carbon 9. The aglycone is inactive and modifications of the amino sugar can also alter antitumor and/or toxic potency (Henry 1979). The amino group on the sugar daunosamine is protonated at physiologic pH. This confers water solubility to the drug. This amphipathic quality of DOX explains its ready penetration of cell membranes.

Doxorubicin HCl is freely soluble in water, slightly soluble in normal saline, and very slightly soluble in alcohol. The aglycone is not water soluble. The glycosidic bond is sensitive to a pH outside the range 3 to 9.8.

■ Antitumor Activity

In experimental animal systems, DOX has shown a wide spectrum of activity in solid tumors such as sarcomas, adenocarcinomas, and melanomas as well as in transplantable and virally induced leukemias and lymphomas (Silverstrini et al 1970, Di Marco 1972). Initial clinical studies confirmed a broad spectrum of activity for DOX in both hematologic cancers and solid tumors (Blum and Carter 1974). Acute leukemias, both lymphocytic and myelogenous, are highly responsive to DOX-containing combinations (McCredie et al 1976). Doxorubicin is a mainstay of conventional regimens for non-Hodgkin's lymphomas including CHOP, MBACOD, BACOP (Schein et al 1976), and MACOP-B. In addition, it is extremely active in Hodgkin's disease as in the "ABVD" combination (with bleomycin, vinblastine, and dacarbazine) (Bonnadonna et al 1974).

Numerous nonhematologic tumors are similarly responsive to DOX. These include (1) sarcomas, including osteogenic sarcoma (Cortes et al 1974, 1978), Ewing's sarcoma, and Wilms' tumor (O'Bryan et al 1973); (2) neuroblastoma (Samuels et al 1971); (3) ovarian carcinoma (Barlow et al 1973); (4) breast carcinoma in various combinations such as "AC" (with cyclophosphamide) (Salmon and Jones 1974) or "FAC" (with fluorouracil and cyclophosphamide) (Hortobagyi et al 1979); and (5) non-small cell lung cancer (Kenis et al 1972) and small cell carcinoma of the lung in combinations such as "VAC" (with vincristine and cyclophosphamide) (Livingston et al 1978); (7) thyroid carcinoma (Gottlieb and Hill 1974); and (8) bladder carcinoma (O'Bryan et al 1973). Hepatocellular carcinomas are also responsive to DOX (Chlebowski et al 1984).

■ Mechanism of Action

DNA Binding. The anthracyclines, including DOX, have several modes of action but seem to share at least one common cytotoxic mechanism with antibiotics such as dactinomycin; intercalation between base pairs in the DNA double helix. With intercalated DOX, the amino sugar projects into the minor groove of DNA and can interact electrostatically with negatively charged phosphate groups in the DNA strand. This tends to stabilize the noncovalent binding of the intercalated aglycone moiety. The anthracycline portion of the molecule appears to intercalate between stacked nucleotide pairs in the DNA helix via pi–pi-type bonds (Di Marco et al 1971). The drug may also bind ionically around certain base pairs of DNA (adlineation). The overall effect of this lesion is interference with nucleic acid synthesis, specifically an inhibition of chain elongation rather than interference with the initiation of DNA synthesis (Painter 1978); however, preribosomal RNA synthesis is also affected by the drug. This thereby prevents DNA-directed RNA and DNA transcription (Driscoll et al 1974).

Doxorubicin–Metal Complexes. Doxorubicin can also form complexes with iron or copper via the hydroquinone moieties (Hasinoff and Davey 1988). These metal–drug complexes have high association constants indicating avid binding for Fe^{2+}–DOX ($10^{33}\,M^{-2}$) and for Cu^{2+}–DOX ($10^{16.7}\,M^{-2}$). Metal–iron DOX complexes may contribute to cardiotoxicity by enhancing redox cycling of the quinone moiety to produce membrane-damaging oxygen free radicals (Myers et al 1982).

Doxorubicin Covalent Binding. Covalent DNA binding by a 7-deoxyaglycone metabolite has also been suggested (Sinha and Sik 1980). In this instance an electrophilic carbon may be formed at the C–7 position following enzymatic or chemical reduction of the glycosidic bond, liberating the amino sugar. The C-7 radical could covalently bind to a variety of nucleophiles including DNA, proteins such as cytochrome P450 reductase, and another DOX molecule, forming a dimer. Thus, although intercalation is well characterized with DOX, other mechanisms may also contribute to the antitumor effect of the molecule. The contribution of alkylation to antitumor effects is not established.

Free Radical Formation. Oxygen free radical intermediates containing an unpaired electron can be formed by DOX in the presence of flavin-dependent oxidoreductases such as cytochrome P450 reductase with the reducing equivalent NADPH (Handa and Sato 1976). In the presence of oxygen and especially metal catalysts such as Fe(II), DOX can undergo a one-electron reduction to the semiquinone radical. This can rapidly react with oxygen to form superperoxide. In the presence of hydrogen peroxide, highly reactive hydroxyl radicals can form. These radicals mediate several effects: membrane lipid peroxidation (Goodman and Hochstein 1977); DNA strand scission; direct oxidation of purine or pyrimidine bases, thiols, and amines (Myers 1982). Free radical mechanisms have most often been associated with cardiotoxicity, possibly because of preferential drug association with negatively charged cardiolipin in cardiac myocyte membranes (Goormatigh et al 1980) and the low level of antioxidant enzymes found in the heart (see Side Effects and Toxicity). Free radical generation is also associated with mitochondrial membrane damage because of the presence of the appropriate reducing enzymes and cofactors. The contribution of membrane effects to antitumor efficacy is unknown although drug complexed to large beads can produce limited cytolysis in vitro, ostensibly via membrane-mediated oxidative effects (Tritton and Yee 1982).

Inhibition of DNA Topoisomerases I and II. Topoisomerases are enzymes capable of covalent binding to DNA, forming transient breaks in one strand (topoisomerase I) or two strands (topoisomerase II). This activity is highly phase dependent for G_2, and in the case of topoisomerase II, enzyme activity normally mediates strand passage to facilitate DNA condensation or decondensation (Glisson and Ross 1987). Doxorubicin inhibits the strand-passing activity of topoisomerase II by increasing and stabilizing initial enzyme–DNA ("cleavable") complexes. This leads to protein-linked DNA double-strand breaks which occur in rough proportion to the cytotoxic potency of the drug in vitro (Tewey et al 1984). Recently, DOX has also been shown to inhibit DNA topoisomerase I enzymes (Fogleson et al 1992).

Cell Cycle Specificity. Doxorubicin can be cytotoxic in all phases of the cell cycle, and although maximally cytotoxic in S phase, it is not cell cycle phase specific (Kim and Kim 1972). Cells exposed to lethal DOX concentrations in G_1 can proceed through S phase but are then blocked and die in G_2. Higher concentrations can also produce an S-phase blockade (Ritch et al 1981).

■ Availability and Storage

Doxorubicin HCl is commercially available from several manufacturers in a ready to use liquid or lyophilized form (see table below). Manufacturers generally report at least 2-year stability for intact vials of lyophilized powder when stored at room temperature and away from direct light. The commercial solution formulations must be stored under refrigeration. One manufacturer includes methylparabens as a solubility enhancer and as an antimicrobial to facilitate multidosing from a single vial (Adriamycin PFS®, Adria Laboratories).

■ Preparation for Use, Stability, and Admixture

Lyophilized drug may be reconstituted with sterile water for injection, D5W, normal saline, and most other common intravenous solutions. For intravenous push doses, reconstitution with either D5W or normal saline is advised to ensure isotonicity of the resultant solution. For this purpose, any convenient amount of diluent is usually sufficient (eg, 10 mL for doses up to 50 mg and 15–20 mL for larger doses). Solutions that will not be used within 8 hours of reconstitution should optimally be protected from light but are otherwise stable for prolonged periods (see table on top of page 398). Although concentrated DOX solutions can be frozen for later use (Hoffman et al 1979), repeated freezing and thawing of dilute solutions can result in self-polymerization of DOX with a resultant loss of biologic activity (Eksborg 1978). Dilute DOX solutions can also support the growth of several types of microorganisms (Gaj et al 1984). Therefore, all DOX solutions should be handled with strict aseptic technique.

Doxorubicin HCl has been found to be physically incompatible with a number of drugs (see table

DOXORUBICIN AVAILABILITY AND STORAGE

Manufacturer	Brand Name	Vial Size (mg)	Formulation	Excipient	Storage
Adria Laboratories Dublin, Ohio	Adriamycin RDF® Adriamycin PFS®	10, 20, 50 10, 20, 50, 200	LP* 2 mg/mL	Lactose Methylparaben	RT[2] Refrigeration
Astra Pharmaceutical Products Westboro, Massachusetts	Doxorubicin HCl	10, 20, 50	LP	Lactose	RT
Cetus Oncology Corporation Emeryville, California	Doxorubicin HCl Doxorubicin HCl	10, 20, 50 20, 50	LP 2 mg/mL	Lactose Lactose	RT Refrigeration
Immunex Corporation Seattle, Washington	Rubex®	50, 100	LP	Lactose	RT

*LP, lyophilized powder; RT, room temperature

STABILITY OF DIFFERENT DOXORUBICIN SOLUTIONS

Diluent	Doxorubicin Concentration (mg/L)	Temperature (°C)	Utility Time (> 90% Drug Remaining)*	Reference
3.3–5% Dextrose	20–100	25	4 wk	Poochikian et al 1981
Normosol®	10, 20	21	24 h	Poochikian et al 1981
Lactated Ringer's injection	10, 20	21	24 h	Poochikian et al 1981
0.9% Sodium chloride	100	25	28 h	Ketchum et al 1981
Water for injection		Frozen†	6 mo	Hoffman et al 1979

*Storage in light reduces stability.
†Multiple freeze–thaw cycles are contraindicated (Eksborg 1978).

below). These interactions involve a pH-mediated degradation of the glycosidic bond, leading to a darkening of the characteristic red solution; a direct stoichiometric complexation of the cationic anthracycline with negative mucopolysaccharide moieties in heparins; and precipitation of certain drug–drug admixtures (eg, cephalothin and furosemide). There is also evidence for significant DOX adsorption to infusion system surfaces or in vitro culture materials including glass tubes, stainless steel, and various plastics (polypropylene, polytetrafluoroethylene, and polyethylene) (Tomlinson and Malspeis 1982). The clinical significance of this phenomenon is unclear as DOX is known to be nearly completely recoverable from typical plastic or glass infusion systems (Trissel 1988).

COMPATIBILITY OF DOXORUBICIN WITH OTHER PARENTERAL MEDICATIONS

Compatible*	Incompatible (Mechanism)
Bleomycin	Aminophylline (pH degradation)
Cisplatin	Cephalothin sodium (precipitation)
Cyclophosphamide#	Dexamethasone sodium phosphate (precipitation)
Dacarbazine	
Droperidol	5-Fluorouracil (pH degradation)
Leucovorin calcium	Furosemide (precipitation)
Methotrexate	Heparin (complexation and precipitation)
Metoclopramide	
Mitomycin-C	
Ondansetron†	
Vinblastine#	
Vincristine	

*Refers to doxorubicin only; drug concentrations and times of incubation vary.
†Trissel et al 1990.
#Lokich et al 1986; 10 days stability at room temperature and light conditions.
Data from Trissel LA. In: Trissel LA, Hale KN, eds. *ASHP Handbook on Injectable Drugs*. 5th ed. Bethesda, MD: American Society of Hospital Pharmacists; 1988:259–264.

■ Administration

Short intravenous push infusions and intravenous bolus injections are common methods for the administration of DOX; however, a slow, controlled intravenous push over several minutes offers several advantages. First, because the drug can cause severe tissue damage if extravasated, a slow intravenous push over 1 to 2 minutes with constant patient and blood return monitoring can potentially minimize serious extravasations. A 5- to 10-mL flush of normal saline or D5W before and after DOX administration is strongly recommended. This will test venous patency and flush any remaining drug from the tubing, respectively. Alternatively, DOX injection into the side port of a running intravenous infusion may also be used. The patient should be asked to report immediately any change in sensation during administration. Previously established venipuncture sites or infusion sites previously used for administering blood, antibiotics, or other medications should not be used to administer DOX.

Note. Heparin locks (unless recently inserted) are not recommended, and the drug is chemically incompatible with sodium heparin.

Continuous intravenous infusion of DOX appears to significantly lessen cardiotoxicity if the infusion is 96 hours or longer (Legha et al 1982). Shorter infusion times of 24, 48, and 72 hours have not been found to lessen cardiotoxicity and all prolonged infusions increase the incidence and severity of stomatitis and dermatologic toxic effects. The concentration of such DOX infusion solutions does not appear to be critical, although again, the utmost care must be used to prevent extravasation. Thus, administration through tunneled central venous catheters or indwelling vascular access ports is mandatory for all prolonged infusions (Gyves et al 1984, Hickman et al 1979). Careful patient monitoring is required for prolonged DOX infusions, as drug extravasation from central vascular access devices can still occur.

■ Dosage

Numerous drug administration schedules have been reported for DOX. Individual DOX doses will vary depending on several clinical variables. These include the total (cumulative) dose administered to date and the potential for interaction with other drugs or radiation (see table below). As a single agent, doses of 60 to 75 mg/m^2 have been used, repeated no more often than every 3 weeks. Investigationally, single doses of up to 120 mg/m^2 have been used. In an alternative scheme, 20 to 30 mg/m^2 is given daily for 3 consecutive days, repeated in 3 weeks (Creasey et al 1976). Several studies have shown that such weekly injections of 20 mg/m^2 can reduce cardiac toxicity and allow for the administration of cumulative doses of 550 to 2500 mg/m^2 (Weiss et al 1976, 1978, Kessinger et al 1983, Valdivieso et al 1984, Mattson et al 1982, Chlebowski et al 1980, Torti et al 1983). Similarly, Legha et al (1979) and others have reported good clinical results with prolonged continuous infusions of 60 to 90 mg/m^2 given over at least 96 hours. Shorter continuous infusions (over 24 or 48 hours) did not reduce cardiotoxicity compared with intravenous bolus dosing (Legha et al 1979). Clinical activity appeared to be retained, and emetogenic and cardiac toxicity dramatically reduced, by this technique.

As defined by Hryniuk et al (1986) the total dose delivered per unit of time (*dose intensity*) can have a significant impact on the antitumor activity of different agents. Clinical studies with DOX show that in breast cancer, greater dose intensity is associated with enhanced response rates (O'Bryan et al 1977, Carmo-Pereira et al 1986, Jones et al 1987). Doses in the latter two trials were 70 mg/m^2/3 wk for eight cycles or 30 mg/m^2/d × 3 days, repeated every 21 days. Dose-intensive therapy may also be applicable to the treatment of sarcoma (Cortes et al 1972, O'Bryan et al 1977). In the latter trial, an advantage was noted for good-risk sarcoma patients who received a dose of 75 mg/m^2 versus 45 or 60 mg/m^2, all given every 3 weeks; however, recent studies from the Eastern Cooperative Oncology Group have demonstrated activity for doses up to 90 mg/m^2. Metastatic bladder cancer may similarly respond to dose-intensive systemic chemotherapy regimens which use doses of 60 mg/m^2 (Hrushesky et al 1987).

Dose adjustments are required in a number of clinical settings (see table on page 400). With compromised hepatobiliary function, doses should be lowered to 50% of the usual dose for mild dysfunction (serum bilirubin 1.2-3.0) and to 25% of the usual dose for severe liver impairment (serum bilirubin ≥ 3.0 mg%) (Benjamin 1975b). Interestingly, dose adjustments appear to be unwarranted for patients with elevated hepatocellular enzyme levels in the absence of hyperbilirubinemia (Chan et al 1980).

For patients with normal cardiac function, a maximum lifetime cumulative DOX dose of 500 mg/m^2 is recommended to prevent cardiac toxicity (Benjamin 1975a). More recent recommendations suggest limiting the cumulative DOX dose to 450 mg/m^2. If DOX is combined with radiation therapy, a 300 mg/m^2 dose is recommended (Bristow et al 1978b). Doxorubicin doses may also need to be based on ideal body weight in obese patients, as drug clearance appears to be lower in this population (Rodvold et al 1988).

The total dose limit must also take into account the doses of any other anthracyclines or DNA-intercalating compounds the patient has received (eg, esorubicin, epirubicin, idarubicin, daunorubicin, and mitoxantrone). Prospective monitoring including cardiac biopsies may be useful to assess if further

DOXORUBICIN INTRAVENOUS DOSING GUIDELINES*

Dose (mg/m^2)	IV Method	Schedule	Reference
60–75	Bolus	Every 3 weeks	
20–30[†]	Bolus	3 successive days, repeat in 3 weeks	
20	Bolus	Weekly	Valdivieso et al 1984
			Chlebowski et al 1980
60	96-h infusion	Every 3–4 weeks	Garnick et al 1983
			Legha et al 1982

*Lower doses for hepatobiliary dysfunction and for poor bone marrow reserve or performance status.
[†]Allows for greater dose intensity in breast cancer (Jones et al 1987). Also, the higher dose level of 30 mg/m^2/d × 3 produces significant toxicity as a single-agent regimen.

SUGGESTED MODIFICATIONS OF DOXORUBICIN DOSES

Condition	Recommended Dose Modification	Reference
Prior doses	Limit total cumulative lifetime doses (by intravenous bolus) to 550 mg/m^2	Von Hoff et al 1979
Prior chest radiotherapy	Reduce total dose limit to 300–350 mg/m^2	Bristow et al 1978a*
Obesity (>30% ideal body weight)	Base doses on ideal body weight	Rodvold et al 1988*
Hepatobiliary dysfunction	Reduce doses for elevated serum bilirubin (given 50% of dose for serum bilirubin of 1.2–2.9 µg/dL and give 25% of dose for serum bilirubin ≥ 3.0 mg/dL	Benjamin 1975a
	Use indocyanine green plasma disappearance rate as an indicator of doxorubicin clearance for individual patients with hepatic dysfunction	Doroshow and Chan 1982*
Infusion method	Greater cumulative (total) dosing may be afforded by weekly bolus doses *or*	Weiss et al 1978
	continuous (96-h) infusions	Legha et al 1982

*Subjective recommendation only because prospective clinical validation of this dose adjustment schema is not available.

DOX doses can be given in an individual patient (see table on Doxorubicin Cardiotoxicity Grading Systems later in this monograph). Fortunately, no dose reductions are required for renal dysfunction.

■ Special Precautions

Inadvertent extravasation of DOX is associated with severe ulceration and soft tissue necrosis (Rudolph et al 1976, Reilly et al 1977). Therefore, venous patency must be ensured before DOX injection. And, all DOX infusions through peripheral veins should be constantly monitored throughout the total administration period (see Administration). To reduce hair loss from DOX, a scalp tourniquet or ice bag has been used during the drug administration period in such diseases as breast cancer wherein cancer dissemination to the scalp is extremely uncommon. This maneuver is not generally recommended and is specifically contraindicated in any widely metastatic cancer and, by definition, in any hematologic malignancy (see Side Effects and Toxicity).

■ Drug Interactions

Doxorubicin may interact with other drugs used in the cancer patient (see table on opposite page); however, most of these interactions have been described only in experimental systems and their clinical significance is therefore unknown. Nonetheless, a number of potentially significant interactions have been documented in cancer patients. Altered DOX disposition is postulated when DOX is administered with interferon alfa and streptozotocin. With interferon alfa, substantial DOX dose reductions are required (Muss et al 1985, Sarosy et al 1986). In contrast, for streptozotocin, the need for DOX dose reduction is unclear (Chang et al 1976). And, although not evaluated clinically, the combination of DOX with H$_2$ antihistamines such as ranitidine (Harris et al 1988) and cimetidine (Brenner et al 1986) could result in significantly increased DOX toxicity.

Despite a large number of studies showing pharmacologic prevention of DOX-induced cardiotoxicity by diverse agents (see table), only one potential antidote has been clinically verified in cancer patients. The metal-chelating compound ICRF-187 at a dose of 1000 mg/m^2 IV before chemotherapy was able to significantly retard the development of DOX cardiotoxicity in patients with breast cancer (Speyer et al 1988). This allowed for the administration of significantly higher cumulative DOX doses without evidence of congestive heart failure; however, DOX-induced myelosuppression may be slightly increased with this drug combination (Speyer et al 1988).

The reversal of DOX-induced multidrug resistance (MDR) has also been clinically tested using a variety of pharmacologic modulators. Most have dose-limiting toxic effects. For example, dosing of phenothiazines such as trifluoperazine has been limited by neurotoxicity at drug levels required for modulation (Miller et al 1988). The calcium channel antagonist verapamil can also reverse the MDR phenomenon in vitro. It is also active in patients, albeit at doses producing significant hypotension and heart conduction blockade (Dalton et al 1989). The

DRUG INTERACTIONS WITH DOXORUBICIN

Agent	Effect on Doxorubicin	Postulated Mechanism	System Evaluated	Reference
Adenosine	Reduced cardiotoxicity	Enhanced coronary blood flow, general hypothermia	Mice	Hacker and Newman 1983
Allopurinol	Antitumor effects	Inhibition of aglycone formation by xanthine oxidase inhibition	Leukemic L-1210 mice	Schwartz 1983
Allyl alcohol	Increased doxorubicinol exposure and myelotoxicity	Reduced hepatocellular volume as a result of additive necrosis	Rabbits	Brenner et al 1986
	Reduced doxorubicin maximum threshold dose by one half to two thirds	Unknown	Cancer patients	Muss et al 1985 Sarosy et al 1986
Amphoteracin B	Reduced resistance	Inhibition of membranes	Cancer patients	Presant et al 1977
Ascorbate	Reduced cardiotoxicity	Blocked lipid peroxidation	Mice, guinea pigs	Fujita et al 1982
Bepridil	Modulation of DOX resistance	Interference with P-glycoprotein	Tumor cell lines	Schuurhuis et al 1987
Buthionine sulfoximine	Potentiation of cytotoxicity	Glutathione depletion	Sensitive and resistant tumor cells	Dusre et al 1989
Caffeine	Blocked cytotoxicity	Unknown	P-388 cells in vitro	Ganapathi et al 1986
Carnitine	Decreased toxicity	Enhanced cellular energy	Normal mice	Alberts et al 1978
Cimetidine	Decreased clearance, increased plasma exposure	Blocked DOX breakdown	Rabbits	Brenner et al 1986
Coenzyme Q	Reduced cardiotoxicity	Enzyme replenishment	Cardiac mitochondria, rats	Kishi and Folkers 1976 Choe et al 1978
Cromolyn sodium	Reduced cardiotoxicity	Blocked histamine release	Rabbits	Bristow et al 1982
Cyclophosphamide	Increased exposure to active alkylating species	Inhibition of cytochrome P-450 enzymes	Rats Children with cancer	Dodion et al 1984 Evans et al 1980
Cyclosporin	Modulation of DOX resistance	Inhibition of P-glycoprotein drug efflux pump	Tumor cell lines	Hait et al 1989
Digitalis glycosides	Reduced cardiotoxicity	Blocked tissue uptake	Perfused cat hearts Cancer patients	Somberg et al 1978 Guthrie and Gibson 1977
Dipyridamole	Increased cytotoxicity	Unknown	Human ovarian cancer cells	Howell et al 1989
Dimethylsulfoxide IV	Increased aglycones in cerebrospinal fluid	Altered blood–brain barrier	Cancer patients	Kaplan et al 1981
Eflornithine (DFMO)	Reduced cytotoxicity	Blocked polyamine synthesis	Human cancer cells	Seidenfeld et al 1986
Gentamicin	Antagonized bactericidal activity	Unknown	*Proteus mirabilis* in vitro	Bossa et al 1981
Iron chelators ICRF-159,187	Reduced cardiotoxicity	Blocked formation of doxorubicin–iron complexes	Beagle dogs Cancer patients	Herman et al 1981 Speyer et al 1992
Others	Blocked cytotoxicity	Blocked formation of oxygen radicals	MCF-7 breast cancer cells	Doroshow 1986

(continued)

DRUG INTERACTIONS WITH DOXORUBICIN (continued)

Agent	Effect on Doxorubicin	Postulated Mechanism	System Evaluated	Reference
Insulin	Enhanced antitumor effects	Reversed nutritional toxicity	Rats with tumors	Peacock et al 1987
Interferon alfa	Cytotoxic synergy		Human tumor cell lines	Green et al 1985
Interleukin-1	Reduced hematologic toxicity	Stimulation of granulopoiesis	Mice	Eppstein et al 1989
Menadione (vitamin K_3)	Reduced cardiotoxicity	Antioxidant effects	Rat heart cells	Dietrich et al 1989
Methylene blue	Reduced cardiotoxicity	NADPH depletion	Rat heart cells and mice	
N-Acetylcysteine	Reduced cardiotoxicity	Sulfhydryl repletion	Mouse heart cells	Doroshow et al 1981
	Ineffective cardio-protection	Antioxidant	Cancer patients	Myers et al 1982
Ouabain	Cardiotonic effects inhibited by doxorubicin	Altered Ca^{2+} in rapid compartment	Guinea pig atria	Villani et al 1978
	Lack of interaction at ouabain receptor	Na, K-ATPase receptor	Isolated rabbit papillary muscle, mouse/fibroblasts	Van Boxtel et al 1978
	Reduced cytotoxicity	Blocked topoisomerase II effect	Human and hamster cells	Lawrence 1988
Phenobarbital	Enhanced doxorubicin clearance	Microsomal enzyme induction	Mice	Reich and Bachur 1976
Phenothiazines				
Prochlorperazine	Reversal of multidrug resistance	Binding to P-glycoprotein inactivates efflux pump	Cell lines	Krishan et al 1985, Helson 1984
Chlorpromazine	No alterations in pharmacokinetics	Lack of enzyme induction	Humans	Riggs et al 1982
Polysorbate 80 (Tween 80®)	Decreased systemic exposure to doxorubicin	Increased volume of distribution twofold and reduced clearance by one half	Cancer patients	Cummings et al 1986a
Prenylamine	Reduced cardiotoxicity	Reduced intracellular Ca^{2+}	Mice	Milei et al 1980
Prochlorperazine	No effect on DOX disposition	—	Cancer patients	
Propranolol	Potentiated cardiotoxicity	Inhibition of coenzyme Q	Mice	Choe et al 1978
Ranitidine	Increased erythrotoxicity as a result of increased exposure to doxorubicin and doxorubicinol	Unknown	Rabbits	Harris et al 1988
Ricin	Synergistic	Unknown	L-1210 leukemic mice	Fodstad and Pihl 1980
Streptozotocin	Increased systemic DOX exposure and toxicity	Reduced DOX clearance	Cancer patients	Chang et al 1976
Taxmoxifen	Modulation of DOX resistance	Inhibition of P-glycoprotein	P-388 leukemia cells	Ramu et al 1984
Trifluoperazine	Modulation of DOX resistance	Inhibition of P-glycoprotein	Cancer patients P-388 leukemia cells	Miller et al 1988 Ganapathi and Grabowski 1983

(continued)

DRUG INTERACTIONS WITH DOXORUBICIN (continued)

Agent	Effect on Doxorubicin	Postulated Mechanism	System Evaluated	Reference
Verapamil	Reversal of DOX resistance	Inhibition of P-glycoprotein	Cancer patients	Dalton et al 1989
	Increased DOX exposure	Increased volume of distribution and half-life, reduced DOX clearance	Cancer patients	Kerr et al 1986
	Possible enhanced cardiotoxicity	Increased DOX levels in myocytes	Rabbits	Stephens et al 1987
	Enhanced lethality	Unknown	Mice	Giri and Marafino 1984
Vitamin E (α-tocopherol)	Reduced cardiotoxicity	Blocked lipoperoxidation	Rat electrocardiographic changes	Sonneveld 1978
	Reduced cardiotoxicity	Blocked lipoperoxidation	Mice	Myers et al 1977
	No effect on cardiotoxicity	—	Cancer patients	Legha et al 1981
	Reduced cardiotoxicity	Blocked lipoperoxidation	Rabbits	Van Vleet and Ferrans 1980
	No effect on cardiotoxicity	—	Rabbits	Breed et al 1980
Warfarin	Lack of pharmacokinetic or antitumor interaction	—	Tumor-bearing mice	Ghersa and Donelli 1980

mechanism for this effect and that of other diverse modulators such as cyclosporin (Sonneveld and Nooter 1990) and tamoxifen-like triphenylethylene compounds such as toremifine (DeGregorio et al 1989) is believed to involve competitive binding to the 170,000- to 180,000-molecular-weight membrane P-glycoprotein. This molecule mediates MDR by acting as an energy-dependent drug efflux pump in the membranes of resistant cells (Rothenberg and Ling 1989). Most MDR modulator compounds lack direct antitumor activity but several may increase DOX-induced toxic effects such as cardiotoxicity (see drug interaction table). An additional interaction with cyclosporin appears to involve reduced clearance of doxorubicin by blockade of P-glycoprotein-mediated biliary secretion of doxorubicin (Erlichman et al 1991).

■ Pharmacokinetics

Intravenous Administration. Doxorubicin's disposition and elimination from the plasma are best described by a two-compartment or three-compartment open model (see table on page 404). The drug is rapidly distributed in body tissues with about 75% binding to plasma proteins, principally albumin (Eksborg et al 1982). In the blood, the free DOX fraction is dependent on the patient's hematocrit, with greater free drug available in patients with a reduced hematocrit (Piazza et al 1981). Also, drug levels in various tissues are roughly proportional to the DNA content of the specific tissue (Terasaki et al 1982). The avid binding of DOX to DNA is believed to explain the prolonged terminal elimination half-life of 30 to 40 hours, the large apparent volume of distribution of up to 28 L/kg, and the incomplete (50%) total recovery of drug in urine, bile, and feces (Benjamin et al 1977; Takanashi and Bachur 1976). Human tissues with high drug concentrations (in descending order) include liver, lymph nodes, muscle, bone marrow, fat, and skin (Lee et al 1980). In animals, high DOX concentrations have been found in the liver, kidney, and heart tissues (Yesair et al 1972). The drug does not distribute into the central nervous system and experimental efforts to increase central nervous system uptake by osmotic disruption produced significant neurotoxicity (Neuwelt et al 1981).

There is also significant distribution of DOX into human breast milk (Egan et al 1985). Doxorubicin levels of 0.24 μM and doxorubicinol levels of 0.2 μM have been measured in a nursing mother following DOX therapy. The cumulative AUCs for DOX and DOXOL in breast milk was 9.9 and 16.5 $\mu M \cdot h$, respectively. Of interest, both of these values were greater than concurrent AUC val-

DOXORUBICIN PHARMACOKINETICS WITH DIFFERENT METHODS OF ADMINISTRATION

Administration Method (Duration)	Dose (mg/m²)	Plasma Level Peaks	Plasma Level Steady State	Half-life α (min)	Half-life β (h)	Half-life γ (h)	AUC	Clearance	Volume of Distribution	Urinary Excretion (% Dose)	Doxorubicinol Level	Doxorubicinol +1/2 (h)	Reference
Bolus	22.5, 60, 90	0.7, 0.8, 1.1 μg/mL	—	1.5	14	21	—	—	1450 L	3.5	—	—	Creasey et al 1976
Infusion: 4, 8, 72, 24, 48, 96 h	30	0.18, 0.09, 0.05, 0.24, 0.13, 0.097 μg/mL	—	2–5	22–58	—	2, 2, 0, 2.5 mg · h/L	—	—	—	—	—	Speth et al 1987b
													Legha et al 1982
Bolus	50	15 mol/L	—	2.4	0.8	23	17.9 ng · min/L	60.4 L/h/1.74 m²	24 L/kg	—	0.05 mol/L	33	Mross et al 1988
96-h Infusion	9/24 h	—	0.016	6	27	—	1478 μg · h/L	—	—	—	6 ng/mL	—	Speth et al 1987a
Bolus	50	3 μM	1	4.8	0.8	19	—	28–98 L/h	—	—	105 nM	—	Robert et al 1982
Bolus	60	5.6 nmol/mL	—	1.1	16.7	—	—	0.64 L/min/m²	1780 L/m²	5.7	1.6 nmol/mL	32	Benjamin et al 1977

Sources: Ertmann et al 1988, Benjamin 1973, 1974, 1975b.

ues achieved in the plasm. In contrast, DOX does not appear to consistently achieve transplacental uptake. Except for one study reporting low drug levels in placental blood of 0.78 to 1.19 nmol/g and no drug in cord blood plasma (Karp et al 1983), several other trials detected no drug in amniotic fluid following DOX administration to pregnant patients (Roboz et al 1979, D'Incalci et al 1983).

Doxorubicin is extensively metabolized and eliminated primarily as glucuronide conjugates of the parent aglycone or its hydroxylated congener doxorubicinol (DOXOL) (Benjamin et al 1977, Bachur 1975). DOXOL is the main circulatory metabolite of DOX and typically constitutes up to 8.5% of total anthracycline levels in the plasma (see table on page 403). DOXOL also appears to be a more potent cardiotoxin than DOX (Olson et al 1988). The metabolic conversion of DOX to DOXOL is mediated by ubiquitous cytoplasmic aldo/keto reductase enzymes in a reaction dependent on NADPH. Doxorubicinol has approximately 1/20th the antitumor activity of DOX (Schott and Robert 1989) but it may be a more potent cardiotoxin (Brenner et al 1986). DOXOL may also follow dose-dependent elimination in humans (Preiss et al 1989). Thus, in regimens producing high DOXOL levels, clearance of DOXOL may be reduced. In contrast, tissue uptake of DOXOL is poor: 4% or less of DOX levels (Peters et al 1981). This may be due to the greater polarity of DOXOL compared with DOX.

Doxorubicin metabolites which have been variably identified in cancer patients' blood include: 1) the 7-deoxyaglycone of DOX (representing 1-5% of total drug in the serum with a half life of 30 min), and 2) the equivalent aglycone of DOXOL which is present only in some patients at 10-20% of DOX levels. The DOXOL aglycone half lives vary from 0.1 to 24 hours (Cummings et al 1986a). Similar variability in the identification of 7-deoxyaglycones in the plasma is reported by Mross et al (1988) and Cummings et al (1986b). The 7-deoxyaglycones are formed by microsomal glycosidases which are found in many tissues but are primarily concentrated in the liver (Takanashi and Bachur 1976). Subsequent 0-demethylation and conjugation reactions produce ester conjugates of glucuronide or sulfate with 7-deoxy DOX or 7-deoxy DOXOL. Alternatively, the 7-deoxyaglycones may form an alkylating carbon at C-7 which could contribute to cytotoxicity (Sinha and Sik 1980). The conjugated metabolites are exclusively excreted in the bile and feces. Overall, biliary excretion accounts for about 40% of an administered dose (Riggs et al 1977). Approximately 42% of the biliary drug is parent DOX, 22% is doxorubicinol and 36% is other metabolites (Riggs et al 1977). Other recent studies suggest that the biliary secretion of DOX is reduced by cyclosporin A, a compound used to reverse P-glycoprotein mediated multidrug resistance (Erlichman et al 1991). Little drug (5-10%) is excreted in the urine. This small urinary fraction is recovered as either DOX (40%), DOXOL (29%) and 31% as other metabolites (Takanashi and Bachur 1976).

Alterations in Doxorubicin Pharmacokinetics. Patients with cholestasis have delayed DOX clearance and clearly experience greater toxicity from standard doses ([See Dose Adjustment] Benjamin 1975a); however, hepatoma patients with either cirrhosis or simple hepatocellular enzyme elevations appear to have normal DOX clearance and no increased toxicity from standard doses (Chan et al 1980). The only pharmacokinetic alteration in this population was a delay in DOXOL formation and elimination (Chan et al 1980). The clinical significance of this finding is unknown but probably is minimal.

Indocyanine green plasma clearance has also been successfully used as an indicator of hepatobiliary function and DOX clearance (Doroshow and Chan 1982). Delayed fractional elimination of an indocyanine green bolus from the plasma correlates with total bilirubin and with DOX systemic clearance. In contrast, hepatic radiation does not alter DOX pharmacokinetics in children (Holcenberg et al 1981).

Other Factors Altering Doxorubicin Disposition

Obesity. Obesity has been found to result in reduced clearance of DOX in adult cancer patients possibly as a result of drug sequestration in fatty tissues (Rodvold et al 1988). Mildly obese patients with 115 to 130% of ideal body weight (IBW) and obese patients with more than 130% IBW experience significantly delayed clearance of DOX, leading to increased systemic drug exposure. The half-life of DOX in nonobese patients was 13 hours, in mildly obese patients 15 hours, and in obese patients 20 hours. The AUC increased proportionally in these three groups: from 1190 to 1455 and 2,209 ng·h/mL in normal to mildly obese and obese patients, respectively. There were no obesity-related changes in the volume of distribution of DOX nor in the disposition of doxorubicinol. Interestingly there were no differences in DOX toxicity in any of the groups.

Repeated Doses. There is some evidence that repeated DOX dosing results in altered pharmacokinetics (Morris et al 1989, Gessner et al 1981, Robert and Hoerni 1983). In these reports, DOX levels were lower after repeated dosing, which suggests increased drug clearance. There also may be a degree of dose dependence in the peak drug concentrations achieved. Thus, higher peak levels may be obtained with successive doses of drug (Piazza et al 1980, Siemann and Sutherland 1979); however, because neither toxicity nor response rates were altered the clinical significance of these observations is not established.

Age. In one trial the highest clearances of DOX were observed in the younger patients (Robert and Hoerni 1983). In this trial early-phase drug clearance was most affected and ranged from 35 to 200 L/h/m². Lower early-phase clearances (<50 L/h/m²) were found in patients over 50 years of age; however, there was considerable variability in the clearances among patients with different tumor types, and the best correlations between age and clearance were found in breast cancer and lymphoma patients. These observations suggest that higher peak DOX levels may be achieved in older patients, a finding compatible with those of Piazza et al (1980).

Intraarterial Administration. The hepatic extraction rate for DOX in humans ranges from 0.45 to 0.50 and systemic drug levels are about 25% lower with intraarterial administration than with intravenous dosing (Garnick et al 1979). Several other studies have shown that, overall, the pharmacokinetics of intraarterially administered DOX are similar to that of intravenous doses (Lee et al 1980, Bern et al 1978). The relatively low hepatic extraction rate and similar overall disposition patterns provide little pharmacokinetic rationale for intraarterial administration as a means of localizing DOX effects to the liver (Chen and Gross 1980).

Intraperitoneal Administration. When administered in 2 L of Inpersol® via a Tenckhoff catheter for 4-hour dwell times, about 85% of an intraperitoneal dose is systemically absorbed. Peak plasma levels of about 0.1 μM are achieved within the first hour of intraperitoneal instillation which are 10-fold lower than after a 60-mg intravenous dose. Peak peritoneal drug concentrations are 474-fold higher than those achieved after intravenous dosing. These intraperitoneal levels were still 166-fold higher than plasma levels at the end of the 4-hour dwell time. The approximate DOX half-life in the intraperitoneal space was 1 hour (Ozols et al 1982); however, considerable pain and adhesions are produced by intraperitoneal administration and this route is not generally recommended.

■ Side Effects and Toxicity

Myelosuppression. The single acute dose-limiting toxic effect of DOX is bone marrow suppression. Leukopenia from DOX has a nadir of approximately 10 to 14 days. Thrombocytopenia is less severe and is rarely dose limiting. Other hematologic toxic effects such as anemia have been reported, but they are rare and generally less severe. Hematologic recovery from myelosuppression is usually prompt, with resolution often within about 1 week of the nadir.

Extravasation Reactions. Doxorubicin is known to produce local skin and deep tissue damage at the site of inadvertent extravasation (Rudolph et al 1976; Reilly et al 1977). Ulcers may result from one third of extravasations (Larson 1982). The lesions undergo a slow, indolent expansion and can occasionally involve tendons and other deep structures. Doxorubicin-induced ulcers characteristically do not heal and are associated with prolonged local drug retention (Sonneveld et al 1984, Dorr et al 1989). Reilly et al (1977) recommend early surgical debridement, with skin grafting and tendon repair for serious infiltrations noted by extensive local tissue breakdown. Recall reactions have also been reported in areas of previous drug infiltration (Cohen et al 1975). Numerous pharmacologic antidotes have been evaluated but few have demonstrated unequivocal efficacy (Dorr 1990). A prospective clinical trial has reported good results with topical 99% dimethylsulfoxide: 1.5 mL applied every 6 hours for 14 days (Olver et al 1988). The application of cold packs has also been shown to be consistently effective in animal models (Dorr et al 1985, Harwood and Bachur 1987) and in several clinical case reports (Larson 1982). Unproven local adjuvants include sodium bicarbonate, vitamin E, β-adrenergic agents, and large doses of glucocorticosteroids given either topically or especially by the intradermal route (Dorr 1990).

Venous Flare Reactions. Etcubanas and Wilbur (1974) and Souhami and Feld (1978) have additionally reported erythematous streaking along the vein used for DOX infusion. It is usually associated with delayed urticaria and pruritus. These reactions are felt to be due to localized histamine release which has been documented systemically in dogs (Bristow et al 1980, Eschalier et al 1988). Symptoms rarely last more than 1 hour after treatment with intravenous antihistamines and glucocorticosteroids. These venous flare reactions can occur on first administration but this does not appear to contraindicate the subsequent use of DOX (Souhami and Feld 1978). The role of prophylactic corticosteroids and antihistamines is unclear but may be useful along with local ice packs after a reaction develops. Typical doses used are 50 to 100 mg hydrocortisone sodium succinate and 25 to 50 mg diphenhydramine.

Cardiotoxicity. Cardiotoxicity from DOX includes both acute toxicity such as a rare pericarditis–myocarditis syndrome with or without electrophysiologic aberrations and a delayed total dose-related cardiomyopathy (Lefrak et al 1975, Lenaz and Page 1976). Nonspecific electrocardiographic changes may be seen during DOX infusion or immediately afterward (Cortes et al 1975). These include T-wave flattening, ST depression, supraventricular tachyarrhythmias, and extrasystolic contractions (Rinehart et al 1974). The conduction abnormalities are generally transient and are not associated with severe morbidity or the need for dose modification. Indeed, careful cardiac monitoring of patients *prior* to receiving DOX may uncover a similar incidence of transient non-life-threatening arrhythmias (de Planque et al 1985).

In contrast, delayed cardiomyopathy from DOX is clearly dose related. The toxicity presents initially as a clinical syndrome identical to classic congestive heart failure. It is usually irreversible but symptoms can be managed with standard medical therapy involving digitalis glycosides and diuretics. Potential risk factors for DOX cardiotoxicity include cumulative doses greater than 550 mg/m^2, prior mediastinal irradiation (≥ 2000 rad), (3) age greater than 70 years, and preexisting cardiovascular diseases such as prior myocardial infarction or long-standing hypertension (Minow et al 1975).

The pathology of DOX-induced cardiac lesions includes myocyte fragmentation, dropout, intracellular inclusion bodies, and severe mitochondrial swelling (Ferrans 1978). The most definitive and quantitative technique for assessing DOX-induced heart damage is the endomyocardial biopsy which is scored on an established pathologic severity scale (see next table). Among various noninvasive grading procedures, serial gated cardiography (MUGA) scans appear to be helpful in predicting anthracycline cardiotoxicity (Ramos et al 1976, Ewy 1978). Nonetheless, the endomyocardial biopsy appears to provide greater predictability for the development of DOX cardiotoxicity after subsequent treatment (Mason et al 1978). Although there is a sound rationale for limiting total doses to less than 550 mg/m^2 (Gottlieb et al 1973), not every patient who receives a larger cumulative dose will develop heart failure, and total doses of more than 1000 mg/m^2 have been tolerated in individual patients. In contrast, the Stanford experience has shown that with age above 70 years and/or previous cardiac radiation, total DOX doses should be reduced from 450 to 300 mg/m^2 (Bristow et al 1978a).

Bristow et al (1978b) have additionally described anthracycline cardiac toxicity occurring after only the first or second dose of either daunorubicin (seven cases) or DOX (one case). Clinical features at presentation included pericarditis and/or classic signs of heart failure. Although these patients were elderly or had some preexisting cardiac disease, histopathologic analyses were consistent with anthracycline-induced myocyte damage and a secondary inflammatory process. Conversely, DOX cardiomyopathy can also occur 4 to 20 years after the drug is stopped at standard dose limits (Steinherz et al 1989). This has rarely resulted in sudden death in asymptomatic patients (Couch et al

DOXORUBICIN CARDIOTOXICITY GRADING SYSTEMS

Method (Reference)	Grade (Criterion)	Incidence of Congestive Heart Failure
Endomyocardial biopsy (Bristow et al 1978b)	0 No change from normal	
	1 Mild myofibrillar loss in <5% of cells	< 1–5%
	2* Marked myofibrillar loss in 16–25% of cells	< 10%
	2.5 Myofibrillar loss in 26–35% of cells	10–25%
	3 Diffuse cell damage with myofibrillar loss in > 35% of cells	> 25%
Radionuclide ejection fraction (Alexander et al 1979)	15–20% absolute decrease*	10%

*Recommended stopping point for further doxorubicin dosing.

1981). Late and progressive cardiac effects are also observed in children who received cumulative DOX doses of at least 228 mg/m^2 for leukemia therapy (Lipshultz et al 1991). The cumulative DOX dose was the single best predictor of heart failure which sometimes occurred 3.7 to 10.3 years after stopping the drug. Increased left ventricular afterload was noted to serially increase in these patients (Lipshultz et al 1991). In contrast, cardiac symptoms and exercise tolerance were poor correlates of DOX cardiotoxicity. Pathologically, a loss of myocytes leading to reduced ventricular wall thickness was a hallmark in these patients (Lipshultz et al 1991).

There is usually a steep dose–response relationship for DOX cardiotoxicity as described by Minow et al (1975): At total doses under 500 mg/m^2 the incidence of cardiomyopathy is low, below 1%; between 501 and 600 mg/m^2, 11% of patients are affected; and the incidence is 30% for doses above 600 mg/m^2. In a retrospective cardiotoxicity study of 4006 patients, Von Hoff et al (1979) described an overall incidence of 2.2%. In this analysis there was no influence of performance status, sex, race, and tumor type on the incidence of congestive heart failure; however, elderly patients were at greater risk even after adjustment for the normally decreased cardiac function in this group. The major determinants were the dose, the schedule of administration, and the age of the patient. Thus, when DOX doses are given weekly up to a cumulative dose of 500 mg/m^2 once every 3 weeks, the cardiotoxic probability is decreased from 0.07 to 0.02. Continuous intravenous infusions over 96 hours can also significantly lessen DOX cardiotoxicity.

Radiosensitization. There is evidence that DOX is radiosensitizing and/or "radiomimetic." DOX can cause reactivation of soft tissue reactions in areas previously irradiated (Donaldson et al 1974). This has been termed the *radiation recall* phenomenon (Greco et al 1976). A particularly sensitive area for serious radiation recall toxicity is the esophagus (Newburger et al 1978).

Other DOX-induced toxic effects are observed in all rapidly proliferating normal tissues. These include marked alopecia in all hairy body areas. For localized tumors scalp hair loss may be minimized by the placement of a scalp tourniquet for 10 to 30 minutes after an injection (Soukop et al 1978) or by use of a scalp ice bag for 5 minutes before and 10 to 30 minutes after bolus chemotherapy injection (Dean et al 1979). This can theoretically decrease high initial drug concentrations in the scalp. These procedures are contraindicated in patients with widely metastatic diseases such as the leukemias and lymphomas wherein scalp relapses can occur as a result of the creation of a local drug sanctuary in the scalp (Witman et al 1981). The procedure is also less efficacious when DOX is combined with systemic cytotoxic agents such as cyclophosphamide which produce prolonged plasma exposure to cytotoxic moieties following an acute treatment (Middleton et al 1985).

Stomatitis from DOX may occur at all doses and is more pronounced when the drug is given on prolonged administration schemes or in dose-intensive regimens. It generally begins in the sublingual and lateral tongue regions as a burning sensation with noticeable erythema. The initial inflammation typically progresses to ulceration after a few days. Anal fissures and/or proctitis are also rarely reported following DOX therapy. Nausea and vomiting are common, but of mild to moderate intensity. Diarrhea is rare. With consecutive daily dosing, the emetic effects of DOX are generally limited to the first day of treatment.

Hyperpigmentation of the skin, especially the nail beds, may occur. Transverse banding corresponding to individual injections is rarely reported (Priestman and James 1975). Conjunctivitis and excessive tearing lasting several days have been described and a single case of probable DOX-induced hypertensive encephalopathy is reported (Patterson 1978).

■ Special Applications

Intraarterial Doxorubicin. Doxorubicin is sometimes administered to well-defined, surgically nonresectable tumors by regional arterial perfusions. In this application, slightly higher DOX doses may be used although systemic toxicity is not significantly minimized (Di Pietro et al 1973, Haskell et al 1975). Conceptual problems with this approach for the treatment of primary liver cancer or disease metastatic to the liver include a relatively low hepatic extraction ratio of 0.4 to 0.5. This blunts any significant pharmacokinetic advantage (DOX localization to the liver) following intraarterial drug administration (see Pharmacokinetics: Intraarterial Administration). Thus, for all intraarterial DOX applications, pretreatment with antiemetics and constant medical supervision of the perfusion are required. Typical doses call for 25 mg/m^2/d × 3 days repeated at 3 weeks or 0.2 to 0.3 mg/kg for 2 to 20 days (Haskell et al 1975).

Bern et al (1978) have recently compared intraarterial and intravenous DOX in hepatocellular carcinoma. In this study, intraarterial administration did not protect patients from systemic DOX toxicity. Gastrointestinal toxicity was noted at DOX plasma levels of 1.2×10^{-7} M. Hepatic and cardiac toxicity was not observed, but some transient liver enzyme elevations were recorded. Myelosuppression and alopecia were also common. Leukopenic nadirs occurred between the 9th and 17th days of the chemotherapy cycle. Toxicity was directly related to peak drug levels.

Pharmacokinetically the drug is distributed similarly after either intravenous or intraarterial administration (Yeu-Tsu et al 1980, Bern et al 1978). A sliding dosage scale has been used for intraarterial studies (see table on page 399) (Bern et al 1978).

In one trial, 50% of evaluable patients with advanced hepatocellular carcinoma showed objective responses to intraarterial DOX. The median duration of response was 11 months in this trial (Haskell et al 1975). Overall, complications were minimal and DOX toxicity was not greater than that anticipated for similarly dosed intravenous therapy; however, greater local catheter complications may be experienced with intraarterial therapy (Haskell et al 1975).

Doxorubicin has also been administered intraarterially via the pulmonary artery (Karakosis et al 1981). In one trial, seven patients with soft tissue sarcomas received a total of 56 injections. Each injection was 10 to 20 mg, given by Swan-Ganz catheter into a temporarily occluded lobar artery. Drug toxicity and surgical complications were minimal, involving only transient local pulmonary infiltrates and one instance of pneumothorax.

Intrapleural Administration. Doxorubicin has been investigationally administered to patients with malignant pleural effusions (Kefford et al 1980). Doses of 30 mg were diluted into 20 mL of saline and administered by paracentesis needle as a bolus intrapleural instillation. Of 11 patients there were 8 responders to DOX, including one patient with complete resolution of fluid reaccumulations. This response rate was superior to that for nitrogen mustard or tetracycline. Toxicity of intrapleural DOX included pain or fever in 20% of patients each and nausea and/or vomiting in 45% of patients. No alopecia or hematologic toxicity was reported (Kefford et al 1980). Markman et al (1984) have combined intrapleural DOX (3 mg) with cytarabine (61 mg) and cisplatin (100 mg/m^2) in seven cancer patients with malignant pleural effusions. Two ovarian cancer patients responded and no significant systemic toxicity was reported. All injections were given in 250 mL of saline with aggressive systemic therapy to counteract cisplatin nephrotoxicity (Markman et al 1984).

Topical Bladder Instillation. The intravesical administration of DOX is an effective treatment for recurrent, superficial transitional cell carcinoma of the urinary bladder (Pavone-Macaluso 1982). Response rates up to 70% are common (Edsmyr 1980, Matsumara 1978), but patients typically achieve a short duration of response.

Banks et al (1977) have described typical uses of topical DOX in instillations of 50 mg in 150 mL of normal saline. The drug was instilled through a No. 18 Robinson catheter and patients were instructed to retain the drug and ambulate for one-half hour prior to voiding. Treatments were given monthly. Leukopenia with intravesical DOX is not a problem (Pavone-Macaluso 1971). Although data on blood levels of DOX are not available, the procedure is well tolerated and can produce responses in 60 to 70% of patients. Many responses are complete. A dose–response relationship has been described for intravesical DOX (Pavone-Macaluso 1982). With doses of 10 to 40 mg, a response rate of 30% is described, whereas doses of 50 to 150 mg produced response rates up to 90%. An escalating schedule for prophylactic DOX dosing to prevent papilloma recurrence is also reported: 70 mg for 3 doses, then 80 mg for 3 doses and 90 mg thereafter (Garnick et al 1984, 1986). These doses were administered in 40 to 50 mL of normal saline and retained for 1 hour before voiding. Of note, no serious toxicity was reported with this technique.

Pharmacokinetic studies of tritiated DOX given intravesically show no systemic uptake but poor drug penetration past the urothelium into the lamina propria and muscularis layers (Jacobi and Kurth 1980). Thus, exophytic papillary tumors are well managed, but deeply invasive bladder tumors may not be responsive to intravesical DOX therapy. Eksborg et al (1980) have also suggested an individualized dosing schema for intravesical DOX that is based on a patient's bladder capacity in milliliters (BC) and a target AUC (ca. 300 µg/mL·h):

$$\text{intravesical doxorubicin dose} = \frac{\text{AUC} \cdot (\text{BC}-50) \cdot \text{BC}}{\text{BC}-25}$$

REFERENCES

Alberts DS, Peng Y-M, Moon TE, Bressler R. Carnitine prevention of Adriamycin toxicity in mice. *Biomedicine.* 1978;**29**:265–268.

Alexander J, Dainiak N, Berger HJ, et al. Serial assessment of doxorubicin cardiotoxicity with quantitative radionuclide angiocardiography. *N Engl J Med.* 1979;**300**:278.

Bachur NR. Adriamycin (NSC-123127) pharmacology. *Cancer Chemother Rep Part 3.* 1975;**6**:153–158.

Banks MD, Pontes JE, Izbicki RM, Pierce JM. Topical instillation of doxorubicin HCl in the treatment of superficial transition cell carcinoma of the bladder. *J Urol.* 1977;**118**:757–760.

Barlow JJ, et al. Adriamycin and bleomycin alone and in combination in gynecologic cancers. *Cancer.* 1973;**32**(4):735–743.

Benjamin RS. Pharmacokinetics of Adriamycin (NSC-123127) in patients with sarcomas. *Cancer Chemother Rep.* 1974;**58**:271–273.

Benjamin RS. A practical approach to Adriamycin (NSC-123127) toxicology. *Cancer Chemother Rep Part 3.* 1975a;**6**:191–194.

Benjamin RS. Clinical pharmacology of Adriamycin (NSC-123127). *Cancer Chemother Rep Part 3.* 1975b;**6**:183–185.

Benjamin RS, Riggs CE Jr, Bachur NR. Pharmacokinetics and metabolism of Adriamycin in man. *Clin Pharmacol Ther.* 1973;**14**:592–600.

Benjamin RS, Riggs CE Jr, Bachur NR. Plasma pharmacokinetics of Adriamycin and its metabolites in humans with normal hepatic and renal function. *Cancer Res.* 1977;**37**:1416–1420.

Benjamin RS, Wiernik PH, Bachur NR. Adriamycin chemotherapy—Efficacy, safety, and pharmacologic basis of an intermittent single high-dose schedule. *Cancer.* 1974; **33**:19–27.

Bern MM, McDermott W Jr, Cady B, et al. Intraarterial hepatic infusion and intravenous Adriamycin for treatment of hepatocellular carcinoma: A clinical and pharmacology report. *Cancer.* 1978;**42**:399–405.

Blum RH, Carter SK. Adriamycin: A new anticancer drug with significant clinical activity. *Ann Intern Med.* **80**:249–259.

Bonnadonna G, DeLena M, Oslenghi C, Zucali R. Combination chemotherapy of advanced Hodgkin's disease (HD) with a combination of Adriamycin (ADM), bleomycin (BLM), vinblastine (VBL), and imidazol carboxamide (DTIC) versus MOPP. 65th Annual Meeting Houston, Texas, March 27–30. *Proc Am Assoc Cancer Res.* 1974;**360**:90.

Bossa R, Galatulas I, Perrone G. Bactericidal and antineoplastic effect of combination of gentamicin and adriamycin. *Chemotherapy.* 1981;**27**:350–353.

Breed JGS, Zimmerman ANE, Dormans JAMA, Pinedo HM. Failure of the antioxidant vitamin E to protect against Adriamycin-induced cardiotoxicity in the rabbit. *Cancer Res.* 1980;**40**:2033–2038.

Brenner DE, Collins JC, Hande KR. The effects of cimetidine upon the plasma pharmacokinetics of doxorubicin in rabbits. *Cancer Chemother Pharmacol.* 1986;**18**:219–222.

Bristow MR, Sageman WS, Scott RH. Acute and chronic cardiovascular effects of doxorubicin in the dog. The cardiovascular pharmacology of drug-induced histamine release. *J Cardiovasc Pharmacol.* 1980;**2**:487–515.

Bristow MR, Billingham ME, Mason JW, Daniels JR. Clinical spectrum of anthracycline antibiotic cardiotoxicity. *Cancer Treat Rep.* 1978a;**62**(6):873–879.

Bristow MR, Kantrowitz NE, Billingham ME. Prevention of subacute anthracycline cardiotoxicity by cromolyn sodium. *Circulation.* 1982;**66**:II-365.

Bristow MR, Mason JW, Billingham ME, Daniels JR. Doxorubicin cardiomyopathy: Evaluation by phonocardiography, endomyocardial biopsy and cardiac catheterization. *Ann Intern Med.* 1978b;**88**:168.

Carmo-Pereira J, Costa FO, Henrigues E, et al. Advanced breast carcinoma: A comparison of two dose levels of Adriamycin. *Proc Am Soc Clin Oncol.* 1986;**5**:56.

Chan KK, Chlebowski RT, Tong M, et al. Clinical pharmacokinetics of Adriamycin in hepatoma patients with cirrhosis. *Cancer Res.* 1980;**40**:1263–1268.

Chang P, Riggs CE Jr, Scheerer MT, et al. Combination chemotherapy with Adriamycin and streptozotocin. II. Clinicopharmacologic correlation of augmented Adriamycin toxicity caused by streptozotocin. *Clin Pharmacol Ther.* 1976;**20**:611–616.

Chen H-SG, Gross JF. Intra-arterial infusion of anticancer drugs: Theoretic aspects of drug delivery and review of responses. *Cancer Treat Rep.* 1980;**64**:31–40.

Chlebowski RT, Brzechwa-Adjukiewicz A, Cowden A, et al. Doxorubicin (75 mg/m^2) for hepatocellular carcinoma: Clinical and pharmacokinetic results. *Cancer Treat Rep.* **68**:487–491.

Chlebowski RT, Paroly WS, Pugh RP, et al. Adriamycin given as a weekly schedule without a loading course: Clinically effective with reduced incidence of cardiotoxicity. *Cancer Treat Rep.* 1980;**64**:47–51.

Choe JY, Combs AB, Folkers K. Potentiation of the toxicity of Adriamycin by propranolol. *Res Commun Chem Pathol Pharmacol.* 1978;**21**:577–579.

Cohen SC, DiBella NJ, Michalak JC. Recall injury from Adriamycin. *Ann Intern Med.* 1975;**83**(2):232.

Cortes EP, Ellison RR, Yates JN. Adriamycin (NSC-123127) in the treatment of acute myelocytic leukemia. *Cancer Chemother Rep.* 1972;**1**:237–243.

Cortes EP, Holland JF, Glidewell O. Amputation and Adriamycin in primary osteosarcoma. A 5-year report. *Cancer Treat Rep.* 1978;**62**:271–277.

Cortes EP, Holland JF, Wany JJ, et al. Amputation and adriamycin in primary osteosarcoma. *N Engl J Med.* 1974;**291**:998–1000.

Cortes EP, Lutman G, Wanka J, et al. Adriamycin (NSC-123127) cardiotoxicity: Clinicopathological correlation. *Cancer Chemother Rep Part 3.* 1975;**6**(2):215–225.

Couch RD, Loh KK, Sugino J. Sudden cardiac death following Adriamycin therapy. *Cancer.* 1981;**48**:38–39.

Creasey WA, McIntosh LS, Brescia T, et al. Clinical effects and pharmacokinetics of different dosage schedules of Adriamycin. *Cancer Res.* 1976;**36**:216–221.

Cummings J, Forrest GJ, Cunningham D, et al. Influence of polysorbate 80 (Tween 80) and etoposide (VP-16-213) on the pharmacokinetics and urinary excretion of Adriamycin and its metabolites in cancer patients. *Cancer Chemother Pharmacol.* 1986a;**17**:80–88.

Cummings J, Milstead R, Cunningham D, Kay S. Marked inter-patient variation in Adriamycin biotransformation to 7-deoxyaglycones: Evidence from metabolites identified in serum. *Eur J Cancer Clin Oncol.* 1986b;**22**:991–1001.

Dalton WS, Grogan TM, Meltzer PS, et al. Drug-resistance in multiple myeloma and non-Hodgkin's lymphoma. Detection of P-glycoprotein and potential circumvention by addition of verapamil to chemotherapy. *J Clin Oncol.* 1989;**7**:415–424.

Dean JC, Griffity KS, Salmon SE. Scalp hypothermia prevents Adriamycin-induced alopecia (abstract C-201). *Proc Am Soc Clin Oncol.* 1979;**20**:340.

DeGregorio MW, Ford JM, Benz CC, Wiebe VJ. Toremifene: Pharmacologic and pharmacokinetic basis of reversing multidrug resistance. *J Clin Oncol.* 1989;**7**:1359–1364.

De Planque MM, Beukers AFEMTh, Benraadt T, et al. Occurrence of rhythm and conduction disturbances before, during, and after anthracyclines. *Proc Am Soc Clin Oncol.* 1985;**4**:25.

Dietrich MF, Lamentzen MP, Gil-Gomez K, Block JB. Modulation of doxorubicin (DR) induced cardiotoxicity by menadione (VK$_3$) in neonatal rat culture. *Proc Am Assoc Clin Res.* 1989;**30**:573.

Di Marco A. Adriamycin: The therapeutic activity on experimental tumors. In: Carter SK, et al, eds. *International Symposium on Adriamycin*. New York: Springer-Verlag; 1972:53–63.

Di Marco A, Zunino F, Silvestrini R, et al. Interaction of some daunomycin derivatives with deoxyribonucleic acid and their biological activity. *Biochem Pharmacol.* 1971;**20**(6):1323–1328.

D'Incalci M, Broggini M, Buscaglia M, Pardi G. Transplacental passage of doxorubicin. *Lancet.* 1983;**1**:75.

Di Pietro S, De Palo G, Gennari L, et al. Cancer chemotherapy by intraarterial infusion with Adriamycin. *J Surg Oncol.* 1973;**5**:421–430.

Dodion P, Riggs CE Jr, Akman SR, et al. Interactions between cyclophosphamide and Adriamycin metabolism in rats. *J Pharmacol Exp Ther.* 1984;**229**:51–57.

Donaldson SS, Glick JM, Wilbur JR. Adriamycin activating a recall phenomenon after radiation therapy. *Ann Intern Med.* 1974;**81**:407–408.

Doroshow JH. Prevention of doxorubicin-induced killing of MCF-7 human breast cancer cells by oxygen radical scavengers and iron chelating agents. *Biochem Biophys Res Commun.* 1986;**135**:330–335.

Doroshow J, Chan K. Relationship between doxorubicin (D) clearance and indocyanine green dye (ICG) pharmacokinetics (PK) in patients with hepatic dysfunction. *Proc Am Soc Clin Oncol.* 1982;**1**:11.

Doroshow JH, Locker GY, Ifrim I, et al: Prevention of doxorubicin cardiac toxicity in the mouse by N-acetylcysteine. *J Clin Invest.* 1981;**68**:1053–1064.

Dorr RT. Antidotes to vesicant chemotherapy extravasations. *Blood Rev.* 1990;**4**:41–60.

Dorr RT, Alberts DS, Stone A. Cold protection and heat enhancement of doxorubicin skin toxicity in the mouse. *Cancer Treat Rep.* 1985;**69**(4):431–437.

Dorr RT, Dordal MS, Koenig LM, et al. High levels of doxorubicin in the tissues of a patient experiencing extravasation during a 4-day infusion. *Cancer.* 1989;**64**:2462–2464.

Driscoll JS, Hazard GF, Wood HB. Structure–activity relationships among quinone derivatives. *Cancer Chemother Rep Part 2.* 1974;**4**(2):1–362.

Dusre L, Mimnaugh EG, Myesr CE, Sinha BK. Potentiation of doxorubicin cytotoxicity by buthionine sulfoximine in multidrug-resistant human breast tumor cells. *Cancer Res.* 1989;**49**:511–515.

Edsmyr F. Intravesical therapy with Adriamycin in patients with superficial bladder tumors. *Eur Urol.* 1980;**6**:132–136.

Egan PC, Costanza ME, Dodion P, et al. Doxorubicin and cisplatin excretion into human milk. *Cancer Treat Rep.* 1985;**69**:1387–1389.

Eksborg S. Extraction of daunorubicin and doxorubicin and their hydroxyl metabolites: Self-association in aqueous solution. *J Pharm Sci.* 1978;**67**(6):782–785.

Eksborg S, Ehrsson H, Ekqvist B. Protein binding of anthraquinone glycosides, with special reference to Adriamycin. *Cancer Chemother Pharmacol.* 1982;**10**:7–10.

Eksborg S, Nilsson S-O, Edsmyr F. Intravesical instillation of Adriamycin. *Eur Urol.* 1980;**6**:218–220.

Eppstein DA, Kurahara CG, Bruno NA, Terrell TG. Prevention of doxorubicin-induced hematotoxicity in mice by interleukin 1. *Cancer Res.* 1989;**49**:3955–3960.

Erlichman C, Bjamason G, Bunting P, et al. Cyclosporin A (CYA) modulation of doxorubicin (D): A pharmacokinetic/pharmacodynamic trial. *Proc Am Soc Clin Oncol.* 1991;**10**:111.

Erttmann R, Erb N, Steinhoff A, Landbeck G. Pharmacokinetics of doxorubicin in man: Dose and schedule dependence. *J Cancer Res Clin Oncol.* 1988;**114**:509–513.

Eschalier A, Lavarenne J, Burtin C, et al: Study of histamine release induced by acute administration of antitumor agents in dogs. *Can Chemother Pharmacol.* 1988;**21**:246–250.

Etcubanas E, Wilbur JR. Uncommon side effects of Adriamycin. *Cancer Chemother Rep Part 1.* 1974;**58**:757–758.

Evans, WE, Crom WR, Yee GC et al: Adriamycin pharmacokinetics in children. *Proc Amer Assoc Cancer Res and ASCO.* 1980;**21**:176.

Ewy GA, Jones SE, Friedman MJ. Noninvasive cardiac evaluation of patients receiving adriamycin. *Cancer Treat Rep.* 1978;**62**(6):915–917.

Ferrans VJ. A review of cardiac pathology in relation to

anthracycline cardiotoxicity. *Cancer Treat Rep.* 1978;**62**: 955–961.

Fodstad O, Pihl A. Doxorubicin and ricin, a strongly synergistic combination in mouse leukemia. *Cancer Treat Rep.* 1980;**64**:1375–1378.

Fogelsong PD, Reckord C, Swinks S. Doxorubicin inhibits DNA topoisomerase I. *Cancer Chemother Pharmacol.* 1992;**30**:123–125.

Fujita K, Shinpo K, Yamada K, et al. Reduction of Adriamycin toxicity by ascorbate in mice and guinea pigs. *Cancer Res.* 1982;**42**:309–316.

Gaj E, Sesin GP, Griffen RE. Evaluation of growth of five microorganisms in doxorubicin and floxuridine media. *Pharm Manufacturing.* 1984;**1**:50, 52–53.

Ganapathi R, Grabowski D. Enhancement of sensitivity to Adriamycin in resistant P388 leukemia by the calmodulin inhibitor trifluoperazine. *Cancer Res.* 1983; **43**:3696–3699.

Ganapathi R, Grabowski D, Schmidt H, et al. Modulation of Adriamycin and N-trifluoroacetylAdriamycin-14-valerate induced effects on cell cycle traverse and cytotoxicity in P388 mouse leukemia cells by caffeine and the calmodulin inhibitor trifluoperazine. *Cancer Res.* 1986;**46**:5553–5557.

Garnick MB, Ensminger WD, Israel M. A clinical–pharmacological evaluation of hepatic arterial infusion of Adriamycin. *Cancer Res.* 1979;**39**:4105–4110.

Garnick MB, Maxwell B, Gibbs RS, et al. Intravesical doxorubicin for prophylaxis in the management of superficial bladder carcinoma—An update. In: *Intra-arterial and Intracavitary Chemotherapy*. Proceedings of the University of California, San Diego Conference on Intra-arterial and Intracavitary Chemotherapy. Hingham: Martinus Nijhoff; 1986.

Garnick MB, Schade D, Israel M, et al. Intravesical doxorubicin for prophylaxis in the management of recurrent superficial bladder carcinoma. *J Urol.* 1984;**131**: 43–46.

Garnick MB, Weiss GR, Stelle GD Jr, et al. Clinical evaluation of long-term, continuous-infusion doxorubicin. *Cancer Treat Rep.* 1983;**67**:133–142.

Gessner T, Rotot J, Bolanowski W, Hoerni B, et al. Effects of prior therapy on plasma levels of Adriamycin during subsequent therapy. *J Med.* 1981;**12**:183–193.

Ghersa P, Donelli MG. Distribution and antitumoral activity of Adriamycin combined with warfarin in mice. *Cancer Chemother Pharmacol.* 1980;**5**:43–47.

Giri SN, Marafino BJ Jr. Effects of verapamil on doxorubicin-induced mortality and electrolyte changes in the mouse heart. *Drug Chem Toxicol.* 1984;**7**:407–422.

Glisson BS, Ross WE. DNA topoisomerase II: A primer on the enzyme and its unique role as a multidrug target in cancer chemotherapy. *Pharmacol. Ther.* 1987;**32**:89–106.

Goodman J, Hochstein P. Generation of free radicals and lipid peroxidation by redox cycling of Adriamycin and daunomycin. *Biochem Biophys Res Commun.* 1977;**77**:797.

Goormatigh E, Chatelain P, Caspers J, et al. Evidence of a complex between Adriamycin derivatives and cardiolipin: Possible role in cardiotoxicity. *Biochem Pharmacol.* 1980;**29**:3003.

Gottlieb JA, Hill CS. Chemotherapy of thyroid cancer with Adriamycin. *N Engl J Med.* 1974;**290**(4):193–197.

Gottlieb JA, Lefrak EA, O'Bryan RM, et al. Fatal Adriamycin cardiomyopathy (CMP): Prevention by dose limitation. *Proc Am Assoc Cancer Res.* 1973;**14**:abstract 352.

Greco FA, Bereton HD, Kent H, et al. Adriamycin and enhanced radiation reaction in normal esophagus and skin. *Ann Intern Med.* 1976;**85**:294–298.

Green MD, Speyer J, Wernz J, et al. Doxorubicin and interferon: Rationale and clinical experience. *Cancer Treat Rev.* 1985;**12**:61–67.

Guthrie D, Gibson AL. Doxorubicin cardiotoxicity: Possible role of digoxin in its prevention. *Br Med J.* 1977;**2**:1447–1449.

Gyves JW, Ensminger WD, Niederhube JE, et al. A totally implanted injection port system for blood sampling and chemotherapy administration. *JAMA.* 1984;**251**:2538–2541.

Hacker MP, Newman RA. Reduction of acute Adriamycin toxicity in mice treated with adenosine. *Eur J Cancer Clin Oncol.* 1983;**19**:1121–1126.

Hait WN, Stein JM, Koletsky AJ, et al. Activity of cyclosporin A and a non-immunosuppressive cyclosporin against multidrug resistant leukemic cell lines. *Cancer Commun.* 1989;**1**:35–43.

Handa K, Sato S. Stimulation of microsomal NADPH oxidation by quinone group containing anticancer chemicals. *Gann.* 1976;**67**:523.

Harris NL, Brenner DE, Anthony LB, et al. The influence of ranitidine on the pharmacokinetics and toxicity of doxorubicin in rabbits. *Cancer Chemother Pharmacol.* 1986;**21**:323–328.

Harwood KVS, Bachur NR. Evaluation of dimethylsulfoxide and local cooling as antidotes for doxorubicin extravasation in a pig model. *Oncol Nurs. Forum.* 1987;**14**:39–44.

Hasinoff BB, Davey JP. Adriamycin and its iron(III) and copper(II) complexes. Glutathione-induced dissociation; cytochrome c oxidase inactivation and protection; binding to cardiolipin. *Biochem Pharmacol.* 1988;**37**:3663–3669.

Haskell CM, Eilber FR, Morton DL. Adriamycin (NSC-123127) by arterial infusion. *Cancer Chemother Rep Part 3.* 1975;**6**(2):187–189.

Helson L. Calcium channel blocker enhancement of anticancer drug cytotoxicity—A review. *Cancer Drug Delivery.* 1984;**1**:353–361.

Henry DW. Structure–activity relationships among daunorubicin and Adriamycin analogs. *Cancer Treat Rep.* 1979;**63**:845.

Herman EH, Ferrans VJ, Waravdekar VS. Marked reduction of chronic doxorubicin cardiotoxicity by pretreatment with ICRF-187 in beagle dogs. *Proc Am Assoc Clin Res.* 1981;**22**:238.

Hickman RO, Buckner CD, Clift RA, et al. A modified

right atrial catheter for access to the venous system in marrow transplant recipients. *Surg Gynecol Obstet.* 1979;**148**:871–875.

Hoffman DM, Grossano DD, Damin LA. Stability of refrigerated and frozen solutions of doxorubicin hydrochloride. *Am J Hosp Pharm.* 1979;**36**:1536–1538.

Holcenberg JS, Kun LE, Ring BJ, Evans WE. Effect of hepatic irradiation on the toxicity and pharmacokinetics of Adriamycin in children. *Int J Rad Oncol Biol Phys.* 1981;**7**:953–956.

Hortobagyi GM, Gutterman JU, Blumenschein GR, et al. Combination chemoimmunotherapy of metastatic breast cancer. *Cancer.* 1979;**44**:1955–1962.

Howell SB, Hom D, Sanga R, et al. Comparison of the synergistic potentiation of etoposide, doxorubicin, and vinblastine cytotoxicity by dipyridamole. *Cancer Res.* 1989;**49**:3178–3183.

Hrushesky WJM, Roemeling RV, Wood PA, et al. High-dose intensity systemic therapy of metastatic bladder cancer. *J Clin Oncol.* 1987;**5**:450–455.

Hryniuk W, Levine MN. Analysis of dose-intensity for adjuvant chemotherapy trials in stage II breast cancer. *J Clin Oncol.* 1986;**4**:1162–1170.

Jacobi GH, Kurth KH. Studies on the intravesical action of topically administered G^{3}H-deoxyrubicin hydrochloride in men: Plasma uptake and tumor penetration. *J Urol.* 1980;**124**:34–37.

Jones RB, Holland JF, Bhardwaj S, et al. A phase I–II study of intensive-dose Adriamycin for advanced breast cancer. *J Clin Oncol.* 1987;**5**:172–177.

Kaplan RS, Riggs CE Jr., Miles LM, et al. Preliminary observations on the effects of dimethyl sulfoxide on the metabolism and distribution of Adriamycin. *Am Soc Clin Oncol.* 1981;**21**:367.

Karakosis CP, Park HC, Sharma SD, Kanter P. Regional chemotherapy via the pulmonary artery for pulmonary metastases. *J Surg Oncol.* 1981;**18**:249–255.

Karp GI, von Oeyen P, Valone F, et al. Doxorubicin in pregnancy: Possible transplacental passage. *Cancer Treat Rep.* 1983;**67**:773–777.

Kefford RF, Woods RL, Fox RM, Tattersall MHN. Intracavitary Adriamycin, nitrogen mustard and tetracycline in the control of malignant effusions. *Med J Aust.* 1980;**2**:447–448.

Kenis Y, Michel J, Rimoldi R, et al. Results of a clinical trial with intermittent doses of Adriamycin in lung cancer. *Eur J Cancer.* 1972;**8**:485–489.

Kerr DJ, Graham J, Cummings J, et al. The effect of verapamil on the pharmacokinetics of Adriamycin. *Cancer Chemother Pharmacol.* 1986;**18**:239–242.

Kessinger A, Lemon HM, Foley JF. Mini-dose weekly Adriamycin™ therapy for patients with malignant disease at increased risk to Adriamycin™ toxicity. *Am J Clin Oncol.* 1983;**6**:113–115.

Ketchum D, Wolf E, Sesin GP. Cost-benefit and stability of study of doxorubicin following reconstitution. *J IV Ther.* 1981;Apr 15–18.

Kim SH, Kim JH. Lethal effect of Adriamycin on the division of HeLa cells. *Cancer Res.* 1972;**32**:323–325.

Kimler BF, Cox GG, Reddy EK. Interaction of radiation, dihydroxyanthraquinone, and Adriamycin on the induction of acute lethality in mice. *Int J Radiat Oncol Biol Phys.* 1984;**10**:1459–1463.

Kishi T, Folkers K. Prevention by coenzyme Q_{10} (NSC-140865) of the inhibition by Adriamycin (NSC-123127) of coenzyme Q_{10} enzymes. *Cancer Treat Rep.* 1976;**60**:223–224.

Krishan A, Sauerteig A, Willham LL. Flow cytometric studies on modulation of cellular Adriamycin retention by phenothiazines. *Cancer Res.* 1985;**45**:1046–1051.

Landolph JR, Bhatt RS, Telfer N, Heidelberger C. Comparison of Adriamycin- and ouabain-induced cytotoxicity and inhibition of ^{86}rubidium transport in wild-type and ouabain-resistant C3H/10T1/2 mouse fibroblasts. *Cancer Res.* 1980;**40**:4581–4588.

Larson DL. Treatment of tissue extravasation by antitumor agents. *Cancer.* 1982;**49**:1796–1799.

Lawrence TS. Reduction of doxorubicin cytotoxicity by ouabain: Correlation with topoisomerase-induced DNA strand breakage in human and hamster cells. *Cancer Res.* 1988;**48**:725–730.

Lee YTN, Chan KK, Harris PA, et al. Distribution of Adriamycin in cancer patients: Tissue uptakes, plasma concentrations after IV and hepatic IA administration. *Cancer.* 1980;**45**:2231–2239.

Lefrak EA, Pitha J, Rosenheim S, et al. Adriamycin (NSC-123127) cardiomyopathy. *Cancer Chemother Rep Part 3.* 1975;**6**(2):203–208.

Legha S, Benjamin R, Wang YM, et al. Evaluation of α-tocopherol against Adriamycin cardiotoxicity in humans. *Proc Am Assoc Cancer Res.* 1981;**22**:176.

Legha SS, Benjamin RS, Mackay B, et al. Reduction of doxorubicin cardiotoxicity by prolonged continuous intravenous infusion. *Ann Intern Med.* 1982;**96**:133–139.

Legha SS, Benjamin RS, Yayo HY, Freireich EJ. Augmentation of Adriamycin's therapeutic index by prolonged continuous IV infusion for advanced breast cancer (abstract 1059). *Proc Am Assoc Cancer Res.* 1979;**20**:261.

Lenaz L, Page JA. Cardiotoxicity of Adriamycin and related anthracyclines. *Cancer Treat Rev.* 1976;**3**:111–120.

Lipshultz SE, Colan SD, Gelber RD, et al. Late cardiac effects of doxorubicin therapy for acute lymphoblastic leukemia in childhood. *N Engl J Med.* 1991;**324**:808–815.

Livingston RB, Moore TN, Heilbrun L, et al. Small cell carcinoma of the lung: Combined chemotherapy and radiation. *Ann Intern Med.* 1978;**88**:194–199.

Markman M, Howell SB, Green MR. Combination intracavitary chemotherapy for malignant pleural disease. *Cancer Drug Delivery.* 1984;**1**(4):333–336.

Mason JW, Bristow MR, Billingham ME, Daniels JR. Invasive and noninvasive methods of assessing Adriamycin cardiotoxic effects in man: Superiority of histopathologic assessment using endomyocardial biopsy. *Cancer Treat Rep.* 1978;**62**(6):857–864.

Matsumura Y. Intravesical infusion therapy with Adriamycin. *Nishi Nihon J.* 1978;**38**:236–237.

Mattsson W, Borgstrom S, Landberg T, Trope C. A weekly schedule of low-dose doxorubicin in the treatment of advanced breast cancer. *Clin Ther.* 1982;**5**(2):193–203.

McCredie KB, Hewlett JS, Kennedy A. Sequential Adriamycin–Ara-C(A-OAP) for remission induction (RI) of adult acute leukemia (AAL). *Proc Am Assoc Cancer Res.* 1976;**17**:239.

McKelvey EM, Gottlieb JA, Wilson HE, et al. Hydroxyldaunorubicin (Adriamycin) combination chemotherapy in malignant lymphoma. *Cancer.* 1976;**38**: 1484–1493.

Middleton J, Franks D, Buchanan RB, et al. Failure of scalp hypothermia to prevent hair loss when cyclophosphamide is added to doxorubicin and vincristine. *Cancer Treat Rep.* 1985;**69**:373–375.

Milei J, Busch L, Marantz H, Bolomo N. Prenylamine inhibition of Adriamycin cardiomyopathy in mice. *Am Soc Clin Oncol.* 1980;**21**:330.

Miller RL, Bukowski RM, Budd GT, et al. Clinical modulation of doxorubicin resistance by the calmodulin-inhibitor, trifluoperazine: A phase I/II trial. *J Clin Oncol.* 1988;**6**:880–888.

Minow RA, Benjamin RS, Gottlieb JA, Adriamycin (NSC-123127) cardiomyopathy—An overview with determination of risk factors. *Cancer Chemother Rep Part 3.* 1975;**6**(2):195–201.

Morris RG, Reece PA, Dale BM, et al. Alteration in doxorubicin and doxorubicinol plasma concentrations with repeated courses to patients. *Ther Drug Monitoring.* 1989;**11**:380–383.

Mross K, Maessen P, van der Vijgh WJF, et al. Pharmacokinetics and metabolism of epidoxorubicin and doxorubicin in humans. *J Clin Oncol.* 1988;**6**:517–526.

Muss HB, Welander C, Caponera M, et al. Interferon and doxorubicin in renal cell carcinoma. *Cancer Treat Rep.* 1985;**69**(6):721–722.

Myers CE. Anthracyclines. In: Chabner B, ed. *Pharmacologic Principles of Cancer Treatment.* Philadelphia: WB Saunders; 1982;416–434.

Myers CE, Gianni L, Simone SB, et al. Oxidative destruction of erythrocyte ghost membranes catalyzed by the doxorubicin–iron complex. *Biochem.* 21:1707–1713.

Myers CE, McGuire W, Young R. Adriamycin: The role of lipid peroxidation in cardiac toxicity and tumor response. *Science.* 1977;**197**:165–167.

Neuwelt EA, Pagel M, Barnett P, et al. Pharmacology and toxicity of intracarotid Adriamycin administration following osmotic blood–brain barrier modification. *Cancer Res.* 1981;**41**:4466–4470.

Newburger PE, Cassady R, Jaffe N. Esophagitis due to Adriamycin and radiation therapy for childhood malignancy. *Cancer.* 1978;**42**:417–423.

O'Bryan RM, Balcer LH, Gottlieb JE, et al. Dose response evaluation of Adriamycin in human neoplasia. *Cancer.* 1977;**39**:1940–1948.

O'Bryan RM, Luce JK, Talley RW. Phase II evaluation of Adriamycin in human neoplasia. *Cancer.* 1973;**32**(1):1–8.

Olson RD, Mushlin PS, Brenner DE, et al. Doxorubicin cardiotoxicity may be caused by its metabolite, doxorubicinol. *Proc Natl Acad Sci USA.* 1988;**85**:3585–3589.

Olver IN, Aisner J, Hament A, et al. A prospective study of topical dimethyl sulfoxide for treating anthracycline extravasation. *J Clin Oncol.* 1988;**6**:1732–1735.

Ozols RF, Young RC, Speyer JL, et al. Phase I and pharmacological studies of Adriamycin administered intraperitoneally to patients with ovarian cancer. *Cancer Res.* 1982;**42**:4265–4269.

Painter RB. Inhibition of DNA replicon initiation by 4-nitroquinoline 1-oxide, Adriamycin and ethyleneimine. *Cancer Res.* 1978;**38**:4445.

Patterson AHG. Hypertensive reaction to Adriamycin (letter). *Cancer Treat Rep.* 1978;**62**(8):1269–1270.

Pavone-Macaluso M. Chemotherapy of vesical and prostatic tumours. *Br J Urol.* 1971;**43**:701–709.

Pavone-Macaluso M. Intravesical chemotherapy in the treatment of bladder cancer. In: Jones SE, ed. *Current Concepts in the Use of Doxorubicin Chemotherapy.* Milan: Farmitalia Carlo Erba; 1982:137–144.

Peacock JL, Gorschboth CM, Norton JA. Impact of insulin on doxorubicin-induced rat host toxicity and tumor regression. *Cancer Res.* 1987;**47**:4318–4322.

Peters JH, Gordon GR, Kashiwase D, Acton EM. Tissue distribution of doxorubicin and doxorubicinol in rats receiving multiple doses of doxorubicin. *Cancer Chemother Pharmacol.* 1981;**7**:65–69.

Piazza E, Broggini M, Trabattoni A, et al. Adriamycin distribution in plasma and blood cells of cancer patients with altered hematocrit. *Eur J Cancer Clin Oncol.* 1981;**17**:1089–1096.

Piazza E, Donelli MG, Broggini M, et al. Early phase pharmacokinetics of doxorubicin (Adriamycin) in plasma of cancer patients during single- or multiple-drug therapy. *Cancer Treat Rep.* 1980;**64**:845–854.

Poochikian GK, Craddock JC, Flora KP. Stability of anthracycline antibiotics in four infusion fluids. *Am J Hosp Pharm.* 1981;**38**:483–486.

Preiss R, Sohr R, Kittelmann B, et al. Investigations on the dose-dependent pharmacokinetics of Adriamycin and its metabolites. *Int J Clin Pharmacol Ther Toxicol.* 1989;**27**:156–164.

Presant CA, Klahr C, Santala R. Amphotericin B induction of sensitivity to Adriamycin 1,3-bis(2-chloroethyl)-1-nitrosourea (BCNU) plus cyclophosphamide in human neoplasia. *Ann Intern Med.* 1977;**86**:47–51.

Priestman TJ, James KW. Adriamycin and longitudinal pigmented banding of fingernails. *Lancet.* 1975;**1**:1337–1338.

Ramos A, Meyer RA, Korfhagen J, et al. Echocardiographic evaluation of Adriamycin cardiotoxicity in children. *Cancer Treat Rep.* 1976;**60**:1281–1284.

Ramu A, Glaubiger D, Fuks Z. Reversal of acquired resistance to doxorubicin in P388 murine leukemia cells by tamoxifen and other triparanol analogues. *Cancer Res.* 1984;**44**:4392–4395.

Reich SD, Bachur NR. Alterations in Adriamycin efficacy by phenobarbital. *Cancer Res.* 1976;**36**:3803–3806.

Reilly JJ, Neifeld JP, Rosenberg SA. Clinical course and management of accidental Adriamycin extravasation. *Cancer.* 1977;**40**(5):2053–2056.

Riggs CE Jr, Benjamin RS, Serpick AA, et al. Biliary disposition of Adriamycin. *Clin Pharmacol Ther.* 1977;**22**:234–241.

Riggs CE, Jr., Engel S, Wesley M, Wiernik PH. Doxorubicin pharmacokinetics: Prochlorperazine and barbiturate effects. *Clin Pharmacol Ther.* 1982;**31**:263.

Rinehart J, Lewis R, Balcerzak SP. Adriamycin cardiotoxicity in man. *Ann Intern Med.* 1974;**81**:475–478.

Ritch PS, Occhipinti SJ, Cunningham RE, Shackney SE. Schedule-dependent synergism of combinations of hydroxyurea with Adriamycin and 1-beta-D-arabinofuranosylcytosine with Adriamycin. *Cancer Res.* 1981;**41**:3881.

Robert J, Hoerni B. Age dependence of the early-phase pharmacokinetics of doxorubicin. *Cancer Res.* 1983;**43**:4467–4469.

Robert J, Illiadis A, Hoerni B, et al. Pharmacokinetics of Adriamycin in patients with breast cancer: Correlation between pharmacokinetic parameters and clinical short-term response. *Eur J Cancer Clin Oncol.* 1982;**18**:739–745.

Roboz J, Gleicher N, Wu K, et al. Does doxorubicin cross the placenta? *Lancet.* 1979;**2**:1381–1383.

Rodvold KA, Rushing DA, Tewksbury DA. Doxorubicin clearance in the obese. *J Clin Oncol.* 1988;**6**:1321–1327.

Rothenberg M, Ling V. Multidrug resistance: Molecular biology and clinical relevance. *J Natl Cancer Inst.* 1989;**81**:907–913.

Rudolph R, Stein R, Patillo RA. Skin ulcers due to adriamycin. *Cancer.* 1976;**38**:1087–1094

Salmon SE, Jones SE. Chemotherapy of advanced breast cancer with a combination of Adriamycin and cyclophosphamide (abstract). *Proc Am Assoc Cancer Res.* 1974;**15**:90.

Samuels L, Newton WA Jr, Heyn R. Daunorubicin therapy in advanced neuroblastoma. *Cancer.* 1971;**27**:831–834.

Sarosy GA, Brown TD, Von Hoff DD, et al. Phase I study of α_2-interferon plus doxorubicin in patients with solid tumors. *Cancer Res.* 1986;**46**:5368–5371.

Schein PS, et al. Bleomycin, Adriamycin, cyclophosphamide, vincristine and prednisone (BACOP): Combination chemotherapy in the treatment of advanced diffuse histiocytic lymphoma. *Ann Intern Med.* 1976;**85**:417–422.

Schott B, Robert J. Comparative activity of anthracycline 13-dihydrometabolites against rat glioblastoma cells in culture. *Biochem Pharmacol.* 1989;**38**:4069–4074.

Schuurhuis GJ, Broxterman HJ, van der Hoeven JJM, et al. Potentiation of doxorubicin cytotoxicity by the calcium antagonist bepridil in anthracycline-resistant and -sensitive cell lines. *Cancer Chemother Pharmacol.* 1987;**20**:285–290.

Schwartz HS. Enhanced antitumor activity of adriamycin in combination with allopurinol. *Cancer Lett.* 1983;**26**:69–74.

Seidenfeld J, Komar KA, Naujokas MF, Block AL. Reduced cytocidal efficacy for Adriamycin in cultured carcinoma cells depleted of polyamines by difluoromethylornithine treatment. *Cancer Res.* 1986;**46**:1155–1159.

Siemann DW, Sutherland RM. A comparison of the pharmacokinetics of multiple and single dose administrations of Adriamycin. *Int J Radiat Oncol Biol Phys.* 1979;**5**:1271–1274.

Silverstrini R, Gambarucci C, Dasdia T. Biological activity of Adriamycin in vitro. *Tumori.* 1970;**56**(3):137–148.

Sinha B, Sik RH. Bindings of Adriamycin to cellular macromolecules in vivo. *Biochem Pharmacol.* 1980;**29**:1867.

Somberg J, Cagin N, Levitt B, et al. Blockade of tissue uptake of the antineoplastic agent, doxorubicin. *J Pharmacol Exp Ther.* 1978;**204**:226–229.

Sonneveld P. Effect of α-tocopherol on the cardiotoxicity of Adriamycin in the rat. *Cancer Treat Rep.* 1978;**62**:1033–1036.

Sonneveld P, Nooter K. Reversal of drug-resistance by cyclosporin-A in a patient with acute myelocytic leukaemia. *Br J Haematol.* 1990;**75**:208–211.

Sonneveld P, Wassenaar HA, Nooter K. Long persistence of doxorubicin in human skin after extravasation. *Cancer Treat Rep.* 1984;**68**:895–896.

Souhami L, Feld R. Urticaria following intravenous doxorubicin administration. *JAMA.* 1978;**240**(15):1624–1626.

Soukop M, Campbell A, Gray MM, Calman KC. Adriamycin, alopecia and the scalp tourniquet (letter). *Cancer Treat Rep.* 1978;**62**(3):489–490.

Speth PAJ, Lissen PCM, Boezeman JBM, et al. Cellular and plasma Adriamycin concentrations in long-term infusion therapy of leukemia patients. *Cancer Chemother Pharmacol.* 1987a;**20**:305–310.

Speth PAJ, Lissen PCM, Holdrinet RSG, Haanen C. Plasma and cellular Adriamycin concentrations in patients with myeloma treated with ninety-six-hour continuous infusion. *Clin Pharmacol Ther.* 1987b;**41**:661–665.

Speyer JL, Green MD, Kramer E, et al. Protective effect of the bispiperazinedione ICRF-187 against doxorubicin-induced cardiac toxicity in women with advanced breast cancer. *N Engl J Med.* 1988;**319**:745–752.

Speyer JL, Green MD, Zeleniuch-Jacquotte A, et al. ICRF-187 permits longer treatment with doxorubicin in women with breast cancer. *J Clin Oncol.* 1992;**10**:117–127.

Steinherz L, Steinherz P, Tan C, Murphy L. Cardiac toxicity 4–20 years after completing anthracycline therapy. *Proc Amer Soc Clin Oncol.* 1989;**8**:296.

Stephens LC, Wang YM. Adriamycin cardiotoxicity in rabbits treated with verapamil. *Proc Am Assoc Cancer Res.* 1985;**26**:218.

Stephens LC, Wang Y-M, Schultheiss TE, Jardine JH. Enhanced cardiotoxicity in rabbits treated with verapamil and Adriamycin. *Oncology* 1987;**44**:302–306.

Takanashi S, Bachur NR. Adriamycin metabolism in man. Evidence from urinary metabolites. *Drug Metab Dispos.* 1976;**4**:79–87.

Terasaki T, Iga T, Sugiyama Y, Hanano M. Experimental evidence of characteristic tissue distribution of Adriamycin. Tissue DNA concentration as a determinant. *J Pharm Pharmacol.* 1982;**34**:597–600.

Tewey KM, Rowe TC, Yang L, et al. Adriamycin-induced DNA damage mediated by mammalian DNA topoisomerase II. *Science*. 1984;**226**:466–468.

Tomlinson E, Malspeis L. Concomitant adsorption and stability of some anthracycline antibiotics. *J Pharm Sci*. 1982;**71**:1121–1125.

Torti F, Bristow M, et al. Reduced cardiotoxicity of doxorubicin on a weekly schedule. *Ann Intern Med*. 1983; **99**(6):745–749.

Trissel LA. In: Trissel LA, Hale KN, eds. *ASHP Handbook on Injectable Drugs*. 5th ed. Bethesda, MD: American Society of Hospital Pharmacists; 1988:259–264.

Trissel LA, Fulton B, Tramonte SM. Visual compatibility of ondansetron with chemotherapeutic agents, antibiotics, and other selected drugs during simulated Y-site injection (abstract #P-468R). In: *25th Annual ASHP Midyear Clinical Meetings and Exhibit, Las Vegas, Nevada*. Bethesda, MD: American Society of Hospital Pharmacists, 1990.

Tritton TR, Yee G. The anticancer agent Adriamycin can be actively cytotoxic without entering cells. *Science*. 1982;**217**:248–251.

Valdivieso M, et al. Increased therapeutic index of weekly doxorubicin in the therapy of NSC lung cancer. A prospective randomized study. *J Clin Oncol*. 1984;**2**(3):207–214.

Van Boxtel CJ, Olson RD, Boerth RC, Oates JA. Doxorubicin: Inotropic effects and inhibitory action on ouabain. *J Pharmacol Exp Ther*. 1978;**207**:277–283.

Van Vleet JF, Ferrans VJ. Evaluation of vitamin E and selenium protection against chronic Adriamycin toxicity in rabbits. *Cancer Treat Rep*. 1980;**64**:315–317.

Villani F, Piccinini F, Merelli P, Favalli L. Influence of Adriamycin on calcium exchangeability in cardiac muscle and its modification by ouabain. *Biochem Pharmacol*. 1978;**27**:985–987.

Von Hoff DD, Layard MW, Basa P, et al. Risk factors for doxorubicin-induced congestive heart failure. *Ann Intern Med*. 1979;91:710–717.

Weiss AJ, Metter GE, Fletcher WS. Studies on Adriamycin using a weekly regimen demonstrating its clinical effectiveness and lack of cardiac toxicity. *Cancer Treat Rep*. 1978;**60**:813–822.

Witman G, Cadman E, Chen M. Missuse of scalp hypothermia. *Cancer Treat Rep*. 1981;**65**:507–508.

Yesair DW, Schwartzbach E, Shuck D, et al. Comparative pharmacokinetics of daunomycin and Adriamycin in several animal species. *Cancer Res*. 1972;**32**:1177–1183.

Yeu-Tsu NL, Chan KK, Harris PA, et al. Distribution of Adriamycin in cancer patients. *Cancer*. 1980;**45**:2231–2239.

Echinomycin

■ Other Names

Quinomycin A; NSC-526417.

■ Chemistry

The cyclic peptide echinomycin is one of a family of quinoxaline antibiotics isolated from *Streptomyces echinatus* (Corbaz et al 1957). It consists of two planar quinoxoline moieties connected by an octapeptide bridge (Martin et al 1975). It is thought to exert its antitumor activity by working as a bifunctional DNA intercalator. This is considered to be secondary to the polar quinoxoline chromophores on opposite sides of the cyclic peptides, both of which can intercalate between DNA base pairs. Echinomycin has a molecular weight of 1119.27 and the formula $C_5H_{64}N_{12}O_{12}S_2 \cdot H_2O$. It is very soluble in chloroform or dioxane and insoluble in hexane and water. An excellent preclinical and early clinical review of the agent was published in 1985 (Foster et al 1985).

Echinomycin is still undergoing phase II clinical trials as an investigational anticancer agent. The drug has had activity against a number of in vivo animal test systems including B-16 melanoma (no cures in that system, however) and P-388. The compound was not active against L-1210, Lewis lung, colon-38, CD8F1 mammary, and human colon, lung, and mammary tumor xenografts tested in athymic mice. The drug had borderline schedule dependency. In other words, continuous tumor exposure produced only modest enhancements in cytotoxic activity. The drug also produced cytotoxic activity in vitro against primary human tumor colony-forming units of the following cancers: breast, sarcoma, and colon (Lathan and Von Hoff 1984).

In phase II clinical trials to date the drug has had no antitumor activity in patients with advanced refractory metastatic breast cancer (Hakes et al 1990, Muss et al 1990b) and minimal activity (7% response rate) in patients with cervical cancer (Muss et al 1990b). The drug had activity including 2 complete responses in 22 patients with advanced cisplatin-refractory ovarian cancer (Muss et al 1990a). The drug appears to be inactive in patients with refractory metastatic malignant melanoma (Kilton et al 1990).

■ Mechanism of Action

The mechanism of action of echinomycin is probably bifunctional intercalation of DNA (Ward et al 1965, Waring and Makoff 1974, Waring and

Structure of echinomycin

Wakelin 1974). The binding is specific for DNA and not RNA (Waring and Wakelin 1974).

■ **Availability and Storage**

Echinomycin is supplied by the Investigational Drug Branch, Division of Cancer Treatment, National Cancer Institute, Bethesda, Maryland. It is supplied as a sterile, 0.4-mg, white, vacuum-dried film in a 3.5-mL flint vial. Each echinomycin vial is packaged with an ampule containing 1 mL of Sterile Diluent 12 composed of equal parts of polyethoxylated castor oil (Cremophor EL®) and ethanol.

The intact packages should be stored in the freezer (−10 to −20°C).

■ **Preparation for Use, Stability, and Admixture**

The contents of the vial are completely dissolved with 0.2 mL of Diluent 12. Then 1.8 mL of Sterile Water for Injection, USP, or 0.9% Sodium Chloride Injection, USP, is added. The resulting solution contains 0.2 mg/mL echinomycin. The pH of this solution is 4 to 7. This solution can then be added to other intravenous solutions. Because of the phlebitis noted in some studies (Kuhn et al 1989) all doses of the drug should be diluted in at least 500 mL of 5% dextrose in half-normal saline. Shelf-life surveillance studies are ongoing.

A vacuum should be present in intact vials. The vial *should not be used* unless a vacuum is present because the sterility may be compromised and the rate of drug decomposition may be increased.

When reconstituted as directed, the solution of echinomycin exhibits little or no decomposition for at least 8 hours both at room temperature (22–25°C) and under refrigeration (2–8°C).

Further dilution with 5% dextrose in 0.9% Sodium Chloride Injection, USP, to a concentration of 0.4 mg/40 mL results in a solution exhibiting little or no decomposition for 24 hours at room temperature (both exposed to light and in the dark) and under refrigeration.

Caution: The single-use vial contains no antibacterial preservatives. Therefore, it is advised that the reconstituted product be discarded 8 hours after initial entry.

■ **Administration**

The most appropriate doses and schedules for administration have not yet been worked out. The administration schedules used are outlined in the table on page 418. Most of the reported phase II studies employed the weekly schedules.

■ **Special Precautions**

Because of the severe nausea and vomiting noted in phase I and II trials of echinomycin, pretreatment with antiemetics is required. Hypersensitivity reactions (believed to be secondary to the Cremophor EL® vehicle) have also been observed and medications and equipment to treat anaphylactic reactions should be available at bedside before echinomycin is administered (Pazdur et al 1987, Harvey et al 1985). A vasculocutaneous reaction consisting of some ulceration over the distribution of the vessel infused has been noted (Garrison et al 1987).

■ **Drug Interactions**

None have been noted to date.

Administration Schedule	Dose Range (μg/m²)	Recommended Dose (μg/m²)	Dose Limiting Toxic Effect	Reference
24-h continuous infusion every 28 days	60–2128	1600	Nausea and vomiting	Kuhn et al 1989
Weekly by 15-min infusion × 4 with 2-wk rest	60–1500	1200	Nausea and vomiting	Pazdur et al 1987
Once every 4 wk	20–1800	1500	Nausea and vomiting	Harvey et al 1985

■ Dosage

The earlier table outlines the phase II suggested doses on the various schedules; however, no absolute dosage recommendations can yet be made. It is possible that with the more effective antiemetic regimens now available, the doses of echinomycin could be escalated.

■ Pharmacokinetics

Unfortunately, an assay for echinomycin that could detect the agent in the very low concentrations achieved in serum has never been developed. Therefore, no clinical pharmacology studies are available on the agent.

■ Side Effects and Toxicity

Toxic effects noted in phase I and II trials (weekly schedule) have included severe or life-threatening nausea and vomiting in 43% of patients and transient elevations in liver function tests is 30% of patients (Schilsky et al 1991). Further evaluation of echinomycin should be possible with the recent availability of more effective antimetics such as ondansetron.

Other toxic effects noted in phase I trials include fever, severe phlebitis with the 24-hour infusion (Kuhn et al 1989), and sporadic thrombocytopenia. A localized skin ulceration along the course of the vein used for infusion is also described in one patient (Garrison et al 1987). Although extravasation of drug did not lead to necrosis, all 24-hour echinomycin infusions produced severe phlebitis along the vein used for infusion. This was more common at higher doses and lasted about 1 to 2 weeks (Kuhn et al 1989). Watery diarrhea was also noted (7% of patients).

Anaphylactic reactions thought to be secondary to the Cremophor EL® vehicle have also been noted (Pazdur et al 1987, Harvey et al 1985).

■ Special Applications

None are known to date.

REFERENCES

Corbaz R, Ettlinger L, Gaumann E, et al. Metabolic products of Actinomycetes. VII. Echinomycin. *Helv Chim Acta.* 1957;**40**:199–204.

Foster BJ, Clagett-Carr K, Shoemaker DD, et al. Echinomycin: The first bifunctional intercalating agent in clinical trials. *Invest New Drugs.* 1985;**3**:403–410.

Garrison J, Marshall ME, MacDonald JS. Unusual skin reaction to echinomycin (letter). *Cancer Treat Rep.* 1987;**71**:433–444.

Hakes T, Markman M, Philips M. A phase II trial of echinomycin in metastatic cervix carcinoma. *Invest New Drugs.* 1990;**8**:311–312.

Harvey JH, McFadden M, Andrews WG, Byrne PJ, Ahlgren JD, Woodley PV. Phase I study of echinomycin administered on an intermittent bolus schedule. *Cancer Treat Rep.* 1985;**69**:1365–1368.

Kilton L, Wade J, Locker G. Phase II trial of echinomycin in metastatic melanoma: An Illinois Cancer Council study. *Proc Am Soc Clin Oncol.* 1990;**9**:200.

Kuhn J, Von Hoff D, Hersh M. Phase I trial of echinomycin (NSC-526417), a bifunctional intercalating agent, administered by 24 hour continuous infusion. *Eur J Cancer Clin Oncol.* 1989;**25**:797–803.

Lathan B, Von Hoff DD. Cytotoxin activity of echinomycin in a human tumor cloning system. *Cancer Drug Delivery.* 1984;**1**:191–198.

Martin DG, Misak SA, Biles C, Stewart JC, Baczynskyj L, Meulman PA. Structure of quinomycin antibiotics. *J Antibiot.* 1975;**28**:332–336.

Muss HR, Blessing JA, Baker VV, Barnhill DR, Adelson MD. Echinomycin (NSC-526417) in advanced ovarian cancer. A phase II trial of the Gynecologic Oncology Group. *Am J Clin Oncol.* 1990a;**13**:299–301.

Muss HR, Blessing JA, Malfetano J. Echinomycin (NSC-526417) in squamous-cell carcinoma of the cervix: A phase II trial of the Gynecologic Oncology Group. *Am J Clin Oncol.* 1990b;**13**:191–193.

Pazdur R, Haas CD, Baker LH, Leichman CG, Decker D. Phase I study of echinomycin. *Cancer Treat Rep.* 1987;**71**:1217–1219.

Schilsky RL, Faraggi D, Korzan A, et al. Phase II study of echinomycin in patients with advanced breast cancer: A report of the Cancer and Leukemia Group B protocol 8641. *Invest New Drugs.* 1991;**9**:2269–2272.

Wakelin LPG, Waring MJ. The binding of echinomycin to deoxyribonucleic acid. *Biochem J.* 1976;**157**:721–740.

Ward DC, Reich E, Goldberg IH. Base specificity in the interaction of polynucleotides with antibiotic drugs. *Science.* 1965;**149**:1259–1263.

Waring M, Makoff A. Breakdown of pulse-labeled ribonucleic acid and polysomes in *Bacillus megaterium*: Actions of streptolydigin, echinomycin, and triostins. *Mol Pharmacol.* 1974;**10**:214–224.

Waring MJ, Wakelin LPG. Echinomycin: A bifunctional intercalating antibiotic. *Nature.* 1974;**252**:653–657.

Edatrexate

Other Names

10-Edam; 10-ethyl-10-deazaaminopterin; CGP 30694 (Ciba-Geigy Corporation).

Chemistry

Structure of edatrexate

The complete chemical name of edatrexate is *N*-[4-1-((2,4-diamino-6-pteridinyl)methylpropyl)benzoyl]-L-glutamic acid. Edatrexate is structurally similar to the folic acid antagonist methotrexate. It differs by an alkyl replacement of the nitrogen at the N^{10}-position of methotrexate. The pteridine and glutamate domains of methotrexate are unchanged. Edatrexate has the molecular formula $C_{22}H_{25}N_7O_5$ and a molecular weight of 485.51 (Sirotnak et al 1984a). The compound is strongly fluorescent, with absorbance peaks at (excitation) 375 nm and (emission) 460 nm (Kinahan et al 1985).

Antitumor Activity

Edatrexate produces superior antitumor effects compared with methotrexate in a variety of transplanted murine tumors (Sirotnak et al 1984b). This may be the result of enhanced uptake and enhanced intracellular retention via increased polyglutamation (see Mechanism of Action).

Mouse tumor cells sensitive to edatrexate include the Tapper carcinosarcoma, EOTII mammary adenocarcinoma, L-1210 leukemia, Ehrlich ascites tumor, and sarcoma-180 wherein the drug is active at submicromolar concentrations. In vivo, edatrexate has produced cures in some mice bearing these same tumors. Edatrexate responses in vivo and in vitro were superior to those obtained with methotrexate in these tumors. High-dose therapy with leucovorin rescue is also more effective than similar methotrexate regimens in tumor-bearing mice (Sirotnak et al 1993).

Edatrexate is also active against a series of human solid tumors grown as subcutaneous xenografts in nude mice (Schmid et al 1985). Highly sensitive tumors include LX-1 lung carcinoma, MX-1 mammary carcinoma (Schmid et al 1985), and head and neck squamous cell carcinoma (Brown et al 1989). The CX-1 human colon carcinoma was moderately sensitive (Schmid et al 1985). Murine ovarian cancer (teratoma) was sensitive to intraperitoneal edatrexate (Sirotnak et al 1989).

In a phase I clinical trial, 4 objective partial responses were observed among 62 patients given a variety of edatrexate doses (Kris et al 1988). Responders included 3 of 36 patients with non-small cell lung cancer (NSCLC) and 1 of 3 patients with breast cancer. A follow-up phase II trial was performed in 20 patients with advanced (stage III or IV) NSCLC. Six of nineteen evaluable patients (32%) responded to edatrexate, including four partial responses and two minor responses (Shum et al 1988). In other phase II trials conducted at Memorial–Sloan Kettering, edatrexate produced 0 of 12 responses in colon cancer, 3 of 7 (43%) responses (including one complete response) in heavily pretreated lymphomas, and 3 of 11 (27%) responses in head and neck cancers. Preliminary European trials in head and neck cancers have also described activity for edatrexate (Schornagel et al 1989).

Combination phase II and III chemotherapy trials with edatrexate in NSCLC are currently underway. Other drugs being evaluated in combination with edatrexate include mitomycin-C, vinblastine, cyclophosphamide, and cisplatin. Clinical results are not available. Nonetheless, edatrexate appears to be an active agent for human hematologic and solid neoplasms. Whether it is clinically superior to methotrexate or significantly active in methotrexate-resistant tumors is unknown.

■ Mechanism of Action

Edatrexate binds stoichiometrically to dihydrofolate reductase (DHFR) enzymes. This blocks the conversion of dihydrofolic acid to the active cofactor, tetrahydrofolic acid. The inhibition of DHFR by edatrexate depletes intracellular reduced folate levels which can block a number of biochemical processes involving 1-carbon transfer reactions. The conversion of uridylate monophosphate to thymidine is one such reaction. This blockade in thymidine synthesis by folate antagonists can inhibit subsequent DNA synthesis, leading to cell death. Other 1-carbon transfer reactions are similarly inhibited by edatrexate. This includes the inhibition of RNA and protein synthesis, albeit to a lesser extent compared with the inhibition of DNA synthesis. All of these biochemical actions are similar to those of methotrexate. Cytotoxicity from edatrexate is cell cycle (phase) specific with maximal but not exclusive activity in S phase (Tattersall 1984).

Although edatrexate shares the common folic acid uptake mechanism with methotrexate, there are several differences in cellular uptake characteristics. First, in murine systems, edatrexate is transported more efficiently than methotrexate into sensitive tumors compared with normal tissue cells (Sirotnak et al 1984b). This property may relate to enhanced formation of highly charged and poorly diffusable polyglutamate forms of edatrexate compared with methotrexate (Sirotnak et al 1984b). The extent of polyglutamation is known to correlate positively with sensitivity to antifols and this may confer enhanced intracellular retention of edatrexate over methotrexate. For unknown reasons, edatrexate polyglutamate formation is reduced in normal target tissues such as the gut but is increased in sensitive tumor cell lines (Sirotnak et al 1984b). Overall, such differential polyglutamation with edatrexate may explain much of the enhanced therapeutic efficacy of edatrexate compared with methotrexate in experimental tumor models.

■ Availability and Storage

Edatrexate is investigationally available as a lyophilized light yellow powder in 50-mg glass vials (Ciba-Geigy Corporation). The vials are stored at room temperature and should be protected from light.

■ Preparation for Use, Stability, and Admixture

Each 50-mg vial is reconstituted with 4 mL of normal saline to yield a 12.5 mg/mL solution. This solution is compatible with 5% dextrose, Ringer's lactate, and bacteriostatic water. Compatibility with other drugs is unknown.

■ Administration

Edatrexate is administered as a brief intravenous infusion, typically over 20 to 30 minutes. It has also been administered by a brief injection into the side port of a freely flowing intravenous infusion (Kris et al 1988).

■ Dosage

Kris et al (1988) reported that the tolerable edatrexate dose was 80 mg/m^2 IV weekly. This dose could be escalated to 100 mg/m^2/wk followed by a 2-week rest period. In NSCLC, a dose of 80 mg/m^2/wk was administered for 5 consecutive weeks. Subsequent courses could be started 1 week later (day 36 after the initiation of therapy) (Shum et al 1988). Dose escalations of 10 mg/m^2 were allowed every 2 weeks if toxicity allowed. For moderate to severe toxicity, the weekly edatrexate dose was halted until toxicity resolved. It was then restarted at doses 20 mg/m^2 lower than the last dose.

■ Drug Interactions

Leucovorin calcium administration antagonizes the myelotoxic effects of edatrexate similarly to methotrexate (Sirotnak et al 1989, 1993). In addition, edatrexate and cisplatin appear to produce synergistic antitumor activity against murine ovarian cancer (Sirotnak et al 1989).

■ Pharmacokinetics

In rats given 50 mg/m^2 edatrexate, elimination was triphasic with a terminal elimination half-life of 18.5 hours and a mean residence time of 0.7 hour. In the rat, biliary secretion is the major route of elimination, with deglutamated species appearing in the feces (Fanucchi et al 1987). Similar disposition patterns have been noted in dogs wherein the terminal plasma half-life was 9.1 hour and the mean residence time 2.5 hours. Again, nonrenal clearance was the main route of elimination. High parent drug and low polyglutamate drug concentrations were recovered in the liver, kidney, and small intestine of rats. In contrast, edatrexate levels in the bone marrow were low (Fanucchi et al 1987).

In adult patients with advanced cancer, a triphasic elimination pattern was again noted (see the table). A dose-independent elimination pattern was observed with edatrexate. Unlike the animal trials, however, urinary edatrexate elimination was more prominent in humans, and at least two metabolites of edatrexate have been observed in the plasma and urine: 7-hydroxyedatrexate and 10-ethyl-10-deaza-2,4-diaminopteroic acid (Kris et al 1988). The 7-hydroxy metabolite of edatrexate is a weak inhibitor of dihydrofolate reductase and represents only a small percentage (0.06–0.38%) of the total edatrexate dose (Kris et al 1988).

Extensive polyglutamate formation was observed in tissue homogenates from skin metastases of patients with kidney cancer and, especially, breast cancer (Kris et al 1988). This retention of polyglutamates was greater in tumor cells than in normal tissues (Kris et al 1988).

The cumulative urinary excretion of edatrexate in cancer patients ranged from 12.5 to 55.3% of a dose (mean, 33%). About 88% of this urinary recovery occurred within the first 4 hours of administration. Furthermore, the relatively high ratio of edatrexate clearance to creatinine clearance (mean, 3.5) suggests that edatrexate is subject to significant renal tubular secretion. Total body clearance of edatrexate also appears to correlate with toxicity. Patients with a clearance of 9 L/m^2/h or less experienced more severe toxicity than those patients with a total body clearance greater than 9 L/m^2/h. Also, several of the patients with slow clearance had significant hepatic metastases, which may explain the impaired edatrexate elimination. Finally, no patient with a 24-hour edatrexate level less than 15 nM experienced early toxicity (Kris et al 1988).

■ Side Effects and Toxicity

The major dose-limiting toxic effect of edatrexate is oral mucositis which is dose-dependent (Kris et al 1988). At doses of 100 mg/m^2 and higher every 3 weeks, 86% of patients experience mild mucositis and 41% experience mild to moderate stomatitis. At weekly doses of 80 mg/m^2, 29% of patients experience severe mucositis. In most cases the mucositis lasted 3 to 7 days but was well managed with general supportive measures (Kris et al 1988).

Mild to moderate myelosuppression is also common with edatrexate. The median nadir for mild myelosuppression occurs on day 12, and only 15% of patients experience moderate to severe leukopenia or thrombocytopenia. These effects are always reversible and occur concomitantly with mucositis.

Hepatic toxicity from edatrexate is common. It is noted by mild to moderate elevations in serum glutamic–oxalacetic acid in most patients. Jaundice is not observed. About one third of patients experience lethargy and/or fatigue at doses of 80 mg/m^2 and greater (Kris et al 1988). In contrast, diarrhea is much less common, although 18% of patients may experience dose-dependent nausea and vomiting. A macular/papular rash was observed in 19% of patients in a phase I trial (Kris et al 1988). A slightly

PHARMACOKINETICS OF EDATREXATE IN HUMANS WITH ADVANCED BREAST CANCER

Dose (mg/m^2)	Number of Patients	Half-life α (min)	Half-life β (h)	Half-life γ (h)	AUC (nM·h)	Steady State Volume of Distribution (L/m^2)	Clearance (L/m^2/h) Total Body	Clearance (L/m^2/h) Renal
5	3	7.2	2.3	—	1.76	26.4	7	2.9
30	3	9.2	1.5	13.1	4.78	44.8	16.8	5.57
100	6	16.5	1.4	11.3	12.56	38.1	17.7	5.73
Mean		12.4	1.7	11.9	—	36.9	14.8	4.98

Data from Kris MG, Kinahan JJ, Gralla RJ, et al. Phase I trial and clinical pharmacologic evaluation of 10-ethyl-10-deazaaminopterin in adult patients with advanced cancer. Cancer Res. 1988;48:5573–5579.

smaller percentage of patients may experience mild abnormalities in coagulation studies, including transient elevations in partial thromboplastin and prothrombin times. While frank hemorrhage and purpura were not observed, a mild epistaxis occurred occasionally. Less than 10% of patients developed mild alopecia, and elevated serum creatinine levels were observed only in three patient courses (Kris et al 1988).

Severe toxic dermatitis has been reported in a European phase I trial in which mucositis was otherwise the dose-limiting toxic effect (Verweij et al 1990). Histologic observations in affected patient specimens demonstrate a toxic dermatitis with infiltrates of histiocytes and lymphocytes around a superficial vascular plexus (Verweij et al 1990). A rash is the most common type of skin reaction. The rash with edatrexate differs from that of methotrexate in that it first appears on the lower portion of the legs. It can also appear anywhere else on the body, especially if edatrexate therapy is continued once the rash appears even if the dose is reduced. Fortunately, discontinuance of edatrexate invariably results in resolution of the dermatitis and healing is complete within days to 1 to 2 weeks.

■ Special Applications

Edatrexate has been administered by the intracavitary route in mice with a murine ovarian teratoma (Sirotnak et al 1989). Antitumor effects were significantly greater than with maximally tolerated doses of intravenously administered drug. In addition, intravenous leucovorin protected animals from systemic edatrexate toxicity.

REFERENCES

Brown DH, Braakhuis BJM, van Dongen GAMS, et al. Activity of the folate analog 10-ethyl-10-deaza-aminopterin (10-EdAM) against head and neck squamous cell carcinoma (HNSCC) (abstract 110). In: Sixth NCI-EORTC Symposium on New Drugs in Cancer Therapy, Amsterdam, March 7–10. *Invest New Drugs.* 1989;7:376.

Fanucchi MP, Kinahan JJ, Samuels LL, et al. Toxicity, elimination, and metabolism of 10-ethyl-10-deazaaminopterin in rats and dogs. *Cancer Res.* 1987;47:2334–2339.

Kinahan JJ, Samuels LL, Farag F, et al. Fluorometric high-performance liquid chromatographic analysis of 10-deazaaminopterin, 10-ethyl-10-deazaaminopterin, and known metabolites. *Anal Biochem.* 1985;150:203–213.

Kris MG, Kinahan JJ, Gralla RJ, et al. Phase I trial and clinical pharmacologic evaluation of 10-ethyl-10-deazaaminopterin in adult patients with advanced cancer. *Cancer Res.* 1988;48:5573–5579.

Schmid FA, Sirotnak FM, Otter GM, DeGraw JI. New folate analogs of other 10-deaza-aminopterin series: Markedly increased antitumor activity of the 10-ethyl analog compared to the parent compound and methotrexate against some human tumor xenografts in nude mice. *Cancer Treat Rep.* 1985;69:551–553.

Schornagel JH, Cappelaere P, Cognetti F, et al. A randomized phase II trial of methotrexate (MTX) vs 10-ethyl-10-deaza-aminopterin (10-EdAM) in patients with advanced squamous cell carcinoma of the head and neck (abstract 462). In: Sixth NCI-EORTC Symposium on New Drugs in Cancer Therapy, Amsterdam, March 7–10. *Invest New Drugs.* 1989;7:464.

Shum KY, Kris MG, Gralla RJ, et al. Phase II study of 10-ethyl-10-deaza-aminopterin in patients with stage III and IV non-small-cell lung cancer. *J Clin Oncol.* 1988;6(3):446–450.

Sirotnak FM, DeGraw JI, Moccio DM, et al. New folate analogs of the 10-deaza-aminopterin series. Basis for structural design and biochemical and pharmacologic properties. *Cancer Chemother Pharmacol.* 1984a;12:18–25.

Sirotnak FM, DeGraw JI, Schmid FA, et al. New folate analogs of the 10-deaza-aminopterin series. Further evidence for markedly increased antitumor efficacy compared with methotrexate in ascitic and solid murine tumor models. *Cancer Chemother Pharmacol.* 1984b;12:26–30.

Sirotnak FM, Schmid FA, DeGraw JI. Intracavitary therapy of murine ovarian cancer with *cis*-diamminedichloroplatinum(II) and 10-ethyl-10-deazaaminopterin incorporating systemic leucovorin protection. *Cancer Res.* 1989;49:2890–2893.

Sirotnak FM, Otter GM, Schmid FA: Markedly improved efficacy of edatrexate compared to methotrexate in a high-dose regimen with leucovorin rescue against metastatic murine solid tumors. *Cancer Res.* 1993;53:587–591.

Tattersall MHN. Clinical utility of methotrexate in neoplastic disease. In: Sirotnak FM, Burchal JJ, Ensminger WB, Montgomery JA, eds. *Folate Antagonists as Therapeutic Agents.* New York: Academic Press; 1984;2:166–189.

Verweij J, Schornagel J, de Mulder P, et al. Toxic dermatitis induced by 10-ethyl-10-deaza-aminopterin (10-EdAM), a novel antifolate. *Cancer.* 1990;66:1910–1913.

Edelfosine

■ Other Names

ET-18-OCH$_3$; alkyllysophospholipid; ALP.

■ Chemistry

$$\begin{array}{l} H_2C-O-(CH_2)_{17}-CH_3 \\ | \\ H_3C-O-C-H \\ | \quad\;\; O \\ | \quad\;\; \| \\ H_2C-O-P-O-(CH_2)_2-N(CH_3)_3 \\ | \\ O^{(-)} \end{array}$$

Structure of edelfosine

Edelfosine is an ether lipid with the chemical name 1-O-octadecyl-2-O-methyl-rac-glycero-3-phosphocholine. This agent is a synthetic derivative of the endogenous alkyllysophospholipid 2-lysophosphatidylcholine (2-LPC) (Eibl et al 1967). It has a molecular weight of 523.76 and is water soluble. At high concentrations ($\geq$ 5 mg/mL) solubility is enhanced at 37°C.

■ Antitumor Activity

Ether lipids are active in a variety of experimental models including Ehrlich ascites carcinoma (Ando et al 1972), metastatic mouse sarcoma (Boeryd et al 1971), and Lewis lung carcinoma (Berdel et al 1979, 1980). In these experiments, the most active lipid analogs had a long aliphatic side chain in the sn-1 position and a substitution such as a methyl group in the sn-2 position (Berdel 1987). Edelfosine was active in each of the systems just described; however, edelfosine was not active at preventing radiation-induced lymphomas in mice (Berdel et al 1983).

Human tumors sensitive to edelfosine concentrations of 1 to 10 µg/mL in vitro include prostate cancer, testicular tumors, bladder cancer, renal cell cancer, astrocytoma, lung cancer, and acute myelogenous or lymphocytic leukemias (Berdel 1987). Antitumor activity is lost if the drug is preincubated with a microsomal tetrahydropteridine-requiring 1-O-alkyl cleavage enzyme (Berdel 1987). In addition, only the D-isomer of edelfosine has antitumor activity in human HL-60 myeloblasts (Berdel et al 1987).

In phase I clinical trials, edelfosine has produced partial responses in two patients with non-small cell lung cancer, a minor response in one patient each with thyroid gland carcinoma and renal cell carcinoma, and a greater than 50% reduction in peripheral blast cells in a patient with acute myeloid leukemia (Berdel et al 1982b). Edelfosine has also been used to purge leukemic cells from human bone marrow prior to autologous bone marrow transplantation (Okamoto et al 1987, Dulisch et al 1985). This selective in vitro antitumor activity was greatest if the edelfosine exposure preceded marrow cryopreservation.

■ Mechanism of Action

Edelfosine is believed to have direct antitumor effects on tumor cell membranes and indirect antitumor effects on normal macrophages. The indirect effect involves activation of macrophages to become cytotoxic effector cells (Berdel et al 1982a); however, mitogenic stimulation from edelfosine in mixed lymphocyte cultures is inconsistently noted in specimens from cancer patients (Berdel et al 1987). Macrophage activation requires preincubation with edelfosine for several hours. Following this exposure, the monocytes and macrophages possess cytostatic activity toward autologous tumor cells from the same patient (Berdel et al 1982a). This effect has been observed in vitro with human leukemic cells, renal cell carcinoma cells, and non-small cell lung cancer cells but not with human brain tumors. Leukemic cells appear to be particularly sensitive to this indirect immunologic effect of edelfosine (Andreesen et al 1979).

The direct antitumor effects of edelfosine include selective membrane lysis noted in human leukemic cells (Berdel et al 1982a) and in human urologic cancers (Berdel et al 1981). This activity may result from an accumulation of drug in tumor cells (Arnold et al 1978) followed by a disturbance of membrane phospholipid turnover (Modolell et al 1979). One explanation for the tumor selectivity is the relative lack of alkyl cleavage enzymes observed in some neoplastic cells compared with normal cells (Soodsma et al 1970, Snyder and Wood 1969, Wykle and Snyder 1976). Another direct effect of edelfosine is the induction of differentiation observed in HL-60 myeloblasts in vitro (Honma et al 1981).

■ Availability and Storage

Edelfosine is investigationally available from Medmark Pharma, Grünwald, Germany. It is supplied as a lyophilized white powder in glass vials containing 300 mg of sterile drug without additives.

The vials are stable for several years at −20°C. The drug should be stored in a desiccator.

■ Preparation for Use, Stability, and Admixture

The contents of the vials are aseptically dissolved in a 20% human albumin solution (Berdel et al 1982b). For infusions of highly concentrated solutions containing 5 mg/mL edelfosine or more, the 20% albumin diluent should be warmed to 37°C as solubility of edelfosine is temperature dependent. To lessen gastrointestinal side effects, the edelfosine concentration should not exceed 5 mg/mL and the infusion rate should be kept below 20 mL/h (Berdel et al 1987).

An oral preparation of edelfosine has been prepared by dissolving the drug in whole cow's milk (3.5% fat content) (Berdel et al 1987). The drug is also soluble at a concentration of 1000 μg/mL in RPMI-1640 culture medium containing 10% (v/v) fetal bovine serum. These preparations have been stored at −20°C for in vitro bone marrow (tumor) purging experiments.

All edelfosine solutions should be prepared immediately prior to use. Further stability and compatibility information is not available.

■ Drug Interactions

None are known at present.

■ Administration

Edelfosine has usually been administered by continuous daily intravenous infusion. Oral doses were administered daily in milk. For in vitro bone marrow purging studies, edelfosine exposures of 1 or 4 hours have been used (Okamoto et al 1987).

■ Dosage

The maximally tolerated dose (MTD) of edelfosine by daily intravenous infusion was 20 mg/kg/d (Berdel et al 1987). Dosing is usually continued for up to 3 weeks. The dose recommended for phase II trials was 16 mg/kg/d × 3 weeks (Berdel et al 1982b). The MTD for a single weekly intravenous injection was 50 mg/kg given over 24 hours (Berdel et al 1987).

An MTD was not achieved in the initial oral dose study because of acute gastrointestinal toxicity. Oral dosing was well tolerated at 5 mg/kg/d for extended periods but severe toxicity including pulmonary edema occurred at oral daily doses of 10 mg/kg/d (Berdel et al 1987).

■ Pharmacokinetics

Pharmacokinetic studies are not available for this compound.

■ Side Effects and Toxicity

Gastrointestinal toxic effects can be acutely dose limiting and are dependent on the drug concentration (ie, the rate of delivery) but not the absolute dose delivered (Berdel et al 1987). Nausea, vomiting, and diarrhea were observed in this trial. These effects could be minimized if the drug concentration was less than 5 mg/mL and the rate of infusion was less than 20 mL/h. Liver toxicity was noted in several patients who experienced increased serum bilirubin and alkaline phosphatase levels. A few patients also experienced transient elevations in serum creatinine levels with concomitant glucosuria and proteinuria. At high daily intravenous doses, life threatening interstitial pulmonary edema occurred. This condition reversed rapidly on drug removal, treatment with glucocorticosteroids, and assisted ventilation(Berdel et al 1987).

Overall, the two primary dose-limiting toxic effects were liver dysfunction and pulmonary edema. Myelosuppression was not reported although a few patients showed evidence of immunosuppression on in vitro testing of lymphocytes obtained during edelfosine treatment. Edelfosine causes local tissue irritation and thrombophlebitis if inadvertently extravasated (Berdel et al 1987). Transient tachycardia and fever are also described in one patient with non-small cell lung carcinoma (Berdel et al 1992b).

REFERENCES

Ando K, Kodama K, Kato A, et al. Antitumor activity of glyceryl ethers. *Cancer Res.* 1972;**32**:125–129.

Andreesen R, Modolell M, Munder PG. Selective sensitivity of chronic myelogenous leukemia cell populations to alkyllysophospholipids. *Blood.* 1979;**54**:519–523.

Arnold B, Reuther R, Weltzien HU. Distribution and metabolism of synthetic alkyl analogs of lysophosphatidylcholine in mice. *Biochem Biophys Acta.* 1978;**530**:47–55.

Berdel WE. Ether lipids and analogs in experimental cancer therapy. A brief review of the Munich experience. *Lipids.* 1987;**22**(1):970–973.

Berdel WE, Bausert WR, Weltzien HU, et al. The influence of alkyllysophospholipids and lysophospholipid-activated macrophages on the development of metastases of 3-Lewis lung carcinoma. *Eur J Cancer.* 1980;**16**:1199–1204.

Berdel WE, Fink U, Egger B, et al. Inhibition by alkyllysophospholipids of tritiated thymidine uptake in cells of human malignant urologic tumors. *J Natl Cancer Inst.* 1981;**66**:813–817.

Berdel WE, Fink U, Rastetter J. Clinical phase I pilot study of the alkyllysophospholipid derivative ET-18-OCH₃. *Lipids.* 1987;**22**(11):967–969.

Berdel WE, Fink U, Thiel E, et al. Purification of human monocytes by adherence to polymeric fluorocarbon. Characterization of the monocyte-enriched cell fraction. *Immunobiology.* 1982a;**163**:511–520.

Berdel WE, Luz A, Rastetter J, et al. Alkyllysophospholipids lack influence on the occurrence of radiation-induced lymphomas and AKR-leukemia. *Cancer Lett.* 1983;**20**:215–221.

Berdel WE, Schlehe H, Fink U, et al. Early tumor and leukemia response to alkyllysophospholipids in a phase I study. *Cancer.* 1982b;**50**:2011–2015.

Boeryd B, Hallgren B, Ställberg G. Studies on the effect of methoxy-substituted glycerol ethers on tumor growth and metastasis formation. *Br J Exp Pathol.* 1971;**52**:221–230.

Dulisch I, Neumann HA, Löhr, Andreesen R. Clonogenicity of normal and malignant hematopoietic progenitor cells after exposure to synthetic alkyllymphospholipids. *Blut.* 1985;**51**:393–399.

Eibl JH, Arnold D, Weltzien HU, et al. Synthesen von cholinphosphatiden. I. Zur synthese von alpha- und beta-lecithinen und ihren atheranaloga. *Liebig's Ann Chem.* 1967;**709**:226–230.

Honma Y, Kasukabe T, Hozumi M, et al. Introduction of differentiation of cultured human and mouse myeloid leukemia cells by alkyllysophospholipids. *Cancer Res.* 1981;**41**:3211–3216.

Modolell M, Andreesen R, Pahlke W, et al. Disturbance of phospholipid metabolism during selective destruction of tumor cells induced by alkyllysophospholipids. *Cancer Res.* 1979;**39**:4681–4686.

Okamoto S, Olson AC, Vogler WR, Winton EF. Purging leukemic cells from simulated human remission marrow with alkyllysophospholipid. *Blood.* 1987;**69**(5):1381–1387.

Snyder F, Wood R. Alkyl- and alk-1-enyl ethers of glycerol in lipids from normal and neoplastic human tissues. *Cancer Res.* 1969;**29**:251–257.

Soodsma JF, Piantadosi C, Snyder F. The biocleavage of alkyl glyceryl ethers in Morris hepatomas and other transplantable neoplasms. *Cancer Res.* 1970;**30**:309–311.

Wykle RL, Snyder F. Microsomal enzymes involved in the metabolism of ether linked glycerolipids and their precursors in mammals. In: Martonosi A, ed. *The Enzymes of Biological Membranes.* New York: Plenum, 1976;**2**:87–117.

Eflornithine

■ Other Names

α-DFMO; α-difluoromethylornithine; RMI 71782A (Merrell Dow Pharmaceuticals, Inc).

■ Chemistry

$$H_2N-CH_2-CH_2-CH_2-\underset{NH_2}{\overset{CHF_2}{\underset{|}{C}}}-COOH$$

Structure of eflornithine

Eflornithine (α-DFMO) has the molecular formula $C_6H_{12}F_2N_2O_2$ and is usually formulated as the hydrochloride–monohydrate salt. The molecular weight is 236.65 and the salt form is freely soluble in water, sparingly soluble in methanol, slightly soluble in ethanol, and insoluble in chloroform. The drug is stable in crystalline form if protected from heat and light and can be frozen for prolonged stability.

■ Antitumor Activity

In cell culture studies eflornithine has inhibited the growth of human oat cell carcinoma, rat hepatoma cells, L-1210 mouse leukemia, human prostate adenocarcinoma (MA-160 cells), B-16 melanoma, EMT6 mouse fibrosarcoma, and rat 9L brain tumor cells (Mamont et al 1978, Prakash et al 1978, 1980, Sunkara et al 1983). The drug has also demonstrated cytotoxic activity against a number of human tumor cell xenografts in vivo including HL60 leukemia, HeLa cells, small cell carcinoma of the lung, and prostate adenocarcinoma (Luk et al 1981, 1983, Sunkara et al 1980). In vitro tests using the human tumor colony-forming assay have additionally suggested that melanoma, ovary, and lung cancer cells may also be sensitive to eflornithine (Meyskens et al 1986). The drug has often been combined experimentally with other antitumor agents (see Drug Interactions).

Eflornithine has been evaluated for clinical antitumor activity in 27 patients with small cell lung cancer (SCLC) and 14 patients with colon cancer (Abeloff et al 1984). There was only one partial response (PR) in SCLC and none in colon cancer. Oral eflornithine was also used as postinduction therapy in non-small cell lung cancer (NSCLC) (Mabry et al

1987). No PRs were converted to complete responses (CRs) by this therapy although there were slight increases in median survival CR > PR.

Partial responses were observed in 3 of 17 patients with malignant melanoma who had been given oral eflornithine and intramuscular interferon alfa (Croghan et al 1987). Eflornithine is also active in patients with refractory gliomas, either as a single agent used at high doses (Levin et al 1992) or in lower doses combined with mitoguazone (Levin et al 1987) or carmustine (Prados et al 1989). As a single agent, eflornithine produced a response rate of 45% in patients with anaplastic gliomas, including minor responses and stable disease (Levin et al 1992). The response rate in glioblastoma multiforme was 17% (Levin et al 1992). These studies suggest that eflornithine is an active agent for the palliative treatment of recurrent anaplastic gliomas.

■ Chemopreventive Activity

Eflornithine can block the promotion step of the carcinogenic process in a variety of experimental animal tumor models. These include colon cancer (Tempero et al 1989, Luk et al 1989), breast cancer (Ip and Thompson 1989, Manni et al 1988), bladder cancer (Homma et al 1987, Uchida et al 1989), and skin cancer (Takigawa et al 1982, 1983, Weeks et al 1982). Because of this activity the compound is currently under evaluation in clinical chemoprevention trials in patients with precancerous disease states.

■ Anti-infective Activity

Eflornithine has marked antiprotozoal activity against *Trypanosoma brucei brucei* (Bacchi et al 1980), Gambian trypanosomiasis (Taelmlan et al 1987), the exoerythrocytic form of *Plasmoslium bergei* (Gillet et al 1982), *Giardia lamblia* (Gillin et al 1984), *Trichomonas vaginalis* (Brenner et al 1987), and *Pneumocystis carinii* (Sahai and Berry 1989). Eflornithine is also active in acquired immunodeficiency syndrome (AIDS) patients with *Pneumocystis carinii* opportunistic infections who could not tolerate or were refractory to sulfas and/or pentamidine. Survival rates of 30 to 60% are described in this population (Sahai and Berry 1989, Gilman et al 1986).

■ Mechanism of Action

Eflornithine is a structural analog of the amino acid L-ornithine. Biochemically it acts as a "suicide" substrate inhibitor of ornithine decarboxylase (EC 4.1.1.17), the rate-limiting enzyme in polyamine synthesis (Metcalf et al 1978). As a result of ornithine decarboxylase inhibition, there is a commensurate depletion in the intracellular levels of putrescine and spermidine but not spermine (Danzin et al 1979, Mamont et al 1984). This results in growth inhibition, as cells are blocked from traversing through G_1 phase into S phase (Sunkara et al 1979). In viral-transformed cells, the cell cycle is halted in S phase (Sunkara et al 1979).

Eflornithine thereby acts to deplete cellular polyamines leading to growth inhibition. Polyamines are also known to bind to the outer helix of DNA and to control the rate of DNA synthesis by modulating the rate of movement of a DNA replication fork (Cohen 1978). In addition, polyamines are required to maintain the integrity of microfilaments and microtubules (Pojanpelto et al 1981) and to modulate the translation of specific ribosomal codons (Tabor and Tabor 1982).

Several structure–activity relationships are known for eflornithine. These involve substitution of fluorine for hydrogens to provide latent leaving groups, which are exchanged at the enzymes's active site as a result of normal catalytic turnover. This results in the formation of a carbanion radical(s) which covalently bind to nucleophilic sites in ornithine decarboxylase and thereby irreversibly inhibit its action. An initial step in the activation of eflornithine is the binding of pyridoxal phosphate (Jung et al 1980). Next, enzymatic decarboxylation yields the carbanion species which leads to loss of one or more fluorines and to alkylation of a nucleophilic site at or near the active site of the enzyme.

The inhibition of ornithine decarboxylase by eflornithine is time- and concentration-dependent, but is irreversible. Inhibitory drug concentrations range from 0.1 to 5 mM and the K_i in rat liver 39 µM. The half-life of inhibition at an infinite concentration of inhibitor is 3.1 minutes; however, the enzyme has a very rapid turnover with a normal biologic half-life of 30 to 60 minutes (Russell and Snyder 1969).

Putrescine is known to antagonize the growth-inhibitory activity of eflornithine. In addition, because of the rapid turnover of ornithine decarboxylase, growth inhibition is generally achieved only when eflornithine concentrations are maintained for prolonged periods.

■ Availability and Storage

Eflornithine is investigationally available in an aqueous solution in a concentration of 3 g/15 mL

(Merrell Dow Pharmaceuticals, Cincinnati, Ohio). The bulk solution should be protected from light and can be stored at room temperature.

An investigational injectable dosage form has also been prepared by Merrell Dow Research Institute. This formulation is supplied as a 100 or 200 mg/mL solution of eflornithine hydrochloride in Sterile Water for Injection, USP. The undiluted sterile solution is stored at room temperature.

■ Preparation for Use, Stability, and Admixture

Eflornithine injection has usually been diluted to deliver the appropriate dose in 100 mL of 5% Dextrose for Injection, USP. This solution is then infused intravenously over 1 hour (Abeloff et al 1984).

■ Dosage

Oral eflornithine doses in cancer chemotherapy studies have ranged from 2.25 to 3.75 g/m^2 every 6 hours for 28 days (Abeloff et al 1984, Griffin et al 1987). Continuous intravenous infusion doses have ranged up to 5.25 g/m^2 × 4 days without producing excessive toxicity (Griffin et al 1987). In another phase I study, drug-refractory leukemic patients were given doses up to 64 g/m^2 by continuous 24-hour infusion (Maddox et al 1985). Of interest, there appeared to be no relationship between the infusion dose and the degree of leukemic blast cell inhibition, which consistently occurred at all daily doses above 8 g/m^2. Gastrointestinal toxic effects and metabolic acidosis were severe at the 64 g/m^2 infusion dose level but were not dose limiting at 32 g/m^2. When combined with interferon alfa-2a (9 × 10^6 U/m^2) the maximally tolerated oral eflornithine dose was 4 g/m^2/d (Croghan et al 1987). In combination with mitoguazone, the daily oral eflornithine dose in refractory glioma patients was 1.8 g/m^2 (Levin et al 1992); however, this combination produced two cases of lethal hepatic necrosis and was terminated early in the trial. As a single agent in gliomas, the eflornithine dose was 3.6 g/m^2 every 8 hours on days 1 to 14, 22 to 35, and 45 to 56 (Levin et al 1992).

In AIDS patients, the intravenous dose of eflornithine for *Pneumocystis carinii* pneumonia has most often been 100 mg/kg every 6 hours for 14 days followed by 4 to 6 weeks of 75 mg/kg orally every 6 hours (Sahai and Berry 1989, Gilman et al 1986, Wordell and Hauptman 1988).

■ Drug Interactions

Eflornithine has been combined with a large number of other anticancer agents to evaluate the effect of polyamine depletion on various drug actions. The table on the top of page 428 summarizes these predominantly in vitro interactions. It is apparent that some drug combinations may produce greater than additive effects, although often this is highly dependent on the sequence of drug administration. The combination of interferon alfa-2a with eflornithine has been clinically evaluated and, although there was no clear evidence of enhancement, the combination was active and tolerable in a small population of patients with malignant melanoma (see Antitumor Activity) (Croghan et al 1987). Mitoguazone, which blocks *S*-adenosylmethionine decarboxylase, and eflornithine have also been extensively evaluated. This combination produces marked synergy in preclinical systems as a result of two-pronged inhibition of polyamine synthesis (Gau and Natale 1982). Early clinical results also suggest enhanced biologic activity for this combination, but whether this produces enhanced antitumor efficacy is unknown. There is, however, an apparent increase in hepatic toxicity that may limit the therapeutic activity of this combination (Levin et al 1992).

■ Pharmacokinetics

Oral eflornithine is well absorbed at low doses with a half-life for absorption of about 1.5 hours (range, 8–195 minutes) (Abeloff et al 1984). An elimination half-life of about 3.5 hours is described in most studies (Abeloff et al 1984, Mildvan et al 1982), although one group reported a longer half-life of 6.3 to 7.6 hours following higher doses of 3.75 to 5.25 g/m^2 (Griffin et al 1987) (see table on bottom of page 428). The latter study also described an absolute oral bioavailability of 1.00 (± 0.29) at dose levels of 3.75 g/m^2, but with lowered availability at doses of 4.5 and 5.25 g/m^2 (46 and 61% of a dose, respectively) (Griffin et al 1987).

The data in the next table suggests that clearance of the drug may decrease with increasing doses (Abeloff et al 1984). Nonetheless, there is still a good correlation between the dose and the maximal plasma level and the area under the plasma concentration × time curve (AUC) (see table). Clearance in AIDS patients also appears to be rapid at 99 (± 26) mL/min/70 kg, with the majority of drug (about 80%) excreted unchanged by the kidneys (Sahai and Berry 1989). The estimated volume of distribution in

DRUG COMBINATIONS WITH EFLORNITHINE IN VITRO

Cytotoxic Agent	Effect of Combination on Cytotoxicity (Comment)	Reference

Bleomycin	Synergistic increase
	  Mouse trypanosomiasis
	  L-1210, 8226 lymphoid tumor cells
		Clarkson et al 1983
		Dorr et al 1986

Interferon alfa	Tolerable and active
	  Human lymphoblastoid cells
	  Malignant melanoma patients
		Rosenblum and Gutterman 1984
		Croghan et al 1987

Carmustine	Increased (rat 9L brain tumor)	Marton et al 1981 Hung et al 1981
Mitoguazone	Enhanced cell kill in vitro (rat prostate tumors) Overcomes intrinsic cell resistance to either drug alone (human tumor cells) Enhanced cellular uptake of mitoguazone Enhanced myelosuppression (human clinical trials)	Herr et al 1984 Gau and Natale 1982 Janne et al 1981 Warrell and Burchenal 1983
Doxorubicin and/or vindesine	Enhanced tumor growth inhibition (animals)	Bartholeyns and Koch-Weser 1981
Cytarabine	Potentiation (HeLa cells)	Sunkara et al 1980
Amsacrine	Enhanced DNA breaks without increased cytotoxicity (L-1210 cells)	Zwelling et al 1985
Cisplatin	Decreased (α-DFMO first) Additive (cisplatin first) Decreased (rat 9L brain tumor)	Chang et al 1984 Oredsson et al 1982
Aziquone, vincristine, methotrexate	Decreased	Alhonen-Hongisto et al 1984a Alhonen-Hongisto et al 1984b

these studies was 0.43 ± 0.10 L/kg. This agrees well with the volumes of distribution reported in cancer patients given intravenous doses of eflornithine (range, 0.3–0.82 L/kg; mean, 0.48 L/kg) (Griffin et al 1987).

■ Side Effects and Toxicity

The dose-limiting toxic effect of eflornithine is thrombocytopenia, which occurs in about 50% of patients treated at therapeutic doses (Abeloff et al 1984, Griffin et al 1987). Leukopenia is described in approximately 20% of patients and anemia in 10%. Pancytopenia has been reported in AIDS patients treated for *Pneumocystis carinii* pneumonia (Golden et al 1984). In continuous daily oral dosing schedules, thrombocytopenia is first noted 2 to 3 weeks after starting therapy and generally resolves 2 weeks after stopping the drug (Abeloff et al 1984). The time courses of anemia and thrombocytopenia tend to occur in tandem.

The second major toxic effect of eflornithine is nausea and vomiting, which occur in up to 90% of patients although the severity is usually only mild to moderate. Diarrhea can also occur in about 20% of patients taking oral drug (Griffin et al 1987). For AIDS patients, a switch to the injectable eflornithine formulation may reduce or eliminate this toxic effect. At high dose levels, anorexia can also be troublesome. In very high infusion doses, severe meta-

PHARMACOKINETICS OF EFLORNITHINE

Dose (g/kg)	Route	Half-life (h)	Peak Level (nmol/mL)	AUC (nmol · h/mL)	Reference
0.1	Oral	3.6	196–318 µg/mL	NL	Sahai and Berry 1989
3.75	Oral	6.4	737	3800	Griffin et al 1987
0.75–2.6		1.3–2.3	292–1936	640–4148	Griffin et al 1987
0.75–3.0		2.5–4.0	230–503	1107–2111	Abeloff et al 1984

bolic acidosis has occurred with serum bicarbonate concentrations as low as 6 mEq/L (Maddox et al 1985).

Other toxic effects include alopecia, a diffuse skin rash, and a bilateral high-frequency hearing loss. The last effect is not permanent and, although it may be cumulative in severity, typically reverses slowly once the drug is halted. Baseline audiograms repeated at monthly intervals are indicated while on this drug. Hearing loss may also be more prominent in patients with preexisting impairment and in those concomitantly receiving aminoglycoside antibiotics (Maddox et al 1985).

Hepatocellular liver enzyme elevations have been described in patients without prior liver injury. These typically reverse rapidly on drug discontinuance. In addition, lethargy and fatigue can occur and fever is described in 3 of 24 patients (Griffin et al 1987).

Eflornithine may be harmful to a developing fetus as polyamines are known to be required for normal embryogenesis (Fozard et al 1980).

■ Special Applications

Eflornithine has been administered by hepatic artery infusion to patients with a variety of cancers metastatic to the liver (Lipton et al 1987). The dose-limiting toxic effect after 7 weeks of therapy was tinnitus and reversible hearing loss at daily infusion doses of 1 g/m² and greater. The drug has also been formulated into an investigational 10% topical cream preparation which has been used to treat psoriasis (Grosshans et al 1980). This was marginally effective perhaps as a result of the poor percutaneous absorption of eflornithine in mice when administered without a topical absorption enhancer such as 1-dodecylazacycloheptan-2-one (Azone®) (McCullough et al 1985). The cream base in the latter experiments included alcohol 47.5%, laureth 4, isopropylalcohol 4%, and propylene glycol.

REFERENCES

Abeloff MD, Slavik M, Luk GD, et al. Phase I trial and pharmacokinetic studies of α-difluoromethylornithine—An inhibitor of polyamine biosynthesis. *J Clin Oncol.* 1984;**2**(2):124–130.

Alhonen-Hongisto L, Deen DF, Marton LJ. Decreased cytotoxicity of aziridinylbenzoquinone caused by polyamine depletion in 9L rat brain tumor cells in vitro. *Cancer Res.* 1984a;**44**:39–42.

Alhonen-Hongisto L, Hung DT, Deen DF, et al. Decreased cell kill of vincristine and methotrexate against 9L rat brain tumor cells in vitro caused by α-difluoromethylornithine-induced polyamine depletion. *Cancer Res.* 1984b;**44**:4440–4442.

Bacchi CJ, Nathan HC, Hunter SH, et al. Polyamine metabolism: A potential therapeutic target in trypanosomes. *Science.* 1980;**180**:210, 332–334.

Bartholeyns J, Koch-Weser J. Effects of α-difluoromethylornithine alone and combined with Adriamycin or vindesine on L-1210 leukemia in mice, EMT6 solid tumors in mice, and solid tumors induced by injection of hepatoma tissue culture cells in rats. *Cancer Res.* 1981;**41**:5158–5161.

Brenner AF, Coombs GH, North MJ. Antitrichomonal activity of a difluoromethylornithine. *J Antimicrob Chemother.* 1987;**20**:405–411.

Chang BK, Black O Jr, Gutman R. Inhibition of growth of human or hamster pancreatic cancer cell lines by α-difluoromethylornithine alone and combined with cis-diamminedichloroplatinum(II). *Cancer Res.* 1984;**44**:5100–5104.

Clarkson AB Jr, Bacchi CJ, Mellow GH, et al. Efficacy of combinations of difluoromethylornithine and bleomycin in a mouse model of central nervous system African trypanosomiasis. *Proc Natl Acad Sci USA.* 1983;**80**:5729–5733.

Cohen SS. What do the polyamines do? *Nature.* 1978;**274**:209.

Croghan M, Booth A, Meyskens F. A phase I trial of recombinant α-interferon (IFN) and difluoromethylornithine (DFMO) in metastatic melanoma (MM) (abstract 825). *Proc Am Soc Clin Oncol.* 1987;**6**:209.

Danzin C, Jung MJ, et al. Effect of α-difluoromethylornithine, an enzyme-activated irreversible inhibitor of ornithine decarboxylase, on polyamine levels in rat tissues. *Life Sci.* 1979;**24**:519–524.

Dorr RT, Liddil JD, Gerner EW. Modulation of etoposide cytotoxicity and DNA strand scission in L-1210 and 8226 cells by polyamines. *Cancer Res.* 1986;**46**:3891–3895.

Fozard JR, Part ML, Prakash NJ, et al. L-Ornithine decarboxylase: An essential role in early mammalian embryogenesis. *Science.* 1980;**208**:505–508.

Gau TC, Natale RB. In vitro activity of methylglyoxal bis(guanylhydrazone) (MGBG) ± α-DFMO using the human tumor clonogenic assay (HTCA). *Proc Am Assoc Cancer Res.* 1982;**23**:183.

Gillet JN, Bone G, Herman HF. Inhibitory action of difluoromethylornithine on rodent malaria (*Plasmodium bergei*). *Trans R Soc Trop Med Hyg.* 1982;**76**:776–777.

Gillin FD, Reiner DS, McCann PP. Inhibition of growth of *Giardia lamblia* by difluoromethylornithine, a specific inhibitor of polyamine biosynthesis. *J Protozool.* 1984;**31**:161–163.

Gilman TM, Paulson YJ, Boylen CT, et al. Eflornithine treatment of *Pneumocystic carinii* pneumonia in AIDS. *JAMA.* 1986;**256**:2197–2198.

Golden WJM, Sjoerdsma A, Santi DV. *Pneumosystic carinii* pneumonia treated with difluoromethylornithine. *West J Med.* 1984;**141**:613–623.

Griffin CA, Slavik M, Chien SC, et al. Phase I trial and pharmacokinetic study of intravenous and oral α-difluoromethylornithine. *Invest New Drugs.* 1987;**5**:177–186.

Grosshans E, Henry M, Tell G, et al. Les plyamines dans le psoriasis. *Ann Dermatol Venereol.* 1980;**107**:377–387.

Herr HW, Kleinert EL, Conti PS, et al. Effects of α-difluoromethylornithine and methylglyoxal bis(guanylhydrazone) on the growth of experimental renal adenocarcinoma in mice. *Cancer Res.* 1984;**44**:4385–4387.

Homma Y, Kakizoe T, Samma S, et al. Inhibition of N-butyl-N-(4-hydroxybutyl)nitrosamine-induced rat urinary bladder carcinogenesis by α-difluoromethylornithine. *Cancer Res.* 1987;**47**:6176–6179.

Hung DT, Deen DF, Seidenfeld J, et al. Sensitization of 9L rat brain glioarcoma cells to 1,3-bis(2-chloroethyl)-1-nitrosourea by α-difluoromethylornithine, an ornithine decarboxylase inhibitor. *Cancer Res.* 1981;**41**:2783–2785.

Ip C, Thompson HJ. New approaches to cancer chemoprevention with difluoromethylornithine and selenite. *J Natl Cancer Inst.* 1989;**81**:839–843.

Janne J, Alhonen-Hongisto L, Seppanen P, et al. Use of polyamine antimetabolites in experimental tumor and in human leukaemia. *Med Biol.* 1981;**59**:448–457.

Jung MJ, Koch-Weser J, Sjoerdsma A. Biochemistry and pharmacology of enzyme-activated irreversible inhibitors of some pyridoxal-phosphate dependent enzymes. In: Sandler M, ed. *Enzyme Inhibitors as Drugs.* Baltimore, MD: University Park Press; 1980.

Levin VA, Chamberlain MD, Prados MD, et al. Phase I–II study of eflornithine and mitoguazone combined in the treatment of recurrent primary brain tumors. *Cancer Treat Rep.* 1987;**71**:459–464.

Levin VA, Prados MD, Yung WKA, et al. Treatment of recurrent gliomas with eflornithine. *J Natl Cancer Inst.* 1992;**84**:1432–1437.

Lipton A, Harvey H, Glenn J, et al. A phase I study of hepatic artery infusion employing DFMO (abstract 308). *Proc Am Soc Clin Oncol.* 1987;**6**:79.

Luk GD, Abeloff MD, Griffin CA, et al. Successful treatment with DL-α-difluoromethylornithine in established human small cell variant lung carcinoma implants in athymic mice. *Cancer Res.* 1983;**43**:439–443.

Luk GD, Goodwin G, Marton LJ, Baylin SB. Polyamines are necessary for the survival of human small cell lung carcinoma in culture. *Proc Natl Acad Sci USA.* 1981;**78**:2355–2358.

Luk GD, Zhang S-Z, Hamilton SR. Effects of timing of administration and dose of difluoromethylornithine on rat colonic carcinogenesis. *J Natl Cancer Inst.* 1989;**81**:421–427.

Mabry M, Abeloff MD, Booker SV, et al. Phase II pilot of α-difluoromethylornithine (DFMO) as post-induction therapy in small cell lung cancer (SCLC) (abstract 690). *Proc Am Soc Clin Oncol.* 1987;**6**:175.

Maddox AM, Keating MJ, McCredie KE, et al. Phase I evaluation of intravenous difluoromethylornithine—A polyamine inhibitor. *Invest New Drugs.* 1985;**3**:287–292.

Mamont PS, Dechesne MC, Grove J, et al. Antiproliferative properties of DL-α-difluoromethylornithine in cultured cells. A consequence of the irreversible inhibition of ornithine decarboxylase. *Biochem Biophys Res Commun.* 1978;**81**:58–66.

Mamont PS, Siat M, Joder Ohlenbusch AM. Effects of (2R, 5R)-6-heptyne-2,5-diamine, a potent inhibitor of L-ornithine decarboxylase, on rat hepatoma cells cultured in vitro. *Eur J Biochem.* 1984;**142**:457–463.

Manni A, Badger B, Luk G, et al. Role of polyamines in the growth of hormone-responsive experimental breast cancer in vivo. *Breast Cancer Res Treat.* 1988;**11**:231–240.

Marton LJ, Levin VA, Hervatin SJ, et al. Potentiation of the antitumor therapeutic effects of 1,3-bis(2-chloroethyl)-1-nitrosourea by α-difluoromethylornithine, an ornithine decarboxylase inhibitor. *Cancer Res.* 1981;**41**:4426–4431.

McCullough JL, Peckham P, Klein J, et al. Regulation of epidermal proliferation in mouse epidermis by combination of difluoromethylornithine (DFMO) and methylglyoxal bis(guanylhydrazone) (MGBG). *J Invest Dermatol.* 1985;**85**:518–521.

Metcalf BW, Bey P, Danzin C, et al. Catalytic irreversible inhibition of mammalian ornithine decarboxylase by substrate and product analogues. *J Am Chem Soc.* 1978;**100**(8):2551–2553.

Meyskens FL, Kingsley EM, Glattke T, et al. A phase II study of α-difluoromethylornithine (DFMO) for the treatment of metastatic melanoma. *Invest New Drugs.* 1986;**4**:257–262.

Mildvan D, Mathur U, Enlow RW, et al. Opportunistic infections and immune deficiency in homosexual men. *Ann Intern Med.* 1982;**96**(pt 1):700–704.

Oredsson SM, Deen DF, Marton LJ. Decreased cytotoxicity of cis-diamminedichloroplatinum(II) by α-difluoromethylornithine depletion of polyamines in 9L rat brain tumor cells in vitro. *Cancer Res.* 1982;**42**:1296–1299.

Pojanpelto P, Virtanen I, Holtta E. Polyamine starvation causes disappearance of actin filaments and microtubules in polyamine autotrophic CHO cells. *Nature.* 1981;**293**:475–476.

Prados M, Rodriguez L, Chamberlain M, et al. Treatment of recurrent gliomas with 1,3-bis(2-chloroethyl)-1-nitrosourea and α-difluoromethylornithine. *Neurosurgery.* 1989;**24**:806–809.

Prakash NJ, Schechter PJ, Grove J, et al. Effect of α-difluoromethylornithine, an enzyme-activated irreversible inhibitor of ornithine decarboxylase, on L-1210 leukemia in mice. *Cancer Res.* 1978;**38**:3059–3062.

Prakash NJ, Schechter PJ, Mamont PS, et al. Inhibition of EMT 6 tumor growth by interference with polyamine biosynthesis: Effects of alpha-difluoromethylornithine, an irreversible inhibitor of ornithine decarboxylase. *Life Sci.* 1980;**26**:181–194.

Rosenblum MG, Gutterman JU. Synergistic antiproliferative activity of leukocyte interferon in combination with α-difluoromethylornithine against human cells in culture. *Cancer Res.* 1984;**44**:2339–2340.

Russell DH, Snyder SH. Amine synthesis in regenerating rat liver: Extremely rapid turnover of ornithine decarboxylase. *Mol Pharmacol.* 1969;**5**:253–262.

Sahai J, Berry AJ. Eflornithine for the treatment of *Pneumocystis carinii* pneumonia in patients with the acquired immunodeficiency syndrome: A preliminary review. *Pharmacotherapy.* 1989;**9**(1):29–33.

Sunkara PS, Fowler SK, Nishioka K, et al. Inhibition of polyamine biosynthesis by α-difluoromethylornithine potentiates the cytotoxic effects of arabinosyl cytosine in HeLa cells. *Biochem Biophys Res Commun.* 1980;**95**:423–430.

Sunkara PS, Nellkunja JP, Mayer GD, et al. Tumor suppression with a combination of alpha difluoromethylornithine and interferon. *Science.* 1983;**219**:851–853.

Sunkara PS, Pargac MB, Nichioka K, et al. Differential effects of inhibition of polyamine biosynthesis on cell cycle traverse and structure of the prematurely condensed chromosomes of normal and transformed cells. *J Cell Physiol.* 1979;**98**:451–458.

Tabor CS, Tabor H. Polyamines in microorganisms. *Microb Rev.* 1982;**49**:81–99.

Taelmlan H, Schechter PJ, Marcells L, et al. Difluoromethylornithine, an effective new treatment of Gambian trypanosomiasis. *Am J Med.* 1987;**82**:607–614.

Takigawa M, Verma AK, Simsiman RC, et al. Polyamine biosynthesis and skin tumor promotion: Inhibition of 12-O-tetradecanoylphorbol-13-acetate-promoted mouse skin tumor formation by the irreversible inhibitor or ornithine decarboxylase α-difluoromethylornithine. *Biochem Biophys Res Commun.* 1982;**105**:969–976.

Takigawa M, Verma AK, Simsiman RC, et al. Inhibition of mouse skin tumor promotion and of promoter-stimulated epidermal polyamine biosynthesis by α-difluoromethylornithine. *Cancer Res.* 1983;**43**:3732–3738.

Tempero MA, Nichioka K, Knott K, et al. Chemoprevention of mouse colon tumors with difluoromethylornithine during and after carcinogen treatment. *Cancer Res.* 1989;**49**:5793–5797.

Uchida K, Seidenfeld J, Rademaker A, et al. Inhibitory action of α-difluoromethylornithine on N-butyl-N-(4-hydroxybutyl)nitrosamine-induced rat urinary bladder carcinogenesis. *Cancer Res.* 1989;**49**:5249–5253.

Warrell RP Jr, Burchenal JH. Methylglyoxal-bis(guanylhydrazone) (methyl-GAG): Current status and future prospects. *J Clin Oncol.* 1983;**1**(1):52–65.

Weeks CE, Herrman AL, Nelson FR, et al. α-Difluoromethylornithine, an irreversible inhibitor of ornithine decarboxylase, inhibits tumor promoter-induced polyamine accumulation and carcinogenesis in mouse skin. *Proc Natl Acad Sci USA.* 1982;**79**:6028–6032.

Wordell CJ, Hauptman SP. Treatment of *Pneumocystic carinii* pneumonia in patients with AIDS. *Clin Pharmacol.* 1988;**7**:514–527.

Zwelling LA, Kerrigan D, Marton LJ. Effect of difluoromethylornithine, an inhibitor of polyamine biosynthesis, on the topoisomerase II-mediated DNA scission produced by 4′-(9-acridinylamino)methanesulfon-*m*-anisidide in L-1210 murine leukemia cells. *Cancer Res.* 1985;**45**:1122–1126.

Elliott's B Solution

■ Other Names

NSC #V-7.

■ Chemistry

Elliott's B solution contains 7.3 mg sodium chloride, 0.3 mg potassium chloride, 0.2 mg calcium chloride·2H$_2$O, 0.3 mg magnesium sulfate·7H$_2$O, 0.2 mg sodium phosphate dibasic·7H$_2$O, 0.8 mg dextrose, 1.9 mg sodium bicarbonate, and 0.1 μg phenol red in each milliliter of solution. The pH is 6.6 to 7.2. Purportedly, the solution will turn pink if the pH significantly exceeds 7.2 (Cradock et al 1978, Duttera et al 1972).

Elliott's B solution approximates the normal ionic composition of cerebrospinal fluid, as is shown in the table on page 432.

■ Use in Oncology and Mechanism of Action

Elliott's B solution is not an antitumor agent. Elliott's B solution is an artificial fluid that approximates the chemical composition of human cerebrospinal fluid (Elliott and Jasper 1949, Lewis and Elliott 1950). Because of the relatively small cerebrospinal fluid volume, the close proximity to vital brain areas, and the poor cerebrospinal fluid buffering system, intrathecally or intraventricularly administered drugs should optimally be given in precise physiologic media. This method is particularly important for reconstitution of the antimetabolites methotrexate and cytosine arabinoside for intrathecal use. It is believed that use of Elliott's B solution for intrathecal administration of these drugs may prevent possible neurotoxicity resulting from a nonphysiologic pH or the osmolality of commercial (preservative-containing) diluents (Geiser et al 1975, Band et al 1973). Preservatives such as methyl- or propylparaben and benzyl alcohol are known to be potent central nervous system irritants following intrathecal injections in primates. In a comparison of the typical intrathecal drug diluents (normal saline, lactated Ringer's, and Elliott's B), Cradock et al

COMPOSITION OF ELLIOTT'S B SOLUTION*

Solution	Na+	K+	Ca²⁺	Mg²⁺	P	HCO₃	Cl⁻	Osmolality (mosmol)	Glucose (mg)
Normal cerebrospinal fluid	117–137	2.3–4.6	2.3	2.2	1.2–2.1	22.9	113–127	281	45–80
Elliott's B	147	4	3	1.2	2.3	22.6	129	288	80

*Values in milliequivalents per liter except as indicated.
From Craddock JC, Kleinman LM, Rahman A. Evaluation of some pharmaceutical aspects of intrathecal methotrexate sodium, cytarabine and hydrocortisone sodium succinate. Am J Hosp Pharm. 1978;35:402–406. Adapted with permission.

(1978) found that Elliott's B solution provided significantly greater buffering capacity for both cytarabine, which is acidic, and methotrexate, which is basic.

■ Availability and Storage

Elliott's B is an investigational agent available in 10-mL, single-use glass ampules from the National Cancer Institute. It may be stored at room temperature. Only clear solutions should be used.

■ Preparation for Use, Stability, and Admixture

The investigational preparation is premixed; however, once the ampule is opened, the pH of the solution can rise as a result of diffusion of carbon dioxide (Cradock et al 1978). Ampules should also be inspected for clarity and lack of color, because turbidity may indicate particulate contamination (seen in the once commercially marketed vials) and a red color indicates an unsatisfactory pH.

The following drugs are chemically stable for at least 24 hours in Elliott's B solution: cytarabine (5 mg/mL), methotrexate (2.5 mg/mL), and hydrocortisone sodium succinate (1 mg/mL). The pH range is maintained at 7.2 to 7.8; however, osmolality is slightly increased (range, 298–305 osmol) with these admixtures (Cradock et al 1978). Prolonged storage of the opened solution alone or these admixtures beyond 8 hours is not recommended. Filtration of the solution through a 5-μm aspiration needle is also recommended before drug admixture. Strict sterile technique under laminar flow conditions is recommended.

■ Administration

Elliott's B is to be used as the vehicle or diluent for methotrexate and cytosine arabinoside for intrathecal use (see Special Applications sections for these specific drugs).

■ Special Precautions

None are known.

■ Drug Interactions

None are known.

■ Dosage

Usual volumes of 5 to 10 mL of Elliott's B are reported; however, total volumes of up to 30 mL (one-fourth the cerebrospinal fluid volume) have been successfully used in adults (Reiselbach et al 1962).

■ Pharmacokinetics

There are no studies with this solution.

■ Side Effects and Toxicity

Adverse reactions to Elliott's B have not been reported; however, particulate matter was reported in some earlier batches of the drug. Special scrutiny for particulate matter is thus important before use.

■ Special Applications

See earlier text.

REFERENCES

Band PR, Holland JF, Bernard J, Weil M, Walker M, Rall D. Treatment of central nervous system leukemia with intrathecal cytosine arabinoside. *Cancer*. 1973;**32**:744–748.

Cradock JC, Kleinman LM, Rahman A. Evaluation of some pharmaceutical aspects of intrathecal methotrexate sodium, cytarabine and hydrocortisone sodium succinate. *Am J Hosp Pharm*. 1978;**35**:402–406.

Duttera MJ, Gallelli JF, Kleinman LM, Tangrea JA, Wittgrove AC. Intrathecal methotrexate. *Lancet*. 1972;**1**:540.

Elliott KAC, Jasper HH. Physiological salt solutions for brain surgery: Studies of local pH and pial vessel reactions to buffered and unbuffered isotonic solutions. *J Neurosurg.* 1949;**6**(2):140–152.

Geiser CF, Bishop Y, Jaffee N, et al. Adverse effects of intrathecal methotrexate in children with acute leukemia in remission. *Blood.* 1975;**45**:189–195.

Lewis RC, Elliott KAC. Clinical uses of an artificial cerebrospinal fluid. *J Neurosurg.* 1950;**7**(3):256–260.

Reiselbach RE, DiChiro G, Freireich EJ, Rall DP. Subarachnoid distribution of drugs after lumbar injection. *N Engl J Med.* 1962;**267**:1273–1278.

Elsamitrucin

■ Other Names

BMY-28090 (Bristol-Myers Oncology Division); Elsamicin, Elsaminicin A.

■ Chemistry

Structure of elsamitrucin

Elsamitrucin is a fermentation product derived from cultures of unidentified actinomycete species. It is a water-soluble analog of the antibiotic chartreusin (Casazza et al 1990). The molecular formula is $C_{33}O_{13}N_1H_{35}$ and the molecular weight 654. The free base has negligible water solubility (< 50 µg/mL), but the investigational formulation as a succinic acid salt is water soluble.

■ Antitumor Activity

Elsamitrucin has shown activity in a large number of preclinical tumor models. These include P-388 and L-1210 leukemia, B-16 melanoma, and M5076 sarcoma. The drug was also active in human HCT-116 colon tumor xenografts in nude mice and against human tumors in cell culture (Schurig et al 1989).

■ Mechanism of Action

Elsamitrucin is believed to inhibit DNA topoisomerase I and topoisomerase II enzymes. This activity is maximal in G_2 phase and leads to protein-linked DNA strand breaks (Casazza et al 1990).

■ Availability and Storage

Elsamitrucin is investigationally available from Bristol-Myers Oncology Division, Princeton, New Jersey, in glass vials containing 5 or 50 mg of drug with 50 and 500 mg mannitol, respectively. The intact vials are stored at room temperature.

■ Preparation for Use, Stability, and Admixture

The 5- and 50-mg vials are reconstituted with 4.9 and 20 mL of Sterile Water for Injection, USP, or 5% dextrose. This results in a clear yellow 1 mg/mL solution which is stable for 48 hours at 4°C and for 24 hours at room temperature. Further dilutions in D5W to 0.1 mg/mL in glass containers are stable for 24 hours at 4°C or 25°C; however, at a concentration of 0.01 mg/mL the elsamitrucin solution is stable for only 4 to 8 hours. There is also no adsorption of drug to Travenol®-type infusion sets.

■ Administration

Elsamitrucin is administered intravenously over 10 to 20 minutes.

■ Dosage

The LD_{10} in CD2F1 male mice was 29 mg/m² as an intravenous single dose. The toxic dose low in the dog was 1.8 mg/m² (Hennik et al 1990). In an initial phase I trial the maximally tolerated dose of elsamitrucin was 36 mg/m² every 3 weeks (Raber et al 1991, 1992).

■ Pharmacokinetics

The terminal-phase half-life for elsamitrucin ranged from 36.5 to 56 hours, with a mean of 47.5 hours (Raber et al 1991). The volume of distribution was 400–1100 L/m² with a mean clearance of 10–19 L/hr/m². Approximately 22% of a dose is excreted in the bile and only 5% of a dose is recovered in the urine (Raber et al 1992). In contrast, another group reported three-phase elimination with a terminal half-life of 2.8 days (Hennik et al 1990). The plasma concentration × time product (AUC) varied from 0.5

to 2 µg·h/mL following intravenous doses of 30 mg/m². In another trial an AUC of 24.7 µmol/L·min was reported after a dose of 9.6 mg/m². Total clearance was 10 to 14 L/h/m², with a volume of distribution of 400 to 625 L/m². Urinary excretion accounts for less than 5% of a dose (Hennik et al 1990); 22% is excreted in the bile after 48 hours (Raber et al 1991). In addition, biliary flow may be slightly increased immediately after drug administration.

■ Side Effects and Toxicity

The dose-limiting toxic effect of elsamitrucin is hepatic enzyme elevation. Serum glutamic–oxalacetic and glutamic–pyruvic transaminase enzyme levels peaked about 3 days after drug administration and returned to normal after 2 weeks. Bilirubin, lactate dehydrogenase, and alkaline phosphatase enzyme levels do not consistently rise after drug administration. Other toxic effects include nausea and vomiting, malaise, phlebitis, and local reactions at the site of administration (Raber et al 1991, 1992). Mucositis was reported in one phase I trial (Hennik et al 1990) and grade I myelosuppression was observed in one patient in another trial (Amato et al 1990). Typically little hematologic toxicity is seen (Raber et al 1992).

REFERENCES

Amato R, Raber M, Schacter L. Phase I clinical trial of elsamicin (abstract). *Invest New Drugs.* 1990;**8**:456.

Casazza AM, Schurig JE, Forenza BH, et al. Novel fermentation derived cytotoxic antitumor agents (abstract). *Invest New Drugs.* 1990;**8**:352.

Hennik MBv, Vermorken JB, Vijgh WJF vd, et al. Phase I study of elsamicin (BMY-28090) (abstract). *Invest New Drugs.* 1990;**8**:456.

Raber MN, Newman RA, Newman BM, et al. Clinical pharmacology study of elsamitrucin (E) (BMY-28090). *Proc Am Assoc Cancer Res.* 1991;**32**:175.

Raber MN, Newman BM, et al. Phase I trial and clinical pharmacology of elsamitrucin. *Cancer Res.* 1992;**52**:1406–1410.

Schurig JE, Bradner WT, Basler GA, et al. Experimental antitumor activity of BMY 28090, a new antitumor antibiotic. *Invest New Drugs.* 1989;**7**:173–178.

Epirubicin

■ Other Names

4'-Epidoxorubicin; 4'-epi-DX; IMI-28; NSC-256942; FI-7701; Farmorubicin® (Farmitalia Carlo Erba).

■ Chemistry

Structure of epirubicin

Epirubicin (EPI) is an epimer of doxorubicin wherein the C-4' hydroxyl group on the amino sugar is in the equatorial position rather than the axial position (Arcamone et al 1975a,b). This increases the lipophilicity of EPI. Epirubicin has the same molecular weight as doxorubicin, 579. The drug has a lower pK_a (8.08) than doxorubicin, and this altered basicity favors the cationic form of the amino sugar required for water solubility and cell uptake.

■ Antitumor Activity

Epirubicin is active in a wide variety of murine tumors (Arcamone et al 1975b, Casazza 1979, Casazza et al 1978). In several murine tumors, EPI, unlike doxorubicin, can be dose escalated to produce increased therapeutic effects in experimental animals without producing enhanced toxicity (Casazza 1979). Human cancers sensitive to EPI in the nude mouse xenograft model include melanoma, breast, lung cancer (both small cell and non-small cell), prostate cancer, and ovarian cancer (Giuliani et al 1981). Similar activity was observed in fresh human tumors tested in colony-forming assays in vitro

(Salmon et al 1981). Compared with doxorubicin, EPI also produces slightly greater experimental immunosuppressive effects such as reduced antibody production and delayed hypersensitivity reactions (Isetta and Trizio 1981).

Epirubicin has demonstrated significant therapeutic activity in a wide variety of solid tumors in humans (see table) (Ganzina 1983, Mouridsen et al 1990). Consistent single-agent activity is observed in advanced breast cancer, with an overall response rate of about 40% (Ganzina 1983). Brambilla et al (1986) report an even higher 62% response in patients who had relapsed after receiving the CMF combination. Antitumor results with epirubicin combinations are equivalent to results for doxorubicin-regimens as in CAF (with doxorubicin) versus CEF (with EPI) (French Epirubicin Study Group 1991). Responses up to 73% were observed in previously untreated patients. Some prospective trials have also reported longer remission durations in EPI-treated patients compared with those receiving doxorubicin (Young 1984).

As a single agent, EPI has limited activity in malignant melanoma, producing a 9% average partial response rate (Ganzina 1983). Colorectal cancer is occasionally sensitive to EPI, with reported response rates of 3 to 25% (Michaelson et al 1982, Wils 1984). A response rate of 17% is described in previously untreated patients with either gastric cancer (Scarffe et al 1985) or hepatocellular carcinoma (Hochster et al 1985). A 19% response rate is reported in pancreatic cancer (Hochster et al 1986). Epirubicin has produced up to 25% objective response rates in renal cell carcinoma in some trials (Bonfante et al 1982), but has been relatively inactive in other studies (Fossa et al 1982). A 20% overall objective response rate is seen in soft tissue sarcoma and an approximately 8% objective response rate is reported in non-small cell lung cancer (Ganzina 1983).

As a single agent, EPI has a low, 16% response rate in previously treated ovarian cancer patients, but when combined with cisplatin, EPI elicits a 50% response rate (Ganzina 1983). Hematologic malignancies are more responsive to EPI and a 76% response rate is reported in non-Hodgkin's lymphoma patients (some previously untreated) (Bonfante et al 1982). In this setting, EPI is also highly effective as a substitution for DOX in multidrug combinations such as CHOP and BACOP

OVERALL OBJECTIVE RESPONSE RATES TO SINGLE-AGENT EPIRUBICIN IN HUMAN CANCER

Tumor Type	Number of Patients	All Evaluable Patients (% Response Rate)	Previous Treatment (% Response Rate) Yes	None
Solid tumors				
Breast cancer	33*	33	24	48
	229†	35	—‡	—
Malignant melanoma	84*	9	—	—
Colorectal carcinoma	88*	3–25	11	18
Renal cell cancer	54*	5	—	—
Gastric, pancreatic, hepatocellular cancer	33*	24	—	—
Pancreatic cancer†	21	8–25		
Soft tissue sarcoma	43*	21	—	—
Ovarian cancer	32*	—	16	30
Non-small cell lung cancer	296†	41	125	66
Small cell lung cancer	191†	18	—	—
Hematologic cancers				
Non-Hodgkin's lymphoma	32*,§	76		
Chronic leukemias	3*	10 (approx)		

*After Ganzina 1983.
†Mouridsen et al 1990.
‡—, Status not mentioned in original citation.
§EPI combined with other agents in nine patients.

(Ganzina 1983). It has also shown some activity in treating chronic leukemias and in relapsing patients with multiple myeloma when combined with a vinca alkaloid and prednisone (Ganzina 1983).

■ Mechanism of Action

Epirubicin intercalates into DNA to inhibit nucleic acid synthesis (DiMarco et al 1976, Plumbridge and Brown 1978). The activity of both DNA and RNA polymerases is inhibited by the drug at a concentration equivalent to that of doxorubicin (DiMarco et al 1976). The affinity constant for EPI binding to DNA, $1.9 \times 10^{-6} M^{-1}$, with about 0.25 binding site per nucleotide, is roughly comparable to that of doxorubicin. Epirubicin also induces protein-linked DNA double-strand breaks in a manner that is compatible with drug-induced inhibition of topoisomerase II enzymes. In the presence of such intercalating drugs, topoisomerase II is believed to form stabilized conformations of an otherwise transient or "cleavable" complex between DNA and subunits of the enzyme.

■ Availability and Storage

Epirubicin is commercially available in Europe from Farmitalia Carlo Erba, Milan. It is investigationally available in the United States from Adria Laboratories, Columbus, Ohio. The drug is supplied in 10- and 50-mg vials of sterile red-orange lyophilized powdered drug. Unopened vials should be stored under refrigeration and protected from light.

■ Preparation for Use, Stability, and Admixture

Epirubicin vials are reconstituted to a concentration of 2 mg/mL in sterile 0.9% sodium chloride or Sterile Water for Injection, USP; however, saline is generally preferred as it may lessen the incidence of acute venous reactions. Once reconstituted, the solution is chemically stable for at least 24 hours if protected from light. At room temperature, solutions lose 43% activity after 20 hours in daylight. A 12% loss may also occur when frozen solutions are thawed (Weenen et al 1983). Detailed admixture data are not available and the reader is referred to the *Doxorubicin* monograph for identifying potential incompatibilities such as with sodium heparin. EPI is compatible with all major types of infusion solutions including 5% dextrose in water, normal saline and lactated Ringer's injection.

■ Administration

Epirubicin is administered by intravenous injection, either through the side port of a running intravenous line or as a brief infusion in 50 to 100 mL of fluid over 15 to 20 minutes. The drug has vesicant potential if extravasated; thus, EPI infusions should be closely monitored. Specific antidotes to extravasation have not been described, although topical cooling and dimethylsulfoxide have been reported to be effective with extravasations of doxorubicin. For investigational intraperitoneal and hepatic intraarterial administration methods, see Special Applications.

■ Dosage

The most frequently recommended EPI dose for phase II studies ranged from 75 to 90 mg/m^2 administered as an intravenous bolus every 3 weeks. An alternate schedule involves giving an intravenous bolus of 40 to 50 mg/m^2/d on two consecutive days every 3 weeks (Kolaric et al 1983). One group has also evaluated high-dose epirubicin (120 mg/m^2) as primary chemotherapy in advanced breast carcinoma (Carmo-Pereira et al 1991). Doses were repeated every 3 weeks. As a 6-hour infusion a dose of 90 mg/m^2 was safely administered every 3 weeks (Hochster et al 1985). Although some clinicians suggest a 50% dose reduction in patients with hepatic metastases with or without hepatic insufficiency, there are no controlled studies to validate this empiric recommendation. If clearance is similar to that of doxorubicin, then EPI doses should be reduced 50% for a serum bilirubin of 1.2 or higher up to 2 mg/dL, and to 75% for a serum bilirubin above 2 mg/dL (Ganzina 1983). No similar dose reductions are recommended in patients with renal dysfunction even though drug clearance may be reduced by about 20% (Ganzina 1983).

■ Pharmacokinetics

The pharmacokinetics of EPI in human cancer patients is summarized in the table on the opposite page. Overall, EPI appears to be eliminated more rapidly than DOX, producing steady-state plasma levels 20 to 40% lower than those of doxorubicin at comparable doses. Both agents exhibit prolonged retention in the body following a rapid distribution phase. The conversion of EPI to at least five metabolites proceeds rapidly. Known metabolites include the C-13 alcohol epirubicinol, which is active, and several inactive aglycones of EPI and epirubicinol that can be conjugated with glucuronide and excreted primarily in the bile (Weenen et al 1983). Sometimes, the level of aglycones exceeds that of the parent drug. Urine excretion accounts for about 11% of a dose over 48 hours, and only three metabolites can be recovered in the urine. These include epirubicinol and the glucuronide–aglycone conjugates of epirubicin and epirubicinol (Weenen et al 1983). Epirubicinol is formed by the ubiquitous cytosolic enzyme aldoketoreductase, as is doxorubicinol.

Of interest, the plasma levels and metabolism of EPI are significantly altered in patients with hepatic metastases, with or without liver impairment (Gazina 1983). In such patients a 50% dose reduction produced levels of EPI and epirubicinol comparable to those in patients without hepatic disease or impairment. In patients with renal impairment, EPI clearance is reduced variably, by about 20%, although no change in dosing was recommended (Ganzina 1983).

■ Side Effects and Toxicity

Myelosuppression is the typical dose-limiting toxic effect of EPI. Leukopenia is more prominent than thrombocytopenia, with nadirs of about 10 and 14 to 20 days, respectively. In phase I trials, a 10% decrease in hemoglobin levels was also observed between 7 and 14 days after dosing (Ganzina 1983). All of the hematologic effects of EPI are usually resolved by 3 weeks.

The incidence and severity of other acute anthracycline toxic effects appear to be decreased with EPI. This includes nausea and vomiting, seen in 50% of patients at a mild to moderate intensity, and alopecia, seen in 25 to 50% of patients (Bonfante et al 1979). Of interest, even high cumulative doses of EPI usually produce only minimal hair loss and over 50% of patients may have no hair loss (Bonfante et al 1979). There were no instances of phlebitis in many trials, although one group reported a 4% incidence of phlebitis. In another trial, pain, swelling, and erythema followed inadvertent extravasation of the drug (Schauer et al 1981). Four extravasations in one study resulted in transient dark-brown staining of the skin but no ulceration (Carmo-Pereira et al 1991). Stomatitis is not usual with EPI and diarrhea has been observed in only 50% of patients receiving relatively high doses of 90 mg/m^2 (Bonfante et al 1979). Renal and hepatic toxic effects have not been described with EPI.

Cardiac toxicity appears to be markedly diminished with EPI. In experimental systems EPI lacked cardiac effects in cultured mouse myocytes and was much more selective for tumor cells over heart cells in a rat myocyte model (Dorr et al 1991). In vivo, EPI was 30% less cardiotoxic than doxorubicin in mice and threefold less cardiotoxic in isolated rabbit heart muscle preparations (Ganzina 1983). Compared with doxorubicin in isolated guinea pig atria, EPI produced fewer negative inotropic effects and less inhibition of intracellular calcium turnover (Villani et al 1980).

Epirubicin is similarly less cardiotoxic in humans, although the same characteristic anthracycline effects do occur after large cumulative doses of EPI have been administered. Acute effects include reversible T-wave flattening and a cumulative dose-dependent increase in systolic time intervals (Bonfante et al 1979). Tachyarrhythmias and premature ventricular beats have also been described (Cuna et al 1983). Clinical signs of congestive heart failure have not been commonly reported even in a few patients receiving large cumulative doses of an-

CLINICAL PHARMACOKINETICS OF EPIRUBICIN

Route of Administration	Plasma Half-life α (min)	Plasma Half-life β (h)	Plasma Half-life γ (h)	Clearance (L/min)	Volume of Distribution at Steady State (L/m^2)	AUC (10^{-8} mol/L/h) EPI	AUC (10^{-8} mol/L/h) EPI-OL
Intravenous bolus*	4–5	2.4	30	1.4 (plasma)	1430	109[†]	70[†]
Hepatic artery	—	—	45	82 (hepatic)	62 L/kg	—	—
Intraperitoneal	—	—	26	131 (IP space)	—		Ratio[‡]

*Bonfante et al 1979, Weenen et al 1983.
[†]Corrected to 60 mg/m^2 (Weenen et al 1983).
[‡]Mean ratio of (AUC metabolite/AUC parent drug) × 100 was 37 (Strocchi et al 1985).

thracyclines before EPI (Hurteloup et al 1983). In another trial, 1 of 18 patients receiving more than 500 mg/m² EPI did develop congestive heart failure (left ventricular ejection fraction [LVEF] of 36%). This occurred at a cumulative EPI dose of 1080 mg/m². A similar event was observed in hepatoma patients who received a cumulative EPI dose of 1460 mg/m² (LVEF drop from 56 to 39%). In another trial, a 20% drop in LVEF in two women given 600 mg/m² of EPI was not associated with clinical signs or symptoms of heart failure (Brambilla et al 1986). Young et al (1984) compared doxorubicin and EPI using serial MUGA scans. A 10% drop in LVEF was found at significantly different cumulative doses of 850 mg/m² for EPI and 360 mg/m² for doxorubicin. Clinical congestive heart failure occurred in four EPI patients at a median dose of 1134 mg/m² compared with a median doxorubicin dose of only 492 mg/m². Overall, EPI is cardiotoxic and requires significantly greater cumulative dosing than doxorubicin to elicit cardiac effects.

■ Special Applications

Intraarterial Administration. Epirubicin has been administered by intrahepatic arterial methods (Strocchi et al 1985). Hepatic arterial doses of 20 to 40 mg were given as a rapid infusion through a subcutaneous Infusaid® access port. Partial responses were observed in 6 of 10 patients with colon cancer or hepatocellular cancer. Doses were administered weekly using intrahepatic epirubicin doses of 40 mg and 750 mg 5-fluorouracil. Leukopenia and alopecia were observed in only one patient who had a hepatopulmonary shunt. And, even in patients with hepatic disease, no clinical or electrocardiographic evidence of toxicity was produced by the intrahepatic EPI therapy. The first-pass effect of EPI removal through the liver was substantial. This produced relatively low plasma levels of EPI and glucuronide conjugates of EPI and epirubicinol (EPI–OL). The earlier table summarizes EPI pharmacokinetics for the intrahepatic route of administration which shows a high apparent plasma clearance rate.

Intraperitoneal Administration. Intraperitoneal epirubicin was administered to six patients with ascites from peritoneal metastases (three each with ovarian cancer and colorectal cancer). A weekly dose of 30 mg was administered in 60 mL of saline after paracentesis. Drug concentrations in the blood were 2000-fold lower than in the intraperitoneal space, although the overall systemic bioavailability of EPI following intraperitoneal administration averaged 0.52. Thus, about half of an intraperitoneal EPI dose was systemically absorbed. Nonetheless, side effects, including peritonitis and systemic toxic effects, were not observed.

Intravesical Administration. Epirubicin has been used to treat superficial bladder cancer (Calais da Silva et al 1988) and as a prophylactic regimen. In the first study, 67% of patients with previously untreated tumors responded compared with 37% of patients with recurrent tumors. An epirubicin dose of 50 mg was diluted into 50 mL of 0.9% sodium chloride and instilled into the bladder for about 2 hours (Calais da Silva et al 1988). Dosing was repeated frequently (up to six instillations in 10 days). Higher doses up to 80 mg have been used by Matsumura et al (1986). Chemical cystitis occurred in 9 of 46 (26%) patients (Calais da Silva et al 1988). As a prophylactic regimen, intravesical epirubicin significantly reduced the tumor recurrence rate in patients with recurrent superficial papillary cancer. Liver enzymes were transiently elevated in 17 of 57 (30%) patients and chemical cystitis occurred in 7 of 57 (12%) patients. Interestingly, addition of the calcium channel antagonist verapamil was felt to enhance EPI efficacy.

REFERENCES

Arcamone F, Penco S, Vigevani A. Adriamycin: New chemical development and analogs. *Cancer Chem Rep.* 1975a;**6**:123–129.

Arcamone F, Penco S, Vigevani A, et al. Synthesis and antitumor properties of new glycosides of daunomycinone and adriamycinone. *J Med Chem.* 1975b;**18**:703–707.

Bonfante V, Bonadonna G, Villani F, et al. Preliminary phase I study of 4'-epi-Adriamycin. *Cancer Treat Rep.* 1979;**63**:915–918.

Bonfante V, Villani F, Bonadonna G. Toxic and therapeutic activity of 4'-Epidoxorubicin. *Tumori.* 1982;**68**:105–111.

Brambilla C, Rossi A, Bonfante V, et al. Phase II study of doxorubicin versus epirubicin in advanced breast cancer. *Cancer Treat Rep.* 1986;**70**:261–266.

Calais da Silva F, Denis L, Bono A, Bollack C, Bouffioux C. Intravesical chemoresection with 4'-epi-doxorubicin in patients with superficial bladder tumors. *Eur Urol.* 1988;**14**:207–209.

Carmo-Pereira J, Costa FO, Miles DW, et al. High-dose epirubicin as primary chemotherapy in advanced breast carcinoma: A phase II study. *Cancer Chemother Pharmacol.* 1991;**27**:394–396.

Casazza AM. Experimental evaluation of anthracycline analogs. *Cancer Treat Rep.* 1979;**63**:835–844.

Casazza AM, Di Marco A, Bertazzoli C, Formelli F. Antitumor activity, toxicity and pharmacological properties of 4'-epi-adriamycin. In: *Current Chemotherapy.* Am Soc Microbiol Intl Soc Chemother, Bethesda, MD; 1978; 1257–1260.

Cuna GRD, Pavesi L, Preti P, Ganzina F. Clinical evaluation of 4'-Epidoxorubicin in advanced solid tumors. *Invest New Drugs.* 1983;**1**:349–353.

DiMarco A, Casazza AM, Gambetta R, et al. Relationship between activity and amino sugar stereochemistry of daunorubicin and Adriamycin derivatives. *Cancer Res.* 1976;**36**:1962–1966.

Dorr RT, Shipp NG, Lee KM. Comparison of cytotoxicity in heart cells and tumor cells exposed to DNA intercalating agents in vitro. *Anti-Cancer Drugs.* 1991;**2**:27–33.

Fossa SD, Wik B, Bae E, Lien HH. Phase II study of 4'-Epidoxorubicin in metastatic renal cancer. *Cancer Treat Rep.* 1982;**66**:1219–1221.

French Epirubicin Study Group. A prospective randomized trial comparing epirubicin monochemotherapy to two fluorouracil, cyclophosphamide, and epirubicin regimens different in epirubicin dose in advanced breast cancer patients. *J Clin Oncol.* 1991;**9**(2):305–312.

Ganzina F. 4'-Epidoxorubicin, a new analogue of doxorubicin: A preliminary overview of preclinical and clinical data. *Cancer Treat Rev.* 1983;**10**:1–22.

Giuliani FC, Coirin AK, Rene Rice M, Kaplan NO. The effect of 4'-Epidoxorubicin analogs on heterotransplantation of human tumors in congenitally athymic mice. *Cancer Treat Rep.* 1981;**65**:1063–1075.

Hochster HS, Green MD, Speyer J, et al. 4'-Epidoxorubicin (epirubicin): Activity in hepatocellular carcinoma. *J Clin Oncol.* 1985;**3**:1535–1540.

Hochster H, Green MD, Speyer JL, et al. Activity of epirubicin in pancreatic carcinoma. *Cancer Treat Rep.* 1986;**70**(2):299–300.

Hurteloup P, Cappelaere P, Armand JP, Mathe G. Phase II clinical evaluation of 4'-Epidoxorubicin. *Cancer Treat Rep.* 1983;**67**:337–341.

Isetta AM, Trizio D. Effect of new anthracyclines antibiotics on humoral and cell mediated immune responses in vivo. *12th International Congress of Chemotherapy, Florence, Italy;* July 19–24, 1981:115.

Kolaric K, Potrebica V, Cervek J. Phase II clinical trial of 4'-Epidoxorubicin in metastatic solid tumors. *J Cancer Res Clin Oncol.* 1983;**106**(2):148–152.

Michaelson R, Kemeny N, Young C. Phase II evaluation of 4'-Epidoxorubicin in patients with advanced colorectal carcinoma. *Cancer Treat Rep.* 1982;**66**:1757–1758.

Mouridsen HT, Alfthan C, Bastholt L, et al. Current status of epirubicin (Farmorubicin) in the treatment of solid tumors. *ACTA Oncol.* 1990;**29**:257–285.

Plumbridge TW, Brown JR. Studies on the mode of interaction of 4'-Epidoxorubicin and 4-demethoxydaunomycin with DNA. *Biochem Pharmacol.* 1978;**27**:1881–1882.

Salmon SE, Liu R, Cassaza AM. Evaluation of new anthracycline analogs with the human tumor stem cell assay. *Cancer Chemother Pharmacol.* 1981;**6**:103–109.

Scarffe JH, Kenny JB, Johnson RJ, et al. Phase II trial of epirubicin in gastric cancer. *Cancer Treat Rep.* 1985;**69**:1275–1277.

Schauer PK, Wittes RE, Gralla RJ, et al. A phase I trial of 4'-epi-Adriamycin. *Cancer Clin Trials.* 1981;**4**:433–437.

Strocchi E, Camaggi CM, Rossi AP, et al. Epirubicin pharmacokinetics after intrahepatic arterial and intraperitoneal administration. *Drugs Exp Clin Res.* 1985;**11**:295–301.

Villani FP, Favalli L, Piccinini F. Relationship between the effect on calcium turnover and early cardiotoxicity of doxorubicin and 4'-Epidoxorubicin in guinea pig heart muscle. *Tumori.* 1980;**66**:689–697.

Weenen H, Lankelma J, Penders, PGM, et al. Pharmacokinetics of 4'-Epidoxorubicin in man. *Invest New Drugs.* 1983;**1**:59–64.

Wils JA. Phase II trial of 4'-Epidoxorubicin in metastatic colorectal carcinoma. *Invest New Drugs.* 1984;**2**:397–399.

Young CW. Evaluation of epirubicin in patients with advanced breast cancer. In: *Advances in Anthracycline Chemotherapy: Epirubicin.* Milan: Masson Italia Editori; 1984:71–74.

Young CW, Casper ES, Geller NL. Clinical and cineangiographic comparison of the cardiotoxic effects of epirubicin and doxorubicin (abstract). In: *International Symposium on Advances in Anthracycline Chemotherapy, Milan, Italy;* 1984:18.

Esorubicin

■ Other Names

4'-deoxydox; 4'-DXDX; NSC-267469; 4'-deoxydoxorubicin; IMI-58; ESO.

■ Chemistry

Structure of esorubicin

Esorubicin (ESO) is an analog of doxorubicin that lacks a hydroxy group in the 4'-position of the amino sugar. The empiric formula is $C_7H_{29}NO_{10} \cdot HCl$ and the molecular weight is 563.98. Removal of the 4'-hydroxyl increases the basicity and lipophilicity of the agent compared with doxorubicin (Cummings et al 1987). This structural change is believed to increase the therapeutic ratio of the compound as a result of the reduced cardiotoxicity.

■ Antitumor Activity

Esorubicin was 1.5 to 2 times more active than doxorubicin in numerous preclinical tumor models including P-388 and L-1210 ascites leukemia and Gross leukemia. It had equivalent activity in murine mammary carcinoma and MS-2 sarcoma. Activity was slightly reduced in B-16 melanoma, its activity was enhanced compared with doxorubicin in murine colon-26 and colon-38 models (Casazza 1980, Casazza et al 1983). Esorubicin was active in human colon tumor xenografts in nude mice but was inactive in rectal cancer xenografts (Giuliani and Kaplan 1980, Giuliani et al 1981). Activity was observed in several types of fresh human tumors in colony-forming assays in vitro including breast cancer, ovarian carcinoma, and melanoma (Salmon et al 1981, 1984). Activity was not seen in fresh human colon cancers, but there was evidence of a lack of cross-resistance with doxorubicin in vitro (Salmon and Durie 1982).

In early clinical trials responses to esorubicin were sporadically observed. Two responses were seen in a phase I trial in patients with advanced adenocarcinoma. The response duration was 7 months in a patient with nasopharyngeal cancer and 5 months in a patient with endometrial cancer (Stanton et al 1985). Minor responses in melanoma, breast cancer, lymphoma, and gastric cancer were observed in another phase I trial (Garewal et al 1984). In a phase II trial 2 of 20 melanoma patients achieved a partial response (Hochster et al 1990). Partial responses have been reported in cancer of the pancreas, colon (Falkson and Vorbiof 1986), anus, and breast (Braich et al 1986, Carlson et al 1987a), as well as in patients with non-Hodgkin's lymphoma (Ferrari et al 1984). Esorubicin appears to have significant therapeutic activity in the last indication (Miller et al 1991). Partial responses have been observed in acute nonlymphocytic leukemia (Kreis et al 1988) and in a phase II trial of patients with adenocarcinoma of the pancreas. Limited activity was observed in gastric cancer, with one partial response in 15 patients in a phase II trial (Somlo et al 1991).

Therapeutic results have been disappointing in non-small cell lung cancer (Kaplan et al 1985) and in one study of advanced breast cancer (Leitner et al 1985). No activity was reported in ovarian cancer (Green et al 1990). Overall, the greatest level of activity for ESO has been observed in hematologic cancers and in lymphomas followed by breast cancer.

■ Mechanism of Action

The mechanism of antitumor action for ESO is believed to be similar to that of doxorubicin and daunorubicin (DiMarco et al 1977). Esorubicin is taken up more rapidly in sensitive tumor cells than is doxorubicin. The drug is also more potent than doxorubicin in assays for DNA intercalation (DiMarco et al 1977). The synthesis of RNA and especially DNA is inhibited by ESO at cytotoxic drug concentrations. Esorubicin may also inhibit strand-passing activity of topoisomerase II enzymes, leading to protein-associated DNA strand breaks primarily in G_2 phase. This has been noted for most intercalators. In contrast, oxygen free radical formation, thought to be associated with doxorubicin cardiotoxicity, may be absent with ESO (Dickinson et al 1984).

■ Availability and Storage

Esorubicin is investigationally available in 5-mg vials of lyophilized red powder from Farmitalia Carlo Erba, Milan, Italy. The vials are stored at room temperature.

■ Preparation for Use, Stability, and Admixture

The ESO vials are reconstituted with 5 mL of Sterile Water for Injection, USP, or normal saline. The latter diluent is felt to produce a lower incidence of acute local venous reactions. Reconstituted solutions are stable for at least 48 hours and, as with doxorubicin, there may be numerous incompatibilities with other drugs including heparin. Specific compatibility information is not reported (refer to *Doxorubicin* monograph for admixture guidelines). Solutions for prolonged infusion (> 24 hours) should be protected from light.

Administration

Esorubicin is administered intravenously only. A brief intravenous infusion over 5 to 20 minutes in 50 to 150 mL of saline or 5% dextrose is most often used. Esorubicin has also been administered as a continuous infusion over 48 hours (Kreis et al 1988). The daily infusion solution was prepared in 1 L of D5W and was protected from light.

Dosage

The recommended single intravenous dose for phase II studies is 30 mg/m² in good-risk patients and 25 mg/m² in heavily pretreated patients (Stanton et al 1985). Slightly higher doses of 35 mg/m² in good-risk patients and 30 mg/m² in poor-risk patients were recommended by others (Rozencweig et al 1983). A single maximum tolerated dose of 40 to 45 mg/m² was recommended by Ferrari et al (1984). In contrast, another group recommended lower doses of 30 and 25 mg/m² in good- and poor-risk patients, respectively (Garewal et al 1984). The recommended total dose for 48-hour continuous infusions of ESO was 45 mg/m². All ESO regimens were typically repeated at 21-day intervals without evidence of cumulative toxicity. Recommended doses for a weekly × 3 schedule were 17.5 and 15 mg/m² in good- and poor-risk patients, respectively (Sessa et al 1984).

Pharmacokinetics

The table below summarizes the pharmacokinetics of ESO in cancer patients given single intravenous doses (Stanton et al 1985) or 48-hour infusions (Kreis et al 1988). The results show that ESO is eliminated similarly to doxorubicin with a triphasic elimination pattern characterized by a significantly long terminal half-life of over 90 hours. Esorubicin is metabolized similarly to doxorubicin forming esorubicinol, an active 13-alcohol, and several inactive 7-deoxy aglycones of both the parent drug and esorubicinol. Little drug is excreted in the urine. Only 2 to 10% of intact drug and 0.6 to 2.5% of esorubicinol are recovered in the urine (Kreis et al 1988) and total urinary elimination averages 4.2% (Stanton et al 1985). Unlike doxorubicin or epirubicin, less glucuronides are formed with ESO, suggesting that the 4'-hydroxyl group is necessary for glucuronide conjugation. Biliary secretion is a major means of drug elimination. Cumulative 5-day biliary excretion of drug was 21% in a patient with a biliary drainage tube (Stanton et al 1985).

Side Effects and Toxicity

The dose-limiting toxic effect of ESO is myelosuppression, mainly leukopenia (Ferrari et al 1984, Garewal et al 1984, Stanton et al 1985). Dose-dependent granulocyte and platelet nadirs typically occur about 2 weeks after drug administration (Garewal et al 1984). Recovery by 3 to 4 weeks is characteristic. Mild nausea and vomiting are reported in one third of patients and are very responsive to antiemetics (Ferrari et al 1984). Alopecia is also seen in most patients but it is usually not complete in contrast to doxorubicin. Renal or hepatic toxic effects are rare with ESO but local reactions may be common.

About 22% of patients may experience acute local venous toxicity following intravenous administration of ESO (Garewal et al 1984). Local reactions

ESORUBICIN PHARMACOKINETICS

Route	Dose (mg/m²)	Half-life α (min)	Half-life β (h)	Half-life γ (h)	AUC (ng·h/mL) ESO	AUC (ng·h/mL) ESO-OL	Steady-State Volume of Distribution (L/min)	Total Body Clearance (L/h/m²)
Intravenous bolus*	10	1.23	1.94	129	550	—	—	—
	30	1.28	1.73	91	1083	—	—	—
Intravenous 48-h infusion†	35	—	—	22	384	291	1814	92
	45	—	—	28	450	310	2425	101
	65	—	—	20	771	566	1639	85
	75	—	—	54	2079	1552	1335	42
	85	—	—	24	1351	1151	1631	63

*Stanton et al 1985.
†Kreis et al 1988.

consisted of hives at the injection site and occasional supravenous erythema along the course of the infusion. Phlebitis is not usually a problem (Stanton et al 1985). The local venous reactions to ESO tend to recur in patients but are not blocked by prophylactic antihistamines and glucocorticosteroids (Lee et al 1987); however, these medications and topical cooling were helpful at alleviating symptoms once a reaction developed. Esorubicin can produce necrosis if extravasated (Hochster et al 1990). One case of ESO extravasation was successfully treated with topical cooling (Lee et al 1987). In experimental models, ESO is a potent vesicant for which corticosteroids were ineffective as antidotes. Rare reactions to ESO include fever, stomatitis, and diarrhea (Rozencweig et al 1983).

Esorubicin produces variable cardiotoxicity in animal models reported as either less than that caused by doxorubicin (Casazza 1980) or equivalent to that caused by doxorubicin (Cummings et al 1987). There was also very little evidence of cardiotoxicity in the initial phase I–II clinical trials with ESO (Garewal et al 1984, Ferrari et al 1984, Rozencweig et al 1983, Stanton et al 1985); however, in a quantitative in vitro model, ESO was significantly less cardiotoxic than doxorubicin (Dorr et al 1991) and was associated with congestive heart failure in one patient at a cumulative ESO dose of 184 mg/m^2 (Blayney 1986). It produced fatal cardiac toxicity in one other study (Dich et al 1988). Routine serial gated heart (MUGA) scans are recommended for patients receiving ESO, and serial histologic changes can be observed in patients undergoing endomyocardial biopsies while receiving ESO (Carlson et al 1987b). In a prospective ESO cardiotoxicity study using serial gated heart scans there were 5 and 10% decreases in left ventricular ejection fractions at cumulative ESO doses of 240 and 488 mg/m^2, respectively. A maximal cumulative dose endpoint of 240 mg/m^2 was recommended (Ringenberg et al 1990).

REFERENCES

Blayney D. Cardiotoxicity associated with 4'-deoxydoxorubicin. *Cancer Treat Rep.* 1986;**70**:433.

Braich TA, Salmon SE, Robertone A, et al. Phase II trial of esorubicin in cancers of the breast, colon, kidney, lung and melanoma. *Invest New Drugs.* 1986;**4**:269–274.

Carlson RW, Billingham M, Kohler M, et al. Esorubicin in refractory metastatic carcinoma of the breast: A NCOG study. *Cancer Treat Rep.* 1987a;**71**:427–438.

Carlson RW, Williams RB, Billingham ME, et al. Phase II trial of esorubicin in the treatment of metastatic carcinoma of the kidney. *Cancer Treat Rep.* 1987b;**71**:767–768.

Cassaza AM. Antitumor activity and cardiac toxicity of 4'-deoxydoxorubicin in mice. In: Mathe G, et al, eds. *Anthracyclines—Current Status and Future Developments.* New York: Masson; 1980;193–197.

Cassaza AM, Savi G, Pratesi G, DiMarco A. Antitumor activity in mice of 4'-deoxydoxorubicin in comparison with doxorubicin. *Eur J Cancer Clin Oncol.* 1983;**19**:411–418.

Cummings J, Willmott N, More I, et al. Comparative cardiotoxicity and antitumor activity of doxorubicin (Adriamycin) and 4'-deoxydoxorubicin and the relationship to in vivo disposition and metabolism in the target tissues. *Biochem Pharmacol.* 1987;**36**:1521–1526.

Dich LF, Banks T, Carter W, et al. Fatal doxorubicin induced cardiomyopathy. *Cancer Chemother Pharmacol.* 1988;**21**:347–350.

Dickinson AC, DeJordy JO, Boutin MG, Teres D. Absence of generation of oxygen-containing free radicals with 4'-deoxydoxorubicin, a non-cardiotoxic anthracycline drug. *Biochem Biophys Res Commun.* 1984;**125**:584–591.

DiMarco A, Casazza AM, Dasdia T, et al. Changes of activity of daunorubicin, Adriamycin, and stereoisomers following the introduction or removal of hydroxyl groups in the amino sugar moiety. *Chem–Biol Interact.* 1977;**19**:191–202.

Dorr RT, Shipp NG, Lee KM. Comparison of cytotoxicity in heart cells and tumor cells exposed to DNA intercalating agents in vitro. *Anti-Cancer Drugs.* 1991;**2**:27–33.

Falkson G, Vorbiof DA. Phase II study of 4'-deoxydoxorubicin in advanced colorectal cancer. *Invest New Drugs.* 1986;**4**:165–169.

Ferrari L, Rossi A, Brambilla C, et al. Phase I study with 4'-deoxydoxorubicin. *Invest New Drugs.* 1984;**2**:287–295.

Garewal HS, Robertone A, Salmon SE, et al. Phase I trial of esorubicin (4'-deoxydoxorubicin). *J Clin Oncol.* 1984;**2**:1034–1039.

Giuliani FC, Kaplan NO. New doxorubicin analogs active against doxorubicin-resistant colon tumor xenografts in the nude mouse. *Cancer Res.* 1980;**40**:4682–4687.

Giuliani FC, Zirvi KA, Kaplan NO, Goldin A. Chemotherapy of human colorectal tumor xenografts in athymic mice with clinically active drugs: 5-Fluorouracil and BCNU. Comparison with doxorubicin derivatives: 4'-deoxydoxorubicin and 4'-O-methyldoxorubicin. *Int J Cancer.* 1981;**27**:5–13.

Green MD, Speyer JL, Wernz JC, et al. Phase II study of esorubicin (4'-deoxydoxorubicin) in anthracycline naive patients with ovarian cancer. *Invest New Drugs.* 1990;**8**:333–336.

Hochster H, Hunt M, Green M, et al. Esorubicin (deoxydoxorubicin) has low grade activity in malignant melanoma. *Invest New Drugs.* 1990;**8**:329–332.

Kaplan S, Sessa C, Joss R, et al. Phase II trial of

4′-deoxydoxorubicin in advanced non-small cell lung cancer. *Cancer Treat Rep.* 1985;**69**:1337–1338.

Kreis W, Rottach C, Budman DR, et al. Pharmacokinetic and phase I evaluation of esorubicin (4′-deoxydoxorubicin) by continuous infusion over forty-eight hours in patients with leukemia. *Cancer Res.* 1988;**48**:5580–5584.

Lee KM, Dorr RT, Robertone A. High incidence of local venous reactions to esorubicin. *Invest New Drugs.* 1987;**5**:31–35.

Leitner SP, Casper ES, Hakes TB, et al. Phase II trial of 4′-deoxydoxorubicin in patients with advanced breast cancer. *Cancer Treat Rep.* 1985;**69**:1319–1320.

Miller TP, Dahlberg S, Salmon SE, et al. Activity of esorubicin in recurrent malignant lymphoma: A Southwest Oncology Group study. *J Clin Oncol.* 1991;**9**(7):1–4.

Ringenberg QS, Propert KJ, Muss HB, et al. Clinical cardiotoxicity of esorubicin (4′-deoxydoxorubicin, DxDx): Prospective studies with serial gated heart scans and reports of selected cases. *Invest New Drugs.* 1990;**8**:221–226.

Rozencweig M, Crespeigne N, Kenis Y. Phase I trial with 4′-deoxydoxorubicin (esorubicin). *Invest New Drugs.* 1983;**1**:309–313.

Salmon SE, Durie BGM. In vitro phase II trial of 4′-deoxydoxorubicin with comparison to doxorubicin. *Proc Am Soc Clin Oncol.* 1982;**1**:9.

Salmon SE, Liu RM, Cassaza AM. Evaluation of new anthracycline analogs with the human tumor stem cell assay. *Cancer Chemother Pharmacol.* 1981;**6**:103–110.

Salmon SE, Young L, Soehnlen B, Liu R. Antitumor activity of esorubicin in human tumor clonogenic assays with comparisons to doxorubicin. *J Clin Oncol.* 1984;**2**:282–286.

Sessa C, Bosia L, Kaplan S, et al. Phase I trial of 4′-deoxydoxorubicin given weekly. *Invest New Drugs.* 1984;**2**:369–374.

Somlo G, Dorosho J, Akman S, et al. Phase II study of 4′-deoxydoxorubicin (esorubicin) in advanced or metastatic adenocarcinoma of the stomach. *Invest New Drugs.* 1991;**9**:83–85.

Stanton GF, Raymond V, Wittes RE, et al. Phase I and clinical pharmacological evaluation of 4′-deoxydoxorubicin in patients with advanced cancer. *Cancer Res.* 1985;**45**:1862–1868.

Estramustine Phosphate

■ Other Names

Estracyte® (Roche Laboratories), NSC-89199, CAS reg. no. 4891-15-0; Emcyt® (Kabi Pharmacia).

■ Chemistry

Structure of estramustine phosphate

Chemically, the drug is estra-1,3,5(10)-triene-3,17-diol(17β)-3-[bis(2-chloroethyl)carbamate] 17-(disodium phosphate). Estramustine in simpler terms is a chemical combination of estradiol phosphate and nitrogen mustard linked via a carbamate at the C-3 position of the steroidal molecule. The oral preparation is the disodium salt of estramustine phosphate, supplied as a stable, slightly hygroscopic, white powder. At physiologic pH the compound exists in an ionized form. The empiric formula is $C_{23}H_{30}Cl_2NN_{92}O_6P$ and the formula weight 582.4.

■ Antitumor Activity

Estramustine was chemically designed for use in advanced carcinoma of the prostate (Nilsson and Muntzing 1972). Approximately 20% of patients with diffuse disease have responded to the drug in several European and American trials (Muntzing et al 1974, Nilsson and Jonsson 1975, Fossa and Miller 1976, Mittelman et al 1975); however, most responses in prostate patients are subjective, characterized by decreased symptoms, and the objective response rate to the drug is only about 10% (Benson et al 1979). A low response rate has similarly been described in patients with advanced breast cancer (Alexander et al 1979, Dawes 1982). In melanoma (Lopez et al 1978) and renal cell cancer (Swanson and Johnson 1981), estramustine is largely inactive.

Mechanism of Action

Estramustine phosphate has bischloroethyl side chains and was presumed to act by chemical alkylation. However, the drug may not act as an alkylating agent. The basic steroidal structure also imparts weak estrogenic activity. Animal experiments have shown antiandrogenic and also antiestrogenic activity for the drug. The estrogenic portion of the molecule was believed to act as a carrier ostensibly to facilitate selective uptake of drug into cells with estradiol hormone receptors (Muntzing et al 1974); however, most studies suggest that the antitumor activity of the drug in prostate cancer relates to its estrogenic effects on hormonally dependent tissues (Yamanaka et al 1977). There is no convincing evidence for selective release of nitrogen mustard in estrogen-dependent tissues (Von Hoff et al 1977). Furthermore, there is no alkylation of target nucleophiles by estramustine in vitro (Tew et al 1986).

More recent studies suggest that estramustine has antimicrotubule activity (Stearns and Tew 1985). The drug appears to bind to high-molecular-weight microtubule-associated proteins to promote microtubule disassembly. Estramustine can kill tumor cells in any phase of the cell cycle and causes cells to accumulate in metaphase (Tew and Stearns 1989). Of further interest, estramustine is not associated with the multidrug resistance phenomenon in vitro (Tew and Stearns 1989). Thus, estramustine does not appear to act like an alkylating agent, but instead has selective activity at enhancing microtubule disassembly.

Availability and Storage

Estramustine phosphate is investigationally available as an injectable compound for intravenous use and commercially as hard, off-white capsules containing 140 mg of drug as the disodium salt (12.5 mg sodium per capsule) from Roche Laboratories, Nutley, New Jersey (Estracyte®), and Kabi Pharmacia, Piscataway, New Jersey (Emcyt®). The drug is weakly hygroscopic and requires storage under refrigeration at temperatures of 2 to 8°C. The commercially available capsules may be stored at room temperature for 24 to 48 hours.

Preparation for Use

The investigational injectable product is dissolved in at least 10 mL sterile water for intravenous injection.

Administration

Oral estramustine doses may be taken with meals and, if necessary, with antacids to lessen gastrointestinal upset. The effect of the antacid on drug absorption is not known; however, decreased drug absorption is possible. Intravenous doses may be given as a slow intravenous push in D5W with especially careful attention to prevent extravasation (significant thrombophlebitis at the injection site has been noted). A flush of 5 to 10 mL D5W before and after injection is recommended.

Dosage

Oral doses have ranged from 1 to 10 capsules (140–1400 mg) daily. According to the manufacturer, doses may be taken with meals to lessen the incidence of nausea and vomiting. Generally, smaller doses are given initially and adjustments made according to response and toxicity. Maximal oral doses of 20 to 25 mg/kg/d have been employed, with more intolerance seen at doses of 30 mg/kg for 7 days of continuous dosing (Muntzing et al 1974). Although oral maintenance doses of as few as 2 capsules per day have been used, the usual oral dose is 560 mg or 2 capsules twice a day. This is one-half the maximally tolerated oral daily dose reported by Nagel and Kolln (1977). The maximum tolerated intravenous estramustine dose appears to be 300 mg/d. Significant gastrointestinal toxicity has been noted at daily doses of 450 mg/kg and above. Initial intravenous doses of 150 mg are recommended by the manufacturer. One month of therapy has been suggested as an adequate therapeutic trial.

Drug Interactions

Drugs that reduce cellular glutathione may enhance the activity of estramustine (Tew et al 1986). The combination of estramustine with vinblastine has also been shown to produce synergistic cytotoxicity in human prostate cancer cells in vitro (vanBell et al 1988).

Special Precautions

Estramustine may increase thromboembolic risks and should not be administered to patients with thrombophlebitis or thromboembolic disorders. The manufacturers list several contraindications to estramustine use: childhood, peptic ulceration, severe liver disease, and cardiac disease. Close monitoring of patients with hypertension or diabetes is also recommended.

Pharmacokinetics

Pharmacokinetic studies in humans have shown that about 75% of orally administered estramustine phosphate is absorbed (Forshell et al 1976); however, Nilsson and Jonsson (1975) demonstrated roughly equivalent results from the intravenous and oral preparations. The compound is excreted as metabolites of both the alkylating and estrogenic moieties into the bile, urine, and feces. Kirdani et al (1974) have studied tritium-labeled estramustine phosphate elimination. Within 48 hours of administration only 23% of the dose could be recovered in the urine. There was only minimal unchanged drug present, indicating nonrenal excretion as the major route of elimination. In the liver the steroidal component is conjugated primarily as the glucuronide and excreted into the bile, feces, and urine.

The pharmacokinetic and biologic half-life of estramustine is long. Studies with radiolabeled drug described a terminal half-life of 20 to 24 hours in humans (Forshell et al 1976). Peak plasma concentrations after multiple-dose studies with 600 mg/m^2 three times daily were 326 ng/mL for estromustine (the dephosphorylated estrone derivative), 82 ng/mL for estramustine phosphate, 36 ng/mL for estramustine, 162 ng/mL for estrone, and 17 ng/mL for estradiol (Kirdani et al 1980). Dephosphorylation of estramustine phosphate is avid, is nonselective for tumor tissues, and probably begins in the gastrointestinal cells on absorption of the tablet.

Side Effects and Toxicity

Dose-limiting adverse effects of estramustine have generally consisted of extreme gastrointestinal and/or local toxicity (for intravenous estramustine). In general, renal and systemic hematologic toxicity has not been encountered. Several patients with preexisting cardiac disease have demonstrated increasing congestive heart failure symptoms during estramustine therapy, presumably because of the salt-retaining effects of the estrogenic portion of the drug. Other rare cardiovascular complications include thromboembolism, ischemic effects, and cerebral effects. The incidence and severity are similar to those with estrogen treatment of prostate cancer. Diarrhea is described in 15 to 30% of patients.

The nausea and vomiting from estramustine can occur soon after administration. Symptoms are generally transient and responsive to phenothiazines. A similar but delayed and often intractable gastrointestinal toxicity is rarely reported. This latter presentation can occur up to 6 to 8 weeks after initiation of continuous therapy and usually necessitates immediate drug discontinuance.

Other reported toxic effects include gynecomastia in 20 to 100% of patients (although initial nipple tenderness may be common). Rare effects include thrombocytopenia and drug allergy with rash or fever and abnormalities of liver function. Myelosuppression is not commonly described.

Patients receiving the intravenous preparation may commonly experience severe thrombophlebitis and transient paresthesias of the mouth. With the investigational parenteral formulation, transient perineal itching and pain have also been noted immediately after injection. Occasionally, arteriovenous shunts have been implemented to reduce the extreme local toxicity of estramustine; however, careful intravenous injection technique may be equally effective.

REFERENCES

Alexander JN, Hancock AK, Masood MB, et al. Estracyt in advanced carcinoma of the breast. *Clin Radiol.* 1979;**30**:139–147.

Alfthan DS, Rush IL. Estracyt in advanced prostatic carcinoma. *Ann Chir Gynaecol Fenn.* 1968;**56**:234.

Benson RC, Wear JB, Gill GM. Treatment of stage D hormone-resistant carcinoma of the prostate with estramustine phosphate. *J Urol.* 1979;**121**:452–454.

Dawes PHDQ. A pilot study of Estracyt in advanced breast cancer. *Cancer Treat Rep.* 1982;**66**:581–582.

Forshell GP, Muntzing J, Ek A, et al. The absorption, metabolism, and excretion of Estracyt (NSC-89199) in patients with prostatic cancer. *Invest Urol.* 1976;**14**:128–131.

Fossa SD, Miller A. Treatment of advanced carcinoma of the prostate with estramustine phosphate. *J Urol.* 1976;**116**:406–412.

Kirdani RY, Karr JP, Murphy GP, et al. Prostate cancer: Plasma concentrations of estramustine phosphate and its metabolites. *NY State J Med.* 1980;**80**:1390–1393.

Kirdani RY, Muntzing J, Varkarakis MJ, et al. Studies on the antiprostatic action of Estracyt, a nitrogen mustard of estradiol. *Cancer Res.* 1974;**34**:1025–1031.

Lopez R, Karakousis CP, Didolkar MS, et al. Estramustine phosphate in the treatment of advanced malignant melanoma. *Cancer Treat Rep.* 1978;**62**:1329–1332.

Mittelman A, Shukle SK, Welvaart K, et al. Oral estramustine phosphate (NSC-89199) in the treatment of advanced stage D carcinoma of the prostate. *Cancer Chemother Rep Part 1.* 1975;**59**(1):219–223.

Muntzing J, Shukla SK, Chu TM, et al. Pharmacologic study of oral estramustine phosphate (Estracyt) in advanced carcinoma of the prostate. *Invest Urol.* 1974;**12**(1):65–68.

Nagel R, Kolln CP. Treatment of advanced carcinoma of the prostate with estramustine phosphate. *Br J Urol.* 1977;**49**:73–79.

Nilsson T, Jonsson G. Clinical results with estramustine phosphate (NSC-89199): A comparison of the intravenous and oral preparations. *Cancer Chemother Rep.* 1975;**59**:229–232.

Nilsson T, Muntzing J. Estracyt in advanced prostatic carcinoma. *Scand J Urol Nephrol.* 1972;**6**:11–16.

Stearns ME, Tew KD. Antimicrotubule effects of estramustine, an antiprostatic tumor drug. *Cancer Res.* 1985;**45**:3891–3897.

Swanson DA, Johnson DE. Estramustine phosphate (Emcyt) as treatment for metastatic renal carcinoma. *Urology.* 1981;**17**:344–346.

Tew KD, Stearns ME. Estramustine—A nitrogen mustard/steroid with antimicrotubule activity. *Pharmacol Ther.* 1989;**43**:299–319.

Tew KD, Woodworth A, Stearns ME. Relationship of glutathione depletion and inhibition of glutathione-S-transferase activity to the antimitotic properties of estramustine. *Cancer Treat Rep.* 1986;**70**(6):715–720.

VanBell SJP, Schalleier D, deWasch G, et al. Broad phase II study of the combination of two microtubular inhibitors: Estramustine and vinblastine. *Proc Am Soc Clin Oncol.* 1988;**7**:207.

Von Hoff DD, Rozencweig M, Slavik M, et al. Estramustine phosphate: A specific chemotherapeutic agent? *J Urol.* 1977;**117**:464–466.

Yamanaka H, Shimazaki J, Imai K, et al. Effect of Estracyt on the rat prostate. *Invest Urol.* 1977;**14**:400–404.

Estrogens

■ Other Names

Chlorotrianisene: TACE®; Premarin; conjugated estrogens, USP: Premarin®; ethinyl estradiol: Estinyl®; diethylstilbestrol (DES), USP.

■ Chemistry

Structures of three estrogens. Premarin is a mixture of estrogens; therefore, no structure is available.

There are two classes of chemicals with estrogenic activity. The estradiol preparations consist of various oral or injectable products (usually in oil), with steroidal structures closely resembling the natural cyclopentanoperhydrophenanthrene compounds. The injectable formulations are generally oil suspensions of estradiol esters associated with slow local absorption and more prolonged effects. The substances used most often, however, are the synthetic nonsteroidal compounds with estrogenic activity. These include chlorotrianisene and diethylstilbestrol (DES).

■ Antitumor Activity

The natural and synthetic estrogenic substances are used primarily palliatively in postmenopausal breast carcinoma and in advanced prostatic carcinoma. Patients with estrogen receptor (ER)-positive breast cancer have a much higher chance of responding to estrogen treatment (Allegra et al 1980, Campbell et al 1981). In unselected patient populations with metastatic breast cancer the response rate is 33%. If ER-positive patients are treated the response rate is about twice as high. The higher the ER value, the greater the chance the patient will respond (Kiang et al 1978, Jensen et al 1976). For treatment of patients with metastatic breast cancer most oncologists typically start therapy with the antiestrogen tamoxifen, even though randomized studies show no survival differences between DES and tamoxifen (Gockerman et al 1986). Estrogens are more conventionally used for second- or third-line therapy for patients who have previously responded to tamoxifen or progestational agents. Of interest, a few breast cancer patients can also have a tumor response when estrogens are stopped.

The estrogen of choice in prostate cancer is diethylstilbestrol (DES), which elicits about an 85% partial objective response rate with 50% survival of 2 years or greater (Leuprolide Study Group 1984).

■ Mechanism of Action

The exact mechanism of antitumor action for estrogens is not known. It is known that the hormonally sensitive tissues that require steroid hormones to maintain optimal growth and function characteristically contain steroid-binding proteins in the nucleus of the cell. For hormonal (estrogenic) activity a two-step process is hypothesized (Jensen et al 1971).

In the first step, the chemically unchanged steroid binds with a receptor protein, whereupon a temperature-dependent conversion of the complex occurs (Korenman 1970). In the second step, this new chemical complex activates to another specific receptor site in the chromatin of the cell nucleus. The result of this nuclear interaction is thought to modulate cell growth; however, the exact mechanism for this final effect is not known. DES can have a direct cytotoxic effect on cells as well as cause chromosomal nondisjunction, resulting in cell death (Reddel and Sutherland 1987, Tsutsui et al 1983). Pharmacologic investigation of estrogen action historically followed the surgical observation that removal of the ovaries in premenopausal breast cancer patients, in some cases, provided a striking response, and it is now established that surgical or chemical hormone deprivation is occasionally beneficial in breast cancer. Thus, in postmenopausal breast cancer patients exogenous estrogens may displace endogenous growth-enhancing estrogens in specific patients (those with the specific estrogen receptors) (Leclercq et al 1975, Wittliff et al 1976). The exact reason for estrogen responsiveness in prostatic tumors similarly remains unclear (Gustafsson et al 1978). Estrogen therapy in males will suppress pituitary secretion of luteinizing hormone and consequently testicular androgen secretion is decreased. A direct estrogenic response on the prostate has not been documented.

■ Availability and Storage, Preparation for Use, Stability, and Admixture

See the table on page 448 and follow manufacturers' recommendations for reconstitution, storage, and administration of these commercially available preparations.

■ Special Precautions

There is some evidence that estrogen administration may result in a higher incidence of endometrial cancer (Ziel and Finkel 1975, Mack et al 1976). Estrogens should not be used during pregnancy. Their use will result in an increased form of clear cell carcinoma of the vagina in the offspring, epithelial changes in the vagina and cervix, congenital heart abnormalities, limb abnormalities, and reproductive organ abnormalities in males (Herbst et al 1971, Greenwald et al

ESTROGENS

Preparations Available:			Indication (Metastatic Cancer)	Dose	Comment
Generic Name	*Trade Name*	Availability			
Estradiols					
Ethinyl estradiol	Estinyl®	Tablets: 0.02, 0.05, 0.1, 0.5 mg	Prostatic and breast	1.5 mg 3×/wk (both men and women)	Orally effective natural product
Estradiol benzoate	Progynon B®	Estradiol (plain) aqueous			
Estradiol cypionate	Depo-Estradiol®	In oil 1, 5 mg	Prostatic	1–5 mg/wk initially, 2–5 mg IM every 3–4 wk maintenance	Oil suspensions intramuscularly only
Estradiol valerate	Delestrogen®	In oil 10, 20, 40 mg/mL	Prostatic	30 mg or greater IM every 1–2 wk	
Conjugates estrogenic substances	Premarin®	Tablets: 0.1, 0.3, 0.625, 1.25, 2.5 mg Injection: 1, 2, 4, 5 mg/mL	Prostatic and breast	1.25–2.5 tid PO 10 mg tid PO	Relatively short-acting Slow intravenous push to avoid flushing
Polyestradiol	Estradurin®	Injection: 40 mg	Prostatic	40 mg IV every 2–4 wk	Deep intramuscular injection only
Diethylstilbestrol (DES), USP		Tablets: 0.1, 0.25, 0.5, 1, 2, 5, 10, 25 mg	Prostatic Breast	1–3 mg PO/d 1–5 mg PO tid	Most potent nonsteroidal compound
Fosfestrol (diethylstilbestrol diphosphate)	Stilphostrol® Honvol®	Tablets: 50 mg Injection: 250 mg/5mL	Prostatic	50–200 mg PO tid 500–1000 IV × 5 d; then 250–1000 mg IV weekly	Give intravenously over at least 30–60 min
Chlorotrianisene	TACE®	Capsules: 12, 25, 72 mg	Prostatic	12–25 mg/d PO	Fat storage, slow onset, long duration

1971, Nora and Nora 1973, Janerich et al 1974, Stenchever et al 1981, Whitehead and Leiter 1981).

■ Drug Interactions

None are known.

■ Dosage

The usual doses of estrogen given to patients with metastatic breast cancer are Premarin® 2.5 mg three times per day, ethinyl estradiol 1 mg three times per day, or DES 5 mg three times daily. It is customary to start out with doses of about one half of the usually prescribed amounts (to decrease side effects) and to escalate to the listed doses in 4 weeks (Carter et al 1977).

In prostate cancer patient therapy, DES at doses greater than 1 mg/d may not achieve increased antitumor responses with survival advantage, but are associated with enhanced risks of cardiovascular and thromboembolic complications (Bailar and Byar 1970, Blackard et al 1970). Nonetheless, one of the most common DES doses is 3 mg/d in prostate cancer (Smith 1981). In 1968 Kaplan reported a historical comparison of three estrogenic preparations used in various long-term estrogen studies. From this literature review it appears that doses of 1.25 to 2.5 mg/d of natural conjugated estrogens produce low to moderate degrees of feminization and little adverse cardiovascular risk (long-term follow-up was not available though). The best care for patients is to use the smallest dose of estrogen which results in a decrease of serum testosterone levels to zero.

■ Pharmacokinetics

The absorption of orally administered synthetic and natural estrogenic substances appears to be prompt and relatively complete. The naturally occurring steroidal derivatives do not possess good oral efficacy because of rapid hepatic biotransformation (the "first-pass" effect) (Kappas 1968). The synthetic preparation ethinyl estradiol and the nonsteroidal estrogenic compounds are hepatically processed at a much slower rate and hence have good bioavailability. Injectable preparations include long-acting (slow-release) esters of estradiol, which produce therapeutic effects for several days. These natural products are inactivated primarily in the liver by conjugation as glucuronides and excretion in the urine. Inactivation of the nonsteroidal synthetic compounds is much slower and not well characterized. Chlortrianisene is extremely fat soluble (nonpolar), and considerable storage in fat probably accounts for its delayed onset and prolonged duration of action. Also, this compound is hepatically biotransformed into a more potent form. The nonsteroidal compounds do not apparently display the high degree of enterohepatic cycling seen with natural derivatives.

A specific radioimmunoassay for DES has been developed (Kemp et al 1981). In patients with prostate cancer receiving 1 mg of DES three times a day plasma concentrations ranged from 0.15 to 6.0 ng/mL.

■ Side Effects and Toxicity

Estrogenic substances are relatively well tolerated even in the large pharmacologic doses commonly employed. Most "side effects" are actually extensions of their natural hormonal activities.

Women appear to experience more nausea and vomiting than men treated with estrogens, but this is probably a function of the higher doses used in women. Estrogen-induced anorexia and nausea are described as resembling "morning sickness." This does not usually interfere with eating nor cause weight loss. Antiemetics may be beneficial, but usually this side effect substantially diminishes or completely disappears with continued treatment. Sometimes initiation of estrogen therapy with low doses followed by slow dosage escalation overcomes the nausea. At other times it may be worthwhile to change to a different estrogen preparation for a specific patient.

Estrogen will of course produce feminization in male patients. This includes the induction of gynecomastia. Pretreatment, low-dose breast irradiation is indicated in males to prevent this side effect. In female patients a decrease in libido as well as some breast tenderness is common.

A variety of metabolic effects can be seen in patients receiving estrogen therapy. The two most significant effects include sodium retention and acute hypercalcemia. Sodium retention is common and can adversely influence cardiovascular status in patients with congestive heart failure. Patients may also develop hypertension. Serious hypercalcemia may occur, usually during initial therapy (Beckett 1969). Symptoms of hypercalcemia include polyuria, polydipsia, weakness, constipation, and mental sluggishness or disorientation. If hypercalcemia is not recognized and treated appropriately, there can be rapid progression to coma and death. Of note, patients with breast cancer who develop hypercalcemia with the initiation of estrogen treatment frequently will have a beneficial antitumor effect if the estrogens are continued. The hypercalcemic response is due to initial estrogenic stimulation of bony metastases which later go on to respond with growth inhibition in the face of continued therapy.

Of great interest is that hypocalcemia can be seen when DES is given to patients with osteoblastic metastatic prostate cancer (Harley et al 1983).

Other complications include uterine bleeding ("breakthrough" and withdrawal bleeding) and increased pigmentation of the nipple. In 5 to 10% of women with metastatic breast cancer, a flare of metastatic lesions can occur (eg, rapid growth of skin nodules and sudden increase in bone pain). Urinary frequency may also occur in some women.

High doses of estrogenic substances definitely predispose patients to increased risk of thromboembolic complications including pulmonary embolus, myocardial infarction, and strokes. In prostatic cancer therapy this risk is greater when more than 1 mg of DES per day is used (Blackard et al 1970, Marmoston et al 1962).

Konturri and Sontaniemi (1970) have noted a

variety of metabolic changes in prostatic cancer patients receiving estrogens. These included transient elevations of serum transaminases, bilirubin, and triglycerides (Kontari and Sontamiemi 1969). Serum cholesterol and blood glucose were inconsistently affected and, depending on when measured, could be increased or depressed initially but tended to normalize over a 4-month observation period. A DES-associated hemolytic anemia (direct positive Coombs') has also recently been described (Rosenfeld et al 1989). Patients receiving intramuscular preparations may become sensitized to the oil carrier and may exhibit painful and erythematous local reactions. Overall, however, estrogens are generally well tolerated and enjoy a wide margin of therapeutic safety.

REFERENCES

Allegra J, Lippman M, Thompson E. Estrogen receptor status: An important variable in predicting response to endocrine therapy in metastatic breast cancer. *Eur J Cancer.* 1980;**16**:323–331.

Bailar JC III, Byar DP, Veterans Administration Cooperative Urological Research Group. Estrogen treatment for cancer of the prostate: Early result with 3 doses of diethylstilbestrol and placebo. *Cancer.* 1970;**26**:257–261.

Beckett VL. Hypercalcemia associated with estrogen administration in patients with breast carcinoma. *Cancer.* 1969;**24**:610–616.

Blackard CE, Doe PR, Mellinger GT, Byar DP. Incidence of cardiovascular disease and death in patients receiving diethylstilbestrol for carcinoma of the prostate. *Cancer.* 1970;**26**:249–256.

Campbell FC, Elston CW, Blamey RW, et al. Quantitative estradiol receptor values in primary breast cancer and response of metastases to endocrine therapy. *Lancet.* 1981;**2**:1317–1319.

Carter AC, Sedransk N, Kelley RM. Diethylstilbestrol: Recommended dosages for different categories of breast cancer patients. *JAMA.* 1977;**237**(19):2079–2085.

Gockerman JP, Spremulli EN, Raney M, Logan T. Randomized comparison of tamoxifen versus diethylstilbestrol in estrogen receptor-positive or unknown metastatic breast cancer: A Southeastern Cancer Study Group trial. *Cancer Treat Rep.* 1986;**70**(10):1199–1203.

Greenwald P, Barlow JJ, Nasca PC, Burnett WF. Vaginal cancer after maternal treatment with synthetic estrogens. *N Engl J Med.* 1971;**285**:390–392.

Gustafsson JA, Ekman P, Snochowski M, Zetterberg A, Pousette A, Högberg B. Correlation between clinical response to hormone therapy and steroid receptor content in prostatic cancer. *Cancer Res.* 1978;**38**:4345–4358.

Harley HA, Mason R, Phillips PJ. Profound hypocalcemia associated with estrogen treatment of carcinoma of the prostate. *Med J Aust.* 1983;**2**:41–42.

Herbst AL, Ulfelder H, Poskanzer DC. Adenocarcinoma of the vagina. *N Engl J Med.* 1971;**284**:878–881.

Israel SL. *Diagnosis and Treatment of Menstrual Disorders and Sterility.* 5th ed. New York/Evanston/London: Hoeber Medical Division, Harper & Row; 1967.

Janerich DT, Piper JM, Gleatis DM. Oral contraceptives and congenital limb-reduction defects. *N Engl J Med.* 1974;**291**:697–700.

Jensen EV, Numata M, Brecher PI, DeSombre ER. Estrogen–receptor interaction as a guide to biochemical mechanism. In: Smellie RMS, ed. *The Biochemistry of Steroid Hormone Action.* London: Academic Press, 1971: 133–159.

Jensen EV, Smith S, DeSombre ER. Hormone dependency in breast cancer. *J Steroid Biochem* 1976;**7**:911–917.

Kaplan L. Cancer of the prostate: Estrogen therapy natural conjugated estrogen vs. stilbestrol. *Rev Surg.* 1968; **25**:323–329.

Kappas A. Studies in endocrine pharmacology: Biologic action of some natural steroids on the liver. *N Engl J Med.* 1968;**278**:378–384.

Kemp HA, Read GF, Riad-Fahmy D, et al. Measurement of diethylstilbestrol in plasma from patients with cancer of the prostate. *Cancer Res.* 1981;**41**(11, pt 1):4693–4697.

Kiang DT, Frenning DH, Goldman AI, Ascensao VF, Kennedy BJ. Estrogen receptors and responses to chemotherapy and hormonal therapy in advanced breast cancer. *N Engl J Med.* 1978;**299**(24):1330–1334.

Kistner RW. Feminine forever? An evaluation of therapy during perimenopause. *Med Sci.* 1968;**18**:42–46.

Kontturi M, Sontaniemi E. Effect of estrogen in liver function of prostatic cancer patients. *Br Med J.* 1969;**4**:204–205.

Konturri M, Sontaniemi E. Estrogen-induced metabolic changes during treatment of prostate cancer. *Scand J Clin Lab Invest.* 1970;**25**:45.

Korenman SG. Specific estrogen binding by the cytoplasm of human breast carcinoma. *J Clin Endocrinol.* 1970;**30**:639–645.

Leclerc G, Heuson JG, Heuson JC, Deboel MC, Mattheiem WH. Oestrogen receptors in breast cancer: A changing concept. *Br Med J.* 1975;**1**:185–189.

Leuprolide Study Group. Leuprolide versus diethylstilbestrol for metastatic prostate cancer. *N Engl J Med.* 1984;**311**:1281–1286.

Mack TM, Pike MC, Henderson BE, et al. Estrogens and endometrial cancer in a retirement community. *N Engl J Med.* 1976;**294**:1262–1267.

Marmoston J, Moore FJ, Hopkins CE, Kuzma OT, Weiner J. Clinical studies of long term estrogen therapy in men with myocardial infarction. *Proc Soc Exp Biol Med.* 1962;**110**:400.

Nora JJ, Nora AH. Birth defects and oral contraceptives. *Lancet.* 1973;**1**:941–942.

Reddel RR, Sutherland RL. Effects of pharmacological concentrations of estrogens on proliferation and cell cycle kinetics of human breast cancer cell lines in vitro. *Cancer Res.* 1987;**47**:5323–5329.

Rosenfeld CS, Winters SJ, Tedrow HE. Diethylstilbestrol-associated hemolytic anemia with a positive direct antiglobulin test result. *Am J Med.* 1989;**86**(5):617–618.

Smith PH. Endocrine and cytotoxic therapy. *Recent Results Cancer Res.* 1981;**78**:143–172.

Stenchever MA, Williamson RA, Leonard J, et al. Possible relationship between in utero diethylstilbestrol exposure and male fertility. *Am J Obstet Gynecol.* 1981;**150**(2):186–193.

Tsutsui T, Maizumi H, McLachlan JA, Barrett J. Aneuploidy induction and cell transformation by diethylstilbestrol: A possible chromosomal mechanism in carcinogenesis. *Cancer Res.* 1983;**43**:3814–3821.

Whitehead ED, Leiter E. Genital abnormalities and abnormal semen analyses in male patients exposed to diethylstilbestrol in utero. *J Urol.* 1981;**125**(1):47–50.

Wittliff JL, Beatty BW, Savlov ED, Patterson WB, Cooper RA. Estrogen receptors and hormone dependency in human breast cancer. *Recent Results Cancer Res.* 1976;**57**:59–77.

Ziel HK, Finkel WD. Increased risk of endometrial carcinoma among users of conjugated estrogens. *N Engl J Med.* 1975;**293**:1167–1170.

Etanidazole

■ Other Names

SR 2508; NSC-301467.

■ Chemistry

Structure of etanidazole

Etanidazole (SR 2508) is a less lipophilic analog of the 2-nitroimidazole, misonidazole. The chemical name is N-(2-hydroxyethyl)-2-(2-nitro-1-imidazolyl)-acetamide. Because it is less lipophilic it was thought the compound might cause less peripheral neuropathy than misonidazole (eg, less central nervous system penetration with more rapid excretion) (Brown 1982, 1984, Brown et al 1981). The molecular formula is $C_7H_{10}N_4O_4$ and the molecular weight 214.2.

■ Antitumor Activity

To date, etanidazole has not been developed as a cytotoxic antitumor agent. Rather, it has been developed as a radiation sensitizer or as a sensitizer to the effects of alkylating agents.

A definitive trial of radiation alone (66.00 Gy in 33 fractions at 2.0 Gy/fraction, 5 fractions/week) versus radiation plus etanidazole (2.0 g/m² IV 30–60 minutes before radiotherapy each Monday, Wednesday, and Friday to a maximum dose of 34 g/m² [17 doses]) in patients with head and neck cancer is ongoing. This important study should define the role of etanidazole in that disease (Marcial et al 1988). At the time of this writing, the final results of this trial are not available.

■ Mechanism of Action

The precise mechanism of action of etanidazole is unknown. The compound has an oxygen-mimetic effect and reacts with the radiation-induced free radicals to produce a lesion in DNA. When hypoxic cells are exposed to etanidazole for longer periods the drug is metabolized and produces enhancement of radiation effects by other, unknown mechanisms.

■ Availability and Storage

Etanidazole is investigationally available from the National Cancer Institute. It is supplied as a sterile lyophilized yellow powder. Each 30-mL vial contains 1 g of drug.

■ Preparation for Use, Stability, and Admixture

The 1-g vials are reconstituted with 19.4 mL of 0.9% Sodium Chloride for Injection, USP. Each milliliter then contains 50 mg of drug at a pH of 5.5 to 7.5. The total dose of drug is diluted in 100 to 200 mL of fluid and infused over 30 minutes. The intact vials are stable for at least 3 years at room temperature. Solutions of drug at pH 4 to 8 are stable for 7 days at temperatures up to 50°C. When diluted to 1 mg/mL in normal saline or D5W (National Cancer Institute 1987), the drug is stable for 14 days at room temperature.

■ Administration

The drug is given by intravenous infusion over 5 to 10 minutes in 100 to 200 mL of fluid. Radiation treatments are given within 30 minutes of beginning the infusion (Coleman et al 1986).

■ Special Precautions

Serum samples should be used to predict the total dose of drug the patient will tolerate (see details later). The toxicity of the compound is clearly related to the total drug exposure (area under concentration–time curve × number of drug administrations).

■ Drug Interactions

Patients with preexisting neuropathies from prior chemotherapy (eg, *cis*-platinum or vincristine) might be more sensitive to the neuropathic effects of etanidazole. Etanidazole may also enhance radiation toxicity and augment the activity of alkylating agents.

■ Dosage

Based on multiple phase I trials (see later) the recommended dose for phase II trials was 2 g/m^2 three times per week over a period of 6 weeks (Coleman et al 1986). On the basis of pharmacokinetic information, the dose should be adjusted in the individual patient (Coleman et al 1986).

■ Pharmacokinetics

Knowledge of the pharmacokinetics of this compound is very important in preventing the neurotoxicity associated with it. A total area under the curve (indicated by AUC for single treatment × number of treatments) of 39 mM · h or less is acceptable. AUCs above that value are associated with substantial neurotoxicity (Coleman et al 1984, 1986). Detailed pharmacokinetic studies done on 71 pooled patients indicated a mean α half-life of 17 minutes, mean β half-life of 280 minutes, a mean plasma clearance of 0.106 L/min, and a mean volume of distribution of 38 L. At a dose of 2 g/m^2, the end-of-infusion plasma serum concentration was 239 µg/mL with a 1-hour concentration of 78 µg/mL (Coleman et al 1987). Biopsies have shown solid tumor levels of 72 µg/g of tumor (Newman et al 1986). Glioma levels have reached 13.5 µg/g of tissue. Normal brain was 4.0 µg/g of tissue (Newman et al 1988). Biopsies of bladder tumors also show high concentrations of etanidazole (Awwad et al 1989). Occasionally, the pharmacokinetics of etanidazole can be erratic (Maughan et al 1990).

■ Side Effects and Toxicity

The most common toxic effect with etanidazole (dose limiting) has been a peripheral neuropathy (Coleman et al 1986, 1987, 1989, 1990) manifested by numbness and tingling, dysesthesias, and pain. Most have resolved over 2 to 6 months. Nausea and vomiting have been seen infrequently (Coleman et al 1986).

A rash has been reported in a few patients by Coleman et al (1986). It is clear that more drug can be given when the duration of treatment is increased (Coleman et al 1986).

■ Special Applications

Etanidazole has also been studied in phase I trials in combination with cyclophospamide. This is based on the ability of etanidazole to enhance the cytotoxicity of alkylating agents, presumably by inhibition of glutathione-dependent detoxifying enzymes or by glutathione depletion. O'Dwyer and colleagues (1988) have administered etanidazole at doses of 2.5 to 4.2 g/m^2 4 hours after a dose of 1 g/m^2

cyclophosphamide. No dose-limiting toxicity was noted. Leukopenia, nausea and vomiting, nasal congestion, and mild to moderate elevations in liver enzymes were noted. No neurotoxicity was reported. Of particular interest was an etanidazole-induced inhibitor of monocyte and red blood cell glutathione-dependent detoxifying enzymes as well as a depletion in monocyte glutathione.

Trump and colleagues (1988) alternated cyclophosphamide and cyclophosphamide + etanidazole in every other cycle to analyze the impact of etanidazole on cyclophosphamide-induced myelosuppression. At the time the abstract was written the effect of etanidazole on cyclophosphamide-induced myelosuppression had not yet been determined.

REFERENCES

Awwad KH, ed Badawy S, abd el Baki H, et al. Pharmacokinetics of etanidazole (SR 2508) in bladder and cervical cancer: Evidence of diffusion from urine. *Int J Radiat Oncol Biol Phys.* 1989;**16**(4):1083–1084.

Brown JM. Clinical perspectives for the use of new hypoxic cell sensitizers. *Int J Radiat Oncol Biol Phys.* 1982;**8**:1491–1497.

Brown JM. Clinical trials of radiosensitizers: What should we expect? *Int J Radiat Oncol Biol Phys.* 1984;**10**:425–429.

Brown JM, Yu NY, Brown DM, Lee WW. Sr 2508: A 2-nitroimidazole amide which should be superior to misonidazole as a radiosensitizer for clinical use. *Int J Radiat Oncol Biol Phys.* 1981;**7**:695–703.

Coleman CN, Halsey J, Cox RS, et al. Relationship between the neurotoxicity of the hypoxic cell radiosensitizer SR 2508 and the pharmacokinetic profile. *Cancer Res.* 1987;**47**:319–322.

Coleman CN, Noll L, Howes AE, Harris JR, Zakar J, Kramer RA. Initial results of a phase I trial of continuous infusion SR 2508 (etanidazole): A Radiation Therapy Oncology Group study. *Int J Radiat Oncol Biol Phys.* 1989;**16**(4):1085–1087.

Coleman CN, Urtasun RC, Wasserman TH, et al. Initial report of the phase I trial of the hypoxic cell radiosensitizer SR 2508. *Int J Radiat Oncol Biol Phys.* 1984;**10**:1749–1753.

Coleman CN, Wasserman TH, Urtasun RC, et al. Phase I trial of the hypoxic cell radiosensitizer SR 2508: The results of the five to six week drug schedule. *Int J Radiat Oncol Biol Phys.* 1986;**12**:1105–1108.

Coleman CN, Wasserman TH, Urtasun RC, et al. Final report of the phase I trial of the hypoxic cell radiosensitizer SR 2508 (etanidazole): A Radiation Therapy Oncology Group study. *Int J Radiat Oncol Biol Phys.* 1990;**18**(2):389–393.

Marcial VA, Pazak TF, Kramer S, et al. Radiation Therapy Oncology Group (RTOG) studies in head and neck cancer. *Semin Oncol.* 1988;**15**:39–60.

Maughan TS, Newman HF, Bleehen NM, Ward R, Workman P. Abnormal clinical pharmacokinetics of the developmental radiosensitizers pimonidazole (Ro 03-8799) and etanidazole (SR 2508). *Int J Radiat Oncol Biol Phys.* 1990;**18**(5):1151–1156.

National Cancer Institute. *NCI Investigational Drugs: Pharmaceutical Data.* NIH Publication 88-2141. Washington, DC: Department of Health and Human Services; 1987:138–139.

Newman HF, Bleehan NM, Ward R, Workman P. Hypoxic cell radiosensitizers in the treatment of high grade gliomas: A new direction using combined RO03-8799 (pimonidazole) and SR 2508 (etanidazole). *Int J Radiat Oncol Biol Phys.* 1988;**15**:677–684.

Newman HFV, Bleehan NM, Workman P. A phase I study of the combination of two hypoxic cell radiosensitizers RO 03-8799 and SR 2508: Toxicity and pharmacokinetics. *Int J Radiat Oncol Biol Phys.* 1986;**12**:113–1116.

O'Dwyer PJ, LaCreta FP, Walczak J, et al. Phase I pharmacology study of nitroimidazole sensitizer SR 25908 in combination with cyclophosphamide. *Proc Am Assoc Cancer Res.* 1988;**29**.

Trump D, Mulcahy RT, Remick S, et al. A phase I trial of SR 2508 and cyclophosphamide (CTX) administered by intravenous injection. *Proc Am Assoc Cancer Res.* 1988;**29**:361.

Ethiofos

■ Other Names

WR-2721; amifostine; Ethyol® (U.S. BioScience); NSC-296961; Gammaphos®.

■ Chemistry

$$H_2N-(CH_2)_3-NH-(CH_2)_2-S-\underset{\underset{OH}{|}}{\overset{\overset{O}{\|}}{P}}-OH$$

Structure of ethiofos

Ethiofos is an organic thiophosphate compound. The chemical name is *S*-[(3-aminopropyl)amino]-ethanethiol, dihydrogen phosphate (ester). It has alternatively been labeled *S*-2-(3 aminopropyl-amino)ethylphosphorothioic acid. The molecular weight is 214.2 and the molecular formula

$C_5H_{15}N_2O_3PS$. Compared with other sulfhydryl-containing molecules, ethiofos has a high degree of hydrophilicity because of the phosphate group. The octanol:water partition coefficient for ethiofos has been estimated to be between 0.00065 and 0.00045, indicating very little partitioning into lipids (Yuhas et al 1982). Ethiofos differs from other sulfhydryl-containing compounds in that the thiol group is protected or "covered" by a phosphate. Thus, ethiofos requires dephosphorylation by an alkaline phosphatase to become active as a sulfhydryl compound (Shaw et al 1986).

■ Antitumor Activity

Ethiofos does not produce cytotoxic effects against tumor cells. Rather, it is used to modulate the hematologic toxicity of ionizing radiation and DNA alkylating agents (Glover et al 1986a, Woolley et al 1983, Yuhas et al 1980) and the nephrotoxicity and neurotoxicity of cisplatin-containing antitumor agents (Glover et al 1986b, Yuhas and Culo 1980). Tumor tissues typically are not protected by ethiofos.

Radiation Therapy. Preclinical studies of ethiofos and ionizing radiation in a variety of animal models show that most normal tissues are protected from lethality to varying degrees (see table). The exceptions were brain and spinal cord (Yuhas et al 1980). A large number of experimental rodent tumors simultaneously treated with ethiofos and radiation were not protected by the drug. Mouse skin appears to be particularly responsive to ethiofos protection. The radioprotective effects are dependent on tissue oxygen concentrations, with the best protection achieved at oxygen levels just above those needed for radiosensitization (Rojas and Denekamp 1984). The maximal effect is obtained if ethiofos is given not less than 30 minutes prior to radiation (Travis et al 1982). Experimental radioprotection of mouse skin was lost if the percentage of oxygen in the inspired gas was less than 21% and was greatly diminished at an inspired gas oxygen percentage greater than 50% (Denekamp et al 1982).

In patients with advanced rectal cancer, pretreatment with intravenous ethiofos at a dose of 340 mg/m^2 20 to 30 minutes before fractionated pelvic radiation reduced the incidence of moderate to severe toxicity by 13% and slightly increased complete response rates by 6% (Kligerman et al 1992). In the canine model, radioprotection from ethiofos is enhanced by the addition of filgrastim (recombinant granulocyte colony-stimulating factor [G-CSF]) (MacVittie et al 1992).

Several phase I clinical trials have evaluated different doses of ethiofos with ionizing radiation with and without concomitant DNA alkylating agents (Kligerman et al 1980, 1981). Ethiofos doses of 750 mg/m^2 and greater significantly enhanced recovery of bone marrow suppression following hemibody irradiation in patients with various metastatic cancers (Constine et al 1986). In patients receiving fractionated radiotherapy for rectal adenocarcinoma (225 cGy/fraction × 20 over 5 weeks), the addition of ethiofos reduced moderate or severe toxicity from 28 to 15% in skin, mucous membrane, genitourinary tract, and gastrointestinal tract (Kligerman et al 1992).

DNA Alkylating Agents. Mechlorethamine (HN$_2$) hematopoietic lethality in mice is reduced by a factor of 2 when ethiofos is administered 15 minutes before the alkylating agent (Yuhas 1979). This experimental protection declined with a half-life of 1.5 to 2.0 hours and did not alter antitumor efficacy in Linel lung carcinoma. Another preclinical study reported a dose-modifying factor (DMF) of 4.6 for mechlorethamine-induced cytotoxicity against normal mouse bone marrow hematopoietic colony-forming units in vitro (see table on the next page) (Wasserman et al 1981). In the clinic, however, ethiofos did not reduce the myelosuppression from

NORMAL TISSUES SHOWING RADIORESISTANCE FOLLOWING ETHIOFOS THERAPY IN ANIMALS

Tissue	Dose-Modifying Factor*
Bone marrow	2.4–3.0
Immune system	1.8–3.4
Skin	2.0–2.4
Colon	1.8
Small intestine	1.8–2.0
Lung	1.2–1.8
Esophagus	1.4
Kidney	1.5
Liver	2.7
Salivary gland	2.0
Oral mucosa	>>1
Testes	2.1

*Fold increase in dose of ionizing radiation with ethiofos to produce equivalent cytotoxicity.
From Yuhas JM, Spellman JM, Culo F. The role of WR-2721 in radiotherapy and/or chemotherapy. Cancer Clin Trials. 1980;3:211–216. Modified with permission.

DOSE MODIFYING FACTORS FOR HEMATOPOIETIC TOXICITY WITH DNA-BINDING ANTITUMOR AGENTS COMBINED WITH ETHIOFOS IN MOUSE BONE MARROW CELLS IN VITRO

Agent	Experimental Dose-Modifying Factor
Mechlorethamine	4.6
Cisplatin	3.2
Cyclophosphamide	2.4
Carmustine	1.5
5-Fluorouracil	2.7

Data from Wasserman TH, Phillips TL, Ross G, et al. Differential protection against cytotoxic chemotherapeutic effects on bone marrow CFUs by WR-2721. Cancer Clin Trials. 1981;4:3–6.

mechlorethamine doses of 10 to 16 mg/m^2 (Glick et al 1982).

Cyclophosphamide has a high DMF in normal hematopoietic cells when combined with ethiofos in vitro (see table). This protective effect of ethiofos can be enhanced in vivo by pretreatment with phenobarbital (Glover et al 1982). In cancer patients, ethiofos pretreatment roughly doubles the mean granulocyte nadir count and shortens the recovery period following a cyclophosphamide dose of 1.5 g/m^2 (Glover et al 1986a). There were no neutropenic fevers in the patients receiving cyclophosphamide plus ethiofos. Glick et al (1984) also describe protection from cyclophosphamide-induced granulocytopenia. A previous trial reported no amelioration of cyclophosphamide toxicity by WR-2721 (Woolley et al 1983). Hematopoietic toxicity from 4-hydroperoxycyclophosphamide in normal bone marrow cells is also reduced by ethiofos in vitro. Antitumor efficacy against acute lymphocytic leukemia cells was unaltered in this study (Rogers et al 1992).

Mitomycin-C-induced thrombocytopenia was reduced by ethiofos in patients with advanced colorectal cancer refractory to fluoropyrimidines (Veach et al 1992). The antitumor activity of mitomycin-C in human PA-1 ovarian cancer cells is also maintained when ethiofos is added in vitro (Ghiorghis et al 1992).

Platinum-Containing Antitumor Agents. Ethiofos administered 30 minutes before cisplatin reduced the degree of nephrotoxicity in rats by a factor of 1.7 (Yuhas and Culo 1980). Antitumor efficacy was unaffected. The protective effect in mice required pretreatment with ethiofos by at least 30 minutes. Simultaneous treatment with cisplatin or the administration of ethiofos after cisplatin was ineffective (Treskes et al 1992a). A similar result was obtained in a phase I–II trial of 100 to 150 mg/m^2 cisplatin plus mannitol diuresis and ethiofos (Glover et al 1986b). At the highest cisplatin dose level, ethiofos prevented serum creatinine elevation in five patients. Cumulative-dose cisplatin-induced neuropathies were also marginally reduced in a few patients receiving concomitant ethiofos (Glover et al 1986b). This combination was reported to be particularly active in malignant melanoma, with an objective response rate of 44% described in one preliminary trial (Glover et al 1987). The mean duration of response was 4.5 months. A follow-up study reported a 35% response rate with the same regimen (Avril et al 1992).

Cisplatin-induced neurotoxicity was also moderately reduced by ethiofos in ovarian cancer patients receiving concomitant cyclophosphamide. Neutropenic sepsis was seen in only 8% of patients receiving ethiofos compared with 28% of control (no ethiofos) patients in this study (Glick et al 1992). Response rates to the cisplatin/cyclophosphamide combination were 36% with ethiofos and 29% without ethiofos (Glick et al 1992). In contrast, Kish et al (1991) described no protection by ethiofos from toxic effects of cisplatin and fluorouracil in patients with recurrent and/or metastatic head and neck cancer. And, the overall response rate of 34% in this trial is not remarkable compared with that obtained by 5-flourouracil/cisplatin combinations without ethiofos.

There is controversy over whether ethiofos can consistently alter the myelotoxic effects of carboplatin. Some recent trials report partial protection from myelotoxicity in mice with some evidence of increased carboplatin antitumor activity with ethiofos (Treskes et al 1992b). Gill et al (1992) also reported that ethiofos-induced myeloprotection was insufficient to allow for dose escalation of either carboplatin or cisplatin. Similarly, ethiofos provided no protection from carboplatin-induced myelotoxicity in a phase II study of ethiofos in 22 patients with advanced tumors (Luginbuhl et al 1992).

Other Antitumor Agents. Other antitumor agents that have shown experimental toxicity modulation with ethiofos include doxorubicin (Green et al 1992,

Ghiorghis et al 1992) and carmustine (Ghiorghis et al 1992, Wasserman et al 1981). In contrast, ethiofos did not alter the experimental hematopoietic toxicity of etoposide, methylprednisolone, or the ether lipid compound ilmofosine in human ovarian cancer cells in vitro (Rogers et al 1992).

■ Mechanism of Action

Ethiofos presumably acts as a prodrug to form the radioprotective thiol N-2-mercaptoethyl-1,3-diaminopropane, which is a free radical scavenger (Tabachnik et al 1980, 1982). The active moiety is believed to be the sulfhydryl, which may be able to supplement endogenous thiol pools and act as a nucleophile to bind electrophilic species from alkylating agents. It is, however, clear that ethiofos does not elevate intracellular glutathione concentrations (Utley et al 1984). The supposed specificity for normal tissues over tumor tissues may relate to the marked hydrophilicity of ethiofos (Yuhas 1980). This physicochemical property appears to favor selective uptake by normal tissues which can occur against a concentration gradient (Yuhas 1980). In contrast, ethiofos uptake in tumor tissues is a passive process. Murine studies with radiolabeled ethiofos have shown that drug levels in solid tumor tissues may be 0.1 to 0.01 that in normal tissues (Yuhas 1980). Although a difference in tumor vascularity has been postulated to explain the poor uptake into tumors, this has not been proven. Nonetheless, the selective concentration of active thiol in normal tissues may explain the radio- and chemoprotective activity of this agent.

In contrast, ethiofos may produce additive or synergistic toxicity with agents that produce oxygen free radicals. This effect has been observed with the experimental oxidative neurotoxin 6-hydroxydopamine (Schor 1988). The mechanism for synergistic toxicity was shown to involve inactivation of γ-glutamylcysteine synthetase (γ-GCS) by a proposed disulfide metabolite of ethiofos (Schor 1988). This inactivation blocked the synthesis of glutathione possibly by a covalent modification of γ-GCS by the active ethiofos metabolite N-2-mercaptoethyl-1,3-diaminopropane.

■ Availability and Storage

Ethiofos is investigationally available from the National Cancer Institute for clinical trials jointly sponsored by U.S. Bioscience, West Conshohocken, Pennsylvania. It is supplied as a lyophilized powder in 500-mg, 10-mL vials which also contain 500 mg of mannitol, USP. The intact vials are stable for at least 2 years frozen (–2 to –10°C), and are much less stable if stored at room temperature.

■ Preparation for Use, Stability, and Admixture

Each 500-mg vial is reconstituted with 9.3 mL of Sterile Water for Injection, USP. This yields a clear solution containing 50 mg (each) of ethiofos and mannitol at a pH of 6.0 to 8.0. The initial solution can be diluted further in D5W or normal saline to a concentration of 10 mg/mL. This solution is stable for at least 24 hours at room temperature and light conditions (National Cancer Institute 1987). For maximal stability, however, the drug has also been diluted with 5% dextrose in lactated Ringer's injection (D5LR) buffered to a pH of 7.2 to 7.4 with sodium bicarbonate (Glover et al 1987). This solution is prepared by adding 20 mL of a 1 mEq/mL sodium bicarbonate solution to 1 L of D5LR. This may prevent degradation of ethiofos under weakly acidic conditions to more toxic dephosphorylated disulfide and thiol metabolites (Glover et al 1984).

■ Administration

Ethiofos is administered intravenously over 15 minutes. Longer infusions over 30 to 60 minutes have also been used (Woolley et al 1983). The short 15-minute infusion time appears to produce significantly less hypotension than longer infusions (Kligerman et al 1984). All ethiofos infusions are given 15 to 30 minutes prior to chemotherapy or radiotherapy to provide adequate time for distribution of active metabolites to normal tissues (Travis et al 1982).

Ethiofos is inactive as a radioprotectant when administered orally to animals (Davidson et al 1980).

■ Special Precautions

Because of the acute hypotensive effects of ethiofos, blood pressures should be measured every 2 minutes during infusions (Glover et al 1984, 1986a,b).

■ Dosage

For single-dose chemotherapy regimens, the recommended ethiofos dose for phase II studies is 740 mg/m^2 (Glover et al 1984). For fractionated-dose chemotherapy or radiotherapy regimens, the recommended dose is 340 mg/m^2, 30 minutes prior to each day's therapy (Kligerman et al 1984). A typical ethiofos schedule with chemo/radiotherapy calls for 340 mg/m² × 4 days/week × 5 weeks (Mehta et al 1991). A higher dose of ethiofos, 910 mg/m², has also been used. This dose was effective as an antagonist of mitomycin-C-induced thrombocytopenia (Veach et al 1992). In contrast, a schedule involving two 910 mg/m² doses of ethiofos was inactive as an antagonist of carboplatin myelotoxicity (Luginbuhl et al 1992). The ethiofos doses were administered prior to and 2 hours after carboplatin to account for the very short plasma half-life of ethiofos (approximately 5 minutes).

Other studies report that ethiofos doses of 750 mg/m² before cisplatin and 340 mg/m² before radiation can facilitate the administration of 90% of the planned cisplatin dose intensity (80 mg/m²) and 85% of the planned 5-fluorouracil dose intensity (800 mg/m²) in patients receiving chemotherapy with simultaneous radiation therapy (4 Gy day 1 plus 2 Gy days 1–5) for advanced head and neck cancer (Taylor et al 1991).

■ Drug Interactions

Because ethiofos is metabolized to active sulfhydryls, a number of potential means of altering drug activation are available. Phenobarbital pretreatment has been shown to enhance the degree of hematologic protection from ethiofos in Fischer rats (Glover et al 1982). This effect was not due to any significant alteration of ethiofos levels in the serum or tissues; however, phenobarbital also enhanced ethiofos toxicity, as noted by an increase in ethiofos-induced hypothermia in the rats.

Levamisole was used as an inhibitor of alkaline phosphatase activity to study the role of dephosphorylation in mediating radioprotection from ethiofos in mice (Brown et al 1986). Levamisole slightly reduced the radioprotection of ethiofos and lowered the levels of the active sulfhydryl metabolite, WR-1065, by 37%; however, levamisole also increased the toxicity of the parent molecule, ethiofos, which may be approximately 3.5-fold more toxic than WR-1065 (Brown et al 1986). Levamisole was also toxic at the dose required to modify ethiofos metabolism.

■ Pharmacokinetics

Ethiofos is rapidly eliminated from the plasma. Following a 150 mg/m² intravenous bolus injection, the mean plasma clearance was 2.17 L/min, with a volume of distribution at steady state of 6.44 L (Shaw et al 1986). The mean volume of the central compartment was 3.5 L. This demonstrates that the drug does not distribute extensively outside the vascular compartment. A biphasic elimination pattern was evident for the parent drug with half-lives of 0.88 minutes (α) and 8.76 minutes (β) (Shaw et al 1986).

There are two known dephosphorylated metabolites of ethiofos, the free sulfhydryl, WR-33278, and the symmetric disulfide, WR-1065 (Shaw et al 1986). When added to blood or plasma, both metabolites decrease in concentration rapidly. This is probably due to the formation of mixed disulfides with other sulfhydryl-containing substances. The hydrolysis of ethiofos in acidic conditions precludes oral administration (Swynnerton et al 1986).

In the mouse, over half of a dose of WR-2721 is converted to the disulfide metabolite within 15 minutes of injection (Utley et al 1984). Similar effects have been observed in monkeys given ethiofos, wherein the levels of WR-1065 are much higher at all time points than those of the parent compound (Swynnerton et al 1986). The levels of WR-1065 vary widely in different tissues, with the highest levels seen in kidney, liver, lung, salivary gland, heart, spleen, muscle, tumor, and brain (in descending order) (Utley et al 1984). WR-1065 levels were reduced most rapidly in tumor specimens, suggesting a different pattern of metabolism and clearance compared with normal tissues. Dephosphorylation activity, which converts ethiofos to WR-1065, is known to be high in the kidney, liver, and small intestine (Mori et al 1984). This may explain the high degree of radioprotection from ethiofos in those tissues.

■ Side Effects and Toxicity

The primary toxic effects of ethiofos are nausea, vomiting and hypotension (Kligerman et al 1980, 1981). The most serious and dose-limiting side effect of ethiofos is the drop in blood pressure, which can involve a 15 to 20 mm Hg decrease in systolic pressure at varying times after drug infusion. The onset has ranged from 30 minutes to 4 hours later (Kligerman et al 1980). Occasionally, some patients may experience a transient hypertensive response to ethiofos (Kligerman et al 1981). The effects on blood pressure typically occur early in the infusion period and are usually rapidly reversed when the infusion is halted (Kligerman et al 1984); however, these hypotensive reactions are not always dose related.

About 55% of patients may experience moderate nausea and vomiting following ethiofos. This is typically of brief duration and highly responsive to antiemetics. In contrast to the hypotensive effects, emesis was clearly increased with high doses of ethiofos.

Somnolence may occur in about 10 to 20% of patients. This is transient, occurring during the infusion, and typically resolves within less than 30 minutes (Glover et al 1986a,b). Approximately 27% of patients also experience a flushed feeling toward the end of infusion. A sensation of "cold hands" is described in some trials but the etiology of this effect is unknown.

Sneezing is reported in 19% of patients. Hiccups are occasionally described. Some patients have also complained of a metallic taste in the mouth during infusion (Kligerman et al 1984).

With repeated doses of ethiofos, an allergic syndrome was described in a few patients in an early trial (Turrisi et al 1983). This reaction consists of chills, fever, rash, and hypotension. Later studies have not reported this constellation of side effects.

REFERENCES

Avril MF, Ortoli JC, Fortier-Beaulieu M, et al. High dose cisplatin (C) and WR 2721 in metastatic melanoma. *Proc Am Soc Clin Oncol.* 1992;**11**:344.

Brown DQ, Shaw LM, Pittock JW III, et al. Modification of WR-2721 toxicity and radioprotection by an inhibitor of alkaline phosphatase. *Int J Radiat Oncol Biol Phys.* 1986;**12**:1491–1493.

Constine LS, Zagars G, Rubin P, et al. Protection by WR-2721 of human bone marrow function following irradiation. *Int J Radiat Oncol Biol Phys.* 1986;**12**:1505–1508.

Davidson DE, Grenan MM, Sweeney TR. Biological characteristics of some improved radioprotectors. In: Brady LW, ed. *Radiation Sensitizers, Their Use in the Clinical Management of Cancer.* New York: Masson; 1980:309–320.

Denekamp J, Michael BD, Rojas A, et al. Radioprotection of mouse skin by WR-2721: The critical influence of oxygen tension. *Int J Radiat Oncol Biol Phys.* 1982;**8**:531–534.

Ghiorghis A, Talebian A, Schein PS, et al. Effect of anticancer drugs against PA-1 human ovarian cancer cells pretreated with the chemoprotective agent WR-2721. *Proc Am Assoc Cancer Res.* 1992;**33**:500.

Gill I, Muggia F, Parker R, et al. WR-2721 (WR) pretreatment protects against the marrow toxicity of carboplatin (CB) and cisplatin (CP). *Proc Am Soc Clin Oncol.* 1992;**11**:132.

Glick JH, Glover DJ, Weiler C, et al. Phase I clinical trials of WR-2721 with alkylating agent chemotherapy. *Int J Radiat Oncol Biol Phys.* 1982;**8**:575–580.

Glick JH, Glover D, Weiler C, et al. Phase I controlled trials of WR-2721 and cyclophosphamide. *Int J Radiat Oncol Biol Phys.* 1984;**10**:1777–1780.

Glick J, Kemp G, Rose P, et al. A randomized trial of cyclophosphamide and cisplatin ± WR-2721 in the treatment of advanced epithelial ovarian cancer. *Proc Am Soc Clin Oncol.* 1992;**11**:109.

Glover D, Glick JH, Weiler C, et al. Phase I trials of WR-2721 and *cis*-platinum. *Int J Radiat Oncol Biol Phys.* 1984;**10**:1781–1784.

Glover D, Glick JH, Weiler C, et al. WR-2721 protects against the hematologic toxicity of cyclophosphamide: A controlled phase II trial. *J Clin Oncol.* 1986a;**4**:584–588.

Glover D, Glick JH, Weiler C, et al. Phase I/II trials of WR-2721 and *cis*-platinum. *Int J Radiat Oncol Biol Phys.* 1986b;**12**:1509–1512.

Glover D, Glick JH, Weiler C, et al. WR-2721 and high-dose cisplatin: An active combination in the treatment of metastatic melanoma. *J Clin Oncol.* 1987;**5**:574–578.

Glover DJ, Yuhas JM, Glick JH. WR-2721: Enhanced chemoprotection by increasing cyclophosphamide activation with phenobarbitol. *Int J Radiat Oncol Biol Phys.* 1982;**8**:571–574.

Green D, Wright A, Schein P, et al. WR-2721 chemoprotection of doxorubicin toxicity in mice. *Proc Am Assoc Cancer Res.* 1992;**33**:490.

Kish JA, Ensley JF, Tilchen E, et al. Evaluation of high dose (HD) WR-2721 (WR) + high dose cisplatin (HD CP) + 5-fluorouracil infusion (5FUI) in recurrent/metastatic (r/M) head and neck cancer (HNC). *Proc Am Soc Clin Oncol.* 1991;**10**:205.

Kligerman MM, Blumberg AL, Glick JH, et al. Phase I trials of WR-2721 in combination with radiation therapy and with the alkylating agents cyclophosphamide and *cis*-platinum. *Cancer Clin Trials.* 1981;**4**:469–474.

Kligerman MM, Glover DJ, Turrisi AT, et al. Toxicity of WR-2721 administered in single and multiple doses. *Int J Radiat Oncol Biol Phys.* 1984;**10**:1773–1776.

Kligerman MM, Liu TF, Moore A, et al. Protection of normal pelvic tissues in patients with advanced rectal cancer: A randomized trial of fractionated radiation therapy ± WR-2721. *Proc Am Soc Clin Oncol.* 1992;**11**:161.

Kligerman MM, Shaw MT, Slavik M, et al. Phase I clinical studies with WR-2721. *Cancer Clin Trials.* 1980;**3**:217–221.

Luginbuhl W, Tester W, Shaw L, et al. One or two doses of WR-2721—Does it protect patients receiving carboplatin? *Proc Am Soc Clin Oncol.* 1992;**11**:123.

MacVittie TJ, Brundenburg R, Farese AM, et al. Enhanced recovery from supralethal radiation exposure using combined modality WR-2721 plus recombinant human (rh) G-CSF. *Proc Am Assoc Cancer Res.* 1992;**33**:505.

Mehta M, Schiller JH, Bastin K, et al. Pilot study of WR-2721/CDDP/VLB and sequential TRT/WR-2721 in stage III NSCLC: Preliminary results. *Proc Am Soc Clin Oncol.* 1991;**10**:263.

Mori T, Nikaido O, Sugahara T. Dephosphorylation of WR-2721 with mouse tissue homogenates. *Int J Radiat Oncol Biol Phys.* 1984;**10**:1529–1531.

Rogers PCJ, Chan KW, Rodriguez WC, et al. Effect of amifostine (WR-2721) on cytotoxicity of pharmacological purging agents used for autologous marrow graft in acute lymphoblastic leukemia. *Proc Am Soc Clin Oncol.* 1992;**11**:284.

Rojas A, Denekamp J. The influence of x ray dose levels on normal tissue radioprotection by WR-2721. *Int J Radiat Oncol Biol Phys.* 1984;**10**:2351–2356.

Schor NF. Mechanisms of synergistic toxicity of the radioprotective agent, WR-2721, and 6-hydroxydopamine. *Biochem Pharmacol.* 1988;**37**:1751–1762.

Shaw LM, Turrisi AT, Glover DJ, et al. Human pharmacokinetics of WR-2721. *Int J Radiat Oncol Biol Phys.* 1986;**12**:1501–1504.

Swynnerton NF, Huelle BK, Mangold DJ. A method for the combined measurement of ethiofos and WR-1065 in plasma: Application to pharmacokinetic experiments with ethiofos and its metabolites. *Int J Radiat Oncol Biol Phys.* 1986;**12**:1495–1499.

Tabachnik NF, Blackburn P, Peterson CM, Cerami A. Protein binding of N-2-mercaptoethyl-1,3-diaminopropane via mixed disulfide formation after oral administration of WR-2721. *J Pharmacol Exp Ther.* 1982;**220**:243–246.

Tabachnik NF, Peterson CM, Cerami A. Studies on the reduction of sputum viscosity in cystic fibrosis using an orally absorbed protected thiol. *J Pharmacol Exp Ther.* 1980;**214**:246–249.

Taylor SG IV, Murthy AK, Showel JL, et al. Phase I dose escalation study of combined cisplatin 5-FU infusion chemotherapy with simultaneous radiation and WR-2721. *Proc Am Soc Clin Oncol.* 1991;**10**:208.

Travis EL, de Luca AM, Fowler JF, et al. The time course of radioprotection by WR-2721 in mouse skin. *Int J Radiat Oncol Biol Phys.* 1982;**8**:843–850.

Treskes M, Boven E, Holwerda U, et al. Time dependence of the selective modulation of cisplatin-induced nephrotoxicity by WR-2721 in the mouse. *Cancer Res.* 1992a;**52**:2257–2260.

Treskes M, Holwerda U, Boven E, et al. Selective modulation of cisplatin and carboplatin-induced toxicities by the modulating agent WR-2721 (amifostine). *Proc Am Assoc Cancer Res.* 1992b;**33**:425.

Turrisi AT, Kligerman MM, Glover DJ, et al. Experience with phase I trials of WR-2721 preceding radiation therapy. In: Nygaard OF, ed. *Radioprotectors and Anticarcinogens.* New York: Academic Press; 1983:681–694.

Utley JF, Seaver N, Newton GL, et al. Pharmacokinetics of WR-1065 in mouse tissue following treatment with WR-2721. *Int J Radiat Oncol Biol Phys.* 1984;**10**:1525–1528.

Veach SR, Poplin EA, MacDonald JS, et al. Randomized clinical trial of mitomycin-C with or without pretreatment with WR-2721 in patients with advanced colorectal cancer whose disease has either failed to respond or progressed on 5-FU or 5-FU + leucovorin. *Proc Am Soc Clin Oncol.* 1992;**11**:185.

Wasserman TH, Phillips TL, Ross G, et al. Differential protection against cytotoxic chemotherapeutic effects on bone marrow CFUs by WR-2721. *Cancer Clin Trials.* 1981;**4**:3–6.

Woolley PV III, Ayoob MJ, Smith FP, et al. Clinical trial of the effect of S-2-(3-aminopropylamino)-ethylphosphorothioic acid (WR-2721) (NSC 296961) on the toxicity of cyclophosphamide. *J Clin Oncol.* 1983;**1**:198–203.

Yuhas JM. Differential protection of normal and malignant tissues against the cytotoxic effects of mechlorethamine. *Cancer Treat Rep.* 1979;**63**:971–976.

Yuhas JM. Active versus passive absorption kinetics as the basis for selective protection of normal tissues by S-2-(3-aminopropylamino)-ethylphosphorothioic acid. *Cancer Res.* 1980;**40**:1519–1524.

Yuhas JM, Culo F. Selective inhibition of the nephrotoxicity of *cis*-dichlorodiammineplatinum(II) by WR-2721 without altering its antitumor properties. *Cancer Treat Rep.* 1980;**64**:57–64.

Yuhas JM, Davis ME, Glover D, et al. Circumvention of the tumor membrane barrier to WR-2721 absorption by reduction of drug hydrophilicity. *Int J Radiat Oncol Biol Phys.* 1982;**8**:519–522.

Yuhas JM, Spellman JM, Culo F. The role of WR-2721 in radiotherapy and/or chemotherapy. *Cancer Clin Trials.* 1980;**3**:211–216.

Etoposide

■ Other Names

NSC-141540; VePesid® (Bristol-Myers Oncology Division); VP-16 VP-16-213; epipodophyllotoxin; EPEG; ethylidene-lignan P.

■ Chemistry

Structure of etoposide

Etoposide (VP-16) is a semisynthetic epipodophyllotoxin derived from the root of *Podophyllum peltatum* (the May apple plant or mandrake) (Kelly and Hartwell 1954). The chemical name is 4′-demethylepipodophyllotoxin 9-(4,6-O-ethylidene-β-D-glucopyranoside). Etoposide has the empiric formula $C_{29}H_{32}O_{13}$ and the molecular weight 588. It is very soluble in methanol and chloroform, slightly soluble in ethanol, and sparingly soluble in water and ether. Because of poor water solubility, the commercial drug is dissolved in an ethanol-based cosolvent system.

Etoposide was originally synthesized by Sandoz Laboratories from *Podophyllum embodi*, a plant native to India, in an effort to produce less toxic cytostatic podophyllum derivatives (Keller-Justin et al 1971). Structure–activity studies show that the hydroxyl group at the C-4′ position is required for activity and that alterations at this site can dramatically alter activity (Loike and Horwitz 1976).

■ Antitumor Activity

Reports of cytotoxic effects produced by podophyllum derivatives are hundreds of years old. The initial citation in the United States was by Bentley in 1861 (Kelly and Hartwell 1954). In 1942, Kaplan revived clinical interest for topical podophyllum in oil, which is useful in treating condyloma acuminata.

Etoposide demonstrated significant preclinical a large number of tumor types, including activity in Ehrlich ascites tumors, sarcoma-37 and -180, Walker carcinosarcoma, and murine L-1210 leukemia (Dombernowsky and Nissen 1973, Stahelin 1973, Venditti 1971). In the L-1210 mouse model, continuous drug administration regimens significantly enhance the antileukemic effects of etoposide (Rozencweig et al 1977). There is also efficacy in this model for etoposide combined with cytarabine (Rivera et al 1975), although an additive rather than synergistic interaction appears likely (Dombernowsky and Nissen 1976).

A phase I clinical trial by Nissen et al (1972) demonstrated significant antitumor activity in lymphosarcoma, Hodgkin's disease, and reticulum cell sarcoma. It is also active in diffuse histiocytic lymphoma (Jacobs et al 1975). Mathe et al (1974) confirmed etoposide activity in lymphoid tumors and against monocytoid leukemias. It is also active in solid tumors (Jungi 1982). Various reports have described substantial drug activity in advanced, previously untreated small cell bronchogenic carcinoma (Eagen et al 1976, Dombernowsky and Nissen 1976, Cohen et al 1977a,b). The drug appears to lack significant activity in patients with melanomas (Cecil et al 1978). In early European studies (European Organization for Research on the Treatment of Cancer [EORTC] 1973), etoposide was similarly ineffective in malignancies involving the brain, bladder, head, and neck and in soft tissue sarcomas. Breast cancer appears to be poorly responsive to the drug (Ahmann et al 1976, Nissen et al 1972), but some activity is observed in combination with doxorubicin (Van Echo et al 1979). Ovarian tumors are similarly resistant (Falkson et al 1975, Jungi and Senn 1975, Slayton et al 1979).

Etoposide is effective in relapsed patients with Hodgkin's disease and other malignant non-Hodgkin's lymphomas (Nissen et al 1980, Cecil et al 1978). Of particular note is the inclusion of etoposide in the effective multidrug combination regimen ProMACE/MOPP (Fisher et al 1983).

Williams and Einhorn (1982) also report a 34% response rate for etoposide used in resistant neoplasms of the testis. The three-drug regimen of etoposide, cisplatin, and bleomycin produces complete responses in 43% of relapsed patients, with long-term survival rates of 37% (Williams et al 1979, 1980). Combinations without bleomycin are also highly effective (Bosl et al 1982).

Overall, etoposide has demonstrated the most consistent activity in leukemias and in small cell (oat cell) carcinoma of the lung (Cohen et al 1977a,b, Greco et al 1979). For the latter indication numerous effective drug combinations including etoposide have been described. Some of these include ACE with Adriamycin® and cyclophosphamide (Aisner et al 1982b); APE with procarbazine and Adriamycin® (Broder et al 1981); ECHO with Cytoxan®, Adriamycin®, and Oncovin® (Valdivieso et al 1979); and an intensive induction called CAVe with Cytoxan® and Adriamycin® (Abeloff et al 1979, Klastersky et al 1982); and cyclophosphamide, methotrexate, and etoposide (Bonomi et al 1983).

In leukemia, drug activity appears to be limited primarily to acute nonlymphocytic histologies. The drug is also active in some childhood acute lymphocytic leukemias wherein Rivera et al (1975) have described good activity for etoposide in phase II studies. In acute nonlymphocytic leukemia, combinations of etoposide with other agents have produced response rates of 20 to 66% in preliminary studies (O'Dwyer et al 1985). As first-line therapy, response rates of 50 to 81% are described for etoposide combined with thioguanine and an anthracycline. Etoposide is also active in patients with refractory multiple myeloma when combined with cytarabine, cisplatin, and dexamethasone in the EDAP regimen (Barlogie et al 1989).

Occasionally responsive tumors include AIDS-related Kaposi's sarcoma (Laubenstein et al 1983), non-small cell lung cancer when combined with cisplatin (Pedersen and Hansen 1983), and neuroblastoma (Schmoll 1982).

See also Special Applications at end of this monograph for high-dose applications with bone marrow transplantation.

■ Mechanism of Action

There is marked schedule dependence for etoposide cell killing and cytotoxic effects are maximal in G_2 phase (Misra and Roberts 1975). There is also some activity on cells in late S phase and the drug can halt cell cycle traverse at the S/G_2 interphase (Krishan et al 1975).

Etoposide produces protein-linked DNA strand breaks by inhibition of DNA topoisomerase II (TOPO-II) enzymes (Ross et al 1984). This normal mammalian enzyme mediates double-strand passing activities in G_2 phase to condense or decondense supercoiled DNA (Glisson and Ross 1987). The expression and activity of TOPO-II are highly phase dependent and minimal or undetectable in nondividing cells. Drug-induced inhibition of TOPO-II is an energy-requiring process dependent on both dose and duration of exposure. Magnesium is also required as an enzymatic cofactor.

Etoposide does not bind directly to DNA but rather "stabilizes" a covalent transition form of the DNA–TOPO-II complex (Ross et al 1984). This intermediate, termed the *cleavable complex,* can, under alkaline (denaturing) conditions, be discerned as two sets of TOPO-II homodimers bound at the 5' end of double-stranded fragments of DNA. Both single and double DNA strand breaks are produced in close proportion to the cytotoxic dose–response curve (Wozniak and Ross 1983). Thus etoposide, as well as intercalative drugs such as doxorubicin, "poison" TOPO-II enzymes by stabilizing an otherwise transient form of TOPO-II covalently linked with DNA (Tewey et al 1984). Normal TOPO-II strand-passing activity is thereby blocked and cell progression out of G_2 phase is halted (Smith et al 1986, Glisson and Ross 1987). Cytotoxicity from etoposide may also be characterized by chromosomal breaks characterized as sister chromatid exchanges (Chatterjee et al 1990).

Another postulated etoposide mechanism includes microsomal activation (Van Maanen et al 1983) to reactive intermediates capable of generating oxygen free radicals (Wozniak et al 1984). The pendant phenol may be important in mediating this activity and changes at this site can dramatically reduce antitumor effects (Loike and Horwitz 1976). Nucleoside transport is also inhibited at high drug concentrations (Yalowich et al 1983), but whether this makes a major contribution to the antitumor effect is unknown.

■ Availability and Storage

Etoposide is commercially available in 100-mg, 5-mL ampules in a nonaqueous solution from Bristol-Myers Oncology Division, Princeton, New Jersey. Each milliliter contains etoposide, 20 mg; citric acid (anhydrous), 2 mg; benzyl alcohol, 30 mg; polysorbate 80, 80 mg; polyethylene glycol 300, 650 mg; and absolute alcohol. The drug should be protected from light and, undiluted, is stable for at least 3 years from date of manufacture at room temperature. The commercial oral formulation is supplied as 50-mg pink capsules (Vepesid®), which also include citric acid, glycerin, purified water, and polyethylene glycol 400. The gelatin capsules also include sorbital, ethyl- and propylparabens, and the dyes iron oxide and titanium dioxide. These capsules should be stored under refrigeration (2–8°C). Several investigational oral formulations have also been evaluated previously (Nissen et al 1975, 1976), including (1) hydrophilic, soft gelatin capsules containing 100 mg of etoposide solution (Lau et al 1979); (2) lipophilic capsules of etoposide suspension (100 mg etoposide, 320 mg miglyol 812, 70 mg bee's wax, 10 mg soya lecithin [Falkson et al 1975]); and (3) special (100 mg/5 mL) drinking ampules (Trink-Ampulles) in which the drug is dissolved in a solution consisting of 20 mg Tween 80, 650 mg polyethylene glycol 300, 30 mg benzyl alcohol, 2 mg citric acid (anhydrous), and absolute alcohol to make 1.0 mL/20 mg etoposide (Nissen et al 1976).

■ Preparation for Use, Stability, and Admixture

The recommended diluent for the commercial formulation is 5% Dextrose in Water, USP, or 0.9% Sodium Chloride for Injection, USP. VP-16 is recommended to be diluted with at least 50 equivalent volumes of solution to yield a concentration of 0.4 mg/mL, which is stable for 48 hours (96 hours if diluted to a concentration of 0.2 mg/mL). (Therefore, to give a 60-mg dose [3 mL of the commercial preparation], the volume of sodium chloride or D5W used must be at least 150 mL. *More concentrated admixtures have much shorter stability times; see table below.*)

Contact with buffered aqueous solutions with a pH above 8 should be avoided. It is also important to observe the solution for clarity before use. Any cloudy solutions should be discarded.

Etoposide is compatible with glass or plastic (polyvinyl chloride) infusion containers (see table); however, undiluted etoposide solutions have been reported to cause cracks and leaks in infusion devices made of acrylic or ABS-type plastic. This has not been observed with diluted solutions of etoposide. The drug is physically compatible for 24 hours with cisplatin (Lokich et al 1989) or carboplatin (Stewart and Hampton 1989), with morphine sulfate (*Wellcome Trends in Hospital Pharmacy* 1986;3:3,15), and with ondansetron for 1 to 4 hours in 5% dextrose (Leak and Woodford 1989). It is also compatible for 72 hours with a solution containing cytarabine and daunorubicin (Seargeant et al 1987) and with ondansetron (Trissel et al 1990).

■ Administration

Intravenous Administration. Etoposide should be diluted as described earlier and given by intravenous infusion over at least 30 minutes. Severe hypotension may occur if the drug is given too rapidly.

UTILITY TIMES FOR ETOPOSIDE SOLUTIONS STORED AT ROOM TEMPERATURE (25°C)

Etoposide Concentration (mg/mL)[†]	Utility Time (h)*			
	D5W	0.9% NaCl	Lactated Ringer's	10% Mannitol
2	0.5[‡]	0.5[‡]	—	—
1	2	2	—	—
0.6	8	8	—	—
0.4	48	48	8	8
0.2	96	96	8	8
0.2	96	96	—	—

*Stability in glass or plastic (PVC) containers except as noted. Utility time represents ≥ 90% original concentration remaining.
[†]Examine all solutions carefully for fine precipitates.
[‡]One-hour stability in polyvinyl chloride (PVC) plastic containers.

Although not a vesicant (Dorr and Alberts 1983), extravasation of the drug should be avoided.

Continuous infusions of etoposide have been used as a means of enhancing the cell cycle (phase)-specific mode of cytotoxic action (Achterrath et al 1982). Most infusions have used 5-day courses (Lokich 1989, Aisner et al 1982a, Steward et al 1984), although 72-hour infusions have also been evaluated either alone (Bennett et al 1987) or in sequence with cisplatin (Krook et al 1989).

Oral Administration. Oral administration of etoposide capsules may be useful whenever patient compliance is high and low emetogenic drug regimens are used. The capsules may be taken all at once to achieve the desired dose. Neither food nor other chemotherapy drugs appear to alter oral absorption of the drug (Harvey et al 1985). Recent studies suggest that the bioavailability of low oral doses of 100 mg is better than of higher oral doses (Hande et al, 1993; see Pharmacokinetics section).

■ Special Precautions

The drug should be administered by slow intravenous infusion over at least 30 minutes to avoid severe hypotension. All solutions should be examined for fine precipitates and mixed prior to use.

■ Dosage

A variety of doses and schedules have been used with etoposide (see table on opposite page). General principles of dosing include more frequent administration to take advantage of cell cycle-dependent cytotoxicity; a rough doubling of oral doses because of the 50% bioavailability for the gelatin capsules; and significant dose reductions for combinations of etoposide with other myelosuppressive drugs or for patients with poor bone marrow reserve and/or poor performance status. In general, etoposide doses can be repeated every 3 to 4 weeks depending on the leukocyte count. With the continuous 21-day oral regimens, dosing can usually resume after 1 to 2 weeks off therapy (Hainsworth et al 1989).

A pharmacokinetic study in patients with obstructive jaundice showed no significant dose reductions are needed if renal function is normal (Hande et al 1990); however, pharmacokinetic studies of unbound etoposide suggest that patients with an increased total bilirubin (> 1 mg/dL) have significantly decreased clearance of unbound (active) drug (Stewart et al 1990). This reinforces the empiric recommendation that etoposide doses be decreased

DOSES AND SCHEDULES FOR ETOPOSIDE

Administration Method	Dose mg/m²/d	Days	Repeat Dosing Interval (wk)	Clinical Application	Reference
IV short infusion	200–250	1	7	Single agent, small cell lung cancer	Cavelli et al 1978
IV short infusion	50–100	1–5	3–4	Testicular cancer	
	100	1, 3, 5	3–4	With other drugs	Einhorn 1986
	45	1–7	3	Phase I	Nissen et al 1972
IV continuous	125	1–5	4	Phase I single agent	Aisner et al 1982a
	30	1–5	4	With cisplatin in advanced cancer	Creagan et al 1988
	80	1–5	4	Phase I, good-risk patients	
	50	1–5	4	Poor-risk patients	Lokich and Corkey 1981
	125	1–3	4	Adult patients with advanced cancer	Bennett et al 1987
	500	1 (24 h)	3	Small cell lung cancer	Slevin et al 1989a
Oral	160	1–5	3–4	Small cell lung cancer	Carney et al 1990
	50	1–21	4–5	Small cell lung cancer	Greco et al 1990, Einhorn et al 1990, Johnson et al 1990
	50	1–21	5	Advanced refractory cancers	Hainsworth et al 1989

by 50% in patients with total bilirubin levels of 1.5 to 3.0 mg/dL and that no drug be administered to patients with a bilirubin level greater than 5 mg/dL (Perry 1982).

Dose reductions in patients with renal dysfunction have also been recommended. One group recommends a 30% dose reduction in patients with serum creatinine levels above 1.47 mg/dL (130 µmol/L) (Joel et al 1991). This adjustment was calculated to equivalent total drug exposure (AUCs) in patients with normal and reduced renal function. By use of a formula provided by Anderson et al (1976), etoposide doses would be similarly reduced by 15, 20, and 25% in patients with normal hepatic function and creatinine clearance values of 60, 45, and 30 mL/min, respectively.

■ Drug Interactions

A number of drug interactions are suggested from work with experimental tumors both in cell culture and in laboratory mice (Dombernowsky and Nissen 1976). Etoposide thus appears to have at least additive antitumor actions in murine L-1210 leukemia when combined with cytarabine (Rivera et al 1975).

Mabel (1979) has also recently reported apparent antitumor synergism for etoposide combined with cisplatin against murine B-16 melanoma and P-388 leukemia. In a Lewis lung cancer model the two drugs were most effective when VP-16 was administered prior to cisplatin (Zupi et al 1985). Nonetheless, the mechanism of the positive antitumor interaction between cisplatin and etoposide is unknown. A number of renally excreted drugs (cisplatin, ifosfamide, cyclosporine) may decrease VP-16 clearance, resulting in increased exposure (see Pharmacokinetics for details).

Both etoposide and teniposide (VM-26) slow the efflux of methotrexate and methotrexate polyglutamates to increase cellular retention of methotrexate in vitro (Yalowich et al 1987). The clinical significance of this effect is unknown.

Etoposide resistance can variably involve the multidrug resistance phenomenon. This form of membrane-mediated cross-resistance to natural products can be experimentally overcome with the calcium channel antagonist verapamil (Yalowich and Ross 1984). Verapamil also appears to potentiate etoposide-induced DNA strand breaks (Slater et al 1985).

■ Pharmacokinetics

Intravenous Dosing. A two-compartment open pharmacokinetic model appears to adequately describe etoposide disposition in cancer patients (Allen and Creaven 1975) (see table below). Older studies with radiolabeled drug showed a longer β half-life than studies with more specific high-performance liquid chromatography assays. The terminal half-life of the drug appears to be about 7 hours and is not dependent on the dose, route, or method of administration (D'Incalci et al 1982). Renal excretion appears to account for about 30% of overall drug elimination (Arbuck et al 1986). Nonetheless, one patient on renal dialysis was found to have normal VP-16 kinetics and no drug accumulation either systemically or in the dialysate fluid (Holthuis et al 1985).

Normally, about 30% of a dose is recovered in the urine (D'Incalci et al 1982). A higher percentage of radiolabeled drug (43%) is recovered, 66% of which is the parent VP-16 (Creaven and Allen 1975).

Biliary secretion of parent drug accounts for 2% or less of the dose, although fecal recovery of drug and metabolites is variable, ranging from 1.5 to 16.3% (Creaven and Allen 1975). In another trial, cumulative biliary excretion accounted for less than 3% of a dose (Arbuck et al 1986); however, patients with obstructive jaundice excrete a larger fraction of a dose in the urine as etoposide (46%) compared with normals (35%) (Hande et al 1990). Urinary excretion of the glucuronide conjugate of etoposide was 29% in control patients and 15% in the jaundiced patients, whereas renal clearance (11 mL/min/m^2) and metabolic clearance (4.9–6.9 mL/min/m^2) were not different (Hande et al 1990). This study suggests that in patients with obstructive jaundice, there is a slight decrease in hepatic drug metabolism with a commensurate increase in renal clearance.

The primary metabolites of etoposide are the *cis/trans* and *picro* hydroxy acids and the *cis (picro)* lactone (Creaven 1982, Evans et al 1982). The major urinary metabolite is 4'-demethylepipodophyllic acid-9-(4,6-O-ethylidene-β-D-glucopyranoside) (Allen et al 1976). These metabolites have been identified in the plasma and urine, but in vitro cytotoxicity assays suggest they are much less active than the parent (Evans et al 1982). A late-appearing metabolite in the saliva has been identified as the etoposide aglycone (Gouyette et al 1987). Overall, the fraction of saliva to plasma concentrations was very low, in the range 0.003 to 0.25.

The plasma protein binding of etoposide is typically high, averaging 95% in normal patients (Stewart et al 1990). The free (unbound) fraction of etoposide can vary from 6 to 37% between patients (Stewart and Hampton 1989). Further study has shown that patients with increased bilirubin and/or decreased albumin may have an increase in the free

Method of Administration (Patients)	Half-life α *(min)*	Half-life β *(hr)*	AUC [Dose: mg/m^2] (μg/mL/min)]	Clearance mL/min/m^2	V$_d$ L/m^2	Reference
IV short infusion (adults)	70	7	4000 (100)	27	15.7	D'Incalci et al 1982
IV short infusion (children)	35	3.4	2500 (100)	39	10	D'Incalci et al 1982
IV short infusion (children with no prior platinum)	48	5.9	—	24	7.8	Sinkule et al 1984
IV short infusion (children with prior platinum)	48	8.3	—	16	6.3	Sinkule et al 1984
IV continuous infusion (adults, with cisplatin)						
(24 hr)	—	—	3200 (200)	19	10.9	Miller et al 1990
(36 hr)	—	—	8000 (400)	13.4	4.2	Miller et al 1990
(24 hr)	—	7.4	7633 (500)	18.9	1.4	Slevin et al 1989

fraction even though systemic clearance is unaltered (Stewart et al 1990). Myelosuppression may also be commensurately increased in these patients (Stewart and Hampton 1989).

Other conditions that may decrease etoposide clearance include prior cisplatin therapy, concurrent cisplatin therapy (Saito et al 1991), obesity, and elevated alkaline phosphatase levels (Pfluger et al 1987). Ifosfamide may also decrease etoposide clearance possibly as a result of renal toxicity. In pediatric sarcoma patients, etoposide clearance decreased by 27% from 25.8 to 18.9 mL/min/m^2 after three ifosfamide/VP-16 courses (Crom et al 1991). Cyclosporin A infusions (18 mg/kg/d) were also recently shown to significantly decrease etoposide clearance, resulting in half-life prolongation by 69 and a 103% increase in AUC (Lum et al 1991).

Oral Dosing. The absolute oral bioavailability of etoposide from the gelatin capsules ranges from 25 to 74% with a mean of 48% (Smyth et al 1985). One author has described dose-dependent bioavailability, suggesting that daily oral doses should be divided (Harvey et al 1984). One recent study showed that oral bioavailability of a 100-mg dose was 76 ± 22%, which is significantly greater than a mean bioavailability of 48 ± 18% for a 400-mg dose (Hande et al 1993). Slevin et al (1989b) similarly observed nonlinear increases in AUC with oral doses above 200 mg. In this trial, the mean increases in AUC from a dose of 100 mg (38.8 μg/mL·h/1.7 m^2) were 8, 145, 173, and 262% for oral doses of 200, 300, 400, and 600 mg, respectively. Significant intrapatient variations in bioavailability are also reported for oral etoposide (Smyth et al 1985). For example, some patients experience a 30% change in overall bioavailability (both increased and decreased) with repeat dosing. In this regard, neither food nor the administration of other chemotherapy agents appears to alter etoposide absorption (Harvey et al 1985). Wide variations in peak levels and AUC values were also described in this trial.

■ Side Effects and Toxicity

The principal toxic effect of etoposide is dose-related bone marrow suppression. Leukopenia and thrombocytopenia occur, but leukopenia consistently predominates, with a nadir of about 16 days and recovery usually by days 20 to 22.

Gastrointestinal complaints of nausea, vomiting, and anorexia are usually minor and are typically much greater with the oral preparations (Rozencweig et al 1977). Other adverse effects include alopecia in 20 to 90% of patients (EORTC 1973, Jungi and Senn 1975), headache, fever, and hypotension. Severe hypotension can occur if the drug is infused too rapidly, that is, in less than 30 minutes (Creaven et al 1974). Stomatitis has been infrequently reported, along with one possible case of drug-induced pancreatitis. Rare instances of generalized allergic reactions and anaphylaxis are reported (Dombernowsky et al 1972). A few episodes of possible cardiotoxicity including myocardial infarction and congestive heart failure have also been described (Aisner et al 1982b).

Bronchospasm with severe wheezing has been rarely observed and has usually been responsive to antihistamines and glucocorticosteroids. There is a single case report of a myocardial infarction occurring in a 27-year-old female who received VP-16 after mediastinal irradiation (Schechter et al 1975). A single case report of radiation recall skin reaction is also associated with the drug (Fontana 1979). In this instance, a female lung cancer patient developed localized erythematous, urticarial eruptions only in skin areas overlying the field. This occurred 18 hours after a first intravenous dose of etoposide and 3 weeks after radiation. There was complete healing in about 10 days; however, with a second dose 3 weeks later the identical toxic reaction developed.

Chemical phlebitis is also reported for etoposide but the drug is not a vesicant once diluted. For inadvertent extravasations of highly concentrated etoposide solution, hyaluronidase was effective in an experimental mouse model (Dorr and Alberts 1983). In each case the various solubilizers in the diluent solution are highly implicated. Immune suppression appears to be minimal with this drug (EORTC 1973).

Neurotoxicity is rarely reported with etoposide. This has consisted of sommolence and fatigue in 3% of patients and peripheral neuropathy in less than 1% of patients. The drug may also exacerbate preexisting neuropathy caused by vincristine (Thant et al 1982). Predisposing factors included advanced age, impaired nutritional status, and poor performance status. Degradation of myelin lamellae was noted in affected nerves.

There are also suggestions that etoposide may be leukemogenic in drug combinations which often include cisplatin (Ratain et al 1987, DeVore et al 1989, Pedersen-Bjergaard et al 1990). Recently, weekly or biweekly VM-26 and/or VP-16 as part of maintenance therapy for acute lymphocytic leukemia in children has been associated with an increased risk (12%) of developing secondary acute myelogenous leukemia (Pui et al 1991). A lower 5.9% risk of secondary leukemia was reported by Winick et al (1993). Other factors such as concomitant radiation and alkylating agents are probable cofactors (Murphy 1993). The prolonged schedules involving weekly or biweekly etoposide dosing was felt to contribute substantially to the increased leukemogenic risk, compared with the 1.6% risk with therapy every 2 weeks during remission induction only. Epipodophyllotoxin-induced secondary leukemias tend to lack a myelodysplastic phase and involve monoblasts or myelomonoblasts and translocation of the long arm of chromosome 11 (11q23) (Pui et al 1989).

■ Special Applications

Intraperitoneal Administration. Despite preclinical data showing peritonitis with intraperitoneal injections (Stahelin 1976), etoposide has been safely administered intraperitoneally with cisplatin. Doses of 350 mg/m^2 VP-16 were directly mixed with 200 mg/m^2 cisplatin and administered intraperitoneally in 2L of normal saline via a Tenckhoff catheter (Zimm et al 1987). A 4-hour dwell time was used. Total peritoneal drug clearance was 12.6 mL/min/m^2, with a AUC in the intraperitoneal space of 470 µg/mL·h. The ratio of peak peritoneal drug levels to plasma drug levels was 6.6:1 for total drug and 188:1 for free (unbound) drug; however, the fractional AUCs for intraperitoneal:plasma compartments was only 1.5 for total drug but 65 for free drug. This indicates a relatively good selective localization of unbound drug in the intraperitoneal space. Peak plasma concentrations of 32 µg/mL were measured and the half-life of drug in the intraperitoneal space was short at about 3 hours (Zimm et al 1987).

Objective responses were noted in 7 of 39 patients, and the primary dose-limiting toxic effect was myelosuppression with a mean nadir granulocyte count of 1000/mm^3. Abdominal pain was reported in one third of patients, but only 3 of 39 patients experienced chemical peritonitis. Nausea and vomiting occurred in all patients but was due mainly to cisplatin.

In another trial, higher maximally tolerated doses of 700 mg/m^2 were instilled intraperitoneally in 2 L of normal saline after drainage of ascites (O'Dwyer et al 1991). The dwell time was 4 hours followed by drainage. Abdominal pain was the principal acute toxic effect and was easily controlled with nonsteroidal anti-inflammatory agents. Neutropenia was the dose-limiting toxic effect. Other toxic effects included thrombocytopenia, nausea and vomiting, and alopecia. Etoposide pharmacokinetics were similar to that in the prior study. The mean plasma half-life was 7.7 hours (range, 4.2–15.6 hours), whereas the harmonic mean half-life of the drug in the peritoneum was 3.5 hours (range, 1.9–7.8 hours). The relative pharmacologic advantage (ratio of peritoneal to plasma AUC) for drug localization in the intraperitoneal space was 2.8 for total drug and 47 for free drug as a result of the minimal protein binding in the intraperitoneal space.

Intrapleural Administration. Ten patients with malignant pleural effusions were treated with a range of etoposide doses diluted in 500 mL of normal saline, which was infused over 2 hours into the pleural space after complete drainage. A monthly course involved three consecutive weekly doses. Myelotoxicity was severe at 225 mg/m^2 and mild at doses of 150 mg/m^2. Clearance from the pleural cavity was 2 mL/min/m^2, and peak pleural drug levels were greater than 300 µg/mL with simultaneous plasma levels less than 10 µg/mL. The intrapleural AUC values ranged from 572 to 2099. Although effusions did not disappear in 9 of 10 patients, there was cytologic evidence of a local response in most patients (Holoye et al 1990). There was no local toxicity, but mild emesis, alopecia, and malaise were common and progressive.

High-Dose Etoposide With or Without Bone Marrow Transplantation. Etoposide is commonly used at high doses to treat a variety of malignancies. The drug has also been used in vitro to purge bone marrow using 2-hour drug incubations at concentrations of 20 to 125 µM (Ciobanu et al 1986). When used as a single agent in patients with solid tumors, etoposide 3.5 g/m^2 produced dose-limiting oropharyngeal mucositis (Postmus et al 1984). Myelosuppression was severe but reversible, with recovery of leukocyte counts to more than 1000/mm^3 and platelet counts to more than 50,000/mm^3 by days 17 to 23 after dosing. Mucositis recovered in the same time frame and was not cumulative with consecutive courses. Skin lesions were observed on the trunk and neck comparable to the recently described case of Stevens–Johnson syndrome with lower-dose etoposide (Holthuis et al 1983). Hypotension was rarely encountered. Partial responses were observed in 9 of 17 evaluable patients with a variety of solid tumors (Postmus et al 1984).

When used with autologous bone marrow transplantation (BMT), lower etoposide doses of 2.4 g/m^2 were recommended for phase II trials (Wolff et al 1983). A subsequent phase II trial of single-agent, high-dose etoposide and autologous BMT in germinal malignancies reported an overall 60% response rate, with complete responses in 2 of 10 patients and partial responses in 4 of 10 evaluable patients (Wolff et al 1984). Unfortunately, response durations were short at a median of 3.5 months. Toxic effects included severe myelosuppression, nausea and vomiting, alopecia, mucositis, and hepatitis. The hepatitis was reversible and was seen in only two patients who received total etoposide doses above 6 g/m^2 (Wolff et al 1984). A compensated metabolic acidosis was documented in 43% of patients, with serum bicarbonate levels dropping to as low as 16 to 18 mM within 1 week of therapy. This was readily reversible and was postulated to be caused by the complex etoposide cosolvent system.

High-dose etoposide doses of 25 to 70 mg/kg and total body irradiation (TBI) have also been combined as a preparatory regimen for bone marrow transplantation in patients with advanced hematologic malignancies (Blume et al 1987). A 60 mg/kg dose was found to be optimal in this study. The 4-hour drug infusions produced peak plasma levels of 100 μg/mL or greater. Unusual toxic effects in this regimen included a transient, somewhat painful rash on the palms, soles, and periorbital areas which lasted 1 to 3 weeks. Hemorrhagic cystitis was noted in patients not given aggressive hydration to maintain a high urine flow for 3 days after the drug infusion. No arrhythmias, serious hypotension, or metabolic acidosis occurred in this trial. This therapy produced a high disease-free survival rate of 43%, with a 32% relapse rate in patients with acute leukemia not in first relapse (Blume et al 1987). Prolonged responses were also obtained in 5 of 14 patients with other hematologic malignancies.

Etoposide has been added to a number of high-dose chemotherapy combination regimens. For example, in the treatment of relapsed Hodgkin's disease, three etoposide doses of 100 to 150 mg/m^2 are given every 12 hours for 3 consecutive days beginning 6 days prior to autologous BMT (Jagannath et al 1989). Four total etoposide doses were evaluated in the dose-escalation schema: 450, 600, 750, and 900 mg/m^2. The cyclophosphamide dose of 1.5 g/m^2/d × 4 was combined with a single carmustine dose of 300 mg/m^2. This produced a 47% complete response rate and an 18% partial response rate among 61 patients (Jagannath et al 1989). Remission durations were longer than 2 years. The authors did recommend limiting the total etoposide dose to 750 mg/m^2, as four patients who received the 900 mg/m^2 dose died within a month of treatment without recovering hematopoietic function. In other patients, the median time to hematologic recovery was 22 days for leukocytes and 26 days for platelets. This same high-dose CBV chemotherapy regimen with autologous BMT has been used successfully in adult patients with a variety of solid tumors (Spitzer et al 1980) and for relapsed acute leukemia.

High-Dose Etoposide Administration. A variety of intravenous infusion schedules have been used to deliver high-dose etoposide. Typically the drug is administered as a 4-hour infusion at a concentration of 1 mg/mL in saline (Blume et al 1987). This usually involves the administration of separate but consecutive hourly fractions of 500 mg/500 mL which are prepared immediately prior to use. This lessens the chance of drug precipitation if more concentrated dilutions are used (Wolff et al 1983). Another group used a final dilution of 0.8 mg/mL in saline administered over 1 to 1.5 hours with six infusions of equal amounts at 12-hour intervals (Postmus et al 1984).

Undiluted high-dose etoposide has also been infused as a single dose by syringe pump through a central venous catheter (Lazarus et al 1986). Fractional doses of 1 g/50 mL were delivered over 1 hour by this method. In some instances, however, cracking of ABS plastic devices occurred during these infusions (Schwinghammer and Reilly 1985). This appeared to be partially related to the weight of filled 50-mL syringes on specific lots of a plastic plenum cassette (Omni-Flow). Chemotherapy venting pins constructed of ABS plastic may also crack when used with undiluted etoposide solutions. Cracking with other types of hard plastic devices has been noted occasionally. Thus, close inspection of all infusion lines is needed when infusing undiluted etoposide.

The infusion of undiluted etoposide solutions has not been associated with hypotension, bronchospasm, or metabolic acidosis in one trial (Lazarus et al 1986); however, another group reported a dose-dependent drop in serum bicarbonate levels with this infusion method but no cracking of plastic infusion devices (Creger et al 1990). This method does seem to safely avoid the administration of large volumes of saline to deliver high-dose etoposide.

REFERENCES

Abeloff MD, Ettinger DS, Khouri N. Intensive induction therapy for small cell carcinoma of the lung (SCC). *Proc Am Assoc Cancer Res.* 1979;**20**:326.

Achterrath W, Niederle N, Raettig R, et al. Etoposide—Chemistry, preclinical and clinical pharmacology. *Cancer Treat Rev.* 1982;**9**:3–13.

Ahmann DL, Bissel HF, Eagan RT, et al. Phase II evaluation of VP-16-213 (NSC-141540) and cytembene (NSC 104801) in patients with advanced breast cancer. *Cancer Chemother Rep.* 1976;**58**:877–882.

Aisner J, Van Echo DA, Whitacre M, Wiernik PH. A phase I trial of continuous infusion VP-16-213 (etoposide). *Cancer Chemother Pharmacol.* 1982a;**7**:157–160.

Aisner J, Whitacre M, VanEcho DA, et al. Doxorubicin cyclophosphamide and VP-16-213 (ACE) in the treatment of small cell lung cancer. *Cancer Chemother Pharmacol.* 1982b;**7**:187–193.

Allen LM, Creaven PJ. Comparison of the human pharmacokinetics of VM-26 and VP-16, two antineoplastic epipodophyllotoxin glucopyranoside derivatives. *Eur J Cancer.* 1975;**11**:697–707.

Allen LM, Marcks C, Creaven PJ. 4'-Demethyl-epipodophyllic acid-9-(4,6-O-ethylidene-β-D-glucopyranoside), the major urinary metabolite of VP-16-213 in man. *Proc Am Assoc Cancer Res.* 1976;**17**:15.

Anderson RJ, Gambertoglio JG, Schrier RW. *Clinical Use of Drugs in Renal Failure.* Springfield, IL: Charles C Thomas; 1976:15–17.

Arbuck SG, Douglass HO, Crom WR, et al. Etoposide pharmacokinetics in patients with normal and abnormal organ function. *J Clin Oncol.* 1986;**4**:1690–1695.

Barlogie B, Velasquez WS, Alexanian R, Cabanillas F. Etoposide, dexamethasone, cytarabine, and cisplatin in vincristine, doxorubicin, and dexamethasone-refractory myeloma. *J Clin Oncol.* 1989;**7**:1514–1518.

Bennett C, Sinkule JA, Schilsky RL, et al. Phase I clinical and pharmacological study of 72-hour continuous infusion of etoposide in patients with advanced cancer. *Cancer Res.* 1987;**47**:1952–1956.

Blume KG, Forman SJ, O'Donnell MR, et al. Total body irradiation and high-dose etoposide: A new preparatory regimen for bone marrow transplantation in patients with advanced hematologic malignancies. *Blood.* 1987;**69**(4):1015–1020.

Bonomi PD, O'Reilly WS, Vogl S, et al. A phase II trial of cyclophosphamide, VP-16 and methotrexate in small cell bronchogenic carcinoma (SCBC): An ECOG pilot study. *Proc Am Soc Clin Oncol.* 1983;**2**:199.

Bosl GJ, Jain K, Dukeman M, et al. VP-16 and cisplatin (DDP) in the treatment of patients (PTS) with advanced germ cell tumors (GCT). *Proc Am Soc Clin Oncol.* 1982;**1**:114.

Broder LE, Selawry OS, Charyulu KN, et al. A controlled clinical trial testing two potentially non-cross-resistant chemotherapeutic regimens in small-cell carcinoma of the lung. *Chest.* 1981;**79**:327–335.

Carney DN, Grogan L, Smit EF, et al. Single-agent oral etoposide for elderly small cell lung cancer patients. *Semin Oncol.* 1990;**17**:49–53.

Cavalli F, Sonntag RW, Jungi F, et al. VP-16-213 monotherapy for remission induction of small cell lung cancer: A randomized trial using three dosage schedules. *Cancer Treat Rep.* 1978;**62**:473–475.

Cecil JW, Quagliana JM, Coltman CA, et al. Evaluation of VP-16-213 in malignant lymphoma and melanoma. *Cancer Treat Rep.* 1978;**62**(5):801–803.

Chatterjee S, Trivedi D, Petzold SJ, Berger NA. Mechanism of epipodophyllotoxin-induced cell death in poly(adenosine diphosphate-ribose) synthesis-deficient V7 Chinese hamster cell lines. *Cancer Res.* 1990;**50**:2713–2718.

Ciobanu N, Paietta E, Andreeff M, et al. Etoposide as an in vitro purging agent for the treatment of acute leukemias and lymphomas in conjunction with autologous bone marrow transplantation. *Exp Hematol.* 1986;**14**:626–635.

Cohen MH, Broder LE, Fossieck BE, et al. Phase II clinical trial of weekly administration of VP-16-213 in small cell bronchogenic carcinoma. *Cancer Treat Rep.* 1977a;**61**:(3):489–490.

Cohen MH, Creaven PJ, Fossieck BE Jr, et al. Intensive chemotherapy of small cell bronchogenic carcinoma. *Cancer Treat Rep.* 1977b;**61**:349–354.

Creagan ET, Richardson RL, Kovach JS. Pilot study of a continuous five-day intravenous infusion of etoposide concomitant with cisplatin in selected patients with advanced cancer. *J Clin Oncol.* 1988;**6**:1197–1201.

Creaven PJ. The clinical pharmacology of VM-26 and VP-16-213: A brief overview. *Cancer Chemother Pharmacol.* 1982;**7**:133–140.

Creaven PJ, Allen LM. EPEG, a new antineo-plastic epipodophyllotoxin. *Clin Pharmacol Ther.* 1975;**18**:221–226.

Creaven PJ, Newman SJ, Selawry OS, et al. Phase I clinical trial of weekly administration of 4'-demethylepipodophyllotoxin 9-(4,6-O-ethylidene-β-D-glucopyranoside) (NSC-141540; VP-16-213). *Cancer Chemother Rep.* 1974;**58**:901–907.

Creger RJ, Fox RM, Lazarus HM. Infusion of high doses of undiluted etoposide through central venous catheters during preparation for bone marrow transplantation. *Cancer Invest.* 1990;**8**(1):13–16.

Crom WR, Kearns CM, Meyer WH, Rodman JH. Changes in etoposide pharmacokinetics during combination chemotherapy with ifosfamide in Ewing sarcoma patients. *Proc Am Assoc Cancer Res.* 1991;**32**:174.

DeVore R, Whitlock J, Hainsworth JD, et al. Therapy-related acute nonlymphocytic leukemia with monocytic features and rearrangement of chromosome 11q. *Ann Intern Med.* 1989;**110**:740–742.

D'Incalci M, Farina P, Sessa C, et al. Pharmacokinetics of VP-16-213 given by different administration methods. *Cancer Chemother Pharmacol.* 1982;**7**:141–145.

Dombernowsky P, Nissen NI. Schedule dependency of the antileukemic activity of the podophyllotoxin derivative VP-16-213 (NSC 141540) in L-1210 leukemia. *Acta Pathol Microbiol Scand.* 1973;**81**:715–724.

Dombernowsky P, Nissen NI. Combination chemotherapy with 4'-demethylepipodophyllotoxin 9-(4,6-O-ethylidene-β-D-glucopyranoside) VP-16-2B(NSC141540) in L-1201 leukemia. *Eur J Cancer.* 1976;**12**:181–188.

Dombernowsky P, Nissen NI, Larsen V. Clinical investigation of a new podophyllum derivative in patients with malignant lymphoma and solid tumors. *Cancer Chemother Rep.* 1972;**56**:71–82.

Dorr RT, Alberts DS. Skin ulceration potential without therapeutic anticancer activity for epipodophyllotoxin commercial diluents. *Invest New Drugs.* 1983;**1**:151–159.

Eagan RT, Fryfak S, Rubin J. VP-16 vs polychemotherapy in small cell lung cancer. *Proc Am Assoc Cancer Res.* 1976;**17**:243.

Einhorn LH. Initial therapy with cisplatin + VP-16 in small cell lung cancer. *Semin Oncol.* 1986;**13**:5–9.

Einhorn LH, Penington K, McClean J. Phase II trial of daily oral VP-16 in refractory small cell lung cancer: A Hoosier Oncology Group study. *Semin Oncol.* 1990;**17**:32–35.

European Organization for Research on the Treatment of Cancer, Clinical Screening Group. Epipodophyllotoxin VP-16-213 in treatment of acute leukemias, haematosarcomas and solid tumors. *Br Med J.* 1973;**3**:199–207.

Evans WE, Sinkule JA, Crom WR, et al. Pharmacokinetics of teniposide (VM-26) and etoposide (VP-16-213) in children with cancer. *Cancer Chemother Pharmacol.* 1982;**7**:145–150.

Falkson G, Van Dyk JJ, Van Eden EB, et al. A clinical trial of the oral form of 4'-demethyl-epipodophyllotoxin-β-D-ethylidene glucoside (NSC-141540) VP-16-213. *Cancer.* 1975;**35**:1141–1144.

Fisher RI, DeVita VT Jr, Hubbard SM, et al. Diffuse aggressive lymphomas: Increased survival after alternating flexible sequences of ProMACE and MOPP chemotherapy. *Ann Intern Med.* 1983;**98**:304–309.

Fontana JA. Radiation recall associated with VP-16-213 therapy (letter). *Cancer Treat Rep.* 1979;**63**(2):224–225.

Glisson BS, Ross WE. DNA topoisomerase II: A primer on the enzyme and its unique role as a multidrug target in cancer chemotherapy. *Pharmacol Ther.* 1987;**32**:89–106.

Gouyette A, Deniel A, Pico J-L, et al. Clinical pharmacology of high-dose etoposide associated with cisplatin. Pharmacokinetic and metabolic studies. *Eur J Cancer Clin Oncol.* 1987;**23**:1627–1632.

Greco A, Johnson DH, Hainsworth JD. Chronic daily administration of oral etoposide. *Semin Oncol.* 1990;**17**:71–74.

Greco FA, Einhorn LH, Hande KE, Oldham RK. Phase II studies in resistant small cell lung cancer. *Proc Am Assoc Cancer Res.* 1979;**20**:28.

Hainsworth JD, Johnson DH, Frazier SR, Greco FA. Chronic daily administration of oral etoposide—A phase I trial. *J Clin Oncol.* 1989;**7**:396–401.

Hande KR, Wedlund PJ, Noone RM. Pharmacokinetics of high dose etoposide (VP-16-213) administered to cancer patients. *Cancer Res.* 1984;**44**:379–382.

Hande KR, Wolff SN, Greco A, et al. Etoposide kinetics in patients with obstructive jaundice. *J Clin Oncol.* 1990;**8**:1101–1107.

Hande KR, Krozely MG, Greco A, et al. Bioavailability of low-dose oral etoposide. *J Clin Oncol.* 1993;**11**:374–377.

Harvey VJ, Slevin ML, Joel SP, et al. The pharmacokinetics of oral etoposide (VP-16-213). *Proc Am Soc Clin Oncol.* 1984;**3**:24.

Harvey VJ, Slevin ML, Joel SP, et al. The effect of food and concurrent chemotherapy on the bioavailability of oral etoposide. *Br J Cancer.* 1985;**52**:363–367.

Holoye PY, Jeffries DG, Dhingra HM, et al. Intrapleural etoposide for malignant effusion. *Cancer Chemother Pharmacol.* 1990;**26**:147–150.

Holthuis JJM, Postmus PE, Sleijfer DTH, et al. Pharmacokinetics of etoposide (VP-16-213) after high-dose intravenous administration (abstract). In: *Second European Conference on Clinical Oncology.* 1983;**13**:2–19.

Holthuis JJM, Van de Vyver FL, van Oort WJ, et al. Pharmacokinetic evaluation of increasing dosages of etoposide in a chronic hemodialysis patient. *Cancer Treat Rep.* 1985;**69**:1279–1282.

Jacobs P, King HS, Saly GRH. Epipodophyllotoxin (VP-16-2B) in the treatment of diffuse histiocytic lymphoma. *S Afr Med J.* 1975;**49**:483–485.

Jagannath S, Armitage JO, Dicke KA, et al. Prognostic factors for response and survival after high-dose cyclophosphamide, carmustine, and etoposide with autologous bone marrow transplantation for relapsed Hodgkin's disease. *J Clin Oncol.* 1989;**7**(2):179–185.

Joel S, Clark P, Slevin M. Renal function and etoposide pharmacokinetics: Is dose modification necessary. *Proc Am Soc Clin Oncol.* 1991;**10**:103.

Johnson DH, Greco FA, Strupp J, et al. Prolonged administration of oral etoposide in patients with relapsed or refractory small-cell lung cancer: A phase II trial. *J Clin Oncol.* 1990;**8**:1613–1617.

Jungi WF. Etoposide single-agent chemotherapy for solid tumors. *Cancer Treat Rev.* 1982;**9**:31–37.

Jungi WF, Senn HJ. Clinical study of the new podophyllotoxin derivative, 4'-demethylepipodophyllotoxin 9-(4,6-O-ethylidene-β-D-glucopyranoside) (NSC-141540; VP-16-213) in solid tumors in man. *Cancer Chemother Rep.* 1975;**59**:737–742.

Kaplan I. Condylomata acuminata. *New Orleans Med Surg J.* 1942;**94**:388–390.

Keller-Justin C, Kuhn M, Von Wartburg A. Synthesis and antimitotic activity of glycosidic lignan derivatives related to podophyllotoxin. *J Med Chem.* 1971;**14**:936–940.

Kelly M, Hartwell J. The biological effects and chemical composition of podophyllin. A review. *J Natl Cancer Inst.* 1954;**14**:967–1010.

Klastersky J, Nicaise C, Longeval E, Stryckmans P. Cisplatinum, Adriamycin, and etoposide (CAV) for remission induction of small-cell bronchogenic carcinoma: Evaluation of efficacy and toxicity and pilot study of a "late intensification" with autologous bone-marrow rescue. *Cancer.* 1982;**50**:652–658.

Krishan A, Paikg K, Frei E III. Cytofluorometric studies on the action of podophyllotoxin and epipodophyllotoxins (VM-26 and VP-16-213) on the cell cycle traverse of human lymphoblasts. *J Cell Biol.* 1975;**66**:521–530.

Krook JE, Jett JR, Little C. A phase I–II study of sequential infusion VP-16 and cisplatin therapy in advanced lung cancer. *Am J Clin Oncol.* 1989;**12**:114–117.

Lau ME, Hansen HH, Nissen NI, Pedersen H. Phase I trial of a new form of an oral administration of VP-16-213. *Cancer Treat Rep.* 1979;**63**(3):485–487.

Laubenstein LJ, Krigel RL, Hymes KB, Muggia FM. Treatment of epidemic Kaposi's sarcoma with VP-16-213 (etoposide) and a combination of doxorubicin, bleomycin, and vinblastine (ABV). *Proc Am Soc Clin Oncol.* 1983;**2**:228.

Lazarus HM, Creger RJ, Diaz D. Simple method for the administration of high-dose etoposide during autologous bone marrow transplantation. *Cancer Treat Rep.* 1985;**70**(6):819–820.

Leak RE, Woodford JD. Pharmaceutical development of ondansetron injection. *Eur J Cancer Clin Oncol.* 1989;**25**(suppl 1):S67–S69.

Loike JD, Horwitz SB. Effect of VP-16-213 on the intracellular degradation of DNA and HeLA cells. *Biochem.* 1976;**15**:5443–5448.

Lokich J, Anderson N, Bern M, et al. Etoposide admixed with cisplatin. Phase I clinical investigation of 72-hour infusion. *Cancer.* 1989;**63**:818–821.

Lokich J, Corkey J. Phase I study of VP-16-213 (etoposide) administered as a continuous 5-day infusion. *Cancer Treat Rep.* 1981;**65**:887–889.

Lum BL, Kaubisch S, Gosland MP, et al. The effect of cyclosporine (CSA) on etoposide (E) pharmacokinetics in a phase I trial of E with CSA as a modulator of multidrug resistance (MDR). *Proc Am Soc Clin Oncol.* 1991;**10**:102.

Mabel JA. Therapeutic synergism in murine tumors for combinations of *cis*-diammine dichloroplatinum with VP-16-2B or BCNU. *Proc Am Assoc Cancer Res.* 1979;**20**:230.

Mathe G, Schwar-Zenberg L, Poillart P, et al. Two epipodophyllotoxin derivatives, VM-26 and VP-16-213, in the treatment of leukemias, hematosarcomas and lymphomas. *Cancer.* 1974;**34**:985–992.

Miller AA, Stewart CF, Tolley EA. Clinical pharmacodynamics of continuous-infusion etoposide. *Cancer Chemother Pharmacol.* 1990;**25**:361–366.

Misra NC, Roberts D. Inhibition by 4'-demethyl-epipodophyllotoxin 9-(4,6-O-2-ethylidene-β-D-glucopyranoside) of human lymphoblast cultures in G_2 phase of the cell cycle. *Cancer Res.* 1975;**35**:99–105.

Murphy SB. Secondary acute myeloid leukemia following treatment with epipodophyllotoxins (Editorial) *J Clin Oncol.* 1993;**11**:199–201.

Nissen NI, Dombernowsky P, Hansen HH, Larsen V. Phase I clinical trial of an oral solution of VP-16-213. *Cancer Treat Rep.* 1976;**60**(7):943–945.

Nissen NI, Hansen HH, Pedersen H, et al. Clinical trial of the oral form of a new podophyllotoxin derivative, VP-16-213(NSC-141540), in patients with advanced neoplastic disease. *Cancer Chemother Rep Part 1.* 1975;**59**(5):1027–1029.

Nissen NI, Larsen V, Pedersen H, et al. Phase I clinical trial of a new antitumor agent. 4'-demethylepipodophyllotoxin-9-(4,6-O-ethylidene-D-glucopyranoside) (NSC-141540; VP-16-213). *Cancer Chemother Rep.* 1972;**56**:769–777.

Nissen NI, Pajak TF, Leone LA, et al. Clinical trial of VP-16-213 (NSC 141540) I.V. twice weekly in advanced neoplastic disease. *Cancer.* 1980;**45**:232–235.

O'Dwyer PJ, LaCreta FP, Daugherty JP, et al. Phase I pharmacokinetic study of intraperitoneal etoposide. *Cancer Res.* 1991;**51**:2041–2046.

O'Dwyer PJ, Leyland-Jones B, Alonso MT, et al. Etoposide (VP-16-213): Current status of an active anticancer drug. *N Engl J Med.* 1985;**312**:692–700.

Pedersen AG, Hansen HH. Etoposide (VP-16) in the treatment of lung cancer. *Cancer Treat Rev.* 1983;**10**:245–264.

Pedersen-Bjergaard J, Philip P, et al. Chromosome aberrations and prognostic factors in therapy-related myelodysplasia and acute nonlymphocytic leukemia. *Blood.* 1990;**76**:1083–1091.

Perry MC. Hepatotoxicity of chemotherapeutic agents. *Semin Oncol.* 1982;**9**:65–74.

Pfluger K-H, Schmidt L, Merkel M, et al. Drug monitoring of etoposide (VP-16-213). Correlation of pharmacokinetic parameters to clinical and biochemical data from patients receiving etoposide. *Cancer Chemother Pharmacol.* 1987;**20**:59–66.

Postmus PE, Holthuis JJM, Haazma-Reiche H, et al. Penetration of VP-16-213 into cerebrospinal fluid after high-dose intravenous administration. *J Clin Oncol.* 1984;**2**(3):215–220.

Postmus PE, Mulder NH, Sleijfer DT, et al. High-dose etoposide for refractory malignancies: A phase I study. *Cancer Treat Rep.* 1984;**68**(12):1471–1474.

Pui C-H, Behm FG, Raimondi SC, et al. Secondary acute myeloid leukemia in children treated for acute lymphoid leukemia. *N Engl J Med.* 1989;**321**:136–142.

Pui C-H, Ribeiro RC, Hancock ML, et al. Acute myeloid leukemia in children treated with epipodophyllotoxins for acute lymphoblastic leukemia. *N Engl J Med.* 1991;**325**:1682–1687.

Ratain MJ, Kaminer LS, Bitran JD, et al. Acute nonlymphocytic leukemia following etoposide and cisplatin combination chemotherapy for advanced non-small-cell carcinoma of the lung. *Blood.* 1987;**70**:1412–1417.

Rivera G, Avery T, Roberts C. Response of L-1210 to combinations of cytosine arabinoside and VM-26 or VP-16-213. *Eur J Cancer.* 1975;**11**:639–647.

Ross W, Towe T, Glisson B, et al. Role of topoisomerase II in mediating epipodophyllotoxin-induced DNA cleavage. *Cancer Res.* 1984;**44**:5857–5860.

Rozencweig M, Von Hoff DD, Henney JE, Muggia FM. VM-26 and VP-16-213: A comparative analysis. *Cancer.* 1977;**40**:334–342.

Saito H, Brown NS, Ho DH, et al. Pharmacokinetic study of 72-hour continuous infusion of cisplatin and etoposide in patients with non-small cell lung cancer. *Proc Am Assoc Cancer Res.* 1991;**32**:173.

Schecter JP, Jones SE, Jackson RA. Myocardial infarction in a 27 year old woman: Possible complication of treatment with VP-16-213 (NSC 141540), mediastinal irradiation or both. *Cancer Treat Rep Part 1.* 1975;**59**(5):887–888.

Schmoll H. Review of etoposide single-agent activity. *Cancer Treat Rev.* 1982;**9**(suppl A):21–30.

Schwinghammer TL, Reilly M. Cracking of ABS plastic devices used to infuse undiluted etoposide injection. 1988; *Am J Hosp Pharm.* **45**:1277.

Seargeant LE, Kobrinsky NL, Sus CJ, Nazeravich DR. In vitro stability and compatibility of daunorubicin, cytarabine, and etoposide. *Cancer Treat Rep.* 1987;**71**:1189–1192.

Sinkule JA, Hutson P, Hayes FA, et al. Pharmacokinetics of etoposide (VP-16) in children and adolescents with refractory solid tumors. *Cancer Res.* 1984;**44**:3109–3113.

Slater L, Murray S, Wetzel M, et al. Verapamil potentiation of VP-16-213 in acute lymphatic leukemia (ALL) in vivo and reversal of pleiotropic drug resistance (PDR). *Proc Am Assoc Cancer Res.* 1985;**26**:336.

Slayton R, Petty W, Blessing J. Phase II trial of VP-16 in treatment of advanced ovarian adenocarcinoma. *Proc Am Assoc Cancer Res.* 1979;**20**:190.

Slevin ML, Clark PI, Joel SP, et al. A randomized trial to evaluate the effect of schedule on the activity of etoposide in small-cell lung cancer. *J Clin Oncol.* 1989a;**7**:1333–1340.

Slevin ML, Joel SP, Whomsley R, et al. The effect of dose on the bioavailability of oral etoposide: Confirmation of a clinically relevant observation. *Cancer Chemother Pharmacol.* 1989b;**24**:329–331.

Smith PJ, Anderson CO, Watson JV. Predominant role for DNA damage in etoposide-induced cytotoxicity and cell cycle perturbation in human SV40-transformed fibroblasts. *Cancer Res.* 1986;**46**:5641–5645.

Smyth RD, Pfeffer M, Scalzo A, Comis RL. Bioavailability and pharmacokinetics of etoposide (VP-16) *Semin Oncol.* 1985;**12**:48–51.

Spitzer G, Dicke KA, Litam J, et al. High-dose combination chemotherapy with autologous bone marrow transplantation in adult solid tumors. *Cancer.* 1980;**45**:3075–3085.

Stahelin H. Activity of new glycosidic lignan derivative (VP-16-213) related to podophyllotoxin in experimental tumors. *Eur J Cancer.* 1973;**9**:215–221.

Stahelin H. Delayed toxicity of epipodophyllotoxin derivatives (VM-26 and VP-16-213) due to a local effect. *Eur J Cancer.* 1976;**12**:925–931.

Steward WP, Thatcher N, Edmundson JM, et al. Etoposide infusions for treatment of metastatic lung cancer. *Cancer Treat Rep.* 1984;**68**:897–899.

Stewart CF, Arbuck SG, Fleming RA, Evans WE. Changes in the clearance of total and unbound etoposide in patients with liver dysfunction. *J Clin Oncol.* 1990;**8**:1874–1879.

Stewart CF, Hampton EM. Stability of cisplatin and etoposide in intravenous admixtures. *Am J Hosp Pharm.* 1989;**46**:1400–1404.

Stewart DJ, Richard M, Hugenholtz H, Dennery J. VP-16 (VP) and VM-26 (VM) penetration into human brain tumors (BT). *Proc Am Assoc Cancer Res.* 1983;**24**:133.

Tewey KM, Chen GL, Nelson EM, Liu LF. Intercalative antitumor drugs interfere with the breakage–reunion reaction of mammalian DNA topoisomerase II. *J Biol Chem.* 1984;**259**:9182–9187.

Thant M, Hawley RJ, Smith MT, et al. Possible enhancement of vincristine neuropathy by VP-16. *Cancer.* 1982;**49**:859–864.

Trissel LA, Fulton B, Tramonte SM. Visual compatibility of ondansetron with chemotherapeutic agents, antibiotics, and other selected drugs during simulated Y-site injection (abstract #P-468R). In: *Twenty-fifty Annual ASHP Midyear Clinical Meeting and Exhibit, Las Vegas, Nevada,* December 1990.

Valdivieso M, Cabanillas F, Bedikian AY, et al. Intensive induction chemotherapy (IIC) of small cell lung cancer (SCLC) with ECHO: E=epipodophyllotoxin VP-16, C=cytoxan, H=hydroxydaunorubicin, O=oncovin. *Proc Am Assoc Cancer Res.* 1979;**20**:382.

Van Echo DA, Aisner J, Wiernik PH, et al. Combination chemotherapy of advanced breast cancer with Adriamycin and VP-16-213. *Proc Am Assoc Cancer Res.* 1979;**20**:228.

Van Maanen JMS, Holthuis JJM, Gobas F, et al. Role of bioactivation in covalent binding of VP-16 to rat liver and HeLa cell microsomal proteins. *Proc Am Assoc Cancer Res.* 1983;**24**:319.

Venditti JM. Treatment schedule dependency of experimentally active antileukemic (L-1210) drugs. *Cancer Chemother Rep.* 1971;**2**(3):35–59.

Williams SD, Einhorn LH. Etoposide salvage therapy for refractory germ cell tumors: An update. *Cancer Treat Rev.* 1982;**9**(suppl A):67–71.

Williams SD, Einhorn LH, Greco FA, et al. VP-16-213 salvage therapy for refractory germinal neoplasms. *Cancer.* 1980;**46**:2154–2158.

Williams SD, Einhorn LH, Greco A, et al. VP-16-213: An active drug in germinal neoplasms. *Proc Am Assoc Cancer Res.* 1979;**20**:72.

Winick NJ, McKenna RW, Shuster JJ, et al. Secondary acute myeloid leukemia in children with acute lymphoblastic leukemia treated with etoposide. *J Clin Oncol.* 1993;**11**:209–217.

Wolff SN, Fer MF, McKay CM, et al. High-dose VP-16-213 and autologous bone marrow transplantation for refractory malignancies: A phase I study. *J Clin Oncol.* 1983;**1**(11):701–705.

Wolff SN, Johnson DH, Hainsworth JD, Greco FA. High-dose VP-16-213 monotherapy for refractory germinal malignancies: A phase II study. *J Clin Oncol.* 1984;**2**(4):271–274.

Wozniak AJ, Glisson BS, Hande KR, Ross WE. Inhibition of etoposide-induced DNA damage and cytotoxicity in L-1210 cells by dehydrogenase inhibitors and other agents. *Cancer Res.* 1984;**44**:626–632.

Wozniak AJ, Ross WE. DNA damage as a basis for 4'-demethylepipodophyllotoxin-9-(4,6-O-ethylidene-β-D-glucopyranoside) (etoposide) cytotoxicity. *Cancer Res.* 1983;**43**:120–124.

Yalowich J, Fry D, Goldman ID. Teniposide (VM-26) and etoposide (VP-16-213) in induced augmentation of methotrexate transport and polyglutamation in Ehrlich ascites tumor cells in vitro. *Cancer Res.* 1987;**42**:3648–3653.

Yalowich JC, Goldman ID, Back N. Analysis of the inhibitory effects of VP-16 and podophyllotoxin (PDT) on thymidine (dThd) transport and metabolism in Ehrlich ascites tumor cells in vitro. *Proc Am Assoc Cancer Res.* 1983;**24**:309.

Yalowich JC, Ross WE. Potentiation of etoposide-induced DNA damage by calcium antagonist in L-1210 cells in vitro. *Cancer Res.* 1984;**44**:3360–3365.

Zimm S, Cleary SM, Lucas WE, et al. Phase I/pharmacokinetic study of intraperitoneal cisplatin and etoposide. *Cancer Res.* 1987;**47**:1712–1716.

Zupi G, Greco C, Sacchi A, Calabresi. Etoposide prior to *cis*-diamminedichloroplatinum in combination chemotherapy: In vitro and in vivo studies. *Eur J Cancer Clin Oncol.* 1985;**21**:1501–1506.

Fadrazole

■ Other Names

CGS 16949A (Ciba Geigy).

■ Chemistry

Structure of fadrazole

Fadrazole is a nonsteroidal tetrahydroimidazopyridine derivative that inhibits the enzyme aromatase. The complete chemical name is 4-[5,6,7,8-tetrahydroimidazo[1,5α]pyridin-5-yl]benzonitrile monohydrochloride. The molecular weight is 259.16.

■ Antitumor Activity

Fadrazole has been shown to significantly suppress circulating levels of estradiol and estrone in postmenopausal patients with breast cancer (Dowsett et al 1990, Lipton et al 1990, Raats et al 1992).

In a phase I trial of fadrazole in 16 heavily pretreated postmenopausal patients with metastatic breast cancer, there were 2 partial responses (13%) and 7 patients (44%) with stable disease (Lipton et al 1990). More recently, two different fadrazole dose schedules were compared in 78 postmenopausal breast cancer patients with metastatic disease (Raats et al 1992). Most patients had relapsed after prior hormonal therapy including tamoxifen. The overall objective response rate was 23%, composed of 10% complete responses and 13% partial responses. Another 45% of patients had stable disease on fadrazole (Raats et al 1992). Response rates did not differ significantly based on estrogen receptor status or with either a 1- or 4-mg daily dose. Median survival was 22.6 months at the 1-mg dose, and the overall median time to treatment failure was 4.4 months (Raats et al 1992). These results indicate that fadrazole has good activity as second-line hormonal therapy in postmenopausal patients with metastatic breast cancer.

Mechanism of Action

Fadrazole is a potent and highly specific inhibitor of the steroidal conversion enzyme aromatase (Steele et al 1987). This mechanism of action blocks the conversion of androstenedione to estrogenic or androgenic sex hormones in female or male animals, respectively. In preclinical studies, fadrazole is approximately 200 to 1000 times more potent than aminoglutethimide (Miller 1989, Dowsett et al 1990, Steele et al 1987). Both agents are competitive inhibitors of the aromatase enzyme. In vitro studies report an inhibition constant (K_i) of 1.6 nM for fadrazole in human placental microsomes (Steele et al 1987).

The reduction in sex hormone levels with fadrazole in humans is dose dependent and maximal after about 4 days of therapy (Dowsett et al 1990). Estrogen levels drop to 30% of pretreatment values and estrone levels fall to approximately 50% of pretreatment values. Of interest, serum aldosterone levels also fall in a dose-dependent fashion to approximately 40% of pretreatment levels after a dose of 2 mg twice daily (Dowsett et al 1990). A higher dose of 4 to 16 mg daily depressed aldosterone levels similarly (Lipton et al 1990). Levels of testosterone, cortisol, and 17-OH-progesterone remained unchanged with low-dose (1–2 mg) fadrazole therapy (Dowsett et al 1990). Higher doses of 4 to 16 mg/d increase the levels of 17-hydroxyprogesterone, testosterone, and Δ_4-androstenedione, suggesting a blockage of the C_{21}-hydroxylase enzyme (Lipton et al 1990). This effect has not been reported at the clinical doses of 1 to 2 mg/d.

The lack of glucocorticoid inhibitory effects with fadrazole contrasts sharply with the nonspecific inhibitory activity of aminoglutethimide, which blocks cortisol production and generally requires glucocorticoid supplementation. Fadrazole also does not produce the weak androgenic effects observed in animals treated with another specific aromatase inhibitor, 4-hydroxyandrostenedione (Brodie et al 1977, 1982).

Availability and Storage

Fadrazole is investigationally available from Ciba-Geigy (Basel, Switzerland). It has been supplied as tablets containing 0.3, 0.5, 1, and 2 mg. The tablets are stored at room temperature.

Administration

Fadrazole is taken orally, usually twice daily (Raats et al 1992, Lipton et al 1990, Dowsett et al 1990).

Dosage

A variety of oral doses have been evaluated in phase I trials with fadrazole. Dowsett et al (1990) compared twice daily doses of 0.3, 1.0, and 2.0 mg. Serum estrogen levels decreased maximally after the 2-mg dose level. The same conclusion was reached by Lipton et al (1990); maximal estrogen suppression is achieved with an oral dose of 2 mg twice daily. Higher dose levels of 4 to 16 mg/d appear to cause more nonspecific hormonal inhibition (see Mechanism of Action).

Pharmacokinetics

Gas chromatography has been used to follow the pharmacokinetics of fadrazole in cancer patients receiving twice daily doses of 2 or 8 mg (Lipton et al 1990). Peak plasma levels of 8 ng/mL and 25 ng/mL were achieved approximately 3 to 4 hours after patients ingested oral doses of 2 and 8 mg, respectively (Lipton et al 1990). The mean terminal-phase half-life was 10.5 hours (± 6.3 hours).

Side Effects and Toxicity

Fadrazole is typically very well tolerated. Reported side effects are non-life threatening and include mild nausea and vomiting (31%), fatigue (13%), leg cramps and lightheadedness (6% each), orthostatic hypotension (13%), and hot flashes (19%) (Lipton et al 1990). Loss of appetite is described in about 5% of patients (Raats et al 1992). No skin toxic effects or allergic effects are observed. Likewise, serum electrolytes and calcium are unchanged (Raats et al 1992). Thyroid-stimulating hormone and luteinizing hormone levels are unchanged, whereas follicle-stimulating hormone levels increase very slightly with fadrazole therapy of postmenopausal females (Raats et al 1992).

REFERENCES

Brodie AMH, Garrett WM, Hendrikson JR, et al. Effects of aromatase inhibitor 4-hydroxyandrostenedione and other compounds in the DMBA-induced breast cancer. *Cancer Res.* 1982;**42**:3360–3364.

Brodie AMH, Schwarzel WC, Shaikh AA, et al. The effect of an aromatase inhibitor 4-hydroxy-4-androstene-3, 17-dione on estrone-dependent processes in reproduction and breast cancer. *Endocrinology.* 1977;**100**:1684–1695.

Dowsett M, Stein RC, Mehta A, et al. Potency and selectivity of the non-steroidal aromatase inhibitor CGS 16949A in postmenopausal breast cancer patients. *Clin Endocrinol.* 1990;**32**:623–634.

Lipton A, Harvey HA, Demers LM, et al. A phase I trial of CGS 16949A. *Cancer.* 1990;**65**:1279–1285.

Miller WR. Aromatase inhibitors in the treatment of advanced breast cancer. *Cancer Treat Rev.* 1989;**16**:83–93.

Raats JI, Falkson G, Falkson HC. A study of fadrazole, a new aromatase inhibitor, in postmenopausal women with advanced metastatic breast cancer. *J Clin Oncol.* 1992;**10**:111–116.

Steele RE, Mellor LB, Sawyer WK, et al. In vitro and in vivo studies demonstrating potent and selective estrogen inhibition with the nonsteroidal aromatase inhibitor CGS 16949A. *Steroids.* 1987;**50**:147–161.

Fazarabine

■ Other Names

NSC-281272; Ara-AC.

■ Chemistry

Structure of fazarabine

Fazarabine is an analog of both 5-azacytidine and cytosine arabinoside and was first synthesized by Beisler and colleagues (1977, 1979). The complete chemical name is 1-β-D-arabinofuranosyl-5-azacytosine, or 4-amino-1-β-D-arabinofuranosyl-1,3,5-triazin-2(1)-one. The compound has a molecular weight of 244.2 and the empiric formula $C_8H_{12}N_4O_5$. The compound has demonstrated a wide spectrum of experimental antitumor activity, including activity against CX-1 colon, LX-1 lung, and MX-1 mammary xenografts, P-388 and L-1210 murine leukemia, Lewis lung carcinoma, and B-16 melanoma (Dalal et al 1986, Grem et al 1987, Wallace et al 1987, Driscoll et al 1985). There was schedule dependency, with multiple small fractions being more effective than less frequent doses.

■ Antitumor Activity

Fazarabine is undergoing phase I trials and early phase II testing. Unfortunately, it is too early to determine if the compound has any antitumor activity in humans.

■ Mechanism of Action

Fazarabine is first phosphorylated by deoxycytidine kinase (Townsend et al 1985). In fact, resistance of tumor cells to fazarabine is usually accomplished by a reduction in the ability of cells to phosphorylate fazarabine (Ahluwalia et al 1986).

Fazarabine, like cytosine arabinoside, inhibits DNA synthesis (Townsend et al 1985, Glazer and Knode 1984). There appears to be no effect on RNA or protein synthesis. The precise mechanism whereby fazarabine inhibits DNA synthesis is unknown.

■ Availability and Storage

Fazarabine is supplied by the National Cancer Institute in Bethesda, Maryland. The drug is supplied as a white lyophilized powder in 250-mg vials. The intact vial should be stored under refrigeration (2–8°C) (National Cancer Institute 1987).

■ Preparation for Use, Stability, and Admixture

The 250-mg vial is reconstituted with 25 mL of Sterile Water for Injection, USP, to yield a 10 mg/mL solution. The dose should immediately be further diluted in the appropriate amount of Lactated Ringer's Injection, USP, to yield a fazarabine concentration between 0.01 and 1 mg/mL. Because of decomposition, the infusion must be completed in 3 hours or less.

For a 24-hour infusion, the 250-mg vial should be reconstituted with 3.5 mL of sterile 70% (v/v) dimethylsulfoxide (DMSO) to yield a 70 mg/mL solution. The dose is further diluted with additional sterile 70% DMSO to yield the appropriate fazarabine concentration. This solution must be administered slowly through the side injection port of a running intravenous infusion of 5% Dextrose Injection, USP, using a syringe pump. A total volume of 12 mL with an infusion rate of 0.5 ml/h is suggested for fazarabine 70% DMSO solution (Mojaverian and Repta 1984). Prior to drug infusion, it is recommended that the accuracy of the syringe pump volume be verified.

Shelf-life studies of the intact vial are ongoing; however, further dilution of fazarabine reconstituted with sterile water to a final concentration of 0.01 to 1 mg/mL in Lactated Ringer's Injection, USP, results in a solution that exhibits about 10% decomposition in 3 hours at room temperature. Therefore, infusion of solutions prepared in lactated Ringer's must be used within 3 hours of mixture.

■ Administration

Fazarabine has been administered on two different schedules in phase I trials: (1) 30 mg/m^2/d × 5 in 100 mL lactated Ringer's solution administered over 45 minutes and repeated every 28 days (Leiby et al 1988); (2) 2.0 mg/m^2/h × 72 hours (Amato et al 1988, Surbone et al 1990). The latter infusion was prepared by reconstituting the 250 mg vial with 9.9 mL of 70% (v/v) DMSO in water (Tera Pharmaceutical), resulting in a final fazarabine concentration of 25 mg/mL. A 24-hour supply of drug was diluted to a final volume of 12 mL with 70% DMSO placed in a 12-mL syringe. The reader is encouraged to read the precise preparation used by Surbone et al (1990).

■ Special Precautions

None are known at this time.

■ Drug Interactions

None have been described.

■ Dosage

The maximally tolerated fazarabine dose in phase I studies was 72 mg/m^2/d × 5 days. This dose was highly myelotoxic. Surbone et al (1990) have recommended that in phase II studies, fazarabine be administered as a 72-hour continuous infusion at a dose of 2.0 mg/m^2/h (48 mg/m^2/d). The Southwest Oncology Group is also pursuing phase II trials using 30 mg/m^2/d for 5 days with each daily infusion given over 45 minutes.

■ Pharmacokinetics

Surbone and colleagues have reported limited pharmacokinetic results. Plasma concentrations at steady state (with the 72-hour continuous infusion) have ranged from 32 ng/mL (0.13 μM) to 137 ng/mL (0.6 μM).

The mean clearance was 647 mL/min/m^2 for patients treated at doses above 1.25 mg/m^2/h. Leiby et al, using the 45-minute infusion daily × 5, noted that the compound exhibited a biphasic decline with an apparent terminal half-life of 0.5 hour.

■ Side Effects and Toxicity

The dose-limiting toxic effects of fazarabine were reversible leukopenia and thrombocytopenia (Surbone et al 1990). Nadir days of leukopenia and thrombocytopenia were days 18 (range, 7–31) and 13 (range, 7–22), respectively. Increases in serum alkaline phosphatase and transaminase were also observed, as were sporadic nausea and vomiting.

Another problem was the odor from the DMSO, which is noted by visitors but not by the patient (Surbone et al 1990).

■ Special Applications

None are known at this time.

REFERENCES

Ahluwalia G, Cohen M, Kang G-J, et al. Arabinosyl-5-azacytosine: Mechanisms of native and acquired resistance. *Cancer Res.* 1986;**46**:4479–4485.

Amato R, Raber M, Newman R, Ho D, Schmidt S, McKelvey E. Phase I study of 5-azacytosine arabinoside (Ara-AC, fazarabine). *Proc Am Assoc Cancer Res.* 1988;**29**:770.

Beisler J, Abbasi MM, Driscoll JS. The synthesis and antitumor activity of arabinosyl-5-azacytosine. *Biochem Pharmacol.* 1977;**26**:2469–2472.

Beisler J, Abbasi M, Driscoll JS. Synthesis and antitumor activity of arabinosyl-5-azacytosine. *J Med Chem.* 1979;**22**:1230–1234.

Dalal M, Plowman J, Breitman TR, et al. Arabinofuranosyl-5-azacytosine: Antitumor and cytotoxic properties. *Cancer Res.* 1986;**46**:831–838.

Driscoll JS, John DG, Plowman J. Comparison of the activity of arabinosyl-5-azacytosine, arabinosyl cytosine, and 5-azacytidine against intracerebrally implanted L-1210 leukemia. *Invest New Drugs.* 1985;**3**:331–334.

Glazer RI, Knode MC. 1-β-D-arabinosyl-5-azacytosine: Cytocidal activity and effects on the synthesis and methylation of DNA in human colon carcinoma cells. *Mol Pharmacol.* 1984;**26**:381–387.

Grem JL, Shoemaker DD, Hoth DF, et al. Arabinosyl-5-azacytosine: A novel nucleoside entering clinical trials. *Invest New Drugs.* 1987;**5**:315–338.

Leiby JM, Malspeis L, Staubus AE, Kraut EH, Grever MR. Fazarabine (NSC 281272) is myelosuppressive at the initial dose level in a phase I study. *Proc Am Soc Clin Oncol.* 1988;**7**:235.

Mojaverian P, Repta AJ. Development of an intravenous formulation for the unstable investigational cytotoxic nucleosides 5-azacytosine arabinoside (NSC 281272) and 5-azacytidine (NSC 102816). *J Pharm Pharmacol.* 1984;**36**:728–733.

National Cancer Institute. *Fazarabine (ARA-AC) IND 29722.* Clinical Brochure. Washington, DC: U.S. Government Printing Office; January 1987.

Surbone A, Ford H, Kelley JA, et al. Phase I and pharmacokinetic study of arabinofuranosyl-5-azacytosine (fazarabine, NSC 281272). *Cancer Res.* 1990;**50**:1220–1225.

Townsend A, Leclerc J-M, Dutschman G, Cooney D, Cheng Y-C. Metabolism of 1-β-D-arabinofuranosyl-5-azacytosine and incorporation into DNA of human T-lymphoblastic cells (Molt-4). *Cancer Res.* 1985;**45**:3522–3528.

Wallace RE, Lindh D, Durr FE. Arabinosyl-5-azacytosine (Ara-AC, fazarabine, NSC-281272): Activity against human tumor xenografts (abstract 1216). *Proc Am Assoc Cancer Res.* 1987;**28**:307.

Fenretinide

■ Other Names

McN-R-1967; 4-HPR.

■ Chemistry

Fenretinide is a synthetic vitamin A derivative. The chemical name is N-4-hydroxyphenyl-all-*trans*-retinamide. It differs from retinol by the substitution of a parahydroxyphenylamide moiety for the alcohol on retinol. This substitution substantially increases the lipophilicity of the molecule compared with retinol.

■ Antitumor Activity

This retinoid has a high degree of therapeutic activity in murine models of bladder cancer (Moon et al 1982) and mammary carcinoma (Moon et al 1983). Experimental ovariectomy has been demonstrated to enhance the antitumor effect, possibly by increasing the expression of cytosolic retinoic acid-binding proteins (CRABPs). Fenretinide has also been shown to block the development of breast cancer in rats treated with a carcinogen (Moon et al 1979). In human tumor cell lines, fenretinide had modest activity against ovarian, lung, and breast cancer and melanoma cells in vitro (Meyskens et al 1983).

Fenretinide was inactive as an anticancer agent in a phase II trial with 15 breast cancer patients and 16 melanoma patients (Modiano et al 1990). All of these patients were heavily pretreated. Currently, the compound is being evaluated for chemopreventive activity in breast cancer patients at high risk of relapse following potentially curative primary therapy (Rotmensz et al 1991).

■ Mechanism of Action

The mechanism of action of fenretinide is felt to involve its binding to specific CRABPs; however, the exact mechanisms responsible for direct cytotoxic effects are unknown. Indeed, retinoids are generally classified as chemopreventive agents that can block tumorigenesis in selected animal models (Sporn and Newton 1978).

Structure of fenretinide

Availability and Storage

Fenretinide is investigationally available in 100- and 300-mg gelatin capsules from McNeil Pharmaceuticals, Fort Washington, Pennsylvania. The capsules are stored at room temperature.

Administration

This agent is administered orally after meals, a schedule associated with more consistent absorption.

Dosage

A tolerable daily dose of fenretinide is 300 to 400 mg/d orally (Modiano et al 1990). A 300-mg dose has been administered daily for over 6 months, but the recommended dose for phase II studies was 200 mg/d (Costa et al 1989). This dose has been safely administered for up to 42 months using a schedule that halted therapy on the last 3 days of each month (Rotmensz et al 1991). One pilot trial evaluated a daily dose of 800 mg in patients with basal cell carcinoma. This dose produced significant nyctalopia (Kaiser-Kupfer et al 1986).

Drug Interactions

Fenretinide increases the antitumor effects of tamoxifen in ovariectomized rats with mammary carcinoma (Ratko et al 1989, Dowlatshahi et al 1989). The mechanism for this enhanced activity is unknown. Fenretinide also reduces endogenous plasma retinol concentration by up to 60% in patients with advanced cancers (Peng et al 1989, Formelli et al 1989). There is also a concomitant drop in plasma retinol-binding protein levels in these patients. Retinol and fenretinide do not complex with each other, so the mechanism for the drop in plasma retinol levels with fenretinide is unknown. The drop in retinol and retinol-binding proteins occurs within 24 hours of starting fenretinide and is reversible on discontinuation of fenretinide (Formelli et al 1989).

Pharmacokinetics

Fenretinide differs from other retinoids in that in animals it accumulates extensively in adipose and other tissues, but not in the liver (Swanson et al 1980, 1981).

In humans, the drug is extensively metabolized by O-methylation to N-(4-methoxyphenyl)retinamide (4-MPR). The pharmacokinetics of an oral fenretinide dose of 300 mg in three cancer patients is summarized in the table. In this study, the parent drug exhibited a biphasic clearance from the plasma with a terminal half-life of approximately 14 hours. The majority of the total plasma retinoid exposure is due to the parent molecule, fenretinide. Clearance of the major metabolite, 4-MPR, is much more rapid than fenretinide's clearance (see table). Steady-state levels of fenretinide and 4-MPR average approximately 400 and 500 ng/mL, respectively, for a 200-mg daily dose administered for 12 months (Formelli et al 1989).

As previously discussed (see Drug Interactions), oral fenretinide significantly lowers plasma retinol and retinol-binding proteins (Peng et al 1989, Formelli et al 1989). This decrease averages 60% for retinol (range, 40–88%) and 47% for retinol-binding proteins (range, 23–65%) after 1 to 2 weeks of therapy. These reductions appear to be cumulative with chronic oral dosing (Peng et al 1989). Thus, after 3 to 4 weeks of fenretinide, plasma retinol levels are decreased by an average of 69% (range, 44–86%) and retinol-binding proteins are decreased by 53% (range, 39–65%).

Side Effects and Toxicity

Fenretinide increases serum triglycerides in 6% of breast cancer patients and elevates cholesterol concentrations by 13% in one fifth of patients (Modiano et al 1990). For unknown reasons, this was observed only in breast cancer patients. By far, the most com-

PHARMACOKINETICS OF FENRETINIDE IN THREE CANCER PATIENTS GIVEN 300 mg/300 mg/m²/d ORALLY

Retinoid	Half-life (h)	AUC (μg·h/mL)	Total Body Clearance (L/h/m²)	Peak Plasma Level* (ng/mL)	Time To Peak* (h)
4-HPR	13.7 (1.9)†	3.49 (0.76)	56.6 (13.3)	509	3–4
4-MPR	23	1.15	239.3	80	8–12

*Values from a single patient.
†Standard deviations in parentheses.
Data from Peng et al 1989.

mon toxic effects are a mild to moderate xerostomia and xerodermia (dry skin condition) (Costa et al 1989, Modiano et al 1990). Abnormal cutaneous photosensitivity (Ferguson and Johnson 1989) and nail dystrophy (Ferguson et al 1983) have been observed with other retinoids but not with fenretinide (Rotmensz et al 1991). This occurs in up to 52% of patients given 300 mg/d. Other toxic effects include cheilitis, blurred or double vision, nyctalopia (nightblindness), and fatigue. These side effects occur in 10% or less of patients given oral doses of 300 to 400 mg/d (Modiano et al 1990).

The nyctalopia from fenretinide has a rapid onset but readily reverses after discontinuation of therapy. At a dose of 300 mg daily for 6 months nightblindness occurred in 1 of 25 patients. Nyctalopia may be accompanied by decreased b-wave amplitude microvoltage on electroretinography (Modiano et al 1990). The higher (67%) incidence with an 800-mg daily dose suggests that this toxic effect is dose dependent (Kaiser-Kupfer et al 1986). This side effect and the pharmacokinetic interaction between retinol and fenretinide suggest that fenretinide significantly alters rod function by blocking vitamin A or by competing with retinol for binding sites on opsin.

Nausea and headache were only rarely reported and there were no changes in renal or hepatic indices. Some menstrual irregularities were described, particularly in patients between the ages of 45 and 55 (Costa et al 1989). This is similar to the effects observed with other retinoids (Halkier-Sorensen 1987). A slight anemia was noted in only 1 of 25 patients receiving 200 to 300 mg daily for 6 months (Costa et al 1989). No other hematologic effects were observed.

Retinoids can also induce skeletal hyperostosis in the long bones following high-dose therapy (Gerber et al 1954). This can lead to bone fractures in hypervitaminosis A (Sower and Wallace 1990). In one series, 4 of 53 fenretinide-treated patients with breast cancer were noted to have abnormal bone densitometric evaluations but without any pathologic sequelae (Rotmensz et al 1991). The clinical significance of this finding, if any, is unclear.

Patients receiving fenretinide do not appear to experience a significantly greater degree of depressive symptoms. Although a general mood index survey may become slightly more negative on therapy (Rotmensz et al 1991), no serious psychologic changes are induced by long-term therapy (Filiberti et al 1988).

REFERENCES

Costa A, Malone W, Perloff M, et al. Tolerability of the synthetic retinoid fenretinide (HPR). *Eur J Cancer Clin Oncol.* 1989;**25**:805–808.

Dowlatshahi K, Mehta RG, Thomas CF, et al. Therapeutic effect of N-[4-hydroxyphenyl]retinamide on N-methyl-N-nitrosourea induced rat mammary cancer. *Cancer Lett.* 1989;**47**(3):187–192.

Ferguson J, Johnson BE. Retinoid associated phototoxicity and photosensitivity. *Pharmacol Ther.* 1989;**40**:123–135.

Ferguson J, Simpson NB, Hammersley N. Severe nail dystrophy associated with retinoid therapy. *Lancet.* 1983;**2**:974.

Filiberti A, Tamburini M, Andreoli C, et al. Psychologic aspects of patients participating in a phase I study with the synthetic retinoid 4-hydroxyphenyl retinamide. *Tumori.* 1988;**74**:353–356.

Formelli F, Carsana R, Costa A, et al. Plasma retinol level reduction by the synthetic retinoid fenretinide: A one year follow-up study of breast cancer patients. *Cancer Res.* 1989;**49**:6149–6152.

Gerber A, Raab AP, Sobel AE. Vitamin A poisoning in adults with description of a case. *Amer J Med.* 1954;**16**:729–734.

Halkier-Sorensen L. Menstrual changes in a patient treated with etretinate. *Lancet.* 1987;**2**:636.

Kaiser-Kupfer MI, Peck GL, Caruso RC, et al. Abnormal retinal function associated with fenretinide, a synthetic retinoid. *Arch Ophthalmol.* 1986;**104**:69–70.

Meyskens FL, Alberts DS, Salmon SE. Effect of 13-*cis*-retinoic acid and 4-hydroxyphenyl-all-*trans*-retinamide on human tumor colony formation in soft agar. *Int J Cancer.* 1983;**32**:295–299.

Modiano MR, Dalton WS, Lippman SM, et al. Phase II study of fenretinide (N-[4-hydroxyphenyl]retinamide) in advanced breast cancer and melanoma. *Invest New Drugs.* 1990;**8**:317–319.

Moon RC, McCormick DL, Brecci PJ, et al. Influence of 15-retinoic acid amides on urinary bladder carcinogenesis in mouse. *Carcinogenesis.* 1982;**3**:1469–1472.

Moon RC, McCormick DL, Mehta RG. Inhibition of carcinogenesis by retinoids. *Cancer Res.* 1983;**43**:2469–2475.

Moon RC, Thompson HJ, Becci PJ, et al. N-(4-hydroxyphenyl)-retinamide, a new retinoid for prevention of breast cancer in the rat. *Cancer Res.* 1979;**39**:1339–1346.

Peng Y-M, Dalton WS, Alberts DS, et al. Pharmacokinetics of N-4-hydroxyphenyl-retinamide and the effect of its oral administration on plasma retinol concentrations in cancer patients. *Int J Cancer.* 1989;**43**:22–26.

Ratko TA, Detrisac CJ, Dinger NM, et al. Chemopreventive efficacy of combined retinoid and tamoxifen treatment following surgical excision of a primary mammary cancer in female rats. *Cancer Res.* 1989;**49**: 4472–4476.

Rotmensz N, De Palo G, Formelli F, et al. Long-term tolerability of fenretinide (4-HPR) in breast cancer patients. *Eur J Cancer.* 1991;**27**(9):1127–1131.

Sower MR, Wallace RB. Retinol, supplemental vitamin A and bone status. *J Clin Epidemiol.* 1990;**43**:683–699.

Sporn MB, Newton DL. Chemoprevention of cancer with retinoids. *Fed Proc.* 1978;**38**:2528–2534.

Swanson BN, Newton DL, Roller PP, Sporn MB. Biotransformation and biological activity of N-(4-hydroxyphenyl) retinamide derivatives in rodents. *J Pharmacol Exp Ther.* 1981;**219**:632–637.

Swanson BN, Zaharevitz DW, Sporn MB. Pharmacokinetics of N-(4-hydroxyphenyl)-all-*trans*-retinamide in rats. *Drug Metab Disp.* 1980;**8**:168–172.

Filgrastim

■ Other Names

Granulocyte colony-stimulating factor; G-CSF; Neupogen® (Amgen Inc); recombinant methionyl human granulocyte colony-stimulating factor (r-metHuG-CSF). (*Note:* other commercial types of G-CSF (Chugai, Kirin) are currently in clinical trials under other brand names.)

■ Chemistry

Human G-CSF is a human granulocyte colony-stimulating factor produced by recombinant DNA technology. The compound is a 175-amino-acid protein produced in *Escherichia coli*. It has a molecular weight of 18,800. The protein is identical to the natural human G-CSF sequence except that an N-terminal methionine has been added for expression in *E. coli*. Human G-CSF shares only 69% amino acid homology with murine G-CSF. The protein is also not glycosylated (as it would be in human cells). The human gene for G-CSF is located on chromosome 17q22 and consists of five exons and four introns (Nagata et al 1986). It is transcribed into a 2.0-kb mRNA which can be alternatively spliced into several different species of G-CSF (Nagata et al 1986). There are two disulfide bonds in the molecule with mostly an α-helical structure and a few β-pleated sheet segments (Lu et al 1989). G-CSF has been shown to enhance both the production of mature myeloid elements and the function of white cells.

Many fine reviews have been written on the role of G-CSF in cancer chemotherapy (Davis and Morstyn 1991, Morstyn et al 1989, Applebaum 1989).

■ Biologic Activity

Human G-CSF promotes both the proliferation and the differentiation of neutrophils. The target cells are thought to be both late precursors to neutrophils and the neutrophils themselves. G-CSF enhances the functional properties of the mature neutrophils

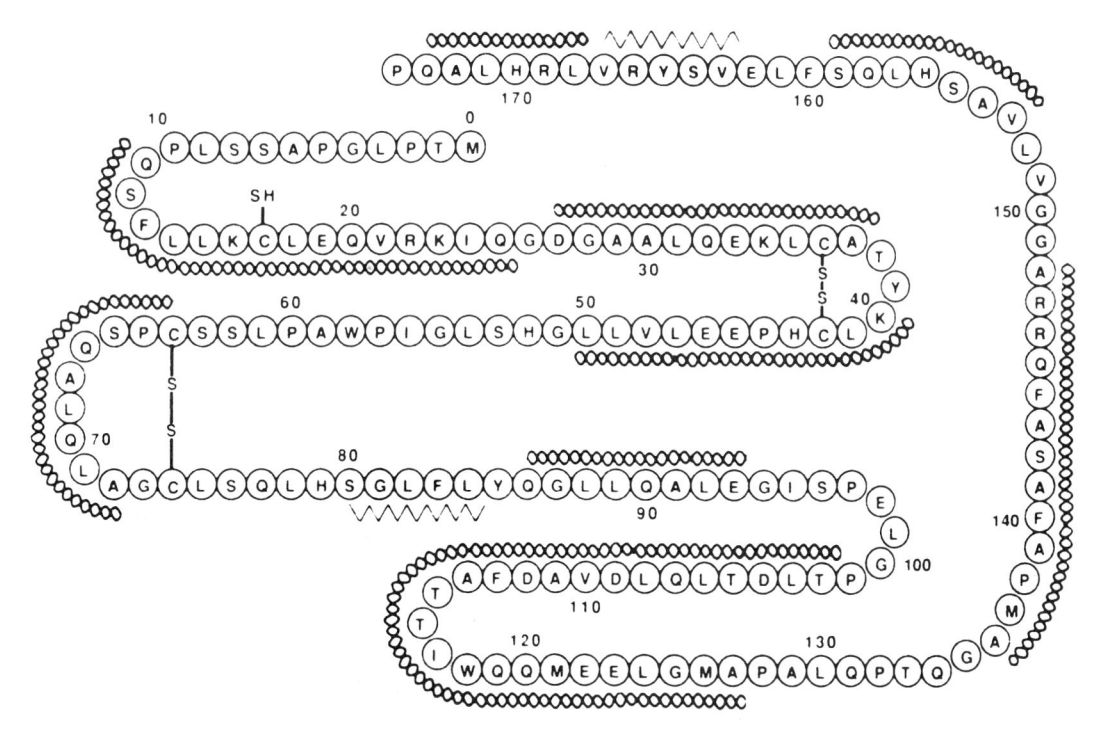

Structure of filgrastim

(eg, increased phagocytic activity, increased antimicrobial killing).

Several early nonrandomized clinical trials have clearly demonstrated a salutary effect of G-CSF on the neutropenia induced by cancer chemotherapy (Ohno et al 1990, Neidhart et al 1989, Bronchud et al 1988, 1989, Morstyn et al 1989, Parker et al 1991, Demetri et al 1991), status post-bone marrow transplant (Sheridan et al 1989), or in patients with malignancy not receiving chemotherapy (Gabrilove et al 1988a, Lindemann et al 1989). These early studies also documented that G-CSF increased functionally competent neutrophils (Lindemann et al 1989).

One of the most definitive studies of G-CSF has been conducted in patients with small cell lung cancer. Patients were treated with cyclophosphamide + doxorubicin + etoposide and randomized to either placebo or G-CSF (given days 4–17 of a 21-day cycle). At least one episode of neutropenia with fever occurred in 77% of the placebo group versus 40% of the G-CSF group (Crawford et al 1991). In addition, the duration of neutropenia (< 500 granulocytes) was 1 day with G-CSF versus 6 days with placebo. The number of days on intravenous antibiotics, the number of days hospitalized, and the incidence of confirmed infections were decreased by 50%.

Other randomized or sequential trials in patients with urogenital malignancies have generated similar results (Kotake et al 1991, Gabrilove et al 1988b, Ogawara et al 1990, Masuda et al 1991, Green et al 1991).

Human G-CSF has been effective in the treatment of cyclic neutropenia (Hammond et al 1989). G-CSF reduced mouth ulcers, fevers, and infections in patients with that disease. G-CSF has had beneficial effects in children with aplastic anemia (Kojima et al 1991). It has also been used in patients with myelodysplastic syndrome, with improvement in neutrophil levels and myeloid maturation and fewer infections (Negrin et al 1989, 1990).

Human G-CSF has been used successfully to treat chronic idiopathic neutropenia (Furukawa et al 1991) as well as severe congenital neutropenia (Weston et al 1991) and congenital agranulocytosis (Bonilla et al 1989). G-CSF has had a salutary effect on AIDS-related neutropenia (Kimura et al 1990). Combined therapy with G-CSF and erythropoietin has been found to decrease the hematologic toxicity of zidovudine (Miles et al 1991).

Human G-CSF has also been found to be useful as an adjunct to the treatment of hairy cell leukemia. It is often combined with interferon or pentostatin (Glaspy et al 1988, 1990).

One major concern about the use of G-CSF was that it might cause accelerated growth of leukemia cells (because of the potential for myeloid leukemia cells to contain receptors for the molecule). In carefully performed studies there has been no evidence of this occurring (Ohno et al 1990).

Some studies have reported a decreased incidence of chemotherapy-induced mucositis in patients receiving G-CSF (Gabrilove et al 1988b). G-CSF has also been shown to increase the number of peripheral blood stem cells (37- to 221-fold) (Toki et al 1990, Peterson et al 1991).

■ Mechanism of Action

Human G-CSF binds to specific cell surface receptors. G-CSF affects primarily neutrophil progenitor proliferation and differentiation (Welte et al 1987, Duhrsen et al 1988, Souza et al 1986). The binding affinity (K_a) of human G-CSF for its receptor ranges from 1 to 5×10^9 M^{-1}. G-CSF receptor is a single-chain molecule of 150 kDa that is present on cells of neutrophil lineage. Very few receptors are expressed on monocytes (Nicola 1987). The normal producer cells of G-CSF are activated monocytes and macrophages, activated neutrophils, fibroblasts, and endothelial cells (Oster et al 1990). Unlike other hematopoietic colony-stimulating factors that are paracrine hormones, G-CSF appears to act in both an endocrine and a paracrine fashion. Thus, circulating G-CSF levels can be detected in response to systemic infections.

The action of G-CSF involves a proliferative stimulus of immature neutrophils as well as functional activation of mature polymorphonuclear neutrophils. These activities include an enhancement of antibody-dependent cellular cytotoxicity, increased and sustained production of oxygen radicals (Weisbart et al 1989), and enhanced expression of FMLP and Fc receptors for immunoglobulin A (Weisbart et al 1989). In addition, G-CSF also acts as a chemotactic signal for phagocytic cells including polymorphonuclear leukocytes and monocytes (Wang et al 1988).

■ Availability and Storage

Human G-CSF (Neupogen®) is supplied by Amgen Inc, Thousand Oaks, California, as a sterile, clear, colorless liquid. It is preservative free. Each 1-mL vial contains 300 µg of G-CSF with a specific activity of $1.0 \pm 0.6 \times 10^8$ U/mg. The 1.6-mL vial contains 480 µg of G-CSF. G-CSF is formulated in a buffer (10 mM sodium acetate buffer) at pH 4.0, with 5% mannitol and 0.004% polysorbate 80. The vials should be stored at refrigeration temperature (4–8°C). The vial should not be frozen or left in direct sunlight. Filgrastim aggregates when frozen at –20°C (–4°F) and at temperatures exceeding 30°C (86°F). Vigorously shaking the vial (which produces a foam that might lead to an inaccurate dose) should be avoided. The undiluted solution is chemically stable in polyvinyl chloride tuberculin syringes for 24 hours at room temperature and 7 days at refrigeration temperatures.

■ Preparation for Use, Stability, and Admixture

The vial is entered with a small needle attached to a syringe. The appropriate amount is withdrawn and injected subcutaneously (or intravenously). Unused portions of the vial can be stored for 24 hours under refrigeration, although no antibacterial preservative is present. For intravenous infusions, filgrastim should only be diluted in 5% dextrose in water. It is incompatible with saline-containing solutions. For dilute infusions in 5% dextrose, no albumin is needed if the final concentration is 15 µg/mL or greater. For more dilute G-CSF infusions of 2 to 15 µg/mL, human serum albumin (2 mg/mL final concentration) should be added to the container first to prevent G-CSF adsorption. These dilute solutions are chemically stable for up to 7 days at 2 to 8°C or at room temperatures of 15 to 30°C (59 to 86°F) (Amgen Inc, data on file, 1992). The drug solution is also compatible with several types of plastic infusion containers including polyvinyl chloride (Abbott, Kendall-McGaw, Baxter, Pharmacia-Deltec, Travenol [Infusor®], Cormed) and polypropylene (Terumo and Becton Dickinson syringes) (Amgen Inc, data on file, 1992).

■ Administration

Prior to injection, G-CSF should be allowed to come to room temperature. The recommended dose (5 µg/kg/d) can then be injected subcutaneously or intravenously. Twice weekly complete blood counts should be obtained while the patient is receiving G-CSF. The package insert for G-CSF cautions against administering G-CSF 24 hours before or after chemotherapy. The agent is usually continued daily for up to 2 weeks or until the absolute neutrophil count has reached 10,000/mm^3 (after the nadir count has been passed).

■ Special Precautions

Human G-CSF should not be given to patients with a history of known hypersensitivity to *E. coli*-derived proteins.

■ Drug Interactions

None have been described to date.

■ Dosage

The recommended dose for Neupogen® is 5 µg/kg/d subcutaneously. Nonetheless, phase I studies have shown a dose-dependent neutrophil increase for daily doses up to 60 µg/kg/d for 6 days (Gabrilove et al 1988). Dosing should not be concurrent with chemotherapy, as severe myelosuppression has been reported with such therapy (Meropol et al 1992). Typically, G-CSF dosing is delayed for 24 hours following the last dose of chemotherapy.

There are also some indications that myelostimulatory activity may be schedule dependent, favoring more frequent drug administration. In this regard, twice daily subcutaneous injections may enhance the degree of myelopoiesis possible from the same total dose given subcutaneously once daily. Definitive trials are clearly needed in this area.

The recommended doses for other preparations of G-CSF are still under investigation.

■ Pharmacokinetics

Pharmacokinetic studies of G-CSF in children after subcutaneous administration of G-CSF demonstrated a one-compartment, first-order absorption model. Peak G-CSF concentrations were achieved after 4 to 8 hours and ranged from 10.3 to 111.6 mg/mL (baselines were below 150 mg/mL). Clearance averaged 0.3 mL/min/d on day 1 and 0.46 on day 10. The AUC was related to the daily dose (Stute et al 1991). Petros and colleagues (1991) have noted (using an ELISA technique) that the clearance of G-CSF increased over the time of administration. Clearance of the molecule was unaffected by renal or hepatic dysfunction.

■ Side Effects and Toxicity

Mild to moderate medullary bone pain (controlled with oral analgesics) has been seen in up to 20% of patients receiving G-CSF (Crawford et al 1991). The bone pain has been more common in patients given higher doses intravenously. Flareup of preexisting eczema (eg, psoriasis) has been reported (Crawford et al 1991). Ross et al (1991) have recently reported a case of bullous pyoderma gangrenosum at a site of prior eczema.

There were no reports of allergic reactions with G-CSF until recently, when a case of acute anaphylaxis was noted (Jaiyesimi et al 1991). No studies of possible antibody formation have been reported.

Some elevations of lactate dehydrogenase and alkaline phosphate have occurred in patients receiving G-CSF.

Splenomegaly has been reported in children receiving G-CSF and in adults receiving long-term (up to 3 years) G-CSF. Careful studies of peripheral blood smears after G-CSF have found increases in large granular lymphocytes (Kerrigan et al 1989).

■ Special Applications

See Biologic Activity.

REFERENCES

Appelbaum FR. The clinical use of hematopoietic growth factors. *Semin Hematol.* 1989;**26**(3):7–14.

Bonilla MA, Gillio AP, Russeiro M, et al. Effects of recombinant human granulocyte colony-stimulating factor on neutropenia in patients with congenital agranulocytosis. *N Engl J Med.* 1989;**320**(24):1574–1580.

Bronchud M, Scarffe JH, Thatchr N, et al. Phase I/II study of recombinant human granulocyte colony-stimulating factor in patients receiving intensive chemotherapy for small cell lung cancer. *Behring Inst Mitt.* 1988;**83**:327–329.

Bronchud MH, Howell A, Crowther D, Hopwood P, Souza L, Dexter TM. The use of granulocyte colony-stimulating factor to increase the intensity of treatment with doxorubicin in patients with advanced breast and ovarian cancer. *Br J Cancer.* 1989;**60**(1):121–125.

Crawford J, Ozer H, Stoller R, et al. Reduction by granulocyte colony-stimulating factor of fever and neutropenia induced by chemotherapy in patients with small-cell lung cancer. *N Engl J Med.* 1991;**315**:164–170.

Davis I, Morstyn G. The role of granulocyte colony-stimulating factor in cancer chemotherapy. *Semin Hematol.* 1991;**28**(2, suppl 2):25–33.

Demetri GD, Younger J, McGuire BW, et al. Recombinant methionyl granulocyte-CSF (r-metG-CSF) allows an increase in the dose intensity of cyclophosphamide, doxorubicin/5-fluorouracil (CAF) in patients with advanced breast cancer. *Proc Am Soc Clin Oncol.* 1991;**10**:70.

Duhrsen U, Villefal JL, Boyd J, Kannourakis G, Morstyn G, Metcalf D. Effects of recombinant human granulocyte colony-stimulating factor on hematopoietic progenitor cells in cancer patients. *Blood.* 1988;**72**:2074–2081.

Furukawa T, Takahashi M, Moriyama Y, Koike T, Kurokawa I, Shibata A. Successful treatment of chronic idiopathic neutropenia using recombinant granulocyte colony-stimulating factor. *Ann Hematol.* 1991;**62**(1):22–24.

Gabrilove JL, Jakubowski A, Fain K, et al. Phase I study of granulocyte colony-stimulating factor in patients with transitional cell carcinoma of the urothelium. *J Clin Invest.* 1988a;**82**(4):1454–1461.

Gabrilove JL, Jakubowksi A, Scher H, et al. Effect of granulocyte colony-stimulating factor on neutropenia and associated morbidity due to chemotherapy for transitional-cell carcinoma of the urothelium. *N Engl J Med.* 1988b;**318**(22):1414–1422.

Glaspy J, Ambersley J, Narachi M, Wyres M, Golde D. Treatment of hairy cell leukemia (HCL) with granulocyte colony stimulating factor (G-SCF) and alpha interferon (IFN-a). *Proc Am Soc Clin Oncol.* 1990;**9**:213.

Glaspy JA, Baldwin GC, Robertson PA, et al. Therapy for neutropenia in hairy cell leukemia with recombinant human granulocyte colony-stimulating factor. *Ann Intern Med.* 1988;**109**(10):789–795.

Green JA, Trillet VN, Manegold C. r-metHuG-CSF (G-CSF) with CED chemotherapy (CT) in small cell lung cancer (SCLC): Interim results from a randomized, placebo controlled trial. *Proc Am Soc Clin Oncol.* 1991;**10**:243.

Hammond WP IV, Price TH, Souza LM, Dale DC. Treatment of cyclic neutropenia with granulocyte colony-stimulating factor. *N Engl J Med.* 1989;**320**(20):1306–1311.

Jaiyesimi I, Giralt SS, Wood J. Subcutaneous granulocyte colony-stimulating factor and acute anaphylaxis (letter). *N Engl J Med.* 1991;**325**(8):587.

Kerrigan DP, Castillo A, Foucar K, Townsend K, Neidhart J. Peripheral blood morphologic changes after high-dose antineoplastic chemotherapy and recombinant human granulocyte colony-stimulating factor administration. *Am J Clin Pathol.* 1989;**92**(3):280–285.

Kimura S, Matsuda J, Ikematsu S, et al. Efficacy of recombinant human granulocyte colony-stimulating factor on neutropenia in patients with AIDS. *AIDS.* 1990;**4**(12):1251–1255.

Kojima S, Fududa M, Miyajima Y, Matsuyama T, Horibe K. Treatment of aplastic anemia in children with recombinant human granulocyte colony-stimulating factor. *Blood.* 1991;**77**(5):937–941.

Kotake T, Miki T, Akaza H, et al. Effect of recombinant granulocyte colony-stimulating factor (rG-CSF) on chemotherapy-induced neutropenia in patients with urogenital cancer. *Cancer Chemother Pharmacol.* 1991;**27**(4):253–257.

Lindemann A, Herrmann F, Oster W, et al. Hematologic effects of recombinant human granulocyte colony-stimulating factor in patients with malignancy. *Blood.* 1989;**74**(8):2644–2651.

Lu HS, Boone TC, Souza LM, Lai PH. Disulfide and secondary structures of recombinant human granulocyte colony stimulating factor. *Arch Biochem Biophys.* 1989;**268**:81–92.

Masuda N, Fukuoka M, Negoro N, et al. Code chemotherapy with or without recombinant human granulocyte colony-stimulating factor (rhG-CSF) in extensive-stage (ES) small cell lung cancer (SCLC). *Proc Am Soc Clin Oncol.* 1991;**10**:254.

Meropol NJ, Miller LL, Korn EL, et al. Severe myelosuppression resulting from concurrent administration of granulocyte colony-stimulating factor and cytotoxic chemotherapy. *J Natl Cancer Inst.* 1992;**84**(15):1201–1204.

Miles SA, Mitsuyasu RT, Moreno J, et al. Combined therapy with recombinant granulocyte colony-stimulating factor and erythropoietin decreases hematologic toxicity from zidovudine. *Blood.* 1991;**77**(10):2109–2117.

Morstyn G, Campbell L, Lieschke G, et al. Treatment of chemotherapy-induced neutropenia by subcutaneously administered granulocyte colony-stimulating factor with optimization of dose and duration of therapy. *J Clin Oncol.* 1989;**7**(10):1554–1562.

Nagata S, Tsuchiya M, Asamo S, et al. The chromosomal gene structure and mRNA's for human granulocyte colony stimulating factor. *Nature.* 1986;**319**:415–418.

Negrin RS, Haeuber DH, Nagler A, et al. Treatment of myelodysplastic syndromes with recombinant human granulocyte colony-stimulating factor. A phase I–II trial. *Ann Intern Med.* 1989;**110**(12):976–984.

Negrin RS, Haeuber DH, Nagler A, et al. Maintenance treatment of patients with myelodysplastic syndromes using recombinant human granulocyte colony-stimulating factor. *Blood.* 1990;**76**(1):36–43.

Neidhart J, Mangalik A, Kohler W, et al. Granulocyte colony-stimulating factor stimulates recovery of granulocytes in patients receiving dose-intensive chemotherapy without bone marrow transplantation. *J Clin Oncol.* 1989;**7**(11):1685–1692.

Nicola NA. Why do hematopoietic growth factors interact with each other? *Immunol Today.* 1987;**8**:134–140.

Ogawara M, Furuse K, Kawahara M, et al. Randomized study of recombinant human granulocyte colony stimulating factor (rhG-CSF) on prevention of infection in leukocytopenia induced by chemotherapy in lung cancer patients (pts). *Proc Am Soc Clin Oncol.* 1990;**9**:225.

Ohno R, Shirakawa A, Hiraoka A, et al. Effect of granulocyte colony stimulating factor (G-CSF) after intensive chemotherapy in refractory acute leukemia: A randomized trial. *Proc Am Assoc Cancer Res.* 1990;**31**:194.

Ohno R, Tomonaga M, Kobayashi T, et al. Effect of granulocyte colony-stimulating factor after intensive induction therapy in relapsed or refractory acute leukemia. *N Engl J Med.* 1990;**323**(13):871–877.

Oster W, Mertelsmann R, Herrmann F. Regulation of cell function by hematopoietic growth factors. In: Mertelsmann R, Herrman F, eds. *Hematopoietic Growth Factors in Clinical Applications.* New York: Marcel Dekker; 1990:25–39.

Parker BA, Anderson JR, Canellos GP, Gockerman JP, Gottlieb AJ, Peterson BA. Dose escalation study of chop plus etoposide (CHOPE) without and with rhG-CSF in untreated non-Hodgkin's lymphoma (NHL). *Proc Am Soc Clin Oncol.* 1991;**10**:283.

Peterson J, Kirkpatrick G, Ross M, Vredenburgh J, Peters WP, Kurtzberg J. Growth factor primed peripheral blood progenitor cells (PBPC) are enriched for hematopoietic progenitor cells (HPC). *Proc Am Soc Clin Oncol.* 1991;**10**:78.

Petros W, Rabinowitz J, Stuart A, Peters WP. Comparative pharmacokinetics of granulocyte colony-stimulating factor (rHuG-CSF) and granulocyte-macrophage colony-stimulating factor (rHuGM-CSF) in patients receiving high-dose chemotherapy and autologous bone marrow support. *Proc Am Soc Clin Oncol.* 1991;**10**:97.

Ross HJ, Moy LA, Kaplan R, Figlin RA. Bullous pyroderma gangrenosum after granulocyte colony-stimulating factor treatment. *Cancer.* 1991;**68**(2):441–443.

Sheridan WP, Morstyn G, Wolf M, et al. Granulocyte colony-stimulating factor and neutrophil recovery after high-dose chemotherapy and autologous bone marrow transplantation. *Lancet.* 1989;**2**:891–895.

Souza LM, Boone TC, Gabrilove J, et al. Recombinant human granulocyte colony-stimulating factor: Effects on normal and leukemic myeloid cells. *Science.* 1986;**232**:61–65.

Stute N, Santana V, Rodman JH, Schell M, Evans WE. Pharmacokinetics of subcutaneous (SC) rmetG-CSF in children with neuroblastoma treated with myelosuppressive chemotherapy. *Proc Am Soc Clin Oncol.* 1991;**10**:98.

Toki H, Shimokawa T, Okabe K, Ishimitsu T. Recombinant human granulocyte colony-stimulating factor (rG-CSF) amplified the number of peripheral blood stem cells (PBSC) of lymphoma patients on chemotherapy. *Proc Am Soc Clin Oncol.* 1990;**9**:188.

Wang JM, Chen ZG, Golella S, et al. Chemotactic activity of recombinant G-CSF. *Blood.* 1988;**72**:1456–1460.

Weisbart RH, Gasson JC, Golde DW, et al. Colony-stimulating factors and host defense. *Ann Intern Med.* 1989;**110**:297–303.

Welte K, Bonilla MA, Gillio AP, et al. Recombinant human G-CSF: Effects on hematopoiesis in normal and cyclophosphamide treated primates. *J Exp Med.* 1987;**165**:941–948.

Weston B, Todd RF III, Axtell R, et al. Severe congenital neutropenia: Clinical effects and neutrophils function during treatment with granulocyte colony-stimulating factor. *J Lab Clin Med.* 1991;**117**(4):282–290.

Finasteride

Other Names

Proscar® (Merck & Co); MK-906.

Chemistry

Structure of finasteride

Finasteride is a 4-azasteroid derivative of testosterone which blocks the conversion of testosterone to dihydrotestosterone. The complete chemical name is N-(1,1-dimethylethyl-3-oxo-(5α,17β)-4-azaandrost-1-ene-17-carboxamide.

Antitumor Activity

Clinical trials in normal volunteers and those with benign prostatic hypertrophy have shown that finasteride consistently suppresses dihydrotestosterone levels to 75 to 85% of control. This results in elevations of serum and prostate gland testosterone levels (Gormley et al 1990). Nonetheless, continuous finasteride therapy for 6 months in these populations results in a mean 28% reduction in the size of the prostate (Gormley 1991). In addition, serum levels of prostatic specific antigen (PSA) are decreased by about 50%.

A pilot study has been performed in 13 patients with stage D prostate cancer treated with oral finasteride daily for 6 weeks. This resulted in a 70 to 75% reduction in serum dihydrotestosterone levels and a 15 to 20% reduction in serum PSA levels. An ongoing placebo-controlled trial is being performed in men with elevated PSA levels following radical prostatectomy. In benign prostatic hypertrophy, prostate volume is reduced by 18% after 12 weeks of finasteride therapy (Stoner 1990). This decrease is maintained over a 6 month period with continued therapy. Current clinical trials in patients with prostate cancer are addressing the effects of finasteride alone and of combinations of finasteride with antiandrogens to produce a more complete or "total" androgen blockade (Gormley 1991).

Mechanism of Action

Finasteride is a competitive inhibitor of the enzyme 5α-reductase (EC 1.3.1.22, 3-oxo-5α-steroid:NADP$^+$ Δ^4-oxidoreductase). This enzyme is associated with the nuclear membrane of androgen-dependent cells. It normally catalyzes the reduction of testosterone to the more active androgenic substance dihydrotestosterone using NADPH as a cofactor. Finasteride binds tightly to 5α-reductase and prevents testosterone reduction intracellularly. This depletes intracellular levels of DHT and thereby prevents formation of the dihydrotestosterone–androgen receptor complex. Normally, it is this complex that mediates the majority of androgen-related stimulation in prostatic tissues (Grino et al 1990). Some studies have shown that prostate tumor tissues may contain less 5α-reductase activity than either normal or benign hyperplastic prostate tissues (Klein et al 1988).

Finasteride does not affect testosterone binding to the androgen receptor. Therefore, all of the other (nonprostatic) hormonal effects of testosterone, such as hair growth, maintenance of muscle mass, spermatogenesis, and libido, are not affected by finasteride. Conversely, finasteride does not produce any hormonal effects of its own including androgenic, estrogenic or progestational effects (Rasmussen 1987).

Availability and Storage

Finasteride is commercially available from Merck & Co (West Point, PA) in 1- and 5-mg tablets. The tablets are stored at room temperature.

Administration

Finasteride is administered orally, usually once per day.

Dosage

The maximally effective dose and schedule of finasteride in any indication have not been established. Early clinical trials evaluated daily oral doses of 25, 50, and 100 mg for 11 days in a high-dose group and 0.04, 0.12, 0.2, and 1.0 mg for 14 days in a low-dose group (Gormley et al 1990). The higher dose levels may not be needed as 5 mg daily for 6 months produced 80% suppression of dihydrotestosterone levels in normal male volunteers (Stoner 1990).

PHARMACOKINETICS OF ORAL FINASTERIDE IN HEALTHY MALE VOLUNTEERS

Dose (mg)	Plasma Half-life (h)	Time to Peak Plasma Level (h)	Maximal Plasma Concentration (μg/mL)	Plasma Concentration (μg/mL) at 24 h	AUC 0–24 h (μg/mL·h)
50	—	4	0.29	0.0015	—
200	17.3	2–4	0.92	0.29	12.9
400	13.4	4–6	2.05	0.72	31.5

Data from Carlin et al 1988.

■ Pharmacokinetics

The above table outlines the pharmacokinetics of three different doses of finasteride in volunteers. Less than 0.1% of a dose is excreted as unchanged drug in the urine. Several polar metabolites have been tentatively identified in the urine. These may represent a series of monohydroxylated finasteride metabolites (Carlin et al 1988). Despite the short plasma half-life of 5 to 6 hours, the half-life of the biologic effect is much longer. In one phase I study, suppression of dihydrotestosterone levels is maintained for up to 14 days after drug discontinuance (Gormley et al 1990).

■ Side Effects and Toxicity

Side effects have been minimal in the early clinical trials of finasteride. In healthy male volunteers given high-dose therapy the only symptoms were mild headache in 3 of 22 patients (Gormley et al 1990). No significant alterations in laboratory chemistry values were described. This included levels of other circulating hormones such as luteinizing hormone, follicle-stimulating hormone, cortisol, estradiol, and serum lipids.

REFERENCES

Carlin JR, Christofalo P, Vandenheuvel WJA. High-performance liquid chromatographic determination of N-(2-methy-2-propyl)-3-oxo-4-aza-5α-androst-1-ene-17β-carboxamide, a 4-azasteroid, in human plasma from a phase I study. *J Chromatogr.* 1988;**427**:79–91.

Gormley GJ. Role of 5α-reductase inhibitors in the treatment of advanced prostatic carcinoma. *Urol Clin N Am.* 1991;**18**(1):93–98.

Gormley GJ, Stoner E, Rittmaster RS, et al. Effects of finasteride (MK-906), a 5α-reductase inhibitor, on circulating androgens in male volunteers. *J Clin Endocrinol Metab.* 1990;**70**:1136–1141.

Grino PB, Griffen JE, Wilson JD. Testosterone at high concentrations interacts with the human androgens receptor similarly to dihydrotestosterone. *Endocrinol.* 1990;**126**:1165–1170.

Klein H, Bressel M, Kastendieck H, et al. Quantitative assessment of endogenous testicular and adrenal sex steroid metabolizing enzymes in untreated human prostatic cancerous tissue. *J Steroid Biochem.* 1988;**30**:119–130.

Rasmusson GH. Biochemistry and pharmacology of 5α-reductase inhibitors. In: Furr BJ, Wakeling AE (eds): *Pharmacology and Clinical Uses of Inhibitors of Hormone Secretion and Action.* London: Baillere Tindall, 1987;308–325.

Stoner E. The clinical development of a 5α-reductase inhibitor, finasteride. *J Steroid Biochem Mol Biol.* 1990;**37**(3):375–378.

Flavone Acetic Acid

■ Other Names

NSC-347512; FAA.

■ Chemistry

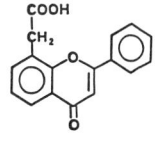

Structure of flavone acetic acid

Flavone acetic acid is a synthetic benzopyrone derivative. The complete chemical name is 4-oxo-2-phenyl-4H-1-benzopyran-8-acetic acid. It has the empiric formula $C_{17}H_{12}O_4$ and a molecular weight of 280. An excellent review article has been published on the preclinical aspects of the agent (O'Dwyer et al 1987).

Antitumor Activity

Flavone acetic acid is an investigational compound that is more active in animal solid tumors than in leukemia models (Plowman et al 1986, Corbett et al 1986). Flavone acetic acid has had phase II clinical trial testing in patients with cancers of the breast, colon, and head and neck and melanoma (Kerr and Kaye 1989, Kaye et al 1990, Kerr et al 1989). To date, no significant antitumor activity has been noted.

Mechanism of Action

The mechanism of action of flavone acetic acid is unknown. DNA damage in the form of nonreparable single-strand breaks occurring in a dose-dependent manner has been documented (Bissery et al 1988). There is, however, a growing body of evidence that the cytotoxicity of flavone acetic acid is at least in part an indirect effect accomplished through immunomodulation, particularly with induction and augmentation of natural killer (NK) cell activity (Ching and Baguley 1987, Wiltrout et al 1988) and/or effects on tumor vasculature (Zwi et al 1989, Bibby et al 1989, Evelhoch et al 1988, Mahadevan et al 1990). Triozzi et al (1990) have observed significant immunologic effects of flavone acetic acid, whereas Zwi et al (1989) report significant reduction in local tumor blood flow in the nude mouse model. This latter effect of impaired skin blood flow may explain the marked and possibly exaggerated antitumor effects of flavone acetic acid seen in subcutaneously implanted mouse tumor models (Plowman et al 1986). One group has suggested that the reduction in tumor blood flow following flavone acetic acid is due to induction of tumor necrosis factor with subsequent hemorrhagic necrosis (Mahadevan et al 1990).

Availability and Storage

Flavone acetic acid is available for authorized investigational studies under the auspices of the National Cancer Institute, Bethesda, Maryland. The drug is supplied as a sterile 250 mg vial, prepared as an off-white to light yellow lyophilized cake or powder with sodium hydroxide to adjust the pH. The intact vials should be stored under refrigeration (2–8°C).

Preparation for Use, Stability, and Admixture

Flavone acetic acid is stable in aqueous phosphate-buffered solutions over the pH range 7.3 to 9.6, exhibiting little or no decomposition over 12 hours at 70°C. At higher pH values, increased rates of decomposition occur. When reconstituted as directed with Sterile Water for Injection, USP, flavone acetic acid solutions exhibit little or no decomposition over 14 days at room temperature. These studies are ongoing. Flavone acetic acid has demonstrated sensitivity to sunlight (Rewcastle et al 1990).

The single-use lyophilized dosage form contains no antibacterial preservatives. Therefore, it is advised that the reconstituted product be discarded 8 hours after initial entry.

Administration

Flavone acetic acid has limited aqueous solubility under acidic conditions. Therefore, most investigators have prehydrated all patients and alkalinized their urine with sodium bicarbonate (1 ampule in 1 L of 0.9% sodium chloride over 4 hours). The goal is to maintain urine pH greater than 6.5. The urine pH should be monitored every 4 hours during the 24 hours following the infusion. The drug must be protected from light with an opaque overwrap during the infusion.

Special Precautions

The patients' urine must be alkalinized to a pH greater than 6.5 (see alkalinization of urine plan above). The drug has also been described to prolong bleeding times (Rubin et al 1987).

Drug Interactions

Flavone acetic acid is synergistic with interleukin-2 in mice bearing experimental renal cell tumors (Wiltrout et al 1988).

Dosage

The doses and schedules listed in the table at the top of the opposite page have been investigated in phase I studies. A phase I trial has also been performed with the parent diethylaminoethyl ester (NSC-293015), with sedation and an acute expressive aphasia noted as the major side effects (Kerr et al 1986, Dodion et al 1987).

Pharmacokinetics

The table at the bottom of the opposite page summarizes the pharmacokinetics of the compound. A hallmark of flavone acetic acid is dose-dependent pharmacokinetics. It appears that there is dose-dependent elimination at the lower dose levels with a shift to first-order elimination at the 2 to 2.3 g/m^2

PHASE I STUDIES INVOLVING FLAVONE ACETIC ACID

Schedule	Dose Range (g/m^2)	Dose-Limiting Toxic Effect	Recommended Phase II Dose (g/m^2)	Reference
Weekly × 4 over 1–6 h every 5 wk	0.33–12.5	Hypotension	8	Havlin et al 1991
Weekly × 4 over 1–3 h every 6 wk	0.33–6.4	Hypotension	—	Weiss et al 1988
1-h infusion	—	—	4.8	Kerr et al 1987
8-h infusion	—	—	8.6	Kerr et al 1987
1–3 h every 3–4 wk	0.10–10.0	Hypotension	None	Grever et al 1988

dose level (Havlin et al 1991, Weiss et al 1988, Gouyette et al 1988). The percentage of flavone acetic acid excreted in the urine has been 29.3 ± 3.6% over 48 hours as parent drug and 28 ± 5.6% as conjugated glucuronide metabolite(s) (well characterized by Cummings et al 1989) for a combined total of 57% (Havlin et al 1991). Cummings et al (1989) have documented that drug biotransformation represents the predominant mechanism for drug clearance. At high doses there appears to be a saturation of glucuronidation pathways with a subsequent overall reduction in drug clearance.

Increasing evidence suggests that flavone acetic acid does not have antitumor activity in patients due to extensive plasma protein binding. Other authors have not agreed with these conclusions (Cassidy et al 1989). Tumor levels of the drug have been measured in patients and are close to the levels noted in animal tumors (wherein the drug was effective) (Damia et al 1990).

■ Side Effects and Toxicity

The dose-limiting toxic effect noted on the weekly schedule was hypotension (Havlin et al 1991, Weiss et al 1988). The hypotension can be orthostatic and related to volume depletion, but that is not always the case. In fact, the hypotension does not always respond to fluids. Prolonging the infusion time from 1 to 6 hours has allowed administration of higher drug doses.

Other toxic effects include mild nausea, vomiting, diarrhea, a flushing or feeling of warmth, reversible blurred vision, and, rarely, severe myalgias (Weiss et al 1988, Havlin et al 1991, Melink et al 1987, Grever et al 1988). A hypersensitivity reaction has been reported with facial angioedema (Havlin et al 1991). An autonomic neuropathy has also been reported with the drug (Lewis et al 1989). A prolonged bleeding time has been noted in some patients (Rubin et al 1987).

PHARMACOKINETICS OF FLAVONE ACETIC ACID

Schedule	Peak Concentration (μg/mL)	Half-life (h) $t_{1/2\alpha}$	Half-life (h) $t_{1/2\beta}$	Volume of Distribution (L/m^2) $V_{d_c}^\dagger$	Volume of Distribution (L/m^2) $V_{d_{ss}}^\ddagger$	Total Body Clearance (L/h/m^2)	Reference
Weekly 1- to 6-h infusion	630*	2.3 ± 0.7	22.4 ± 7.5	12.1 ± 5.2	24.3 ± 12.9	3.0 ± 1.3	Havlin et al 1991
1-h infusion	—	—	14.7 ± 1.3	—	52 ± 4	2.6 ± 0.2	Damia et al 1990
Weekly over 1–3 h	>300	2	—	—	—	—	Weiss et al 1988
1-h infusion	650*	—	2.5–6.7	—	11.8–44.2	2.0–7.7	Kerr et al 1987
6-h infusion	338*	—	3.4–5.9	—	12.7–21.6	2.1–2.9	Kerr et al 1987
Children	—	—	13.7–25.4	—	7.7–23.1	1.32–2.55	Relling et al 1990

*Varied with the dose.
†V_{d_c} = volume of distribution in the central compartment.
‡$V_{d_{ss}}$ = steady state volume of distribution.

■ Special Applications

Some investigators have found suggestive evidence, on one of three patients studied, that flavone acetic acid can increase Leu-19-positive (natural killer lymphocyte) cells with a resultant increase in K562 cytotoxicity (Havlin et al 1991). In other patients there is no evidence that flavone acetic acid increases LAK cells in patients (Havlin et al 1991, Triozzi et al 1990).

REFERENCES

Bibby MC, Double JA, Loadman PM, Duke CV. Reduction of tumor blood flow by flavone acetic acid: A possible component of therapy. *J Natl Cancer Inst.* 1989;**81**:216–220.

Bissery MC, Valeriote FA, Chabot GG, Crissman JD, Yost C, Corbett TH. Flavone acetic acid (NSC 347512)-induced DNA damage in Glasgow osteogenic sarcoma in vivo. *Cancer Res.* 1988;**48**:1279–1285.

Brodfuehrer J, Valeriote F, Chan K, Heilbruin L, Corbett T. Flavone acetic acid and plasma protein binding. *Cancer Chemother Pharmacol.* 1990;**27**(1):27–32.

Cassidy J, Kerr DJ, Setanoians A, Zaharko DS, Kaye SB. Could interspecies differences in the protein binding of flavone acetic acid contribute to the failure to predict lack of efficacy in patients? *Cancer Chemother Pharmacol.* 1989;**23**(6):397–400.

Ching LM, Baguley BC. Induction of natural killer cell activity by the antitumor compound flavone acetic acid (NSC 347512). *Eur J Cancer Clin Oncol.* 1987;**23**:1047–1050.

Corbett TH, Bissery MC, Wozniak A, et al. Activity of flavone acetic acid (NSC-347512) against solid tumor of mice. *Invest New Drugs.* 1986;**4**:207–220.

Cummings J, Double JA, Bibby C, et al. Characterization of the major metabolites of flavone acetic acid and comparison of their disposition in humans and mice. *Cancer Res.* 1989;**49**:3587–3593.

Damia G, Freschi A, Sorio R, et al. Flavone acetic acid distribution in human malignant tumors. *Cancer Chemother Pharmacol.* 1990;**26**:67–70.

Dodion PF, Abrams J, Gerard B, et al. Clinical and pharmacokinetic phase I trial with the diethylaminoester of flavone acetic acid (LM985, NSC-293-15). *Eur J Cancer Clin Oncol.* 1987;**23**(6):837–842.

Evelhoch JL, Bissery MC, Chabot GG, et al. Flavone acetic acid (NSC 347512)-induced modulation of murine tumor physiology monitored by in vivo nuclear magnetic resonance spectroscopy. *Cancer Res.* 1988;**48**:4749–4755.

Gouyette A, Kerr DJ, Kaye SB, et al. Flavone acetic acid: A nonlinear pharmacokinetic model. *Cancer Chemother Pharmacol.* 1988;**22**(2):114–119.

Grever MR, Leiby JM, Kraut EH, Balcerzak SP, Staubus AE, Malspeis L. A phase I investigation of flavone acetic acid (NSC-347512). *Proc Am Soc Clin Oncol.* 1988;**7**:62.

Havlin KA, Kuhn JG, Craig JB, et al. Phase I clinical and pharmacokinetic trial of flavone acetic acid. *J Natl Cancer Inst.* 1991;**83**:124–128.

Kaye SB, Clavel M, Dodion P, et al. Phase II trials with flavone acetic acid (NCS-347512, LM975) in patients with advanced carcinoma of the breast, colon, head and neck and melanoma. *Invest New Drugs.* 1990;**8**: S95–S99.

Kerr DJ, Kaye SB. Flavone acetic acid—Preclinical and clinical activity. *Eur J Cancer Clin Oncol.* 1989;**25**:1271–1272.

Kerr DJ, Kaye SB, Cassidy J, et al. Phase I and pharmacokinetic study of flavone acetic acid. *Cancer Res.* 1987;**47**:6776–6781.

Kerr DJ, Kaye SB, Graham J, et al. Phase I and pharmacokinetic study of LM985 (flavone acetic acid ester). *Cancer Res.* 1986;**46**(6):3142–3146.

Kerr DJ, Maughan T, Newlands E, et al. Phase II trials of flavone acetic acid in advanced malignant melanoma and colorectal carcinoma. *Br J Cancer.* 1989; **60**:104–106.

Lewis CR, Jardine A, Rankin EM, Kaye SB. Autonomic neuropathy following treatment with flavone acetic acid. *Eur J Cancer Clin Oncol.* 1989;**25**(3):573–574.

Mahadevan V, Meager A, Lewis GP, Hart IR. Flavone acetic acid-induced tumor blood flow reduction. A possible role for tumor necrosis factor. *Proc Am Soc Clin Oncol.* 1990;**31**:2376.

Melink T, Egorin M, Conley B, et al. Phase I trial and pharmacokinetics of flavone acetic acid (NSC-347512) (FAA) administered by 1-hour infusion. *Proc Am Soc Clin Oncol.* 1987;**6**:39.

O'Dwyer PJ, Shoemaker D, Zaharko DS, et al. Flavone acetic acid (LM 975, NSC-347512). A novel antitumor agent. *Cancer Chemother Pharmacol.* 1987;**19**(1):6–10.

Plowman J, Narayanan VL, Dykes D, et al. Flavone acetic acid: A novel agent with preclinical antitumor activity against colon adenocarcinoma 38 in mice. *Cancer Treat Rep.* 1986;**70**:631–635.

Relling MV, Maupin J, Evans WE, Pratt CB. Flavone acetic acid (FAA) pharmacokinetics (PK) in children with cancer. *FASEB J.* 1990;**4**(3):A739.

Rewcastle GW, Kestell P, Bauley BC, Denny WA. Light-induced breakdown of flavone acetic acid and zanthenone analogues in solution. *J Natl Cancer Inst.* 1990;**82**:528–529.

Rubin J, Ames MM, Schutt AJ, Nichols WL, Bowie EJ, Kovach JS. Flavone-8-acetic acid inhibits ristocetin-induced platelet agglutination and prolongs bleeding time. *Lancet.* 1987;**2**:1081–1082.

Triozzi PL, Rinehart JJ, Malspeis L, Young DC, Grever MR. Immunological effects of flavone acetic acid. *Cancer Res.* 1990;**50**:6483–6485.

Weiss RB, Greene RF, Knight RD, et al. Phase I and clinical pharmacology study of intravenous flavone acetic acid (NSC-347512). *Cancer Res.* 1988;**48**:5878–5882.

Wiltrout RH, Boyd MR, Back TC, Salup RR, Arthur JA, Hornung RL. Flavone-8-acetic acid augments systemic natural killer cell activity and synergizes with IL-2 for treatment of murine renal cancer. *J Immunol.* 1988;**140**:3261–3265.

Zwi LJ, Baguley BC, Gavin JB, Wilson WR. Blood flow failure as a major determinant in the antitumor action of flavone acetic acid. *J Natl Cancer Inst.* 1989;**81**:1005–1013.

Floxuridine

■ Other Names

FUDR® (Ro 5-0360) (Roche Laboratories); NSC-27640; NDC 4-1935-08.

■ Chemistry

Structure of floxuridine

Floxuridine is a fluorinated pyrimidine with structural and functional similarities to its prodrug form, fluorouracil (Heidelberger 1967). Floxuridine is 2'-deoxy-5-fluorouridine and has the chemical formula $C_9H_{11}FN_2O_5$. Floxuridine differs from tegafur (ftorafur) by the presence of hydroxymethyl and hydroxyl groups in the ribose moiety. It has a molecular weight of 246.21 and is soluble in water, 50 g/100 mL; in alcohol, 8.1 g/100 mL; in chloroform, 0.3 g/100 mL; in propylene glycol, 12 g/100 mL; and in dimethyl acetamide, >50 g/100 mL (Roche Laboratories 1971).

■ Antitumor Activity

Floxuridine is used in the continuous intraarterial (or less frequently intravenous) chemotherapy of advanced adenocarcinomas of the gastrointestinal tract (Moore and Loike 1960). These include oral cancers (Couture 1968), and tumors of the colon (Moertel 1978), pancreas (Barone 1975), liver, and biliary tract (Davis et al 1974). Some activity has also been observed in adenocarcinoma of the breast (Papac and Calabresi 1966). Most often, continuous hepatic artery infusions over several days are used to treat metastatic adenocarcinoma involving the liver (Oberfield et al 1979, Sullivan et al 1964, 1967), often as an adjunct to surgery in cancer of the large bowel (Dwight et al 1975).

Reitemeier et al (1965) and a large Eastern Cooperative Group study (1967) could find no demonstrable differences between fluorouracil and floxuridine when used in colorectal adenocarcinoma and in breast carcinoma, respectively; however, fluoropyrimidines remain the mainstay of the chemotherapeutic management of colon cancer (Moertel 1978).

In animal models, floxuridine has marked activity in the locoregional management of cancers metastatic to the liver (Bartkowski et al 1986). Kemeny et al (1987) compared 14-day continuous infusions of floxuridine given arterially via the hepatic artery or systemically by the cephalic vein. In patients with liver metastases from colorectal carcinoma, intrahepatic therapy produced a significantly higher overall response rate of 50%, compared with only 20% in the systemic (intravenous) therapy arm. When crossed over to the intrahepatic route, patients who had relapsed on intravenous therapy still achieved a 25% partial response rate (Kemeny et al 1987). In another trial, 1-year survival was 64% for hepatic arterial floxuridine compared with 44% for a control population (Rougier et al 1992). Survival times at 2 years were 23 and 13% for the floxuridine and control groups, respectively; however, the development of extrahepatic metastases was common. These results suggest that intraarterial infusions of floxuridine are superior to intravenous regimens for treating hepatic metastases of colorectal cancer. In addition, intraarterial floxuridine can be combined with systemic 5-fluorouracil in patients with metastatic colorectal cancer (Seiter et al 1992). A 64% partial response rate was described in this trial. Also, a decreased incidence of systemic relapse was reported for the combination of intraarterial floxuridine with concomitant intravenous floxuridine in metastatic colon carcinoma (Safi et al 1989).

■ Mechanism of Action

Floxuridine is an antimetabolite whose structure and cytotoxic mechanisms are similar to those of ftorafur and 5-fluorouracil (Karnofsky and Young 1967). Floxuridine may be thus considered to be a preactivated form of 5-fluorouracil differing by the addition of the deoxyribose sugar moiety at the

1-position of the pyrimidine nucleus in floxuridine. After injection, floxuridine is either catabolized primarily to fluorouracil (if a large bolus dose is given) or metabolized to the active monophosphorylated nucleotide, 5-fluoro-2′-deoxyuridine-5′-monophosphate (FdUMP) when small doses are given (eg, as with continuous infusion). Ultimately the FdUMP metabolite binds to and inhibits thymidylate synthetase in concert with reduced folate cofactors, including N^5,N^{10}-methylenetetrahydrofolate.

Floxuridine is a cell cycle phase-specific agent with marked cytotoxic activity in S phase (DNA synthesis). The basic biochemical block produced by the drug involves inhibition of DNA synthesis. This effect may be enhanced by continuous drug infusion over several days (Sullivan and Miller 1965, Miller and Sullivan 1962, 1967). Secondarily, phosphorylated metabolites of floxuridine, including fluorouracil, can also interrupt RNA synthesis. These latter metabolites fraudulently enter RNA synthetic reactions and can ultimately be incorporated into RNA, causing miscoding and cell death.

Floxuridine has significant advantages over fluorouracil when given by intrahepatic artery perfusions. These include a much higher first-pass hepatic extraction rate, which helps to localize cytotoxic effects to the liver. Furthermore, the drug requires an alternate metabolic step for activation compared to 5-fluorouracil.

Resistance to floxuridine has been shown to involve reduced metabolism to FdUMP (Mulkins and Heidelberger 1982), decreased binding to thymidylate synthetase (Bapat et al 1983), and increased levels of thymidylate synthetase (Baskin et al 1975, Rosanna et al 1982). The last effect may be mediated by amplification of the thymidylate synthetase gene (Berger et al 1985).

■ Availability and Storage

Floxuridine is commercially available from Roche Laboratories, Nutley, New Jersey. It is supplied in 500-mg glass vials as a white lyophilized powder. The vials may be stored at room temperature for up to 36 months after manufacture.

■ Preparation for Use, Stability, and Admixture

Each 500 mg, 5-mL vial may be reconstituted with 5 mL of Sterile Water for Injection, USP, yielding a 100 mg/mL solution at a pH of 4.0 to 5.5. If necessary, this solution may be stored under refrigeration for up to 2 weeks.

For intraarterial or intravenous use the solution may then be added to a convenient volume of either D5W or normal saline. Properly diluted solutions (at room temperature and in normal light conditions) are chemically stable for up to 2 weeks (Lokich et al 1988). Caution must be exercised, though, as microbial contamination is possible when prolonged infusions or nonbacteriostatic diluents are used.

Floxuridine is known to be compatible with sodium heparin (Trissel 1988) and does not appear to bind to fluid surfaces in implantable infusion pumps wherein the drug was stable for at least 12 days (Keller and Ensminger 1982). When floxuridine (10 mg/mL) was admixed with cisplatin (0.5 mg/mL) in polyvinyl chloride bags containing normal saline, there was a 13% loss of floxuridine after 7 days and an 18% loss after 14 days (Lokich et al 1988). The appearance of a new peak on the chromatogram suggests complexation between floxuridine and cisplatin. Overall, the admixture of floxuridine and cisplatin in saline for less than 7 days was deemed feasible (Lokich et al 1988). Floxuridine has also been mixed directly with fluorouracil (10 mg/mL each) in polyvinyl chloride bags of 60 mL normal saline. No decomposition of either drug was observed over 14 days (Anderson et al 1989). The drug is also physically compatible for 4 hours with ondansetron (Trissel et al 1990).

■ Administration

The manufacturer recommends that floxuridine be given only intraarterially, but it can also be administered intravenously (Sullivan et al 1962, Kemeny et al 1987). For intraarterial regimens, an H_2 antihistamine such as ranitidine is administered (150 mg PO twice daily) to prevent the development of peptic ulcer disease while on therapy.

Intraarterial administration is facilitated through a surgically placed catheter directed to the major artery supplying a well-defined tumor (eg, in the liver, head and neck region, gallbladder). By the use of various infusion pumps, very slow flow rates may be achieved that can deliver the desirable doses of 0.1 to 0.6 mg/kg/24 h. Typically, heparin (10,000 U/50 mL of solution) is added to the floxuridine infusate to prevent localized clotting complications

(Seiter et al 1992). Often the catheter is kept in place for weeks or months, and generally, treatments are given over 1 to 6 weeks with continuous infusion of a sterile isotonic fluid, such as heparinized normal saline, between courses.

Floxuridine has been given intravenously in solid tumor therapy by dilution into 500 to 1000 mL of D5W or normal saline. For this use it has been administered continuously over 24 hours for several days per course (Sullivan and Miller 1965).

■ Dosage

Intraarterial doses of floxuridine have ranged from 100 to 600 μg (0.1 to 0.6 mg)/kg/d for between 1 and 6 weeks. The higher dose range of 0.4 to 0.6 mg/kg/d × 14 days is generally used in intrahepatic administration, as the liver can detoxify more of a given dose and thus reduce systemic toxicity. Therapy is usually continued for at least 2 weeks or until severe toxic effects become apparent. Intraarterial floxuridine doses of 0.3 mg/kg/d × 14 days have also been combined with systemic 5-fluorouracil (800 mg/m^2/d × 5) administered by continuous intravenous infusions beginning on day 15 (Seiter et al 1992). Despite the low dose of 5-fluorouracil, 100% of patients required dose reductions within 6 months to yield 59% of the planned dose intensity (Seiter et al 1992). A mean 74% dose reduction was reported in another trial using 0.3 mg/kg/d × 14 days when hepatic and gastrointestinal complications ensued (Rougier et al 1992). Safi et al (1989) have also combined intraarterial floxuridine (0.2 mg/kg/d × 14 days) with concomitant intravenous floxuridine (0.09 mg/kg/d × 14 days).

Intravenous doses of 0.5 to 1.0 mg/kg/d for 6 to 15 days by continuous infusion have been used in certain solid tumors. Alternately, a bolus induction dose schedule has employed single daily doses of 30 mg/kg/d for up to 5 days. Following induction as described earlier, a maintenance regimen of 15 mg/kg given every other day has been continued until a relapse or significant toxicity becomes apparent.

When combined in a 14-day infusion with cisplatin, the recommended phase II doses were 0.075 mg/kg/d for floxuridine and 7.5 mg/m^2/d for cisplatin (Lokich et al 1988). When combined in a 14-day intravenous infusion with 5-fluorouracil the recommended phase II doses were 350 mg/m^2 5-fluorouracil and 0.1 mg/kg/d floxuridine (Anderson et al 1989).

■ Drug Interactions

Floxuridine has been administered by intravenous infusion with thymidine to reduce its toxicity (Miller et al 1961). A high thymidine dose of 30 mg/kg/d was used to block otherwise lethal intravenous infusion floxuridine doses of 1.5 to 3 mg/kg/d for 15 to 20 days. Floxuridine has also been combined with cytarabine in patients with solid tumors. The dose-limiting toxic effect was myelosuppression with a 2-hour intravenous infusion of low-dose floxuridine (0.04–0.05 mg/kg or 1.6–2 mg/m^2) given prior to cytarabine (100 mg/m^2/d for 5 consecutive days) (Cummings et al 1979). This clinical trial was based on experimental observations of sensitization of L5178Y cells to cytarabine cell killing when low-dose floxuridine preceded cytarabine (Chu et al 1976). The mechanism of the observed synergy was believed to involve floxuridine-mediated inhibition of cytidine uptake without affecting cytarabine (Chu et al 1976).

Dipyridamole has also been combined with floxuridine in an effort to block cellular efflux. Although this interaction achieves potentiation in vitro (Alberts et al 1987), clinical potentiation could not be demonstrated because of the low free dipyridamole fraction in human plasma (Buzaid et al 1989). Floxuridine's antitumor activity can also be modulated with leucovorin, which acts to increase the affinity of binding to and inhibition of thymidylate synthetase (Yin et al 1983). Optimal dosing schedules have not been established for this interaction but the low toxicity of leucovorin allows exploration of a variety of dose levels; however, as with fluorouracil, more severe diarrhea may be anticipated when leucovorin is given with floxuridine.

Floxuridine has been directly admixed with fluorouracil (Anderson et al 1989) or with cisplatin for prolonged 14-day intravenous infusions (Lokich et al 1988) (see Preparation for Use, Stability, and Admixture and Dosage sections for compatibility and specific dosing recommendations). The rationale for the dual fluoropyrimidine infusions is based on slight quantitative differences in the cytotoxic mechanisms of action of 5-fluorouracil and floxuridine: greater RNA incorporation with 5-fluorouracil and greater conversion of floxuridine to FdUMP, which inhibits thymidine synthesis (Anderson et al 1989). The combination of floxuridine with cisplatin is based on observations of in vitro antitumor synergy (Schabel et al 1979).

■ Pharmacokinetics

Floxuridine is poorly absorbed by the oral route. Following intravenous dosing, about 29% of a dose is excreted renally as inactive metabolites (Clarkson et al 1964). The fraction excreted in the urine decreases with continuous infusions. When floxuridine is injected intravenously (30 mg/kg over 1 minute), high initial plasma concentrations are followed by an estimated elimination half-life of about 15 minutes (determined by nonspecific bioassay) (Clarkson et al 1964).

Both floxuridine and its metabolite fluorouracil are metabolized in the liver (Mukherjee et al 1963). Continuous infusion appears to decrease the rate of metabolic degradation of floxuridine. The manufacturer suggests that continuous infusion thereby favors conversion of floxuridine to the monophosphorylated active metabolite FdUMP, whereas bolus injections of large doses favors metabolic conversion back to 5-fluorouracil.

Ensminger et al (1978) have recently compared hepatic arterial infusions of fluorouracil and floxuridine. The results demonstrate a very high hepatic extraction ratio for floxuridine (0.69–0.92) compared with fluorouracil (hepatic extraction ratio 0.22–0.45). Thus, when given by hepatic artery infusion, up to 92% of floxuridine and approximately 22 to 45% of fluorouracil are removed from the circulation on one pass through the liver. Correspondingly, peripheral venous floxuridine levels after arterial infusion are one-fourth those obtained after intravenous administration (Ensminger et al 1978). These results may explain (1) the reduced systemic toxicity often reported for (hepatic) arterially administered drug (Sullivan and Miller 1965) and (2) the increased toxicity possible from prolonged peripheral infusions of the drug (DeConti et al 1973).

Ultimately, the metabolic products of the fluorinated pyrimidines are largely excreted through the lungs as carbon dioxide (about 60%). The fraction excreted in the urine probably approaches 10 to 30% at 24 hours. The excreted species include urea, a small amount of unchanged floxuridine, some 5-fluorouracil, and a large number of inactive 5-fluorouracil metabolites.

■ Side Effects and Toxicity

The intraarterial route of administration may produce less systemic toxicity with floxuridine but is not devoid of toxic complications. Most of these relate to the prolonged use of an arterial catheter and include arterial ischemia, thrombosis, and bleeding at the catheter site. Blocked catheters, leakage at the site, embolism, and infection at the catheter site can also occur (Oberfield et al 1979, Sterchi et al 1989). Other than these procedural complications, adverse drug reactions are limited mostly to bone marrow suppression, mucositis, and organ-specific complications at the principal site perfused (hepatic dysfunction with intrahepatic infusion). Typical signs of hepatic toxicity include elevation in lactate dehydrogenase, alkaline phosphatase, serum glutamic–oxalacetic transaminase, and, rarely, serum bilirubin levels. When administered by intrahepatic infusion, floxuridine can produce frank gastric ulceration and biliary sclerosis. These effects have been reported to occur in 17 and 8% of patients, respectively (Kemeny et al 1987). The 1-year rate of sclerosing cholangitis was 9% at 6 months and 25% at 1 year in another trial of floxuridine administered by hepatic artery infusion (Rougier et al 1992). This led to the interruption of therapy in 80% of patients.

Careful surgical technique can reduce or even eliminate these toxic effects. Hohn et al (1985) have shown that gastritis is completely prevented by division and ligation of the hepatic arteries distal to the point of cannulation that supply the superior border of the distal stomach and proximal duodenum. The manufacturer warns that drug doses be reduced in patients with any of the following: a history of high-dose pelvic irradiation or alkylating agent therapy, abnormal kidney function, and (especially) abnormal liver function. Compromised nutritional and/or hematologic status is also a consideration for reducing dosage as it is for any type of chemotherapy.

Significant myelosuppression can be expected with intravenous floxuridine doses and, to a lesser extent, with intraarterial doses (Curreri and Ansfield 1959, Ansfield and Curreri 1960). These effects are generally comparable to those observed with fluorouracil. Hematologic toxicity manifests as leukopenia and to a lesser extent thrombocytopenia. Anemia is also observed after several courses of therapy, especially in heavily pretreated patients.

Gastrointestinal toxic effects are also common with floxuridine. These include nausea, vomiting, anorexia, abdominal cramps, and some pain. Severe secretory diarrhea has also been noted especially with continuous intravenous infusions (Kemeny et al 1987). This is typically the dose limiting toxic effect of prolonged infusions and usually necessitates immediate dose reduction in most settings. Sigmoid ulcerations can be observed if sigmoidoscopy is performed.

Mucositis is noted in about 10% of patients receiving prolonged, intrahepatic infusions of floxuridine. As with 5-fluorouracil the appearance of severe glossitis or stomatitis usually indicates the need to either reduce doses or discontinue therapy.

Dermatologic toxic effects, including alopecia, edema, dermatitis, rashes and pruritis, and hyperpigmentation of veins, have been infrequently reported.

Rare central nervous system toxic effects are associated with floxuridine, including blurred vision, depression, nystagmus, vertigo, and lethargy. These effects can have both an acute and a delayed (months) onset. Convulsions have been seen rarely, as have a few instances of paralysis. Other than drug discontinuance at the earliest sign, little can therapeutically be done to alleviate these effects. Fortunately, most cases of floxuridine neurotoxicity resolve rapidly after discontinuation of the drug.

■ Special Applications

Circadian-Timed Floxuridine Administration. Studies in rats have shown that a sine wave infusion pattern of floxuridine was better than a constant infusion regimen. The least toxic regimen had maximal drug delivery, occurring during the last portion of the activity cycle of the animal and continuing into the early rest phase (von Roemeling et al 1987). This infusion pattern also produced the best antitumor response in Fischer rats bearing the FN-13762 adenocarcinoma. These circadian schedules do not appear to alter floxuridine pharmacokinetic patterns in the rats (von Roemeling et al 1989). In patients with renal cell carcinoma, two types of 14-day floxuridine intravenous infusions have been compared: a flat-rate continuous infusion or a time-modified pattern in which the majority of the daily dose was given between 3:00 PM and 9:00 PM to reduce GI tract sensitivity. Very little drug was administered thereafter (between 3:00 AM and 9:00 AM). Both regimens were delivered by implanted programmable pumps and the dose of 0.15 mg/kg was increased or decreased by 0.025 mg/kg increments depending on toxicity (von Roemeling et al 1988). Toxicity, particularly diarrhea, nausea, and vomiting, was reduced significantly with the time-modified delivery regimen. Fewer dose reductions and treatment delays were also noted with the time-modified regimen, although similar response rates were observed in both groups.

In a follow-up trial, floxuridine was delivered by implanted Synchromed® pumps using the same general circadian flow rate described earlier: maximal flow rates occurred in the late afternoon/early evening. Gastrointestinal toxic effects were reduced compared with constant-rate infusions, and clinical activity (complete or partial response) was noted in 7 of 30 patients with lung metastases from renal cell carcinoma (von Roemeling and Hrushesky 1989). Although greater floxuridine dose intensity may be achieved with this approach, the benefits in terms of higher response rates remain unclear.

Intraventricular Floxuridine. Floxuridine has been experimentally administered by the intraventricular route in three patients with meningeal neoplasia (Dakhil et al 1981). Doses of 4 to 16 mg were administered using a Rickham reservoir surgically connected to the lateral ventricle. The elimination half-life of floxuridine was about 32 minutes, which is roughly double the rate accounted for by bulk cerebrospinal fluid flow. Levels of floxuridine in ventricular cerebrospinal fluid were dose dependent: 8 to 31 μM at 4 mg/d and 4.1 to 14 μM at 1 mg/d. These cerebrospinal fluid levels are over 1000-fold higher than those achievable using systemic floxuridine infusions.

Intracavitary Floxuridine. Floxuridine has also been administered intrapleurally and intraperitoneally at 30 mg/kg doses (Clarkson et al 1964). There was delayed elimination of drug from effusions in these compartments. The approximate half-lives in ascites fluid and pleural fluid were 2 to 6 and 1 to 8 hours, respectively. This indicates that very prolonged cumulative local exposures to floxuridine are obtained following intracavitary administration (Clarkson et al 1964). In some cases, this regimen produced objective therapeutic responses in patients with malignant effusions (Clarkson 1964).

REFERENCES

Alberts DS, Einspahr J, Peng Y-M, Spears P. Dipyridamole (D) potentiation of FUDR antitumor activity (abstract IIID-I). *Clin Pharmacol Ther.* 1987;**41**(2):247.

Anderson N, Lokich J, Bern M, et al. Combined 5-fluorouracil and floxuridine administered as a 14-day infusion. A phase I study. *Cancer.* 1989;**63**:825–827.

Ansfield FJ, Curreri AR. Clinical studies with 5-fluoro-2'-deoxyuridine. *Cancer Chemother Rep.* 1960;**6**:21–25.

Bapat AR, Zarow C, Danenberg PV. Human leukemic cells resistant to 5-fluoro-2′-deoxyuridine contain a thymidylate synthetase with lower affinity for nucleotides. *J Biol Chem*. 1983;**258**:4130–4136.

Barone RM. Treatment of carcinoma of the pancreas with radon seed implantation and intra-arterial infusion of 5-FUDR. *Surg Clin North Am*. 1975;**55**(1):117–128.

Bartkowski R, Berger MR, Aguiar JLA, et al. Experiments on the efficacy and toxicity of locoregional chemotherapy of liver tumors with 5-fluoro-2′-deoxyuridine (FUDR) and 5-fluorouracil (5-FU) in an animal model. *J Cancer Res Clin Oncol*. 1986;**111**:42–46.

Baskin F, Carlin SC, Kraus P, et al. Experimental chemotherapy of neuroblastoma II. Increased thymidylate synthetase activity in a 5-fluorodeoxyuridine-resistant variant of mouse neuroblastoma. *Mol Pharmacol*. 1975;**11**:105–117.

Berger SH, Jenh C-H, Johnson LF, Berger FG. Thymidylate synthetase overproduction and gene amplification in fluorodeoxyuridine-resistant human cells. *Mol Pharmacol*. 1985;**28**:461–467.

Buzaid AC, Alberts DS, Einspahr J, et al. Effect of dipyridamole on fluorodeoxyuridine cytotoxicity in vitro and in cancer patients. *Cancer Chemother Pharmacol*. 1989;**25**(2):124–130.

Chu MY, Hoovis ML, Fischer GA. Effects of 5-fluorodeoxyuridine on cell viability and uptake of deoxycytidine and [^{3}H]cytosine arabinoside in L5178 cells. *Biochem Pharmacol*. 1976;**25**:355–357.

Clarkson B. Relationship between cell type, glucose concentration and response to treatment in neoplastic effusions. *Cancer*. 1964;**17**:914–928.

Clarkson B, O'Connor A, Winston L, Hutchison D. The physiologic disposition of 5-fluorouracil and 5-fluoro-2′-deoxyuridine in man. *Clin Pharmacol Ther*. 1964;**5**:581.

Couture J. Intra-arterial infusion therapy for oral cancer. *Can J Surg*. 1968;**11**:420–423.

Cummings FJ, Hoovis ML, Calabresi P. Phase I study of 5-fluorodeoxyuridine plus cytosine arabinoside infusions in patients with solid tumors. *Cancer Treat Rep*. 1979;**63**(8):1371–1374.

Curreri AR, Ansfield F. Toxicity and preliminary clinical studies with 5-fluoro-2′-deoxyuridine (5-FUDR). *Cancer Chemother Rep*. 1959;**2**:8–11.

Dakhil S, Ensminger W, Strother V, Kindt G, et al. Pharmacokinetics of intraventricular 5-fluoro-2′-deoxyuridine (FUDR) in patients with meningeal neoplasia (abstract 706). *Proc Am Assoc Cancer Res*. 1981;**21**:178.

Davis HL, Guillermo R, Ansfield FJ. Adenocarcinomas of stomach, pancreas, liver and biliary tracts. *Cancer*. 1974;**33**:105–197.

DeConti RC, Kaplan SR, Papac RJ, Calabresi P. Continuous intravenous infusions of 5-fluoro-2′-deoxyuridine in the treatment of solid tumors. *Cancer*. 1973;**31**:894–898.

Dwight RW, Humphrey EW, Higgins GA, et al. FUDR as an adjuvant to surgery in cancer of the large bowel. *J Surg Oncol*. 1975;**5**:243–249.

Eastern Cooperative Group in Solid Tumor Chemotherapy. Comparison of antimetabolites in the treatment of breast and colon cancer. *JAMA*. 1967;**200**:770–778.

Ensminger WD, Rosowsky A, Raso V, et al. A clinical pharmacological evaluation of hepatic arterial infusions of 5-fluoro-2′-deoxyuridine and 5-fluorouracil. *Cancer Res*. 1978;**38**:3784–3792.

Heidelberger C. Cancer chemotherapy with purine and pyrimidine analogues. *Annu Rev Pharmacol*. 1967;**7**:101–124.

Hohn DC, Stagg RJ, Price DC, Lewis BJ. Avoidance of gastroduodenal toxicity in patients receiving hepatic arterial 5-fluoro-2′-deoxyuridine. *J Clin Oncol*. 1985;**3**(9):1257–1260.

Karnofsky DA, Young CW. Comparative aspects of the pharmacology of the antimetabolites. *Fed Proc*. 1967;**26**:1139–1145.

Keller JH, Ensminger WD. Stability of cancer chemotherapeutic agents in a totally implanted drug delivery system. *Am J Hosp Pharm*. 1982;**39**:1321–1323.

Kemeny N, Daly J, Reichman B, Geller N, et al. Intrahepatic or systemic infusion of fluorodeoxyuridine in patients with liver metastases from colorectal carcinoma. *Ann Intern Med*. 1987;**107**:459–465.

Lokich J, Anderson N, Bern M, et al. Combined floxuridine® and cisplatin in a fourteen day infusion. Phase I study. *Cancer*. 1988;**62**:2309–2312.

Miller E, Sullivan RD. Clinical effects of the continuous intravenous infusion of cancer chemotherapeutic compounds. In: Vermel YM, Wollfson KG, eds. *VIII International Cancer Congress*. Moscow: Medgiz Publishing House; 1962:338–339.

Miller E, Sullivan RD. The alteration of biologic activity of cancer chemotherapy agents by prolonged infusion. In: Brodsky I, Kahn SB, Moyer JH, eds. *Cancer Chemotherapy: Basic and Clinical Applications, 15th Hahnemann Symposium*. New York: Grune & Stratton; 1967:331–337.

Miller E, Sullivan R, Young C, Burchenal JH. Clinical effects of the continuous infusion of antimetabolites—Prevention of toxicity of 5-fluoro-2′-deoxyuridine by thymidine (abstract 192). *Proc Am Assoc Cancer Res*. 1961;**3**:251.

Moertel CG. Chemotherapy of gastrointestinal cancer. *N Engl J Med*. 1978;**299**(19):1049–1052.

Moore GE, Loike A. Clinical experience with 5-fluoro-2′-deoxyuridine. *Cancer Chemother Rep*. 1960;**6**:26–28.

Mukherjee KL, et al. Studies on fluorinated pyrimidines. XVII. Tissue distribution of 5-fluorouracil-2C^{14} and 5-fluoro-2′-deoxyuridine in cancer patients. *Cancer Res*. 1963;**23**:67–77.

Mulkins MA, Heidelberger C. Biochemical characterization of fluoropyrimidine-resistant murine leukemic cell lines. *Cancer Res*. 1982;**45**:965–973.

Oberfield RA, McCaffrey JA, Polio J, Clouse ME, et al. Prolonged and continuous percutaneous intra-arterial hepatic infusion chemotherapy in advanced metastatic

liver adenocarcinoma from colorectal primary. *Cancer.* 1979;**44**:414–423.
Papac RJ, Calabresi P. Infusion of floxuridine in the treatment of solid tumors. *JAMA.* 1966;**197**:237–241.
Reitmeier RJ, Moertel CG, Hahn RG. Comparison of 5-fluorouracil (NSC-19893) and 2'-deoxy-5-fluorouridine (NSC-27640) in treatment of patients with advanced adenocarcinoma of colon or rectum. *Cancer Chemother Rep.* 1965;**44**:39–43.
Roche Laboratories. *FUDR*™ (*Floxuridine*) *Roche*®: Comprehensive Product Information. Booklet No. FUDR-RL-1071. Nutley, NJ: Roche Laboratories, 1971.
Rosanna C, Rao LG, Johnson LF. Thymidylate synthetase overproduction in 5-fluorodeoxyuridine-resistant mouse fibroblasts. *Mol Cell Biol.* 1982;**2**:1118–1125.
Rougier P, Laplanche A, Huguier M, et al. Hepatic arterial infusion of floxuridine in patients with liver metastases from colorectal carcinoma: Long-term results of a prospective randomized trial. *J Clin Oncol.* 1992;**10**(7):1112–1118.
Safi F, Bittner R, Roscher R, et al. Regional chemotherapy for hepatic metastases of colorectal carcinoma (continuous intraarterial versus continuous intraarterial/intravenous therapy). *Cancer.* 1989;**64**:379–387.
Schabel FM Jr., Trader MW, Laster WR, et al. *cis*-Dichlorodiammineplatinum(II): Combination chemotherapy and cross resistance studies with tumors of mice. *Cancer Treat Rep.* 1979;**63**:1459–1473.
Seiter K, Kemeny N, Sigurdson E, et al. A phase I trial of hepatic artery fluorodeoxyuridine combined with systemic 5-fluorouracil for the treatment of metastases from colorectal cancer. *Reg Cancer.* 1992;**4**:166–169.
Sterchi JM, Richards F, White DR, et al. Chemoinfusion of the hepatic artery for metastases to the liver. *Surg Gynecol Obstet.* 1989;**168**(4):291–295.
Sullivan RD, Miller E. The clinical effects of prolonged intravenous infusion of 5-fluoro-2'-deoxyuridine. *Cancer Res.* 1965;**25**:1025–1033.
Sullivan RD, Miller E, Watkins E. Effects of the continuous intravenous and intra-arterial infusion of fluorinated pyrimidines. *Proc Am Assoc Cancer Res.* 1962;**3**:365.
Sullivan RD, Norcross JW, Watkins E Jr. Chemotherapy of metastatic liver cancer by prolonged hepatic-artery infusion. *N Engl J Med.* 1964;**270**:321–327.
Sullivan RD, Watkins E Jr., Oberfield RA, Khazei AM. Current status of protracted arterial infusion cancer chemotherapy for the treatment of solid tumors. *Surg Clin North Am.* 1967;**47**:769–783.
Trissel LA, ed. *ASHP Handbook on Injectable Drugs.* 5th ed. Bethesda, MD: American Society of Hospital Pharmacists.
Trissel LA, Fulton B, Tramonte SM. Visual compatibility of ondansetron with chemotherapeutic agents, antibiotics, and other selected drugs during simulated Y-site injection (abstract #P-468R). In: *25th Annual ASHP Midyear Clinical Meetings and Exhibit, Las Vegas, Nevada.* Bethesda, MD: American Society of Hospital Pharmacists, 1990.

Von Roemeling R, Mormont MC, Walker K, et al. Cancer control depends on the circadian shape of continuous FUDR infusion. *Proc Am Assoc Cancer Res.* 1987;**28**:326.
Von Roemeling RV, Fukuda E, Fudin J, et al. Are FUDR pharmacokinetics circadian stage dependent? (abstract 2345) *Proc Am Assoc Cancer Res.* 1989;**30**:589.
Von Roemeling R, Hrushesky WJM. Circadian patterning of continuous floxuridine infusion reduces toxicity and allows higher dose intensity in patients with widespread cancer. *J Clin Oncol.* 1989;**7**(11):1710–1719.
Von Roemeling R, Rabatin JT, Fraly EE, Hrushesky WJM. Progressive metastatic renal cell carcinoma controlled by continuous 5-fluoro-2'-deoxyuridine infusion. *J Urol.* 1988;**139**:259–262.
Yin MB, Zakrzewski SF, Hakala MT. Relationship of cellular folate pools to the activity of 5-fluorouracil. *Mol Pharmacol.* 1983;**23**:190–199.

Fludarabine Phosphate

■ Other Names

NSC-312887; 2-fluoro-Ara-AMP; FLAMP, Fludara® (Berlex Laboratories).

■ Chemistry

Structure of fludarabine phosphate

Fludarabine phosphate is a novel nucleotide analog of the antiviral agent adenine arabinoside (Ara-A). The complete chemical name is 9-β-D-arabinofuranosyl-2-fluoroadenine 5'-monophosphate. It has the empiric formula $C_{10}H_{11}FN_5O_7PF$ and a molecular weight of 365.2. The compound was synthesized to overcome two deficiencies of Ara-A as an antitumor agent. Fludarabine phosphate is less readily deaminated and more water soluble than Ara-A (Montgomery 1982). These properties are imparted by the fluorine substitution on the purine ring. The solubility of fludarabine in water is pH dependent: 9.2 mg/mL in water, 27.6 mg/mL in pH 4 buffer, and 57 mg/mL in pH 9 buffer (Chun et al 1991).

■ Antitumor Activity

Fludarabine phosphate is commercially available for the treatment of chronic lymphocytic leukemia (Keating et al 1989). It is still undergoing active phase II testing in other tumors. To date, however, the compound has produced consistent antitumor activity in patients with three diseases including chronic lymphocytic leukemia (CLL), low-grade lymphomas, and mycosis fungoides.

Fludarabine phosphate has remarkably good activity in patients with advanced CLL. Bolus daily × 5 doses of 20 to 25 mg/m^2/d given every 28 days have resulted in hematologic improvements in 39 to 52% of patients (Grever et al 1986, Keating et al 1987). Some responses have been dramatic, with marked improvement in quantitative serum immunoglobulins. Eradication of all disease in the bone marrow (complete remission) occurs in up to 33% of patients (Keating et al 1989, 1991). The response rates for CLL patients vary by stage: 64% for Rai stages 0 to II, 58% for Rai stage III, and 50% for Rai stage IV (Keating et al 1989). Survival is similarly correlated with the final disease stage achieved after fludarabine treatment. Responses to fludarabine in CLL are rapid, with 92% of responses obtained after three courses of therapy. The median time to response in the CLL trials of alkylator-refractory patients was 7 weeks. Complete peripheral responses in the blood, liver, spleen, and lymph nodes are obtained in 48 to 69% of patients. The time to recurrence after treatment is discontinued in complete responders ranges from 9 to 26 months (Keating et al 1991). Overall, 50% survival is greater than 30 months for all CLL patients treated with fludarabine. For patients with Rai stages 0 to II there is 85% survival at 30 months compared with 70% survival for stages III and IV (Keating et al 1991).

Doses of 25 to 30 mg/m^2/d × 5 days repeated every 3 to 5 weeks produce response rates ranging from 33% in diffuse small cell lymphoma to 64% in follicular small/cleaved cell lymphoma (Redman et al 1988). Similar response rates were noted with a loading dose of 20 mg/m^2 followed by a continuous infusion of 30 mg/m^2/24 h for 48 hours (Leiby et al 1987).

Doses of 18 to 25 mg/m^2/d × 5 have produced responses in 20% of patients with cutaneous T-lymphocyte malignancy (Von Hoff et al 1989).

Fludarabine phosphate has definite activity against acute nonlymphocytic leukemia and acute lymphocytic leukemia (Warrell and Berman 1986, Spriggs et al 1986); however, these responses were achieved at highly toxic doses of 150 mg/m^2/d × 5 days and 125 mg/m^2/d × 7 days. At those doses, severe central nervous system toxicity consisting of blindness, encephalopathy, and progressive neurologic deterioration was noted (see later text). It is clear that the drug cannot be used at dose levels active in acute leukemia. Doses of 125 mg/m^2/d × 5 or less did not produce any tumor responses.

Initial phase II trials have indicated that fludarabine phosphate has some activity in patients with gliomas (Taylor and Eyre 1987); however, other trials have not confirmed this activity (Cascino et al 1988).

Fludarabine phosphate is not active in several types of solid tumors (as reviewed by Chun et al 1991). It has undergone phase II trials in patients with colorectal carcinoma, multiple myeloma (Kraut et al 1990), malignant melanoma (Kish et al 1991), carcinoma of the pancreas, breast cancer, non-small cell and small cell lung cancer, astrocytomas (Taylor et al 1991) ovarian cancer, head and neck cancer, hepatoma, endometrial cancer (Von Hoff et al 1988), renal cell cancer, and sarcoma. No substantial antitumor activity was noted in any of these patient groups.

■ Mechanism of Action

Studies in humans and animals have shown that fludarabine phosphate is rapidly dephosphorylated by serum phosphates in vivo and converted to 2-fluoro-Ara-AMP (2-FLAA) (Hersh et al 1986). Like other nucleosides the active prodrug 2-FLAA enters cells by a carrier-mediated transport process (Sirotnak et al 1983). The metabolite is phosphorylated intracellularly by the pyrimidine salvage enzyme deoxycytidine kinase (Tseng et al 1982). The 2-FLAA undergoes intracellular phosphorylation to 2-fluoro-Ara-ATP by deoxycytidine kinase. This intracellular phosphorylation to 2-fluoro-Ara-ATP is necessary for cytotoxicity (Brockman et al 1980). Studies done on leukemic cells in patients showed that reduced DNA synthesis is proportional to the 2-fluoro-Ara-ATP concentration (Danhauser et al 1986). Ultimately, fludarabine inhibits DNA synthesis by inhibition of ribonucleotide reductase (Tseng et al 1982, Chang and Cheng 1980). DNA synthesis is also blocked by fludarabine-induced inhibition of the repair enzyme DNA polymerase (Tseng et al 1982).

▪ Availability and Storage

Fludarabine phosphate is available from Berlex Laboratories, Richmond, California, as a sterile white powder (50 mg) in 6-mL-capacity sterile vials. Each vial contains 50 mg of lyophilized drug, 50 mg mannitol, and sodium hydroxide to adjust pH to 7.7. The intact vials should be stored under refrigeration (2–8°C).

▪ Preparation for Use, Stability, and Admixture

Each 50-mg vial is reconstituted with 2 mL of Sterile Water for Injection, USP. The resulting solution is clear and colorless and contains 25 mg/mg fludarabine phosphate. The pH range of the solution is 7.2 to 8.2. When reconstituted as directed, the solution exhibits little or no decomposition for at least 8 hours at room temperature (22–25°C) and under refrigeration (2–8°C); however, the single-use vial contains no antibacterial preservatives. Therefore, it is advised that the reconstituted product be discarded 8 hours after initial entry. After removal from the vial, the appropriate dose of the agent can be further diluted in 100 to 125 mL of 5% dextrose in water or 0.9% sodium chloride solution.

▪ Administration

Fludarabine phosphate has been given as a short intravenous infusion over 30 minutes (in 100 mL 0.9% NaCl) (Hutton et al 1984) or as a rapid loading dose/continuous infusion for 48-hour schedules (Leiby et al 1987). The drug should be administered through a well-running intravenous line. No episodes of extravasation necrosis have been reported with fludarabine phosphate.

▪ Special Precautions

Patients with preexisting neurologic disorders should be cautiously treated with fludarabine. Severe neurologic toxic effects including blindness, encephalopathy, seizures, and coma have been noted with fludarabine phosphate given at doses 96 mg/m^2/d or greater for 5 to 7 days (Warrell and Berman 1986, Spriggs et al 1986, Merkel et al 1986, Chun et al 1986). A progressive process of demyelination appears to be the mechanism for this neurologic deterioration. It may be caused by the toxic metabolite 2-fluoro-ATP (Avramis and Plunkett 1983). The toxicity has been seen in only one patient receiving conventional (25 mg/m^2/d × 5) doses of the agent (Merkel et al 1986).

Allopurinol should be prophylactically administered to patients with bulky CLL prior to fludarabine therapy. This should prevent the tumor lysis symptoms noted previously in a few patients who did not receive allopurinol (Chun et al 1991).

Patients with extensive prior therapy involving marrow-suppressive drugs should be cautiously followed if large cumulative fludarabine doses are administered. Fludarabine phosphate causes dose-limiting granulocytopenia and leukopenia (Hutton et al 1984). Patients who receive multiple doses of the agent may develop cumulative myelosuppression (Leiby et al 1987).

▪ Dosage

Usual doses of fludarabine phosphate range from 18 to 30 mg/m^2/d × 5 given as a 30-minute infusion each day. The recommended dose for CLL treatment is 25 mg/m^2/d for 5 consecutive days. Doses are repeated at 28- to 35-day intervals (Hutton et al 1984, Redman et al 1988). Typically, three courses are administered after a response is obtained and then the drug is discontinued.

Another important schedule is a loading dose of 20 mg/m^2 as a rapid intravenous infusion followed by 30 mg/m^2/d by continuous infusion for 48 hours (Leiby et al 1988). Doses may be reduced or dosing delayed in patients experiencing neurologic toxicity and/or severe cumulative myelosuppression (see Special Precautions).

▪ Drug Interactions

Pretreatment of human leukemia cells or lymphocytes with fludarabine in vitro potentiates the activation of cytarabine to its triphosphorylated form, cytarabine triphosphate. This has been evaluated in patients with CLL who were given fludarabine 30 mg/m^2 over 30 minutes followed in 4 hours by a 2-hour cytarabine infusion of 0.5 g/m^2 (Gandhi et al 1992). This sequential regimen increased the levels of cytarabine triphosphate by 15-fold in circulating CLL cells.

Five patients receiving fludarabine and pentostatin developed severe pulmonary toxicity requiring respirator support.

Pharmacokinetics

In patients receiving doses of 18 or 25 mg/m² daily × 5 over 30 minutes, and assuming fludarabine phosphate is instantaneously converted to 2-FLAA, the levels of 2-FLAA decline in a biexponential fashion with an average distribution (α) half-life of 0.60 hour and a terminal (β) half-life of 9.3 hours. The estimated plasma clearance of 2-FLAA is 9.07 ± 26.0 L/m². Of interest, there is an inverse correlation between the area under the 2-FLAA plasma concentration curve (AUC) and the absolute granulocyte count. Approximately 24 ± 3% of 2-FLAA is excreted in the urine over 5 days (Hersh et al 1986).

Side Effects and Toxicity

As noted earlier, the dose-limiting toxic effect of fludarabine phosphate is myelosuppression (granulocytopenia and thrombocytopenia). Boldt et al (1984) noted lymphocytopenia was also quite common in patients receiving the agent. Total T-lymphocyte counts fell by 90%, with decreases in all major T-lymphocyte subsets. By contrast, B-lymphocyte counts declined an average of 50%. The myelosuppression noted with fludarabine phosphate can be cumulative.

Transient nausea, vomiting, and diarrhea have been noted in about 30% of patients but treated with fludarabine. Hepatic transaminase and serum creatinine levels are occasionally elevated slightly.

Severe central nervous system toxicity and interstitial pneumonitis have been described. Most of the severe central nervous system toxicity of fludarabine has been observed only in leukemic patients receiving very high doses in phase I studies (Chun et al 1991). Most patients had also received prior chlorambucil, which is toxic to the lungs. Pulmonary toxicity has been described in six CLL patients (Hurst et al 1987). Patients present with fever, dyspnea, cough, and hypoxia (45–55 mm Hg at room air). The onset ranges from 3 to 28 days after starting the third to fifth course of therapy. Bilateral interstitial infiltrates and effusions are observed. The carbon dioxide diffusing capacity is also reduced. Limited lung biopsy results have suggested fibrosing interstitial pneumonitis, alveolitis, or centrilobular emphysema (Hurst et al 1987). Typically, respiratory function resolves spontaneously over several weeks with or without administration of corticosteroids. Rare side effects include skin rash, somnolence with administration, anemia, and, very occasionally, mild increases in hepatic enzymes. Tumor lysis syndrome was described in three patients with bulky CLL and included hyperuricemia, hyperphosphatemia, hypocalcemia, hyperkalemia, uratecrystalluria, and renal failure. Symptoms include flank pain and hematuria.

Special Applications

Fludarabine phosphate has been explored in a phase I and pharmacokinetic study utilizing the intraperitoneal route. Intraperitoneal administration of 4 to 25 mg/m² every 28 days resulted in peritoneal AUC/plasma AUC ratios of 8.1 to 12.7. Toxic effects included mild granulocytopenia, lymphopenia, anemia, thrombocytopenia, and elevations in serum alkaline phosphatase amylase and lactate dehydrogenase elevations (Weiss et al 1990). No antitumor responses were observed in six patients with metastatic peritoneal malignancy.

REFERENCES

Avramis VL, Plunkett W. 2-Fluoro-ATP: A toxic metabolite of 9-β-D-arabinoyl-2-fluoroadenine. *Biochem Biophys Res Commun.* 1983;**113**:35–43.

Boldt DH, Von Hoff DD, Kuhn JG, Hersh M. Effects on human peripheral lymphocytes of in vivo administration of 9-β-D-arabinofuranosyl-2-fluoroadenine-5′-monophosphate (NSC 312887), a new purine antimetabolite. *Cancer Res.* 1984;**44**:4661–4666.

Brockman RW, Cheng YC, Schable FM Jr, Montgomery TA. Metabolism and chemotherapeutic activity of 9-β-D-arabinofuranosyl-2-fluoroadenine against murine leukemia L-1210 and evidence for its phosphorylation by deoxycytidinekinase. *Cancer Res.* 1980;**40**:3610–3615.

Cascino TL, Brown LD, Morton RF, et al. Evaluation of fludarabine phosphate in patients with recurrent glioma. *Am J Clin Oncol.* 1988;**11**:586–588.

Chang C-H, Cheng Y-C. Effects of deoxyadenosine triphosphate and 9-β-D-arabinofuranosyladenine-5′-triphosphate on human ribonucleotide reductase from Molt-4F cells and the concept of "self-potentiation." *Cancer Res.* 1980;**40**:3555–3558.

Chun HG, Leyland-Jones BR, Caryk SM, Hoth DF. Central nervous system toxicity of fludarabine phosphate. *Cancer Treat Rep.* 1986;**70**:1225–1228.

Chun HG, Leyland-Jones B, Cheson BD. Fludarabine

phosphate: A synthetic purine antimetabolite with significant activity against lymphoid malignancies. *J Clin Oncol.* 1991;9(1):175–188.

Danhauser L, Plunkett W, Keating R, Cabanillas F. 9-Beta-D-arabinofuranosyl-2-fluoroadenine 5′-monophosphate pharmacokinetics in plasma and tumor cells of patients with relapsed leukemia and lymphoma. *Cancer Chemother Pharmacol.* 1986;18:145–152.

Gandhi V, Kemena A, Keating MJ, Plunkett W. Fludarabine infusion potentiates arabinosylcytosine metabolism in lymphocytes of patients with chronic lymphocytic leukemia. *Cancer Res.* 1992;52:897–903.

Grever MR, Coltman CA, Fileo JC, et al. Fludarabine monophosphate in chronic lymphocytic leukemia. *Blood.* 1986;68:223a.

Hersh MR, Kuhn JG, Phillips JL, Clark G, Ludden TM, Von Hoff DD. Pharmacokinetic study of fludarabine phosphate (NSC-312887). *Cancer Chemother Pharmacol.* 1986;17:277–280.

Hurst PG, Habib MP, Garwal H, Bluestein M, Paguin M, Greenberg BR. Pulmonary toxicity associated with fludarabine monophosphate. *Invest New Drugs.* 1987;5:207–210.

Hutton JJ, Von Hoff DD, Kuhn J, Phillips J, Hersh M, Clark G. Phase I clinical investigation of 9-β-D-arabinofuranosyl-2-fluoroadenine 5′-monophosphate (NSC 312887), a new purine antimetabolite. *Cancer Res.* 1984;44:4183–4186.

Keating MJ, Kantarjian H, O'Brien S, et al. Fludarabine: A new agent with marked cytoreductive activity in untreated chronic lymphocytic leukemia. *J Clin Oncol.* 1991;9(1):44–49.

Keating MJ, Kantarjian H, Talpaz M, et al. Fludarabine: A new agent with major activity against chronic lymphocytic leukemia. *Blood.* 1989;74(1):19–25.

Keating M, Redman J, Plunkett W, et al. Fludarabine (FAMP) has major antitumor activity in chronic lymphocytic leukemia (CLL). *Proc Am Soc Clin Oncol.* 1987;6:152.

Kish JA, Kopecky K, Samson MK, et al. Evaluation of fludarabine phosphate in malignant melanoma. *Invest New Drugs.* 1991;9:105–108.

Kraut EH, Crowley JJ, Grever MR, et al. Phase II study of fludarabine phosphate in multiple myeloma. *Invest New Drugs.* 1990;8:199–200.

Leiby JM, Grever MR, Staubus AE, et al. Phase I clinical investigation of fludarabine phosphate by a loading-dose and continuous infusion schedule. *J Natl Cancer Inst.* 1988;80:447–449.

Leiby JM, Snider KM, Kraut EH, Metz FN, Malspeis L, Grever MR. Phase II trial of 9-β-D-arabinofuranosyl-2-fluoroadenine 5′-monophosphate in non-Hodgkin's lymphoma: Prospective comparison of response with deoxycytidine kinase activity. *Cancer Res.* 1987;47:2719–2722.

Merkel DE, Griffin NL, Kagan-Hallet K, Von Hoff DD. Central nervous system toxicity with fludarabine. *Cancer Treat Rep.* 1986;70:1449–1450.

Montgomery JA. Has the well gone dry? The First Cain Memorial Award Lecture. *Cancer Res.* 1982;42:3911–3917.

Redman J, Cabarillas F, McLaughlin P. et al. Fludarabine phosphate: A new agent with major activity in low grade lymphoma. *Proc Am Assoc Cancer Res.* 1988;29:211.

Sirotnak FM, Chello PL, Dorick DM, et al. Specificity of systems mediating transport of adenosine, 9-β-D-arabinofuranosyl-2-fluoroadenosine, and other purine nucleoside analogues in L-1210 cells. *Cancer Res.* 1983;43:104–109.

Spriggs DR, Stopa E, Mayer RJ, Schoene W, Kufe DW. Fludarabine phosphate (NSC 312878) infusions for the treatment of acute leukemia: Phase I and neuropathological study. *Cancer Res.* 1986;46:5953–5958.

Taylor SA, Crowley J, Vogel FS, et al. Phase II evaluation of fludarabine phosphate in patients with central nervous system tumors. *Invest New Drugs.* 1991;9:195–197.

Taylor S, Eyre HJ. Randomized phase II Trials of acivicin (AT125, NSC 16350) and fludarabine (2-fluoro-Ara-AMP, NSC 31288) (2-Flamp) in recurrent gliomas: A SWOG study. *Proc Am Soc Clin Oncol.* 1987;6:71.

Tseng W-C, Derse D, Cheng Y-C, et al. In vitro biological activity of 9-β-D-arabinofuranosyl-2-fluoroadenine and the biochemical actions of its triphosphate on DNA polymerases and ribonucleotide reductase from HeLa cells. *Mol Pharmacol.* 1982;21:474–477.

Von Hoff DD, Dahlberg S, Hartsock RJ, Eyre H. Activity of fludarabine phosphate in patients with advanced mycosis fungoides. A Southwest Oncology Group study. *Proc Am Soc Clin Oncol.* 1989;8:289.

Von Hoff DD, Green S, Alberts DS, et al. Phase II study of fludarabine phosphate (NSC-312887) in patients with advanced endometrial cancer. *Am J Clin Oncol (CCT).* 1988;11:146–148.

Warrell RP, Berman E. Phase I and II study of fludarabine phosphate in leukemia: Therapeutic efficacy with delayed central nervous system toxicity. *J Clin Oncol.* 1986;4:74–79.

Weiss GR, Phillips JL, Kuhn JG, et al. A clinical–pharmacological study of the intraperitoneal administration of fludarabine phosphate. *Reg Cancer Treat.* 1990;3:158–162.

5-Fluorouracil

■ Other Names

5-FU; fluorouracil; NSC-19893; Efudex® (topical, Roche Dermatologics); Adrucil® (Adria Laboratories); Fluorouracil Injection (Roche Laboratories).

■ Chemistry

Structure of 5-fluorouracil

5-Fluorouracil (5-FU) is a fluorinated pyrimidine differing from the normal RNA and DNA base uracil by a fluorinated No. 5 carbon. The complete chemical name is 5-fluoro-2,4(1H,3H)-pyrimidinedione. 5-FU has a pK_a of 8.1, and the commercially available solution is buffered with sodium hydroxide to obtain an alkaline solution with a pH of around 9.0. The drug is light sensitive and will precipitate at low temperatures or occasionally with prolonged standing at room temperature. The melting range of the solid is 280 to 284°C. At 25°C the solubility is 12.2 mg/mL in water, 5.5 mg/mL in 95% ethanol, and less than 0.1 mg/mL in chloroform. The sodium content is 8.35 mg/mL sodium ions. The molecular weight is 130.08.

■ Antitumor Activity

Fluorouracil was originally discovered by Heidelberger et al (1958) and since that time has been found useful in a wide variety of solid tumors. The drug is approved for use in a wide variety of gastrointestinal malignancies including those of the colon, rectum, stomach (used in combination with doxorubicin and mitomycin-C (in the FAM regimen MacDonald et al 1976), and pancreas as well as for breast cancer patients (Bonadonna et al 1976). In oncology practice the drug is currently used for head and neck cancer, renal cell carcinoma, squamous cell carcinoma of the esophagus, and prostate cancer. For patients with colorectal cancer, 5-FU is occasionally combined with a nitrosourea (Baker et al 1976, Kaufman 1973), with cisplatin (Kemeny et al 1990a). It is currently combined most often with levamisole or leucovorin (see later). Topical 5-FU therapy has been curative in the treatment of basal cell carcinomas and a variety of other malignant dermatoses (Eaglestein et al 1970, Dillaha et al 1965).

There has been a tremendous explosion of investigative activity in the use (and rediscovery) of 5-FU over the last 10 years. The following briefly summarizes those data.

Colorectal Cancer. In an important study by Lokich et al (1987, 1989) standard bolus 5-FU (500 mg/m^2/d × 5 every 5 weeks) and protracted-infusion 5-FU (350 mg/m^2/d continuously × 12 weeks) were compared. Six responses were noted in the 76 patients on the daily × 5 arm (all were partial responses), whereas 4 complete and 21 partial responses were noted in the 82 patients on the infusion arm. Median survivals were comparable.

5-Fluorouracil + levamisole, when used in an adjuvant situation, has resulted in significant increases in disease-free and overall survival (Grem 1990, Moertel et al 1990, Laurie et al 1989, Windle et al 1987) (see *Levamisole* for details).

The combination of interferon alfa-2 with 5-FU has been reported to elicit responses in 40 to 73% of patients (Fornasiero et al 1990, Wadler et al 1989, 1990, Wadler and Wiernik 1990). Other investigators have felt the combination provides no advantage over single-agent 5-FU (Ajani et al 1989). Kemeny et al (1990b) have found the combination of 5-FU + interferon alfa-2a to be quite toxic (52% incidence of stomatitis, 43% diarrhea, and 34% neurotoxicity). They felt the observed response rate of 20% was not substantially superior to those in other 5-FU programs.

5-Fluorouracil in combination with cisplatin has been tested by a number of investigators. At present, although some investigators report an improved response rate there is no evidence the combination improves patient survival over what can be achieved with 5-FU alone (Kemeny et al 1990a, Labianca et al 1988). Loehrer and colleagues (1987, 1988) have also demonstrated no advantage of cisplatin + 5-FU over 5-FU alone for treatment of patients with colorectal carcinoma.

Most recently, there has been tremendous interest in the use of leucovorin to modulate the clinical activity of 5-FU (see *Leucovorin Calcium* in this book and Dosage later in this monograph). There is evidence that 5-FU + leucovorin improves response rate and survival over the use of 5-FU alone in patients with advanced colorectal cancer.

Bladder Cancer. 5-Fluorouracil has been used as a radiation sensitizer (Byfield 1989). The use of 5-FU infusion + irradiation for prospective treatment of transitional cell carcinoma of the bladder has been reported by Russell et al (1990). This approach has achieved complete responses with no histologic evidence of tumor in the resected specimen.

Gastric Cancer. 5-Fluorouracil has significant antitumor activity in combinations used to treat gastric cancer. Unfortunately, most regimens do not significantly enhance survival in a majority of patients. Active 5-FU-containing regimens include FAM with doxorubicin and mitomycin-C (Biran et al 1989), and the sequential combination FAMTX, where methotrexate (1.5 g/m^2) is given 1 hour before 5-FU (1.5 g/m^2) followed by 24 hours by oral leucovorin (15 mg/m^2 every 6 hours × 12 doses) and on day 15 by doxorubicin 30 mg/m^2 IV (Wils et al 1991). A response rate of 41% with 42 weeks' survival was reported in this trial (Wils et al 1991).

Pancreatic Cancer. There is some evidence that surgery + 5-FU + radiation therapy versus surgery alone results in improved overall survival (Gastrointestinal Tumor Study Group 1987). 5-FU is also occasionally used in three-drug combinations with doxorubicin and mitomycin-C (FAM) (Smith et al 1980) or with doxorubicin and cisplatin (FAP) (Cullinan et al 1990).

Anal Carcinoma. Use of 5-FU combined with radiation therapy has demonstrated this combined modality can allow preservation of the rectal sphincter along with achievement of excellent survival (Sischy et al 1989).

Head and Neck Cancer. 5-Fluorouracil in combination with cisplatin gives tumor responses in up to 68% of patients (Al-Sarraf 1989, Toohill et al 1987).

Breast Cancer. Testing of 5-FU by continuous infusion has shown activity in patients refractory to standard 5-FU (Jabboury et al 1989, Chang et al 1989, Huan et al 1989). Combinations of 5-FU + leucovorin in refractory patients have also shown significant responses (Doroshow et al 1989).

■ Mechanism of Action

5-Fluorouracil basically acts as a "false" pyrimidine or antimetabolite to ultimately inhibit the formation of the DNA-specific nucleoside base thymidine. The mechanisms of action of 5-FU are at least three, including (1) inhibition of thymidylate synthase by FdUMP, the active metabolite of 5-FU; (2) incorporation of FUTP into cellular RNA; and (3) incorporation of FUTP into cellular DNA (Rustum 1990). 5-Fluorouracil is a cell cycle phase-specific agent with maximal cytotoxic effects in S phase.

■ Availability and Storage

5-Fluorouracil is available as a clear yellow aqueous solution containing 500 mg/10 mL drug in glass ampules (Fluorouracil Injection, Roche Laboratories, Nutley, New Jersey). The pH of the solution is about 9.0 (adjusted with sodium hydroxide). The vials should be protected from light and stored at room temperature (59–86°F). Precipitates will form at lower temperatures and occasionally on prolonged standing. Slight discolorations that occur with storage do not usually denote decomposition. 5-Fluorouracil is also available in 2% (w/w) and 5% (w/w) 10-mL solutions (in propylene glycol, hydroxymethyl cellulose, paraben preservatives, and disodium edetate). A 25-g 5% 5-fluorouracil cream in white petrolatum, stearyl alcohol, propylene glycol, polysorbate 80, and parabens is available for topical use (Efudex®, Roche Dermatologics, Nutley, New Jersey). An investigational 250-mg capsule of 5-fluorouracil has also been studied (Meeker et al 1976). From earlier work, however, drug absorption from a capsule may be less than from a solution (Khung et al 1966).

■ Preparation for Use, Stability, and Admixture

All doses should be visually inspected for signs of a precipitate. If apparent, the vials may be vigorously agitated and/or gently heated to not more than 140°F in a water bath (do not heat directly as the sealed ampules may explode).

As glass particles may drop into the solution during opening of the ampules, filtration with an aspiration needle (5-μm pore size) is recommended. This filtered solution may then be added to infusion solutions or given directly into the vein. No compatibility problems have been encountered with either D5W or normal saline. Infusion solutions have been successfully used for up to 24 hours.

Oral doses have historically been mixed in water, juice, and carbonated beverages. Because stability data are lacking, oral doses made from the injection form of the agent should optimally be prepared immediately before use (see Special Applications for oral usage recommendations).

Several physical incompatibilities for fluorouracil are reported. 5-Fluorouracil forms a milky precipitate when directly admixed with diazepam (Valium®). Complete intravenous line flushing in between injections of these two drugs is recommended. Fluorouracil forms a deep purple-colored product on direct admixture with doxorubicin; a fine precipitate is also noted. Complete intravenous line flushing between injections of these two drugs is recommended, and direct admixture of the two drugs should be avoided.

Careful study of the stability of 5-FU + cisplatin in 0.9% sodium chloride has been performed by Stewart and Fleming (1990). They found admixtures must be used within 1 hour of preparation. For prolonged intravenous infusions of the agents, the drugs cannot be in the same container. Coughenour et al (1988) have documented that 5-FU and heparin are compatible in the same infusion solution. The stability of 5-FU administered through four different portable infusion pumps has been studied by Stiles and colleagues (1989). All tested brands of 5-FU were found to be stable over a 7-day period at 37°C.

These are the results of spectrophotometric analysis of 5-FU admixed with several agents (McRae and King 1976). Compatible combinations (no change in spectrum of either drug and no physical alterations noted) were observed for 5-fluorouracil and prednisolone sodium phosphate, sodium cephalothin, or vincristine sulfate; nonetheless, direct admixture of these drugs with 5-fluorouracil is not recommended.

5-Fluorouracil causes a change in the spectrophotometric spectrum of cytarabine when mixed in the same solution. This probably evidences a chemical change in cytarabine which may alter its effectiveness, and again, direct admixture is not recommended; complete intravenous line flushing between injections of these two drugs is recommended. 5-Fluorouracil was additionally found to be absolutely incompatible with methotrexate. A significant alteration in the spectra of both drugs occurred; however, no physical alterations were noted. Because of the alkaline nature of the drug, admixture with any acidic agent (amino acids, penicillin, multivitamins, insulin, tetracycline, etc.) represents a theoretical (physical) incompatibility.

■ Administration

Intravenous Push. Doses to be given by the intravenous push route do not require further dilution from the commercial solution. Vein patency should be ensured before giving a dose, with a 5- to 10-mL flush of normal saline or D5W given prior to 5-FU administration and another flush following the dose to rinse the remaining drug from the tubing. The rate of administration is not critical, and the dose should be given at a rate compatible with the particular vein selected. The patient should be continuously monitored to guard against extravasation. Most doses can be conveniently given over 1 to 2 minutes in this fashion.

Infusions. Continuous infusions may maximize efficacy of this cycle-specific drug and lessen hematologic toxicity (Lemon 1960, Seifert et al 1975, Hum and Bateman 1975, Moertel et al 1972, Lokich et al 1987, 1989). Infusions of the drug may be added to a convenient volume of either D5W or normal saline and administered over 24 hours (for each reconstituted daily dose). Commonly, the daily dose of the drug is added to a liter although volume is not critical. Only unquestionable, patent, new intravenous sites should be used, and the administration of other drugs through this line is not recommended.

With recent advances in catheters as well as in infusion devices the continuous infusion (for > 6 weeks) of 5-FU has been explored. There is evidence this method of administration provides for a good quality of life (low toxicity) with a respectable response rate (Hansen et al 1989a, Chang et al 1989, Jabboury et al 1989; Huan et al 1989, Lockich et al 1987, 1989).

Lokich and colleagues (1989) have conducted a randomized trial of continuous-infusion 5-FU (× 10 weeks) versus 5-FU daily bolus × 5 repeated every 5 weeks. Response rates in the bolus arm were 7%, whereas response rates in the continuous-infusion arm were 30%. Toxicity was lower in the continuous infusion arm. Overall survival was the same for both groups. In addition, rare tumors such as metastatic sweat gland tumors and nonfunctioning islet cell tumors have been found to respond to 5-FU by continuous 96-hour infusion (Swanson et al 1989, Hansen et al 1988).

Circadian Rhythm Considerations. Hrushesky (1990) has advocated administration of 5-FU based on the patients' circadian rhythm to lessen gastrointestinal and bone marrow toxicity. Early studies in laboratory rodents suggested that host tolerance to 5-FU was greatest when the drug was administered in the first half of the animal's normal rest period (ie, early morning). In humans this would correlate to the early evening. This has been followed up by a number of investigators but the impact of circadian-based dosing on the clinical utility of 5-FU is still not clear. However, Petit et al (1988) have shown that plasma drug levels in humans do vary on a circadian schedule with a 5-day continuous intravenous infusion. The mean lowest levels of 254 ng/mL were obtained at 1:00 PM and the mean highest levels of 584 ng/ML were obtained at 1:00 AM.

■ Special Precautions

See also Drug Interactions. 5-FU should never be given during pregnancy. However, two patients inadvertently treated with topical 5-FU for papillomavirus lesions while they were pregnant did deliver healthy normal children (Odom et al 1990). Patients with a familial deficiency of dihydropyrimidine dehydrogenase (familial pyrimidinemia) should not receive 5-FU because they may develop severe neurotoxicity (Diasio et al 1988). It is claimed that 5-FU increases the cortisone requirement in patients who have had an adrenalectomy (eg, for breast cancer) and consideration should be given to increased doses of cortisone for patients receiving 5-FU.

■ Dosage

Various regimens are reported for the use of 5-fluorouracil. These include the use of a loading dose, weekly intravenous bolus, continuous infusions over 4 to 5 days or over 6 weeks, and oral dosing (see Special Applications). The dosing of 5-FU should be based on lean body weight (excluding fat and edematous weight from calculations).

The *conventional bolus dose* scheme calls for one course of 400 to 500 mg/m^2 (12 mg/kg) (maximum 800 mg) daily for 4 days given as either a single daily bolus injection or a 4-day continuous infusion. This is then followed by a weekly maintenance regimen. Horton et al (1970) and Jacobs et al (1971), however, have strongly associated the use of the loading dose with significant morbidity and occasional fatalities, and suggest that it offers no greater antitumor efficacy over a weekly bolus injection of 15 mg/kg IV.

Maintenance 5-FU dosing schedules include the following regimens: (1) 200–250 mg/m^2 (6 mg/kg) every other day for 4 days, repeated in 4 weeks (if toxicity has resolved); (2) 500–600 mg/m^2 (15 mg/kg) IV weekly as a continuous infusion or bolus injection (this has been given with and without the use of the loading dose).

The manufacturer recommends no daily dose greater than 800 mg regardless of the patient's weight although higher doses of up to 1 to 2 g/day are routinely administered by continuous infusion. Again, the work of Horton et al (1970) should be considered: Intravenous bolus doses of 20 to 25 mg/kg generally produced severe toxicity, and some deaths from hemorrhagic colitis or bone marrow failure have been reported. By continuous infusion, higher daily doses have been successfully used, and many investigators have reported lessened hematologic toxicity and enhanced efficacy.

Note: As most of a dose is eliminated by the liver and the remainder by the kidney, marked dysfunction in either system probably requires a lower dose adjustment; however, 5-FU dose adjustments based on age are not warranted (Milano et al 1992).

When 5-FU is used with leucovorin, the most commonly used doses and schedules are listed below:

1. 5-FU 370 mg/m^2/d × 5 days by intravenous bolus plus leucovorin given as a continuous infusion of 500 mg/m^2/d beginning 24 hours before the first dose of 5-FU and continuing for 12 hours after completion of therapy (Doroshow et al 1990).
2. 5-FU 500 to 1000 mg/m^2 as an intravenous bolus (about 1 g/min infusion rate) every 2 weeks preceded by calcium leucovorin at a dose of 20 mg/m^2 given as a 10-minute infusion (Bruckner et al 1990).
3. 5-FU 600 mg/m^2 by intravenous push plus 500 mg/m^2 immediately after leucovorin by 2-hour infusion weekly × 6 weeks, or 5-FU 600 mg/m^2 + 25 mg/m^2 leucovorin weekly × 6 weeks (high-dose arm was more active) (Petrelli et al 1990).
4. 5-FU 370 mg/m^2 daily × 5 given as a rapid intravenous bolus immediately after an intravenous bolus of high-dose leucovorin (200 mg/m^2/d × 5), or 5-FU 370 mg/m^2 daily × 5 intravenous bolus given immediately after an intravenous bolus of low-dose leucovorin (20 mg/m^2/d × 5). In this study, the 5-FU + low-dose leucovorin arm was as active as the high-dose leucovorin and gave an improvement in quality of life and lower drug costs (Poon et al 1989).

■ Drug Interactions

As a result of the alkaline chemical nature of 5-fluorouracil, several pH-affected admixture interactions with a number of drugs are possible (see Preparation for Use, Stability, and Admixture). There are also a number of potential pharmacologic drug interactions, some with laboratory documentation; however, none has established clinical relevance. A rat study by Ambre and Fischer (1971) discussed the alteration of 5-FU catabolism by prednisolone. Additionally, Kuwano et al (1973) have found that the antifungal agent amphotericin B and the antibiotic polymixin B potentiated the activity of fluorouracil, but again clinical relevance is not established. Osborne et al (1989) have shown that tamoxifen antagonizes the activity of 5-FU in breast cancer cell cultures.

Allopurinol. There is a report that allopurinol may modulate the hematologic toxicity of high-dose 5-fluorouracil (Fox et al 1979). The proposed mechanism involves oxipurinol inhibition of thymidine phosphorylase, one of three enzymes that activates 5-FU. Experimentally, these authors suggest that concurrent allopurinol may allow a twofold increase in 5-FU dose. When allopurinol has been used clinically to modulate the toxicity of 5-FU, the data do not consistently report increased efficacy (Tsavaris et al 1990).

Thymidine. Vogel et al (1979) described synergism for the combination of thymidine + fluorouracil in patients with advanced colorectal carcinoma. In this study, thymidine ($8 g/m^2/d \times 5$) concurrent with allopurinol ($5-20 mg/kg/d \times 5$) reduced the minimal toxic dose level of 5-FU by two thirds (reduced to 7.5 mg/kg/day) and favored myelosuppression as the dose-limiting toxic effect over the usual gastrointestinal toxic effects, stomatitis and diarrhea. Ensminger and Frei (1977) have described clinical protection from 5-fluorouracil toxicity with thymidine infusions. Mechanistically, however, thymidine appears to slow 5-fluorouracil clearance and prolong the serum half-life probably by competition for identical pyrimidine-degradative enzymes. Enhanced antitumor efficacy for the combination is not yet established but has been noted in several experimental animal systems (Martin et al 1978).

Methotrexate. In vitro and in vivo studies by Tattersall et al (1973) and Bruckner and Creasey (1974) indicate that under certain conditions 5-fluorouracil and methotrexate can mutually antagonize the activity of each other. Inasmuch as these studies were conducted on isolated cell preparations, the clinical relevance of the interaction is unknown; however, it does place methotrexate–fluorouracil combinations under some suspicion.

Tattersall et al (1973) and others have demonstrated that 5-FU, through the active metabolite 5-F-dUMP, antagonizes the antipurine effects of methotrexate (necessary for cytotoxicity in the presence of excess thymidine) by inhibiting the utilization of reduced folates into thymidine biosynthesis. Conversely, methotrexate causes a buildup of the natural substrate dUMP, which can compete with the false inhibitor 5-F-dUMP and/or (2) reduce cellular activation of 5-fluorouracil by dUMP-mediated feedback inhibition. The clinical significance of the interaction is unclear and schedule dependency is suggested. If methotrexate is given before or at the same time as 5-FU, the irreversible effects on the thymidine cofactor necessary for expression of 5-FU cytotoxicity would be reduced. If given after the effects of 5-FU have peaked, further methotrexate–thymidine inhibition could be additive or even synergistic. Clinical trials of this combination have not definitely answered the question of synergism versus antagonism (Poon et al 1989).

Leucovorin Calcium. This area is covered in more depth in the *Leucovorin Calcium* monograph. Preclinical studies have shown that the antitumor activity of 5-FU can be potentiated by using reduced folates at concentrations of 1 µM or greater. These reduced folates raise the level of $N_5,N/O$-methylenetetrahydrofolate and thus form a stable tertiary complex of thymidylate synthase, the folate coenzyme, and 5-FU (in the form of 5-fluorodeoxyuridylate). (See Mini et al [1990] for an excellent review of this area.) There is now definitive evidence this combination provides higher response rates (and sometimes longer survival) for patients with metastatic gastrointestinal malignancies than 5-FU treatment alone (Erlichman 1990, Laufman et al 1987, Doroshow et al 1990, Petrelli et al 1987, 1990, Poon et al 1989; Erhlichman et al 1988). The combination is also being extensively tested in other malignancies (Vokes et al 1990, Doroshow et al 1989, Allegra et al 1987). It is important to remember that severe and fatal toxic effects have been seen with the combination (Grem et al 1987).

Uridine. Other potential modulators include uridine (Darnowski and Handschumaker 1989, Klubes and Leyland-Jones 1989). Van Groeningen et al (1989) have treated patients with 5-FU plus intravenous infusions of uridine ($2 g/m^2/h \times 72$ hours). They found leukopenia was reversed but thrombocytopenia was not. The major side effect of the uridine was fever.

Dipyridamole. Dipyridamole appears to increase the in vitro cytotoxicity of 5-FU by blocking the pyrimidine salvage pathway for nucleoside synthesis (Grem and Fischer 1989, Darnowski and Handschumacher 1989). Dipyridamole accentuates the inhibition of DNA synthesis by the FdUMP metabolite of 5-FU, as cells cannot use the salvage pathway to maintain thymidine concentrations; however, the very high degree of protein binding by dipyridamole significantly lessens its ability to effectively modulate 5-FU cytotoxicity. Dipyridamole coadministration results in increased total body clearance of 5-FU and a lower new steady-state 5-FU plasma level (Remick et al 1990).

***N*-Phosphonoacetyl-L-aspartate + Thymidine.** *N*-Phosphonoacetyl-L-aspartate (PALA) has been used to modulate the efficacy of 5-FU by Ardalan et al (1988). They found higher response rates in the combination arm (PALA + 5-FU) than for 5-FU alone. PALA and thymidine have also been advocated as biochemical modulators to improve the cytotoxicity of 5-FU (Windschitl et al 1990).

■ Pharmacokinetics

A summary of the pharmacokinetic parameters of 5-FU on various schedules appears in the table on page 506. Methodologies for determination of levels have included high-performance liquid chromatography, gas chromatography–mass spectrometry, radiolabeling techniques, and microbiologic and nuclear magnetic resonance methods. There is disagreement over whether 5-FU is eliminated by a two- or three-compartment model (McDermott et al 1982, Collins et al 1980, 1988). Some of the first measurements of the disposition of 5-FU in humans were made by Clarkson et al (1964). They performed microbiologic assays to measure the agent. Fraile et al (1980) have demonstrated that plasma levels of 5-FU are quite erratic after oral administration. Schaaf and colleagues (1987) have clearly documented that the pharmacokinetic characteristics of 5-FU are nonlinear. Doubling of the dose was accompanied by a decrease in nonrenal clearance. The half-life from the high dose was twice as long as that for the low dose of 5-FU. Their data were compatible with a product-inhibition model. They also postulated pulmonary clearance for 5-FU. Yoshida et al (1990) have recently found there were positive correlations between the dose and serum steady-state levels (SSC) and area under the concentration × time curve (AUC). Patients who developed toxic effects had greater SSCs and AUCs; however, there were no correlations between serum level and patient response to therapy. The same findings were noted by Thyss et al (1986) in patients with head and neck cancer.

5-Fluorouracil is extensively metabolized in the liver (up to 80% detoxified); however, there is no absolute documentation that patients with impaired liver function require dose reductions (Floyd et al 1982, MacMillan et al 1978). Up to 15% of a dose may be found intact in the urine by 6 hours, with 90% of this excreted in the first hour. Depressed renal function does not generally require dosage adjustment for 5-FU. Clarkson et al (1964) found that when 5-FU is given as a continuous infusion (40–60 mg/kg/24 h), stable plasma levels are attained and less intact drug appears in the urine. This could indicate either more complete degradation to inactive metabolites or enhanced conversion to the active nucleoside.

The clearance of 5-FU is significantly lower in women (median, 155 L/h/m^2; range, 56–466) compared with men (median, 179 L/h/m^2; range, 29–739) (Milano et al 1992). This same trial reported no significant effect of age on 5-FU clearance in either sex. Indeed, the older patients (>70 years) maintained the ability to clear 5-FU doses ranging from 500 to 1000 mg/m^2 (Milano et al 1992).

Heggie and colleagues (1987) carefully studied the pharmacokinetics of 5-FU and its metabolites in plasma, bile, and urine. Dihydrofluorouracil was found as a metabolite in most patients. Between 60 and 90% of the administered dose was excreted in the urine within 24 hours as α-fluoro-β-alanine. Biliary excretion amounted to 2 to 3% of the total radioactivity. The chemical nature of the metabolites was not reported.

5-Fluorouracil distributes to all areas of body water apparently by simple diffusion (Mukherjee et al 1963). Thus, significant quantities of the drug may enter the central nervous system. After 15 mg/kg is given intravenously, cerebrospinal fluid levels of 6 to 8×10^{-6} M are obtained after 30 minutes. These levels persist for several hours and only slowly subside. Although distribution to brain tissue is less rapid, abnormal areas such as those with neoplasms may take up drug more readily. Intracarotid and intrathecal administration has led to augmented formation of the neurotoxic metabolites fluoroacetate and fluorocitrate, and therefore those types of infusion are not recommended (Koenig and Patel 1970, Bourke et al 1973).

5-Fluorouracil achieves high and persistent lev-

PHARMACOKINETICS OF 5-FLUOROURACIL

Dose/Method of Administration	Number of Patients	β Half-life (min)	Volume of Distribution (L/m²)	Steady-State Volume of Distribution (L)	AUC (μg/h/mL)	Clearance (mL/min/m²)	MRT (min)	Concentration at Steady State (μg/mL)	Reference
190–600 mg/m²/d CI*	19	—	—	—	0.65 – 19.80	—	—	0.05–0.317	Yoshida et al 1990
300–500 mg/m²/d CI*	25	—	—	—	—	—	—	0.7–1.4 ng/mL	Spicer et al 1988
500 mg/m² bolus	10	12.9 ± 7.3	8.84 ± 3.9	—	7125 ± 2371 μM min L⁻¹	594 ± 198	—	—	Heggie et al 1987
7.5 mg/kg bolus	6	6.2 ± 1.3	—	21.4 ± 6.5	225 ± 56.8 mg min L⁻¹	2.3 ± 0.48 L/min	6.1 ± 1.5	—	Schaaf et al 1987
15 mg/kg bolus	6	12.3 ± 4.7	—	36.3 ± 3.9	753 ± 203 mg min L⁻¹	1.48 ± 0.71 L/min	18.7 ± 7.8	—	Schaaf et al 1987
7.2–14.4 mg/kg bolus	12	12.1 ± 1.0	—	—	12.7 ± 1.9 mg · h/mL	—	—	—	McDermott et al 1982
500 mg IV bolus	11	8.3 ± 0.45	—	12.6 ± 1.5	507 ± 32.8	—	—	—	Finch et al 1979
500 mg/m2 bolus	3	9.4 ± 2.2	0.24 ± 0.16 L/kg	—	—	17.3 ± 8.7 mL/kg/min	—	—	Fraile et al 1980
10.9 ± 0.1 mg/kg	8	11.4 ± 1.5	—	—	128.5 ± 204 μg·min mL⁻¹	—	—	—	MacMillan et al 1978

*CI, continuous infusion.

els in effusions after intravenous administration. Hepatic administration through the portal vein or artery also achieves high concentrations in the liver parenchyma and produces relatively low systemic levels (see later). A similar argument in support of oral 5-FU in liver cancer has been advanced because oral dosing may produce higher portal vein concentrations; however, there is little evidence favoring oral over parenteral use even in the specific instance of hepatic cancer.

Yoshida and colleagues (1990) have carefully examined serum levels of 5-FU when the drug is given by continuous infusion. Toxicity was inversely related to clearance. Of note is that high serum concentrations did not correlate with response in the patient. Santini and colleagues (1989) have shown that therapeutic monitoring of 5-FU levels in patients with head and neck cancer can be used to improve the therapeutic index of the drug (less toxicity with maximal efficacy). No correlation between 5-FU blood levels and cardiotoxicity could be established (Thyss et al 1988, and see later). Recent developments in nuclear magnetic resonance spectroscopy have enabled assays of metabolites of 5-FU in biologic samples. Correlation studies of levels of metabolites with assessment of patient responses are just surfacing (Hull et al 1988).

Ensminger and colleagues (1978) have studied the hepatic extraction of both 5-FU and 5-fluoro-2'-deoxyuridine given by intrahepatic arterial infusion. They found the hepatic extraction ratio of 5-FU ranged from 0.22 to 0.45, whereas the hepatic extraction ratio of 5-fluoro-2'-deoxyuridine ranged from 0.69 to 0.92.

Schwartz et al (1985) found that allopurinol could be used to allow administration of higher doses of 5-FU. The steady-state plasma levels ranged from 3.37 to 7.49 μM, with clearances from 1.79 to 2.41 L/min/m^2 (Erlichman et al 1986). Benz et al (1985) found that sequential infusions of methotrexate followed by 5-FU caused delays in achieving a steady-state concentration of 5-FU. This effect did not appear to be the result of altered drug clearance, as the α half-life and clearance of 5-FU and methotrexate did not appear to be substantially different from previous reported values.

■ Side Effects and Toxicity

Gastrointestinal Effects. The most pronounced and dose-limiting toxic effects of 5-fluorouracil are on the normal, rapidly proliferating tissues of the bone marrow and the lining of the gastrointestinal tract. Some nausea and vomiting can be expected. This may respond relatively well to antiemetic treatment. Stomatitis, however, is usually an early sign of impending severe toxicity and may become evident after 5 to 8 days of therapy. Symptoms include a soreness, erythema, or ulceration of the oral cavity or dysphagia. Other reported gastrointestinal symptoms are diarrhea, proctitis, and esophagitis. The use of allopurinol mouthwash as prophylaxis against 5-FU-induced mucositis has not been shown to be effective (Loprinzi et al 1990). Pazdur and LoRusso (1988) demonstrated that continuous-infusion 5-FU (200–300 mg/m^2/d $\times$ 1 month) can cause gastric ulcerations (not associated with mucositis or diarrhea) in 19% of patients.

Myelosuppression. Leukopenia, primarily granulocytopenia, and thrombocytopenia occur with a nadir of 9–14 days for the granulocytes, and 7–14 days for platelets. Patients who are poor candidates to receive 5-FU therapy are those with a total white cell count of 2,000/mm^2 or less and/or platelets of 100,000/mm^2 or less, or those with poor nutritional status at the outset of therapy.

Dermatologic Effects. Some degree of alopecia is a frequent event although hair regrowth has occurred even when successive doses are given. Partial loss of nails and hyperpigmentation of the nail beds and other body areas (face, hands) have been reported. These may resemble the syndrome of Addison's disease in terms of the hyperpigmentation. A maculopapular rash occurring on the extremities and sometimes the trunk may occur. The rash is usually reversible. Sunlight may heighten or initiate many dermatologic reactions to fluorouracil. Pigmented nevi have been noted in patients treated with systemic 5-FU (Cho et al 1988). Contact dermatitis has also been reported (Tennstedt et al 1987).

Palmar–Plantar Erythrodysethesias. Palmar–plantar erythrodysethesias have been noted associated with continuous infusion 5-FU (42–82% of patients). The syndrome is progressive and causes disruption of treatment (Curran and Luce 1989a). Treatment with 50 or 150 mg of pyridoxine per day has been associated with a reversal of the syndrome in 4 of 5 patients (Fabian et al 1990, Vukelja et al 1989).

Vein Toxicity. Hyperpigmentation has been noted over the veins used for fluorouracil administration (Hrushesky 1976). The veins remained patent but showed marked darkening of the skin immediately over the vein, particularly when infusions were employed. Kuzel et al (1990) have recently described increased thrombogenicity of the combination of 5-FU plus platinum infusions.

Neurotoxicity. 5-Fluorouracil may also cause an acute cerebellar syndrome which can persist beyond the period of actual treatment (Boileau et al 1971, Gottlieb and Luce 1971). Neurotoxicity may be evidenced by headache, minor visual disturbances, cerebellar ataxia, or all three. This complication is generally rare (see distribution to central nervous system under Pharmacokinetics). The neurotoxic metabolite is probably fluorocitrate.

Cardiotoxicity. There are over 65 cases in the world literature of cardiotoxicity attributable to 5-FU (Pottage et al 1978, Ensley et al 1989, Lomeo et al 1990). These include cases of myocardial infarction (Misset et al 1990), angina, dysrhythmias, cardiogenic shock, sudden death, and electrocardiographic changes (Jakubowski and Kemeny 1988, Mancuso 1987, Ensley et al 1989, Freeman and Costanza 1988). An elegant study by Rezkalla and colleagues (1988, 1989) found that asymptomatic ST segment changes were very common (68% of patients), which suggests ischemia. These changes were more common in patients with a prior history of coronary artery disease. The mechanism of the cardiotoxicity is unknown. An autoimmune mechanism has been proposed (Lomeo et al 1990), as has 5-FU-induced depletion of high-energy phosphate in the myocardium (Misset et al 1990) or 5-FU activation of the coagulation system with thrombogenesis (Kuzel et al 1990). Use of a calcium channel blocker to mitigate against coronary artery spasm is being explored (Oleksowicz and Bruckner 1988).

Exposure of Personnel to 5-Fluorouracil. Accidental splashing of 5-FU on the skin or eye should be treated immediately with saline or water irrigation. There have been no long-term sequelae of these accidents (Curran and Luce 1989b). In addition, inhalation of 5-FU caused by the material burning in a truck fire has not caused unusual reactions (Curran and Luce 1989b).

■ Special Applications

Intrathecal Administration. Intrathecal administration of 5-FU is *contraindicated* because of neurotoxicity.

Oral Administration. 5-Fluorouracil is generally administered intravenously as either a bolus, rapid injections, or continuous infusion. Oral doses of up to 15 to 20 mg/kg/d for 5 to 8 days have been used (Hahn et al 1975, Lahiri et al 1971, Khung et al 1966, Nadler 1968); however, recent reports conflict with earlier favorable bioavailability data, and the efficacy of oral 5-FU has not been confirmed at this time. The bioavailability of 5-FU following oral administration (which is an unapproved use of the drug by FDA) varies widely between different patients (50–80%). This has therefore necessitated the use of generally higher doses and subsequently an increased risk of gastrointestinal side effects (Cohen et al 1974). Bruckner and Creasy (1974) found that oral absorption was poorer in patients with metastases to the bowel or with congestive heart failure. Responses produced by oral administration have also tended to be of shorter duration or fewer compared with intravenously administered doses (Bateman and Moertel 1974, Bateman et al 1971, Stolinsky et al 1975). Various authors have suggested that hepatic metastases may receive larger drug fractions with oral dosing; however, this remains unproven. Therefore, the oral route of 5-FU administration should be considered highly experimental at present. Pharmaceutically, greater absorption has been noted when either 4 fluid ounces of water or a $0.2\ M$ (pH 9) bicarbonate buffer solution is used rather than orange juice or another fruit juice. This may relate to precipitation of the alkaline drug in the acidic fruit juice medium (pH $\simeq 4.0$) and hence slowed dissolution and absorption of 5-FU. To enhance absorption, patients may be instructed not to eat for 2 hours before and after ingesting the drug.

Topical Administration. Topical 5-fluorouracil in either solution or cream is occasionally used in the treatment of various neoplastic keratoses (Klein et al 1970, Honeycutt et al 1970). The drug apparently achieves significant penetration only into areas of damaged or diseased (neoplastic) skin. The onset of action is reported to be 2 to 3 days. The use of an occlusive dressing can increase the inflammatory reaction and penetration. The same is true for exposure of treated areas to sunlight, which is therefore to be avoided. The manufacturer reports slight, systemic absorption of about 6% of a topically applied dose (Dillaha et al 1965). If the hands and fingers are used in application they should be immediately washed afterward, and extra care used if the drug is applied near the eyes, nose, and mouth. When 5-FU is applied to hemorrhagic ulcerated tissues, absorption is so rapid that classic toxic symptoms can develop (Miller 1971).

Generally, a nonmetal applicator or glove

should be used with enough solution or cream to cover the lesion. The expected response progresses from erythema to vesiculation, erosion, ulceration, necrosis, and epithelization. Generally, normal skin is not affected to the same extent as diseased areas. Therapy is usually continued to reach the erosion, necrosis, and ulceration stage (2–4 weeks), after which healing can occur over the next 1 to 2 months.

Topical reactions include local pain, pruritis, hyperpigmentation (Hrushesky 1976), and burning at the site of application. These can be common. Other reactions include alopecia, dermatitis (in 5–20% of patients), swelling, tenderness, scarring, insomnia, stomatitis, medicinal taste in the mouth, photosensitivity (Falkson and Schulz 1962), and excessive lacrimation.

Intraarterial Administration. 5-Fluorouracil is occasionally perfused intraarterially in the palliative management of advanced carcinomas of the head and neck (Oberfield 1975), for bladder cancer (Hatch and Fuchs 1989), and for hepatic metastases of colorectal malignancies (Tandon et al 1973, Fortuny et al 1975). Ansfield et al (1971, 1975) used intrahepatic 5-FU doses of 20 to 30 mg/kg/d × 4, then 15 mg/kg/d × 17 days, followed by systemic therapy with good results for patients with progressive liver metastases of gastrointestinal origin. Daily doses were diluted in 1 L of D5W with 5000 U of heparin added. In patients with head and neck cancer, intraarterial 5-FU doses of 5 to 7.5 mg/kg/24 h have been employed with some success (Oberfield 1975). Adenocarcinomas of the stomach, pancreas, liver, and biliary tract have also been somewhat amenable to intraarterial 5-FU: 12 to 15 mg/kg/d × 4 to 5 days followed by 6 to 7.5 mg/kg/d every other day to slight toxicity; or by a continuous regimen as before: 4 days of 30 mg/kg and 17 days of 15 mg/kg again followed by systemic therapy (Davis et al 1974).

Ensminger et al (1978) have described hepatic 5-FU extraction ratio of 0.22 to 0.45 (clearance 0.24–0.45 L/min) after intraarterial dosing. Thus in one pass, 22 to 45% of 5-FU is extracted by the liver, producing only 60% of the corresponding systemic levels seen with comparable peripheral venous infusion; however, some pharmacologic data suggest that floxuridine is preferentially metabolically activated with continuous administration, whereas continuous 5-FU may be preferentially metabolized (to inactive products). Thus, floxuridine may be the fluorpyrimidine of choice for continuous therapy regimens (Mukherjee et al 1963). Over the last 10 years this area has been well investigated. The conclusion of this work is that indeed the response rate is higher for intraarterial floxuridine versus systemic 5-FU, but the overall survival is no different (Martin et al 1990).

Portal Vein Infusion. Wolmark et al (1990) have recently reported a randomized trial of adjuvant portal vein infusion of 5-FU for 7 days postsurgery versus surgery alone. They noted an improvement in disease-free and overall survival; however, as the infusion failed to decrease the evidence of hepatic metastases it was felt the positive effect was really due to a systemic effect of the 5-FU. Beart and colleagues in the North Central Cancer Treatment Group (1990) have found no improvement in time to progression or survival in patients treated with intraportal 5-FU postoperatively versus surgery alone (median followup is 5.5 years).

Intraperitoneal Administration. Speyer et al (1979) investigated intraperitoneal 5-fluorouracil in patients with ovarian and colon carcinomas. Through a Tenckhoff catheter, patients received either repeated 36-hour courses of eight 2-L exchanges, each 4 hours in length, or a 3- to 5-day course of single daily 2-L instillations. 5-Fluorouracil concentrations ranged from 10^{-6} M ($\simeq$ 130 µg/liter) to 8×10^{-3} M (1 g/liter). The procedure was relatively well tolerated locally, although there were two instances of catheter-related bacterial peritonitis which were easily managed. Concentrations of 4×10^{-3} M produced only nausea and vomiting, whereas higher doses, 5×10^{-3} M for 36 hours, caused mucositis, pancytopenia, and alopecia. The systemic toxic effects were quite severe with the highest dose tested (8×10^{-3} M). Pharmacokinetic studies revealed first-order drug elimination with an intraperitoneal half-life of 72 to 112 minutes. Peritoneal permeability ranged from 13 to 18 mL/min and total body clearance of 5-FU was 3 to 6 L/min. Although plasma drug levels peaked 30 to 45 minutes after intraperitoneal instillation, at 4 hours afterward intraperitoneal levels greater than 3×10^{-6} M in toxic patients were still 300-fold greater than simultaneous plasma levels. Thus, intraperitoneal 5-FU administration appears to produce high drug concentrations with minimal systemic toxicity. Objective responses were documented in two of the seven patients studied in this phase I investigation. The authors recommended further intraperitoneal 5-FU investigation at initial drug concentrations of 4×10^{-3} M (500 mg/L) for 36 hours.

Sugarbaker et al (1990) have shown high ratio AUCs of peritoneal versus intravenous 5-FU if the 5-FU is given immediately after surgery (to effect better distribution before adhesions form). Of note is the report by Walton et al (1989) regarding the difficulty with this procedure (catheter problems, etc).

Intracavitary Administration. Suhrland and Weisberger (1965) used intracavitary 5-FU to manage malignant pleural effusions from carcinoma of the breast and lung tumors and to control malignant ascites from ovarian carcinoma. Approximately 38% of patients responded to a single intracavitary dose of 2.0 to 3.0 g. For pericardial effusions, doses of 500 to 1000 mg were used. Repeat dosing was not necessary. Patients with pleural effusions tended to respond better than those with ascites. Although side effects were minimal in this study, some systemic toxicity was consistently produced.

Other Special Applications. 5-Fluorouracil is currently being evaluated for its effect on proliferative vitreoretinopathy and for the control of scarring after glaucoma filtration procedures (Panek 1990). Krebs (1990) reported that topical 5-FU can be successfully used to treat extensive condylomata acuminata. 5-FU has been used to treat refractory psoriasis (Abernethy et al 1989) and to significantly reduce blood loss in transurethral resection of the prostate (Yang and Cheng 1989). 5-FU has also been explored for treatment of systemic sclerosis with improvement in skin and vasculature (Casas et al 1987). Topical 5-FU has been used to treat hard skin thickening or "corns" on the feet (Swain 1986).

REFERENCES

Abernethy DR, Alper JC, Wiemann MC, McDonald CJ, Calabresi P. Oral 5-fluorouracil in psoriasis: Pharmacokinetic–pharmacodynamic relationships. *Pharmacology.* 1989;**39**(2):78–88.

Ajani JA, Rios AA, Ende K, et al. Phase I and II studies of the combination of recombinant human interferon-gamma and 5-fluorouracil in patients with advanced colorectal carcinoma. *J Biol Response Mod.* 1989;**8**(2):140–146.

Allegra CJ, Chabner BA, Sholar PW, Bagley C, Drake JC, Lippman ME. Preliminary results of a phase II trial for the treatment of metastatic breast cancer with 5-fluorouracil and leucovorin. *NCI Monogr.* 1987;**5**:199–202.

Al-Sarraf M. Clinical trials with fluorinated pyrimidines in patients with head and neck cancer. *Invest New Drugs.* 1989;**7**(1):71–81.

Ambre JJ, Fischer LJ. The effect of prednisolone and other factors on the catabolism of 5-fluorouracil in rats. *J Lab Clin Med.* 1971;**78**:343–353.

Ansfield FJ, Ramirez G, Davis L. et al. Further clinical studies with intrahepatic arterial infusion with 5-fluorouracil. *Cancer.* 1975;**36**:2413–2417.

Ansfield FJ, Ramirez G, Skibba JL, Bryan GT, Davis HL, Wirtanen GW. Intrahepatic arterial infusion with 5-fluorouracil. *Cancer.* 1971;**28**:1147–1151.

Ardalan B, Singh G, Silberman H. A randomized phase I and II study of short-term infusion of high-dose fluorouracil with or without N-(phosphonacetyl)-L-aspartic acid in patients with advanced pancreatic and colorectal cancers. *J Clin Oncol.* 1988;**6**(6):1053–1058.

Baker LH, Talley RW, Matter R. Phase III comparison of the treatment of advanced gastrointestinal cancer with bolus weekly 5-FU vs methyl-CCNU plus bolus weekly 5-FU. *Cancer.* 1976;**38**:1–7.

Bateman JR, Moertel CG. Oral vs intravenous administration of fluorouracil. *JAMA.* 1974;**229**(8):1109.

Bateman JR, Pugh RP, Cassiday FR, Marshall JG, Irwin LE. 5-Fluorouracil given once weekly: Comparison of intravenous and oral administration. *Cancer.* 1971;**28**:907–913.

Beart RW Jr, Moertel CG, Wieand HS, et al. Adjuvant therapy for resectable colorectal carcinoma with fluorouracil administered by portal vein infusion. A study of the Mayo Clinic and the North Central Cancer Treatment Group. *Arch Surg.* 1990;**125**(7):897–901.

Benz C, DeGregorio M, Saks S, et al. Sequential infusions of methotrexate and 5-fluorouracil in advanced cancer: Pharmacology, toxicity, and response. *Cancer Res.* 1985;**45**:3354–3358.

Biran H, Sulkes A, Biran S. 5-Fluorouracil, doxorubicin (Adriamycin) and mitomycin-C (FAM) in advanced gastric cancer: Observations on response, patient characteristics, myelosuppression and delivered dosage. *Oncology.* 1989;**46**:83–87.

Boileau G, Piro AJ, Lahiri SR, Hall TC. Cerebellar ataxia during 5-fluorouracil (NSC-19893) therapy. *Cancer Chemother Rep.* 1971;**55**:595–598.

Bonadonna GG, Brusamolino E, Valgussa P. Combination chemotherapy as an adjuvant treatment in operable breast cancer. *N Engl J Med.* 1976;**294**:405–410.

Bourke RS, West CR, Chheda G, Tower DB. Kinetics of entry and distribution of 5-fluorouracil in cerebrospinal fluid and brine following intravenous injection in a primate. *Cancer Res.* 1973;**33**:1735–1746.

Bruckner HW, Creasey WA. The administration of 5-fluorouracil by mouth. *Cancer.* 1974;**33**:14–18.

Bruckner HW, Glass LL, Chesser MR. Dose-dependent leucovorin efficacy with an intermittent high-dose 5-fluorouracil schedule. *Cancer Invest.* 1990;**8**(3/4):321–326.

Byfield JE. 5-Fluorouracil radiation sensitization—A brief review. *Invest New Drugs.* 1989;**7**(1):111–116.

Casas JA, Subauste CP, Alarcon GS. A new promising

treatment in systemic sclerosis: 5-Fluorouracil. *Ann Rheum Dis.* 1987;**46**(10):763–767.

Chang AY, Most C, Pandya KF. Continuous intravenous infusion of 5-fluorouracil in the treatment of refractory breast cancer. *Am J Clin Oncol.* 1989;**12**(5):453–455.

Cho KH, Chung JH, Lee AY, Lee YUS, Kim NK, Kim CW. Pigmented macules in patients treated with systemic 5-fluorouracil. *J Dermatol.* 1988;**15**(4):342–346.

Clarkson B, O'Connor A, Winston L, Hutchinson D. The physiologic disposition of 5-fluorouracil and 5-fluoro-2'-deoxyuridine in man. *Clin Pharmacol Ther.* 1964;**5**:581–610.

Cohen JL, Irwin LE, Darvey H, Batemann JR. Clinical pharmacology of oral and intravenous 5-fluorouracil (NSC 19893). *Cancer Chemother Rep Part I.* 1974;**58**(5):723–731.

Collins JM, Dedrick RL, King FG, Speyer JL, Myers CE. Nonlinear pharmacokinetic models for 5-fluorouracil in man; Intravenous and intraperitoneal routes. *Clin Pharmacol Ther.* 1980;**28**(2):235–246.

Collins JM, Russell KJ, Boileau MA, Higano C. A pilot study of neo-adjuvant 5-fluorouracil (5-FU) and irradiation (XRT) in the treatment of bladder cancer. *Proc Annu Meet Am Soc Clin Oncol.* 1988;**7**:122.

Coughenour M, Slavik M, Fabian C, Brown N, Cheng CC. Clinical and compatibility studies of 5-fluorouracil (5-FU) and heparin (HN) administered by continuous iv infusion. *Proc Annu Meet Am Assoc Cancer Res.* 1988;**29**:191.

Cullinan S, Moertel CG, Wieand HS, et al. A phase III trial on the therapy of advanced pancreatic carcinoma: Evaluations of the Mallinson regimen and combined 5-fluorouracil, doxorubicin, and cisplatin. *Cancer.* 1990;**65**:2207–2212.

Curran CF, Luce JK. Fluorouracil and palmar–plantar erythrodysesthesia. *Ann Intern Med.* 1989a;**111**(10):858.

Curran CF, Luce JK. Accidental acute exposure to fluorouracil. *Oncol Nurs Form.* 1989b;**16**:1468.

Darnowski JW, Handschumacher RE. Enhancement of fluorouracil therapy by the manipulation of tissue uridine pools. *Pharmacol Ther.* 1989;**41**(1/2):381–392.

Davis HL, Ramirez G, Ansfield FJ. Adenocarcinomas of stomach, pancreas, liver and biliary tracts. *Cancer.* 1974;**33**:193–197.

Diasio RB, Beavers TL, Carpenter JT. Familial deficiency of dihydropyrimidine dehydrogenase. Biochemical basis for familial pyrimidinemia and severe 5-fluorouracil-induced toxicity. *J Clin Invest.* 1988;**81**(1):47–51.

Dillaha J, Jansen GT, Honeycott WM, Holt GA. Further studies with topical 5-fluorouracil. *Arch Dermatol.* 1965;**92**:410–417.

Doroshow JH, Leong L, Margolin K, et al. Refractory metastatic breast cancer: Salvage therapy with fluorouracil and high-dose continuous infusion leucovorin calcium. *J Clin Oncol.* 1989;**7**(4):439–444.

Doroshow JH, Multhauf P, Leong L, et al. Prospective randomized comparison of fluorouracil versus fluorouracil and high-dose continuous infusion leucovorin calcium for the treatment of advanced measurable colorectal cancer in patients previously unexposed to chemotherapy. *J Clin Oncol.* 1990;**8**(3):491–501.

Eaglestein W, Weinstein G, Frost P. Topical fluorouracil. *Arch Dermatol.* 1970;**101**:132.

Ensley JF, Patel B, Kloner R, Ish JA, Wynne J, al-Sarraf M. The clinical syndrome of 5-fluorouracil cardiotoxicity. *Invest New Drugs.* 1989;**7**(1):101–109.

Ensminger WD, Frei E III. The prevention of methotrexate toxicity by thymidine infusions in humans. *Cancer Res.* 1977;**37**:1857–1863.

Ensminger WF, Rosowsky A, Raso V, et al. A clinical–pharmacological evaluation of hepatic arterial infusions of 5-fluoro-2'-deoxyuridine and 5-fluorouracil. *Cancer Res.* 1978;**38**:3784–3792.

Erlichman C. Fluorouracil and leucovorin for metastatic colorectal cancer. *J Chemother.* 1990;**1**(suppl 2):38–40.

Erlichman C, Fine S, Elhakim T. Plasma pharmacokinetics of 5-FU given by continuous infusion with allopurinol. *Cancer Treat Rep.* 1986;**70**(7):903–904.

Erlichman C, Fine S, Wong A, Elhakim T. A randomized trial of fluorouracil and folinic acid in patients with metastatic colorectal carcinoma. *J Clin Oncol.* 1988;**6**(3):469–475.

Fabian CJ, Molina R, Slavik M, Dahlberg S, Giri S, Stephens R. Pyridoxine therapy for palmar–plantar erythrodysesthesia associated with continuous 5-fluorouracil infusion. *Invest New Drugs.* 1990;**8**(1):57–63.

Falkson G, Schulz EJ. Skin changes in patients treated with 5-fluorouracil. *Br J Dermatol.* 1962;**24**:229–236.

Finch RE, Bending MR, Lant AF. Plasma levels of 5-fluorouracil after oral and intravenous administration in cancer patients. *Br J Clin Pharmacol.* 1979;**7**:613–617.

Floyd FA, Hornbeck CL, Byfield JE, Griffiths JC, Frankel SS. Clearance of continuously infused 5-fluorouracil in adults having lung or gastrointestinal carcinoma with or without hepatic metastases. *Drug Intell Clin Pharm.* 1982;**16**:665–667.

Fornasiero A, Daniele O, Ghiotto C, Aversa SM, Morandi P, Fiorentino MV. Alpha-2 interferon and 5-fluorouracil in advanced colorectal cancer. *Tumori.* 1990;**76**(4):385–388.

Fortuny IE, Theologide A, Kennedy BJ. Hepatic arterial infusion for liver metastases from colon cancer. *Cancer Chemother Rep Part I.* 1975;**59**:401–404.

Fox RM, Woods RL, Tattersall MHN. Allopurinol modulation of high-dose fluorouracil toxicity. *Lancet.* 1979;**1**:677.

Fraile RJ, Baker LW, Buroker TR, Horwitz J, Vaitkevicius VK. Pharmacokinetics of 5-fluorouracil administered orally, by rapid intravenous and by slow infusion. *Cancer Res.* 1980;**40**:2223–2228.

Freeman NJ, Costanza ME. 5-Fluorouracil-associated cardiotoxicity. *Cancer.* 1988;**61**(1):36–45.

Gastrointestinal Tumor Study Group. Further evidence of effective adjuvant combined radiation and chemotherapy following curative resection of pancreatic cancer. *Cancer.* 1987;**59**(12):2006–2010.

Gottlieb JA, Luce JK. Cerebellar ataxia with weekly 5-fluorouracil administration. *Lancet.* 1971;**1**:138–139.

Grem JL. 5-Fluorouracil and levamisole in colorectal carcinoma. *Cancer Invest.* 1990;**8**(2):283–284.

Grem JL, Fischer PH. Enhancement of 5-fluorouracil's anticancer activity by dipyridamole. *Pharmacol Ther.* 1989;**40**(3):349–371.

Grem JL, Shoemaker DD, Petrelli NJK, Douglass HO Jr. Severe and fatal toxic effects observed in treatment with high- and low-dose leucovorin plus 5 fluorouracil for colorectal carcinoma. *Cancer Treat Rep.* 1987;**71**(11):1122.

Hahn RG, Moertel CG, Schultz AJ. A double-blind comparison of intensive course 5-fluorouracil by oral vs intravenous route in the treatment of colorectal carcinoma. *Cancer.* 1975;**33**:1031–1033.

Hansen R, Helm J, Wilson JF, Wilson S. Nonfunctioning islet cell carcinoma of the pancreas. Complete response to continuous 5-fluorouracil infusion. *Cancer.* 1988;**62**(1):15–17.

Hansen RM, Quebbeman E, Anderson T. 5-Fluorouracil by protracted venous infusion. A review of current progress. *Oncology.* 1989a;**46**(4):245–250.

Hansen R, Quebbeman E, Ausman R, et al. Continuous systemic 5-fluorouracil infusion in advanced colorectal cancer: Results in 91 patients. *J Surg Oncol.* 1989b;**40**(3):177–181.

Hatch TR, Fuchs EF. Intra-arterial infusion of 5-fluorouracil for recurrent adenocarcinoma of bladder. *Urology.* 1989;**33**(4):311–312.

Heggie GD, Sommadossi J, Cross DS, Huster WJ, Diasio RB. Clinical pharmacokinetics of 5-fluorouracil and its metabolites in plasma, urine, and bile. *Cancer Res.* 1987;**47**:2203–2206.

Heidelberger C, Chaudhuri N, Weston E. The metabolism of 5-fluorouracil-2-C14 in humans. *Proc Am Assoc Cancer Res.* 1958;**2**:306.

Honeycutt W, Jansen G, Dillaha C. Topical fluorouracil. *Cutis.* 1970;**6**:63.

Horton J, Olson JB, Sullivan J, Reilly C, Schnider B, Eastern Cooperative Oncology Group. 5FU in cancer: An improved regimen. *Ann Intern Med.* 1970;**73**:897–900.

Hrushesky WJ. Serpentine supravenous 5-fluorouracil (NSC-19893) hyperpigmentation (letter). *Cancer Treat Rep.* 1976;**60**(50):639.

Hrushesky WJ. More evidence for circadian rhythm effects in cancer chemotherapy: The fluorpyrimidine story. *Cancer Cells.* 1990;**2**(3):65–68.

Huan S, Pazdur R, Singhakowinta A, Samal B, Vaitkevicius VK. Low-dose continuous infusion 5-fluorouracil. Evaluation in advanced breast carcinoma. *Cancer.* 1989;**63**(3):419–422.

Hull WE, Port RE, Herrmann R, Britsch B, Kunz W. Metabolites of 5-fluorouracil in plasma and urine, as monitored by ^{19}F nuclear magnetic resonance spectroscopy, for patients receiving chemotherapy with or without methotrexate pretreatment. *Cancer Res.* 1988;**48**(6):1680–1688.

Hum GJ, Bateman JR. 5 day IV infusion with 5-fluorouracil (5-FU; NSC-19893) for gastroenteric carcinoma after failure on weekly 5-FU therapy. *Cancer Chemother Rep Part I.* 1975;**59**(6):1177–1179.

Jabboury K, Holmes FA, Hortobagyi G. 5-Fluorouracil rechallenge by protracted infusion in refractory breast cancer. *Cancer.* 1989;**64**(4):793–797.

Jacobs EM, Reeves WJ Jr, Wood DA, Pugh R, Braunwald J, Bateman JR. Treatment of cancer with weekly intravenous 5-fluorouracil. *Cancer.* 1971;**27**:1302–1305.

Jakubowski AA, Kemeny N. Hypotension as a manifestation of cardiotoxicity in three patients receiving cisplatin and 5-fluorouracil. *Cancer.* 1988;**62**(2):266–269.

Kaufman S. 5-Fluorouracil in the treatment of gastrointestinal neoplasia. *N Engl J Med.* 1973;**288**:199–201.

Kemeny N, Israel K, Niedzwiecki D, et al. Randomized study of continuous infusion fluorouracil versus fluorouracil plus cisplatin in patients with metastatic colorectal cancer. *J Clin Oncol* 1990a;**8**(2):313–318.

Kemeny N, Younes A, Seiter K, et al. Interferon alpha-2a and 5-fluorouracil for advanced colorectal carcinoma. *Cancer.* 1990b;**66**:2470–2475.

Khung CL, Hall TC, Piro AJ, Dederick MM. A clinical trial of oral 5-fluorouracil. *Clin Pharmacol Ther.* 1966;**7**:527–533.

Klein E, Stoll HL, Miller E, Milgrom H, Hel F, Burgess G. The effects of 5-fluorouracil (5-FU) ointment in the treatment of neoplastic dermatoses. *Dermatologica.* 1970;**140**(suppl I):21–33.

Klubes P, Leyland-Jones B. Enhancement of the antitumor activity of 5-fluorouracil by uridine rescue. *Pharmacol Ther.* 1989;**41**(1/2):289–302.

Koenig H, Patel A. Biochemical basis for fluorouracil neurotoxicity. *Arch Neurol.* 1970;**23**:155–160.

Krebs HB. Treatment of extensive vulvar condylomata acuminata with topical 5-fluorouracil. *South Med J.* 1990;**83**(7):761–764.

Kuwano M, Kamiya T, Endo H, Komiyama S. Potentiation of 5-fluorouracil, chromomycin A3, and blenomycin and amphotericin B or polymixin B in transformed fibroblastic cells. *Antimicrob Agents Chemother.* 1973;**2**:580–584.

Kuzel T, Esparaz B, Green D, Kies M. Thrombogenicity of intravenous 5-fluorouracil alone or in combination with cisplatin. *Cancer.* 1990;**65**(4):885–889.

Labianca R, Pancera G, Cesana B, Clerici M, Montinari F, Luporini G. Cisplatin + 5-fluorouracil versus 5-fluorouracil alone in advanced colorectal cancer: A randomized study. *Eur J Cancer Clin Oncol.* 1988;**24**(10):1579–1581.

Lahiri SR, Boileau G, Hall TC. Treatment of metastatic colorectal carcinoma with 5-fluorouracil (5-FU) by mouth. *Dermatologica.* 1971;**29**:902–906.

Laufman LR, Krzeczowski KA, Roach R, Sesal M. Leucovorin plus 5-fluorouracil: An effective treatment for metastatic colon cancer. *J Clin Oncol.* 1987;**5**(9):1394–1400.

Laurie JA, Moertel CG, Fleming TR, et al. Surgical adjuvant therapy of large-bowel carcinoma: An evaluation of levamisole and the combination of levamisole and fluorouracil. *J Clin Oncol.* 1989;**7**(10):1447–1456.

Lemon HM. Reduction of 5-fluorouracil toxicity in man with retention of anticancer effects by prolonged intravenous administration in 5% dextrose. *Cancer Chemother Rep.* 1960;**8**:97–101.

Loehrer PJ, Turner S, Kubilis P, et al. A prospective randomized study of 5-fluorouracil (5-FU) alone or with cisplatin (p) in the treatment of metastatic colorectal cancer: A Hoosier Oncology Group trial. *Proc Am Soc Clin Oncol.* 1987;**6**:76.

Loehrer PJ Sr, Turner S, Kubilis P, et al. A prospective randomized trial of fluorouracil versus fluorouracil plus cisplatin in the treatment of metastatic colorectal cancer: A Hoosier Oncology Group trial. *J Clin Oncol.* 1988;**6**(4):642–648.

Lokich J, Ahlgren J, Gullo J, Phillips J, Fryer J. A randomized trial of standard bolus 5-FU vs protracted infusional 5-FU in advanced colon cancer. *Proc Am Soc Clin Oncol.* 1987;**6**:81.

Lokich JJ, Ahlgren JD, Gullo JJ, Philips JA, Fryer JG. A prospective randomized comparison of continuous infusion fluorouracil with a conventional bolus schedule in metastatic colorectal carcinoma: A Mid-Atlantic Oncology Program Study. *J Clin Oncol.* 1989;**7**:425–432.

Lomeo AM, Avolio C, Iacobellis G, Manzione L. 5-Fluorouracil cardiotoxicity. *Eur J Gynaecol Oncol.* 1990;**11**(3):237–241.

Loprinzi CL, Cianflone SG, Dose AM, et al. A controlled evaluation of an allopurinol mouthwash as prophylaxis against 5-fluorouracil-induced stomatitis. *Cancer.* 1990;**65**(8):1879–1882.

MacDonald J, Schein P, Nemo W, Wooley P. 5-Fluorouracil (5-FU), mitromycin C (MMC) and Adriamycin (ADR-FAM): A new combination chemotherapy program for advanced gastric carcinoma (abstract C-111). *Proc Am Soc Clin Oncol.* 1976;**17**:264.

MacMillan WE, Wolberg WH, Welling PG. Pharmacokinetics of fluorouracil in humans. *Cancer Res.* 1978;**38**:3479–3482.

Mancuso L. Prinzmetal's angina during 5-fluorouracil chemotherapy. *Ann J Med.* 1987;**83**(3):602.

Martin DS, Stolfi RL, Spiegelman S. Striking augmentation of the in vivo anticancer activity of 5-fluorouracil (FU) by combination with pyrimidine nucleosides: An RNA effect. *Proc Am Assoc Cancer Res.* 1978;**19**:221.

Martin JK Jr, O'Connell MJ, Wieand HS, et al. Intra-arterial floxuridine vs systemic fluorouracil for hepatic metastases from colorectal cancer. A randomized trial. *Arch Surg.* 1990;**125**(8):1022–1027.

McDermott BJ, van den Berg HW, Murphy RF. Nonlinear pharmacokinetics for the elimination of 5-fluorouracil after intravenous administration in cancer patients. *Cancer Chemother Pharmacol.* 1982;**9**:173–178.

McRae MP, King JC. Compatibility of antineoplastic, antibiotic and corticosteroid drugs in intravenous admixtures. *Am J Hosp Pharm.* 1976;**33**:1010–1013.

Meeker WR, Godfrey J, Levick S, Dollinger MR, Serpick AA, Miller E. Phase III study of oral fluorouracil capsules (abstract C123). *Proc Am Assoc Cancer Res Am Soc Clin Oncol.* 1976;**17**:276.

Milano G, Etienne MC, Cassuto-Viguier E, et al. Influence of sex and age on fluorouracil clearance. *J Clin Oncol.* 1992;**10**(7):1171–1175.

Miller E. The metabolism and pharmacology of 5-fluorouracil. *J Med.* 1971;**299**(19):1049–1052.

Mini E, Trave F, Rustum YM, Bertino JR. Enhancement of the antitumor effects of 5-fluorouracil by folinic acid. *Pharmacol Ther.* 1990;**47**(1):1–19.

Misset B, Escudier B, Leclercq B, Rivara D, Rougier P, Nitenberg G. Acute myocardiotoxicity during 5-fluorouracil therapy. *Intensive Care Med.* 1990;**16**(3):210–211.

Moertel CG. Chemotherapy of gastrointestinal cancer. *N Engl J Med.* 1978;**299**(19):1049–1052.

Moertel CG, Fleming TR, Macdonald JS, et al. Levamisole and fluorouracil for adjuvant therapy of resected colon carcinoma. *N Engl J Med.* 1990;**322**(6):352–358.

Moertel CG, Schutt AJ, Reitemeier RJ, Hahn R. A comparison of fluorouracil administered by slow infusion and rapid injection. *Cancer Res.* 1972;**32**:2717–2719.

Mukherjee KL, Curreri, AR, Javid M, Heidelberger C. Studies on fluorinated pyrimidines. XVII. Tissue distribution of 5-fluorouracil-2C14 and 5-fluoro-2′-deoxyuridine in cancer patients. *Cancer Res.* 1963;**23**:67–77.

Nadler SH. Oral administration of fluorouracil, a preliminary trial. *Arch Surg.* 1968;**97**:654–656.

Oberfield RA. Current status of regional arterial infusion chemotherapy. *Med Clin N Am.* 1975;**59**:411–424.

Odom LD, Plouffe L Jr, Buttler WJ. 5-Fluorouracil exposure during the period of conception: Report on two cases. *Am J Obstet Gynecol.* 1990;**163**(1):76–77.

Oleksowicz L, Bruckner HW. Prophylaxis of 5-fluorouracil-induced coronary vasospasm with calcium channel blockers. *Am J Med.* 1988;**85**(5):750–751.

Osborne CK, Kitten L, Arteaga CL. Antagonism of chemotherapy-induced cytotoxicity for human breast cancer cells by antiestrogens. *J Clin Oncol.* 1989;**7**(6):710–717.

Panek W. Using fluorouracil in surgical therapy for glaucoma. *West J Med.* 1990;**153**(2):190.

Pazdur R, LoRusso P. Toxicity report: 290 patient-months of continuous infusion low dose 5-fluorouracil. *Proc Am Soc Clin Oncol.* 1988;**7**:113.

Petit E, Milano G, Levi F, Thyss A, Bailleul F, Schneider M. Circadian rhythm-varying plasma concentration of 5-fluorouracil during a five-day continuous venous infusion at a constant rate in cancer patients. *Cancer Res.* 1988;**48**(6):1676–1679.

Petrelli N, Douglass HO Jr, Herrera L, et al. The modulation of fluorouracil with leucovorin in metastatic colorectal carcinoma: A prospective randomized phase III trial. Gastrointestinal Tumor Study Group. *J Clin Oncol.* 1990;**8**(1):185.

Petrelli N, Herrera L, Rustum Y, et al. A prospective randomized trial of 5-fluorouracil versus 5-fluorouracil and high-dose leucovorin versus 5-fluorouracil and methotrexate in previously untreated patients with advanced colorectal carcinoma. *J Clin Oncol.* 1987;**5**(10):1559–1565.

Poon MA, O'Connell MJ, Moertel CG, et al. Biochemical modulation of fluorouracil: Evidence of significant improvement of survival and quality of life in patients with advanced colorectal carcinoma. *J Clin Oncol.* 1989;**7**(10):1407–1418.

Pottage A, Holt S, Ludgate S, Langlands AO. Fluorouracil cardiotoxicity. *Br Med J.* 1978;**1**:547.

Remick SC, Grem JL, Fischer PH, et al. Phase I trial of 5-fluorouracil and dipyridamole administered by seventy-two-hour concurrent continuous infusion. *Cancer Res.* 1990;**50**(9):2667–2672.

Rezkalla S, Ensley J, Turi Z, et al. 5-Fluorouracil (5-FU) cardiotoxicity: A controlled, prospective investigation of ischemic changes during 5-FU infusion. *Proc Am Soc Clin Oncol.* 1988;**7**:150.

Rezkalla S, Kloner RA, Ensley J, et al. Continuous ambulatory ECG monitoring during fluorouracil therapy: A prospective study. *J Clin Oncol.* 1989;**7**(4):509–514.

Russell KJ, Boileau MA, Higano C, et al. Combined 5-fluorouracil and irradiation for transitional cell carcinoma of the urinary bladder. *Int J Radiat Oncol Biol Phys.* 1990;**19**(3):693–699.

Rustum YM. Biochemical rationale for the 5-fluorouracil leucovorin combination and update of clinical experience. *J Chemother.* 1990;**1**(suppl 2):5–11.

Santini J, Milano G, Thyss A, et al. 5-FU therapeutic monitoring with dose adjustment leads to an improved therapeutic index in head and neck cancer. *Br J Cancer.* 1989;**59**(2):287–290.

Schaaf LJ, Dobbs BR, Edwards IR, Perrier DG. Nonlinear pharmacokinetic characteristics of 5-fluorouracil (5-FU) in colorectal cancer patients. *Eur J Clin Pharmacol.* 1987;**32**:411–418.

Schwartz PM, Turek PJ, Hyde CM, Cadman EC, Handschumacher RE. Altered plasma kinetics of 5-FU at high dosage in rat and man. *Cancer Treat Rep.* 1985;**69**(1):133–136.

Seifert P, Baker LH, Reed ML, Vaitkevicius VK. Comparison of continuously infused 5-fluorouracil with bolus injection in treatment of patients with colorectal carcinoma. *Cancer.* 1975;**36**:123–128.

Sischy B, Doggett RL, Krall JM, et al. Definitive irradiation and chemotherapy for radiosensitization in management of anal carcinoma: Interim report on Radiation Therapy Oncology Group Study No. 8314. *J Natl Cancer Inst.* 1989;**81**(11):850–856.

Smith FP, Hoth DF, Levin B, et al. 5-Fluorouracil, Adriamycin, and mitomycin-C (FAM) chemotherapy for advanced adenocarcinoma of the pancreas. *Cancer.* 1980;**46**:2014–2018.

Speyer JL, Collins JM, Dedrick RL, et al. Phase I and pharmacological studies of intraperitoneal (IP) 5-fluorouracil (5-FU) (abstract C-251). *Proc Am Assoc Cancer Res Am Soc Clin Oncol.* 1979;**20**:352.

Spicer DV, Ardalan B, Daniels JR, Silberman H, Johnson K. Reevaluation of the maximum tolerated dose of continuous venous infusion of 5-fluorouracil with pharmacokinetics. *Cancer Res.* 1988;**48**:459–461.

Stewart CF, Fleming RA. Compatibility of cisplatin and fluorouracil in 0.9% sodium chloride injection. *Am J Hosp Pharm.* 1990;**47**(6):1373–1377.

Stiles ML, Allen LV Jr, Tu YH. Stability of fluorouracil administered through four portable infusion pumps. *Am J Hosp Pharm.* 1989;**46**(10):2036–2040.

Stolinsky DC, Pugh RP, Bateman JR. 5-Fluorouracil (NSC-19893) therapy for pancreatic carcinoma: Comparison of oral and intravenous routes. *Cancer Chemother Rep.* 1975;**59**:1031–1033.

Sugarbaker PH, Graves T, DeBruijn EA, et al. Early postoperative intraperitoneal chemotherapy as an adjuvant therapy to surgery for peritoneal carcinomatosis from gastrointestinal cancer: Pharmacological studies. *Cancer Res.* 1990;**50**(18):5790–5794.

Suhrland LG, Weisberger AS. Intracavitary 5-fluorouracil in malignant effusions. *Arch Intern Med.* 1965;**116**:431–433.

Swain R. Topical 5-fluorouracil for corns—An effective new treatment. *Clin Exp Dermatol.* 1986;**11**(4):396–397.

Swanson JD Jr, Pazdur R, Sykes E. Metastatic sweat gland carcinoma: Response to 5-fluorouracil infusion. *J Surg Oncol.* 1989;**42**(1):69–72.

Tandon RN, Bunnel IL, Copper RG. The treatment of metastatic carcinoma of the liver by the percutaneous selective hepatic artery infusion of 5-fluorouracil. *Surgery.* 1973;**73**:118–121.

Tattersall MHN, Jackson RC, Connors TA, Harrap KR. Combination chemotherapy: The interaction of methotrexate and 5-fluorouracil. *Eur J Cancer.* 1973;**9**:733–739.

Tennstedt D, Lachapelle JM. Allergic contact dermatitis to 5-fluorouracil. *Contact Dermatitis.* 1987;**16**(5):279–280.

Thyss A, Milano G, Renee N, Vallicioni J, Schneider M, Demard F. Clinical pharmacokinetic study of 5-FU in continuous 5-day infusions for head and neck cancer. *Cancer Chemother Pharmacol.* 1986;**16**:64–66.

Thyss A, Milano G, Schneider M, Demard F. Circulating drug levels in patients presenting cardiotoxicity to 5-FU. *Eur J Cancer Clin Oncol.* 1988;**24**(10):1675–1676.

Toohill RJ, Anderson T, Byhardt RW, et al. Cisplatin and fluorouracil as neoadjuvant therapy in head and neck cancer. A preliminary report. *Arch Otolaryngol Head Neck Surg.* 1987;**113**(7):758–761.

Tsavaris N, Karagiaouris P, Vonorta K, et al. Concomitant adminstration of 4-hydroxypyrazolopyrimidine (allopurinol) and high-dose continuous infusion 5-fluorouracil. *Oncology.* 1990;**47**(1):70–74.

Van Groeningen CJ, Peters GJ, Leyva A, Laurensse E, Pinedo HM. Reversal of 5-fluorouracil-induced myelosuppression by prolonged administration of high-dose uridine. *J Natl Cancer Inst.* 1989;**81**(2):157–162.

Vogel SE, Greenwald E, Kaplan BH. The "CHAD" regimen (cyclophosphamide, hexamethylmelamine, Adriamycin and diamminedichloroplatinum) in advanced ovarian cancer. *Proc Am Soc Clin Oncol.* 1979;**20**:385.

Vokes EE, Schilsky RL, Weichselbaum RR, Kozloff MF, Panje WR. Induction chemotherapy with cisplatin, fluorouracil, and high-dose leucovorin for locally advanced head and neck cancer: A clinical and pharmacologic analysis. *J Clin Oncol.* 1990;**8**(2):241–247.

Vukelja SJ, Lombardo FA, James WD, Weiss RB. Pyroxidine for the palmar–plantar erythrodysesthesia syndrome. *Ann Intern Med.* 1989;**111**(8):688–689.

Wadler S, Goldman M, Lyver A, Wiernik PH. Phase I trial of 5-fluorouracil and recombinant alpha 2a-interferon in patients with advanced colorectal carcinoma. *Cancer Res.* 1990;**50**(7):2056–2059.

Wadler S, Schwartz EL, Goldman M, et al. Fluorouracil and recombinant alfa-2a-interferon: An active regimen against advanced colorectal carcinoma. *J Clin Oncol.* 1989;**7**(12):1764–1765.

Wadler S, Wiernik PH. Clinical update on the role of fluorouracil and recombinant interferon alfa-2a in the treatment of colorectal carcinoma. *Semin Oncol.* 1990b;**17**(1, suppl 1):16–21.

Walton LA, Blessing JA, Homesley HD. Adverse effects of intraperitoneal fluorouracil in patients with optimal residual ovarian cancer after second-look laparotomy: A Gynecologic Oncology Group study. *J Clin Oncol.* 1989;**7**(4):466–470.

Wils JA, Klein HO, Wagener DJTh, et al. Sequential high dose methotrexate and fluorouracil combined with doxorubicin—A step ahead in the treatment of advanced gastric cancer: A trial of the European Organization for Research and Treatment of Cancer, Gastrointestinal Tract Cooperative Group. *J Clin Oncol.* 1991;**9**(5):827–831.

Windle R, Bell PR, Shaw D. Five-year results of a randomized trial of adjuvant 5-fluorouracil and levamisole in colorectal cancer. *Br J Surg.* 1987;**74**(7):569–572.

Windschitl HE, O'Connell JH, Wieand HS, et al. A clinical trial of biochemical modulation of 5-fluorouracil with N-phosphonoacetyl-L-aspartate and thymidine in advanced gastric and anaplastic colorectal cancer. *Cancer.* 1990;**66**(5):853–856.

Wolmark N, Rockette H, Wickerham DL, et al. Adjuvant therapy of Dukes' A, B, and C adenocarcinoma of the colon with portal-vein fluorouracil hepatic infusion: Preliminary results of National Surgical Adjuvant Breast and Bowel Project Protocol C-02. *J Clin Oncol.* 1990;**8**(9):1466–1475.

Yang OB, Cheng JY. Preoperative use of 5-fluorouracil to reduce operative bleeding in transurethral resection of prostate. *Urology.* 1989;**33**(5):407–409.

Yoshida T, Araki E, Iigo M, et al. Clinical significance of monitoring serum levels of 5-fluorouracil by continuous infusion in patients with advanced colonic cancer. *Cancer Chemother Pharmacol.* 1990;**26**:352–354.

Fluosol®

■ Other Names

Fluosol DA®; 20% Intravascular Perfluorochemical Emulsion (Alpha Therapeutic Corporation.)

■ Chemistry

Fluosol is a perfluorocarbon emulsion containing perfluorodecalin and perfluorotri-*n*-propylamine in a 7:3 ratio. The solution is stabilized by phospholipids, glycerol, and the mixture of the nonionic surfactant poloxamer 188 (Pluronic F-68®) with polyethylene–polyoxypropylene polymers. The natural phospholipids are isolated from egg yolks. The average particle size is 0.175 μm and the material is supplied in three parts: (1) the emulsified perfluorochemicals; (2) a sodium bicarbonate buffer solution; and (3) a physiologic salt solution to maintain isotonicity (see Availability and Storage). The compositions of the final and component Fluosol® solutions are listed in the table on page 516. Once properly reconstituted, emulsion particles form around a perfluorocarbon core which is coated by the egg yolk phospholipids and poloxamer 188. The viscosity of Fluosol® at 37°C is about 3 cP, which is lower than that of blood at low shear rates. The final emulsion is slightly hypertonic at 450 mosmol/kg. This is due primarily to the glycerol stabilizer.

■ Antitumor Activity

Fluosol does not produce antitumor effects but is being investigated for use as a chemotherapy-modulating agent.

Hypoxic tumors (3–20 mm Hg oxygen partial pressure) tend to resist the effects of both radiotherapy and most cytotoxic agents (Rockwell et al 1982). Fluosol® in combination with carbogen (95% O_2 5% CO_2) breathing has been shown to improve the oxygenation of experimental hypoxic tumors (Song et al 1987, Hasegawa et al 1987). Fluosol® infused into rats prior to single-dose radiation with carbogen breathing improves the radiosensitivity of Lewis lung cancer and EMT6 fibrosarcoma (Teicher and Rockwell 1983, Teicher and Rose 1984). Fluosol® alone and carbogen breathing alone do not delay tumor cell growth and only slightly increase normal bone marrow toxicity. The BA1112 rhabdomyosarcoma also responds to Fluosol® plus radiation, although the Fluosol® effect was not dose depen-

COMPOSITION OF FLUOSOL SOLUTION

Ingredient	Stem Solution	Annex Solution C	Annex Solution H	Final
Perfluorodecalin	17.5			14
Perfluorotri-*n*-propylamine	7.5			6
Poloxamer 188 (Pluronic F-68®)	3.4			2.7
Glycerol	1.0			0.8
Egg yolk phospholipid	0.5			0.4
Potassium oleate	0.04			0.032
Sodium chloride			4.26	0.6
Potassium chloride		0.567		0.034
Calcium chloride			0.2	0.028
Magnesium chloride			0.144	0.020
Sodium bicarbonate		3.5		0.21
Glucose			1.28	0.18
Water for injection, USP				q.s

Concentration (g/100mL)

dent (Rockwell 1985). Fluosol® does not appear to increase radiation toxicity in normally hypoxic tissues such as jejunal epithelium and sperm, although skin erythema and dry desquamation are slightly enhanced.

A large number of cytotoxic chemotherapy agents have shown enhanced antitumor effects with Fluosol®/carbogen breathing. Studies were performed in experimental animals bearing the FSa-IIc fibrosarcoma (Teicher and Holden 1987). The list of agents active with Fluosol® includes melphalan, cyclophosphamide, busulfan, carmustine, semustine, lomustine, chlorozotocin, procarbazine, bleomycin, vincristine, and etoposide. The most significant enhancement was with procarbazine (15-fold increase in tumor growth delay) and busulfan (8-fold increase in tumor growth delay). In contrast, the experimental activity of mitomycin-C was significantly decreased by Fluosol®/carbogen breathing. Several drugs were not significantly altered by Fluosol®/carbogen breathing; these include methotrexate, 5-fluorouracil, dacarbazine, and cisplatin.

Fluosol® and 100% oxygen breathing have been clinically combined with radiation therapy in patients with squamous cell carcinoma of the head and neck and in patients with non-small cell lung cancer. In head and neck cancer, all treated patients had some evidence of tumor regression, with a complete response rate of 83% (21/26 evaluable patients). Complete responses were also observed in nonsmall cell lung cancer patients. In contrast, a much lower response rate was observed in solid tumor patients treated with 5-fluorouracil and Fluosol®/oxygen therapy. Numerous controlled trials are underway to validate the preliminary positive radiation studies and prospectively compare the results of chemotherapy/Fluosol® with those of chemotherapy alone.

Currently, Fluosol® is approved as an adjunct to prevent ischemia during transluminal coronary angioplasty. It may also be useful in the postmyocardial infarction setting and possibly in the treatment of various types of cerebral ischemia.

■ Mechanism of Action

Fluosol® acts principally as an easily perfused ischemic modifier or hypoxic cell sensitizing agent. Perfluorocarbon particles in the emulsion act to absorb, transport, and release oxygen and carbon dioxide dependent on the partial pressure of each gas in the surrounding medium. Oxygen and carbon dioxide are very soluble in Fluosol® which acts as a gas carrier to facilitate reoxygenation of ischemic cells in the myocardium during transluminal coronary angioplasty, or investigationally to reoxygenate and sensitize hypoxic tumor cells to the effects of cytotoxic chemotherapy drugs or ionizing radiation.

■ Availability and Storage

Fluosol® (Alpha Therapeutic Corporation, Los Angeles, California) is now commercially available as a 400-mL frozen stem emulsion of perfluorocarbon with two annex solutions C and H (see Chemistry for composition). The stem emulsion is stored frozen and the two annex solutions are stored at room temperature.

■ Preparation for Use, Stability, and Admixture

The frozen stem solution stored in a polyethylene bag is thawed in a water bath (not > 37°C) and accessed aseptically via the multipurpose port. Thirty milliliters of annex solution C (sodium bicarbonate buffer) is added to the thawed stem emulsion and gently mixed. Next, 35 mL of annex solution H (electrolytes) is added to the emulsion bag and mixed. This is repeated once (a total of 75 mL of solution H is added to the emulsion bag). The resulting final emulsion should be used within 8 hours of thawing if stored at temperatures up to 37°C. Refreezing or refrigeration is contraindicated and the solution must be warmed to 37°C prior to administration. No information is available concerning admixture with other drugs.

■ Administration

Fluosol® is administered intravenously by an infusion pump. A 0.5-mL test dose is initially infused and the patient is observed for 10 minutes to rule out hypersensitivity reactions. In some applications, the Fluosol® emulsion is first oxygenated with carbogen through a special 0.2-μm filter/vent attachment. Saline or 5% dextrose in water may be used to flush the intravenous line and to infuse the 0.5-mL intravenous test dose.

■ Drug Interactions

Fluosol® may prolong the duration of action of lipid-soluble anesthetics. In animals Fluosol® enhances the hepatotoxicity of carbon tetrachloride and may similarly enhance the liver toxicity of anesthetics, alcohol, and other hepatotoxic drugs.

■ Dosage

The optimal Fluosol® dose as a chemotherapy modulator is not known. An initial intravenous test dose of 0.5 mL is required to rule out acute Fluosol® hypersensitivity reactions. Low intracoronary doses of 15 mL/kg have been used investigationally to reduce myocardial infarct size. In angioplasty procedures, a fixed dose of Fluosol® was administered at flow rates between 15 and 120 mL/min with a maximum dose of 283 mL or about 4.6 mL/kg. In cancer patients receiving radiation therapy and carbogen breathing, Fluosol® doses ranged from 8 to 49 mL/kg. Weekly doses of 7 mL/kg were also used in some patients. For use as a contrast agent to enhance splenic or hepatic echogenicity for tumor scanning by ultrasound, a dose of 10 mL/kg is recommended.

■ Pharmacokinetics

There are two primary paths of Fluosol® elimination: rapid expiration as a gas and slower uptake by the reticuloendothelial system. The perfluorocarbon ingredients do not appear to be metabolized and are excreted unchanged. Other natural ingredients, glycerol and the phospholipids, are highly metabolized by normal catabolic pathways.

In rodents, the circulating half-life of intravenous Fluosol® is dose and species dependent, with half-lives of 13 hours in the rat, 25 hours in the dog, and 29 hours in the rabbit. Clearance of the perfluorocarbon ingredients is more rapid at low doses. Thus, removal is complete after 17 hours with a 10 mL/kg dose but requires up to 25 hours with a dose of 80 mL/kg in rats. The primary distribution sites for the emulsion particles are the liver and spleen and, to a lesser extent, the bone marrow. Some perfluorocarbons are also distributed into the breast milk of lactating animals. Very small amounts are taken up in other tissues. In all tissues, the perfluorocarbons are taken up primarily by fixed macrophages or "foam cells" wherein they are stored in the cell membrane. The uptake of perfluorocarbons into liver and spleen is cumulative over 7 to 14 days after Fluosol® infusion. In dogs this peaks about 1 week after administration but only small amounts remain 4 to 6 months after administration.

Greater than 98% of the perfluorocarbons in Fluosol® are expired from the body as a gas. The rate of excretion is maximal between 6 and 8 hours after administration. There is no urinary excretion of the perfluorocarbons.

■ Side Effects and Toxicity

Acute hypersensitivity reactions include chest pain, shortness of breath, chills, facial flushing, nausea and vomiting, back pain, fever, and hypertension. Both tachycardia and bradycardia are also reported, and if an acute reaction occurs after the test dose, a single intravenous injection of methylprednisolone is recommended. Diphenhydramine has also been used to prevent recurrent reactions. In patients undergoing transluminal coronary angioplasty there is a low rate of acute cardiotoxic effects, including ventricular tachycardia or fibrillation and a transient increase in angina with ST segment elevations. If not adequately warmed prior to administration, Fluosol® solutions may produce an increased incidence of cardiac rhythm disturbances.

REFERENCES

Hasegawa T, Rhee JG, Levitt SH, Song CW. Increase in tumor pO_2 perfluorochemicals and carbogen. *Int J Radiat Oncol Biol Phys.* 1987;**13**:569–574.

Rockwell S. Use of perfluorochemical emulsion to improve oxygenation in a solid tumor. *Int J Radiat Oncol Biol Phys.* 1985;**11**:97–103.

Rockwell S, Kennedy KA, Sartorelli AC. Mitomycin-C as a prototype bioreductive alkylating agent: In vitro studies of metabolism and cytotoxicity. *Int J Radiat Oncol Biol Phys.* 1982;**8**:753–755.

Song CW, Lee I, Hasegawa T, et al. Increase in pO_2 and radiosensitivity of tumors by Fluosol®-DA and carbogen. *Cancer Res.* 1987;**47**:442–446.

Teicher BA, Holden SA. Survey of the effect of adding Fluosol®-DA 20%/O_2 to treatment with various chemotherapeutic agents. *Cancer Treat Rep.* 1987;**71**:173–177.

Teicher B, Rockwell S. Increased efficacy of radiotherapy in mice treated with perfluorochemical emulsions plus oxygen. *Proc Am Assoc Cancer Res.* 1983;**24**:267.

Teicher B, Rose CM. Enhancement of anticancer drug efficiency by a PFC emulsion. *Proc Am Assoc Cancer Res.* 1984;**25**:316.

Flutamide

■ Other Names

Eulexin® (Schering Corporation); SCH-13521.

■ Chemistry

Structure of flutamide

Flutamide is an aniline-based nonsteroidal antiandrogen. The chemical names for flutamide include 2-methyl-*N*-[4-nitro-3-(trifluoromethyl)phenyl]propanamide and 4'-nitro-3'-trifluoromethylisobutyranilide. The molecular formula is $C_{11}H_{11}F_3N_2O_3$ and the formula weight is 276.2. The yellow to buff-colored powder is insoluble in water but is soluble in chloroform, diethyl ether, and propylene glycol. It is also freely soluble in acetone, alcohol, dimethylformamide, dimethylsulfoxide, ethyl acetate, methanol, and propylene glycol 400.

■ Antitumor Activity

Flutamide is officially indicated for use in advanced prostate cancer when combined with an inhibitor of gonadotropin-releasing hormone (GnRH) such as leuprolide. In a placebo-controlled clinical trial of 617 previously untreated patients, the addition of flutamide to leuprolide increased survival from 27.9 to 34.9 months. This represents a 25% (7-month) increase in overall survival and a 19% (2.6-month) increase in progression-free survival (Crawford et al 1989). Similar results were reported in earlier uncontrolled trials of flutamide combined with leuprolide (Labrie et al 1985b). When used alone (eg, without GnRH inhibitors), flutamide demonstrated palliative efficacy similar to that of diethylstilbestrol in double-blind studies of previously untreated stage D prostate cancer patients (Jacobo et al 1976, Airhart et al 1978). In a placebo-controlled trial, about half of previously treated patients symptomatically improved on flutamide therapy (Stoliar and Albert 1974). A smaller percent of responders (23%) was described in another trial (Sogani et al 1979). Clearly, the best symptomatic responses are produced in previously untreated patients (Sogani and Whitmore 1979).

In benign prostatic hypertrophy, flutamide produces no gland shrinkage, no histologic improvement in prostate biopsy scores, nor any objective improvements in urinary retention, hesitancy, or residual volume (Caine et al 1975). This trial used a double blind, placebo-control design in 30 patients. Although no objective responses were obtained, some patients nonetheless reported symptomatic improvement in urinary flow while on flutamide.

Flutamide does not appear to be effective in other endocrine-sensitive tumors. In 33 patients with metastatic breast cancer, flutamide produced only one partial response of 8 weeks' duration (Perrault et al 1988). This may discount a role for antiandrogen therapy in advanced breast cancer.

■ Mechanism of Action

Flutamide is an androgen receptor antagonist. Flutamide is believed to inhibit the uptake and binding of the androgens testosterone and, especially, dihydrotestosterone to specific receptors in hormonally dependent prostate cells. It does not appear to possess other hormonal activities, specifically estrogenic, progestational, androgenic, glucocorticoid, and mineralocorticoid activities (Neri et al 1972).

The administration of flutamide to normal male animals causes a prompt reduction in the size of the prostate gland and the seminal vesicles (Neri and Monahan 1972). In the rat, flutamide does not significantly inhibit prostatic 5-α-reductase and arginase activities (Varkarakis et al 1975). Thus, flutamide does not appear to impair the prostatic conversion of testosterone to its active form, dihydrotestosterone.

■ Availability and Storage

Flutamide (Eulexin®, Schering Corporation, Kenilworth, New Jersey) is available in two-toned, brown 125-mg capsules. The capsules are imprinted "Schering 525" and also contain the inactive ingredients lactose (360.6 mg/capsule), povidone, cornstarch, sodium lauryl sulfate, and magnesium stearate. Eulexin® capsules can be stored at room temperature. Flutamide bulk powder in the solid state is reported to be stable for at least 5 years when stored between 2 and 30°C (Schering Corporation 1989a,b).

An investigational 400-mg sustained-release tablet has also been studied for use in a once daily dosing regimen (Asade et al 1991).

■ Administration

Flutamide capsules are administered orally. It is not known if food affects flutamide absorption.

■ Dosage

In prostate cancer, the approved oral dose in adult men is 250 mg (two capsules), taken three times daily, preferably at 8-hour intervals. Thus, the approved total daily dose is 750 mg taken continuously. A 300-mg daily dose of flutamide (100 mg three times daily) was relatively inactive in patients with benign prostatic hypertrophy (Caine et al 1975). In prostate cancer a higher dose of 500 mg three times daily (1.5 g/d) apparently does not produce greater toxicity and has occasionally been associated with increased response rates (Jacobo et al 1976, Sogani and Whitmore 1979, Stoliar and Albert 1974, Airhart et al 1978). Overall, however, a clear dose–response relationship has not yet been established for this drug at daily dose levels greater than 750 mg.

■ Pharmacokinetics

Pharmacokinetic studies of ^{3}H-labeled flutamide show that peak plasma levels are achieved within 2 to 4 hours of dosing (Katchen and Buxbaum 1975). The absolute bioavailability of the agent has not been reported. Flutamide is extensively metabolized, and the major species identified is an α-hydroxylated active metabolite, hydroxyflutamide. One hour after dosing, only 2.5% of flutamide in the plasma is unchanged drug. Up to 23% of the plasma radiolabel is represented by the metabolite hydroxyflutamide. The half-time of formation of hydroxyflutamide from flutamide is estimated to be 0.9 hour (Symchowicz et al 1986).

In the urine, the major metabolite observed is 2-amino-5-nitro-4-(trifluoromethyl)phenol. Only 4.2% of a dose is recovered as unchanged flutamide. Both the parent drug and its metabolites are highly bound to plasma proteins, in the range 86 to 94%. The half-lives for flutamide at steady state are 0.8 hour (α) and 7.8 hours (β).

In normal older male patients, the plasma half-life of the active metabolite, hydroxyflutamide, was 8 hours after a single dose and 9.6 hours at steady state (Symchowicz et al 1986). When flutamide is given three times daily, steady-state levels of 24 to 78 ng/mL are achieved after the fourth dose. This compares with simultaneous hydroxyflutamide levels of 1680 and 720 ng/mL (maximum and minimum), respectively.

Pharmacokinetic studies of hydroxyflutamide have shown that the investigational 400-mg sustained-release tablet produces higher levels, but similar formation and elimination patterns, as compared to the 250-mg tablets (Asade et al 1991).

■ Side Effects and Toxicity

Flutamide is normally well tolerated. Like most hormonal agents it produces non-life-threatening toxic effects at effective doses. When it was combined with the luteinizing hormone-releasing hormone (LHRH) agonist leuprolide, the most common adverse effects were hot flashes (60%), loss of libido (36%), impotence (33%), diarrhea (12%), nausea or vomiting (10–12%), and gynecomastia (9%) (Crawford et al 1989). Many of these effects were also produced in the concurrent patient control group receiving leuprolide plus a placebo; however, the incidence of diarrhea was greater with flutamide.

When flutamide is used alone, the most common complaints are gynecomastia and frank pain in the nipple. These effects have been noted in most patients receiving the drug (Caine et al 1975, Jacobo et al 1976). As flutamide has an aniline-based chemical structure, there were worries that methemoglobinemia could occur, as was observed in high-dose studies in cats; however, methemoglobinemia has not been observed in several prospectively monitored trials (Airhart et al 1978, Caine et al 1975).

Rare flutamide toxic effects include mild and transient liver enzyme elevations and anorexia. The following symptoms were reported in less than 1% of the patient population: hypertension, photosensitivity, edema, genitourinary symptoms, and mild central nervous system excitation or depression. The causal relationship between these effects and flutamide is not established.

Gastrointestinal side effects occur in 1 to 21% of patients and can be severe in 1 to 10% of patients (Crawford et al 1989, Labrie et al 1985a, Dekernion et al 1988). Yagoda (1989) has recently described severe diarrhea in four prostate cancer patients receiving flutamide who had documented lactose intolerance. Symptoms included abdominal discomfort, borborygmi, flatulence, and multiple watery bowel movements daily. Typically the symptoms halted immediately after stopping drug therapy. Lactose intolerance was suspected, as each 125-mg tablet contains 360.5 mg of lactose (more than 2 g of lactose per day at the approved dose in prostate cancer) (Yagoda 1989).

REFERENCES

Airhart RA, Barnett TF, Sullivan JW, Levine RL, Schlegel JU. Flutamide therapy for carcinoma of the prostate. *South Med J.* 1978;**71**(7):798–801.

Asade RH, Prizont L, Muino JP, Tessler J. Steady-state hydroxyflutamide plasma levels after the administration of two dosage forms of flutamide. *Cancer Chemother Pharmacol.* 1991;**27**:401–405.

Caine M, Perlberg S, Gordon R. The treatment of benign prostatic hypertrophy with flutamide (SCH 13521): A placebo-controlled study. *J Urol.* 1975;**114**:564–568.

Crawford DE, Eisenberger M, McLeod D, et al. A comparison of leuprolide with and without flutamide in previously untreated patients with disseminated prostatic carcinoma: A placebo-controlled randomized trial. *N Engl J Med.*

DeKernion JN, Murphy GR, Priore R. Comparison of flutamide and Emcyt in hormone-refractory metastatic prostatic cancer. *Urology.* 1988;**31**:312–317.

Jacobo E, Schmidt JD, Weinstein SH, Flocks RH. Comparison of flutamide (SCH-13521) and diethylstilbestrol in untreated advanced prostatic cancer. *Urology.* 1976;**8**(3):231–233.

Katchen B, Buxbaum S. Disposition of a new nonsteroid antiandrogen, alpha, alpha, alpha-trifluoro-2-methyl-4′-nitro-*m*-propionotoluidide (flutamide) in men following a single oral 200 mg dose. *J Clin Endocrinol Metab.* 1975;**41**:373–379.

Labrie F, DuPont A, Belanger A. Complete androgenic blockade for the treatment of prostate cancer. In: DeVita VT, Hellman S, Rosenberg SH, eds. *Important Advances in Oncology.* Philadelphia, PA: Lippincott; 1985a:193–217.

Labrie F, DuPont A, Belanger M, et al. Combination therapy with flutamide and copstration (LHRH agonist or orchiectomy) in advanced prostate cancer: A marked improvement in response and survival. *J Steroid Biochem.* 1985b;**23**:833–841.

Neri R, Florance K, Koziol P, Van Cleave S. A biological profile of a nonsteroidal antiandrogen, SCH 13521 (4′-nitro-3′-trifluoromethylisobutyranilide). *Endocrinology.* 1972;**91**:427–437.

Neri RO, Monahan M. Effects of a novel nonsteroidal antiandrogen on canine prostatic hyperplasia. *Invest Urol.* 1972;**10**;123–130.

Perrault DJ, Logan DM, Stewart DJ, Bramwell VHC, et al. Phase II study of flutamide in patients with metastatic breast cancer. A National Cancer Institute of Canada Clinical Trials Group study. *Invest New Drugs.* 1988;**6**:207–210.

Prout GR Jr, Irwin RJ Jr, Kliman B, Daly JJ, et al. Prostatic cancer and SCH-13521. II. Histological alterations and the pituitary gonadal axis. *J Urol.* 1975;**113**:834–840.

Schering Corporation. *Eulexin*® Brand of Flutamide Capsules. Product Information Sheet. Kenilworth, NJ: Schering Corporation; 1989a.

Schering Corporation. *Eulexin*®, Hospital Formulary Monograph. Kenilworth, NJ: Schering Corporation; 1989b:14.

Sogani PC, Whitmore WF Jr. Experience with flutamide in previously untreated patients with advanced prostatic cancer. *J Urol.* 1979;**122**:640–643.

Stoliar B, Albert DJ. SCH 13521 in the treatment of advanced carcinoma of the prostate. *J Urol.* 1974;**111**:803–807.

Symchowicz S, Radwanski E, Affrime M, et al. Single and multiple dose pharmacokinetics of flutamide (Eulexin) in normal geriatric volunteers. *Acta Pharmacol Toxicol (Copenhagen).* 1986;**58**:301.

Varkarakis MJ, Kirdani RY, Yamanaka H, Murphy GP, Sandberg AA. Prostatic effects of a nonsteroidal antiandrogen. *Invest Urol.* 1975;**12**(4):275–284.

Yagoda A. Flutamide-induced diarrhea secondary to lactose intolerance. *J Natl Cancer Inst.* 1989;**81**(23):1839–1840.

Gallium Nitrate

■ Other Names

NSC-15200; Ganite® (Fujisawa USA).

■ Chemistry

Gallium nitrate is an anhydrous salt produced by a reaction of nitric acid and the naturally occurring group IIIa heavy metal gallium. It has a molecular weight of 256 and the simple empirical formula Ga(NO$_3$)$_3$. The clinical material is made from a white nonahydrate (Ga(NO$_3$)$_3$·9H$_2$O) crystalline powder with a molecular weight of 417.87. It is soluble in water. The preclinical and clinical aspects of gallium nitrate were reviewed in 1986 by Foster et al.

■ Biologic Activity

Gallium nitrate was originally developed as an anticancer agent. In phase I trials, antitumor activity was noted in patients with lymphoma, melanoma, thyroid carcinoma, ovarian cancer, and osteogenic sarcoma (Bedikian et al 1978, Valdivieso et al 1978, Brown et al 1978). Follow-up studies in the phase II stage showed antitumor activity for patients with lymphoma (Keller et al 1986, Weick et al 1983, Warrell et al 1983) and a hint of antitumor activity in patients with bladder cancer (Seidman et al 1991, Seligman and Crawford 1991). The compound has given a 10% response rate in patients with advanced prostate cancer with a more impressive decrease in bone pain (unfortunately of short duration) (Scher et al 1987). Modest activity has also been noted in patients with refractory ovarian cancer (Malfetano et al 1991); however, the drug has not been found to be active for patients with non-small cell lung cancer (Olver et al 1991), sarcoma (Saiki et al 1982), melanoma (Casper et al 1985), colon cancer (Canfield and Lyss 1991), breast cancer (Fabian et al 1982, Jabboury et al 1989), hypernephroma (Vugrin et al 1987, Schwartz and Yogoda 1984), and head and neck cancer (Decker et al 1984).

The approved use for gallium nitrate is for the treatment of cancer-related hypercalcemia. In a randomized double-blind trial, gallium nitrate was compared with calcitonin. Serum calcium was normalized in 75% of patients receiving gallium nitrate (lasted 6.0 days) versus 31% of those patients receiving calcitonin (lasted 1 day) (Warrell et al 1988). In similar studies, Warrell et al (1990b, 1991) demonstrated that gallium nitrate is also superior to etidronate for acute control of modest to severe hypercalcemia.

Warrell and colleagues (1987) documented that gallium nitrate reduces the biochemical parameters (eg, hydroxyproline) associated with bone turnover in patients with bone metastases. This is being further explored for treatment of patients with bone metastases.

Of additional interest is that the radioactive metal ^{67}Ga shows selective localization in neoplastic tissue (Hayes et al 1970, Dudley et al 1950).

■ Mechanism of Action

Gallium nitrate probably works in hypercalcemia by inhibiting calcium resorption from bone; however, the precise mechanism of action of gallium nitrate for causing resolution of hypercalcemia is unknown.

■ Availability and Storage

Gallium nitrate is supplied by Fujisawa USA, Deerfield, Illinois, as 500 mg (25 mg/mL) in a 20-mL single-dose, flip-top vial. Each milliliter of gallium nitrate for injection (Ganite®) contains gallium nitrate 25 mg (on an anhydrous basis) and sodium citrate dihydrate 28.75 mg. The solution may contain sodium hydroxide for pH adjustment to 6.0 to 7.0. The vials should be stored at room temperature (15–30°C, 59–86°F).

■ Preparation for Use, Stability, and Admixture

The daily dose should be diluted in 1000 mL of 0.9% Sodium Chloride Injection, USP, or in 5% Dextrose Injection, USP, for administration as a 24-hour infusion. Each of these solutions is stable for 48 hours at room temperature or for 7 days under refrigeration (2–8°C). The product contains no preservatives. Any unused portion should be discarded.

■ Administration

The usual dose for gallium nitrate is 200 mg/m^2/d × 5 days. The daily dose should be administered as an intravenous infusion over 24 hours. Each daily dose should be diluted in 1000 mL of 0.9% Sodium Chloride Injection, USP, or 5% Dextrose Injection, USP, for infusion over 24 hours. The patients should be receiving adequate hydration throughout the time they are receiving gallium nitrate. Use of the agent as a continuous infusion has greatly decreased its nephrotoxicity (Leyland-Jones et al 1983).

■ Specific Precautions

Gallium nitrate should not be given to patients with a serum creatinine above 2.5 mg/dL. In addition, adequate hydration should be used before gallium nitrate is started and should be maintained throughout the gallium nitrate treatment period.

■ Drug Interactions

The package insert for Ganite® cautions against the use of highly nephrotoxic drugs (eg, aminoglycosides, amphotericin B) in combination with gallium nitrate (with the possibility of synergistic nephrotoxicity); however, there is no published literature in this area.

■ Dosage

The recommended dosage for treatment of patients with hypercalcemia is 200 mg/m² daily × 5 (or fewer days). Lower doses can be used for less severe hypercalcemia (eg, 100 mg/m²/d × 5).

In phase II trials of gallium nitrate as an antitumor agent, the doses included 700 mg/m² as a 30-minute infusion with prehydration every 2 weeks (Olver et al 1991); up to 350 mg/m²/d as a continuous infusion × 5 days (Seidman et al 1991); and 300 mg/m²/d as a continuous infusion × 7 days (Seligman and Crawford 1991). Use of the drug as a continuous infusion has decreased the nephrotoxicity seen with the agent (Leyland-Jones et al 1983).

■ Pharmacokinetics

Krakoff et al (1979) administered a single dose of gallium nitrate to patients with cancer. They noted the drug had a biphasic half-life with an α half-life of 87 minutes and β half-life of 24.5 hours. Recovery of the drug in the urine was approximately 65% in the first 24 hours. Mannitol-induced diuresis did not significantly increase the urinary excretion of the drug.

Kelsen et al (1980) studied the kinetics after a rapid intravenous infusion and after a continuous infusion. During continuous infusion, plasma levels ranged from 0.9 ± 0.2 to 1.9 ± 0.4 µg/mL. After rapid infusion, the α half-life ranged from 8.3 to 26 minutes, and the β half-life, 6.3 to 196 hours. Between 69 and 91% of the administered dose was recovered in the urine.

More recently Olver et al (1991) demonstrated a biphasic elimination for gallium nitrate with a β half-life of 6.2 to 11.9 hours, a plasma clearance of 169 to 244 mL/min, and a volume of distribution for free gallium of 128 to 186 L.

■ Side Effects and Toxicity

When used as an agent to treat patients with hypercalcemia, side effects can include hypocalcemia (up to 38% of patients according to package insert); hypophosphatemia (Scher et al 1987, Warrell et al 1991); decreased serum bicarbonate; and asymptomatic decreases in blood pressure. In patients receiving gallium nitrate for treatment of their malignancies, dose-limiting toxic effects were nephrotoxicity (Krakoff et al 1979) and hypocalcemia (Canfield and Lyss 1991). Other toxic effects have included anemia (Krakoff et al 1979, Malfetano et al 1991), hypomagnesemia (Canfield and Lyss 1991), tinnitus and decreased hearing (Jabboury et al 1989), mucositis (Jabboury et al 1989), optic neuropathy (Olver et al 1991), an offensive metallic taste (Krakoff et al 1979, Olver et al 1991, Canfield and Lyss 1991), nausea and vomiting (Krakoff et al 1979, Olver et al 1991), retinal hemorrhage (Canfield and Lyss 1991), and fever and diarrhea (Canfield and Lyss 1991).

In very recent studies (Seidman et al 1991) a bilateral optic neuropathy was dose limiting (it did resolve) in a patient receiving 400 mg/m²/d × 5 days.

■ Special Applications

Warrell et al (1990a) noted that gallium nitrate can correct some of the parameters of disease (eg, serum alkaline phosphatase) activity in patients with Paget's disease. This initial finding is being further investigated in larger studies.

REFERENCES

Bedikian AY, Valdivieso M, Bodey GP, et al. Phase I clinical studies with gallium nitrate. *Cancer Treat Rep.* 1978;**62**(10):1449–1453.

Brown J, Santos E, Rosen G, Helson L, Young C, Tan C. Phase I study of gallium nitrate in patients with advanced cancer. *Proc Am Assoc Cancer Res.* 1978;**19**:198.

Canfield V, Lyss AP. Gallium nitrate (GaN) in metastatic colorectal cancer (ca): Preliminary results of a phase II study. *Proc Am Soc Clin Oncol.* 1991;**10**(159):504.

Casper ES, Stanton GF, Sordillo PP, Parente R, Michaelson RA, Vinceguerra V. Phase II trial of gallium nitrate in patients with advanced malignant melanoma. *Cancer Treat Rep.* 1985;**69**(9):1019–1020.

Decker DA, Costanzi JJ, McCracken JD, Baker LH. Evaluation of gallium nitrate in metastatic or locally recurrent squamous cell carcinoma of the head and neck: A Southwest Oncology Group study. *Cancer Treat Rep.* 1984; **68**(7/8):1047–1048.

Dudley HC, Imrie W, Istock JT. Deposition of radiogallium (GA-72) in proliferating tissues. *Radiology.* 1950;**55:** 571–578.

Fabian CJ, Baker LH, Vaughn CB, Hynes HE. Phase II evaluation of gallium nitrate in breast cancer: A Southwest Oncology Group study. *Cancer Treat Rep.* 1982; **66**(7):1591.

Foster BJ, Clagett-Carr K, Hoth D, Leyland-Jones B. Gallium nitrate: The second metal with clinical activity. *Cancer Treat Rev.* 1986;**70**(11):1311–1319.

Hayes RL, Nelson B, Swartendruber DC, Carlton JE, Byrd BL. Gallium-67 localization in rat and mouse tumors. *Science.* 1970;**167**:289–290.

Jabboury K, Frye D, Holmes FA, Fraschini G, Hortobagyi G. Phase II evaluation of gallium nitrate by continuous infusion in breast cancer. *Invest New Drugs.* 1989;**7**(2/3): 225–229.

Keller J, Bartolucci A, Carpenter JT Jr, Feasler J. Phase II evaluation of bolus gallium nitrate in lymphoproliferative disorders: A Southeastern Cancer Study Group trial. *Cancer Treat Rep.* 1986;**70**(10):1221–1223.

Kelsen DP, Alcock N, Yeh S, Brown J, Young C. Pharmacokinetics of gallium nitrate in man. *Cancer.* 1980;**46**(9): 2009–2013.

Krakoff IH, Newman RA, Goldberg RS. Clinical toxicologic and pharmacologic studies of gallium nitrate. *Cancer.* 1979;**44**:1722–1727.

Leyland-Jones B, Bhalla RB, Farag F, Williams L, Coonley CJ, Warrell RP Jr. Administration of gallium nitrate by continuous infusion: Lack of chronic nephrotoxicity confirmed by studies of enzymuria and beta 2-macroglobulinuria. *Cancer Treat Rep.* 1983;**67**(10):941–942.

Malfetano JH, Blessing JA, Adelson MD. A phase II trial of gallium nitrate (NSC #15200) in previously treated ovarian carcinoma. *Am J Clin Oncol (CCT).* 1991;**14**(4):349–351.

Olver IN, Webster LK, Sephton RG, Bishop JF, Ball DL. A phase II study with pharmacokinetics of gallium nitrate in non-small cell lung cancer. *Proc Am Assoc Cancer Res.* 1991;**32**(190):1132.

Saiki JH, Baker LH, Stephen RL, Fabian CJ, Kraut EH, Fletcher WS. Gallium nitrate in advanced soft tissue and bone sarcomas: A Southwest Oncology Group study. *Cancer Treat Rep.* 1982;**66**(8):1673–1674.

Scher HI, Curley T, Geller N, et al. Gallium nitrate in prostatic cancer: Evaluation of antitumor activity and effects of bone turnover. *Cancer Treat Rep.* 1987;**71**(10):887–893.

Schwartz S, Yogoda A. Phase I–II trial of gallium nitrate for advanced hypernephroma. *Anticancer Res.* 1984;**4**(4/5):317–318.

Seidman A, Scher H, Sternberg C, et al. Gallium nitrate (GaN): An active agent in patients (PTS) with advanced refractory transitional cell carcinoma (TCC) of the urothelium. *Proc Am Soc Clin Oncol.* 1991;**10**(164):520.

Seligman PA, Crawford ED. Treatment of advanced transitional cell carcinoma (TCC) of the bladder with constant infusion gallium nitrate. *Proc Am Soc Clin Oncol.* 1991;**10**(168):534.

Valdivieso M, Bodey GP, Freireich EJ. Initial clinical studies of gallium nitrate. *Proc Am Assoc Cancer Res.* 1978;**19**:215.

Vugrin D, Einhorn LH, Brich R. Phase II trial of gallium nitrate in patients with metastatic renal carcinoma. A SECSG study (abstract). *Proc Am Assoc Cancer Res.* 1987;**28**:203.

Warrell RP, Alcock NW, Bockman RS. Gallium nitrate inhibits accelerated bone turnover in patients with bone metastases. *J Clin Oncol.* 1987;**5**(2):292–298.

Warrell RP Jr, Bosco B, Weinerman S, Levine B, Lane J, Bockman RS. Gallium nitrate for advanced Paget disease of bone: Effectiveness and dose–response analysis. *Ann Intern Med.* 1990a;**113**:847–851.

Warrell RP Jr, Coonley CJ, Straus DJ, Young DW. Treatment of patients with advanced malignant lymphoma using gallium nitrate administered as a seven-day continuous infusion. *Cancer.* 1983;**51**(11):1982–1987.

Warrell RP Jr, Israel R, Frisone M, Synder T, Gaynor JJ, Bockman RS. Gallium nitrate for acute treatment of cancer-related hypercalcemia. *Ann Intern Med.* 1988;**108:** 669–674.

Warrell RP Jr, Murphy WK, Schulman P, O'Dwyer PJ. Gallium nitrate for treatment of cancer-related hypercalcemia: A randomized double-blind comparison to etidronate. *Proc Am Soc Clin Oncol.* 1990b;**9**:250.

Warrell RP, Murphy WK, Schulman P, O'Dwyer PJ, Heller G. A randomized double-blind study of gallium nitrate compared with etidronate for acute control of cancer-related hypercalcemia. *J Clin Oncol.* 1991;**9**(8): 1467–1475.

Weick JK, Stephens RL, Baker LH, Jones SE. Gallium nitrate in malignant lymphoma: A Southwest Oncology Group study. *Cancer Treat Rep.* 1983;**67**(9):823–825.

Gemcitabine

■ Other Names

LY 188011; difluorodeoxycytidine; dFdC.

■ Chemistry

Structure of gemcitabine

Gemcitabine is a deoxycytidine analog antimetabolite (structurally related to cytosine arabinoside). It was originally synthesized as an antiviral agent; however, the agent was found to have excellent in vivo activity against a variety of animal tumors (Plunkett et al 1988, Boven et al 1991). The chemical name is 2',2'-difluorodeoxycytidine.

■ Antitumor Activity

Gemcitabine is highly active in several experimental tumor models including ccRF-CEM human leukemic blast cells (Hertel et al 1990), M5 ovarian cancer cells, X5563 myeloma, 6C3HED lymphosarcoma, and carcinoma-755 (Grindey et al 1986). Of note, several of these tumors were resistant to cytarabine. Marginal activity was noted in subcutaneous B-16 melanoma in mice (Grindey et al 1986).

Gemcitabine is still undergoing phase I testing to try to optimize the dose and schedule of the agent. In phase I trials, responses have been noted in patients with non-small cell lung, pancreatic, breast, and colon cancers (Weeks et al 1989, Poplin et al 1989, Tanis et al 1990, O'Rourke et al 1989, Brown et al 1991). Preliminary phase II studies have also reported significant antitumor activity for gemcitabine. Objective responses have been described in patients with non-small cell lung cancer (17% partial response rate [Lund et al 1992b, Abratt et al 1992]), small cell lung cancer (3/8 responders, 1 complete [Eisenhauer et al 1992]), head and neck cancer (Clavel et al 1992), previously cisplatin-treated ovarian cancer patients (20% partial response rate [Lund et al 1992a]), renal cancer (10% of patients [Weisbach et al 1992]), and breast cancer patients (4/18 patients [Carmichael et al 1992]).

Additionally early phase II trials have documented a 20% response rate in patients with non-small cell lung cancer (Anderson et al 1991) and a 15% response rate in patients with advanced pancreatic cancer (Casper et al 1991). The drug has been found to be inactive in one schedule in patients with advanced colorectal cancer (Abbruzzese et al 1991b).

■ Mechanism of Action

Gemcitabine is an antimetabolite that acts as an inhibitor of DNA synthesis. Gemcitabine is triphosphorylated in tumor cells by the enzyme deoxycytidine kinase (Heinemann et al 1988). There is subsequent inhibition of DNA polymerase activity (Burke et al 1990). There is also recent evidence that gemcitabine may inhibit ribonucleotide reductase. This would block the conversion of ribonucleotides to deoxyribonucleotides. In Chinese hamster ovary cells, the 5'-triphosphate of gemcitabine is the major metabolite, constituting 85 to 90% of total intracellular drug content. Gemcitabine achieves 20-fold higher intracellular concentrations compared with equimolar exposures to cytarabine. The reason for the increase in accumulation involves increased membrane permeation, greater affinity of deoxycytidine kinase for gemcitabine (K_M = 3.6 μM), and slower and biphasic elimination of intracellular drug with half-lives of (α) 3.9 minutes at low drug concentrations and (β) more than 16 hours at higher concentrations of 100 to 600 μM (Heinemann et al 1988). The enhanced accumulation and more avid, nonsaturable activation of gemcitabine may explain the prolonged inhibition of DNA synthesis seen following a short-term exposure to the drug. The cytotoxic activity of gemcitabine can be completely reversed by excess deoxycytidine, which confirms that deoxycytidine kinase is absolutely necessary for antitumor activity (Heinemann et al 1988). The drug appears to be cell cycle specific for S phase, causing cells to accumulate at the G_1–S phase boundary (Chubb et al 1987).

■ Availability and Storage

The drug is available for investigational use from Eli Lilly & Company, Indianapolis, Indiana. It is provided as a lyophilized powder in vials containing either 20 or 100 mg of active drug as the hydrochloride salt, mannitol, and sodium acetate. The vials are stored at room temperature.

■ Preparation for Use, Stability, and Admixture

Gemcitabine vials must be reconstituted with 2 mL (20-mg vial) or 10 mL (100-mg vial) of normal saline to make a solution containing 10 mg/mL. After reconstitution, an appropriate amount of drug is diluted in 100 to 1000 mL of saline and infused over 30 minutes to 4 hours. **Caution:** Because of drug solubility problems, doses of 2500 mg/m^2 and greater must be diluted in at least 1000 mL of normal saline and infused over 4 hours or longer.

■ Administration

The optimal method(s) (dose and schedule) for administration of gemcitabine is only now being worked out. The most common method of administration is a 30-minute infusion weekly × 3 followed by a 1-week rest (Casper et al 1991).

Because of drug solubility problems at doses over 2500 mg/m^2 the drug should be infused in no less than 4 hours.

■ Special Precautions

None are known at this time.

■ Drug Interactions

None are known at this time.

■ Dosage

The current dose recommended for ongoing phase II trials is 800 mg/m^2 weekly × 3 weeks every 4 weeks. A twice weekly dose of 90 mg/m^2 is not tolerated as well as the weekly dose (Lund et al 1992b). A weekly × 3 dose of 1000 mg/m^2 has also been reported to be active in lung cancer (Abratt et al 1992, Eisenhauer et al 1992); however, there is a push for a more intensive dose schedule such as 3600 mg/m^2 every 2 weeks (Brown et al 1991).

■ Pharmacokinetics

Pharmacokinetic studies with gemcitabine are ongoing. Peters et al (1990), using a 30-minute infusion, noted that gemcitabine and its deaminated uridine metabolite, difluorodeoxyuridine (dFdU), reached peak levels of 50 to 100 μM after doses of 1500 mg/m^2. Gemcitabine has a β half-life of 4 to 20 minutes (Peters et al 1990) or 27 minutes (Abbruzzese et al 1991a), whereas dFdU was still present after 24 hours (± 20 μM). Peak dFdU levels of about 10 mM are achieved within 5 to 15 minutes of infusion. Renal clearance of dFdU is rapid at about 157 mL/min (Abbruzzese et al 1991a). A median of 77% of gemcitabine dose is excreted in the urine and only about 5% is recovered as intact drug. The table below summarizes the dose-dependent plasma AUC values for gemcitabine and the principal metabolite dFdU.

■ Side Effects and Toxicity

Toxic effects have included dose-limiting myelosuppression characterized by thrombocytopenia with relative sparing of leukocytes (Abbruzzese et al 1991a). Anemia has rarely been noted. The myelosuppressive effects of the drug are not cumulative and typically resolve rapidly when the drug is discontinued. There is also a reversible skin rash (which may be somewhat alleviated by steroids),

MEAN PLASMA PHARMACOKINETICS OF GEMCITABINE AND DIFLUORODEOXYURIDINE

	Gemcitabine					Difluorodeoxyuridine		
Dose (mg/m^2)	Number of Patients	Peak (μmol/L)	Half-life (min)	AUC (mg/L/h)	Clearance (L/h/m^2)	Peak (μmol/L)	β Half-life (h)	AUC (μg/L/h)
53	3	1.3	14.6	0.43	406.3	NA*	NA	NA
80	3	3	8.7	0.63	203.6	NA	NA	NA
120	3	7	6.3	1.6	69.3	17.3	>24	183.7
180	3	8	19.3	1.53	111	23	>24	230.7
350	3	19	18.7	2.93	99.7	35.7	14.6	125.6
790	5	57	5.8	8.75	213.5	92.7	14.2	207.6
1000	5	56.4	8.2	10.6	408.4	118.2	10.4	293.2

* Data not available.
From Abbruzzese JL, Grunewald R, Weeks EA, et al. A phase I clinical, plasma, and cellular pharmacology study of gemcitabine. *J Clin Oncol.* 1991;9(3):491–498. Reprinted with permission.

fever, mild nausea and vomiting, and a flulike syndrome (particularly with the daily × 5 schedule). Transient febrile episodes are seen in about 50% of patients within 6 to 12 hours of receiving the first dose. The fevers were responsive to acetaminophen and did not recur with subsequent doses (Abbruzzese et al 1991a). The generalized rash caused by gemcitabine was seen within 48 to 72 hours in 5 of 42 patients who received doses above 525 mg/m²/wk. It presented as an erythematous, pruritic, maculopapular rash involving the neck and extremities. Topical corticosteroids and dose reductions allowed continued dosing in these patients (Abbruzzese et al 1991a).

In careful studies, Pollera et al (1991) have found a significant negative effect of gemcitabine on erythropoiesis. Increases in serum iron and ferritin with a drop in reticulocyte count were noted.

■ **Special Applications**

None are known at this time.

REFERENCES

Abbruzzese JL, Grunewald R, Weeks EA, et al. A phase I clinical, plasma, and cellular pharmacology study of gemcitabine. *J Clin Oncol.* 1991a;**9**(3):491–498.

Abbruzzese T, Pazdur R, Ajani T, Daugherty K, Tarassoff P, Levin B. A phase II trial of gemcitabine (dFdc) in patients (Pts) with advanced colorectal cancer. *Proc Am Soc Clin Oncol.* 1991b;**10**:147.

Abratt R, Bezwoda W, Falkson G, et al. Efficacy and safety of gemcitabine in non-small cell lung cancer. *Proc Am Soc Clin Oncol.* 1992;**11**:311.

Anderson H, Lund B, Hansen HH, Walling J, Thatcher N. Phase II study of gemcitabine in non-small cell lung cancer (NSCLC). *Proc Am Soc Clin Oncol.* 1991;**10**:247.

Boven E, Erkelens CAM, Pinedo HM, Hatty SA. The new cytidine analog gemcitabine (GEM) has schedule rather than dose-related activity in human tumor xenografts. *Proc Am Assoc Cancer Res.* 1991;**32**:382.

Brown T, O'Rourke T, Burris H, et al. A phase I trial of gemcitabine (LY 188011) administered intravenously every two weeks. *Proc Am Soc Clin Oncol.* 1991;**10**:115.

Burke T, Grindey GB, Hertel L, Rinzal S, Worzalla J, Boder GB. Cellular distribution of gemcitabine (LY188011). *Proc Am Assoc Cancer Res.* 1990;**31**:344.

Carmichael J, Philip P, Rea D, et al. Gemcitabine: An active drug in advanced breast cancer. Results of a phase II study. *Proc Am Soc Clin Oncol.* 1992;**11**:77.

Casper ES, Green MR, Brown TD, et al. Phase II trial of gemcitabine (2′,2′-difluorodeoxycitadine) in patients with pancreatic cancer. *Proc Am Soc Clin Oncol.* 1991;**10**:143.

Chubb S, Heinemann V, Novotny L, et al. Metabolism and action of 2′-2′-difluorodeoxycitidine in human leukemic cells. *Proc Am Assoc Cancer Res.* 1987;**28**:324.

Clavel M, Vermorken JB, Judson I, et al. Gemcitabine is an active drug in patients with squamous cell carcinoma of the head and neck. *Proc Am Soc Clin Oncol.* 1992;**11**:249.

Eisenhauer E, Cormier Y, Gregg R, et al. Gemcitabine is active in patients (PTS) with previously untreated extensive small cell lung cancer (SCLC)—A phase II study of the National Cancer Institute of Canada Clinical Trials Group (NCIC CTG). *Proc Am Soc Clin Oncol.* 1992;**11**:309.

Grindey GB, Boder GB, Hertel LW, et al. Antitumor activity of 2′,2′-difluorodeoxycitidine (LY188011). *Proc Am Assoc Cancer Res.* 1986;**27**:296.

Heinemann V, Hertel LW, Grindey GB, et al. Comparison of the cellular pharmacokinetics and toxicity of 2′,2′-difluorodeoxycitidine and 1-β-D-arabinofuranosylcytosine. *Cancer Res.* 1988;**48**:4024–4031.

Hertel LW, Boder GB, Kroin S, et al. Evaluation of the antitumor activity of gemcitabine (2′,2′-difluoro-2′-deoxycytidine). *Cancer Res.* 1990;**50**:4417–4422.

Lund B, Hansen OP, Neijt JP, et al. Phase II study of gemcitabine in previously treated ovarian cancer patients. *Proc Am Soc Clin Oncol.* 1992a;**11**:222.

Lund B, Ryberg M, Anderson H, et al. A phase II study of gemcitabine in non-small cell lung cancer (NSCLC) using a twice weekly schedule. *Proc Am Assoc Cancer Res.* 1992b;**33**:226.

O'Rourke T, Brown T, Havlin K, et al. Phase I trial and immunologic assessment of difluorodeoxycitidine (LY 188011). *Proc Am Soc Clin Oncol.* 1989;**8**:82.

Peters G, Tanis B, Clavel M, et al. Pharmacokinetics of gemcitabine (LY 188011; difluorodeoxycitidine) administered every two weeks in a phase I study. *Proc Am Assoc Cancer Res.* 1990;**31**:180.

Plunkett W, Chubb S, Nowak B, Hertel L, Grindey GB. Increased cytotoxicity and therapeutic activity of 2,2′-difluorodeoxycitidine (dFdc) over cytosine arabinoside (ara-C) in L1210 leukemia. *Proc Am Assoc Cancer Res.* 1988;**29**:352.

Pollera CF, Amgelio F, Giannarelli D, Sabino F, Gandolfo GM, Calabresi F. Gemcitabine-induced erythropoiesis impairment. *Proc Am Assoc Cancer Res.* 1991;**32**:175.

Poplin E, Redman B, Flaherty L, Wozniak A, Valdevieso M, Baker L. Difluorodeoxycitidine (DRdc): A phase I study. *Proc Am Assoc Cancer Res.* 1989;**30**:282.

Tanis B, Clavel M, Guastalla J, et al. Phase I study of gemcitabine (difluorodeoxycitidine; dFdc; LY 188011) administered in a two week schedule. *Proc Am Assoc Cancer Res.* 1990;**31**:207.

Weeks A, Abbruzzese J, Gravel D, et al. Phase I clinical and pharmacology study of difluorodeoxycitidine. *Proc Am Assoc Cancer Res.* 1989;**30**:273.

Weisbach L, de Mulder P, Osieka R, et al. Phase II study of gemcitabine in renal cancer. *Proc Am Soc Clin Oncol.* 1992;**11**:219.

Goserelin Acetate

■ Other Names

Zoladex® (ICI Pharma); ICI 118630.

■ Chemistry

Goserelin is a synthetic decapeptide analog of luteinizing hormone-releasing hormone (LH-RH). It is commercially available as the acetate salt of pyro-Glu–His–Trp–Ser–Tyr–D-Ser(Bu^t)–Leu–Arg–Pro–Azgly- NH$_2$ (Coy and Schally 1978). Substitution of the butylated D-serine at position 6 and the altered glycine at position 10 significantly increases the pharmacologic activity over that of the natural LH-RH protein. The goserelin depot formulation is a dispersion of the protein into a matrix of DL-lactic acid–glycolic acid copolymer (C$_2$H$_4$O$_2$)$_{1-2.4}$, which is completely biodegradable, providing continuous drug release over 28 days. The molecular formula of goserelin is C$_{59}$H$_{84}$N$_{18}$O$_{14}$ and the molecular weight of 1269 as the free base. This material is freely soluble in glacial acetic acid and is soluble in water. The base is not soluble in acetone, chloroform, or ether. About 13.3 to 14.3 mg of the DL-lactic acid–glycolic acid copolymer is in each depot dose containing 3.6 mg of goserelin acetate and less than 2.5% acetic acid.

■ Antitumor Activity

Goserelin is used in the palliative management of advanced prostate cancer, as a medical alternative to orchiectomy and/or estrogen therapy. Clinical trials indicate an objective partial response rate of about 40%, with over half of treated patients showing stabilization of disease (Ahmann et al 1987). Subjective improvement is noted in up to 60 to 80% of patients (Van Cangh and Opsomer 1987), with partial response rates of up to 86% in some trials (Emtage et al 1987, Holdaway et al 1988).

The agent has also been investigationally tested in women with breast cancer, treated at various stages of the menstrual cycle (Nicholson et al 1984). This treatment was able to reduce plasma estradiol concentrations to postmenopausal levels. In one fifth of the women, some residual follicle-stimulating hormone (FSH) activity was present until the third menstrual cycle. These data suggest that goserelin might be useful in premenopausal women with hormonally dependent breast cancer.

■ Mechanism of Action

Goserelin acts as a slow-release form of a potent inhibitor of gonadotropin release from the pituitary (Coy and Schally 1978). As with leuprolide, goserelin is technically a superpotent agonist of LH-RH. Thus, on initiation of therapy, FSH and LH release is stimulated, causing a brief surge in gonadal synthesis of sex hormones including testosterone, progesterone, 17-hydroxyprogesterone, and estrogen; however, the continuous stimulation produced by goserelin leads to near-complete inhibition of FSH and LH release. This subsequently reduces testosterone, progesterone, and estradiol to castrate levels (Nicholson et al 1984). Gonadal steroid suppression is generally achieved within 2 to 4 weeks of starting goserelin in prostate cancer patients. Fortunately, suppression to castrate sex steroid levels can be maintained for prolonged periods of up to 2 years with chronic monthly subcutaneous goserelin dosing.

■ Availability and Storage

Goserelin is supplied as a sterile dispersion of 3.6 mg drug in the biodegradable DL-glycolic acid–lactic acid matrix. (Zoladex®, ICI Pharma, Wilmington, Delaware). It is provided premixed in a disposable syringe. The syringe comes fitted with a 16-gauge needle, and the unit is sealed in a light-protective and moisture-proof foil pack which also contains a desiccant packet. The drug-filled syringe in its packet can be stored at room temperature for prolonged periods.

■ Preparation for Use, Stability, and Admixture

The drug-filled syringe is supplied ready for injection. Admixture with any other drug or solution is not recommended and could alter the drug's stability and/or the dissolution characteristics of the slow-release matrix. The packet should not be opened until the day the drug is to be administered.

■ Administration

Goserelin acetate is administered by a single subcutaneous injection into abdominal body fat. The syringe cannot be used for aspiration; however, blood will appear in the syringe chamber if a blood vessel is inadvertently penetrated. A new syringe and alternate injection site should then be used. After the skin is pierced, the needle should be tunneled parallel to the skin and fat until the hub touches the skin. The needle is then partially withdrawn (about 1 cm) to leave a space for the drug/matrix. A single push on the syringe plunger is typically adequate to deliver the dose. The site is then covered with a sterile bandage. Local anesthesia with lidocaine may also be used prior to goserelin injection.

■ Dosage

A fixed adult dose of 3.6 mg (one syringe) is administered subcutaneously every 28 days. Usage in children is not reported.

■ Pharmacokinetics

When a solution of goserelin is administered subcutaneously, the drug exhibits a short plasma half-life (see table below). Steady-state plasma levels after a 120 µg/d SC infusion ranged from 2.1 to 2.7 ng/mL (Clayton et al 1985). This is slightly lower than the peak plasma levels 6 to 8 ng/mL obtained 12 to 15 days after subcutaneous injection of the 3.6-mg goserelin depot matrix formulation (Clayton et al 1985). Thus, goserelin acetate absorption is slightly slower during the first 8 days after depot injection. Plasma levels thereafter fall to 1 ng/mL or less at 29 days, just prior to the next injection. There is no evidence of drug accumulation with repeated monthly doses in patients with normal renal function (creatinine clearance ≥ 70 mL/min). In patients with reduced renal function (creatinine clearance ≤ 20 mL/min), however, the goserelin half-life increases from the normal 4.2 hours to a mean of 12.1 hours. Nonetheless, there was no evidence of excess drug toxicity in this group of patients.

■ Side Effects and Toxicity

The primary toxic effects of goserelin are due to its endocrine effects. These include hot flashes seen in 50%, decreased libido in 9%, and gynecomastia in 9% of male prostate cancer patients (Ahmann et al 1987). Transient acute increases in bone pain may be seen in up to 17% of patients starting the drug. This is thought to be related to the initial increase in FSH and LH release induced by the drug; however, patients with preexisting bony metastases may experience a slightly higher incidence of increased bone pain. Fortunately, increased analgesic doses are typically not necessary and the effect is usually transient on initiation of therapy.

Other side effects noted in 10% or less of patients include edema, lethargy, pain and/or rash at the injection site, anorexia, and nausea. Dizziness and sweating are also rarely observed. Unlike estrogens, goserelin does not lower antithrombin III concentrations (Varenhorst et al 1986). This reduces the risk of thrombosis seen with diethylstilbestrol therapy in prostate cancer patients.

REFERENCES

Ahmann FR, Citrin DL, deHaan HA, et al. Zoladex: A sustained-release, monthly luteinizing hormone-releasing hormone analogue for the treatment of advanced prostate cancer. *J Clin Oncol.* 1987;**5**:912–917.

Clayton RN, Bailey LC, Cottam J, et al. A radioimmunoassay for GnRH agonist analogue in serum of patients with prostate cancer treated with D-Ser (tBu)^{6}A$_{ZA}$ Gly^{10} GnRH. *Clin Endocrinol.* 1985;**22**:453–462.

Coy DH, Schally AV. Gonadotrophin releasing hormone analogues. *Ann Clin Res.* 1978;**10**:139–144.

Emtage LA, Perren TJ, Stuart NSA, et al. Phase II study of Zoladex depot in advanced prostatic cancer with special reference to criteria of response and survival. *Br J Urol.* 1987;**60**:436–442.

Holdaway IM, Ibberston HK, Croxson MS, et al. Zoladex treatment of symptomatic prostatic carcinoma. *Am J Clin Oncol.* 1988;**11**(2):S123–S126.

Nicholson RI, Walker KJ, Turkes A, et al. Therapeutic significance and the mechanism of action of the LH-RH agonist ICI 118630 in breast and prostate cancer. *J Steroid Biochem.* 1984;**20**(1):129–135.

Van Cangh PJ, Opsomer RJ. Treatment of advanced carcinoma of the prostate with a depot luteinizing hormone-releasing hormone analogue (ICI-118630). *J Urol.* 1987;**137**:61–64.

Varenhorst E, Svensson M, Hjertberg H, Malmqvist E. Antithrombin III concentration, thrombosis, and treatment with luteinizing hormone releasing hormone agonist in prostatic carcinoma. *Br Med. J.* 1986;**292**:935–936.

CLINICAL PHARMACOKINETICS OF GOSERELIN*

Half-life	4.9 h
Total body clearance	32.4 mL/min
Volume of distribution	13.7 L

*250-µg subcutaneous bolus of goserelin solution (not depot) measured by a nonspecific radioimmunoassay (Clayton et al 1985).

Hepsulfam

■ Other Names

NSC-329680; sulfamin.

■ Chemistry

$$H_2N-O-\underset{\underset{O}{\|}}{\overset{\overset{O}{\|}}{S}}-O-(CH_2)_7-O-\underset{\underset{O}{\|}}{\overset{\overset{O}{\|}}{S}}-O-NH_2$$

Structure of hepsulfam

Hepsulfam (1,7-heptanediol bis-sulfamate or 1,7-heptanediol sulfamic acid ester) is one of a series of bis-sulfamic acid esters synthesized by Sterling-Winthrop in an attempt to improve the antitumor efficacy of busulfan through introduction of a more polar leaving group. The project was successful in obtaining a derivative with a broader spectrum of preclinical in vivo activity. The compound has the chemical formula $H_2NO_2SOCH_2(CH_2)_5CH_2OSO_2NH_2$ and a molecular weight of 290. The empiric formula is $C_9H_{18}N_2O_6S_2$.

■ Antitumor Activity

In preclinical tumor models, hepsulfam demonstrated activity superior to busulfan in L-1210 and P-388 leukemias (Sladek et al 1991). The drug was also active in human tumor xenografts in nude mice (Berger et al 1990). Responsive tumors included breast and colon carcinomas. Other murine solid tumors responsive to hepsulfam include B-16 melanoma, colon-38 carcinoma, and CD8F mammary carcinoma. Hematologic responses to hepsulfam have been observed in patients with refractory leukemias who were given multiple courses of high-dose therapy (Geller et al 1992). One response was obtained in a patient with blast-phase chronic myelogenous leukemia.

■ Mechanism of Action

Hepsulfam is a DNA alkylating agent (Hincks et al 1990, Pacheco et al 1989, 1990). The potential alkylating activity of hepsulfam was evaluated by the nitrobenzylpyridine assay and the alkaline elution assay. Hepsulfam was 10- and 1.6 fold less reactive than mechlorethamine and busulfan, respectively, in the nitrobenzylpyridine assay. The ability of hepsulfam to cause interstrand crosslinks was examined in P-388 cells following exposure to drug for 1 hour. After being washed, the drug-treated cells were reincubated in fresh medium for 4 hours to allow for formation of crosslinks, irradiated with 500 rad, and examined in the alkaline elution assay. DNA from cells treated with hepsulfam eluted more slowly than DNA from irradiated, untreated controls, indicating the formation of DNA interstrand crosslinks and DNA–protein crosslinks. Inclusion of proteinase K in the assay increased the elution of DNA, indicating the predominance of DNA–protein crosslinks. Similar elution profiles were obtained with equimolar concentrations of busulfan. Nonetheless, hepsulfam is about fourfold more potent than busulfan in terms of DNA alkylating activity (Pacheco et al 1989, 1990). This correlates with a two- to threefold greater cytotoxic potency in human HL-60 and K-562 leukemia cells in vitro (Pacheco et al 1990). Of interest, hepsulfam induced DNA interstrand crosslinks in these cell lines in vitro whereas busulfan did not (Pacheco et al 1990). In preclinical systems the drug does not exhibit schedule dependency and is not cell cycle specific in cytotoxic activity.

■ Availability and Storage

Hepsulfam is available as an investigational drug from the Investigational Drug Branch of the National Cancer Institute. The vials should be stored under refrigeration (2–8°C).

■ Preparation for Use, Stability, and Admixture

A two-component formulation has been developed for the clinic consisting of (1) 150 mg of hepsulfam freeze-dried from 40% t-butanol in a 10-mL flint vial and (2) 5 mL of a vehicle composed of 10% ethanol, 40% propylene glycol, and a sufficient quantity of 0.05 M, pH 7.4 phosphate buffer. The drug is dissolved by adding 5.0 mL of the special vehicle to the 150-mg hepsulfam powder vial. This yields a 30 mg/mL solution of hepsulfam. For phase I studies the drug is placed in 150 mL of D5W and infused over 30 minutes.

The shelf-life surveillance of the two vials is ongoing. The solution is stable for 24 hours at room temperature. Ten percent decomposition is noted in approximately 8 days. After a tenfold dilution with either D5W or 0.9% sodium chloride injection, a 10%

PHASE I TRIALS WITH HEPSULFAM

Schedule	Dose Range Explored (mg/m^2)	Maximally Tolerated Dose (mg/m^2)	Recommended Phase II Dose (mg/m^2)	Reference
Single every 21–35 d	30–360	360	210	Ravdin et al 1991
Single every 28 d	30–270	—	210	Hendricks et al 1991
Single every 21–35 d	30–360	—	—	Sladek et al 1991

loss was noted at 38 hours at 25°C. The difference in observed stability in the diluted solution is probably due to the decreased organic portion in the infusion fluid.

■ Administration

The drug, diluted in 150 mL of normal saline, is usually administered over 30 minutes; however, the optimal dose and schedule have yet to be determined (see Dosage).

■ Special Precautions

On the basis of results from the initial clinical trial it appears that the bone marrow-suppressive effects of hepsulfam are cumulative.

■ Drug Interactions

None are known at this time, but the use of the agent to date has been limited.

■ Dosage

The phase I trials described in the above table have been completed or are ongoing.

As can be seen, the drug cannot be given any more often than every 28 to 35 days because of late (and possibly cumulative) myelosuppression. Clinical trials with escalating doses of hepsulfam are ongoing with the appropriate marrow support. In refractory leukemias, hepsulfam doses of 640 mg/m^2 have been administered (Geller et al 1992). Some of these patients tolerated multiple courses of hepsulfam repeated at 4- to 6-week intervals.

■ Pharmacokinetics

The data in the table below summarize the currently available pharmacokinetic information on hepsulfam. Urinary secretion of hepsulfam in the first 48 hours has been 21 to 23 ± 9.3% (Marshall et al 1991, Sladek et al 1991). Of interest is that penetration of hepsulfam into the cerebral spinal fluid compartment in baboons has been shown to be between 35 and 60% (Marshall et al 1991).

■ Side Effects and Toxicity

The dose-limiting toxic effects of hepsulfam are leukopenia and thrombocytopenia. Both appear to be cumulative (Ravdin et al 1991, Hendricks et al 1991). These effects have been noted only in second or subsequent courses. The median day of leukopenia onset is day 22 and the median day of recovery is day 44 after dosing (Hendricks et al 1991). Thrombocytopenia is less common but often more severe. It is similar to neutropenia in onset and delayed recovery. Hepsulfam has been found to be sequestered in red blood cells and could contribute to the delayed neutropenia and thrombocytopenia (Marshall et al 1991). Of interest, both toxic effects are not more common in extensively pretreated patients. Some patients may also experience a drop in hemoglobin, which is not dose related (Hendricks et al 1991).

PHARMACOKINETIC DATA FOR HEPSULFAM

Schedule	Half-life (h) α	Half-life (h) β	Volume of Distribution (L/m^2)	Clearance (L/h/m^2)	Reference
Single dose	—	Plasma 15.9 (4.6)*	—	6.0 (1.7)	Marshall et al 1991
	—	Blood 90 (15.5)	—	0.09 (0.04)	
Single dose	0.10	3.87	25 (15)	0.23 (0.18)	Hendricks et al 1991
Single dose	—	20.5 (10.2)	—	0.08 (0.02)	Sladek et al 1991

*Standard deviations are given in parentheses.

Other toxic effects noted are mild nausea and vomiting and elevated liver function tests (Ravdin et al 1991, Hendricks et al 1991). The increases in serum aminotransferases were seen in about one third of patients, most of whom had documented hepatic involvement with tumor. Of note, pulmonary toxicity, alopecia, and rashes were not reported in phase I hepsulfam studies (Hendricks et al 1991). Facial flushing and perioral numbness were noted and were thought to be related to the propylene glycol and alcohol vehicle used in the hepsulfam infusion (Sladek et al 1991).

■ Special Applications

Use of hepsulfam to prepare the bone marrow for bone marrow transplantation is currently being explored. With appropriate hematologic stem cell support, dose escalation above 480 mg/m² is envisioned (Hendricks et al 1991).

REFERENCES

Berger DP, Winterhalter BR, Widmer KH, et al. Activity of hepsulfam and busulfan in combined in vitro/in vivo screening system with human tumor xenografts. *Proc Am Assoc Cancer Res.* 1990;**31**:415.

Geller RB, Janisch L, Kampmeier P, et al. Phase I trial of hepsulfam in patients (PTS) with refractory leukemias. *Proc Am Soc Clin Oncol.* 1992;**11**:264.

Hendricks CB, Brochow LB, Rowinsky EK, et al. Phase I and pharmacokinetic study of hepsulfam (NSC-329680). *Cancer Res.* 1991;**51**:5781–5785.

Hincks JR, Adlakha A, Cook CA, et al. In vitro studies in the mechanism of action of hepsulfam in chronic myelogenous leukemia patients. *Cancer Res.* 1990;**50**:7559–7563.

Marshall MV, Von Hoff DD, Ravdin PM, et al. Pharmacokinetics of hepsulfam (sulfamic acid heptanediyl ester) in patients following a brief infusion. *Proc Am Soc Clin Oncol.* 1991;**10**:95.

Pacheco DY, Cook C, Hincks JR, et al. Mechanisms of toxicity of hepsulfam in human tumor cell lines. *Cancer Res.* 1990;**50**:7555–7558.

Pacheco DY, Stratton NK, Gibson NW. Comparison of the mechanism of action of busulfan with hepsulfam, a new antileukemic agent, in the L1210 cell line. *Cancer Res.* 1989;**49**:5108–5110.

Ravdin PM, Havlin KA, Marshall MV, et al. A phase I trial with pharmacokinetics of hepsulfam. *Proc Am Assoc Cancer Res.* 1991;**32**:201.

Sladek G, Dearing MP, Ihde D, et al. Phase I clinical and pharmacokinetic study of hepsulfam. *Proc Am Soc Clin Oncol.* 1991;**10**:107.

Hexamethylene Bisacetamide

■ Other Names

HMBA; NSC-955580.

■ Chemistry

$$CH_3-\overset{O}{\underset{\|}{C}}-NH-(CH_2)_6-NH-\overset{O}{\underset{\|}{C}}-CH_3$$

Structure of hexamethylene bisacetamide

Hexamethylene bisacetamide (HMBA) is a polar-alkyl compound structurally related to N-methylformamide (NMF) (Chun et al 1986). The chemical name is N,N'-hexamethylene bisacetamide. The molecular formula is $C_{10}H_{20}N_2O_2$ with formula weight of 200.3. The pH of the 5% sterile solution is 4.5 to 6.5 and the osmolality is 250 mosmol/kg.

■ Antitumor Activity

Hexamethylene bisacetamide has been shown to induce the differentiation of tumor cells into nonmalignant phenotypes (Chun et al 1986). It has not produced direct antitumor activity in a number of experimental murine cancers including P-388 and L-1210 leukemia, B-16 melanoma, colon-38 cancer, CD8F1 mammary cancer, Lewis lung cancer, and M-5076 sarcoma. It is also inactive against human tumor xenografts in mice (Chun et al 1986). Furthermore, the compound is not cytotoxic at concentrations that induce differentiation in vitro.

This agent induces differentiation in a number of tumor cell lines including HL-60 promyelocytic leukemia (Collins et al 1980), Friend erythroleukemia cells (Tanaka et al 1971, Reuben et al 1976, 1978, 1980, Reuben 1979, Fibach et al 1977, Marks and Rifkind 1978), mouse neuroblastoma cells (Palfrey et al 1977), Madin–Darby canine kidney (MDCK) cells (Lever 1979), and human glioblastoma cells (Rabson et al 1977). Histologic or functional signs of differentiation include the development of mature myeloid markers in HL-60 cells, normal erythroid differentiation in Friend cells, expression of extended neurites and excitable membranes in neuroblastoma cells, procollagen synthesis in glioblastoma cells, and formation of special epithelial transport "domes" in MDCK cells.

Exposure of tumors to HMBA in vivo may also

decrease tumor formation in certain rodent models such as methylnitrosourea-induced tumors in Sprague-Dawley rats (Chun et al 1986).

In vitro, 5 mM HMBA has produced inhibition in tumor colony formation in soft agar assays. Inhibition of colony formation to less than 30% of control was noted in four of seven human ovarian tumors, one Hodgkin's lymphoma, one of four human melanomas, and one of two other specimens (Chun et al 1986). There is one report of a synergistic increase in survival for the combination of HMBA with cyclophosphamide in nude mice inoculated with human HL-60 cells (Bogden et al 1985). No objective antitumor responses have been observed in two phase I clinical trials involving 23 cancer patients (Rowinsky et al 1986) and 20 cancer patients (Egorin et al 1987a). The compound was similarly inactive in 15 patients with severe myelodysplastic syndrome when administered on a 5-day schedule (Rowinsky et al 1990).

■ Mechanism of Action

A variety of polar-alkyl compounds have differentiating effects on tumor cells. Although their precise mechanism of action is unknown, structure–activity studies with different bisacetamides do show that polar head groups (eg, the acetamide moieties) need to be six carbons apart for optimal differentiating activity (Reuben et al 1978). The polar amides on HMBA tend to act as Lewis bases, accepting protons, and this property is related to the differentiating effect (Matsuo et al 1984).

Cells treated with differentiating agents such as dimethylsulfoxide exhibit prolongation of G_1 phase or inhibition of progression into S phase (Levy et al 1975, Terada et al 1977); however, cell cycle arrest has not been directly correlated to the differentiating effect (Friedman and Schildkraut 1978) and in HL-60 cells there is no correlation of G_1 arrest to differentiation (Ferrero et al 1982).

Chromatin and DNA are altered by HMBA. The changes include reduced stability to heat denaturation and the development of DNase 1- and S-1 nuclease-sensitive sites on chromatin near globin genes (Sheffery et al 1983). There is also a temporal association between the accumulation of α-globin mRNA and the differentiating effect following HMBA treatment of murine erythroleukemia cells (Reuben 1979, Reuben et al 1980). This activity appears to be controlled at the level of DNA transcription (Profou-Juchelka et al 1983).

■ Availability and Storage

Hexamethylene bisacetamide is investigationally available from the National Cancer Institute as a 5% (50 mg/mL) sterile solution in water. The drug is supplied in 500-mL infusion bottles containing 25 g of HMBA. The infusion bottles are stored at room temperature and should *not* be refrigerated or frozen. The drug was previously supplied in 500-mL bottles as a 3% solution in 0.154 M sodium chloride. This formulation was used in the initial phase I 5-day infusion trials in cancer patients (Rowinsky et al 1986, Egorin et al 1987a).

■ Preparation for Use, Stability, and Admixture

The HMBA sterile solutions can be administered intravenously directly as supplied using a self-venting administration set. The solution is also compatible with polyvinyl chloride plastic infusion systems for up to 90 days and can be filtered without loss of activity (National Cancer Institute 1977).

■ Administration

Hexamethylene bisacetamide has been administered intravenously as a continuous infusion for 5 consecutive days (Rowinsky et al 1986, Egorin et al 1987a) and 10 consecutive days (Young et al 1988).

■ Dosage

The recommended phase II dose of HMBA by continuous intravenous infusion is 24 g/m^2/d (Rowinsky et al 1986, Egorin et al 1987a).

■ Drug Interactions

Hexamethylene bisacetamide has shown experimental therapeutic synergism with cyclophosphamide (Bogden et al 1985) and 5-fluorouracil (Waxman et al 1990). The proposed mechanisms for the latter effect include (1) enhanced HMBA differentiating activity by 5-fluorouracil, itself a weak differentiator, and (2) inhibition of repair of 5-fluorouracil-induced DNA strand breaks by HMBA (Waxman et al 1990).

Sodium bicarbonate is currently recommended by some groups to alleviate HMBA-induced metabolic acidosis (Conley et al 1988). A bicarbonate solution is concurrently infused to maintain a urine pH of 7.0 or higher. Neurotoxicity induced by high HMBA levels has also been shown to be aggravated by the concomitant use of narcotic analgesics (Conley et al 1988). For this reason, the use of narcotic analgesics should be minimized in patients receiving HMBA.

■ Pharmacokinetics

Preclinical pharmacokinetic studies in dogs and rats showed that the half-life of HMBA is relatively short, about 2 hours. Also, a majority of drug was excreted renally (Chun et al 1986). High HMBA concentrations up to 4 mM were well tolerated. Importantly, the levels produced by parenteral administration were within the range of concentrations that produce differentiating effects on tumor cells in vitro (Marks et al 1978, Collins et al 1980, Fibach et al 1977). Similar concentrations can also inhibit human tumor colony formation in vitro (Chun et al 1986). The animal studies showed that tolerable oral doses of HMBA could produce drug levels of about 2 mM with up to 97.5% bioavailable.

The table below compares the pharmacokinetic parameters of two studies in which HMBA was administered to cancer patients as a continuous intravenous infusion for 5 days (Rowinsky et al 1986, Egorin et al 1987a). A monophasic pattern of elimination was noted in both studies. Urinary excretion of HMBA accounted for 34% of the dose as unchanged drug (Egorin et al 1987a, b). In another study 66 to 93% of the dose was excreted into the urine as HMBA and the 6-acetoamidohexanoic acid (6-AHA) metabolite (Rowinsky et al 1986). Total body clearance of HMBA was equal to $0.87 \times$ creatinine clearance + 59. The steady-state levels attained with HMBA were also roughly proportional to the dose: 0.45 mM after 9.6 g/m^2, 0.9 mM after 16 g/m^2, 1.3 mM after 24 g/m^2, and 2.03 mM after 33.6 mg/m^2 (Egorin et al 1987a, b).

Orally administered HMBA solution (given every 4 hours for 5 days via a nasogastric tube; see Special Applications) showed that HMBA absorption is rapid and complete (Chun et al 1988). Total body clearance of orally administered drug averaged 69 mL/min/m^2, and the percentages excreted in the urine were 42% for HMBA and 32% for the 6-AHA metabolite. This is quite similar to the pharmacokinetics of continuously infused drug.

The major metabolite of HMBA is 6-AHA and this accounts for about 13% of the dose excreted in the urine. It reaches a steady-state level in the plasma of 0.12 to 0.72 mM following HMBA doses of 4.8 and 43.2 g/m^2/d, respectively (Egorin et al 1987a, b); however, the ratio of 6-AHA to HMBA steady-state levels decreases with increasing HMBA doses.

The initial metabolite of HMBA, N-acetyl-1,6-diaminohexane (NADAH), achieves steady-state levels of 0.14 to 0.19 mM following HMBA infusions of 24 to 43.2 g/m^2/d (Egorin et al 1987a, b). The ratio of steady-state levels of HMBA to NADAH is only 0.18 to 0.31 over the dosing range 24 to 43.2 g/m^2. The cumulative total of both metabolites is still insufficient to account for the anion gap in patients experiencing metabolic acidosis following high-dose HMBA infusions. Other minor metabolites include 1,6-diaminohexane, 6-acetoamidohexanol, and 6-aminohexanoic acid (Egorin et al 1987b). In HL-60 promyelocytic leukemia cells in vitro, intracellular levels of these latter metabolites can actually exceed those of 6-AHA and NADAH (Egorin et al 1988). All of these HMBA metabolites have been identified in the urine (Callery et al 1986), and some appear to have differentiating activity (Snyder et al 1988). Indeed, NADAH appears to be two- to threefold more potent than HMBA at differentiating HL-60 cells. In contrast, the major metabolite, 6-AHA, fails to induce differentiation in vitro (Snyder et al 1988).

There appears to be a good correlation between the area under the plasma concentration × time curve (AUC) for HMBA and one of the major toxic effects, thrombocytopenia. This relationship is described by the equation (Egorin et al 1987b)

HUMAN PHARMACOKINETIC PARAMETERS OF HEXAMETHYLENE BISACETAMIDE

Dose Range* (g/m^2/d)	Half-life (h)	AUC (mM/L·min)	Volume of Distribution (L/m^2)	Systemic Clearance (mL/min/m^2)	Reference
9.6–33.6	2.4	2.035–13,872	1.1–30.2 (mean, 17)	57–121	Rowinsky et al 1986
4.8–43	2–5.7	26–24,300	—	87–150	Egorin et al 1987b

*Five-day continuous intravenous infusion.

$$\% \text{ decrease in platelets} = 100(1-e^{-0.000652(\text{AUC})})$$

or

$$\% \text{ decrease in platelets} = \frac{100(\text{AUC}^{1.55})}{(1033)^{1.55} + (\text{AUC})^{1.55}}$$

Other pharmacodynamic observations conclude that with concurrent urine alkalinization, the maximally tolerable steady-state plasma concentration of HMBA ranges between 1.5 and 2.0 mM (Conley et al 1990). Achievement of maximally tolerated exposures in most patients would require infusions for 6 to 8 days at plasma levels of 350 to 400 mg/L (Forrest et al 1988).

■ Side Effects and Toxicity

Preclinical toxicology studies in rats and dogs consistently identified the central nervous system as the primary target of HMBA toxicity (Chun et al 1986). This toxicity was characterized by convulsions, nervousness, agitation, and fine body tremors. In the dog, it was both dose dependent and reversible. Male rats additionally showed evidence of irreversible damage to reproductive organs.

In the initial phase I clinical trial of HMBA, dose-limiting toxic effects included renal insufficiency, hyperchloremic metabolic acidosis, and excitatory central nervous system toxicity (Rowinsky et al 1986). This manifested as agitation and delirium, which progressed to coma in a patient with concomitant renal insufficiency. Metabolic toxicity was noted by acute increases in serum creatinine, increases in serum chloride concentrations to 95 to 106 mEq/L, decreases in bicarbonate concentrations to 20 mEq/L or lower, and an anion gap of 13 to 17 (Rowinsky et al 1986). Central nervous system toxicity occurred concomitantly with the development of metabolic acidosis and renal insufficiency. It typically became severe on the fourth day of infusion with initial symptoms of delirium and combativeness; however, most electroencephalograms showed either no changes or only mild runs of nonspecific alpha slowing, diffuse delta activity, or theta wave slowing.

Hematologic suppression included infrequent leukopenia with a nadir of 2600/μL on day 15 and recovery by day 22. Thrombocytopenia was more prominent with nadirs of 50,000 to 90,000/μL on days 15 to 22 after dosing. Resolution was generally complete after 22 to 29 days. This toxic effect is dose related and has been correlated to the particular AUC achieved in a particular patient (Egorin et al 1987a) (see preceding section).

Other toxic effects include mild nausea and vomiting which peaked on days 3 to 5 of a 5-day infusion. Mild mucositis was also commonly noted near the end of the infusion period (Rowinsky et al 1987). Rarely observed toxic effects include elevations of liver enzymes, bilirubin, and alkaline phosphatase; malaise; and anorexia. Cutaneous herpes infections have been seen in about 20% of patients (Egorin et al 1987a). Vasculitis has also been described (Rowinsky et al 1987).

■ Special Applications

Hexamethylene bisacetamide has been administered through a nasogastric tube as a 5% (w/v) solution to determine the feasibility of long-term oral drug delivery (Chun et al 1988, Ward et al 1991). Doses of 12 to 30 g/m^2/d (same solution as the injectable) were administered every 4 hours for 5 days followed in 21 days by a 5-day continuous intravenous infusion. Neurotoxicity and nausea and vomiting were dose limiting at 30 g/m^2 per nasogastric tube. The drug was rapidly absorbed with nearly 100% oral bioavailability. Pharmacokinetic and metabolic patterns were comparable to those for the intravenous routes, and a plasma concentration of 1 mM was achieved with oral doses of 24 g/m^2/d. Other toxic effects included mucositis, renal toxicity, thrombocytopenia, hypocalcemia, and leukopenia. About 27 to 60% of the dose was excreted intact in the urine. On the basis of this study, oral HMBA doses of 24 to 30 g/m^2/d are tolerable and produce blood levels comparable to those produced by intravenous doses; however, a more palatable oral formulation will be needed for broad phase I–II trials.

REFERENCES

Bodgen AE, Cobb WR, Breitman TR, et al. HL-60/ascites tumors: A transplantable human tumor model for in vivo testing of differentiation inducers (DI's). *Proc Am Assoc Cancer Res*. 1985;**26**:34.

Callery PS, Egorin MJ, Geelhaar LA, Balachandran Nayar MS. Identification of metabolites of the cell-differentiating agent hexamethylene bisacetamide in humans. *Cancer Res*. 1986;**46**:4900–4903.

Chun HG, Leyland-Jones B, Hoth D, et al. Hexamethylene bisacetamide: A polar-planar compound entering clinical trials as a differentiating agent. *Cancer Treat Rep*. 1986;**70**(8):991–996.

Chun HG, Roth JS, Kelley JA, et al. Phase I bioavailability and pharmacokinetics or oral hexamethylene bisacetamide (HMBA; NSC-95580) (abstract #757). *Proc Am Assoc Cancer Res.* 1988;**29**:191.

Collins SJ, Bodner A, Ting R, et al. Induction of morphological and functional differentiation of human promyelocytic leukemia cells (HL-60) by compounds which induce differentiation of murine leukemia cells. *Int J Cancer.* 1980;**25**:213–218.

Conley BA, Forrest A, Egorin M, et al. Adaptive control phase I trial of hexamethylene bisacetamide (HMBA) with & without concurrent alkalinization (abstract #232). *Proc Am Soc Clin Oncol.* 1988;**7**:61.

Conley BA, Forrest A, Sinibaldi V, et al. Factors associated with the acute dose-limiting toxicities of hexamethylene bisacetamide (HMBA) (abstract #283). *Proc Am Soc Clin Oncol.* 1990;**9**:73.

Egorin MJ, Sigman LM, Van Echo DA, et al. Phase I clinical and pharmacokinetic study of hexamethylene bisacetamide (NSC-95580) administered as a five-day continuous infusion. *Cancer Res.* 1987a;**47**:617–623.

Egorin MJ, Snyder SW, Cohen AS, et al. Metabolism of hexamethylene bisacetamide and its metabolites in leukemic cells. *Cancer Res.* 1988;**48**:1712–1716.

Egorin MJ, Zuhowski EG, Cohen AS, et al. Plasma pharmacokinetics and urinary excretion of hexamethylene bisacetamide metabolites. *Cancer Res.* 1987b;**47**:6142–6146.

Ferrero D, Tarella C, Gallo E, et al. Terminal differentiation of the human promyelocytic leukemia cell line, HL-60, in the absence of cell proliferation. *Cancer Res.* 1982;**42**:4421–4422.

Fibach E, Reuben RD, Rifkind RA, et al. Effect of hexamethylene bisacetamide on the commitment to differentiation of murine erythroleukemia cells. *Cancer Res.* 1977;**37**:440–444.

Forrest A, Conley BA, Egorin MJ, et al. Adaptive control of hexamethylene bisacetamide (HMBA) pharmacodynamics (abstract 230). *Proc Am Soc Clin Oncol.* 1988;**7**:61.

Friedman EA, Schildkraut CL. Lengthening of the GI phase is not strictly correlated with differentiation in Friend erythroleukemia cells. *Proc Natl Acad Sci USA.* 1978;**75**:3813–3817.

Lever JE. Inducers of mammalian cell differentiation stimulate dome formation in a differentiated kidney epithelial cell line (MDCK). *Proc Natl Acad Sci USA.* 1979;**76**:1323–1327.

Levy J, Terada M, Rifkind RA, et al. Induction of erythroid differentiation by dimethylsulfoxide in cells infected with Friend virus: Relationship to the cell cycle. *Proc Natl Acad Sci USA.* 1975;**72**:28–32.

Marks PA, Reuben R, Epner E, et al. Induction of murine erythroleukemia cells to differentiate: A model for the detection of new anti-tumor drugs. *Antibiot Chemother.* 1978;**23**:33–41.

Marks PA, Rifkind RA. Erythroleukemic differentiation. *Annu Rev Biochem.* 1978;**47**:419–448.

Matsuo T, Imamura T, Fujita K, et al. Differentiation of murine erythroleukemia mice analogues. *Acta Haematol Jpn.* 1984;**47**:926–937.

National Cancer Institute, Pharmaceutical Resources Branch, Division of Cancer Treatment. *5% HMBA in Sterile Water for Injection. NSC-95580.* Washington, DC: U.S. Government Printing Office; 1977:43–44.

Palfrey C, Kimhi Y, Littauer UZ, et al. Induction of differentiation in mouse neuroblastoma cells by hexamethylene bisacetamide. *Biochem Biophys Res Commun.* 1977;**76**:937–942.

Profou-Juchelka HR, Reuben RC, Marks PA, et al. Transcriptional and post-transcriptional regulation of globin gene accumulation in induced murine erythroleukemia cells. *Mol Cell Biochem.* 1983;**3**:229–232.

Rabson AS, Stern R, Tralka TS, et al. Hemamethylene bisacetamide induces morphologic changes and increased synthesis of procollagen in cell lines from glioblastoma multiforme. *Proc Natl Acad Sci USA.* 1977;**74**:5060–5064.

Reuben RC. Studies on the mechanism of action of hexamethylene bisacetamide, a potent inducer of erythroleukemic differentiation. *Biochim Biophys Acta.* 1979;**588**:310–321.

Reuben RC, Khanna PL, Gazitt Y, et al. Inducers of erythroleukemic differentiation: Relationship of structure to activity among planar-polar compounds. *J Biol Chem.* 1978;**253**:4214–4218.

Reuben RC, Rifkind RA, Marks PA. Chemically induced murine erythroleukemic differentiation. *Biochim Biophys Acta.* 1980;**605**:325–346.

Reuben RC, Wife RL, Breslow R, et al. A new group of potent inducers of differentiation in murine erythroleukemia cells. *Proc Natl Acad Sci USA.* 1976;**73**:862–866.

Rowinsky EK, Conley BA, Jones RJ, et al. Efficacy of hexamethylene bisacetamide (HMBA) in myelodysplastic syndromes (MDS): 5-day exposure to maximal levels (abstract #1132). *Proc Am Assoc Cancer Res.* 1990;**31**:190.

Rowinsky EK, Ettinger DS, Grochow LB, et al. Phase I and pharmacologic study of hexamethylene bisacetamide in patients with advanced cancer. *J Clin Oncol.* 1986;**4**(12):1835–1844.

Rowinsky EK, Ettinger DS, McGuire WP, et al. Prolonged infusion of hexamethylene bisacetamide: A phase I and pharmacologic study. *Cancer Res.* 1987;**47**:5788–5795.

Sheffery M, Rifkind RA, Marks PA. Hexamethylene-bisacetamide-resistant murine erythroleukemia cells have altered patterns of inducer-mediated chromatin changes. *Proc Natl Acad Sci USA.* 1983;**80**:3349–3353.

Snyder SW, Egorin MJ, Geelhaar LA, et al. Induction of differentiation of human promyelocytic leukemia cells (HL60) by metabolites of hexamethylene bisacetamide. *Cancer Res.* 1988;**48**:3613–3616.

Tanaka M, Levy J, Terada M, et al. Induction of erythroid differentiation in murine cells by highly polar compounds. *Proc Natl Acad Sci USA.* 1971;**68**:378–382.

Terada M, Fried J, Nudel U, et al. Transient inhibition of initiation of S-phase associated with dimethyl sulfoxide induction of murine erythroleukemia cells to erythroid differentiation. *Proc Natl Acad Sci USA.* 1977;**74**:248–252.

Ward FT, Lelley JA, Roth JS, et al. A phase I bioavailability and pharmacokinetic study of hexamethylene bisacetamide (NSC 95580) administered via nasogastric tube. *Cancer Res.* 1991;**51**:1803–1810.

Waxman S, Wang S, Tan I, Scher W. Combination cytotoxic-differentiation therapy with 5-fluorouracil, leucovorin and hexamethylene bisacetamide (abstract #2551). *Proc Am Assoc Cancer Res.* 1990;**31**:430.

Young CW, Fanucchi MP, Walsh TD, et al. Phase I trials and clinical pharmacologic evaluation of hexamethylene bisacetamide administered by ten-day continuous intravenous infusion at twenty-eight day intervals. *Cancer Res.* 1988;**48**:7304–7309.

Homoharringtonine

■ Other Names

NSC-141633

■ Chemistry

Structure of homoharringtonine

Homoharringtonine (HHT) is an alkaloidal natural product isolated from the needles and bark of the Chinese evergreen, *Cephalotoxus fortueni* (Powell et al 1970, 1972). The complete chemical name is cephalotaxine, 4-methyl-2-hydroxy-2-(4-hydroxy-4-methylpentyl) butanediocate ester. It has the molecular formula $C_{29}H_{39}N_1O_9$ and the formula weight of 545.6.

■ Antitumor Activity

Homoharringtonine has a long history of clinical use in acute leukemia in China (Chinese Liberation Army 187th Hospital 1977, Huang and Xue 1984). In preclinical models, the drug is active against L-1210 and P-388 leukemia and colon-38 and CD8F mammary carcinoma (O'Dwyer et al 1986). In human tumor colony-forming assays, HHT demonstrated significant antitumor activity in ovarian cancer, endometrial cancer, sarcoma, and breast cancer. In these continuous drug exposure studies, HHT was more potent than the congener, harringtonine (Jiang et al 1983). Activity for HHT has also been observed in a variety of human tumors studied in the murine subrenal capsule assay (Cobb et al 1983). Lymphomas and leukemias were most sensitive, and in HL-60 promyelocytic leukemia, the drug may act as a differentiating agent (Boyd and Sullivan 1984).

In an initial Chinese trial of a mixture of alkaloids (harringtonine:homoharringtonine 1:3 or 2:1) objective complete responses were noted in 5 of 35 (14%) patients with acute nonlymphocytic leukemia (ANLL). A careful retrospective review of other subsequent Chinese trials of *Cephalotoxus* alkaloid mixtures in ANLL patients reported an overall complete response rate of 24% (95% confidence interval of 19–29%) (Grem et al 1988). In patients with chronic myelogenous leukemia (CML) a 37% hematologic complete response rate was described (95% confidence interval of 25–49%). The duration of complete responses was short in ANLL (1–7 months), whereas more durable responses of 6 to 20 months were obtained in CML (Grem et al 1988).

Response rates in leukemia trials in the United States have been lower than those in China and are dependent on the dose and schedule as well as on prior therapy. With daily dosing for 7 to 9 days, complete response rates in ANLL ranged from 25% (Warrell et al 1985) to 16% (Arlin et al 1985, 1987); however, a number of trials have reported only rare responses in ANLL patients (Kantarjian et al 1989, Tan et al 1987, Ekert and Richards 1980, Ekert et al 1982). Response rates in ANLL are not much higher in trials combining HHT with etoposide (5% complete responses) (Warrell and Berman 1986), with amsacrine (15% complete responses) (Haines et al 1987), or with cytarabine (Grem et al 1988). Homoharringtonine alone does not appear to be effective in patients with refractory acute myelogenous leukemia (Kantarjian et al 1989). The drug has also been used in the treatment of polycythemia vera in China in patients refractory to busulfan or cyclophosphamide (Lu et al 1983). In heavily pretreated patients, however, HHT is inactive in solid tumors such as ovarian cancer (Kavanaugh et al

1984) and in malignant melanoma, sarcoma, head and neck cancer, breast cancer, and colorectal cancer (Ajani et al 1986).

■ Mechanism of Action

Homoharringtonine and other *Cephalotoxus* alkaloids inhibit protein synthesis after the initiation step. On a subcellular level there is a delay in HHT-induced inhibition of protein synthesis. This is noted by degradation of polyribosomes and release of recently synthesized protein chains (Huang 1975). The most likely biochemical sites of action for HHT are the early steps in chain elongation involving aminoacyl-tRNA binding and peptide bond formation (Fresno et al 1977).

In L-1210 cancer cells in vitro, HHT cytotoxicity correlates well with both the degree of protein synthesis inhibition and the amount of radiolabeled drug retained by the cells (Chou et al 1983). DNA synthesis and, to a lesser degree, RNA synthesis were also inhibited after near-complete cessation of protein synthesis. The cell-killing activity of HHT is cell cycle specific, with maximal cytotoxicity expressed in the G_1 and G_2 phases (Baaske and Heinstein 1977). This correlates well with enhanced cytotoxic activity in more rapidly growing leukemia cells which are also more sensitive to prolonged drug exposures in vitro (Takemura et al 1985).

Resistance to HHT is seen in cell lines developed for resistance to other natural products such as doxorubicin and vincristine (Chou et al 1983). Drug retention is commensurately decreased in HHT-resistant cells, suggesting involvement of the P-glycoprotein-mediated form of multidrug resistance.

■ Availability and Storage

Homoharringtonine is investigationally available from the National Cancer Institute as a 10-mg vial of lyophilized powder. Mannitol (50 mg) and hydrochloric acid are added during final formulation (National Cancer Institute 1987). The intact vials are stored frozen (−10 to −20°C).

■ Preparation for Use, Stability, and Admixture

The 10-mg vial of HHT is reconstituted with 4.9 mL of 0.9% Sodium Chloride for Injection, USP. This yields a final solution of pH 3 to 5 containing 2 mg/mL HHT as the hydrochloride salt. This solution is stable for 96 hours at room temperature and room light conditions. Further dilution in 5% Dextrose for Injection, USP, or saline (to concentrations of 0.01 to 0.05 mg/mL) are also stable for 96 hours.

■ Administration

In leukemia studies performed in China, the drug has most often been administered as a brief intravenous infusion over 4 to 6 hours. Similar brief infusions over 10 to 360 minutes were used in the initial U.S. trials (O'Dwyer et al 1986). To counter acute cardiovascular toxicity (hypotension and tachycardia) and, theoretically, to enhance cytotoxicity, HHT has been given by continuous intravenous infusion over 5 to 30 days (O'Dwyer et al 1986).

■ Dosage

The recommended phase II doses from U.S. continuous intravenous infusion trials are 3.5 mg/m^2/d on day 1 with 6 mg/m^2 on days 2 to 8 for a total of 45.5 mg/m^2 (Stewart et al 1988). Other schedules include 4 mg/m^2/d for 10 days (Coonley et al 1983) and 1 mg/m^2/d for 30 days (Neidhart et al 1986). In acute leukemia, a regimen of 5 mg/m^2/d × 9 days was found to be the maximal dose (Warrell et al 1985). Of note, lowering the HHT dose to 3.5 mg/m^2/d for 9 to 12 days (in combination with other myelosuppressive agents) resulted in an apparent loss of HHT antileukemic activity. Similarly, a dose of 2.5 to 3.0 mg/m^2/d for 15 days was ineffective in acute myelogenous leukemia (Kantarjian et al 1989). In the Chinese trials, typical dosing regimens involved 2 to 4 mg/d for 9 to 50 days given intravenously over 15 minutes or intramuscularly in adults (Grem et al 1988). In pediatric patients, 0.15 mg/d was given by the same schedule. An alternate schedule involved a dose of 0.05 to 0.5 mg/kg for 5 to 10 days by slow infusions.

■ Drug Interactions

Homoharringtonine is not synergistic against human myeloid leukemia cells when combined with doxorubicin, cytarabine, dexamethasone, 5-fluorouracil, or methotrexate (Okano et al 1983). Indeed, the drug was antagonistic in this model when combined singly or with two other drugs known to block protein synthesis, specifically acivicin and L-asparaginase. In contrast, HHT and 5-fluorouracil were synergistic in mice bearing a cytarabine-resistant subline of P-388 leukemia (Laster et al 1982). The combination of etoposide and HHT were nonsynergistic in mice bearing standard P-388 leukemia cells (O'Dwyer et al 1986).

Pharmacokinetics

The clinical pharmacokinetics of HHT has been studied in patients given 3 to 4 mg/m² tritiated HHT by continuous 6-hour intravenous infusion (Savaraj et al 1986). The parent HHT molecule was cleared from the plasma in a biphasic manner with half-lives of 0.5 and 9.3 hours. Total clearance was 177 mL/h/kg and the apparent volume of distribution was 2.4 L/kg. The clearance of total radioactivity (parent drug plus metabolites) was 5.5 times slower than with HHT (terminal half-life of total radioactivity of 67 hours); however, the volume of distribution for total radioactivity was similar at 2.7 L/kg. Total (cumulative) urinary excretion of radiolabeled drug amounted to 28% of the dose, but only one third of this amount was excreted as unchanged HHT. Thus, urinary excretion is a relatively minor route of HHT elimination, accounting for only 11% of a dose. Therefore, hepatic metabolism probably represents the major route of HHT elimination. At least two known HHT metabolites are observed in the plasma. One major metabolite peaks in concentration 2 to 6 hours after HHT administration and has an average half-life of 84 hours.

In dogs, biliary HHT excretion accounts for 14% of a dose, only 2% as unchanged HHT (Lu et al 1988). At autopsy (5 hours after HHT dosing) the drug was found to be widely distributed: 7.4% in liver, 2.5% in small intestine, 1% in stomach, 0.8% each in pancreas and kidneys, and 0.7% in lungs. A high uptake into cerebrospinal fluid (40% of the plasma concentration) is also noted 4 hours after drug administration in dogs. Drug penetration into human brain tumors is also documented (Savaraj et al 1985).

Side Effects and Toxicity

In the early trials of brief HHT infusions, delayed hypotension and reflex tachycardia were the dose-limiting and dose-dependent toxic effects of the drug (Neidhart et al 1983, O'Dwyer et al 1986, Zhang et al 1979). These effects were most prominent at doses above 3 mg/m² and appeared 4 hours after drug administration. Occasionally, fatal tachyarrhythmias and cardiovascular collapse occurred after a brief intravenous infusion, even in the face of emergency treatment with fluids and pressors. Peripheral vasodilation by HHT binding to calcium channel receptor sites has been suggested as an explanation for the HHT-induced hypotension and reflex stimulation of cardiac output to 30 to 80% over resting values. When HHT continuous infusions are used, myelosuppression becomes dose limiting. Myelosuppression has occasionally been prolonged in patients receiving prolonged infusions for leukemia therapy.

Nonmyelosuppressive toxicities include gastrointestinal effects such as nausea, vomiting, mucositis, diarrhea, and hepatic toxicity (Tan et al 1987). Most of these effects are mild and transient. Skin lesions are also seen in a number of patients. These involve alopecia and erythema on the abdomen, groin, and extremities during HHT infusions. A generalized maculopapular rash with peeling generally follows and then slowly resolves. Diffuse myalgic pain is also noted during HHT infusions. This often requires treatment with pain medications. Transient elevations of liver enzymes are observed, most often involving serum glutamic–oxalacetic transaminase (SGOT) and bilirubin. Preexisting elevations in SGOT and bilirubin have also been implicated as possible predisposing factors for HHT-induced hypotension.

Rare toxic effects with prolonged HHT infusions include an elevation in serum creatinine and hyperglycemia. The latter phenomenon has been associated with doses greater than 5 mg/m² in adult patient populations. The hyperglycemia has also been associated with increased plasma insulin levels which is consistent with HHT-induced insulin resistance (Sylvester et al 1989). This may persist several weeks after discontinuing the drug and is no doubt more profound in patients with preexisting diabetes. Insulin may thus be required in about 60% of cases.

Special Applications

In Chinese patients with central nervous system leukemia, HHT has been administered intrathecally (Hou and Zhang 1981). For this experimental application, the drug was diluted into 4 to 5 mL of normal saline and injected intrathecally over 2 to 3 minutes, every 5 to 7 days, until the leukemia cells were cleared. It was then given intrathecally every 2 weeks. Toxic effects included fever, headache, nausea, and vomiting within 2 to 5 hours of treatment (Grem et al 1988). Cytoreductive responses were noted in the cerebrospinal fluid of 12 of 18 (66%) patients with acute nonlymphocytic leukemia and in 5 of 8 (63%) of patients with chronic myelogenous leukemia.

REFERENCES

Ajani JA, Dimery I, Chawla SP, et al. Phase II trial of homoharringtonine in patients with advanced malignant melanoma; sarcoma; and head and neck, breast, and colorectal carcinomas. *Cancer Treat Rep.* 1986;**70**:375–379.

Arlin Z, Feldman E, Biguzzi S. Phase I/II trial of homoharringtonine in acute leukemia. *Proc Am Soc Clin Oncol.* 1987;**6**:160.

Arlin Z, Gaddipati J, Mittelman A, et al. Phase I–II trial of homoharringtonine (HHT) in acute myelogenous leukemia (AML). *Proc Am Soc Clin Oncol.* 1985;**4**:173.

Baaske DM, Heinstein P. Cytotoxicity and cell cycle specificity of homoharringtonine. *Antimicrob Agents Chemother.* 1977;**12**:298–300.

Boyd AW, Sullivan JR. Leukemic cell differentiation in vivo and in vitro: Arrest of proliferation parallels the differentiation induced by the antileukemic drug harringtonine. *Blood.* 1984;**63**:384–392.

Chinese Liberation Army 187th Hospital, Leukemia Research Section. The therapeutic effectiveness study of 99 leukemic patients treated with four alkaloids of *Cephalotoxus fortunei*. In: Hook F. *Chin Herbal Med Rep.* 1977;**5**:12,25–29.

Chou T-C, Schmid FA, Feinberg A, et al. Uptake, initial effects, and chemotherapeutic efficacy of harringtonine in murine leukemic cells sensitive and resistant to vincristine and other chemotherapeutic agents. *Cancer Res.* 1983;**43**:3074–3079.

Cobb WR, Bogden AE, Reich SD, et al. Activity of two phase I drugs, homoharringtonine and tricyclic nucleotide, against surgical explants of human tumors in the 6-day subrenal capsule assay. *Cancer Treat Rep.* 1983;**67**:173–178.

Coonley CJ, Warrell RP Jr, Young CW. Phase I trial of homoharringtonine administered as a 5-day continuous infusion. *Cancer Treat Rep.* 1983;**67**:693–696.

Ekert H, Richards M. Experience with homoharringtonine in one patient with acute myeloid leukemia. *Proc Clin Oncol Soc Aust.* 1980;**8**:152.

Ekert H, Sullivan J, Waters K. Treatment of acute myeloid leukemia with harringtonine. *Proc Clin Oncol Soc Aust.* 1982;**9**:122.

Fresno M, Jimenez A, Vasquez D. Inhibition of translation in eukaryotic systems by harringtonine. *Eur J Biochem.* 1977;**72**:323–330.

Grem JL, Cheson BD, King SA, et al. Cephalotaxine esters: Antileukemic advance or therapeutic failure? *J Natl Cancer Inst.* 1988;**80**:1095–1103.

Haines IE, Lowethal DA, Warrel RP. Homoharringtonine and amsacrine in pretreated patients with acute non-lyphoblastic leukemia. *Proc Am Soc Clin Oncol.* 1987;**6**:163.

Hou C-H, Zhang Z-Y. Chinese Peoples Liberation Army 187th Hospital: Intrathecal injection of harringtonine and homoharringtonine in treating central nervous system leukemia—Clinical analysis in 26 cases. *J Chin Acad.* 1981;**61**:530–532.

Huang L, Xue Z. Cephalotaxus alkaloids. In: Broosi A, ed. *The Alkaloids.* Orlando FL: Academic Press; 1984;**23**:157–226.

Huang M-T. Harringtonine, an inhibitor of initiation of protein biosynthesis. *Mol Pharmacol.* 1975;**11**:511–519.

Jiang TL, Liu RH, Salmon SE. Comparative in vitro antitumor activity of homoharringtonine and harringtonine against clonogenic human tumor cells. *Invest New Drugs.* 1983;**1**:21–25.

Kantarjian HM, Keating MJ, Walters RS, et al. Phase II study of low-dose continuous infusion homoharringtonine in refractory acute myelogenous leukemia. *Cancer.* 1989;**63**:813–817.

Kavanagh JJ, Gershenson DM, Copeland LJ, et al. Intermittent IV homoharringtonine for the treatment of refractory epithelial carcinoma of the ovary: A phase II trial. *Cancer Treat Rep.* 1984;**68**:1503–1504.

Laster WR, Trader MW, Schabel FM Jr, et al. Therapeutic synergism of homoharringtonine plus 5-fluorouracil against leukemia P388 (P388/0) and Ara-C resistant P388 (P388/Ara-C). *Proc Am Assoc Cancer Res.* 1982;**23**:199.

Lu K, Savaraj N, Feun LG, et al. Pharmacokinetics of homoharringtonine in dogs. *Cancer Chemother Pharmacol.* 1988;**21**:139–142.

Lu L-H, Lin S-P, Liang Y-Y, et al. Harringtonine in treatment of polycythemia vera. *Chin Med J.* 1983;**96**:533–535.

National Cancer Institute. *NCI Investigational Drugs: Homoharringtonine. NSC-141633.* Washington, DC: U.S. Department of Health and Human Services; 1987:75–76.

Neidhart JA, Young DC, Derocher D, et al. Phase I trial of homoharringtonine. *Cancer Treat Rep.* 1983;**67**:801–804.

Neidhart JA, Young DC, Kraut E, et al. Phase I trial of homoharringtonine administered by prolonged continuous infusion. *Cancer Res.* 1986;**46**:967–969.

O'Dwyer PJ, King SA, Hoth DF, et al. Homoharringtonine—Perspectives on an active new natural product. *J Clin Oncol.* 1986;**4**:1563–1568.

Okano T, Ohnuma T, Holland JF, et al. Effects of harringtonine in combination with acivicin, Adriamycin, L-asparaginase, cytosine arabinoside, dexamethasone, fluorouracil or methotrexate on human acute myelogenous leukemia cell line KG-1. *Invest New Drugs.* 1983;**1**:145–150.

Powell RG, Weisleder D, Smith CR Jr. Antitumor alkaloids from *Cephalotaxus harringtonia*: Structure and activity. *J Pharm Sci.* 1972;**61**:1227–1230.

Powell RG, Weisleder D, Smith CR Jr, et al. Structures of harringtonine, isoharringtonine, and homoharringtonine. *Tetrahedron Lett.* 1970;**11**:815–818.

Savaraj N, Lu K, Dimery I, et al. Clinical pharmacology of homoharringtonine. *Cancer Treat Rep.* 1986;**70**:1403–1407.

Savaraj N, Lu K, Feun LG, et al. Central nervous system (CNS) penetration of homoharringtonine (HHT). *Proc Am Soc Clin Oncol.* 1985;**4**:50.

Stewart JA, Cassileth PA, Bennett JM, O'Connell MJ. Continuous infusion homoharringtonine (NSC-141633) in refractory acute nonlymphocytic leukemia. *Am J Clin Oncol.* 1988;**11**:627–629.

Sylvester RK, Lobell M, Ogden W, Stewart JA. Homoharringtonine-induced hyperglycemia. *J Clin Oncol.* 1989;**7**:392–395.

Takemura Y, Ohnuma T, Chou T-C, et al. Biologic and pharmacologic effects of harringtonine on human leukemia–lymphoma cells. *Cancer Chemother Pharmacol.* 1985;**14**:206–210.

Tan CTC, Luks E, Bacha DM, et al. Phase I trial of homoharringtonine in children with refractory leukemia. *Cancer Treat Rep.* 1987;**71**:1245–1248.

Warrell RP Jr, Berman E. Etoposide (VP-16) does not increase remission induction with homoharringtonine (HHT) in patients with acute nonlymphoblastic leukemia (ANLL). *Proc Am Assoc Cancer Res.* 1986;**27**:192.

Warrell RP Jr, Coonley CJ, Gee TS. Homoharringtonine: An effective new drug for remission induction in refractory nonlymphoblastic leukemia. *J Clin Oncol.* 1985;**3**:617–621.

Zhang Y-JY, Hui L, Zheng X-Y, et al. Toxicity of harringtonine and homoharringtonine. *Acta Pharm Sin.* 1979;**14**:135–140.

Hydrazine Sulfate

■ Other Names

NSC-150014; CAS Registry No. 10034-93-2.

■ Chemistry

The empiric formula is $H_6N_2O_4S$, the chemical formula $H_2NNH_2 \cdot H_2SO_4$, and the molecular weight 130.12. It is freely soluble in hot water and in 33 parts of water at room temperature. It is insoluble in alcohol, and a 0.2 M solution has a pH of 1.3.

■ Antitumor Activity

Hydrazine sulfate has had a long and controversial history as an anticancer agent and is currently under study as a metabolic inhibitor of cancer-associated cachexia (Chlebowski et al 1987). Hydrazine sulfate has shown experimental antitumor activity in a variety of animal tumor systems. These include Walker 256 intramuscular carcinosarcoma, B-16 melanoma, L-1210 leukemia, and Murphy–Sturm lymphosarcoma (Gold 1973); however, other researchers could not demonstrate any activity for hydrazine in some of the same animal tumor models including sarcoma 180, meth A sarcoma, B-16 melanoma, and Ridgway osteogenic sarcoma (Ochoa et al 1975). When hydrazine sulfate was combined with vitamin K_3 (menadione), antitumor synergy was noted in experimental tumors in vivo (Gold 1986b). In patients with advanced malignancies, however, little objective antitumor activity has been produced with this agent despite a promising pilot study by Gold (1974). For example, there were no objective responses in 29 patients treated at Memorial-Sloan Kettering (Ochoa et al 1975). The majority of tumors in this trial were adenocarcinomas (ovary 5, colon 4, breast 3, lung and pancreas 2 each). Other diagnoses included tumors of the cervix, larynx, bladder, esophagus, kidney, mesothelioma (all 1 each), and melanoma (3). Appetite improvement was described in four patients, and one patient had significant relief of bone pain from prostate cancer. In another U.S. trial from the Pennsylvania Hospital, no objective responses were seen in 25 patients with a variety of solid tumors (Lerner and Regelson 1976). Indeed, all of the 25 patients had disease progression on hydrazine sulfate therapy. In 4 patients, weight loss was halted, whereas a slow weight loss continued unabated in the remaining 21 patients (Lerner and Regelson 1976). In a large clinical trial in the Soviet Union, hydrazine sulfate produced partial responses in 3 of 95 evaluable patients (lung cancer, Hodgkin's disease, and a recurrent desmoid tumor of the anterior abdominal wall) (Gershanovich et al 1976). Disease stabilization was noted in 20 of 95 (21%) patients in this trial. There were also positive subjective responses in half of the patients. These effects included a slight euphoria, "improved stamina" and appetite, and reduced pain (Gershanovich et al 1976).

A single response has been reported in a patient with giant cell tumor metastatic to the lung (Gold 1987). In patients with non-small cell lung cancer, the addition of hydrazine increased survival by about 100 days over the same "PVB" combination regimen used alone (cisplatin, vinblastine, and bleomycin) (Chlebowski et al 1987). The overall response frequency was not, however, increased by hydrazine and survival advantages were noted only in patients with good performance status.

These results suggested that the beneficial effect of hydrazine on survival was not mediated by direct antitumor activity and might instead be a result of improved metabolic or nutritional indices in responding patients. A subsequent metabolic study in lung cancer patients preliminarily confirmed this hypothesis: patients receiving hydralazine had improved glucose turnover and tolerance and reduced turnover of protein (Chlebowski et al 1989). Another study in patients with solid tumors showed that hydrazine sulfate increased calorie intake in 58% of the population. This was associated with significant weight gain, especially in patients with lung cancer (Chlebowski et al 1985). Thus, overall, hydrazine appears to lack efficacy as an antitumor agent, but may be useful as a nutritional adjunct to prevent cachexia in patients with advanced solid tumors, especially those with non-small cell lung cancer.

■ Mechanism of Action

The precise mechanism of action for hydrazine sulfate is not known. It is proposed to inhibit the breakdown of proteins to form glucose (gluconeogenesis) (Gold 1968). One postulate was that hydrazine blocked gluconeogenesis by inhibiting phosphoenolpyruvate carboxykinase (Gold 1968).

In animals, hydrazine has been shown to induce liver and muscle glycogenolysis (Taylor 1966) and hyperglycemia (Underhill 1911); however, if the animals are fasted to deplete liver glycogen stores, hydrazine then induces a prompt hypoglycemia (Fortney et al 1967). Later studies in rats conclusively showed that hydrazine inhibited gluconeogenesis in liver and renal tissues. It also simultaneously caused hypoglycemia and elevations in serum lactate and pyruvate levels. These effects are compatible with a metabolic blockade of the conversion of oxalacetate to phosphoenolpyruvate (Ray et al 1970). This inhibition of phosphoenolpyruvate carboxykinase is noncompetitive with respect to oxalacetate (Ray et al 1970).

Metabolic studies in human cancer patients have shown that oral hydrazine therapy for 1 month can correct abnormal glucose tolerance characterized by prolonged glucose elevation after challenge. Hydrazine also decreased a heightened rate of glucose production in these patients (Chlebowski et al 1984). There were no significant endocrine alterations in these patients (including levels of the hormones insulin, glucagon, and cortisol). An improvement in body weight was noted in 7 of 9 patients whose oral glucose tolerance improved on hydrazine therapy. In contrast, there was no weight gain in four patients whose oral glucose tolerance did not improve on hydralazine. These results suggest that an inhibition of gluconeogenesis is related to the drug's positive effect on body weight in cachectic patients with advanced cancers.

Conversely, there is no information on possible direct antitumor mechanisms of action for hydrazine, although this class of drugs is known to form reactive DNA-degrading binding intermediates following oxidative metabolism in some experimental systems (Gutterman et al 1969). The lack of an alkyl side group(s) on hydrazine sulfate may obviate this possible mechanism.

■ Availability and Storage

Hydrazine sulfate was originally provided for investigation as a nonsterile powder (Eastman Kodak Company, others) which was then transferred to gelatin capsules (Ochoa et al 1975). The drug was subsequently formulated into 60-mg capsules for investigational trials (Calbiochem, San Diego, California) (Lerner and Regelson 1976).

■ Administration

Hydrazine sulfate capsules are taken orally, usually 0.5 to 2 hours prior to meals (Gershanovich et al 1976, Ochoa et al 1975).

■ Dosage

A controlled dose-finding phase I trial of hydrazine sulfate (used for any indication) has not been performed. Thus, most of the dosing recommendations are based on poorly detailed anecdotes (Gold 1974) or fixed dosing schedules of 60 mg three times daily, not adjusted for weight or body surface area (Lerner and Regelson 1976, Chlebowski et al 1982, 1985, 1989, Gershanovich et al 1976). This schedule (total dose of 180 mg per day) appears to be well tolerated in patients with advanced cancer. One other tolerable schedule involved an initial dose of 35 $mg/m^2/d \times 4$, then twice daily on days 5 to 8 (Ochoa et al 1975). Usually, dosing is continued daily without interruption unless significant toxicity occurs. In one study, when side effects were observed, the daily dose was reduced to 120 mg (60-mg capsule twice daily).

■ Drug Interactions

Several studies from one laboratory have reported antitumor potentiation or synergy for the combination of vitamin K_3 (menadione) and hydrazine sulfate and for this combination plus several other cytotoxic chemotherapeutic agents (Gold 1987, 1988). In rats bearing Walker 256 carcinosarcoma, hydrazine or menadione enhanced the antitumor activity of etoposide (Gold, 1988). Vitamin K_2 (menadiol sodium diphosphonate) also enhanced the antitumor activity of hydrazine sulfate and the folic acid antagonist methotrexate (Gold, 1986). In this regard, vitamin K_2 was superior to its K_3 (menadione) analog as a result of lower host toxicity.

In adrenalectomized rats, hydrocortisone can further increase the accumulation of malate and citrate following hydrazine therapy. Conversely, glucose suppresses this accumulation, thereby confirming a role for hydrazine in modulating gluconeogenesis (Ray et al 1970).

■ Pharmacokinetics

The pharmacokinetic properties of hydrazine sulfate have not been studied.

■ Side Effects and Toxicity

The major side effects of hydrazine sulfate are gastrointestinal and neurologic in nature. Gastrointestinal toxic effects occur in about 15 to 20% of patients (Gershanovich et al 1976). They are typically mild, mostly nausea with rare vomiting and anorexia (Ochoa et al 1975). Diarrhea and hunger have been reported in a few patients. The time of onset ranges from 3 to 30 days, and these effects do not impair food intake. Gastrointestinal toxic effects typically subside within 24 hours of stopping hydrazine therapy (Ochoa et al 1975).

Neurologic toxicity from hydrazine sulfate is much more common and includes a wide array of symptoms. Paresthesias can occur in a third of patients and affect both upper and lower extremities (Ochoa et al 1975). These may persist for months after the drug is discontinued and often affect fine motor functions such as writing. Central nervous system toxic effects are also reported. These effects usually resolve within 1 week of drug discontinuance. Symptoms include dizziness, confusion, lethargy, and somnolence. Blurred vision, slurred speech, vertigo, and a palpebral tic have also been described (Ochoa et al 1975).

The most common abnormal laboratory finding (about 70% of patients receiving hydrazine) has been hypoglycemia, which becomes prominent within 10 days of starting therapy. In most affected patients, fasting hypoglycemia is mild (fasting blood glucose of 80–89 mg/dL); however, some patients may experience more profound hypoglycemia with fasting blood glucose below 69 mg/dL and, rarely, below 50 mg/dL (Ochoa et al 1975). This resolves rapidly on drug discontinuance. Other abnormal laboratory findings include transient elevations in serum alkaline phosphatase in 8 of 25 patients (32%) and elevations in serum bilirubin, serum glutamic-oxalacetic transaminase, or lactate dehydrogenase levels in 2 of 25 patients (8%) (Ochoa et al 1975).

Rare hydrazine toxic effects include pruritus, auditory hallucination, diaphoresis, and headache.

REFERENCES

Chlebowski RT, Bulcavage L, Grosvenor M, et al. Influence of hydrazine sulfate on survival in non-small cell lung cancer: A randomized, placebo-controlled trial (abstract 688). *Proc Am Soc Clin Oncol.* 1987;**6**:175.

Chlebowski RT, Bulcavage L, Tayek J, et al. Metabolic "response frequency" associated with hydrazine sulfate (HS) vs placebo use in patients with advanced non-small cell lung cancer (NSCLC) (abstract 49). *Proc Am Assoc Cancer Res.* 1989;**30**:13.

Chlebowski RT, Grosvenor M, Scrooc M, et al. Influence of hydrazine sulfate on food intake and weight maintenance in patients with cancer (abstract C-1029). *Proc Am Soc Clin Oncol.* 1985;**4**:265.

Chlebowski RT, Heber D, Richardson B. Influence of hydrazine sulfate (HS) on carbohydrate metabolism in cancer cachexia: A randomized, placebo controlled trial. *Proc Am Soc Clin Oncol.* 1982;**1**:59.

Chlebowski RT, Heber D, Richardson B, Block JB. Influence of hydrazine sulfate on abnormal carbohydrate metabolism in cancer patients with weight loss. *Cancer Res.* 1984;**44**:857–861.

Fortney SR, Clark DA, Stein E. Inhibition of gluconeogenesis by hydrazine administration in rats. *J Pharmacol Exp Ther.* 1967;**156**(2):277–284.

Gershanovich ML, Danova LA, Kondratyev VB. Clinical data on the antitumor activity of hydrazine sulfate. *Cancer Treat Rep.* 1976;**60**(7):933–935.

Gold J. Remission of metastatic giant cell tumor (GCT) by hydrazine sulfate and vitamin K_3 therapy (abstract 915). *Proc Am Assoc Cancer Res.* 1987;**28**:230.

Gold J. Combination effect of VP-16, vitamin K_3 (menadione) and hydrazine sulfate in tumor bearing animals (abstract 1296). *Proc Am Assoc Cancer Res.* 1988; **29**:326.

Gold J. Proposed treatment of cancer by inhibition of gluconeogenesis. *Oncology.* 1968;**22**:185–207.

Gold J. Inhibition by hydrazine sulfate and various hydrazides of in vivo growth of Walker 256 intramuscular carcinoma, β-16 melanoma, Murphy-Sturm lymphosarcoma L-1210 solid leukemia. *Oncology.* 1973;**27**:69–80.

Gold J. Use of hydrazine sulfate in advanced cancer patients: Preliminary results. *Proc Amer Assoc Cancer Res and ASCO.* 1974;**15**:83.

Gold J. In vivo synergy of vitamin K_3 and methotrexate in tumor-bearing animals. *Cancer Treat Rep.* 1986;**70**:1433–1435.

Gutterman J, Huang A, Hochstein P. The mode of action of N-isopropyl-α-(2-methylhydrazine)-*p*-toluamide. *Exp Biol Med.* 1969;**130**:797.

Lerner HJ, Regelson W. Clinical trial of hydrazine sulfate in solid tumors. *Cancer Treat Rep.* 1976;**60**(7):959–960.

Ochoa M Jr, Witters RE, Krakoff IH. Trial of hydrazine sulfate (NSC-150014) in patients with cancer. *Cancer Chemother Rep Part 1.* 1975;**59**(6):1151–1154.

Ray PD, Hanson RL, Lardy HA. Inhibition by hydrazine of gluconeogenesis in the rat. *J Biol Chem.* 1970;**245**(4):690–696.

Taylor GD. Effects of hydrazine on blood glucose and muscle and liver glycogen in the anesthetized dog. *School Aerosp Med Tech Rep.* 1966;**12**:66.

Underhill FP. The influence of hydrazine upon the organism, with special reference to the blood sugar content. *J Biol Chem.* 1911;**10**:159–168.

4-Hydroxyandrostenedione

■ Other Names

4-OHA; CGP-32349 (Ciba-Geigy Pharmaceuticals); HAD.

■ Chemistry

Structure of 4-hydroxyandrostenedione

4-Hydroxyandrostenedione (4-OHA) has the complete chemical name 4-hydroxyandrost-4-ene-3,17-dione. It is an analog of the normal androgenic precursor to estrogens which blocks aromatase enzymes. The melting point of 4-OHA is between 205 and 206°C, and the ultraviolet extinction coefficient is 10,811 at the λ_{max} of 278 nm (Coombes et al 1984).

■ Antitumor Activity

4-Hydroxyandrostenedione acts as a hormonal inhibitor to block the conversion of androgen to estrogens in peripheral tissues. Thus, the drug has most often been used in the treatment of disseminated postmenopausal breast cancer (Coombes et al 1984, Cunningham et al 1987, Stein et al 1990, Dowsett et al 1987). In an initial clinical trial, intramuscular 4-OHA produced objective partial responses (PRs) in 4 of 11 (36%) patients with breast cancer refractory to other hormonal manipulations including oophorectomy and tamoxifen (Coombes et al 1984). In a phase II trial, 14 of 52 (27%) breast cancer patients with measurable disease had partial responses to the drug. Disease stabilization was noted in another 19% (Goss et al 1986b). After 1 month of therapy, plasma estradiol levels were suppressed from a mean of 7.2 to 2.6 pg/mL (Goss et al 1986b). There was no significant fall in the level of other hormones including estrone, dehydroepiandrosterone, sex hormone-binding globulin, testosterone, and follicle-stimulating hormone (FSH).

Orally administered 4-OHA is also active in patients with disseminated breast cancer. Partial responses have been noted in 8 of 29 (28%) patients in one trial (Cunningham et al 1987). A median response duration of 12 months is typical in postmenopausal patients, and the overall response rate of 33% is similar to those of tamoxifen and aminoglutethimide in this patient population (Stein et al 1990).

■ Mechanism of Action

4-Hydroxyandrostenedione binds to and inhibits the activity of aromatase enzymes, blocking the conversion of androgens to estrogens (peripheral aromatization) (Schwarzel et al 1973). Aromatases mediate the conversion of androstenedione to estrone and estradiol and of testosterone to estradiol. Inhibitors like 4-OHA inhibit the enzyme at its active site (Brodie et al 1981). Indeed, 4-OHA is one of the most selective of several such inhibitors and aromatase enzymes from human placental tissues have a K_i for inhibition by 4-OHA of only 0.15 μM (Brodie et al 1977).

Studies of 4-OHA in animals show that the drug suppresses ovarian estrogen secretion in rats (Brodie et al 1976) and can block the estrogen-dependent development of mammary tumors in carcinogen-treated rats (Brodie et al 1982). 4-OHA can also block peripheral aromatization in rhesus monkeys (Brodie and Longcope 1980).

The aromatase-inhibitory activity of 4-OHA differs from that of aminoglutethimide which is dependent on the general inhibition of steroidogenesis via an interaction with cytochrome P450 enzymes.

In contrast, 4-OHA binds directly and irreversibly to aromatases, acting as a suicide substrate inhibitor. 4-OHA does not block the synthesis or release of other hormones including luteinizing hormone, FSH, testosterone, and sex hormone-binding globulin (Goss et al 1986b). Unexpectedly, 4-OHA suppresses estrone levels only slightly in humans (Goss et al 1986b). This differs from the marked suppression by aminoglutethimide. Unlike, aminoglutethimide, 4-OHA does not suppress the adrenal gland, as normal levels of dehydroepiandrostenedione are maintained in patients.

■ Availability and Storage

4-Hydroxyandrostenedione is investigationally available as a microcrystalline powder in glass ampules (Ciba-Geigy Corporation, Basel, Switzerland), The intact ampules are stored under refrigeration (4°C).

■ Preparation for Use, Stability, and Admixture

For parenteral injection the microcrystalline powder is reconstituted in 0.9% Sodium Chloride for Injection, USP, to a concentration of 125 mg/mL. Intramuscular injections of 4-OHA have also been prepared in 0.5% caboxymethylcellulose in water (Coombes et al 1984). All doses were administered immediately after preparation. Stability and admixture data are not currently available.

For oral administration, the powder has been initially reconstituted as described and then diluted in water or saline to a concentration of 50 mg/mL (Dowsett et al 1987).

■ Dosage

Preclinical toxicology studies in mice showed that the LD_{50} and LD_{10} were 4.325 and 2.9 g/kg, respectively (Coombes et al 1984). Initial clinical trials used a weekly intramuscular dose of 500 mg (Coombes et al 1984, Dowsett et al 1987). A higher intramuscular dose of 1000 mg (500 mg in each buttock) was evaluated in patients who failed to respond initially (Goss et al 1986b); however, Stein et al (1990) have suggested that the optimal intramuscular dose of 4-OHA is 250 mg every 2 weeks. This was based on serial measurements of serum estradiol levels showing equivalent suppression (to a mean of 37% of normal) 1 week after intramuscular doses of 500 and 250 mg (Stein et al 1990).

With oral administration much higher doses of 4-OHA are recommended because of significant hepatic first-pass metabolism. Thus, an oral dose of 500 mg was recommended for *daily* administration to patients with disseminated breast cancer (Cunningham et al 1987).

■ Pharmacokinetics

The pharmacokinetics of 4-OHA in plasma have been studied in cancer patients using the drug's crossreactivity with a radioimmunoassay for androstenedione (Dowsett et al 1984). A chromatographic separation on Lipidex® columns was used prior to analysis using the radioimmunoassay procedure. Following a single intramuscular dose of 500 mg, peak 4-OHA levels of 10 to 30 ng/mL were obtained in six patients with breast cancer (Dowsett et al 1987). The half-life was approximately 8 days, except in one patient in whom plasma levels declined much more rapidly. Of interest, this patient also showed rapid (< 2 weeks) escape from estradiol suppression while on 4-OHA. In other patients, serum estradiol levels were suppressed for 14 to 21 days after a 500-mg dose. At that time, serum 4-OHA levels had fallen to 3 ng/mL or less (Dowsett et al 1987). Furthermore, the degree of estradiol suppression was equal following a 125-mg dose but escape from suppression was more rapid. These data provided the rationale for a 250-mg intramuscular dose given every 2 weeks (Stein et al 1990).

With an oral dose of 250 mg, the highest serum levels of 44.6 ng/mL were measured 1 to 3 hours after dosing (Dowsett et al 1987). Twenty-four hours after oral dosing, 4-OHA levels were below 0.3 ng/mL in three patients and 0.8 ng/mL in one patient.

A wide variety of more hydrophilic 4-OHA metabolites have been identified in rats (Foster et al 1986). Only one such metabolite, 2-hydroxy-4-OHA, also demonstrated aromatase-inhibitory activity. This metabolite is 45% as active as 4-OHA (Foster et al 1986). The major urinary metabolite in humans has been identified as the 4-glucuronide conjugate (Goss et al 1986a). No intact 4-OHA was recovered in the urine.

■ Side Effects and Toxicity

The main side effect of 4-OHA is pain at the intramuscular injection site (Coombes et al 1984). Hot flashes are also reported in about 50% of patients. With very high intramuscular doses of 1000 mg, sterile abscesses at the injection site were frequent (Goss et al 1986b). This has necessitated drug discontinuation in some patients. Anaphylactoid reactions have been reported in a few patients who received the drug for 6 months. Perioral edema, which resolved within 24 to 48 hours was described in another patient (Goss et al 1986b).

Other reported reactions include a transient, mild lethargy. Nausea has rarely been reported (Stein et al 1990). One patient developed a morbiliform rash which required drug discontinuance (Stein et al 1990). With oral therapy, side effects are rare and one study described no toxicity in 90% of treated patients (Cunningham et al 1987).

REFERENCES

Brodie AMH, Garrett WM, Hendrickson JR, et al. Inactivation of aromatase in vitro by 4-hydroxyandrostenedione and 4-acetohydroxyandrostenedione and sustained effects in vivo. *Steroids.* 1981;**38**:693–702.

Brodie AMH, Garrett WM, Hendrikson JR, et al. Effects of aromatase inhibitor 4-hydroxyandrostenedione and other compounds in the DMBA-induced breast carcinoma model. *Cancer Res.* 1982;**42**:3360s–3364s.

Brodie AMH, Longcope C. Inhibition of peripheral aromatization by aromatase inhibitors, 4-hydroxy- and 4-acetoxy-androstene-3,17-dione. *Endocrinology.* 1980;**106**:19–21.

Brodie AMH, Schwarzel WC, Brodie HJ. Studies on the mechanisms of estrogen biosynthesis in the rat ovary. *J Steroid Biochem.* 1976;**7**:787–793.

Brodie AMH, Schwarzel WC, Shaikh AA, et al. The effect of an aromatase inhibitor 4-hydroxy-4-androstene-3,17-dione, on estrogen-dependent processes in reproduction and breast cancer. *Endocrinology.* 1977;**100**:1684–1695.

Coombes RC, Goss P, Dowsett M, et al. 4-Hydroxyandrostenedione in treatment of postmenopausal patients with advanced breast cancer. *Lancet.* 1984;**2**:1237–1239.

Cunningham D, Powles TJ, Dowsett M, et al. Oral 4-hydroxyandrostenedione, a new endocrine treatment for disseminated breast cancer. *Cancer Chemother Pharmacol.* 1987;**20**:253–255.

Dowsett M, Goss PE, Powles TJ, et al. Use of the aromatase inhibitor 4-hydroxyandrostenedione in postmenopausal breast cancer: Optimization of therapeutic dose and route. *Cancer Res.* 1987;**47**:1957–1961.

Dowsett M, Harris AL, Smith IE, et al. Endocrine changes associated with relapse in advanced breast cancer patients on aminoglutethimide therapy. *J Clin Endocrinol Metab.* 1984;**58**:99–104.

Foster AB, Jarman M, Mann J, et al. Metabolism of 4-hydroxyandrost-4-ene-3,17-dione by rat hepatocytes. *J Steroid Biochem.* 1986;**24**(2):607–617.

Goss PE, Jarman M, Wilkinson JR, et al. Metabolism of the aromatase inhibitor 4-hydroxyandrostenedione in vivo. Identification of the glucuronide as a major urinary metabolite in patients and biliary metabolite in the rat. *J Steroid Biochem.* 1986a;**24**(2):619–622.

Goss PE, Powles TJ, Dowsett M, et al. Treatment of advanced postmenopausal breast cancer with an aromatase inhibitor, 4-hydroxyandrostenedione: Phase II report. *Cancer Res.* 1986b;**46**:4823–4826.

Schwarzel WC, Kruggel W, Brodie HJ. Studies on the mechanism of estrogen biosynthesis. VIII. The development of inhibitors of the enzyme system in human placenta. *Endocrinology.* 1973;**92**:866–880.

Stein RC, Dowsett M, Hedley A, et al. Treatment of advanced breast cancer in postmenopausal women with 4-hydroxyandrostenedione. *Cancer Chemother Pharmacol.* 1990;**26**:75–78.

Hydroxyurea

■ Other Names

NSC-32065; hydroxycarbamide; HU; Hydrea® (Immunex Corporation); Litalir® (Chemische Fabrik von Heyden).

■ Chemistry

$$\underset{H_2N-\underset{\underset{\|}{O}}{C}-\underset{\underset{|}{H}}{N}-OH}{}$$

Structure of hydroxyurea

Hydroxyurea is a hygroscopic white crystalline powder with a molecular weight of 76. It has the empiric formula $CH_4N_2O_2$ and is freely soluble in water and slightly soluble in alcohol.

■ Antitumor Activity

Hydroxyurea is most often used for the treatment of chronic phases of chronic myelogenous leukemia (CML) (Kennedy 1972, Schwartz and Cannellos, 1975, Rushing et al 1982). It is rarely used in the blast phase of CML. The drug is now being used in CML in combination with interferon alfa with promising results (Anger et al 1989, Taylor et al 1992, Talpaz et al 1992). The drug is modestly active in the treatment of patients with malignant melanoma (Bloedow 1964) and refractory ovarian cancer and in combination with radiation therapy for patients with head and neck cancer (Lerner et al 1969, Ariel 1970). The drug has had hints of activity for patients with advanced prostate cancer (Lerner and Malloy 1977, Loening et al 1981, Mundy 1982). Stephens et al (1984) have not confirmed that level of activity. The drug has minimal activity against renal cell carcinoma (Stolbach et al 1981) and transitional cell carcinoma of the urinary bladder (Beckloff et al 1976).

There is intriguing evidence that hydroxyurea is an effective radiation sensitizer. Piver and colleagues (1987) reported a dramatic decrease in recurrence of cervical cancer when hydroxyurea was added to radiation therapy versus when placebo was added to radiation therapy. This work is being followed up by several groups (Stehman et al 1988).

Recently, high-dose regimens of hydroxyurea achieving serum levels above 1 mM were assessed and some efficacy was noted (Veale et al 1988) in patients with non-small cell lung cancer glioblastoma multiforme (Dennison et al 1990) and in a patient with an unknown primary tumor (Blumenreich et al 1990). Hydroxyurea has also been added to autologous marrow transplant regimens (Vaughan et al 1991, Ariel 1975).

■ Mechanism of Action

The exact mechanism(s) of action, even after years of study of hydroxyurea, has not been established but the drug appears to diffuse passively into cells to block the ribonucleotide reductase system. This enzyme normally consists of two subunits that contain the substrate and allosteric binding sites M_1 and M_2; M_2 is the catalytic subunit (Donehower 1982). Hydroxyurea is believed to inactivate the free tyrosyl radical on the M_2 subunit. This inhibition can be partially reversed by ferrous iron (Moore 1969) and enhanced by iron chelating agents (Satyamoorthy et al 1986), suggesting that a nonheme iron cofactor is involved in hydroxyurea's cytotoxic activity. Hydroxyurea causes immediate inhibition of DNA synthesis without interfering with the synthesis of RNA or protein. Thus, hydroxyurea acts as a DNA-selective antimetabolite by interfering with the enzymatic conversion of ribonucleotides to deoxyribonucleotides. It appears that the drug may also inhibit the incorporation of thymidine into DNA and, additionally, may directly damage DNA. The repair of spontaneous DNA lesions may also be inhibited by hydroxyurea (Li and Kaminskas 1987). This leads to progressive DNA lesions in cultured Ehrlich ascites carcinoma cells. Hydroxyurea also decreases the binding of vitamin B_{12} to transcobalamin II, thereby causing a secondary type of B_{12} deficiency (Vu et al 1992). How this relates to antitumor cytotoxicity is unclear.

In vitro studies indicate that hydroxyurea exerts lethal effects on cells in S phase. Thus, cytotoxicity from hydroxyurea is both cell cycle dependent and schedule dependent, favoring enhanced cytotoxicity with prolonged drug exposures. It may also cause synchronization of cells in the cell cycle at the G_1/S phase (Krakoff et al 1968). Some of this cell cycle activity may result from inhibition of ornithine decarboxylase induction which blocks polyamine synthesis (Cress and Gerner 1979).

■ Availability and Storage

Hydroxyurea is commercially available in 500-mg capsules for oral use (Immunex Corporation, Seattle, Washington). It is also available from the Investigational Drug Branch of the National Cancer Institute as a lyophilized powder in 50-mL vials containing 2 g of hydroxyurea with anhydrous citric acid (56 mg) and anhydrous sodium phosphate (144 mg). Both of these formulations may be stored at room temperature. Because the drug is degraded by moisture, the capsules should be kept in a tightly sealed container with a desiccant included.

■ Preparation for Use, Stability, and Admixture

The investigational vial should be diluted with 18.6 mL of Sterile Water for Injection, USP. The pH of this solution is 6.1. The initial dilutions may be further diluted with up to 500 mL of D5W or normal saline. These solutions are stable for at least 72 hours in the refrigerator or at room temperature; however, as no bacteriostatic agent is added, any unused portion should be discarded after 24 hours.

■ Administration

Hydroxyurea is usually administered orally in a single daily dose. For patients who experience difficulty swallowing capsules, the content of the capsules may be emptied into a glass of water. Hydroxyurea readily dissolves but some inert vehicle residue may float on the surface. The investigational injectable form may be given intravenously by slow push or infusion (which may maximize activity). Daily infusions over 8 hours for 4 to 5 days have also been successfully employed (Moertel et al 1965).

■ Special Precautions

Hydroxyurea is secreted in human breast milk (Sylvester et al 1987). Hydroxyurea has been found to interfere negatively with triglyceride measurement by a glycerol oxidase method (McPherson et al 1985).

Drug Interactions

Lokich et al (1975) noted a lack of therapeutic effect with the combination of hydroxyurea and 5-fluorouracil in patients with gastrointestinal cancer. This was attributed to an inability to convert 5-fluorouracil to its active metabolite, 5-fluorodeoxyuridylate monophosphate (FdUMP), because of the presence of hydroxyurea. Additionally, an unusually high incidence of neurotoxicity was noted, suggesting accumulation of neurotoxic 5-fluorouracil catabolites such as fluoroacetate.

The addition of hydroxyurea to 5-fluorouracil/leucovorin regimens is postulated to enhance 5-fluorouracil activity by reducing the pool of deoxyuridylate monophosphate. Hydroxyurea doses of 1 g/m^2 have reversed resistance to 5-fluorouracil/leucovorin therapy in patients with metastatic colorectal carcinoma (de Gramont et al 1992, Jones et al 1992). Other investigators have frequently used hydroxyurea with 5-fluorouracil and leucovorin ± radiation therapy with acceptable toxicity (no neurotoxic effects) (Vokes et al 1990). More recently, iododeoxyuridine (IUdR) has been added to this combination to take advantage of this drug's radiation-sensitizing activity (Vokes et al 1992); however, significant myelosuppression and mucositis with low-dose IUdR may limit the efficacy of this hydroxyurea-containing combination. Hydroxyurea can also modulate cytarabine metabolism and cytotoxicity (Robichard and Fram 1987). This involves an increase in ara-CTP formation (Kubota et al 1988) with enhanced uptake into DNA. The mechanism for the enhanced activity of cytarabine may ultimately involve a hydroxyurea-induced decrease in deoxycytidine triphosphate levels; however, reduced levels of deoxycytidine, the normal substrate for the enzyme deoxycytidine kinase, may also explain the enhancement in cytarabine activity with concomitant hydroxyurea (Kubota et al 1988). Because of this interaction, cytarabine doses must be lowered when combined with hydroxyurea (Zittoun et al 1985).

Because hydroxyurea may also block DNA repair (Li and Kaminskas 1987), it is being evaluated in combination with cytotoxic drugs that damage DNA as their mechanism of action.

Dosage

When the dose of hydroxyurea is calculated by patient weight, the lean body weight should be calculated and used if the patient is obese or has fluid retention. The drug is most effective in chronic myelogenous leukemia when titrated according to effects on normal peripheral white blood cells. A starting intravenous dose of 50 to 75 mg/kg is recommended by Schwartz and Cannellos (1975) when the white count is greater than 100,000/mm^3. With lower initial blast counts, a daily oral dose of 10 to 20 mg/kg is recommended. For resistant CML a continuous daily dose of 20 to 30 mg/kg is recommended by the manufacturer.

Careful dosage adjustments must be individualized to each patient. Older patients and children may be particularly sensitive to hydroxyurea.

Hydroxyurea may be administered orally either continuously or intermittently. When it is given in continuous daily doses, the dosage range is about 20 to 30 mg/kg/d. An intermittent dose regimen for patients with solid tumors is 80 mg/kg every third day (Lerner and Malloy 1977). The intermittent approach may offer some reduction of myelosuppressive toxicity. Therapy, however, should be interrupted if the white blood count falls below 2500/mm^3 or the platelets below 100,000/mm^3. Moertel et al (1965) used daily infusions of up to 100 mg/kg/d for 4 to 5 days without undue hematologic toxicity, although gastrointestinal side effects were common at that dose. All oral doses are typically taken as a single oral dose.

Veale et al (1988) have explored high-dose hydroxyurea (up to 48 g in 48 hours) achieving blood levels greater than 1 mM, which were sustained when the drug was administered by continuous intravenous infusion. Belt et al (1980) compared intravenous and oral hydroxyurea. They found the maximally tolerated dose was 800 mg/m^2 every 4 hours for the oral route and 3.0 mg/m^2/min for the 72-hour continuous intravenous infusion. Trump et al (1991) are conducting a phase I trial of a 24-hour infusion of the drug. A maximally tolerated dose was not reached at the time of their report.

Pharmacokinetics

Pharmacokinetic studies of hydroxyurea have all been performed using a spectrophotometric assay which has had limited sensitivity (5 µg/mL). Additional methods for measurement of hydroxyurea are needed.

On the basis of data obtained in the 1960s and 1970s with a nonspecific spectrophotometric assay, hydroxyurea appears to be well absorbed from the gastrointestinal tract and produces peak serum levels of 0.3 to 2 mM about 1 to 2 hours after administration (Belt et al 1980). Continuous infusions of 1 g/h can produce steady-state levels of 1 mM (Veale et al 1988). Hydroxyurea readily passes the blood–brain barrier achieving peak cerebrospinal fluid levels 3 hours after administration. The plasma/cerebrospinal fluid concentration ratios range from 4:1 to 2:1. In addition, hydroxyurea distributes well into peritoneal or pleural effusions. The plasma:ascites concentration ratios range from 2:1 to 7.5:1 (Beckloff et al 1963). About 50% of an oral dose is degraded in the liver and excreted into the urine as urea and as respiratory carbon dioxide. Hydroxyurea is degraded by the enzyme urease, which is found in intestinal bacteria. A major metabolite in humans is acetohydroxamic acid (Fishbein and Carbone 1963). The direct conversion of hydroxyurea to urea is documented in mice. The elimination half-life appears to range from 3.5 to 4.5 hours (Belt et al 1980). The remaining portion is excreted intact in the urine. Eighty percent of an oral or intravenous dose may therefore be recovered in the urine as hydroxyurea or urea in 12 hours (Fishbein 1967).

In a recent study of intravenous hydroxyurea given as a continuous infusion of 2 to 4 g/m^2/d, plasma levels of 0.6 mM were sustained (Dennison et al 1990). Blumenreich et al (1990) have given from 0.5 to 2.5 g/m^2/d for up to 10 weeks. They noted plasma levels ranging from 3.6 ± 0.8 to 11 ± 6.4 µg/mL. Fetal hemoglobin levels rose two- to fivefold.

■ Side Effects and Toxicity

The major adverse effect of hydroxyurea is bone marrow depression which is dose related in both severity and onset. Leukopenia occurs with a median onset at 10 days at doses of 60 mg/kg/d. These effects are more rapid in onset in patients with myeloproliferative syndromes. Significant thrombocytopenia and anemia are less common and have an onset at about 10 days. At doses above 40 mg/kg/d, Thurman et al (1964) described a consistent megaloblastosis, unresponsive to vitamin B$_{12}$ or folate.

Gastrointestinal symptoms include nausea, vomiting, diarrhea or constipation, and, rarely, stomatitis. These are common (> 80% incidence) in patients receiving doses greater than 60 to 75 mg/kg/d (Moertel et al 1965).

Dermatologic reactions consisting of a maculopapular rash, facial erythema, and acral erythema have been reported (Silver et al 1983). Hydroxyurea may aggravate the inflammation of mucous membranes secondary to irradiation. Hydroxyurea can cause a recall of erythema and hyperpigmentation in previously irradiated tissues (Sears 1965). Long-term use has been associated with thinning of the skin with erythema (Burns et al 1980). Some of the skin lesions have been felt to mimic chronic dermatomyositis (Richard et al 1989). In addition, extensive skin ulceration has been associated with continuous administration of the compound (Montefusco et al 1986). Alopecia is noted rarely.

Hydroxyurea may also cause dysuria or impairment of renal tubular function, resulting in azotemia (elevated blood urea nitrogen and serum creatinine) (Sharon et al 1986). Rare neurologic disturbances including headache, dizziness, disorientation, hallucinations, and convulsions have been reported.

Fever has been noted with hydroxyurea treatment for patients with psoriasis (Bauman et al 1981). Hydroxyurea has been reported to cause a self-limited hepatitis (Heddle and Calvert 1980). A drug-induced alveotitis in a patient with CML has also been reported (Jackson et al 1990).

A controversial finding is that when hydroxyurea is used to treat patients with polycythemia vera, there may be a high risk of leukemic transformation (Nand et al 1990).

■ Special Applications

Hydroxyurea has been used to treat patients with sickle cell anemia (Rodgers et al 1990, Platt et al 1984). Hydroxyurea increases the production of fetal hemoglobin which is associated with a decreased incidence of hemolysis in these patients.

Hydroxyurea has occasionally been noted to decrease myelofibrosis (Löfvenberg et al 1990).

Hydroxyurea has been used, with some success, in the treatment of psoriasis (Layton et al 1989). Of great interest is that hydroxyurea can be used to inhibit bacterial urease. Inhibition of bacterial urease aids in the control of very chronic urinary tract infections (with subsequent struvite stones) caused by urea-splitting bacteria (Carmignani et al 1980).

Recently, hydroxyurea has been found to reverse drug resistance by causing elimination of amplified drug resistance genes located in extrachromosomal sites (Von Hoff et al 1992, Christen et al 1990, 1991). Hydroxyurea has also been shown to eliminate amplified oncogenes in an extrachromosomal compartment (Von Hoff et al 1990b). This work is being explored clinically (Odajnyk et al 1986).

REFERENCES

Anger B, Porzsolt F, Leichtle R, Heinze B, Bartram C, Heimpel H. A phase I/II study of recombinant interferon alpha 2a and hydroxyurea for chronic myelocytic leukemia. *Blut.* 1989;**58**(6):275–278.

Ariel IM. Therapeutic effects of hydroxyurea: Experience with 118 patients with inoperable tumors. *Cancer.* 1970;**25**:705–714.

Ariel JM. Treatment of disseminated cancer by intravenous hydroxyurea and autogenous bone-marrow transplants: Experience with 35 patients. *J Surg Oncol.* 1975;**7**(5):331–335.

Bauman JL, Shulfuff S, Hasegawa GR, Roden R, Hartsough N, Bauernfeind RA. Fever caused by hydroxyurea. *Arch Intern Med.* 1981;**141**(2):260–261.

Beckloff GL, Lerner HJ, Cole DR, et al. Hydroxyurea in bladder carcinoma. *Invest Urol.* 1976;**6**:530–534.

Beckloff GL, Lerner HJ, Frost D, et al. Hydroxyurea in biologic fluids: Dose–concentration relationship. *Cancer Chemother Rep.* 1963;**48**:57–58.

Belt RJ, Haas CD, Kennedy J, Taylor S. Studies of hydroxyurea administered by continuous infusion: Toxicity, pharmacokinetics, and cell synchronization. *Cancer.* 1980;**46**(3):455–462.

Bloedow CE. Phase II studies of hydroxyurea in adults: Miscellaneous tumor. *Cancer Chemother Rep.* 1964;**40**:39.

Blumenreich MS, Joseph UG, Woodcock TM, et al. Long-term hydroxyurea intravenous infusion in patients with advanced cancer. A phase I trial (meeting abstract). *Proc Annu Meet Am Assoc Cancer Res.* 1990;**31**:204.

Burns DA, Sarkany I, Gaylarde P. Effects of hydroxyurea therapy on normal skin: A case report. *Clin Exp Dermatol.* 1980;**5**(4):447–449.

Carmignani G, Belgrano E, Puppo P, Cichero A, Gluliani L. Hydroxyurea in the management of chronic urea-splitting urinary infections. *Br J Urol.* 1980;**52**(4):316–320.

Christen RD, Shalinsky DR, Howell SB. Hydroxyurea (HU) accelerates the rate of loss of resistance to vinblastine (VBL) in KBV$_1$ cells, but does not change the sensitivity to cisplatin in cisplatin resistant human ovarian carcinoma cells. *Proc Am Soc Clin Oncol.* 1990;**9**:255.

Christen RD, Shalinsky DR, Howell SB. Enhancement of the loss of multiple drug resistance by hydroxyurea. *Proc Am Soc Clin Oncol.* 1991;**10**:209.

Cress AR, Gerner EW. Hydroxyurea inhibits ODC induction but not the G$_1$ to S-phase transition. *Biochem Biophys Res Commun.* 1979;**87**:773–780.

De Gramont A, Louvet C, Varette C, et al. Reversal of resistance to high-dose folinic acid (LV) and 5-fluorouracil (5-FU) in metastatic colorectal cancer by hydroxyurea. *Proc Am Soc Clin Oncol.* 1992;**11**:178.

Dennison D, Vaughan WP, Moss S. Pharmacokinetics of parenteral hydroxyurea (HU) in rat and man (meeting abstract). *Proc Annu Meet Am Assoc Cancer Res.* 1990;**31**:3831.

Donehower RC. Hydroxyurea. In: Chabner B, ed. *Pharmacologic Principles of Cancer Treatment.* Philadelphia: WB Saunders, 1982:269–275.

Fishbein WN. Excretion and hematologic effects of single intravenous hydroxyurea infusions in patients with chronic myeloid leukemia. *Johns Hopkins Med J.* 1967;**121**:1–8.

Fishbein WN, Carbone PP. Hydroxyurea: Mechanism of action. *Science.* 1963;**142**:1069–1070.

Heddle R, Calvert AF. Hydroxyurea induced hepatitis. *Med J Aust.* 1980;**1**(3):121.

Jackson GH, Wallis J, Ledingham J, Lennard A, Proctor SJ. Hydroxyurea-induced alveolitis in a patient with chronic myeloid leukemia. *Cancer Chemother Pharmacol.* 1990;**27**(2):168–169.

Jones JJ, Laufman LR, Spiridonidis CH. Sequential 5-fluorouracil (5-FU), methotrexate (MTX), hydroxyurea (HU) and leucovorin (LV) in refractory carcinomas (CA). *Proc Am Soc Clin Oncol.* 1992;**11**:188.

Kennedy BJ. Hydroxyurea therapy in chronic myelogenous leukemia. *Cancer.* 1972;**29**:1052–1056.

Krakoff IH, Brown NC, Reichard P. Inhibition of ribonucleoside diphosphate reductase by hydroxyurea. *Cancer Res.* 1968;**28:1559–1565.**

Kubota M, Takimoto T, Tanizawa A, et al. Differential modulation of 1-beta-D-arabinofuranosylcytosine metabolism by hydroxyurea in human leukemic cell lines. *Biochem Pharmacol.* 1988;**37**:1745–1749.

Layton AM, Sheeham-Dare RA, Goodfield MJ, Cottrill JA. Hydroxyurea in the management of therapy resistant psoriasis. *Br J Dermatol.* 1989;**121**(5):647–653.

Lerner HF, Malloy TC. Hydroxyurea in stage D carcinoma of the prostate. *Urology.* 1977;**10**(1):35–38.

Lerner HJ, Beckloff GL, Godwin MC. Hydroxyurea intermittent therapy in malignant disease. *Cancer Chemother Rep.* 1969;**53**:385–395.

Li JC, Kaminskas E. Progressive formulation of DNA lesions in cultured Ehrlich ascites tumor cells treated with hydroxyurea. *Cancer Res.* 1987;**47**:2755–2758.

Loening SA, Scott WE, deKernion J, et al. A comparison of hydroxyurea, methyl chlorethyl-cyclohexy-nitrosourea and cyclophosphamide in patients with advanced carcinoma of the prostate. *J Urol.* 1981;**125**(6):812–816.

Löfvenberg E, Wahlin A, Roos G, Ost A. Reversal of myelofibrosis of hydroxyurea. *Eur J Haematol.* 1990;**44**(I): 33–38.

Lokich JJ, Pitman SW, Skarin AT. Combined 5-fluorouracil and hydroxyurea therapy for gastrointestinal cancer. *Oncology.* 1975;**32**(1):34–37.

McPherson RA, Brown KD, Agarwal RP, Threatte GA, Jacobson RJ. Hydroxyurea interferes negatively with triglyceride measurement by a glycerol oxidase method. *Clin Chem.* 1985;**31**(8):1355–1357.

Moertel CG, Reitemeier RJ, Hahn RG. Evaluation of hydroxyurea (NSC-32065) by parenteral infusion. *Cancer Chemother Rep.* 1965;**49**:27–29.

Montefusco E, Alimena G, Gastaldi R, Charlesimo OA, Valesini G, Mandelli F. Unusual dermatologic toxicity of long-term therapy with hydroxyurea in chronic myelogenous leukemia. *Tumori.* 1986;**72**(3):317–321.

Moore EC. The effects of ferrous iron and dithiothreitol on inhibition by hydroxyurea of ribonucleotide reductase. *Cancer Res.* 1969;**29**:291–295.

Mundy AR. A pilot study of hydroxyurea in hormone "escaped" metastatic carcinoma of the prostate. *Br J Urol.* 1982;**54**(1):20–25.

Nand S, Meesmore H, Fisher SG, Bird JL, Schulz W, Fisher RI. Leukemic transformation in polycythemia vera: Analysis of risk factors. *Am J Hematol.* 1990;**34**(1):32–36.

Odajnyk C, Green M, Muggia F. Phase I trial of an oral regimen of simultaneous methotrexate (MIX) and hydroxyurea (HU) (meeting abstract). *Proc Annu Meet Am Soc Clin Oncol.* 1986;**5**:43.

Piver MS, Vongtama V, Emrich LJ. Hydroxyurea plus pelvic radiation versus placebo plus pelvic radiation in surgically staged stage IIIB cervical cancer. *J Surg Oncol.* 1987;**35**(2):129–134.

Platt OS, Orkin SH, Dover G, Beardsley GP, Miller B, Nathan DG. Hydroxyurea enhances fetal hemoglobin production in sickle cell anemia. *J Clin Invest.* 1984;**74**(2):652–656.

Richard M, Truchetet F, Friedel J, Leclech C, Heid E. Skin lesions simulating chronic dermatomyositis during long-term hydroxyurea therapy. *J Am Acad Dermatol.* 1989;**21**(4):797–799.

Robichard NJ, Fram PJ. Potentiation of Ara-C-induced cytotoxicity by hydroxyurea in LoVo colon carcinoma cells. *Biochem Pharmacol.* 1987;**36**:1673–1677.

Rodgers GP, Dover GJ, Noguchi CT, Schechter AN, Nienhuis AW. Hematologic responses of patients with sickle cell disease to treatment with hydroxyurea. *N Engl J Med.* 1990;**322**(15):1037–1045.

Rushing D, Goldman A, Gibbs G, Howe R, Kennedy BJ. Hydroxyurea versus busulfan in the treatment of chronic myelogenous leukemia. *Am J Clin Oncol.* 1982;**5**(3):307–313.

Satyarmoothy K, Chitnis M, Basrur VS, et al. Potentiation of hydroxyurea cytotoxicity in human chronic myeloid leukemia cells by iron-chelating agents. *Leukemia Res.* 1986;**10**:1327–1330.

Schwartz JH, Cannellos GP. Hydroxyurea in the management of hematologic complications of chronic granulocytic leukemia. *Blood.* 1975;**46**(1):11–16.

Sears ME. Erythema in areas of previous irradiation in patients treated with hydroxyurea. *Cancer Chemother Rep.* 1965;**40**:31–32.

Sharon R, Tatarsky I, Ben-Arieh Y. Treatment of polycythemia vera with hydroxyurea. *Cancer.* 1986;**57**(4):718–720.

Silver FS, Espinoza LR, Hartman RC. Acral erthyema and hydroxyurea (letter). *Ann Intern Med.* 1983;**98**(5):675.

Stehman FB, Bundy BN, Keys H, Currie JL, Mortel R, Creasman WT. A randomized trial of hydroxyurea versus misonidazole adjunct to radiation therapy in carcinoma of the cervix. A preliminary report of a Gynecologic Oncology Group study. *Am J Obstet Gynecol.* 1988;**159**(1):87–94.

Stephens RL, Vaughn C, Lane M, et al. Adriamycin and cyclophosphamide versus hydroxyurea in advanced prostatic cancer. A randomized Southwest Oncology Group study. *Cancer.* 1984;**53**(3):406–410.

Stolbach LL, Begg CB, Hall T, Horton J. Treatment of renal carcinoma: A phase III randomized trial of oral medroxyprogesterone (Provera), hydroxyurea, and nafoxidine. *Cancer Treat Rep.* 1981;**65**(7/8):689–692.

Sylvester RK, Lobell M, Teresi ME, Brundage D, Dubowy R. Excretion of hydroxyurea into milk. *Cancer.* 1987;**60**(90):2177–2178.

Talpaz M, O'Brien S, Kurzrock R, et al. Alpha interferon (IFN-α) and chemotherapy combination in early chronic myelogenous leukemia (CML)—A summary of 3 M.D. Anderson studies. *Proc Am Soc Clin Oncol.* 1992;**11**:274.

Taylor K, Eliadis P, Elliott S, et al. Alpha-interferon (α-IFN)/hydroxyurea (HU) therapy in newly diagnosed chronic myeloid leukemia (CML) between age 20 and 50. *Proc Am Soc Clin Oncol.* 1992;**11**:268.

Thurman WG, Watlins WL. Study of serum B_{12} and folate in patients treated with hydroxyurea. *Cancer Chemother Rep.* 1964;**40**:23.

Trump DL, Smith DC, Ellis PG, et al. Phase I trial of high dose, 24 hour continuous infusion hydroxyurea. *Proc Am Assoc Cancer Res.* 1991;**32**:200.

Vaughan WP, Bierman PJ, Reed EC, Vose J, Kessinger A, Armitage JO. High dose hydroxyurea (HU) incorporation into autologous marrow transplant (ABMT) regimens. *Proc Am Soc Clin Oncol.* 1991;**10**:119.

Veale D, Cantwell BM, Kerr N, Upfold A, Harris AL. Phase I study of high-dose hydroxyurea in lung cancer. *Cancer Chemother Pharmacol.* 1988;**21**(1):53–56.

Vokes E, Krishnasamy S, Dolan E, et al. 5-Fluorouracil (5-FU), hydroxyurea (HU) with escalating doses of iododeoxyuridine (IUdR) and concomitant radiotherapy (XRT) for malignant gliomas (MGL): A clinical and pharmacologic analysis. *Proc Am Assoc Cancer Res.* 1992;**33**:212.

Vokes EE, Vijayakumar S, Hoffman PC, et al. 5-Fluorouracil with oral leucovorin and hydroxyurea and concomitant radiotherapy for stage III non-small cell lung cancer. *Cancer.* 1990;**66**(3):437–442.

Von Hoff DD, McGill JR, Forseth BJ, et al. Elimination of extrachromosally amplified Mycgenes from human tumor cells reduces their tumorigenicity. *Proc Natl Acad Sci.* 1992;**89**:8165–8169.

Von Hoff D, VanDevanter D, Forseth B, Davidson K, Waddelow T, Wahl G. Hydroxyurea can decrease drug resistance gene copy number in tumor cell lines (meeting abstract 2243). *Proc Am Assoc Cancer Res.* 1990b;**31**:378.

Vu T, Amin J, Tisman G. Hydroxyurea decreases holotranscobalamin II: Possible case of a drug self-modulating its direct effects on DNA synthesis by causing secondary B_{12} deficiency. *Proc Am Assoc Cancer Res.* 1992;**33**:247.

Zittoun R, Marie JP, Zittoun J, et al. Modulation of cytosine arabinoside (ara-C) and high dose ara-C in acute leukemia. *Semin Oncol.* 1985;**12**:139–143.

Idarubicin HCl

Other Names

Idamycin® (Adria Laboratories); 4-demethoxy-daunorubicin; IDA; IMI-30; 4-dm-DNR; 4-DMDR; 4DDM; NSC-256439.

Chemistry

Structure of idarubicin

Idarubicin is an anthracycline antibiotic that differs from daunorubicin by the lack of a methoxy group at the 4-position of the D ring on the aglycone (Arcamone 1985). This increases the lipophilicity of the compound compared with doxorubicin and may facilitate deeper penetration into the DNA helix by the A, B, and C rings of the aglycone (Plumbridge and Brown 1978). The molecular formula of idarubicin is $C_{26}H_{27}NO_9$. Idarubicin HCl has a molecular weight of 533.96. The complete chemical name is 5,12-naphthacenedione, 9-acetyl-7-{(3-amino-2,3,6-trideoxy-α-L-lyxo-hexopyranosyl)oxy}-7,8,9,10-tetrahydro-6,9,11-trihydroxy hydrochloride, (7S-cis). The melting point is 173 to 174°C, and a solution in water has a pH of 5.0 to 6.5 with a pK_a of 8.5. Idarubicin occurs as an orange powder which at room temperature is soluble in sodium chloride and water, slightly soluble in water, sparingly soluble in methanol, and practically insoluble in nonpolar organic solvents.

Antitumor Activity

Idarubicin is highly active in numerous preclinical models (Ganzina et al 1986). Sensitive tumors include L-1210 leukemia, sarcoma 180, and, to a lesser extent, C3H mammary carcinoma. Intravenous idarubicin is approved by the U.S. Food and Drug Administration for remission induction therapy of acute nonlymphocytic leukemia (ANLL) in combination with cytarabine (Vogler et al 1989, Lambertenghi-Deliliers et al 1989; Berman et al 1989a,b, 1991, Wiernik et al 1989, Arlin 1989). In the Italian study by the cooperative group Grupo Italiano Malattie Emetologiche Maligna del Adulto (GIMEMA), idarubicin induced complete remissions in 40% of previously untreated acute myelocytic leukemia patients with the first course of therapy. This compares with a 39% complete response (CR) rate for daunorubicin and cytarabine in the same trial (Petti and Mandelli 1989). Second-course CR rates of about 40% and median remission durations of 8 to 9 months were roughly equal for doxorubicin and idarubicin. Three randomized controlled studies comparing cytarabine + daunorubicin or idarubicin were performed in the United States; a trial at Memorial Sloan-Kettering (Berman et al 1991), one by the Southeastern Group (Vogler et al 1989), and one other multicenter trial (Wiernik et al 1989). Two of these three trials showed higher first-course remission induction rates and longer median durations of survival for idarubicin compared with daunorubicin. In one trial, overall survival was 19.5 months with idarubicin versus 13.5 months with daunorubicin (Berman et al 1991).

Idarubicin has also demonstrated activity in patients in the blast phase of chronic myelogenous leukemia. A single trial has reported that a second chronic phase could be achieved in 4 of 10 patients treated with idarubicin (Berman et al 1989a). Remissions were also obtained in this same trial in 2 of 3 patients with relapsed acute lymphocytic leukemia (ALL). Another European trial demonstrated a high response rate in ALL (Lambertenghi-Deliliers et al 1987). The CR rates were 15/18 in ANLL (acute non-lymphocytic leukemia) and 4/4 in T-cell ALL. A similar complete remission rate of 56% was reported in adult and pediatric patients with refractory ALL (Meloni et al 1987). A lower response rate of 25% was described in 16 pediatric ALL patients (Madon et al 1987). In patients with previously treated ANLL, response rates to idarubicin and cytarabine range from 22% (Berman et al 1989a) to 68% with etoposide added (Carella 1988). A 60% CR rate was reported for the combination of idarubicin and intermediate to high-dose cytarabine (Harousseau et al 1989). Oral idarubicin is also active in non-Hodgkin's lymphoma (Lopez et al 1986a).

Idarubicin has some activity in solid tumors. In postmenopausal women with untreated advanced breast cancer, oral idarubicin produces objective responses in about one third of patients (Bastholt and Dalmark 1987, Bastholt et al 1987; Lionetto et al 1986). Response rates of 23% have been reported by Lopez et al (1989) and by Kolaric et al (1987); however, when compared with doxorubicin in advanced breast cancer, idarubicin was substantially less active (21% versus 46%) (Lopez et al 1989). Likewise, Bonfante et al (1985, 1986) described only 3 partial responses in 22 evaluable patients, a 14% response rate. Casper et al (1987) reported no responses to idarubicin in 22 anthracycline-naive patients. Similarly, a very low response rate was reported by the EORTC in previously untreated breast cancer patients (Ganzina et al 1986). In other solid tumors, idarubicin has demonstrated very little activity. The compound is inactive in gastric cancer (MacCormick et al 1991, Abad-Esteve et al 1989). A few patients with extensive non-small cell lung cancer have also responded to oral idarubicin (Umsawasdi et al 1989); however, the objective response rates were only 1/15 in a follow-up trial (Umsawasdi et al 1990), 1/30 in a second trial (Kris et al 1985) and 0/20 in a third trial (Ardizzoni et al 1988). Idarubicin is similarly inactive in malignant melanoma (Lopez et al 1986b) and in Kaposi's sarcoma (Chachoua et al 1987).

■ Mechanism of Action

Idarubicin produces lesions in DNA that are similar to those produced by other anthracycline antibiotics. The DNA double helix is stabilized against heat denaturation to a greater degree with idarubicin than with daunorubicin (Zunino et al 1976). These and other findings suggest that idarubicin has a stronger intercalative binding affinity for DNA. The number of "binding sites" in DNA for idarubicin is roughly comparable to that for daunorubicin (Plumbridge and Brown 1978). Thus, the higher binding affinity of idarubicin may result from the lack of the 4-methoxy group which otherwise blocks coplanarity in the four rings of the aglycone (Neidle 1977). Anthracycline binding to DNA leads to direct inhibition of both DNA and RNA polymerase in vitro (Zunino et al 1976). Uptake of thymidine into tumor cells and normal fibroblasts is also inhibited by idarubicin. This activity occurs at lower idarubicin concentrations compared with daunorubicin and other anthracyclines (Supino et al 1977, Casazza et al 1980).

In addition to DNA intercalation and the inhibition of macromolecule synthesis, idarubicin may also degrade double-stranded DNA by an inhibition of topoisomerase II enzymes. This interference results in the formation of protein-associated DNA double-strand breaks which predominate if drug exposure is in the G_2 phase of cell division (Capranico et al 1989). At low drug concentrations the lesions are relatively stable, suggesting that removal or repair of idarubicin-induced strand breaks is difficult (Capranico et al 1989). In resistant cells, higher drug concentrations are required to achieve both equitoxic inhibition of growth and equivalent levels of DNA strand breaks. There was little evidence of non-protein-associated DNA strand breaks with idarubicin. Thus, oxygen free radical generation may be less prominent than with other anthracyclines such as daunorubicin and, especially, doxorubicin.

■ Availability and Storage

Idarubicin is commercially available in single-dose vials containing 5 or 10 mg of orange lyophilized powder (Idamycin® Package Insert, Adria Laboratories, Columbus, OH, 1990). The vials are stored at room temperature and should be protected from light. Investigational oral capsules contain 1, 5, and 10 mg of powdered drug (Kaplan et al 1984).

■ Preparation for Use, Stability, and Admixture

The 5- and 10-mg vials are reconstituted with 5 and 10 mL of Sodium Chloride for Injection, USP, respectively. This yields a 1 mg/mL solution. The use of bacteriostatic solutions for reconstitution is not recommended by the drug manufacturer. Intact vials are filled under negative pressure and should possess a slight vacuum when initially penetrated. This is done to reduce potential aerosolization of drug solution during reconstitution. Idarubicin is compatible with 5% dextrose, and either saline or dextrose can be used for infusion of the reconstituted drug.

Reconstituted idarubicin solutions are chemically stable for at least 7 days under refrigeration and 72 hours at room temperature. The drug is unstable in prolonged contact with highly alkaline solutions and can precipitate with heparin. The table below lists those drugs that have been found to be physically compatible with a 1 mg/mL solution of idarubicin. It is important to note that chemical compatibility of these admixtures is not established. Drugs found to be physically incompatible with idarubicin are listed in the table at the top of this page. Most of these admixtures resulted in precipitation within minutes and therefore must be strictly avoided.

DRUGS PHYSICALLY COMPATIBLE WITH IDARUBICIN

Agent	Concentration Tested (mg/mL)
Amikacin	5
Cimetidine	6
Cyclophosphamide	4
Cytarabine	6
Diphenhydramine	1, 50
Droperidol	0.04, 2.5
Erythromycin	2
Magnesium sulfate	2
Mannitol	12.5
Metoclopramide	5
Potassium chloride	0.03 mEq
Ranitidine	1
Hyperalimentation, solution	
Dextrose	250 g/L
Amino acids	60 g/L
Calcium gluconate	1 g/L
Sodium chloride	100 mEq/L
Potassium chloride	30 mEq/L
Phytonadione	1 mg/L
Multivitamins	1 unit/L
Magnesium sulfate	2 g/L

Data from Adria Laboratories Idamycin Product Monograph, Columbus, OH: Erbamont, Inc; 1991.

DRUGS INCOMPATIBLE WITH IDARUBICIN*

Acyclovir (P)	Hydrocortisone (P)
Ampicillin/sublactans (P)	Imipenem/cilastin (P)
Cefazolin (P)	Lorazepam (C)
Ceftazidime (P)	Meperidine (C)
Clindamycin (P)	Methotrexate (C)
Dexamethasone (P)	Mezlocillin (P)
Etoposide (G)	Sodium bicarbonate (P)
Furosemide (P)	Vancomycin (C)
Gentamicin (C)	Vincristine (C)
Heparin (P)	

*P = precipitate within minutes up to 24 hours, C = color change of solution, G = gas formation.

■ Administration

Idarubicin solutions are administered intravenously as a brief infusion over 10 to 15 minutes. Caution should be used to prevent extravasation, as the drug is a potent vesicant if delivered outside of the vein. The drug has also been administered as a 4-hour infusion (Speth et al 1986). Investigational oral (capsule) doses were administered with 8 to 12 oz of water on an empty stomach.

■ Dosage

The dose of idarubicin in the remission induction therapy of ANLL is 12 mg/m^2/d for 3 consecutive days. If a CR is not obtained, a second induction course may be given. The dose of the second course is the same, 12 mg/m^2/d × 3, unless severe mucositis is present. In that case, the dose should be reduced by 25%. Doses should also be reduced for severe hepatic or renal dysfunction, but specific guidelines have not been established. In one phase III trial, doses were reduced 50% for serum bilirubin levels of 2.6 to 5.0 mg/dL. This appeared to prevent severe myelotoxicity with preserved antitumor activity. The manufacturer recommends that for a serum bilirubin of 2.5 mg/dL or higher, a 50% dose reduction is indicated, and if the bilirubin exceeds 5 mg% the drug should not be administered. The investigational oral dose of idarubicin ranged from 30 to 45 mg/m^2 because of the low and variable bioavailability of the capsular dosage form (Stewart et al 1990).

■ Pharmacokinetics

Intravenous Idarubicin. Idarubicin has a pharmacologic disposition similar to that of other anthracycline antibiotics. This involves a multi-compartment disposition pattern with a long terminal elimination half-life, extensive tissue uptake, and primary biliary elimination. Unlike the other anthracyclines, however, idarubicin is extensively metabolized to the 13-hydroxylated metabolite, idarubicinol. This metabolite is unique in that it has equipotent cytotoxic activity compared with the parent molecule, and is 29- to 103-fold more potent than the alcohol derivatives daunorubicinol, doxorubicinol, and epirubicinol against human leukemia cells in vitro (Kuffel et al 1992). Thus, the majority of a plasma or systemic anthracycline exposure is to idarubicinol, which has a mean plasma exposure ratio 3- to 4-fold greater than that of the parent drug. This is largely due to a significantly longer half-life for idarubicinol (about 50 hours) compared with idarubicin (about 18 hours) (see next table). Both compounds are also 97% bound to plasma proteins. In one trial, concomitant cytarabine did not appear to significantly alter idarubicin or idarubicinol clearance (Berman et al 1989a); however, inter- and intrapatient variation in pharmacokinetic disposition patterns were large and could possibly obscure the effect of a small interaction. The total anthracycline exposure following idarubicin in this trial ranged from 153 to 3355 mg/min/mL. The AUC values for unchanged idarubicin ranged from 7.0 to 403 µg/min/mL. Unfortunately, AUC values showed no correlation with the degree of marrow hypoplasia or with the CR induction rate (Berman et al 1989a).

Only about 13% of the total dose is recovered as anthracyclines in the urine 24 hours after idarubicin administration. Thus, renal elimination is relatively minor for idarubicin (Kaplan et al 1982, Berman et al 1983). The major route for idarubicin and idarubicinol elimination is via the hepatobiliary system, where it is conjugated to either glucuronide or sulfate. These conjugates are slowly eliminated by biliary secretion into feces. For this reason, dose adjustments are probably indicated for patients with mild to moderate elevations in serum bilirubin levels (see Dosage).

The systemic clearance of idarubicin is two- to threefold higher than hepatic plasma flow, suggesting avid metabolism of idarubicin to idarubicinol. Both hepatic metabolism and nonhepatic metabolism are important in clearing drug from the systemic circulation. This is probably due to the wide tissue distribution of aldoketoreductase enzymes which convert idarubicin to idarubicinol. There may also be a slight autoinduction of idarubicin clearance with successive doses. This was suggested by a 50% decrease in the 24-hour AUC for the third daily idarubicin dose compared with the 24-hour AUC for the first daily dose in one trial (Robert et al 1987). This trend has not been observed in several other studies which report similar pharmacokinetics for idarubicin given on different days or for different courses of therapy.

Idarubicin and idarubicinol both concentrate in nucleated blood cells (Speth et al 1986). The release of drug from nucleated blood cells is also significantly slower than elimination of drug and metabolite from the plasma. Thus, the half-lives of idarubicin and idarubicinol in blood cells are 100% and 35% longer than their comparable plasma half-lives, respectively. Furthermore, idarubicinol appears to be more efficiently metabolized intracellularly than idarubicin. This is evidenced by the fourfold lower AUC_{IDA-OL}/AUC_{IDA} ratio in nucleated cells relative to plasma (Speth et al 1989).

Idarubicinol has been found in the cerebrospinal fluid of 19 of 21 children with leukemia who were given intravenous idarubicin doses of 12 mg/m^2 (Reid et al 1989). Idarubicinol levels of 0.14 to 1.05 (mean 0.29) ng/mL were recovered from the cerebrospinal fluid 18 to 30 hours after dosing. Overall, the disposition of drug in pediatric patients is similar to that in adults. Adult patients with solid

MEAN HUMAN PHARMACOKINETICS OF INTRAVENOUS IDARUBICIN (IDA) AND IDARUBICINOL (IDA-OL) IN ADULT LEUKEMIA PATIENTS

Half-life (h)		Idarubicin			Exposure Ratio:	
IDA	IDA-OL	Clearance (L/h/m^2)	AUC (µg/min/mL)	Volume of Distribution (L/m^2)	AUC_{IDA}/AUC_{IDA-OL}	Reference
13 (22)*	49 (42)	109 (23)	28†	1,837 (21)	4.8 (6)	Berman et al 1989a
22 (72)	54 (78)	43 (17)	—	910 (44)	2.7 (56)	Daghestani et al 1985

*Value in parentheses is % coefficient of variation.
†AUC for a dose of 10 mg/m^2/d.

tumors also report pharmacokinetics similar to that of leukemic patients (Smith et al 1987).

Oral Idarubicin. Following an oral dose of 50 mg/m² in two leukemic patients, the AUC values for total anthracycline species from idarubicin were 234 and 746 µg/h/L (Berman et al 1983). These compare with mean AUCs of 204 and 344 µg/h/L for idarubicin and idarubicinol (respectively) following an intravenous dose of 12.5 mg/m². With oral dosing, idarubicinol again was the only metabolite detected in the plasma. The absorption of oral idarubicin appears to be rapid, with peak levels achieved after about 3 hours (see table below) (Stewart et al 1991, Kaplan et al 1984). A smaller portion of an oral dose is excreted in the urine, averaging only 2.3% of total drug in one study (Lu et al 1986). In this same trial, the oral bioavailability of idarubicin was about 39% based on plasma AUC levels (Lu et al 1986). Bioavailability was only 24% in another trial (Smith et al 1987). As noted in the table, the plasma elimination of idarubicinol after oral idarubicin is similar to that following intravenous dosing. The apparent half-life of 34.8 hours for idarubicin is longer with oral dosing than with intravenous doses. Furthermore, the clearance of 9.2 L/kg/h is faster and the apparent volume of distribution of 410 L/kg greater than with intravenous dosing (Lu et al 1986). Again, hepatobiliary elimination predominates, as noted by the very prolonged idarubicin half-life of up to 112 hours following oral dosing in a patient with progressively severe liver dysfunction (Lu et al 1986). Thus, overall bioavailability is low for idarubicin, and the apparent terminal idarubicin half-life is not sufficiently extended to offer a significant pharmacokinetic advantage over intravenous dosing.

■ Side Effects and Toxicity

Myelosuppression, specifically leukopenia, is the principal dose-limiting toxic effect of idarubicin. The median day of nadir white blood cells counts is 10 days, with recovery evident after 15 to 20 days (Kaplan et al 1984). Thrombocytopenia is both less common and less severe than leukopenia. The platelet nadir typically occurs on days 10 to 15. The median duration of thrombocytopenia has been about 25 days. Anemia is very rarely observed with idarubicin.

Mild to moderate nausea and vomiting are common with idarubicin and occur in up to 90% of patients. At least one group has also reported more severe emesis after oral dosing (Berman et al 1983). Fortunately, the emetic effects of idarubicin are typically well controlled with antiemetics. The onset of vomiting is about 2 hours after oral doses and 15 to 30 minutes after intravenous dosing. Other common gastrointestinal toxic effects include diarrhea and mucositis. Both effects are described in about 60% of patients. Mucositis can occasionally by severe, especially if repeated remission induction courses are administered to leukemic patients. Mild anorexia is also described in about 70% of patients.

Elevated liver function tests are described in 20 to 40% of patients receiving idarubicin plus cytarabine. In one trial 38% of leukemic patients receiving idarubicin and cytarabine developed a serum bilirubin level greater than 2 mg/dL (Berman et al 1991). The median range of elevation was to 3.2 mg/dL. Hepatic enzyme levels can also rise in over half of patients. The median increase of SGOT was to 111 U/mL in this trial. Both results are similar to the results for the combination of daunorubicin and cytarabine (Berman et al 1991). Renal function tests are altered in only 2% of patients receiving either agent.

Preclinical trials have suggested that there is reduced cardiotoxicity for idarubicin in the mouse, rat, rabbit, and dog (Casazza et al 1979). In vitro studies in rat heart myocytes confirm a good therapeutic/toxic ratio for idarubicin compared with other anthracyclines (Dorr et al 1991). In human leukemia trials about 17% of patients demonstrate a significant (> 10%) decrease in left ventricular ejection fraction (LVEF) following induction therapy

MEAN HUMAN PHARMACOKINETICS OF ORAL IDARUBICIN

Oral Dose (mg/m²)	Peak Plasma Level (ng/mL) IDA	Peak Plasma Level (ng/mL) IDA-OL	Time to Peak (h) IDA	Time to Peak (h) IDA-OL	Half-life (h) of IDA-OL	Total AUC (µg/mL/h)
40–60	8.2	26.1	3.2	4.4	39	1.16

Data from Kaplan et al 1984.

(Berman et al 1991); however, only 1 of 30 patients developed frank congestive heart failure in this trial. In other comparative trials, a 10% or greater decrease in LVEF was noted at cumulative idarubicin doses greater than 150 mg/m^2. A more complete hazard function curve for cardiotoxicity has not been reported for idarubicin. Nonetheless, the agent is clearly cardiotoxic and produces (1) cumulative cardiotoxic effects with other anthracyclines and (2) synergistic toxicity with preexisting heart disease or with previous irradiation of the chest.

Dermatologic side effects of idarubicin include mild alopecia in approximately 70% of patients (near complete in about 40%) and a generalized rash in 64% of patients (possibly from concomitant antibiotics or other drugs). Although idarubicin is a potent vesicant in preclinical models, there have been few reported clinical extravasations. They have generally produced local lesions that did not require skin grafting (Lu et al 1986). Topical ice packs and elevation are recommended by the manufacturer as therapy for idarubicin extravasation (Adria Laboratories Package Insert). Topical dimethylsulfoxide has shown efficacy with other anthracyclines (Olver et al 1988) and might be similarly useful for idarubicin extravasations.

Other local reactions to idarubicin include erythematous streaking along the vein and urticaria or hives. This is probably due to local histamine release and does predispose patients to extravasation or repeat reactions.

REFERENCES

Abad-Esteve A, Diaz-Rubio E, Jimeno JM, et al. Oral idarubicin in measurable gastric cancer. *Am J Clin Oncol.* 1989;**12**(1):14–16.

Arcamone F. Properties of antitumor anthracyclines and new developments in their application: Cain Memorial Award Lecture. *Cancer Res.* 1985;**45**:5995–5999.

Ardizzoni A, Pronzato P, Repetto L, et al. Phase II trial of oral idarubicin in advanced non-small cell lung cancer (NSCLC). *Cancer Invest.* 1988;**6**(4):409–411.

Arlin ZA. Idarubicin in acute leukemia: An effective new therapy for the future. *Semin Oncol.* 1989;**16**(1, suppl 2):35–36.

Bastholt L, Dalmark M. Phase II study of idarubicin given orally in the treatment of anthracycline-naive advanced breast cancer patients. *Cancer Treat Rep.* 1987;**71**(5):451–454.

Bastholt L, Dalmark M, Jakobsen A, et al. Weekly idarubicin by oral route in postmenopausal women with advanced breast cancer. *Proc ECCO.* 1987;**4**:443.

Berman E, Heller G, Santorsa J, et al. Results of a randomized trial comparing idarubicin and cytosine arabinoside with daunorubicin and cytosine arabinoside in adult patients with newly diagnosed acute myelogenous leukemia. *Blood.* 1991;**77**(8):1666–1674.

Berman E, Raymond V, Daghestani A, et al. 4-Demethoxydaunorubicin (idarubicin) in combination with 1-β-D-arabinofuranosylcytosine in the treatment of relapsed or refractory acute leukemia. *Cancer Res.* 1989a;**49**:477–481.

Berman E, Raymond V, Gee T, et al. Idarubicin in acute leukemia: Results of studies at Memorial Sloan-Kettering Cancer Center. *Semin Oncol.* 1989b;**16**(1, suppl 2):30–34.

Berman E, Wittes RE, Leyland-Jones B, et al. Phase I and clinical pharmacology studies of intravenous and oral administration of 4-demethoxydaunorubicin in patients with advanced cancer. *Cancer Res.* 1983;**43**:6096–6101.

Bonfante V, Ferrari L, Brambilla C, et al. New anthracycline analogs in advanced breast cancer. *Eur J Cancer Clin Oncol.* 1986;**22**(11):1379–1385.

Bonfante V, Rossi A, Brambilla C, et al. Comparative activity and toxicity of Adriamycin (ADM) and new anthracycline analogs in advanced breast cancer. *Proc Am Assoc Cancer Res.* 1985;**26**:165.

Capranico G, Tinelli S, Zunino F. Formation, resealing and persistence of DNA breaks produced by 4-demethoxydaunorubicin in P388 leukemia cells. *Chem–Biol Interact.* 1989;**72**:113–123.

Carella AM. Idarubicin in acute non-lymphoblastic leukaemia. The Genoa experience. *Haematologica.* 1988;**73**:50.

Casazza AM, Bertazzoli C, Pratesi G, et al. Antileukemic activity and cardiac toxicity of 4-demethoxydaunorubicin (4-DMD). *Proc Am Assoc Cancer Res.* 1979;**20**:16.

Casazza AM, Di Marco A, Bonadonna G, et al. Effects of modifications in position 4 of the chromophore or in position 4' of the amino sugar, on the antitumor activity and toxicity of daunorubicin and doxorubicin. In: Crook ST, Reich S, eds. *Anthracyclines: Current Status and New Developments.* New York: Academic Press; 1980:403–430.

Casper ES, Raymond V, Hakes TB, et al. Phase II evaluation of orally administered idarubicin in patients with advanced breast cancer. *Cancer Treat Rep.* 1987;**71**(12):1289–1290.

Chachoua A, Green M, Laubenstein L, et al. Phase II study of oral idarubicin in patients with AIDS-associated Kaposi's sarcoma. *Cancer Treat Rep.* 1987;**71**(7/8):775–776.

Daghestani AN, Zalmen AA, Leyland-Jones B, et al. Phase I and II clinical and pharmacological study of 4-demethoxydaunorubicin (idarubicin) in adult patients with acute leukemia. *Cancer Res.* 1985;**45**:1408–1412.

Dorr RT, Shipp NG, Lee KM. Comparison of cytotoxicity in heart cells and tumor cells exposed to DNA intercalating agents in vitro. *Anti-Cancer Drugs.* 1991;**2**:27–33.

Ganzina F, Pacciarini MA, Di Pietro N. Idarubicin(4-

demethoxydaunorubicin). *Invest New Drugs.* 1986;**4**:85–105.

Harousseau JL, Reiffers J, Hurteloup P, et al. Treatment of relapsed acute myeloid leukemia with idarubicin and intermediate-dose cytarabine. *J Clin Oncol.* 1989;**7**(1):45–49.

Kaplan S, Martini A, Varini M, et al. Phase I trial of 4-demethoxydaunorubicin with single i.v. doses. *Eur J Cancer Clin Oncol.* 1982;**18**:1303–1306.

Kaplan S, Sessa C, Willems Y, et al. Phase I trial of 4-demethoxydaunorubicin (idarubicin) with single oral doses. *Invest New Drugs.* 1984;**2**:281–286.

Kolaric K, Mechl Z, Potrebica V, Sopkova B. Phase II study of oral 4-demethoxydaunorubicin in previously treated (except anthracyclines) metastatic breast cancer patients. *Oncology.* 1987;**44**:82–86.

Kris MG, Burke MT, Gralla RJ, et al. Phase II trial of oral 4-demethoxydaunorubicin in patients with non-small cell lung cancer. *Am J Clin Oncol.* 1985;**8**:377–379.

Kuffel MJ, Reid JM, Ames MM. Anthracyclines and their C-13 alcohol metabolites: Growth inhibition and DNA damage following incubation with human tumor cells in culture. *Cancer Chemother Pharmacol.* 1992;**30**:51–57.

Lambertenghi-Deliliers G, Annaioro C, Colombi M, et al. Therapeutic efficacy of idarubicin in induction therapy for adults with untreated acute leukemia. In: Mandelli F, Polli E, Clarkson B, eds. *Proceedings, 4th International Symposium on Therapy of Acute Leukemia, Rome, February 7–12,* 1987;3–9.

Lambertenghi-Deliliers G, Annaioro C, Cortelezzi A, et al. Idarubicin plus cytarabine as first-line treatment of acute nonlymphoblastic leukemia. *Semin Oncol.* 1989;**16**(2, suppl 2):16–20.

Lionetto R, Pronzato P, Conte PF, et al. Idarubicin in advanced breast cancer: A phase II study. *Cancer Treat Rep.* 1986;**70**(12):1439–1440.

Lopez M, Contegiacomo A, Vici P, et al. A prospective randomized trial of doxorubicin versus idarubicin in the treatment of advanced breast cancer. *Cancer.* 1989;**64**:2431–2436.

Lopez M, Di Lauro L, Papaldo P. Oral idarubicin in non-Hodgkin's lymphomas. *Invest New Drugs.* 1986a;**4**:263–267.

Lopez M, Di Lauro L, Papaldo P, et al. Phase II evaluation of oral idarubicin (4-demethoxydaunorubicin) in patients with disseminated malignant melanoma. *Cancer Treat Rep.* 1986b;**70**(7):911–912.

Lu K, Savaraj N, Kavanagh J, et al. Clinical pharmacology of 4-demethoxydaunorubicin (DMDR). *Cancer Chemother Pharmacol.* 1986;**17**:143–148.

MacCormick R, Hirsch G, Gupta S, et al. A phase II study of idarubicin in the treatment of measurable gastric cancer. *Cancer.* 1991;**67**:2988–2989.

Madon E, Grazia G, De Bernardi B, et al. Phase II study of idarubicin administered IV to pediatric patients with acute lymphoblastic leukemia. *Cancer Treat Rep.* 1987;**71**(9):855–856.

Meloni G, Amadori S, Carella AM, et al. High-dose cytarabine and idarubicin for the treatment of advanced acute lymphoblastic leukemia. In: Mandelli F, Polli E, Clarkson B, eds. *Proceedings, 4th International Symposium on Therapy of Acute Leukemia, Rome, February 7–12,* 1987;18–25.

Neidle S. A hypothesis concerning possible new derivatives of daunorubicin and Adriamycin with enhanced DNA binding properties. *Cancer Treat Rep.* 1977;**61**:928–929.

Olver IN, Aisner J, Hament A. A prospective study of topical dimethylsulfoxide for treating authracycline extravasation. *J Clin Oncol.* 1988;**6**:1732–1735.

Petti MC, Mandelli F. Idarubicin in acute leukemias: Experience of the Italian cooperative group GIMEMA. *Semin Oncol.* 1989;**16**(1):10–15.

Plumbridge TW, Brown JR. Studies on the mode of interaction of 4'-epi-adriamycin and 4-demethoxydaunomycin with DNA. *Biochem Pharmacol.* 1982;**27**:1881.

Reid JM, Kuffel MJ, Pendergrass TW, et al. Cytotoxic concentrations of idarubicinol, the alcohol metabolite of idarubicin, are present in CSF following administration of idarubicin to children with relapsed leukemia (abstract 994). *Proc Am Assoc Cancer Res.* 1989;**30**:250.

Robert J, Rigal-Huguet F, Harousseau JL, et al. Pharmacokinetics of idarubicin after daily intravenous administration in leukemic patients. *Leukemia Res.* 1987;**11**(11):961–964.

Smith DB, Margison JM, Lucas SB, et al. Clinical pharmacology of oral and intravenous 4-demethoxydaunorubicin. *Cancer Chemother Pharmacol.* 1987;**19**:138–142.

Speth PAJ, Minderman H, Haanen C. Idarubicin v daunorubicin: Preclinical and clinical pharmacokinetic studies. *Semin Oncol.* 1989;**16**(1, suppl 2):2–9.

Speth PAJ, van de Loo FAJ, Linssen PCM, et al. Plasma and human leukemic cell pharmacokinetics of oral and intravenous 4-demethoxydaunomycin. *Clin Pharmacol.* 1986;**40**:643–649.

Stewart DJ, Grewaal D, Green RM, et al. Bioavailability and pharmacology of oral idarubicin. *Cancer Chemother Pharmacol.* 1991;**27**:308–314.

Stewart DJ, Verma S, Maroun JA, et al. Phase I study of idarubicin administered orally on a daily × 3 schedule. *Invest New Drugs.* 1990;**8**:275–281.

Supino R, Necco A, Dasdia J, et al. Relationship between effects on nucleic acid synthesis in cell cultures and cytotoxicity of 4-demethoxy derivatives of daunorubicin and Adriamycin. *Cancer Res.* 1977;**37**:4523–4528.

Umsawasdi T, Felder TB, Jeffries D, Newman RA. Phase II study of 4-demethoxydaunorubicin in previously untreated extensive disease non-small cell lung cancer. *Invest New Drugs.* 1990;**8**:S73–S78.

Umsawasdi T, Holoye P, Jeffries D, Carr D. Phase II study of idarubicin in extensive disease non-small cell lung cancer. *Am J Clin Oncol.* 1989;**12**(6):519–520.

Vogler WR, Velez-Garcia E, Omura G, Raney M. A phase-three trial comparing daunorubicin or idarubicin combined with cytosine arabinoside in acute myelogenous leukemia. *Semin Oncol.* 1989;**16**(1, suppl 2):21–24.

Wiernik PH, Case DC Jr, Periman PO, et al. A multicenter trial of cytarabine plus idarubicin or daunorubicin as induction therapy for adult nonlymphocytic leukemia. *Semin Oncol.* 1989;**16**(1, suppl 2):25–29.

Zunino F, Gambetta R, Di Marco A, et al. Effects of stereochemical configuration on the interaction of some daunomycin derivatives with DNA. *Biochem Biophys Res Commun.* 1976;**69**:744–750.

Ifosfamide

■ Other Names

IFEX® (Bristol-Myers Oncology Division); Holoxan® (Astra-Werke Chemical Company); isophosphamide; Z4942; NSC-10924.

■ Chemistry

Structure of ifosfamide

Chemically, ifosfamide is a structural analog of cyclophosphamide. It differs only in the position of one of the two chloroethyl groups which is transposed to the endocyclic (ring) nitrogen. The empiric formula is $C_7H_{15}Cl_2N_2O_2P$, and the compound has a molecular weight of 261. The complete chemical name is 3-(2-chloroethyl)-2-[(2-chloroethyl)amino]-tetrahydro-2*H*-1,3,2-oxazaphosphorine-2-oxide.

■ Anti-Tumor Activity

Ifosfamide, although similar to cyclophosphamide, has actually shown superiority in animal (L-1210) leukemia and is active in a variety of other experimental tumor systems, including Lewis lung and various mouse sarcomas and ascites models (Brock et al 1973). Phase I clinical trials in the United States and Germany also demonstrated good activity in a number of nonhematologic tumors, especially bronchogenic carcinoma (Morgan et al 1976, Scheef 1972). The FDA approved indication for ifosfamide in the United States is as third-line combination chemotherapy of germ cell testicular cancer (Loehrer et al 1986). The drug is also highly active in soft tissue sarcoma (Antman et al 1985). About 20 to 40% of sarcoma patients respond to ifosfamide. In the only randomized comparative trial in adult soft tissue sarcoma, ifosfamide produced a response rate of 18% compared with 8% for cyclophosphamide (Bramwell et al 1987). Myelosuppression was also reduced on the ifosfamide arm of this trial. The unique dose-intensive nature of ifosfamide/mesna schedules may explain some of the enhanced activity in sarcoma, which has been shown to be a dose-responsive malignancy.

In non-small cell lung cancer, combinations including ifosfamide have produced significant response rates but not enhanced long-term survival (Costanzi et al 1982). Other human tumors in which significant activity has been noted include Hodgkin's disease (Rodriguez et al 1978), ovarian carcinoma (Bruhl et al 1976), breast carcinoma (Ahmann et al 1974), and both acute and chronic leukemias. Ifosfamide is highly effective in combination salvage regimens for non-Hodgkin's lymphomas (Cabanillas et al 1982). A particularly effective regimen is the "MIME" regimen containing ifosfamide with mitoguazone, methotrexate, and etoposide (Cabanillas et al 1987). In advanced breast carcinoma, Buzdar et al (1979) have recently reported no advantage for ifosfamide over cyclophosphamide, both in combination with 5-fluorouracil, doxorubicin, and bacillus Calmette–Guérin. In fact, ifosfamide appeared to be much more toxic compared to cyclophosphamide in this setting.

■ Mechanism of Action

Ifosfamide is an alkylating agent that is metabolically activated in the liver (Norpoth 1976). Thus, similar to cyclophosphamide, it must first undergo hydroxylation by microsomal (mixed function oxidase) enzyme systems (Allen and Creaven 1972a). The activation of ifosfamide occurs more slowly than that of cyclophosphamide. Studies in rat liver have shown that although the maximal velocity of enzymatic activation (V_{max}) is similar for the two drugs, the concentration required for half-maximal reaction velocity (K_m) is five times greater for ifosfamide (Allen and Creaven 1975). This may explain the ability to use larger total doses of ifosfamide than cyclophosphamide.

Metabolic activation of ifosfamide is slightly augmented by enzyme-inducing drugs such as phenobarbital pretreatment in rat models. The activating process leads to the formation of highly reactive metabolites capable of covalent binding to protein and to DNA (Allen and Creaven 1973). A defined sequence of steps leads to alkylation. Following hydroxylation at the 4-position, an equilibrium forms with the ring-opened aldehyde form of the drug, aldoifosfamide. This metabolite can spontaneously break down to yield the bladder irritant acrolein and the active alkylating moiety ifosforamide mustard (Allen and Creaven 1975).

Crosslinking of DNA strands proceeds from ifosforamide mustard, whereas acrolein binds nonspecifically and covalently to bladder epithelia. Chain scission of DNA inhibition of thymidine uptake also occur with ifosfamide (Allen and Creaven 1972b). The primary mechanism of action, alkylation, is not particularly cell cycle (phase) specific.

■ Availability and Storage

Ifosfamide is commercially available in 1- and 3-g vials as an off-white lyophilized powder (Ifex®, Bristol-Myers Oncology Division, Princeton, New Jersey). The intact vials may be stored at room temperature or under refrigeration for prolonged periods. At temperatures above 35°C the drug can liquefy and undergo accelerated decomposition.

■ Preparation for Use, Stability, and Admixture

The 1-g vial should be diluted with at least 20 mL sterile water and the 3-g vial with 60 mL. For prolonged sterility, bacteriostatic water containing benzyl alcohol or parabens should be used for initial reconstitution and the vials stored under refrigeration. When so diluted, the solution is stable for at least 1 week at room temperature and for at least 3 weeks under refrigeration. Otherwise, solutions should be used within 8 hours of reconstitution. Each milliliter of the solution will then contain 50 mg of drug. The pH of the initial reconstituted solution ranges from 5.5 to 6.5. Sterile saline may also be used as a diluent. The initial saline- or water-diluted ifosfamide solutions and any further dilutions are chemically stable for 7 days at room temperature. Compatible infusion vehicles include 0.9% sodium chloride, 5% dextrose in water, and lactated Ringer's injection. Glass or plastic infusion containers may be used. Ifosfamide is also compatible with mesna for up to 9 days at temperatures up to 27°C (Radford et al 1990). Thus, the two drugs may be infused simultaneously without a loss of alkylating or uroprotectant activity for the ifosfamide and mesna, respectively. Use within 8 hours of reconstitution is recommended, however, because of the lack of bacteriostatic preservative. Ifosfamide is physically compatible for 4 hours with ondansetron (Trissel et al 1990).

■ Administration

Ifosfamide is administered intravenously, usually by a short infusion in 5% dextrose or normal saline. Doses may also be given by slow intravenous push (in 75-mL minimal volume of sterile saline but not water), infused over at least 30 minutes or by continuous infusion over 5 days. Adequate hydration of the patient both before and for 72 hours after ifosfamide therapy is recommended to reduce the incidence of drug-induced hemorrhagic cystitis. The use of concurrent mesna is required to prevent severe hematuria from high-dose ifosfamide (see Special Precautions). Enough fluid (at least 2 L/d) is recommended to produce a copious urine output with frequent bladder emptying.

Continuous infusions of ifosfamide over 24 hours have also been given every 3 weeks (Stuart-Harris et al 1983); however, renal toxic effects may be increased with a single large infusion dose schedules (see Side Effects and Toxicity). Mesna can be given either concurrently in the same infusion container (Klein et al 1983, Shaw and Rose 1984) or as a 4 hour intermittent intravenous bolus. Extravasation of the drug should not cause severe tissue necrosis, as the agent is inactive prior to hepatic metabolism. However, a mouse study documented ulcerogenic effects for ifosfamide given intradermally (Marnocha and Huston 1992).

■ Special Precautions

The patient must be kept well hydrated during ifosfamide therapy to reduce the potential for hemorrhagic cystitis. Mesna given intravenously and/or orally is required to prevent hemorrhagic cystitis. The table on page 560 outlines the recommended mesna schedule for ifosfamide uroprotection. In older trials hemorrhagic cystitis was managed with bladder catheterization and continuous irrigation with 1% N-acetyl-L-cysteine (Mucomyst®) 2000 mL, during and after administration of ifosfamide, to prevent this complication (Cohen et al 1975). This is probably not necessary if adequate hydration and mesna are used.

Patients who have received previous or concur-

MESNA DOSING SCHEDULE TO PREVENT IFOSFAMIDE UROTOXICITY

Route of Mesna Administration	Dose (mg/kg) as a Percentage of Ifosfamide at Times Before and After Ifosfamide		
	15 Minutes Before	4 Hours After	8 Hours After
IV	20%	20%	20%
PO	Not recommended, use IV route	40%	40%
IV	(Mixed with ifosfamide 1:1 for 6- to 24-hour infusions for 5 consecutive days[†])		

*Mesna solution diluted in juice or water for highly compliant (reliable) patients who are not experiencing nausea or vomiting.
[†]Data from Klein et al 1983.

rent therapy with radiation and/or other cytotoxic drugs may require significant ifosfamide dosage reductions.

■ Dosage

Ifosfamide has been used at varying dosing schedules, generally at higher (milligram) doses than cyclophosphamide (Zalupski and Baker 1988). Creaven et al (1974) stated that the alkylating activity ratio of the two drugs is about 1:5, implying that an ifosfamide dose of 5000 mg/m^2 would be tolerated equivalently to 1000 to 1500 mg/m^2 cyclophosphamide. The FDA-approved dose for testicular cancer is 1.2 g/m^2/d for 5 consecutive days in combination with vinblastine and cisplatin (Loehrer 1990) or with cisplatin and etoposide (Loehrer et al 1986).

Other schedules have also been evaluated. Nelson et al (1976) found 2400 mg/m^2/d IV push for 3 consecutive days to be a maximally tolerated dose as a single agent. In another phase I study by Cohen et al (1975), single intravenous push doses of 200 to 10,000 mg/m^2 given every 3 weeks were explored. For phase II studies these authors recommended a single dose of 5000 mg/m^2; however, large single doses of ifosfamide produce much more toxicity than fractionated schedules which are therefore preferred in solid tumor regimens (Morgan et al 1982). Morgan et al (1976) evaluated several intravenous push and infusion dose schedules: (1) 700 to 900 mg/m^2/d IV push × 5 days repeated every 3 weeks; (2) 700 to 1000 mg/m^2/d × 5 days repeated every 3 weeks plus oral ascorbic acid (1 g/d PO) to acidify the urine; (3) 4 g/m^2 as a 24-hour slow infusion repeated every 3 weeks; and (4) 900 mg/m^2 IV push weekly. There appeared to be less hematuria with the sequential 5-day schedule (number 2, with concomitant ascorbic acid).

In addition, a study by Schnitker (1976) again showed the clinical superiority of fractionated dosing (50–60 mg/kg on 5 consecutive days) over a single intravenous bolus. This effect was independent of tumor type. Brock et al (1973) described the clinical superiority of a divided dosing schedule, giving the drug daily for 2 to 5 days. Accordingly, Rodriguez et al (1978) recently described good therapeutic results with continuous infusions of ifosfamide at 1200 mg/m^2/d × 5. Significant genitourinary toxicity was not encountered and myelosuppression predominated as the dose-limiting toxic effect. In combination with other cytotoxic drugs such as doxorubicin or lomustine, a single intravenous push dose of 1 g/m^2 (not to exceed 1.25 g total) has been recommended.

■ Drug Interactions

Several drug interactions are possible with ifosfamide. Because the compound undergoes hepatic "activation" by microsomal enzymes, induction is potentially possible by pretreatment with various enzyme-inducing drugs such as phenobarbital, phenytoin, and chloral hydrate.

In rat models such barbiturate-induced activation appears to be more significant for ifosfamide than for cyclophosphamide (Allen and Creaven 1972b). Morgan et al (1976) suggested that ascorbic acid prevents bladder toxicity from ifosfamide by keeping the drug in a reduced state. Although it is reported that acetylcysteine reduces cyclophosphamide bladder toxicity in experimental animals (Primack 1971), this is not clinically documented for ifosfamide. Indeed the apparent protective effects of acetylcysteine (1%, 2000 mL) bladder irrigations may be simply explained by dilutional effects rather than specific pharmacologic antagonism (Creaven et al 1974). This conclusion is supported by an in vitro acetylcysteine/ifosfamide incubation study by Creaven et al (1976). Thus, mesna appears to be the preferred uroprotectant for ifosfamide (Hilgard and Burkert 1984). Conversely, other nephrotoxic drugs such as cisplatin may significantly increase ifosfamide renal damage (Goren et al 1987).

Other drug interactions reported for cyclophosphamide that may also occur with ifosfamide include reactions with metabolic alteration of H_2 antihistamines such as cimetidine and other agents such as allopurinol (see *Cyclophosphamide, Drug Interactions*). Although these remain speculative associations, in both instances, increased ifosfamide toxicity might be anticipated.

Pharmacokinetics

The pharmacokinetics of ifosfamide appear to be qualitatively similar to that of cyclophosphamide. Creaven et al (1974) found a plasma half-life for radioactively labeled ifosfamide (5000 mg/m^2) of 13.8 hours with 82% urinary (radioactivity) recovery.

The plasma decay pattern appears to be described biexponentially (two-compartment model) for large bolus doses and monoexponentially (one-compartment model) for fractionated doses. The compartment volumes in adults in the study by Allen et al (1976) were noted to be about 0.65 L/kg for the central compartment and about 0.2 L/kg for the peripheral compartment. Thus, in contrast to single-dose pharmacokinetic studies, Allen et al (1976) found that with sequential daily administration of 2.4 g/m^2/d × 3 days, ifosfamide appears to be handled in the same way as cyclophosphamide. There is an apparent half-life of 7 hours and a urinary recovery of 73%. This finding suggested that the metabolic disposition of the drug may be dose dependent. Sixty-two percent of the urinary fraction was excreted as unchanged drug. Similarly, Allen et al (1976) describe a longer plasma half-life of 15.2 hours after a single (bolus) dose. These half-lives are approximately twice those reported for cyclophosphamide. Allen et al (1976) also determined that only about half of an ifosfamide dose is metabolized compared with about 90% for cyclophosphamide. This reflects a substantial difference in the metabolic clearance capacities for the two analogs.

In contrast, recent pharmacokinetic studies in children have shown no evidence of dose-dependent urinary excretion and, instead, wide interpatient differences in urinary elimination were reported (Heideman et al 1991). Total urinary ifosfamide excretion averaged 31% (± 17%) and was about equally made up of the *R*- and *S*-enantiomers.

Creaven et al (1974) additionally demonstrated that because unchanged ifosfamide, but not metabolites, penetrates the blood–brain barrier, alkylating activity in the cerebrospinal fluid may occur but should be negligible.

At least two alkylating metabolites are found in the urine after bolus dosing. Although more intact (inactive) ifosfamide than cyclophosphamide is renally excreted, the recovery of urine with alkylating activity occurs over longer periods after ifosfamide. The renal clearance of ifosfamide is about twice that for cyclophosphamide, 21.3 versus 10.7 mL/min in bolus dosing, and 18.7 versus 10.7 mL/min with fractionated doses.

A longer ifosfamide half-life may also be seen in obese patients (> 20% over ideal body weight). This prolongation appeared to result from an increase in the volume of distribution from 34 L in the nonobese to 43 L in the obese patients (Lind et al 1989). Total plasma drug clearance in the two groups was unchanged at about 74 mL/min.

Side Effects and Toxicity

Creaven et al (1976) reviewed the clinical toxicity of ifosfamide given as a large bolus injection (200–10,000 mg/m^2) and in a fractionated 3-day (2400 mg/m^2/d) schedule. Urinary tract toxicity is the dose-limiting toxicity with both schedules. The clinical hallmark is hemorrhagic cystitis. It is related to the excretion of active alkylating metabolites into the urinary bladder. This appears to be greater with the bolus regimen and is definitely higher after ifosfamide than after equivalent doses of cyclophosphamide. Therefore, vigorous hydration with oral and intravenous fluids and concomitant mesna is needed to prevent serious ifosfamide-induced bladder damage. Nelson et al (1976) used intravenous furosemide 20 to 40 mg to maintain adequate urine flow. Diuretic responses usually occurred within 1 hour.

Symptoms of dysuria and urinary frequency appear to closely parallel those of hematuria. The onset of symptoms is 1 to 2 days after injection with an average duration of 9 days (range, 1–41 days) (Van Dyk et al 1972). Dose-related ifosfamide-induced nephrotoxicity was noted by elevation of the blood urea nitrogen, producing a subsequent dose-related uremia in 66% of patients receiving 150 mg/kg. Other lesions seen at autopsy (in four of seven patients) included evidence of acute tubular necrosis and pyelonephritis. At low daily doses granular cylinduria was seen in all patients, denoting marked tubular damage. The cylinduria cleared within 10 days of drug discontinuance (Van Dyk et al 1972). De Fronzo et al (1974) described glomerular dysfunction and a Fanconi-type picture in a patient treated with ifosfamide. Prior cisplatin therapy may also increase ifosfamide-induced nephrotoxicity (Goren et al 1987, Hacke et al 1983).

Nausea and vomiting appear to be common and are more severe after rapid injection of large ifosfamide doses. Emesis typically begins within a few hours of administration and persists an average of 3 days (range, 1–28 days) (Van Dyk et al 1972).

Hematologic toxicity from ifosfamide usually involves only a mild to moderate degree of leukopenia in most patients. In the review by Creaven et al (1976), significant thrombocytopenia was not encountered at any of the dose schedules used; however, at the 10,000 mg/m^2 single dose, two early deaths occurred possibly as a result of leukopenia. An insignificant but consistent fall in hemoglobin was noted by Van Dyk et al (1972). It is also important to note that increased myelotoxicity is consistently reported in nephrectomized patients (Fossa and Talle 1980).

Lethargy and confusion are seen with high doses of ifosfamide. Nelson et al (1976) noted that this lasted from 1 to 8 hours and was spontaneously reversible and related to the passage of intact drug into the central nervous system. Seizures, ataxia, stupor, and weakness are all reported after ifosfamide. These effects may be increased by concomitant neurotoxic drugs such as certain antiemetics, tranquilizers, narcotics, and antihistamines. Although active (alkylating) metabolites do appear to significantly penetrate the blood–brain barrier, the levels achieved are too low to be useful in the treatment of central nervous system tumors (Creaven et al 1974). Central nervous system toxicity may be significantly greater in nephrectomized patients as a result of the accumulation of chloracetaldehyde, a dechloroethylated ifosfamide metabolite with neurotoxic properties (Goren et al 1986). Large single doses or oral dosing appear to increase the incidence of neurotoxicity from ifosfamide.

Alopecia is usually seen with ifosfamide, especially when large bolus doses are employed. In the study by Van Dyk et al (1972), the average onset to maximal hair loss was 19 days (range, 11–32 days) after the start of treatment. Cohen et al (1975) noted alopecia in about half of patients receiving high bolus doses.

Hepatic enzyme elevations have been described in some patients. The elevations in alkaline phosphatase and serum transaminase are transient and typically resolve rapidly without sequelae.

A sterile phlebitis at the injection site is reported. Therefore, the injection site should be continuously monitored during drug infusion. Extravasation necrosis has not been described for ifosfamide in humans, but is reported in an experimental mouse model (Marnocha and Huston 1992).

REFERENCES

Ahmann DL, Bisel HF, Hahn RG. Phase II clinical trial of isophosphamide (NSC-109724) in patients with advanced breast cancer. *Cancer Chemother Rep.* 1974;**58**: 861–865.

Allen LM, Creaven PJ. In vitro liver activation of isophosphamide (NSC-109724): A new axazaphosphorine. *Cancer Chemother Rep.* 1972a;**56**:603–610.

Allen LM, Creaven PJ. The effect of microsomal activation on the interaction between isophosphamide and DNA. *J Pharm Sci.* 1972b;**61**:2009–2011.

Allen LM, Creaven PJ. Interaction of mechlorethamine and isophosphamide with bovine serum albumin and rat liver microsomes. *J Pharm Sci.* 1973;**62**:854–856.

Allen LM, Creaven PJ. Human pharmacokinetic model for isophosphamide (NSC-109724). *Cancer Chemother Rep.* 1975;**59**:877–882.

Allen LM, Creaven PJ, Nelson RL. Studies on the human pharmacokinetics of isophosphamide (NSC-109724). *Cancer Treat Rep.* 1976;**60**:451–458.

Antman KH, Montella D, Rosenbaum C, et al. Phase II trial of ifosfamide with mesna in previously treated metastatic sarcoma. *Cancer Treat Rep.* 1985;**69**:499–504.

Bramwell VHC, Mouridsen HT, Santoro A, et al. Cyclophosphamide versus ifosfamide: Final report of a randomized phase II trial in adult soft tissue sarcomas. *Eur J Cancer Clin Oncol.* 1987;**23**(3):311–321.

Brock NN, Hoefer-Janker H, Hohorst H-J, et al. Die aktivierung von ifosfamide an mensch und tier. *Arzneim-Forsch.* 1973;**23**:1–14.

Bruhl P, Gunther U, Hoefer-Janker H, et al. Results obtained with fractionated ifosfamide massive dose treatment in generalized malignant tumours. *Int J Clin Pharmacol.* 1976;**14**:29–39.

Buzdar AV, Legha SS, Tashima CK, et al. Ifosfamide versus cyclophosphamide in combination drug therapy for metastatic breast cancer. *Cancer Treat Rep.* 1979;**65**(1): 115–120.

Cabanillas F, Hagemeister FB, Bodey GP, et al. IMVP-16: An effective regimen for patients with lymphoma who have relapsed after initial combination chemotherapy. *Blood.* 1982;**60**:693–697.

Cabanillas F, Hagemeister FB, McLaughlin P, et al. Results

of MIME salvage regimen for recurrent or refractory lymphoma. *J Clin Oncol.* 1987;**5**:407–412.

Cohen MH, Creaven PJ, Tejada F, et al. Phase I clinical trial of isophosphamide (NSC-109724). *Cancer Chemother Rep.* 1975;**59**:751–755.

Costanzi JJ, Morgan LH, Hokanson J. Ifosfamide in the treatment of extensive non-oat cell carcinoma of the lung. *Semin Oncol.* 1982;**9**(suppl 1):61–65.

Creaven PJ, Allen LM, Alford DA, et al. Clinical pharmacology of isophosphamide. *Clin Pharmacol Ther.* 1974;**16**:77–86.

Creaven PJ, Allen LM, Cohen MH, Nelson RL. Studies on the clinical pharmacology and toxicology of isophosphamide (NSC-109724). *Cancer Treat Rep.* 1976;**60**(4):445–449.

De Fronzo RA, Abeloff M, Braine H, et al. Renal dysfunction after treatment with ifosfamide (NSC-109724). *Cancer Chemother Rep.* 1974;**58**:375–382.

Fossa SK, Talle K. Treatment of metastatic renal cancer with ifosfamide and mesnum with and without irradiation. *Cancer Treat Rep.* 1980;**64**:1103–1108.

Goren MP, Wright RK, Pratt CB, et al. Dechlorethylation of ifosfamide and neurotoxicity. *Lancet.* 1986;**2**:1219–1220.

Goren MP, Wright RK, Pratt CB, et al. Potentiation of ifosfamide neurotoxicity, hematotoxicity, and tubular nephrotoxicity by prior *cis*-diamminedichloroplatinum(II) therapy. *Cancer Res.* 1987;**47**:1457–1460.

Hacke M, Schmoll H, Alt JM, et al. Nephrotoxicity of *cis*-diamminedichloroplatium with or without ifosfamide in cancer treatment. *Clin Physiol Biochem.* 1983;**1**:17–26.

Heideman RL, Kearns CM, Crom WR, et al. Total ifosfamide excretion in the urine of pediatric patients and enantiomeric composition. *Proc Am Assoc Cancer Res.* 1991;**32**:176.

Hilgard P, Burkert H. Sodium-2-mercaptoethane sulfonate (mesna) and ifosfamide nephrotoxicity. *Eur J Cancer Clin Oncol.* 1984;**20**:1451–1452.

Klein HO, Dias Wickramanayake P, Coerper CL, et al. High dose ifosfamide and mesna as continuous infusion over five days—A phrase I/II trial. *Cancer Treat Rev.* 1983;**10**(suppl A):167–173.

Lind MJ, Margison JM, Cerny T, et al. Prolongation of ifosfamide elimination half-life in obese patients due to altered drug distribution. *Cancer Chemother Pharmacol.* 1989;**25**:139–142.

Loehrer PJ. Ifosfamide in testicular cancer. *Semin Oncol.* 1990;**17**(2, suppl 4):2–5.

Loehrer PJ, Einhorn LH, Williams SD. VP-16 plus ifosfamide plus cisplatin as salvage therapy in refractory germ cell cancer. *J Clin Oncol.* 1986;**4**:528–536.

Marnocha RSM, Huston PR. Intradermal carboplatin and ifosfamide extravasation in the mouse. *Cancer.* 1972;**70**:850–853.

Morgan LR, Harrison EF, Hawke JE, et al. Toxicity of single vs. fractionated-dose ifosfamide in non-small cell lung cancer: A multicenter study. *Semin Oncol.* 1982;**9**(suppl 1):66–70.

Morgan LR, Posey LE, Hite S, et al. Ifosfamide in the treatment of carcinoma of the lung. *Clin Res.* 1976;**24**(3):512.

Nelson RI, Creaven PJ, Cohen MH, Fossiek BE Jr. Phase I clinical trial of a 3-day divided dose schedule of ifosphamide (NSC-109724). *Eur J Cancer.* 1976;**12**:195–198.

Norpoth K. Studies on the metabolism of isophosphamide (NSC-109724) in man. *Cancer Treat Rep.* 1976;**60**:437–443.

Primack A. Amelioration of cyclophosphamide-induced cystitis. *J Natl Cancer Inst.* 1971;**47**:223–227.

Radford JA, Margison JM, Swindell R, et al. The stability of ifosfamide in aqueous solution and its suitability for continuous 7-day infusion by ambulatory pump. *Cancer Chemother Pharmacol.* 1990;**26**:144–146.

Rodriguez V, McCredie KB, Keating MJ, et al. Isophosphamide therapy for hematologic malignancies in patients refractory to prior treatment. *Cancer Treat Rep.* 1978;**62**(4):493–497.

Scheef W. Problems, experience, and results of clinical investigations with ifosfamide. In: Hejzlar M, et al, eds. *Proceedings of the Seventh International Congress on Chemotherapy.* Munich: Urban & Schwarzenberg; 1972.

Schnitker J. Evaluation of the cytostatic agent ifosfamide. *Arzneim-Forsch.* 1976;**26**:1783–1793.

Shaw IC, Rose JW. Infusion of ifosfamide plus mesna. *Lancet.* 1984;**1**:1353–1354.

Stuart-Harris RC, Harper PG, Parsons CA, et al. High dose alkylation therapy using ifosfamide infusion with mesna in the treatment of adult advanced soft tissue sarcoma. *Cancer Chemother Pharmacol.* 1983;**11**:69–72.

Trissel LA, Fulton B, Tramonte SM. Visual compatibility of ondansetron with chemotherapeutic agents, antibiotics, and other selected drugs during simulated Y-site injection (abstract #P-468R). In: *25th Annual ASHP Midyear Clinical Meetings and Exhibit, Las Vegas, Nevada;* 1990.

Van Dyk JJ, Falkson HC, Van der Merwe AM, et al. Unexpected toxicity in patients treated with iphosphamide. *Cancer Res.* 1972;**32**:921–924.

Zalupski M, Baker LH. Ifosfamide. *J Natl Cancer Inst.* 1988;**80**:556–566.

Interferon Alfa

■ Other Names

Intron® A (recombinant human interferon alfa-2b, Schering Corporation); Roferon®-A (recombinant human interferon alfa-2a, Roche Laboratories); alpha-interferon; leukocyte interferon, type I (pH 2-stable interferon); Alferon® N Injection (multispecies, natural human leukocyte interferon alfa-n3, The Purdue Frederick Company); interferon alfa C (Interpharm); natural interferon alfa-n2 (Wellferon®, Burroughs Wellcome).

■ Chemistry

Alpha interferons represent a group of related proteins produced by a family of at least 16 genes located on human chromosome 9 (Sehgal 1982). "Natural" (leukocyte) alpha interferon is typically derived in a partially purified state from human blood "buffy coat" white blood cells exposed to an inducer such as Sendai virus. The purity of this latter material, at least as obtained from the Finnish Red Cross (Finnferon®), is 1% or less, or about 1×10^6 antiviral units/mg protein (Cantell et al 1975). This "natural" alpha interferon is glycosylated and has multispecies proteins with molecular weights that can vary from 35,000 to 37,000. The nonglycosylated protein has a molecular weight of approximately 19,000 and consists of 165 amino acids in a tertiary structure of four alpha-helical coils, interspersed by two beta-"pleated sheet" arrangements with two intramolecular disulfide bonds (see figure). The isoelectric point of the commercial alpha interferons is approximately 6.0.

Alpha interferons produced by recombinant DNA techniques are nonglycosylated and may have substituted amino acids at position 23: arginine in interferon alfa-2a (Roferon®-A) versus methionine in interferon alfa-2b (Intron® A). Over 90% of the α-2b molecules contain an N-terminal methionine residue. These changes do not appear to significantly affect the antiviral or antitumoral activities of this protein.

Alpha interferons and beta interferons were

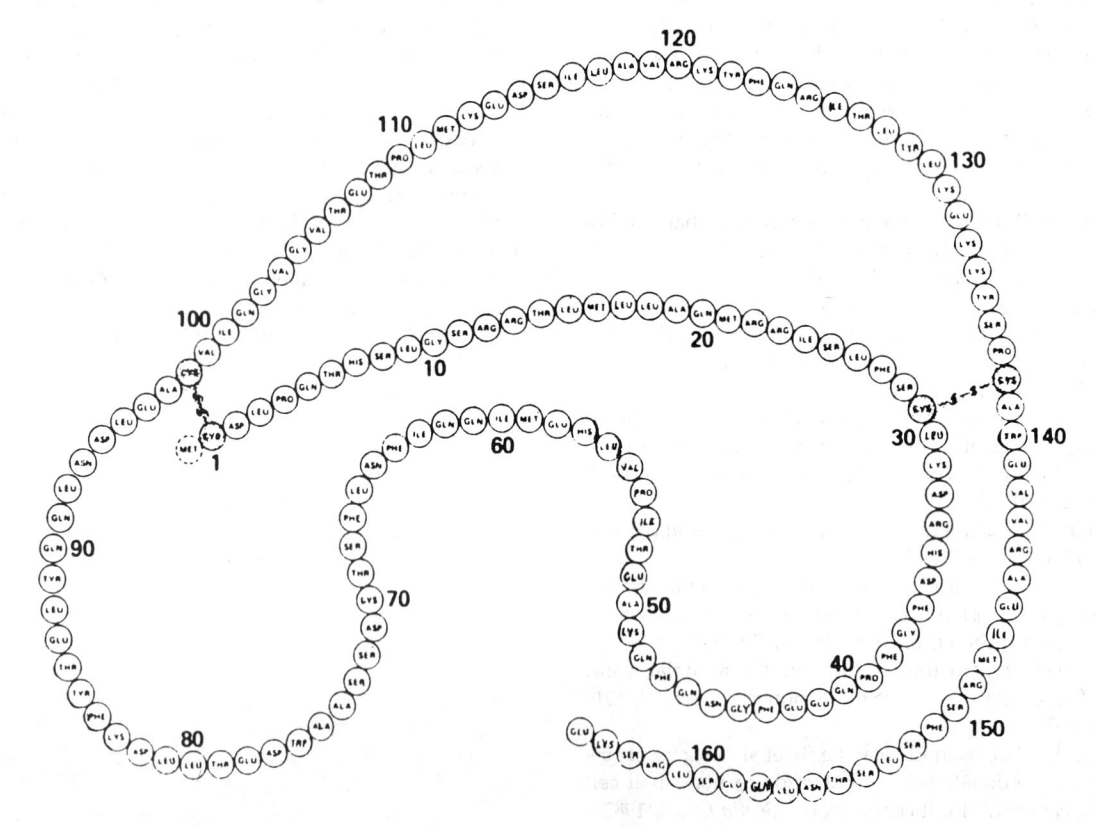

Amino acid sequence of interferon-alfa

originally called type I interferons because of their relative stability at an acid pH (2.0). This compares with the acid instability of interferon gamma (type II interferon). The two recombinant commercial alpha interferons are prepared from *Escherichia coli* bacteria into which the human α-2 gene has been transfected. Purification of bacterial cell supernatants containing interferon is by standard column chromatography (Intron® A) or by affinity chromatography using murine monoclonal antibodies specific to human interferon A (Roferon®-A). Purity by either means is 99% or greater based on final protein content. Human interferon alfa C (Interpharm) is also a bacterially derived recombinant protein with a high relative specific (antiviral) activity of 1 to 2×10^9 U/mg protein (Merimsky et al 1991).

Interferon alfa-n3 is derived from pooled buffy coat leukocytes from fresh human blood. The donors are screened for hepatitis B, human immunodeficiency virus type 1 (HIV-1), human T-lymphotropic virus type 1 (HTLV-1), cytomegalovirus (CMV), and Epstein–Barr virus (EBV) negativity. Sendai virus is used to induce interferon production from these leukocytes and the resultant material is then purified by immunoaffinity chromatography with a murine monoclonal antibody (NK-2 column, Cell Tech, Slough, England). The antibody binds multiple species of human alpha interferon. Subsequent steps involve incubation at 4°C, pH 2, for 5 days to inactivate any viruses followed by gel filtration chromatography. A slight amount of murine IgG remains in the preparation (0.9–5.6 ng/10^6 IU), but otherwise the product has over 95% purity of mixed alpha interferons. The specific activity of this product is approximately 2×10^8 IU/mg of protein.

Because of slightly different chemical compositions, interferon content has been standardized using World Health Organization International Units (IU). This is based on biological antiviral activity, specifically a cytopathic effect inhibition assay using human foreskin diploid fibroblasts exposed to encephalomyocarditis virus. The specific activity of recombinant alpha interferons is then compared with the activity from an international reference standard of human leukocyte interferon. Thusly defined, the specific activity of commercial recombinant alpha interferons is 2×10^8 IU of antiviral activity per milligram of protein determined by the Lowry method.

■ Antitumor Activity

Alpha interferons are active in several hematologic and solid tumors (Goldstein and Laszlo 1986) (see table below). The U.S. Food and Drug Administration-approved labeling indications for alpha interferons are hairy cell leukemia and acquired immunodeficiency syndrome (AIDS)-associated Kaposi's sarcoma. Some nonmalignant conditions also respond to alpha interferons including condyloma acuminata (venereal warts) (Eron et al 1986), cervical papillomas (Seto et al 1984), laryngeal papillomas (McCabe and Clark 1983, Leventhal et al 1991), and certain forms of chronic hepatitis B (Eddleston 1986) and chronic hepatitis C (Davis et al 1989).

Hematologic Malignancies. In hairy cell leukemia, alpha interferon produces partial response rates of

RESPONSE RATES TO SYSTEMIC INTERFERON ALFA

	Typical Response Rate (%)	Reference
Hematologic malignancies		
Hairy cell leukemia	85 (90)*	Quesada et al 1984
Chronic lymphocytic leukemia	33 (100)	Misset et al 1982
Chronic myelogenous leukemia	88 (100)	Talpaz 1988
Multiple myeloma	30 (100)	Cooper et al 1986
Lymphoma	25 (75)	Louie et al 1981
Mycosis fungoides	45 (100)	Bunn et al 1986
Solid tumors		
Kaposi's sarcoma	25 (100)	Krown et al 1990
Malignant melanoma	18 (100)	Kirkwood and Ernstoff 1984
Malignant carcinoid	65 (100)	Oberg et al 1987
Renal cell carcinoma	15–26 (80–90)	Neidhart et al 1985, Figlin et al 1988, Quesada et al 1985
Laryngeal papilloma	71 (50)	Goepfert et al 1982

*Total (partial).

75 to 85% (Quesada et al 1984). Responses to alpha interferon typically involve hematologic improvement in peripheral blood levels of platelets, leukocytes, and erythrocytes and a decreased incidence of infection within 2 to 3 months of starting therapy. There is usually not complete eradication of the malignant hairy cell clone in the bone marrow following alpha interferon treatment. Therefore, alpha interferon therapy must be administered continuously for at least 6 months to obtain a response. Alpha interferon is not curative in this disease but responses have a relatively long duration and survival is significantly improved in responding patients (Golomb et al 1985).

Chronic myelogenous leukemia (CML) also responds to alpha interferon with partial response rates of up to 80% (Talpaz et al 1983). Like hairy cell leukemia, CML patients usually achieve only partial hematologic remissions of their disease. Occasionally, response is associated with the loss of the Ph[1] chromosome. Responses can generally be maintained for 2 to 3 years. When patients become interferon resistant, their disease is usually in a chronic phase. More uncommonly, an accelerated phase or acute blast crisis occurs which is lymphoblastoid only approximately 15% of the time and sensitive to hydroxyurea. In CML, thrombocytosis appears to be effectively controlled by a mechanism independent of the effect on granulocytes. Alpha interferon has also been found to be highly effective in the treatment of essential thrombocytosis (Giles et al 1988).

Non-Hodgkin's lymphomas of a more indolent nature (low grade, favorable prognosis) are responsive to alpha interferon. These include nodular, poorly differentiated lymphomas in previously treated patients. Response rates of up to 70% are reported with remission durations of 6 to 12 months (Louie et al 1981). Other histologies such as diffuse histiocytic lymphoma (intermediate grade) rarely respond to interferon.

Multiple Myeloma. Overall response rates in multiple myeloma are reported in 20 to 30% of previously treated patients (Cooper et al 1986). When interferon is combined with alkylators such as melphalan or cyclophosphamide and prednisone in previously untreated patients, much higher response rates of up to 78% are described but the effect of alpha interferon in the combination is unclear (Cooper et al 1986). Importantly, substantial alkylator drug dose reductions are required in such protocols (see Dosage and Drug Interactions sections).

Interferon alfa-2b has also been shown to increase response durations and survival when used as maintenance treatment for multiple myeloma in remission after cytotoxic therapy (Mandelli et al 1990). Therapy was given three times weekly at doses similar to those used in hairy cell leukemia.

Solid Tumors

Kaposi's Sarcoma. Response rates to alpha interferon are generally lower in solid tumors. In renal cell carcinoma and in Kaposi's sarcoma, a dose–response relationship has been evident in some studies. Very high doses are reportedly effective in patients with stage II or III, epidemic, AIDS-related Kaposi's sarcoma (Groopman et al 1984); however, the severe toxicity of these regimens limit their efficacy in this patient population (see Dosage for tolerable dose escalation schemes). Importantly, alpha interferon can be safely combined with zidovudine (AZT) in AIDS patients with Kaposi's sarcoma (Krown et al 1990).

Malignant Melanoma. Response rates in malignant melanoma vary from 5 to 29% with a median of 18% (Goldstein and Laszlo 1986). Of interest, alpha interferon is highly active when given intralesionally in this disease (Von Wussow et al 1988). Unfortunately, early descriptions of synergy with oral cimetidine (Borgstrum et al 1983) or greater response rates with high doses (often given intravenously) have not been reproduced in follow-up studies (Goldstein and Laszlo 1986).

Renal Cell Carcinoma. The response rate in renal cell carcinoma ranges from 15 to 31%, with a majority being partial responses (80–90%) (Figlin et al 1988, Quesada et al 1985, Neidhart et al 1985). A large percentage of additional patients may have minor responses but neither these nor the partial responses confer greater survival. Some studies suggest that higher doses are required to obtain responses in renal cell cancer (see Dosage) (Kirkwood et al 1985, Quesada et al 1985). As with interleukin-2, responses to alpha interferon in renal cell carcinoma occur predominantly in lung parenchyma or mediastinal lymph node metastases (Quesada et al 1985). Up to 30% of 41 renal cell carcinoma patients receiving a high-dose regimen achieved a partial response (PR) or complete response (CR) in contrast to no responses in 15 patients treated at the low dose level, 2.0 versus 20×10^6 U/m^2 IM daily (Quesada et al 1985).

Locoregional Applications. Alpha interferon is active when administered locoregionally or intralesionally in a variety of malignancies (see table below). Notably, these include bladder carcinoma, wherein multiple superficial tumors are not as responsive to intravesical interferon as is carcinoma in situ (Torti et al 1984). In ovarian carcinoma, high-dose intraperitoneal therapy is highly effective for patients with small residual tumors (< 5 mm) after surgery (Berek et al 1985). Alpha interferon is also active when administered intralesionally into malignant melanoma (von Wussow et al 1988) and condyloma acuminata (Eron et al 1986, Friedman-Kien et al 1988). Recombinant interferon alfa-2b (Intron® A) and natural leukocyte interferon alfa-n3 (Alferon® N Injection) are both approved for the intralesional therapy of venereal warts or condyloma acuminata. Although not curative, these therapies are associated with eradication of lesions in about one third of patients and more than 50% shrinkage in wart areas in over half of patients receiving one to three weekly intralesional injections of interferon alfa-2b (Eron et al 1986). Twice weekly injections of naturally derived interferon alfa-n3 (about 1×10^6 IU) have been associated with wart eradication in 62% of patients and wart shrinkage in all patients (Friedman-Kien et al 1988). The drug has some topical activity against cervical carcinoma, although response rates are low and the duration of partial remissions is short (Seto et al 1984).

In patients with advanced head and neck cancer, intralesional therapy (3×10^5 IU/d × 14) was highly effective in 10 of 30 patients with a variety of histologic diagnoses and avoided more extensive surgeries in a number of patients (Ikic 1982). A similar regimen has been used in a small number of breast cancer patients treated with local daily injections of 2×10^6 units for 2 months (Ikic 1982). Local tumor regressions were observed in 4 of 4 patients who also received three systemic (intramuscular) (IM) alpha interferon injections of 2×10^6 IU each week (Ikic 1982).

Antiviral Therapies. Clearly, the major physiologic role of alpha interferon is that of an antiviral cytokine. Thus, it is not surprising that the drug has significant antiviral efficacy against a variety of diseases (see table on page 568). The majority of these applications are for prophylaxis (rhinovirus, cytomegalovirus, herpes simplex). In addition, alpha interferon has impressive activity against human papillomavirus diseases of the larynx in children and the uterine cervix in adults (Strander 1986). The use of alpha interferon in the latter setting often spares the patient multiple surgeries, which produce significant local trauma and scarring. Another important antiviral role for alpha interferon is in the treatment of chronic hepatitis B (Eddleston 1986) and hepatitis C (Davis et al 1989). These uses can lead to significant reductions in long-term morbidity and possibly mortality. Finally, alpha interferon can decrease the frequency of viral isolation in patients with asymptomatic human immunodeficiency virus infection (Lane et al 1990).

■ Mechanism of Action

For antitumor activity, alpha interferon must first interact with specific high-affinity cell surface receptors. These receptors are the same as used for beta interferon internalization (Aguet and Mogenson 1983). Most human cells possess alpha/beta interferon receptors, and receptor densities range from 100 to 10,000 per cell; however, receptor quantities do not directly correlate with alpha interferon activ-

RESPONSE RATES TO LOCOREGIONAL OR TOPICAL INTERFERON ALFA

Disease	Administration Route	Response Rate, Comment	Reference
Superficial bladder cancer	Intravesical	20–40 (higher in carcinoma in situ)	Torti et al 1984
Ovarian carcinoma	Intraperitoneal	5/7 (71% in residual tumor < 5 mm) 0/4 (0% if residual tumors > 5 mm)	Berek et al 1985
Cervical carcinoma in situ	Topical	5/5 (100%)	Seto et al 1984
Condyloma acuminata (venereal warts)	Intralesional	40–60% reduction in wart areas 36% CRs* in treated warts	Eron et al 1986; Friedman-Kien et al 1988
Malignant melanoma	Intralesional	2/51 (4% systemic CRs) 6/51 (12% systemic PRs) 23/51 (45% local lesions PRs)	Von Wussow et al 1988

*CR, complete response; PR, partial response.

ANTIVIRAL EFFECTS OF INTERFERON ALFA

Viral Infection	Route of Administration	Response Rate, Comment	Reference
Rhinovirus	Intranasal	Up to 90%, prophylactic use needed	Douglas et al 1986
Cytomegalovirus		Prophylaxis in transplant patients	Cheeseman et al 1979
Human immunodeficiency virus (HIV)	Systemic (SC)	> 75% p24 HIV antigen reduction in 40% of patients	Lane et al 1988
Herpes simplex			Pazin et al 1979
Herpes zoster			Merigan et al 1978
Human papillomavirus*		(For review see Strander 1986)	
Chronic hepatitis B	Systemic (IM, SC)		Eddleston 1986

*See entries for Laryngeal papilloma and Cervical Carcinoma in situ in first and second tables, respectively.

ity. The binding affinity for alpha interferon to its receptor is quite high with K_D's in the range 10^{-10} to 10^{-12} M.

Following binding, the alpha interferon/receptor complex is internalized, the complex is degraded partially, and the receptor is returned to the cell surface. Unidentified intracellular signals between the receptor complex and the nucleus then produce rapid but transient changes in gene transcription. Increased gene transcription following alpha interferon is not dependent on new protein synthesis, but it does lead to the induction of several new proteins (see table on the opposite page). Clearly, the major physiologic role of many of these proteins is the production of an enhanced antiviral state in the cell. This is characterized by the activation of other immune system cells and the release of other cytokines, some with direct antitumor cytolytic potential (eg, interleukin-2[IL-2] and tumor necrosis factor [TNF]). Biochemical changes in the cell include the enhanced expression of 2′, 5′-oligoadenylate synthetase (2′, 5′-A), an enzyme that forms long polyadenylated nucleotide strands. Of interest, the levels of 2′, 5′-A in malignant lymphoid cells have been found to correlate with response in patients with chronic myelogenous leukemia (Rosenblum et al 1986). The increase in 2′, 5′-A levels acts in concert with any double-stranded (viral) RNA (dsRNA) to induce several endonucleases which can halt synthesis of new mRNA and rRNA with a subsequent blockade of protein synthesis (Williams and Kerr 1980). A specific protein kinase is also induced when alpha interferon and dsRNA are present and a subunit on the elongation/initiation factor 2 (eIF-2) is phosphorylated, leading to a blockade in the delivery of RNA to the ribosome (Samuel 1979). New protein synthesis is thereby halted.

In contrast, some genes and proteins are not induced but are inhibited by alpha interferon. These include the oncogenes *c-myc, c-H-ras,* and *c-fos* (Contente et al 1990) and the protein ornithine decarboxylase, which is the rate-limiting enzyme involved in polyamine synthesis (Taylor-Papadimitriou and Rozengurt 1985). The downregulation of the *c-myc* gene by alpha interferon has been used to explain the cell cycle-inhibitory effect of alpha interferon (Einat and Kimchi 1988). Other repressed genes include those for the receptors for insulin, transferrin, and epidermal growth factor (EGF) (Faltynek and Kung 1988). In renal cell carcinoma, alpha interferon reduces EGF receptors by a posttranscriptional mechanism, possibly a block in translational elongation (Eisenkraft et al 1991). These effects arrest cells in the G_0/G_1 interphase, although alpha interferon also slows cell cycle progression through all phases of division (Balkwill and Taylor-Papadimitriou 1978).

Overall, the antitumor activity of alpha interferon may relate to a composite of several of the effects described earlier and probably differs in different tumor cell lines. Principally, the antitumor effect appears to involve cytostatic mechanisms that relate to direct or indirect regulation of cell growth. Direct regulation of tumor cell growth by alpha interferon may involve inhibition of growth signal production as a result of oncogene and growth receptor downregulation, induction of maturation or differentiation factors, or general inhibition of protein synthesis. This last effect can be profound and is probably responsible for several drug interactions involving microsomal enzyme metabolism. Perhaps the strongest argument for some direct antitumor effects from alpha interferon comes from studies showing broad-spectrum inhibition of human tumor colon formation in vitro when alpha interferon is added to the growth medium in the absence of any immune effector cells (Salmon et al 1983).

GENES AND PROTEINS ALTERED IN INTERFERON ALFA-RESPONSIVE CELLS

Genes and Proteins Induced	Physiologic Role	Therapeutic Implication
2′,5′-oligoadenylate synthetase	Activates a latent cellular endonuclease (in concert with viral double-stranded RNA)	Reduced transcription of mRNA and rRNA to block protein synthesis, also a marker of therapeutic activity in CML cells (Rosenblum et al 1986)
M_X protein	Inhibition of flu virus replication	Unknown
Indoleamine 2,3-dioxygenase	Catabolism of tryptophan	Tryptophan deprivation
Thymosin B_4	Lymphocyte maturation	Enhanced cytotoxicity in lymphocytes
Class I and II major histocompatibility (MHC) loci	Increased antigen expression and antigen presenting capability	Stimulation of host recognition of and host response to tumor cells
Tumor necrosis factor (TNF)	Activation of cellular proteases and phospholipases; activation of macrophages, neutrophils, and lymphocytes	Direct tumor cell lysis, recruitment of LAK and NK cells
Interleukin-2 (IL-2)	Stimulation of LAK or TIL cell production	Tumor cell lysis
Neopterin (a pyrazinopyrimidine)	Results from a GTP degradation pathway leading to the synthesis of tetrahydrobiopterin (Fuchs et al 1988)	A therapeutic marker of interferon alfa activity in monocytes and macrophages (Gastl et al 1989)

Data from Balkiwill 1989.

Indirect (immune) mechanisms of alpha interferon involve primarily stimulation of host responses to tumor cells. This has excellent experimental evidence: (1) enhancement of natural killer (NK) cell activity; (2) release of other toxic cytokines such as IL-2 and TNF; and (3) enhanced antigen expression in some tumor cells from an effect on major histocompatibility complex (MHC) proteins (although this effect is generally greater for interferon gamma) (Boyer et al 1989, Maio et al 1989).

■ **Availability and Storage**

There are two commercial formulations of recombinant interferon alfa, and one natural source mixture of alpha interferons is available (see table on page 570). The recombinant formulations differ in the use of a protein carrier and the availability of a premixed solution (both Roferon®-A, Roche Laboratories, Nutley, New Jersey). The latter solution contains phenol as a preservative and human serum albumin to reduce drug adsorption to infusion containers. Interferon alfa-2b (Intron® A, Schering Corporation, Kenilworth, New Jersey) uses a mixture of human albumin and glycine to suppress hydrophobic and ionic characteristics, which otherwise can lead to binding to siliconized glass and polypropylene infusion surfaces.

The natural-source alpha interferon, interferon alfa-n3 (Alferon® N Injection; The Purdue Frederick Company, Norwalk, Connecticut), is derived from human leukocytes and is a mixture of different species of alpha interferon. It is officially indicated for the treatment of genital warts.

■ **Preparation for Use, Stability, and Admixture**

Lyophilized alpha interferon powders are reconstituted by gentle aspiration with the diluent provided or Bacteriostatic Water for Injection, USP. Freezing and vigorous agitation of the vials are discouraged to avoid possible drug breakdown. A final alpha interferon concentration of 3 to 5×10^6 IU/mL is desired. Alpha interferon solutions slowly decompose in strong light or at room temperatures; however, they generally retain greater than 90% potency for at least 7 days at room temperature, and the commercial formulations do not significantly bind to glass or plastic large-volume parenteral infusion system surfaces or sterilizing (0.22 μm size) membrane filters.

Alpha interferon solutions are compatible and stable (at least 24 hours) with all standard infusion fluids including 0.9% sodium chloride, diluted amino acid solutions, and Lactated Ringers Injec-

COMMERCIAL INTERFERON ALFA FORMULATIONS

Parameter	Interferon Alfa-2a (Roferon®-A)	Interferon Alfa-2b (Intron®A)	Interferon Alfa-n3 (Alferon®)
Vial size (million IU)	3 (1 mL), 18 (3 mL)	3, 5, 10, 25	5 (1 mL)
Diluent provided	(In solution)	Bacteriostatic water for injection	(In phosphate-buffered saline solution)
Additives (per mL)	NaCl 9 mg, human serum albumin 5 mg, phenol 3 mg	Phosphate pH buffer, glycine, and human albumin	Containing 8 mg sodium chloride, 1.74 mg sodium phosphate dibasic, 0.2 mg potassium phosphate dibasic and monobasic (each), 0.2 mg potassium chloride, 3.3 mg phenol as a preservative, and 1 mg human serum albumin as a stabilizer
Chemistry and production	Recombinant DNA, non-glycosylated, amino acid No. 23 = arginine	Recombinant DNA, non-glycosylated, amino acid No. 23 = methionine	Supernatant from human white blood cells, mixture of glycosylated proteins
Visual	Clear solution	Lyophilized powder; clear to yellow solution after reconstitution	Clear solution
Storage	Refrigeration (2–8°C [36–46°F])	Refrigeration (2–8°C [36–46°F])	Refrigeration (2–8°C [36–46°F])
Stability	30 days after reconstitution if stored at 2–8°C	30 days after reconstitution if stored at 2–8°C	Dated on each vial
Precautions	Avoid freezing and vigorous shaking		Discard if discolored (dark solution) or if particulate matter is present
Preparation source	Recombinant DNA in *E. coli* using human α2a gene	Recombinant DNA in *E. coli* using human α-2b gene	Virus-induced human leukocyte cultures followed acidification immunoaffinity
Purification process	Affinity chromatography using a murine monoclonal antibody	Acidification, ethanol extraction, and gel chromatography	Chromatography using a murine monoclonal antibody

tion, USP; however, the commercial alpha interferons are not compatible in 5% Dextrose for Injection, USP, because of short stability (less than 8 hours). Interferon alfa-2b (Intron® A) has been shown to be compatible with the following infusion systems: Volumetric Infusion Pump (McGaw Laboratories, San Diego, CA); Provider 2000® peristaltic infusion pump (Pancretec, Inc, San Diego, California); Porta-A-Cath® implantable access port (Pharmacia-Deltec, St. Paul, Minnesota). Intron® A was *not* compatible with the Infusor® elastomeric infusion pump (Travenol Laboratories, Deerfield, Illinois).

Subcutaneous alpha interferon doses can be reconstituted in highly concentrated solutions (≥ 6 × 10^6 IU/mL) for either bolus or prolonged subcutaneous infusions (Dorr et al 1988).

■ Administration

Systemic Administration. Alpha interferon can be administered by intravenous, subcutaneous, and intramuscular routes. These routes are favored because of the ease of administration with nearly complete bioavailability and the avoidance of high peak plasma levels. Oral administration is inefficient because of avid breakdown in the gut. A review of different routes of administration has been published (Bocci 1984).

Intralesional Administration. In malignant melanoma alpha interferon has been administered both intralesionally and perilesionally. Doses up to 10 × 10^6 IU are diluted into 1 to 2 mL of saline for these treatments. For intralesional therapy of condyloma acuminata, doses of 1×10^6 IU are injected in a volume of 0.1 mL of diluent.

Other investigational intralesional applications of alpha interferon include the injection of 3×10^5 units daily for 2 weeks, then three times weekly to patients with advanced head and neck cancers (Ikic 1982).

Other Types of Administration. See Special Applications for investigational topical, intraventricular/intrathecal, intravesical, intrapleural, and intraperitoneal uses of alpha interferon.

■ Special Precautions

Patients receiving alpha interferon should be evaluated for adequate fluid balance to prevent serious dehydration brought on by the fever, chills, and general flulike syndrome elicited by the drug. Similarly, the drug should be used cautiously in patients with a history of cardiovascular disease, pulmonary disease, or diabetes mellitus.

■ Dosage

A wide range of dose schedules are reported for alpha interferon used in various indications (see table). The approved (package insert) dose levels in hairy cell leukemia range from 3×10^6 IU/d (Roferon®-A) to 2×10^6 IU/m² SC or IM three times per week (Intron® A). Lower doses of 0.2×10^6 IU/m² three times per week are less effective in patients with hairy cell leukemia. Response rates of 54% (18% complete) are described in one study (Moormeier et al 1989). This dose was ineffective for treating patients who relapsed following previous alpha interferon therapy (Thompson et al 1989); however, in one series this dose was effective and produced little toxicity but consistent elevation in the biomarker protein neopterin (Gastl et al 1989). In solid tumors, extremely high doses have been evaluated, up to 50×10^6 IU/m² as a daily single injection. For most alpha interferon-responsive diseases, however, the dose–response curve is flat beyond a dose of 5×10^6 IU/m² (Goldstein and Lazlo 1986). The three disease states in which dose–response relationships have been critically evaluated include renal cell carcinoma, AIDS-associated Kaposi's sarcoma, and lymphoma. The data are most persuasive for Kaposi's sarcoma wherein clinical response rates are maximal after daily dose levels of 10×10^6 IU/m² or greater are achieved (Goldstein and Lazlo 1986). Because the toxicity of high-dose alpha interferon can be severely debilitating in patients with AIDS-related Kaposi's sarcoma, it is advisable to escalate dose levels slowly in 3×10^6 IU/m² increments up to 20 to 30×10^6 IU/m² over several weeks and to immediately reduce doses by 50% when serious toxicity is encountered.

For the treatment of non-A, non-B hepatitis (hepatitis C), an effective dose was 3×10^6 IU given subcutaneously three times per week for 6 months. A lower dose of 1×10^6 IU was not effective in this disease, thereby demonstrating a dosing threshold effect for this antiviral indication (Davis et al 1989). In renal cell carcinoma, lymphoma, and malignant melanoma, response rates are maximal at intermediate dose levels of 5 to 10×10^6 IU/m² three times weekly. With the exception of intravesical therapy

DOSE LEVELS OF INTERFERON ALFA

Indication	Route	Dose Level	Reference
Hairy cell leukemia	SC, IM	3 IU × 10⁶/m² daily (Roferon®-A) or 2 IU × 10⁶/m² 3 times/wk (Intron®A)	Quesada et al 1984 Golumb et al 1985
Chronic myelogenous leukemia	SC, IM	3–9 IU × 10⁶/m² daily	Talpaz et al 1983
Solid tumors Renal cell, malignant Melanoma, carcinoid Syndrome, multiple myeloma	SC, IM	5–10 IU × 10⁶/m² daily to 3 times/wk	Goldstein and Lazlo 1986
Kaposi's sarcoma	SC, IM	Escalate slowly to 20–30 IU × 10⁶/m² daily	Groopman et al 1984
Condyloma acuminata	IL*	1 IU × 10⁶	Eron et al 1986
Hepatitis C	SC	3 IU × 10⁶, 3 times/wk × 24 wk	Davis et al 1989

*IL, intralesional.

for bladder cancer or intraperitoneal therapy for ovarian cancer, few diseases require alpha interferon doses greater than 15×10^6 IU/m^2. An exception is Kaposi's sarcoma in which the recommended dose is 20×10^6 IU/m^2/d. When alpha interferon was combined with zidovudine (100–200 mg every 4 hours) in AIDS patients with Kaposi's sarcoma, dose-limiting toxic effects occurred with continuous alpha interferon doses of 9×10^6 IU/d (Krown et al 1990). The maximally tolerated daily interferon doses with 100 and 200 mg of zidovudine (every 4 hours) were 4.5×10^6 and 18×10^6 IU.

Most alpha interferon dosing regimens repeat daily doses every 2 to 3 days. This is based on the known antitumor activity of these schedules as well as recent pharmacodynamic data showing that 2 to 3 days of antiviral activity follow the administration of single doses in normal volunteers (Barouki et al 1987). In addition to antiviral activity (inhibition of infectivity of vesicular stomatitis virus), the induction of the antiviral protein 2′, 5′-A begins within 6 hours and returns to baseline 96 to 104 hours after dosing (Barouki et al 1987). Indeed this enzyme may act as a biologic marker of alpha interferon response in patients with hairy cell leukemia (Rosenblum et al 1986).

The pharmacodynamic studies also show that antiviral activity and 2′, 5′-A induction are elevated in a true dose–response fashion (Witter et al 1987). Near-maximal elevations of both activities are achieved with doses of 3×10^6 IU given intramuscularly. Of interest, higher intravenous doses are not associated with significantly greater biologic effects in healthy volunteers (Witter et al 1987); however, high daily doses of 17.5×10^6 IU were effective at reducing the frequency of viral isolation in asymptomatic AIDS patients (Lane et al 1990). In patients with hairy cell leukemia, very low dose therapy of 0.3×10^6 IU/m^2 given three times weekly is associated with a 54% overall response rate (18% CR + PR); however, longer treatment durations are required to achieve responses, and in one fourth of the patients, disease progressed rapidly, indicating a poor-quality response (Moormeier et al 1989). In addition, response rates to such low doses are less frequent. This suggests that there is a very low threshold for alpha interferon biologic activity which may not necessarily correlate with the intensity of clinical toxicity (Witter et al 1987). At high dose levels there is clearly a correlation with severe toxicity. Thus, for most disease states the antitumor dose–response curve is flat, whereas serious toxic effects increase in proportion to the dose.

■ Drug Interactions

Alpha interferon has been combined experimentally with a number of other agents (see table). Most drug interactions are limited to tumor cell culture studies in vitro or studies in non-tumor-bearing rodents (Smyth et al 1987). Singh and Renton (1981) showed that inbred mice given injections of polyinosinic and cytidylic acid double-stranded oligomers to induce interferon had significantly lower activities of hepatic biotransforming enzymes. The enzymes affected included cytochrome P450 and aminopyrene N-demethylase. This inhibition appears to be a common property of interferon-inducing agents (Mannering et al 1980) as well as natural (Singh and Renton 1982) and recombinant interferons (Parkinson et al 1982). Commensurate with hepatic enzyme inhibition, drug-metabolizing activity is reduced in mice (Parkinson et al 1982). Similar effects in humans receiving alpha interferon and other drugs metabolized by P450 microsomal enzymes may be anticipated, and this may explain the reduced tolerance to some interferon–anticancer drug combinations. For example, cyclophosphamide is an alkylating agent whose activation and inactivation are both dependant on hepatic P450 metabolism. When alpha interferon and cyclophosphamide are administered concurrently to multiple myeloma patients, substantially reduced doses of cyclophosphamide are required if the concomitant interferon dose is greater than 3×10^6 IU (Durie et al 1986).

Similarly, Sarosy et al (1986) have noted that patients with solid tumors could tolerate only relatively low doxorubicin doses of 30 mg/m^2 in combination with an alpha interferon dose of 10×10^6 IU/m^2 three times per week. In another trial, alpha interferon did not alter the pharmacokinetics of a related anthracycline, epirubicin. Doxorubicin also did not enhance alpha interferon's antitumor efficacy in renal cell cancer (Muss et al 1985). Similar nonadditive efficacy has been reported for tolerable combinations of alpha interferon with vinblastine in renal cell cancer. In this instance, partial response rates ranged from 16% (Figlin et al 1986, Martinelli and Cavalli 1987) to 32% (Fossa et al 1986). The combination of cisplatin and alpha interferon produced unacceptable toxicity in a phase I trial of 5×10^6 IU/m^2 alpha interferon and 20 mg/m^2 cisplatin given daily for five doses (Martinelli and Cavalli 1987).

In animal trials, positive antitumor effects have been noted for alpha interferon combined with carmustine, cyclophosphamide, cisplatin, and eflorni-

DRUG COMBINATIONS WITH INTERFERON ALFA

Drug	Dose (mg/m^2)	Type of Study	α-IFN Dose (μg/m^2/d)	Effects	Reference
Aspirin/ acetaminophen	650 mg	Clinical trial, normal volunteers	18	No effect on clinical side effects nor on interferon antiviral activity	Witter et al 1988
Azidothymidine (AZT)	200 mg 100 mg	HIV patients with Kaposi's sarcoma	9/day	Tolerable combination with antiviral/antiproliferative activity	Krown et al 1990
Carmustine	—	Mouse leukemia	—	Additive or synergistic antitumor effects	Balkwill et al 1984
Chlorambucil	—	Clinical, lymphomas	—	14/23 (61%) response rate	Rohatiner et al 1987
Cisplatin		Human lung cancer, xenografts in mice		Additive or synergistic antitumor effects	Smyth et al 1987
	20 × 5 d	Clinical phase I	5	High toxicity, schedule not tolerated well	Martinelli and Cavalli 1987
	25/wk	Clinical phase I	5 tiw*	Moderate myelosuppression and fatigue	Dhingra et al 1991
Cyclophosphamide	—	Mouse lymphoma, neuroblastoma, and myeloma	—	Additive or synergistic antitumor effects	Balkwill and Moodie 1984
		Human breast and bowel cancer, xenografts in mice		Synergistic antitumor effect	Smyth et al 1987
		Human lung cancer, xenografts in mice		Synergistic antitumor effect	Smyth et al 1987
	150 × 4 d	Clinical multiple myeloma	3–5	Added toxicity especially with α-IFN doses > 3 × 10^6 μg/m^2	Durie et al 1986
Dexamethasone	—	Human leukocyte cell lines	—	Maintained antiproliferative action and enhanced HLK antigen expression	Pan and Guyre 1988
Doxorubicin		Human breast and lung, xenografts in mice		Synergistic antitumor effect	Balkwill and Moodie 1984
	20–40	Clinical phase I in solid tumors	10	Low doxorubicin MTD of 30 mg/m^2 due primarily to myelosuppression, 2/14 (14%) partial response rate	Sarosy et al 1986
Eflornithine		Daudi lymphoblastoid cells	—	Synergistic antitumor effects	Rosenblum and Gutterman 1984
	1500	Clinical phase I in melanoma	0.4–3.2	2/12 (17%) partial response rate	Talpaz et al 1986
Epirubicin	100	Clinical pharmacokinetic study	6	No change in epirubicin pharmacokinetics	Eksborg and Mattson 1988
Fluorouracil		Clinical phase I in colon cancer		1/6 (16%) partial responses	Cooper et al 1986
Fluoruro-pyrimidines[†]	—	Human colon cancer cell lines	—	Enhanced 5-fluorouracil cytotoxicity in vitro	Elias and Crissman 1988
Interferons beta and gamma		Human melanoma tumor cell lines		Additive or synergistic cytotoxicity (16%)	Schiller et al 1986

(*continued*)

DRUG COMBINATIONS WITH INTERFERON ALFA (continued)

Drug	Dose (mg/m^2)	Type of Study	α-IFN Dose (μg/m^2/d)	Effects	Reference
Indomethacin	25 mg	Clinical trial	10–20	Significant reduction of interferon side effects	
Melphalan/ prednisone				23/30 partial response rate	Wadler et al 1989a
Prednisone	40 mg	Clinical trial in normal volume	18	No effect on clinical side effects nor antiviral activity, halved induction of 2′,5′-oligoadenylate	Witter et al 1988
Vinblastine	0.15 (mg/kg)	Clinical, renal cell	3	3/24 (13%) partial response rate	Figlin et al 1986
	0.15 (mg/kg)	Carcinoma	18	4/25 (16%) partial response rate	Martinelli and Cavalli 1987
	0.1–0.15 (mg/kg)	Phase I in solid tumors	36	5/16 (32%) partial response rate	Fossa et al 1986

*tiw, three times weekly.
[†]5-Fluorouracil, floxuridine.

thine (Balkiwill 1989). The last combination produced dramatic synergy in human lymphoblastoid (Daudi) cells tested in vitro (Rosenblum and Gutterman 1984). In a phase I trial in patients with malignant melanoma, alpha interferon and eflornithine produced 2 partial responses in 12 patients (Talpaz et al 1986).

Other clinical studies have evaluated the impact of common anti-inflammatory agents on alpha-interferon activity or toxicity. When tested in vitro, glucocorticosteroids such as dexamethasone did not block alpha interferon's inhibition of tumor cell proliferation and enhancement of HLA antigen expression on several human lymphoblastic cell lines (Pan and Guyre 1988). A careful clinical trial by Witter et al (1988) has shown no inhibition of antiviral activity when high-dose interferon (18 × 10^6 IU) was combined with prednisone and aspirin or acetaminophen in normal volunteers; however, prednisone reduced by 50% the degree of alpha interferon induction of 2′, 5′-A synthetase in peripheral blood mononuclear cells. Interestingly, none of these agents significantly reduced alpha interferon side effects (chills, headache, myalgia, fatigue, *and* temperature elevation). In patients with malignant melanoma, indomethacin has been shown to reduce the fever associated with alpha interferon without interfering with its therapeutic or immunomodulatory activities (Miller et al 1989). The oral indomethacin dose in this study was 25 mg three times daily.

Interferons have been shown to interact experimentally with halogenated pyrimidines in human and murine tumor cell models. The synergistic cytotoxic effect is greatest for interferon gamma over interferon beta and for floxuridine over 5-fluorouracil (Elias and Crissman 1988). Because this interaction was inhibited by thymidine, the mechanism was postulated to involve enhanced inhibition of thymidylate synthetase by alpha interferon (Elias and Crissman 1988). Alternatively, alpha interferon can decrease thymidine uptake in tumor cells (Brouty-Boye and Tovey 1978, and Gewert et al 1981) and may also inhibit thymidine kinase activity (Gewert et al 1983). Wadler et al (1989a, b) observed therapeutic synergism for alpha interferon and 5-fluorouracil in vitro and in vivo. In a clinical trial, 5-fluorouracil (750 mg/m^2/d × 5) as a continuous infusion was followed by weekly bolus alpha interferon therapy (9 × 10^6 IU subcutaneously three times per week). Responses were observed in 15 of 36 (42%) previously untreated patients but in none of 13 previously treated patients (Wadler et al 1991); however, several follow-up trials have not confirmed results (Chun et al 1992, Cortesi et al 1992). Pharmacokinetic studies similarly show no effect of alpha-interferon on the disposition of 5-fluorouracil and methylene tetrahydrofolate in cancer patients (Patel et al 1992).

■ Pharmacokinetics

Alpha interferon is rapidly eliminated from the vascular compartment following parenteral administration (Wills et al 1984). The table below in this monograph summarizes the plasma pharmacokinetics for this agent when given by three different routes. In general, there are no significant pharmacokinetic differences between the forms of commercial alpha interferon. Both agents are slowly but nearly completely absorbed following intramuscular and subcutaneous administration (Wills et al 1984, Radwanski et al 1987). The subcutaneous and intramuscular routes may be associated with rate-limited absorption, which extends the apparent plasma elimination half-life (Wills et al 1984, Radwanski et al 1987). Disposition of intravenous alpha interferon appears to be adequately described by a two-compartment model with an initial distributive half-life of about 7 minutes (Radwanski et al 1987). The elimination half-life averages 4 to 5 hours in normal volunteers and clearance is brisk at 2.8 mL/min/kg (Wills et al 1984). There is also no evidence of drug accumulation or zero-order alpha interferon clearance in cancer patients receiving high-dose therapy on repetitive dosing regimens (Gutterman et al 1982).

Interferon alfa C (Interpharm) produces peak plasma levels of 53.2 U/mL following an intramuscular injection of 10×10^6 IU (Merimsky et al 1991). The area under the plasma concentration × time curve (AUC) for this dose was 1259 U · h/mL and the terminal half-life was 3 to 4 hours. As with the other interferons, the presence of renal failure did not alter interferon alfa C disposition (Merimsky et al 1991).

When it is given as a 14-day continuous intravenous infusion to leukemic patients, the clearance of interferon alfa-2a is lowered to about one third that in normal volunteers (Wills and Spiegel 1985). The apparent steady-state volume of distribution is also increased in this patient population; however, the elimination half-life is not significantly altered. Alpha interferon has been administered as a subcutaneous daily infusion continuously for several months and extremely high AUCs were obtained with this therapy (Dorr et al 1988). The estimated 24-hour AUC (AUC_{24}) ranged from 480 to 1464 IU/mL · h^{-1}, and the time needed to reach steady-state levels of 20 to 60 IU/mL was prolonged at 40 to 72 hours. These observations suggest that continuous subcutaneous infusions produce high exposures, possibly as a result of delayed drug clearance.

Alpha interferon does not effectively cross the blood–brain barrier, even when extremely high doses are administered intravenously (Smith et al 1985). Following intraventricular administration, interferon levels in the cerebrospinal fluid approach 3500 U/mL with no serious central nervous system toxicity (Smith et al 1982). The clearance of interferon from the cerebrospinal fluid is slow, with an

MEAN PHARMACOKINETIC PARAMETERS FOR INTERFERON ALFA ADMINISTERED INTRAVENOUSLY, INTRAMUSCULARLY, OR SUBCUTANEOUSLY

Route of Administration	Peak Concentration (IU/mL)*	t_{max} (h)	Area Under Curve (IU·h/mL)	Terminal Phase Half-life (h)	Volume of Distribution (L/kg)	Clearance (mL/min/kg)	Bioavailability (%)
IV infusion (over 40 min)	2950	—	2933	5.1	0.4	216	NR[†]
Continuous IV infusion[‡]	—	—	7756 (per day)	7.3	9.5	71.5	NR
IM[§]	337	3.8	2433	2.3	NR	NR	83
SC[§]	288	7.3	2650	3.5	NR	NR	90
SC (continuous infusion)[#]	19–61	40–72	480–1464	NR	NR	NR	NR

*The data were converted to IU using a factor of 6 pg/IU.
[†]Not reported.
[‡]Modified after Wills and Spiegel 1985; n = 4 leukemia patients.
[§]Modified after Dorr et al 1988; dose levels were 2.5–3.6 × 10^6 IU/m^2/d × 28.
[#]Modified after Wills et al 1984; n = 6 normal volunteers (36 × 10^6 IU fixed dose).

initial half-life of 2 hours and persistence of detectable drug levels for several days (Bocci 1984). In contrast, no interferon could be detected in the ventricular cerebrospinal fluid of patients receiving 1×10^6 IU of alpha interferon by intrathecal (lumbar) administration.

The major route of alpha interferon clearance involves renal elimination (Bino et al 1982, Bocci et al 1982a, b). Alpha interferon undergoes glomerular filtration and subsequent proteolytic degradation during renal tubular reabsorption (Bocci et al 1982a). As catabolism of the molecule is nearly complete, very little if any alpha interferon is returned to the circulation or excreted in the urine (Wills et al 1984). Patients with chronic renal failure have alpha interferon pharmacokinetics similar to that of patients with normal renal function (Hirsch et al 1983). There was also no effect of hemodialysis on alpha interferon pharmacokinetics. Data from animal studies show that very little alpha interferon is metabolized in the liver (Bocci et al 1982b); however, the fact that clearance values (up to 216 mL/min; see table) are generally much higher than glomerular filtration suggests that, in addition to tubular secretion and catabolism, some nonrenal elimination must also occur.

■ Side Effects and Toxicity

The major acute toxic effects of alpha interferon involve a flulike syndrome consisting of fever, chills, slight tachycardia, malaise, myalgias, and headaches (Quesada et al 1986). In up to 40% of patients, chills usually precede the fever, which peaks within 4 to 6 hours of intramuscular or subcutaneous drug administration. Large doses or intravenous administration significantly increases the intensity of such reactions. For severe flu symptoms, indomethacin may be most useful (Miller et al 1989), and although acetaminophen is commonly used, its efficacy may be minimal (Witter et al 1988). Transient hypotension and syncope are rarely encountered unless high doses and/or intravenous administration is used. Luckily, a slow tachyphylaxis (tolerance) to the flu syndrome develops on continued dosing over several months.

Fatigue is typically the most common reason for alpha interferon dose reductions (Quesada et al 1986). Tolerance is improved with late-night administration and intermittent dosing schedules.

Gastrointestinal effects of alpha interferon are usually limited to anorexia in 20 to 30% of patients and an altered taste sensation in some patients. Again, the most severe toxic effects occur after dose levels of 10×10^6 IU or greater are administered. At these dose levels, weight loss and nausea with some vomiting can occur. A watery type of severe diarrhea is also described following high-dose therapy.

Hepatic and renal toxic effects are rare with alpha interferon. Approximately 25 to 30% of patients will have a slight elevation in transaminase levels, and some proteinuria is described in 15 to 20% of patients. The incidence and severity of hepatic enzyme elevation are clearly dose related and more commonly involve serum glutamic–oxalacetic and glutamic–pyruvic transaminases rather than lactate dehydrogenase. In contrast, proteinuria and increases in serum creatinine are infrequent and apparently not dose dependent.

Alpha interferons produce very mild and transient myelosuppressive toxic effects. Leukopenia to 40 to 60% of baseline levels can be observed within hours of drug administration. This is associated with reduced granulocyte/monocyte colony-forming units (GM-CFUs) in the bone marrow (Ernstoff et al 1985). The rapid reversal of leukopenia when interferon is stopped suggests that part of the effect is due to redistribution of leukocytes rather than a direct cytotoxic effect (Quesada et al 1986). Both the granulocyte and lymphocyte levels decrease rapidly after interferon, then plateau and recover briskly after a day. There is also some suggestion of a reversible block in the release of mature cells from the bone marrow. Mild, asymptomatic thrombocytopenia and normochromic normocytic anemia also occur in patients receiving prolonged therapy. Rarely, immune-related hemolytic anemia or thrombocytopenia may occur. This is usually responsive to corticosteroids (Quesada et al 1986).

Neurotoxic effects are typically described only in patients receiving very high doses of alpha interferon ($> 20 \times 10^6$ IU). Both central and peripheral nervous system toxic effects are described. Patients given very large single doses of alpha interferon ($\geq 50 \times 10^6$ IU) have experienced marked somnolence, lethargy, confusion, and diffuse motor slowing, rarely producing seizures or dysphagia. Paresthesias have been described in the same high-dose patients. The distribution is usually distal and rarely has a circumoral presentation. It is believed to represent a mild reversible sensory motor neuropathy. As anticipated, this toxicity is more common in patients treated concomitantly or previously with vinca alkaloids.

Alpha interferon is not a vesicant and only rarely causes skin toxicity, usually manifested as a maculopapular rash on the trunk and extremities. Rarely, diffuse erythema and urticaria can occur. Continuous subcutaneous infusions were also associated with local site erythema and rarely cellulitis if injection sites were not rotated every 1 to 2 days (Dorr et al 1988). Alpha interferon does produce a mild degree of alopecia if therapy continues longer then a few months.

The effects of alpha interferon on the cardiovascular system are primarily indirect. Signs include tachycardia, peripheral vasoconstriction, and distal cyanosis. Diaphoresis and hypotension are usually related to the severity of the acute febrile reaction to the drug (Quesada et al 1986). Although myocardial infarctions have been reported in patients receiving alpha interferon, this toxic effect has not been unequivocally associated directly with the drug. Likewise, AIDS patients receiving high-dose alpha interferon therapy for Kaposi's sarcoma have experienced reversible congestive heart failure (Deyton et al 1989); however, congestive heart failure has been noted in AIDS patients who were not receiving alpha interferon (Calabrese et al 1987), and in vitro, alpha interferon does not damage isolated beating rat heart myocytes (Dorr et al 1988). Other rare toxic effects reported following alpha interferon include an increase in urinary 11-hydroxycorticosteroids, decreases in serum estrogen and progesterone, and a decrease in high-density lipoproteins. The last effect may produce a 34% decrease in plasma cholesterol levels without altering triglyceride concentrations (Massaro et al 1986). This has led some to speculate that alpha interferon may act in vivo as a down regulator of cholesterol by inducing the activity of lipoprotein lipases.

Glycosuria, hyperkalemia, and hypercalcemia have been described although diabetic patients can usually tolerate alpha interferon therapy without problems. Hyponatremia resulting from the syndrome of inappropriate antidiuretic hormone secretion was reported in a few patients with amyotrophic lateral sclerosis given very high doses (100–200 $\times 10^6$ IU) of alpha interferon therapy. Tumor lysis syndrome and prolonged coagulation times are also described in some patients (Mirro et al 1985). Although alpha interferons are not specifically approved for use in pregnant or nursing females, the drug was not teratogenic, mutagenic, or carcinogenic in preclinical test screens.

Alpha-Interferon Antibodies. Like all protein-based drugs, alpha interferon can induce the formation of antibodies in some patients. Two different types of alpha interferon antibodies can be produced, neutralizing and nonneutralizing antibodies. Of these, the loss of alpha interferon activity is associated only with the rarer neutralizing type of antibody. The incidence of alpha interferon antibody formation may also vary with dose intensity, the specific patient population, the type of assay used for antibody detection, and the specific alpha interferon formulation.

With these considerations in mind there appear to be significant differences reported in the overall incidence of antibody formation with interferon alfa-2a, Roferon®-A (27%) (Jones and Itri 1986), and interferon alfa-2b, Intron® A (2.4%) (Spiegel et al 1986). In one clinical trial of interferon alfa-2a in renal cell carcinoma, neutralizing antibodies developed in 20 of 53 patients (38%) and was associated with the loss of antitumor activity in 7 of 12 initially responding patients (58%). In another trial in renal cell cancer, however, neutralizing antibodies had no effect on response rates or response durations (Figlin et al 1988).

A loss of response with antibody development has also been noted in hairy cell leukemia patients treated with either interferon alfa-2a (Steis et al 1988) or interferon alfa-2b (Von Wussow et al 1987). These antibodies may be lost with continuous interferon alfa-2a therapy (Steis et al 1990). In patients with chronic hepatitis, a significantly higher incidence of neutralizing antibodies was noted with interferon alfa-2a (20.2%) compared with interferon alfa-2b (6.9%) (Antonelli and Currenti 1991). The occurrence of antibodies to interferon alfa-2a has also been associated with reactivation of hepatitis B viral replication in white adults (Porres et al 1989) and Asians (Lok et al 1990).

It is clear that on prolonged therapy, neutralizing antibodies and the development of drug resistance can occur in a small fraction of patients receiving either commercial formulation of alpha interferon. Once a neutralizing antibody has developed, patients typically become resistant to both recombinant alpha interferons (2a or 2b), but not to natural leukocyte-derived alpha interferon such as Finnferon® (produced by the Finnish Red Cross) or Alferon® N Injection (produced by Interferon Sciences and distributed by The Purdue Frederick Company).

Special Applications

Topical Rhinovirus Prophylaxis. Alpha interferon has been administered topically to the nose in a solution containing 2.5×10^7 IU/mL. Each aerosol "puff" contained 1.25×10^6 IU, and two puffs were administered to each nostril daily for 7 days to normal family members of an individual with cold symptoms for 2 days (Douglas et al 1986). This regimen was effective at reducing the number of days of definite respiratory illness and the number of days with any nasal symptoms. Similar results have been described for volunteers challenged with intranasal rhinovirus after beginning a prophylactic regimen of aerosol leukocyte interferon (Scott et al 1982).

Intrathecal and Intraventricular Administration. Alpha interferon has been successfully given by intrathecal injections in patients with gliomas and other malignant brain tumors (Ueda et al 1982). Human leukocyte interferon alfa (Green Cross Corporation, 10^6 IU activity/mg protein) was dissolved in saline and administered intraventricularly via an Omaya reservoir daily or weekly for 1 to 6 months. Doses ranged from 5 to 10×10^5 IU/d to 2.8×10^7 IU/wk. The injections were well tolerated and produced a few responses in patients who had failed systemic interferon therapy. In contrast, intrathecal drug administration produces much lower ventricular cerebrospinal fluid concentrations of alpha interferon (Smith et al 1982; see Pharmacokinetics). Both routes of central nervous system drug administration are, however, well tolerated. Ventricular doses produce fever, chills and malaise and anorexia which resolves after 24 hours (Ueda et al 1982). There can also be some sterile cerebrospinal fluid pleocytosis and, rarely, meningitis, which is probably bacterial in etiology, following repeated intraventricular administrations.

Intravesical Administration. Alpha interferon has been instilled intravesically to experimentally treat bladder carcinoma and to reduce the recurrence of superficial bladder tumors (Williams 1988). Treatments of $1-1,000 \times 10^6$ IU diluted in saline were given twice a week for 5 weeks and responses are noted in 30 to 100% patients. Torti et al (1984) observed high response rates in patients with carcinoma in situ wherein large weekly intravesical alpha interferon doses of 50 to 200×10^6 IU were well tolerated.

Intrapleural Administration. Human leukocyte interferon has been administered by the intrapleural route to breast cancer patients with malignant pleural effusions (Ikic 1982). Patients received two to five instillations of several million International Units of interferon, with doses repeated every 3 to 5 days. Although this regimen eliminated malignant cells after the second or fourth dose, the effusions nonetheless persisted.

Intraperitoneal Administration. Berek et al (1985) described good activity for high doses of alpha interferon (50×10^6 IU) administered intraperitoneally to patients with advanced ovarian cancer. Five of seven patients with small residual peritoneal masses (< 5 mm in size) had surgically documented responses to the drug. Patients with larger residual masses did not respond. The primary toxic effect was fever, which was moderate in 60% and severe in 18% of patients. Abdominal pain occurred in 22% but peritonitis occurred in only one patient. High intraperitoneal alpha interferon levels of 5×10^4 IU/mL were obtained. These are generally 30- to 1000-fold higher than the levels that can be obtained by intramuscular, intravenous, or subcutaneous administration of standard doses. The alpha interferon doses were administered one to three times weekly in 250 mL saline following the instillation of 1750 mL of dialysis fluid.

REFERENCES

Aguet M, Mogenson KE. Interferon receptors. In: Gresser I, ed. *Interferon*. London: Academic Press; 1983:1–22.

Antonelli G, Currenti M. Neutralizing antibodies to interferon-α: Relative frequency in patients treated with different interferon preparations. *J Infect Dis.* 1991;**163**:882–885.

Balkwill FR. *Cytokines in Cancer Therapy*. Oxford: Oxford Press; 1989:23–47.

Balkwill FR, Moodie EM. Positive interactions between human interferon and cyclophosphamide or Adriamycin in a human tumor model system. *Cancer Res.* 1984;**44**:904–908.

Balkwill FR, Mowshowitz S, Seilman SS, et al. Positive interactions between interferon and chemotherapy due to direct tumor action rather than effects on host drug-metabolizing enzymes. *Cancer Res.* 1984;**44**:5249–5255.

Balkwill FR, Taylor-Papadimitriou J. Interferon affects both G_1 and $S + G_2$ in cells stimulated from quiescence to growth. *Nature.* 1978;**274**:798–800.

Barouki FM, Witter FR, Griffin DE, et al. Time course of interferon levels, antiviral state, 2′,5′-oligoadenylate synthetase and side effects in healthy men. *J Interferon Res.* 1987;**7**:29–39.

Berek JS, Hacker NF, Lichtenstein A, et al. Intraperitoneal

recombinant α-interferon for "salvage" immunotherapy in stage III epithelial ovarian cancer: A Gynecologic Oncology Group study. *Cancer Res.* 1985;**45**:4447–4453.

Bino T, Madar F, Gertler A, Rosenberg H. The kidney is the main site of interferon degradation. *J Interferon Res.* 1982;**2**:301–308.

Bocci V. Evaluation of routes of administration of interferon in cancer: A review and a proposal. *Cancer Drug Delivery.* 1984;**1**(4):337–351.

Bocci V, Pacini A, Bandinelli L, et al. The role of liver in the catabolism of human α- and β-interferon. *J Gen Virol.* 1982a;**60**:397–400.

Bocci V, Pacini A, Muscettola M, et al. The kidney is the main site of interferon catabolism. *J Interferon Res.* 1982b;**2**:309–314.

Borgstrum S, Von Eyben FE, Flodgren P, et al. Human leukocyte interferon and cimetidine for metastatic melanoma. *N Engl J Med.* 1983;**307**:1080–1081.

Boyer CM, Dawson DV, Neal SE, et al. Differential induction by interferons of major histocompatibility complex-encoded and non-major histocompatibility complex-encoded antigens in human breast and ovarian carcinoma cell lines. *Cancer Res.* 1989;**49**:2928–2934.

Brouty-Boye D, Tovey MG. Inhibition by interferon of thymidine uptake in chemostat cultures of L-1210 cells. *Intervirology.* 1978.**9**:243–252.

Bunn PA Jr, Ihde DC, Foon KA. The role of recombinant interferon in the therapy of cutaneous T-cell lymphomas. *Cancer.* 1986;**57**:1689–1695.

Calabrese LH, Proffitt MR, Yen-Lieberman B, et al. Congestive cardiomyopathy and illness related to the acquired immunodeficiency syndrome (AIDS) associated with isolation of retrovirus from myocardium. *Ann Intern Med.* 1987;**107**:691–692.

Cantell K, Hervonen S, Morgensen KE. Human leukocyte interferon production purification, and animal experiments. In: Waymouth C, ed. *In Vitro.* Baltimore: Baltimore Tissue Culture Association; 1975:35–38.

Cheeseman S, Rubin R, Steward J, et al. Controlled clinical trial of prophylactic human leukocyte interferon in renal transplantation. *N Engl J Med.* 1979;**300**:1345–1349.

Chun H, Mittelman A, Puccio C, et al. A combination of 5-fluorouracil (FU), alpha interferon (IFN-A) and interleukin-2 (IL-2) in patients (PTS) with advanced colorectal adenocarcinoma (ACA). *Proc Am Soc Clin Oncol.* 1992;**11**:188.

Contente S, Kenyon K, Rimoldi D, et al. Expression of gene *rrg* is associated with reversion of NIH 3T3 transformed by LTR-c-H-*ras*. *Science.* 1990;**249**:796–798.

Cooper MR, Fefer A, Thompson J, et al. Alpha-2 interferon/melphalan/prednisone in previously untreated patients with multiple myeloma: A phase I–II trial. *Cancer Treat Rep.* 1986;**70**:473–476.

Cortesi E, D'Aprile M, De Palma M, et al. Advanced colorectal cancer: A phase II study of chemoimmunotherapy with IFN alpha 2B + 5-FU C.I. or 5-FU + F.A. *Proc Am Soc Clin Oncol.* 1992;**11**:183.

Davis GL, Balart LA, Schiff ER, et al. Treatment of chronic hepatitis C with recombinant interferon alfa: A multicenter randomized, controlled trial. *N Engl J Med.* 1989;**321**:1501–1506.

Deyton LR, Walker RE, Kovacs JA, et al. Reversible cardiac dysfunction associated with interferon alfa therapy in AIDS patients with Kaposi's sarcoma. *N Engl J Med.* 1989;**321**:1246–1249.

Dhingra K, Talpaz M, Dhingra HM, et al. A phase I trial of recombinant alpha-2a interferon (Roferon-A) with weekly cisplatin. *Invest New Drug.* 1991;**9**:37–39.

Dorr RT, Salmon SE, Robertone A, Bonnem E. Phase I–II trial of interferon-$α_{2b}$ by continuous subcutaneous infusion over 28 days. *J Interferon Res.* 1988;**8**:717–725.

Douglas RM, Moore BW, Miles HB, et al. Prophlactic efficacy of intranasal alpha$_2$-interferon against rhinovirus infections in the family setting. *N Engl J Med.* 1986;**314**:65–70.

Durie BGM, Clouse L, Braich T, et al. Interferon alfa-2b–cyclophosphamide combination studies: In vitro and phase I–II clinical results. *Semin Oncol.* 1986;**13**(3):84–88.

Eddleston A. Interferons in the treatment of chronic hepatitis B virus infection. *Med Clin North Am.* May 1986(suppl):25–30.

Einat M, Kimchi A. Transfection of fibroblasts with activated c-*myc* confers resistance to antigrowth effects of interferon. *Oncogene.* 1988;**2**:485–491.

Eisenkraft BL, Nanus DM, Albino AP, Pfeffer LM. α-Interferon downregulates epidermal growth factor receptors on renal carcinoma cells: Relation to cellular responsiveness to the antiproliferative action of α-interferon. *Cancer Res.* 1991;**51**:5881–5887.

Eksborg S, Mattson K. Pharmacokinetics of epirubicin in man. Noninfluence of alpha interferon. *Med Oncol Tumor Pharmacother.* 1988;**5**(2):131–133.

Elias L, Crissman HA. Interferon effects upon the adenocarcinoma 38 and HL-60 cell lines: Antiproliferative responses and synergistic interactions with halogenated pyrimidine antimetabolites. *Cancer Res.* 1988;**48**:4868–4873.

Ernstoff MS, Gallicchio V, Kirkwood JM. Analysis of granulocyte macrophage progenitor cells in patients treated with recombinant interferon-2. *Am J Med.* 1985;**79**:167–171.

Eron LJ, Judson F, Tucker S, et al. Interferon therapy for condyloma acuminata. *N Engl J Med.* 1986;**315**:1059–1964.

Faltynek CR, Kung H. The biochemical mechanisms of action of the interferons. *Biofactors.* 1988;**1**:227–235.

Figlin RA, Dekernion JB, Maldazys J, Sarna G. Treatment of renal cell carcinoma with (human leukocyte) interferon and vinblastine in combination: A phase I–II trial. *Cancer Treat Rep.* 1986;**69**:263–267.

Figlin RA, Dekernion JB, Mukamel E, et al. Recombinant interferon alfa-2a in metastatic renal cell carcinoma: Assessment of antitumor activity and anti-interferon antibody formation. *J Clin Oncol.* 1988;**6**(10):1604–1610.

Fossa SD, et al. Recombinant interferon α/2A with or

without vinblastine in metastatic renal cell carcinoma. *Cancer.* 1986;**57**:1700–1704.

Friedman-Kien AE, Eron LJ, Conant M, et al. Natural interferon alfa for treatment of condylomata acuminata. *JAMA.* 1988;**259**(4):5330–5338.

Fuchs D, Hausen A, Reibnegger G, et al. Neopterin as a marker for activated cell-mediated immunity. *Immunol Today.* 1988;**5**:150–155.

Gastl G, Werter M, De Pauw B, et al. Comparison of clinical efficacy and toxicity of conventional and optimum biological response modifying doses of interferon alpha-2C in the treatment of hairy cell leukemia: A retrospective analysis of 39 patients. *Leukemia.* 1989;**3**(6):453–460.

Gewert DR, Moore G, Clemens MJ. Inhibition of cell division by interferons. The relationship between changes in utilization of thymidine for DNA synthesis and control of proliferation in Daudi cells. *Biochem J.* 1983;**214**:983–990.

Gewert DR, Shah S, Clemens MJ. Inhibition of cell division by interferons: Changes in the transport and intracellular metabolism of thymidine in human lymphoblastoid (Daudi) cells. *Eur J Biochem.* 1981;**116**:487–492.

Giles FJ, Gray AG, Brozovic M, et al. Alpha-interferon therapy for essential thrombocythaemia. *Lancet.* 1988;**2**:70–72.

Goepfert H, Sessions RB, Gutterman JV, et al. Leukocyte interferon in patients with juvenile laryngeal papillomatosis. *Ann Otol Rhinol Laryngol.* 1982;**91**:413–436.

Goldstein D, Laszlo J. Interferon therapy and cancer: From imaginon to interferon. *Cancer Res.* 1986;**46**:4315–4329.

Golomb H, Fefer A, Ratain M. Intron A, recombinant α-2 interferon for induction of remission in hairy cell leukemia. *Proc Am Soc Clin Oncol.* 1985;**4**:225.

Gresser I, Burke D, Cantell K, et al. In: Gresser I, ed. *Interferon 7.* New York: Academic Press; 1986.

Groopman JE, Gottlieb MS, Goodman J, et al. Recombinant alpha-2-interferon therapy for Kaposi's sarcoma associated with the acquired immunodeficiency syndrome. *Ann Intern Med.* 1984;**100**:671–676.

Gutterman JU, Fine S, Quesada J, et al. Recombinant leukocyte A interferon: Pharmacokinetics, single-dose tolerance, and biologic effects in cancer patients. *Ann Intern Med.* 1982;**96**:549–556.

Hirsch MS, Tolkoff-Rubin NE, Kelly AP, Rubin RH. Pharmacokinetics of human and recombinant leukocyte interferon in patients with chronic renal failure who are undergoing hemodialysis. *J Infect Dis.* 1983;**148**(2):335.

Ikic D. Intralesional therapy. In: Sikora K, ed. *Interferon and Cancer.* New York: Plenum Press; 1982:169–181.

Jones GJ, Itri LM. Safety and tolerance or recombinant interferon alfa-2a (Roferon®-A) in cancer patients. *Cancer.* 1986;**57**:1709–1715.

Kirkwood JM, Ernstoff MS. Interferons in the treatment of human cancer. *J Clin Oncol.* 1984;**2**:336–352.

Kirkwood JM, Harris JE, Vera R, et al. Randomized trial of low and high doses of leukocyte interferons in metastatic renal cell carcinoma. *Cancer Res.* 1985;**45**:863–871.

Krown SE, Gold JWM, Niedzwiecki D, et al. Interferon-α with zidovudine: Safety, tolerance, and clinical and virologic effects in patients with Kaposi sarcoma associated with the acquired immunodeficiency syndrome (AIDS). *Ann Intern Med.* 1990;**112**:812–821.

Lane HC, Davey V, Kovacs JA, et al. Interferon-α in patients with asymptomatic human immunodeficiency virus (HIV) infection. *Ann Intern Med.* 1990;**112**(11):805–811.

Lane HC, Feinberg J, Davey V, et al. Anti-retroviral effects of interferon-α in AIDS-associated Kaposis' sarcoma. *Lancet.* 1988;**1**:1218–1222.

Leventhal BG, Kashima HK, Mounts P, et al. Long-term response of recurrent respiratory papillomatosis to treatment with lymphoblastoid interferon alfa-n1. *N Engl J Med.* 1991;**325**:613–617.

Lok AS-F, Lai C-L, Leung EK-Y. Interferon antibodies may negate the antiviral effects of recombinant α-interferon treatment in patients with chronic hepatitis B virus infection. *Hepatology.* 1990;**12**:1266–1270.

Louie AC, Gallagher JG, Sikora K, et al. Follow-up observations on the effect of human leukocyte interferon in non-Hodgkin's lymphoma. *Blood.* 1981;**58**:712–718.

Maio M, Gulwani B, Langer JA, et al. Modulation by interferons of HLA antigen, high-molecular-weight melanoma-associated antigen, and intercellular adhesion molecule 1 expression by cultured melanoma cells with different metastatic potential. *Cancer Res.* 1989;**49**:2980–2987.

Mandelli F, Avvisati G, Amadori S, et al. Maintenance treatment with recombinant interferon alfa-2b in patients with multiple myeloma responding to conventional induction chemotherapy. *N Engl J Med.* 1990;**322**:1430–1434.

Mannering GJ, Renton KW, El Azhary R, et al. Effects of interferon-inducing agents on hepatic cytochrome P-450 drug metabolizing systems. *Ann NY Acad Sci.* 1980;**350**:314–331.

Martinelli G, Cavalli F. α-Interferon alone or in combination with chemotherapy in the treatment of malignant melanoma, renal cell carcinoma and other solid tumours. In: Veronesi U, ed. *Interferons in Oncology, Current Status and Future Direction.* Berlin: Springer-Verlag; 1987:33–38.

Massaro ER, Borden EC, Hawkins MJ, et al. Effects of recombinant interferon-α_2 treatment upon lipid concentrations and lipoprotein composition. *J Interferon Res.* 1986;**6**:655–662.

McCabe BF, Clark KF. Interferon and laryngeal papillomatosis. *Ann Otol Rhinol Laryngol.* 1983;**92**:2–7.

Merigan TC, Pollard RB, Abdallah PS, et al. Human leukocyte interferon for the treatment of herpes zoster in patients with cancer. *N Engl J Med.* 1978;**298**:981–987.

Merimsky O, Rubinstein M, Fischer D, et al. Pharmacokinetics of recombinant interferon alpha-C. *Cancer Chemother Pharmacol.* 1991;**27**:406–408.

Miller RL, Steis RG, Clark JW, et al. Randomized trial of recombinant α2b-interferon with or without indomethacin in patients with metastatic malignant melanoma. *Cancer Res.* 1989;**49**:1871–1876.

Misset JL, Mathe G, Gastiaburu J, et al. Traitement des leucemies et des lymphomes par les interferons. II. Essai phase II de traitement de la leucemie lymphoid chronique par l'interferon de humain. *Biomedicine.* 1982;**36**:112–116.

Moormeier JA, Ratain MJ, Westbrook CA, et al. Low-dose interferon alfa-2b in the treatment of hairy cell leukemia. *J Natl Cancer Inst.* 1989;**81**:1172–1174.

Muss HB, Welander C, Caponera M, et al. Interferon and doxorubicin in renal cell carcinoma. *Cancer Treat Rep.* 1985;**69**(6):721–722.

Neidhart J, Gagen MM, Young D, et al. Interferon-α therapy of renal cancer. *Cancer Res.* 1985;**45**:863–871.

Oberg K, Eriksson B, Norheim I. Interferon treatment of neuroendocrine gut tumors. *Proc Am Soc Clin Oncol.* 1987;**6**:80.

Pan L, Guyre PM. Individual and combined tumoricidal effects of dexamethasone and interferons on human leukocyte cell lines. *Cancer Res.* 1988;**48**(3):567–571.

Parkinson A, Lasker J, Kramer MJ, et al. Effects of three recombinant human leukocyte interferons on drug metabolism in mice. *Drug Metab Dispos.* 1982;**10**:579–585.

Patel N, Joel SP, Seymour MT, et al. Lack of pharmacokinetic interaction when interferon-α2a is added to a combination of 5-fluorouracil and folinic acid. *Proc Am Soc Clin Oncol.* 1992;**11**:134.

Pazin G, Armstrong J, Lam MT, et al. Prevention of reactivated herpes simplex infection by human leukocyte interferon after operation on the trigeminal root. *N Engl J Med.* 1979;**301**:225–229.

Porres JC, Carreno V, Ruiz M, et al. Interferon antibodies in patients with chronic HBV infection treated with recombinant interferon. *J Hepatol.* 1989;**8**:351–357.

Quesada JR, Hersh DM, Rueben J, Gutterman JV. α-Interferon for induction of remission of hairy cell leukemia. *N Engl J Med.* 1984;**310**:15–18.

Quesada JR, Rios A, Swanson D, et al. Antitumor activity of recombinant-derived interferon alpha in metastatic renal cell carcinoma. *J Clin Oncol.* 1985;**3**:1522–1528.

Quesada JR, Talpaz M, Rios A, et al. Clinical toxicity of interferons in cancer patients: A review. *J Clin Oncol.* 1986;**4**:234–243.

Radwanski E, Perentesis G, Oden E, et al. Pharmacokinetics of α-2b interferon in healthy volunteers. *J Clin Pharmacol.* 1987;**27**(5):432–435.

Rohatiher AZS, Richards MA, Barnett MJ, et al. Chlorambucil and interferon for low grade non-Hodgkin's lymphoma. *Brit J Cancer.* 1987;**55**:225–226.

Rosenblum MG, Gutterman JU. Synergistic antiproliferative activity of leukocyte interferon in combination with α-difluoromethylornithine against human cells in culture. *Cancer Res.* 1984;**44**:2339–2340.

Rosenblum MG, Maxwell BL, Talpaz M, et al. In vivo sensitivity and resistance of chronic myelogenous leukemia cells to α-interferon: Correlation with receptor binding and induction of 2′,5′-oligoadenylate synthetase. *Cancer Res.* 1986;**46**:4848–4852.

Salmon SE, Durie BGM, Young L, et al. Effects of cloned human leukocyte interferons in the human tumor stem cell assay. *J Clin Oncol.* 1983;**1**(3):217–225.

Samuel CE. Mechanisms of interferon action: Phosphorylation of protein synthesis initiation factor eIF-2 in interferon-treated cells by a ribosome-associated kinase possessing site specificity similar to hemin-regulated rabbit reticulocyte kinase. *Proc Natl Acad Sci USA.* 1979;**76**:600–607.

Sarosy GA, Brown TD, Von Hoff DD, et al. Phase I study of α$_2$-interferon plus doxorubicin in patients with solid tumors. *Cancer Res.* 1986;**46**:5368–5371.

Schiller JH, Willson JKV, Bittner G, et al. Antiproliferative effects of interferons on human melanoma cells in the human tumor colony-forming assay. *J Interferon Res.* 1986;**6**:615–625.

Scott GM, Phillpotts RJ, Wallace J, et al. Purified interferon as protection against rhinovirus infection. *Br Med J.* 1982;**284**:1822–1825.

Sehgal PB. The interferon gene. *Biochim Biophys Acta.* 1982;**695**:17–33.

Seto WH, Choo YC, Merrigan TC, et al. Local IFN treatment of intraepithelial neoplasia. *Antiviral Res.* 1984;**3**:35–90.

Singh G, Renton KW. Interferon-mediated depression of cytochrome P-450-dependent drug biotransformation. *Mol Pharmacol.* 1981;**20**:681–684.

Singh G, Renton KW. Homogeneous interferon from *E. coli* depresses hepatic cytochrome P-450 and drug biotransformation. *Biochem Biophys Res Commun.* 1982;**106**:1256–1261.

Smith RA, Kingsbury D, Alksne J, et al. Distribution of interferon in cerebrospinal fluid after systemic, intrathecal, and intraventricular administration. *Ann Neurol.* 1982;**12**:81.

Smith RA, Norris F, Palmer D, et al. Distribution of alpha interferon in serum and cerebrospinal fluid after systemic administration. *Clin Pharmacol Ther.* 1985;**37**:85–88.

Smyth JF, Balkwill FR, Fergusson RJ. Interferons combined with other anticancer agents: Studies in experimental systems. In: Veronesi U, ed. *Interferons in Oncology: Current Status and Future Directions,* Berlin: Springer-Verlag; 1987:39–42.

Spiegel RJ, Spicehandler JR, Jacobs SL, Oden EM. Low incidence of serum neutralizing factors in patients receiving recombinant alfa-2b interferon (Intron A). *Am J Med.* 1986;**80**:223–228.

Steis RG, Smith JW II, Ewel C, et al. Loss of serum interferon alpha-2a (IFN-α2a) antibodies (ABS) during continuous long-term interferon therapy of hairy cell leukemia (HCL). *Proc Am Soc Clin Oncol.* 1990;**9**:182.

Steis RG, Smith JW, Urba WJ, et al. Resistance to recombinant interferon alpha-2a in hairy-cell leukemia associated with neutralizing anti-interferon antibodies. *N Engl J Med.* 1988;**318**:1409–1413.

Strander HA. Interferon in the treatment of human papilloma virus. *Med Clin North Am.* 1986;May(suppl):19–23.

Talpaz M. Clinical studies of alpha-interferons in chronic myelogenous leukemia. *Cancer Treat Rev.* 1988;**15**(suppl):49–53.

Talpaz M, McCredie KB, Mavligit GM, Gutterman JU. Leukocyte interferon induced myeloid cytoreduction in chronic myelogenous leukemia. *Blood.* 1983;**62**:689–692.

Talpaz M, Plager C, Quesada J, et al. Difluoromethylornithine and leukocyte interferon: A phase I study in cancer patients. *Eur J Cancer Clin Oncol.* 1986;**22**(6):685–689.

Taylor-Papadimitriou J, Rozengurt E. Interferons as regulators of cell growth and differention. In: Taylor-Papadimitriou J, ed. *Interferons, Their Impact in Biology and Medicine.* Oxford: Oxford Medical Publications; 1985:81–98.

Thompson JA, Kidd P, Rubin E, Fefer A. Very low dose α-2b interferon for the treatment of hairy cell leukemia. *Blood.* 1989;**73**(6):1440–1443.

Torti F, Shortliffe LN, Williams RD, et al. Superficial bladder cancers are responsive to α2-interferon administered intravesically. *Proc Am Soc Clin Oncol.* 1984;**3**:160.

Ueda S, Hirakawa K, Nakagawa Y, et al. Brain tumors. In: Sikora K, ed. *Interferon and Cancer.* New York: Plenum Press; 1982;129–139.

Von Wussow P, Block B, Hartmann F, Deicher H. Intralesional interferon-alpha therapy in advanced malignant melanoma. *Cancer.* 1988;**61**:1071–1074.

Von Wussow P, Freund M, Block B, et al. Clinical significance of anti-IFN-α antibody titres during interferon therapy. *Lancet.* 1987;**2**:635–636.

Wadler S, Lenbersky B, Atkins M, et al. Phase II trial of fluorouracil and recombinant interferon alfa-2a in patients with advanced colorectal carcinoma: An Eastern Cooperative Oncology Group study. *J Clin Oncol.* 1991;**9**:1806–1810.

Wadler S, Schwartz EL, Goldman M, et al. Fluorouracil and recombinant alfa-2a-interferon: An active regimen against advanced colorectal carcinoma. *J Clin Oncol.* 1989a;**7**(12):1769–1775.

Wadler S, Schwartz EL, Wersto R, et al. Interferon (IFN) modulates the activity of 5-fluorouracil (5FU) against two human colon cancer cell lines (abstract 2264). *Proc AACR.* 1989;**30**:569.

Williams BRG, Kerr I. The 2-5A (pppA2'P5', A2'P5'A) system in interferon-treated and control cells. *Trends Biochem Sci.* 1980:138–140.

Williams RD. Intravesical interferon alfa in the treatment of superficial bladder cancer. *Semin Oncol.* 1988;**5**:10–13.

Wills RJ, Dennis S, Spiegel HE, et al. Interferon kinetics and adverse reactions after intravenous, intramuscular, and subcutaneous injection. *Clin Pharmacol Ther.* 1984;**35**(5):722–727.

Wills RJ, Spiegel HE. Continuous intravenous infusion pharmacokinetics of interferon to patients with leukemia. *J Clin Pharmacol.* 1985;**25**:616–619.

Witter F, Barouki F, Griffin D, et al. Biologic response (antiviral) to recombinant human interferon alpha 2a as a function of dose and route of administration in healthy volunteers. *Clin Pharmacol Ther.* 1987;**42**:567–575.

Witter FR, Woods AS, Griffin MD, et al. Effects of prednisone, aspirin, and acetaminophen on an in vivo biologic response to interferon in human. *Clin Pharmacol Ther.* 1988;**44**:239–243.

Interferon Beta

■ Other names

Recombinant human interferon beta; Betaseron; interferon β_{ser17}; IFN-β_{ser17}.

■ Chemistry

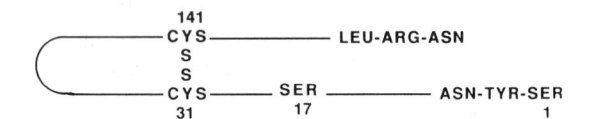

```
          141
         CYS ─────────── LEU-ARG-ASN
          S
          S
         CYS ──── SER ──────── ASN-TYR-SER
          31      17                     1
```

Partial amino acid and sequence of interferon beta

Interferon beta (IFN-β_{ser17}) is a recombinant molecule made by Mark and colleagues (1984) by substituting a serine for cysteine at the 17-position using the techniques of site-specific mutagenesis. This substitution allowed for a proper folding of the molecule with retention of the biologic activity of native interferon beta that was stable during storage at −70°C. The molecule is produced in *Escherichia coli*. It has a molecular weight of approximately 18,500 and consists of 166 amino acids. It has a specific activity of 100×10^6 IU/mg protein (as measured in antiviral units). IFN-β_{ser17} is not glycosylated and it also lacks the N-terminal methionine found on the native interferon beta. The predicted tertiary structure involves about 50% alpha-helix content which is less than that of alpha interferon.

■ Antitumor Activity

To date, IFN-β_{ser17} has shown antitumor activity in patients with renal cell carcinoma (approximately a 20% response rate) (Rinehart et al 1986, Borden et al 1988, Kinney et al 1990). Of note is that responses are noted most often in patients with small tumor burden and predominantly pulmonary disease (Kinney et al 1990). Attempts to use in vitro immunologic assays to predict response have not been successful (Rinehart et al 1987). Miles et al (1990) noted a 16% response rate in Kaposi's sarcoma. In addition, there was a suggestion of antiviral activity as well as a decrease in the expected incidence of opportunistic infections. No responses were noted in a phase II trial in patients with malignant melanoma (Sarna et al 1987). A complete response in only one of 17 patients with colon cancer was reported by Lillis and colleagues (1987).

Interferon beta has been extensively tested in vitro against primary human tumor colony-forming units and against human tumor cell lines (Von Hoff and Huong 1988, Vita et al 1988, Borden et al 1984). In those systems it has been found to have activity against several tumor types (eg, mesothelioma). In addition, IFN-β_{ser17} has been found to be synergistic in vitro with interferon gamma, vinblastine, and other agents as well as radiation therapy (Chang et al 1987).

■ Mechanism of Action

As with the other interferons the mechanism of action of this agent is unknown. IFN-β_{ser17} may mediate its antiproliferative effect via the *c-myc* gene. IFN-β has been reported to decrease expression of *c-myc* in Daudi cells (Knight et al 1985). Many alternative explanations for the antiproliferative effects are available.

■ Availability and Storage

Available from Triton Biosciences, Inc, Alameda, California, IFN-β_{ser17} is supplied as a lyophilized cake in 5-mL vials. The lyophilized product contains Human Albumin, USP, and 50% Dextrose Injection, USP, for solubilization and stabilization. The unopened vials should be stored at 2 to 8°C (36 to 48°F).

■ Preparation for Use, Stability, and Admixture

The reconstitution procedure has varied according to the clinical protocol used. In one common method, the material is placed in 200 mL normal saline and administered over 2 hours. The reconstituted product should be inspected visually for particulate matter and discoloration. After reconstitution with diluent the solution should be stored at 2 to 8°C for up to 3 hours before use.

■ Administration

See Dosage.

■ Special Precautions

Interferon beta should not be given to patients with a history of sensitivity to the agent or to human albumin (present in the formulations). The agent should be administered with caution (if at all) to patients with a history of serious cardiac disorders, as arrhythmias, myocardial infarctions, and congestive heart failure have been reported with the agent.

■ Drug Interactions

None have been reported to date.

■ Dosage

The table on page 584 summarizes the phase I clinical trials with IFN-β_{ser17}. As can be seen in that table, the precise recommended dose is uncertain. Patients frequently can be started on lower doses with escalation to higher doses. Three regimens are used most often in phase II trials:

1. 2.5 mg three times per week as a 2-hour intravenous infusion (Kinney et al 1990); however, the variability in patient tolerance is described as quite wide.
2. 30×10^6 units in an intravenous bolus 5 days a week for 2 weeks followed by 2 weeks of rest (Sarna et al 1987).
3. 30×10^6 units in an intravenous bolus daily for 5 days in week 1, 60×10^6 units daily for 5 days in week 2, and then twice weekly doses escalating from 90 to 270×10^6 units (Sarna et al 1987).

There is some evidence to indicate that biologic responses (eg, increased natural killer activity) are more impressive when IFN-β_{ser17} is given by the subcutaneous route (Goldstein et al 1988).

■ Pharmacokinetics

Sarna and colleagues (1986) have evaluated the pharmacokinetics of IFN-β_{ser17} using an antiviral cytopathic technique. The kinetics followed a biphasic curve with an α half-life of 9 minutes and a β half-life of 103 minutes. Mean peak interferon levels were 1508 to 8286 units/mL 1 minute after the intravenous push injection. Hawkins et al (1985)

PHASE I CLINICAL TRIALS WITH IFN-$\beta_{ser\ 17}$

Schedule	Route	Dose Range (10^6/IU)	Reference
Single dose	IM	60–300	Hawkins et al 1985
	IV	10–400	
Twice weekly	IV	0.006–500	Sarna et al 1986
Twice weekly 4-h infusion	IV	0.01–150	Rinehart et al 1986
Daily × 14	IV	3–30	Borden et al 1988
Twice weekly 4-h infusion	IV	0.01–400	Grunberg et al 1987
Three times per week 10-min bolus	IV	3–300	Hu and Horning 1987
Five times per week	SC	45–360	Chang et al 1987

found that serum concentrations were not dose related by the intravenous route and IFN-β_{ser17} was barely detectable after high-dose intramuscular administration. Their conclusion was that serum levels (detectable by present techniques) were not a prerequisite for biologic activity.

■ Side Effects and Toxicity

Many of the toxic effects of IFN-β_{ser17} are ameliorated after repeated doses. The side effects include a flulike syndrome consisting of fever (2–10 hours postinjection), malaise, myalgias, chills, anorexia, and headaches (Sarna et al 1986, Borden et al 1988, Rinehart et al 1986). Acetaminophen has been useful in controlling the flulike symptoms. Nausea and vomiting can occur (Sarna et al 1986, Lillis et al 1987).

Neurologic effects have included fatigue, dizziness, confusion, decreased concentration, and an exacerbation of seizure disorders (Borden et al 1988, Rinehart et al 1987). Leukopenia and/or thrombocytopenia may occur but have only occasionally been dose limiting (Borden et al 1988). Other unusual toxic effects include skin rashes, increase in serum glutamic–oxalacetic or glutamic–pyruvic transaminase or alkaline phosphatase, mild to moderate but reversible proteinuria, hypotension and brachycardia, and angina (Sarna et al 1986, Borden et al 1988, Rinehart et al 1986, Kinney et al 1990). There are variable reports of anti-interferon antibody formation in patients (ranging from 0 to 47%); however, the presence of antibodies does not appear to correlate with response or toxicity (Sarna et al 1986, Borden et al 1988).

■ Special Applications

Interferon beta has been given through an Ommaya reservoir into the tumors of 20 patients with recurrent malignant gliomas (Fetel et al 1990). The incidence of obstruction and infection of the reservoir was high. Side effects attributable to IFN-β_{ser17} were noted in only one patient (fever, chills, nausea, and vomiting). The agent may also be used in the future as a radiation sensitizer based on convincing preclinical data (Chang and Keng 1987).

REFERENCES

Borden EC, Groveman DS, Nasu T, Reznikoff C, Bryan GT. Antiproliferative activities of interferon against human bladder carcinoma cell lines in vitro. *J Urol.* 1984;**132**:800–803.

Borden EC, Hawkins MJ, Sielaffe KM, Storer BM, Schiesel JD, Smalley RV. Clinical and biological effects of recombinant interferon-β administered intravenously daily in phase I trial. *Interferon Res.* 1988;**8**:357–366.

Chang AMC, Keng PC. Potentiation of radiation cytotoxicity by recombinant interferon, a phenomenon associated with increased blockage at the G_2M phase of the cell cycle. *Cancer Res.* 1987a;**47**:4338–4341.

Chang AYC, Pandya KJ, Woll J, Smith B, Bennett J. Phase I study of subcutaneous (SC) injection of recombinant interferon data (rHuIFN-Bser) with dose escalation in each patient. *Proc Am Soc Clin Oncol.* 1987b;**6**:249.

Fetel MR, Housespran EM, Oster MW, et al. Intratumor administration of beta-interferon in recurrent malignant gliomas. *Cancer.* 1990;**65**:78–83.

Goldstein D, Sielaff K, Storer B, et al. Effect of route on biological response modification by interferon β_{ser}. *Proc Am Assoc Cancer Res.* 1988;**29**:184.

Grunberg SM, Kempf RA, Venturi CL, Mitchell MS. Phase I study of recombinant β-interferon given by four-hour infusion. *Cancer Res.* 1987;**47**:1174–1178.

Hawkins M, Horning S, Konrad M, et al. Phase I evaluation of a synthetic mutant of β-interferon. *Cancer Res.* 1985;**45**:5914–5919.

Hu E, Horning SJ. Phase I study of recombinant interferon

beta in patients with advanced cancer. *J Biol Response Mod.* 1987;**6**:21–129.

Kinney P, Triozzi P, Young D, et al. Phase II trial of interferon-beta serine in metastatic renal cell carcinoma. *J Clin Med.* 1990;**8**:881–885.

Knight E, Anton ED, Fahey D, Friedland BK, Jonak GJ. Interferon regulates *c-myc* gene expression in Daudi cell at the post-transcriptional level. *Proc Natl Acad Sci USA.* 1985;**82**:1151–1154.

Lillis PK, Brown TD, Beougher K, Koeller J, Marcus SG, Von Hoff DD. Phase I trial of recombinant beta interferon in advanced colorectal cancer. *Cancer Treat.* 1987;**71**:965–967.

Mark DF, Lu SD, Creasy AA, Yamamoto R, Lin LS. Site specific mutagenesis of the human fibroblast interferon gene. *Proc Natl Acad Sci USA.* 1984;**81**:5662–5666.

Miles SA, Wang H, Cortes F, Corden J, Marcus S, Mitsuyasu TR. Beta interferon therapy in patients with poor prognosis Kaposi's sarcoma related to the acquired immunodeficiency syndrome (AIDS). *Ann Intern Med.* 1990;**112**:582–589.

Rinehart J, Malspeis L, Young D, Merdhart T. Phase I/II trial of human recombinant β-interferon serine in patients with renal cell carcinoma. *Cancer Res.* 1986;**46**:5364–5367.

Rinehart JJ, Young D, Laforge J, Colburn D, Medhart JA. Phase I/II trial of interferon-β-serine in patients with renal cell carcinoma: Immunological and biological effects. *Cancer Res.* 1987;**47**:2481–2487.

Sarna G, Pertcheck M, Figlin R, Ardalon B. Phase I study of recombinant β$_{ser17}$ interferon in the treatment of cancer. *Cancer Treat Rep.* 1986;**70**:1365–1372.

Sarna GP, Figlin RA, Pertcheck M. Phase II study of Betaserom (β$_{ser17}$-interferon) as treatment of advanced malignant melanomas. *J Biol Response Mod.* 1987;**6**:375–378.

Vita JR, Edwalds GM, Gorey T, et al. Enhanced *in vitro* growth suppression of human glioblastoma cultures treated with the combination of recombinant fibroblast and immune interferon. *Anticancer Res.* 1988;**8**:297–302.

Von Hoff DD, Huong AM. Effect of recombinant interferon β$_{ser}$ on primary human tumor colony forming units. *J Interferon Res.* 1988;**8**:813–820.

Interferon Gamma

■ Other Names

Recombinant gamma interferon; rGIFN.

■ Chemistry

Interferon gamma has weak antiviral properties yet is a relatively immunomodulatory agent (Epstein 1983, Wallach et al 1982, Rubin and Gupta 1980, Sonnenfeld et al 1978). Interferon gamma has a molecular weight of 17,000 and 146 amino acids, of which only 18 are homologous with interferon alfa. One gene coding for interferon gamma has been identified, but several subspecies exist as a result of posttranslational modifications including variable degrees of glycosylation. Human interferon gamma has an acid-labile Asp–Pro bond between positions 2 and 3. This bond is broken at pH 2.3 with a resultant loss of biologic activity.

■ Antitumor Activity

Interferon gamma demonstrated some activity against B-cell malignancies in phase I trials (Vadhan-Raj et al 1986b) as well against malignant melanoma (Smith et al 1990). Intraperitoneal interferon gamma for patients with minimal ovarian cancer has been tested in uncontrolled series with some evidence that the drug had an effect (Pujade-Lauraine et al 1990, 1991, Piccart et al 1990).

The addition of interferon gamma to chemotherapy regimens appears to consolidate complete responses in patients with small cell lung cancer (uncontrolled trial—Bitran et al 1990). A definitive adjuvant trial of treatment postresection of patients with stage I or II malignant melanoma shows no effect of the drug in decreasing recurrence (Meyskens et al 1991). Of interest is that ex vivo incubation of chronic myelogenous leukemia-affected marrow with interferon gamma appears to eradicate Ph[1] positive cells which can be used for autologous bone marrow transplants (McGlave et al 1990).

In phase II studies the drug has been found to be inactive or to have very low levels of activity ($\leq 10\%$ response rate) in patients with renal cell carcinoma (Kuebler et al 1990, Bruntsch et al 1990), melanoma (Creagan et al 1990) squamous cell head and neck cancer (Richtsmeier et al 1990), nasopharyngeal carcinoma (Dimery et al 1989, Mahjoubi et al

```
  1                                          10                                              20
Cys Tyr Cys Gln Asp Pro Tyr Val Lys Glu Ala Glu Asn Leu Lys Lys Tyr Phe Asn Ala Gly His
                                  30                                  40
Ser Asp Val Ala Asp Asn Gly Thr Leu Phe Leu Gly Ile Leu Lys Asn Trp Lys Glu Glu Ser
                      50                                          60
Asp Arg Lys Ile Met Gln Ser Gln Ile Val Ser Phe Tyr Phe Lys Leu Phe Lys Asn Phe Lys Asp
                  70                                      80
Asp Gln Ser Ile Gln Lys Ser Val Glu Thr Ile Lys Glu Asp Met Asn Val Lys Phe Phe Asn Ser
              90                                  100
Asn Lys Lys Lys Arg Asp Asp Phe Glu Lys Leu Thr Asn Tyr Ser Val Thr Asp Leu Asn Val
      110                                 120                                 130
Gln Arg Lys Ala Ile His Glu Leu Ile Gln Val Met Ala Glu Leu Ser Pro Ala Ala Lys Thr Gly Lys
                      140
Arg Lys Arg Ser Gln Met Leu Phe Arg Gly Arg Arg Ala Ser Gln
```

Amino acid sequence of interferon gamma

1991), and Kaposi's sarcoma (Krigel et al 1985, Green et al 1988).

■ Mechanism of Action

Interferon gamma augments major histocompatibility antigens (HLA class I) in tumor cells as well as increases the cytotoxicity of tumor-associated macrophages (Allavena et al 1990). The drug also induces 2',5'-oligoadenylate synthetase, increases natural killer cells, and increases helper:suppressor T-cell ratios (Kirkwood et al 1990). The drug is linked with macrophage stimulation, with enhanced oxidative metabolism and production of tumor necrosis factor. Interferon gamma can also induce the "terminal" differentiation of human leukemic cells to a normal phenotype (Ball et al 1984). Gamma interferons may help regulate lipid metabolism by inhibiting lipoprotein lipase, which results in a significant rise in serum triglycerides and very low density lipoproteins (Kurzrock et al 1986b).

■ Availability and Storage

Interferon gamma is supplied as an investigational anticancer agent by Schering Corporation, Kenilworth, New Jersey. It is packaged in vials in lyophilized form to be reconstituted with sterile water (preservative free) for injection. The Schering product has a specific activity of 2.6×10^6 IU/mg protein. The drug is also supplied as an investigational agent by Biogen Inc, Cambridge, Massachusetts, and Genentech, South San Francisco, California.

The lyophilized powder must be stored in a refrigerator at 2 to 8°C (36 to 46°F). Reconstituted solution must be stored at −20 to 30°C (−4 to 86°F) and must be used within 24 hours.

■ Preparation for Use, Stability, and Admixture

Vials containing 2×10^6 U of interferon gamma (Schering) are reconstituted with 1.0 mL of Sterile Water for Injection, USP. Further dilution prior to administration may be performed with either D5W or saline. Reconstitution of interferon gamma with further dilution as directed results in a solution that is stable at room temperature for at least 24 hours.

■ Administration

The optimal dose and schedule for administration of interferon gamma have not yet been determined. (see Dosage for schedules that have been explored.)

■ Special Precautions

None described to date.

■ Drug Interactions

In vitro, there is experimental synergy between interferon alfa or beta and interferon gamma (Zerial et al 1982). This activity has been noted for antiviral effects, for natural killer cell induction, and for antiproliferative effects against transformed human tumor cells (Czarniecki et al 1984). Interferon gamma can also sensitize resistant tumor cells to the cytotoxic effects of tumor necrosis factor by increasing cellular receptors for tumor necrosis factor

(Tsujimoto et al 1986). There is also a data report describing ablation of γ-IFN flu-like symptoms with oral diazepam (Beattie and Smyth 1988).

■ Dosage

The table below describes some of the doses and schedules explored. A recommended dose has not yet been determined.

Kirkwood et al (1990) have determined the optimal biologic response-modifying dose for Biogen interferon gamma to be 300 to 1000 µg/m^2/d.

■ Pharmacokinetics

Vadhan-Raj et al (1986a) noted peak serum interferon levels within 30 minutes to 1 hour of infusion of the agent. Serum levels were dose dependent. The agent was rapidly cleared from the serum with no detectable levels 2 hours after infusion. Brown et al (1987) could not detect serum levels when interferon gamma was given on a continuous infusion × 5 days schedule. Using an α half-life of 60 minutes, blood levels were related to dose in that study. Kurzrock et al (1985) noted longer half-lives (227–462 minutes) after intramuscular injection than after intravenous injection (25–35 minutes).

■ Side Effects and Toxicity

Dose-limiting toxic effects have generally consisted of fever, flulike symptoms (rigors, diaphoresis, myalgias, arthralgias, headaches, malaise) and hypotension (Vadhan-Raj et al 1986a, b, Kurzrock et al 1985, 1986a, Rinehart et al 1986, Brown et al 1987). The observed toxic effects may be schedule dependent. The drug was much less toxic when given as a 2-hour bolus daily × 5 than when it was given as a continuous infusion daily × 5 (Brown et al 1987).

Other toxic effects noted include lethargy, confusion, and rarely seizures. Chest pain and pulmonary edema have also been reported. Leukopenia has been described by Creagan et al (1990). Reversible renal failure has been noted in a pediatric population (Mahmoud et al 1990).

■ Special Applications

In preclinical systems, interferon gamma acts as a radiation sensitizer (Kwok et al 1991). The agent has been shown to have antiangiogenesis properties (Sato et al 1990). As interferon alfa has been used effectively to treat patients with hepatitis C, interferon gamma was also tried. Unfortunately, interferon gamma has been shown not to be active against the disease (Saez-Royuela et al 1991).

Interferon gamma has been shown to partially correct the metabolic defect in phagocytes of patients with chronic granulomatous disease and to decrease the frequency of serious infections in patients with that disease (International Chronic Granulomatous Disease Group 1991).

Intralesional injections of interferon gamma have been used to treat keloids with some success (Granstein et al 1990). The drug has also been used to treat patients with myelodysplastic syndrome with some success (Maiolo et al 1990).

The drug has been found to be ineffective for treatment of patients with allergic rhinitis (Li et al 1990) or rheumatoid arthritis (Cannon et al 1989). Other investigators felt interferon gamma was active against rheumatoid arthritis (Lemmel et al 1988).

Agent	Schedule	Dose Range	Maximally Tolerated Dose	Dose-limiting Toxic Effect	Reference
Biogen	Daily × 5 (2-h bolus)	3–300 µg/m^2	—	—	Kirkwood et al 1990
Biogen	Continuous infusion × 16 days	—	—	—	Kirkwood et al 1990
Biogen	4-h infusion twice per week	0.01–1.50 µg/m^2	75 µg/m^2	Constitutional	Rinehart et al 1986
Genentech	1-h infusion three times per week	0.1–2.0 mg/m^2	1.0 mg/m^2	Constitutional	Vadhan-Raj et al 1986b
Genentech	Daily × 14	0.1–0.75 mg/m^2	0.75 mg/m^2/d	Renal failure	Mahmoud et al 1990
Schering	Continuous infusion × 5 d	0.5 × 10^6 U/m^2 2.0 × 10^6	0.5 m^2/d	Neurotoxicity Hypotension Constitutional	Brown et al 1987
Genentech	Daily × 42	0.01–2.5 mg/m^2	0.5 mg/m^2	Constitutional	Kurzrock et al 1986a

REFERENCES

Allavena P, Peccatori F, Maggioni D, et al. Intraperitoneal recombinant gamma-interferon in patients with recurrent ascitic ovarian carcinoma: Modulation of cytotoxicity and cytokine production in tumor-associated effectors and of major histocompatibility antigen expression on tumor cells. *Cancer Res.* 1990;59(22):7318–7323.

Ball ED, Guyre PM, Shen L, et al. Gamma interferon induces monocytoid differentiation in the HL-60 cell line. *J Clin Invest.* 1984;73:1072–1077.

Beattie GJ, Smyth JF. Diazepam ablates the constitutional side-effects of gamma interferon. *Med Oncol Tumor Pharmacother.* 1988;5:129–130.

Bitran J, Goutsou M, Clamon J, Perry M, Green M. A test of gamma interferon (γ-INF) after initial chemotherapy for previously untreated extensive disease (PUED), small cell lung cancer (SCLC). *Proc Am Soc Clin Oncol.* 1990;9:231.

Brown TD, Koeller J, Beougher K, et al. A phase I clinical trial of recombinant DNA gamma interferon. *J Clin Oncol.* 1987;5:790–798.

Bruntsch U, de Mulder PH, ten Bokkel Huinink WW, et al. Phase II study of recombinant human interferon-gamma in metastatic renal cell carcinoma. *J Biol Response Mod.* 1990;9(3):335–338.

Cannon GW, Pincus SH, Emkey RD, et al. Double-blind trial of recombinant gamma-interferon versus placebo in the treatment of rheumatoid arthritis. *Arthritis Rheum.* 1989;32(8):964–973.

Creagan ET, Schaid DJ, Ahmann DL, Frytak S. Disseminated malignant melanoma and recombinant interferon: Analysis of seven consecutive phase II investigations. *J Invest Dermatol.* 1990;95(6, suppl):188S–192S.

Czarniecki CW, Fennie CW, Powers DB, et al. Synergistic antiviral and antiproliferative activities of *E. coli*-derived human alpha, beta, and gamma interferons. *J Virol.* 1984;49:490–496.

Dimery IW, Jacobs C, Tseng A Jr, et al. Recombinant interferon-gamma in the treatment of recurrent nasopharyngeal carcinoma. *J Biol Response Mod.* 1989;8(3):221–226.

Epstein LB. Interferon gamma: Success, structure and speculation. *Nature.* 1983;295:453–454.

Granstein RD, Rook A, Flotte TJ, et al. A controlled trial of intralesional recombinant interferon-gamma in the treatment of keloidal scarring. Clinical and histologic findings. *Arch Dermatol.* 1990;126(10):1295–1302.

Green M, Chachoua A, Laubenstein L, Ward C, Flanagan S, Fischl M. Randomized study of gamma interferon (IFN) in patients (pts) with AIDS related Kaposi's saroma (KS) (meeting abstract). *Proc Am Soc Clin Oncol.* 1988;7:3.

International Chronic Granulomatous Disease Cooperative Study Group. A controlled trial of interferon gamma to prevent infection in chronic granulomatous disease. *N Engl J Med.* 1991;324(8):509–516.

Kirkwood JM, Ernstoff MS, Trautman T, et al. In vivo biological response to recombinant interferon-gamma during a phase I dose–response trial in patients with metastatic melanoma. *J Clin Oncol.* 1990;8(6):1070–1082.

Krigel RL, Odajnyk CM, Laubenstein LJ, et al. Therapeutic trial of interferon-gamma in patients with epidemic Kaposi's sarcoma. *J Biol Response Mod.* 1985;4(4):358–364.

Kuebler JP, Goodman PJ, Brown TD, et al. Phase II study of continuous infusion recombinant gamma interferon in renal carcinoma. A Southwest Oncology Group study. *Invest New Drugs.* 1990;8(3):307–309.

Kurzrock R, Quesada JR, Talpaz M, et al. Phase I study of multiple dose intramuscularly administered recombinant gamma interferon. *J Clin Oncol.* 1986a;4:1101–1109.

Kurzrock R, Rohde MF, Quesada JR, et al. Recombinant gamma interferon induces hypertriglyceridemia and inhibits post-heparin lipase activity in cancer patients. *J Exp Med.* 1986b;164:1093–1101.

Kurzrock R, Rosenblum MG, Sherwin SA, et al. Pharmacokinetics, single-dose tolerance, and biological activity of recombinant gamma interferon in cancer patients. *Cancer Res.* 1985;45:2866–2872.

Kwok CS, Lee S, Mitchel REJ. Parameters of sensitization of human cells to low dose rate radiation by recombinant human interferon-γ (rhIFN-γ). *Proc Am Assoc Cancer Res.* 1991;32:389.

Lemmel EM, Brackertz D, Franke M, et al. Results of a multicenter placebo-controlled double-blind randomized phase III clinical study of treatment of rheumatoid arthritis with recombinant interferon-gamma. *Rheumatol Int.* 1988;8(2):87–93.

Li JT, Yunginger JW, Reed CE, Jaffe HS, Nelson DR, Gleich GJ. Lack of suppression of IgE production by recombinant interferon gamma: A controlled trial in patients with allergic rhinitis. *J Allergy Clin Immunol.* 1990;85(5):934–940.

Mahjoubi R, Bachouchi M, Munch JN, et al. Phase II trial of recombinant interferon (INT) gamma in undifferentiated carcinoma of nasopharyngeal type (UCNT). *Proc Am Assoc Cancer Res.* 1991;32:257.

Mahmoud H, Pui C-H, Kennedy W, Jaffe HS, Murphy SB. Phase I study of human recombinant interferon gamma in children with refractory leukemia. *Proc Am Assoc Cancer Res.* 1990;31:198.

Maiolo AT, Cortelezzi A, Calori R, Polli EE. Recombinant gamma-interferon as first line therapy for high risk myelodysplastic syndromes. Italian MDS Study group. *Leukemia.* 1990;4(7):480–485.

McGlave PB, Arthur D, Miller WJ, Lasky L, Kersey J. Autologous transplantation for CML using marrow treated ex vivo with recombinant human interferon gamma. *Bone Marrow Transplant.* 1990;6(2):115–120.

Meyskens FL Jr, Kopecky K, Samson M, et al. A phase II trial of recombinant human interferon-gamma (IFN) as adjuvant therapy of high risk malignant melanoma (MM). *Proc Am Soc Clin Oncol.* 1991;10:291.

Piccart M, Marth C, Hochster H, et al. Phase I–II trial of escalating doses of intraperitoneal (ip) γ interferon (IFN) ± cisplatin (DDP) in refractory ovarian cancer patients (OVCA pts). *Proc Am Soc Clin Oncol.* 1990;**9**:166.

Pujade-Lauraine E, Colombo N, Namer N, et al. Intraperitoneal human r-IFN gamma in patients with residual carcinoma (OC) at second look laparotomy (SLL). *Proc Am Soc Clin Oncol.* 1990;**9**:156.

Pujade-Lauraine E, Guastella JP, Colombo N, et al. Intraperitoneal human r-IFN gamma as treatment of residual carcinoma (OC) at second look laparotomy (SLL). *Pro Am Soc Clin Oncol.* 1991;**20**:195.

Richtsmeier WJ, Koch WM, McGuire WP, Poole ME, Chang EH. Phase I–II study of advanced head and neck squamous cell carcinoma patients treated with recombinant human interferon gamma. *Arch Otolaryngol Head Neck Surg.* 1990;**116**(11):1271–1277.

Rinehart JJ, Malspeis L, Young D, Neidhart JA. Phase I/II trial of human recombinant interferon gamma in renal cell carcinoma. *J Biol Response Mod.* 1986;**5**:300–308.

Rubin BY, Gupta SL. Differential efficacies of human type I and type II interferons as antiviral and antiproliferative agents. *Proc Natl Acad Sci USA.* 1980;**77**:5928–5932.

Saez-Royuela F, Porres JC, Moreno A, et al. High doses of recombinant alpha-interferon or gamma-interferon for chronic hepatitis C: A randomized, controlled trial. *Hepatology.* 1991;**13**(2):327–331.

Sato N, Beitz J, Kato J, Clark J, Calabresi P, Frackelton AR Jr. Inhibitory effects of gamma-interferon (IFN-γ) on angiogenesis *in vitro*. *Proc Am Assoc Cancer Res.* 1990;**31**:78.

Smith J II, Longo D, Steis R, et al. An immunomodulatory trial of three different doses of IFNγ in patients with metastatic malignant melanoma. *Proc Am Assoc Cancer Res.* 1990;**9**:199.

Sonnenfeld G, Mandel AD, Merigan TC. Time and dosage dependence of immunoenhancement by murine type II interferon preparations on antibody production. *Cell Immunol.* 1978;**40**:285–293.

Tsujimoto M, Yip YK, Vilcek J. Interferon gamma enhances expression of cellular receptors for tumor necrosis factor. *J Immunol.* 1986;**136**:2441–2444.

Vadhan-Raj S, Al Katib A, Bhalla R, et al. Phase I trial of recombinant interferon gamma in cancer patients. *J Clin Oncol.* 1986a;**4**:137–146.

Vadhan-Raj S, Nathan CF, Sherwin SA, Oettgen HF, Krown SE. Phase I trial of recombinant interferon gamma by 1-hour infusion. *Cancer Treat Rep.* 1986b;**70**:609–614.

Wallach D, Fellous M, Revel M. Preferential effect of gamma interferon on the synthesis of HLA antigens and their mRNAs in human cells. *Nature.* 1982;**299**:833–836.

Zerial A, Hovanessian AG, Stafanos S. Synergistic activities of type I (α,β) and type II (gamma) murine interferons. *Antiviral Res.* 1982;**2**:227–229.

Interleukin-1, Alpha and Beta

■ Other Names

IL-1α; IL-1β; lymphocyte-activating factor (LAF); endogenous pyrogen (EP); β cell-activating factor (BAF); mononuclear cell factor (MCF); leukocyte endogenous mediator (LEM); tumor-inhibitory factor 2.

■ Chemistry

Recombinant interleukin-1 alpha (IL-1α) and interleukin-1 beta (IL-1β) are related protein families with molecular weights of about 17,500. There is 26% amino acid sequence homology between the two distinct protein families. Both proteins nonetheless share the same cell surface receptor on lymphocytes. The natural proteins are produced primarily in monocytes and have molecular weights ranging from 12,000 to 17,000 with a median of 15,000 (Dinarello et al 1974). The isoelectric point of the protein is near neutrality. The usual bioassay for IL-1 is the lymphocyte-activating factor (LAF) assay, which measures stimulation of juvenile murine thymocytes in the presence of suboptimal concentrations of phytohemagglutinin (PHA) or concanavalin A (Gery et al 1972).

The human IL-1 cDNA is 1560 base pairs long and encodes a precursor polypeptide of 269 amino acids and a molecular weight of 30,747 (Auron et al 1984). The mature final protein (molecular weight 17,000) curiously lacks the hydrophobic amino acid "signal" sequence typically associated with secreted proteins. The biologic activity also appears to be associated with the carboxyl-terminal portion of the precursor protein (Lomedico et al 1984).

■ Antitumor Activity

In Vitro Studies. The IL-1 proteins are primarily immunoregulatory but also exhibit some direct antiproliferative effects in vitro. The proliferation of the human ovarian carcinoma cell line NIH:OVCAR-3 is half-maximally inhibited in the presence of 2 to 3 units of IL-1α or IL-1β (Kilian et al 1991). A maximal (80%) inhibitory effect is achieved at concentrations of 10 U/mL or greater for 3 days. This activity can be inhibited by recombinant human IL-1 receptor antagonist (Antril®, Synergen Inc, Boulder, Colorado). Conversely, synergistically increased antiproliferative effects are achieved with IL-1 and alpha interferon. Interleukin-1 is also directly

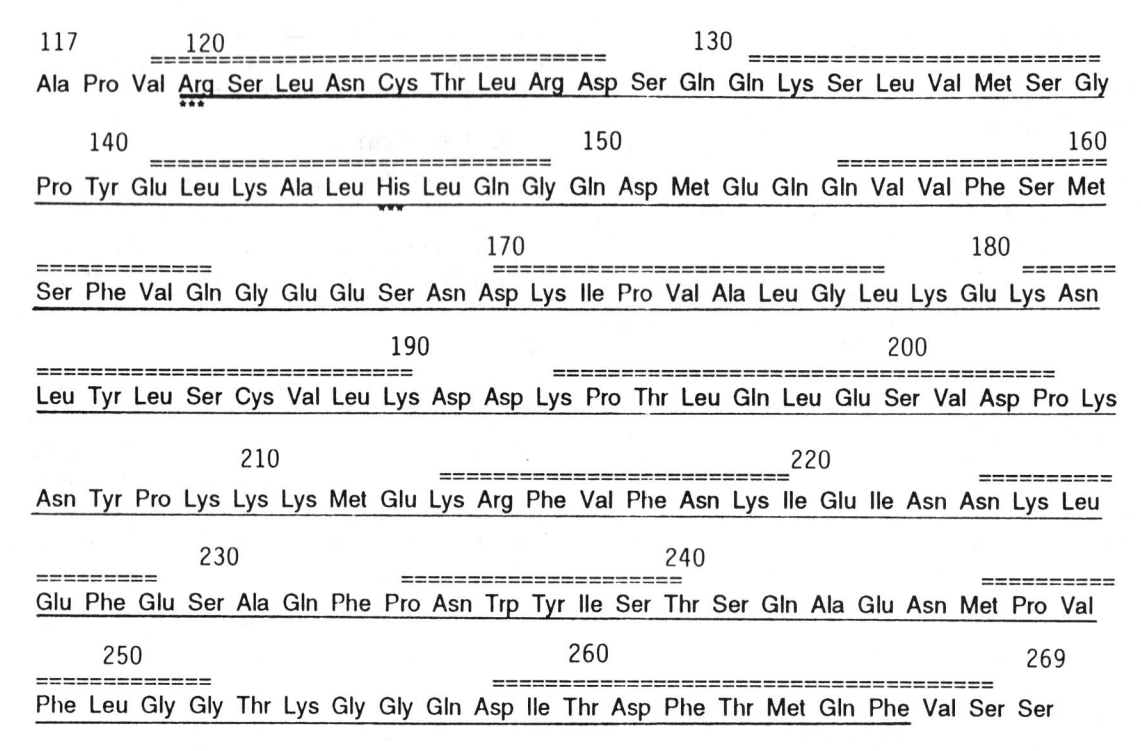

```
117         120                              130
          =====================================    ===========================
Ala Pro Val Arg Ser Leu Asn Cys Thr Leu Arg Asp Ser Gln Gln Lys Ser Leu Val Met Ser Gly
            ***
         140                              150                              160
===================================                           ======================
Pro Tyr Glu Leu Lys Ala Leu His Leu Gln Gly Gln Asp Met Glu Gln Gln Val Val Phe Ser Met
                                   ***
                                          170                              180
==============                ================================       =======
Ser Phe Val Gln Gly Glu Glu Ser Asn Asp Lys Ile Pro Val Ala Leu Gly Leu Lys Glu Lys Asn
                         190                              200
==============================    ========================================
Leu Tyr Leu Ser Cys Val Leu Lys Asp Asp Lys Pro Thr Leu Gln Leu Glu Ser Val Asp Pro Lys
              210                              220
                                 ===========================        ==========
Asn Tyr Pro Lys Lys Lys Met Glu Lys Arg Phe Val Phe Asn Lys Ile Glu Ile Asn Asn Lys Leu
              230                              240
=========        =======================                            ==========
Glu Phe Glu Ser Ala Gln Phe Pro Asn Trp Tyr Ile Ser Thr Ser Gln Ala Glu Asn Met Pro Val
         250                      260                         269
==============        =========================================
Phe Leu Gly Gly Thr Lys Gly Gly Gln Asp Ile Thr Asp Phe Thr Met Gln Phe Val Ser Ser
```

The minimum amino acid sequence of human interleukin-1β required for full activity spans residues 120 to 266. Underlined amino acids represent the minimum sequence required for complete activity. Asterisks indicate amino acids important for binding to the receptor. Double broken lines indicate sequences corresponding to beta-pleated sheet configuration. *Data from Gubler et al 1989.*

cytocidal or cytostatic for human A375 melanoma cells in vitro (Lachman et al 1986, Onozaki et al 1985). Other human tumors inhibited by IL-1 in vitro include myeloid leukemic cell lines (Onozaki et al 1989), rhabdomyosarcoma A673 cells, human mammary carcinomas, and adenocarcinoma of the lung (Fryling et al 1989).

Animal Studies. Animal tumors inhibited by IL-1 in vivo include malignant glioma in the rat (Rice and Merchant 1990) and, to a slight degree, $CD8F_1$ breast cancer in mice (Moore et al 1990). In one preliminary study, however, IL-1 increased B-16 melanoma metastases to the lung (Garofalo et al 1990).

The IL-1 proteins also act like early hematopoietic growth factors with chemoprotectant and radioprotectant properties. Interleukin-1α enhances the survival of hematopoietic stem cells and can lessen experimental neutropenia following cyclophosphamide or 5-fluorouracil treatment of mice (Moore et al 1990). In this trial, the combination of 5-fluorouracil with rHuIL-1β and granulocyte–macrophage colony-stimulating factor (GM-CSF) or granulocyte colony-stimulating factor (G-CSF) produced superior tumor growth inhibition in mice with spontaneous $CD8F_1$ breast tumors (Moore et al 1990). In normal mice recombinant human IL-1β alone produced neutrophilia and lymphopenia and, in combination with 5-fluorouracil, can reduce high-dose 5-fluorouracil lethality. This effect was further enhanced with the addition of GM-CSF. In all studies, the effect of IL-1β on neutrophils was biphasic. An initial decrease in neutrophils on day 4 after 5-fluorouracil was followed by enhanced white blood cell recovery by day 14. Indeed, IL-1 can stimulate both granulopoiesis and megakaryocytopoiesis following repetitive cycles of cyclophosphamide. This acts to accelerate the recovery of normal hematopoiesis following myelosuppressive anticancer drug therapy. There is also evidence of partial protection from anemia with IL-1 in 5-fluorouracil-treated animals.

Clinical Trials. In a phase I clinical trial of IL-1β (Syntex) in solid tumor patients, a nonmaximally toxic dose of 0.3 μg/kg transiently elevated white blood cell counts after an initial drop. There was a minor drop in platelets which was followed by a delayed increase in platelet counts (Steis et al 1991). Bone marrow examinations showed a 20% increase in cellularity, increased myeloid/erythroid ratios, and increased numbers of osteoclasts and osteoblasts. Serum IL-2 and IL-6 levels were also increased, but circulating CD34-positive stem cell numbers did not change.

More recently, IL-1α doses of 0.3 μg/kg IV × 5 days have been shown to limit the thrombocytopenic effect of high-dose carboplatin (800 mg/m^2) when IL-1α was administered after carboplatin (Smith et al 1992a). Similar thrombopoietic effects were observed with carboplatin (400 mg/m^2 day 1) and IL-1α given as a continuous intravenous infusion on days 1 to 4 at doses up to 3.0 μg/m^2/d (Vadhan-Raj et al 1992). Leukocyte and platelet increases are noted on days 1 to 6 and 14 to 28, respectively, in cancer patients receiving single-agent IL-α therapy at doses up to 2 μg/m^2 as a daily 2-hour infusion (Dennis et al 1992). Hematologic recovery following high-dose chemotherapy is accelerated by 7 days of pretreatment with IL-1α doses up to 0.2 μg/kg/d as a 3-hour infusion daily (Wilson et al 1992). In this trial, recombinant IL-1α enhanced autologous bone marrow engraftment noted by earlier recovery of granulocyte and platelet counts. The optimal dose and schedule in this setting are unknown.

Objective responses to 5-day IL-1β infusions were reported in three of nine patients with malignant melanoma (Starnes et al 1991). There were two partial responses and one partial response lasting from 6 to 12 months in this preliminary trial; however, in another phase II trial of IL-1 with indomethacin no objective responses were observed in eight patients with malignant melanoma (Smith et al 1991) or other advanced tumors such as gastrointestinal cancer (Smith et al 1992b). Recombinant IL-1β has also been evaluated in patients with metastatic colorectal cancer (Crown et al 1989). The results of this phase I–II clinical trial show that IL-1β somewhat reduces 5-fluorouracil myelosuppression but does not alter the days of febrile neutropenia nor the total number of days that antibiotics are required. IL-1β dose escalation is ongoing in this trial.

■ Mechanism of Action

Interleukin-1 has diverse activities which may contribute to more effective treatment of cancer. Broadly, these actions include hematopoietic (growth factor) stimulation of early bone marrow precursors, stimulation of growth factor production and release (eg, IL-2 and others), augmentation of T-cell cytotoxicity and β-cell differentiation, and mediation of inflammatory response including antitumor interactions.

Interleukin-1 activities are mediated by binding to two types of cell surface receptors. Both IL-1α and IL-1β bind to these same receptors (Kilian et al 1986). The first type of IL-1 receptor is found on T cells and fibroblasts (Sims et al 1988). The second type is found on B lymphocytes and macrophages. The mechanism of direct cytotoxicity in NIH:OVCAR-3 cells is known to be receptor dependent but does not involve prostaglandin E_2 synthesis as in febrile reactions (Kilian et al 1991). Cell division is halted by IL-1 in these cells, noted by rapid changes in the size and density of the nucleus (Kilian et al 1991).

There are a number of IL-1 mechanisms other than direct inhibition of tumor cell growth. Interleukin-1 is a potent stimulator of IL-2 (T-cell growth factor) production (Smith et al 1980). It thus can enhance thymocyte proliferation, particularly in response to stimulation with T-cell mitogens such as phytohemagglutinin (Krakauer 1986). IL-1 may also cause the differentiation of immature thymocytes in helper (CD4+) T cells. In B lymphocytes, IL-1 directly stimulates proliferation and differentiation (Howard and Paul 1983).

All of the IL-1 proteins are also highly active in the rabbit pyrogen test which measures fever production resulting from the strong endogenous pyrogen activity of the molecule. The natural sources of IL-1 include all types of mononuclear phagocytes including leukemic cells and a variety of other cells such as keratinocytes, exudate cells, astrocytes and glial cells, corneal epithelial cells, mesangial cells, and renal carcinoma cells (Dinarello 1984). Potent inducers of IL-1 production and secretion include microorganisms, microbial cell wall products and lipopolysaccharides (LPS), and asbestos and ultraviolet light exposure (Blyden and Handschumacher 1977, Krakauer 1986). The febrile effect of IL-1 involves an interaction with receptors clustered in thermosensitive cells of the preoptic anterior hypothalamus. This interaction leads to arachidonic acid metabolism by cyclooxygenase enzymes. Several prostaglandins, especially prostaglandin E_2, are rapidly produced. This leads to resetting of the thermoregulatory center and, consequently, the induction of a fever by normal heat generation mechanisms in the muscle and other tissues (Dinarello 1984). Of interest, IL-1 has greater biologic activity at temperatures elevated above 37°C, although the biologic significance of this effect is unknown.

The effect of IL-1 on hematopoietic cells is complex. First, the protein is known to stimulate the production of several hematopoietic growth factors including IL-2, IL-4, IL-6, GM-CSF, G-CSF, and CSF-1, along with the acute-phase reactants fibrinogen, haptoglobin, ceruloplasmin, and serum amyloid A protein (Dinarello 1984). In contrast, the acute effects of IL-1 on circulating white blood cells appear to be the result of alterations in leukocyte migration (Moore et al 1990). In response to IL-1, leukocytes adhere avidly to endothelium and migrate to extravascular spaces. Leukocyte release from bone marrow is also enhanced (Dinarello and Savage 1989). In humans, myeloid progenitor cells are increased in the peripheral blood. These include CFU-G, M, GM, GEMM, and BFU-E cells (Dennis et al 1992). The lymphopenia induced by IL-1 may be caused by increased production of glucocorticosteroids which causes lympholysis (Morrissey et al 1988). The lack of prolonged hematopoietic stimulation with continued IL-β administration may result in part from the induction of the negative hematopoietic factor tumor necrosis factor (Gasparetto et al 1989).

Interleukin-1 synergizes with tumor-derived G-CSF to stimulate neutrophil production in the bone marrow (Moore et al 1990). Interleukin also induces the production of GM-CSF in a variety of cell types such as fibroblasts, endothelial cells, and macrophages (Moore 1988, Moore and Warren 1987). Overall, these findings suggest that hematopoiesis due to IL-1 results from augmented growth factor production and enhanced migration of leukocytes out of bone marrow and into the vascular compartment and extravascular tissues.

■ Availability and Storage

Interleukin-1α is investigationally available as a sterile preparation through the Biological Response Modifiers Program of the National Cancer Institute. Interleukin-1α from *Escherichia coli* is also available from Dainippon Pharmaceutical Company, Ltd, Osaka, Japan. It is investigationally supplied as 10 μg of lyophilized powder in single-use vials containing human serum albumin as a stabilizer and no antibacterial preservative (Smith et al 1992b). This material has a purity of 99% or greater and a specific activity of approximately 2×10^7 lymphocyte-activating factor units/mg of protein. Commercial human interleukin-1β (rhIL-1β) is produced by recombinant DNA techniques in *E. coli*. It is supplied as a sterile lyophilized powder from Syntex Research (Palo Alto, California) and is investigationally available through the National Cancer Institute. Each vial of rhIL-1β (Syntex) contains 100 μg in a 5-mL glass vial with mannitol, sucrose, and tromethamine buffer (355 mosmol/L). The pH is adjusted to 7.5 using HCl or NaOH. Investigational IL-1 preparations are also available from the Genetics Institute (Boston, Massachusetts) and Immunex Corporation (Seattle, Washington).

■ Preparation for Use, Stability, and Admixture

The 10-μg IL-1α (Dainippon) vials are reconstituted with 5 mL of 0.9% Sodium Chloride for Injection, USP. This results in a clear solution containing 2 μg/mL IL-1α and 2 μg/mL human serum albumin.

Each 100-μg vial of rhIL-1β is reconstituted with 1 mL of either Sterile Water for Injection, USP, or 5 mL of Sodium Chloride for Injection, USP. At low doses, 1% (v/v), human serum albumin should be added to the IL-β solution to reduce adsorption of the protein to infusion system surfaces. The reconstituted solution can be stored for 8 hours at 2 to 8°C.

■ Administration

Both of the investigational IL-1 preparations have been administered intravenously as a brief infusion (over 15 minutes) in normal saline.

■ Dosage

The maximally tolerated dose (MTD) of IL-1α combined with indomethacin (25 mg orally or rectally every 8 hours) was 0.1 μg/kg/d for 7 days, repeated at 2-week intervals (Smith et al 1991). When IL-β was used alone (without indomethacin), the MTD of IL-1α was 0.3 μg/kg/d × 7 days (Smith et al 1992a). These treatments were not repeated. The MTD of IL-β (Syntex) is unknown but is greater than 0.3 μg/kg/d for 7 days (Steis et al 1991). An alternate schedule comprised five daily intravenous infusions of doses ranging from 1 to 100 ng/kg (0.1 μg/kg) (Starnes et al 1991).

■ Drug Interactions

Indomethacin has been used to partially reduce IL-1α flulike symptoms (Smith et al 1991b) but appears to actually lower the MTD of IL-1α (Smith et al 1992a). The effect of indomethacin on IL-1 antitumor activity is unknown. Both indomethacin and dexamethasone block IL-1β expression in astrocytomas exposed to lipopolysaccharide (Velasco et al 1990).

Dexamethasone also blocks IL-1-induced potentiation of mitomycin-C antitumor activity in solid tumor models (Braunschweiger et al 1991); however, the clinical use of indomethacin does not abrogate dose-limiting hypotension but does lessen myalgias and arthralgias slightly (Smith et al 1992b). Dexamethasone appears to selectively decrease gene transcription and destabilize mRNA specific to the IL-1β gene (Velasco et al 1990). Conversely, the antitumor agent hydroxyurea is known to enhance IL-1 production in vitro (Luger and Oppenheim, 1983). IL-1 is known to act in an additive or superadditive fashion with exogenous G-CSF to reduce chemotherapy-induced myelosuppression (Moore et al 1990). The specific interaction of IL-1 with the other numerous hematopoietic growth factors induced by IL-1 is unknown. This includes IL-2, GM-CSF, and especially IL-6 (Smith et al 1992b). In the case of tumor necrosis factor, however, a reduction in IL-1 bone marrow stimulation is known to occur (Gasparetto et al 1989).

Pharmacokinetics

The plasma pharmacokinetics of IL-1β has been studied in cynomolgus monkeys given intravenous doses of 1, 2, and 10 µg/kg. Mean plasma elimination half-lives were 25, 51, and 99 minutes, respectively. The area under the plasma concentration × time curve (AUC) was proportional to the dose administered. Mean systemic clearance was not, however, dose dependent.

Side Effects and Toxicity

Fever is the most common toxic effect of IL-1. The fever induced by IL-1 is monophasic and can be partially abrogated by nonsteroidal anti-inflammatory agents such as indomethacin (Smith et al 1991). Rigors may be common and can be alleviated by meperidine (Dennis et al 1992). Other toxic effects noted in phase I clinical trials of IL-1β included rigors, headache, mild nausea and vomiting, myalgias, and arthralgias (Steis et al 1991). Hypotension with IL-1α tends to be the dose-limiting toxic effect. This is due to a profound drop in systemic vascular resistance with reflex tachycardia (Smith et al 1992a). There are biphasic blood pressure changes noted by an increase over the first 60 minutes followed by dose-dependent hypotension afterward. Hypotension can be quite prolonged and has resulted in myocardial infarction; however, one patient also developed severe hypertension with acute pulmonary edema and left ventricular failure. Pulmonary infiltrates and weight gain can develop in the absence of left ventricular failure (Smith et al 1992b). This suggests noncardiogenic pulmonary edema secondary to a capillary leak syndrome. The pulmonary effects are usually not severe (Smith et al 1992b). Atrial fibrillation was noted in another patient (Steis et al 1991). The blood pressure changes from IL-1 are responsive to intravenous fluids, although 4 of 19 patients required phenylephrine therapy for acute hypotension in one trial (Smith et al 1991). This is typically most severe with the first course of IL-1 therapy.

As noted earlier, white blood cell and platelet counts show an initial decrease 1 hour after administration followed by dose-dependent elevations which are apparent after 24 hours. Prolonged elevation of the white blood cell level for more than 1 to 2 weeks is not possible, however, because of the induction of tumor necrosis factor in monocytes (Gasparetto et al 1989). The myeloid/erythroid ratio and the degree of bone marrow cellularity increased in 7 of 10 patients in one phase I trial of IL-α alone (Dennis et al 1992). The number of bone marrow progenitor cells in the peripheral blood is also increased following IL-1α therapy. Nonetheless, IL-1α did not increase the colony-forming ability of bone marrow cells (Smith et al 1992b).

Interleukin-1 also causes minor transient elevations in serum creatinine, bilirubin, and serum glutamic-oxalacetic transaminase levels (Steis et al 1991). Other toxic effects include mild nausea and vomiting (Wilson et al 1992) phlebitis at the intravenous site, and abdominal/back pain (Crown et al 1990). No long-term or cumulative toxicity has been noted following IL-1 therapy and most effects resolve rapidly when the drug is discontinued.

Metabolic effects of IL-1 include elevated C-reactive protein and transient hypoglycemia followed by rebound hyperglycemia (Crown et al 1990). The blood urea nitrogen and creatinine levels also increase consistent with prerenal azotemia. These effects are typically mild and transient.

Central nervous system effects of IL-1α include agitation, somnolence, confusion, and delusional ideation in a few patients (Smith et al 1992b).

REFERENCES

Auron PE, Webb AC, Rosenwasser LJ, et al. Nucleoside sequence of human monocyte interleukin 1 precursor cDNA. *Proc Natl Acad Sci USA.* 81:7–7911.

Blyden G, Handschumacher RE. Purification and properties of human lymphocyte-activating factor (LAF). *J Immunol.* 1977;**118**:1631.

Braunschweiger PG, Jones SA, Johnson CS et al. Potentiation of mitomycin-C and porfiromycin antitumor activity in solid tumor models by recombinant human interleukin 1α. *Cancer Res.* 1991;**51**:5454–5460.

Crown J, Gabrilove J, Kemeny N, et al. Phase I–II trial of recombinant human interleukin 1β (IL-1) in patients (PTS) with metastatic colorectal cancer (MCC) receiving myelosuppressive doses of 5-fluorouracil (5-FU). *Proc Am Soc Clin Oncol.* 1990;**9**:183.

Crown J, Kemeny N, Jakubowski A, et al. Phase I–II trial of recombinant human interleukin-1β (IL-1) in patients (PTS) with metastatic colorectal cancer (MCC) receiving 5-fluorouracil (5FU). *Blood.* 1989;**74**(suppl 1):15.

Dennis D, Chachoua A, Caron D, et al. Biologic activity of interleukin 1 (IL-1) alpha in patients with refractory malignancies. *Proc Am Soc Clin Oncol.* 1992;**11**:255.

Dinarello CA. Interleukin-1. *Rev Infect Dis.* 1984;**6**(1):51–95.

Dinarello CA, Goldin NP, Wolff SM. Demonstration and characterization of two distinct human leukocytic pyrogens. *J Exp Med.* 1974;**139**:1369–1381.

Dinarello CA, Savage N. Interleukin-1 and its receptor. *CRC Crit Rev Immunol.* 1989;**9**:1–20.

Fryling C, Dombalagian M, Burgess W, et al. Purification and characterization of tumor inhibitory factor-2: Its identity to interleukin 1. *Cancer Res.* 1989;**49**:3333–3337.

Garofalo A, Bani MR, Giavazzi R. Augmentation of metastases induced by interleukin-1 in different tumor systems. *Proc Am Assoc Cancer Res.* 1990;**31**:71.

Gasparetto C, Laver J, Abboud M, et al. Effects of interleukin 1 on hematopoietic progenitors: Evidence of stimulatory and inhibitory activities in a primate model. *Blood.* 1989;**74**:547–550.

Gery I, Gershon RK, Waksman BH. Potentiation of the T-lymphocyte response to mitogens. I. The responding cell. *J Exp Med.* 1972;**136**:128–142.

Gubler U, Chua AO, Lugg DK. Cloning and expression of interleukin-1. In: Bomford R, Henderson B, eds. *Interleukin-1, Inflammation and Disease.* Amsterdam: Elsevier; 1989:40.

Howard M, Paul WB. Regulation of B cell growth and differentiation by soluble factors. *Annu Rev Immunol.* 1983;**1**:307.

Kilian PL, Kaffka KL, Stern AS, et al. Interleukin 1 alpha and interleukin 1 beta bind to the same receptor on T cells. *J Immunol.* 1986;**136**:4509–4514.

Kilian PL, Kaffka KL, Biondi DA, et al. Antiproliferative effect of interleukin-1 on human ovarian carcinoma cell line (NIH:OVCAR-3). *Cancer Res.* 1991;**51**:1823–1828.

Krakauer T. Human interleukin 1. *CRC Crit Rev Immunol.* 1986;**6**(3):213–244.

Lachman BL, Dinarello CA, Llansa ND, et al. Natural and recombinant human interleukin 1-beta is cytotoxic for human melanoma cells. *J Immunol.* 1986;**136**:3098–3102.

Lomedico PT, Gubler U, Hellmann CP, et al. Cloning and expression of murine interleukin-1 cDNA in *Escherichia coli. Nature (London).* 1984;**312**:458.

Luger TA, Oppenheim JJ. Characteristics of interleukin-1 and epidermal cell-derived thymocyte activating factor. In: Weissman G, ed. *Advances in Inflammation Research.* New York: Raven Press; 1983;**5**:1–22.

Moore MAS. The use of hematopoietic growth and differentiation factors for bone marrow stimulation. In: DeVita VT Jr, Hellman S, Rosenberg SA, eds. *Important Advances in Oncology.* Philadelphia: Lippincott; 1988:31–54.

Moore MAS, Stolfi RL, Martin DS. Hematologic effects of interleukin-1β, granulocyte colony-stimulating factor, and granulocyte–macrophage colony-stimulating factor in tumor-bearing mice treated with fluorouracil. *J Natl Cancer Inst.* 1990;**82**:1031–1037.

Moore MAS, Warren DJ. Synergy of interleukin 1 and granulocyte colony-stimulating factor: In vivo stimulation of stem-cell recovery and hematopoietic regeneration following 5-fluorouracil treatment of mice. *Proc Natl Acad Sci USA.* 1987;**84**:7134–7138.

Morrissey PJ, Charrier K, Alpert A, et al. In vivo administration of IL-1 induces thymic hypoplasia and increased levels of serum corticosterone. *J Immunol.* 1988;**141**:1456–1463.

Onozaki K, Akiyama Y, Okamo A, et al. Synergistic regulatory effects of interleukin 6 and interleukin 1 on the growth and differentiation of human and mouse myeloid leukemic cell lines. *Cancer Res.* 1989;**49**:333–337.

Onozaki K, Matsushima K, Aggarwal BB, et al. Human interleukin 1 is cytocidal for several tumor cell lines. *J Immunol.* 1985;**135**:3962–3968.

Rice CD, Merchant RE. The influence of murine recombinant interleukin-1 (rIL-1) on the survival of rats with malignant glioma. *Proc Am Assoc Cancer Res.* 1990;**31**:298.

Sims JE, Marsh CJ, Cosman D, et al. cDNA expression cloning of the IL-1 receptor, a member of the immunoglobin superfamily. *Science.* 1988;**241**:585–589.

Smith J II, Longo D, Alvord W, et al. Thrombopoietic effects of IL-1α in combination with high-dose carboplatin. *Proc Am Soc Clin Oncol.* 1992a;**11**:252.

Smith JW II, Urba WJ, Curti BD, et al. The toxic and hematologic effects of interleukin-1 alpha administered in a phase I trial to patients with advanced malignancies. *J Clin Oncol.* 1992b;**10**(7):1141–1152.

Smith J II, Urba W, Steis R, et al. Phase II trial of interleukin-1 alpha (IL-1α) in combination with indomethacin (IND) in melanoma patients (pts). *Proc Am Soc Clin Oncol.* 1991;**10**:293.

Smith KA, Lachman LB, Oppenheim JJ, Favata MF. The functional relationship of the interleukins. *J Exp Med.* 1980;**151**:1551.

Starnes HF Jr, Hartman G, Torti F, et al. Recombinant human interleukin-1β (IL-1β) has anti-tumor activity and acceptable toxicity in metastatic malignant melanoma. *Proc Am Soc Clin Oncol.* 1991;**10**:292.

Steis R, Smith J II, Janik J, et al. Phase I study of recombinant IL-1 beta (Syntex). *Proc Am Soc Clin Oncol.* 1991;**10**:211.

Vadhan-Raj S, Kudelka A, Garrison L, et al. Interleukin-1α (IL-1α) increases circulating platelet (PLT) counts and reduces carboplatin (CBDCA)-induced thrombocytopenia. *Proc Am Soc Clin Oncol.* 1992;**11**:224.

Velasco S, Tarlow M, McCracken G, Nisen P. Modulation of interleukin-1 gene expression in astrocytomas in vitro. *Proc Am Assoc Cancer Res.* 1990;**31**:81.

Wilson WH, Bryant G, Jain V, et al. Phase I study of infusional interleukin-1α (IL-1) with ifosfamide (I), CBDCA (C) and etoposide (E) (ICE) and autologous bone marrow transplant (BMT). *Proc Am Soc Clin Oncol.* 1992;**11**:335.

Interleukin-3

■ Other Names

IL-3; SDZ IL-E964 (Sandoz Inc); rhuIL3; Multi CSF.

■ Chemistry

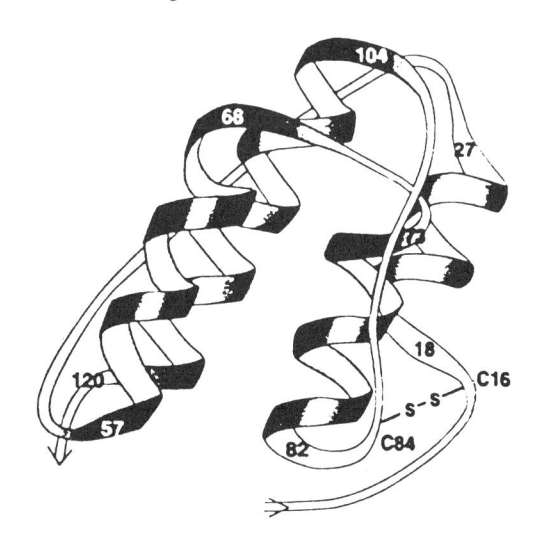

Structure of interleukin-3

Interleukin-3 (IL-3) is produced by recombinant DNA techniques from *Escherichia Coli* bacteria (Sandoz, Inc) *Saccharomyces* yeast (Hoechst-Roussel Pharmaceuticals Inc) or *Bacillus licheniformis* (Gist-brocades, NV, Delft, The Netherlands) engineered to express the human gene for IL-3. Human IL-3 contains 133 amino acids and has a molecular weight ranging from 14,000 to 16,000 (Yang et al 1986). While the natural protein is glycosylated, the recombinant molecule from *E. coli* is nonglycosylated and typically contains an additional terminal methionine residue. It is as active biologically as the native glycosylated protein. The original Immunex/Hoechst protein differs from the natural protein by the substitution of aspartic acid for asparagine at positions 15 and 70 to preclude possible N-linked glycosylation in yeast (Cantrell et al 1985).

The potency of IL-3 preparations is nominally rated between 0.5 to 6.0×10^8 U/mg in colony-forming assays and 1 to 8×10^{10} U/mL in receptor binding assays. The material produced by Immunex/Behringwerke AG has a specific activity of 1×10^7 units/mg of protein and a wider molecular weight range as a result of partial glycosylation by the host yeast organism.

■ Mechanism of Action

Interleukin-3 is a species-specific multilineage stimulator of early bone marrow progenitors known as CFU-GEMM (colony-forming units—granulocyte, erythrocyte, megakaryocyte, macrophage). It is normally produced in activated T lymphocytes and binds to a 140-kDa receptor on hematopoietic precursor cells. The receptor becomes phosphorylated on a tyrosine after binding (Isfort et al 1988). The proliferative effect of IL-3 may be mediated by protein kinase C (He et al 1988). The hematopoietic stimulation by IL-3 is relatively broad spectrum, affecting bone marrow progenitors of the granulocyte, monocyte, erythrocyte, and megakaryocyte series (Kindler et al 1986, Metcalf et al 1986a,b). This stimulation occurs prior to S phase (Kelvin et al 1986), and the effect stimulates hexose uptake, enhances asparaginase activity, and enhances intracellular calcium mobilization (Oster et al 1990). Following administration of IL-3, the peripheral blood count increases with a shift favoring the myelocytic series. This includes platelets, erythrocytes, leukocytes, and monocytes. In cynomolgus monkey models, this increase becomes prominent within 1 to 2 weeks after initiating treatment. The increase in neutrophils is particularly prominent and is synergistic when given after GM-CSF (Williams et al 1988); however, in contrast to G-CSF and GM-CSF, IL-3 does not stimulate mature neutrophil activity (Lopez et al 1988).

In patients with preserved hematopoietic function, eosinophil stimulation may be the most prominent and profound change (Lindemann et al 1990, 1991). However, a sustained, dose-dependent increase in platelet counts is also reported (Ganser et al 1991). This ranged from 1.3-fold at 250 μg/mL to 1.9-fold at 500 μg/m² (Ganser et al 1991, Lindemann et al 1991). Basophils are stimulated to a lesser degree. The platelet stimulatory effect is significant and long lasting, but onset is delayed. A peak of thrombopoiesis was noted 15 to 20 days after starting 15 daily subcutaneous injections of IL-3 (125 to 250 μg/m²/d [Lindemann et al 1990]).

Recombinant human IL-3 can release histamine from human basophils in vitro and in monkeys but not in humans (Lindemann et al 1991). IL-3 also increases the tumoricidal activity of human peripheral blood monocytes against human A375 malignant melanoma cells. A number of other cytokines are released following IL-3 injection, including the B-lymphocyte growth factor IL-6 (Lindemann et al 1991). Soluble interleukin-2 receptors are also increased. These other proteins may mediate some of the activity of IL-3. IL-3 enhances myeloid cell functions including antibody-dependent cellular cytotoxicity, and oxidative metabolism in eosinophils (Rothenberg et al 1988), but not neutrophils, which are known to lack the IL-3 receptor (Lopez et al 1988). Monocyte cytotoxicity is also enhanced by IL-3 through a tumor necrosis factor-dependent mechanism (Cannistra et al 1988).

Excess IL-3 may be produced in some B-cell lymphocytic leukemia cells (Meeker et al 1990). This was found to be caused by a chromosomal translocation joining the IgH gene with the IL-3 gene: t(5:14)(q31:q32). Serum levels of IL-3 ranged up to 7995 (pg/mL) in the affected patient (Meeker et al 1990).

■ Antitumor Activity

Interleukin-3 does not appear to possess antitumor activity although it can suppress human tumor colony formation in vitro in about 10% of specimens from patients with solid tumors (Von Hoff et al 1992). However, opposite (tumor stimulatory) effects have been observed in a few human pancreas or lung cancer cell lines (Dippold et al 1992, Vellenga et al 1991). One of eight small cell lung cancer cell lines was stimulated to proliferate by IL-3 (Vellenga et al 1990). This effect has not been observed in other in vitro studies with human ovarian cancer cell lines (Hirte 1990). In leukemic blasts, IL-3 may enhance the incorporation of cytarabine triphosphate into DNA to block cell division (Bhalla et al 1990). Overall, there is no clear role for IL-3 as either a tumor stimulant or inhibitor. One minor response to IL-3 alone has been reported in melanoma (Bhatia et al 1992). Interleukin-3 is mainly a potent, broad-spectrum myelotopoietic factor which may be useful in certain cases of bone marrow failure or as an adjunct to counteract the effects of myelosuppressive chemotherapy drugs. Preclinical studies show that IL-3 is an effective stimulator of myelopoiesis, erythropoiesis, and thrombopoiesis in murine models (Kindler et al 1986, Metcalf et al 1986a,b) as well as in nonhuman primate models (Donahue et al 1988, Krumwich and Seiler 1989, Mayer et al 1989). Similarly, it is relatively active on undifferentiated human hematopoietic cells (Ottmann et al 1989).

Several phase I/II clinical trials have shown that recombinant human IL-3 (rHuIL-3) can induce significant hematopoietic effects in patients with bone marrow failure secondary to chemotherapy (Ganser et al 1990a, Lindemann et al 1991) or in patients with myelodysplastic syndromes (Ganser et al 1990b, Kurzrock et al 1991a,b). In patients with advanced tumors and normal or depressed hematopoiesis, rHuIL-3 produces dose-dependent increases in the levels of neutrophils and platelets. Erythropoiesis is variable and delayed, and was least responsive to IL-3 in both patient populations. There was also no dose–response apparent for the increase in reticulocytes following IL-3 (Ganser et al 1990a, Kurzrock et al 1991a,b).

Overall, patients with secondary hematopoietic failure respond much more slowly to IL-3. The median time to peak neutrophil counts in these patients was 19 days compared with 15 days in cancer patients with preserved hematopoietic function. This effect was dose dependent. The time to an increased platelet count was also dose dependent, generally peaking between days 15 and 25 after starting a 15-day single daily injection schedule (Ganzer et al 1990a). In a patient with chronic myelomonocytic leukemia, Kurzrock et al (1991a,b) observed maturation of monocytes. Another patient with refractory anemia and excess blasts did experience an increase in bone marrow blast cells (from 9 to 24%) which necessitated drug discontinuance. In mice, IL-3 is effective at enhancing leukocyte recovery following irradiation (Kindler et al 1986, Metcalf et al 1986a). When given after cyclophosphamide and carboplatin, IL-3 was slightly more effective at blocking thrombocytopenia than granulocytopenia (Biesma et al 1992, Speyer et al 1992). With carboplatin, IL-3 at 10 μg/kg/d allows a 45% dose intensification as a result of decreased chemotherapy postponement (de Vries et al 1992). IL-3 doses of 250 µg/m² were also effective for preventing low-dose carboplatin (350 µg/m²-induced thrombocytopenia (Rusthoven et al 1992). IL-3 lessens the hematologic toxicity of ifosfamide, carboplatin, and etoposide (ICE) therapy for non-small cell lung cancer (Tepler et al 1992) and of etoposide, carboplatin, and epirubicin for small cell lung cancer (D'Hont et al 1992). IL-3 also blocks the myelotoxicity of ifosfamide, epirubicin, and etoposide therapy in patients with aggressive lymphomas (Gerhartz et al 1992).

In nine patients with myelodysplastic syndromes, IL-3 increased leukocytes 1.3- to 3.6-fold including lymphocytes, neutrophils, eosinophils, basophils, and monocytes (Ganser et al 1990b, Kurzrock et al 1991a,b). An increase in platelets was noted in two of four profoundly thrombocytopenic patients and the need for red blood cell transfusions temporarily improved in one patient. Both studies show that IL-3 is an effective stimulant of granulocytepoiesis, thrombopoiesis, and, to a lesser degree, erythropoiesis.

In patients with AIDS, IL-3 doses of up to 5 µg/kg/day were ineffective at stimulating hematopoiesis, and there was no enhanced viral (HIV) activity (Scadden et al 1992).

■ Availability and Storage

Interleukin-3 is investigationally available as a lyophilized white powder in 250-µg vials also containing 10 mg sucrose, 40 mg mannitol, and 1.2 mg tris(hydroxymethyl)aminomethane buffer (Hoechst-Roussel Pharmaceuticals Inc, Somerville, New Jersey). The material is stable at room temperatures for short periods, but biologic activity is reduced when it is stored at 37°C for 3 months or at 56°C for 1 month. The IL-3 supplied by Sandoz, Inc, East Hanover, New Jersey, is packaged in 5-mL clear glass vials containing 0.15 mg (150 µg) of white lyophilized IL-3 powder. These vials and the 2-mL sterile water ampule are stored at 4°C. The material from Gist-brocades is supplied in vials containing 200 µg, 500 µg, or 1,000 µg.

■ Preparation for Use, Stability, and Admixture

When reconstituted with 1 to 3 mL Sterile Water for Injection, USP, a pH of 7.4 is achieved. This solution can be further diluted with 0.9 and 0.45% sodium chloride and in D5W. Such dilutions of the stock solution should also include human serum albumin at a 0.1% final concentration to prevent significant adsorption of the protein to the infusion system surfaces.

■ Administration

In the initial clinical trials, rHuIL-3 was administered as an intravenous bolus and as a single daily subcutaneous injection. Because of acute acrocyanosis and chills, the intravenous bolus was subsequently dropped (Ganser et al 1990b). A 4-hour daily infusion was studied by Kurzrock et al (1991a,b). Indeed, the short plasma half-life suggests that prolonged infusions or depot injections may be most effective (Kurzrock et al 1991a). IL-3 has also been administered as a 120-hour continuous intravenous infusion (Ceribelli et al 1992). In patients with advanced cancer treated with cytotoxic agents, there was no difference in the hematopoietic efficacy of intravenous compared to subcutaneous doses (Biesma et al 1992).

■ Dosage

The dose range explored in early phase I–II studies in cancer patients was 30 to 500 µg/m²/d for 15 consecutive days (Ganser et al 1990a,b, Lindemann et al 1991). Kurzrock et al (1991a,b) have found that IL-3 is tolerable and active at doses up to 1000 µg/m²/d for 28 consecutive days. Significant, dose-dependent hematopoietic effects are produced at daily doses above 60 µg/m²/d (1.1-fold leukocyte elevation) up to 500 µg/m²/d for 15 days (2.8-fold leukocyte elevation) (Ganser et al 1990a).

In patients with myelodysplastic syndromes daily subcutaneous doses of 20 to 500 µg/m²/d × 15 days produced leukocyte increases of 1.3- to 3.6-fold (Ganser et al 1990b). Daily doses greater than 5 µg/kg by a 2-hour intravenous infusion are not well-tolerated in patients undergoing autologous bone marrow transplantation following high dose chemotherapy (Nemunaitis et al 1992). In patients with advanced ovarian cancer, headache is dose-limiting at 15 mg/kg/d and tolerable at 10 µg/kg/d given intravenously or subcutaneously on days 5 through 11 after a day 1 chemotherapy regimen (Biesma et al 1992). Another phase I trial found that IL-3 was active and tolerable at daily doses of 8 µg/kg for 14 consecutive days in patients being treated with chemotherapy for relapsed small cell lung cancer (Postmus et al 1992). At 16 µg/kg/d, headache became intolerable with the *Bacillus licheniformis* preparation (Postmus et al 1992).

Drug Interactions

Interleukin-3 is synergistic in hematopoietic activity when given prior to granulocyte–macrophage colony-stimulating factor (GM-CSF) but it is antagonistic if given simultaneously with GM-CSF (Broxmeyer et al 1987, Donahue et al 1988). There is also significant overlap in the hematopoietic activity of GM-CSF and IL-3. Indeed, the fusion protein (PIXY-321®, Immunex) combining the active (binding) subunits of IL-3 and GM-CSF has been synthesized and is highly active in preclinical systems. Sequential IL-3 and GM-CSF were effective at increasing granulocyte and platelet counts, but were not synergistic in patients with advanced cancers (Bretti et al 1992).

Interleukin-3 has been clinically combined with other hematopoietic proteins. When combined with GM-CSF in three patients with "CAF" chemotherapy-induced neutropenia and in two cases of aplastic anemia, IL-3 alone at 250 µg/m² for 15 days was compared with the same IL-3 dose plus GM-CSF 250 µg/m², both started 1 day after chemotherapy (Lindemann et al 1990). In this preliminary report, IL-3 alone did not shorten the period of neutropenia and the combination did not appear to be synergistic. In lymphoma patients, the sequential use of IL-3 followed by GM-CSF appeared to stimulate multilineage hematopoietic cells (Fay et al 1992); however, the sequential use of IL-3 before GM-CSF did not aid in engraftment of granulocyte or platelet producing cells (Wheeler et al 1992). Clearly, more trials and patients are needed to firmly delineate the role for IL-3 as a hematopoietic growth factor in cancer patients. Another pilot trial compared filgrastim (G-CSF) with filgrastim plus IL-3 (given 4 days prior to G-CSF). The combination produced significant protection from thrombocytopenia in non-small cell lung cancer patients receiving ifosfamide, etoposide, and carboplatin (Hamm et al 1992).

Interleukin-3 may also block some deleterious effects of IL-2 on macrophages, including the induction of tumor necrosis factor production (Lissoni et al 1992). IL-3 may also be useful in recruiting quiescent refractory myeloid leukemic cells into a chemotherapy-sensitive state in patients with acute myeloid leukemia (Andreef et al 1992). In another preliminary report, IL-3 was shown to selectively recruit leukemic cells into the cell cycle in patients with acute myelogenous leukemia (Andreef et al 1992). If verified, this could lead to greater cell kill with the sequential use of antileukemic agents such as anthracyclines and cytarabine (Andreef et al 1992).

Pharmacokinetics

In cynomolgus monkeys given an intravenous bolus of 100 µg/kg rHuIL-3, the plasma half-life ranged between 4 and 8 minutes. Elimination appeared to be first order in the monkeys. In human patients with primary or secondary bone marrow failure, IL-3 disposition has been rapid and is possibly complex (see the table below) (Kurzrock et al 1991a,b). The results in the table show that the smallest apparent volume of distribution was achieved at the highest IL-3 dose tested (500 µg/m²), although clearance was relatively rapid at all doses, resulting in a half-life of less than 20 minutes. A one-compartment model seemed to fit the data best. Similar results were described by Lindemann et al (1991): half-lives of 20 minutes after intravenous administration and 210 minutes following subcutaneous administration. Peak serum levels for 60 and 125 µg/m² doses range from 15 to 30 ng/mL for an intravenous bolus and 2 to 10 ng/mL for a subcutaneous injection. The time to the peak is delayed 2 to 4 hours after the subcutaneous injection (Lindemann et al 1991). Two hours after a 0.5 µg/kg subcutaneous dose, a peak plasma level of 346 ng/mL was described in leukemic patients (Andreef et al 1992). The apparent half-life was 3.2 hours in this study.

CLINICAL PHARMACOKINETICS OF RECOMBINANT INTERLEUKIN-3

Dose* (µ/m²)	Number of Patients	Half-life (min) α	Half-life (min) β	Volume of Distribution (L)	AUC (ng/mL·min)
60	3	—	19	66.6	77.7
125	1	11.3	101	30	900
250	3	5	66	43	807
500	1	—	17.3	13	1512

*Doses administered daily × 28 as a 4-hour infusion.
Data from Kurzrock et al 1991.

■ Side Effects and Toxicity

The major toxic effect of IL-3 is fever, which is typically not higher than 39°C and is more intense on initiation of therapy. The fever lasts from 2 to 16 hours after dosing in the first 4 days of therapy. Other common toxic effects include headache and a stiff neck, which rarely led to dose reductions. This may be related to a release of kinins from mature hematopoietic cells. Specifically, the headaches may relate to marked elevations in circulating histamine levels (Bhatia et al 1992). Propranolol was recommended as an antidote in this trial. Occasional side effects include facial flushing, mild local edema, and erythema at the injection site (Ganser et al 1990a). Moderate bone pain is occasionally reported (Ganser et al 1990b, Lindemann et al 1991). In myelodysplastic patients, an early mild thrombocytopenia is sometimes noted. Infections are also rarely seen, and one patient with refractory anemia progressed to refractory anemia with excess blasts while undergoing IL-3 therapy (Ganser et al 1990b). With a continuous intravenous infusion, IL-3 produces flulike symptoms, hypotension, skin rash, headache, and a vasculitis-like purpura (Ceribelli et al 1992).

Interleukin-3 is a potent stimulator of leukemic blast cells in vitro (Delwel et al 1987) and did stimulate excess blast formation in one myelodysplastic patient with refractory anemia (Ganser et al 1990b). However some stimulation was observed in another trial (Kurzrock et al 1991a).

Blood chemistry studies show no consistent changes in liver or renal enzymes; however, acute-phase reactants can increase in a dose-dependent fashion (Lindemann et al 1990). This includes two- to fourfold increases in the acute-phase reactants, C-reactive protein, haptoglobin, β_2-microglobulin, and IgM. This may explain some of the initial mild inflammatory effects of IL-3. Other Ig subclasses are not affected (Lindemann et al 1990).

Rare toxic effects include one instance each of transaminase elevation, atrial fibrillation, and dose dependent nausea, vomiting, bone pain, and peripheral edema (Kurzrock et al 1991a). These effects were observed in less than half of the patients receiving daily doses of 500 to 750 $\mu g/m^2$ and greater. Urticaria on the trunk following a 4-hour infusion of IL-3 has also been described. This reaction subsided without treatment several hours following each infusion (Kurzrock et al 1991a,b). Diphenhydramine did not prevent these reactions, which were not associated with dyspnea or wheezing.

On intravenous injection, there is a transient decrease in circulating monocytes and eosinophils (Lindemann et al 1991). These cell levels reach a nadir 20 minutes after IL-3 injection, return to pre-treatment levels after about 5 to 6 hours, and become elevated thereafter. The immediate decrease does not affect neutrophils and does not appear to involve enhanced expression of adhesion molecules on monocytes or eosinophils (Lindemann et al 1991). Furthermore, the transient decrease does not appear to produce any overt toxic sequelae. In patients undergoing autologous bone marrow transplantation (ABMT) therapy following high-dose chemotherapy, IL-3 is reported to lower circulating levels of several cytokines including IL-6, M-CSF and GM-CSF (Gupton et al 1992). The toxicologic or pharmacologic significance of this finding is as yet unknown. In contrast, another trial with bacterial IL-3 reported a dose-related increase in C-reactive protein, TNF-α and IL-6 (Postmus et al 1992). Cholesterol levels also decreased at the end of a 14-day dosing period as a result of a decrease in LDL cholesterol with high-dose bacterial-derived IL-3 (Postmus et al 1992).

REFERENCES

Andreef M, Drach J, Tafuri A, et al. Interleukin-3 (IL-3) before and during idarubicin/ARA-C in acute myeloblastic leukemia (AML): Phase I clinical and laboratory study. *Blood.* 1992;**80**(suppl 1):111a.

Bhalla K, Kommor M, Grant S, Lutzky J. Improved selectivity of ara-C against AML blasts by a combined treatment with rGM-CSF and rIL-3 (abstract 2505). *Proc Am Assoc Cancer Res.* 1990;**31**:422.

Biesma B, Willemse PHB, Mulder NH, et al. Effects of interleukin-3 after chemotherapy for advanced ovarian cancer. *Blood.* 1992;**80**(5):1141–1148.

Bhatia A, Olencki T, Murthy S, et al. Phase IA/IB trial of rhIL-3 in patients with refractory malignancies: Hematologic and immunologic effects. *Blood.* 1992;**80**(suppl 1): 410a.

Bretti S, Kamthan A, Hicks F, et al. Phase I study of sequential IL-3 and GM-CSF by continuous intravenous infusion. *Proc Am Soc Clin Oncol.* 1992;**11**:181.

Broxmeyer HE, Williams D, Hangoc G, et al. Synergistic myelopoietic actions in vivo after administration to mice of combinations of purified natural murine colony-stimulating factor 1, recombinant murine interleukin-3, and recombinant murine granulocyte/macrophage colony-stimulating factor. *Proc Natl Acad Sci USA.* 1987; **84**:3871.

Cannistra SA, Vellenga E, Groshek P, et al. Human granulocyte–monocyte colony-stimulating factor and interleukin 3 stimulate monocyte cytotoxicity through a tumor necrosis factor-dependent mechanism. *Blood.* 1988;**71**:672.

Cantrell MA, Anderson D, Cerretti DP, et al. Cloning, sequence, and expression of a human granulocyte–macrophage colony stimulating factor. *Proc Natl Acad Sci USA.* 1985;**82**:6250.

Ceribelli A, Fossati C, Gamucci T, et al. Interleukin-3 (IL-3) by 120-hour continuous infusion (c.i.) after myelosuppressive chemotherapy (CT): A phase I study. *Proc Am Assoc Cancer Res.* 1992;**33**:231.

Delwel R, Dorssers L, Touw I, et al. Human recombinant multilineage colony stimulating factor: Stimulator of acute myelocytic leukemia progenitor cells in vitro. *Blood.* 1987;**70**:333.

De Vries EGE, Biesma B, Vellenga E, et al. Recombinant human interleukin-3 (rhIL-3) for chemotherapy (CT) dose intensification in advanced ovarian cancer (OC). *Proc Am Soc Clin Oncol.* 1992;**11**:230.

D'Hont V, Canon JL, Humblet Y, et al. Dose-dependent IL3 stimulation of thrombopoiesis and neutropoiesis in patients with small cell lung carcinoma (SCLC) before and after chemotherapy (CT): A placebo controlled randomized phase 1b study. *Proc Am Soc Clin Oncol.* 1992;**11**:381.

Dippold WG, Klingel R, Kerlin M, et al. Stimulation of pancreas and gastric carcinoma cell growth by interleukin 3 and granulocyte-macrophage colony-stimulating factor. *Gastroenterology.* 1991;**100**:1338.

Donahue RE, Seehra J, Metzger M, et al. Human IL-3 and GM-CSF act synergistically in stimulating hematopoiesis in primates. *Science.* 1988;**241**:1820.

Fay J, Bernstein S, Herzig R, et al. A phase I study of sequential rhIL-3 (SDZ ILE 964) and rhGM-CSF (Leucomax) following autologous bone marrow transplantation therapy for lymphoma. *Blood.* 1992;**80**(suppl 1): 86a.

Ganser A, Lindemann A, Seipelt G, et al. Effects of recombinant human interleukin-3 in patients with normal hematopoiesis and in patients with bone marrow failure. *Blood.* 1990a;**76**(4):666–676.

Ganser A, Lindemann A, Seipelt G, et al. Clinical effects of recombinant human interleukin-3. *Am J Clin Oncol (CCT).* 1991;**14**(suppl 1):S51–S63.

Ganser A, Seipelt G, Lindemann A, et al. Effect of recombinant human interleukin-3 in patients with myelodysplastic syndromes. *Blood.* 1990b;**76**(3):455–462.

Gerhartz HH, Walther J, Bunica O, et al. Clinical hematological and cytokine response to interleukin-3 (IL-3) supported chemotherapy in resistant lymphomas: A phase II study. *Proc Am Soc Clin Oncol.* 1992;**11**:329.

Gupton C, Rabinowitz J, Petros W, et al. Interleukin-3 therapy suppresses endogenous cytokine concentrations following high-dose chemotherapy and autologous bone marrow transplantation (ABMT). *Blood.* 1992;**80** (suppl 1)85a.

Hamm JT, Tepler I, Ritch P, et al. Sequential use of recombinant human interleukin-3 (IL-3) and granulocyte colony stimulating factor (G-CSF) after chemotherapy for non-small cell lung cancer (NSCLC). *Blood.* 1992;**80** (suppl 1):414a.

He Y, Hewlett E, Temeles D, Quesenberry P. Inhibition of interleukin-3 and colony-stimulating factor 1-stimulated marrow cell proliferation by pertussis toxin. *Blood.* 1988;**71**:1187–1195.

Hirte HW. Effect of granulocyte–macrophage colony stimulating factor (GM-CSF) and interleukin-3 (IL-3) on the in vitro growth of human ovarian carcinoma cells (abstract 297). *Proc Am Assoc Cancer Res.* 1990;**31**:50.

Isfort RJ, Stevens D, May WS. Interleukin-3 binds to 140-kDa phosphotyrosine-containing cell surface protein. *Proc Nat Acad Sci USA.* 1988;**85**:7982–7986.

Kelvin DJ, Chance S, Shreeve M, et al. Interleukin-3 and cell cycle progression. *J Cell Physiol.* 1986;**127**:403–409.

Kindler V, Thorens B, de Kossodo S, et al. Stimulation of hematopoiesis in vivo by recombinant bacterial murine interleukin 3. *Proc Natl Acad Sci USA.* 1986;**83**:1001–1005.

Krumwieh D, Seiler FR. In vivo effects of recombinant colony stimulating factors on hematopoiesis in cynomolgus monkeys. *Transplant Proc.* 1989;**21**:379.

Kurzrock R, Estrov Z, Talpaz M, Gutterman JU. Interleukin-3. *Am J Clin Oncol (CCT).* 1991a;**14**(suppl 1):S45–S50.

Kurzrock R, Talpaz M, Estrov Z, et al. Phase I study of recombinant human interleukin-3 in patients with bone marrow failure. *J Clin Oncol.* 1991b;**9**:1241–1250.

Lindemann A, Ganser A, Herrmann F, et al. Biologic effects of recombinant human interleukin-3 in vivo. *J Clin Oncol.* 1991;**9**(12):2120–2127.

Lindemann A, Herrmann F, Mertelsmann R, et al. Human recombinant interleukin 3: A phase I/II clinical trial. In: Mertelsmann R, Herrmann F, eds. *Hematopoietic Growth Factors in Clinical Applications.* New York: Marcel Dekker; 1990;149–159.

Lissoni P, Pittalis S, Rovelli F, et al. Modulation of IL-2–induced macrophage activation by IL-3. *Proc Am Soc Clin Oncol.* 1992;**11**:250.

Lopez AF, Dyson PG, To LB, et al. Recombinant human interleukin-3 stimulation of hematopoiesis in humans: Loss of responsiveness in differentiation in the neutrophilic myeloid series. *Blood.* 1988;**72**:1797–1804.

Mayer P, Valent P, Schmidt G, et al. The in vivo effect of recombinant human interleukin-3: Demonstration of basophil differentiation factor, histamine-producing activity and priming of GM-CSF-responsive progenitors in nonhuman primates. *Blood.* 1989;**74**:613.

Meeker TC, Hardy D, Willman C, et al. Activation of the interleukin-3 gene by chromosome translocation in acute lymphocytic leukemia with eosinophilia. *Blood.* 1990;**76**(2):285–289.

Metcalf D, Begley CG, Johnson GR, et al. Effects of purified bacterially synthesized murine multi-CSF (IL-3) on hematopoiesis in normal adult mice. *Blood.* 1986a;**68**:46–57.

Metcalf D, Begley CG, Johnson GR. Hemopoietic effects of purified bacterially synthesized multi-CSF in normal and marrow-transplanted mice. *Immunobiology.* 1986b;**172**:158–167.

Nemunaitis I, Buckner CD, Appelbaum FR, et al. Phase I trial with recombinant human interleukin-3 (rhIL-3) in patients with lymphoid cancer undergoing autologous bone marrow transplantation (ABMT). *Blood.* 1992;**80**(suppl 1):85a.

Oster W, Mertelsmann R, Herrmann F. Regulation of cell function by hematopoietic growth factors. In: Mertelsmann R, Herrmann F, eds. *Hematopoietic Growth Factors in Clinical Applications.* New York: Marcel Dekker; 1990: 25–39.

Ottmann OG, Abboud M, Welte K, et al. Stimulation of human hematopoietic progenitor cell proliferation and differentiation by recombinant human interleukin 3. Comparison and interactions with recombinant human granulocyte–macrophage and granulocyte colony-stimulating factors. *Exp Hematol.* 1989;**17**:191–197.

Postmus PE, Gietema JA, Damsma O, et al. Effects of recombinant human interleukin-3 in patients with relapsed small-cell lung cancer treated with chemotherapy: A dose-finding study. *J Clin Oncol.* 1992;**10**(7): 1131–1140.

Rothenberg ME, Owen WF Jr, Silberstein DS, et al. Human eosinophils have prolonged survival, enhanced functional properties, and become hypodense when exposed to human interleukin 3. *J Clin Invest.* 1988;**81**:1986.

Rusthoven JJ, Eisenhauer E, Mazurka J, et al. Phase I clinical trial of escalating doses of interleukin-3 (IL-3) in patients with relapsed ovarian cancer receiving carboplatin. *Proc Am Soc Clin Oncol.* 1992;**11**:237.

Scadden DT, Levine JD, Hammer S, et al. Recombinant human interleukin-3 for cytopenia in AIDS: A phase I study. *Blood.* 1992;**80**(suppl 1):515a.

Speyer J, Cohen C, Runowicz C, et al. Phase I trial of interleukin 3 (IL3)/cytoxan (CY)/carboplatin (CP) in women with ovarian cancer (OC). *Proc Am Soc Clin Oncol.* 1992;**11**:227.

Tepler I, Elias A, Young D, et al. Use of recombinant human interleukin-3 (IL-3) after "ice" chemotherapy for non-small cell lung cancer (NSCLC): Effect on hematologic recovery. *Proc Am Soc Clin Oncol.* 1992;**11**:296.

Vellenga E, Biesma B, Meyer C, et al. The effects of five hematopoietic growth factors on human small cell lung carcinoma cell lines: Interleukin 3 enhances the proliferation in one of the eleven cell lines. *Cancer Res.* 1991;**51**:73.

Vellenga E, Biesma B, Willemse P, et al. IL-3 stimulates proliferation of a SCLC cell line and modulates action of cytostatic agents in this line (abstract 325). *Proc Am Assoc Cancer Res.* 1990;**31**:55.

Von Hoff DD, Degen D, Myers LA, et al. Effect of hematopoietic growth factors GMCSF, IL3 and IL6 on colony-forming units of tumors taken directly from patients. *Blood.* 1992;**80**(suppl 1):421a.

Wheeler C, Guinan E, Sieff C, et al. Interleukin 3 (IL-3) before marrow harvest and GM-CSF post-autotransplant (ABMT) in patients with relapsed lymphoma: No enhancement of hematopoietic recovery. *Blood.* 1992;**80**(suppl 1):85a.

Williams DE, Bicknell DC, Park LS, et al. Purified murine granulocyte/macrophage progenitor cells express a high-affinity receptor for recombinant murine granulocyte/macrophage colony stimulating factor. *Proc Natl Acad Sci USA.* 1988;**85**(2):487–491.

Yang YC, Ciarletta AB, Temple PA, et al. Human IL-3 (multi-CSF): Identification by expression cloning of a novel hematopoietic growth factor related to murine IL-3. *Cell.* 1986;**47**:3–10.

Interleukin-4

■ Other Names

IL-4; B-cell growth factor (BCGF); B-cell stimulatory factor 1 (BSF-1); BB-IND 2861 (Sterling Drug, Inc).

■ Chemistry

Recombinant human IL-4 (rHuIL-4) has been produced in yeast cells using a modified complementary (c)DNA to the human IL-4 gene located on the long arm of chromosome 5 (Laver and Moore 1989). The recombinant product has a molecular weight of approximately 15,385 and its 129 amino acids are not glycosylated. The Sterling product differs from natural human IL-4 by six amino acids. These include a four-amino-acid leader sequence (Glu–Ala–Glu–Ala) used in the yeast protein expression system and the substitution of aspartic acid for asparagine at positions 38 and 105 to prevent glycosylation. There are six cysteine residues at positions 3, 24, 46, 65, 99, and 127 which facilitate the formation of up to three intramolecular disulfide bonds. Another IL-4 product (Immunex Corporation) is also produced by recombinant DNA techniques.

Interleukin-4 activity is defined by the ability of the protein to stimulate the proliferation of human tonsillar B lymphocytes in the presence of antibodies to human immunoglobulin. One unit of rHuIL-4 activity will stimulate [^{3}H-]thymidine uptake to 50% maximal levels in the tonsillar B cells in vitro.

■ Antitumor Activity

Interleukin-4 has broad immunostimulatory effects that can potentiate the antitumor activity from lymphokine-activated killer (LAK) lymphocytes and/or other effector cells (see Mechanism of Action). Interleukin-4 alone stimulates LAK cell antitu-

```
        -4                  1                              10
        **  **  **  **      *
        Glu Ala Glu Ala His Lys Cys Asp Ile Thr Leu Gln Glu Ile Ile Lys Thr Leu Asn Ser

                            20                      30
                                            *
        Leu Thr Glu Gln Lys Thr Leu Cys Thr Glu Leu Thr Val Thr Asp Ile Phe Ala Ala Ser

                #           40                              50
                                                    *
        Lys Asp Thr Thr Glu Lys Glu Thr Phe Cys Arg Ala Ala Thr Val Leu Arg Gln Phe Tyr

                            60                              70
                                            *
        Ser His His Glu Lys Asp Thr Arg Cys Leu Gly Ala Thr Ala Gln Gln Phe His Arg His

                            80                              90
        Lys Gln Leu Ile Arg Phe Leu Lys Arg Leu Asp Arg Asn Leu Trp Gly Leu Ala Gly Leu

            *               100                 #           110
        Asn Ser Cys Pro Val Lys Glu Ala Asp Gln Ser Thr Leu Glu Asn Phe Leu Glu Arg Leu

                            120                             129
                                                    *
        Lys Thr Ile Met Arg Glu Lys Tyr Ser Lys Cys Ser Ser
```

Proposed amino acid sequence of recombinant human interleukin-4. Double asterisks mark segment −4 to −1 (Glu–Ala–Glu–Ala), which is not part of the normal human protein but is derived from the leader sequence used in the yeast expression system. The single asterisks indicate the six cysteine residues available for disulfide bonding. Aspartic acid is substituted for asparagine at positions 38 and 105 (see pound signs) to prevent glycosylation.

mor activity directed against fresh tumor cells (Mule et al 1987) and can also inhibit the in vitro growth of some human gastric cancers that express IL-4 receptors (Morisaki et al 1992). In vitro combinations of human IL-3 with rHuIL-4 have produced synergistic generation of LAK cells with tumor-lysing capability. These dual-stimulated LAK cells have been shown to be much more potent at mediating tumor lysis than those produced by either agent alone. Furthermore, LAK cells produced in vitro by the combination of IL-2 and IL-4 were highly active in C57BL/6 mice given intravenous fibrosarcoma cells (Mule et al 1985). These cells reduced pulmonary metastases significantly better than similar numbers of LAK cells stimulated in vitro by either IL-2 or IL-4 alone. In addition, injections of IL-2 combined with IL-4, but without LAK cells, are much more active at reducing experimental pulmonary metastases than are injections of either agent alone. Phase I studies of IL-2 with IL-4 have shown a fourfold elevation in LAK cell precursors; CD3+ T cells, CD56+ cells, CD4+ T cells, and CD8+ cytotoxic T cells. No antitumor responses have been seen (Whitehead et al 1992, Sosman et al 1992a). The platelet count may also increase by 40% with the IL-2, IL-4 combination (Olencki et al 1992). IL-4 also induces a dose-dependent increase in eosinophils in cancer patients (Sosman et al 1992b). This increase was in addition to that of IL-2. The role of systemic eosinophil activation in mediating antitumor effects by IL-4 is not known.

These studies suggest that IL-4 alone or in combination with IL-2 may produce antitumor effects by stimulating LAK cell generation in vivo. This would obviate the need for infusing large numbers of exogenously generated LAK cells as has been recommended for IL-2. No responses have been reported in Phase I studies of IL-4 in patients with advanced, refractory malignancies (Sosman et al 1992a, Atkins et al 1992).

Mechanism of Action

Interleukin-4 is normally produced by non-antigen-stimulated T lymphocytes. It is taken up via species-specific cell surface receptors that distinguish between human and murine forms of the protein. This has precluded studying human IL-4 in the mouse. However, human and mouse IL-4 have similar reactivities in vitro suggesting that studies of murine IL-4 in vivo will have relevance to studies of rHuIL-4 in humans.

Interleukin-4 was originally identified as an agent that could enhance the proliferation of purified mouse B lymphocytes in vitro in a dose-dependent fashion (Howard et al 1982). Class II major histocompatibility antigen expression and antibody secretion are also enhanced following IL-4 exposure to murine or human B lymphocytes (Matis et al 1983). IL-4 also stimulates the proliferation of murine and human T lymphocytes. Furthermore, antigen-specific, tumor-cytolytic T lymphocytes can be generated from mixed leukocyte cultures exposed to IL-4 over periods up to 14 days. This effect occurs even when the cultures are specifically depleted of CD4-positive helper-T-cell populations. The proliferation of mitogen-stimulated T cells and the expression of IL-2 receptors are also enhanced by IL-4.

Human peripheral blood monocytes cultured in the presence of IL-4 have enhanced antitumor activity as a result of macrophage-mediated tumor cell lysis. In addition, IL-4 can induce the expression of myeloid hematopoietic colony-stimulating factor(s) from irradiated rat fibroblasts grown in vitro. This results in a predominance of macrophage colonies (80%) over granulocytic colonies (20%). Similar but more broad spectrum effects have been noted in human cells exposed to IL-4: T cells were stimulated to secrete GM-CSF and IL-3, monocytes secreted M-CSF and G-CSF, and endothelial cells secreted GM-CSF, G-CSF, and M-CSF (Herrmann et al 1989). Recent studies, however, show that IL-4 suppresses M-CSF-induced antibody-dependent cytotoxicity in vitro (Munn and Armstrong 1992). IL-4 also suppresses production of the immunomodulators IL-1 and tumor necrosis factor (Nishioka et al 1991). This down regulation of specific cytokines may explain the blockade in colony growth of bone marrow specimens from some patients with acute myelogenous leukemia and/or the myelodysplastic syndrome (Wetzler et al 1992). Conversely, administration of the IL-1 receptor antagonist can augment IL-4 production (Orino et al 1992).

Other studies in human cells have shown that IL-4 does not stimulate resting human lymphocytes but does activate the proliferation of cells stimulated by mitogen or antigen (Treisman et al 1989). Similarly, Higuchi et al (1989) have shown that IL-4 does not induce LAK cells in normal human lymphocytes and can actually inhibit their induction by IL-2 (Higuchi et al 1989). Thus, the type of lymphocyte treated *and* the sequence of cytokine exposure are highly critical for IL-4 activity. For example, IL-4 given following IL-2 provides enhanced tumor LAK cell production, whereas co-incubation in normal lymphocytes inhibits LAK cell generation (Higuchi et al 1989).

Overall these results show that LAK cells are regulated by several interrelated and independent interleukin pathways involving IL-4. Ultimately, however, enhanced LAK cell generation in lymphocytes from cancer patients' blood may constitute the major mechanism of antitumor action for IL-4 in humans.

Availability and Storage

Interleukin-4 is supplied in two commercial dosage forms. The material from Sterling Drug, Inc, is supplied as a lyophilized powder in 5-mL vials containing 100 or 500 µg of rHuIL-4. This formulation also contains sucrose, mannitol, and tris(hydroxymethyl)aminomethane, and a pH buffer. An alternate lyophylized preparation is supplied by Immunex Corp. The activity of these preparations is approximately 1.8×10^6 U/100 µg. The intact vials are stored under refrigeration (2–8°C) and are stable as such for at least 12 months.

Preparation for Use, Stability, and Admixture

The lyophilized powder is reconstituted with 0.5 or 1.0 mL of Sterile Water for Injection, USP. The pH of this solution is 7.4. To reduce possible adsorption to glass and a loss of activity, the use of plastic syringes and limiting dilution to at least 20 µg/mL is recommended for all IL-4 dose preparations. Once reconstituted, the IL-4 solution is stable for at least 24 hours if stored under refrigeration. There is, however, no antibacterial preservative in this preparation. This solution may be diluted into 0.9% sodium chloride for intravenous administration.

Administration

In phase I trials of IL-4 with IL-2, IL-4 has been administered as a continuous intravenous infusion for

7 days (Sosman et al 1992a) or over 120 hours (Ceribelli et al 1992) and as an intravenous bolus over 5 minutes (Atkins et al 1992). A 5-day subcutaneous IL-4 regimen has also been evaluated (Whitehead et al 1992a).

■ Dosage

Interleukin-4 is just entering phase I clinical testing in humans; thus little human dosing information is currently available. In cynomolgus monkeys, doses of 1, 10, and 100 µg/kg/d were not toxic when given for 14 consecutive days. Initial clinical trials in cancer patients suggest that the maximally tolerated dose may be in the range of 500 µg/m^2/d given subcutaneously for 5 to 7 consecutive days (Sosman et al 1992a). The maximum tolerated dose for an intravenous bolus schedule was 10 µg/kg given every 8 hours on days 1 to 5 and 15 to 19 of a 31-day study period (Atkins et al 1992).

■ Drug Interactions

Interleukin-4 may need to be administered separately from IL-2 to avoid inhibition of LAK cell stimulation (see Mechanism of Action). Such a sequential IL-4/IL-2 regimen has been evaluated clinically in cancer patients (Sosman et al 1992b). Of interest, interleukin-1 can reverse IL-4 suppression of LAK cells (Shau et al 1989).

■ Pharmacokinetics

In primates given doses of 100 µg/kg as an intravenous bolus injection, rHuIL-4 was rapidly eliminated from the vascular compartment. The IL-4 half-life in these studies ranged from 14 to 17 minutes; however, a second intravenous bolus study observed biexponential elimination of rHuIL-4 in monkeys with estimated half-lives of 10 minutes (α) and 45 minutes (β). When IL-4 was administered subcutaneously, systemic bioavailability was reduced by about half and the apparent terminal half-life was increased to about 3 hours.

■ Side Effects and Toxicity

The toxicity of rHuIL-4 was initially evaluated in cynomolgus monkeys given intravenous bolus injections of 100 µg/kg for 14 days. No significant organ toxic effects or behavioral effects were noted. Mean body temperatures also did not change while on this drug.

Initial clinical trials suggest that fatigue and diarrhea may be dose limiting after 5-day drug regimens involving subcutaneous dosing. Other acute effects include fever, chills, weight gain, and headache (Sosman et al 1992a). Fever may be lessened with the intravenous bolus schedule (Atkins et al 1992). IL-4 significantly enhances IL-2-induced eosinophilia and basophilia and may also increase the platelet count by approximately 40% (Olencki et al 1992). Decreases are noted in the lymphocyte count, serum bicarbonate, sodium, albumin, and fibrinogen (Atkins et al 1992). In contrast, the hematocrit, partial thromboplastin, and prothrombin times increase with IL-4 therapy. Less frequent increases were observed in serum creatinine and hepatic transaminase levels (Atkins et al 1992). Orthostatic hypotension is reported, but usually resolves rapidly with drug discontinuance and pressor therapy is typically not required. The combination of IL-4 and IL-2 has produced hyponatremia myocarditis and duodenal ulcers (Whitehead et al 1992). There is also a suggestion that prostaglandins may mediate the diarrhea which is occasionally severe, requiring fluid and electrolyte replacement. A flulike syndrome is also observed after dosing. This consists of fever and myalgia and is partially reduced by acetaminophen. An unusual periorbital edema is observed following IL-4. Of interest, this excess fluid accumulation was not readily mobilized with diuretic therapy.

REFERENCES

Atkins MB, Vachino G, Tilg HJ, et al. Phase I evaluation of thrice-daily intravenous bolus interleukin-4 in patients with refractory malignancy. *J Clin Oncol.* 1992;**10**(11): 1802–1809.

Ceribelli A, Fossati C, Gamucci T, et al. Interleukin-3 (IL-3) by 120-hour continuous infusion (c.i.) after myelosuppressive chemotherapy (CT): A phase I study. *Proc Am Assoc Cancer Res.* 1992;**33**:231.

Herrmann F, Wieser M, Riedel D, et al. Interleukin-4 (IL-4) is a major inducer of hematopoietic growth factors. *Proc Am Assoc Cancer Res.* 1989;**30**:68 (abstract 268).

Higuchi C, Thompson J, Gillis S, et al. Induction of lymphokine activated killer activity in human cells by interleukin-4. *Proc Am Assoc Cancer Res.* 1989;**30**:324 (abstract 1283).

Howard M, Farrar J, Hilfiker M, et al. Identification of a T cell-derived B cell growth factor distinct from interleukin 2. *J Exp Med.* 1982;**155**:914–923.

Laver J, Moore MAS. Clinical use of recombinant human hematopoietic growth factors. *J Natl Cancer Inst.* 1989;**81**: 1370–1382.

Matis LA, Glimcher LH, Paul WE, et al. Magnitude of response of histocompatibility-restricted T-cell clones is a function of the product of the concentrations of antigen and Ia molecules. *Proc Natl Acad Sci USA.* 1983;**80**:6019–6023.

Morisaki T, Hoon DSB, Yuzuki D, et al. Expression of IL4 receptors (IL4R) and response to IL4 by human gastric cancer cells. *Proc Am Assoc Cancer Res.* 1992;**33**:73.

Mule JJ, Shu S, Rosenberg SA. The anti-tumor efficacy of lymphokine-activated killer cells and recombinant interleukin 2 in vivo. *J Immunol.* 1985;**135**:646–652.

Mule JJ, Smith CA, Rosenberg SA. Interleukin 4 (B cell stimulatory factor 1) can mediate the induction of lymphokine-activated killer cell activity directed against fresh tumor cells. *J Exp Med.* 1987;**156**:792–797.

Munn DH, Armstrong E. Coordinate regulation of M-CSF-induced anti-tumor cytotoxicity and cell cycle progression by IL-4 during human macrophage differentiation in vitro. *Proc Am Assoc Cancer Res.* 1992;**33**:301.

Nishioka Y, Sone S, Orino E, et al. Down-regulation by interleukin 4 of activation of human alveolar macrophages to the tumoricidal state. *Cancer Res.* 1991;**51**:5526–5531.

Olencki T, Netaji B, Budd GT, et al. Phase I trial of rIL-2 and rHuIL-4 in patients with refractory malignancy: Hematologic and immunologic effects. *Proc Am Assoc Cancer Res.* 1992;**33**:245.

Orino E, Sone S, Nii A, et al. Augmentation by IL-4 of production of IL-1 receptor antagonist by human monocytes. *Proc Amer Assoc Cancer Res.* 1992;**33**:347.

Shau H, Gallardo D, Ebina N, et al. Reversion of interleukin 4 suppression of lymphokine-activated killer induction with interleukin 1. *Proc Am Assoc Cancer Res.* 1989;**30**:328 (abstract 1302).

Sosman JA, Ellis T, Bodner B, et al. A phase IA/IB trial of continuous infusion (CI) interleukin-4 alone and following interleukin-2 in cancer patients. *Proc Am Assoc Cancer Res.* 1992a;**33**:347.

Sosman J, Bartemes K, Fisher S, et al. Biologic effects of interleukin-4 (IL-4) alone and following interleukin-2 (IL-2) in human cancer patients: Evidence for eosinophil activation. *Blood.* 1992b;**80**(suppl 1):185a.

Treisman J, Kern D, Thompson J, et al. Interleukin-4 augments the proliferative response of human lymphocytes to anti-CD3 and anti-CD28 after activation by interleukin-2. *Proc Am Assoc Cancer Res.* 1989;**30**:323 (abstract 1282).

Wetzler M, Kurzrock R, Estrov Z, et al. Interleukin-4 modulates aberrant cytokine expression in adherent layers derived from myelodysplastic and acute myelogenous leukemia patients. *Blood.* 1992;**80**(suppl 1):463a.

Whitehead RP, Friedman KD, Clark DA. A phase I trial of subcutaneous interleukin 2 and interleukin 4. *Proc Am Assoc Cancer Res.* 1992;**33**:231.

Interleukin-6

■ Other Names

IL-6; interferon-β_2; BSF-2; B-cell stimulatory factor-2; hepatocyte stimulatory factor 2; plasmacytoma growth factor.

■ Chemistry

Natural interleukin-6 (IL-6) is a 21- to 30-kDa glycoprotein containing 212 amino acids and variable degrees of glycosylation (Matsuda and Hirano 1990). In the natural protein there is a 28-residue hydrophobic signal sequence that is not present in the recombinant molecule. The investigational product for clinical use is a purified nonglycosylated protein prepared by recombinant DNA technique in *Escherichia coli* (Sandoz Pharmaceuticals). Internal disulfide bonds are found between residues 51 and 74 and between 74 and 84 (see figure). The N-terminal region of the molecule does not appear to be important for biologic activity (Brakenhoff et al 1989).

■ Antitumor Activity

Interleukin-6 has produced antitumor effects in mice bearing a variety of metastatic carcinomas and colon-38 carcinoma (Mulé et al 1990). Inhibition of pulmonary metastases was observed in this trial. IL-6 was also active against transplantable murine erythroleukemia (Kitahara et al 1990). When admixed with murine tumor cells, IL-6 augments the production of therapeutically active tumor-infiltrating lymphocytes (Mulé et al 1992a,b). IL-6 is directly cytotoxic to human MCF-7, T47D, and HTB-133 breast and to U-937 leukemia/lymphoma cell lines grown in nude mice (Chen et al 1988). THe cytokine is also active in murine acute myeloid leukemias induced by radiation or transplanted from donor cultures (Givon et al 1992).

In the initial phase I study, there were no responses among 11 patients with advanced malignancies (Wever et al 1993). Similar results are described by Olencki et al (1992) in 10 patients with a variety of solid tumors. In vitro studies with fresh human tumors have shown that IL-6 can inhibit colony formation from melanoma, ovarian cancer, and unknown primary cancers (Von Hoff et al 1992). IL-6 has also been administered following cytotoxic chemotherapy drugs to produce hematopoietic protection from myelosuppression and immunosuppression. In sarcoma patients given 10 days of IL-6

Met-Asn-Ser-Phe-Ser-Thr-Ser-Ala-Phe-Gly-Pro-Val-Ala-Phe-
-27   -25   -20   -15

Ser-Leu-Gly-Leu-Leu-Leu-Val-Leu-Pro-Ala-Ala-Phe-Pro-Ala
        -10   -5   1

Pro-Val-Pro-Pro-Gly-Glu-Asp-Ser-Lys-Asp-Val-Ala-Ala-Pro-His-
         5   10   15

Arg-Gln-Pro-Leu-Thr-Ser-Ser-Glu-Arg-Ile-Asp-Lys-Gln-Ile-Arg-
         20   25   30

Tyr-Ile-Leu-Asp-Gly-Ile-Ser-Ala-Leu-Arg-Lys-Glu-Thr-
         35   40

Cys-Asp-Lys-Ser-Asp-Met-Cys-Glu-Ser-Ser-Lys-Glu-Ala-Leu-Ala-
 45   50   55

Glu-Asn-Asn-Leu-Asn-Leu-Pro-Lys-Met-Ala-Glu-Lys-Asp-Gly-
 60   65   70

Cys-Phe-Gln-Ser-Gly-Phe-Asn-Glu-Glu-Thr-Cys-Leu-Val-Lys-Ile-
 75   80   85

Ile-Thr-Gly-Leu-Leu-Glu-Phe-Glu-Val-Tyr-Leu-Glu-Tyr-Leu-
         90   95   100

Gln-Asn-Arg-Phe-Glu-Ser-Ser-Glu-Glu-Gln-Ala-Arg-Ala-Val-Gln-
        105   110   115

Met-Ser-Thr-Lys-Val-Leu-Ile-Gln-Phe-Leu-Gln-Lys-Lys-Ala-
        120   125   130

Lys-Asn-Leu-Asp-Ala-Ile-Thr-Thr-Pro-Asp-Pro-Thr-Thr-Asn-
        135   140   145

Ala-Ser-Leu-Thr-Thr-Lys-Leu-Gln-Ala-Gln-Asn-Gln-Trp-Leu-
        150   155

Gln-Asp-Met-Thr-Thr-His-Leu-Ile-Leu-Arg-Ser-Phe-Lys-Glu-
        160   165   170

Phe-Leu-Gln-Ser-Ser-Leu-Arg-Ala-Leu-Arg-Gln-Met-COOH
        175   180   185

Amino acid sequence of human interleukin-6 as deduced from the cytoplasmic DNA. Underlined portion −27 to −1 indicates the signal sequence. Internal disulfide bonds are indicated between cysteines 45 and 51 and between 74 and 84. Potential *N*-glycosylation sites are noted by asterisks. Data are from Van Snick 1990.

for 7 days before receiving the MAID regimen (mesna, doxorubicin [Adriamycin]), ifosfamide, and dacarbazine), low-dose IL-6 increased platelet counts but not leukocyte counts. Dose escalation was planned in this trial (Demetri et al 1992). Similar effects were described for IL-6 given 14 days after ICE chemotherapy (ifosfamide, carboplatin, etoposide) (Chang et al 1992).

Of patients with myelodysplasias, about one third develop a significant increase in platelet count midway through a 28-day consecutive dosing period (Gordon et al 1992); however, as with the trials in cancer patients, an increase in anemia was observed following IL-6 therapy.

■ Mechanism of Action

Interleukin-6 is produced by T cells, monocytes, fibroblasts, keratinocytes, and endothelial cells (Van Snick 1990). It has also been isolated from cultures of human multiple myeloma cells and is believed to act as an paracrine B-cell growth factor (Klein et al 1989, Van Damme et al 1987). IL-6 binds to an 80-kDa transmembrane receptor (Yamasaki et al 1988), which mediates signal transduction in concert with a second 130-kDa membrane glycoprotein, gp130 (Taga et al 1989).

Although IL-6 may have some direct antitumor effects, it appears to act primarily as a cofactor for the proliferation and differentiation of special populations of cytotoxic T cells (Mulé et al 1992a). T-cell activation by IL-6 may not always proceed via IL-2-dependent pathways. Antitumor effects in tumor-bearing mice appear to involve both helper (CD-4) and suppressor (CD-8) populations of T lymphocytes (Mulé et al 1990). In humans, however, the ratio of CD-4/CD-8 lymphocytes and the total number of lymphocytes remain unchanged by IL-6 (Weber et al 1993). Thus, one of the main effects of IL-6 is T-lymphocyte activation and not T-cell proliferation. This is substantiated by an IL-6-induced increase in the expression of ICAM-1 adhesion molecules and low-affinity IL-2 (Tac) receptors on T cells (Weber et al 1993).

Interleukin-6 also produces a number of hematopoietic effects that do not directly involve antitumor activity. These include stimulation of megakaryocyte differentiation (thrombopoiesis). In vivo, this results in higher numbers of platelets in the peripheral blood (Ishibabshi et al 1989, Asano et al 1990). This appears to be a result of augmented platelet production and release without an increase in the number of megakaryocyte precursors in the bone marrow. Many of these hematopoietic effects of IL-6 involve augmentation of IL-3 activities (Ikebuchi et al 1987).

Other biologic effects of IL-6 include activation of acute-phase protein genes (Geiger et al 1988, Morrone et al 1988), increased secretion of adrenocorticotropin (Naitoh et al 1989), and increased osteoclast activation which promotes bone absorption (Jilka et al 1992).

■ Availability and Storage

Interleukin-6 is investigationally available as a lyophilized protein supplied in glass vials. It is produced by Sandoz Pharmaceuticals, East Hanover, New Jersey. The vials are stable for up to 6 months when stored at –25°C. The vials also contain a phosphate buffer, sucrose, and glycine. Refrigerated storage of intact vials is recommended.

■ Preparation for Use, Stability, and Admixture

Interleukin-6 vials are reconstituted with 1.0 mL Sterile Water for Injection, USP, prior to use. The final volume should not be greater than 2 mL per dose and all solutions should be used within 24 hours of reconstitution as no bacteriostatic agent is included in the formulation. Admixture data are not available.

■ Administration

In early phase I trials, IL-6 has been administered by subcutaneous injection (Weber et al 1993).

■ Dosage

The effective dose of IL-6 as a tumor inhibitor or hematopoietic agent is unknown. The maximally tolerated dose of IL-6 in the initial phase I trial was 30 µg/kg/d SC for 7 days followed by a 7-day rest period for two cycles (Weber et al 1993); however, some serious toxic effects were reported at this dose level and further refinement of IL-6 doses and schedules is required. At least six patients in the initial phase I trial could tolerate six cycles of daily IL-6 injections for 1 week each (Weber et al 1993). When IL-6 was used as a potential hematopoietic stimulant, doses of 2.5 to 5.0 µg/kg/d produced moderate platelet increases without causing dose-limiting toxic effects (Demetri et al 1992, Chang et al 1992). Thus, further dose escalations are being planned in these populations. Similar daily doses of 2.5 to 5.0 µg/kg are being evaluated in patients with myelodysplasia (Gordon et al 1992).

■ Special Precautions

Patients with preexisting heart disease may be poor candidates for IL-6 because of reports of atrial fibrillation at a dose of 30 µg/kg (Weber et al 1993). Also, patients with diabetes, any B- or T-cell malignancy, and especially multiple myeloma should not receive IL-6 until further data become available.

In phase I studies, prophylactic anti-inflammatory and antipyretic agents were routinely administered to patients experiencing severe fever and chills on inital dosing. Meperidine was occasionally required to control severe chilling on the first dose.

■ Pharmacokinetics

By use of ELISA, IL-6 demonstrated a biphasic elimination pattern with a mean β half-life of 4.2 hours (Weber et al 1993). There is some evidence for a third, more prolonged elimination phase based on the persistence of measurable levels up to 24 hours after dosing. A peak serum level of approximately 2 ng/mL is achieved 5 hours after administration of a subcutaneous dose of 30 µg/kg. The area under the serum concentration × time curve (AUC) for this IL-6 dose was 20.3 ng/h/mL. Another patient treated with 30 μg/kg/d also had a large hepatic tumor burden and developed a peak concentration of 7.8 ng/mL and a serum AUC of 67 ng/h/mL (Gunn et al 1992).

■ Side Effects and Toxicity

In phase I studies of Il-6 alone in patients with advanced malignancies, fever and chills are the most common toxic effects. Anorexia and arthralgias are also common (Olencki et al 1992). There were transient low-level increases in alkaline phosphatase, transaminases, creatinine and fasting glucose levels (Weber et al 1993). Moderate to severe headaches within 4 hours of administration are reported in most patients. These symptoms are typically very responsive to prophylactic antipyretic and anti-inflammatory agents.

Interleukin-6 consistently induces anemia even as platelet counts increase and leukocyte counts remain unchanged (Weber et al 1993, Demetri et al 1992, Chang et al 1992). The onset for hemoglobin decrease is several days and recovery occurs within 1 week of stopping IL-6. This toxic effect may be particularly troublesome in patients with myelodysplasias (Gordon et al 1992). The moderate drop in hemoglobin levels is dose dependent and is not accompanied by changes in the reticulocyte count, erythrocyte size, or evidence of hemolysis. Thus, the mechanism for this brief decrease is unknown but may involve transient sequestration of erythrocytes. With high-dose IL-6 therapy, atrial fibrillation has occurred in two patients given only a few doses of 30 μg/kg/d. One patient also developed centrilobular hepatic necrosis heralded by significant increases in alkaline phosphatase and serum bilirubin (Weber et al 1993).

As anticipated, IL-6 induces a rapid and significant elevation in acute-phase reactants. Within days of initiating IL-6 therapy, levels of C-reactive protein, haptoglobin, and fibrinogen increase to levels commonly seen in patients with sepsis or severe burns (Weber et al 1993). Albumin was noted to decrease in these patients. Overall, the level of C-reactive protein elevations appears to closely follow other biologic actions of IL-6. Antinuclear antibody titers are unchanged following IL-6 and no M-spike proteins are observed; however, IL-6 does increase adrenocorticotropin and cortisol levels in all patients given subcutaneous doses of 30 μg/kg/d (Weber et al 1993).

REFERENCES

Asano S, Okano A, Ozawa K, et al. In vivo effects of recombinant human interleukin-6 in primates: Stimulated production of human platelets. *Blood.* 1990;**75**:1602–1608.

Brakenhoff JPJ, Hart M, Aarden LA. Analysis of human IL-6 mutants expressed in *Escherichia coli*—Biologic activities are not effected by deletion of amino acids 1–28. *J Immunol.* 1989;**143**:1115–1128.

Chang A, Mittelman A, Boros L, et al. Phase I study of interleukin-6 (IL-6) in cancer patients treated with ifosfamide, carboplatin, and etoposide (ICE). *Blood.* 1992;**80**(10, suppl 1):89a.

Chen L, Zilberstein A, Revel M. Growth inhibition of breast carcinoma and leukemia/lymphoma cell lines by recombinant interferon-β2. *Proc Natl Acad Sci USA.* 1988;**85**:8037–8041.

Demetri GD, Samuels B, Gordon M, et al. Recombinant human interleukin-6 (IL-6) increases circulating platelet counts and C-reactive protein levels in vivo: Initial results of a phase I trial in sarcoma patients with normal hemopoiesis. *Blood.* 1992;**80**(10, suppl 1):88a.

Geiger T, Andus T, Klapproth J, et al. Induction of rat acute phase proteins by interleukin-6 in vivo. *Eur J Immunol.* 1988;**18**:717–721.

Givon T, Slavin S, Haran-Ghera N, et al. Anti-tumor effects of human recombinant interleukin-6 on acute myeloid leukemia in mice and cell cultures. *Blood.* 1992;**79**:2392–2396.

Gordon MS, Nemunaitis J, Hoffman R, et al. Phase I trial of subcutaneous (SC) recombinant human interleukin-6 (IL-6) in patients (PTS) with myelodysplasia (MDS) and thrombocytopenia (TP). *Blood.* 1992;**80**(10, suppl 1):249a.

Gunn HC, Weber J, Myers LA, et al. Pharmacokinetic profile of rhIL-6 in four patients. *Blood.* 1992;**80**(10, suppl 1):414a.

Ikebuchi K, Wong GG, Clark S, et al. Interleukin-6 enhancement of interleukin-3 dependent proliferation of multipotential hematopoietic progenitors. *Proc Natl Acad Sci USA.* 1987;**84**:9035–9039.

Ishibabshi T, Kimura H, Uchida T, et al. Human interleukin-6 as a direct promoter of the maturation of megakaryocytes in vitro. *Proc Natl Acad Sci USA.* 1989;**86**:5953–5957.

Jilka RL, Hangoc G, Grasole G, et al. Increased osteoclast development after estrogen loss: Mediation by interleukin-6. *Science.* 1992;**257**:88–91.

Kitahara M, Kishimoto S, Hirano T, et al. The in vivo antitumor effect of human recombinant interleukin-6. *Jpn J Cancer Res.* 1990;**81**:1032–1038.

Klein B, Zhang XC, Jourdan M, et al. Paracrine rather than autocrine regulation of myeloma cell growth and differentiation by interleukin-6. *Blood.* 1989;**73**:517–526.

Matsuda T, Hirano T. Interleukin-6 (IL-6). *Biotherapy.* 1990;**2**:363–373.

Morrone G, Cilberto G, Olwero S, et al. Recombinant interleukin-6 regulates the transcriptional activation of a set of human acute phase genes. *J Biol Chem.* 1988;**236**: 12554–12558.

Mulé JJ, Custer MC, Travis WD, et al. Cellular mechanisms of the antitumor activity of recombinant IL-6 in mice. *J Immunol.* 1992a;**148**:2622–2626.

Mulé JJ, Marcus SG, Yang JC, et al. Clinical applications of IL-6 in cancer therapy. *Res Immunol.* 1992b;**143**:777–779.

Mulé JJ, McIntosh JK, Jablons DM, et al. In vivo administration of recombinant interleukin-6 mediates tumor regression in mice. *J Exp Med.* 1990;**171**:629–637.

Naitoh Y, Fukata J, Tominaga T, et al. Interleukin-6 stimulates potent thrombopoietic factor in vivo in mice. *Blood.* 1989;**74**:1241–1244.

Olencki T, Budd GT, Murthy S, et al. Phase 1A/1B trial of rhIl-6 in patients with refractory malignancy: Hematologic and immunologic effects. *Blood.* 1992;**80**(10, suppl 1): 89a.

Taga T, Hibi M, Hirata Y, et al. Interleukin-6 triggers the association of its receptor with a possible signal transducer gp130. *Cell.* 1989;**58**:573–581.

Van Damme J, Opdenakker G, Simpson RJ. Identification of the human 26kD protein, interferon beta-2 (IFN β2) as a B cell hybridoma/plasmacytoma growth factor induced by interleukin and tumor necrosis factor. *J Exp Med.* 1987;**165**:914–920.

Van Snick J. Interleukin-6: An overview. *Annu Rev Immunol.* 1990;**8**:253–278.

Von Hoff DD, Degen D, Myers LA, et al. Effect of hematopoietic growth factors GFMCSF, IL3 and IL6 on colony-forming units of tumors taken directly from patients. *Blood.* 1992;**80**(10, suppl 1):421a.

Weber J, Yang JC, Topalian SL, et al. Phase I trial of subcutaneous interleukin-6 in patients with advanced malignancies. *J Clin Oncol.* 1993;**11**(3):499–506.

Yamasaki K, Taga T, Hirata Y, et al. Cloning and expression of the human interleukin-6 (BSF-2/IFNβ2) receptor. *Science.* 1988;**241**:825–828.

4-Ipomeanol

■ Other Names

IPO; NSC-349438.

■ Chemistry

Structure of 4-ipomeanol

The chemical name of 4-ipomeanol is 1-(3-furyl)-4-hydroxy-1-pentanone. It has a molecular formula of $C_9H_{12}O_3$ and formula weight of 168.2 (National Cancer Institute 1987). The substance occurs naturally in sweet potato slice cultures of *Ipomoea galatas* infected with the fungus *Fusarium solani* (Boyd and Wilson 1972). The compound can also be obtained from a furanoterpenoid precursor which is catabolized to 4-ipomeanol in infected *Ipomoea batatas* species. The furan ring is known to be essential for pulmonary binding and toxicity. Ipomeanol was originally isolated in chemical studies of lung toxicity in cattle fed moldy sweet potatoes (Boyd et al 1974).

■ Antitumor Activity

4-Ipomeanol is inactive in murine mouse tumor models including P-388 and L-1210 leukemias as well as other "solid" tumor models tested in vivo (Christian et al 1989); however, the drug has shown activity in human tumor colony-forming assays in vitro. Continuous exposure to a concentration of 100 µg/mL was active (> 70% inhibition of colony formation) in 20% of cell lines derived from patients with cancers of the breast, lung, ovary, and malignant melanoma (Shoemaker et al 1985). Cytotoxic 6-day drug concentrations that resulted in greater than 50% growth inhibition in an automated cell culture system ranged from 2 to 8 mM or 336 to 841 µg/mL (Christian et al 1989). At these high concentrations, sensitive human tumors included adenocarcinomas such as human MCF-7 breast cancer and its multidrug-resistant variant MCF-7/ADR.

The drug has also been shown to be active in two non-small cell lung cancer cell lines but not in the small cell lung cancer lines NCI-H128 and NIC-H69 (Falzon et al 1986). The sensitive lung cancer cell lines NCI-H322 and NCI-H358 both have significant P450 microsomal enzyme activity and thus can metabolize 4-ipomeanol to its active form. Inhibition of tumor colony formation was demonstrated in these two cell lines at 4-day drug concentrations of 0.01 to 10 mM (1.68 to 1682 µg/mL). The more sensitive NCI-H322 cells morphologically resembled bronchiolar Clara cells with smooth endoplasmic reticulum and electron-dense granules (Falzon et al 1986). This cell line has shown sensitivity to ipomeanol in a nude mouse model (McLemore et al 1987) and in the murine subrenal capsule assay (Christian et al 1989). Other in vivo models showing sensitivity to 4-ipomeanol include a microencapsulated intraperitoneal lung tumor model treated with intravenous drug injections (Gorelik et al 1988) and an intrabronchial human lung tumor model in nude mice (McLemore et al 1988). No responses have been noted in early clinical trials of 4-ipomeanol (Rowinsky et al 1992).

Mechanism of Action

4-Ipomeanol is inactive until it is metabolized to products that can covalently bind to target tissues (Boyd 1976). As such, 4-ipomeanol appears to be a pulmonary-specific monofunctional alkylating agent. The ultimate active moiety has been too unstable to isolate as yet, but a furan ring epoxide intermediate is hypothesized (Boyd 1976). The furan ring is known to be essential for activity, as furan analogs lacking the hydroxypentanone moiety are also active. All of the active compounds in this class appear to produce highly unstable unsaturated dialdehydes which may constitute the ultimate cytotoxic species.

Cells with low metabolic activity are completely resistant to 4-ipomeanol. Metabolism presumably occurs via cytochrome P450 enzymes and there is an absolute requirement for reduced nicotinamide dinucleotide phosphate (NADPH) (Boyd et al 1978). Microsomes prepared from both liver and lung cells can metabolize 4-ipomeanol; however, covalent binding is greatest in the lung, primarily in bronchiolar Clara cells (Boyd and Wilson 1972). Pulmonary alveolar type II cells are also affected but to a lesser extent.

Specific cytochrome P450 isoenzymes that can activate 4-ipomeanol include forms 2 and 5. As both forms are distributed in liver and lung, other isoenzymes or factors may be needed to explain the relative pulmonary specificity of the drug. Cytochrome b_5 appears to be involved in the metabolic activation of the drug in both liver and lung. The activation and covalent attachment by ipomeanol metabolite(s) appear to occur in the same tissue, thereby discounting a role for a circulating active metabolite(s) (Boyd 1977). Furthermore, alterations of mixed function oxidase or cellular glutathione content dramatically affect 4-ipomeanol toxicity and organ specificity (see Drug Interactions).

Availability and Storage

4-Ipomeanol is investigationally available from the National Cancer Institute in 20-mg, 2-mL vials. The clear ipomeanol solution contains 0.9% sodium chloride and sodium hydroxide to adjust pH to 4 to 7. The vials are stored under refrigeration (2–8°C) (National Cancer Institute 1987).

Preparation for Use, Stability, and Admixture

4-Ipomeanol can be diluted into 0.9% Sodium Chloride Injection, USP, and 5% Dextrose Injection, USP, for intravenous infusion. Such solutions of 0.1 mg/mL 4-ipomeanol in either glass or polyvinyl chloride plastic containers are chemically stable for at least 14 days at temperatures ranging from 4 to 37°C (National Cancer Institute 1987). As no bacteriostatic agent is included in the formulation, prolonged storage of reconstituted solutions should be avoided unless sterility can be assured.

Administration

In phase I clinical trials, 4-ipomeanol has been administered as a 30-minute intravenous infusion in 100 mL of 0.9% Sodium Chloride Injection, USP, or 5% Dextrose Injection, USP (Rowinsky et al 1989, 1992).

Special Precautions

4-Ipomeanol is a potent lung toxin. Precautions against direct inhalation or other contact with the solution by medical personnel should be observed. A mask, gloves, and biological safety cabinet should be routinely used when working with this agent. Likewise, patients with pulmonary insufficiency may be poor candidates to receive this agent.

Dosage

The initial phase I clinical trial has evaluated intravenous doses ranging from 6.5 to 22 mg/m^2 given every 21 days (Rowinsky et al 1989). A later phase I study evaluated doses of 6.5 to 1612 mg/m^2 every 21 days (Rowinsky et al 1992). Severe hepatic toxicity is seen at doses ≥1032 mg/m^2, which is the maximally tolerated dose on an every-21-day schedule. The maximally tolerated dose and optimal schedule for this agent are, however, currently unknown.

Drug Interactions

Drugs that alter cytochrome P450 enzyme activity can influence 4-ipomeanol toxicity. Mice given the mixed function oxidase inhibitor piperonyl butoxide had reduced covalent binding of 4-ipomeanol in the lung along with increased blood and lung levels of unmetabolized drug (Boyd 1977). This inhibitor blocked 4-ipomeanol renal toxicity in mice (Boyd and Dutcher 1981). Other cytochrome P450 inhibitors can also reduce 4-ipomeanol lung binding and toxicity in rats (Boyd 1980).

Unexpectedly, rats given microsomal enzyme inducers such as 3-methylcholanthrene and phenobarbital experience significantly reduced acute lethality, possibly as a result of enhanced hepatic clearance of unmetabolized drug. In addition, 3-methylcholanthrene increased liver binding and cytotoxicity of 4-ipomeanol, whereas phenobarbital reduced binding and toxicity to both the lung and the liver (Statham et al 1982a).

Finally, drugs that alter tissue glutathione (GSH) concentrations significantly affect 4-ipomeanol toxicity. For example, the depletion of pulmonary GSH by diethylmaleate markedly enhances covalent binding and cytotoxicity of 4-ipomeanol metabolite(s) (Statham et al 1982b). In addition, at least two GSH adducts with 4-ipomeanol metabolites have been identified in vitro (Buckpitt et al 1982). Furthermore, 4-ipomeanol does transiently reduce pulmonary GSH concentrations (Boyd et al 1981). In contrast, pretreating rats with the sulfhydryls cysteine and cysteamine blocks 4-ipomeanol binding and toxicity.

Overall, these preclinical findings suggest that 4-ipomeanol should not be combined clinically with agents that alter cytochrome P450 or GSH metabolism.

■ Pharmacokinetics

Rats given radiolabeled 4-ipomeanol intraperitoneally rapidly distribute the compound to the lungs, gut, liver, kidney, and blood, in decreasing order of magnitude. After 4 hours, tissue concentrations of radiolabel reach a plateau which persists up to 24 hours. These latter levels represent radiolabel that is tightly bound to tissues (Boyd et al 1975). At least 50% of the radiolabel is excreted in the urine by 24 hours. And, almost half of this amount is 4-ipomeanol metabolites, with the major species being ipomeanol-4-glucuronide (Statham et al 1982b). Pretreatment of rats with phenobarbital increases this fraction considerably while at the same time decreasing drug distribution into and binding in the lung (Statham et al 1982a).

Pharmacokinetic studies in rats and dogs show that the terminal plasma half-life of intact drug is short at 6 and 10 minutes, respectively (Christian et al 1989). Drug clearance rates were 0.047 and 0.92 L/min·kg^{-1} in rats and dogs, and the volumes of distribution were 0.4 and 1.4 L/kg, respectively.

Preliminary pharmacokinetic studies in four patients have been performed with the same gas chromatography method used in the preclinical studies (Rowinsky et al 1989). The mean pharmacokinetic values in this preliminary study report were as follows: initial half-life of 8.5 minutes, terminal half-life of 140 minutes, clearance of 10.6 L/min/m^2, and a volume of distribution of 128 L/m^2. A later study reported central and steady-state volumes of distribution of 306 and 1074 L/m^2, respectively (Rowinsky et al 1992). The AUCs increased nonlinearly with the dose, suggesting saturable elimination. Clearance rates were 27.6 L/min/m^2 at a dose of 216 mg/m^2 and 8.6 L/min/m^2 at a dose of 1290 mg/m^2. Plasma concentrations averaged 0.265 µmol/L after intravenous doses of 13.6 to 22 mg/m^2 and 32 µM at the maximally tolerated dose of 1032 mg/m^2 (Rowinsky et al 1992).

■ Side Effects and Toxicity

4-Ipomeanol is known to be an environmental lung toxin in cattle fed moldy sweet potatoes (Wilson et al 1971). These animals typically develop pulmonary edema and emphysema. Histologically, there is marked necrosis of nonciliated bronchiolar (Clara) cells 16 hours after ingestion. Ciliated bronchiolar cells and adjacent lung parenchyma appear to be spared (Boyd 1977). In avian species the liver is the major organ of toxicity (Buckpitt et al 1982). These organ- and species-dependent differences probably relate to specific P450 isoenzyme patterns in the tissues of different species (Dutcher and Boyd 1979).

The cellular dynamics of 4-ipomeanol-induced lung injury has been described in mice given LD$_{30}$ doses of the drug. At 2 hours, interstitial edema is observed around damaged bronchiolar endothelial cells. After 12 to 24 hours endothelial cell damage is maximal and is associated with marked alveolar edema. In contrast, Clara cell damage is first noted at 4 hours and is maximal after 36 to 48 hours. Repair and resolution of the resultant necrosis and sloughing are usually not complete up to 10 days after dosing (Durham et al 1985).

In dogs, respiratory changes are noted on day 2 after 4-ipomeanol administration. These effects include an increase in respiratory rate and decreases in tidal volume, pulmonary capacity, and carbon monoxide diffusing capacity (Christian et al 1989). Histopathologic examinations demonstrate severe inflammation of the lungs, an infiltration of neutrophils and monocytes, a proteinaceous alveolar exudate, capillary congestion, and necrosis of alveolar cells (Christian et al 1989).

The LD_{10}, LD_{50}, and LD_{90} doses for 4-ipomeanol in mice were 33 and 23 mg/kg, 35 and 26 mg/kg, and 37 and 30 mg/kg for males and females, respectively. The mouse studies also showed little evidence for cumulative toxicity when the drug was administered every 7 days; however, in the dog there was some evidence for cumulative toxicity (Elhawari et al 1987). In contrast, chronic dosing has been shown to lead to tolerance to otherwise lethal doses in the mouse. Other toxic effects noted in the preclinical dog studies were weight loss, roughened hair, lethargy, nasal discharge, and, rarely, emesis and diarrhea.

Preliminary studies in humans show that 4-ipomeanol can produce significant increases in pulmonary densities noted on computerized tomography scans performed 4 to 7 days after treatment. Of interest, clinical pulmonary toxicity was observed in these same two patients who received 4-ipomeanol doses of 6.4 and 22 mg/m^2. Thus, 4-ipomeanol dose escalation studies are ongoing, and the spectrum and intensity of clinical toxic effects will likely increase significantly as the maximally tolerated dose is discovered.

REFERENCES

Boyd MR. Role of metabolic activation in the pathogenesis of chemically induced pulmonary disease: Mechanism of action of the lung-toxic furan, 4-ipomeanol. *Environ Health Perspect.* 1976;**16**:127–138.

Boyd MR. Evidence for the Clara cell as a site of cytochrome P450-dependent mixed-function oxidase activity in lung. *Nature.* 1977;**269**:713–715.

Boyd MR. Effects of inducers and inhibitors on drug metabolizing enzymes and drug toxicity in extrahepatic tissues. *Ciba Found Symp.* 1980;**76**:43–66.

Boyd MR, Burka LT, Harris TM, et al. Lung-toxic furanoterpenoids produced by sweet potatoes following microbial infection. *Biochim Biophys Acta.* 1974;**337**:184–195.

Boyd MR, Burka LT, Wilson BJ. Distribution, excretion, and binding of radioactivity in the rat after intraperitoneal administration of the lung-toxic furan [^{14}C]4-ipomeanol. *Toxicol Appl Pharmacol.* 1975;**32**:147–157.

Boyd MR, Burka LT, Wilson BJ, et al. In vitro studies on the metabolic activation of the pulmonary toxin, 4-ipomeanol, by rat lung and liver microsomes. *J Pharmacol Exp Ther.* 1978;**207**:677–686.

Boyd MR, Dutcher JS. Renal toxicity due to reactive metabolites formed in situ in the kidney. *J Pharmacol Exp Ther.* 1981;**216**:640–646.

Boyd MR, Stiko, Statham CN, et al. Protective role of endogenous pulmonary glutathione and other sulfhydryl compounds against lung damage by alkylating agents: Investigations with 4-ipomeanol in the rat. *Biochem Pharmacol.* 1981;**31**:1579–1583.

Boyd MR, Wilson BJ. Isolation and characterization of 4-ipomeanol, lung-toxic furanoterpenoid produced by sweet potatoes (*Ipomoea batatas*). *J Agric Food Chem.* 1972;**20**:428–430.

Buckpitt RA, Statham CN, Boyd MR. In vivo studies on the target tissue metabolism, covalent binding, glutathione depletion, and toxicity of 4-ipomeanol in birds, species deficient in pulmonary enzymes for metabolic activation. *Toxicol Appl Pharmacol.* 1982;**65**:38–52.

Christian MC, Wittes RE, Leyland-Jones B, et al. 4-Ipomeanol: A novel investigational new drug for lung cancer. *J Natl Cancer Inst.* 1989;**81**:1113–1143.

Durham SK, Boyd MR, Castleman WL. Pulmonary endothelial and bronchiolar epithelial lesions induced by 4-ipomeanol in mice. *Am J Pathol.* 1985;**118**:66–75.

Dutcher JS, Boyd MR. Species and strain differences in target organ alkylation and toxicities by 4-ipomeanol: Predictive value of covalent binding in studies of target organ toxicities by reactive metabolites. *Biochem Pharmacol.* 1979;**28**:3367–3372.

Elhawari M, Barrett D. Preclinical toxicology of 4-ipomeanol (NSC-349438) (abstract). *Proc Am Assoc Cancer Res.* 1987;**28**:440.

Falzon M, McMahon JB, Schuller HM, et al. Metabolic activation and cytotoxicity of 4-ipomeanol in human non-small cell lung cancer lines. *Cancer Res.* 1986;**46**:3483–3489.

Gorelik E, Ovejera A, Shoemaker R, et al. Investigation of 4-ipomeanol in an in vivo microencapsulated tumor model. *Proc Am Assoc Cancer Res.* 1988;**29**:490.

McLemore T, Coudert B, Adelberg S, et al. Metabolic activation and cytotoxicity of 4-ipomeanol in human non-small cell lung cancer lines. *Cancer Res.* 1988;**46**:3483–3489.

McLemore TL, Liu MC, Blacker PC, et al. Novel intrapulmonary model for orthotopic propagation of human lung cancers in athymic nude mice. *Cancer Res.* 1987;**47**:5121–5140.

National Cancer Institute. *NCI Investigational Drugs: Ipomeanol* (NSC-349438). Washington, DC: U.S. Department of Health and Human Services; 1987:166–168.

Rowinsky EK, Ettinger DS, Noe DA, et al. Phase I and pharmacologic study of 4-ipomeanol in patients with lung cancer (abstract). *Proc Am Soc Clin Oncol.* 1989;**8**:72.

Rowinsky EK, Lubejko BG, Noe DA, et al. Phase I & pharmacologic study of 4-ipomeanol (IPO), a lung toxin, on a single dose schedule: Hepatotoxicity is dose-limiting in humans. *Proc Am Soc Clin Oncol.* 1992;**11**:115.

Shoemaker RH, Wolpert-DeFilippes MK, Kern DH, et al. Application of a human tumor colony-forming assay to new drug screening. *Cancer Res.* 1985;**45**:2145–2153.

Statham CN, Ducher JS, Kim SH, et al. Effects of phenobarbital and 3-methylcholanthrene on the in vivo distribution, metabolism and covalent binding of 4-ipomeanol in the rat: Implications for target organ toxicity. *Biochem Pharmacol.* 1982a;**31**:3973–3977.

Statham CN, Dutcher JS, Kim SH, et al. Ipomeanol 4-glucuronide, a major urinary metabolite of 4-ipomeanol in the rat. *Drug Metab Dispos.* 1982b;**10**:264–267.

Wilson BJ, Boyd MR, Harris TM, et al. Toxicity of mould-damaged sweet potatoes (*Ipomoea batatas*). *Nature.* 1971;**231**:52–53.

Iproplatin

■ Other Names

CHIP; JM-9; NSC-256927.

■ Chemistry

Structure of iproplatin

The complete chemical name for iproplatin is dichlorodihydroxybis(2-propylamine) platinum(IV). The molecular weight of iproplatin is 418 with a molecular formula of $C_6H_{20}C_{12}N_2O_2Pt$. The solubilities of iproplatin (mg/mL) in dimethylsulfoxide, dimethylacetamide, water, and ethanol are 5, 2.5, 1 to 2, and less than 0.2, respectively. Iproplatin has an octahedral structure that differs significantly from the planar coordinate configuration of cisplatin. This is afforded by the positive tetravalency of the platinum in iproplatin compared with the positive bivalent platinum in cisplatin and carboplatin.

■ Antitumor Activity

In preclinical studies iproplatin had activity comparable to that of cisplatin in L-1210 leukemia, B-16 melanoma, Lewis lung cancer, and a few human tumor xenografts growing in nude mice (Bradner et al 1980, Wolpert-DeFillippes 1980, Mihich et al 1979). Iproplatin was, however, inferior to cisplatin in CD8F and mammary carcinoma and was inactive in colon-38 carcinoma (Wolpert-Defillippes 1979). It was also inactive against cisplatin-resistant L-1210 leukemia cells in vitro (Burchenal et al 1978) but had good activity against L-1210 cells resistant to carmustine and cyclophosphamide (Bradner et al 1980, Connors et al 1979). Initially, there was also evidence for incomplete cross-resistance with cisplatin in fresh human tumors tested in the Hamberger–Salmon colony-forming assay in vitro (Anton et al 1983).

In clinical trials, iproplatin demonstrated significant antitumor activity in advanced ovarian cancer (Bramwell et al 1985, Sessa et al 1988, Weiss et al 1989). In 10 patients who had not received prior chemotherapy there were 6 complete responses and 2 partial responses (Bramwell et al 1985). In 16 patients previously treated with alkylating agents there was 1 complete response and 3 partial responses for a 25% overall response rate (Bramwell et al 1985). Lower response rates are reported in patients with advanced ovarian cancer resistant to cisplatin or carboplatin. In this setting, responses were observed in 11 of 79 resistant patients previously treated with cisplatin and in 2 of 18 resistant patients previously treated with carboplatin (Weiss et al 1989). Follow-up phase II studies have confirmed a high iproplatin response rate of 78% in untreated patients, an intermediate response rate of 42% in patients previously treated without cisplatin (42%), and a low response rate of 22% in patients previously treated with cisplatin (Sessa et al 1988). When there was evidence of tumor resistance to prior platinum therapy, the response rate to iproplatin was only 6.4% (Sessa et al 1988).

Iproplatin demonstrated minor activity in a variety of other solid tumors. In cervix cancer, iproplatin produced a response rate of 11%, which was equivalent to that for carboplatin (15%) but inferior to historical results with cisplatin (McGuire et al 1986). When used in a nonrandomized study as a single agent, iproplatin produced an overall response rate of 20.6% in cervix cancer (McGuire et al 1989). The response rate to first-line iproplatin in non-small cell lung cancer was only 9% (Bonomi et al 1989). As second-line therapy in advanced breast cancer, iproplatin produced a response rate of only 8% (Casper et al 1988). Stable disease has also been described in a phase I trial in pediatric patients with brain tumors and retinoblastoma (Pratt et al 1987).

Overall, iproplatin is an active drug in advanced ovarian cancer but it has reduced efficacy in previously treated patients. Unfortunately, it is relatively inactive in ovarian tumors that develop resistance to other platinum-containing agents. Similarly, it has poor activity in a number of other solid tumors that characteristically respond to cisplatin.

Mechanism of Action

Iproplatin has been reported to induce the breakage of covalently closed circular PM2 DNA (Bocian et al 1983). This breakage has been correlated to cytotoxicity in vitro and in vivo (Mong et al 1980). Similar effects are not seen with cisplatin, as only iproplatin with the platinum(IV) has the axial *trans* bonds. The axial bonds are believed to be responsible for the breakage of DNA which does not occur with the equatorial *cis* bonds in cisplatin.

In addition to this unique mechanism, it is also probable that iproplatin forms adducts with mammalian DNA that act to impair DNA and RNA synthesis. Platinum–DNA adducts have been shown to result from the loss of the chlorides, which exposes two sites for potential interactions. These may form DNA–DNA or DNA–protein bifunctional adducts and may involve both inter- and intrastrand DNA crosslinks.

Availability and Storage

Iproplatin was investigationally available from Bristol-Myers Company, Princeton, New Jersey. It was formulated as 50 mg of lyophilized powder with 125 mg of mannitol in 15-mL vials. The vials may be stored at room temperature (22–25°C) and protected from light (National Cancer Institute 1987).

Preparation for Use, Stability, and Admixture

The 50-mg vials are reconstituted with 10.3 mL of Sterile Water for Injection, USP, to yield 10-mL (deliverable dose) of iproplatin solution (5 mg/mL). Iproplatin solutions in water, 5% Dextrose Injection, USP, or 0.2 to 0.9% Sodium Chloride Injection, USP, are stable for at least 24 hours in room temperature and light conditions (Cheung et al 1987). There was only about 5% drug decomposition over this time period and there was no difference between storage in glass or polyvinyl chloride plastic containers. No light protection precautions are needed for iproplatin solutions stored for up to 24 hours.

It is possible that like cisplatin, iproplatin may react with aluminum metal in needles and infusion sets. Direct exposure to such metals is therefore not recommended.

Administration

Iproplatin is administered intravenously as a brief infusion in 100 to 1000 mL of infusate. Specific regimens include brief infusions in 100 mL of 5% Dextrose in Water, USP, over 30 minutes (Chawla et al 1988) or in 250 mL of normal saline over 30 minutes (Casper et al 1988) and also infusions over 1 to 2 hours in 1 L of normal saline (Bramwell et al 1985, Sessa et al 1988). Unlike cisplatin, iproplatin infusions do not require prehydration or diuretics (Bramwell et al 1985, Sessa et al 1988).

Dosage

The recommended iproplatin doses from phase I–II studies are 300 mg/m^2 IV every 4 weeks in untreated, good-performance-status patients and 240 mg/m^2 IV every 4 weeks in heavily pretreated patients (Bramwell et al 1985, Sessa et al 1988). In patients previously treated with other platinum-containing agents, a dose of 270 mg/m^2 has been used (Weiss et al 1989). The recommended dose for phase II solid tumor studies in children was 325 mg/m^2 IV every 4 weeks (Pratt et al 1987).

A weekly dosing schedule for iproplatin has been described with a recommended phase II dose of 95 mg/m^2/wk (Chawla et al 1988). These doses could be repeated for 4 consecutive weeks followed by a 6-week rest period. However, this schedule was not active in a variety of solid tumors and does not appear to have advantages over a monthly infusion.

Pharmacodynamic observations suggest that there are linear correlations (1) between total body clearance of iproplatin and creatinine clearance and (2) between the percentage reduction in platelets and the area under the plasma iproplatin concentration × time curve (Pendyala et al 1985a). Thus, patients with reduced renal function require commensurate dose reductions to prevent severe thrombocytopenia; however, specific dose reduction guidelines for iproplatin in patients with compromised renal function have not been established.

Pharmacokinetics

In the rat, iproplatin (10 mg/kg) displayed a biphasic elimination pattern with a β half-life of 14

IPROPLATIN PHARMACOKINETICS IN CANCER PATIENTS*

Dose (mg/m^2) as a 30-min Infusion	Average Peak Plasma Level (µg/mL)	% Urinary Excretion of Platinum	Platinum Half-life (h) α	Platinum Half-life (h) β	Iproplatin Half-life (h)	Volume of Distribution Central Compartment (L) Iproplatin	Volume of Distribution Central Compartment (L) Total Platinum	Clearance (L·h^{-1}) Iproplatin	Clearance (L·h^{-1}) Total Platinum
20	1	42	—	—					
120	4	42	—	—					
270	15	33	—	—					
350	18	27	—	—					
Mean	—	16–63	0.4–2.2	58–103	0.9	23.4	10.4	18	0.77

*Data from Pendyala et al 1983.

hours. Renal excretion accounted for most of the drug's clearance. The amounts of drug recovered in rat urine were 44% at 5 hours and 57% at 26 hours. A substantial amount of drug was bound to kidney tissues, with platinum concentrations ranging from 6 to 42 µg/g of tissue (Pfister et al 1978). More prolonged elimination was observed in dogs, with half-lives of (α) 0.6 hour and (β) 39 hours (Pendyala et al 1976). Renal clearance was similar to that in the rat, with 57% of a dose recoverable in the urine in 24 hours (Pendyala and Creaven 1980).

Iproplatin elimination patterns in humans are summarized in the table on page 615 (Pendyala et al 1983). A biphasic elimination pattern was again observed with rapid but variable urinary recovery of drug. The terminal elimination half-life of iproplatin was quite prolonged; however, iproplatin is bound much more loosely to plasma proteins than is cisplatin, so renal elimination is more rapid. Two platinum-containing metabolites have been identified in the blood and five in the urine of iproplatin-treated patients (Pendyala et al 1983). Of interest, one of the major urinary metabolites was tentatively identified as *cis*-dichlorobis(isopropylamine) platinum(II) (JM-6). This less polar metabolite can result from exposing iproplatin to chemical reducing agents and it has some antitumor activity (Bradner et al 1980, Wolpert-DeFillippes 1979).

Pharmacokinetic findings suggest that creatinine clearance may be an important determinant for predicting severe thrombocytopenia from iproplatin and this may be helpful in individualizing the dose of the agent (Monfardini et al 1986).

■ Side Effects and Toxicity

The dose-limiting toxic effect of iproplatin is thrombocytopenia which is both dose related and cumulative (Bramwell et al 1985). The median platelet nadir after a 300 mg/m² dose is about 25×10^9/L. This consistently occurs on day 14 after dosing, with recovery by day 21 in early courses and days 28 to 42 in later courses (Bramwell et al 1985). Leukopenia is typically mild, with a nadir on days 21 to 28 and slow recovery over 4 to 6 weeks. Most patients also show a progressive fall in hemoglobin levels following iproplatin with a simultaneous increase in mean corpuscular volume (Bramwell et al 1985). Transfusions are typically required in previously treated patients.

Nausea and vomiting occur consistently but are much less severe and not as prolonged as with cisplatin. With iproplatin, emesis typically ensues within 1 hour of drug administration. It is rarely present after the first day. In contrast, however, diarrhea can be much more intense with iproplatin and is clearly dose related. This frequently requires treatment with narcotic analgesics and sometimes drug discontinuation.

Renal toxicity is usually not observed with iproplatin even without the use of prehydration (Pendyala et al 1985b). Occasionally, the serum creatinine will be transiently and mildly elevated. Rarely, renal marker enzymes such as β_2-microglobulin, α_1-microglobulin, or urinary albumin are elevated (Bramwell et al 1985).

Mild peripheral neuropathy is either rarely reported (Sessa et al 1988) or not observed at all following iproplatin (Bramwell et al 1985). Other rare toxic effects include serum electrolyte disturbances (Sessa et al 1988) and alopecia. Hearing loss is not observed with iproplatin. There have been several reports of allergic reactions to the drug (Bramwell et al 1985, Sessa et al 1988). These typically manifest as an itchy erythematous rash which occurs briefly and immediately after iproplatin infusion (Bramwell et al 1985). Occasionally, purpuric rashes on the shins occur 1 to 2 weeks after drug administration.

REFERENCES

Anton A, Paricia L, Rozencweig M, et al. Comparative effect of cisplatin (DDP), TNO-6, carboplatin (CBDCA), CHIP and JM40 in human myeloid and human tumor clonogenic assays. *Proc Am Assoc Cancer Res*. 1983;23:292.

Bocian E, Laverick M, Nias AH. The mode of action of *cis*-dichloro-*trans*-dihydroxy-bis-isopropylamine platinum IV (CHIP) studied by the analysis of chromosome aberration production. *Br J Cancer*. 1983;47:503–509.

Bonomi PD, Finkelstein DM, Ruckdeschel JC, et al. Combination chemotherapy versus single agents followed by combination chemotherapy in stage IV non-small-cell lung cancer: A study of the Eastern Cooperative Oncology Group. *J Clin Oncol*. 1989;7(11):1602–1613.

Bradner WT, Rose WC, Huftalen JB. Antitumor activity of platinum analogs. In: Prestayko AW, Crooke ST, Carter SK, eds. *Cisplatin: Current Status and New Developments*. New York: Academic Press; 1980:171–182.

Bramwell VHC, Crowther D, O'Malley S, et al. Activity of JM9 in advanced ovarian cancer: A phase I–II trial. *Cancer Treat Rep*. 1985;69(4):409–416.

Burchenal JH, Kalaher B, Dews K, Loys L, et al. Studies of cross-resistance, synergistic combinations and blocking of activity of platinum derivatives. *Biochemie*. 1978;60:961–965.

Casper ES, Smart TC, Hakes TB, et al. Clinical trial of iproplatin (*cis*-dichloro-*trans*-dihydroxy-bis-isopropylamine platinum IV, CHIP) in patients with advanced breast cancer. *Invest New Drugs.* 1988;**6**:87–91.

Chawla SP, Yap B-S, Tenney DM, et al. Phase I study of weekly-administered iproplatin [*cis*-dichloro-*trans*-dihydroxy-bis-isopropylamine platin (CHIP, JM9]. *Invest New Drugs.* 1988;**6**:311–317.

Cheung YM, Cradock JC, Vishnuvajjala BR, et al. Stability of cisplatin, iproplatin, carboplatin, and tetraplatin in commonly used intravenous solutions. *Am J Hosp Pharm.* 1987;**44**:124–130.

Connors TA, Cleare MJ, Harrap KR. Structure–activity relationships of the antitumor platinum coordination complexes. *Cancer Treat Rep.* 1979;**63**:1499–1502.

Creaven PJ, Madajewicz S, Pendyala L, et al. Phase I clinical trial of *cis*-dichloro-*trans*-dihydroxy-bis-isopropylamine platinum(IV) (CHIP). *Cancer Treat Rep.* 1983;**67**:795–800.

McGuire WP III, Arseneau J, Blessing JA, et al. A randomized comparative trial of carboplatin and iproplatin in advanced squamous carcinoma of the uterine cervix: A Gynecologic Oncology Group study. *J Clin Oncol.* 1989;**7**(10):1462–1468.

McGuire WP, Blessing JA, Hatch K, et al. A phase II study of CHIP in advanced squamous cell carcinoma of the cervix (a Gynecologic Oncology Group study). *Invest New Drugs.* 1986;**4**:181–186.

Mihich E, Bullard G, Pavelic Z, et al. Preclinical studies of dihydroxy-*cis*-dichloro-bis-isopropylamine platinum IV (CHIP) (abstract #C-559). *Proc Am Assoc Cancer Res.* 1979;**20**:426.

Monfardini S, Renard J, Pinedo HM, et al. Iproplatin (CHIP) and carboplatin (CBDCA) induced thrombocytopenia: Analysis of risk factors (abstract). *Proc Am Assoc Cancer Res.* 1986;**27**:165.

Mong S, Prestayko AW, Crooke ST. In vitro interaction of covalently linked closed circular DNA with second generation platinum compounds. In: Prestayko A, Crooke S, Carter S, eds. *Cisplatin: Current Status and New Developments.* New York: Academic Press; 1980:213–226.

National Cancer Institute. *NCI Investigational Drugs: Iproplatin.* NIH Publication 88-2141. Washington, DC: U.S. Department of Health and Human Services; 1987:113–115.

Pendyala L, Cowens JW, Creaven PJ. Studies on the pharmacokinetics and metabolism of *cis*-dichloro-*trans*-dihydroxy-bis-isopropylamine platinum(IV) in the dog. *Cancer Treat Rep.* 1976;**66**:509–516.

Pendyala L, Creaven PJ. Disposition of *cis*-dichloro-*trans*-dihydroxy-bis-isopropylamine platinum IV (CHIP) in the dog. *Pharmacologist.* 1980;**22**:240.

Pendyala L, Greco W, Cowens JW, et al. Pharmacokinetics of *cis*-dichloro-*trans*-dihydroxy-bis-isopropylamine platinum IV (CHIP) in patients with advanced cancer. *Cancer Chemother Pharmacol.* 1983;**11**:23–28.

Pendyala L, Madajewicz S, Creaven PJ. Effect of renal function impairment on iproplatin pharmacokinetics and relation to toxicity. *Cancer Res.* 1985a;**45**:5936–5938.

Pendyala L, Madajewicz S, Lele SB, et al. Evaluation of the nephrotoxicity of iproplatin (CHIP) in comparison to cisplatin by measurement of urinary enzymes. *Cancer Chemother Pharmacol.* 1985b;**15**:203–207.

Pfister M, Pavelic ZP, Bullard GA, et al. Dichloro-dihydroxy-bis-isopropylamine platinum IV a new antitumor platinum complex. Pharmacokinetics in the rat: Relation to renal toxicity. *Biochimie.* 1978;**60**:1057.

Pratt CB, Kamen BA, Winick N, et al. Phase I study of iproplatin in pediatric patients: A Pediatric Oncology Group study. *Cancer Treat Rep.* 1987;**71**:87–88.

Sessa C, Vermorken J, Renard J, et al. Phase II study of iproplatin in advanced ovarian carcinoma. *J Clin Oncol.* 1988;**6**:98–105.

Weiss GR, Green S, Stock-Novak D. A phase II study of the second-line treatment of advanced ovarian cancer with iproplatin: A Southwest Oncology Group study (abstract #317). *Invest New Drugs.* 1989;**7**:428.

Wolpert-DeFillippes MD. Antitumor activity of *cis*-dichlorodiammineplatinum(II). *Cancer Treat Rep.* 1979;**63**: 1453–1458.

Wolpert-DeFillippes MK. Antitumor activity of cisplatin analogs. In: Prestayko AW, Crooke ST, Carter SK, eds. *Cisplatin: Current Status and New Developments.* New York: Academic Press; 1980:183–191.

Isotretinoin

■ Other Names

13-*cis*-Retinoic acid; cRA; Accutane®; Ro 4-3780 (Roche Dermatologics).

■ Chemistry

Structure of isotretinoin

Isotretinoin is a photoisomer of all-*trans*-retinoic acid in which the terminal carbon is in the *cis* configuration. Otherwise, the molecules are identical. The molecular formula of isotretinoin is $C_{20}H_{28}O_2$ and the formula weight is 300.44. It occurs naturally as a yellow to orange crystalline powder and has very limited aqueous solubility.

Antitumor Activity

In preclinical cancer models, retinoids are known to induce the differentiation of a variety of malignant tumor cell types toward a normal phenotype (Lippman et al 1987). This has been demonstrated for myeoblasts from acute myelocytic leukemia (Lawrence et al 1987), human lung cancer cells (Saccomanno et al 1982), pulmonary adenomas in mice (Frasca and Garfinkel 1981), and a variety of other malignant cell types (as reviewed by Meyskens et al 1987). Carcinogen-induced lung cancer in mice is blocked by isotretinoin (Port et al 1975). In contrast, isotretinoin did not prevent carcinogen-induced bladder cancer in rats (Croft et al 1981). Isotretinoin can also be directly cytotoxic to these same cell types (Meyskens et al 1987).

Leukemia and Myelodysplastic Syndromes. Isotretinoin is active in patients with similar types of cancer. Like its isomer, *trans*-retinoic acid, isotretinoin can produce a high degree of complete remissions in patients with acute promyelocytic leukemia (Fontana et al 1986); however, remission durations are not long and *trans*-retinoic acid has become the preferred retinoid in this disease. Responses to isotretinoin are achieved without inducing disseminated intravascular coagulation (DIC), as is common when cytotoxic agents are used to treat acute promyelocytic leukemia (APL). Clinical improvement in APL is brisk following retinoids and is evident within 1 to 2 weeks. Remission durations average about 6 to 10 months. Retinoic acid therapy can be combined with cytotoxic agents, which are often used for remission maintenance therapy. There are no conclusive data to suggest that chronic maintenance therapy with retinoic acid is beneficial in this disease.

There are a number of anecdotal reports of activity for isotretinoin in patients with myelodysplastic syndromes (Hellstrom et al 1988, List et al 1990, Picozzi et al 1986). In one phase I–II trial, partial responses were obtained in 2 of 18 patients (Greenberg et al 1985). Most often, isotretinoin has been combined with other agents such as low-dose cytarabine (Clark et al 1987a) and interferon alfa (Besa et al 1990). The efficacy of low-dose cytarabine and isotretinoin has not been consistently reported (Hellstrom et al 1988). Furthermore, a placebo-controlled trial could not substantiate any statistically significant benefits for isotretinoin in this disease (Koeffler et al 1988). In contrast, a subset of myelodysplastic patients with refractory anemia and less than 5% blasts did appear to improve with isotretinoin therapy in a trial of isotretinoin alone (Clark et al 1987b) or with cytarabine (Clark et al 1987a). There is also a suggestion that prolonged isotretinoin therapy may enhance response rates when α-tocopherol is added to reduce retinoid toxicity (Besa et al 1990). The response rate in this trial was 26% in transfusion-dependent myelodysplastic syndrome patients (Besa et al 1990).

In a small pilot trial, complete responses to isotretinoin were reported in two of eight patients with juvenile chronic myelogenous leukemia (Castleberry et al 1991).

Patients with mycosis fungoides, a helper-T-lymphocyte malignancy, are also responsive to isotretinoin. In pretreated patients, responses were obtained in 11 of 25 (44%) patients. Six patients achieved a complete response (Kessler et al 1987). A similar 46% overall response rate was reported in a Scandinavian trial of isotretinoin in mycosis fungoides. Interestingly, clinical improvement is typically noted within 2 to 4 weeks of starting isotretinoin, and about one half of the responses may be complete (Molin et al 1985). Isotretinoin is also active in refractory cutaneous Ki-1 lymphoma (Chow et al 1991).

Patients with acute myelogenous leukemia (AML) have responded to isotretinoin therapy, although objective response rates are low. In one trial with 41 pediatric patients, one complete and two partial responses were obtained for a 7% overall response rate (Bell et al 1991). Limited efficacy was also noted in adult patients treated with isotretinoin combined with low-dose cytarabine (Kramer et al 1991). There is a description of a partial response to isotretinoin in one of two patients with chronic myelomonocytic leukemia (Greenberg et al 1985).

Head and neck carcinoma patients have been treated with isotretinoin as a chemopreventive to reduce the recurrence of the development of secondary squamous cell carcinomas. In one trial, a 12-month course of isotretinoin reduced the incidence of second epithelial tumors from 24 to 4% without affecting recurrence or metastatic spread of the primary cancer (Hong et al 1990). Patients with surgically unresectable head and neck cancer may also achieve partial responses to isotretinoin, although remission durations are quite short (Meyskens et al 1982). A response rate of 15% was described in one randomized phase II trial of patients with locally advanced or metastatic squamous cell head and neck cancer (Lippman et al 1988).

The premalignant condition oral leukoplakia is responsive to isotretinoin (Hong et al 1986). Major decreases in the size of the lesions were achieved in 67% of patients receiving oral isotretinoin for 3 months compared with 10% in the placebo group.

Retinoids have produced conflicting evidence of antitumor activity in patients with a variety of malignant skin cancers. Topical isotretinoin is reported to produce partial or complete regression of basal cell carcinoma lesions in most patients (Sankowski et al 1987). Oral isotretinoin has produced a 10% complete response rate in patients with multiple basal cell carcinomas; however, there is conflicting evidence that isotretinoin can prevent basal cell carcinoma and recent results of a double-blind multicenter trial show that low-dose oral isotretinoin does not reduce the occurrence of new lesions among high-risk patients (Tangrea et al 1992, Robinson and Salasche 1992). This contrasts with earlier smaller studies showing reduced rates of new tumor development in high-risk patients (Peck et al 1988, Goldberg et al 1989, Kraemer et al 1988).

For patients with advanced squamous cell carcinoma of the skin, oral isotretinoin and subcutaneous interferon alfa-2a were highly effective (Lippman et al 1992b). The overall response rate among 28 assessable patients was 68%, with 25% achieving a complete response. The median duration of response following 2 months of therapy was more than 5 months. In a subset analysis, responses were obtained in 13 of 14 patients with advanced local disease, 4 of 6 patients with regional disease, and 2 of 8 patients with distant metastases. Thus, response rates were adversely affected in patients with more advanced disease. This confirms a prior pilot study of oral isotretinoin (without interferon alfa) in a few patients with advanced squamous cell skin cancer (Meyskens et al 1982). This same uncontrolled pilot trial also described a partial response in 1 of 13 patients with malignant melanoma.

Other Solid Tumors. Preclinical breast cancer studies have shown that isotretinoin can inhibit human tumor cell growth in vitro, whereas isotretinoin did not inhibit human breast tumor xenograft growth in athymic mice (Halter et al 1988). Of interest, the isomer *trans*-retinoic acid was active in vivo. Likewise, isotretinoin was also inactive in breast cancer patients studied in phase II clinical trials (Cassidy et al 1982). Isotretinoin was similarly inactive in patients with advanced nonseminomatous germ cell tumors (Gold et al 1984) although a few patients did experience disease stabilization for several months. Oral isotretinoin was also ineffective in six patients with acquired immunodeficiency syndrome-related Kaposi's sarcoma.

Bone marrow involvement from neuroblastoma has been reported to respond to isotretinoin therapy but without objective evidence of primary tumor shrinkage (Reynolds et al 1990, 1991). Another potentially responsive tumor is squamous cell carcinoma of the cervix. A pilot trial of isotretinoin and interferon alfa reported more than 50% tumor regression in 13 of 26 patients with locally advanced disease (Lippman et al 1992). In contrast, isotretinoin appears to be relatively ineffective in patients with non-small cell lung cancer (Grunberg and Itri 1987).

■ Mechanism of Action

Isotretinoin interacts with two types of cytoplasmic retinoic acid-binding proteins (CRABPs I and II), which are distinct from those that bind retinol (Chytil and Ong 1984). These binding proteins may aid in the translocation of isotretinoin to the nucleus where it interacts with three types of nuclear retinoic acid receptors, RARs α, β, and γ (Petkovich et al 1987). These receptors, particularly RARα, appear to directly mediate the myeloid differentiating activity of retinoic acid. A number of genes are expressed following retinoic acid stimulation. These include genes that direct the synthesis of (1) proteins that can differentiate myeloid and some epithelial cells and (2) proteins that can block the growth of different epithelial cell types (as reviewed by Smith et al 1992). Retinoic acid also induces both types of CRABP in several different types of cancer cells, with particularly good documentation in skin treated with topical but not oral isotretinoin (Hirschel-Scholz et al 1989).

The differentiating effect of retinoids in acute leukemia cells is maximal in vitro at drug concentrations of 0.1 to 1.0 μmol/L (Koeffler and Amatruda 1985). In acute promyelocytic leukemia, the differentiating effect has an onset of 2 to 4 days and is accompanied by the acquisition of normal morphology in the granulocyte with the exception of secondary granule production (Koeffler and Amatruda 1985). Cell growth in the malignant cells typically ceases by day 4 following retinoic acid exposure. Similar inhibition of clonal proliferation is observed in acute myelocytic leukemia cells.

Retinoid-induced differentiation is observed in

neuroblastoma cell lines (Sidell 1982), teratocarcinoma cell lines (Strickland and Sawey 1980), and normal epithelium of the oral mucosa and tracheobronchial lining that has undergone squamous cell differentiation because of either vitamin A deficiency or as a response to toxic and/or mechanical injury. This latter effect is the rationale for isotretinoin use in smoking-induced oral leukoplakia or bronchial metaplasia.

Retinoids may produce direct growth inhibition of cancer cells without differentiation. This effect also requires nuclear RAR and is greater for *trans*-retinoic acid over isotretinoin in some cell types such as rhabdomyosarcoma (Crouch and Helman 1991). About 20% of freshly isolated human tumors were sensitive to isotretinoin-induced inhibition of colony formation in one study (Meyskens et al 1983). The mechanism for both growth inhibition and differentiation by retinoids may involve the production and local (paracrine) secretion of transforming growth factor β (TGF-β), a normal inhibitor of epithelial cell growth (Wakefield and Sporn 1990). TGF-β in turn may induce apoptosis or programmed cell death (as reviewed by Smith et al 1992). Cell death as a result of apoptosis is known to involve, in sequence, Ca^{2+}/Mg^{2+} influx, activation of endonuclease(s), and degradation of DNA (Kerr et al 1972). Of interest, HL-60 promyelocytic leukemia cells induced into terminal (lethal) differentiation appear to die by a process that involves apoptosis (Martin et al 1990).

■ Availability and Storage

Isotretinoin is commercially available in 10-, 20-, and 40-mg soft gelatin capsules (Accutane®, Roche Dermatologics, Nutley, New Jersey). The capsules also contain butylated hydroxytoluene as an antioxidant preservative, soybean oil, disodium edetate, beeswax, hydrogenated vegetable oil, colorants, and methyl/propylparabens as antibacterial preservative. The capsules are stored at room temperature and should be protected from light.

■ Special Precautions

Pregnant women should not receive isotretinoin and women should be advised to avoid pregnancy while on isotretinoin because of the drug's marked teratogenic potential. A period of at least 1 to 3 months off isotretinoin is advised before becoming pregnant to allow for clearance of drug and metabolites.

■ Dosage

The only current FDA-approved use for isotretinoin is in the treatment of severe, recalcitrant cystic acne at a typical dose of 0.5 to 1.0 mg/kg orally once daily for 15 to 20 weeks. A maximum dose of 2.0 mg/kg is recommended in this indication (Peck et al 1979).

The table on the next page summarizes the investigational doses of isotretinoin when used as a differentiating agent in leukemia or as a tumor growth inhibitor for other malignancies. The most common dose in these trials is 2 to 3 mg/kg/d orally for 1 to 3 months. Phase I studies of oral isotretinoin show that chronic daily doses greater than 60 mg/m² are not well tolerated because of intense headache and desquamative dermatitis (Band et al 1982). In addition, acute oral doses above 400 mg/m² (up to 1800 mg/m²) were very poorly absorbed, thereby limiting the ability to deliver short-term dose-intensive oral therapy with isotretinoin (Clamon et al 1985) (see Pharmacokinetics). Finally, although there is an apparent dose dependency in the severity of symptoms, even low-dose oral isotretinoin therapy of 0.11 to 0.14 mg/kg/d produces significant toxicity over a 9-month treatment period (Edwards et al 1986).

■ Drug Interactions

Several additive or synergistic cytotoxic drug combinations with isotretinoin in experimental differentiation models have been described. These include the combination of isotretinoin with 5-fluorouracil in human transitional cell carcinoma (Recondo et al 1991). The differentiating effect of retinoids is also enhanced in experimental tumor cell systems (in vitro) by combination with hematopoietic cytokines such as interferon alfa, tumor necrosis factor, granulocyte–macrophage colony-stimulating factor, interleukins-1 and -4, and, especially, granulocyte colony-stimulating factor (Peck and Bollag 1991). Patients should be cautioned about the use of other drugs, especially alcohol, that might potentiate an increase in serum triglycerides.

■ Pharmacokinetics

Isotretinoin is 99.9% bound to albumin in plasma. This binding remains constant over a wide range of serum concentrations. The time to peak isotretinoin plasma levels following an oral dose of 3 mg/kg is 192 minutes (Goodman et al 1982). This dose produced peak plasma levels of 0.2 to 0.86 µg/mL with

INVESTIGATIONAL DOSES OF ISOTRETINOIN AS A TUMOR DIFFERENTIATOR OR GROWTH INHIBITOR

Disease	Dose	Reference
Hematologic cancers		
Myelodysplastic syndrome	2.5–4 mg/kg/d PO × 8 wk	Picozzi et al 1986
Acute myelogenous leukemia	100 mg/m^2/d × 6 mo	Koeffler et al 1988
	100 mg/m^2/d × 8 wk	Kramer et al 1991
Solid tumors		
Head and neck cancer		
Prevention	50–100 mg/m^2/d PO × 12 mo	Hong et al 1990
Established disease	3 mg/kg/d PO × 6 wk	Lippman et al 1988
Non-small cell lung cancer	2–3 mg/kg/d PO × 1+ mo	Meyskens et al 1982
Breast cancer	0.5–8 mg/kg/d PO × 1 mo	Cassidy et al 1982
Neuroblastoma	100 mg/m^2/d	Reynolds et al 1991
Oral leukoplakia	1–2 mg/kg/d	Hong et al 1986
Skin cancers		
Basal cell carcinoma	3.1 mg/kg/d topical	Sankowski et al 1987
	3.1 mg/kg/d PO	Peck et al 1988
Squamous cell cancer	1 mg/kg/d PO × 4 wk	Lippman and Meyskens 1987
Malignant melanoma	2–3 mg/kg/d PO	Meyskens et al 1982

a mean of 0.5 µg/mL. The mean terminal plasma half-life for the second (β) phase of elimination was 121 minutes. The longer terminal (γ) phase could not be determined accurately in all patients but ranged from 716 to 4089 minutes (Goodman et al 1982). In most studies, however, the terminal half-life of isotretinoin is reported to range between 10 and 20 hours (Brazzell and Colburn 1982). Mean concentration × time products for the 3 mg/kg dose were 221.5 ± 113.5 µg·min/mL compared with 368 µg·min/mL for doses of 4 to 5 mg/kg (Goodman et al 1982). No intact drug was recovered in the urine.

With higher doses of 200 and 400 mg/m^2, mean peak plasma isotretinoin levels increased to 1.5 and 3.8 µg/mL, respectively (Clamon et al 1985); however, at doses above 400 mg/m^2, there was no further increase in mean peak plasma levels or area under the curve, possibly indicating saturable absorption. Food may also alter isotretinoin oral bioavailability (Colburn et al 1983). There is also consistent evidence of a secondary peak in plasma concentration which might represent enterohepatic circulation of isotretinoin (Goodman et al 1982, Clamon et al 1985).

In a phase I study of high doses, mean plasma isotretinoin clearance rates were 164 and 403 mL/m^2/min for doses of 200 and 400 mg/m^2, respectively. Higher doses of 100 and 1400 mg/m^2 produced higher mean clearances of 294 and 1533 mL/m^2/min, respectively (Clamon et al 1985). At the lower dose levels, the volume of distribution ranged from 173 to 403 L/m^2 and was significantly elevated at the higher dose ranges, from 1510 to 2001 L/m^2 (Clamon et al 1985).

With chronic isotretinoin therapy the 4-oxo metabolite accumulates in the plasma to produce a concentration × time product five times that of the parent molecule (Meyskens et al 1987). The elimination half-life of this metabolite ranges from 11 to 50 hours, with a mean of 29 hours. This explains the plasma accumulation of the 4-oxo metabolite with chronic daily dosing of isotretinoin.

There are significant pharmacokinetic differences between isotretinoin and *trans*-retinoic acid: (1) Isotretinoin steady-state levels do not decrease with chronic dosing; (2) there is significant accumulation of the 4-oxo metabolite of isotretinoin, whereas only 10% of *trans*-retinoic acid doses are converted to the 4-oxo metabolite; (3) isotretinoin has a much longer terminal half-life; and (4) there is evidence of dose-dependent oral bioavailability for isotretinoin.

■ Side Effects and Toxicity

Isotretinoin produces the same general toxic effects as an excess of vitamin A (Kamm et al 1984). Compared with *trans*-retinoic acid, the incidence of central nervous system side effects is higher with isotretinoin but still much less than with retinol (Smith et al 1992). Following an average daily isotretinoin dose of 109 mg (approximately 1.5

mg/kg) the most common toxic effect is cheilitis or dry lips, occurring in up to 90% of patients. Occasionally this can become severe, warranting dose reduction or temporary discontinuation. About one third of patients experience moderate xerosis with inflammation and, in general, have very dry mucous membranes (Windhorst and Nigra 1982). This can lead to pruritus and epistaxis in about one fourth of patients. Brittle nails are also a common complaint. Some patients may also complain of increased sensitivity to the sun, often resulting in sunburn.

Central nervous system side effects of isotretinoin include headache, lethargy, and fatigue, seen in about 10% of patients. Dizziness is reported along with occasional visual disturbances; however, even at very high dose levels, these symptoms are not dose limiting (Clamon et al 1985). Ocular findings include conjunctivitis, eye irritation, and, rarely, the development of corneal ulcers and opacities. The latter findings were noted only after years of chronic daily isotretinoin therapy.

Nausea and vomiting are described in approximately 20% of patients and are typically of mild intensity. Rare side effects include weight loss, alopecia, and liver enzyme elevation, typically alkaline phosphatase and aspartate aminotransferase (Clamon et al 1985); however, triglycerides are consistently elevated to a slight degree (approximately 10–20%) in most patients. Only a few patients have experienced elevations to twice normal values, and these rapidly reverse on drug discontinuance. One trial also reported unexplained microscopic hematuria (one to five red blood cells per high-power field) during a high-dose isotretinoin phase I trial (Clamon et al 1985). Mild proteinuria may also be observed in 10% of patients taking isotretinoin.

Musculoskeletal toxic effects may occur in about 20% of patients. Symptoms include arthralgias (17%), bone and joint pain, and muscle aches or stiffness (15% of patients). In children, premature closure of the epiphyses has been described (Williams and Elias 1981). And, 40% of adults receiving very low dose isotretinoin (0.14 mg/kg/d for 3 years) have developed skeletal hyperostosis. This involves ossification along the anterior margins of vertebral bodies and/or disk spaces (Tangrea et al 1992).

Hematologic effects of isotretinoin are minimal. Reported alterations include a 50% increase in the sedimentation rate, a 10% decrease in both white and red blood cell counts, and a 10 to 14% increase in the platelet count (Windhorst and Nigra 1982).

All retinoids have marked teratogenic activity and are known to alter embryonic morphogenesis. Therefore, patients must not be pregnant or become pregnant while receiving isotretinoin and for 1 to 3 months thereafter (*Physicians' Desk Reference* 1993).

REFERENCES

Band PR, Besner JG, Leclaire R, et al. Phase I study of 13-*cis*-Retinoic acid toxicity. *Cancer Treat Rep.* 1982;**66**:1759–1761.

Bell B, Findley H, Krischer J, et al. Phase II study of 13-*cis*-Retinoic acid in pediatric patients with acute nonlymphocytic leukemia—A Pediatric Oncology Group study. *J Immunother.* 1991;**10**:77–83.

Besa E, Abrahm J, Bartholomew M, et al. Treatment with 13-*cis*-Retinoic acid in transfusion-dependent patients with myelodysplastic syndrome and decreased toxicity with addition of alpha-tocopherol. *Am J Med.* 1990;**89**:739–747.

Brazzell R, Colburn WA. Pharmacokinetics of the retinoids isotretinoin and etretinate. *J Am Acad Dermatol.* 1982;**6**:643–651.

Cassidy J, Lippman M, LaCroix A, et al. Phase II trial of 13-*cis*-Retinoic acid in metastatic breast cancer. *Eur J Cancer Clin Oncol.* 1982;**18**:925–928.

Castleberry R, Emanuel P, Gualtieri R, et al. Preliminary experience with 13-*cis*-Retinoic acid (cRA) in the treatment of juvenile chronic myelogenous leukemia (JCML). *Blood.* 1991;**78**:170a.

Chow JM, Cheng AL, Su IJ, Wang CH. 13-*cis*-Retinoic acid induces cellular differentiation and durable remission in refractory cutaneous Ki-1 lymphoma. *Cancer.* 1991;**67**:2490–2494.

Chytil F, Ong D. Cellular retinoid-binding proteins. In: Sporn M, Roberts A, Goodman D, eds. *The Retinoids.* Orlando, FL: Academic Press; 1984;**2**:90–125.

Clamon G, Chabot GG, Valeriote F, et al. Phase I study and pharmacokinetics of weekly high-dose 13-*cis*-Retinoic acid. *Cancer Res.* 1985;**45**:1874–1878.

Clark R, Ismail S, Jacobs A, et al. A randomized trial of 13-*cis*-Retinoic acid with or without cytosine arabinoside in patients with the myelodysplastic syndrome. *Br J Haematol.* 1987a;**66**:77–83.

Clark R, Lush C, Jacobs A, et al. Effect of 13-*cis*-Retinoic acid on survival of patients with myelodysplastic syndrome. *Lancet.* 1987b;**1**:763–765.

Colburn W, Vane F, Shorter H. Pharmacokinetics of isotretinoin and its major blood metabolite following a single oral dose to man. *Eur J Clin Pharmacol.* 1983;**24**:689–694.

Croft WA, Croft MA, Paulus KP, et al. 13-*cis*-Retinoic acid: Effect on urinary bladder carcinogenesis by *N*-[4-(5-

nitro-2-furyl)-2-thiazolyl]-formamide in Fischer rats. *Cancer Lett.* 1981;**12**:355–360.

Crouch G, Helman L. All-*trans*-retinoic acid inhibits the growth of human rhabdomyosarcoma cell lines. *Cancer Res.* 1991;**51**:4882–4887.

Edwards L, Alberts DS, Levine N. Clinical toxicity of low-dose isotretinoin. *Cancer Treat Rep.* 1986;**70**:663–664.

Fontana J, Rogers J, Durham J. The role of 13-*cis*-Retinoic acid in the remission induction of a patient with acute promyelocytic leukemia. *Cancer.* 1986;**57**:209–217.

Frasca JM, Garfinkel L. 13-*cis*-Retinoic acid and murine pulmonary adenomas: A preliminary report. *Nutr Cancer.* 1981;**3**:64–72.

Gold E, Bosl G, Itri L. Phase II trial of 13-*cis*-Retinoic acid in patients with advanced nonseminomatous germ cell tumors. *Cancer Treat Rep.* 1984;**68**:1287–1288.

Goldberg L, Hsu S, Alcalay J. Effectiveness of isotretinoin in preventing the appearance of basal cell carcinomas in basal cell nevus syndrome. *J Am Acad Dermatol.* 1989;**21**:141–145.

Goodman GE, Einspahr JG, Alberts DS, et al. Pharmacokinetics of 13-*cis*-Retinoic acid in patients with advanced cancer. *Cancer Res.* 1982;**42**:2087–2091.

Greenberg BR, Durie BGM, Barnett TC, et al. Phase I–II study of 13-*cis*-Retinoic acid in myelodysplastic syndrome. *Cancer Treat Rep.* 1985;**69**:1369–1374.

Grunberg S, Itri L. Phase II study of isotretinoin in the treatment of advanced non-small cell lung cancer. *Cancer Treat Rep.* 1987;**71**:1097–1098.

Halter S, Fraker L, Adcock D, et al. Effects of retinoids on xenotransplanted human mammary carcinoma cells in athymic mice. *Cancer Res.* 1988;**488**:3733–3736.

Hellstrom E, Robert K, Gahrton G, et al. Therapeutic effects of low-dose cytosine arabinoside, alpha-interferon, 1α-hydroxyvitamin D3 and retinoic acid in acute leukemia and myeloblastic syndromes. *Eur J Haematol.* 1988;**40**:449–459.

Hirschel-Scholz S, Siegenthaler G, Saurat J-H. Isotretinoin differs from other synthetic retinoids in its modulation of human cellular retinoic acid binding protein (CRABP). *Br J Dermatol.* 1989;**120**:639–644.

Hong WK, Endicott J, Itri LM, et al. 13-*cis*-Retinoic acid in the treatment of oral leukoplakia. *N Engl J Med.* 1986;**315**:1501–1505.

Hong W, Lippman S, Itri L, et al. Prevention of secondary primary tumor with isotretinoin in squamous-cell carcinoma of the head and neck. *N Engl J Med.* 1990;**323**:795–801.

Kamm J, Ashenfelter K, Ehmann C. Preclinical and clinical toxicology of selected retinoids. In: Sporn M, Roberts A, Goodman D, eds. *The Retinoids.* Orlando, FL: Academic Press; 1984;**2**:287–326.

Kerr J, Wyllie A, Currie A. Apoptosis: A basic biological phenomenon with wide-ranging implications in tissue kinetics. *Br J Cancer.* 1972;**26**:239–257.

Kessler J, Jones S, Levine N, et al. Isotretinoin and cutaneous helper T-cell lymphoma (mycosis fungoides). *Arch Dermatol.* 1987;**123**:201–204.

Koeffler H, Amatruda T. The effect of retinoids on haemopoiesis—Clinical and laboratory studies. In: Nugent J, Clark S, eds. *Retinoids, Differentiation, and Disease.* London: Ciba Foundation; 1985;252–273.

Koeffler H, Heitjan D, Mertelsmann R, et al. Randomized study of 13-*cis*-Retinoic acid versus placebo in the myelodysplastic disorders. *Blood.* 1988;**71**:703–708.

Kraemer K, DiGiovanna J, Moshell A, et al. Prevention of skin cancer in xeroderma pigmentosum with the use of oral isotretinoin. *N Engl J Med.* 1988;**318**:1633–1637.

Kramer Z, Boros L, Wiernik P, et al. 13-*cis*-Retinoic acid in the treatment of elderly patients with acute myeloid leukemia. *Cancer.* 1991;**67**:1484–1486.

Lawrence H, Conner K, Kelly M, et al. *cis*-Retinoic acid stimulates the clonal growth of some myeloid leukemia cells in vitro. *Blood.* 1987;**69**:302–307.

Lippman S, Kavanagh J, Paredes-Espinoza M, et al. 13-*cis*-Retinoic acid plus interferon-alpha-2a: Highly active systemic therapy for squamous cell carcinoma of the cervix. *J Natl Cancer Inst.* 1992a;**84**:241–245.

Lippman S, Kessler J, Al-Sarraf M, et al. Treatment of advanced squamous cell carcinoma of the head and neck with isotretinoin: A phase II randomized trial. *Invest New Drugs.* 1988;**6**:51–56.

Lippman S, Kessler J, Meyskens J. Retinoids as preventive and therapeutic anticancer agents. *Cancer Treat Rep.* 1987;**71**:391–405, 493–515.

Lippman S, Meyskens F. Treatment of advanced squamous cell carcinoma of the skin with isotretinoin. *Ann Intern Med.* 1987;**107**:499–502.

Lippman S, Parkinson D, Itri L, et al. 13-*cis*-Retinoic acid and interferon alpha-2a: Effective combination therapy for advanced squamous cell carcinoma of the skin. *J Natl Cancer Inst.* 1992b;**84**:235–241.

List A, Garewal H, Sandberg A. The myelodysplastic syndromes: Biology and implications for management. *J Clin Oncol.* 1990;**8**:1424–1441.

Martin S, Bradley J, Cotter T. HL-60 cells induced to differentiate towards neutrophils subsequently die via apoptosis. *Clin Exp Immunol.* 1990;**79**:448–453.

Meyskens F, Alberts D, Salmon S. Effect of 13-*cis*-Retinoic acid and 4-hydroxyphenyl-all-*trans*-retinamide on human tumor colony formation in soft agar. *Int J Cancer.* 1983;**32**:295–299.

Meyskens F, Gilmartin E, Alberts D, et al. Activity of isotretinoin against squamous cell cancers and preneoplastic lesions. *Cancer Treat Rep.* 1982;**66**:1315–1319.

Meyskens F, Goodman G, Alberts D. 13-*cis*-Retinoic acid: Pharmacology, toxicology, and clinical applications for the prevention and treatment of human cancer. *Crit Rev Oncol Hematol.* 1987;**3**:75–101.

Molin L, Thomsen K, Volden G, et al. 13-*cis*-Retinoic acid in mycosis fungoides. In: Saurat, ed. *Retinoids: New Trends in Research and Therapy.* Basel: Karger; 1985:341–344.

Peck R, Bollag W. Potentiation of retinoid-induced differentiation of HL-60 and U937 cell lines by cytokines. *Eur J Cancer.* 1991;**27**:53–57.

Peck G, DiGiovanna J, Sarnoff D, et al. Treatment and prevention of basal cell carcinoma with oral isotretinoin. *J Am Acad Dermatol.* 1988;**19**:176–185.

Peck GL, Olsen TG, Yoder FW, et al. Prolonged remissions of cystic and conglobate acne with 13-*cis*-Retinoic acid. *N Engl J Med.* 1979;**300**:329–333.

Petkovich M, Brand N, Krust A, et al. A human retinoic acid receptor which belongs to the family of nuclear receptors. *Nature.* 1987;**330**:444–450.

Physicians' Desk Reference. 47th ed. Oradell, NJ: Medical Economics Company; 1993:1960–1962.

Picozzi V, Swanson G, Morgan R, et al. 13-*cis*-Retinoic acid treatment for myelodysplastic syndromes. *J Clin Oncol.* 1986;**4**:589–595.

Port CD, Sporn MB, Kaufman DG. Prevention of lung cancer in hamsters by 13-*cis*-retinoic acid. *Proc Am Assoc Cancer Res.* 1975;**16**:21.

Recondo G, Kilbourn RG, Logothetis C. Evidence for synergistic antitumor effect of 5-fluorouracil (5-FU) with alpha-interferon and 5-FU with 13-*cis*-Retinoic acid or 4-hydroxyphenylretinamide in human transitional cell carcinoma cell lines. *Proc Am Assoc Cancer Res.* 1991;**32**:341.

Reynolds C, Kane D, Einhorn P, et al. Response of neuroblastoma to retinoic acid in vitro and in vivo. In: Evans A, D'Angio G, Knudson A, et al, eds. *Advances in Neuroblastoma Research.* New York: Liss; 1991;**3**:203–211.

Reynolds C, Matthay K, Crouse V, et al. Response of neuroblastoma bone marrow metastases to 13-*cis*-Retinoic acid. *Proc Am Soc Clin Oncol.* 1990;**9**:54.

Robinson JK, Salasche SJ. Isotretinoin does not prevent basal cell carcinoma. *Arch Dermatol.* 1992;**128**:975–976.

Saccomanno G, Moran P, Schmidt R, et al. Effects of 13-*cis*-retinoids on premalignant and malignant cells of lung origin. *Acta Cytol.* 1982;**26**:78–85.

Sankowski A, Janik P, Jeziorska M, et al. The results of topical application of 13-*cis*-Retinoic acid on basal cell carcinoma. A correlation of the clinical effect with histopathological examination and serum retinol level. *Neoplasma.* 1987;**34**:485–489.

Sidell N. Retinoic acid-induced growth inhibition and morphologic differentiation of human neuroblastoma cells in vitro. *J Natl Cancer Inst.* 1982;**68**:589–593.

Smith MA, Parkinson DR, Cheson BD, et al. Retinoids in cancer therapy. *J Clin Oncol.* 1992;**10**:839–864.

Strickland S, Sawey M. Studies on the effect of retinoids on the differentiation of teratocarcinoma stem cells in vitro and in vivo. *Dev Biol.* 1980;**78**:76–85.

Tangrea JA, Kilcoyne RF, Taylor PR, et al. Skeletal hyperostosis in patients receiving chronic, very-low-dose isotretinoin. *Arch Dermatol.* 1992;**128**:921–925.

Wakefield L, Sporn M. Suppression of carcinogenesis: A role for TFG-β and related molecules in prevention of cancer. In: Klein G, ed. *Tumor Suppressor Genes.* New York: Dekker; 1990:217–243.

Williams M, Elias P. Nature of skin fragility in patients receiving retinoid for systemic effect. *Arch Dermatol.* 1981;**117**:611–619.

Windhorst D, Nigra T. General clinical toxicology of oral retinoids. *J Am Acad Dermatol.* 1982;**6**:675–682.

Leucovorin Calcium

■ Other Names

NSC-3590; calcium folinate; citrovorum Factor; N^5-formyltetrahydrofolate; 5-formyl-FH$_4$; folinic acid; folinic acid-SF; (6RS)-folinic acid; leucovorin calcium tablets, Wellcovorin® (Burroughs Wellcome); Leucovorin Calcium for Injection® (Lederle Laboratories).

■ Chemistry

Structure of leucovorin

Leucovorin calcium is chemically known as calcium N-[4-[[2-amino-5-formyl-1,4,5,6,7,8-hexahydro-4-oxo-6-pteridinyl)methyl]amino]benzoyl]-L-glutamic acid or calcium 5-formyl-5,6,7,8-tetrahydrofolate. It is the reduced (active) derivative of folic acid, having a molecular weight of 483. The term *citrovorum factor* actually refers to the natural product (1,5-formyl-tetrahydrofolate), which on a molar basis is approximately twice as active as synthetic leucovorin (folinic acid or d-l,5-formyl-tetrahydrofolate) or the commercially available calcium salt (Cosulich et al 1952). Physically, it exists as a yellow to white microcrystalline powder that is very soluble in water and practically insoluble in alcohol. Commercial leucovorin is a racemic mixture of SR-formyl-tetrahydrofolic acid, and only the S⁻ isomer is active (L-leucovorin).

■ Antitumor Activity

Leucovorin is not a cytotoxic agent but rather a nutritional supplement. The first experimental use of leucovorin in animals given antifolates dates to

Goldin et al (1954). Early clinical trials reported benefits from leucovorin "rescue" after high-dose methotrexate in acute lymphocytic leukemia in children (Djerassi et al 1966), in head and neck cancer (Merlano et al 1990, Lefkowitz et al 1967), and in other solid tumors such as osteogenic sarcoma (Jaffe 1974). High-dose methotrexate with leucovorin rescue has also begun to play a prominent role in treatment of patients with non-Hodgkin's lymphoma in such regimens as the M-BACOD regimen (high-dose methotrexate + bleomycin, doxorubicin, cyclophosphamide, vincristine, and dexamethasone) (Skarin and Canellos 1987). Recently, the racemic form has been shown to be compatible to one-half the dose of the *l*-form as an antidote to high-dose methotrexate in children (Etienne et al 1992).

More recently, leucovorin has been used to modulate the activity and toxicity of 5-fluorouracil (5-FU). There is now definitive evidence that this combination provides higher response rates (and sometimes longer survival) for patients with metastatic gastrointestinal malignancies than 5-FU treatment alone (Grem et al 1987, Erlichman 1990, Laufman et al 1987, Doroshow et al 1990, Poon et al 1989, Erlichman et al 1988; Petrelli et al 1986, 1987). The combination is also being extensively tested in other malignancies. Severe and fatal toxic effects have been seen with the combination (Vokes et al 1990, Doroshow et al 1989, Allegra et al 1987).

■ Mechanism of Action

Leucovorin calcium is a reduced form of folic acid. As such it competes effectively with methotrexate (MTX) for transport into mammalian cells and, presumably, human target tissues such as bone marrow and gastrointestinal epithelium. In the cancer patient, calcium leucovorin is used to circumvent the effects of methotrexate when given in high, otherwise lethal, doses. The (6S)-leucovorin isomer is biologically active whereas the (6R)-leucovorin isomer has 1/4000th the activity at blocking cell cytotoxicity from methotrexate. The 6R isomer is also not a substrate for folyl-polyglutamate synthetase and, hence, is not converted to a polyglutamated from (McGuire and Heitzman 1992). This may contribute to the relative lack of biologic activity of the 6R isomer.

Methotrexate, by binding to dihydrofolic acid reductase, inhibits the production of reduced folates (Bertino 1977). Subsequently, thymidylate synthesis is halted, and DNA, RNA, and protein synthesis may be interrupted. The affinity of dihydrofolate reductase for methotrexate is greater than its affinity for folic acid or dihydrofolic acid; therefore, large doses of folic acid must be given to reverse the effects of methotrexate. Leucovorin calcium is metabolized to tetrahydrofolate, thereby bypassing the enzymatic block induced by methotrexate (Nixon et al 1973) and allowing resumption of DNA synthesis. Leucovorin thus prevents, and in certain instances can "rescue," cells from the adverse effects of methotrexate. Leucovorin also reduces stomatitis following administration of the newer antifol edatrexate in patients with non-small cell lung cancer (Lee et al 1992).

Preclinical studies have shown the antitumor activity of 5-FU can be potentiated by using reduced folates at concentrations of 1 μM or greater. These reduced folates raise the level of N_5,N_{10}-methylenetetrahydrofolate which takes part in the formation of a stable ternary complex of thymidylate synthetase, the folate cofactor, and 5-FU in the form of 5-fluorodeoxyuridylate (see Mini et al [1990] for an excellent review of this area). For optimal modulation of fluoropyrimidines, a leucovorin plasma concentration of 1 to 10 μM (6S isomer) should be maintained for a minimum of 5 to 8 hours (Zhang et al 1992).

■ Availability and Storage

Leucovorin calcium, 50 mg/10-mL vial, is available as a pale yellow powder in vials containing in each vial 4 mg methylparaben, 1 mg propyl paraben, and 45 mg sodium chloride. The intact vials are stable for at least 2 years at room temperature. Leucovorin calcium is commercially supplied in a 3 mg/mL ampule in sterile water for injection, paraben preserved, with its pH adjusted to about 7.6 with sodium hydroxide. Tablets containing 5 or 25 mg of calcium leucovorin are available, as are 1 and 10-mL ampules containing 5 mg leucovorin per milliliter (Burroughs Wellcome, Research Triangle Park, North Carolina), or 1-mL ampules containing 3 mg/ml, or vials containing 100 mg of leucovorin, or 10- or 15-mg tablets (Lederle Laboratories, A Division of American Cyanamid, Wayne, New Jersey). It is also available as 5- and 25-mg vials. De Vito et al (1989) have noted no significant difference in the areas under the serum concentration × time curve for two different 25-mg oral formulations of leucovorin calcium.

An investigational L-leucovorin formulation is

available from Lederle Laboratories. It is supplied in 5-mg tablets.

■ Preparation for Use, Stability, and Admixture

Typically, the 50-mg lyophilized powder is reconstituted with at least 2.5 to 5 mL of sterile water for injection. The resultant (10 mg/mL) solution (pH 7.0 to 8.0) is stable for at least 7 days at room temperature.

Admixture stability studies performed by the manufacturer at room temperature, protected from light, have noted 24-hour stability in the following intravenous solutions: 10% dextrose, 10% dextrose in normal saline, Ringer's, and lactated Ringer's injection. The study demonstrated constant pH maintenance at 5.0 to 5.4 for Ringer's and 10% dextrose, 4.5 for 10% dextrose in normal saline, and 6.8 for lactated Ringer's.

Inasmuch as bioavailability is good, oral solutions of leucovorin may be used, and milk, liquid antacids, or other buffered alkaline vehicles are recommended. Solutions in water may also be used.

Highly acidic solutions should be avoided as the compound degrades at a pH less than 3.0 (Lauper et al 1978).

■ Administration

Leucovorin calcium may be administered orally; intravenously, by either push or continuous infusion; or intramuscularly. Bioavailability studies in methotrexate-toxic patients have not been done; thus there is a question as to the relative absorption in that critical patient population.

■ Special Precautions

There is increasing evidence that 5-methyltetrahydrofolate can accumulate in the cerebrospinal fluid (Thyss et al 1989). Progressive accumulation of that metabolite could decrease the antitumor activity of methotrexate against meningeal leukemia cells. Also see Dosage.

■ Drug Interactions

See Dosage.

■ Dosage

Leucovorin rescue is the term applied to methotrexate therapy followed by or concomitant with leucovorin calcium. Various dosing schedules have been employed depending on the dose and route of methotrexate, as well as the tumor type. There are some general dosing considerations: (1) Leucovorin should be used at doses sufficient to block methotrexate cellular influx and promote efflux (ie, larger leucovorin doses than required for larger methotrexate doses). (2) Leucovorin protection should be provided for the time period in which serum methotrexate concentrations are greater than 10^{-8} M (Chabner and Young 1973) monitored by creatinine clearance) and serum methotrexate determinations should be made. (3) A substantial delay in leucovorin administration after methotrexate should be avoided inasmuch as rescue is very difficult after a prolonged delay of $\simeq$ 40 hours. Generally, leucovorin doses of 15 mg/m^2 every 6 hours for 1 to 2 days have been sufficient to prevent toxicity from methotrexate levels of about 10^{-7} M at 24 hours (Nirenberg et al 1977) but not those above 10^{-5} M at 24 hours (Stoller et al 1975). The relative merits of different leucovorin delay periods after methotrexate are not well established; however, the longer the delay, the more critical the leucovorin dosing schedule must be. Delay periods have ranged in ongoing studies from 6 to 36 hours, usually with every-6-hour dosing continuing for 26 to 94 hours (see the table on the top of the opposite page). Occasionally, doses as high as 100 mg/m^2 are given every 3 hours for 12 to 24 doses. In addition, the use of leucovorin "rescue" in high-dose methotrexate therapy should always be accompanied by intensive hydration and urinary alkalinization, to reduce the nephrotoxic potential of methotrexate (Stoller et al 1975) (see *Methotrexate*). The table lists several of the reported methotrexate–leucovorin rescue schemes. In general, the dose of the purified *l*-isomer of leucovorin is one-half that of the commercially available racemic mixture (Etienne et al 1992).

Recent studies of 5-FU with leucovorin have used the following doses and schedules:

1. 5-FU 370 mg/m^2/d × 5 days plus leucovorin calcium as a daily continuous infusion of 500 mg/m^2/d beginning 24 hours before the first dose of 5-FU and continuing for 12 hours after completion of therapy (Doroshow et al 1990).
2. 5-FU at 500 to 1000 mg/m^2 every 2 weeks preceded by calcium leucovorin at mg/m^2 given as a 10-minute infusion (Bruckner et al 1990).
3. 5-FU 600 mg/m^2 + 500 mg/m^2 leucovorin weekly × 6 weeks versus 5-FU 600 mg/m^2

METHOTREXATE–LEUCOVORIN SCHEDULES

Tumor Type	Dose of Methotrexate	Infusion Time (h)	Methotrexate Treatment Interval	Leucovorin Rescue Delay (h)	Leucovorin Rescue Scheme
Osteogenic sarcoma	15–600 mg/kg	6	Every 2 wk to 200 mg/kg, then every 3 wk at >200 mg/kg	2	6–15 mg every 6 h × 12 (higher dose to match higher MTX doses)
Other solid tumors Epidermoid tumors	240 mg/m² increased by same to toxicity	36	Varies	Immediately	40 mg/m² over 6 h, then 25 mg every 6 h for four doses
Lung tumors	100 mg to 12 g	2–18	10 d to 3 wk	1–6	
Various refractory tumors (multiple myeloma, lung, ovarian, breast, etc.)	1–3 g/m²	IV push	Varies (often weekly)	24	10 mg/m² every 6 h × 12 and if MTX level at 24 h is 10^{-6} M, 100 mg/m² every 3 h × 24 (or until MTX levels fall below 10^{-8} M)

Data from Bender JF, Grove WR, Fortner CL. High-dose methotrexate with folinic acid rescue. Am J Hosp Pharm. 1977;34:961–965.

+ 25 mg/m² of leucovorin weekly × 6 weeks (high-dose arm was more active) (Petrelli et al 1989).
4. 5-FU 500 mg/m² daily × 5 plus leucovorin 200 mg/m²/d × 5.
5. 5-FU 600 to 800 mg/m²/day × 5 plus leucovorin 25 mg/m²/d, both administered as a continuous infusion for 5 days (Lokich et al 1992).
6. 5-FU 1.5 to 1.8 g/m² plus 2.5 g/m² leucovorin as a continuous infusion over 24 hours (Creaven et al 1992). Leucovorin has also been used to reduce the toxicity of the new antifol edatrexate. The leucovorin dose was 15 mg orally every 6 hours for four doses beginning 24 hours after edatrexate (Lee et al 1992).
7. 5-FU 500 mg/m² daily × 5 + low-dose leucovorin (20 mg/m²/d × 5). In this study the 5-FU low-dose leucovorin arm was as active as the high-dose leucovorin arm and was associated with an improvement in quality of life and lower drug costs (Poon et al 1989).

■ Pharmacokinetics

Studies have demonstrated leucovorin calcium to be about 90% absorbed after oral administration of tablets or injectable solution (Nixon and Bertino 1972). Oral leucovorin appears to be extensively converted by the gastrointestinal tract to the active form 5-methyltetrahydrofolate (MeTHF) (Whitehead et al 1970). This is the form that effectively reverses methotrexate toxicity in humans. Pharmacokinetic studies of radioactive MeTHF given in the absence of methotrexate have shown biphasic and rapid plasma disappearance; 10 to 20% radioactivity loss is noted 6 to 8 hours after dosing and 1% per day thereafter. This indicates that tissue uptake is substantial (Kirschner et al 1968). When given 24 to 48 hours after methotrexate infusion, the plasma disappearance was slower and urinary excretion greater, and more of the drug was eliminated as unchanged

CLINICAL PHARMACOKINETICS OF LEUCOVORIN DIASTEREOISOMERS

Formyl-tetrahydrofolate Diastereoisomer	α Half-life (h)	Peak Plasma Concentration* (μg/mL)	AUC* (μg/mL · h)	Protein Binding (%)
R	6.74	38.5	185.4	88
S	0.77	16.3	10.4	59

*200 mg/m² IV racemic leucovorin calcium (Schleyer et al 1992).

MeTHF. Studies with leucovorin have shown that both intact drug and MeTHF are renally excreted, with some hint that the kidney may preferentially retain the activated form (MeTHF) over leucovorin.

Mehta et al (1978) have compared serum levels and distribution of oral tablets and solution versus intramuscular leucovorin calcium. Serum half-lives of about 34 to 45 minutes for leucovorin and 2 hours for MeTHF were observed for both intramuscular and oral leucovorin calcium doses. Levels of active folates after oral dosing were generally comparable to those after intramuscular dosing. The tablets and an oral solution made from the injection showed no significant differences in bioavailability.

After intravenous administration of leucovorin, both intact drug and MeTHF rapidly enter the cerebrospinal fluid; in contrast, intravenous methotrexate does not achieve significant cerebrospinal fluid levels after systemic dosing. Therefore *low doses* of intravenous leucovorin must be used after intrathecal methotrexate to retain the antileukemic effects of the methotrexate (3 to 6 mg leucovorin given at least 12 to 24 hours after intrathecal methotrexate) (Bertino 1977).

With the availability of new high-performance liquid chromatography methodologies, the pharmacokinetics of the diastereoisomers of (6RS)-folinic acid has been studied in elegant detail by Newman et al (1989). Following a 6-day continuous infusion, patients had a median steady-state plasma concentration of 3.25 μM of the bioactive diastereoisomer, (6S)-folinic acid. The bioactive metabolite, (6S)-5-methyltetrahydrofolic acid, had a steady-state concentration of 5.7 μM. The steady-state plasma concentration of (6R)-folinic acid was 38.2 μM. Following a dose of 500 mg/m^2 as a 2-hour infusion, the concentration × time product (AUC) of the biologically active 6S isomer was 45 $\mu M \cdot h$ (Creaven et al 1992). A higher dose of 2.5 g/m^2 as a 24-hour continuous infusion produced mean steady-state 6S-isomer plasma concentrations of 9.75 to 10.74 μM. This is in the concentration range necessary for optimal modulation of 5-FU. (See the table on the bottom of page 627.)

Median terminal half-lives were 45, 446, and 338 minutes for (6S)-folinic acid, (6S)-5-methyltetrahydrofolic acid, and (6R)-folinic acid, respectively. The renal clearance for the two diastereoisomers was quite different. The (6R)-folinic acid has low plasma clearance, which is felt to result from extensive plasma protein binding of the compound. Both the commercial racemic mixture and the purified *l*-isomer (at one-half the racemic dose) produced comparable levels of 5-methylenetetrahydrofolate in pediatric patients receiving high-dose methotrexate (Etienne et al 1992). This indicates that comparable degrees of MTX rescue are provided by the *l*-isomer. There was also no difference in the MTX elimination half-life (13.9 hours) with either form of leucovorin (Etienne et al 1992).

In another study Schilsky and Ratain (1990) determined that intravenous administration of leucovorin results in equivalent AUCs for leucovorin and its bioactive metabolite, (6S)-5-methyltetrahydrofolic acid. There were also high AUCs for (6R)-folinic acid. Oral administration of leucovorin over 24 hours results in an AUC for the bioactive metabolite equivalent to that obtained after intravenous dosing. With oral dosing, however, much smaller amounts of the less active (6R)-folinic acid species are produced. Even so it is still not certain whether intravenous or oral administration is preferable (Schilsky and Ratain 1990). Thus, Bertrand and Jolivet (1989) have suggested that it is unlikely the (6R)-folinic acid will interfere with cellular uptake of the 6S isomer sufficiently to have an impact on the clinical situation.

Fiore and colleagues (1987) have studied the absorption of leucovorin when it is given as a mouthwash. They noted small increases in 5-methyltetrahydrofolate but no increase in plasma citrovorum factor. They concluded the agent could reduce mucositis without systemic absorption significant enough to reduce methotrexate efficacy.

■ Side Effects and Toxicity

Allergic sensitization has been reported after both oral and parenteral administration of folic acid, and, it is assumed that it may also occur with leucovorin calcium. In general, however, this drug is remarkably free of side effects.

■ Special Applications

Leucovorin has also been used to treat children with dihydropteridine deficiency (Woody et al 1989). It has actually controlled seizures in a child with that deficiency.

Leucovorin has been given intraperitoneally along with 5-FU in an attempt to increase the efficacy of 5-FU. Doses were 1200 mg/m^2 5-FU and 50 mg/m^2 leucovorin (Budd et al 1986).

Leucovorin has been added to a continuous intraarterial infusion into the liver along with 5 floxuridine. The amount of leucovorin given was constrained to 120 mg/m²/d because of pump problems. Sclerosing cholangitis was noted in some patients (Kemeny et al 1990).

Leucovorin has also been used to treat methotrexate-induced leukoencephalopathy with limited success (Cohen et al 1990).

REFERENCES

Allegra CJ, Chabner BA, Sholar PW, Bagley C, Drake JC, Lippman ME. Preliminary results of a phase II trial for the treatment of metastatic breast cancer with 5-fluorouracil and leucovorin. *NCI Monogr.* 1987;**5**:199–202.

Bertino JR. "Rescue" techniques in cancer chemotherapy. Use of leucovorin and other rescue agents after methotrexate treatment. *Semin Oncol.* 1977;**4**(2):203–216.

Bertrand R, Jolivet J. Lack of interference by the unnatural isomer of 5-formyltetrahydrofolate with the effects of the natural isomer in leucovorin preparations. *J Natl Cancer Inst.* 1989;**81**(15):1175–1178.

Bruckner HW, Glass LL, Chesser MR. Dose-dependent leucovorin efficacy with an intermittent high-dose 5-fluorouracil schedule. *Cancer Invest.* 1990; 3/4:321–326.

Budd GT, Schreiber MJ, Steiger E, Bukowski RM, Weick JK. Phase I trial of intraperitoneal chemotherapy with 5-fluorouracil and citrovorum factor. *Invest New Drugs.* 1986;**4**(2):155–158.

Chabner B, Young R. Threshold methotrexate concentration for in vivo inhibition of DNA synthesis in normal and tumorous target tissues. *J Clin Invest.* 1973;**52**:1804–1811.

Cohen IJ, Stark B, Kaplinsky C, et al. Methotrexate-induced leukoencephalopathy is treatable with high-dose folinic acid: A case report and analysis of the literature. *Pediatr Hematol Oncol.* 1990;**7**:79–87.

Cosulich DB, Roth B, Smith JM Jr, Hultquist ME, Parker RP. Chemistry of leucovorin. *J Am Chem Soc.* 1952;**74**: 3252–3263.

Creaven PJ, Rustum YM, Petrelli NJ, et al. A pharmacokinetically directed phase I/II study of 5-fluorouracil/high dose leucovorin in colorectal carcinoma resistant to standard doses. *Proc Am Assoc Cancer Res.* 1992;**33**:218.

De Vito JM, McGuire BW, De Lap RJ, Weiss AI. Bioequivalence of two leucovorin calcium tablet formulations. *Drug Intell Clin Pharm.* 1989;**23**(2):153–154.

Djerassi L, Abir E, Roger GL Jr. Long term remission in childhood acute leukemia: Use of infrequent infusions of methotrexate: Supportive role of platelet transfusions and citrovorum factor. *Clin Pediatr.* 1966;**5**:502–509.

Doroshow JH, Leong L, Margolin K, et al. Refractory metastatic breast cancer: Salvage therapy with fluorouracil and high-dose continuous infusion leucovorin calcium. *J Clin Oncol.* 1989;**7**(4):439–444.

Doroshow JH, Multhauf P, Leong L, et al. Prospective randomized comparison of fluorouracil versus fluorouracil and high-dose continuous infusion leucovorin calcium for the treatment of advanced measurable colorectal cancer in patients previously unexposed to chemotherapy. *J Clin Oncol.* 1990;**8**(3):491–501.

Erlichman C. Fluorouracil and leucovorin for metastatic colorectal cancer. *J Chemother.* 1990;1(suppl):38–40.

Erlichman C, Fine S, Wong A, Elhakim T. A randomized trial of fluorouracil and folinic acid in patients with metastatic colorectal carcinoma. *J Clin Oncol.* 1988;**6**(3):469–475.

Etienne M-C, Thyss A, Bertrand Y, et al. L-Folinic acid versus D,L-folinic acid in rescue of high-dose methotrexate therapy in children. *J Natl Cancer Inst.* 1992;**84**(15):1190–1195.

Fiore JJ, Kemeny NE, Mehta BM, Geller N, Grossano D, Murphy D. Systemic absorption of a leucovorin mouth wash: A pharmacologic study. *Cancer Invest.* 1987;**5**(2): 109–111.

Goldin A, Mantel N, Greenhouse SW, Venditti JM, Humphreys SR. Effect of delayed administration of citrovorum factor on the antileukemic effectiveness of aminopterin in mice. *Cancer Res.* 1954;**14**:43–48.

Grem JL, Hoth DF, Hamilton JM, King SA, Leyland-Jones B. Overview of current status and future direction of clinical trials with 5-fluorouracil in combination with folinic acid. *Cancer Treat Rep.* 1987;**71**:1249–1264.

Jaffe N. Progress report on high dose methotrexate (NSC-740) with citrovorum rescue in the treatment of metastatic bone tumors. *Cancer Chemother Rep.* 1974;**58**:275–280.

Kemeny N, Cohen A, Bertino JR, Sigurdson ER, Botet J, Oderman P. Continuous intrahepatic infusion of floxuridine and leucovorin through an implantable pump for the treatment of hepatic metastases from colorectal carcinoma. *Cancer.* 1990;**65**(11):2446–2450.

Kirschner EA, Nixon PF, Bertino JR. Metabolism of methyltetrahydrofolate in man. *Clin Res.* 1968;**16**:537.

Laufman LR, Krzeczowski KA, Roach R, Segal M. Leucovorin plus 5-fluorouracil: An effective treatment for metastatic colon cancer. *J Clin Oncol.* 1987;**5**(9):1394–1400.

Lauper RD. Leucovorin calcium administration and preparation (letter). *Am J Hosp Pharm.* 1978;**35**:377–378.

Lee JS, Fossella FV, Libshitz HI, et al. Improved therapeutic index by leucovorin of edatrexate, cyclophosphamide, and cisplatin regimen for non-small cell lung cancer. *Proc Am Assoc Cancer Res.* 1992;**33**:266.

Lefkowitz E, Papac RJ, Bertino JR. Head and neck cancer. III. Toxicity of 24 hour infusions of methotrexate and protection by leucovorin in patients with epidermoid carcinomas. *Cancer Chemother Rep.* 1967;**51**:305–311.

Lokich J, Zipoli T, Bern M, et al. Platinum (P)–leucovorin (L)–5-fluorouracil (F) (PLF) infusion: Analysis of the optimal leucovorin dose with all 3 agents infused simultaneously over 4 days. *Proc Am Soc Clin Oncol.* 1992;**11**:132.

McGuire JJ, Heitzman KJ. Biological properties of (6S)-, (6R)-, and (6R, S)-leucovorin. *Proc Am Assoc Cancer Res.* 1992;**33**:406.

Mehta BM, Gisolfi AL, Hutchison DJ, Nirenberg A, Kellick MG, Rosen G. Serum distribution of citrovorum factor and 5-methyltetrahydrofolate following oral and in administration of calcium leucovorin in normals. *Cancer Treat Rep.* 1978;**62**(3):345–350.

Merlano M, Bacigalupo A, Benasso M, et al. 5-Fluorouracil and high-dose folinic acid as second-line chemotherapy in head and neck cancer. *Am J Clin Oncol.* 1990;**13**(1):1–3.

Mini E, Trave F, Rustum YM, Bertino JR. Enhancement of the antitumor effects of 5-fluorouracil by folinic acid. *Pharmacol Ther.* 1990;**47**(1):1–19.

Newman EM, Straw JA, Doroshow JH. Pharmacokinetics of diastereoisomers of (6R, S)-folinic acid (leucovorin) in humans during constant high-dose intravenous infusion. *Cancer Res.* 1989;**49**(20):5755–5760.

Nirenberg A, Mosende C, Mehta B, et al. High dose methotrexate with citrovorum factor rescue: Predictive value of serum methotrexate concentrations and corrective measures to avert toxicity. *Cancer Treat Rep.* 1977;**61**:779–783.

Nixon PF, Bertino TR. Effective absorption and utilization of oral formyltetrahydrofolate in man. *N Engl J Med.* 1972;**286**(4):175–179.

Nixon PF, Slutsky G, Nahas A et al. The turnover of folate coenzymes in murine lymphoma cells. *J Biol Chem.* 1973;**248**:5932–5936.

Petrelli N, Douglass HO Jr, Herrera L, et al. The modulation of fluorouracil with leucovorin in metastatic colorectal carcinoma: A prospective randomized phase III trial. *J Clin Oncol.* 1989;**7**(10):1419–1426.

Petrelli NJ, Madajewicz S, Herrera L, et al. Biologic modulation of 5-fluorouracil with high-dose leucovorin and combination chemotherapy of 5-fluorouracil and cisplatin in metastatic colorectal adenocarcinoma. *NCI Monogr.* 1987;**5**:189–192.

Poon MA, O'Connell MJ, Moertel CG, et al. Biochemical modulation of fluorouracil: Evidence of significant improvement of survival and quality of life in patients with advanced colorectal carcinoma. *J Clin Oncol.* 1989;**7**:1407–1418.

Schilsky RL, Ratain MJ. Clinical pharmacokinetics of high-dose leucovorin calcium after intravenous and oral administration. *J Natl Cancer Inst.* 1990;**82**(17):1411–1415.

Schleyer E, Reinhardt J, Grimm M, et al. Pharmacokinetics and protein binding of leucovorin diastereoisomers. *Proc Am Assoc Cancer Res.* 1992;**33**:532.

Skarin AT, Canellos GP. Methotrexate–leucovorin factor rescue regimens in diffuse large cell lymphoma. *NCI Monogr.* 1987;**5**:71–76.

Stoller RG, Jacobs SA, Drake JC, Lutz RJ, Chabner BA. Pharmacokinetics of high-dose methotrexate (NSC-740). *Cancer Chemother Rep.* 1975;**6**:19–24.

Thyss A, Milano G, Etienne MC, et al. Evidence for CSF accumulation of 5-methyltetrahydrofolate during repeated courses of methotrexate plus folinic acid rescue (comment). *Br J Cancer.* 1989;**60**(5):799.

Vokes EE, Schilsky RL, Weichselbaum RR, Kozloff MF, Panje WR. Induction chemotherapy with cisplatin, fluorouracil, and high-dose leucovorin for locally advanced head and neck cancer: A clinical and pharmacologic analysis. *J Clin Oncol.* 1990;**8**(2):241–247.

Whitehead VM, Pratt R, Viallet A, Cooper BA. Intestinal conversion of folinic acid to 5-methyltetrahydrofolate in man. *Blood.* 1970;**36**:857.

Woody RC, Brewster MA, Glasier C. Progressive intracranial calcification in dihydropteridine reductase deficiency prior to folinic acid therapy. *Neurology.* 1989;**39**(5):673–675.

Zhang ZG, Rustum YM, Shane B. Role of dose and schedule of leucovorin (LV) treatment in the modulation of 5,10-methylenetetrahydrofolate (CH_2FH_4) level, polyglutamate chain length distribution, and fluorodeoxyuridine (FdUrd) cytotoxicity. *Proc Am Soc Clin Oncol.* 1992;**11**:110.

Leuprolide Acetate

■ Other Names

Lupron® (TAP Pharmaceuticals Inc); leuprorelin acetate; D-Leu^6–des-Gly^{10}–Pro^9-N-ethyl-LHRH; Abbott-43818; TAP-144.

■ Chemistry

Leuprolide is a D-amino acid-substituted peptide analog of human gonadotropin-releasing hormone (GnRH) also called luteinizing hormone-releasing hormone (LH-RH) (Schally et al 1983). The chemical name is 5-oxo-L-prolyl-L-histidyl-L-tryptophanyl-L-seryl-L-tyrosyl-D-leucyl-L-leucyl-L-arginyl-N-ethyl-L-prolinamide. This molecule differs from natural GnRH by the substitution of D-leucine for L-glycine in the 6-position and an ethylamine moiety for glycine in the 10-position. The molecular formula of the acetate salt is $C_{59}H_{84}N_{16}O_{12} \cdot CH_3COOH$ and the molecular weight 1209.4. It is soluble in water and other aqueous solutions including lower alcohols.

■ Antitumor Activity

The current official (U.S. Food and Drug Administration) indication for leuprolide is the palliative treatment of prostate cancer. Leuprolide produces a "medical castration" in prostate cancer patients (Smith and May 1983, Tolis et al 1982). It is active in previously untreated patients (Santen et al 1984, Trachtenberg 1983) and in patients who relapse after or are unable to tolerate estrogenic therapy and/or orchiectomy (Smith et al 1985). Compared

Structure of leuprolide acetate

with the standard therapy of diethylstilbestrol, leuprolide produces comparable partial response rates of about 80% with fewer serious side effects (Leuprolide Study Group 1984).

Leuprolide is also active in patients with metastatic breast cancer (Harvey et al 1985) and refractory ovarian cancer (Kavanaugh et al 1989). A 44% partial response rate was described in premenopausal patients with breast cancer and a 17% partial response was reported in ovarian cancer, primarily in patients with stage I disease (Kavanaugh et al 1989). In the breast cancer study the median disease remission was 39 weeks in responders and an additional 20% of patients remained stable on leuprolide (Harvey et al 1985).

■ Mechanism of Action

Leuprolide acts initially as a superpotent GnRH agonist which binds to cell surface receptors in the pituitary (Sharpe and Fraser 1980); however, the prolonged agonist activity ultimately leads to complete blockade of GnRH. The initial stimulatory effect causes the release of follicle-stimulating hormone (FSH) and luteinizing hormone (LH) from the pituitary. In males, LH stimulates the testis to produce and release testosterone systemically. Testosterone is converted in tissues into dihydrotestosterone, which stimulates or maintains the growth of androgen-dependent tissues including most prostate tumors (Santen and Warner 1985); however, because the normal release of FSH and LH is cyclical and is regulated by feedback inhibition, the continual agonist activity of leuprolide at the pituitary chronically suppresses LH and FSH release (Belchtez et al 1978). This is mediated by downregulation of pituitary GnRH receptors. Ultimately, leuprolide deprives the testis of LH stimulation. This ultimately blocks the rate-limiting step in the conversion of cholesterol to testosterone in the Leydig cell of the testes. Thus, the lack of LH in prostate cancer patients treated with leuprolide results in a loss of testosterone production.

Plasma levels of testosterone and the active metabolite dihydrotestosterone initially rise but then precipitously fall to castrate levels of 20 ng/dL or less after about 1 to 2 weeks of continual leuprolide therapy (Leuprolide Study Group 1984). Similar effects mediate a decrease in estrogenic hormones in female patients treated with leuprolide. Levels remain low as long as leuprolide is administered, but a residual low androgen or estrogen level is provided through steroidal metabolism by aromatase enzyme activity in peripheral tissues. There may also be some direct inhibition of testicular cells by GnRH agonists, as a related analog, buserelin, decreases testosterone levels without lowering LH levels (Hsueh 1982). The contribution of such direct testicular inhibitory activity, if any, to the efficacy of leuprolide is unknown.

■ Availability and Storage

Leuprolide is commercially available in a multidose vial containing 2.8 mL of a 5 mg/mL sterile solution (Lupron®, TAP Pharmaceuticals Inc, Deerfield, Illinois). Sodium chloride and 9 mg/mL benzyl alcohol are added for isotonicity and bacteriostatic activity, respectively. The vials are stored at 4°C and should be protected from light. Once dispensed, leuprolide is stable at room temperature until the expiration date on the vial. The vials should not be frozen or vigorously shaken for prolonged periods. (TAP Pharmaceuticals 1985).

A depot formulation has been developed with leuprolide microcapsules in a biodegradable copolymer of DL-lactic acid/glycolic acid (Toguchi 1990). Lupron® depot (TAP Pharmaceuticals Inc) is available in a single-dose vial containing lyophilized microspheres of 7.5 mg leuprolide acetate, 1.3 mg purified gelatin, 66.2 mg of DL-lactic acid/glycolic acid copolymer, and 13.2 mg D-mannitol. An accompanying diluent ampule contains 7.5 mg carboxymethylcellulose sodium, 75 g D-mannitol, and 1.5 mg polysorbate 80 dissolved in Sterile Water for Injection, USP. The unmixed drug and diluent may be stored at room temperature.

■ Preparation for Use, Stability, and Admixture

Individual doses of the 5 mg/mL solution for subcutaneous administration are given undiluted. Specific data on stability and admixture under different conditions are not available. For the depot formulation 1 mL of the provided diluent is added to the 7.5-mg leuprolide vial to form a milky suspension. The suspension should be shaken well to thoroughly disperse the particles into a uniform, milky appearing suspension. This suspension is chemically stable for at least 24 hours but contains no antibacterial preservative.

■ Administration

Leuprolide is not effective orally. The commercial 5 mg/mL solution (Lupron®) is administered subcutaneously into areas on the arm, thigh, or abdomen. The site should be swabbed with alcohol before and after injection. Injection sites should be varied daily and all solutions should be clear and free of any particulate matter.

Reconstituted Lupron® depot suspension is intended for intramuscular injection only. A 21- or 22-gauge needle is used, and the intramuscular injection site should be rotated with each monthly dose.

The drug has investigationally been administered transdermally by iontophoresis (Meyer et al 1988). In this instance, a current of 0.22 µA was used to deliver 5-mg doses through the positive iontophoretic electrode patch on the skin (Drug Delivery Systems, Inc, New York). A related GnRH agonist, buserelin, has been administered intranasally as a spray of 200 to 500 µg/d (Faure et al 1982). If these pilot studies can be confirmed, other routes of leuprolide administration may be feasible.

■ Dosage

The dose of leuprolide in prostate cancer is fixed at 1 mg (0.2 mL) daily by subcutaneous injection. Increasing the daily dose to 5 or 10 mg in breast cancer produced objective responses in only 10% of patients (Harvey et al 1985). The standard 1-mg daily dose was used in ovarian cancer (Kavanaugh et al 1989).

The monthly adult dose of the leuprolide depot formulation is 7.5 mg by intramuscular injection (Sharifi et al 1990). It is concluded that the constant blockade of LH-RH receptors by the depot formulation lowers the monthly dose from 30 mg (1 mg/d SC) to 7.5 mg (Toguchi 1990).

■ Pharmacokinetics

The bioavailability of a 1-mg subcutaneous dose of leuprolide is 0.94 compared with an intravenous injection. The mean half-life of intact drug in the plasma is 2.9 hours. The metabolism, distribution, and excretion of leuprolide in humans are not known.

The depot intramuscular formulation of leuprolide microspheres reduces serum testosterone to castrate levels within 4 days. Testosterone remains at castrate levels for at least 30 days (Sharifi et al 1990). Mean serum luteinizing hormone levels initially rise but then fall to about 4 mIU/mL for 24 to 30 days after dosing. This allows for monthly intramuscular dosing of the depot formulation.

Pharmacokinetic studies in rats show a slow release of leuprolide acetate from an intramuscular injection site (Toguchi 1990). In this trial, about 20 to 25% of the dose is lost each week from the intramuscular injection site.

Leuprolide pharmacokinetic studies following the intramuscular depot injection show that mean levels of 1.0 ng/mL are obtained initially. The levels then decline to steady-state levels of about 0.5 ng/mL by week 8 or just after the second monthly intramuscular dose is administered.

■ Side Effects and Toxicity

The most common adverse reaction to leuprolide in males is hot flashes, occurring in about 50% of patients (Leuprolide Study Group 1984). This symptom ranges from mild discomfort and flushing to recurrent sweats. Also, on initiation of therapy, there may be temporary intensification of disease symptoms, especially bone pain, in about 10% of patients. Other symptoms include dysuria, weakness, and paresthesias of the lower extremities. These acute reactions probably relate to the transient initial increase in testosterone levels when leuprolide is started. Peripheral edema is reported in 8% of patients, but thrombophlebitis or pulmonary emboli are rare, reported in less than 1% of patients. Some central nervous system effects are reported in less than 10% of patients. These include dizziness, headache, and, rarely, paresthesias.

Gynecomastia is described in only 3% of patients and impotence in only 2%. Nausea, vomiting, constipation, and anorexia are rarely noted (< 5% of patients) and typically do not require dose reduction or aggressive antiemetic therapy.

Female patients experience similar side effects. Most commonly they include hot flashes and bilateral pedal edema. Amenorrhea is induced in all premenopausal patients who receive the drug for 10 weeks or longer (Harvey et al 1985). Local site reactions are very rare in both male and female patients. Overall, the incidence and severity of side effects with leuprolide are significantly lower than with diethylstilbestrol. This includes important reductions in potentially life-threatening thromboembolic disorders, edema, and nausea and vomiting. Hot flashes are the only side effect more common with leuprolide than with diethylstilbestrol (Leuprolide Study Group 1984).

Toxic effects of the depot formulation are qualitatively similar to those of the solution. Hot flashes occur in 57% of patients, with sweating described in 11% (Sharifi et al 1990). There are no reported local toxic effects at the intramuscular injection site.

REFERENCES

Belchtez PE, Plant TM, Nakai Y, et al. Hypophysical responses to continuous and intermittent delivery of hypothalamic gonadotropin-releasing hormone. *Science.* 1978;**202**:631–633.

Faure N, Labrie F, Lemay A, et al. Inhibition of serum androgen levels by chronic intranasal and subcutaneous administration of a potent luteinizing hormone-releasing hormone (LH-RH) agonist in adult men. *Fertil Steril.* 1982;**37**:416–424.

Harvey HA, Lipton A, Max DT, et al. Medical castration produced by the GnRH analogue leuprolide to treat metastatic breast cancer. *J Clin Oncol.* 1985;**3**:1068–1072.

Hsueh AJW. Direct effects of gonadoptropin-releasing hormone on testicular Leydig cell functions. *Ann NY Acad Sci.* 1982;**383**:249–271.

Kavanaugh JJ, Roberts W, Townsend P, Hewitt S. Leuprolide acetate in the treatment of refractory or persistent epithelial ovarian cancer. *J Clin Oncol.* 1989;**17**:115–118.

Leuprolide Study Group. Leuprolide versus diethylstilbestrol for metastatic prostate cancer. *N Engl J Med.* 1984;**311**:1281–1286.

Meyer BR, Kreis W, Eschbach J, et al. Successful transdermal administration of therapeutic doses of a polypeptide to normal human volunteers. *Clin Pharmacol Ther.* 1988;**44**:607–612.

Santen RJ, Demeris LM, Max DT, et al. Long-term effects of administration of a gonadotropin-releasing hormone superagonist analog in men with prostatic carcinoma. *J Clin Endocrinol Metab.* 1984;**58**:397–400.

Santen RJ, Warner B. Evaluation of synthetic agonist analogue of gonadotropin-releasing hormone (leuprolide) on testicular androgen production in patients with carcinoma of prostate. *Urology.* 1985;**25**:53–57.

Schally AV, Redding TW, Comaru-Schally AM. Inhibition of prostate tumors by agonistic and antagonistic analogues of LH-RH. *Prostate.* 1983;**4**:545–552.

Sharifi R, Soloway M, Leuprolide Study Group. Clinical study of leuprolide depot formulation in the treatment of advanced prostate cancer. *J Urol.* 1990;**143**:68–71.

Sharpe RM, Fraser HM. Leydig receptors for luteinizing hormone-releasing hormone and its agonists and their modulation by administration or depression of the releasing hormone. *Biochem Biophys Res Commun.* 1980;**95**:256–262.

Smith JA, Glode LM, Wettlauffer JN, et al. Clinical effects of gonadotropin-releasing hormone analogue in metastatic carcinoma of prostate. *Urology.* 1985;**25**:106–114.

Smith JA Jr, May DT. Clinical effects of a new GnRH analogue in metastatic carcinoma of the prostate. Prostatic cancer. In: *Proceedings, 13th International Congress of Chemotherapy.* 1983;**242**:45–58.

TAP Pharmaceuticals. *Package Insert: Lupron™ (Leuprolide Acetate Injection).* Abbott Labs Brochure No. 3626-01-2372-R1, Rev. April 1985.

Toguchi H. Pharmaceutical manipulation of leuprorelin acetate to improve clinical performance. *J Int Med Res.* 1990;**18**:35–41.

Tolis G, Ackman D, Stellos A, et al. Tumor growth inhibition in patients with prostatic carcinoma treated with luteinizing hormone-releasing hormone agonists. *Proc Natl Acad Sci USA.* 1982;**79**:1658–1662.

Trachtenberg J. The treatment of metastatic prostatic cancer with a potent luteinizing hormone releasing hormone analogue. *J Urol.* 1983;**129**:1149–1152.

Levamisole

■ Other Names

Levamisole hydrochloride; Ergamisol® (Janssen Pharmaceutica Inc.); NSC-177023; R 12564.

■ Chemistry

Structure of levamisole

Levamisole is a thiazole derivative with antihelminthic and antianergic properties. The complete chemical name is (−)-(S)-2,3,5,6-tetrahydro-6-phenylimidazo[2,1-b]thiazole monohydrochloride. It has a molecular weight of 241 and the molecular formula $C_{11}H_{12}N_2S \cdot HCl$.

■ Antitumor Activity

Levamisole is inactive in animal tumors (Potter et al 1974). When used alone, levamisole has not been documented to have any antitumor activity in colon cancer (Arnaud et al 1989), glioma (Mahaley et al 1981), ovarian cancer (Khoo et al 1984), and gastric cancer (Niimoto et al 1984). There is inconsistent evidence of antitumor activity in the adjuvant therapy of human malignant melanoma. It was inactive in one trial (Spitler 1991), despite early reports of activity (Gonzalez et al 1978); however, one study reported a 29% decrease in the death rate and recurrence rate with levamisole compared with untreated controls (Quirt et al 1991). Similar mixed results have been reported in leukemia (Lehtinen 1980). Levamisole is inactive in head and neck cancer (Olivari et al 1979, Wanebo et al 1978), transitional cell carcinoma of the bladder (Smith et al 1978), and lung cancer (Amery 1978, Davis et al 1982). Inconsistent results are also reported in breast cancer (Vogel et al 1978, Klefström 1980) and acute leukemia (Stevenson et al 1991); however, levamisole is consistently active when administered in combination with 5-fluorouracil. This combination decreases the recurrence rate and improves the survival rate of patients with resected Dukes' C stage adenocarcinoma of the colon (Mayer 1990).

In a large intergroup study (1269 patients), randomizing patients with either locally invasive (Dukes' stage B_2) or with regional lymph node involvement (Dukes' stage C) to either observation, levamisole, or levamisole + 5-fluorouracil, Moertel and colleagues (1990) demonstrated that levamisole plus 5-fluorouracil reduced the risk of cancer recurrences in patients with Dukes' C disease by 41% ($p < 0.0001$) and reduced the death rate by 33% ($p = 0.006$). Treatment with levamisole alone had no effect. The median follow-up time for patients on this study was 3 years. The results of the study did not allow for the assessment of the impact of levamisole + 5-fluorouracil (5-FU) in patients with Dukes' stage B_2 disease. In addition, this study did not include patients with rectal carcinoma.

In 1989 the North Central Cancer Treatment Group (NCCTG) (Laurie et al 1989) also showed that for patients with Dukes' stage C disease the combination of levamisole + 5-FU significantly reduced cancer recurrence rate (versus no treatment). The use of levamisole alone in that study produced only a borderline advantage (versus no treatment). Levamisole + 5-FU did confer a survival advantage when given postoperatively to patients with stage C disease (but that finding was based on a subset analysis).

Unfortunately, there has never been an adequate trial comparing levamisole + 5-FU versus 5-FU alone versus an untreated control group. The one study that was performed suggested an advantage for the combination; however, the group of patients with stage C disease was too small (41 patients) (Windle et al 1987).

Levamisole + 5-FU should be given no earlier than 1 week and no later than 5 weeks after surgery.

■ Mechanism of Action

Levamisole acts as an anthelminthic by serving as an agonist of the acetylcholine receptor in the worm. It also inhibits fumarate reductase in helminths to block ATP synthesis (Stevenson et al 1991). (See Grem [1990] for an excellent review.) There are at least two functional moieties in the drug: (1) the thiol group, which can be liberated by hydrolysis, and (2) the imidazole moiety, which has cholinergic-like properties (Stevenson et al 1991). The latter group may mediate the in vitro potentiation of interleukin-2-induced T-lymphocyte proliferation (Hadden et al 1975). The precise mechanism whereby the combination of levamisole + 5-FU is effective for patients with Dukes' C resected colon cancer is unknown. In vitro studies by Grem and Allegra (1989) have shown no *in vitro* synergism for levamisole + 5-FU against colon cancer cells grown in culture. Levamisole does restore the function of macrophages and T lymphocytes after immunosuppression in mice and humans (Lewinski et al 1980). As noted by Grem (1990), more than 15 different immunologic effects have been attributed to levamisole in preclinical models. In these immunology studies, a threshold amount of levamisole is required for the immunostimulatory effects, whereas higher concentrations can cause immunosuppression.

Recent in vitro studies in human cancer cell lines have suggested that a levamisole metabolite, *p*-hydroxytetramisole, may potentiate 5-FU antiproliferative activity by inhibiting tyrosine phosphatases (Kovach et al 1992). The potentiation could be mimicked by orthovanadate, another inhibitor of tyrosine phosphatase. These preliminary findings suggest that the mechanism for the 5-FU–levamisole interaction may involve inhibited dephosphorylation of cellular regulatory phosphoproteins leading to enhanced 5-FU cytotoxicity (Kovach et al 1992).

In patients with hepatocellular cancer levamisole produced no increased natural killer activity or increase in interferon (Sone et al 1982). Increased colony-stimulating factor activity has been documented to occur after oral administration. This is of interest because levamisole + 5-FU appears to produce more neutropenia than 5-FU alone. Of great interest is that although there is a great deal of in vitro information on the immunologic effects, there are very few studies describing the in vivo immunologic effects of levamisole in patients.

■ Availability and Storage

Levamisole hydrochloride (Ergamisol®) is available from Janssen Pharmaceutica Inc, Titusville, New Jersey, in tablets for oral administration containing the equivalent of 50 mg of levamisole base. Fifty-nine milligrams of levamisole hydrochloride is equivalent to 50 mg of levamisole. The inactive ingredients include colloidal silicon dioxide, hydrogenated vegetable oil, hydroxypropyl methylcellulose, lactose, microcrystalline cellulose, polyethylene glycol 6000, polysorbate 80, and talc. The white-coated tablets embossed "Janssen" and "L"/"50" are supplied in blister packages of 36 tablets. They should be stored at room temperature (15–30°C [59–86°F]) and protected from moisture.

■ Preparation for Use, Stability, and Admixture

No preparation for use is necessary. The tablets are stable in the aforementioned storage conditions for 5 years (National Cancer Institute data).

■ Administration

The only current approved indication for the use of levamisole is in combination with 5-FU for patients with resected Dukes' C colon cancer. Initial therapy includes levamisole 50 mg PO every 8 hours for 3 days (starting 7–30 days post surgery) followed by 50 mg PO every 8 hours for 3 days every 2 weeks for 1 year. 5-Fluorouracil is given at a dose of 450 mg/m^2/d by rapid intravenous infusion for 5 days concomitant with a 3-day course of levamisole (starting 21–34 days post surgery), followed by a dose of 5-FU 450 mg/m^2 intravenously once a week for 48 weeks, beginning 28 days after initiating the 5-day course (Moertel et al 1990).

If stomatitis, diarrhea, or leukopenia develops, weekly 5-FU is deferred until the side effects subside. If the side effects are moderate to severe, the dose of 5-FU should be reduced by 20% (see package insert for details).

■ Special Precautions

Levamisole administration has been associated with agranulocytosis which, on occasion, has been fatal. This may or may not be accompanied by a flulike syndrome (fever, chills, etc). Routine monitoring should be performed on all patients receiving levamisole. When levamisole is given with 5-FU, neutropenia, anemia, and thrombocytopenia are frequently noted.

■ Drug Interactions

When levamisole is given with alcohol, a disulfiram-like syndrome develops. Levamisole + 5-FU has been shown to increase plasma levels of phenytoin. In addition, levamisole appears to increase the myelotoxic effects of numerous cytotoxic agents, including 5-FU, carmustine, and antileukemic combination regimens (Symoens et al 1978).

■ Dosage

See Administration.

Pharmacokinetics

The pharmacokinetics of levamisole alone were studied in the late 1970s. After oral administration the compound is rapidly absorbed with peak plasma levels of 0.5 to 0.7µg/µL 1 to 4 hours after a dose of 150 mg. The elimination half-life is about 4 hours. Metabolism of levamisole takes place in the liver, while less than 5% of the unmetabolized drug is detected in the urine and feces (Adams 1978, Graziani and Demartin 1977). Approximately 12% is recovered in the urine as the glucuronide of p-hydroxylevamisole.

Unfortunately, the pharmacokinetics of levamisole in combination with 5-FU have never been studied.

Side Effects and Toxicity

The toxic effects noted in patients receiving levamisole + 5-FU include nausea and vomiting (20–65% of patients), diarrhea (52%), and, less commonly, anorexia and abdominal pain (5–6%). Significant leukopenia (white blood cells < 2000/mm^3) and thrombocytopenia (< 50,000/mm^3) are noted in 1 and 0% of patients, respectively. Rash (occasionally pruritic) has been noted in 23% of patients, with alopecia occurring in 22% of patients. Agranulocytosis is noted more frequently in women, in those with rheumatic disorders, and in those with the HLA-B27 genotype (Symoens et al 1978). Erythrocyte, megakaryocyte, and lymphocyte counts are usually normal.

Most of the preceding effects (except the nausea, diarrhea, and skin rash) can be attributed to the 5-FU. Hallucinations, impaired concentration ability, periorbital edema, an encephalopathy, convulsions, confusion, renal failure, and elevated creatinine and alkaline phosphatase have also been reported occasionally. Nonetheless, levamisole typically does not cause renal or liver toxicity.

REFERENCES

Adams JG. Pharmacokinetics of levamisole. *J Rheumatol.* 1978;5(suppl 4):137–142.

Amery WK. Final results of a multicenter placebo-controlled levamisole study of resectable lung cancer. *Cancer Treat Rep.* 1978;62:1677–1683.

Arnaud JP, Buyse M, Nordlinger B, et al. Adjuvant therapy of poor prognosis colon cancer with levamisole: Results of an EORTC double blind randomized clinical trial. *Br J Surg.* 1989;76:284–289.

Davis S, Mietlowski W, Rohwedder JJ, et al. Levamisole as an adjuvant to chemotherapy in extensive bronchogenic carcinoma. A Veterans Administration Lung Cancer Group study. *Cancer.* 1982;50:646–651.

Gonzalez RL, Spitler LE, Sagebiel RW. Effect of levamisole as a surgical adjuvant therapy for malignant melanoma. *Cancer Treat Rep.* 1978;62:1703–1707.

Graziani G, DeMartin GL. Pharmacokinetics studies on levamisole: On the pharmacokinetics and relative bioavailability of levamisole in man. *Drug Exp Clin Res.* 1971;2:235–239.

Grem JL. Levamisole as a therapeutic agent for colorectal carcinoma. *Cancer Cells.* 1990;2:131–137.

Grem JL, Allegra CJ. Toxicity of levamisole and 5-fluorouracil in human colon carcinoma cells. *J Natl Cancer Inst.* 1989;81:1413–1417.

Hadden JW, Coffey RG, Hadden EM, et al. Effects of levamisole and midazole on lymphocyte proliferation and cyclic nucleotide levels *Cell Immunol.* 1975;20:98–103.

Khoo SK, Whitaker SV, Jones ISC, et al. Levamisole as adjuvant to chemotherapy of ovarian cancer. Results of a randomized trial and 4-year followup. *Cancer.* 1984;54:986–990.

Klefström P. Combination of levamisole immunotherapy and polychemotherapy in advanced breast cancer. *Cancer Treat Rep.* 1980;64(1):65–72.

Kovach JS, Svingen PA, Schaid DJ. Levamisole potentiation of fluorouracil antiproliferative activity mimicked by orthovanadate, an inhibitor of tyrosine phosphatase. *J Natl Cancer Inst.* 1992;84:515–519.

Laurie JA, Moertel CG, Fleming TR, et al. Surgical adjuvant therapy of large-bowel carcinoma: An evaluation of levamisole and the combination of levamisole and fluorouracil. *J Clin Oncol.* 1989;7:1447–1456.

Lehtinen M. Levamisole and leukaemia. *Cancer Immunol Immunother.* 1980;9:137.

Lewinski UH, Mavligit GM, Hersh EM. Cellular immune modulation after a single high dose of levamisole in patients with carcinoma. *Cancer.* 1980;46:2185–2194.

Mahaley MS, Steinbok B, Aronin P, et al. Immunobiology of primary intracranial tumors. Part 4: Levamisole as an immune stimulant in patients and in the ASV glioma model. *J Neurosurg.* 1981;54:220–227.

Mayer RJ. Does adjuvant therapy work in colon cancer? *N Engl J Med.* 1990;322:399–401.

Moertel CG, Fleming TR, Macdonald JS, et al. Levamisole and fluorouracil for adjuvant therapy of resected colon carcinoma. *N Engl J Med.* 1990;322:352–358.

Niimoto M, Hattori T, Ito I, et al. Levamisole in postoperative adjuvant immunochemotherapy for gastric cancer. *Cancer Immunol Immunother.* 1984;18:13–18.

Olivari AJ, Glait HM, Guardo A, et al. Levamisole in squamous cell carcinoma of the head and neck. *Cancer Treat Rep.* 1979;63:983–990.

Potter CW, Carr I, Jennings R, et al. Levamisole inactive in treatment of four animal tumours. *Nature.* 1974;249:567–569.

Quirt IC, Shelley WE, Pater JL, et al. Improved survival in

patients with poor-prognosis malignant melanoma treated with adjuvant levamisole: A phase III study by the National Cancer Institute of Canada Clinical Trials Group. *J Clin Oncol.* 1991;**9**(5):729–735.

Smith RB, deKernion J, Lincoln B, et al. Preliminary report of the use of levamisole in the treatment of bladder cancer. *Cancer Treat Rep.* 1978;**62**:1709–1714.

Sone K, Kew M, Rabson AR. Depressed natural killer cell activity in patients with hepatocellular carcinoma: In vitro effects of interferon and levamisole. *Cancer.* 1982;**50**:2820–2825.

Spitler LE. A randomized trial of levamisole versus placebo as adjuvant therapy in malignant melanoma. *J Clin Oncol.* 1991;**9**(5):736–740.

Stevenson HC, Green I, Hamilton JM, et al. Levamisole: Known effects on the immune system, clinical results, and future applications to the treatment of cancer. *J Clin Oncol.* 1991;**9**(11): 2052–2066.

Symoens J, Veys E, Mielants M, et al. Adverse reactions to levamisole. *Cancer Treat Rep.* 1978;**62**:1721–1730.

Vogel CL, Lipscomb DL, Silverman MA, et al. Levamisole granulocytopenia in patients receiving an adjuvant chemoimmunotherapy program after surgery for breast carcinoma with axillary lymph node involvement. *Cancer Treat Rep.* 1978;**62**(10):1587–1589.

Wanebo HJ, Hilal EY, Pinsky CM, et al. Randomized trial of levamisole in patients with squamous cancer of the head and neck: A preliminary report. *Cancer Treat Rep.* 1978;**62**:1663–1669.

Windle R, Bell PR, Shaw D. Five-year results of a randomized trial of adjuvant 5-fluorouracil and levamisole in colorectal cancer. *Br J Surg.* 1987;**74**:569–572.

Liposomal Daunorubicin

■ Other Names

DaunoXome® (Vestar, Inc); VS103.

■ Chemistry

Liposomal daunorubicin consists of free daunorubicin encapsulated into small unilamellar vesicles about 100 nm in diameter. In this preparation the anthracycline is ionically entrapped within the aqueous interior of the vesicles. The liposomes are composed of distearoylphosphatidylcholine:cholesterol:daunorubicin in a mole ratio of 10:5:1. Citrate is used in the formulation as a counterion to entrap daunorubicin inside the vesicle.

■ Antitumor Activity

Prior evidence suggests that small unilamellar liposomes with a distearylphosphatidylcholine:cholesterol mole ratio of 2:1 can selectively target solid tumors in animals (Profitt et al 1983) and humans (Turner et al 1988). In the animal trials, unilamellar phospholipid vessicles accumulated in an EMT6 tumor on the flank of BALB/c mice to significantly higher levels than in normal tissues. It was hypothesized that alterations in tumor capillary permeability or vascular structure mediated the selective enhancement of liposome uptake (Profitt et al 1983). In humans, indium-111-labeled liposomes were shown to distribute homogenously to normal liver and spleen. There was enhanced uptake of radioactivity in tumor tissues when compared with normal tissues 48 hours after intravenous injection of the labeled liposomes (Turner et al 1988).

Intravenous liposomal daunorubicin has shown activity in mice bearing subcutaneous Ma16c murine mammary adenocarcinoma. Doses of 2 to 35 mg/kg increased survival compared with untreated controls or equivalent doses of free daunomycin. Cures were obtained in at least 70% of mice given liposomal daunorubicin doses greater than 15 mg/kg. The drug is also active in the P-1798 lymphosarcoma tumor model in mice (Forssen et al 1992).

In preliminary clinical trials, liposomal daunorubicin has produced responses in patients with acquired immunodeficiency syndrome (AIDS)-related Kaposi's sarcoma (Gill et al 1991). For example, three of seven Kaposi's sarcoma patients had objective partial responses to liposomal daunorubicin in one trial (Sharma et al 1990). Minor responses have been recorded in a phase I trial of liposomal daunorubicin in patients with a variety of advanced malignancies (Guaglianone et al 1992).

■ Availability and Storage

Liposomal daunorubicin (DaunoXome®) is an investigation agent available from Vestar, Inc, San Dimas, California. It is supplied as a translucent red emulsion in rubber-stoppered glass vials. Each milliliter in the vial contains 1.87 mg of daunorubicin, which is equivalent to 2.0 mg of daunorubicin hydrochloride. In addition to the lipids distearoylphosphatidylcholine (28.16 mg/mL) and cholesterol (6.72 mg/mL), other excipients (per 1.0 mL) include sucrose (85 mg), glycine (3.75 mg), citric acid (0.32 mg), calcium chloride·2H$_2$O (0.294 mg), and Sterile Water for Injection, USP (sufficient quantity 1.0 mL). Hydrochloric acid is used to adjust pH. The vials must be stored at refrigerated temperatures (2–8°C) and are stable for at least 3 months after manufacture. Longer-duration shelf-life stability studies are in progress.

■ Preparation for Use, Stability, and Admixture

Doses are prepared for intravenous administration by aseptically removing the appropriate volume of liposome solution from the vial. This solution is then diluted into 50 to 100 mL of 5% dextrose in a plastic infusion container (either a flexible bag or volumetric gravity infusion set). Only dextrose should be used for diluting liposomal daunorubicin. These solutions are compatible with 5-μm filters which may be used to reduce phlebitis.

■ Administration

Liposomal daunorubicin solutions are administered intravenously over 10 to 60 minutes. Although care should be taken to prevent inadvertent extravasation, the liposomal solution has not produced vesicant reactions in experimental animal models or in humans (Guaglianone et al 1992, Sharma et al 1990).

■ Dosage

The initial phase I clinical trial of liposomal daunorubicin for solid tumors recommended intravenous doses of 100 and 120 mg/m^2 for poor-risk and good-risk patients, respectively. Doses are repeated at 3-week intervals, with dose adjustments based on the degree of neutropenia (Guaglianone et al 1992). In patients with AIDS-related Kaposi's sarcoma the recommended dose for phase II studies was 40 mg/m^2 at 2-week intervals (Sharma et al 1990).

■ Drug Interactions

None are known.

■ Pharmacokinetics

The pharmacokinetics of liposomal daunorubicin appears to differ significantly from that of non-liposomal (free) daunorubicin. With liposomal daunorubicin, the initial plasma half-life is longer and the volume of distribution is between 200- and 400-fold smaller (Forssen et al 1990). These features lead to enhanced peak serum concentrations and AUCs for the liposomal drug. Clearance of liposomal daunorubicin appears to be dose dependent, noted by decreasing clearance and increased AUCs with each increasing dose. Saturation appears to be most prominent at liposomal daunorubicin doses of 60 mg/m^2 and greater. These liposomes slowly yield free drug; thus, only low levels of daunorubicin aglycone and daunorubicinol are detectable following liposomal daunorubicin therapy (Forssen et al 1990). The table summarizes these data. Of course, once liberated from the liposome, free daunorubicin exhibits its standard triphasic elimination characterized by a longer terminal plasma half-life of approximately 20 to 30 hours and clearance via conjugation and biliary secretion.

Clearance of the liposomes may be mediated by reticuloendothelial cells with a selective enhancement of uptake in tumor cells (Forssen et al 1992). The higher AUCs and selective liposomal localization in tumor cells may explain the enhanced antitumor efficacy of liposomal daunorubicin in experimental tumor models.

■ Side Effects and Toxicity

The dose-limiting toxic effect of liposomal daunorubicin is myelosuppression, principally neutropenia. Grade 3 and 4 neutropenia is consistently observed at doses of 120 mg/m^2 or greater. In patients with solid tumors unrelated to AIDS, no hematologic toxicity was observed at doses up to 60 mg/m^2 every 2 weeks (Sharma et al 1990). In patients with

PHARMACOKINETICS OF LIPOSOMAL DAUNORUBICIN

Mean Pharmacokinetic Parameter	Dose (mg/m^2)* 10–40	60	80
Peak level (μg/mL)	4.6–18.2	36.2	47.1
Half-life (h)	2.8–3.8	8.3	5.2
AUC (ng · h/mL)	16.9–120.1	301.2	375.3
Volume of distribution (L)	2.5–2.8	2.9	2.9
Clearance (mL/min)	15.7–8.9	6.9	6.6

*Equivalent dose to free daunorubicin hydrochloride.
Data from Forssen et al (1990).

AIDS-related Kaposi's sarcoma, transient granulocytopenia was noted at all dose levels (20–60 mg/m^2). Thrombocytopenia is much less common (Guaglionone et al 1992). Stomatitis is noticeably absent following liposomal daunorubicin. Similarly, nausea and vomiting are greatly reduced compared with much lower doses of free daunorubicin. Alopecia is also mild or nonexistent. Liposomal daunorubicin extravasation is not associated with toxicity both in preclinical studies and following several inadvertent clinical occurrences (Guaglianone et al 1992, Sharma et al 1990). A low-grade fever is reported in 10% of patients, and about 35% of patients may experience transient fatigue.

Cardiotoxicity has not been noted in patients receiving liposomal daunorubicin. This is similar to preclinical studies showing markedly reduced cardiac toxicity for other liposomally entrapped anthracyclines (Rahman et al 1982); however, relatively few patients have been treated to high cumulative doses of liposomal daunorubicin. Thus, the true cardiotoxic potential of the drug in humans is not yet known.

REFERENCES

Forssen E, Chan KK, Muggia FM, et al. Clinical pharmacokinetics (PK) of liposomal daunorubicin (VS103). *Proc Am Assoc Cancer Res.* 1990;**31**:181.

Forssen EA, Coulter DM, Proffitt RT. Selective in vivo localization of daunorubicin small unilamellar vesicles in solid tumors. *Cancer Res.* 1992;**52**:3255–3261.

Gill P, Sharma D, Levine A, et al. Phase I/II trials with liposomal daunorubicin (DaunoXome) in AIDS-related Kaposi's sarcoma (abstract 358a). *Proc Am Soc Hematol.* 1991;**78**:1423.

Guaglianone P, Chan K, Hanisch R, et al. Phase I clinical trial of liposomal daunorubicin (Daunoxome) in advanced malignancies. *Proc Am Soc Clin Oncol.* 1992;**11**:135.

Profitt RT, Williams LE, Presant CA, et al. Liposomal blockade of the reticuloendothelial system: Improved tumor imaging with small unilamellar vesicles. *Science.* 1983;**220**:502–505.

Rahman A, More N, Schein PS. Doxorubicin-induced chronic cardiotoxicity and its protection by liposomal administration. *Cancer Res.* 1982;**42**:1817–1825.

Sharma D, Muggia F, Lucci L, et al. Liposomal daunorubicin (VS103): Tolerance and clinical effects in AIDS-related Kaposi's sarcoma (KS) during a phase I study. *Proc Am Soc Clin Oncol.* 1990;**9**:4.

Turner AF, Presant CA, Profitt RT, et al. In-111-labeled liposomes: Dosimetry and tumor depiction. *Radiology.* 1988;**166**:761–765.

Liposome Encapsulated Doxorubicin

■ Other Names

NSC-620212; LED; TLC-D99 (Liposome Company).

■ Chemistry

Georgetown LED. Several formulations of liposome-encapsulated doxorubicin (LED) are available. The best characterized to date is the positively charged small unilamellar vesicle preparation made by mixing 280 mg of doxorubicin with 420 mg of cardiolipin (LED, Georgetown, Fujisawa/Lyphomed) (Rahman et al 1990). This mixture is evaporated to dryness under nitrogen and the following lipids are added: 1050 mg of phosphatidylcholine, 350 mg of cholesterol, and 140 mg of stearylamine. This mixture is then evaporated to dryness, sonicated at 37°C for 90 minutes, and dialyzed at 4°C for 20 hours to remove non-entrapped doxorubicin. The resulting unilamellar formulation has a size range of 0.9 to 1.2 μm and contains 5% or less free doxorubicin. It has approximately 14 mg of total lipid per milligram of doxorubicin (Rahman et al 1990).

Liposome Company LED. A second preparation of neutral large unilamellar vesicles is also available. This LED formulation is prepared by hydrating a dry film of an egg phosphatidylcholine/cholesterol (55:45, mol:mol) in 150 mM citric acid (pH 4.0) followed by five cycles of freezing and thawing. The resultant multilamellar vesicles are extruded through polycarbonate filters (pore size, 200 nm) and doxorubicin is then entrapped by pH-driven incubation in a sodium hydroxide (pH 7.8) medium with a drug:lipid ratio of 0.25:1 (w:w). The sample is heated at 60°C for 5 minutes to entrap over 98% of the doxorubicin. This final solution can then be diluted into sterile sodium chloride (Balazsovits et al 1989).

■ Antitumor Activity

Preclinical Activity. Negatively charged (cardiolipin-based) LED has demonstrated antitumor efficacy in a variety of preclinical models including P-388 leukemia (Rahman et al 1985), gross leukemia and mammary carcinoma (Rahman et al 1986a), and Lewis lung carcinoma (Rahman et al 1980). In the last tumor model, other formulations of anionic liposomes have significantly greater antitumor efficacy than does the free drug (Forssen and Tokes 1983b). The free drug showed antitumor activity equivalent to that of LED against sarcoma 180. The cardiolipin-based formulation is also active in vitro against several human tumor cell lines (Dusre et al 1989). For example, the LED formulation displayed up to fivefold greater potency against MCF-7 breast cancer with lesser degrees of enhanced potency against OVCAR (human ovarian cancer cells) and HT-29 colon cancer cells (Dusre et al 1989). Of interest, doxorubicin cellular uptake with the liposomal formulation was roughly comparable to that of the free drug in this study.

There is also evidence that other multilamellar LED formulations have activity in fibrosarcoma cells that are cultured for resistance to doxorubicin (Fan et al 1989). This activity was enhanced by increasing phosphatidylserine concentrations. In contrast, others have reported that antitumor activity is not influenced dramatically by alterations in the lipid composition, whereas variations in vesicle size strongly influenced antitumor activity (Mayer et al 1989). In this regard, small vesicle systems (< 100 nm) were much more active than free drug and opposite effects occurred with larger systems. Finally, LED formulations show activity in multidrug (doxorubicin)-resistant tumors in transgenic mice (Mickisch et al 1992).

Clinical Activity

Georgetown LED. An initial phase I trial reported no responses in patients with advanced solid tumors (primarily adenocarcinomas of the lung, breast, or unknown origin) (Rahman et al 1990). In a subsequent phase II trial in patients with advanced breast cancer, objective responses were observed in 9 of 20 (45%) patients, with complete disappearance of the index tumor sites in 5 of 9 responders (Treat et al 1990). The median duration of response was 7 months.

Liposome Company LED. Two phase I clinical trials of the phosphatidylcholine-based formulation have been performed (Cowens et al 1989, 1990a). As might be expected, no antitumor responses were observed in these initial dose-finding studies. In preclinical studies this LED formulation has shown antitumor activity equal to that of doxorubicin in P-815 mastocytoma in mice (Balazsovits et al 1989).

In a phase II trial of the Liposome Company TLC-D99 formulation in previously untreated patients with metastatic breast cancer, responses were observed in 9 of 17 patients (Batist et al 1992). The nine responses included one complete response.

■ Mechanism of Action

Non-drug-containing liposomes are inert in terms of antitumor activity. Thus, LED formulations serve as enhanced drug delivery vehicles. These are believed to differentially alter the pharmacodynamics of drug presentation to tumor and normal tissues. In general, drug uptake in the kidney, heart, and lung is decreased, whereas uptake into liver and spleen is equal to or higher than that obtained with free doxorubicin (Parker et al 1982). With the liposome, there is increased drug uptake into the lymphatic circulation. This may explain enhanced efficacy for LED in tumors that metastasize through the lymphatics (eg, Lewis lung cancer, in vivo). A slower rate of cellular uptake and release of free doxorubicin from LED formulations (Ganapathi et al 1982) may thus simulate continuous drug infusions which are associated with both acute toxicity and cumulative chronic toxicity, for example, cardiotoxicity (Herman et al 1983, Rahman et al 1982). Thus, myelotoxicity is not usually reduced with LED in experimental systems (Rahman et al 1985), whereas animal trials conclusively show that significantly less doxorubicin reaches the heart with the LED formulations (Rahman et al 1985).

Other unique mechanistic aspects of LED involve an altered means of cellular uptake. This may include pinocytosis or membrane fusion which could theoretically overcome membrane-mediated forms of drug resistance. Some vesicles are also removed by active phagocytosis in macrophages. This may explain a large degree of the drug distribution to reticuloendothelial system tissues.

■ Availability and Storage

Unilamellar, small positively charged LED is investigationally available from Fujisawa/Lyphomed (Deerfield, Illinois; Georgetown preparation). A second investigational preparation of neutral, large unilamellar vesicles is available from the Liposome Company (Princeton, New Jersey). The latter preparation is supplied by the Division of Cancer Treatment, National Cancer Institute, as a three-vial injection kit containing (1) the vehicle—3.9 mL of egg phosphatidylcholine cholesterol liposomes less than

1 μm in size (concentration of 100 mg lipid/mL of citric acid buffer, pH 3.7–4.5); (2) the alkalinization agent—sodium carbonate 53 ng/mL (0.5 M, pH 10.8–12.0); and (3) the active agent–Adriamycin RDF® (Adria Laboratories, Columbus, Ohio) in a 50-mg vial containing lactose and methylparaben. The sterile liposome vehicle and the alkalinization agent vials are stored under refrigeration (2–8°C).

■ Preparation for Use, Stability, and Admixture

Overall, the stability of LED formulations is problematic as time- and medium-dependent drug leakage from vesicles is well documented with all formulations. Physiologic factors affecting LED stability include antibodies, lysosomes, macrophages, and lipoproteins (especially high-density lipoproteins). Some liposomal components such as phosphatidylcholine can also lead to vesicle lipid degradation by peroxidation over time in storage. Thus, shelf-life, uniformity of size, and maintenance of lipid composition are all significant limitations with current LED formulations.

Georgetown LED. The chemical preparation of this LED formulation is outlined under Chemistry (Rahman et al 1986b). The prepared LED is reconstituted in 0.9% Sodium Chloride for Injection, USP, and used immediately for subsequent infusion.

Liposome Company LED. This preparation is also prepared freshly before use by a complex procedure involving serial heating and shaking steps. The 50-mg doxorubicin vial is first reconstituted with 22 mL of saline and shaken. Next, 2.7 mL of the sodium carbonate solution is added to the egg phosphatidylcholine/cholesterol liposome vial (both at room temperature). Three milliliters of the alkalinized liposomes is added to the doxorubicin vial. This vial is shaken for 10 seconds, heated in a water bath (55–60°C) for 1 minute, and shaken for 10 seconds for three consecutive times. This is followed by a 7-minute heating period with a final vigorous shaking. The final preparation can be stored at room temperature and should be used within 8 hours.

■ Administration

Both LED formulations are infused intravenously over 10 to 45 minutes (Rahman et al 1990) or 1 hour (Cowens et al 1990a). Because of a significantly lower vesicant potential (Forssen and Tokes 1983a, Balazsovits et al 1989), LED can be administered through peripheral veins. Nonetheless, caution should still be taken to avoid extravasation.

■ Dosage

The maximum tolerated dose (MTD) of the cardiolipin-based LED (Georgetown preparation) was 90 mg/m^2 (Rahman et al 1990). The same 90 mg/m^2 MTD was recommended for the other LED formulation (Liposome Company) (Cowens et al 1990). Recommended doses for phase II studies have ranged from 30 mg/m^2/wk × 4 as a 1-hour infusion (Brown et al 1991) to 60 mg/m^2 IV every 3 to 4 weeks (Embree et al 1991) to 75 mg/m^2 (Batist et al 1992).

■ Drug Interactions

Specific interactions with liposomes are unknown. For drug interactions with doxorubicin refer to the *Doxorubicin* monograph.

■ Pharmacokinetics

Georgetown LED. Levels of free doxorubicin have been followed in cancer patients receiving the Georgetown (cardiolipin-based) LED formulation (see table on page 642) (Rahman et al 1990). The results show that free doxorubicin clearance may be dose dependent (zero-order elimination). Thus, doxorubicin clearance was actually highest with the lowest doses of LED. The table shows that overall, free drug levels decay in a biexponential fashion with half-lives of 4 to 7 min and 5 to 9 hours. There was also a noticeably slow rate of metabolic conversion to doxorubicinol. The cumulative urinary excretion of doxorubicin over 24 hours was less than 10% of the dose.

As noted earlier, preclinical drug distribution studies have shown that LED preferentially distributes to liver, spleen, and lymphatic tissues with markedly reduced uptake in heart tissues (Rahman et al 1985). The plasma levels of doxorubicin are 10- to 20-fold higher with the LED formulations than would be anticipated following the intravenous administration of equivalent free doxorubicin doses (Rahman et al 1990). Furthermore, doxorubicin clearance values are 3- to 4-fold lower, the steady-state volume of distribution is lower, and the rate and extent of conversion to metabolites are much lower than with free drug. The lack of an observed third phase of elimination with this LED doxorubicin formulation may relate to the truncated

MEAN PHARMACOKINETIC PARAMETERS OF FREE DOXORUBICIN IN PATIENTS GIVEN LIPOSOMAL ENCAPSULATED DOXORUBICIN

Parameter	LED Dose [mg/m^2 over 10 min except as noted]			
	30	4.5	60	90*
Number of patients	2	2	3	3
Half-life				
α (min)	5.5	4.8	4.1	4.4
β (h)	5.1	6.7	8.7	7.7
Peak level (mg/L)	3.2	5.0	15	4.65
AUC (mg·h/mL)	119	623	979	1192
Clearance (L/min)	0.63	0.148	0.196	0.182
Volume of distribution				
Central (L)	18	9.1	3.4	16.4
Steady state (L)	164	75	62	88

*Infused over 15 to 45 minutes.
Data from Rahman et al 1990 (positively charged small unilamellar liposomes).

blood sampling times used in the study (Rahman et al 1990).

Preclinical studies with the Georgetown LED formulation showed a preferential retention of drug in the liver, spleen, and lungs (Rahman et al 1980). This effect is due largely to filtration rather than active uptake. Nonetheless, cellular uptake in the heart is dramatically lessened with this preparation (Rahman et al 1985). This heightened distribution of LED into reticuloendothelial system tissues probably explains most of the saturable, nonlinear pharmacokinetics of LED formulations.

Liposome Company LED. In BALB/c mice the plasma clearance of doxorubicin from this formulation was 2.7 mL/h with an AUC of 73.4 µg·h/mL (Gabizon and Papahadjopoulos 1989). These values were one-fifth and 19 times those of the unencapsulated drug, respectively. This indicates significantly slowed elimination and higher systemic drug exposure with the LED formulation.

The table on the opposite page describes the pharmacokinetics of total doxorubicin in patients (free plus liposomal drug) (Cowens et al 1990b). These results show a heterogenous spread of clearance and AUC values. Doxorubicin metabolites were variably observed beginning 8 hours after drug administration. These included doxorubicinol and the 7-deoxy and doxorubicin aglycones; however, no specific metabolite pattern was immediately apparent (Cowens et al 1990b). When LED was administered as a brief infusion at a dose of 25 mg/m^2, a plasma AUC for encapsulated doxorubicin was 0.6 µg·h/mL compared with 2.9 µg·h/mL for free doxorubicin liberated from the liposomes produced by the Liposome Company (TLC-D99) (Brown et al 1991). The half-life of LED was 4.6 hours compared with 67.9 hours for the free drug. The peak level of LED was 332 µg·h/mL (doxorubicin content in liposomes) versus 243 ng/mL for free doxorubicin. Clearance was 42.8 L/h/m^2 for LED compared with 8.7 L/h/m^2 for free drug. Similar findings were reported by Embree et al (1991). Both studies suggest that LED serves as a slow-release depot for free doxorubicin. The doxorubicinol peak was only 6% that of doxorubicin following administration of LED (Embree et al 1991).

■ Side Effects and Toxicity

The dose-limiting toxic effect for both LED formulations has been myelosuppression (Rahman et al 1990, Cowens et al 1989, 1990a, Brown et al 1991). Granulocytopenia is the predominant effect, with a nadir of 10 to 15 days (Rahman et al 1990). Thrombocytopenia and a normochromic, normocytic anemia are also observed (Brown et al 1991). The latter effect tended to be cumulative as long as treatment continued (Rahman et al 1990).

Alopecia is common and can be total at doses greater than 60 mg/m^2; however, descriptions of other effects such as stomatitis, extravasation necrosis, and cardiotoxicity have been limited (Treat et al 1990) or significantly absent with the LED formulations. With a weekly × 4 schedule, mucositis, fever,

PHARMACOKINETIC PARAMETERS FOR TOTAL (FREE PLUS LIPOSOMAL) DOXORUBICIN*

Dose (mg/m^2)	Number of Patients	AUC ($\mu M \cdot$ h)	Clearance (L/h)
20	3	2.05, 2.68, 13.7	35.7, 26.4, 5.44
90	7	18.9, 88.6, 23.9, 31.3, 117, 326, 6.96	13.8, 3.19, 10.5, 8.43, 2.36, 8.38, 32.8

*Liposome Company LED.
Data from Cowens et al 1990b.

fatigue, and hepatotoxicity have been observed (Brown et al 1991, Batist et al 1992). Renal and hepatic toxicity is also not observed; however, mild nausea and vomiting were common but easily controlled with antiemetics. Anorexia is also reported with LED (Brown et al 1991, Cowens et al 1990a).

Idiosyncratic reactions from both LED formulations are reported (Rahman et al 1990, Cowens et al 1990a). With the Liposome Company preparation, fevers occur 2 to 13 hours after drug infusion (Cowens et al 1990a), whereas with the Georgetown preparation, chills lasting 30 minutes are reported in the absence of fever or changes in blood pressure (Rahman et al 1990). Patients experiencing the latter toxic effects were subsequently pretreated with diphenhydramine and hydrocortisone which blocked further reactions. Lower back pain, substernal chest pain, and a transient slight elevation in lactate dehydrogenase were described in one patient receiving the Georgetown formulation (Rahman et al 1990). Some patients treated to high cumulative LED doses have also developed slight decreases (13–17%) in left ventricular ejection fractions without evidence of significant pathology on endomyocardial biopsy (Rahman et al 1990, Batist et al 1992). Asymptomatic ventricular fibrillation has also been described in one patient.

■ Special Applications

The Georgetown LED formulation has been administered intraperitoneally to patients with advanced ovarian cancer (Potkul et al 1989). Doses up to 100 mg have been administered in 2 L of normal saline with a 4-hour dwell time. Repeat doses were given at 21 days. This dose produced a peak doxorubicin intraperitoneal level of 32 µg/mL, which decreased to 14 µg/mL after 1 hour. Simultaneous blood levels ranged from 0.7 to 0.9 µg/mL. Five of thirteen (38%) of patients responded. Toxic effects included chemical peritonitis in one patient and nausea or vomiting in three patients. No myelosuppression, alopecia, hepatotoxicity, or local tissue necrosis was reported.

REFERENCES

Balazsovits JAE, Mayer LD, Bally MB, et al. Analysis of the effect of liposome encapsulation on the vesicant properties, acute and cardiac toxicities, and antitumor efficacy of doxorubicin. *Cancer Chemother Pharmacol.* 1989;**23**:81–86.

Bally MB, Jayar B, Masin D, et al. Studies on the myelosuppressive activity of doxorubicin entrapped in liposomes. *Cancer Chemother Pharmacol.* 1990;**27**:13–19.

Batist G, Ahlgren P, Panasci L, et al. Phase II study of liposomal doxorubicin (TLCD99) in metastatic breast cancer. *Proc Am Soc Clin Oncol.* 1992;**11**:82.

Brown T, Kuhn J, Marshall M, et al. A phase I clinical and pharmacokinetic trial of liposomal doxorubicin (NSC-620212). *Proc Am Soc Clin Oncol.* 1991;**10**:93.

Cowens JW, Creaven PJ, Brenner DE, et al. Phase I study of doxorubicin encapsulated in liposomes. *Proc Am Soc Clin Oncol.* 1990a;**9**:87.

Cowens JW, Greco W, Ginsberg R, Creaven PJ. Pharmacokinetics of doxorubicin encapsulated in liposomes in patients with advanced cancer. *Proc Am Soc Clin Oncol.* 1990b;**9**:87.

Cowens JW, Kanter P, Brenner DE, et al. Phase I study of doxorubicin encapsulated in liposomes. *Proc Am Soc Clin Oncol.* 1989;**8**:69.

Dusre L, Forst D, Rahman A. A comparative therapeutic study of free doxorubicin and doxorubicin entrapped in cardiolipin liposomes in human breast, ovarian and colon tumors. *Proc Am Assoc Cancer Res.* 1989;**30**:556.

Embree L, Gelmon LK, Cullis MP, et al. Liposome encapsulated doxorubicin (TLC D-99) pharmacokinetics in patients with non-small cell lung cancer. *Proc Am Soc Clin Oncol.* 1991;**10**:102.

Fan D, Seid C, Bucana CD, Fidler IJ. Reversal of tumor cell resistance to Adriamycin by presentation of the drug incorporated in liposomes. *Proc Am Assoc Cancer Res.* 1989;**30**:522.

Forssen EA, Tokes ZA. Improved therapeutic benefits of doxorubicin by entrapment in anionic liposomes. *Cancer Res.* 1983a;**43**:546–550.

Forssen EA, Tokes ZA. Attenuation of dermal toxicity of doxorubicin by liposome encapsulation. *Cancer Treat Rep.* 1983b;**67**:481–484.

Gabizon A, Papahadjopoulos D. Encapsulation of doxorubicin in stable liposomes with long circulation times in mice: Changes in pharmacokinetics and tissue distribution. *Proc Am Assoc Cancer Res.* 1989;**30**:605.

Ganapathi R, Krishan A, Zubrod CG. Mechanism for reduced toxicity of liposome-encapsulated Adriamycin. *Proc Am Assoc Cancer Res.* 1982;**23**:175.

Herman EH, Rahman A, Ferrans VJ, et al. Prevention of chronic doxorubicin cardiotoxicity in beagles by liposomal encapsulation. *Cancer Res.* 1983;**43**:5427–5432.

Mayer LD, Tai LCL, Ko DSC, et al. Influence of vesicle size, lipid composition, and drug-to-lipid ratio on the biological activity of liposomal doxorubicin in mice. *Cancer Res.* 1989;**49**:5922–5930.

Mickisch GH, Rahman A, Pastan I, et al. Increased effectiveness of liposome-encapsulated doxorubicin in multidrug-resistant-transgenic mice compared with free doxorubicin. *J Natl Cancer Inst.* 1992;**84**(10):804–805.

Parker RJ, Priester ER, Sieber SM. Effect of route administration and liposome entrapment on the metabolism and disposition of Adriamycin in the rat. *Drug Metab Dispos.* 1982;**10**:499–504.

Potkul R, Treat J, Forst D, et al. A phase I–II study of intraperitoneal (IP) administered liposome encapsulated doxorubicin (LED). *Proc Am Soc Clin Oncol.* 1989;**8**:80.

Rahman A, Fumagalli A, Barbieri B, et al. Antitumor and toxicity evaluation of free doxorubicin and doxorubicin entrapped in cardiolipin liposomes. *Cancer Chemother Pharmacol.* 1986a;**16**:22–27.

Rahman A, Joher A, Neefe JR. Immunotoxicity of multiple dosing regimens of free doxorubicin and doxorubicin entrapped in cardiolipin liposomes. *Br J Cancer.* 1986b;**54**:401–408.

Rahman A, Kessler A, More N, et al. Liposomal protection of Adriamycin-induced cardiotoxicity in mice. *Cancer Res.* 1980;**40**:1532–1537.

Rahman A, More N, Schein PS. Doxorubicin-induced chronic cardiotoxicity and its protection by liposomal administration. *Cancer Res.* 1982;**42**:1817–1825.

Rahman A, Treat J, Roh J-K, et al. A phase I clinical trial and pharmacokinetic evaluation of liposome-encapsulated doxorubicin. *J Clin Oncol.* 1990;**8**:1093–1100.

Rahman A, White G, More N, Schein PS. Pharmacological, toxicological, and therapeutic evaluation in mice of doxorubicin entrapped in cardiolipin liposomes. *Cancer Res.* 1985;**45**:796–803.

Treat J, Greenspan A, Forst D, et al. Antitumor activity of liposome-encapsulated doxorubicin in advanced breast cancer: Phase II study. *J Natl Cancer Inst.* 1990;**82**:1706–1710.

Lomustine

■ Other Names

NSC-79037; CCNU; CeeNU® (Bristol-Myers Oncology Division).

■ Chemistry

Structure of lomustine

1-(2-Chloroethyl)-3-cyclohexyl-1-nitrosourea (lomustine) is a nitrosourea related to carmustine. With lomustine, the chlorethyl moiety is replaced by a cyclohexyl group. Lomustine is more lipid soluble than carmustine with a log P (octanol/water) partition coefficient of 2.83 (Mellett 1977). It is unionized at physiologic pH. It exists as a yellow powder and has a molecular weight of 234. It is also slightly soluble in water, saline, or alcohol. The molecular formula is $C_9H_{16}N_3Cl_1O_2$.

■ Antitumor Activity

Similar to the other nitrosoureas, lomustine has marked activity against L-1210 leukemia in mice (Chirigos et al 1965). In humans, however, the drug is used primarily in solid tumors and lymphomas (Wasserman et al 1974a, b, 1975). The official clinical indications for lomustine are the management of primary or metastatic brain tumors (Fewer et al 1972, Rosenblum et al 1973) and advanced Hodgkin's disease (Hoogstraten et al 1973, DeConti et al 1973, Selawry and Hansen 1972). In advanced Hodgkin's disease, lomustine has been shown to be superior to carmustine when both drugs were used as single agents. The response rate to lomustine was 60% compared with 28% for carmustine (Hansen et al 1981). Lomustine combined with vincristine is also active in children with recurrent gliomas (Lefkowitz et al 1988). Although not curative, this treatment results in relatively long-term disease stabilization. The drug also has activity in combination chemotherapy regimens for multiple myeloma (Salmon 1976) and advanced gastrointestinal carcinoma (Klaassen and Rapp 1973, Moertel 1973). Other solid tumors that are occasionally sensitive to lomustine are advanced non-small cell lung carcinoma (Takita and Brugarolas 1973, Eagan et al 1974) and prostate cancer. Breast cancer, however, is relatively insensitive to the drug (Gottlieb et al 1974, Hoogstraten et al 1973, Cunningham et al 1973). In malignant melanoma, nitrosoureas show modest but consistent antitumor effects, comparable to the effects of other single agents (Ahmann 1976).

■ Mechanism of Action

Lomustine is rapidly converted to monohydroxylated derivatives which produce most, if not all, of the DNA alkylation and protein carbamoylation associated with the drug's cytotoxic activity (Reed and May 1975, Wheeler et al 1977). The cytotoxic effect of lomustine involves the inhibition of both DNA and RNA synthesis through DNA alkylation (Ewig and Kohn 1978). Lomustine slowly forms both DNA–DNA and DNA–protein crosslinks in L-1210 cells exposed to the drug in vitro for short periods. Like the other haloethyl nitrosoureas, lomustine can also carbamoylate lysine residues in cellular proteins. Antitumor activity appears to correlate best with interstrand crosslinking, although some of the drug's cytotoxic activity may be the result of other effects (Erickson et al 1980). There is also biochemical interference with histidine utilization, thereby upsetting the 1-carbon metabolic transfer process (Cheng et al 1972, Woolley et al 1976, Kann et al 1974). Lomustine may lower the amount of reduced glutathione in tissues. This is similar to the effects of carmustine and is due to inhibition of glutathione reductase (McConnell et al 1979).

Alkylation of DNA by the chloroethyl moiety in lomustine may not occur in the same fashion as it does with conventional alkylating agents. Indeed, cells resistant to nitrosoureas may still retain sensitivity to classic alkylating agents (Bodell et al 1985). Conversely, some experimental rat tumors resistant to other bifunctional alkylating agents may remain sensitive to nitrosoureas because of their protein-carbamoylating actions (Tew and Wang 1982).

Similar to the other nitrosoureas, lomustine has been shown to affect a number of cellular processes including RNA, protein synthesis, and the processing of ribosomal and nucleoplasmic messenger RNA (Kann et al 1974); DNA base component structure (Cheng et al 1972, Ludlum et al 1975); the rate of DNA synthesis (Wheeler and Alexander 1974); and DNA polymerase activity (Wheeler and Bowden 1975). Lomustine does not exhibit true cell cycle phase specificity, although the cell cycle can be arrested in G_2 phase by the drug and/or metabolites in some cases (Bray et al 1970, Tobey and Crissman 1975).

■ Availability and Storage

Lomustine is commercially available in an oral dose pack of six capsules (CeeNu®, Bristol-Myers Oncology Division, Princeton, New Jersey). This commercial kit contains a total of 300 mg of drug: 2×100 mg, 2×40 mg, and 2×10 mg. The unopened, tightly sealed bottles of drug retain stability for 2 years at room temperature. Care must be taken to avoid exposure to excessive heat (>40°C).

■ Preparation for Use, Stability, and Admixture

The appropriate dose should be dispensed to the nearest 10 mg for use by the patient. The dispensing of more than one treatment course at a time is not wise because of the possibility of an accidental overdose by an unsupervised outpatient (Foon and Haskell 1982). All lomustine doses should be protected from excess heat (>40°C) and prolonged exposure to moisture (humidity).

■ Administration

All doses of lomustine are intended for oral administration. Taking the drug on an empty stomach is recommended, as nausea and vomiting may occur after drug ingestion. Alcohol should be avoided for short periods after taking a dose of lomustine. Absorption of the drug is reportedly fairly rapid (30–60 minutes); therefore, vomiting after this period may not significantly reduce drug efficacy. To maximize lomustine absorption, other drugs that cause vomiting should not be concurrently administered.

■ Dosage

The recommended dose of lomustine as a single agent for both adults and children is 100–130 mg/m² as a single oral dose. This dose should not be given more often than every 6 weeks (Broder and Hansen 1973). Reduced dosages are recommended if significant and/or prolonged myelosuppressive effects were observed with previous doses. With compromised marrow function, 100 mg/m² every 6 weeks is recommended as the initial dose.

When combined with other cytotoxic agents, lomustine doses have ranged from 30 mg/m^2 (Chahinian et al 1989) to 75 mg/m^2 for an "eight drugs in one day" protocol in pediatric brain tumor therapy (Pendergrass et al 1987). When combined with vincristine in childhood gliomas, lomustine doses of 100 mg/m^2 were given every 6 weeks for eight cycles (Lefkowitz et al 1988).

■ Drug Interactions

In rats, pretreatment with phenobarbital, a microsomal enzyme-inducing agent, significantly reduces the antitumor activity of lomustine (Levin et al 1979). Similar effects have been described in tumor-bearing mice (Siemann 1983). Pretreatment with phenytoin, methylprednisolone, and dexamethasone did not affect lomustine activity (Levin et al 1979). The basis for the interaction with phenobarbital may involve a markedly enhanced rate of drug elimination from plasma. This has been documented with the related nitrosourea carmustine (Levin et al 1979). Conversely, inhibitors of microsomal enzyme metabolism such as SKF-525A can significantly increase the experimental antitumor activity of lomustine in mice (Siemann 1983). The radiosensitizer misonidazole can also enhance lomustine experimental activity (Siemann 1981), as can the more lipophilic congener benznidazole (Siemann et al 1983). This potentiation was found to be greater in tumor tissues compared with normal tissues.

The H$_2$ antihistamine cimetidine has been shown to potentiate lomustine myelotoxicity in a patient receiving a 120-mg dose of lomustine with cimetidine (300 mg every 6 hours) for glioblastoma. This patient experienced a profound leukopenia (900 WBC/mm^3) and neutropenia (< 5%) which led to an emergency hospitalization for a severe bronchopneumonia (Hess and Kornblith 1985).

Experimentally, lomustine has also produced synergistic antileukemic activity when combined with chlorozotocin (Wheeler et al 1981). One explanation for this effect involves preferential binding of lomustine and chlorozotocin to DNA in L-1210 cells compared to normal murine bone marrow DNA (Green et al 1979).

■ Pharmacokinetics

Lomustine appears to have the same basic pharmacokinetic characteristics as the other nitrosoureas: high lipid solubility facilitating rapid transport across biologic membranes (including the gastrointestinal mucosa and the blood–brain barrier); rapid decomposition by nonenzymatic processes that are dependent on pH temperature and different media; and the rapid biotransformation to products which are extensively bound to cellular macromolecules through alkylation of nucleic acids and also by carbamoylation of cellular proteins (Oliverio 1976; Oliverio et al 1970a, b).

The physiologic disposition of radioactively labeled lomustine has been studied in humans. Sponzo et al (1973) demonstrated relatively rapid oral absorption which was nearly complete after 30 minutes. This produced peak plasma levels of lomustine metabolites 3 hours after administration. Significant metabolite levels are noted as early as 10 minutes after injection. Peak levels of radioactivity, however, accounted for only less than 0.1% of the administered dose. In contrast, plasma levels of lomustine degradation products are prolonged, and urinary excretion is fairly slow. About 60% of a dose is recovered after 48 hours, with 50% recovered in the first 12 hours. There are also different elimination patterns for the cyclohexyl and chloroethyl moieties. Other 2-chloroethyl metabolites include thiodiacetic acid and *S*-carboxylmethyl-1-cysteine. Overall, most of a lomustine dose is metabolized by ring hydroxylation at the 4-position of the cyclohexy group.

Following the administration of unlabeled oral lomustine in humans, no parent drug is detectable in the plasma. This is due to rapid conversion to the *cis*- and *trans*-4-hydroxy metabolites (Lee et al 1985). This conversion occurs during the drug's "first pass" through the liver. Peak concentrations of the *cis* and *trans* isomers of ring hydroxylated lomustine are achieved 2 to 4 hours after dosing. Plasma levels at this time range from 0.8 to 0.9 μg/mL. Formation of the *trans* metabolite is slightly favored over the *cis* metabolite by a 6:4 ratio. The elimination half-lives of these active metabolites range from 1.3 to 2.9 hours (see table on the opposite page).

Reed and May (1975) have shown that part of lomustine metabolism in rats is mediated through hepatic microsomal enzymes. The primary metabolic pattern involved hydroxylation at three separate positions of the cyclohexyl ring, primarily at the 3- and 4-positions. This activity was cytochrome P450 dependent. Further studies also demonstrated quantitative differences in phenobarbital-treated animals favoring the *cis*-4-hydroxy compound over the usually predominant *cis*-3-hydroxy derivative.

MEAN CLINICAL PHARMACOKINETICS OF LOMUSTINE METABOLITES*

CCNU Species	Peak Concentration (μg/mL)	Half-life (h)	AUC$_{0-}$ (μg · h/mL)
trans-4-Hydroxy	0.53	1.81	2.05
cis-4-Hydroxy	0.32	1.91	1.48
Total nitrosoureas	0.85	—	3.37

*n = 4 patients given 130 mg/m^2.
Data from Lee et al 1985.

Drug penetration into the central nervous system is relatively good with absolute cerebrospinal fluid levels approximating 15 to 30% of simultaneous plasma levels. As with the other nitrosoureas, intact drug cannot be recovered from physiologic body fluids including cerebrospinal fluid and urine.

■ Side Effects and Toxicity

Similar to carmustine, the dose-limiting toxic effect for lomustine is delayed and potentially cumulative myelosuppression. Thrombocytopenia is reported with a nadir of 26 to 34 days and a duration of 6 to 10 days. Leukopenia is described with a nadir of 41 to 46 days and a duration of 9 to 14 days (Hansen et al 1971). An inadvertent lomustine overdose (550 mg/m^2, 1120 mg total dose) was followed by severe bone marrow aplasia but with full hematologic recovery (Foon and Haskell 1982). This patient took four 40-mg capsules each night for 7 nights in a row instead of only 1 night every 6 weeks. No liver, lung, or renal toxicity was apparent and only minimal nausea was reported. Bone marrow recovery was complete after 4 weeks.

Nausea and vomiting often occur 2 to 6 hours after lomustine administration. Diarrhea is less common, although anorexia may last several days. Antiemetics may reduce these symptoms.

Neurologic toxic effects such as confusion, lethargy, and ataxia have been noted rarely. Permanent cortical blindness has been reported in three patients treated with lomustine and low-dose cranial irradiation for glioblastoma multiforme or small cell lung cancer (Wilson et al 1987). In these cases, there was a sudden onset of total blindness followed by optic atrophy. Blindness was permanent in each case, suggesting synergy between lomustine and radiotherapy.

Other toxic effects include stomatitis, alopecia, and transient hepatic enzyme elevations. These are rarely dose limiting.

Chronic nitrosourea therapy has been associated with CCNU dose-dependent nephrotoxicity, particularly with the related analog semustine. Silver and Morton (1979) have recently described a single case of drug-induced nephrotoxicity in a patient with small cell carcinoma of the lung. After a cumulative lomustine dose of 2.3 g (100–130 mg/m^2 every 6 weeks), frank renal failure requiring chronic dialysis ensued. The clinical findings were consistent with toxic nephritis. In addition, interstitial nephritis has been described in lomustine toxicity studies in primates. Some reports suggest a causal relationship between renal failure and a long remission duration of 11 months which allows for high cumulative doses to be given. Renal failure has been ultimately fatal in some cases.

All of the nitrosoureas have been found to be mutagenic, teratogenic, and carcinogenic in experimental systems. An increased risk of myelodysplasia is reported for lomustine combined with alkylating agents in patients with Hodgkin's disease (Brusamolino et al 1992). To date, however, significant hepatic and cardiopulmonary toxic effects have not been encountered. Pulmonary fibrosis has, however, been associated with lomustine in one patient with an astrocytoma (Vats et al 1982); the total dose of lomustine was 1170 mg/m^2 given as individual courses of 130 mg/m^2 every 6 weeks. The fibrosis was fatal in this patient even though the maximum damage presented 2 years after discontinuation of therapy.

Overall, the major toxic effect of lomustine is prolonged myelosuppression, which may be cumulative with repeated dosing. Sequential dosing must therefore be based on laboratory determination of adequate bone marrow reserve.

■ Special Applications

Lomustine has been tried experimentally as a topical treatment for psoriasis (Peck et al 1972) and for the cutaneous T-cell lymphoma mycosis fungoides. In the latter instance, a 95% alcohol solution of lomustine, 0.17 to 0.4% was applied once or twice daily to individual plaques. Although lomustine was less irritating than carmustine, a higher dose of lomustine solution was required and carmustine was favored for investigational topical nitrosourea applications.

REFERENCES

Ahmann DL. Nitrosoureas in the management of disseminated malignant melanoma. *Cancer Treat Rep.* 1976;60(6):747–751.

Bodell WJ, Gerosa M, Aida T, et al. Investigation of resistance to DNA cross-linking agents in 9L cell lines with different sensitivities to chloroethylnitrosoureas. *Cancer Res.* 1985;45:3460–3464.

Bray D, Oliverio V, Adamson R, DeVita F. Cell cycle effects produced by 1-(2-chloroethyl)-3-cyclohexyl-1-nitrosourea (CCNU) and its decomposition products. *Proc Am Assoc Cancer Res.* 1970;11:12.

Broder LE, Hansen HH. 1-(2-Chloroethyl)-3-cyclohexyl-1-nitrosourea (CCNU, NSC-79037): A comparison of drug administration at four-week and six-week intervals. *Eur J Cancer.* 1973;9:147–152.

Brusamolino E, Pagnucco G, Castelli G, et al. The risk of secondary myelodysplasia and acute non-lymphoid leukemia in Hodgkin's disease is related to combined modality therapy and to the use of nitrosourea derivatives. *Proc Am Soc Clin Oncol.* 1992;11:329.

Chahinian AP, Propert KJ, Ware JH, et al. A randomized trial of anticoagulation with warfarin and of alternating chemotherapy in extensive small-cell lung cancer by the cancer and leukemia group B. *J Clin Oncol.* 1989;7:993–1002.

Cheng CJ, Fujimuar S, Grunberger D, Weinstein IB. Interaction of 1-(2-chloroethyl)-3-cyclohexyl-1-nitrosourea (NSC-79037) with nucleic acids and proteins in vivo and in vitro. *Cancer Res.* 1972;32:22–27.

Chirigos MA, Humphreys SR, Goldin A. Duration of effective levels of three antitumor drugs in mice with leukemia L-1210 implanted intracerebrally and subcutaneously. *Cancer Chemother Rep.* 1965;49:15–19.

Cunningham TJ, Rosner D, Olson KB, et al. A comparison of 5-azacytidine (5AC) with CCNU in breast cancer (abstract 356). *Proc Am Assoc Cancer Res.* 1973;14:89.

DeConti RC, Hubbard SP, Pinch P, Bertino JR. Treatment of advanced neoplastic disease with 1-(2-chloroethyl)-3-cyclohexyl-1-nitrosourea (CCNU; NSC-79037). *Cancer Chemother Rep.* 1973;57:201–207.

Eagan RT, Carr DT, Coles DT, et al. Randomized study comparing CCNU (NSC-79037) and methyl-CCNU (NSC-95441) in advanced bronchogenic carcinoma. *Cancer Chemother Rep.* 1974;58(pt 1):913–918.

Erickson LC, Bradley MO, Ducore JM, et al. DNA cross-linking and cytotoxicity in normal and transformed human cells treated with antitumour nitrosoureas. *Proc Natl Acad Sci USA.* 1980;77:467.

Ewig RAG, Kohn KW. DNA-protein cross-linking and DNA interstrand crosslinking by haloethylnitrosoureas in L1210 cells. *Cancer Res.* 1978;38:3197–3203.

Fewer D, Wilson CB, Boldrey EB, Enot JK. Phase II study of 1-(2-chloroethyl)-3-cyclohexyl-1-nitrosourea (CCNU; NSC-79037) in the treatment of brain tumors. *Cancer Chemother Rep.* 1972;56:421–427.

Foon KA, Haskell CM. Inadvertent overdose with lomustine (CCNU) followed by hematologic recovery. *Cancer Treat Rep.* 1982;66(5):1241–1242.

Gottlieb JA, Rivkin S, Spigel SC, et al. Superiority of Adriamycin over oral nitrosoureas in patients with advanced breast carcinoma. *Cancer.* 1974;35:519–526.

Green D, Smulson ME, Schein PS. Differential binding of chlorozotocin (Clz) and CCNU to murine bone marrow chromatin (abstract). *Proc Am Assoc Cancer Res ASCO.* 1979;20:253.

Hansen HH, Selawry OS, Muggia FM, et al. Clinical studies with 1-(2-chloroethyl)-3-cyclohexyl-1-nitrosourea (NSC-79037). *Cancer Res.* 1971;31:223–227.

Hansen HH, Selawry OS, Pajak TF, et al. The superiority of CCNU in the treatment of advanced Hodgkin's disease: Cancer and leukemia group B study. *Cancer.* 1981;47:14–18.

Hess WA, Kornblith PL. Combination of lomustine and cimetidine in the treatment of a patient with malignant glioblastoma: A case report. *Cancer Treat Rep.* 1985;69(6):733.

Hoogstraten B, Gottlieb JA, Caoili E, et al. CCNU (1-[2-chloroethyl]-3-cyclohexyl-1-nitrosourea, NSC-79037) in the treatment of cancer. *Cancer.* 1973;32:38–43.

Kann HE Jr, Kohn KW, Wilderlite L. Effects of 1,3-bis(2-chloroethyl)-1-nitrosourea and related compounds on nuclear RNA metabolism. *Cancer Res.* 1974;34:1982–1988.

Klaassen D, Rapp E. Phase II study of CCNU in the treatment of advanced gastrointestinal malignancy (abstract 90). *Cancer Chemother Rep.* 1973;57:112.

Lee FYF, Workman P, Roberts JT, Bleechen NM. Clinical pharmacokinetics of oral CCNU (lomustine). *Cancer Chemother Pharmacol.* 1985;14:125–131.

Lefkowitz IB, Packer RJ, Sutton LN, et al. Results of the treatment of children with recurrent gliomas with lomustine and vincristine. *Cancer.* 1988;61:896–902.

Levin VA, Stearns J, Byrd A, et al. The effect of phenobarbital pretreatment on the antitumor activity of 1,3-bis(2-chloroethyl)-1-nitrosourea (BCNU), 1-(2-chloroethyl)-3-cyclohexyl-1-nitrosourea (CCNU) and 1-(2-chloroethyl)-3-(2,6-deoxo-3-piperidyl-1-nitrosourea (PCNU), and on the plasma pharmacokinetics and biotransformation of BCNU. *J Pharmacol Exp Ther.* 1979;208(1):1–11.

Ludlum DB, Kramer BS, Wang J, et al. Reaction of 1,3-

bis(2-chloroethyl)-1-nitrosourea with synthetic polynucleotides. *Biochemistry.* 1975;**14**:5480–5485.

McConnell WR, Kari P, Hill DL. Reduction of glutathione levels in livers of mice treated with N,N'-bis(2-chloroethyl)-N-nitrosourea. *Cancer Chemother Pharmacol.* 1979;**2**:221–223.

Mellett LB. Physicochemical considerations and pharmacokinetic behavior in delivery of drugs to the central nervous system. *Cancer Treat Rep.* 1977;**61**:527–531.

Moertel CG. Clinical management of advanced gastrointestinal cancer. *Semin Drug Treat.* 1973;**3**:55–68.

Oliverio VT. Pharmacology of the nitrosoureas: An overview. *Cancer Treat Rep.* 1976;**60**(6):703–707.

Oliverio VT, Vietzke WM, Williams MK, et al. The absorption, distribution, excretion, and biotransformation of the carcinostatic 1-(2-chloroethyl)-3-cyclohexyl-1-nitrosourea in animals. *Cancer Res.* 1970a;**30**:1330–1337.

Oliverio VT, Walker MD, Hayes SL, DeVita VT. The physiologic distribution of radioactive 1-(2-chloroethyl)-3-cyclohexyl-1-nitrosourea (CCNU) in man. *Proc Am Assoc Cancer Res.* 1970b;**11**:61.

Peck GL, Guss SB, Key DJ. Topical lomustine in the treatment of psoriasis. *Arch Dermatol.* 1972;**106**:172–176.

Pendergrass TW, Milstein JM, Geyer JR, et al. Eight drugs in one day chemotherapy for brain tumors: Experience in 107 children and rationale for preradiation chemotherapy. *J Clin Oncol.* 1987;**5**:1221–1231.

Reed DJ, May HE. Alkylation and carbamoylation intermediates from the carcinostatic 1-(2-chloroethyl)-3-cyclohexyl-1-nitrosourea (CCNU). *Life Sci.* 1975;**16**:1263–1270.

Rosenblum ML, Reynolds AF, Smith KA, et al. Chloroethyl-cyclohexyl-nitrosourea (CCNU) in the treatment of malignant brain tumors. *J Neurosurg.* 1973;**39**:306–314.

Salmon SE. Nitrosoureas in multiple myeloma. *Cancer Treat Rep.* 1976;**60**(6):789–794.

Selawry OS, Hansen HH. Superiority of CCNU (1-(2-chloroethyl)-3-cyclohexyl-1-nitrosourea; NSC-79037) over BCNU (1,3-bis(2-chloroethyl)-1-nitrosourea; NSC-40962) in treatment of advanced Hodgkin's disease. Acute leukemia group B protocol 6753 report (abstract 182). *Proc Am Assoc Cancer Res.* 1972;**13**:46.

Siemann DW. In vivo combination of misonidazole and the chemotherapeutic agent CCNU. *Br J Cancer.* 1981;**43**:367–377.

Siemann DW. Effect of pretreatment with phenobarbital or SKF 525A on the toxicity and antitumor activity of lomustine. *Cancer Treat Rep.* 1983;**67**:259–265.

Siemann DW, Morrissey S, Wolf K. In vivo potentiation of 1-(2-chloroethyl)-3-cyclohexyl-1-nitrosourea by the radiation sensitizer benznidazole. *Cancer Res.* 1983;**43**:1010–1013.

Silver HKB, Morton DL. CCNU nephrotoxicity following sustained remission in oat cell carcinoma (letter). *Cancer Treat Rep.* 1979;**63**(2):227–228.

Sponzo RW, DeVita VT, Oliverio VT. Physiologic disposition of 1-(2-chloroethyl)-3-cyclohexyl-1-nitrosourea (CCNU) and 1-(2-chloroethyl)-3-(4-methyl cyclohexyl)-1-nitrosourea (McCCNU) in man. *Cancer.* 1973;**31**:1154–1159.

Takita H, Brugarolas A. Effect of CCNU (NSC-79037) on bronchogenic carcinoma. *J Natl Cancer Inst.* 1973;**50**:49–53.

Tew KD, Wang AL. Selective cytotoxicity of haloethyl-nitrosoureas in a carcinoma cell line resistant to bifunctional nitrogen mustards. *Mol Pharmacol.* 1982;**21**:729–738.

Tobey RA, Crissman HA. Comparative effects of three nitrosourea derivatives on mammalian cell cycle progression. *Cancer Res.* 1975;**35**:460–470.

Vats TS, Trueworthy RC, Langston CM. Pulmonary fibrosis associated with lomustine (CCNU): A case report. *Cancer Treat Rep.* 1982;**66**(10):1881–1882.

Wasserman TH, Slavik M, Carter SK. Review of CCNU in clinical cancer therapy. *Cancer Treat Rev.* 1974a;**1**:131–151.

Wasserman TH, Slavik M, Carter SK. Methyl CCNU in clinical cancer therapy. *Cancer Treat Rev.* 1974b;**1**:251–269.

Wasserman TH, Slavik M, Carter SK. Clinical comparison of the nitrosoureas. *Cancer.* 1975;**36**:1258–1268.

Wheeler GP, Alexander JA. Duration of inhibition of synthesis of DNA in tumours and host tissues after single doses of nitrosoureas. *Cancer Res.* 1974;**34**:1957–1964.

Wheeler GP, Bowden BJ. Effects of 1,3-bis(2-chloroethyl)-1-nitrosourea and related compounds upon the synthesis of DNA by cell free systems. *Cancer Res.* 1975;**35**:460–470.

Wheeler GP, Johnston TP, Bowdon BJ, et al. Comparison of the properties of metabolites of CCNU. *Biochem Pharmacol.* 1977;**26**:2331.

Wheeler GP, Schabel FM Jr, Trader MW. Synergistic antileukemic activity of combinations of two nitrosoureas. *Cancer Treat Rep.* 1981;**65**:591–599.

Wilson WB, Perez GM, Kleinschmidt-Demasters BK. Sudden onset of blindness in patients treated with oral CCNU and low-dose cranial irradiation. *Cancer.* 1987;**59**:901–907.

Woolley PV, Dion RL, Kohn KW, et al. Binding of 1-(2-chloroethyl)-3-cyclohexyl-1-nitrosourea to L-1210 cell nuclear proteins. *Cancer Res.* 1976;**36**:1470–1474.

Lonidamine

■ Other Names

Dichlondazolic acid; AF-1890.

■ Chemistry

Structure of lonidamine

Lonidamine is a 1-substituted indazole-3-carboxylic acid which was originally developed as an inhibitor of spermatogenesis. The complete chemical name is 1-(2,4-dichlorobenzyl)-1*H*-indazole-3-carboxylic acid. The compound was synthesized at the Angelini Research Institute, Rome, Italy. Lonidamine has a molecular weight of 321.18 and the empiric formula $C_{15}H_{10}Cl_2N_2O_2$. The compound has poor solubility in organic solvents and in water or alkaline solutions.

■ Antitumor Activity

Lonidamine has only moderate antitumor activity in in vivo murine systems (Silvestrini et al 1983). The table below summarizes the phase II data for lonidamine. As can be seen, there have been hints of antitumor activity for the compound against a number of different histologic types of malignancies; however, no definitive studies have yet indicated lonidamine has a place in the routine treatment of patients. Lonidamine has been shown to reverse doxorubicin resistance in experimental models (Citro et al 1991). A pilot clinical trial reported reversal of epirubicin resistance by lonidamine in adult patients with advanced sarcomas (Lopez et al 1992).

Because lonidamine has an effect on the testis, one patient with a metastatic Leydig cell tumor was treated and reported to have a subjective response to lonidamine (Grem et al 1986).

Breau and colleagues (1988) conducted a randomized study of cisplatin + bleomycin with or without lonidamine versus cisplatin + bleomycin + etoposide with and without lonidamine. The lonidamine arms showed higher response rates but were not *statistically* different. Multiple combinations of lonidamine plus other agents have been tested by Battelli and colleagues (1984). The details of those studies are too voluminous to mention here, and for further details, the reader is referred to their work.

Lonidamine has been combined with radiotherapy in a number of studies. The two can be used safely in combination (Maroun et al 1986a, Robins et al 1988). Privitera and colleagues (1987) conducted a randomized trial of radiotherapy + lonidamine in patients with squamous cell lung cancer. They found a higher response rate and improved survival in patients with stage III disease; however, that analysis was a subset analysis and the results of an ongoing larger multicenter study will be important to confirm those initial findings. A similar study by Magno et al (1987) in patients with head and neck

PHASE II TRIALS WITH LONIDAMINE

Tumor Type	Prior Chemotherapy	Number of Patients Evaluable	Number of Responses Complete	Number of Responses Partial	Reference
Breast	Yes	30	0	5	Band et al 1986
Breast	Yes	25	0	4	Lionetto et al 1988
Renal cell	Yes	25	0	2	Weinerman et al 1986
Non-small cell lung	No	31	0	3	Kokron et al 1984
Small cell lung	Yes	20	0	2	Murray et al 1987
Non-small cell lung	No	29	0	1	Maroun et al 1986b
Melanoma	Yes and no	10	0	2	Clamon et al 1988
Sarcoma	Yes	21	0	1	Wissel et al 1984
Chronic lymphocytic leukemia	Yes and no	19	0	2	Tura et al 1984

cancer also suggests that lonidamine + radiotherapy can produce superior local control ($p = 0.037$) and improved survival ($p = 0.087$).

Finally, Robins and colleagues (1988) conducted a phase I study of lonidamine + hyperthermia. Toxic effects included myalgia and, in one patient, anxiety and depression. Responses were noted in patients with nodular lymphoma, adenocarcinoma of the lung, and adenocarcinoma of the appendix.

■ Mechanism of Action

As noted earlier, lonidamine was originally intended to inhibit spermatogenesis in a variety of mammalian species (Corsi et al 1976). The compound was found to exert that effect by inhibition of germ cell respiration in vitro and in vivo with an effect on aerobic glycolysis. These findings extended over into tumor cells (Floridi et al 1981); however, lonidamine decreased tumor cell aerobic glycolysis as opposed to the increase in aerobic glycolysis seen in rat germ cells. The inhibition of aerobic glycolysis in tumor cells appears to result from the effect of lonidamine on mitochondria-bound hexokinase, which is present at much higher levels on rapidly growing tumor cells than in normal tissue (Pederson 1978).

The drug has recently been shown to release intracellular Ca^{2+} stores in tumor cells by a nonionophoretic mechanism unrelated to ATP depletion (Castiglione et al 1992). Additionally, lonidamine significantly increases antitumor activity when it is combined with hyperthermia or radiation. It is felt lonidamine displays synergism with hyperthermia (particularly under acidic conditions), because hyperthermia makes the mitochondria "susceptible" to the effects of lonidamine (causes condensation of tumor cell mitochondria) (Kim et al 1984, Floridi et al 1983).

Lonidamine also appears to inhibit the recovery of radiation-induced potentially lethal damage (Hahn et al 1984). Lonidamine has also been found to reduce plasma testosterone levels in males, which results in a rise in luteinizing hormones (Evans et al 1984).

■ Availability and Storage

The drug is available as tablets containing 150 mg of lonidamine. Lonidamine should be stored at room temperature.

■ Preparation for Use, Stability, and Admixture

No preparation for use is necessary. Currently, there are no data on the stability of the compound.

■ Administration

The drug is most commonly given daily orally in two divided doses, 12 hours apart (Band et al 1986, Weinerman et al 1986), every day (median duration was 174 days in some studies). Many investigators have used an escalating schedule beginning with 60 mg/m^2 day 1 (total daily use), 120 mg/m^2 day 2, 180 mg/m^2 days 3 to 7, 270 mg/m^2 days 8 to 14, 360 mg/m^2 days 15 to 21, and, if tolerated, 450 mg/m^2 days 22+ (Murray et al 1987). As can be seen from these rather complicated schedules, the precise doses and schedules are still a matter of investigation. Division of the daily dose into two or three doses and a gradual escalation in dose appear to improve the gastrointestinal tolerance and decrease the severity of myalgia and other side effects.

Several authors have used prednisone (5 mg orally twice daily) when moderate or severe myalgias have occurred (Murray et al 1987, Band et al 1986).

■ Special Precautions

None are known at this time.

■ Drug Interactions

Lonidamine has been shown to reverse doxorubicin resistance in experimental systems (Citro et al 1991) and in some patients given the related anthracycline epirubicin (Lopez et al 1992). Reversal of experimental cisplatin resistance by lonidamine is also described (Zaffaroni et al 1992). Cells were exposed to lonidamine following cisplatin. This was associated with enhanced cisplatin accumulation and an increased frequency in cisplatin-induced DNA cross-links (Zaffaroni et al 1992). An additive or synergistic cell kill in MCF-7 breast cancer cells is also described for lonidamine combined with other alkylating agents. These included melphalan, 4-hydroxy-cyclophosphamide, and carmustine (Rosbe et al 1989). Synergy was described for lonidamine exposures concurrent with the alkylating agent and for 12 hours afterward.

■ Dosage

As noted earlier, dosages have been quite variable. In a phase I study Band et al (1984) gave patients doses ranging from 45 to 275 mg/m² twice daily. They noted somnolence, myalgia, headache, and diarrhea. They recommended a dose of 135 mg/m² twice daily.

Young et al (1984) treated patients with doses from 180 to 520 mg/m² for 28 days. They noted myalgia, testicular pain in males, and a reversible ototoxicity. Conjunctivitis and photophobia were also noted. They recommended a dose of 430 mg/m²/d (divided into three doses) as a phase II dose. They too felt gradual escalation of the dose from 100 mg/m² on day 1 to 430 mg/m² on days 4 and 5 kept the muscular discomfort to a minimum.

■ Pharmacokinetics

Somewhat abbreviated studies have been performed describing the pharmacology of lonidamine. Young et al (1984) noted 12-hour trough levels at a dose of 360 mg/m²/d were 3 ± 6 µg/mL. When samples were drawn one and two hours postadministration, serum levels were 15.5 ± 5.1 and 13.5 ± 3.5 µg/mL, respectively. Of note was that even within a patient, the 1- or 2-hour levels were quite variable when measured from day to day.

Besner et al (1984) found the plasma kinetics to be highly variable, indicating a variable first-pass effect. The maximum plasma concentrations ranged from 4.5 to 25 µg/mL. On modeling the data, they felt the pharmacokinetics for the compound best fit an open, two-compartment model with first-order absorption and a lag time. The time for achieving maximal plasma concentration ranged from 0.75 to 10 hours (mean, 3.5 ± 3.3 hours). The distribution half life (α) was 0.37 ± 0.25 hours and the β half-life was 12.1 ± 5.46 hours. More than 70% of the drug was eliminated in the urine after 48 hours in the form of free (7.5%) and conjugated metabolites. These data indicate that hepatic metabolism is mainly responsible for lonidamine elimination. These investigators felt an intravenous form of lonidamine would be an improvement as it would avoid a first-pass effect and likely result in more consistent plasma levels.

Weinerman and colleagues (1986) also noted extremely variable plasma levels in their phase II study, indicating variable absorption of lonidamine from patient to patient.

■ Side Effects and Toxicity

Lonidamine administration has not been associated with myelosuppression or stomatitis. The most common toxic effect has been myalgias (made somewhat better by prednisone 5 mg PO twice daily). Other toxic effects have included nausea and vomiting, testicular pain (severe enough to cause discontinuation in some patients), somnolence, fatigue, hyperesthesias, alopecia, diarrhea, apathy, conjunctivitis, photophobia, headache, dizziness, chills and fever (up to 39°C), and moderate alopecia. Decreased hearing on audiometry has also been noted (Wissel et al 1984).

Very uncommon toxic effects include mastalgia, ataxia, tremor, scotomata, precordial discomfort (probably a form of myalgias), urinary frequency, decreased libido, hot flashes, and arthritis (Weinerman et al 1986, Band et al 1984, 1986, Murray et al 1987, Clamon et al 1988, Kokron et al 1984, Battelli et al 1984).

Santiemma and colleagues (1984) have found that when lonidamine is given to males, the serum follicle-stimulating and luteinizing hormone levels are significantly higher as compared with pretreatment values, whereas levels of testosterone, prolactin, and thyroid-stimulating hormone levels remain unchanged.

■ Special Applications

Please see the data under Antitumor Activity regarding the use of lonidamine in conjunction with radiation therapy and hyperthermia.

REFERENCES

Band PR, Deschamps M, Besner JG, Leclaire R, Gervais P, De Sanctis A. Phase I toxicologic study of lonidamine in cancer patients. *Oncology*. 1984;**41**(suppl 1):56–59.

Band PR, Maroun J, Pritchard K, et al. Phase II study of lonidamine in patients with metastatic breast cancer: A National Cancer Institute of Canada Clinical Trials Group Study. *Cancer Treat Rep*. 1986;**70**:1305–1310.

Battelli T, Manocchi P, Guistini L, et al. A long term clinical experience with lonidamine. *Oncology*. 1984;**41**(1):39–47.

Besner J-G, Leclaire R, Band PR, Deschamps M, De Sanctis AJ, Catanese B. Pharmacokinetics of lonidamine after oral administration in cancer patients. *Oncology*. 1984;**41**:48–52.

Breau JL, Morere JF, Israel L. Chemotherapy with or without lonidamine for induction therapy in squamous cell carcinoma of the lung. A randomized study comparing cisplatinum–bleomycin or cisplatinum–bleomycin–VP16 213 (± lonidamine). *Proc Am Soc Clin Oncol*. 1988;**7**:212.

Castiglione S, Floridi A, Fiskum G. Lonidamine releases intracellular Ca^{2+} stores from tumor cells by a non-ionophorectic mechanism. *Proc Am Assoc Cancer Res.* 1992;**33**(abstr):A2515.

Citro G, Cucco C, Verdina A, et al. Reversal of Adriamycin resistance by lonidamine in a human breast cancer cell line. *Br J Cancer.* 1991;**64**:534–536.

Clamon G, Traves M, Bowen K. Activity of lonidamine in metastatic melanoma: A phase II trial. *Proc Am Soc Clin Oncol.* 1988;**7**:251.

Corsi G, Palazzo G, Germani C, Scorza Barcellona P, Silvestrini B. 1-Halobenzyl-1H-indazol-3-carboxylic acid. A new class of anti-spermatogenic agents. *J Med Chem.* 1976;**19**:778–782.

Evans WK, Shepard FK, Mullis B. Phase II evaluation of lonidamine in patients with advanced malignancy. *Oncology.* 1984;**41**(1):69–77.

Floridi A, Lehningher A. Action of the antitumor and anti-spermatogenic agent lonidamine on electron transport in Ehrlich ascites tumor mitochondria. *Arch Biochem Biophys.* 1983;**226**:73–83.

Floridi A, Paggi MG, D'Atri S, et al. Effect of lonidamine on the energy metabolism of Ehrlich ascites tumor cells. *Cancer Res.* 1981;**41**:4661–4666.

Grem JL, Robins HI, Wilson KS, Gilchrist K, Trump DL. Metastatic Leydig cell tumor of the testis. *Cancer.* 1986;**58**:2116–2119.

Hahn GM, Van Kersen I, Silvestrini B. Inhibition of the recovery from potentially lethal damage by lonidamine. *Br J Cancer.* 1984;**50**:657–660.

Kim JH, Kim S, Alfieri A, Young CW, Silvestrini B. Lonidamine: A hyperthermic sensitizer of HeLa cells in culture and of the Meth-A-tumor in vivo. *Oncology.* 1984;**41**(1):30–35.

Kokron O, Maca S, Scheiner W, DeGregorio M, Ciottoli GB. Phase II study of lonidamine in inoperable non-small cell lung cancer. *Oncology.* 1984;**41**:86–89.

Lionetto R, Pronzato P, Cusimano MP, et al. Phase II trial of lonidamine in advanced breast cancer. *Proc Am Soc Clin Oncol.* 1988;**7**:20.

Lopez M, Carpeno S, D'Aprile M, et al. High-dose epirubicin (HD-EPI) ± lonidamine (LND) in adult patients with advanced sarcomas. *Proc Am Soc Clin Oncol.* 1992;**11**:414.

Magno L, Terraneo F, Scandolaro L, Bertoni F, DeGregorio M, Ciottoli GB. Lonidamine (L) and radiotherapy in head and neck cancer: A preliminary report. *Proc Am Soc Clin Oncol.* 1987;**6**:126.

Maroun JA, Danjoux C, Stewart DJ, et al. Phase I study of lonidamine (LND) used as a radio-potentiator in limited disease non-small cell lung cancer (NSCLC). *Proc Am Assoc Clin Res.* 1986a;**27**:180.

Maroun JA, Stewart DJ, Young V, Band P. Phase II study of lonidamine (NDL) in non-small cell lung cancer (NSCLC). *Proc Am Soc Clin Oncol.* 1986b;**5**:182.

Murray N, Shah A, Band P. Phase II study of lonidamine in patients with small cell carcinoma of the lung. *Cancer Treat Rep.* 1987;**71**:1283–1284.

Pederson PL. Tumor mitochondria and bioenergetics of cancer cells. *Prog Exp Tumor Res.* 1978;**22**:190–274.

Privitera G, Ciottoli GB, Patane C, et al. Phase II double-blind randomized study of lonidamine and radiotherapy in epidermoid carcinoma of the lung. *Radiother Oncol.* 1987;**10**:285–290.

Robins HI, Longo WL, Lagoni RK, et al. Phase I trial of lonidamine with whole body hyperthermia in advanced cancer. *Cancer Res.* 1988;**48**:6587–6592.

Rosbe KW, Brann TW, Holden SA, et al. Effect of lonidamine on the cytotoxicity of four alkylating agents in vitro. *Cancer Chemother Pharmacol.* 1989;**25**:32–36.

Santiemma V, Tullio G, Iapadre G, Fabbrini A. Effects of lonidamine on pituitary-gonadal axis in man. *Oncology.* 1984;**41**:53–55.

Silvestrini B, Hahn GM, Cioli V, et al. Effects of lonidamine alone or combined with hyperthermia is some experimental cell and tumor systems. *Br J Cancer.* 1983;**47**:221–231.

Tura S, Cavo M, Gobbi M, Franchi P. Lonidamine in the treatment of chronic lymphoid leukemia. *Oncology.* 1984;**41**:90–93.

Weinerman BH, Eisenhauer EA, Besner JG, Coppin CM, Stewart D, and Band PR. Phase II study of lonidamine in patients with metastatic renal cell carcinoma: A National Cancer Institute of Canada Clinical Trials Group Study. *Cancer Treat Rep.* 1986;**70**:751–754.

Wissel P, Magill G, Welt S, O'Hehir M, Sordillo P, Currie V. Phase II trial of lonidamine (1,-2,4-dichlorophenyl)-1H-indazol-3-carboxylic acid) (LON) in advanced soft tissue sarcomas. *Proc Am Soc Clin Oncol.* 1984;**3**:258.

Young CW, Currie VE, Kim JH, O'Hehir MA, Farag FM Kinahan JE. Phase I and clinical pharmacologic evaluation of lonidamine in patients with advanced cancer. *Oncology.* 1984;**41**(suppl 1):60–65.

Zaffaroni N, Silvestrini R, Villa R, et al. Reversal of cisplatin resistance by lonidamine in human ovarian carcinoma cells. *Proc Am Assoc Cancer Res.* 1992;**33**:486.

Maytansine

Other Names

Maitansine; NSC-153858.

Chemistry

Structure of maytansine

Maytansine is a naturally occurring ansa macrolide isolated by Kupchan et al (1972) from the wood or bark of the African shrub *Maytenus ovatus*. It belongs to the ansamycin class of antibiotics, which have large complex structural formulas consisting of an aromatic nucleus attached at two nonadjacent ring carbons to a macrocyclic aliphatic bridge. Three functional or unique side groups include an aryl chloride, an epoxide, and a carbonolamine. The empiric formula is $C_{34}H_{46}ClN_3O_{10}$. It has some structural similarity to the vinca alkaloids vincristine and vinblastine. Maytansine has a molecular weight of 692.21. A review article summarizing the preclinical and clinical data on maytansine was published by Issell and Crooke (1978).

Antitumor Activity

Experimentally, maytansine showed significant activity against a variety of animal tumors including B-16 melanoma and P-388 lymphocytic leukemia. It was inactive against a vincristine-resistant leukemia (Sieber et al 1976). Unfortunately, maytansine was not highly active in human cancers.

In limited phase I human studies, responses have been noted in patients with acute lymphocytic leukemia (including two vincristine-resistant patients), non-Hodgkin's lymphoma and ovarian carcinoma (Chabner et al 1978, Chahinian et al 1979), advanced breast carcinoma (Blum and Kahlert 1978, Cabanillas et al 1978), thymoma (Chahinian et al 1979, Jaffrey et al 1980), as well as in a few other solid tumor patients (Cabanillas et al 1978.) In phase II studies Eagen et al (1978a) described very limited activity for maytansine in patients with metastatic lung cancer, and O'Connell et al (1978) were unable to detect any significant drug activity in patients with advanced colorectal carcinoma. Creagan et al (1979) found the drug inactive against head and neck cancer. The drug was also inactive against refractory childhood acute lymphocytic leukemia (Sabio et al 1983), melanoma (Ahmann et al 1980), small cell lung cancer (Creech et al 1982), pancreatic cancer (Gastrointestinal Tumor Study Group 1985), cervical cancer (Thigpen et al 1983a), sarcomas (Edmonson et al 1983, Borden et al 1982), ovarian cancer (Thigpen et al 1983b) non-Hodgkin's lymphoma (Ratanatharathorn et al 1982, Rosenthal et al 1980), and breast cancer (Edmonson et al 1981, Neidhart et al 1980). Other phase II studies in a variety of different tumors were also disappointing (Ravry et al 1985).

Mechanism of Action

Maytansine has both structural and mechanistic similarities to the vinca alkaloids. Cytotoxic activity appears to relate to polymerization of tubulin and, thus, inhibition of proper formation of the mitotic spindle (Wolpert-DeFilippes et al 1975, Remillard et al 1975). This produces a blockade of the cell cycle in late G_2 phase or early M phase (metaphase arrest). In these respects, the action is similar to that of vincristine but is irreversible. Maytansine also appears to be more avidly bound than vincristine and perhaps occupies an additional tubulin binding site (Mandelbaum-Shavit et al 1976).

Rao et al (1979) confirmed that maytansine is a potent mitotic inhibitor, producing the greatest effects in G_2 phase cells, the least in G_1. No effects on macromolecular synthesis were noted.

Availability and Storage

Maytansine was previously available as an investigational agent from the National Cancer Institute as a lyophilized white powder in 10-mL vials containing 0.25 mg maytansine and 100 mg mannitol. The vials should be stored under refrigerated temperatures (2–8°C) (Helman et al 1976).

■ Preparation for Use, Stability, and Admixture

Initially, the vials are reconstituted with 4.9 mL of Sterile Water for Injection, USP, 5% Dextrose, USP, or Normal Saline, USP. Each milliliter of solution will then contain 0.05 mg maytansine and 20 mg mannitol.

A solution of 0.01 to 0.05 mg/mL maytansine is chemically stable for at least 4 days in room light and temperature or at refrigerated temperatures. Reconstituted solutions, however, should optimally be used within 8 hours as no preservative is included in the lyophilized preparation.

■ Administration

Maytansine may be given as a slow intravenous push in 50 mL of diluent through a running (new) intravenous line. Alternatively, a new, small-vein intravenous site may be started and the drug given as a slow intravenous push with a flush of 10 mL D5W or normal saline before administration (to test vein patency) and another flush afterward to clear the vein and tubing. Extravasation of this drug can produce necrosis. Mild inflammation, fibrosis, and edema have been noted after subcutaneous administration of maytansine in animals. Cabanillas et al (1978) noted that a superficial phlebitis could be eliminated if more than a 250-mL dilution volume were used: they recommend 250- to 500-mL dilution volumes. In contrast Blum and Kahlert (1978) recommend a careful bolus injection, which in their population also reduced phlebitis. This may be preferred as it would eliminate the possibility of extravasating an unattended infusion.

■ Special Precautions

This drug should not be used concomitantly with a vinca alkaloid such as vincristine or vinblastine because of the potential for overlapping neurotoxicity. Patients are poor candidates for full-dose maytansine if liver function is abnormal. Dosage reduction is required if the serum bilirubin, alkaline phosphate, serum glutamic–oxalacetic transaminase, lactic dehydrogenase, or prothrombin level is significantly elevated. Specific dose reduction guidelines are not available.

Eagen et al (1978a) have described apparently cumulative neurotoxicity including severe constipation and peripheral neuropathy. These effects were relatively unresponsive to dosage reduction or discontinuance, respectively.

■ Drug Interactions

Rao et al (1979) suggested that antitumor synergy may be possible if maytansine is given after a cell cycle-synchronizing course of an S-phase antimetabolite. They were able to demonstrate this when maytansine was administered to HeLa cells following cytarabine exposure. No cycle-dependent effects were noted when maytansine was combined with doxorubicin.

■ Dosage

The optimal dosing regimen of maytansine is not currently known. Chabner et al (1978) recommended initial doses for phase II studies of 1.6 to 2.0 mg/m^2 given every 3 weeks. For a consecutive 3-day regimen Cabanillas et al (1978) recommend 0.5 mg/m^2/d × 3.

Chahinian et al (1979) used a weekly dose and recommended 1 mg/m^2/wk by intravenous bolus × 6 weeks. In their study neurotoxicity was dose limiting. Similar findings were noted by Franklin et al (1980) in their phase I study with the same schedule.

■ Pharmacokinetics

To date pharmacokinetics studies have not been reported with maytansine.

■ Side Effects and Toxicity

Toxicity in human studies has generally been gastrointestinal, hepatic, and neurologic (at high doses). Chabner et al (1978) noted that nausea, vomiting, diarrhea, and profound lethargy were dose limiting after a single injection of 2 mg/m^2. These symptoms persisted for up to 2 weeks after drug administration. With a 5-day regimen, dose-related nausea and vomiting were seen on days 3 to 10, and diarrhea was noted on days 3 to 7 along with transiently elevated serum glutamic–oxalacetic transaminase (Blum and Kahlert 1978). With higher doses, neurotoxicity similar to vincristine axonal neurotoxicity has occurred. Symptoms included paresthesias, jaw pain, loss of deep tendon reflexes, and distal extremity weakness. Blum and Kahlert also found that patients with pretreatment vinca alkaloid neuropathy were at substantially greater risk of developing serious maytansine neurotoxicity.

Gastrointestinal toxicity seems to predominate at most dosage levels employed. Nausea, vomiting, severe cramps, and diarrhea (Eagen et al 1978b) leading to dehydration appear to be the common dose-limiting toxic effects in humans. Stomatitis has been reported along with alopecia and a superficial phlebitis at the injection site (Cabanillas et al 1978). Some mild hepatic dysfunction has been described with maytansine (Cabanillas et al 1978, Blum and Kahlert 1978).

■ Special Applications

None are known.

REFERENCES

Ahmann DL, Frytak S, Kvols LK, et al. Phase II study of maytansine and chlorozotocin in patients with disseminated malignant melanoma. *Cancer Treat Rep.* 1980; **64**(4/5):721–723.

Blum RH, Kahlert J. Maytansine: A phase I study of an ansa macrolide with antitumor activity. *Cancer Treat Rep.* 1978;**62**(3):435–438.

Borden EC, Ash A, Enterline HT, et al. Phase II evaluation of dibromodulcitol, ICRF-159, and maytansine for sarcomas. *Am J Clin Oncol.* 1982;**5**(4):417–420.

Cabanillas F, Rodriguez V, Hall S, Burgen MA, Bodej BE, Freireich EJ. Phase I study of maytansine using a 3-day schedule. *Cancer Treat Rep.* 1978;**62**(3):425–428.

Chabner BA, Levine AS, Johnson BL, Young RC. Initial clinical trials of maytansine, an antitumor plant alkaloid. *Cancer Treat Rep.* 1978;**62**(3):429–433.

Chahinian AP, Nogeire C, Ohnuma T, et al. Phase I study of weekly maytansine given by IV bolus or 24-hour infusion. *Cancer Treat Rep.* 1979;**63**:1953–1960.

Creagan ET, Fleming TR, Edmonson JH, Ingle JN. Phase II evaluation of maytansine in patients with advanced head and neck cancer. *Cancer Treat Rep.* 1979;**63**(11/12):2061.

Creech RH, Stanley K, Vogl SE, Ettinger DS, Bonami PD, Salazar O. Phase II study of cisplatin, maytansine and chlorozotocin, in small cell lung carcinoma. *Cancer Res Rep.* 1982;**6**:1417–1419.

Eagan RT, Creagan ET, Ingle JN, Frytalk S, Rubin R. Phase II evaluation of maytansine in patients with metastatic lung cancer. *Cancer Treat Rep.* 1978a;**62**(10):1577–1579.

Eagan RT, Ingle JN, Rubin J, Frytalk S, Moertel CG. Early clinical study of an intermittent schedule for maytansine (NSL-153858). *J Natl Cancer Inst.* 1978b;**60**:93–96.

Edmonson JH, Hahn RG, Creasan ET, O'Connell MJ. Phase II study of maytansine in advanced sarcomas. *Cancer Treat Rep.* 1983;**67**(4):401–402.

Edmonson JH, Rubin J, Kvols LK, O'Connell MJ, Frytalk S, Green SJ. Phase II study of maytansine in advanced breast cancer (letter). *Cancer Treat Rep.* 1981;**65**(5/6):536–537.

Franklin R, Samson MK, Fraile RJ, Abu-Zahra H, O'Bryan R, Baker LH. A phase III study of maytansine utilizing a weekly schedule. *Cancer.* 1980;**46**(5):1104–1108.

Gastrointestinal Tumor Study Group. Phase II trials of maytansine, low-dose chlorozotocin, and high-dose chlorozotocin as single agents against advanced measurable adenocarcinoma of the pancreas. *Cancer Treat Rep.* 1985;**69**(4):417–420.

Helman L, Henney J, Slavik M. *Maytansine (NSC-153858): Clinical Brochure,* Bethesda, MD: National Cancer Institute; 1976.

Issell CB, Crooke T. Maytansine. *Cancer Treat Rev.* 1978;**5**:199–207.

Jaffrey IS, Denefrio JM, Chahinian P. Response to maytansine in a patient with malignant thymoma (letter). *Cancer Treat Rep.* 1980;**64**(1):193–194.

Kupchan SM, Komoda Y, Court WA. Maytansine, a novel antileukemia ansa macrolide from *Maytensus ovatus.* *J Am Chem Soc.* 1972;**94**:1354–1356.

Mandelbaum-Shavit F, Wolpert-DeFilippes MK, Johns DG. Binding of maytansine to rat brain tubulin. *Biochem Biophys Res Commun.* 1976;**72**:47–54.

Neidhart JA, Laufman LR, Vaughn C, McCracken JD. Minimal single-agent activity of maytansine in refractory breast cancer: A Southwest Oncology Group study. *Cancer Treat Rep.* 1980;**64**(4/5):675–677.

O'Connell MJ, Shani A, Rubin J, Moertel CG. Phase II trial of maytansine in patients with advanced colorectal carcinoma. *Cancer Treat Rep.* 1978;**62**(8):1237–1238.

Rao RN, Freireich EJ, Smith ML, Loo TL. Cell cycle phase-specific cytotoxicity of the antitumor agent maytansine (abstract). *Proc Am Assoc Cancer Res ASCO.* 1979;**20**:42.

Ratanatharathorn V, Gad-el-Mawla N, Wilson HE, Bonnet JD, Rivkin SE, Mass R. Phase II evaluation of maytansine in refractory non-Hodgkin's lymphoma: A Southwest Oncology Group study. *Cancer Treat Rep.* 1982;**66**(7):1687–1688.

Ravry MJ, Omura GA, Birch R. Phase II evaluation of maytansine (NSC-153858) in advanced cancer. A Southeastern Cancer Study Group trial. *Am J Clin Oncol.* 1985;**8**(2):148–150.

Remillard S, Rebhun LI, Howie GA, Kupchan M. Antimitotic activity of the potent tumor inhibitor maytansine. *Science.* 1975;**189**:1002–1005.

Rosenthal S, Harris DT, Horton J, Glick JH. Phase II study of maytansine in patients with advanced lymphomas: An Eastern Cooperative Oncology Group pilot study. *Cancer Treat Rep.* 1980;**64**(10/11):1115–1117.

Sabio H, Frankel L, Sexauer C, Falletta J, Kim TH. Maytansine in refractory childhood acute lymphocytic leukemia: A Pediatric Oncology Group study. *Cancer Treat Rep.* 1983;**67**(11):1045.

Sieber SM, Wolpert MK, Adamson RH, Cysykrl BVH,

Johns DG. Experimental studies with maytansine—A new antitumor agent. *Bibl Haematol.* 1976;**43**:495–500.

Thigpen JT, Ehrlich CE, Conroy J, Blessing JA. Phase II study of maytansine in the treatment of advanced or recurrent squamous cell carcinoma of the cervix. A Gynecologic Oncology Group study. *Am J Clin Oncol.* 1983a;**6**(4):427–430.

Thigpen JT, Ehrlich CE, Creasman WT, Curry S, Blessing JA. Phase II study of maytansine in the treatment of advanced or recurrent adenocarcinoma of the ovary. A Gynecologic Oncology Group study. *Am J Clin Oncol.* 1983b; 6(3):273–275.

Wolpert-DeFilippes MK, Adamson RH, Cysyk RL, Johns DG. Initial studies on the cytotoxic action of maytansine, a novel ansa macrolide. *Biochem Pharmacol.* 1975;**24**:751–753.

Mechlorethamine Hydrochloride

■ Other Names

NSC-762; Mustargen® (Merck & Company); nitrogen mustard; HN2.

■ Chemistry

$$CH_3-N \begin{cases} CH_2CH_2Cl \\ CH_2CH_2Cl \end{cases}$$

Structure of mechlorethamine hydrochloride

Mechlorethamine hydrochloride is an analogue of mustard gas. It has the chemical name 2,2′-dichloro-N-methyldiethylamine hydrochloride. It is very soluble in both water and alcohol. As a powder it occurs as a hygroscopic white crystalline solid. The molecular weight is 192.52, and the empiric formula is $C_5H_{11}Cl_2N \cdot HCl$. An aqueous solution has a pH between 3.0 and 5.0.

■ Antitumor Activity

Mechlorethamine is an alkylating agent derived from toxic gas warfare research (Krumbhaar and Krumbhaar 1919). Gilman and Philips (1946) noted dissolution of lymphoid tissue by nitrogen mustard and followed with positive studies on transplanted lymphosarcoma in mice. The first clinical trials took place in the early 1940s (Goodman et al 1946, Gilman 1963).

The major indication for mechlorethamine is the combination chemotherapy of Hodgkin's and non-Hodgkin's lymphomas (Nicholson et al 1970), most notably in the MOPP regimen (with oncovin, procarbazine, and prednisone) (DeVita et al 1970). Bronchogenic carcinoma has also been responsive to the drug (Green et al 1969).

Intracavitary mechlorethamine is often effective as a sclerosing chemotherapeutic agent to control pleural and other malignant effusions (Weisberger 1958, Fracchia et al 1970, Dollinger 1972, Levison 1961, Kinsey et al 1964).

The topical application of mechlorethamine investigationally has been useful in managing psoriasis (Zackheim et al 1972) and the diffuse skin lesions produced by the cutaneous lymphoma mycosis fungoides (Van Scott and Kalmanson 1973). Skin lesions from chronic granulocytic leukemia have also been treated with topical mechlorethamine ointment (Murphy et al 1985).

■ Mechanism of Action

Mechlorethamine is the prototypical bifunctional alkylating agent. The spectrum of biologic activity of this agent includes cytolytic, mutagenic, and radiomimetic actions. The basic process of alkylation involves the chemical attachment of an alkyl group to important cell nucleophiles such as phosphate, amino, hydroxyl, sulfhydryl, carboxyl, and imidazole groups (Wheeler 1962, Warwick 1963). The nitrogen and oxygen heteroatoms in DNA bases are good nucleophiles for this type of covalent bond formation.

In neutral or alkaline solution the mustard molecule ionizes to a positively charged nitrogen, an aziridine intermediate. This unstable intermediate rapidly rearranges to yield a positively charged carbonium ion. This ion can then attach to susceptible nucleic acids, specifically at the N-7 position of the DNA nucleoside guanine. Recent evidence suggests that linking occurs preferentially at strand positions where one guanine is separated from cytosine by one nucleotide (Walton et al 1991). The cytotoxic result of this interaction can be fourfold: (1) abnormal base pairing of guanine with thymine, causing DNA miscoding; (2) cleavage of the imidazole ring of guanine; (3) cross-linking of DNA by guanine–guanine pairs; and (4) depurination of DNA, causing single-strand breakage (Salmon and Apple 1972). The ultimate outcome of any of these reactions is lethal to the cell. In addition to these actions on DNA, other cellular processes are also inhibited. These include glycolysis, respiration, protein (RNA-directed) synthesis, and other membrane and metabolic processes (Karnofsky and Clarkson 1963). Of these various effects, DNA crosslinking is felt to constitute the predominant cytotoxic lesion. This blocks the ability of DNA to act as a template for DNA and RNA synthesis at concentrations of 5 and 10 µM, respectively (Johnson and Ruddov 1967). At higher concentrations (≥ 1 mM), numerous other biochemical lesions are produced including inhibition of protein synthesis, DNA polymerase activity, and RNA polymerase activity (Johnson and Ruddov 1967).

The cytotoxic effects of polyfunctional agents such as mechlorethamine have not been shown to be cell cycle phase specific, although cytotoxicity is significantly greater in rapidly growing cell populations.

Tumor cell lines resistant to mechlorethamine often express high levels of glutathione (GSH) and related GSH transferase enzymes (Wang and Tew 1985). These enzymes are also inducible in normal tissues following exposure to electrophilic drugs such as mechlorethamine.

■ Availability and Storage

Mechlorethamine hydrochloride is commercially available (Mustargen®, Merck & Company, West Point, Pennsylvania) as a triturate in glass vials containing 10 mg of drug with 90 mg of anhydrous sodium chloride. The undiluted vials may be stored at room temperature.

■ Preparation for Use, Stability, and Admixture

When the contents of a 10-mg vial are diluted with 10 mL of Sterile Water for Injection, USP (without preservatives), the final concentration is 1 mg/mL. The manufacturer states that the drug should be diluted immediately before administration. Other data indicate that mechlorethamine may be stable in solution for longer periods. Until confirmatory studies are completed, it is advisable to use the drug within at least an hour of mixing, although the manufacturer reports only 15 minutes of stability after reconstitution. Also, the drug is known to be more unstable in neutral and alkaline than in acidic solutions. Mechlorethamine was shown to be physically stable for 4 hours with a 1 mg/mL solution of ondansetron (Trissel et al 1990).

Note: Mechlorethamine is a powerful vesicant and should be prepared and administered with great care. The use of rubber gloves, mask, and splash protection is recommended when handling this drug. Extreme caution should be used to avoid inhalation of dust or vapors or contact with the skin or mucous membranes, especially the eyes. See Special Precautions for treatment.

■ Administration

Mechlorethamine hydrochloride is administered by intravenous push. The drug may be given directly in a suitable vein if the "double-needle technique" is used (the use of one syringe needle for reconstitution and direct venipuncture, respectively); however, the preferable means of administering the drug is by slow injection through a side port of an established intravenous line. Venous patency should be confirmed by flushing the vein with a small volume of D5W or normal saline before drug administration. Mechlorethamine should be carefully injected with care to check for blood return before, during, and after injection. The intravenous line should then again be flushed with a small volume of normal saline or D5W to wash in any residual drug from the tubing and proximal vein lumen.

Dilution of mechlorethamine in a large volume of intravenous solution for administration is not recommended because a certain number of patients become sensitized. In these instances, the mechlorethamine injection may be preceded by an intravenous corticosteroid such as 100 to 200 mg of hydrocortisone sodium succinate (Solu-Cortef®). The mechlorethamine dose is then given by intravenous push through a running intravenous infusion. The infusion may be continued after injection so that a total of 150 to 250 mL of D5W or normal saline is delivered.

Direct drug contact by the person administering mechlorethamine should be avoided. Rubber gloves should be used in case any leakage occurs. If the drug accidentally comes in contact with the skin or mucous membranes, the procedure under Special Precautions should be followed.

(For intracavitary, topical, and intralesional administration, see Special Applications.)

■ Dosage

The dose of mechlorethamine will vary with each clinical situation but a typical intravenous dose is 0.4 mg/kg given as a single dose or four separate (0.1 mg/kg) injections on successive days. With higher doses of up to 0.8 mg/kg, significant leukopenia and thrombocytopenia may result. Usually, dosing can be repeated at 4- to 6-week intervals if appropriate bone marrow recovery has been demonstrated.

In the classic MOPP regimen for Hodgkin's lymphoma, DeVita et al (1970) recommended intravenous injections of 6.0 mg/m^2 on days 1 and 8 of a 14-day combination drug program. There are numerous modifications of this original regimen.

For intracavitary applications mechlorethamine doses of 0.2 to 0.4 mg/kg have been reported (0.2 mg/kg for pericardial applications). In controlling pleural effusions, Fracchia et al (1970) suggested that 15 to 20 mg is the optimal dose; however, Anderson et al (1974) and Leininger et al (1969) successfully used doses up to 30 mg (based on the 0.4 mg/kg basis). Because systemic toxicity is a definite hazard with intracavitary dosing, appropriate dose reduction in hematologically compromised patients is required.

■ Drug Interactions

Glutathione-depleting agents can increase the alkylating activity of nitrogen mustard in experimental settings. This has been demonstrated for diethylmaleate and misonidazole in mouse sarcoma tumors in vivo (Murray and Meyn 1984). Similar effects might be anticipated with buthionine sulfoximine.

■ Special Precautions

Extravasation. Mechlorethamine hydrochloride is a powerful vesicant. If any of the drug comes in contact with the skin or mucous membrane, the area should initially be flushed with large amounts of water. The remaining mechlorethamine can be neutralized by applying a 1/6 M sodium thiosulfate solution to the area (preparation of this solution is described next). Sodium thiosulfate also blocks the systemic toxic effects of mechlorethamine (Bonadonna and Karnofsky 1965) with the exception of central nervous system toxic effects.

If extravasation of the drug into tissues surrounding the intravenous site occurs, the area will usually become initially indurated with eventual sloughing of necrotic tissue. If the infiltrate is observed promptly, a solution of sodium thiosulfate, 1/6 M, can be instilled in the area purportedly to neutralize a large portion of the active drug. A recent animal study suggests that thiosulfate should be injected locally in a 200:1 molar excess (thiosulfate:mechlorethamine hydrochloride on a milligram basis). Thus, for an extravasation of 1 mg mechlorethamine hydrochloride, at least 2 mL of the 10% thiosulfate solution should be used (Dorr et al 1988). Treatment should be rapid as delayed thiosulfate was ineffective in the mouse skin model (Dorr et al 1988). Despite this experimental finding, the delayed use of intramuscular thiosulfate was apparently effective in one case involving accidental intramuscular injection of mechlorethamine hydrochloride (Owen et al 1980).

Preparation of Sodium Thiosulfate 1/6 Solution. This solution may be prepared most conveniently by diluting 4 mL Sodium Thiosulfate Injection, USP (10%), with 6 mL of Sterile Water for Injection, USP. Alternatively, 4.14 g reagent-grade sodium thiosulfate (Na$_2$S$_2$O$_3$·5H$_2$O) or 2.64 g anhydrous sodium thiosulfate/100 mL may be used. Speed is essential in the use of thiosulfate for mechlorethamine infiltration.

The manufacturer has recommended that for the safety of those handling the equipment used in preparing and injecting mechlorethamine, this equipment (needles, gloves, syringes, etc) be soaked for 45 minutes in 10% thiosulfate before discarding.

Pharmacokinetics. The pharmacokinetics of mechlorethamine has not been studied. When diluted in water or body fluids, mechlorethamine undergoes chemical transformation to the highly reactive electrophilic ethylenimonium derivative. This active form reacts rapidly with various cellular components so the active drug is no longer present in the blood within minutes of administration. Thus, rapid drug disappearance may make it possible to protect tissues by blocking their blood supply for a few minutes. Also, a localizing effect may be obtained by injecting the drug directly into the arterial blood supply of the tumor to be treated.

Less than 0.01% of the active drug is recovered in the urine. This is understandable because the drug is chemically altered very rapidly after injection; however, more than 50% of the inactive metabolites are excreted in the urine in the first 24 hours.

Side Effects and Toxicity. Myelosuppression is the principal dose-limiting toxic effect of mechlorethamine. Granulocytes and platelets decline in 8 to 14 days. Fortunately, the granulocytopenia and thrombocytopenia typically last 10 to 20 days. Erythrocyte depression is usually not significant, although persistent pancytopenia has been reported rarely. Severe thrombocytopenia may occasionally lead to overt clinical bleeding noted by petechiae, subcutaneous hemorrhages, and bleeding from the gums and gastrointestinal tract. As with other cytotoxic drugs, patients who have had prior antineoplastic therapy or radiation are prone to have more severe bone marrow depression.

Thrombosis or thrombophlebitis may occur when the drug comes in direct contact with the intima of the vein used for injection. Thus, severe phlebitis sometimes occurs despite all precautions, and this has often become a dose-limiting factor in some patients. Extravasation produces pain, swelling, erythema, induration, and eventual tissue sloughing. Again, these conditions should be treated with sodium thiosulfate and cold compresses as described under Special Precautions.

Nausea and vomiting occur in over 90% of patients treated with mechlorethamine, usually within the first 3 hours. Rarely, the onset is delayed for up to 8 hours. Severe vomiting generally does not persist longer than 8 hours. Anorexia, nausea, and vomiting may be controlled by aggressive antiemetic therapy or prophylaxis with combination regimens. Other reported gastrointestinal side effects include a metallic taste just after drug injection and diarrhea for up to several days after administration.

An apparent idiosyncratic maculopapular skin eruption also infrequently occurs. This reaction does not necessarily recur after subsequent injections and generally does not contraindicate further therapy.

Amenorrhea in the female and impaired spermatogenesis in the male should be anticipated.

Other adverse reactions include weakness, drowsiness, fever, and headache after drug administration. Tinnitus, deafness, and temporary aphasia and paresis have also been reported. Severe cerebral toxicity is reported after intravenous dosing (Bethlenfalvay and Bergin 1972). In this case, hyperpyrexia and coma were related to acute internal hydrocephalus which responded to ventricular decompression. The chemical similarity of mechlorethamine to choline, a neurotransmitter precursor, may explain this uncommon event. With intracarotid therapy, however, central nervous system toxic effects become much more common and severe (French et al 1952). Severe allergic reactions and analphylaxis are rare but have been continuously reported in the literature since the drug was commercially released.

Even though nitrogen mustard has been used without teratogenic effects in pregnancy (Deuschle and Wiggans 1953), the potential for such effects on the fetus is high and, therefore, routine use during pregnancy should not be considered.

■ Special Applications

Intracavitary Administration. Mechlorethamine has been administered by intracavitary injection to control malignant pleural, peritoneal, and pericardial effusions. This technique should obviously not be used when the fluid is chylous in nature. The technique most often involves prior removal of excess fluid from the cavity before drug instillation. The dose recommended for these procedures is 0.2 to 0.4 mg/kg (10 to 30 mg) (Anderson et al 1974). The drug has been instilled as the 1 mg/mL concentration by some and further diluted to 50 or 100 mL in normal saline by others. During drug instillation, it is important that the fluid flow freely to ensure adequate intracavitary drug distribution. Frequent aspiration, observing easy fluid return, should be done during injections. This will help ensure that the drug has been instilled. The patient's postural position should be changed frequently (every 5 to 10 minutes) to allow maximum distribution of the drug in the cavity.

After drug instillation, the fluid cavity should be drained at 12 to 24 hours and daily for several days thereafter. Although intracavity treatment is effective in malignant effusions (eg, those with tumor cells present), it may also be effective for effusions without tumor cells, presumably because of the local inflammatory reactions to the drug which obliterate the space and thereby prevent fluid recurrence.

Pain is the primary local adverse effect and prior administration of analgesics is required. Because intrapericardial injection of mechlorethamine may cause transient cardiac irregularities, continuous monitoring of the electrocardiogram during the procedure is highly recommended.

Systemic absorption after intracavitary injection is unpredictable but probably not complete because of rapid intracavitary deactivation. Systemic side effects, nausea, vomiting, and bone marrow depression are observed but are generally much milder than when the drug is administered intravenously. Hypovolemia also is reported after intraperitoneal dosing (Brown and Wright 1965).

Topical and Intralesional Application. Mechlorethamine has been applied topically with good response in electron beam-refractory mycosis fungoides confined to the skin (stages I–III) (Van Scott and Kalmanson 1973). The mechanism for topical activity involves direct toxicity to the lymphoreticular tumor cells or an alteration in the environment of the surrounding tissue causing unfavorable growth conditions for the tumor.

The solution for topical use is prepared by dissolving 10 mg mechlorethamine in 60 mL tap water. This is applied to the entire body surface. The solution may be prepared and applied by the patient with gloved hands. It is recommended that the perineum of men and women and the inframammary areas of women be only lightly moistened. Care must also be taken to avoid direct contact with the eye. For areas the patient cannot reach, another person wearing rubber or plastic gloves may help in the application. An ointment formulation of mechlorethamine has also been used to treat skin lesions from chronic granulocytic leukemia (Murphy et al 1985). Mechlorethamine powder 10 mg was either mixed in 1.0 mL Sterile Water for Injection, USP, and blended into 100 g of soft white paraffin or dissolved into 2 mL absolute ethanol and blended into 100 g of wool alcohol ointment (British Pharmacopoeia Codex). The ointment was applied each day using a wooden spatula up to a total dose of 15 mg over a 3-week period. Surrounding normal skin was protected by a coating of petroleum jelly. The ointment was active and did not appear to cause myelosuppression or local ulceration (Murphy et al 1985).

Initially, this cutaneous application is carried out two to three times a week until lesions disappear. Maintenance is then performed on a once-a-week basis.

Additionally intralesional injection into heavily infiltrated plaques of mycosis fungoides may be of benefit in selected patients. The intralesional preparation is made by diluting 0.1 mg of a 1 mg/mL stock preparation with 1 mL of 2% triamcinolone acetamide suspension and 1 mL of 1% lidocaine. The addition of triamcinolone and lidocaine helps to decrease local pain and inflammation. Injections of 0.1–mL volume per injection site are used with a maximum of 2 mL per treatment (20 injections).

Delayed hypersensitivity to topical mechlorethamine is a frequent occurrence. Minute daily intravenous doses of mechlorethamine (desensitization) may completely abolish this adverse reaction. Systemic toxicity secondary to topical mechlorethamine appears to be minimal; however, hyperpigmentation may occur, and some patients develop urticaria and generalized pruritis. The reactions are nearly universal with repeated topical mechlorethamine applications (Daughters et al 1973). Ross and Chabner (1977) have also reported a case of probable mechlorethamine-induced allergic cross-reaction to cyclophosphamide.

REFERENCES

Anderson CB, Philpott GW, Ferguson TB. The treatment of malignant pleural effusions. *Cancer.* 1974;**33**:916–922.

Bethlenfalvay NC, Bergin JJ. Severe cerebral toxicity after intravenous nitrogen mustard therapy. *Cancer.* 1972;**29**:366–369.

Bonadonna G, Karnofsky DA. Protection studies with sodium thiosulfate against methyl bis(β-chloroethyl)-amine hydrochloride (HN$_2$) and its ethylenimonium derivative. *Clin Pharmacol Ther.* 1965;**6**(1):50–64.

Brown FE, Wright HK. Hypovolemia following intraperitoneal nitrogen mustard therapy. *Surg Gynecol Obstet.* 1965;**121**:528–530.

Daughters D, Zackheim HS, Maibach H. Urticaria and anaphylactoid reactions after an application of mechlorethamine. *Arch Dermatol.* 1973;**107**:429–430.

Deuschle KW, Wiggans WS. Use of nitrogen mustard in management of two pregnant lymphoma patients. *Blood.* 1953;**8**:576–579.

DeVita VT, Serpick AA, Carbon PP. Combination chemotherapy in the treatment of advanced Hodgkin's disease. *Ann Intern Med.* 1970;**73**:881–895.

Dollinger MR. Management of recurrent malignant effusions. *CA.* 1972;**22**:138–147.

Dorr RT, Soble M, Alberts DS. Efficacy of sodium thiosulfate as a local antidote to mechlorethamine skin toxicity in the mouse. *Cancer Chemother Pharmacol.* 1988;**22**:299–302.

Fracchia A, Knapper W, Carey J, Farrow J. Intrapleural chemotherapy for effusion from metastatic breast carcinoma. *Cancer.* 1970;**26**:626–629.

French JD, West PM, von Amerongen FK, Magoun HW. Effects of intracarotid administration of nitrogen mustard on normal brain and brain tumors. *J Neurosurg.* **9**:379–389.

Gilman A. The initial clinical trial of nitrogen mustard. *Am J Surg.* 1963;**105**:574–578.

Gilman A, Philips FS. The biological actions and therapeutic applications of the β-chloroethylamines and sulfides. *Science.* 1946;**103**:409–415.

Goodman LS, Wintrobe M, Dameshek W, et al. Nitrogen mustard therapy: Use of methylbis(β-chloroethyl)amino hydrochloride for Hodgkin's disease, lymphosarcoma, leukemia and certain allied and miscellaneous disorders. *JAMA.* 1946;**132**:126–132.

Green R, Humphrey E, Close H, Patno ME. Alkylating agents in bronchogenic carcinoma. *Am J Med.* 1969;**46**:516–525.

Johnson JM, Ruddov RW. Interaction of nitrogen mustard with polyribonucleotides, ribosomes and enzymes involved in protein synthesis in a cell-free system. *Mol Pharmacol.* 1967;**3**:195–198.

Karnofsky DA, Clarkson BD. Cellular effects of anticancer drugs. *Annu Rev Pharmacol.* 1963;**3**:357–428.

Kinsey DL, Carter D, Klassen KP. Simplified management of malignant pleural effusion. *Arch Surg.* 1964;**89**:389–392.

Krumbhaar EB, Krumbhaar HD. The blood and bone marrow in yellow cross (mustard gas) poisoning: Changes in the bone marrow of fatal cases. *J Med Res.* 1919;**40**:497–507.

Leininger B, Barker W, Langston H. A simplified method for management of malignant pleural effusion. *J Thorac Cardiovasc Surg.* 1969;**58**(5):758–763.

Levison VB. Nitrogen mustard in palliation of malignant effusions. *Br Med J.* 1961;**1**:1143–1145.

Murphy WG, Fotheringham GH, Busuttil A, Allan NC. Skin lesions in chronic granulocytic leukemia: Treatment of a patient with topical nitrogen mustard. *Cancer.* 1985;**55**:2630–2633.

Murray D, Meyn RE. Enhancement of the DNA cross-linking activity of nitrogen mustard by misonidazole and diethyl maleate in a mouse fibrosarcoma tumor in vivo. *Cancer Res.* 1984;**44**:91–96.

Nicholson WM, Beard MEJ, Crowther D, et al. Combination chemotherapy in generalized Hodgkin's disease. *Br Med J.* 1970;**3**:7–10.

Owen OE, Dellatorre DL, Van Scott EJ, Cohen MR. Accidental intramuscular injection of mechlorethamine. *Cancer.* 1980;**45**:2225–2226.

Ross WE, Chabner BA. Allergic reaction to cyclophosphamide in a mechlorethamine-sensitive patient (letter). *Cancer Treat Rep.* 1977;**61**(3):495–496.

Salmon SE, Apple M. Cancer chemotherapy. In: Meyers FH, Goldfien JE, eds. *Review of Medical Pharmacology.* Los Altos, CA: Lange Medical; 1972:448–450.

Trissel LA, Fulton B, Tramonte SM. Visual compatibility of ondansetron with chemotherapeutic agents, antibiotics, and other selected drugs during simulated Y-site injection (abstract #P-468R). In: 25th Annual ASHP Midyear Clinical Meetings and Exhibit, Las Vegas, Nevada; 1990.

Van Scott EJ, Kalmanson JD. Complete remission of mycosis fungoides lymphoma induced by topical nitrogen mustard (HN$_2$). *Cancer.* 1973;**32**:18–30.

Walton MI, O'Connor PM, Kohn KW. Interstrand cross-linking of oligodeoxyribonucleotide duplexes by nitrogen mustards. *Proc Am Assoc Cancer Res.* 1991;**32**:320.

Wang AL, Tew KD. Increased glutathione-S-transferase activity in a cell line with acquired resistance to nitrogen mustards. *Cancer Treat Rep.* 1985;**69**:677–682.

Warwick GP. The mechanism of action of alkylating agents. *Cancer Res.* 1963;**23**:1315–1333.

Weisberger AS. Direct instillation of HN$_2$ in the management of malignant effusions. *Ann NY Acad Sci.* 1958;**68**:1091–1096.

Wheeler GP. Studies related to the mechanisms of action of cytotoxic alkylating agents. *Cancer Res.* 1962;**22**:651–688.

Zackheim HS, Arnold JE, Farber BM, et al. Topical therapy of psoriasis with mechlorethamine. *Arch Dermatol.* 1972;**105**:702–706.

Melphalan

■ Other Names

Alkeran® (Burroughs-Wellcome Company); L-PAM; phenylalanine mustard; L-sarcolysine; CB 3025; NSC-8806.

■ Chemistry

Structure of melphalan

Melphalan is the L-isomer of the synthetic product formed from the amino acid phenylalanine and mechlorethamine. The complete chemical name is 4-[bis(2-chloroethyl)amino]-L-phenylalanine monohydrochloride. The molecular weight is 305 and the empiric formula is $C_{13}H_{18}Cl_2N_2O_2$. It is practically insoluble in water and only slightly soluble in alcohol. A less potent D-isomer of melphalan, medphalan, has also undergone preliminary preclinical evaluation (Vistica 1979). Another chemically related agent is Peptichemio®, which is actually a mixture of six peptides of DL-phenylalanine mustard (Schmid et al 1977).

■ Antitumor Activity

Melphalan has significant activity in multiple myeloma (Hoogstraten et al 1967, Alexander 1968), most often in combination with prednisone (Costa et al 1973) or investigationally by intravenous injection (McIntyre et al 1978). In advanced refractory myeloma it is often combined with vincristine and other alkylating agents such as cyclophosphamide (eg, VMCP) (Alexanian et al 1969). As a single agent, high-dose melphalan produced high response rates (6/11 complete responses [CRs] 5/11 partial responses [PRs]) but short response durations (median, 16 months) in patients with high-risk multiple myeloma (Lokhorst et al 1992). In the adjuvant chemotherapy of breast cancer, melphalan has limited activity as a single agent dosed in a continuous fashion (Fisher et al 1975). The drug also has activity in testicular and ovarian carcinoma (Smith and Rutledge 1974). There is activity for injectable melphalan in the regional (isolated) perfusion of nonresectable malignant melanoma of the extremities (Bulman and Jamieson 1980, Sugarbaker and McBride 1976) (see Special Applications).

The investigational intravenous formulation also has activity in sarcomas and other solid tumors when used as a single agent (see table above). Especially good activity is reported in newly diagnosed rhabdomyosarcoma (Horowitz et al 1988). Human cancers insensitive to intravenous melphalan include Ewing's sarcoma and small cell and non-small cell lung cancer (Sarosy et al 1988) (see Special Applications for the activity of high dose melphalan with bone marrow transplantation).

There is good activity for melphalan combined with other drugs without bone marrow transplantation (BMT) in various solid tumors (see table on page 664). Multiple myeloma, ovarian cancer, and testicular cancer appear to be especially responsive to intravenous melphalan. Melanomas are also highly responsive to regional intravenous melphalan (see Special Applications).

■ Mechanism of Action

Melphalan has alkylating activity and a spectrum of pharmacologic actions similar to those of mechlor-

SINGLE-AGENT ACTIVITY OF INTRAVENOUS MELPHALAN

Sensitive Tumors	Overall Response Rate (%)
Pancreatic cancer	13
Colon cancer	7
Anaplastic glioma	11
Medulloblastoma	22
Multiple myeloma	65
Sarcomas	
Rhabdomyosarcoma	42
Osteosarcoma	11
Ovarian cancer	78

Data from Sarosy et al 1988.

ethamine (nitrogen mustard). The alkylation process involves the transfer of the ethylamine groups to susceptible (nucleophilic) atoms in proteins and nucleic acids. Bifunctional alkylating activity is facilitated through the two bis(chloroethyl) side chains. Experimentally, melphalan forms DNA crosslinks by a delayed two-step (SN_2) type of reaction characteristic of haloethyl alkylating agents. The rate of DNA crosslink formation with melphalan is considerably slower than with mechlorethamine. In L-1210 cells, peak crosslink formation occurs 8 to 12 hours after drug exposure compared with 30 minutes with mechlorethamine. The removal of crosslinks is also slower with melphalan than with mechlorethamine (Ross et al 1978). This finding suggests that the second alkylating step is quite slow with melphalan.

Melphalan also differs in other ways from the other alkylating agents because of its amino acid structure. Begleiter and Goldenberg (1979) have confirmed special melphalan cellular transport by at least two amino acid carrier systems. They further demonstrated nonlinear (Michaelis–Menten) uptake kinetics for drug uptake and competition for cellular uptake by similar amino acid-type compounds. Both features strongly suggest a carrier-mediated transport mechanism for melphalan uptake into cells.

Further experimental studies have shown that two amino acid transport systems are responsible for melphalan uptake: a sodium-independent system, which normally transports leucine, and a monovalent cation dependent system, which can transfer alanine, serine, or cysteine (Goldenberg et

RESPONSE TO INTRAVENOUS MELPHALAN-CONTAINING DRUG COMBINATIONS WITHOUT AUTOLOGOUS BONE MARROW TRANSPLANTATION

Type of Cancer	Melphalan (mg)	Other Agents	Clinical Response Rate*	Reference
Colon	0.3/kg	5-Fluorouracil	0	Gough and Furnival 1983
Lung (non-small cell lung cancer)	0.6/kg	Misonidazole	14	Carlson et al 1987
Melanoma	60/m^2	Vincristine	17	Tchekmedyian et al 1986
	30/m^2	Dacarbazine, bacillus Calmette–Guérin	17	Schwartz et al 1980
Myeloma	16/m^2	Peptichemio®, prednisone	67	Franchi et al 1986
Ovarian	12/m^2	Cisplatin, altretamine	58	Goldhirsch et al 1985
Testicular	0.5–1.0/kg	Vinblastine	46	Samuels and Howe 1970

*Complete response rate + partial response rate.

al 1979). Byfield et al (1979) have recently determined that melphalan acts primarily on "cycling" cell populations but is not particularly cell cycle phase specific.

■ Availability and Storage

Melphalan is available commercially from Burroughs-Wellcome Company (Research Triangle Park, North Carolina) as 2-mg tablets (Alkeran®) for oral use. These may be stored at room temperature away from direct sunlight. The drug has also been available investigationally as a preparation kit for injection. This kit contains an ampule of 100 mg of melphalan equivalent, a 1-mL ampule of acid–alcohol solution, and a 9-mL ampule of the final diluent containing dipotassium phosphate 108 mg, propylene glycol 5.4 mL, Sterile Water for Injection, USP, sufficient quantity, 9.0 mL. This kit should be stored at room temperature and protected from light.

■ Preparation for Use, Stability, and Admixture

The 100-mg injectable formulation is put into solution initially with the addition of the 1-mL acid–alcohol solution. When dissolution is complete, the 9 mL of aqueous diluent is added. This final solution has a pH of approximately 7 and should be used promptly. According to the manufacturer there is 8.5% hydrolysis 24 hours after mixing. A further dilution in D5W is also reportedly stable for 24 hours (Trissel 1977).

Melphalan is known to be more stable in normal saline solution than in water; hydrolysis to mono- or dihydroxy (inactive) species may rapidly occur in water (Chang et al 1979). A 20 μg/mL solution in 0.9% sodium chloride injection loses 5% of its activity in 1.5 hours at room temperature, but requires 20 hours at 5°C and up to 12 months at –20°C to lose similar activity (Bosanquet 1985). The half-life of melphalan in RPMI-1640 medium containing 10% fetal bovine serum at 37°C was 1.13 hours. The table on the opposite page summarizes the stability of melphalan in various infusion solutions.

■ Administration

The total daily oral dose of melphalan may be taken at one time. When ingested with food, the drug is poorly absorbed compared to when taken on an empty stomach (Alberts et al 1979b) (also see Pharmacokinetics). Nausea and vomiting from oral dosing have generally not been a significant clinical problem.

The injectable product is given intravenously as a slow infusion (in 100–200 mL D5W over 15–30 minutes) and is also investigationally given by an arterial "isolated" perfusion technique. It may also be administered by continuous infusion (working within the stability constraints) (see Special Applications for regional arterial perfusion and intraperitoneal administration).

STABILITY OF MELPHALAN IN DIFFERENT INFUSION FLUIDS AND TEMPERATURES

Temperature (°C)	Stability Time (h) for >90% Activity		
	5% Dextrose	Lactated Ringer's Injection	Normal Saline
15	1.9	4.8	5.5
20	1.5	2.9	4.5
25	0.6	1.5	2.4
37	0.3	0.4	0.6

Data from Tabibi and Cradock 1984.

■ Dosage

Multiple Myeloma. Melphalan is most often given in combination with other chemotherapeutic drugs. In the treatment of multiple myeloma, it is generally given intermittently for 4 to 7 days at doses of 9 mg/m² or 0.25 mg/kg/d, and for 7 days at doses of 0.15 mg/kg. These doses can be repeated at 4- to 6-week intervals, when bone marrow toxicity has resolved. If used as a single agent, one-time doses of 1 mg/kg repeated at 4- to 6-week intervals are generally well tolerated. Although the manufacturer reports equal effects from either intravenous or oral doses, the major bioavailability differences and the potential for lessened hepatic clearance of intravenous doses strongly suggest that intravenous doses should be reduced. Although not generally recommended, continuous daily maintenance doses of 2 to 4 mg have been occasionally used in multiple myeloma to maintain the desired level of hematologic control after an initial loading dose was administered (McArthur et al 1970). Frequent and careful hematologic monitoring is essential if continuous daily maintenance therapy is used. This regimen may also connote a heightened risk of leukemogenesis.

Intravenous high-dose melphalan has been used as a single agent for patients with high-risk multiple myeloma. A dose of 140 mg/m² was administered.

Breast and Ovarian Cancer. In a well-known adjuvant trial for high-risk postmastectomy breast carcinoma patients, Fisher et al (1975) used a dose of 0.15 mg/kg/d for 5 days, repeated at 6-week intervals. In a similar surgical adjuvant setting for ovarian carcinoma, melphalan has been used in large cyclical doses: 1 mg/kg IV over 8 hours, repeated in 4 weeks. Alternatively, 1 mg/kg was given orally over 5 days. Each day's dose of 0.2 mg/kg was further split into three fractions per day. The cycle was repeated in 4 weeks (Rutledge 1968). The apparently equivalent therapeutic results with intravenous and oral dosing are interesting and surprising in light of the recently reported poor oral absorption of the compound (see Pharmacokinetics).

Dose Adjustments. Dose reduction is recommended in patients with renal dysfunction although no specific guidelines are available for the oral drug (see Pharmacokinetics). For the intravenous formulation, a 50% dose reduction is recommended for patients with blood urea nitrogen elevated to 30 mg/dL or higher (Cornwell et al 1982). Others have recommended that no drug be administered to patients with a creatinine clearance below 40 mL/min or a serum creatinine above 2 mg/dL.

■ Drug Interactions

Misonidazole. Melphalan has been combined with various agents to modify its activity or to block cellular resistance pathways. The nitroimidazole misonidazole has been shown to enhance DNA crosslinking from melphalan (Murray and Meyn 1983, 1984). This effect did not appear to be caused by reduced repair of crosslinks (Murray and Meyn 1983) but may involve intracellular glutathione depletion (Taylor et al 1982). Importantly, cytotoxicity was also enhanced by concomitant melphalan with misonidazole (Horsman et al 1982). In a phase I clinical trial, misonidazole (4 g/m²) was combined with 0.6 mg/kg melphalan. The results showed that occasionally severe melphalan-induced myelosuppression was the predominant dose-limiting toxic effect, although mild misonidazole peripheral neurotoxicity was seen in 4 of 30 patients (Coleman et al 1983). Misonidazole did not alter melphalan's pharmacokinetics. There were 2 responders among 33 evaluable patients with solid tumors. From this trial it appeared that both drugs could be administered concomitantly at their individual maximum tolerated doses.

L-Buthionine Sulfoximine. Resistance to alkylating agents like melphalan is commonly associated with enhanced glutathione (GSH) levels (Suzukake et al 1982) and/or with enhanced glutathione S-transferases (Wang and Tew 1985). The depletion of GSH by the antimetabolite L-buthionine sulfoximine (L-BSO) has been shown to sensitize resistant cells to melphalan in vitro (Green et al 1984, Suzukake et al 1982) and slightly in vivo (Soble and Dorr 1988). L-BSO also enhances melphalan-induced DNA–DNA crosslinks in L-1210 cells in vitro (Dorr 1987). There was no effect on the rate of removal (repair) of these crosslinks. On the basis of these findings, melphalan has recently been combined with L-BSO in cancer patients in a phase I clinical trial (Bailey et al 1991, Hamilton et al 1990). The results of this trial show that the two agents can be safely combined at doses up to 3.0 g/m^2 of oral L-BSO with 15 mg/m^2 of melphalan given as a 30-minute intravenous infusion. Myelosuppression was dose limiting and significant GSH depletion was documented in peripheral blood mononuclear cells (for a complete discussion, see *Buthionine Sulfoximine* monograph.) Remaining questions are whether significant melphalan dose escalation can be achieved or if there is utility for the combination in patients resistant to melphalan alone.

Corticosteroids. There is evidence for enhanced melphalan antitumor effects with concomitant glucocorticosteroids (Selby et al 1981). In this experimental trial, prednisolone was observed to increase melphalan activity against mice with melanoma xenografts. Lethality was also increased by the combination, although there was no enhancement in gut cell or bone marrow toxicity. When melphalan was combined with methylprednisolone in patients with multiple myeloma, the pharmacokinetic data for melphalan were similar to previously reported data. Conversely, methylprednisolone absorption was apparently unaffected by concurrent melphalan (Taha et al 1982).

L-Leucine and Cimetidine. A number of other interactions involve alterations in the oral bioavailability of melphalan tablets. The ingestion of melphalan with food is known to reduce significantly the bioavailability of melphalan (see Pharmacokinetics). Further experiments have shown that the amino acid L-leucine (2 g orally) can also reduce melphalan absorption by an average of 17% (Reece et al 1987). As with food, the extent of the effect of leucine varied greatly in different individuals. The H$_2$ antagonist cimetidine decreased oral melphalan bioavailability by approximately 30% (Sviland et al 1987). There was also a slight increase in the elimination rate of melphalan reflected in a decrease in half-life from 1.94 to 1.57 hours. Cimetidine at a dose of 200 mg three times daily and 400 mg at night appeared to lower patient-to-patient variation in melphalan absorption at the cost of reduced overall bioavailability.

Hematopoietic Colony-Stimulating Factors. Finally, Morstyn et al (1989) have shown a dramatic reduction in melphalan-induced neutropenia but not thrombocytopenia with granulocyte colony-stimulating factor (G-CSF). In this trial G-CSF was administered subcutaneously on days 1 to 5 and 10 to 18 and melphalan was administered intravenously on day 9 at a dose of 25 mg/m^2. It was found that the pretreatment G-CSF doses were probably unnecessary because C-CSF was effective even when started 8 days after melphalan and continued for 7 days in patients with no prior therapy.

■ Pharmacokinetics

Intravenous Melphalan. Several groups have studied the disposition of oral and intravenous melphalan in humans (see table on the opposite page). There is no significant first-pass effect with melphalan and most of the drug's inactivation is explained by nonenzymatic hydrolysis to the mono- or dihydroxy derivatives (Evans et al 1982). There is also some conjugation to glutathione mediated by glutathione S- transferases (Dulik and Fenselau 1987). The volume of distribution appears to approximate total body water (44 L). The drug appears to have a biphasic elimination pattern with half-lives of (α) 6 to 8 minutes and (β) 40 to 60 minutes (Alberts et al 1979a). The summary results in the table show that there is no evidence of dose-dependent pharmacokinetics. The majority of the drug is cleared by nonrenal mechanisms, although renal elimination is still important. The fraction of drug excreted unchanged in the urine averaged 21 to 34% in one study (Reece et al 1988). Myelosuppression is greatly enhanced in patients with renal dysfunction (Cornwell et al 1982). This effect is possibly due to a significant increase in melphalan systemic exposure (Adair et al 1986). Similar changes have been observed in nephrectomized dogs (Alberts et al 1981). The fraction of melphalan unbound to plasma protein ranges from 21 to 26% (Reece et al 1988). In myeloma patients, over 90% of melphalan was bound in plasma, with 60% bound to albumin and 20% to α_1-acid glycoprotein (Gera et al 1989). Only 30% of the drug was bound covalently in the plasma.

Oral Melphalan. Similar half-lives are seen with oral and intravenous doses; however, oral absorption was both erratic and incomplete, peaking in 2 hours (Alberts et al 1979b). In a separate investigation of oral melphalan, Alberts et al (1978) noted extremely variable oral absorption, including fourfold differences in amounts absorbed from a standard 0.6 mg/kg dose. Absolute bioavailability ranged from 0.25 (25%) to 0.89 with a mean of 0.56. When melphalan is taken with food, oral absorption is decreased even further because of enhanced drug degradation at the alkaline pH in the upper small bowel prior to systemic absorption (Alberts et al 1984, Bosanquet and Gilby 1984). This difference was twofold in the latter trial wherein oral bioavailability was 0.95 in the fasting state and 0.49 in the fed state (Bosanquet and Gilby 1984). The absorption delay increased from 0.3 to 1.1 hour and peak levels of 65 ng/mL were 33% of those in the fasting state (195 ng/mL) after an oral dose of 7 mg/m^2. In one patient no drug was detected in the plasma after observed oral ingestion of melphalan tablets.

■ Side Effects and Toxicity

Hematologic suppression is the dose-limiting toxic effect of melphalan. It is characterized by both leukopenia and thrombocytopenia, which peak 14 and 21 days, respectively, after intermittent dosing schedules. This suppression can sometimes have a delayed onset and may be cumulative, extending the nadir 5 to 6 weeks in older patients. Many investigators feel that optimal results with oral melphalan are not obtained unless there is a significant degree of suppression (3000–3500 lymphocytes/cm^3) and unless therapy is gradual and continuous. The administration of large single oral doses occasionally produces nausea and vomiting. Gastrointestinal side effects are generally not seen with lower continuous dosing; however, there is mounting evidence to suggest that long-term oral dosing programs can increase the chance of developing acute myelogenous leukemia or myelodysplasia as a late consequence of melphalan treatment. Secondary leukemia may be especially important in ovarian cancer (Greene et al 1986), multiple myeloma (Einhorn 1978), and breast cancer (Fisher et al 1985). According to Rosner (1979), acute myelocytic and myelomonocytic types of leukemia predominate. They are often heralded by a preleukemic pancytopenia of several weeks' to months' duration. Various chromosomal abnormalities are also typically noted. Recent reports highlight a 1 to 2% yearly incidence in such melphalan-treated multiple myeloma patients.

Other infrequent toxic effects include alopecia, dermatitis, stomatitis, and pulmonary fibrosis (Codling and Chakera 1972, Taetle et al 1978). Pulmonary infiltrates resulting from interstitial pneumonitis

CLINICAL PHARMACOKINETICS OF INTRAVENOUS MELPHALAN

Dose (mg/m^2)	Clearance Renal	Clearance Nonrenal	Steady-State Volume of Distribution	Half-life (min)	AUC (min · µg/mL)	Reference
0.6 (mg/kg)	0.73 mL/min/kg	4.23 mL/min/kg	0.06 L/kg	108	148	Alberts et al 1979a
5	70 mL/min/m^2)	111 mL/min/m^2	9.93 L/m^2	62	—	Reece et al 1988
140–180	500 mL/min/m^2 (total)	—	—	48	433	Gouyette et al 1986
140	415 mL/min/m^2 (total)	—	17 L/m^2	41	375	Ardiet et al 1986
180	6.7 mL/min/kg (total)	—	0.48 L/kg	61	—	Hersh et al 1983

have also been reported in patients receiving low-dose melphalan for multiple myeloma (Westerfield et al 1980). Pulmonary fibrosis has been rarely observed in patients with multiple myeloma (Codling and Chakera 1972, Major et al 1980). These effects are generally associated with long-term administration of the drug. Serious hypersensitivity reactions with hypotension, diaphoresis, and even cardiac arrest following intravenous drug administration have been reported. In four of five patients, rechallenge with oral melphalan produced rash, itching, and chest pain (Cornwell et al 1979). Anaphylaxis has been described with oral melphalan although this is quite rare (Lawrence et al 1980).

■ Special Applications

Regional Perfusion. Regionally perfused melphalan has been used investigationally for years in the management of localized but nonresectable malignant melanomas of the extremities (Krementz and Ryan 1972, Sugarbaker and McBride 1976, Koops et al 1977, Bulman and Jamieson 1980). A 49% overall response rate was reported in this trial. The 5-year survival rate of 52% is reported for this treatment in stage II melanoma patients (Bulman and Jamieson 1980). The complicated technique involves general anesthesia and an oxygenated peristaltic blood pump for the arterial bypass circuit. Often, the perfusate is heated. Melphalan doses of up to 1.2 mg/kg have been used without producing the usual systemic toxic effects (Stehlin et al 1975). Serious local complications (infections, palsies, hematomas) are possible and only experienced surgical oncology teams should attempt the procedure. Golomb et al (1979) suggested that efficacy for this procedure is limited to patients with lymph node involvement noted at the time of standard surgical excision. Response rates of up to 80% in melanoma have recently been reported for melphalan doses of 0.75 mg/kg by the axillary/popliteal arteries and 1.2 mg/kg by the femoral artery (Minor et al 1985). In another trial a dose of 1.5 mg/kg was administered by the femoral artery in three divided doses at 0, 20, and 40 minutes (Bulman and Jamieson 1980).

The pharmacokinetics of melphalan and regional hyperthermia has been reported by Briele et al (1985). In 16 patients with malignant melanoma, the decrease in drug concentrations sampled in the venous return line during perfusion occurred in two phases, with half-lives of 5 to 10 minutes and 35 to 50 minutes. These phases may correspond to the initial rapid uptake of drug into tissues (first phase) and the slower hydrolysis of melphalan in the heated perfusate (second phase). In this regard, melphalan was found to be more stable in a perfusate containing electrolytes and protein (Plasma Lyte A® [Travenol Laboratories] and 8% albumin). The regional AUC estimate for an arterial dose of 1 to 1.5 mg/kg was 448 µg·min/mL, and little additional uptake is noted after 30 minutes of isolated limb perfusion (Briele et al 1985). Peak perfusate melphalan concentrations ranged between 6.1 to 115 µg/mL in another trial (Minor et al 1985). These levels are 1 to 2 logs higher than those obtained with systemic melphalan. Another trial of regional arterial administration also showed that perfusion-circuit melphalan levels were about 100-fold higher than systemic levels (Rauschecker et al 1991). Peripheral blood melphalan levels were highest in the first 20 minutes, ranging from 0.28 to 0.37 µg/mL. The coadministration of cisplatin did not significantly alter these levels (Rauschecker et al 1991).

Melphalan with Bone Marrow Transplantation. Melphalan has been combined with other agents and BMT in the treatment of a variety of advanced refractory malignancies (Maraninchi et al 1984) (see table on the opposite page). When used alone at 180 mg/m^2 with autologous BMT, high-dose melphalan achieved a 45% overall response rate, with 3 of 20 (15%) colon cancer patients achieving a complete response (Leff et al 1986). Median survival was 198 days. Toxic effects included myelosuppression with granulocytopenia lasting 5 to 35 days and thrombocytopenia (to 20,000/µL or less and requiring transfusions) lasting a median of 8 days (range, 3 to 23 days). Fortunately, prior 5-fluorouracil therapy did not increase the probability of toxicity. There was also mild stomatitis, esophagitis, and diarrhea. Nausea and vomiting were short-lived. There was one treatment-related death as a result of massive gastrointestinal bleeding from intratumoral necrosis (Leff et al 1986). High-dose therapy has also been associated with one case of the syndrome of inappropriate antidiuretic hormone secretion (SIADH) (Greenbaum-Lefkoe et al 1985)

Activity for melphalan-containing drug combinations and BMT has also been observed in a few patients with refractory testicular cancer, ovarian cancer, uterine leiomyosarcoma, thymoma, and malignant melanoma (Maraninchi et al 1984). Response durations were relatively short, however, with a median of 7 weeks (range 4–38 weeks). The

DRUG COMBINATIONS USING HIGH-DOSE MELPHALAN WITH BONE MARROW TRANSPLANTATION

Type of Cancer	Melphalan (mg/m^2)	Other Agent	Overall Response Rate* (%)	Reference
Neuroblastoma	140–200	Vincristine	86	Philip et al 1985
Melanoma	40–130	Cisplatin, cyclophosphamide	67	Peters et al 1986
Lymphoma	140	Carmustine, vindesine, cytarabine	67	Mascret et al 1986
Myeloma	140	Prednisolone	86	Selby et al 1987
Colon	40/d × 5 d or 50/d × 3 d	Misonidazole	60	Spitzer et al 1987
Breast	40–120	Cisplatin, cyclophosphamide	50	Peters et al 1986

*Complete response rate + partial response rate.

melphalan dose was 140 to 240 mg/m^2 given as an intravenous bolus during continuous intravenous hydration. Furosemide (20 mg) was administered afterward to ensure a rapid diuresis (Maraninchi et al 1984). Profound myelosuppression occurred in all patients with a median white blood cell count nadir on day 8 (range, 6–16 days). Two treatment-related deaths were due to neutropenic sepsis. Whether hematopoietic colony-stimulating factors can prevent or reduce this occurrence as has been the case with lower-dose melphalan combined with G-CSF remains to be determined (Morstyn et al 1989) (also see Drug Interactions).

A review of combination drug trials of high-dose melphalan with BMT shows that there are numerous active regimens for both solid tumors and hematologic malignancies (see last table). In these trials, a melphalan doses ranged from 140 to 200 mg/m^2 (Sarosy et al 1988). At these doses, the primary nonhematologic toxic effects involve mucositis, nausea and vomiting, diarrhea, and alopecia. Rare toxic effects in such high-dose/BMT regimens include elevations in liver function tests (Pritchard et al 1982), vasculitis (Skehan and Bernath 1978), SIADH (Greenbaum-Lefkoe et al 1985), interstitial pneumonitis (Westerfield et al 1980), and secondary acute leukemias (Hartmann et al 1984).

Use of a Test Dose to Individualize High-Dose Therapy. Because of interpatient variability in melphalan pharmacokinetics, there is a proposal to use a 0.5 to 1 mg/kg test dose given 24 hours prior to the second maximal dose (total dose of 140 mg/m^2) (Tranchand et al 1989). Within each patient, the pharmacokinetics of the test dose and that of the main dose were similar in terms of steady-state volume of distribution (14.6 L/m^2), clearance (0.44 L/min/m^2), and half-life (44.5 minutes). This allowed for projections of systemic exposure (AUC) that would be achievable by dosing modifications in individual patients. If not adjusted, the fixed doses produced values that ranged from 109 to 691 mg/L· min (n = 10 patients), but with the expected overall mean AUC of about 425 mg/L × min. A prospective evaluation of this methodology will be required to validate this approach to pharmacokinetics-based high-dose individualization with melphalan.

Intraperitoneal Administration. Melphalan has significant cytotoxic potency against ovarian cancer cells in vitro (Alberts et al 1985). In a phase I clinical trial, the maximally tolerated dose of intraperitoneal melphalan was 70 mg/kg. The dose was instilled in 2 L of normal saline using a 4-hour dwell time (Howell et al 1984). The primary toxic effect was myelosuppression with mild nausea and vomiting seen in 22 of 32 courses. There was no local toxicity. Melphalan disappearance from the peritoneal cavity was first order with a mean half-life of 1 hour and an intraperitoneal AUC of 43,000 μg·min/mL after a 60 mg/kg dose. This level represented a 63-fold intraperitoneal pharmacokinetic advantage over intravenous dosing (Howell et al 1984). Peak melphalan levels in the intraperitoneal space ranged from 10 to 100 μg/mL compared with less than 1 μg/mL in the plasma. In addition, some responses were observed in patients with advanced ovarian or gastric cancer.

Intraperitoneal melphalan has been combined with glutaminase enzymes from *Acinebacter* to deplete glutamine and thereby increase melphalan cellular uptake (Holcenberg et al 1983). Doses of 1000 to 2000 IU of glutaminase enzymes were administered in 2 L of Dianeal® solution 1 hour before intraperitoneal melphalan was given (12–32 mg/m^2).

The half-lives of melphalan and glutaminase in the intraperitoneal cavity were 1.2 and 8 hours, respectively. Toxic effects included fever, nausea, and abdominal pain, but no myelosuppression was observed. One objective response was obtained among three ovarian cancer patients treated in this trial (Holcenberg et al 1983).

REFERENCES

Adair CG, Bridges JM, Desai ZR. Renal function in the elimination of oral melphalan in patients with multiple myeloma. *Cancer Chemother Pharmacol.* 1986;**17**:185–188.

Alberts DS, Chang SY, Chen H-SG, et al. Variability of melphalan (M) absorption in man. *Proc Am Assoc Cancer Res ASCO.* 1978;**19**:334.

Alberts DS, Chang SY, Chen H-SG, et al. Kinetics of intravenous melphalan. *Clin Pharmacol Ther.* 1979a;**26**(1):73–80.

Alberts DS, Chang SY, Chen H-SG, et al. Oral melphalan kinetics. *Clin Pharmacol Ther.* 1979b;**26**(6):737–745.

Alberts DS, Chen H-SG, Benz D, Mason NL. Effect of renal dysfunction in dogs on the disposition and marrow toxicity of melphalan. *Br J Cancer.* 1981;**43**:330–334.

Alberts DS, Peng YM, Fisher B. Minimal melphalan (L-PAM) systemic availability (SA): A potential cause for failure of adjuvant breast cancer trials (abstract C-149). *Proc Am Soc Clin Oncol.* 1984;**3**:38.

Alberts DS, Young L, Mason NL, et al. In vitro evaluation of anticancer drugs against ovarian cancer at concentrations achievable by intraperitoneal administration. *Semin Oncol.* 1985;**12**(suppl 4):38–42.

Alexander R, Bergsagel DE, Migliore PJ, et al. Melphalan therapy for plasma cell myeloma. *Blood.* 1968;**31**:1.

Alexanian R, Haut A, Talley RW, et al. Treatment for multiple myeloma—Combination chemotherapy with different melphalan dose regimens. Cooperative Study of Adult Division SWCCSG. *JAMA.* 1969;**203**:1680.

Ardiet C, Tranchand B, Biron P, et al. Pharmacokinetics of high-dose intravenous melphalan in children and adults with forced diuresis. Report in 26 cases. *Cancer Chemother Pharmacol.* 1986;**16**:300–305.

Bailey H, Mulcahy RT, Tutsch K, et al. Phase I trial of intravenous L-buthionine sulfoximine (BSO) and melphalan (L-PAM): An attempt at modulation of glutathione (GSH) chemoprotection (abstract). *Proc Am Soc Clin Oncol.* 1991;**10**:100.

Begleiter A, Goldenberg GJ. Transport of melphalan by amino acid carriers in MCF-7 human breast cancer cells in vitro (abstract 970). *Proc Am Assoc Cancer Res ASCO.* 1979;**20**:240.

Bosanquet AG. Stability of melphalan solutions during preparation and storage. *J Pharm Sci.* 1985;**74**(3):348–351.

Bosanquet AG, Gilby ED. Comparison of the fed and fasting states on the absorption of melphalan in multiple myeloma. *Cancer Chemother Pharmacol.* **12**:183–186.

Briele HA, Djuric M, Jung DT, et al. Pharmacokinetics of melphalan in clinical isolation perfusion of the extremities. *Cancer Res.* 1985;**45**:1885–1889.

Bulman AS, Jamieson CW. Isolated limb perfusion with melphalan in the treatment of malignant melanoma. *Br J Surg.* 1980;**67**:660–662.

Byfield JE, Calabro-Jones J, Murname J, et al. Transport-dependent cytotoxicity of water versus lipid soluble alkylating agents: Origins of cumulative marrow toxicity (abstract 547). *Proc Am Assoc Cancer Res ASCO.* 1979;**20**:136.

Carlson RW, Coleman CN, Kohler M, et al. A randomized phase II study of L-PAM versus L-PAM + the chemosensitizer misonidazole (MISO) for non-small-cell lung cancer (NSCLC): A Northern California Oncology Group study (abstract). *Proc Am Soc Clin Oncol.* 1987;**6**:28.

Chang SY, Evans TL, Alberts DS. The stability of melphalan in the presence of chloride ion. *J Pharm Pharmacol.* 1979;**31**:853–854.

Codling BW, Chakera TMH. Pulmonary fibrosis following therapy with melphalan for multiple myeloma. *J Clin Pathol.* 1972;**25**:668–673.

Coleman CN, Friedman MK, Jacobs C, et al. Phase I trial of intravenous L-phenylalanine mustard plus the sensitizer misonidazole. *Cancer Res.* 1983;**43**:5022–5025.

Cornwell GG, Pajak TF, McIntyre OR. Hypersensitivity reactions to IV melphalan during treatment of multiple myeloma: Cancer and Leukemia Group B experience. *Cancer Treat Rep.* 1979;**63**(3):399–403.

Cornwell GG III, Pajak TF, McIntyre OR, et al. Influence of renal failure on myelosuppressive effects of melphalan: Cancer and Leukemia Group B experience. *Cancer Treat Rep.* 1982;**66**:475–481.

Costa G, Engle RL Jr, Schilling A, et al. Melphalan and prednisone: An effective combination for the treatment of multiple myeloma. *Am J Med.* 1973;**54**:589–599.

Dorr RT. Reduced thiol content in L1210 cells treated with BSO increases DNA crosslinking by melphalan. *Biochem Biophys Res Commun.* 1987;**144**(1):47–52.

Dulik DM, Fenselau. Conversion of melphalan to 4-(glutathionyl)phenylalanine. A novel mechanism for conjugation by glutathione-S-transferases. *Drug Metab Dispos.* 1987;**15**(2):195–199.

Einhorn N. Acute leukemia after chemotherapy (melphalan). *Cancer.* 1978;**44**:444–447.

Evans TL, Chang SY, Alberts DS, et al. In vitro degradation of L-phenylalanine mustard (L-PAM). *Cancer Chemother Pharmacol.* 1982;**8**:175–178.

Fisher B, Carbone P, Economou SG, et al. L-Phenylalanine mustard (L-PAM) in the management of breast cancer: A report of early findings. *N Engl J Med.* 1975;**292**:117–122.

Fisher B, Rockette H, Fisher ER, et al. Leukemia in breast cancer patients following adjuvant chemotherapy or postoperative radiation: The NSABP experience. *J Clin Oncol.* 1985;**3**:1640–1658.

Franchi F, Seminara P, Fanelli FR. Alternating intravenous courses of melphalan and Peptichemio in high-risk multiple myeloma (preliminary results). *Anticancer Res.* 1986;**6**:297–298.

Gera S, Musch E, Osterheld HKO, Loos U. Relevance of the hydrolysis and protein binding of melphalan to the treatment of multiple myeloma. *Cancer Chemother Pharmacol.* 1989;**23**:76–80.

Goldenberg GJ, Lam H-YP, Begleiter A. Active carrier-mediated transport of melphalan by two separate amino acid transport systems in LPC-1 plasmacytoma cells in vitro. *J Biol Chem.* 1979;**254**:1057–1064.

Goldhirsch A, Griener R, Dreher E, et al. The treatment of ovarian cancer by a multimodality approach: Remission induction with chemotherapy—HexaPAMP and RAMP regimens—followed by whole-abdominal radiation. *Onkologie.* 1985;**6**:383–387.

Golomb FM, Bromberg J, Dubin N. A controlled study of isolated perfusion as an adjunct to surgical therapy for primary melanoma of the distal extremities (abstract C-92). *Proc Am Assoc Cancer Res ASCO.* 1979;**20**:313.

Gough IR, Furnival CM. High-dose intermittent IV 5-FU and melphalan in advanced colorectal carcinoma. *Cancer Treat Rep.* 1983;**67**:595–596.

Gouyette A, Hartmann O, Pico J-L. Pharmacokinetics of high-dose melphalan in children and adults. *Cancer Chemother Pharmacol.* 1986;**16**:184–189.

Green JA, Vistica DT, Young RC, et al. Potentiation of melphalan cytotoxicity in human ovarian cancer cell lines by glutathione depletion. *Cancer Res.* 1984;**44**:5427–5431.

Greenbaum-Lefkoe B, Rosenstock JG, Belasco JB. Syndrome of inappropriate antidiuretic hormone secretion: A complication of high dose intravenous melphalan. *Cancer.* 1985;**55**:44–46.

Greene MH, Harris EL, Gershenson DM, et al. Melphalan may be a more potent leukemogen than cyclophosphamide. *Ann Intern Med.* 1986;**105**:360–367.

Hamilton T, O'Dwyer P, Young R, et al. Phase I trial of buthionine sulfoximine (BSO) plus melphalan (L-PAM) in patients with advanced cancer (abstract). *Proc Am Soc Clin Oncol.* 1990;**9**:73.

Hartmann O, Oberlin O, Lemerle J. Acute leukemia in two patients treated with high dose melphalan and autologous marrow transplantation for malignant solid tumors. *J Clin Oncol.* 1984;**2**:1424–1425.

Hersh MR, Ludden TM, Kuhn JG, Knight WA III. Pharmacokinetics of high dose melphalan. *Invest New Drugs.* 1983;**1**:331–334.

Holcenberg J, Anderson T, Ritch P, et al. Intraperitoneal chemotherapy with melphalan plus glutaminase. *Cancer Res.* 1983;**43**:1381–1388.

Hoogstraten B, Sheehe PR, Cuttner J, et al. Melphalan in multiple myeloma. *Blood.* 1967;**30**:74–83.

Horowitz ME, Etcubanas E, Christensen ML, et al. Phase II testing of melphalan in children with newly diagnosed rhabdomyosarcoma: A model for anticancer drug development. *J Clin Oncol.* 1988;**6**:308–341.

Horsman MR, Brown JM, Schelley SL. The effect of misonidazole on the cytotoxicity and repair of potentially lethal damage from alkylating agents in vitro. *Int J Radiat Oncol Biol Phys.* 1982;**8**:761–765.

Howell SB, Pfeifle CE, Olshen RA. Intraperitoneal chemotherapy with melphalan. *Ann Intern Med.* 1984;**101**:14–18.

Koops HS, Oldhoff T, Van der Ploeg E, et al. Some aspects of the treatment of primary malignant melanoma of the extremities by isolated regional perfusion. *Cancer.* 1977;**39**:27–33.

Krementz ET, Ryan RF. Chemotherapy of melanoma of the extremities by perfusion: Fourteen years clinical experience. *Ann Surg.* 1972;**175**:900–917.

Lawrence BV, Harvey HA, Lipton A. Anaphylaxis due to oral melphalan (letter). *Cancer Treat Rep.* 1980;**64**(4/5):731–732.

Leff RS, Thompson JM, Johnson DB, et al. Phase II trial of high-dose melphalan and autologous bone marrow transplantation for metastatic colon carcinoma. *J Clin Oncol.* 1986;**4**(11):1586–1591.

Lokhorst HM, Meuwissen OJAT, Verdonck LF, et al. High-risk multiple myeloma treated with high-dose melphalan. *J Clin Oncol.* 1992;**10**:47–51.

Major PP, Laurin S, Bettez P. Pulmonary fibrosis following therapy with melphalan: Report of two cases. *CMA.* 1980;**123**:197–202.

Maraninchi D, Abecasis M, Gastaut J-A, et al. High-dose melphalan with autologous bone marrow rescue for the treatment of advanced adult solid tumors. *Cancer Treat Rep.* 1984;**68**:471–474.

Mascret B, Maraninchi D, Gastaut JA, et al. Treatment of malignant lymphoma with high dose of chemo or chemoradiotherapy and bone marrow transplantation. *Eur J Cancer Clin Oncol.* 1986;**22**:461–471.

McArthur JR, Athens JW, Wintrobe MM. Melphalan and myeloma: Experience with a low-dose continuous regimen. *Ann Intern Med.* 1970;**72**:665–670.

McIntyre OR, Leone L, Pajak TF. The use of intravenous melphalan (L-PAM) in the treatment of multiple myeloma. *Blood.* 1978;**52**(suppl 1):274.

Minor DR, Allen R, Alberts D, et al. A clinical and pharmacokinetic study of isolated limb perfusion with heat and melphalan for melanoma. *Cancer.* 1985;**55**:2638–2647.

Morstyn G, Campbell L, Lieschke G, et al. Treatment of chemotherapy-induced neutropenia by subcutaneously administered granulocyte colony-stimulating factor with optimization of dose and duration of therapy. *J Clin Oncol.* 1989;**7**:1554–1562.

Murray D, Meyn RE. Enhancement of the DNA cross-linking activity of melphalan by misonidazole in vivo. *Br J Cancer.* 1983;**47**:195–203.

Murray D, Meyn RE. Enhancement of the DNA cross-linking activity of nitrogen mustard by misonidazole and diethyl maleate in a mouse fibrosarcoma tumor in vivo. *Cancer Res.* 1984;**44**:91–96.

Peters WP, Olsen GA, Gockerman JP, et al. High dose combination cyclophosphamide (C), cisplatin (P), and melphalan (M) with autologous bone marrow support (ABMS). A phase I trial (abstract). *Proc Am Soc Clin Oncol.* 1986;**5**:133.

Philip T, Biron P, Philip I, et al. Autologous bone marrow transplantation for very bad prognosis neuroblastoma. In: Evans AE, D'Angio GJ, Seeger RC, eds. *Advances in Neuroblastoma Research.* New York: Liss; 1985:569–586.

Pritchard J, McElwain TJ, Graham-Pole J. High-dose melphalan with autologous marrow for treatment of advanced neuroblastoma. *Br J Cancer.* 1982;**45**:86–94.

Rauschecker HF, Foth H, Michaelis HC, et al. Kinetics of melphalan leakage during hyperthermic isolation perfusion in melanoma of the limb. *Cancer Chemother Pharmacol.* 1991;**27**:379–384.

Reece PA, Dale BM, Morris RG, et al. Effect of L-leucine on oral melphalan kinetics in patients. *Cancer Chemother Pharmacol.* 1987;**20**:256–258.

Reece PA, Hill HS, Green RM, et al. Renal clearance and protein binding of melphalan in patients with cancer. *Cancer Chemother Pharmacol.* 1988;**22**:348–352.

Rosner F. Multiple myeloma and acute leukemia: A review of 104 cases (abstract C-28). *Proc Am Assoc Cancer Res ASCO.* 1979;**20**:299.

Ross WE, Ewig RAG, Kohn KW. Differences between melphalan and nitrogen mustard in the formation and removal of DNA cross-links. *Cancer Res.* 1978;**38**:1502–1506.

Rutledge F. Chemotherapy of ovarian cancer with melphalan. *Clin Obstet Gynecol.* 1968;**11**:354.

Samuels ML, Howe CD. Vinblastine in the management of testicular cancer. *Cancer.* 1970;**25**:1009–1017.

Sarosy G, Leyland-Jones B, Soochan P, Cheson BD. The systemic administration of intravenous melphalan. *J Clin Oncol.* 1988;**6**:1768–1782.

Schmid FA, Banks SE, Stock CC. Comparative antitumor effects of Peptichemio and other alkylating agents. *Cancer Treat Rep.* 1977;**61**(3):473–475.

Schwartz MA, Gutterman JU, Burgess MA, et al. Chemoimmunotherapy of disseminated melanoma with DTIC-BCG, transfer factor + melphalan. *Cancer.* 1980;**46**:2506–2515.

Selby PJ, McElwain TJ, Nandi AC, et al. Multiple myeloma treated with high dose intravenous melphalan. *Br J Haematol.* 1987;**66**:55–62.

Selby PJ, Millar JL, Phelps TA, et al. The combination of melphalan with prednisolone. Anti-tumor effect and normal tissue toxicity in laboratory systems. *Cancer Chemother Pharmacol.* 1981;**6**:169–173.

Skehan MW, Bernath AM. Vasculitis and melphalan (letter). *JAMA.* 1978;**240**:2733–2734.

Smith JP, Rutledge FN. Chemotherapy in advanced ovarian cancer. *Natl Cancer Inst Monogr.* 1974;**42**:141.

Soble MJ, Dorr RT. Lack of enhanced antitumor efficacy for L-buthionine sulfoximine in combination with carmustine, cyclophosphamide, doxorubicin or melphalan in mice. *Anticancer Res.* 1988;**8**:17–22.

Spitzer TR, Lazarus HM, Berger NA. High dose melphalan (MEL), misonidazole (MIS) and autologous bone marrow transplantation (ABMT) for metastatic colorectal carcinoma (abstract). *Proc Am Soc Clin Oncol.* 1987;**6**:82.

Stehlin JS, Piovanella BC, De Ipolyi D, et al. Results of hyperthermic perfusion for melanoma of the extremities. *Surg Gynecol Obstet.* 1975;**140**:339–348.

Sugarbaker EV, McBride CM. Survival and regional disease control after isolation perfusion for invasive stage I melanoma of the extremities. *Cancer.* 1976;**37**:188–198.

Suzukake K, Petro BJ, Vistica DT. Reduction in glutathione content of L-PAM resistant L1210 cells confers drug sensitivity. *Biochem Pharmacol.* 1982;**31**(1):121–124.

Sviland L, Robinson A, Proctor SJ, Bateman DN. Interaction of cimetidine with oral melphalan. A pharmacokinetic study. *Cancer Chemother Pharmacol.* 1987;**20**:173–175.

Tabibi SE, Cradock JC. Stability of melphalan in infusion fluids. *Am J Hosp Pharm.* 1984;**41**:1380–1382.

Taetle R, Dickman PS, Feldman PS. Pulmonary histopathologic changes associated with melphalan therapy. *Cancer.* 1978;**42**:1239–1245.

Taha A-K, Ahmad RA, Gray H, et al. Plasma melphalan and prednisolone concentrations during oral therapy for multiple myeloma. *Cancer Chemother Pharmacol.* 1982;**9**:57–60.

Taylor YC, Bump EA, Brown JM. Studies on the mechanism of chemosensitization by misonidazole in vitro. *Int J Radiat Oncol Biol Phys.* 1982;**8**:705–708.

Tchekmedyian NS, Tait N, VanEcho D, et al. High-dose chemotherapy without autologous bonemarrow transplantation in melanoma. *J Clin Oncol.* 1986;**4**:1811–1818.

Tranchand B, Ploin Y-D, Minuit M-P, et al. High-dose melphalan dosage adjustment: Possibility of using a test-dose. *Cancer Chemother Pharmacol.* 1989;**23**:95–100.

Trissel LA. *Handbook on Injectable Drugs.* Washington, DC: American Society of Hospital Pharmacists; 1977:413.

Vistica DT. Cytotoxicities of the L and D isomers of phenylalanine mustard in the L-1210 cell (abstract 283). *Proc Am Assoc Cancer Res.* 1979;**20**:70.

Wang AL, Tew KD. Increased glutathione-S-transferase activity in a cell line with acquired resistance to nitrogen mustards. *Cancer Treat Rep.* 1985;**69**:677–682.

Westerfield BT, Michalski JP, McCombs C, Light RW. Reversible melphalan-induced lung damage. *Am J Med.* 1980;**68**:767–771.

Menogaril

■ Other Names

Menogarol; NSC-269148; 7-(R)-O-methylnogarol; 7-OMEN.

■ Chemistry

Structure of menogaril

Menogaril is a semisynthetic anthracycline antibiotic synthesized from nogalamycin. The compound has a molecular weight of 541.54 and the empiric formula $C_{28}H_{31}NO_{10}$ (Wiley et al 1979, 1982; Bhuyan et al 1980). The complete chemical name is 7-con-O-methylnogarol. Of interest, the compound is active when administered orally to animals (McGovren, 1989).

■ Antitumor Activity

Menogaril has substantial antitumor activity in a number of animal tumor systems (Neil et al 1979, Li et al 1979, McGovren 1989); however, it is not approved for treatment of any malignancies in patients. In phase I studies responses were noted in patients with glioma, renal cell carcinoma, bladder cancer (when treated with a once-weekly dose schedule), acute lymphocyte leukemia, and acute myelogenous leukemia. Minor responses have been noted in patients with glioma and prostate cancer (Stephens et al 1990, Dutcher et al 1991, Stewart et al 1989).

Phase II trials in patients with solid tumors are outlined in the table below. As can be seen, the compound does have antitumor activity in patients with metastatic breast cancer (even when given orally), as long as those patients have not had prior treatment with an anthracycline.

SUMMARY OF PHASE II RESULTS WITH MENOGARIL

Tumor Type	Route and Schedule	Number of Responses/Number Evaluable	Reference
Pancreas	IV every 3 wk	0/15	Sternberg et al 1988
Breast (no prior chemo)	Oral, weekly	2CR,9PR/48*	Stewart et al 1991
Breast (no prior chemo)	IV, days 1 and 8 every 28 d	1CR,2PR/18	Kennedy et al 1990
Breast (no prior chemo)	IV every 2 h every 28 d	6PR/24	Eisenhauer et al 1990
Breast (no prior regimen)	IV every 1 h every 28 d	4PR/25	Long et al 1988
Breast (no prior anthracyclines)	IV every 2 h every 28 d	6PR/36	Sessa et al 1988
Breast (no prior anthracyclines)	IV every 1 h every 28 d	4PR/25	Long et al 1988
Colon (no prior chemo)	IV every 2 h every 28 d	0/27	Holdener et al 1988
Non-Hodgkin's lymphoma (no prior chemo)	IV every 28 d	9PR/26	Skillings et al 1991
Sarcoma (no prior chemo)	IV every 1 h every 21–28 d	1PR/21	Buckner et al 1989
Ovary (prior chemo)	IV every 4 wk	2/19	Long et al 1991b
Lung, non-small cell (no prior chemo)	IV every 2 h every 28 d	0/44	Joss et al 1988
Colorectal (no prior chemo)	IV, single every 28 d	1CR,1PR/21	Whitehead et al 1990
Cervix (no prior chemo)	IV every 1 h every 28 d	0/14	Long et al 1991c
Kidney (no prior chemo)	IV every 1 h every 28 d	0/15	Long et al 1991a
Lung, non-small cell (no prior chemo)	IV every 1 h every 28 d	1PR/45	Vance et al 1991
Renal	IV every 28 d	3PR/56	Stephens et al 1990

*CR, complete response; PR, partial response.

Mechanism of Action

Even though menogaril is an anthracycline, it appears to have a different mechanism of action than daunorubicin and doxorubicin. Daunorubicin and doxorubicin strongly bind to DNA and then intercalate, whereas menogaril is cytotoxic at concentrations at which menogaril binds minimally to DNA. In addition, menogaril accumulates in the cytoplasm rather than in the nucleus (like doxorubicin) (Bhuyan et al 1981, Krueger et al 1981). These data suggest that DNA is not a primary molecular target for menogaril.

Availability and Storage

Menogaril is an investigational agent manufactured by the Upjohn Company and supplied by the National Cancer Institute, Bethesda, Maryland. It is available as a sterile powder in a vial containing 50 mg of menogaril. The intact vials should be refrigerated at 2 to 8°C. The agent is supplied for injection in 5-mg vials, with meglumine 100 mg. The final product is prepared as a lyophilized powder in 10-mL amber vials. The intact vials should be stored at refrigeration temperature (2–8°C) and protected from light.

Preparation for Use, Stability, and Admixture

For intravenous injections the contents of the 50-mg vial should be dissolved in 10 mL Sterile Water for Injection, USP, and then added to 500 mg of 5% dextrose in water for infusion. Solutions contain no preservatives and must be administered within 8 hours. For oral trials, the preferred method of administration has been menogaril in grape juice (Stewart et al 1991).

Administration

Menogaril may be given as a 1-hour infusion in 500 mL of D5W. The schedules listed in the table below have been tested in phase I clinical trials. It is recommended that menogaril be administered via a central vein to avoid the attended phlebitis. Menogaril can also be administered orally. Dodion et al (1988) have given the drug orally daily × 3 every 4 weeks in doses ranging from 50 to 175 mg/m^2/d. The dose they recommended for phase II trials was 150 mg/m^2/d × 3. Taguchi et al (1991) were able to administer a compound formulation of 100 mg of menogaril daily × 14 days.

Special Precautions

None are known.

Drug Interactions

None are known.

Dosage

The usual dosage for menogaril is 160 mg/m^2 given intravenously × 1 and repeated every 28 days (if the

PHASE I CLINICAL TRIALS WITH MENOGARIL

Schedule	Route	Dose Range (mg/m^2)	Recommended Phase II Dose (mg/m^2)	Dose-Limiting Toxic Effect	Reference
Single infusion every 1 h every 28 d	IV	16–256	160–200	Granulocytopenia	Dorr et al 1986
Single 2-h infusion every 4–5 wk	IV	17–250	160–200	Leukopenia	Dodion et al 1986
Weekly	IV	5–115	115	Granulocytopenia	Stewart et al 1989
1- to 2-h infusion daily × 5 every 28 d	IV	3.5–56	50	Granulocytopenia	Sigman et al 1986
Days 1 and 8 every 28 d	IV	8–140	140 (for no prior treatment)	Granulocytopenia	Brown et al 1987
72-h continuous infusion	IV	—	None	Phlebitis	Long et al 1987
90-min infusion daily × 5 (leukemia)	IV	50–130	100	Mucositis	Dutcher et al 1991
Weekly	PO	20–150	250–300	Granulocytopenia	Stewart et al 1990
Daily × 3 every 4 wk	PO	50–175	150	Granulocytopenia	Dodion et al 1988

MENOGARIL PHARMACOKINETICS

Schedule	Route	Half-life (h) α	Half-life (h) β	Half-life (h) γ	Peak Concentration	Total Clearance (L/h/m²)	Steady-State Volume of Distribution (L/m²)	Bioavailability (%)	Reference
2-h infusion	IV	—	—	29.5	0.13–1.11 μg/mL	20.2	1056		Dodion et al 1986
1-h infusion daily × 5	IV	0.19 ± 0.04	13.22 ± 1.54			28.18 ± 3.33	370 ± 25.7		Egorin et al 1986
2-h infusion	IV	—	38 ± 3			14 ± 21	805 ± 91		Zanette et al 1987
Daily × 3	PO		—	11.3	0.206 μM			32	Dodion et al 1988

675

patient has recovered from drug-related toxic effects). However, the table on page 674 details the recommended doses on other schedules explored in phase I trials.

Pharmacokinetics

Plasma concentrations were best fit to a three-compartment model by some investigators (Dodion et al 1986) and a two-compartment model by others (Egorin et al 1986, Zanette et al 1987) (see table on page 675). Of great interest is that the pharmacokinetics of menogaril in patients with abnormally low liver function tests appears to be no different from that in patients with no hepatic abnormalities (Egorin et al 1987). There are good correlations between the AUC for menogaril and the percentage decrease in white blood cells (Dodion et al 1986) and between the AUC and absolute neutrophil count (Egorin et al 1986). N-Demethyl-menogaril has been detected as a metabolite in plasma (Dodion et al 1986, Egorin et al 1986). Urinary excretion of the drug accounts for about 5% of the administered dose (Egorin et al 1986). Biliary excretion accounts for 2 to 4% of the daily dose (Egorin et al 1986).

Side Effects and Toxicity

Toxic effects consistently noted with menogaril administration include dose-limiting leukopenia (usually a nadir at 2 weeks after administration and recovery by week 4), concentration-dependent phlebitis, alopecia, occasional thrombocytopenia, mild nausea and vomiting, orange discoloration of the skin, mucositis (dose-limiting for patients with leukemia), and local urticaria (Dorr et al 1986, Dodion et al 1986, Dutcher et al 1991, Sigman et al 1986).

McGovren et al (1979) reported that menogaril was one fifteenth as potent as doxorubicin in inducing cardiotoxicity in rabbits. In humans, possible drug-induced cardiac side effects include atrial fibrillation, sinus bradycardia, myocardial infarction, and premature ventricular contractions. Temporary decreases in ejection fractions have been seen in some patients (Dorr et al 1986; Dodion et al 1988, Stewart et al 1989, Kennedy et al 1990). None of these cardiac findings have been definitely related to the use of menogaril. Of note, when the drug is given orally, dose-related leukopenia is the dose-limiting toxic effect (Dodion et al 1988, Taguchi et al 1991, Stewart et al 1990).

Special Applications

None are known.

REFERENCES

Bhuyan BK, McGovren JP, Crampton SL. Intracellular uptake of 7-con-O-methylnogarol and Adriamycin by cells in culture and its relationship to cell survival. *Cancer Res.* 1981;**41**:882–887.

Bhuyan BK, Neil GL, Li LH, McGovren JP, Wiley PF. Chemistry and biological activity of 7-con-O-methylnogarol (7-con-OMEN). In: *Anthracyclines: Current Status and New Developments.* New York: Academic Press; 1980:365–395.

Brown TD, Donehower RC, Grochow LB, Rice AP, Ettinger DS. A phase I study of menogaril in patients with advanced cancer. *J Clin Oncol.* 1987;**5**:92–99.

Buckner JC, Edmonson JH, Ingle JN, Schaid DJ. Evaluation of menogaril in patients with metastatic sarcomas and no prior chemotherapy exposure. *Am J Clin Oncol.* 1989;**12**:384–386.

Dodion P, DeValeriola D, Crespeigne N, et al. Phase I clinical and pharmacokinetic trial of oral menogaril administered on three consecutive days. *Eur J Cancer Clin Oncol.* 1988;**24**:1019–1026.

Dodion P, Sessa C, Joss R, et al. Phase I study of intravenous menogaril administered intermittently. *J Clin Oncol.* 1986;**4**:767–774.

Dorr FA, Von Hoff DD, Kuhn JG, Schwartz R, Kisner DL. Phase I clinical investigation of 7-con-O-methylnogaril, a new anthracycline antibiotic. *Cancer Res.* 1986;**46**:2562–2565.

Dutcher JP, Schwartz EL, Wiernik PH, Brechbuhl AB, Benson L, Garl S. Phase I study of menogaril (M) with pharmacokinetics (PK) in acute leukemia (AL). *Proc Am Assoc Cancer Res.* 1991;**32**:179.

Egorin MJ, Conley BA, Forrest A, Zuhowski EG, Sinibaldi V, Van Echo DA. Phase I study and pharmacokinetics of menogaril (NSC-269148) in patients with hepatic dysfunction. *Cancer Res.* 1987;**47**:6104–6110.

Egorin MJ, Van Echo DA, Whitacre MY, et al. Human pharmacokinetics, excretion, and metabolism of the anthracycline antibiotic menogaril (7-OMEN, NSC-269148) and their correlation with clinical toxicities. *Cancer Res.* 1986;**46**:1513–1520.

Eisenhauer EA, Pritchard KI, Perrault DJ, Verma S, Pater JL. Activity of intravenous menogaril in patients with previously untreated metastatic breast cancer. *Invest New Drugs.* 1990;**8**:283–287.

Holdener EE, ten Bokkel Huinink WW, Decoster G, Ludwig C, Renard G, Pinedo HM. Phase II trial of menogaril in advanced colorectal cancer. *Invest New Drugs.* 1988;**6**:227–230.

Joss RA, Monfardini S, Hansen M, Dombernowsky P,

Renard J, Pinedo H. Negative phase II trial of menogaril in advanced squamous, adeno- and large cell carcinoma of the lung. *Eur J Cancer Clin Oncol.* 1988;**24**:263–265.

Kennedy MJ, Donehower RC, Grochow LB, Ettinger DS, Fetting JH, Abeloff MD. Phase II trial of menogaril as initial chemotherapy for metastatic breast cancer. *Invest New Drugs.* 1990;**8**:289–294.

Krueger WC, Pschigoda LM, Schpok SLF, et al. The interaction of nogalamycin and analogs with DNA and other biopolymers. *Chem–Biol Interact.* 1981;**36**:1–18.

Li HL, Kuentzel SL, Murch LL, Pschigoda LM, Krueger WC. Comparative biological and biochemical effects of nogalamycin and its analogs on L1210 leukemia. *Cancer Res.* 1979;**39**:4816–4822.

Long HJ III, Hauge MD, Therneau TM, Buckner JC, Frytak S, Hahn RG. Phase II evaluation of menogaril in patients with advanced hypernephroma. *Invest New Drugs.* 1991a;**9**:261–262.

Long HJ III, Laurie JA, Wieand HS, et al. A phase II evaluation of menogaril in cisplatin-refractory advanced ovarian carcinoma. A collaborative trial of the North Central Cancer Treatment Group and the Mayo Clinic. *Cancer.* 1991b;**68**:730–732.

Long HJ III, Wieand HS, Foley JF, et al. Phase II evaluation of menogaril in patients with advanced cervical carcinoma. A collaborative trial of the North Central Cancer Treatment Group and Mayo Clinic. *Invest New Drugs.* 1991c;**9**:349–351.

Long HJ, Powis G, Schutt AJ, Moertel CG. Phase I pharmacokinetics study of menogaril administered as a 72-hour continuous i.v. infusion. *Cancer Treat Rep.* 1987;**71**:593–598.

Long HJ, Schaid DJ, Schutt AJ, Ingle JN, Loprinzi CL, Edmonson JH. Phase II evaluation of menogaril in women with metastatic breast cancer after failure of firstline chemotherapy. *Am J Clin Oncol* 11:524–527, 1988.

McGovren JP. Activity of the anthracycline agent, 7-*con-O*-methylnogarol (7-OMEN) administered orally to mice bearing P388 or L1210 leukemia. *Cancer Treat Rep.* 1989;**64**:727–729.

McGovren JP, Neil GL, Denlinger RH, Hall TL, Crampton SL, Swenberg JA. Chronic cardiotoxicity studies in rabbits with 7-*con-O*-methylnogarol, a new anthracycline antitumor agent. *Cancer Res.* 1979;**39**:4849–4855.

Neil GL, Kuentzel SL, McGovren JP. Treatment of mouse tumors with 7-*con-O*-methylnogarol and other analogs of the anthracycline antibiotics, nagalamycin. *Cancer Treat Rep.* 1979;**63**:1971–1978.

Sessa C, Gundersen S, ten Bokkel Huinink W, Renard J, Cavalli F. Phase II study of intravenous menogaril in patients with advanced breast cancer. *J Natl Cancer Inst.* 1988;**80**:1066–1069.

Sigman LM, Van Echo DA, Egorin MJ, Whitacre MY, Aisner J. Phase I trial of menogaril administered as an intermittent daily infusion for 5 days. *Cancer Treat Rep.* 1986;**70**:721–725.

Skillings J, Cripps C, Eisenhauer E, Pater J, Verma S, Walde D. A phase II study of menogaril in low-grade non-Hodgkin's lymphoma. An NCI Canada Clinical Trials Group study. *Invest New Drugs.* 1991;**9**:79–82.

Stephens RL, Goodman P, Crawford ED, et al. Evaluation of menogaril in renal cell carcinoma. A Southwest Oncology Group phase II study (8504). *Invest New Drugs.* 1990;**8**:S69–71.

Sternberg CN, Magill GB, Cheng EW, Hollander P. Phase II trial of menogarol in the treatment of advanced adenocarcinoma of the pancreas. *Am J Clin Oncol.* 1988;**11**:174–176.

Stewart DJ, Maroun JA, Verma S, Perrault D, Earhart RH. Phase I study of weekly intravenous administration of menogaril to adults with solid tumors. *Am J Clin Oncol.* 1989;**12**:511–518.

Stewart D, Verma S. NCI Canada phase II study of weekly oral menogaril (M) as first line chemotherapy for recurrent breast cancer (BC). *Proc Am Soc Clin Oncol.* 1991;**10**:74.

Stewart DJ, Verma S, Maroun JA, Robillard L, Earhart RH. Phase I study of oral menogaril administered on a once weekly schedule. *Invest New Drugs.* 1990;**8**:43–52.

Taguchi T, Wakui A, Majima H, et al. A phase I study and pharmacokinetics of oral menogaril (TUT-7) administered on 14 consecutive days. *Proc Am Soc Clin Oncol.* 1991;**10**:109.

Vance RB, Crowley JJ, Macdonald JS, Ahmann FR. Phase II evaluation of menogaril (NSC-269148) in non-small cell lung carcinoma. A Southwest Oncology Group study. *Invest New Drugs.* 1991;**9**:73–75.

Whitehead RP, Earhart RH, Fleming T, et al. A phase II study of menogaril (NSC-269148) in colorectal carcinoma. A Southwest Oncology Group study. *Invest New Drugs.* 1990;**8**:295–297.

Wiley PF, Elrod DW, Houser DJ, Johnson JL, Pschigoda LM, Krueger WC. Nogalamycin. Stereochemistry and chemical modification. *J Org Chem.* 1979;**44**:4030–4038.

Wiley PF, Elrod DW, Houser DJ, Richard FA. Structure–activity relationships of nogalamycin analogues. *J Med Chem.* 1982;**25**:560–567.

Zanette ML, Tirelli U, Sorio R, et al. Pharmacokinetics of 7-*con-O*-methylnogarol in patients with solid tumors. *Cancer Chemother Pharmacol.* 1987;**20**:67–70.

Merbarone

Other Names

NSC-336628.

Chemistry

Structure of merbarone

Merbarone was submitted to the National Cancer Institute by Uniroyal, Ltd. It is a nonsedating derivative of thiobarbituric acid. Antitumor activity has been observed among the barbiturates (Driscoll et al 1978) and merbarone clearly showed antitumor activity against L-1210 and P-388 mouse leukemia as well as B-16 melanoma and M-5076 carcinoma (Brewer et al 1985, Plowman et al 1985). The antitumor effects were schedule dependent. The complete chemical name is 5-(N-phenylcarboxamido)-2-thiobarbituric acid, or hexahydro-4,6-dioxy-N-phenyl-2-thioxo-5-pyrimidine-carboxamide. The compound has a molecular weight of 263.3 and the empiric formula $C_{11}H_9N_3O_3$. An excellent review of merbarone has been published by Glover et al (1987).

Antitumor Activity

Merbarone has significant anticancer activity in several murine tumor models. These include P-388 and L-1210 leukemias, B-16 melanoma, and M-5076 sarcoma. Merbarone is also active in some multidrug-resistant, P-glycoprotein-positive tumor cell lines in vitro (Glover et al 1987). The antitumor activity of merbarone in experimental models is schedule dependent, favoring more frequent administration to enhance cytotoxicity. The drug is inactive in CD8F breast cancer and in colon-38 adenocarcinoma (Glover et al 1987).

Merbarone is now undergoing phase I and II clinical trials. Therefore, the antitumor activity of the compound has not yet been defined.

Mechanism of Action

The mechanism of action of merbarone may involve DNA damage, but the agent does not bind to DNA. Cooney et al (1985) demonstrated dose-related DNA single-strand breaks following merbarone administration. Recently, Drake et al (1989), Woessner et al (1990), and others documented that merbarone inhibits topoisomerase II activity. There is increasing evidence that this may indeed be the mechanism of action of merbarone. In fact, merbarone is a very novel topoisomerase II inhibitor (not in the epipodophyllin or novobiocin class). There is also electron spin resonance evidence that merbarone can generate oxygen radicals in the presence of reducing equivalents such as NADPH. In addition, the drug can induce hepatic microsomes and generate lipid peroxidation therein. This activity appears to be more potent than the membrane lipid peroxidation induced by doxorubicin (Cooney et al 1986).

Availability and Storage

Merbarone is supplied for investigational use only by the Division of Cancer Treatment, National Cancer Institute. The agent is supplied for injection in 50- and 200-mg vials, with meglumine 100 mg. The final product is prepared as a lyophilized powder in 10-mL amber vials. The intact vials should be stored at refrigeration temperature (2–8°C) and protected from light.

Preparation for Use, Stability, and Admixture

When the vial with 50 mg liquid is reconstituted with 5 mL of Sterile Water for Injection, USP, each milliliter contains 10 mg of merbarone and 20 mg of meglumine at pH 9.0 to 10.5. The 200-mg vial contains 400 mg of meglumine and is reconstituted with 19.5 mL of Sterile Water for Injection, USP. The solution may be light yellow, peach-colored, or light pink in color. Shelf-life surveillance of the intact vials is ongoing. Reconstitution, as directed, results in a solution that is stable, exhibiting no decomposition after 15 days of storage at 0°C, room temperature, and 37°C. This initial solution can be diluted to a concentration of 0.1 mg/mL with 5% dextrose in glass or polyvinyl chloride plastic infusion containers with a resultant stability time of 2 weeks at 0°C or room temperature.

Merbarone is incompatible with metal ions such as Na^+, K^+, Ca^{2+}, and Mg^{2+}. A precipitate may form if the drug is diluted in solutions containing these ions. Dilution of merbarone with isotonic sodium chloride solution has resulted in the formation of crystals in 30 minutes. Therefore, merbarone should not be diluted with solutions that contain metal ions.

■ Administration

The drug is given intravenously. Dimaggio et al (1990) explored both a 2-hour infusion and a 24-hour continuous infusion schedule. They then explored a daily × 5 schedule of administration. Phlebitis was dose limiting at 150 mg/m^2/d × 5. The schedule was then switched to a 5-day *continuous* infusion in which renal insufficiency was dose limiting at 1500 mg/m^2/d. Kraut et al (1988) reached a dose on the same continuous infusion schedule of 1000 mg/m^2/day; using a 2-hour infusion schedule they reached a dose of 336 mg/m^2/d.

■ Special Precautions

See Preparation for Use, Stability, and Admixture for cautions regarding incompatibility of merbarone with metal ions.

■ Drug Interactions

None are known to date.

■ Dosage

The precise recommended dose and schedules for merbarone administration are not yet certain. The recommended dose on the daily × 5 schedule as a continuous infusion is 1000 mg/m^2/d (Dimaggio et al 1990).

■ Pharmacokinetics

Dimaggio et al (1990) noted that steady-state plasma concentrations of merbarone are reached within 24 to 48 hours of beginning a 5-day continuous infusion. Elimination is via a two-compartment model with an α half-life of 4.2 hours and β half-life of 15.3 hours. Renal excretion was 20 to 40% of the administered dose. Only about 0.2 to 2.8% is excreted intact. Kraut et al (1988) have also reported some kinetic studies in an abstract form. The mean clearance was 11.8 mL/m^2/d and was independent of dose. The mean steady-state plasma concentrations at 1000 mg/m^2/d × 5 was 60.5 µg/mL. Supko et al (1988) have identified the major urinary metabolite of merbarone to be 2-oxo-2-desthiomerbarone, 4'-hydroxymerbarone (the predominant species), and 4'-hydroxy-2-oxo-2-desthiomerbarone. Levels of these metabolites are very low in the plasma.

■ Side Effects and Toxicity

As noted earlier, dose-limiting toxic effects have included phlebitis (when the drug is given through a peripheral vein) and renal insufficiency (when the drug is given centrally). Another toxic effect is marked hypouricemia. This is due to a major uricosuric effect as well as inhibition of xanthine oxidase. With respect to the latter, merbarone is much less potent than allopurinol (Warrell et al 1988, 1989). Other mild side effects have included nausea, fatigue, leukopenia, thrombocytopenia, anorexia, and alopecia. Warrell et al (1988, 1989) and Grever et al (1988) have shown that hypouricemia is due to an increase in urinary uric acid excretion.

■ Special Applications

Although not yet used clinically, merbarone might have potential as a uricosuric agent.

REFERENCES

Brewer AD, Minatelli JA, Plowman J, Paull KD, Narayanan VL. 5-(*N*-phenylcarboxyamido)-2-thiobarbituric acid (NSC-336628), a novel potential antitumor agent. *Biochem Pharmacol.* 1985;**34**:2047–2050.

Cooney DA, Covey JM, Dalal M, et al. Mechanistic studies with merbarone (MB; NSC-336628). *Proc Am Assoc Cancer Res.* 1986;**27**:276.

Cooney DA, Covey JM, Kang GJ, Dalal M, McMahon JB, Johns DG. Initial mechanistic studies with merbarone (NSC-336628). *Biochem Pharmacol.* 1985;**34**:3395–3398.

Dimaggio JJ, Warrell RP Jr, Muindi J, et al. Phase I clinical and pharmacological study of merbarone. *Cancer Res.* 1990;**50**:1151–1155.

Drake FH, Hofmann GA, Mong SM, et al. In vitro and intracellular inhibition of toposomerase II by the antitumor agent merbarone. *Cancer Res.* 1989;**49**:2578–2583.

Driscoll JS, Melnick NR, Quinn FR, et al. Psychotropic drugs as potential antitumor agents: A selective screening study. *Cancer Treat Rep.* 1978;**62**:45–74.

Glover A, Chun HG, Kleinman LM, et al. Merbarone: An antitumor agent entering clinical trials. *Invest New Drugs.* 1987;**5**:137–143.

Grever MR, Kraut EH, Supko JG, Trewyn RW, Staubus AE, Malspeis L. Merbarone (NSC-336628) enhances the urinary excretion of uric acid of cancer patients (abstract 752). *Proc Am Assoc Cancer Res.* 1988;**29**:189.

Kraut EH, Grever MR, Staubus AE, Malspeis L. Phase I clinical trial of merbarone (NSC-336628) (abstract 760). *Proc Am Assoc Cancer Res.* 1988;**29**:191.

Plowman J, Paull KD, Narayanan VL, Brewer AD, Minatelli JA. A novel experimental antitumor agent:

5-*N*-phenylcarboxamido)-2-thiobarbituric acid, NSC-336628. *Proc Am Assoc Cancer Res.* 1985;**26**:251.

Supko JG, Grever MR, Balcerzak SP, Kraut EH, Staubus AE, Malspeis L. Spectral characterization and quantitation of the principal metabolites of merbarone (336628) in the urine of patients (abstract 751). *Proc Annu Meet Am Assoc Cancer Res.* 1988;**29**:189.

Warrell RP Jr, Muindi J, Stevens Y-W, et al. Clinical pharmacology of the potent hypouricemic effect induced by merbarone. *Proc Am Soc Clin Oncol.* 1988;**7**:65.

Warrell RP Jr, Muindi J, Stevens YW, Isaacs M, Young CW. Introduction of profound hypouricemia by a non-sedating thiobarbiturate. *Metabolism.* 1989;**38**:550–554.

Woessner RD, Chung TD, Hofmann GA, et al. Differences between normal and *ras*-transformed NIH-3T3 cells in expression of the 170kD and 180kD forms of topoisomerase II. *Cancer Res.* 1990;**50**:2901–2908.

6-Mercaptopurine

■ Other Names

Purinethol® (Burroughs-Wellcome Company); NSC-755; mercaptopurine; 6-MP.

■ Chemistry

Structure of 6-mercaptopurine

6-Mercaptopurine (6-MP) is purine-6-thiol monohydrate and differs from purine by the presence of a sulfhydryl group rather than a hydroxyl group at the 6-position of the purine ring. 6-MP has a pK_a of 7.6 and exists as a yellow crystalline powder. It is insoluble in water but soluble in hot alcohol. The injectable preparation is a water-soluble sodium salt. The molecular weight of 6-MP is 170.23.

■ Antitumor Activity

6-Mercaptopurine has been useful in the treatment of acute leukemia in both children (Henderson, 1967) and adults (Wiernik and Serpick, 1972, Ellison et al 1972). It has also been useful as second-line therapy in chronic granulocytic leukemia. In chronic myelogenous leukemia, 6-MP has been used as both maintenance therapy and a primary treatment for patients in blast crisis. Similar applications have been described in diffuse histiocytic and undifferentiated lymphomas (Lister et al 1978). In various advanced refractory cancers (mostly solid tumors) Esterhay et al (1978) found mercaptopurine to be ineffective.

The more common clinical use of mercaptopurine is in combination chemotherapy for remission induction and maintenance of acute lymphocytic leukemia in children (Henderson 1976). One of the more popular induction regimens in this regard is POMP, wherein mercaptopurine is cyclically combined with methotrexate, vincristine, and prednisone (Rodriguez et al 1975). For remission maintenance, mercaptopurine is often given daily by mouth with other agents such as weekly methotrexate (Aur et al 1979). Note that the oral bioavailability of 6-MP is low. Absorption is also variable and can significantly affect response rates in leukemia (see Pharmacokinetics). Brecher et al (1979) have additionally reported good results in pediatric non-Hodgkin's lymphomas using mercaptopurine, vincristine, prednisone, and cyclophosphamide.

6-MP is also used as an immunosuppressant for a variety of autoimmune conditions such as Crohn's disease (Present et al 1980).

■ Mechanism of Action

6-Mercaptopurine is thought to act as an "anti-" or "false" metabolite because of its close chemical similarity to the purine base hypoxanthine. Similarly to other antimetabolites, 6-MP is not active until it is metabolized to a phosphorylated nucleotide. It can compete with endogenous ribotides for the enzymes that convert iosinic acid to adenine and xanthine-based ribonucleotides. Ribonucleotides of 6-MP can be incorporated into RNA to halt further RNA synthesis. 6-MP can also be metabolized to 6-methyl mercaptopurine ribotide (MMPR) (Zimm et al 1984), a potent inhibitor of de novo purine synthesis by blocking inosinic acid reactions (Henderson and Patterson 1973). Ultimately, 6-MP halts both DNA and RNA synthesis and is considered cell cycle phase specific for S phase.

■ Availability and Storage

Mercaptopurine is commercially available as a 50-mg oral tablet that may be stored at room temperature and should be protected from light. An injectable 6-MP formulation is investigationally available in 500-mg vials containing the sodium salt of mercaptopurine from Burroughs-Wellcome Company (Research Triangle Park, North Carolina). The lyophilized powder may be stored at room temperature.

■ Preparation for Use, Stability, and Admixture

The 500-mg injectable vial is diluted with 49.8 mL of Sterile Water for Injection, USP. The resultant solution contains 10 mg of 6-MP/mL and has a pH of 10.0 to 11.0. For administration to the patient this solution should be further diluted with D5W or normal saline to a final concentration of 12 mg/mL. Mercaptopurine sodium is stable for 4 hours after dilution if kept in the refrigerator.

6-Mercaptopurine is physically incompatible if mixed with sodium allopurinol or with prednisolone sodium succinate. It reportedly is compatible in solution with methotrexate sodium (Trissel 1977).

One reported test of stability (500 mg drug in 150 mL diluent) revealed the following stability characteristics when the solution was stored at 5°C. In normal saline or D5W, the drug retained over 99% of its potency even after 7 days of storage. The pH range for the drug diluted in normal saline was 9.5 to 9.85, and for D5W, 9.5 to 9.6. Because of the lack of antibacterial preservative the manufacturer states that reconstituted vials be used within 8 hours when stored at room temperature or under refrigeration. Nonetheless, the drug has been given as a continuous intravenous infusion for 12 to 48 hours. These solutions contained 1 mg/mL 6-MP in either D5W or 0.9% sodium chloride solution (Zimm et al 1985).

■ Administration

The tablets are administered orally as a single daily dose. The sodium salt of mercaptopurine is administered intravenously by a slow intravenous push over several minutes. Injectable 6-MP may also be given by continuous infusion over 12 to 48 hours (Zimm et al 1985).

■ Dosage

Oral mercaptopurine doses of 80 to 100 mg/m^2/d or 2.5 mg/kg/d (calculated to the nearest 25 mg) are typically used. In the absence of toxicity and with good clinical response, the dose may be increased cautiously to 5 mg/kg/d. The drug can be administered on a daily basis with "titration" of dose against blood counts and response. Some intermittent or weekly IV dosing schedules have also been employed (Regelson et al 1975). Allopurinol blocks the metabolism of 6-MP by xanthine oxidase and, if used concomitantly, requires a 67 to 75% dose reduction of 6-MP. In the POMP combination regimen, mercaptopurine is given at 500 to 700 mg/m^2/d × 5 days for each induction course. Depending on effects and/or toxicity, subsequent courses may escalate this dose by as much as 40%. Combined with methotrexate in the remission maintenance therapy of acute lymphocytic leukemia a typical daily oral dose of 6-MP is 50 mg/m^2/d given for several consecutive days. High-dose oral 6-MP (1 g/m^2/d × 5) was not effective in patients with advanced solid tumors (Esterhay et al 1978).

The recommended dose for continuous intravenous infusions in phase II studies was 50 mg/m^2/h for durations not greater than 48 hours (Zimm et al 1985). Significant liver and renal impairment also requires lower doses. With renal failure, the use of the following prolonged dosing intervals has been suggested: 24 to 36 hours for creatinine clearance of 50 to 80 mL/h and 48 hours for creatinine clearances of 10 to 50 mL/h (Avery 1976).

■ Drug Interactions

Concomitant administration of allopurinol creates a metabolic blockade in mercaptopurine metabolism (detoxification) (Coffey et al 1972). Thus, when allopurinol is given concurrently, the dose of mercaptopurine must be reduced to between one fourth and one third of the usual dose. The long half-life (14 hours) of an active allopurinol metabolite (oxipurinol) should be kept in mind in this instance. In contrast, with intravenous 6-MP allopurinol does not alter 6-MP clearance or increase steady-state drug levels. Instead, allopurinol roughly doubles (from 21 to 41%) the amount of unchanged 6-MP that is recovered in the urine following infusions of 6-MP (Zimm et al 1985).

In vitro studies suggest that mercaptopurine may decrease the cellular uptake of methotrexate and thereby decrease its effect. The clinical significance of this potential interaction is not established; however, oral methotrexate (20 mg/m^2) given simultaneously with oral 6-MP (75 mg/m^2) produces a profound increase in systemic 6-MP exposure (Balis et al 1987). In a study in children, methotrexate increased peak plasma 6-MP levels by 26% and increased the area under the concentration × time curve (AUC) by 31%. This may relate to an inhibition of xanthine oxidase activity by methotrexate, but the clinical significance of this effect is minimal because of the overall variability in 6-MP bioavailability.

The anticoagulant effects of warfarin have been reported to be antagonized by mercaptopurine via an unknown mechanism. In contrast, adenosine may block 6-MP toxicity selectively in normal cells (Jackson et al 1980).

When 6-MP is combined with doxorubicin in adult acute leukemia, toxic synergy is suggested, as the incidence of hepatotoxicity in this group is greater than 50% (Minow et al 1976). In most series, however, the hepatotoxic signs gradually return to normal on discontinuance of 6-MP.

■ Pharmacokinetics

Oral 6-MP is very poorly absorbed but does not damage the gastrointestinal epithelium during intestinal transit. It is also clear that a significant "first-pass" effect (extensive initial liver metabolism) can occur after oral 6-MP dosing. Peak plasma levels of approximately 70 ng/mL are obtained 1 to 2 hours after the ingestion of an oral 6-MP dose of 75 mg/m^2 (Balis et al 1987). In contrast, an equal 6-MP dose given intravenously produces peak levels of about 5000 ng/mL within minutes of a bolus injection (Zimm et al 1983).

The table below compares the pharmacokinetic values for these two routes of administration. These findings show a very low oral bioavailability of 6-MP, averaging only 16%. There is also enormous interindividual variability in 6-MP absorption which can result in fivefold variations in the AUC for 6-MP following a standard oral dose (Zimm et al 1982). The latter effect probably reflects a highly variable first-pass hepatic metabolism of 6-MP (Zimm et al 1983). This variability in intravenous drug exposure has been used as an argument against using fixed intravenous dose conversions from oral drug regimens (Rundles and Elion 1984). One other variable influencing oral 6-MP absorption is simultaneous food intake, which lowers the already poor oral absorption of the drug by another 50% (Riccardi et al 1985). In another trial, the coadministration of oral antioxidants such as glutathione and ascorbic acid did not alter systemic 6-MP exposures in patients (Endresen et al 1990). This latter study also recommended monitoring urinary excretion of parent drug as a more convenient means of quantitating systemic drug exposure in individual patients.

With prolonged infusion regimens, mean steady-state plasma 6-MP levels of 6.9 μM are obtained (Zimm et al 1985). Of interest, these values did not vary greatly from patient to patient and were unaffected by the coadministration of oral allopurinol. Furthermore, the fractional steady-state 6-MP level in the cerebrospinal fluid compared with plasma was 0.27. This suggests potential efficacy for continuous infusion of 6-MP in managing central nervous system cancer (Zimm et al 1985).

The variable systemic exposure following oral 6-MP remission maintenance therapy has been associated with a poor prognosis in children with acute lymphocytic leukemia (Koren et al 1990). Patients who relapsed following oral 6-MP achieved a low AUC of 1.64 μM · min following a 1 mg/m^2 dose. In contrast, those remaining in remission had an average AUC of 2.4 μM · min. Overall, this led to 40% lower daily drug exposures in relapsing patients. This suggests a need for pharmacokinetic monitor-

PHARMACOKINETIC VARIABLES FOR ORAL AND INTRAVENOUS 6-MERCAPTOPURINE IN CHILDREN WITH LEUKEMIA*

Variable	Intravenous	Oral
AUC (μM · min)	993 ± 493	132 ± 79
Apparent body clearance (mL/min/m^2)	719 ± 610	4832 ± 2562
Elimination half-life (h)	0.9 ± 0.3	1.5 ± 0.5
Volume of distribution (L/kg)	0.9 ± 0.8	—
Bioavailability	—	0.16 ± 0.11
Peak plasma concentration (μM)[†]	—	0.29–1.82 (x = 0.89)
Time to peak (h)[†]	—	0.5–4 (x = 2.2)

*Seven patients studied with a specific high-performance liquid chromatography assay for 6-MP.
[†]Monkey data.
Data from Zimm et al 1983.

ing to facilitate dose escalations early in the course of remission maintenance therapy in childhood acute lymphocytic leukemia.

After an intravenous injection, the short half-life of the drug in the plasma is due to rapid renal excretion, hepatic metabolism, and cellular uptake. After 24 hours, more than 50% of a dose can be recovered in the urine as intact drug and metabolites. There are apparently two major pathways for hepatic drug metabolism: (1) methylation of the sulfhydryl group (ultimately yielding the active metabolite 6-methylsulfinyl-8 hydroxypurine and some inorganic sulfate); (2) oxidation to the inactive metabolite 6-thiouric acid by the enzyme xanthine oxidase (Elion 1967, Loo et al 1968). With infusion regimens, a small amount of the 6-mercaptopurine riboside metabolite can be recovered in the urine; this accounted for only 15% of the dose (Zimm et al 1984). A small amount of both nonrenal and nonhepatic drug degradation is also thought to occur. Approximately 30% of a given dose is protein bound, but the drug is dialyzable. Irreversible drug binding to human serum proteins is blocked by reducing agents (Sjoholm and Stjerna 1981). Irreversible protein binding of 6-MP metabolites has also been observed in human liver preparations. It appears to involve drug activation by cytochrome P450 enzymes (Hyslop and Jardine 1981).

Tterlikkis et al (1977) have studied mercaptopurine distribution in rats, finding significant drug uptake in liver, kidney, spleen, muscle, and gut lumen (in descending order of selective uptake).

A key determinant of 6-MP antileukemic activity may be intracellular phosphorylation by hypoxanthine–guanine phosphoribosyl transferase (HGPRT) and the intrinsic concentration of phosphoribosylpyrophosphate (PRPP), which is a cofactor for HGPRT activity. In some 6-MP-resistant cells, there is a loss of HGPRT activity (Higuchi et al 1976).

■ Side Effects and Toxicity

Hematologic toxicity is usually mild with typical doses. It consists of leukopenia and thrombocytopenia and, in high doses, anemia. After a 5-day 6-MP regimen, the average nadir occurred at day 15 (range, 12–21 days) for thrombocytopenia and on day 16 (range, 11–23 days) for leukopenia.

Gastrointestinal toxic effects are uncommon but include anorexia, nausea, and only occasional vomiting. Mucositis and stomatitis are commonly seen with large 6-MP doses. Profound diarrhea and a spruelike condition are also rarely observed. In the study by Esterhay et al (1978), diarrhea was occasionally severe enough to necessitate parenteral rehydration.

Other side effects include a dry scaling rash, drug fever, and eosinophilia. Jaundice and hepatitis have also been reported (McIlvanie and MacCarthy 1959) and may occasionally be dose limiting. Liver function tests should be monitored to detect biliary stasis or direct liver damage (Clark et al 1960, Einhorn and Davidson 1964). The most common clinical sign of 6-MP-induced liver damage is cumulative hyperbilirubinemia. This is usually accompanied by sequential increases in alkaline phosphatase and serum glutamic-oxalacetic transaminase. Pathologic findings consist predominantly of intrahepatic cholestasis invariably associated with mild focal centrolobular necrosis (Minow et al 1976).

Hematuria and crystalluria are also observed following high-dose intravenous bolus therapy (1 g/m^2 in 50 mL of dextrose) (Duttera et al 1972). Hematuria is noted on the second or third day of therapy and is occasionally accompanied by flank pain without dysuria, fever, or alterations in serum creatinine or platelet counts. Symptoms normally disappear within 24 hours. A renal tubule defect may occur in adults with nephrosis (Butler et al 1965). In contrast to bolus dosing, prolonged continuous-infusion regimens produce dose-limiting mucositis (Zimm et al 1985). Mucositis is particularly severe if the infusion is longer than 48 hours. Hematologic suppression and mild liver enzyme elevations are transient with the infusions; however, one instance of severe jaundice was observed with a 60-hour infusion (Zimm et al 1985). This resolved after 2 weeks. Mild nausea and vomiting have been seen in only a few patients and no central nervous system or renal toxic effects (including hematuria) are described with the continuous infusions.

■ Special Applications

A phase I/II clinical trial of intrathecal mercaptopurine has been performed in nine pediatric patients with refractory chronic meningeal leukemia (Adamson et al 1991). All patients had previously failed to respond to numerous other treatments including intrathecal cytarabine and/or methotrexate and cranial/spinal radiotherapy. The intrathecal dose of 6-MP was 10 mg twice weekly for 4 weeks (eight intrathecal injections). The complete and partial response rates were 4/9 and 3/9, respectively. Durations of response ranged from 7 to 22 weeks. Mild toxic effects, which were not dose limiting, included nausea (2/9 patients) and headache (3/9 patients).

Pharmacokinetic studies of intrathecal mercaptopurine showed that drug levels in the cerebrospinal fluid were greater than 1 µM for 12 hours after an intrathecal dose. Mean peak 6-MP levels of 1882 µM were achieved in the cerebrospinal fluid compared with approximately 0.37 µM measured simultaneously in the plasma. The AUC for an intrathecal 6-MP dose of 10 mg in the cerebrospinal fluid was 2.68 µM·h. Clearance of drug from the cerebrospinal fluid averaged 0.071 mL/min with a monophasic elimination half-life of 1.8 hours (Adamson et al 1991).

The intrathecal 6-MP doses were prepared using the investigational sodium salt formulation. The powdered drug was initially reconstituted in Elliott's B solution to a concentration of 10 mg/12 mL. An equivalent volume of cerebrospinal fluid was removed prior to instillation of the 12-mL 6-MP solution.

REFERENCES

Adamson PC, Balis FM, Arndt CA, et al. Intrathecal 6-mercaptopurine: Preclinical pharmacology, phase I/II trial, and pharmacokinetic study. *Cancer Res.* 1991;**51**: 6079–6083.

Aur RJA, Barker LF, Simone JV. Influence of drug dosage in combination therapy during remission in childhood acute lymphocytic leukemia (ALL) (abstract 321). *Proc Am Assoc Cancer Res ASCO.* 1979;**20**:80.

Avery GS. *Drug Treatment.* Sydney, Australia: ADIS Press; 1976:973.

Balis FM, Holcenberg JS, Zimm S, et al. The effect of methotrexate on the bioavailability of oral 6-mercaptopurine. *Clin Pharmacol Ther.* 1987;**41**:384–387.

Brecher ML, Thomas PRM, Sinks LM, Freeman AI. Updated results on the treatment of childhood non-Hodgkin's lymphoma (abstract C-613). *Proc Am Assoc Cancer Res ASCO.* 1979;**20**:438.

Butler HE Jr, Morgan JM, Smythe CM. Mercaptopurine and acquired tubular dysfunction in adult nephrosis. *Ann Intern Med.* 1965;**116**:853–856.

Clark PA, Hsia YE, Huntsman RG. Toxic complications of treatment with 6-mercaptopurine: Two cases with hepatic necrosis and intestinal ulceration. *Br Med J.* 1960;**1**:393–395.

Coffey JJ, White CA, Lesk AB. Effect of allopurinol on the pharmacokinetics of 6-mercaptopurine (NSC-755) in cancer patients. *Cancer Res.* 1972;**32**:1283–1289.

Duttera MJ, Carolla RL, Gallelli JF, et al. Hematuria and crystalluria after high-dose 6-mercaptopurine administration. *N Engl J Med.* 1972;**287**(6):292–294.

Einhorn M, Davidson I. Hepatoxicity of mercaptopurine. *JAMA.* 1964;**188**:802–806.

Elion GB. Biochemistry and pharmacology of purine analogues. *Fed Proc.* 1967;**26**:893–904.

Ellison RR, Hoogstraten B, Holland JF, et al. Intermittent therapy with 6-mercaptopurine (NSC-755) and methotrexate (NSC-740) given intravenously to adults with acute leukemia. *Cancer Chemother Rep.* 1972;**56**:535–542.

Endresen L, Lie SO, Storm-Mathisen I, et al. Pharmacokinetics of oral 6-mercaptopurine: Relationship between plasma levels and urine excretion of parent drug. *Ther Drug Monitoring.* 1990;**12**:227–234.

Esterhay RJ Jr, Aisner J, Levi JA, Wiernik PH. High-dose 6-mercaptopurine in advanced refractory cancer. *Cancer Treat Rep.* 1978;**62**(8):1229–1231.

Henderson ES. Combination chemotherapy of acute lymphocytic leukemia of childhood. *Cancer Res.* 1967;**27**: 2570–2572.

Henderson JF, Patterson ARP. *Nucleotide Metabolism: An Introduction.* New York: Academic Press; 1973:48.

Higuchi T, Nakamura T, Wakisaka G. Metabolism of 6-mercaptopurine in human leukemic cells. *Cancer Res.* 1976;**36**:3779–3783.

Hyslop RM, Jardine I. Metabolism of 6-thiolpurines. I. Irreversible binding of a metabolite of 6-thiolpurine to mammalian hepatic protein in vitro. *J Pharmacol Exp Ther.* 1981;**218**(3):621–628.

Jackson RC, Ross DA, Harkrader RJ, Epstein J. Biochemical approaches to enhancement of antitumor drug selectivity: Selective protection of cells from 6-thioguanine and 6-mercaptopurine by adenosine. *Cancer Treat Rep.* 1980;**64**:1347–1353.

Koren G, Ferrazini G, Sulh H, et al. Systemic exposure to mercaptopurine as a prognostic factor in acute lymphocytic leukemia in children. *N Engl J Med.* 1990;**323**:17–21.

Lazo JS, Hwang KM, Sartorelli AC. Inhibition of L-fucose incorporation into glycoprotein of sarcoma 180 ascites cells by 6-thioguanine. *Cancer Res.* 1977;**37**:4250–4257.

Lister TA, Cullen MH, Brearley RB, et al. Combination chemotherapy in advanced non-Hodgkin's lymphoma of unfavorable histology. *Cancer Chemother Pharmacol.* 1978;**1**:107–113.

Loo TL, Luce JK, Sullivan MP, Frei E III. Clinical pharmacologic observations on 6-mercaptopurine and 6-methyl thiolpurine ribonucleoside. *Clin Pharmacol Ther.* 1968;**9**: 180–194.

McIlvanie SK, MacCarthy JD. Hepatitis in association with prolonged 6-mercaptopurine therapy. *Blood.* 1959;**14**:80–90.

Minow RA, Stern MH, Casey JH, et al. Clinico-pathologic correlation of liver damage in patients treated with 6-mercaptopurine and Adriamycin. *Cancer.* 1976;**38**:1524–1528.

Present DH, Korelitz BI, Wisch N, et al. Treatment of

Crohn's disease with 6-mercaptopurine. A long-term, randomized, double-blind study. *N Engl J Med.* 1980;**302**(18):981–987.

Regelson W, Holland JF, Gold GL, et al. 6-Mercaptopurine (NSC-755) given intravenously at weekly intervals to patients with advanced cancer. *Cancer Chemother Rep.* 1967;**51**(5):277–280.

Riccardi R, Balis F, Ferrara P, et al. Influence of food intake on the absorption of orally administered 6-mercaptopurine (6-MP). *Proc Am Soc Clin Oncol.* 1985;**4**:34.

Rodriguez V, Bodey GP, McCredie K, et al. Combination of 6-mercaptopurine–Adriamycin in refractory acute leukemia. *Clin Pharmacol Ther.* 1975;**18**:462–466.

Rundles RW, Elion GB. Mercaptopurine "bioavailability." *N Engl J Med.* 1984;**310**(14):929.

Sjoholm I, Stjerna B. Binding of drugs to human serum albumin. XII. Irreversible binding of mercaptopurine to human serum proteins. *J Pharm Sci.* 1981;**70**(11):1290–1291.

Trissel A. *Handbook on Injectable Drugs.* Washington, DC: American Society of Hospital Pharmacists; 1977:414.

Tterlikkis L, Ortega E, Solomon R, Day JL. Pharmacokinetics of mercaptopurine. *J Pharm Sci.* 1977;**66**(10):1454–1457.

Wiernik PH, Serpick AA. A randomized clinical trial of daunorubicin and a combination of prednisone, vincristine, 6-mercaptopurine and methotrexate in adult acute nonlymphocytic leukemia. *Cancer Res.* 1972;**32**:2023–2026.

Zimm S, Collins JM, Riccardi R, et al. Variable bioavailability of oral mercaptopurine: Is maintenance chemotherapy in acute lymphoblastic leukemia being optimally delivered? *N Engl J Med.* 1983;**308**(17):1005–1009.

Zimm S, Ettinger LJ, Holcenberg JS, et al. Phase I and clinical pharmacological study of mercaptopurine administered as a prolonged intravenous infusion. *Cancer Res.* 1985;**45**:1869–1873.

Zimm S, Grygiel JJ, Strong JM, et al. Identification of 6-mercaptopurine riboside in patients receiving 6-mercaptopurine as a prolonged intravenous infusion. *Biochem Pharmacol.* 1984;**33**(24):4089–4092.

Zimm S, Narang PK, Riccardi R, et al. The pharmacokinetics of oral (p.o.) 6-mercaptopurine (6-MP). *Proc Am Soc Clin Oncol.* 1982;**1**:16.

Zimm S, Reaman G, Murphy R, Poplack DG. Mercaptopurine (MP) resistance in patients with acute lymphoblastic leukemia (ALL). *Proc Am Soc Clin Oncol.* 1985b;**4**:34.

Mesna

■ Other Names

Asta D 7093; Uromitexan® (Asta-Werke AG-Chemische Fabrik); Mesnex® (Bristol-Myers Oncology Division); NSC-113891; UCB 3938; Mistabron® (UCB Pharmaceuticals, Paris, France).

■ Chemistry

$$HS-CH_2-CH_2-SO_3^--Na^+$$

Structure of mesna

Mesna is the sodium salt of 2-mercaptoethanesulfonic acid. The chemical name is 2-mercaptoethanesulfonatic acid sodium salt. It has a molecular weight of 164.18 and the empiric formula $C_2H_5SO_3Na$. The commercial 100 mg/mL clear solution has a pH range of 6.5 to 8.5. Mesna powder is hygroscopic and freely soluble in water. It is sparingly soluble in ethanol and may be insoluble in other organic solvents.

■ Antitumor Activity

Mesna does not have antitumor activity but rather is a selective urinary tract protectant for oxazophosphorine-type alkylating agents (Burkert 1983). In the urinary bladder, the mesna monomer binds directly to the toxin acrolein via an active sulfhydryl moiety on mesna. Mesna thus blocks bladder damage from the major toxic metabolites of both ifosfamide and cyclophosphamide (Brock et al 1982, Scheef et al 1979, Shaw and Graham 1987). This agent does not block the antitumor activity of oxazophosphorines nor other classes of antitumor agents (see Drug Interactions). Mesna is superior to previous urinary prophylaxis regimens that used increased fluid intake, administration of diuretics, alkalinization of the urine, and intravesical administration of other sulfhydryl-containing compounds such as N-acetylcysteine (Burkert 1983). Among a large series of SH-based uroprotectants, mesna had the greatest efficacy and the least toxicity of any of the agents tested (Brock et al 1981).

■ Mechanism of Action

Mesna uses its free sulfhydryl group to bind and thereby inactivate the toxic oxazophosphorine metabolite acrolein in the urine. Selectivity of mesna for the urinary tract is provided by dimerization of the compound in the blood to the inactive disulfide dimesna. Dimerization appears to be enhanced in the presence of various transition or heavy metals such as copper and lead in the plasma. Much of the reaction is spontaneous and some mixed disulfides may also form. These include mesna–protein sulfur adducts such as mesna–cysteine and mesna–glutathione conjugates. Dimesna distributes poorly outside the vascular compartment and cell uptake is minimal because of its high charge and low lipophilicity.

Dimesna is filtered by the glomerulus and partially reduced back to mesna in the renal tubules. About one third of the original drug dose is secreted back into the urine as mesna where it binds to both acrolein and 4-hydroxycyclophosphamide. The latter reaction interrupts the subsequent breakdown to acrolein and phosphoramide mustard, which is the active crosslinking metabolite from cyclophosphamide (Shaw and Graham 1987).

■ Availability and Storage

Mesna is supplied as a 100 mg/mL clear solution in glass ampules containing 200 mg, 400 mg, or 1 g (Mesnex®, Bristol-Myers Oncology Division, Princeton, New Jersey). Each milliliter of the solution may also contain 0.25 mg disodium edetate and sodium hydroxide to adjust pH to 6.5 to 8.5. The ampules may be stored at room temperature and intact ampules are stable for at least 5 years after manufacture.

■ Preparation for Use, Stability, and Admixture

For intravenous infusions, mesna doses can be diluted in 5% Dextrose Injection, USP; 5% Dextrose and Sodium Chloride Injection, USP; 0.9% Sodium Chloride Injection, USP; or Lactated Ringer's Injection, USP, wherein it is stable for at least 48 hours with 5% decomposition after 24 hours at room temperature. Light protection is not required. Storage of mesna solutions in glass or plastic syringes longer than 10 days does not result in a loss of drug unless air is present. This produces about 10% oxidation to dimesna after 6 to 9 days.

Mesna is stable for 8 days in a 1:1 or 1:5 admixture with grape- or orange-flavored syrups. The stability time of 1:1 to 1:100 mesna admixtures in carbonated cola drinks is at least 24 hours. Mesna is compatible with ifosfamide and cyclophosphamide in the same infusion container; however, mesna can bind to cisplatin to inhibit cisplatin's antitumor activity in vivo (see Drug Interactions).

■ Administration

Mesna can be administered intravenously and orally at twice the intravenous dose. Mesna is usually administered as a brief intravenous infusion in 50 to 100 mL of diluent. The drug is not known to be a vesicant or an irritant. Nonetheless, care should be taken to prevent extravasation. Mesna can also be directly admixed with solutions containing ifosfamide or cyclophosphamide for continuous intravenous infusion over 24 hours or longer (Klein et al 1983).

Because of a disagreeable sulfur odor, mesna solutions for oral administration should be diluted prior to ingestion. Mesna solutions are typically diluted from 1:1 to 1:10 in carbonated cola drinks or in chilled fruit juices including apple, grape, tomato, and orange juice. Dilution into plain or chocolate milk has also been used. Vomiting within 1 hour of oral mesna ingestion should be reported to the physician so that intravenous mesna can be given.

■ Dosage

A variety of mesna/ifosfamide dosing regimens have been explored (see table on the opposite page). Intravenous mesna is typically given in three divided doses, each at 20% of the ifosfamide or cyclophosphamide dose on a milligram/kilogram basis. The first mesna dose is administered 15 minutes before the oxazophosphorine and the second and third doses are administered 4 and 8 hours later. Because of limited bioavailability (Burkert et al 1984) (see Pharmacokinetics), each oral mesna dose should be doubled to 40% of the oxazophosphorine dose (Araujo and Tessler 1983). Oral mesna is not recommended for the first dose (before ifosfamide/cyclophosphamide) and should be used only in patients with good compliance and when there is absolute control of any emetic complications from the chemotherapy. For continuous infusions, mesna doses equal to those of ifosfamide or cyclophosphamide have been used.

■ Drug Interactions

Mesna is physically incompatible with cisplatin. Mesna can also inhibit the experimental systemic antitumor activity of cisplatin if administered simultaneously with cisplatin (Dorr and Lagel 1989).

REPORTED MESNA/IFSOFAMIDE DOSING REGIMENS IN DIFFERENT TUMOR TYPES

Ifosamide Regimen		Mesna Regimen		Tumor Type	References
Dose	*Administration Method*	*Dose*	*Frequency After Ifosfamide*		
85 mg/kg/24 h × 5	Continuous infusion	85 mg/kg/24 h × 5	Concomitant infusion	Various	Klein et al 1983
Various	Continuous infusion	70% of ifosfamide dose	Initial bolus hourly by infusion (6%/h)	Various, phase I/II clinical trial	Hilgard et al 1983
5.0–8.0 g/m²	24-h infusion	400–600 mg/m²	IV bolus initially and every 4 h × 9	Advanced soft tissue sarcoma	Stuart-Harris et al 1983
1.5 g/m²	4-h infusion	20% of ifosfamide dose	Before and 4 h and 8 h after ifosfamide	Soft tissue sarcoma	Hartlapp et al 1985
40–60 mg/kg/d × 5	IV bolus	12 mg/kg IV	0, 4, and 8 h	Sarcomas and germ cell tumors	Niederle et al 1983
3.0 g/m²/d × 5	1-h infusion	20% of ifosfamide dose	15 min prior and every 4 h × 3 d	Pediatric solid tumors	DeKraker and Voute 1983
1.6 g/m²/d × 5	15-min infusion	400 mg/m²	Immediately and 4 and 6 h after	Pediatric solid tumors	Pratt et al 1986
2.5 g/m²/d × 3	4-h infusion	20% of ifosfamide dose	Every 4-h infusion × 5 doses	Untreated advanced sarcoma	Elias and Antman 1986
1.25 g/m²/d × 5	IV bolus	250 mg/m²	15 min before ifosfamide, then every 4 h × 5 d	Non-Hodgkin's lymphoma	Case et al 1986
1.5 g/m²/d × 5	IV bolus	300 mg/m²	Every 4 h × 3 doses, days 1–5	Advanced pelvic malignancies	Sutton et al 1987
2 g/m²/d × 4	4-h infusion	400–500 mg	Every 4 h × 5 doses	Sarcoma	Antman et al 1985
1.2–1.5 g/m²/d × 5	IV bolus	120 mg/m²	IV × 5 d	Testicular, refractory germ cell, extragonadal	Lauer et al 1987
1.8 g/m²/d × 5	IV bolus	2.88 g/m²	IV × 5 d	Pediatric sarcoma	Magrath et al 1987

In contrast, mesna does not affect the antitumor activity of most antitumor agents including the oxazophosphorine alkylating agents ifosfamide and cyclophosphamide, doxorubicin, carmustine, methotrexate, and vincristine (Pohl et al 1981).

■ Pharmacokinetics

The pharmacokinetics of intravenous and oral mesna is summarized in the table on page 688. The primary form of mesna in the plasma is the disulfide dimesna, which is inactive. Both compounds are rapidly cleared from the plasma and excreted in the urine. The excretion of cysteine is also enhanced as a result of the breakdown of mesna–protein mixed disulfides in the renal tubules. About half of an oral mesna dose is absorbed, as reflected in cumulative plasma levels of mesna and dimesna (James et al 1987) or by the extent of urinary thiol excretion (Burkert et al 1984). A slightly lower percentage of a mesna dose may be excreted as urinary thiols in cancer patients (33%) compared with healthy volunteers (40%) (Burkert et al 1984). Maximal urinary thiol levels of 3.2 to 4.1 mg/mL can be achieved from oral mesna doses of 20 to 40 mg/kg, respectively. The time to the peak urinary thiol level averages about 3 hours following oral doses. In contrast, an intravenous mesna dose of 20 mg/kg achieves a peak urinary thiol level of 5.8 mg/mL within 1 hour of administration (Burkert et al 1984). This suggests that oral mesna provides lower but more prolonged urinary thiol levels compared with intravenous doses. And, when the oral mesna dose is doubled, roughly comparable peak urinary thiol concentra-

MESNA PHARMACOKINETICS FOLLOWING INTRAVENOUS AND ORAL DOSES*

Route	Dose (mg)	Half-life (min)	Volume of Distribution (L/kg)	Clearance (L/kg/h) Total Body	Clearance (L/kg/h) Urinary	AUC (nmol/mL/h)	Peak Plasma Level (nmol/mL)	Peak Time (h)
IV	800	22	0.65	1.23	0.41	59.4	111	—
PO	800	—	—	—	—	32.9	19.6	2.7
PO	(Dimesna)	0.7–2.2	—	—	—	51.4	25.3	2.4

Data from James et al 1987.

tions are achieved with the advantage of keeping thiol levels of 100 µg/mL or greater in the urine for a significantly longer period, for example, 13 hours for an oral 20 mg/kg dose compared with 6 hours for an intravenous 20 mg/kg dose (Burkert et al 1984).

The half-life of mesna in the plasma is short at 18 minutes, as measured by a nonspecific calorimetric assay (Pohl et al 1981), or 22 minutes, as measured by a specific high-performance liquid chromatography assay (see first table) (James et al 1987). With oral dosing, there is much more variability in plasma levels of mesna but total urinary recovery is comparable to that following intravenous dosing. About a third of a dose is recovered in the urine as mesna and another third as dimesna, 24 hours after an intravenous dose (James et al 1987). After oral dosing the total urinary availability of mesna averages 42 to 53% of the dose, with total urinary dimesna accounting for another 21% of the dose (James et al 1987). Approximately 25% of the mesna dose is excreted as free thiols (Jones et al 1985). These urinary excretion results are similar to those of Ikeuchi and Amano (1985).

■ Side Effects and Toxicity

As mesna does not produce any antineoplastic effects it has a very low propensity to produce significant side effects. After very high doses of 2.4 g/m² (10 times the recommended dose) in a phase I study, intravenous and oral mesna was associated with headache (50%), fatigue (33%), nausea (33%), diarrhea (83%), limb pain (50%), hypotension (17%), and allergy (17%) (Mesnex® Package Insert, Bristol-Myers Oncology Division, 1989). Other reported effects include a bad taste in the mouth (100%) and soft stools (70%). At standard clinical dose levels, however, mesna appears to be relatively nontoxic, with only minor gastrointestinal complaints reported.

Undiluted oral mesna solutions may have a disagreeable sulfur odor (rotten egg smell), which could lead to nausea and vomiting (see Administration).

Mesna can falsely elevate the level of urinary ketones as measured by standard test strips (Chemstrip®, Boehringer-Mannheim). In this study, a 3+ ketonuria by urinary test strip correlated to a urinary mesna level of about 4.3 nmol/L (Goren and Pratt 1990). Indeed, urinary ketone strips have been advocated as a potential means of following urinary mesna levels using a simple bedside technique.

Mesna was nonmutagenic in a variety of in vitro test systems and was nonteratogenic in pregnant rats and rabbits.

REFERENCES

Antman KH, Montella D, Rosenbaum C, Schwen M. Phase II trial of ifosfamide with mesna in previously treated metastatic sarcoma. *Cancer Treat Rep.* 1985;**69**:499–504.

Araujo CE, Tessler J. Treatment of ifosfamide-induced urothelial toxicity by oral administration of sodium 2-mercaptoethane sulphonate (mesna) to patients with inoperable lung cancer. *Eur J Cancer Clin Oncol.* 1983;**19**:195–201.

Brock N, Pohl J, Stekar J. Studies on the urotoxicity of oxazophosphorine cytostatics and its prevention. II. Comparative study on the uroprotective efficacy of thiols and other sulfur compounds. *Eur J Cancer Clin Oncol.* 1981;**17**:1155–1163.

Brock N, Pohl J, Stekar J, Scheef W. Studies on the urotoxicity of oxazophosphorine cytostatics and its prevention. III. Profile of action of sodium 2-mercaptoethane sulfonate (mesna). *Eur J Cancer Clin Oncol.* 1982;**18**:1377–1387.

Burkert H. Clinical overview of mesna. *Cancer Treat Rev.* **10**:175–181.

Burkert H, Lucker PW, Wetzelsberger N, Breuel HP. Bioavailability of orally administered mesna. *Arzneimforsch.* 1984;**34**:1597–1600.

Case D, Ervin T, Gottlieb A, Anderson J. Phase II trial of ifosfamide and mesna in non-Hodgkin's lymphoma. *Proc Am Soc Clin Oncol.* 1986;**5**:189.

DeKraker J, Voute PA. Ifosfamide (IF) in pediatric soft tissue sarcomas (STS) (abstract). *Proceedings of Eur Org Res Treat Cancer Meeting, Amsterdam, 1983.*

Dorr RT, Lagel K. Interaction between cisplatin and mesna in mice. *J Cancer Res Clin Oncol.* 1989;**115**:604–605.

Elias AD, Antman KH. Doxorubicin, ifosfamide, and dacarbazine (AID) with mesna uroprotection for advanced untreated sarcoma: A phase I study. *Cancer Treat Rep.* 1986;**70**:827–833.

Goren MP, Pratt CB. False-positive ketone tests: A bedside measure of urinary mesna. *Cancer Chemother Pharmacol.* 1990;**25**:371–372.

Hartlapp JH, Iliger HJ, Wolter H, et al. Alternatives to CVADIC-combination therapy of soft tissue sarcomas. *Klin Wochenschr.* 1985;**63**:1160–1162.

Hilgard P, Herdrich K, Brade W. Ifosfamide—Current aspects and perspectives. *Cancer Treat Rep.* 1983;**10**(suppl A):183–192.

Ikeuchi I, Amano T. Simultaneous determination of 2-mercaptoethanesulfonate and its disulphide in human urine by isotachophoresis. *Chem Pharm Bull.* 1985;**33**:3016–3019.

James CA, Mant TG, Rogers HJ. Pharmacokinetics of intravenous and oral sodium 2-mercaptoethane sulphonate (mesna) in normal subjects. *Br J Clin Pharmacol.* 1987;**23**:561–568.

Jones MS, Murrell RD, Shaw IC. Excretion of sodium 2-mercaptoethane sulphonate (mesna) in the urine of volunteers after oral dosing. *Eur J Cancer Clin Oncol.* 1985;**21**:553–555.

Klein HO, Wickrammanayake PD, Coerper CL, et al. High dose ifosfamide and mesna as continuous infusion over 5 days—A phase I/II trial. *Cancer Treat Rev.* 1983;**10**(suppl A):167–173.

Lauer RC, Roth R, Loehrer PJ, et al. Cisplatin and ifosfamide and either VP-16 or vinblastine (VIP) as third line therapy for metastatic testicular cancer. *Proc Am Soc Clin Oncol.* 1987;**6**:99.

Magrath I, Sundlund J, Raynor A, et al. A phase II study of ifosfamide in the treatment of recurrent sarcomas and pediatric tumors. *Contrib Oncol.* 1987;**26**:114–124.

Niederle N, Scheulen ME, Schutte J, et al. Ifosfamide and mesna in combination chemotherapy of sarcomas and germ cell tumors (abstract). *Proceedings of Eur Org Res Treat Cancer Meeting, Amsterdam, 1983.*

Pohl J, Brock N, Schneider B, Wetzelsberger K. Zur Pharmacokinetik von Uromitexan®. *Methods Find Exp Clin Pharmacol.* 1981;**3**:955–1015.

Pratt CB, Green AA, Horowitz ME, et al. Central nervous system toxicity following the treatment of pediatric patients with ifosfamide/mesna. *J Clin Oncol.* 1986;**4**:1253–1266.

Scheef W, Klein HO, Brock N, et al. Controlled clinical studies with an antidote against the urotoxicity of oxazaphosphorines: Preliminary results. *Cancer Treat Rep.* 1979;**63**:501–505.

Shaw IC, Graham MI. Mesna—A short review. *Cancer Treat Rev.* 1987;**14**:67–86.

Stuart-Harris RC, Harper PG, Parsons CA, et al. High-dose alkylation therapy using ifosfamide infusion with mesna in the treatment of adults advanced soft-tissue sarcoma. *Cancer Chemother Pharmacol.* 1983;**11**:69–72.

Sutton G, Blessing J, Malfetano J, Berman M. Phase II trial of ifosfamide and mesna in patients with epithelial ovarian carcinomas resistant to combination chemotherapy. *Proc Am Soc Clin Oncol.* 1987;**6**:115.

Methanol Extraction Residue of Bacillus Calmette–Guérin

■ Other Names

BCG-MER, MER-BCG, NSC-143769.

■ Chemistry

The chemical structure of MER-BCG is unknown. MER is the methanol extraction residue of Phipps strain bacillus Calmette–Guérin (BCG). This derivation process involves exhaustive extraction of phenol-killed, acetone-washed bacteria using methyl alcohol. It is assayed to standard potency using an antibacterial protection assay in mice and by tests measuring immune response to antigen challenge in mice.

MER is not water soluble. The MER component exists in an amorphous form and retains some acid-fast staining potential. Bacterial bodies and fragments are present in the MER fraction. MER offers a better pharmaceutical product than BCG; however, the fraction remains a chemically crude and uncharacterized substance. The nonviable nature of the fraction, its stability, and fairly consistent batch standardization appear to offer distinct pharmacologic advantages over BCG. Whether these properties offer any immunotherapeutic advantage remains to be determined.

■ Antitumor Activity

MER BCG has been evaluated in a large number of phase II and III trials (most still unreported at this time). There is no evidence the compound adds anything to the treatment of patients with leukemia, lymphoma, neuroblastoma, soft tissue sarcoma, breast cancer, lung cancer, and head and neck cancer (formal report to Food and Drug Administration from Division of Cancer Treatment, National Cancer Institute, July 1986, and also Cuttner et al 1976, Robinson et al 1975, 1979, Weiss et al 1975, Gastrointestinal Tumor Study Group 1984, Aisner et al 1981, Kostinas et al 1979, Tormey et al 1983, Britell et al 1979). Indeed, some studies have indicated MER-BCG may be detrimental (Higgins et al 1984; Vinciguerra et al 1981, Aisner and Wiernik 1980, Cooper et al 1982, Gastrointestinal Tumor Study Group 1984, Aisner et al 1981, Kostinas et al 1979, Tormey et al 1983).

■ Mechanism of Action

MER acts as a nonspecific immunostimulant or immunomodulator (also known as an immunologic adjuvant). MER has diverse and diffuse activities on the intact immune system: (1) augmented immunologic activity against normally weak antigenic materials in the reticuloendothelial system; (2) augmented phagocytic activity of macrophages; (3) augmented induction of blastic transformation of lymphoid cells in the presence of various mitogens; (4) amplified delayed hypersensitivity responses.

In cancer patients, MER was investigated for its application as a nonspecific immunomodulator to immunologically augment effects of other treatment (eg, surgery, chemotherapy) (Mikulski and Muggia 1977, Weiss et al 1976). Some degree of restoration of immunocompetence in certain patients with advanced malignancies has been shown to occur. MER induces a delayed hypersensitivity reaction to tuberculin and is not pyrogenic in a tuberculin-negative individual.

■ Availability and Storage

The MER fraction of BCG for human use is provided as a sterile, surfactant-stabilized suspension containing 9 mg sodium chloride, 5 mg sodium carboxymethylcellulose, 0.004 mL of polysorbate 80, and 2 mg of MER/mL of sterile water. The MER fraction is chemically stable for a number of years at refrigerated temperatures. It retains activity after freezing and thawing and after exposure to elevated temperatures.

■ Preparation for Use, Stability, and Admixture

See below. No stability data are available.

■ Administration

The optimal administration technique and route for MER are not known at this time. Clinical trials have used subcutaneous and intradermal administration. Administration by intratumoral scarification and intravenous routes has been considered but not tested. Generally, subcutaneous or intradermal doses are administered by rotating sites, using the upper arms and legs of the patient. Some authors report that injections into the back and flanks seem to cause a less severe local reaction. Repeat injections at a particular site should be spaced far enough apart to prevent overlap of the new and old inflammatory reactions.

■ Special Precautions

None are known.

■ Drug Interactions

None are known.

■ Dosage

The optimal dosage of MER in cancer patients is not known. Subcutaneous and intradermal doses ranging from 0.5 to 2.5 mg (total dose given in multiple sites) have been given at each injection time and continued according to a variety of schemes (usually once per week or once per month). It is generally recommended that the total dose of MER given at any single injection site not be greater than 0.2 mg. Individual subcutaneous doses from 0.1 to 1.0 mg/m^2 have been used but with significant local toxicity at all doses greater than 0.1 mg/m^2. More frequent injections or larger doses of MER per site probably favor increased local toxicity.

Most clinical studies are employing a once-monthly intradermal injection of not more than 1.0 mg total dose, using simultaneous injections of not more than 0.2 mg at each site (Weiss et al 1976).

■ Pharmacokinetics

No studies have been performed with this material.

■ Side Effects and Toxicity

Generalized systemic reactions are not common with MER. Occasional transient episodes of moderate fever and mild to moderate malaise may occur (Moertel et al 1975). It is not pyrogenic in tuberculin-negative patients. With subcutaneous administration, the formation of sterile abscesses at the injection site(s) has been the dose-limiting toxic effect. These ulcers may be deep and characteristically heal slowly (average 4 months). They may cause noticeable discomfort and often become infected. Local reactions to intradermal MER generally evolve as shallow draining lesions which heal over several weeks, usually without superinfection. Old injection sites may "flare" strongly with subsequent dosing at distant sites. Preclinical studies of MER given intravenously to animals have shown granulomatous reactions in the lungs and liver (Vogl et al 1977). Human studies have not yet been reported; however, two cases of pulmonary epithelioid granulomata have been reported in patients receiving MER intradermally (Denefrio 1979).

The most common and significant patient complaint is that of pain at the injection site. Once-monthly dosing and limitation of the intradermal dose per site appear to offer a "tolerable" regimen. Narcotics may sometimes be required to control pain from the local reactions. Significant changes in hematologic, hepatic, or renal function have not been noted to date.

■ Special Applications

None are known.

REFERENCES

Aisner J, Weinberg V, Perloff M, et al. Chemoimmunotherapy for advanced breast cancers. A randomized comparison of 6 combinations (CMF, CAF vs CAFVP and with and without MER immunotherapy). *Proc Am Assoc Cancer Res ASCO.* 1981;**22**:443.

Aisner J, Wiernik PH. Chemotherapy versus chemoimmunotherapy for small-cell undifferentiated carcinoma of the lung. *Cancer.* 1980;**46**:2543–2549.

Britell JC, Ahmann DL, Bisel HF, et al. Treatment of advanced breast cancer with cyclophosphamide, 5-fluorouracil, and prednisone with and without methanol-extracted residue of BCG. *Cancer Clin Trial.* 1979;**2**:345–350.

Cooper MR, Pajak TF, Nissen NI, et al. Effect of the methanol extraction residue of bacillus Calmette–Guérin in advanced Hodgkin's disease. *Cancer.* 1982;**49**:2226–2230.

Cuttner J, Bedesi JG, Holland JF. Chemoimmunotherapy of acute leukemia using MER. *Proc Am Assoc Cancer Res ASCO.* 1976;**17**:196.

Denefrio J. Systemic epithelioid granulomata following immunotherapy with methanol extraction residue of bacillus Calmette–Guérin (MER). *Proc Am Assoc Cancer Res ASCO.* 1979;**20**:386.

Gastrointestinal Tumor Study Group. Adjuvant therapy of colon cancer. Results of a prospectively randomized trial. *N Eng J Med.* 1984;**310**:737–743.

Higgins GA, Donaldson RL, Rogers LS, Juler GL, Keehan RO. Efficacy of HER immunotherapy when added to a regimen of 5-fluorouracil and methyl-CCNU following reaction of the large band. A Veterans Administration Surgical Oncology Group report. *Cancer.* 1984;**54**:193–198.

Kostinas JE, Leone LA, Cuttner J, et al. Procarbazine, vinblastine, and actinomycin D in stage III and IV melanoma with or without methanol-extracted residue of bacillus Calmette–Guérin. *Cancer Treat Rep.* 1979;**63**(2):197–200.

Mikulski S, Muggia F. The biologic activity of MER-BCG in experimental systems and preliminary clinical studies. *Cancer Treat Rev.* 1977;**4**:103–117.

Moertel CG, Ritts RE, Schutt AJ, Hahn RG. A phase I study of methanol extraction residue of BCG (BCG-MER). *Proc Am Assoc Cancer Res ASCO.* 1975;**16**:143.

Robinson E, Bartel A, Cohen Y, Haasz R. A preliminary report on the effects of methanol extraction residue of BCG (MER) on cancer patients. *Br J Cancer.* 1975;**32**:1–4.

Robinson E, Bartel A, Cohen Y, Mekori T. Adjuvant therapy in colorectal cancer (a randomized trial comparing radio-chemotherapy and radio-chemotherapy combined with the methanol extraction residue of BCG, MER). *Proc Am Assoc Cancer Res ASCO.* 1979;**20**:408.

Tormey DC, Weinberg VE, Holland JF, et al. A randomized trial of five and three drug chemotherapy and chemoimmunotherapy in women with operable node positive breast cancer. *J Clin Oncol.* 1983;**1**(2):138–145.

Vinciguerra V, Coleman M, Pajak TF, et al. MER immunotherapy and combination chemotherapy for advanced, recurrent Hodgkin's disease. Cancer and Leukemia Group B study. *Cancer Clin Trials.* 1981;**4**:99–105.

Vogl SE, Lumb G, Bekes JG, Holland JF. Preclinical study of IV administration of mer-methanol extraction residue of bacillus Calmette–Guérin. *Cancer Treat Rep.* 1977;**61**(5):901–903.

Weiss DW. MER and other mycobacterial fractions in the immunotherapy of cancer. *Med Clin North Am.* 1976;**60**(3):473–497.

Weiss DW, Stapp Y, Mowy N, Izak G. Treatment of acute myelocytic leukemia (AML) patients with the MER tubercle bacillus fraction: A preliminary report. *Transplant Proc.* 1975;**7**(suppl):545–552.

Methotrexate

■ Other Names

NSC-740; MTX; amethopterin; sodium methotrexate; Folex®; Mexate®; Methotrexate Tablets®, for Injection®, and LPF® (Lederle Laboratories); Rheumatrex® (Lederle Laboratories).

■ Chemistry

Structure of methotrexate

Methotrexate (MTX) is a mixture containing at least 95% N-[4-[[(2,4-diamino-6-pteridinyl)methyl]methylamino]benzoyl]-L-glutamic acid, the primary product, and at least seven impurities including 4-amino-N^{10}-methylpteroic acid and N^{10}-methylfolic acid, which constitute a small fraction of the commercial product (Hignite et al 1978). These inactive species are believed to represent synthetic by-products rather than degradation products. Methotrexate differs from folic acid in two substitutions: (1) an amino group for a hydroxyl in the pteridine portion of the molecule and (2) a methyl group on the amino nitrogen between the pteridine nucleus and the benzoyl group (see structure) or 4-amino-10-methylfolic acid. MTX is a weak acid with a molecular weight of 454.5 and a molecular formula of $C_{20}H_{22}N_8O_5$. It is only slightly soluble in water and alcohol. Sodium methotrexate is water soluble and is used in injectable preparations. The injectable form has a pH of 8.5 and pK_a's of 4.8 and 5.5.

■ Antitumor Activity

Methotrexate has broad-spectrum antineoplastic activity. Most frequently it is used in combination with other chemotherapeutic agents. Cancers in which activity has been established include acute lymphoblastic and myeloblastic leukemia (including intrathecal administration for leukemic meningeal infiltration); trophoblastic tumors such as chorioepithelioma, choriocarcinoma, chorioadenoma destruens, and hydatidiform mole (Smith et al 1982); Burkitt's lymphoma (Ramirez et al 1979); and, rarely, mycosis fungoides (McDonald and Bertino 1978). In high-dose schedules, MTX has activity in osteogenic sarcoma (Frei et al 1975), epidermoid carcinoma of the head and neck (Capizzi et al 1970), and lung, breast, and ovarian carcinoma.

Methotrexate is used in a number of potentially curable regimens for non-Hodgkin's lymphoma such as ProMACE (Fisher et al 1983), m-BACOD (Skarin and Canellos 1987), and COMLA (Levitt et al 1972). Effective methotrexate-containing remission-induction regimens in acute lymphoblastic leukemia of adults include the VMP regimen (Omura et al 1980) and MOAD (Esterhay et al 1982). Active solid tumor combinations include CMF in breast cancer (Bonadonna et al 1976); CAMP in non-small cell lung cancer (Bitran et al 1978); APE in limited small cell lung cancer (Broder et al 1981); with radiation, cyclophosphamide, and vincristine in extensive small cell lung cancer (Maurer et al 1980); and with cisplatin and bleomycin in head and neck cancer (Von Hoff et al 1981). High-dose methotrexate with leucovorin rescue has demonstrated good activity as primary therapy in metastatic osteogenic sarcoma (Pratt et al 1980) and as preoperative adjuvant chemotherapy (Rosen et al 1982).

Methotrexate is also active in several nonmalignant diseases characterized by rapid cell growth. In psoriasis, MTX is used to treat severe refractory disease. It is often combined with psoralens and ultraviolet-A light (PUVA) (Morison et al 1982) or with ultraviolet-B light (Paul et al 1982). Rheumatoid arthritis is responsive to the drug in patients refractory to standard first-line therapy (Weinblatt et al 1985).

■ Mechanism of Action

Free intracellular MTX tightly binds to dihydrofolate reductase (DHFR) thereby blocking the reduction of dihydrofolate to tetrahydrofolic acid, the active form of folic acid (Goldman 1975a,b). Thymidylate synthetase as well as various steps in de novo purine synthesis is inhibited, resulting in an arrest of DNA, RNA, and protein synthesis.

The binding of MTX to DHFR is stoichiometric (one drug per enzyme molecule) and very tight with a binding affinity in *S. faecium* of 5.8×10^{-11} M (Charlton et al 1979).

Amino acid syntheses blocked by MTX include those requiring 1-carbon transfer, such as the conversion of glycine to serine and homocysteine to methionine. Experimental studies have shown that thymidylate synthetase is inhibited at MTX concentrations of 10^{-8} M or greater, whereas inhibition of purine synthesis requires concentrations of 10^{-7} M or greater (Chabner and Young 1973, Zaharko et al 1977). The antipurine effect is highly correlated with rapid cell growth (Jackson and Weber 1976) and with high N^5, N^{10}-methylenetetrahydrofolate dehydrogenase activity (Tattersall et al 1974).

Methotrexate undergoes a variable degree of polyglutamation intracellularly. The polyglutamated forms of the drug do not readily pass through cell membranes. Thus methotrexate polyglutamates form an intracellular pool of active drug that is retained for long periods (up to months after a single dose) (Jolivet et al 1982). The ability of tumor cells to add γ-glutamyl residues to MTX may be a key determinant of antitumor activity.

The effects of MTX are rapidly reversible, as free MTX leaves the cells. The normal intracellular levels of dihydrofolate are very low (10^{-8} M) but increase greatly following MTX administration (Goldman 1977).

Resistance. Resistance to MTX may develop as a result of elevated dihydrofolate reductase activity or defective transport of MTX into malignant cells. If resistance is used to an increase in dihydrofolate reductase, thymidylate synthetase becomes the rate-limiting step for MTX action. Increased DHFR enzyme levels may also result from amplification of the DHFR gene, a process associated with homogeneously stained regions of chromosomes and an unstable inheritance mediated by double minutes or extra chromosomal DNA fragments (episomes) (Alt et al 1978). Certain quinazolines have been shown to be effective inhibitors of thimidylate synthetase and may be useful clinically in overcoming this type of resistance (Calvert et al 1979). In vitro studies (Rosowsky et al 1979) and clinical experimentation with high-dose therapy suggest that a major mechanism of resistance is secondary to decreased cellular uptake.

High-dose therapy. The apparent enhanced toxicity in tumors compared with normal tissues exposed to high-dose MTX with "leucovorin rescue" may result from diffusion of drug into cells bypassing normal carrier-mediated cell membrane transport of MTX (Bender et al 1977). Leucovorin and its metabolite, 5-methyltetrahydrofolate, share a common influx transport site with MTX. There appear to be at least two active transport carrier systems involved in the influx and efflux of MTX and folates (Chello et al 1979a). Drug uptake is not achieved in some tumor cells following normal doses of MTX or leucovorin. This is possibly due to a lack of folate carrier transport proteins (Bender 1975). Leucovorin may enter normal cells, blocking the toxic effects of MTX. When given in high doses (MTX concentration > 20 μM) (Hill et al 1979), MTX may enter these tumor cells by passive diffusion and thereby attain lethal concentrations (Goldman 1975b). If normal cells are "rescued" with leucovorin calcium, MTX can then exert a relatively greater toxic effect on the tumor cells. It is also possible that selective rescue of normal cells may be mediated by lower rates of DNA synthesis in normal hematopoietic cells rather than tissue-specific differences in transmembrane transport (Kessel et al 1968). The affinity of the influx carrier for MTX in various tumor cell lines is reported to range from 1 to 6 μM, whereas it has much lower affinity (87 μM) in normal intestinal epithelium (Chello et al 1977).

Methotrexate is classified as a cell cycle phase-specific antimetabolite with activity primarily in S phase. Experimentally, MTX synchronizes tumor cells in S phase about 36 to 72 hours after administration (Weinstein et al 1979); however, a study of pulse doses of MTX given during S phase did not prove to be therapeutically advantageous (Moran and Straus 1975).

■ Availability and Storage

Methotrexate is available in 2.5-mg tablets for conventional uses and, investigationally, in 50-mg tablets for high-dose therapy (Methotrexate Tablets®, Rheumatrex® Dose Pack, Lederle Laboratories, Wayne, New Jersey). The injectable form is prepared as the sodium salt and labeled in milligrams of base MTX. The preparations available for conventional use are solutions containing either 2.5 or 25 mg/mL in 2-mL vials. Some of these preparations are preserved with 0.9% benzyl alcohol and also contain 0.861% sodium chloride and sodium hydroxide for pH adjustment (Methotrexate for Injection®, Lederle). A 20-mL vial containing 20 mg of sterile lyophilized sodium MTX powder without preservatives is also commercially available for intravenous or intrathecal use (Methotrexate LPF®, Lederle).

High-dose injectable forms are available in 100-mg, 500-mg and 1000-mg 20- and 30-mL vials, respectively. These contain the lyophilized powder of sodium MTX with no preservatives.

For intrathecal use, a 50-mg lyophilized powder of sodium MTX containing no preservative is commercially available (Methotrexate Sodium for Injection®, Lederle). Both the tablets and the intact vials may be stored at room temperature and are stable for at least 2 years after manufacture. It has been shown that commercially available products of MTX are only 85 to 93.4% pure. Many of the contaminants have been identified, and some have been shown to be biologically active. The clinical importance of these contaminants has not been studied although it is postulated that significant amounts of these chemicals may be inadvertently given in some of the high-dose treatments (Hignite et al 1978).

■ Preparation for Use, Stability, and Admixture

The lyophilized dosage forms may be reconstituted with sterile water for injection, sodium chloride injection, or D5W. Elliott's B solution is the preferred vehicle for intrathecal administration (see *Elliott's B Solution*).

The 20-mg vial may be diluted with 20 mL or less of a suitable diluent (eg, Sodium Chloride for Injection, USP).

The 50-mg vial, when reconstituted with 5 mL normal saline, contains 10 mg/mL MTX base and has a pH of 7.8 to 8.8.

The 500-mg vial, when reconstituted with 9.6 mL sterile water for injection, contains 50 mg/mL MTX base and has a pH of 7.7 to 8.8.

The 1-g vial, when reconstituted with 20 mL sterile water for injection, yields a solution containing 50 mg/mL MTX base with a pH of 7.8 to 8.8.

All of these solutions are chemically stable for at least 7 days at room temperature; however, because they contain no preservatives they should optimally be used within 24 hours of mixing.

5-Fluorouracil, prednisolone sodium phosphate, and cytarabine have been shown to alter the spectrophotometric absorption pattern of MTX when added to the same intravenous mixture. This change probably indicates a chemical interaction that may alter the effectiveness of therapy (McRae and King 1976). For example, the pH of some generic cytarabine solutions has previously produced MTX precipitation when three drug admixtures for intrathecal use were compounded (hydrocortisone, methotrexate, and cytarabine). Methotrexate (15 mg/mL in D5W) is physically stable for at least 4 hours with 1 mg/mL ondansetron (Trissel et al 1990).

■ Administration

For intrathecal and high-dose MTX, refer to Special Applications. MTX may be given by the oral, intramuscular, intravenous (intravenous infusion or push), intraarterial, or intrathecal route.

■ Dosage

Methotrexate has been given by numerous dosing schedules (see the table below). In some solid tumors, dose intensity can have a profound impact on outcome, and arbitrary dose reductions may lead to therapeutic failures (Bonadonna and Valagussa 1981).

In psoriasis, a commonly used regimen calls for oral doses of 2.5 to 5.0 mg every 12 hours for three doses, repeated weekly (Weinstein et al 1970). A

METHOTREXATE DOSING SCHEDULES

Dose (mg/m^2)	Route	Frequency	Leucovorin Rescue
Conventional dose			
15–20	PO	Twice per week	–
30–50	PO, IV	Weekly	–
15 × 5 d	IV, IM	Every 2–3 wk	–
Intermediate dose			
50–150	IV push	Every 2–3 wk	–
240	IV infusion	Every 4–7 d	+
0.5–1 g/m^2	IV infusion (36–48 h)	2–3 wk	+
High dose			
1–12 g/m^2	IV (1–24 h)	Every 1–3 wk	+

similar schedule has been recommended in patients with rheumatoid arthritis: 2.5 to 7.5 mg MTX orally every 12 hours for three doses, repeated weekly (Wilkens and Watson 1982).

Because of extensive renal clearance of MTX, dose adjustments should be considered in patients with impaired renal function. For patients over the age of 65 who are receiving CMF (cyclophosphamide, methotrexate, 5-fluorouracil) therapy for breast cancer, an adjustment equation has been prospectively evaluated by the Eastern Cooperative Oncology Group (Gelman and Taylor 1984):

$$\text{MTX dose in mg/m}^2 \text{ (IV on days 1 and 8)} = 40 \text{ mg/m}^2 \times \frac{\text{creatinine clearance}}{70}$$

This equation arbitrarily assumes that an "ideal" pretreatment creatinine clearance is 70 mL/min. Although this is clearly a simplified model, it nonetheless can suggest higher doses for elderly patients than when a fixed one-third dose reduction is applied (Gelman and Taylor 1984).

All patients with significantly reduced renal function are candidates for MTX dose reduction based on measured or estimated creatinine clearance. By the use of a standard formula for estimating doses in various degrees of renal insufficiency (Anderson et al 1976), a dosing nomogram is suggested (see table on this page). It is important to note that this formula has not been prospectively or retrospectively evaluated with methotrexate, and extreme caution should be used in administering MTX in patients with any renal impairment. Intermediate- and high-dose MTX is typically contraindicated in patients with creatinine clearance of less than 50 mL/min. Similarly, patients with effusions should be cautiously treated to preclude drug accumulation in these slowly equilibrating third-space fluids. Optimally, pleural and/or peritoneal effusions should be drained prior to MTX dosing.

■ Drug Interactions

Potential drug interactions have been postulated to occur with other protein-bound drugs such as salicylates, sulfonamides, phenytoin, and p-aminobenzoic acid (see table on page 696). These drugs displace MTX from its protein binding site in the blood, causing a small increase in the levels of free drug; however, the overall degree of binding is probably not high enough for major displacement interactions. And, in one study, indomethacin did not alter meth-

SUGGESTED METHOTREXATE DOSE ADJUSTMENTS IN PATIENTS WITH RENAL INSUFFICIENCY

Creatinine Clearance (mL/min)	% Standard Dose to Administer
> 80	Full dose
80	75
60	63
50	56
> 50	Use alternate chemotherapy

*Assumes normal creatinine clearance of 120 mL/min and 75% MTX urinary excretion according to the formula of Anderson et al 1976. *Note:* This monogram has not been prospectively or retrospectively tested for MTX.

otrexate binding (Taylor and Halprin 1977). In the kidney, probenecid is known to block MTX tubular secretion, which can increase the activity of a given dose (Gangji et al 1979). Salicylates also compete with MTX for renal tubular secretion and cause an increase in its serum half-life. The nonsteroidal anti-inflammatory ketoprofen also delays MTX elimination and enhances toxicity incidence (Thyss et al 1986).

Antibiotics used in gut sterilization may also alter MTX pharmacokinetics in humans, eliminating the slow phase of excretion (Creaven and Morgan 1975). The macrolide antibiotic pristinamycin also appears to simiarly retard MTX elimination and this combination is therefore contraindicated (Thyss et al 1993).

Ethyl alcohol has been proposed to increase MTX-induced hepatotoxicity. Oral anticoagulants such as warfarin may be greatly potentiated by MTX. It has also been suggested that MTX may alter the liver metabolism of these drugs.

5-Fluorouracil and floxuridine have been reported to be experimentally antagonistic to MTX (Bruckner et al 1975) or synergistic with MTX. Experimental synergism has been described when MTX is given before 5-fluorouracil in high-dose regimens (Trisman et al 1979). The mechanism appears to be related to a MTX-induced increase in intracellular phosphoribosylpyrophosphate (PRPP) levels which enhances 5-fluorouracil nucleotide formation (Cadman and Eiferman 1979, Cadman et al 1979).

Several drug interactions are described for MTX with other chemotherapeutic agents (see table on page 696). For example, a clinically significant interaction between MTX and L-asparaginase involves the administration of MTX 3 to 24 hours prior to L-asparaginase (Capizzi 1975, Yap et al 1978). The MTX treatment is believed to block protein synthesis and thereby reduce asparaginase toxicity, allowing larger doses to be given. The table at the top of

METHOTREXATE INTERACTIONS WITH OTHER AGENTS

Added Drug	Interaction (Experimental System)*	Reference
Allopurinol	Decreased MTX therapeutic effect (T; allopurinol 1 h before MTX)	Grindey and Moran 1975
Cephalothin	Decreased MTX uptake	Bender et al 1975
	Enhanced MTX toxicity (V; cephalothin administered 48 h before MTX)	Bruckner 1969
Chloramphenicol	Enhanced MTX toxicity (V)	Dixon 1968
Dexamethasone	No interference with cytotoxicity (T)	Bruckner 1969
Hydrocortisone	Reduced blockade of thymidylate synthesis by MTX (T)	Bruckner et al 1975
	Decreased MTX uptake (T)	
	Decreased cytotoxicity of MTX (T)	Zager et al 1973
Ketoprofen	Decreased MTX elimination (H)	Thyss et al 1986
Penicillin G	Enhanced MTX toxicity (V)	Bruckner 1969
Phenytoin	Enhanced MTX toxicity (V; phenytoin given 24 h before MTX)	Dixon 1968
Prednisone	Blocked inhibition of DNA synthesis	Bruckner et al 1975
Prednisolone	No interference with MTX cytotoxicity (T)	Bruckner et al 1975
Pristinamycin	Decreased MTX elimination (H)	Thyss et al 1993
Probenecid	Increased MTX uptake (T)	Fry et al 1982
	Decreased cerebrospinal fluid clearance of MTX (H)	Bode et al 1980
Salicylate	Decreased MTX renal clearance (H)	Liegler et al 1970
Sulfasoxazole	No interference with MTX (H)	Liegler et al 1970
Tetracycline	Enhanced MTX toxicity (V)	Dixon 1968
Thymidine	Enhanced antitumor activity (V)	Semon and Grindey 1978
	Reduced MTX toxicity (T, V)	Tattersall et al 1975
		Ensminger and Frei 1977
Tolbutamide	Enhanced MTX toxicity (V)	Dixon 1968
Vincristine	Enhanced MTX uptake (T)	Chello et al 1979b

*T = in vitro cell culture studies, concomitant exposure unless otherwise noted; V = in vivo animal studies; H = human clinical trials.

page 697 describes other sequential drug interactions with MTX. Of these, some sequential MTX combinations may produce enhanced therapeutic activity. For example, MTX given 4 to 9 hours before 5-fluorouracil has produced enhanced antitumor activity in breast cancer (Cadman et al 1979) but with a commensurate increase in toxicity (Wiemann et al 1982). The mechanism of this interaction is reported to involve a significant increase in 5-fluorouracil nucleotides if MTX precedes 5-fluorouracil by at least 3 hours (Cadman et al 1979). Of interest, the reverse sequence (MTX after 5-fluorouracil) results in decreased therapeutic activity (Bowen et al 1978).

A similar mechanism is postulated for the combination of MTX given 1 to 72 hours before cytarabine (Cadman and Eiferman 1979, Edelstein et al 1975). Apparently, MTX increases the formation of cytarabine triphosphate nucleosides, thereby enhancing therapeutic effects in vitro (Cadman and Eiferman 1979). Of interest, the reverse sequence, cytarabine followed in 48 hours by MTX, is highly active in recurrent childhood acute lymphocytic leukemia (Rivera et al 1976). Another clinical observation involves reduced cyclophosphamide bioactivation to alkylating metabolites in patients pretreated with MTX (Mouridsen et al 1976). The therapeutic significance of this interaction is unknown.

Amphotericin B may alter cell membrane structure and permeability and thereby increase cellular uptake of MTX and cytotoxicity (Cundiff and Dietrich 1979). The enzyme carboxypeptidase G can also block MTX toxicity by cleaving the molecule to inactive fragments (Chabner et al 1972).

In vitro studies suggest that the presence of other drugs may alter the cellular uptake of MTX by the active transport system of the tumor cells (see earlier table on interactions with nonchemotherapeutic agents). Increases or decreases in uptake are dependent on the particular drug and its concentration (Fyfe and Goldman 1973). The clinical significance of these findings is not established:

Drugs that *decrease* in vitro cellular uptake of MTX include (% decrease) hydrocortisone sodium succinate (20–63%), cephalothin (6–47%), methylprednisolone sodium succinate (14–45%), and L-asparaginase (7–28%).

SEQUENCE-DEPENDENT ANTICANCER DRUG INTERACTIONS WITH METHOTREXATE

Order of Administration		Interval (h) Between Administrations	Interaction (Experimental System)*	Reference
Drug 1	Drug 2			
MTX	5-Fluorouracil	4–9	Enhanced cytotoxicity (T) or toxicity (H)	Cadman et al 1979 Wiemann et al 1982
5-Fluorouracil or floxuridine	MTX	0–24	Decreased cytotoxicity (T)	Bowen et al 1978
MTX	Vincristine	8–48	Enhanced therapeutic effect (H) Increased MTX uptake (T)	Rivera et al 1976 Fry et al 1982
Vincristine	MTX	0–1	Blocked MTX efflux (T)	Zager et al 1973
MTX	Cytarabine	1–6	Enhanced cytotoxicity (T)	Cadman and Eiferman 1979
Cytarabine	MTX	48	Enhanced therapeutic effect (H)	Rivera et al 1976
MTX	Teniposide or etoposide	C[†]	Decreased MTX efflux (T)	Yalowich et al 1982
MTX	L-Asparaginase	3–24	Decreased L-asparaginase toxicity (T, V, H)	Yap et al 1978 Capizzi et al 1970
MTX	6-Mercaptopurine	C	31% increase in 6-MP levels (H)	Balis et al 1987
MTX	Cyclophosphamide	15	Decreased cyclophosphamide activation (H)	Mouridsen et al 1976

*T = in vitro cell culture studies; V = in vivo experimental studies in animals; H = clinical trials in humans.
[†]C = concomitant.

Drugs that experimentally *increase* the cellular uptake of MTX in vitro (Fyfe and Goldman 1973) include vincristine (2–66% increase) and vinblastine (15–94% increase) (Chello et al 1979b).

■ Pharmacokinetics

Orally administered MTX is rapidly but incompletely absorbed from the gastrointestinal tract. It reaches peak blood levels in about 1 hour (Henderson et al 1965) (see table at the bottom of this page). Approximately 50 to 60% of the drug present in the blood is bound to plasma proteins. MTX is widely distributed to body tissues. In conventional doses, MTX is excreted unchanged in the urine. In high doses it is partially metabolized to 7-hydroxymethotrexate, which is only slightly soluble in acid solution (Leme et al 1975). About 1 to 11% of a dose is excreted as the 7-hydroxy metabolite, which may constitute up to 35% of the drug level in the terminal elimination phase. A minor metabolite is 4-amino-4-deoxy-N^{10}-methylpteroic acid (APA). Only about one third of an oral dose is absorbed but intramuscular absorption is nearly 100% (Campbell et al 1985).

The hepatic extraction coefficient for MTX appears to be very low and intraarterial hepatic doses show metabolism and pharmacokinetics similar to those of intravenous doses (Igroffo et al 1979). MTX is both filtered at the glomerulus and actively secreted by the renal tubule. Drugs that interfere with renal excretion of weak acids, such as probenecid, sulfinpyrazone, and salicylates, may be expected to reduce the rate of MTX excretion. Probenecid has been used successfully in one study to produce a prolonged elevation of plasma MTX levels from otherwise low doses of MTX (Aherne et al 1978).

Plasma decay of MTX levels has been reported to be biphasic and possibly triphasic (Bischoff et al 1977) (see table on pharmacokinetics). Huffman et al (1973) reported half-lives following a 30 mg/m²

CLINICAL PHARMACOKINETICS OF METHOTREXATE IN CANCER PATIENTS

Volume of distrubtion (L)	
Initial	13.8
Steady state	182
Plasma half-life (h)	
α	< 1
β	3–4
γ*	8–10
Route of excretion	
Renal clearance (mL/min)	70–100
Urinary (% of a dose)	60–100
Fecal (% of a dose)	1–9
Biliary (% of a dose)	< 20

*Not observed in some pharmacokinetic studies.
Data from Stoller et al 1975, Nirenberg et al 1977, and Isacoff et al 1977.

dose to be triphasic: 0.75 ± 0.11, 3.49 ± 0.55, and 26.99 ± 4.44 hours. Stoller et al (1975) reported a biphasic plasma decay for high-dose therapy of 2.06 ± 0.16 and 10.4 ± 1.8 hours. Wang et al (1979) reported age-dependent biphasic elimination of high-dose MTX. The half-life of the first phase was 1.2 hours in children and 2.2 hours in adults; the second phase was 10.4 hours in children and 8.4 hours in adults. The elimination rate constants were 0.578/h and 0.306/h in children and adults, respectively. In this study the apparent volume of distribution varied markedly between populations and was 1.1 L/kg in children and 0.5 L/kg in adults.

Peritoneal dialysis of MTX does not appear to be an effective means of reducing drug levels (Ahmad et al 1978). Conflicting reports appear regarding the efficacy of hemodialysis to increase the clearance of MTX. Djerassi et al (1977) suggests that both hemodialysis and charcoal filtration will substantially reduce MTX levels. Other attempts to hemodialyze MTX have failed to significantly increase the clearance of the drug (Howell et al 1978).

Cerebrospinal fluid levels after conventional oral or parenteral doses are normally only 3 to 10% of the plasma level and are not clinically significant; however, when high doses of MTX are used, cerebrospinal fluid levels within the cytotoxic range may be obtained, and the hope has been that separate central nervous system prophylaxis may not be required under conditions of high-dose MTX (this remains to be proven, however). Patients given a MTX dose of 500 mg/m^2 over 24 hours (one third by intravenous push and the remainder by intravenous infusion) exhibited lumbar cerebrospinal fluid levels of 1.2×10^{-7} M at 0.5 hour after infusion. These levels were maintained for 24 hours thereafter (Wang et al 1976).

Vincristine may enhance the MTX cerebrospinal fluid concentration when given after systemic high-dose MTX therapy (Tejada and Zubrod 1979). After intrathecal administration of MTX, the drug is initially redistributed rapidly in the cerebrospinal fluid and then declines in a biphasic manner with reported half-lives of 4.5 and 14 hours (Bleyer and Dedrick 1977) or 1.7 and 6.6 hours (Bode et al 1979).

The second phase of MTX decline in the cerebrospinal fluid of animals has been shown to be slowed significantly by pretreatment with probenecid (Ramu et al 1978). It is also slowed in humans (Bode et al 1979).

From the cerebrospinal fluid, MTX diffuses back into the plasma, reaching peak concentrations of 2×10^{-7} M 3 to 12 hours after a 12 mg/m^2 intrathecal dose. Thus, some myelosuppressive effects may be observed after intrathecal administration (Jacobs et al 1975), particularly after repeated doses. Pneumonitis has even been reported following intrathecal therapy.

Patients with any third-space fluids such as pleural effusions may accumulate MTX, which then slowly distributes from this compartment back into the plasma, increasing systemic exposure and the risk of toxicity (Evans and Pratt 1978). It is recommended that large pleural or peritoneal effusions be drained prior to administration of MTX.

■ Side Effects and Toxicity

Hematologic effects of MTX include leukopenia, thrombocytopenia, and anemia. They occur rapidly and are dependent on the dose and schedule used. The nadir of hemoglobin depression occurs after 6 to 13 days: Reticulocytes reach a nadir at 2 to 7 days, with rebound between 9 and 19 days. The leukocytes nadir occurs in 4 to 7 days and is followed by partial recovery and, then again rarely, a second phase at 12 to 21 days. The platelet nadir is reached in 5 to 12 days. Hypogammaglobulinemia may also rarely occur following MTX.

Nausea, vomiting, and anorexia are usually the earliest gastrointestinal symptoms noted. Gingivitis, glossitis, pharyngitis, stomatitis, and bleeding from ulcerations of the mucosal membranes of the mouth or other portions of the gastrointestinal tract may occur. If ulcerative stomatitis or diarrhea occurs, MTX therapy must be interrupted to prevent severe hemorrhagic enteritis or intestinal perforation.

Hepatotoxicity may occur and is more common in patients receiving high-dose therapy and in those receiving frequent small doses on a chronic basis. Evidence for hepatocellular injury has been detected by rises in serum glutamic–oxalacetic transaminase and ornithine carbamyltransferase levels, usually within the first 12 hours of high-dose methotrexate. Prothrombin times may rise as a result of decreased plasma factor VII activity and indirect hyperbilirubinemia may develop. All of these abnormalities usually return to normal within 1 week. Interestingly, hepatocytes appear to be protected by fractionated high-dose MTX treatments with leucovorin rescue when treatments are administered in less than 1-week intervals. It is postulated that this may be the result of leucovorin activity remaining from prior doses. Further studies are needed to determine whether tumor cells may be similarly protected

(Warkentin et al 1979). Various pathologic hepatic changes can occur, including atrophy, necrosis, fatty changes, fibrosis, and cirrhosis. Liver biopsy is the only reliable means of assessing the degree of MTX hepatotoxicity (Closky et al 1955, Hersh et al 1966). In psoriasis patients, pretreatment liver biopsies and follow-up biopsies at a cumulative dose of 1.5 g are recommended.

Dermatologic side effects include erythematous rashes, pruritus, urticaria, folliculitis, vasculitis, photosensitivity, depigmentation, and hyperpigmentation. Alopecia may occur, with several months required for regrowth.

Central nervous system effects include dizziness, malaise, and blurred vision. Encephalopathy is also reported (Kay et al 1972). Intrathecal administration has been followed by increased cerebrospinal fluid pressure, convulsions, paresis, and a syndrome resembling the Guillain–Barré syndrome (Bleyer et al 1974). Deaths are also reported after intrathecal therapy (Back 1969).

Renal failure may occur in patients receiving MTX, especially at high doses. The risk of renal failure may be decreased by alkalinization of the urine to increase MTX solubility and intensive hydration (Condit et al 1969) (see High-Dose Methotrexate under Special Applications).

Other reactions have been reported rarely and include chills and fever, osteoporosis, and pulmonary reactions—mainly fibrosis (Clarysse et al 1969, Everts et al 1973) and, rarely, pneumonitis (Sostman et al 1976).

■ Special Applications

High-dose Methotrexate. Very high doses of MTX have been administered for a variety of tumors. Although leucovorin "rescue" reduces toxicity, it is still not absolutely established that high-dose therapy is superior to more conventional dosing without leucovorin. Specific dosing schemes vary but, in general, a high dose of MTX is usually administered intravenously (protocols using oral doses have been reported [Christophidis et al 1979]) and is followed by leucovorin calcium 24 to 36 hours after initiation of therapy to prevent toxicity (see first table and table below for specific dosing recommendations).

In patients receiving massive doses (> 20 g), Djerassi et al (1979) have used plasma exchange and charcoal filtration in conjunction with early leucovorin rescue. The dose range of MTX is 100 mg/m^2 to 10 g/m^2 given every 1 to 3 weeks. The lower end of this dosing spectrum has been administered in four divided oral doses over a 24-hour period. Most frequently, the dose is given by intravenous infusion in 1 to 2 L of fluid either as a rapid infusion or over 6 to 24 hours. Higher peak MTX levels occur with more rapid intravenous infusions and this may be theoretically more efficacious. There does not appear to be a difference in clinical toxicity between rapid and prolonged infusions (Lichter et al 1979). Only the nonpreserved 500- and 1000-mg vials should be used for this purpose. Further dilution of the MTX is necessary and can be accomplished in either normal saline or D5W.

High-dose MTX has been associated with a reversible nephrotoxicity and other toxic effects (see table on page 700). At high concentrations MTX may precipitate in the renal tubule, causing tubular dilation and damage. The pK_a of MTX is 5.4. When the urine pH is near this value, MTX is present predominantly in its insoluble form and is likely to precipitate. Renal toxicity may be prevented by increasing urine alkalinity and flow. Sodium bicarbonate, 3 g

LEUCOVORIN DOSING IN HIGH-DOSE METHOTREXATE REGIMENS*

Methotrexate Dose	Methotrexate Level at 48 h (M)*	Time (h) After MTX	Leucovorin Dosing mg/m^2 Every 6 h	Number of Doses
50–250 mg/kg over 6 h	$< 5 \times 10^{-7}$	48	15	7
	$\geq 5 \times 10^{-7}$	48	15	8
	$\geq 1 \times 10^{-6}$	48	100	8
	$\geq 2 \times 10^{-6}$	48	200	8
	$\geq 5 \times 10^{-6}$	96	Continue prior regimen until level is $\leq 5 \times 10^{-7}$	

*Includes prehydration for 12 hours to establish an alkaline diuresis using 1.5 L/m^2 fluid containing 10 mEq bicarbonate and 20 mEq KCl/L (urine should be $\geq$ pH 7.0).
Data from Jaffe 1972 as cited in Chabner 1982.

every 3 hours for 12 hours before therapy, is usually sufficient to induce an alkaline urine (in adults). The sodium bicarbonate should be continued with frequent urine pH checks (> 7.0) during the therapy and for 48 hours after the dose has been delivered. MTX serum levels are useful in predicting toxicity and appropriately adjusting rescue doses of leucovorin (Stoller et al 1977, 1979). Serum creatinine and creatinine clearance should be determined before initiation of therapy and after the infusion is completed. If there is a significant change, the leucovorin calcium dosage should be increased.

Yap et al (1978) have reported the use of high-dose MTX (up to 400 mg/m^2) in patients with acute leukemia followed by L-asparaginase (40,000 IU/m^2) without leucovorin rescue. These patients did not experience significant myelosuppression and stomatitis, which suggests that L-asparaginase, given after MTX, may provide relative protection from MTX toxicity. Thymidine rescue of MTX has also been used. The minimum dose required is reported to be approximately 1 g/m^2/d (Howell et al 1979). Thymidine and other purines may act by a feedback mechanism to lower the rate of thymidylate synthesis. Thymidine would then block both the lethal and growth-inhibitory effects of MTX (Morgan and Mulkins 1979). In an effort to achieve sustained high cerebrospinal fluid levels, MTX has been given in doses of 10 g/m^2 over 6 hours in conjunction with carboxypeptidase G (CPDG) given 50 IU/kg IV push at 24, 36, and 48 hours. CPDG hydrolyzes the C-terminal glutamate from MTX but it cannot pass into the cerebrospinal fluid because of its high molecular weight (92,000). Therefore, use of

COMMON TOXIC EFFECTS AFTER ADMINISTRATION OF HIGH-DOSE METHOTREXATE WITH LEUCOVORIN CALCIUM

Days After HDMTX* Administration	Toxic Effect	Medical and Nursing Intervention
1–3	Nausea and vomiting	Measurement of intake and output and serum electrolytes; intravenous hydration; antiemetics as necessary; test for occult blood; parenteral leucovorin; encourage fluids; small frequent feedings if tolerated
1–5	Maculopapular rash	Observation of color and distribution; observation of any surgical scar for inflammation or wound breakdown; prevention of bullous eruption with skin breakdown, especially pressure areas
1–14	Fever	Acetaminophen orally or rectally as necessary every 4 h; cool mist tent or cooling blanket
3–5	Oral stomatitis	Intravenous hydration; good oral hygiene with sprays of H_2O_2, mouthwash, water, or saline; nystatin suspension (swish and swallow) and/or vaginal suppositories or lozenge; mouth and throat cultures for bacteria and fungus; appropriate antibiotics if indicated; encourage fluid intake; intravenous morphine for severe pain; combination mouthwashes (diphenhydramine, viscous lidocaine, Mylanta®)
7–10	Myelosuppression	Observe for bleeding from mucous membranes or gastrointestinal tract; transfusion of packed erythrocytes if low hemoglobin; platelet transfusion if thrombocytopenia < 20,000 cells/mm^3; prevention of infection (reverse isolation); prophylactic antibiotics (Bactrim®) and/or colony-stimulating factors (G-CSF, GM-CSF)
1–2	Pneumothorax	Closed thoracotomy; insertion of chest tube; instruct patient and parents as to necessity of reporting dyspnea or chest pain; daily auscultation of chest; chest roentgenogram
1–10	Elevated serum glutamic–oxalacetic transaminase	Transient in most patients; careful check of liver chemistries necessary
2–7	Elevated serum creatinine	Follow-up of serum creatinine levels; sodium bicarbonate for 3 days orally to alkalinize urine; intravenous hydration

*HDMTX, high-dose methotrexate; CFR, leucovorin calcium (citrovorum factor) rescue.
Data from Nirenberg et al 1977.

CPDG provides relative protection from MTX except in the cerebrospinal fluid, where it does not penetrate (Abelson et al 1979).

High-dose MTX with rescue is complicated, potentially extremely toxic, and still investigational. Only experienced teams following carefully designed protocols should attempt this treatment. Immediate MTX levels should be readily available. Fatal renal or myelotoxic toxic effects have occurred at major treatment centers despite the prophylactic precautions described herein (Von Hoff et al 1977).

For onset of typical toxic effects and their management refer to the last table.

Intrathecal Methotrexate. Methotrexate given systemically in conventional doses either orally or intravenously does not enter the cerebrospinal fluid in concentrations sufficient to produce significant antitumor effects (Mellett 1977). To achieve adequate cerebrospinal fluid concentrations MTX is given directly into the cerebrospinal fluid by lumbar puncture or directly into the ventricle by techniques such as the Ommaya reservoir (Blasberg et al 1977). Intraventricular drug appears to distribute better than intrathecally administered drug. Once in the cerebrospinal fluid, MTX diffuses out into the general circulation at a relatively slow rate. The usual cerebrospinal fluid half-life is between 12 and 18 hours, but it may be prolonged up to 48 hours (Shapiro et al 1975). A blockage in MTX elimination from the central nervous system has been correlated with prolonged blood levels and severe systemic toxicity in some patients (Jacobs et al 1975).

Doses from 10 to 15 mg/m² are given intrathecally at 2- to 5-day intervals until cerebrospinal fluid cell counts return to normal, and are then followed by one additional dose or doses once weekly for 2 weeks and a month thereafter. MTX should be injected intrathecally only if there is easy flow of blood-free spinal fluid. Bleyer and Dedrick (1977) suggest dosing according to age-related standards, not strictly according to body surface area; however, in adults single intrathecal doses larger than 15 mg total are not recommended.

Because MTX preparations containing preservatives have been associated with a greater incidence of neurotoxicity, it is recommended that the 50-mg nonpreserved vial be used for intrathecal administration. Absolute sterility is necessary for intrathecal drug administration; therefore, it is recommended that the dose be prepared under laminar air flow using mask and gloves, with final filtration of the solution through a 0.22-μm filter if possible. Elliott's B solution is the preferred diluent; however, normal saline, lactated Ringer's, 5% dextrose–lactated Ringer's, and the patient's own cerebrospinal fluid have been used (Duttera et al 1972). Dilution should result in a final volume that approximates the volume of cerebrospinal fluid removed (usually between 4 and 12 mL).

Reported toxic effects include headache, vomiting, and fever. Other central nervous system toxic effects are meningismus and, rarely, convulsions or parethesias (Bleyer et al 1974). A case of cardiac arrest after administration has been reported. The neurotoxicity associated with intrathecal MTX may be secondary to prolonged exposure to excessive drug concentrations in the central nervous system. Impaired elimination of the drug from the cerebrospinal fluid may also occur in two other settings: advanced age and the presence of meningeal leukemia. Cerebrospinal fluid MTX concentrations may be helpful in dosing to reduce toxicity. There are also consistent reports of increased acute and chronic MTX toxicity in patients receiving concomitant cranial irradiation. Cumulative chronic effects of this combination include lower IQs in pediatric patients and, rarely, an acute, progressive degeneration of the brain.

REFERENCES

Abelson HT, Ensminger WD, Rosowsky A. Serum and cerebrospinal fluid (CSF) pharmacokinetic studies of high-dose methotrexate (MTX)–carboxypeptidase G (CPDG). *Proc Am Assoc Cancer Res ASCO.* 1979;**20**:213.

Aherne GW, Piall E, Marks V, et al. Prolongation and enhancement of serum methotrexate concentrations by probenecid. *Br Med J.* 1978;**1**:1097–1099.

Ahmad S, Shen F, Bleyer WA. Methotrexate-induced renal failure and ineffectiveness of peritoneal dialysis. *Arch Intern Med.* 1978;**138**:1146–1147.

Alt FW, Kellems RE, Bertino JR, et al. Selective multiplication of dihydrofolate reductase genes in methotrexate-resistant variants of cultured murine cells. *J Biol Chem.* 1978;**253**:1357.

Anderson RJ, Gambertoglio JG, Schrier RW. *Clinical Use of Drugs in Renal Failure.* Springfield, IL: CC Thomas; 1976:173–184.

Back EH. Death after intrathecal methotrexate. *Lancet.* 1969;**2**:1005.

Balis FM, Holcenberg JS, Zimm S, et al. The effect of methotrexate on the bioavailability of oral 6-mercaptopurine. *Clin Pharmacol Ther.* 1987;**41**(4):384–387.

Bender JF, Grove WR, Fortner CL. High-dose methotrexate with folinic acid rescue. *Am J Hosp Pharm.* 1977;**34**:961–965.

Bender RA. Membrane transport of methotrexate in human neoplastic cells. *Cancer Chemother Rep Part 3.* 1975;**6**(1):73–82.

Bender RA, Bleyer WA, Frisby SA, et al. Alteration of methotrexate uptake in human leukemia cells by other agents. *Cancer Res.* 1975;**35**:1305–1308.

Bischoff KB, Dedrick RL, Zaharko DS, et al. Methotrexate pharmacokinetics. *J Pharm Sci.* 1971;**60**:1128–1133.

Bitran JD, Desser RK, DeMeester T, et al. Metastatic non-oat-cell bronchogenic carcinoma: Therapy with cyclophosphamide, doxorubicin, methotrexate and procarbazine (cAMP). *JAMA.* 1978;**240**:2745–2746.

Blasberg RG, Patlak CS, Shapiro WR. Distribution of methotrexate in the cerebrospinal fluid and brain after intraventricular administration. *Cancer Treat Rep.* 1977;**61**:633–641.

Bleyer W, Dedrick R. Clinical pharmacology of intrathecal methotrexate. I. Pharmacokinetics in non-toxic patients after lumbar injection. *Cancer Treat Rep.* 1977;**61**(4):703–708.

Bleyer WA, Drake JC, Chabner BA. Methotrexate neurotoxicity. *N Engl J Med.* 1974;**290**:57.

Bode U, Magrath I, Bleyer W, et al. Mechanism for methotrexate (MTX) efflux from cerebrospinal fluid (CSF) in man. *Proc Am Assoc Cancer Res ASCO.* 1979;**20**:375.

Bode U, Magrath IT, Bleyer WA, et al. Active transport of methotrexate from cerebrospinal fluid in humans. *Cancer Res.* 1980;**40**:2184–2187.

Bonadonna G, Brausamolino E, Valagussa P, et al. Combination chemotherapy as an adjuvant treatment in operable breast cancer. *N Engl J Med.* 1976;**234**:405–410.

Bonadonna G, Valagussa P. Dose–response effect of adjuvant chemotherapy in breast cancer. *N Engl J Med.* 1981;**304**:10–15.

Bowen D, White JC, Goldman ID. Basis for fluoropyrimidine-induced antagonism to methotrexate in Ehrlich ascites tumor cells in vitro. *Cancer Res.* 1978;**38**:219–222.

Broder LE, Selawry OS, Charyulu KN, et al. A controlled clinical trial testing two potentially non-cross-resistant chemotherapeutic regimens in small-cell carcinoma of the lung. *Chest.* 1981;**79**:327–335.

Bruckner H. Penicillin G: Evaluation of effect on toxicity of antitumor drugs. *Proc Am Assoc Cancer Res.* 1969;**10**:10.

Bruckner HW, Schreiber C, Waxman S. Interaction of chemotherapeutic agents with methotrexate and 5-fluorouracil and its effect on de novo DNA synthesis. *Cancer Res.* 1975;**35**:801–806.

Cadman E, Eiferman F. Mechanism of synergistic cell killing when methotrexate precedes cytosine arabinoside. *J Clin Invest.* 1979;**65**:788–797.

Cadman E, Heimer R, Davis L. Enhanced 5-fluorouracil nucleotide formation after methotrexate administration: Explanation for drug synergism. *Science.* 1979;**205**:1135–1137.

Calvert AH, Jones TR, Jackman AL, et al. 2-Amino-4-hydroxyquinazolines with dual metabolic loci in methotrexate resistant cells. *Proc Am Assoc Cancer Res ASCO.* 1979;**20**:24.

Campbell MA, Perrier DG, Dorr RT, Alberts DS, Finley PR. Methotrexate: Bioavailability and pharmacokinetics. *Cancer Treat Rep.* 1985;**69**(7/8):833–838.

Capizzi RL. Improvement in the therapeutic index of methotrexate (NSC-740) by L-asparaginase (NSC-109229). *Cancer Chemother Rep.* 1975;**6**(3):37–41.

Capizzi RL, DeConti RC, Marsh JC, et al. Methotrexate therapy of head and neck cancer: Improvement in the therapeutic index by the use of leucovorin rescue. *Cancer Res.* 1970;**30**:1782–1788.

Chabner BA. Methotrexate. In: Chabner BA (ed). *Pharmacologic Principles of Cancer Treatment.* Philadelphia: WB Saunders; 1982:229–255.

Chabner BA, Johns DG, Bertino JR. Enzymatic cleavage of methotrexate provides a method for prevention of drug toxicity. *Nature.* 1972;**239**:395–397.

Chabner BA, Young RC. Threshold methotrexate concentration for in vivo inhibition of DNA synthesis in normal and tumorous target tissues. *J Clin Invest.* 1973;**52**:1804–1811.

Charlton PA, Young DW, Birdsall B, et al. Stereochemistry of reduction of folic acid using dihydrofolate reductase. *Chem Commun.* 1979;**20**:922–924.

Chello PL, Sirotnak FM, Dorick DM. Kinetics and growth phase dependence of methotrexate and folic acid transport by L1210 leukemia cells. *Proc Am Assoc Cancer Res ASCO.* 1979a;**20**:219.

Chello PL, Sirotnak FM, Dorick DM, et al. Therapeutic relevance of differences in the structural specificity of the transport systems for folate analogs in L1210 tumor cells and in isolated murine intestinal epithelial cells. *Cancer Res.* 1977;**37**:4297–4303.

Chello PL, Sirotnak FM, Dorick DM. Different effects of vincristine on methotrexate uptake by L1210 cells and mouse intestinal epithelia in vitro and in vivo. *Cancer Res.* 1979b;**39**:2106–2112.

Christophidis N, Vajda FJE, Lucas I, et al. Comparison of intravenous and oral high-dose methotrexate in treatment of solid tumors. *Br Med J.* 1979;**1**:298–300.

Clarysse AM, Cathey WJ, Cartwright GE, et al. Pulmonary disease complicating intermittent therapy with methotrexate. *JAMA.* 1969;**209**:1861–1868.

Closky J, Greenspan EM, Warren TN. Hepatic fibrosis in children with acute leukemia after therapy with folic acid antagonists. *Arch Pathol.* 1955;**59**:198–206.

Condit PT, Chanes RE, Joel W. Renal toxicity of methotrexate. *Cancer.* 1969;**23**:123–131.

Creaven GB, Morgan RG. Alteration of methotrexate (MTX) pharmacokinetics by gut sterilization in man. *Proc Am Assoc Cancer Res.* 1975;**16**:134.

Cundiff D, Dietrich M. Procaine (P) and amphotericin-B (Ampho-B; Fungizone) effects in vitro on a human melanoma cell line. *Proc Am Assoc Cancer Res ASCO.* 1979;**20**:157.

Dixon RL. The interaction between various drugs and methotrexate. *Toxicol Appl Pharmacol.* 1968;**12**:308.

Djerassi I, Ciesielka W, Kim JS. Removal of methotrexate by filtration-absorption using charcoal filters or by hemodialysis. *Cancer Treat Rep.* 1977;**61**(4):751–752.

Djerassi I, Ohanissian H, Kim JS. A new approach to massive methotrexate–citrovorum rescue—A non-toxic dose schedule for methotrexate resistant tumors in poor risk patients. *Proc Am Assoc Cancer Res ASCO.* 1979;**20**:398.

Duttera MJ, Galleli JF, Kleinman LM, et al. Intrathecal methotrexate. *Lancet.* 1972;**1**:540.

Edelstein M, Vietti T, Valeriote F. The enhanced cytotoxicity of combinations of 1-α-D-arabinofuranosylcytosine and methotrexate. *Cancer Res.* 1975;**35**:1555–1558.

Ensminger WD, Frei E III. The prevention of methotrexate toxicity by thymidine infusions in humans. *Cancer Res.* 1977;**37**:1857–1863.

Esterhay RJ, Jr., Wiernik PH, Grove WR, et al. Moderate dose methotrexate, vincristine, asparaginase, and dexamethasone for treatment of adult acute lymphocytic leukemia. *Blood.* 1982;**59**:334–345.

Evans WE, Pratt CB. Effect of pleural effusion on high-dose methotrexate kinetics. *Clin Pharmacol Ther.* 1978;**24**(1):68–72.

Everts CS, Westcott JL, Bragg DG. Methotrexate therapy and pulmonary disease. *Radiology.* 1973;**107**:539–543.

Fisher RI, DeVita VT, Hubbard SM, et al. Diffuse aggressive lymphomas: Increased survival after alternating flexible sequences of ProMACE and MOPP chemotherapy. *Ann Intern Med.* 1983;**98**:304–309.

Frei E, Jaffe N, Tattersal M, et al. New approaches to cancer chemotherapy with methotrexate. *N Engl J Med.* 1975;**292**(16):846–851.

Fry DW, Yalowich JC, Goldman ID. Augmentation of the intracellular levels of polyglutamyl derivatives of methotrexate by vincristine and probenecid in Ehrlich ascites tumor cells. *Cancer Res.* 1982;**42**:2532–2536.

Fyfe MJ, Goldman ID. Characteristics of the vincristine-induced augmentation of methotrexate uptake in Ehrlich ascites tumor cells. *J Biol Chem.* 1973;**243**:5067–5073.

Gangji D, Ross WE, Poplack DG, et al. (1979) Effect of probenecid (P) on methotrexate (MTX) cytotoxicity. *Proc Am Assoc Cancer Res ASCO.* 1979;**20**:244.

Gelman RS, Taylor SG IV. Cyclophosphamide, methotrexate, and 5-fluorouracil chemotherapy in women more than 65 years old with advanced breast cancer: The elimination of age trends in toxicity by using doses based on creatinine clearance. *J Clin Oncol.* 1984;**2**:1404–1413.

Goldman ID. Analysis of the cytotoxic determinants for methotrexate (NSC-740): Role for "free" intracellular drug. *Cancer Chemother Rep.* 1975a;**6**:51–61.

Goldman ID. The membrane transport of methotrexate (NSC-740) and other folate compounds: Relevance to rescue protocols. *Cancer Chemother Rep Part 3.* 1975b;**6**(1):63–72.

Goldman ID. Effects of methotrexate on cellular metabolism: Some critical elements in the drug–cell interaction. *Cancer Treat Rep.* 1977;**71**(4):549–558.

Grindey GB, Moran RE. Effects of allopurinol on the therapeutic efficacy of methotrexate. *Cancer Res.* 1975;**35**:1702–1705.

Henderson ES, Adamson RH, Oliverio VT. The metabolic fate of tritiated methotrexate. II. Absorption and excretion in man. *Cancer Res.* 1965;**25**:1018–1024.

Hersh EM, Wong VG, Henderson ES, et al. Hepatotoxic effects of methotrexate. *Cancer.* 1966;**19**:600–606.

Hignite CE, Shen DD, Azarnoff DL. Separation and identification of impurities in parenteral methotrexate dosage forms. *Cancer Treat Rep.* 1978;**63**(3):405–410.

Hill BT, Bailey BD, White JC, et al. Characteristics of transport of 4-amino antifolates and folate compounds by two lines of L5178Y lymphoblasts, one with impaired transport of methotrexate. *Cancer Res.* 1979;**39**:2440–2446.

Howell SB, Blair HE, Uren J, Frie E. Hemodialysis and enzymatic cleavage of methotrexate in man. *Eur J Cancer.* 1978;**14**:787–792.

Howell SB, Herbst K, Boss G, Frei E III. Thymidine (TdR) rescue of methotrexate (MTX) in man. *Proc Am Assoc Cancer Res ASCO.* 1979;**20**:399.

Huffman DH, Wan SH, Azarnoff DL, et al. Pharmacokinetics of methotrexate. *Clin Pharmacol Ther.* 1973;**14**:572–579.

Igroffo RJ, Friedman MA, Carter SK. The pharmacology of methotrexate (MTX) administered via the hepatic artery in patients with liver tumors. *Proc Am Assoc Cancer Res ASCO.* 1979;**20**:306.

Isacoff WH, Morrison PF, Aroesty J, et al. Pharmacokinetics of high-dose methotrexate with citrovorum factor rescue. *Cancer Treat Rep.* 1977;**61**:1665–1674.

Jackson RC, Weber G. Enzyme pattern directed chemotherapy: The effects of combinations of methotrexate, 5-fluorodeoxyuridine and thymidine on rat hepatoma cells in vitro. *Biochem Pharmacol.* 1976;**25**:2613–2618.

Jacobs SA, Bleyer WA, Chabner BA, et al. Altered plasma pharmacokinetics of methotrexate administered intrathecally. *Lancet.* 1975;**1**:465–466.

Jaffe N. Recent advances in the chemotherapy of metastatic osteogenic sarcoma. *Cancer.* 1972;**30**:1627–1631.

Jolivet J, Schilsky RL, Bailey BD, et al. Synthesis, retention, and biological activity of methotrexate polyglutamates in cultured human breast cancer cells. *J Clin Invest.* 1982;**70**:351–360.

Kay HEM, Kapton PJ, O'Sullivan JP, et al. Encephalopathy in acute leukemia associated with methotrexate therapy. *Arch Dis Child.* 1972;**47**:344–354.

Kessel D, Hall TC, Roberts D. Modes of uptake of methotrexate by normal and leukemic human leukocytes in vitro and their relation to drug response. *Cancer Res.* 1968;**28**:564–570.

Leme PR, Creaven PJ, Allen LM, et al. Kinetic model for the disposition and metabolism of moderate and high-dose methotrexate (NSC-740) in man. *Cancer Chemother Rep.* 1975;**59**:811–817.

Levitt M, Marsh JC, DeConti RC, et al. Combination sequential chemotherapy in advanced reticulum cell sarcoma. *Cancer.* 1972;**29**:630–635.

Lichter JG, Santicky MA, Jacobs SA. A pharmacological comparison of high-dose methotrexate (HD-MTX) administered in 1 hour and 18 hour infusions. *Proc Am Assoc Cancer Res ASCO.* 1979;**20**:411.

Liegler DG, Henderson ES, Hahn MA, et al. The effect of organic acids on renal clearance of methotrexate in man. *Clin Pharmacol Ther.* 1970;**10**:849–857.

Maurer LH, Tulloh M, Weiss RB, et al. A randomized combined modality trial in small cell carcinoma of the lung: Comparison of combination chemotherapy–radiation therapy versus cyclophosphamide–radiation therapy effects of maintenance chemotherapy and prophylatic whole brain irradiation. *Cancer.* 1980;**45**:30–39.

McDonald CJ, Bertino J Jr. Treatment of mycosis fungoides lymphoma: Effectiveness of infusions of methotrexate followed by oral citrovorum factor. *Cancer Treat Rep.* 1978;**62**:1009–1014.

McRae MP, King JC. Compatibility of antineoplastic, antibiotic and corticosteroid drugs in intravenous admixtures. *Am J Hosp Pharm.* 1976;**33**:1010–1013.

Mellett LB. Physiochemical considerations and pharmacokinetic behavior in delivery of drugs to the central nervous system. *Cancer Treat Rep.* 1977;**61**(4):527–531.

Moran RE, Straus MJ. Cell cycle synchronization prior to phase-specific therapy with increased survival. *Proc Am Assoc Cancer Res ASCO.* 1975;**20**:123.

Morgan RG, Mulkins M. The role of thymidylate synthetase (TS) activity in the development of methotrexate (MTX) cytotoxicity. *Proc Am Assoc Cancer Res ASCO.* 1979;**20**:95.

Morison WL, Momtaz K, Parrish JA, et al. Combined methotrexate–PUVA therapy in the treatment of psoriasis. *J Am Acad Dermatol.* 1982;**6**:46–51.

Mouridsen HT, Jacobsen E, Faber O. The pharmacokinetics of cyclophosphamide in man following treatment with methotrexate. *Acta Pharmacol Toxicol.* 1976;**38**:508–512.

Nirenberg A, Mosende C, Mehta BM, et al. High-dose methotrexate with citrovorum factor rescue: Predictive value of serum methotrexate concentrations and corrective measures to avert toxicity. *Cancer Treat Rep.* 1977;**61**(5):779–783.

Omura GA, Moffitt S, Vogler WR, et al. Combination chemotherapy of adult acute lymphoblastic leukemia with randomized central nervous system prophylaxis. *Blood.* 1980;**55**:199–204.

Paul BS, Momtaz K, Stern RS, et al. Combined methotrexate–ultraviolet B therapy in the treatment of psoriasis. *J Am Acad Dermatol.* 1982;**7**:758–762.

Pratt CB, Howarth C, Ransom JL, et al. High-dose methotrexate used alone and in combination for measurable primary or metastatic osteosarcoma. *Cancer Treat Rep.* 1980;**64**:11–20.

Ramirez I, Sullivan MP, Wang Y-M, et al. Effective therapy for Burkett's lymphoma. High-dose cyclophosphamide/high-dose methotrexate with coordinated intrathecal therapy: Plasma and cerebrospinal fluid methotrexate levels. *Cancer Chemother Pharmacol.* 1979;**3**: 103–109.

Ramu A, Fusner JE, Blaschke T, Glaubiger DL. Probenecid inhibition of methotrexate–cerebrospinal fluid pharmacokinetics in dogs. *Cancer Treat Rep.* 1978;**62**(10):1465–1470.

Rivera G, Pratt C, Aur R, et al. Schedule dependence of cystosine arabinoside (Ara-C) and methotrexate (MTX) for recurrent childhood lymphocytic leukemia (ALL). *Proc Am Assoc Cancer Res.* 1976;**17**:270.

Rosen G, Caparros B, Huvos AG, et al. Preoperative chemotherapy for osteogenic sarcoma: Selection of postoperative adjuvant chemotherapy based on the response of the primary tumor to preoperative chemotherapy. *Cancer.* 1982;**49**:1221–1230.

Rosowsky A, Lazarus A, Yuan GC, Beltz WR. Effect of methotrexate (MTX) esters and other lipophilic antifolates on MTX-resistant human leukemic cells. *Proc Am Assoc Cancer Res ASCO.* 1979;**20**:327.

Semon JH, Grindey GB. Potentiation of the antitumor activity of methotrexate by concurrent infusion of thymidine. *Cancer Res.* 1978;**38**:2905–2911.

Shapiro WR, Young DF, Mehta BM. Methotrexate distribution in cerebrospinal fluid after intravenous ventricular and lumbar injections. *N Engl J Med.* 1975;**293**:161–166.

Skarin A, Canellos GP. Methotrexate–leucovorin factor rescue in large cell lymphoma. *NCI Monogr.* 1987;**5**:71–76.

Smith EB, Weed JC Jr, Tyrey L, Hammond CB. Treatment of nonmetastatic gestational trophoblastic disease: Results of methotrexate alone versus methotrexate–folinic acid. *Am J Obstet Gynecol.* 1982;**144**:88–92.

Sostman HD, et al. Methotrexate-induced pneumonitis. *Medicine (Baltimore)* 1976;**55**:371–388.

Stoller R, Hande K, Jacobs S, et al. Use of plasma pharmacokinetics to predict and prevent methotrexate toxicity. *N Engl J Med.* 1977;**297**:630–634.

Stoller RG, Jacobs SA, Drake JC, et al. Pharmacokinetics of high-dose methotrexate (NSC-740). *Cancer Chemother Rep.* 1975;**6**:19–24.

Stoller RG, Kaplan HG, Cummings FJ, Calabresi P. A clinical and pharmacological study of high-dose methotrexate with minimal leucovorin rescue. *Cancer Res.* 1979;**39**:908–912.

Tattersall MH, Brown B, Frei E III. The reversal of methotrexate toxicity by thymidine with maintenance of antitumor effects. *Nature.* 1975;**253**:198–200.

Tattersall MH, Jackson RC, Jackson ST, et al. Factors determining cell sensitivity to methotrexate: Studies of folate and deoxyribonucleotide triphosphate pools in five mammalian cell lines. *Eur J Cancer.* 1974;**10**:819–826.

Taylor JR, Halprin KM. Effect of sodium salicylate and indomethacin on methotrexate–serum albumin binding. *Arch Dermatol.* 1977;**113**:588–591.

Tejada F, Zubrod CG. Vincristine effect on methotrexate cerebrospinal fluid concentration. *Cancer Treat Rep.* 1979;**63**(1):143–145.

Thyss A, Milano G, Kubar J, et al. Clinical and pharmacokinetic evidence of a life-threatening interaction between methotrexate and ketoprofen. *Lancet* 1986;**1**:256–258.

Thyss A, Milano G, Renée N, et al. Severe interaction between methotrexate and a macrolide-like antibiotic. *J Natl Cancer Inst.* 1993;**85**:582–583.

Trisman G, Isacoff WH, Drakes T. Salvage of breast cancer adjuvant treatment failures with high dose methotrexate and 5-FU. *Proc Am Assoc Cancer Res ASCO.* 1979;**20**:140.

Trissel LA, Fulton B, Tramonte SM. Visual compatibility of ondansetron with chemotherapeutic agents, antibiotics, and other selected drugs during simulated Y-site injection (abstract #P-468R). *25th Annual ASHP Midyear Clinical Meetings and Exhibit, Las Vegas, Nevada;* 1990.

Von Hoff D, Penta JS, Hellman LJ, et al. The incidence of drug related deaths secondary to high dose methotrexate and citrovorum factor rescue. *Cancer Treat Rep.* 1977;**61**:745–748.

Von Hoff DD, Alberts DS, Mattx De, et al. Combination chemotherapy with cisplatin, bleomycin, and methotrexate in patients with advanced head and neck cancer. *Cancer Clin Trials.* 1981;**4**:215–218.

Wang JJ, Freeman AI, Sinks LF. Treatment of acute lymphocytic leukemia by high-dose intravenous methotrexate. *Cancer Res.* 1976;**36**:1441–1444.

Wang Y, Sutow WW, Romsdahl MM, Perez C. Age-related pharmacokinetics of high-dose methotrexate in patients with osteosarcoma. *Cancer Treat Rep.* 1979;**63**(3):405–410.

Warkentin P, Hasegawa D, Nesbit M, et al. High dose methotrexate (MTX) hepatotoxicity: Significance of frequency of administration. *Proc Am Assoc Cancer Res ASCO.* 1979;**20**:98.

Weinblatt ME, Coblyn JS, Fox DA, et al. Efficacy of low-dose methotrexate in rheumatoid arthritis. *N Engl J Med.* 1985;**312**:818–822.

Weinstein G, Newburger A, Troner M, Colton A. Cell kinetic synchronization of human malignant melanoma (MM) with low dose methotrexate (MTX) in vivo. *Proc Am Assoc Cancer Res ASCO.* 1979;**20**:403.

Weinstein GD, Cox JW, Suringa DWR, et al. Evaluation of possible chronic hepatotoxicity from methotrexate for psoriasis. *Arch Dermatol.* 1970;**102**:613–618.

Weimann MC, Cumming FJ, Kaplan HG, et al. Clinical and pharmacological studies of methotrexate–minimal leucovorin rescue plus fluorouracil. *Cancer Res.* 1982;**42**:3896–3900.

Willkens RF, Watson MA. Methotrexate: A perspective of its use in the treatment of rheumatic diseases. *J Lab Clin Med.* 1982;**100**:314–321.

Yalowich JC, Fry DW, Goldman ID. Teniposide (VM-26)- and etoposide (VP-16-213)-induced augmentation of methotrexate transport and polyglutamylation in Ehrlich ascites tumor cells in vitro. *Cancer Res.* 1982;**42**:3648–3653.

Yap B-S, McCredie KB, Benjamin RS, et al. Refractory acute leukaemia in adults treated with sequential collapse and high-dose methotrexate. *Br Med J.* 1978;**2**:791–793.

Zager RF, Frisby SA, Oliverio VT. The effects of antibiotics and cancer chemotherapeutic agents on the cellular transport and antitumor activity of methotrexate in L1210 murine leukemia. *Cancer Res.* 1973;**33**:1670–1676.

Zaharko DS, Fung W-P, Yang K-H. Relative biochemical aspects of low and high doses of methotrexate in mice. *Cancer Res.* 1977;**37**:1602–1607.

N-Methylformamide

■ Other Names

NMF; NSC-3051.

■ Chemistry

Structure of N-methylformamide

N-Methylformamide (NMF) is a metabolite of the industrial solvent dimethylformamide (DMF). It has a simple chemical formula with a molecular weight of 59.1. N-Methylformamide is a polar solvent as is DMF. Both compounds have good lipophilicity but are also water miscible. NMF occurs as a colorless liquid with a specific gravity of 1.0 and a pH of 7.0 (Myers et al 1956).

■ Antitumor Activity

Both DMF and NMF produce two types of antitumor effects: (1) maturation of malignant cells to a more normal phenotype (differentiation); (2) direct growth inhibition of experimental tumors (Spremulli and Dexter 1984). The monomethyl derivative NMF appeared to produce the greatest antitumor efficacy against human colon tumor xenografts in athymic (nude) mice (Dexter et al 1982). NMF also showed good antitumor activity against lung and mammary cancer xenografts and marginal activity against P-388 and L-1210 leukemia in mice

(O'Dwyer et al 1985). The drug was active against sarcoma 180, M-5076 ovarian cancer, and TLX5 lymphoma in mice (Spremulli and Dexter 1984). The parent molecule, DMF, also sensitizes tumor cells to the effects of ionizing radiation in vitro (Leith et al 1981, 1982) and in the nude mouse model (Dexter et al 1984).

Several clinical trials with NMF have been conducted. In a phase I trial of intravenous and oral NMF, partial responses were obtained in 2 of 15 patients with solid tumors (prostate and cervix cancer). There were also two minor responses in ovarian carcinoma and hypernephroma (McVie et al 1984); however, the drug was inactive in phase II trials in renal cell carcinoma (Sternberg et al 1986), in advanced colorectal cancer (Tchekmedyian et al 1987), in advanced head and neck cancer (Vogel et al 1987), in cervix cancer (McGuire et al 1990b), and in metastatic melanoma (Eton et al 1991). In advanced epithelial ovarian cancer NMF produced partial responses in 3 of 44 (6.8%) of patients (McGuire et al 1990a).

■ Mechanism of Action

Most mechanistic investigations have focused on DMF, the metabolic precursor of NMF. In cell culture, DMF-treated cells lose the ability to grow in soft agar. Saturation densities are reduced and cell doubling times increase (Dexter et al 1979). In human colon cancers grown in vitro, DMF alters the expression of cell surface antigens toward a more differentiated (nonmalignant) phenotype (Spremulli and Dexter 1984). There is also an increase in the levels of adenosine deaminase and adenosine monophosphate kinase in DMF-treated colon cancer cells (Dexter et al 1981).

Nonetheless, the principal mechanism of the antitumor action of these polar solvents is unknown. The radiation synergy effect has been postulated to involve a decreased capability to repair sublethal radiation damage (Leith et al 1982). There may be a link between the radiosensitization effect and the differentiating effect of the drug. Hill et al (1976) and Lavin et al (1976) have shown that tumor cells induced to differentiate by DMF are significantly more sensitive to ionizing radiation. One major caveat with NMF is that the drug levels required for tumor cell differentiating activity in vitro (Tanaka et al 1975) are much higher than those that can be achieved in vivo (Orr et al 1983, Rowinsky et al 1988, McVie et al 1984).

■ Availability and Storage

N-Methylformamide is investigationally available from the National Cancer Institute in 2-mL glass ampules containing 800 mg of drug (400 mg/mL) in 0.9% Sodium Chloride for Injection, USP. The intact ampules are stable at room temperature for at least 4 years after manufacture and for 1 year at 50°C.

■ Preparation for Use, Stability, and Admixture

The 40% NMF solution is diluted into 500 mL of 5% dextrose or 0.9% sodium chloride to a final concentration of 10 mg/mL (1%). A 1.6 mg/mL solution (800 mg in 500 mL) shows negligible decomposition for 96 hours at 22°C in fluorescent (room) lighting. The compatibility of NMF with different plastic infusion systems components is unknown; however, studies at the National Cancer Institute have shown that the drug does not leach significant amounts of plasticizers from polyvinyl chloride (Viaflex®) or other (Venoset®-60) administration sets (Vishnuvajjala and Cradock 1984). Compatibility with other plastic infusion devices (filters, tubing, etc) is unknown. Therefore, glass syringes and infusion containers should be used during all NMF preparations and infusions.

■ Administration

N-Methylformamide solutions are infused intravenously as a rapid infusion (O'Dwyer et al 1985). The injectable solution has also been mixed with orange juice for oral administration (McVie et al 1984). A dilution into 4 oz of orange juice was used in another trial (Eisenhauer et al 1986).

■ Dosage

The maximally tolerated dose of intravenous NMF given weekly × 6 is 1500 mg/m^2, and the recommended dose for phase II trials was 1125 mg/m^2 (O'Dwyer et al 1985). The recommended dose for weekly oral NMF is 800 mg/m^2/d for 5 days, repeated every 2 to 3 weeks (McVie et al 1984). Eisenhauer et al (1986) used an oral dose of 800 mg/m^2 three times a week for 4 weeks, repeated every 6 weeks. This schedule was quite toxic, however, and therefore a dose of 600 mg/m^2 was recommended for further studies (Rowinsky et al 1987). Other parenteral NMF schedules have been developed from phase I trials such as 1000 mg/m^2 IV × 5 days, repeated every 4 weeks (Sternberg et al 1986,

Tchekmedyian et al 1987), and 2000 mg/m²/wk × 3 (Ettinger et al 1985).

■ Drug Interactions

As with DMF (Lyle et al 1979), NMF also produces a disulfiram-type effect when combined with alcohol (McVie et al 1984). This reaction involves severe facial flushing and nausea. Vomiting may result if a severe reaction ensues. Thus, alcohol should be absolutely avoided when taking NMF.

■ Pharmacokinetics

Preliminary pharmacokinetic studies suggest that plasma NMF clearance is biphasic with an α half-life of 10 minutes and a mean terminal elimination half-life of 9 hours (range, 5–16 hours [Orr et al 1983]) to 12 hours (Rowinsky et al 1988). The volume of distribution of NMF approximates that of total body water. The mean volume of the central compartment was 13.8 L/m², and that at steady state was 18.7 L/m² (Rowinsky et al 1988). The mean plasma NMF clearance in this study was 19.1 mL/min/m² (Rowinsky et al 1988). A peak plasma concentration of 1715 μM was achieved after an intravenous dose of 1125 mg/m² (Orr et al 1983). Importantly, the levels of NMF obtained after intravenous or oral doses (2.78 and 0.46 mmol/L, respectively) are significantly lower than drug concentrations needed for antineoplastic activity in vitro (Rowinsky et al 1988). This probably explains the consistent lack of clinical antitumor activity for this compound. Less than 10% of a dose is excreted into the urine over the first 24 hours after dosing. No plasma or urinary metabolites of NMF were observed. The drug does not appear to be excreted by renal or pulmonary routes (Rowinsky et al 1988). Drug levels in ascites fluid equal those in the plasma 24 hours after dosing (Orr et al 1983).

The bioavailability of oral doses in the range of 1 g/m²/d given in 100 mL of orange juice was 87 to 95% (McVie et al 1983, Rowinsky et al 1988). Accumulation of the drug over a 5-day dosing period was also observed. In contrast, the extent of absorption and drug clearance remained constant on each day of dosing (McVie et al 1983).

■ Side Effects and Toxicity

Hepatotoxicity was well recognized following very early clinical trials or oral NMF (Myers et al 1956, Spremulli et al 1983). Toxicity is noted by elevated hepatic transaminase levels, occasional hypoalbuminemia, and hyperbilirubinemia (Myers et al 1956, O'Dwyer et al 1985). This effect overlaps with a syndrome of fatigue, malaise, nausea, and anorexia best characterized as a drop in performance status (O'Dwyer et al 1985). The median drop in performance status was 30% in this trial. These symptoms resolve rapidly once drug administration stops. The nausea and vomiting with NMF appear to be dose dependent and of moderate intensity at its peak. Fortunately, antiemetics are very effective at controlling this toxic effect. Myelosuppression is generally not observed.

Similar toxic effects are described with oral NMF (McVie et al 1984). These include elevations of alkaline phosphatase, serum glutamic–pyruvic and glutamic-oxalacetic transaminases, and hyperbilirubinemia. Liver biopsies of toxic patients show swollen hepatocytes, some pyknosis, and nonspecific periportal inflammatory infiltrates (McVie et al 1984). Jaundice has been reported rarely and hepatomegaly is uncommon. Peripheral neuropathy has been observed in some patients and could prove to be a consistent side effect if chronic NMF treatments are administered.

REFERENCES

Dexter DL, Barbosa JA, Calabresi P. N,N-Dimethylformamide-induced alteration of cell culture characteristics and loss of tumorigenicity in cultured human colon carcinoma cells. *Cancer Res.* 1979;**39**:1020–1025.

Dexter DL, Crabtree GW, Stoeckler JD, et al. N,N-Dimethylformamide and sodium buyrate modulation of the activities of purine-metabolizing enzymes in cultured human colon carcinoma cells. *Cancer Res.* 1981;**41**:808–812.

Dexter DL, Lee ES, Bliven SF, et al. Enhancement by N-methylformamide of the effect of ionizing radiation on a human colon tumor xenografted in nude mice. *Cancer Res.* 1984;**44**:4942–4946.

Dexter DL, Spremulli EN, Matook GM, et al. Inhibition of growth of human colon cancer xenografts by polar solvents. *Cancer Res.* 1982;**42**:5018–5022.

Eisenhauer EA, Weinerman BH, Kerr I, Quirt I. Toxicity of oral N-methylformamide in three phase II trials: A report from the National Cancer Institute of Canada Clinical Trials Group. *Cancer Treat Rep.* 1986;**70**(7):881–883.

Eton O, Bajorin DF, Casper ES, Houghton AN. Phase II trial of N-methylformamide in patients with metastatic melanoma. *Invest New Drugs.* 1991;**9**:97–100.

Ettinger DA, Orr DW, Rice AP, Donehower RC. Phase I

trial of N-methylformamide in patients with advanced cancer. *Cancer Treat Rep.* 1985;**69**:489–493.

Hill HZ, Hill GJ, Miller CF, et al. Radiation and melanoma: Response of B16 mouse tumor cells and clonal lines to in vitro irradiation. *Radiat Res.* 1976;**80**:259–276.

Lavin MF, McCombe P, Kidson C. DNA replication and post-replication repair in U.V.-sensitive mouse neuroblastoma cells. *Int J Radiat Biol Relat Stud Phys Chem Med.* 1976;**30**:31–40.

Leith JT, Brenner HJ, DeWyngaert JK, et al. Selective modification of the x-ray survival response of two mouse mammary adenocarcinoma sublines of N,N-dimethylformamide. *Int J Radiat Oncol Biol Phys.* 1981;**7**:943–946.

Leith JT, Gaskins LA, Dexter DL, et al. Alteration of the survival response of two human colon carcinoma subpopulations to X-irradiation by N,N-dimethylformamide. *Cancer Res.* 1982;**42**:30–34.

Lyle WH, Spence TWM, McKinnely WM, et al. Dimethylformamide and alcohol intolerance. *Br J Ind Med.* 1979;**36**:63–66.

McGuire WP III, Blessing JA, Berek JS, Munoz A. Phase II study of N-methylformamide (N-MF) (NSC-3051) in patients with advanced epithelial ovarian cancer. *Invest New Drugs.* 1990a;**8**:191–194.

McGuire WP III, Blessing JA, Hatch KD, German ML. Phase II study of N-methylformamide (N-MF) (NSC-3051) in patients with advanced squamous cancer of the cervix. *Invest New Drugs.* 1990b;**8**:195–197.

McVie JG, Ten Bokkel Huinink WW, Newlands E, et al. Phase I studies and clinical pharmacology of N-methylformamide (NSC-3051, NMF) (abstract C-134). *Proc Am Soc Clin Oncol.* 1983;**12**:34.

McVie JG, Ten Bokkel Huinink WW, Simonetti G, Dubbelman R. Phase I trial of N-methylformamide. *Cancer Treat Rep.* 1984;**68**:607–610.

Myers WPL, Karnofsky DA, Burchenal JH. The hepatotoxic action of N-methylformamide in man. *Cancer.* 1956;**9**:949–954.

O'Dwyer PJ, Donehower M, Sigman LM, et al. Phase I trial of N-methylformamide (NMF, NSC-3051). *J Clin Oncol.* 1985;**3**:853–857.

Orr DW, Ettinger DS, Rice AP, et al. Phase I and pharmacokinetic study of N-methylformamide (NMF) (abstract C-93). *Proc Am Soc Clin Oncol.* 1983;**2**:34.

Rowinsky E, Grochow LB, Hantel A, et al. Assessment of N-methylformamide (NMF) administered orally on a three times weekly schedule: A phase I study. *Invest New Drugs.* 1987;**7**:317–325.

Rowinsky EK, Noe DA, Orr DW, et al. Clinical pharmacology of oral and IV N-methylformamide: A pharmacologic basis for lack of clinical antineoplastic activity. *J Natl Cancer Inst.* 1988;**80**:671–678.

Spremulli EN, Dexter DL. Polar solvents: A novel class of antineoplastic agents. *J Clin Oncol.* 1984;**2**(3):227–241.

Spremulli EN, Dexter DL, Cummings FJ, et al. Phase I clinical and pharmacological studies of monomethylformamide (N-MF) (abstract). *Proc Am Soc Clin Oncol.* 1983;**2**:24.

Sternberg CN, Yagoda A, Scher HI, Hollander P. Phase II trial of N-methylformamide for advanced renal cell carcinoma. *Cancer Treat Rep.* 1986;**70**(5):681–682.

Tanaka M, Levy J, Terada M, et al. Induction of erythroid differentiation in murine virus infected erythroleukemia cells by highly polar compounds. *Proc Natl Acad Sci USA.* 1975;**72**:1003–1006.

Tchekmedyian NS, Kaplan RS, Eisenberger M, et al. Phase II study of N-methylformamide in patients with advanced colorectal cancer. *Cancer Treat Rep.* 1987;**71**(5):541–542.

Vishnuvajjala BR, Cradock JC. Compatibility of plastic infusion devices with diluted N-methylformamide and N,N-dimethylacetamide. *Am J Hosp Pharm.* 1984;**41**:1160–1163.

Vogel WC, Forastiere AA, Natale RB, et al. Phase II trial of N-methylformamide in advanced head and neck cancer. *Invest New Drugs.* 1987;**5**:203–206.

Mifepristone

■ Other Names

RU-486, RU-38486 (Hoechst-Roussel-Uclaf Pharmaceuticals Inc); 17β-hydroxy-11β-(4-dimethylaminophenyl)-17α-(1-propynyl)estra-4,9-dien-3-one.

■ Chemistry

Structure of mifepristone

Mifepristone is a synthetic 19-nor aminophenyl derivative of progesterone. It acts as an antiprogestin and antiglucocorticoid (Herrmann et al 1982). The third phenyl ring at position 11β resembles other synthetic triphenylethylene antiestrogens such as tamoxifen (Chobert et al 1983).

■ Antitumor Activity

Mifepristone has both antiprogestational and antiglucocorticoid activities. Thus, the primary clinical use has been as a contraceptive or abortifacient (Couzinet et al 1986). The drug has also been used to treat excess corticosteroid production associated with Cushing's syndrome (Nieman et al 1985). In addition, mifepristone has been shown to reduce intraocular pressure in rabbits and could be useful in glaucoma (Phillips et al 1984). Because of the known hormonal dependence of some breast cancers for growth, mifepristone has been evaluated for antitumor activity in a number of preclinical studies and in two pilot clinical trials. The drug inhibits the growth of human MCF-7 and T47D breast cancer cells in vitro in a dose-dependent fashion (Bardon et al 1985). The magnitude of inhibition correlates with the number of unoccupied progesterone receptors (PRS) present in each cell line. Breast cancer cell growth is also diminished by mifepristone in experimental animals. Drug-sensitive models include the MXT(+) mammary cancer in the mouse and rat mammary tumors induced by the carcinogens DMBA or methylnitrosourea (Schneider et al 1990). In experimental rat prostatic carcinoma, mifepristone significantly depressed tumor growth when concomitant diethylstilbestrol was used to maintain high PR levels (Mobbs and Johnson 1991).

Antitumor effects have also been observed in nude mice given human meningioma cells subcutaneously (Olson et al 1987). Similar inhibitory results are reported for mifepristone added to PR-positive meningioma cells in vitro (Olson et al 1986, Blankenstein et al 1989). Some rationale for mifepristone use has been described in lymphoma (Palca 1987).

Two preliminary clinical trials have reported efficacy for chronic mifepristone therapy in patients with unresectable benign meningiomas. Objective responses were observed in 6 of 14 patients (Grunberg et al 1991) and in 4 of 10 patients (Lamberts et al 1992). In addition, a number of other patients in these trials described subjective improvements in headache and extraocular muscle function. Stable disease was observed in about one third of patients and toxicity was mild in all patients. These preliminary findings suggest that long-term oral mifepristone therapy is effective in up to one half of patients with unresectable meningiomas. Other responsive cell lines include human pituitary cells (Lamberts et al 1985), adrenal tumor cells (Contreras et al 1987), and hepatoma cells (Chasserot-Golaz and Beck 1986).

Pilot clinical trials have been performed in postmenopausal patients with metastatic breast cancer. In one trial, 12 of 22 patients achieved a partial response or disease stabilization after 3 months of chronic mifepristone therapy; however, only 4 of 22 remained in response at 6 months (Romieu et al 1987). In another trial, short-term disease stabilization was achieved in 6 of 11 patients (Klijn et al 1989).

■ Mechanism of Action

Mifepristone exerts its antitumor actions by binding to nuclear PR to inhibit subsequent progestin actions (Baulieu 1991); however, unlike some second-generation antiprogestins such as onapristone, mifepristone also binds to glucocorticoid receptors (GRS) to block corticosteroid-mediated effects (Baulieu 1991). This feature may limit the clinical utility of mifepristone as a chronic antihormonal therapy. Mifepristone is only weakly antiandrogenic and does not bind to mineralocorticoid receptors, estrogen receptors, or specific steroid transport proteins such as transcortin and sex hormone-binding globulin.

The PR and GR are members of the superfamily of DNA-binding receptors modeled originally on thyroid hormone (Evans 1988). Mifepristone has both high affinity for PR and GR, as well as a long metabolic half-life. In this fashion, it efficiently displaces the normal progestin agonist from its receptor sites (Baulieu and Segal 1985). The affinity of mifepristone for PR is five times higher than that of progesterone, and its affinity for GR is two to three times that of dexamethasone (Hermmann et al 1982). After binding, mifepristone slows the transformation of the 8 S form of the PR to its active, DNA-binding form (Groyer et al 1987). There is also a conformational change in the ligand-binding domain of the receptor that blocks transcriptional activity of the drug–receptor complex at progesterone-response elements (PRES) in the DNA. Thus, even though some binding to DNA may occur, the drug–receptor complex does not allow for normal hormonal transcription to occur (Baulieu 1991). In addition, mifepristone blocks the normal down-regulation of PR induced by progestins.

In breast cancer cells, mifepristone reduces the number of cells in S phase by causing a cell cycle arrest in G_0 or G_1 phase (Schneider et al 1990). As a result of mifepristone binding of PR, these cells undergo terminal differentiation, leading to increased cell death.

■ Availability and Storage

Mifepristone (RU-486) is investigationally available as 50- and 200-mg tablets from Roussel-Uclaf, France. The tablets are stored at room temperature.

Drug Interactions

The combination of an antiestrogen such as tamoxifen with mifepristone enhances experimental antitumor effects in rats (Bardon et al 1987). This combination may also block the increase in estradiol levels seen with mifepristone alone. Some clinical trials have used concomitant dexamethasone (1.0 mg/d for 14 days) to initially lessen the antiglucocorticoid effects of the drug (Grunberg et al 1991). Oral prednisone 7.5 mg/d has been used similarly to reduce nausea and vomiting during the initial week of therapy (Lamberts et al 1992).

Administration

Mifepristone has been administered orally twice daily for 1 to 3 months in breast cancer (Romieu et al 1987, Klijn et al 1989) and for up to 1 year in meningioma (Grunberg et al 1991).

Dosage

The active dose and schedule for antitumor activity are not known. Doses used in pilot studies in breast cancer range from 100 mg twice daily (200 mg/d total) (Romieu et al 1987) to 100 to 200 mg twice daily (200–400 mg/d total) (Klijn et al 1989). A similar dose range of 200 mg/d continuously for up to 1 year has been shown to be active in patients with meningiomas (Grunberg et al 1991, Lamberts et al 1992).

Pharmacokinetics

A half-life of 20 hours is reported for mifepristone in humans (Klijn et al 1989).

Side Effects and Toxicity

Mifepristone is usually well tolerated for several months of continuous daily administration (Romieu et al 1987). Slight nausea, anorexia, and general tiredness are the most frequent complaints (Lamberts et al 1992, Klijn et al 1989). Anorexia and exhaustion may be severe in up to one third of patients on initiation of therapy for meningioma (Lamberts et al 1992).

Weight loss (1–7 kg) was reported in one trial (Klijn et al 1989) but was not encountered in others (Lamberts et al 1992). Hypotension has not been observed in any of the pilot clinical trials. A grand mal seizure is described in one breast cancer patient who did not have evidence of cerebral metastases (Klijn et al 1989). Dizziness was described in 2 of 22 patients in another breast cancer trial (Romieu et al 1987).

Endocrine effects of mifepristone in breast cancer patients include a consistent two- to threefold elevation in plasma adrenocorticotropin and cortisol concentrations. These increased cortisol levels could not be suppressed by dexamethasone. Similar elevations are described for plasma levels of estradiol and androstenedione (Klijn et al 1989). There were no changes in levels of steroid-binding globulin, luteinizing hormone, or follicle-stimulating hormone.

A slight, but statistically significant increase in plasma creatinine was described in one trial (Klijn et al 1989). There were no changes in glucose, sodium, or potassium levels. Premenopausal patients may experience hot flashes, and gynecomastia is reported in about half of male meningioma patients (Grunberg et al 1991); however, no patients have reported changes in sexual function or libido with mifepristone. Mild thinning of hair is rarely described.

REFERENCES

Bardon S, Vignon F, Chalbos D, et al. RU486, a progestin and glucocorticoid antagonist, inhibits the growth of breast cancer cells via the progesterone receptor. *J Clin Endocrinol Metab.* 1985;60(4):692–697.

Bardon S, Vignon F, Mountcourrier P, et al. Steroid receptor-mediated cytotoxicity of an antiestrogen and an antiprogestin in breast cancer cells. *Cancer Res.* 1987;47:1441–1448.

Baulieu EE. The steroid hormone antagonist RU486. Mechanism of the cellular level and clinical applications. *Endocrinol Metab Clin North Am.* 1991;20(4):873–891.

Baulieu EE, Segal SJ, eds. *The Antiprogestin Steroid RU486 and Human Fertility Control.* New York: Plenum Press; 1985.

Blankenstein MA, van der Meulen-Dijk C, Thijssen JHH. Effects of steroids and antisteroids on human meningioma cells in primary culture. *J Steroid Biochem.* 1989;34(1–6):419–421.

Chasserot-Golaz S, Beck G. Metabolism and antiproliferative effect of the glucocorticoid antagonist RU 38486 in cultured liver and hepatoma cells. *J Steroid Biochem.* 1986;24:423–426.

Chobert MN, Barouki R, Finidori J, et al. Antiglucocorticoid properties of RU38486 in a differentiated hepatoma cell line. *Biochem Pharmacol.* 1983;32:3481.

Contreras P, Caviedes R, Rojas A, et al. Adrenal cancer: Tumor regression with ketoconazole or mifepristone (RU 486). In vivo and in vitro evidence supporting tumoral hormone-dependency. In: *Proceedings, 69th An-*

nual *Endocrine Society Meeting, Indianapolis;* 1987: Abstract 8, p 23.

Couzinet B, Le Strat N, Uhlmann A, et al. Termination of early pregnancy by the progesterone antagonist RU 486 (mifepristone). *N Engl J Med.* 1986;**315**:1565–1570.

Evans RM. The steroid and thyroid hormone receptor family. *Science.* 1988;**240**:889.

Groyer A, Schweizer-Groyer G, Cadepond F, et al. Antiglucocorticosteroid effects suggest why steroid hormone is required for receptors to bind DNA in vivo but no in vitro. *Nature.* 1987;**328**:624.

Grunberg SM, Weiss MH, Spitz IM, et al. Treatment of unresectable meningiomas with the antiprogesterone agent mifepristone. *J Neurosurg.* 1991;**74**:861–866.

Herrmann W, Wyss R, Riondel A, et al. The effect of an antiprogesterone steroid on women: Interruption of the menstrual cycle and of early pregnancy. *CR Hebd Seances Acad Sci.* 1982;**284**:933–937.

Klijn JGM, de Jong FH, Bakker GH, et al. Antiprogestins, a new form of endocrine therapy for human breast cancer. *Cancer Res.* 1989;**49**:2851–2856.

Lamberts SWJ, Bons EG, Uitterlinden P. Studies on the glucocorticoid-receptor blocking action of RU 38486 in cultures ACTH-secreting human pituitary tumour cells and normal rat pituitary cells. *Acta Endocrinol.* 1985;**109**:64–69.

Lamberts SWJ, Tanghe HLJ, Avezaat CJJ, et al. Mifepristone (RU 486) treatment of meningiomas. *J Neurol Neurosurg Psychiatry.* 1992;**55**:486–490.

Mobbs BG, Johnson IE. Suppression of the growth of the androgen-insensitive R3327 HI rat prostatic carcinoma by combined estrogen and antiprogestin treatment. *J Steroid Biochem Mol Biol.* 1991;**39**(5A):713–722.

Nieman LK, Chrousos GP, Kelner C, et al. Successful treatment of Cushing's syndrome with the glucocorticoid antagonist RU 486. *J Clin Endocrinol Metab.* 1985;**61**:536–540.

Olson JJ, Beck DW, Schlechte J, et al. Hormonal manipulation of meningiomas in vitro. *J Neurosurg.* 1986;**65**:99–107.

Olson JJ, Beck DW, Schlechte JA, et al. Effect of the antiprogesterone RU-38486 on meningioma implanted into nude mice. *J Neurosurg.* 1987;**66**:584–587.

Palca J. Abortion-inducing drug alarms the right-to-life lobby. *Nature.* 1987;**325**:185.

Phillips CI, Gore SM, Green K, et al. Eye drops of RU 486-6, a peripheral steroid blocker, lower intraocular pressure in rabbits. *Lancet.* 1984;**I**:767–768.

Romieu G, Maudelonde T, Ulmann A, et al. The antiprogestin RU486 in advanced breast cancer: Preliminary clinical trial. *Bull Cancer.* 1987;**74**:455–461.

Schneider MR, Michna H, Nishino Y, et al. Antitumor activity and mechanism of action of different antiprogestins in experimental breast cancer models. *J Steroid Biochem Mol Biol.* 1990;**37**(6):783–787.

Mitoguazone

■ Other Names

Methylglyoxal bis(guanylhydrazone); MGBG; NSC-32946; methyl-GAG.

■ Chemistry

Structure of mitoguazone

Mitoguazone was synthesized in 1898 by Thiele and Dralle. The complete chemical name is 2,2'-(1-methyl-1,2-ethanediylidene)bis(hydrazinecarboximidamide). The compound has a molecular weight of 275 and the empiric formula $C_5H_{12}N_8 \cdot 2HCl$ and is water soluble in excess of 100 mg/mL. The compound is structurally similar to the polyamine spermidine as well as to antihelminthics such as hydroxystilbamidine.

■ Antitumor Activity

Mitoguazone is not yet approved for treatment of any malignancy; however, the agent has demonstrated antitumor activity in patients with *refractory* non-Hodgkin's lymphoma and Hodgkin's disease, head and neck cancer, endometrial cancer, leukemia (Bernard 1967, Schwarzenberg et al 1966, Shaw et al 1964), and prostate cancer (see the table on page 712). The agent also has hints of antitumor activity in a variety of other histologic types of cancer (see table on page 712). This agent should undergo further phase II testing.

Mitoguazone has been employed in a number of combination regimens. In advanced non-small cell lung cancer, a recent Southwest Oncology Group phase III trial of cisplatin and etoposide versus cisplatin, etoposide, and mitoguazone showed that there was a significantly higher response rate ($p < 0.01$) with the three-drug combination regimen (Weick et al 1991); however, toxicity was greater and patient survival was not improved. Other combination regimens used to treat patients with refractory Hodgkin's and non-Hodgkin's lymphoma have given response rates up to 84% (eg, the MIME regimen consisting of mitoguazone, ifosfamide, methotrexate, and etoposide and other combina-

SUMMARY OF PHASE II ACTIVITY OF MITOGUAZONE

Tumor Type	Number of Responses/Number Evaluable (%)	Reference
Non-Hodgkin's lymphoma	21/73 (29%)	Knight et al 1983b Warrell et al 1985
Hodgkin's disease	10/25 (40%)	Knight et al 1983b Warrell et al 1985 Hart et al 1982
Head and neck	26/166 (16%)	Luedke et al 1986 Kaplan et al 1983 Perry et al 1983 Urba et al 1990 Thonprasert et al 1984 Chapman et al 1981a Forastiere et al 1986, 1987 Mitchell et al 1981
Prostate	6/50 (12%)	Scher et al 1985 Moore et al 1987 Knight et al 1979
Esophagus	7/64 (11%)	Knight et al 1979 Falkson 1971 Ravry et al 1986 Kelsen et al 1982
Renal	10/119 (8%)	Todd et al 1980 Knight et al 1979, 1983a Hart et al 1982
Non-small cell lung	14/238 (6%)	Mitchell et al 1981 Chapman et al 1981b Christian et al 1988 Vance et al 1983 Samson et al 1982 Knight et al 1979
Small cell lung	0/22 (0%)	Scher et al 1984
Endometrial	3/21 (14%)	Slayton and Faraggi 1986
Pancreas	6/71 (8%)	Inamasu et al 1986 Ravry et al 1986 Knight et al 1979
Stomach	1/31 (3%)	Ravry et al 1986
Breast	7/96 (7%)	Knight et al 1979, 1984 Yap et al 1981
Sarcoma	0/17 (0%)	Welt et al 1982
Colon	15/193 (8%)	Myers et al 1981 Douglass et al 1988 Knight et al 1979 Hart et al 1982 Mitchell et al 1981
Bladder	3/66 (5%)	Von Hoff et al 1990 Knight et al 1979 Barrett et al 1989

tions) (Hagemeister et al 1987, Cabanillas et al 1987, Dana et al 1986, Ferme et al 1991, Warrell et al 1982, Vogel et al 1986, Dabich and Leipman 1988). Impressive response rates of up to 64% have been reported in squamous cell esophageal cancer for mitoguazone-containing combinations (Chapman et al 1987, Kelsen et al 1983, Berenzweig et al 1983, Forastiere et al 1987).

■ Mechanism of Action

Mitoguazone probably has a unique mechanism of action, namely, interference with polyamine biosynthesis. Polyamines are thought to be important in the stabilization of DNA and polyamine levels increase in rapidly dividing cells, especially in tumors. The figure below depicts polyamine biosynthesis. Mitoguazone is similar in structure to spermidine and can act as a competitive inhibitor of S-adenosylmethionine decarboxylase (SAM-DC) (Corti et al 1974, Mihich et al 1975). Overall, mitoguazone does not appear to be a cell cycle-specific agent.

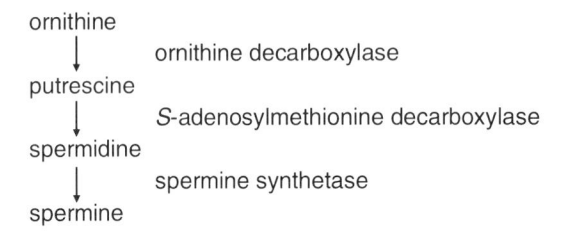

```
ornithine
   ↓      ornithine decarboxylase
putrescine
   ↓      S-adenosylmethionine decarboxylase
spermidine
   ↓      spermine synthetase
spermine
```

Biosynthesis of polyamines

As can be seen, if an inhibitor of ornithine decarboxylase such as eflornithine (α-difluoromethylornithine) were used in conjunction with mitoguazone there may be a more complete and long-lasting inhibition of polyamine biosynthesis. A number of investigators have described potentiation of the antitumor activity of mitoguazone by the ornithine decarboxylase inhibitor α-difluoromethylornithine (α-DFMO) (Warrell and Burchenal 1983, Herr et al 1984, 1986). This combination has been pursued clinically (Siimes et al 1981, Scher et al 1988, Maddox et al 1988) (see Drug Interactions).

In vitro, the antiproliferative effects of mitoguazone can be directly blocked by spermidine (Pegg 1973). The drug also inhibits mitochondria, which become swollen and vacuolized 10 to 12 hours following exposure to mitoguazone (Pleshkewych et al 1980). This effect cannot be inhibited by the addition of spermine or spermidine (Mikles-Robertson et al 1979). Some of these effects may result from an uncoupling of oxidative phosphorylation that shifts cells to anerobic glycolysis for energy product ion (Pine and DiPaolo 1966). Mitoguazone also binds weakly to DNA by ionic forces (Sartorelli et al 1965). DNA synthesis is inhibited by mitoguazone; however, this activity does not appear to contribute greatly to the drug's antitumor activity which is highly specific for actively dividing cells.

■ Availability and Storage

Mitoguazone is an investigational agent available from the National Cancer Institute. It is available in 1.0-g vials as a sterile lyophilized powder. It can be stored at room temperature. It is stable in the vials at room temperature for at least 6 years.

■ Preparation for Use, Stability, and Admixture

For intravenous or intramuscular use, each 1.0-g, 30-mL vial is reconstituted with 10 mL Sterile Water for Injection, USP, providing a solution containing 100 mg/mL. These reconstituted solutions are chemically stable for at least 20 days at room temperature (22°C). Intravenous infusion solutions are further diluted in D5W or normal saline. These admixtures are stable in polyvinyl chloride containers for at least 14 days at room temperature or under refrigeration (Kleinberg et al 1989).

■ Administration

Mitoguazone may be given as a 30-minute intravenous infusion in D5W or normal saline. The intravenous push method is not recommended because of possible orthostatic hypotension. Intravenous drug that extravasates will cause a severe local reaction with pain, inflammation, edema, and eventual tissue sloughing. Subcutaneous administration has produced severe local reactions and is therefore not recommended (Warrell and Burchenal 1983).

In general, a 30-minute infusion is preferred; however, patients with inadequate veins may receive the drug by deep intramuscular injections. Doses of 1 to 4 mg/kg have also been given by deep intramuscular injection into the outer quadrant of the buttocks (Shnider et al 1974). These patients may experience a transient, moderately severe local burning sensation spreading from the face over the entire body. Dizziness and weakness for 15 minutes after intramuscular dosing is reported along with inflammatory skin lesions with high doses of mitoguazone.

■ Special Precautions

See Drug Interactions.

■ Drug Interactions

As noted earlier, investigations (phases I, II, and III) with mitoguazone plus α-DFMO are ongoing. In those trials thrombocytopenia (possibly from the α-DFMO) has been observed (Scher et al 1985, Siimes et al 1981, Maddox et al 1988). In addition, the Investigational Drug Branch of the National Cancer Institute has recently reported two cases of fulminant hepatic necrosis with the combination of α-DFMO and mitoguazone. Investigators were informed that patients who developed the hepatic necrosis were also on the anticonvulsant carbamazepine (Tegretol®).

■ Dosage

The optimal dose and schedule for mitoguazone as an antitumor agent are not entirely certain; however, the preferred dosage schedule is 500 to 600 mg/m^2 intravenously repeated every week for 2 weeks and then every other week. The dose may be escalated by 100 mg/m^2 increments in the absence of substantial toxicity (Knight et al 1979). In leukemic patients, the most effective mitoguazone regimen involved daily doses of 126 to 150 mg/m^2 (Levin et al 1964); however, two or three divided doses per week (same cumulative total dose) were better tolerated (Boiron et al 1965).

The maximally tolerated dose for oral mitoguazone was 20 mg/kg/d for 14 days in adults and up to 50 mg/kg/d for 5 days in children (Warrell and Burchenal 1983). A deep intramuscular injection of 120 to 160 mg/m^2 twice weekly was tolerated with moderate toxicity (Warrell and Burchenal 1983).

■ Pharmacokinetics

Early pharmacokinetic studies with ^{14}C-labeled mitoguazone in humans showed that the agent had a biphasic drug elimination, with an initially rapid half-life followed by a prolonged terminal elimination phase (Oliverio et al 1963). Sixty percent of the dose was excreted intact in the urine and less than 20% in the feces over 3 weeks. Similar results were obtained by Hart et al (1980). After a rapid infusion schedule they noted a triphasic decay with a γ half-life of 100 hours. Stewart et al (1981) had similar findings. Marsh and colleagues (1981) found the urinary excretion of unchanged drug to be 10% at 10 hours and 40% after 2 weeks, noting high drug concentrations in cerebral and cerebellar gray matter. Jensen and associates (1983) observed that mitoguazone is dialyzable and recommend full doses for anephric patients who are being dialyzed. Additionally, dialysis should be considered in patients who develop toxic effects requiring rapid drug elimination. Rosenblum and colleagues (1981) have documented good penetration of mitoguazone into intracerebral tumors in humans.

■ Side Effects and Toxicity

The toxic effects of mitoguazone are dependent on both dose and schedule. Daily dosing produces severe mucositis, vasculitis, painful skin lesions, and anorexia with significant weight loss (Freireich et al 1962). Hematologic suppression is rarely dose limiting, even with daily dosing. Given as a continuous infusion for 5 days, the drug also produces severe mucositis, with pharyngitis and esophagitis. Prolonging the infusion days produced, in addition, severe diarrhea, a few hypoglycemic reactions, and worsening anemia, but not leukopenia.

Intermittent dosing regimens (weekly) produce anorexia with weight loss, muscular weakness, malaise, myalgia, nausea and vomiting (≤ 33% of patients), mild myelosuppression, and mucositis (Knight et al 1979). The myopathy can be reversed if mitoguazone is switched from a weekly to an every-other-week schedule of administration.

Vasculitis may occur with a blotchy erythematous eruption and fat necrosis. Extravasation of this drug causes pain, swelling, and eventual tissue sloughing (seen with inadvertent subcutaneous doses). Intramuscular doses have produced local burning and a transient whole-body "flushing" syndrome with some weakness and dizziness for 5 to 15 minutes after administration.

Orthostatic hypotension has been documented but only after a rapid intravenous push of the drug, not during infusions or with intramuscular dosing. Other infrequent side effects include neuropathy, ileus, and facial paresthesias. Repeated administration, particularly weekly, can result in cumulative toxicity.

Hypoglycemia has been noted in an occasional patient receiving mitoguazone. Interestingly, the hypoglycemic agent phenformin has a structure similar to that of mitoguazone. Mitoguazone has very little effect on bone marrow elements.

Special Applications

Mitoguazone has activity against Cocksackie virus and cytomegalovirus (Ferrari et al 1964, Tyms and Williamson 1982). In addition, the compound has activity against trypanosomiasis (Ulrich et al 1982).

REFERENCES

Barrett JT, Orofiamna B, Khandekar JI, Carbone PP, Comis RL, Davis TE. A Phase II study of mitoguazone and vinblastine in advanced transitional cell carcinoma of the urinary tract. *Cancer.* 1989;**64**:2445–2447.

Berenzweig M, Vogel S, Camacho F, Ruckdeschel J. Esophageal squamous cancer chemotherapy with methylglyoxal bis-guanylhydrazone (MGBG), methotrexate (M), Bleomycin (B) & diamminedichloroplatinum (D)—"MGBG–MBD." *Proc Am Soc Clin Oncol.* 1983; **2**:125.

Bernard J. Acute leukemia treatment. *Cancer Res.* 1967;**27**:2565–2569.

Boiron M, Jacquillat C, Weil M, et al. Combination of methylglyoxal bis(guanylhydrazone) [NSC-32946] and 6-mercaptopurine (NSC-755) in acute granulocytic leukemia. *Cancer Chemother Rep.* 1965;**45**:69–73.

Cabanillas F, Hagemeister FB, McLaughlin P, et al. Results of MIME salvage regimen for recurrent or refractory lymphoma. *J Clin Oncol.* 1987;**5**:407–412.

Chapman R, Fleming TR, Van Damme J, MacDonald T. Cisplatin, vinblastine, and mitoguazone in squamous cell carcinoma of the esophagus: A Southwest Oncology Group study. *Cancer Treat Rep.* 1987;**71**:1185–1187.

Chapman R, Kelsen D, Gralla R, Itri L, Wittes R, Young C. Phase II trials of methylglyoxal bis (guanylhydrazone) (MGBG) in three solid tumors. *Proc Am Assoc Cancer Res ASCO.* 1981a;**22**:526.

Chapman R, Kelsen D, Gralla R, et al. Phase II trial of methylglyoxal bis(guanylhydrazone) in non-small cell lung cancer. *Cancer Clin Trials.* 1981b;**4**:389–391.

Christian ES, Schreeder M, Salter MM, Stephens SB, Carpenter JT Jr, Wheeler RH. Phase I–II study of cisplatin, VP16, MGBG, mitomycin and vinblastine with radiation therapy for non-small cell lung cancer. *Am J Clin Oncol (CC).* 1988;**11**(4):502–505.

Corti A, Dave C, Williamson-Ashman HG, Mihich F, Schenone A. Specific inhibition of the enzymatic decarboxylation of S-adenosylmethionine by methylglyoxal bis(guanylhydrazone) and related substances. *Biochem J.* 1974;**139**:351–357.

Dabich L, Leipman MK. Cisplatin, VP-16213 and MGBG (methylglyoxal bis guanylhydrazone) combination chemotherapy in refractory lymphoma, a phase II study. *Invest New Drugs.* 1988;**6**:231–237.

Dana BW, Jones SF, Coltman CA, Stuckey WJ. Salvage treatment of unfavorable non-Hodgkin's lymphoma with cisplatin, amsacrine and mitoguazone: A Southwest Oncology Group Pilot study. *Cancer Treat Rep.* 1986;**70**:291–292.

Douglass HO, Lefkopoulou M, Davis HL, et al. ECOG phase II trial of MGBG, chlorozotocin COM multidrug therapy in advanced measurable colorectal cancer. *Am J Clin Oncol (CCT).* 1988;**11**(6):646–649.

Falkson G. Methyl-gag (NSC-32946) in the treatment of esophagus cancer. *Cancer Chemother Rep.* 1971;**55**:209–212.

Ferme C, Oberlin O, Bouabdallah K, et al. Methyl-GAG, ifosfamide, navelbine, etoposide (MINF) as salvage therapy for refractory or relapsed Hodgkin's disease. *Proc Am Soc Clin Oncol.* 1991;**10**:378.

Ferrari W, Loddo B, Gessa GL, Spanedda A, Bratzu G. In vitro antipolio activity of methylglyoxal bis-(guanylhydrazone). *Life Sci.* 1964;**3**:755–758.

Forastiere AA, Gennis M, Orringer MB, Agha FP. Cisplatin, vinblastine and mitoguazone chemotherapy for epidermal and adenocarcinoma of the esophagus. *J Clin Oncol.* 1987;**5**:1143–1149.

Forastiere AA, Natale RB, Wheeler RR. Phase II trial of methylglyoxal bis(guanylhydrazone) (MGBG) in advanced head & neck cancer. *Cancer.* 1986;**58**:2585–2588.

Forastiere AA, Perry DJ, Wolf GT, Wheeler RH, Natale RB. Cisplatin and mitoguazone: An induction regimen in advanced head and neck cancer. *Cancer.* 1988;**62**:2304–2308.

Freireich E, Frei E III, Karon M. Methylglyoxal bis(guanylhydrazone): A new agent active against acute myelocytic leukemia. *Cancer Chemother Rep.* 1962;**16**:183–186.

Hagemeister FB, Tannir N, McLaughlin P, et al. MIME chemotherapy (methyl-GAG, ifosfamide, methotrexate, etoposide) as treatment for recurrent Hodgkin's disease. *J Clin Oncol.* 1987;**5**:556–561.

Hart RD, Ohnuma T, Holland JF, Bruckner H. Methyl-GAG in patients with malignant neoplasms: A phase II evaluation. *Cancer Treat Rep.* 1982;**66**:65–71.

Hart RD, Roboz J, Wu K, Bruckner H, Ohnuma T, Holland JF. Clinical and pharmacologic studies with weekly and bi-weekly methylglyoxal bisguanylhydrazone. *Proc Am Assoc Cancer Res ASCO.* 1980;**21**:181.

Herr HW, Kleinert EL, Relya NM, Whitmore WF. Potentiation of methylglyoxal-bisguanylhydrazone by alpha-difluoromethylornithine in rat prostate cancer. *Cancer.* 1984;**53**:1294–1298.

Herr HW, Warrell RP, Buchenal JH. Phase I trial of alpha-difluoromethyl ornithine (DFMO) and methylglyoxal bis(guanylhydrazone) (MGBG) in patients with advanced prostatic cancer. *Urology.* 1986;**28**(6):508–511.

Inamasu MS, Oishi N, Chen TT, et al. Phase II study of mitoguazone in pancreatic cancer: A Southwest Oncology Group study. *Cancer Treat Rep.* 1986;**70**:531–532.

Jensen B, Williams RD, Ohnuma T, Roboz J. Dialyzability of methyl-GAG. *Cancer Treat Rep.* 1983;**67**:283–284.

Kaplan DH, Vogel SE, Amato R, Earhart R, Lerner H. Single agent chemotherapy of advanced head and neck cancer: Methylglyoxal bis-guanylhydrazone (MGBG) and N-phosponacetyl L-asparatate (PALA). *Proc Am Soc Clin Oncol.* 1983;**2**:164.

Kelsen DP, Chapman R, Bains M. Phase II study of methyl GAG in the present treatment of esophageal carcinoma. *Cancer Treat Rep.* 1982;**66**:1427–1429.

Kelsen DP, Coonley C, Bains M, Hilaris B. Cisplatin (D), vindesine (V), and methylglyoxal bis(guanylhydrazone) (M) combination chemotherapy of esophageal carcinoma. *Proc Am Soc Clin Oncol.* 1983;**2**:128.

Kleinberg ML, Oberdier J, Muller RT, et al. Stability of gallium nitrate and mitoguazone dihydrochloride in commonly used intravenous fluids. *Hosp Pharm.* 1989;**24**:929–934.

Knight WA III, Drelichman A, Fabian C, Bukowski RM. Mitoguazone in advanced renal carcinoma: A phase II trial of the Southwest Oncology Group. *Cancer Treat Rep.* 1983a;**67**:1139–1140.

Knight WA III, Fabian C, Costanzi JT, Jones SE, Coltman CA Jr. Methylglyoxal bis-guanylhydrazone (methyl GAG, MGBG) in lymphoma and Hodgkin's disease. *Invest New Drugs.* 1983b;**1**:225–237.

Knight WA III, Livingston RB, Fabian C, Costanzi J. Phase I–II trial of MGBG: A Southwest Oncology Group Pilot study. *Cancer Treat Rep.* 1979;**63**:1933–1937.

Knight WA III, O'Bryan RM, Samal B, Constanzi JJ. Methylglyoxal bis-guanylhydrazone (methyl-GAG, MGBG) in advanced breast cancer. *Invest New Drugs.* 1984;**2**:71–73.

Levin RH, Henderson E, Karon M, Freireich EJ. Treatment of acute leukemia with methylglyoxal bis(guanylhydrazone) (methyl-GAG). *Clin Pharmacol Ther.* 1964; **6**:31–42.

Levin VA, Chamberlain MC, Prados MD, et al. Phase I/II study of DFMO and MGBG for the treatment of recurrent brain tumors. *Proc Am Assoc Cancer Res.* 1987;**28**:218.

Luedke DW, Maddox W, Birch R, Velez-Garcia E, Schleuter J. Mitoguazone in advanced squamous cell carcinoma of head and neck origin: A phase II trial of the Southeastern Cancer Study Group. *Cancer Treat Rep.* 1986;**70**:529–530.

Maddox AM, Freireich EJ, Keating MJ, Maddox MK. Alterations in bone marrow and blood mononuclear cell polyamines and methylglyoxal bis(guanylhydrazone) levels: Phase I evaluation of 2-difluoromethylornithine and methylglyoxal bis(guanylhydrazone) treatment of human hematological malignancies. *Cancer Res.* 1988;**48**:1367–1373.

Marsh KC, Liesmann J, Patton TF, Fabian CJ, Sternson LA. Plasma levels and urinary excretion of methy-GAG following IV infusion in man. *Cancer Treat Rep.* 1981;**65**:253–257.

Mihich F, Simpson CL, Mulhern M. Bis(guanylhydrazones). In: Sartosell AC, Johns DG, eds. *Handbook of Experimental Pharmacology.* New York: Springer-Verlag, 1975;**37**:766–788.

Mikles-Robertson F, Feuerstein B, Dave C, Porter CW. The generality of methylglyoxal bis(guanylhydrazone)-induced mitochondrial damage and the dependence of this effect on cell proliferation. *Cancer Res.* 1979;**39**:1919–1926.

Mitchell E, Killen J, Korsmeyer S, et al. Phase II studies with methylglyoxal bis(guanylhydrazone) (methy-G). *Proc Am Assoc Cancer Res ASCO.* 1981;**22**:166.

Moore MR, Graham SD, Brich R, Irwin L. Phase II evaluation of mitoguazone in metastatic hormone-resistant prostate cancer. A Southeastern Cancer Study Group trial. *Cancer Treat Rep.* 1987;**71**:89–90.

Myers JW, Knight WA III, Livingston RB, Fabian C, Costanzi J. Phase I–II trial of methyl GAG in advanced colon cancer. *Cancer Clin Trials.* 1981;**4**:277–279.

Oliverio V, Adamson R, Henderson E, Davidson J. The distribution, excretion and metabolism of methylglyoxal bisguanylhydrazone-C^{14}. *J Pharmacol.* 1963;**141**:149–156.

Pegg AE. Inhibition of spermidine formation in rat liver and kidney by methylglyoxal bis(guanylhydrazone). *Biochem J.* 1973;**132**:537–540.

Perry DJ, Crain SM, Weltz MD, et al. Phase II trial of mitoguazone in patients with advanced squamous cell carcinoma of the head and neck. *Cancer Treat Rep.* 1983;**67**:91–92.

Pine MJ, DiPaolo J. The antimitochondrial actions of 2-chloro-4′, 4″-bis(2-imidazolin 2-yl)-terephthalanilide and methylglyoxal bis(guanylhydrazone). *Cancer Res.* 1966;**26**:18–25.

Pleshkewych A, Kramer DL, Kelly E, Porter CW. Independence of drug action on mitochondria and polyamines in L1210 leukemia cells treated with methylglyoxal-bis(guanylhydrazone). *Cancer Res.* 1980;**40**:4533–4540.

Ravry MJR, Omura GA, Hill GJ, Bartolucci AA, Velez-Garcia E. Phase II evaluation of mitoguazone in cancer of the esophagus, stomach, and pancreas: A Southeastern Cancer Study Group trial. *Cancer Treat Rep.* 1986;**70**:533–534.

Rosenblum MG, Stewart DJ, Yap BS, Leavens M, Benjamin R, Loo TL. Penetration of methylglyoxal bis(guanylhydrazone) into intracerebral tumors in humans. *Cancer Res.* 1981;**41**:459–462.

Samson MK, Baker LH, Cummings G, Talley RW. Phase II trial of methyl-GAG (NSC-32946) in squamous cell and adenocarcinoma of the lung. *Am J Clin Oncol (CCT).* 1982;**5**:631–633.

Sartorelli AC, Ianotti AT, Booth BA, et al. Complex formation with DNA and inhibition of nucleic acid synthesis by methylglyoxal-bis(guanylhydrazone). *Biochim Biophys Acta.* 1965;**103**:173–176.

Scher H, Chapman R, Kelsen D, Gralla R, Wittes R. Phase II trial of mitoguazone in patients with relapsed small cell carcinoma of the lung. *Cancer Treat Rep.* 1984;**68**:561–562.

Scher H, Smart-Curley T, Heston WDW, et al. Phase I–II trial of alpha-difluoromethylornithine (DFMO) (MDL 71,782) and mitoguazone (MGBG) in hormone refractory prostate cancer. *Proc Am Assoc Cancer Res.* 1988;**29**:204.

Scher HI, Yagoda A, Ahmed T, Watson RC. Methylglyoxal-bis(guanylhydrazone) in hormone-resistant adenocarcinoma of the prostate. *J Clin Oncol.* 1985;**3**:224–228.

Schwarzenberg L, Schneider M, Cattan A, Amiel JL, Schlumberger JR, Mathe G. Le traitement des leucemies aigues par la methyl-glyoxol bis-(guanylhydrazone) et son association avec la 2-hydroxysuibamidine. *Semin Hop Paris.* 1966;**42**:2955–2957.

Shaw RK, Creger WP. Methylglyoxal bis(guanylhydrazone), NSC-32946, in the treatment of acute myeloblastic and monoblastic leukemia in adults. *Cancer Chemother Rep.* 1964;**36**:63–71.

Shnider B, Colsky J, Jones R, Carbone P. Effectiveness of methyl-GAG administered intramuscularly. *Cancer Chemother Rep.* 1974;**58**:689.

Siimes M, Seppanen P, Alhonen-Hongisto L, Janne J. Synergistic action of two polyamine antimetabolites leads to a rapid therapeutic response in childhood leukemia. *Int J Cancer.* 1981;**28**:567–570.

Slayton R, Faraggi D. A phase II clinical trial of methylglyoxal bis-guanylhydrazone (MGBG) in advanced endometrial cancer. *Proc Am Soc Clin Oncol.* 1986;**5**:119.

Stewart DJ, Rosenblum MG, Luna M, Loo TL. Disposition of methylglyoxal bis(guanylhydrazone) (MGBG, NSC-32946) in man. *Cancer Chemother Pharm.* 1981;**7**:31–35.

Thiele J, Dralle F. Zur Kenntnis des amino gunidins. I. Condensations-produkte de amidoguanidins mit aldehyden and ketonen der fettreihe. *Ann Chem.* 1898;**302**:275–299.

Thonprasert S, Bosl GJ, Geller NL, Wittes, RF. Phase II trial of mitoguazone in patients with advanced head and neck cancer. *Cancer Treat Rep.* 1984;**68**:1301–1302.

Todd RF, Garnick HD, Canellos GP. Chemotherapy of advanced renal adenocarcinoma with methyl-GAG. *Proc Am Assoc Cancer Res.* 1980;**21**:340.

Tyms AS, Williamson JD. Inhibitors of polyamine biosynthesis block human cytomegalovirus replication. *Nature.* 1982;**297**:690–691.

Ulrich PL, Grady RW, Cerami A. Trypanocidal activity of aromatic bis-guanylhydrazones. *Drug Dev Res.* 1982;**2**:219–228.

Urba S, Forastiere AA, Wolf GT, Sullivan M, Thornton A, Husted S. Induction chemotherapy (CT) with intensive continuous infusion high dose cisplatin (CDDP), 5-fluorouracil (5-FU) and mitoguazone (MGBG) for advanced head and neck cancer (H&N CA). *Proc Am Soc Clin Oncol.* 1990;**9**:171.

Vance RB, Knight WA III, Chen TT, Costanzi JJ, LoBuglio AF. Phase II evaluation of MGBG in non-small cell carcinoma of the lung. *Invest New Drugs.* 1983;**1**:89–93.

Vogel SE, Chang A, Oken M, Glick J, Knospe W. Methylglyoxal bis-guanylhydrazone (MGBG) in combination with cyclophosphamide (C), vincristine (V), prednisone (P), and Adriamycin (A) for poor prognosis non-Hodgkin's lymphoma—"MEGA–COPA." An Eastern Cooperative Oncology Group (ECOG) pilot trial. *Proc Am Assoc Cancer Res.* 1986;**27**:199.

Von Hoff DD, Blumenstein BA, Pollock TW, et al. Methylglyoxal bis-guanylhydrazone in advanced bladder cancer. *Eur J Cancer.* 1990;**26**:848–849.

Warrell RP, Burchenal JH. Methylglyoxal-bis(guanylhydrazone) (methyl GAG): Current studies and future prospects. *J Clin Oncol.* 1983;**1**:52–65.

Warrell RP, Lee BJ, Kempin ST, Lacher MJ, Straus DJ, Young CW. Effectiveness of methyl-GAG (methylglyoxal-bis[guanylhydrazone]) in patients with advanced malignant lymphoma. *Blood.* 1985;**57**:1011–1014.

Warrell RP, Straus DJ, Young CW. Combination chemotherapy for patients with relapsed malignant lymphoma using methyl GAG and teniposide (VM-26). *Cancer Treat Rep.* 1982;**66**:1121–1125.

Weick JK, Crowley J, Natale RB, et al. A randomized trial of five cisplatinum-containing treatments in patients with metastatic non-small cell lung cancer: A Southwest Oncology Group Study. *J Clin Oncol.* 1991;**9**:1157–1162.

Welt S, Magill GB, Sordillo PP, Brenner J. Phase II studies of methyl-GAG (methylglyoxal-bis[guanylhydrazone]) in patients with advanced sarcoma. *Proc Am Soc Clin Oncol.* 1982;**1**:146.

Yap, HY, Blumenschein GR, Schell FC, Bodey CP. Phase II evaluation of methyl-GAG in patients with refractory metastatic breast cancer. *Cancer Treat Rep.* 1981;**65**:465–467.

Mitomycin-C

■ Other Names

Mutamycin® (Bristol-Myers Oncology Division); mitomycin; NSC-26980.

■ Chemistry

Structure of mitomycin-C

Mitomycin-C is a purple-colored antibiotic (molecular weight 334) isolated from *Streptomyces caespitosus*. The complete chemical name is [1aR]-6-amino-8-[[(aminocarbonyl)oxy]methyl]-1,1a,2,8,8a,8b-hexahydro-8a-methoxy-5-methylazirino[2′,3′:3,4]-pyrrolo[1,2-a]indole-4,7-dione. It is heat stable, soluble in water and other organic solvents, and has a unique absorption peak at 365 nm (Crooke and Bradner 1976). Once in solution it is slowly inactivated by visible but not ultraviolet light. It is very unstable at acidic and highly basic pH. Mitosene breakdown products from mitomycin-C have an ultraviolet absorption peak at approximately 313 nm. The aziridine and carbamate groups on mitomycin-C are known to be necessary for alkylating activity but not for antibacterial activity. The compound can be activated by reduction of the quinone moiety, which releases a methanol residue from the molecule. This allows the aziridine ring to open, exposing an elecrophilic carbon at C_1 (alkylating site). The second (crosslinking) site for alkylation is exposed at C_{10} following an enzymatic or chemically mediated loss of the carbamate side chain.

■ Antitumor Activity

Mitomycin has activity in adenocarcinoma of the stomach, pancreas, colon (Whittington and Close 1970), and breast (Wise et al 1976). Using a regimen of 0.15 mg/kg/d × 5, Moertel et al (1968) produced an objective response rate of about 18% in 45 patients with different gastrointestinal adenocarcinomas. The mean remission duration was slightly over 3 months, and responses were noted in patients with tumors of the colon (11%), pancreas (25%), stomach (43%), and gallbladder (60%). One of three hepatoma patients also responded (Moertel et al 1968). One of the most common mitomycin-C combinations is the FAM regimen (mitomycin with 5-fluorouracil and doxorubicin) for treating gastric cancer (MacDonald et al 1976) and pancreatic carcinoma. This regimen is associated with a 42% partial response rate in gastric cancer, although long-term survival is usually not significantly enhanced. As a continuous intravenous infusion for 7 days, mitomycin-C was relatively inactive (9% response rate) in patients with colorectal carcinoma refractory to 5-fluorouracil (Anderson et al 1992).

Mitomycin-C response rates average 25% in advanced breast cancer and the compound is occasionally useful in second- or third-line regimens for refractory breast cancer (Lenaz 1985, Buzdard et al 1978b).

In non-small cell lung cancer, mitomycin-C produces single-agent response rates of 25% in adenocarcinoma and 13% in large cell carcinoma (Doll et al 1985). Mitomycin-C combination regimens such as FOMI (5-fluorouracil, vincristine, and mitomycin) have produced higher response rates of up to 42% in non-small cell lung cancer (Miller et al 1980). The drug has also been used effectively in some head and neck cancers and in chronic myelogenous leukemia (Crooke and Bradner 1976). Recent studies from Yale University show that mitomycin-C can be used safely as an adjunct to radiation therapy and head and neck cancer (Weissberg et al 1989).

Mitomycin-C has activity in superficial bladder tumors when administered topically (Mishina et al 1975, Early et al 1973). It has systemic activity in advanced biliary, ovarian, and cervical squamous cell carcinoma (Baker et al 1976). The combination of mitomycin-C and bleomycin is particularly active in uterine cervix cancer, producing response rates of up to 80% (Doll et al 1985). Mitomycin-C has been used as an adjuvant following Wertheim's hysterectomy for stage IB cervical cancer (Sivanesaratnam and Jayalakshmi 1989). It is also active in the MOB combination with vincristine and bleomycin.

Besides having antitumor activity, the compound is bactericidal against a variety of gram-positive and gram-negative bacteria (including *Bacillus subtilis* and *Escherichia coli*) as well as rickettsias and some viruses (Crooke and Bradner 1976); however, the drug's marked hematologic toxicity precludes therapeutic use as an antibiotic.

■ Mechanism of Action

Mitomycin-C is activated in vivo to an alkylating agent which crosslinks complementary DNA strands, thereby halting DNA synthesis. DNA is the major site of mitomycin-C activity, although at extremely high concentrations, RNA synthesis may also be affected. The active metabolites of mitomycin-C result from reduction of the quinone moiety to yield an opened aziridine ring and an alkylating site at C_1. A second alkylating site at C_{10} is exposed with the enzymatic loss of the carbamate side chain (Lown and Weir 1978). The molecular site of DNA binding has recently been identified at the N_2 and O_6 positions of adjacent guanines in the minor groove of DNA (Tomasz et al 1986).

Activation of the drug can be mediated by chemical reducing agents, by microsomal enzymes, or even by brief exposure to an acidic pH. The extent of DNA binding appears to relate to the guanine and cytosine content of the particular DNA. The compound does not inhibit DNA polymerase activity and does not alter nucleotide pools as would an antimetabolite. Thus, cytotoxicity probably results directly from DNA synthesis inhibition secondary to alkylation.

In addition to alkylation, several authors have suggested that oxygen free radicals may contribute to cytotoxicity from mitomycin-C by producing DNA strand breaks (Dusre et al 1989, Lown, 1978). These effects are postulated to involve oxygen free radicals produced by cyclic redox reactions of the quinone moiety. This could explain the production of hydrogen peroxide from DNA-bound mitomycin-C (Tomasz 1976). In most systems, however, DNA crosslinking, which is slowly repaired, appears to constitute the predominant cytotoxic lesion (Dorr et al 1985). In addition, the reduction potential of the compound (–0.45 V) is outside the metabolic capability of most mammalian reductases (Powis 1989).

Mitomycin-C's cytotoxic action is not cell cycle phase specific but cytotoxic effects are maximized if cells are treated in late G_1 and early S phase. In addition to the direct cytotoxic effects of the drug, mitomycin-C also causes chromosomal aberrations (mutagenic activity), and in experimental systems it is a potent carcinogen and teratogen.

Kennedy et al (1979) have described selective activation of mitomycin-C by hypoxic cells, suggesting perhaps some drug selectivity for hypoxic tumors. Resistance to mitomycin-C has been noted to involve an increase in specific cytosolic proteins (possibly a glutathione transferase) (Taylor et al 1985) as well as collateral resistance with anthracyclines (Matsumoto et al 1987) and actinomycin D (Biedler and Riehm 1970). The latter type of mitomycin C-induced "multidrug resistance" phenotype may be mediated by P-glycoprotein expression with resultant enhanced drug efflux as noted in mitomycin-C-resistant L-1210 cells (Dorr et al 1987).

■ Availability and Storage

Mitomycin-C (Mutamycin®, Bristol-Myers Oncology Division, Princeton, New Jersey) is available as a purplish to gray, flocculent lyophilized powder in 5- and 20-mg vials. The vials may be stored at room temperature. The 5-mg vial contains 10 mg of mannitol and the 20-mg vial contains 40 mg of mannitol.

■ Preparation for Use, Stability, and Admixture

To each 5-mg vial, 10 mL of Sterile Water for Injection, USP, should be added. If after gentle shaking undissolved drug remains, the vial should be allowed to stand at room temperature until complete dissolution is achieved. The resultant solution usually appears purple and contains 500 µg of mitomycin-C and 1 mg of mannitol per milliliter. The reconstituted solution requires protection from light if not used within 24 hours. It is stable for 14 days when refrigerated and at least 7 days at room temperature. Solutions diluted into 5% Dextrose for Injection, USP, have short stability (2.6 hours) because of the low pH of autoclaved dextrose solutions. When diluted into normal saline mitomycin-C is stable for at least 1 day. In lactated Ringer's injection mitomycin-C is stable for up to 43 hours (Beijnen et al 1985). Concentrated mitomycin-C solutions may be frozen in plastic minibags for at least 4 weeks for rethawing by microwave (Stolk et al 1986). Freezing at –30°C or lower is recommended to prevent crystallization of mitomycin-C from solutions frozen at –20°C or less (Stolk et al 1986).

Mitomycin-C (0.5 mg/mL) is physically compatible with ondansetron (1 mg/mL) for at least 4 hours (Trissel et al 1990). It is also comparable with heparin.

■ Administration

Mitomycin-C is intended for intravenous or intravesical administration. Severe local tissue necrosis occurs on extravasation of the drug (Argenta and Manders 1983). The drug is usually given by a slow intravenous push with continuous patient monitoring to lessen the chance of causing extravasation. Short infusions in 100 to 150 mL of D5W or normal saline have also been used. Vein patency should be checked before the administration of any dose using 5 to 10 mL of fluid (not containing drug solution). The same procedure should follow the dose. This will act to flush any remaining drug from the tubing and the venipuncture site.

Continuous Infusion. Mitomycin-C has been administered as a continuous intravenous infusion for 30 days or longer (Lokich et al 1982), 7 days (Anderson et al 1992), or 5 days (Lokich et al 1982, Miller et al 1962, Yap et al 1983). The drug has also been infused by a regional intraarterial infusion (Tseng et al 1984) and as a peritoneal perfusion (Koga et al 1988) (see Special Applications).

■ Dosage

The recommended dose of mitomycin-C when used as a single agent is 20 mg/m^2 given intravenously every 6 to 8 weeks. In combination with other myelosuppressive drugs, mitomycin-C doses are typically limited to 10 mg/m^2 every 6 to 8 weeks. Bolus doses greater than 20 mg/m² produce severe toxicity without greatly enhanced efficacy. Occasionally, larger doses have been given. These are initiated as a one-time dose which is reduced thereafter to 10 to 20 mg/m².

Early schedules used mitomycin-C at 0.05 mg/kg/d IV × 6 days, then alternating days until a total of 50 mg had been given. Another regimen involved a 5-day course of 0.15 mg/kg repeated at 8- to 12-week intervals. Both of these schedules produce severe bone marrow toxicity and are not generally recommended.

Repeat dosing of mitomycin-C should be based on adequate marrow recovery including leukocytes, platelets, and red blood cells. Mitomycin-C doses are usually not administered more frequently than every 6 to 8 weeks to allow for marrow recovery.

Continuous infusions have been used at 0.75 mg/m²/d for 50 consecutive days and at 3 mg/m²/d × 5 days every 4 to 6 weeks (Lokich et al 1982). These regimens are believed to deliver greater dose intensity by reducing myelosuppressive toxicity (Miller et al 1962). Intraarterial perfusion doses of 20 mg/m² have been given every 6 to 8 weeks (Tseng et al 1984).

Very high doses of mitomycin-C have also been administered by hepatic artery infusions followed by autologous bone marrow transplantation (Corringham et al 1984). Doses in these settings have ranged from 40 to 50 mg/m² given once (Corringham et al 1984) or from 20 to 40 mg/m²/d × 3 (Distefano et al 1980).

■ Special Precautions

Myelosuppression may be cumulative with successive mitomycin-C doses. Serious local ulceration may occur if the drug is delivered outside the vein. Extravasation of mitomycin-C must be avoided.

■ Drug Interactions

The cytotoxic effects of mitomycin-C are experimentally enhanced in preclinical models by combination therapy with dextran sulfate or urokinase (Niitani et al 1974). In animal models, mitomycin-C pharmacokinetics did not change with the coadministration of other anticancer agents including 5-fluorouracil and doxorubicin or with microsomal enzyme-modifying agents such as phenobarbital and 3-methylcholanthrene (Kerpel-Fronius et al 1988). An inhibitor of quinone reductase, dicoumarol, has been shown to sensitize hypoxic tumor cells to mitomycin-C (Rockwell et al 1988). Fumaric acid is also reported to block some toxic effects of mitomycin-C in vivo by an unknown mechanism (Kuroda and Akao 1980); however, fumaric acid was ineffective as a local extravasation antidote (Dorr et al 1986). Finally, depletion of glutathione by the experimental buthionine sulfoximine or by diethylmaleate does not appear to significantly alter mitomycin-C DNA crosslinking and cellular cytotoxicity in vitro (McGurl and Kennedy 1989). This indirectly suggests that glutathione is not of major importance in mediating mitomycin-C's activity.

In experimental animal tumors, mitomycin-C has shown antitumor synergy with vincristine or thioguanine (in L-1210 leukemia) and with dactinomycin (in spontaneous mammary tumors) (Crooke and Bradner 1976). Clinically significant antitumor drug synergy in humans has not been demonstrated for mitomycin-C.

■ Pharmacokinetics

Mitomycin-C is cleared from the vascular compartment rapidly (see table below). Peak concentrations of about 1 µg/mL are typically achieved following intravenous bolus doses of 10 mg/m² (van Hazel et al 1983). Less than 10% of a dose is excreted into the urine and this is complete within a few hours of administration. Mitomycin-C has been detected in the bile and feces, although animal studies demonstrate that the highest drug levels occur in the kidneys. Detectable levels were found in muscle, lung, intestine, stomach, and eye but not in the brain, spleen, or liver (Crooke and Bradner 1976).

The primary means of mitomycin-C elimination is by liver metabolism but the specific enzymes responsible are unknown; however, the enzymes re-

MITOMYCIN-C PHARMACOKINETICS

Parameter	Mean Value
Peak level*	1–1.5 µg/mL
Plasma Half-life	
α	8.0 min
β	48 min
Volume of distribution	41 L/m²
Clearance	400 mL/min/m²
Excretion	
Urinary	11%
Hepatic	23%

*Based on an intravenous bolus dose of 10 to 15 mg/m2 (van Hazel et al 1983).

sponsible for metabolism do not appear to involve P450 mixed function oxidases. In vitro studies show drug inactivation on contact with tissue preparations from the spleen, liver, kidney, brain, and heart. Such inactivation is further augmented by anaerobic conditions (Crooke and Bradner 1976).

There is no detectable change in mitomycin-C pharmacokinetics in patients with altered hepatic function (van Hazel et al 1983), nor when other drugs including furosemide are given concurrently (Verweij et al 1987). Schilcher et al (1984) have shown that the pharmacokinetics of mitomycin-C does not change following the administration of high doses. This clearly discounts the early descriptions of dose-dependent pharmacokinetics of mitomycin-C (Fujita 1971).

Mitomycin-C distribution into bile and ascites fluids has been quantitated in patients receiving standard intravenous doses. The maximum biliary levels of 0.5 µg/mL were achieved after 2 hours and were five- to eightfold higher than simultaneous plasma levels during the elimination phase (den Hartigh et al 1983). Mitomycin-C rapidly penetrated into ascites and reached maximal concentrations of 0.05 µg/mL 1 hour after administration. This distribution represented about 40% of the total plasma exposure. The drug also appears to slightly concentrate in cervical tissues following intravenous administration (Malviya et al 1986).

With intraarterial administration, the hepatic extraction of mitomycin-C averages only 23% (Hu and Howell 1983). Thus, the calculated relative advantage for hepatic arterial infusions is only 2.5 to 3.6-fold. This discounts a significant improvement in mitomycin-C delivery to tumors for this regional method of drug administration.

■ Side Effects and Toxicity

Bone marrow suppression involving platelets, leukocytes, and red blood cells is the most serious toxic effect and can continue for long periods after drug administration (up to 3–8 weeks) (Crooke and Bradner 1976). Myelosuppression, particularly anemia, can be cumulative. This has reportedly been minimized by keeping total lifetime doses under 50 to 60 mg/m^2.

Gastrointestinal disturbances in the form of nausea, vomiting, and anorexia occasionally develop. These reactions are usually not severe and have an onset within 1 to 2 hours of administration. They may persist for several hours. Stomatitis may also occur, but is generally not severe.

Renal toxicity noted by increasing serum blood urea nitrogen and creatinine levels along with glomerular dysfunction is occasionally seen (Early et al 1973). This does not appear to be dose or treatment duration related, and is usually not severe (Liu et al 1971); however, mitomycin-C can also induce a microangiopathic hemolytic anemia (MAHA) with progressive renal failure and cardiopulmonary decompensation (Liu et al 1971). This disease is ultimately fatal within 3 to 4 weeks of diagnosis, although the onset is typically delayed for months following mitomycin-C (Hanna et al 1981). The incidence of this toxic effect may approach 10% in patients given large cumulative doses (Hanna et al 1981). In one series, renal complications from mitomycin-C developed in 1.6% of 63 patients receiving a total dose of 50 mg/m^2 or greater, in 10.8% of 37 patients receiving 50 to 69 mg/m^2, and in 27.8% of 18 patients receiving total doses above 70 mg/m^2 (Valavaara and Nordman 1985). This suggests that a threshold for mitomycin-C-induced MAHA may be a cumulative dose of about 50 mg/m^2. Signs of MAHA include thrombocytopenia, circulating schistocytes, and acute renal failure. Histopathologic examination of the kidneys reveals fibrin thrombi in arterioles, tubular atrophy, and widespread glomerular necrosis. Importantly, there are now several cases of successful treatment of mitomycin-C-induced MAHA with serial blood perfusions over protein A columns (Korec et al 1987).

Veno-occlusive disease of the liver has been reported after high-dose mitomycin-C therapy and autologous bone marrow transplantation (Lazarus et al 1982). Signs include progressive hepatic dysfunction, abdominal pain, and ascites.

Alopecia may occur following mitomycin-C but it is usually not severe. Rarely, purple-colored bands in the nail beds can appear that correspond to sequential doses of the drug. Lethargy or weakness may occur and can last for several days up to as long as 3 weeks. Fatigue and some drowsiness or confusion have also been observed (Baker et al 1976). Dose-related skin reactions and fever with drug administration are occasionally seen.

Severe soft tissue ulcers may also be expected if the drug escapes the vein during administration (Moertel et al 1968). Mitomycin-C extravasation injuries can result in chronic ulcers which can expand over months (Argenta and Manders 1983). Particularly distressing aspects of some mitomycin-C extravasations include occasional delayed (3–4 months) and sometimes distal occurrence of a soft tissue ulceration following uneventful injections in a peripheral vein (Wood and Ellerhorst-Ryan 1984, Johnston-Early et al 1981). In an animal model, the only effective antidote to mitomycin-C skin toxicity was topical dimethylsulfoxide (99% v/v DMSO) (Dorr et al 1986). Thus, mitomycin-C extravasations may be empirically treated using the same regimen described for the anthracyclines (Olver et al 1989). This involves the topical application of 1.5 mL of DMSO every 6 hours for 14 days (Olver et al 1988). Ludwig et al (1987) have treated one patient with 90% DMSO/10% α-tocopherol and no ulceration occurred following the extravasation of 0.32 mg of drug into forearm tissues.

Interstitial pneumonia thought to be secondary to mitomycin-C has been reported in a small number of patients (Orwoll et al 1978). These patients present with dyspnea, cough, and occasionally with fever. Chest x-rays showed reticular infiltrates. These patients showed rapid improvement when treated with corticosteroids (Chang et al 1986).

Possible cardiotoxicity has also been suggested for mitomycin-C in humans and experimental animals (Ravry 1979); however, there is no conclusive evidence of mitomycin-C cardiotoxicity in humans. In most reports there is possible cardiotoxic synergism with anthracyclines (Buzdar et al 1978a). Importantly, no studies report cardiotoxicity in patients receiving only mitomycin-C. There is one report of possible mitomycin-C-induced neurotoxicity in a patient also receiving 5-fluorouracil (Nichols et al 1976).

■ Special Applications

Topical Bladder Instillation. Mitomycin-C has been successfully used for the local treatment of small bladder papillomas (transitional cell carcinoma of the bladder). Topical instillations of 20 mg/20 mL mitomycin-C in distilled water are typically used. The solution is retained as long as possible, usually 3 hours. The procedure can be performed three times weekly, for up to 20 procedures per course.

Mitomycin-C is poorly absorbed by bladder tissues and this is a decided advantage over other intravesical cytotoxic agents such as thiotepa. Myelosuppression has not been noted in mitomycin-C topical bladder trials; however, 3 of 20 (6%) patients in one series developed frequent painful urination following intravesical mitomycin-C. This necessitated a 1-week interruption of therapy in one patient. Of interest, normal bladder tissues appear to be resistant to the effects of mitomycin-C according to these authors (Mishina et al 1975).

Other effective topical bladder regimens involve a single instillation of 40 mg of mitomycin-C in 40 mL of water (Tolley et al 1988). This regimen appears to be particularly effective in patients with noninvasive bladder cancer who have failed thiotepa (Issell et al 1984). Overall response rates range from 50 to 70% and often include complete remission rates of up to 45% (DeFuria et al 1980).

Intraarterial Administration. Hepatic artery infusions of mitomycin-C in colon cancer (1 mg/kg divided into 15-mg doses over 2–3 days) are reported to be less effective than intraarterial 5-fluorouracil infusions (Fortuny et al 1975). In addition, there may be a significant risk of arterial thrombosis with mitomycin-C. In primary and metastatic liver cancer, however, regional hepatic intraarterial mitomycin-C and 5-fluorouracil have demonstrated substantial antitumor effects in some studies (Donegan 1985). Doses in these trials range from 4 to 10 mg of mitomycin-C as a bolus to 10 to 15 mg/m^2 as a 48-hour continuous arterial infusion every 8 weeks (Donegan 1985). The drug has also been given by bronchial artery infusions as an adjuvant procedure before surgery although complications are significant (Neyazaki and Suzuki 1971). In locally advanced breast cancer, intermittent mitomycin-C (with continuous 5-fluorouracil) has produced minor responses when given intraarterially via subclavian or internal mammary veins before mastectomy (Koyama et al 1975).

Arterial mitomycin-C (20 mg/m^2 in 100 mL D5W) every 4 to 8 weeks was effective at palliating pelvic pain in patients with recurrent or metastatic colorectal cancer (Tseng and Park 1985). Therapy was delivered via the regional hypogastric or gluteal artery. The major side effect was necrotizing cellulitis in the buttock. Myelosuppression was also common. In this trial 14 of 26 evaluable patients had stabilization of disease with good pain relief following intraarterial therapy (Tseng and Park 1985).

More recent preliminary reports continue to suggest that intraarterial regimens containing mitomycin-C are active. Campos et al (1979) successfully used intraarterial vincristine, 5-fluorouracil, and mitomycin-C (10 mg/m^2) plus oral lomustine to reduce early hepatic recurrences from Duke's C colon cancer. Patt et al (1979) were also able to demonstrate a high response rate in colon cancer metastatic to the liver with an intraarterial regimen of mitomycin-C (15 mg/m^2) on day 1 and floxuridine (1 g/m^2) by continuous infusion for 5 days. Ten of 22 patients (45%) achieved a partial response and median survival increased from 6 to 14 months in the responders (Patt et al 1979). Hepatic arterial occlusion occurred in equal numbers of responders and nonresponders.

In a variety of metastatic liver cancers, Zatzkin et al (1979) used intraarterial infusions of 5-fluorouracil (15–20 mg/kg/24 h, days 1–3) followed by a 24-hour arterial infusion of mitomycin-C, 0.15 mg/kg (best tolerated dose), on day 4; however, with higher doses of intraarterial mitomycin-C (up to 0.3 mg/kg/24 h), severe myelosuppression and stomatitis were produced.

Intraperitoneal Administration. Mitomycin-C has been administered intraperitoneally to patients with peritoneal carcinomatosis from colon cancer (three patients) and gastric cancer (one patient) (Adams et al 1984). Mitomycin-C (7 mg/m^2) was administered in 1000 mL of 1.5% dialysate solution with a dwell time of 24 hours. This achieved a high intraperitoneal:plasma drug level ratio of 71:1 with intraperitoneal levels in the range of 3.1 µg/mL. Intraperitoneal mitomycin-C was cleared with a half-life of 2.3 hours. This therapy was well tolerated with minimal pain and myelosuppression. Ascites was reduced in all patients.

In another series, mitomycin-C and intraperitoneal hyperthermia were combined to prophylactically treat patients with gastric cancer (Koga et al 1988) or advanced ovarian cancer (Harari et al 1989). In gastric cancer patients mitomycin-C (8–10 mg) was administered continuously in bags containing 2000 mL of heated saline solution (40–45°C). The total perfusion was 8 to 12 L over 50 to 60 minutes, constituting a mitomycin-C dose of 64 to 100 mg. Low peak plasma levels (only 0.1 µg/mL) were produced and approximately 39% of the administered dose was retained intraperitoneally. The half-lives of mitomycin-C in the perfusate are 10 to 17 minutes (α) and 70 to 120 minutes (β) (Fujimoto et al 1989). Serum protein levels decrease significantly during and following the procedure. This indicates that serum protein reaccumulates in the peritoneal space as a result of this procedure.

Mitomycin-C (5–10 mg) has been given every 28 days combined with cisplatin (100 mg/m^2) using the intraperitoneal route. Mitomycin-C was always given 1 week after cisplatin and the dose was diluted in 2 L of normal saline. In 11 patients with malignant peritoneal mesothelioma 5 of 8 previously untreated patients had reduced fluid reaccumulation lasting from 2 to 32 months (median five months) (Markman and Kelsen 1989). The major toxic effects were pain and catheter failure related to the intraperitoneal mitomycin-C.

Intrapleural Administration. Mitomycin-C has been combined with cisplatin for intrapleural therapy of malignant mesothelioma. Sequential 15-minute infusions of cisplatin (100 mg/m^2) and mitomycin-C (8 mg/m^2) were instilled via a chest tube placed immediately after surgical pleurectomy/decortication (Rusch et al 1992). The tubes were not drained for 4 hours and the patient's position was changed every 30 minutes. The mean AUC for mitomycin-C in the pleural fluid was 128,995 µg/mL/h compared with 659 µg/mL/h in the plasma; mean half-lives were 2.3 and 5.5 hours in the pleural space and plasma, respectively. This represents a fivefold advantage (log scale) favoring greater local mitomycin-C exposure with intrapleural therapy.

REFERENCES

Adams SC, Patt YZ, Rosenblum MG. Pharmacokinetics of mitomycin C (MMC) following intraperitoneal (I.P.) administration of MMC and floxuridine (FUDR) for peritoneal carcinomatosis (PC) (abstract #1432). *Preclin Pharmacol Exp Ther*. 1984;**25**:361.

Anderson N, Lokich J, Moore C, et al. Infusional mitomycin-C (MMC) for treatment of measurable colorectal carcinoma (CRC) resistant to 5-fluorouracil (FU). *Proc Am Soc Clin Oncol*. 1992;**11**:191.

Argenta LC, Manders EK. Mitomycin C extravasation injuries. *Cancer*. 1983;**51**:1080–1082.

Baker LH, Opipari MI, Izbicki RM. Phase II study of mitomycin C, vincristine, and bleomycin in advanced squamous cell carcinoma of the uterine cervix. *Cancer*. 1976;**38**:2222–2224.

Biedler JL, Riehm H. Cellular resistance to actinomycin D in Chinese hamster ovary cells in vitro: Cross resistance, radioautographic and cytogenetic studies. *Cancer Res*. 1970;**30**:1174–1184.

Beijnen JH, Rosing H, Underberg WJM. Stability of mitomycins in infusion fluids. *Arch Pharm Chem Sci Ed*. 1985;**13**:58–66.

Buzdar AU, Legha SS, Tashima CK, et al. Adriamycin and mitomycin C: Possible synergistic cardiotoxicity. *Cancer Treat Rep*. 1978a;**62**:1005–1008.

Buzdar AU, Tashima KT, Blumenschein GR, et al. Mitomycin-C and megestrol acetate in treatment of breast cancer refractory to hormonal and combination chemotherapy. *Cancer.* 1978b;**41**:392–395.

Campos LT, Frantz VP, Dossey JE, Khera HC, Boulefindis D, Arkus RL. Adjuvant therapy by intra-arterial infusion and BCG for adenocarcinoma of the colon, stage Duke's C (abstract #C-247). *Proc Am Assoc Cancer Res ASCO.* 1979;**20**:351.

Carter SK. Mitomycin-C (NSC-26980) clinical brochure. *Cancer Chemother Rep.* 1968;**1**(1):99.

Chang AY-C, Kuebler JP, Pandya KJ, Israel RH, Marshall BC, Tormey DC. Pulmonary toxicity induced by mitomycin C is highly responsive to glucocorticoids. *Cancer.* 1986;**57**:2285–2290.

Corringham RET, Dick R, Gilmore MJML, Prentice HG, Boesen EM. Intravenous and hepatic arterial infusion of high dose mitomycin C with autologous bone marrow transplantation in patients with tumour metastatic to the liver. *Br J Cancer.* 1984;**50**:841–842.

Crooke ST, Bradner WT. Mitomycin C: A review. *Cancer Treat Rev.* 1976;**3**:121–139.

DeFuria MD, Bracken RB, Johnson DE, et al. Phase I–II study of mitomycin C topical therapy for low-grade, low-stage transitional cell carcinoma of the bladder: An interim report. *Cancer Treat Rep.* 1980;**64**:225–230.

Den Hartigh J, McVie JG, van Oort WJ, Pinedo HM. Pharmacokinetics of mitomycin C in humans. *Cancer Res.* 1983;**43**:5017–5021.

Distefano A, Spitzer G, Schell F. Phase I study of high dose mitomycin C (MM) with autologous bone marrow transfusion (ABMT) in resistant breast adenocarcinoma. *Proc Am Assoc Cancer Res ASCO.* 1980;**21**:408.

Doll DC, Weiss RB, Issell BF. Mitomycin: Ten years after approval for marketing. *J Clin Oncol.* 1985;**3**(2):276–286.

Donegan W. Hepatic artery infusion chemotherapy for colorectal metastases: A personal experience. *J Surg Oncol.* 1985;**30**:177–183.

Dorr RT. New findings in the pharmacokinetic, metabolic, and drug-resistance aspects of mitomycin C. *Semin Oncol.* 1988;**15**(3, suppl 4):32–41.

Dorr RT, Bowden GT, Alberts DS, et al. Interactions of mitomycin C with mammalian DNA detected by alkaline elution. *Cancer Res.* 1985;**45**:3510–3516.

Dorr RT, Liddil JD, Trent JM, Dalton WS. Mitomycin C resistant L1210 leukemia cells: Association with pleiotropic drug resistance. *Biochem Pharmacol.* 1987;**36**:3115–3120.

Dorr RT, Soble MJ, Liddil JD, et al. Mitomycin C skin toxicity studies in mice: Reduced ulceration and altered pharmacokinetics with topical dimethyl sulfoxide. *J Clin Oncol.* 1986;**4**(9):1399–1404.

Dusre L, Covey JM, Collins C, Sinha BK. DNA damage, cytotoxicity and free radical formation by mitomycin C in human cells. *Chem–Biol Interact.* 1989;**71**:63–78.

Early K, Elias EG, Mittelman A, et al. Mitomycin C in the treatment of metastatic transitional cell carcinoma of urinary bladder. *Cancer.* 1973;**31**:1150–1153.

Falkson G, Schulz EJ. Changes in hair pigmentation associated with cancer chemotherapy. *Cancer Treat Rep.* 1981;**65**(5/6):529.

Fortuny IE, Theologides A, Kennedy BJ. Hepatic arterial infusion for liver metastases from colon cancer: Comparison of mitomycin C (NSC-26980) and 4-fluorouracil (NSC-19893). *Cancer Chemother Rep.* 1975;**59**(2):401–404.

Fujimoto S, Shrestha RD, Kokubun M, et al. Pharmacokinetic analysis of mitomycin C for intraperitoneal hyperthermic perfusion in patients with far-advanced or recurrent gastric cancer. *Reg Cancer Treat.* 1989;**2**:198–202.

Fujita H. Comparative studies on the blood level, tissue distribution, excretion and inactivation of anticancer drugs. *Jpn J Clin Oncol.* 1971;**12**:151–162.

Godfrey TE, Wilbur DW. Clinical experience with mitomycin-C in large infrequent doses. *Cancer.* 1972;**29**:1647.

Hanna WT, Krauss S, Regester RF, Murphy WM. Renal disease after mitomycin C therapy. *Cancer.* 1981;**48**:2583–2588.

Harari PM, Shimm DS, Gerner EW, et al. Intraperitoneal chemotherapy plus regional/systemic hyperthermia in the treatment of advanced ovarian cancer. *Reg Cancer Treat.* 1989;**2**:54–58.

Hu E, Howell SB. Pharmacokinetics of intraarterial mitomycin C in humans. *Cancer Res.* 1983;**43**:4474–4477.

Issell BF, Prout GR Jr, Soloway MS, et al. Mitomycin C intravesical therapy in noninvasive bladder cancer after failure on thiotepa. *Cancer.* 1984;**53**:1025–1028.

Iyer V, Szybalski N. Mitomycin and porfiromycin: Chemical mechanism of activation and cross-linking of DNA. *Science.* 1964;**145**:55–58.

Johnston-Early A, Cohen MH. Mitomycin C-induced skin ulceration remote from infusion site. *Cancer Treat Rep.* 1981;**65**(5/6):529.

Kennedy KA, Rockwell S, Sartorelli AC. Selective metabolic activation of mitomycin C by hypoxic tumor cells in vitro (abstract #1129). *Proc Am Assoc Cancer Res.* 1979;**20**:278.

Kerpel-Fronius S, Verwey J, Stuurman M, Kanyar B, Lelieveld P, Pinedo HM. Pharmacokinetics and toxicity of mitomycin C in rodents, given alone, in combination, or after induction of microsomal drug metabolism. *Cancer Chemother Pharmacol.* 1988;**22**:104–108.

Koga S, Hamazoe R, Maeta M, Shimizu N, Murakami A, Wakatsuki T. Prophylactic therapy for peritoneal recurrence of gastric cancer by continuous hyperthermic peritoneal perfusion with mitomycin C. *Cancer.* 1988;**61**:232–237.

Korec S, Lesesne B, Fuertes B, et al. Treatment of C-HUS with plasma perfusion over staph A filters (abstract #941). *Proc Am Soc Clin Oncol.* 1987;**6**:239.

Koyama H, Wada T, Takahaski Y, Iwanga T, Aoki Y, Wada A. Intra-arterial infusion chemotherapy as a preoperative treatment of locally advanced breast cancer. *Cancer.* 1975;**36**(5):1603–1612.

Kuroda K, Akao M. Reduction by fumaric acid of side effects of mitomycin C. *Biochem Pharmacol.* 1980;**29**:2839–2844.

Lazarus HM, Gottfried MR, Herzig RH, et al. Veno-occlusive disease of the liver after high-dose mitomycin C therapy and autologous bone marrow transplantation. *Cancer.* 1982;**49**:1789–1795.

Lenaz L. Mitomycin C in advanced breast cancer. *Cancer Treat Rev.* 1985;**23**:235–249.

Liu K, Mittelman A, Sproul EE, Elias EG. Renal toxicity in man treated with mitomycin C. *Cancer.* 1971;**28**(5):1314–1320.

Lokich J, Perri J, Fine N, et al. Mitomycin C: Phase I study of a constant infusion ambulatory treatment schedule. *Cancer Clin Trials.* 1982;**5**:443–447.

Lown JW, Sim S-K, Chen H-H. Hydroxyl radical production by free and DNA-bound aminoquinone antibiotics and its role in DNA degradation. Electron spin resonance detection of hydroxyl radicals by spin trapping. *Cancer J Biochem.* 1978;**56**:1042–1047.

Lown JW, Weir G. Studies related to antitumor antibiotics. Part XIV. Reactions of mitomycin B with DNA. *Cancer J Biochem.* 1978;**56**:296–304.

Ludwig CU, Stoll H-R, Obrist R, et al. Prevention of cytotoxic drug induced skin ulcers with dimethyl sulfoxide (DMSO) and α-tocopherol. *Eur J Cancer Clin Oncol.* 1987;**23**(3):327–329.

MacDonald J, Schein P, Nemo W, Wooky P. 5-Fluorouracil (5-FU), mitomycin-C (MMC) and Adriamycin (ADR)—FAM: A new combination chemotherapy program for advanced gastric carcinoma (abstract C-11). *Proc Am Soc Clin Oncol.* 1976;**17**:244.

Malviya VK, Young JD, Boike G, Gove N, Deppe G. Pharmacokinetics of mitomycin-C in plasma and tumor tissue on cervical cancer patients and in selected tissues of female rats. *Gynecol Oncol.* 1986;**25**:160–170.

Markman M, Kelsen D. Intraperitoneal cisplatin and mitomycin as treatment for malignant peritoneal mesothelioma. *Reg Cancer Treat.* 1989;**2**:49–53.

Matsumoto S, Shigeoka T, Takakura Y, Hashida M, Sezaki H. Cellular interaction and in vitro antitumor effect of various mitomycin C prodrugs in mitomycin C-resistant L1210 leukemia cell lines. *Chem Pharm Bull.* 1987;**35**(9):3792–3799.

McGurl J, Kennedy KA. Effect of glutathione (GSH) depletion by diethyl maleate (DEM) or buthionine S, R-sulfoximine (BSO) on mitomycin C (MC) toxicity towards EMT6 mouse mammary tumor cells (abstract 2160). *Proc Am Assoc Cancer Res.* 1989;**30**:543.

Miller E, Sullivan RD, Chryssochoos T. The clinical effects of mitomycin C by continuous intravenous administration. *Cancer Chemother Rep.* 1962;**21**:129–135.

Miller TP, McMahon LJ, Livingston RB. Extensive adenocarcinoma and large cell undifferentiated carcinoma of the lung treated with 5-FU, vincristine, and mitomycin C (FOMI). *Cancer Treat Rep.* 1980;**64**:1241–1245.

Mishina T, Oda K, Muratha S, Ooe H, Muri Y, Takahashi T. Mitomycin C bladder instillation therapy for bladder tumor. *J Urol.* 1975;**114**:217–219.

Miura T, Ishida M. 5-Fluorouracil–mitomycin combination cancer chemotherapy by regional intra-arterial or intra-aortic infusion with or without radiation. In: *Proceedings of the 10th International Cancer Congress, Houston, Texas;* 1970:828.

Moertel CG, Reitemier RJ, Hahn RG. Mitomycin C therapy in advanced gastrointestinal cancer. *JAMA.* 1968;**204**:1045–1048.

Neyazaki T, Suzuki C. Bronchial artery infusion therapy for lung cancer in man. *Panminerva Med.* 1971;**13**:305–307.

Nichols M, Bergevin P, Vyas AC, et al. Neurotoxicity from fluorouracil (NSC-19893) administration reproduced by mitomycin-C (NSC-26980). *Cancer Treat Rep.* 1976;**60**:293–294.

Niitani H, Suzuki A, Taniguchi T, Saijo N, Kawase I, Kimura K. Effect of combination treatment with mitomycin C and lysosome labilizers on nodular pulmonary metastases. *Gann.* 1974;**65**:403–409.

Ogata J, Migita N, Nakamura T. Treatment of carcinoma of the bladder by infusion of the anticancer agent (mitomycin C) via the internal iliac artery. *J Urol.* 1973;**110**:667–670.

Olver IN, Aisner J, Hament A, Buchanan L, Bishop JF, Kaplan RS. A prospective study of topical dimethyl sulfoxide for treating anthracycline extravasation. *J Clin Oncol.* 1988;**6**(11):1732–1735.

Orwoll ES, Kiessling PJ, Patterson JR. Interstitial pneumonia from mitomycin. *Ann Intern Med.* 1978;**89**:352–355.

Patt YZ, Chuang V, Johnson PS, et al. Hepatic arterial infusion (HAT) of mitomycin C (MTC) and floxuridine (FUDRO)—An effective treatment for metastatic colorectal carcinoma to the liver (abstract #C-104). *Proc Am Assoc Cancer Res ASCO.* 1979;**20**:316.

Patton AJ, Knight EW, Tennant JD. Mitomycin C administered by a high dose induction regimen in the treatment of cancer (abstract #C-397). *Proc Am Assoc Cancer Res ASCO.* 1979;**20**:387.

Powis GA. Free radical formation by antitumor quinones. *Free Radicals Biol Med.* 1989;**6**:63–101.

Ravry MJR. Cardiotoxicity of mitomycin C in man and animals (letter). *Cancer Treat Rep.* 1979;**63**(4).

Rockwell S, Keyes SR, Sartorelli AC. Modulation of the cytotoxicity of mitomycin C to EMT6 mouse mammary tumor cells by dicoumarol in vitro. *Cancer Res.* 1988;**48**:5471–5474.

Rusch VW, Niedzwiecki D, Tao Y, et al. Intrapleural cisplatin and mitomycin for malignant mesothelioma following pleurectomy: Pharmacokinetic studies. *J Clin Oncol.* 1992;**10**(6):1001–1006.

Schilcher RB, Young JD, Ratanatharathorn V, Karanes C, Baker LH. Clinical pharmacokinetics of high-dose mitomycin C. *Cancer Chemother Pharmacol.* 1984;**13**:186–190.

Sivanesaratnam V, Jayalakshmi P. Mitomycin C adjuvant chemotherapy after Wertheim's hysterectomy for stage 1B cervical cancer. *Cancer.* 1989;**64**:798–800.

Stolk LML, Fruitier A, Umans R. Stability after freezing and thawing of solutions of mitomycin C in plastic minibags for intravesical use. *Pharm Weekblad Sci Ed.* 1986;**8**:286–288.

Taylor CW, Brattain MG, Yeoman LC. Occurrence of cytosolic protein and phosphoprotein changes in human colon tumor cells with the development of resistance to mitomycin C. *Cancer Res.* 1985;**45**:4422–4427.

Tolley DA, Hargreave TB, Smith PH, et al. Effect of intravesical mitomycin C on recurrence of newly diagnosed superficial bladder cancer: Interim report from the Medical Research Council Subgroup on Superficial Bladder Cancer (Urological Cancer Working Party). *Br Med J.* 1988;**296**:1759–1761.

Tomasz M. H_2O_2 generation during the redox cycle of mitomycin C and DNA-bound mitomycin C. *Chem–Biol Interact.* 1976;**13**:89–97.

Tomasz M, Chowdary D, Lipman R, et al. Reaction of DNA with chemically or enzymatically activated mitomycin C: Isolation and structure of the major covalent adduct. *Proc Natl Acad Sci USA.* **83**:6702–6706.

Trissel LA, Fulton B, Tramonte SM. Visual compatibility of odansetron with chemotherapeutic agents, antibiotics, and other selected drugs during simulated Y-site injection (abstract #P-468R). In: *25th Annual ASHP Midyear Clinical Meetings and Exhibit, Las Vegas, Nevada;* 1990.

Tseng MH, Luch J, Mittelman A. Regional intra-arterial mitomycin C infusion in previously treated patients with metastatic colorectal cancer and concomitant measurement of serum drug level. *Cancer Treat Rep.* 1984;**68**:1319–1324.

Tseng MH, Park HC. Pelvic intra-arterial mitomycin C infusion in previously treated patients with metastatic, unresectable, pelvic colorectal cancer and angiographic determination of tumor vascularity. *J Clin Oncol.* 1985;**3**(8):1093–1100.

Valavaara R, Nordman E. Renal complications of mitomycin C therapy with special reference to the total dose. *Cancer.* 1985;**55**:47–50.

Van Hazel GA, Scott M, Rubin J, et al. Pharmacokinetics of mitomycin C in patients receiving the drug alone or in combination. *Cancer Treat Rep.* 1983;**67**(9):805–810.

Verweij J, den Hartigh J, Stuurman M, de Vries J, Pinedo HM. Relationship between clinical parameters and pharmacokinetics of mitomycin C. *J Cancer Res Clin Oncol.* 1987;**113**:91–94.

Weissberg JB, Son YH, Papac RJ, et al. Randomized clinical trial of mitomycin C as an adjunct to radiotherapy in head and neck cancer. *Int J Radiat Oncol Biol Phys.* 1989;**17**:3–9.

Whittington RM, Close HP. Clinical experience with mitomycin-C (NSC-26980). *Cancer Chemother Rep.* 1970;**54**(3): 195.

Wise GR, Kuhn IN, Godfrey TE. Mitomycin C in large infrequent dosages in breast cancer. *Med Pediatr Oncol.* 1976;**2**:55–60.

Wood HA, Ellerhorst-Ryan JM. Delayed adverse skin reaction associated with mitomycin-C administration. *Oncol Nurs Forum.* 1984;**11**(4):14–18.

Yap H-Y, Valdivieso M, Blumenschein G. A phase I–II study of continuous 5-day infusion mitomycin-C. *Am J Clin Oncol.* 1983;**6**:109–112.

Zatzkin J, Wheeler R, Ensminger W, Bull FE. Phase I study of hepatic artery infusion with 5-FU and mitomycin-C (MITO) (abstract C-323). *Proc Am Assoc Cancer Res ASCO.* 1979;**20**:369.

Mitotane

■ Other Names

o,p'-DDD; NSC-38721; Lysodren® (Bristol-Myers Oncology Division).

■ Chemistry

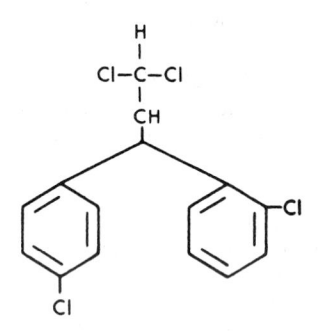

Structure of mitotane

Mitotane is an isomer of the insecticide DDD, a close chemical relative of DDT. Chemically, it is 1,1-dichloro-2-(o-chlorophenyl)-2-(p-chlorophenyl)-ethane. The compound exists as a white solid condensed from clear colorless crystals. It is tasteless but has a slight aromatic odor. The drug is insoluble in water. Gutierrez and Crooke (1980) published a review article on mitotane.

■ Antitumor Activity

The primary clinical indication for mitotane is the palliative treatment of inoperable adrenal cortical carcinoma. Historically, Bergenstal et al (1960) were the first to describe the antitumor action of the compound. More recently reported response rates after 2 months of therapy range from 35 to 60%, with a mean survival of 10.3 months versus 2.4 months in nonresponders (Harrison and Mahoney 1973, Lubitz et al 1973). There are additionally four case reports describing mitotane use which resulted in cure of metastatic disease (Becker and Schumacher 1975, Helson et al 1971, Ostumi and Roginsky 1975). Recently, mitotane has been combined with streptozocin to treat adrenocortical cancer (Eriksson et al 1987).

Southern et al (1961) were the first to report efficacy for the drug in Cushing's disease. Luton et al (1979), Kuhn et al (1989), and Schteingart (1989) confirmed this activity, achieving moderate symptomatic disease control in about 63% of patients. Azer and Braunstein (1981) and Knyrim et al (1981) described the treatment of Leydig cell carcinomas of the testicle with mitotane. The drug has not shown activity against renal and prostate cancer (Hogan et al 1981).

■ Mechanism of Action

Nelson and Woodard (1949) first noted severe adrenal cortex atrophy when DDD was fed to dogs. The cytotoxic effect appears to be specifically directed to the mitochrondria of adrenocortical cells, producing focal lesions in both the fascicular and reticular zones. The onset of cell changes may be noted by 12 hours after administration; with chronic administration, dog lesions are complete in 12 days (Kaminsky et al 1962). Additionally, steroid secretions are markedly reduced by the drug. The exact mechanism for this effect is not known; however, several have been suggested in the literature. These include glucose-6-phosphate dehydrogenase inhibition (Cazorla and Moncloa, 1962) and reduced triphosphopyridine synthesis or incorporation in adrenal cell metabolism (Hart 1970).

In human studies, large daily doses (0.5–3.0 g/d) are required to produce similar changes including blockage of 11β-hydroxylation and alterations in zona fasciculata mitochondrial morphology (Brown et al 1973). Above a 3.0-g daily dose adrenal atrophy results, reducing both glucocorticoid and mineralocorticoid production (Bergenstal et al 1960, Helson et al 1971, Lubitz et al 1973).

Bradlow et al (1973), Hellman et al (1973), and Schein (1972) have additionally documented altered peripheral cortisol and androgen metabolism following mitotane administration. Thus, mitone causes increased excretion of unconjugated 6β-hydroxy derivatives; consequently, urinary 17-hydroxycorticosteroid excretion can initially fall even as plasma cortisol and the cortisol secretory rate remain constant (Bledsoe et al 1964).

■ Availability and Storage

Mitotane is commercially available from Bristol-Myers Oncology Division, Evansville, Indiana, as 500-mg scored tablets (Lysodren®). These may be stored at room temperature.

■ Preparation for Use, Stability, and Admixture

The commercially available material needs no additional preparation.

■ Administration

Mitotane is administered orally. As blood levels do not appear to correlate with therapeutic and/or toxic effects, the patient should not be required to be in a fasting state to maximize absorption. As the drug tends to concentrate in fat, it should not be taken with a "fatty" meal. In a detailed study, Moolenaar and colleagues (1981) noted that the best way to give the drug was as granules in milk; however, the granules are not commercially available.

■ Special Precautions

Mitotane can cause complete adrenal suppression. The drug may need to be discontinued in cases of sepsis, shock, or severe trauma. In addition, supplemental corticosteroids and mineral corticosteroids may be required. Leiba et al (1989) noted that mitotane was toxic to the fetus of a patient receiving the agent.

■ Drug Interactions

Kupfer and Peets (1966) and Street (1969) observed that mitotane consistently stimulates hepatic microsomal oxidases and could thus potentially alter the metabolism of a number of other drugs, including cortisol, barbiturates, phenytoin, warfarin (greater hypoprothrombinemic effect [Cuddy and Loftus 1986]), and perhaps cyclophosphamide as well as others. The microsomal enzyme induction can also lead to adrenal crisis because of the alteration of metabolism of exogenous steroid. This leads to a requirement for increased exogenous steroid supplementation to avoid an adrenal crisis (Hague et al 1989, Robinson et al 1987).

■ Dosage

Initial daily oral doses from 8 to 10 g are commonly given as three to four divided doses per day. The maximum tolerated dose range may vary from 2 to 16 g/d. Treatment is often continued for long periods. Usually, 3 months of treatment constitutes an adequate trial, although 10% of patients show a response only after 3 months or more of continuous therapy. Maximum daily doses of 18 to 19 g have been reported. With beneficial results and a lack of severe toxicity, therapy may be continued indefinitely. Doses are adjusted on the basis of degree of acceptable toxicity and clinical status.

Hogan et al (1978) have recommended limiting daily doses to 5 to 6 g/d because the drug steadily accumulates and responses are noted at this level.

They recommend initiating therapy at 2 g/d PO concurrent with full glucocorticoid replacement and, with daily doses greater than 3.0 g, adding mineralocorticoid replacement.

Because this drug can cause complete adrenal suppression, dosage reduction or discontinuance is necessary in the face of severe trauma, shock, or infection, and supplemental corticosteroids and mineralocorticoids may be required. Doses should also be reduced in the presence of depressed renal and, especially, hepatic function. Liver function should be monitored while the patient is on mitotane therapy.

■ Pharmacokinetics

Approximately 40% of single oral doses are absorbed. Only 10 to 25% appears to be excreted in the urine as an unidentified water-soluble metabolite and up to 60% is excreted unchanged in the stool (Hogan et al 1978). A small fraction of a dose is excreted in the bile, whereas the large remaining fraction is stored primarily in fatty tissues throughout the body (Moy 1961).

Pharmacokinetic studies in humans have not shown either a dose–response or a dose–toxicity relationship (Leiba et al 1989). After administering doses of 5 to 15 g/d, peak blood levels varied from 7 to 90 µg/mL for unchanged drug and from 29 to 54 µg/mL for metabolites. The primary metabolites are oxidation products: the ethene derivative o,p'-DDE and the acetate o,p'-DDA. Several polar metabolites are also produced and can be detected in the urine for up to 1 month after stopping therapy.

With a newly available gas chromatography/mass spectroscopy technique o,p'-DDA has been found to be present in plasma at a concentration 10 times higher than that of o,p'-DDD or o,p'-DDE (Inouye et al 1987). A rapid micromethod employing gas chromatography with electron-capture detection also has been used (Bennecke et al 1987).

The drug can be found in all body tissues but primarily in the fat (Leiba et al 1989, von Slooten et al 1982). Blood levels are detectable for up to 10 weeks after therapy discontinuation. Mitotane can be detected in adipose tissue 20 months after discontinuing the agent (Leiba et al 1989). This is probably related to slow, persistent release of drug from lipid storage sites.

Hogan et al (1978) have followed plasma levels of o,p'-DDD in several patients, noting that measurable drug levels remain for up to 8 months after stopping therapy. Urinary metabolites are still detectable 18 months after discontinuing the drug. With typical daily dosing, plasma levels steadily increase with median levels around 10 µg/mL and metabolite levels 10 times this amount.

The bile appears to clear only the metabolite but is a significant organ of drug elimination. A small portion of metabolite has been noted in cerebrospinal fluid samples. Both the kidney and the liver appear to metabolize relatively small portions of the drug.

■ Side Effects and Toxicity

Eighty percent of patients experience gastrointestinal disturbances such as anorexia, nausea, vomiting, and occasional diarrhea. Forty percent of patients exhibit central nervous system toxic effects of lethargy, sedation, vertigo, and dizziness. Long-term use may cause brain dysfunction, and repeated neurologic and behavioral assessments are recommended when treatment is prolonged.

Acute adrenal insufficiency can be precipitated by stress such as shock, trauma, or infection. Because increased steroid metabolism is affected by mitotane, doses larger than a replacement dose of exogenous steroids are required in therapy.

Allergic rashes are infrequent. Visual disturbances (blurring, double vision, opacification of the lens, toxic retinopathy), genitourinary toxicity (hemorrhagic cystitis, albuminuria, hematuria), and cardiovascular toxicity (hypertension, orthostatic hypotension) have been observed. Minor aches and fever may also be related to drug administration.

In a man receiving mitotane, Sparagana (1987) has described impotence secondary to the cytotoxicity of the agent in the testes.

■ Special Applications

See discussion of treatment of Cushing's disease under Antitumor Activity.

REFERENCES

Azer PC, Braunstein GD. Malignant Leydig cell tumor: Objective tumor response to o,p'-DDD. *Cancer*. 1981;**15:** 47(6):1251–1255.

Becker D, Schumacher OP. o,p' DDD therapy in invasive adrenocortical carcinoma. *Ann Intern Med*. 1975;**82:**677–679.

Bennecke R, Vetter B, De Zeeuw RA. Rapid micromethod for the analysis of mitotane and its metabolite in plasma by gas chromatography with electron-capture detection. *J Chromatogr*. 1987;**417:**287–294.

Bergenstal DM, Hertz R, Lipsett MB, Moy RH. Chemotherapy of adrenocortical cancer with o,p'-DDD. Ann Intern Med. 1960;53:672–679.

Bledsoe TD, Island DP, Ney RL, Liddle GW. An effect of o,p'-DDD on the extraadrenal metabolism of cortisol in man. J Clin Endocrinol Metab. 1964;24:1303.

Bradlow HL, Zumoff B, Fukushima DK, Hellman L. Drug induces alterations of steroid hormone metabolism in man. Ann NY Acad Sci. 1973;212:148.

Brown RD, Nicholson WE, Chick WT, Stott CA. Effect of o,p'-DDD on human adrenal steroid 11-β-hydroxylation activity. J Clin Endocrinol Metab. 1973;36:730.

Carzola A, Moncloa F. Action of 1,1,dichloro-2-p-chlorophenyl-2-o-chlorophenylethane on dog adrenal cortex. Science. 1962;136:47.

Cuddy PG, Loftus LS. Influence of mitotane on the hypoprothrombinemic effect of warfarin. South Med J. 1986;79(3):387–388.

Eriksson B, Oberg K, Curstedt T, et al. Treatment of hormone producing adrenocortical cancer with o,p'-DDD and streptozocin. Cancer. 1987;59(8):1398–1403.

Gutierrez ML, Crooke ST. Mitotane (o,p'-DDD). Cancer Treat Rev. 1980;7(1):49–55.

Hague RV, May W, Cullen DR. Hepatic microsomal enzyme induction and adrenal crisis due to o,p'-DDD therapy for metastatic adrenocortical carcinoma. Clin Endocrinol. 1989;31(1):51–57.

Harrison JH, Mahoney EM. Adrenal cortex and medulla. In: Holland JF, Frie E, eds. Cancer Medicine. Philadelphia: Lea and Febiger; 1973:1646.

Hart M. Effects on steroid synthesis. In: Brader LE, Carter SK, eds. Proceedings of the Chemotherapy Conference on o,p'-DDD. Bethesda, MD: Cancer Therapy Evaluation Branch, National Cancer Institute; 1970.

Hellman L, Bradlou HL, Zumoff B. Decreased conversion of androgens to normal 17-keto steroid metabolites as a result of treatment with o,p'-DDD. J Clin Endocrinol Metab. 1973;36:801.

Helson L, Wollner N, Murphy ML, Schwartz MK. Metastatic adrenal cortical carcinoma: Biochemical changes accompanying clinical regression during therapy with o,p'-DDD. Clin Chem. 1971;17:1191.

Hogan TF, Citrin DL, Freeberg BL. A preliminary report of mitotane therapy of advanced renal and prostate cancer (letter). Cancer Treat Rep. 1981;65(5/6):539–540.

Hogan TF, Citrin DL, Johnson BM, Nakamura S, Danis TE, Borden EC. o,p'-DDD (mitotane) therapy of adrenal cortical carcinoma. Cancer. 1978;42:2177–2181.

Inouye M, Mio T, Sumino K. Use of GC/MS/SIM for rapid determination of plasma levels of o,p'-DDD, o,p'-DDE and o,p'-DDA. Clin Chim Acta. 1987;170(2/3):305–314.

Kaminsky N, Luse S, Hartroft P. Ultrastructure of adrenal cortex of the dog during treatment with DDD. J Natl Cancer Inst. 1962;29:127–159.

Knyrim K, Higi M, Hossfeld DK, Seeber S, Schmidt CG. Autonomous cortisol secretion by a metastatic Leydig cell carcinoma associated with Klinefelter's syndrome. J Cancer Res Clin Oncol. 1981;100(1):85–93.

Kuhn JM, Proeschel MF, Seurin DJ, Bertangna XY, Luton JP, Girard FL. Comparative assessment of ACTH and lipotropin plasma levels in the diagnosis and follow-up of patients with Cushing's syndrome: A study of 210 cases. Am J Med. 1989;86:678–684.

Kupfer D, Peets L. The effect of o,p'-DDD on cortisol and hexobarbital metabolism. Biochem Pharmacol. 1966;15:573.

Leiba S, Weinstein R, Shindel B, et al. The protracted effect of o,p'-DDD in Cushing's disease and its impact on adrenal morphogenesis of young human embryo. Ann Endocrinol. 1989;50(1):49–53.

Lubitz JA, Freeman L, Okun R. Mitotane use in inoperable adrenal cortical carcinoma. JAMA. 1973;223:1109.

Luton JP, Mahoudeau JA, Bouchard PH, et al. Treatment of Cushing's disease by o,p'-DDD. N Engl J Med. 1979;300(9):459–464.

Moolenaar AJ, van Slooten H, van Seters AP, et al. Blood levels of o,p'-DDD following administration in various vehicles after a single dose and during long-term treatment. Cancer Chemother Pharmacol. 1981;7:51–54.

Moy RH. Studies of the pharmacology of o,p'-DDD in man. J Lab Clin Med. 1961;58:296.

Nelson AA, Woodard G. Severe adrenal cortical atrophy (cytotoxic) and hepatic damage produced in dogs by feeding 2,2-bis(para-chlorophenyl)-1,1-dichloroethane (DDD or TDE). Arch Pathol. 1949;48:387–394.

Ostumi JA, Roginsky MS. Metastatic adrenal cortical carcinoma—Documented cure with combined chemotherapy. Arch Intern Med. 1975;135:1257.

Robinson BG, Hales IB, Henniker AJ, et al. The effect of o,p'-DDD on adrenal steroid replacement therapy requirements. Clin Endocrinol. 1987;27(4):437–444.

Schein PS. Chemotherapeutic management of the hormone-secreting endocrine malignancies. Cancer. 1972;30:1616–1626.

Schteingart DE. Cushing's syndrome. Endocrinol Metab Clin North Am. 1989;18(2):311–338.

Southern AL, Weisenfeld S, Laufer A, et al. Effect of o,p'-DDD in a patient with Cushing's syndrome. J Clin Endocrinol Metab. 1961;21:201–208.

Sparagana M. Primary hypogonadism associated with o,p'-DDD (mitotane) therapy. J Toxicol Clin Toxicol. 1987;25(6):463–472.

Street JC. Organochlorine insecticides and the stimulation of liver microsomal enzymes. Ann NY Acad Sci. 1969;160:274.

Von Slooten H, van Seters AP, Smeenk D, Moolenaar AJ. o,p'-DDD (mitotane) levels in plasma and tissues during chemotherapy and at autopsy. Cancer Chemother Phamacol. 1982;9(2):85–88.

Mitoxantrone Hydrochloride

■ Other Names

Novantrone™ (Lederle Laboratories); dihydroxyanthracenedione dihydrochloride; DHAD; NSC-301379; CL-232315; free base compound, DHAQ.

■ Chemistry

Structure of mitoxantrone hydrochloride

Mitoxantrone's chemical name is 1,4-dihydroxy-5,-8-bis[(2-[(2-hydroxyethyl)amino]ethyl)amino]-9,10-anthracenedione dihydrochloride. Its molecular weight is 517.4 and its molecular formula $C_{22}H_{28}N_4O_6 \cdot 2HCl$. The blue powder is hygroscopic and soluble in water and ethanol (Murdock et al 1979).

■ Antitumor Activity

Mitoxantrone is approved for remission-induction therapy in acute nonlymphocytic leukemia (ANLL) (Arlin et al 1985, Paciucci et al 1983). It is typically used in combination with pyrimidine antimetabolites such as cytarabine (Dutcher et al 1985). Response rates of 50 to 70% are common in patients initially treated with such regimens. Mitoxantrone is also active in acute lymphoblastic leukemia, in chronic myelogenous leukemia (Arlin et al 1985), and in pediatric leukemias (Vietti et al 1983).

Mitoxantrone has activity in solid tumors including advanced or recurrent breast cancer (Landys et al 1985, Allegra et al 1985, Yap et al 1981, Cowan et al 1985). As a single agent, mitoxantrone has an overall response rate of up to 22% in metastatic breast cancer and the drug is also active in combination with alkylating agents such as cyclophosphamide (Ehninger et al 1984) or antimetabolites such as 5-fluorouracil (Yap et al 1983). Mitoxantrone has been shown to be active in advanced breast cancer patients treated in combination with mitomycin-C, vincristine, or vinblastine and prednisone. The drug has shown significant antitumor activity in ovarian cancer, although it has limited antitumor activity in hepatocellular cancer, prostate cancer, head and neck cancer, small cell lung cancer, pancreatic adenocarcinoma, colon cancer, renal cell cancer, cervical carcinoma, endometrial carcinoma, various sarcomas, melanoma, pediatric solid tumors, and finally multiple myeloma (Shenkenberg and Von Hoff 1986). There is no evidence of activity in non-small cell lung cancer, malignant mesothelioma, gastric cancer, advanced bladder cancer, germ cell tumors, and Kaposi's sarcoma (Shenkenberg and Von Hoff 1986).

■ Mechanism of Action

Mitoxantrone is believed to produce antitumor activity by interacting with DNA. Several types of interactions have been postulated. First, the drug is known to intercalate into DNA in a process similar to that of anthracyclines such as doxorubicin. Positively charged nitrogens on the two alkyl side chains of mitoxantrone also interact electrostatically with negatively charged ribose phosphates on DNA to stabilize the intercalation process (Durr 1984). This effect may also explain the lacelike linking of chromatin observed in vitro (Lown et al 1983). In addition, mitoxantrone has been shown to inhibit the activity of the enzyme DNA topoisomerase II (Crespi et al 1986). This leads to protein associated double-strand breaks (Bowden et al 1985), which are most prominent in the premitotic G_2 phase of cell division (Traganos et al 1980). The drug has shown specific binding to the intracellular cytoskeletal protein cytokeratin 8. This may also help to impair cell division (Cress et al 1988).

Importantly, mitoxantrone is not a substrate for reductases and does not undergo redox cycling to form oxygen free radicals. It may actually inhibit microsomal oxidative-reductive drug metabolism (Kharasch and Novak 1982). The molecule is very difficult to reduce, with a reduction potential of −0.79 V, a value outside the metabolic capability of mammalian reductases. Mitoxantrone is decidedly different from intercalating agents such as doxorubicin that can undergo redox cycling to produce oxygen free radicals; however, the production of a cationic (electrophilic) free radical metabolite capable of covalent binding has also been observed when mitoxantrone is incubated with horseradish peroxidase in vitro (Kolodziejczyk et al 1988). An air-stable free radical can also be formed in the presence of horseradish peroxidase and hydrogen peroxide (Fisher and Patterson 1991). This product was shown to form extensive crosslinks with plasmid DNA in vitro and may contribute to the cytotoxic activity of the compound.

Overall, mitoxantrone is cytotoxic against both proliferating and nonproliferating cells (Traganos et al 1980); however, rapidly proliferating tissues are more sensitive. Although it is not generally thought to be a cell cycle phase-specific agent, mitoxantrone does induce cell cycle arrest in G_2 phase (Traganos et al 1980).

■ Availability and Storage

Mitoxantrone is supplied as a sterile solution in vials containing 10, 12.5, or 15 mL of a 2mg/mL solution (20, 25, and 30 mg, respectively). Although the solution does not contain preservatives, it is chemically stable for years at room temperature, under refrigeration, or on freezing. Commercial mitoxantrone solutions also contain sodium chloride, sodium acetate, and acetic acid as inactive ingredients. The solution has a pH of approximately 3.7 and contains 0.14 mEq of sodium per milliliter.

■ Preparation for Use, Stability, and Admixture

Mitoxantrone solutions are compatible with 5% dextrose, 0.9% sodium chloride, lactated Ringer's injection, and various combinations of these physiologic solutions. The drug is incompatible with heparin and may form a precipitate if admixed. Although mitoxantrone solutions lack a preservative, in vitro studies have shown that the solution has bacteriostatic activity, and after initial aseptic use, solutions may be stored refrigerated for several weeks. Solutions diluted into 5% dextrose, sodium chloride, or lactated Ringer's injection are chemically stable for at least 2 weeks at room temperature, but should be used within 24 hours because of the possibility of microbial growth if inadvertently contaminated during preparation. The drug is not sensitive to pH manipulations in the range 3 to 9. Mitoxantrone is physically compatible with hydrocortisone sodium phosphate at concentrations up to 2 mg/mL for at least 24 hours. The drug is also physically compatible with 1 mg/mL of ondansetron for at least 4 hours (Trissel et al 1990) and with cytarabine for at least 7 days. The activity of cytarabine is maintained throughout this time period. Mitoxantrone is physically incompatible with heparin and this admixture should be avoided.

■ Administration

Mitoxantrone is approved for administration as an infusion into a freely running intravenous line over a period of not less than 3 minutes. Usually the drug has been diluted into at least 50 mL of Sodium Chloride for Injection, USP, or 5% Dextrose for Injection, USP. Most leukemia studies have used a 15 to 30-minute infusion of mitoxantrone in 50 mL of physiologic solution; however, there are a number of reports of bolus injection of the drug dose in 10 to 20 mL over 1 to 2 minutes without adverse incidents. Mitoxantrone is not generally believed to be a vesicant (Dorr 1990), although every precaution should be made to prevent the solution from extravasating (see Side Effects and Toxicity).

Mitoxantrone has also been administered as a continuous infusion in patients with acute leukemia in relapse. Doses were mixed daily for continuous 24-hour infusions for 5 days (Kaminer et al 1990). A 14-day continuous infusion has also been evaluated (Kreisle et al 1991).

■ Dosage

For therapy of ANLL the recommended dose is 12 mg/m^2 daily for three consecutive days (total dose 36 mg/m^2). These doses have also been combined with 100 mg/m^2 cytarabine for 7 days given as a bolus or as a continuous 24-hour infusion for 1 to 7 days (Dutcher et al 1985). A very high dose experimental regimen has also been reported to be active in ANLL and is also well tolerated with high-dose cytarabine (Arlin et al 1991). In this trial mitoxantrone was administered (at 80 mg/m^2) once or on 2 consecutive days (40 mg/m^2/d). This therapy did not cause an increase in deaths from aplasia and could be combined with daily cytarabine infusions at 3 g/m^2. As a single agent for advanced solid tumors, the typical dose has been 12 to 14 mg/m^2 once every 3 weeks given as a brief intravenous infusion (Shenkenberg and Von Hoff 1986). In autologous bone marrow transplantation programs, mitoxantrone has been given in 12 mg/m^2 doses for up to 3 to 4 consecutive days in combination with other agents. This same dose has been given as a continuous 24-hour infusion for 5 days in patients with acute leukemia in relapse (Kaminer et al 1990). A dose of 1.5 mg/m^2/d × 14 days was the maximally tolerated continuous infusion dose in a phase I trial (Kreisle et al 1991).

■ Drug Interactions

In leukemia cells, the combination of mitoxantrone and high-dose cytarabine produces a synergistic enhancement in DNA strand breaks (Heinemann et al 1988). Although the molecular mechanism is unknown, this may explain the therapeutic synergy noted in patients receiving these two agents (Arlin et al 1985).

■ Pharmacokinetics

Mitoxantrone pharmacokinetics have been studied by specific high-performance liquid chromatography assays (Alberts et al 1985a,b, Savaraj et al 1982). The drug has been shown to be bound up to 78% to human plasma proteins in the concentration range 26–450 ng/mL. This binding is independent of the drug concentration and is not affected by the presence of other highly bound drugs such as phenytoin, doxorubicin, methotrexate, prednisone, heparin, and aspirin.

Mathematical analyses of the serum concentration–time profile show that three compartments are required to adequately describe the elimination of the drug. The initial α-phase half-life ranges from 2.4 to 15 minutes, due primarily to the distribution of mitoxantrone into formed blood elements (Alberts et al 1985a,b). Uptake has been documented in erythrocytes, leukocytes, and platelets. The second or β phase of drug elimination ranges from 17 minutes to 3 hours. This phase is believed to result from the redistribution of mitoxantrone from the formed elements back into the blood and into various tissues. The reported terminal or γ half-life of mitoxantrone has varied from 2.9 to 298 hours, with a median value in the range of 12 days (Savaraj et al 1982, Alberts et al 1985a,b). Serum concentrations produced following high doses of the drug range from several hundred nanograms to one microgram per milliliter and are lower than simultaneous concentrations taken in tissues. With a continuous intravenous infusion over 14 days, mean steady-state plasma concentrations were 3.2 ± 0.7 ng/mL. Mean total body clearance was 340 ± 79 mL/min/m^2, with a mean AUC of 955 ± 185 µg/h/L for a daily dose of 1.5 mg/m^2 (Kreisle et al 1991).

The mean plasma clearance of the drug ranges from 210 to 600 mL/min. Renal clearance of mitoxantrone is minimal at 15 to 20 mL/min and generally accounts for less than 10% of the total mitoxantrone dose. This means that dose adjustments in patients with impaired renal function may not be necessary.

The highest concentrations of drug are found in the liver, pancreas, thyroid, spleen, and heart. Bone marrow is also a major site of distribution of mitoxantrone (Stewart et al 1982). Large amounts of drug may be retained in these organs for prolonged periods, sometimes accounting for up to 15% of an administered dose. At least two minor metabolites have been noted: the monocarboxylic and dicarboxylic acids formed by oxidation of the terminal hydroxyl groups on the alkyl side chain. Neither of these metabolites has antineoplastic activity in vitro and they represent a small fraction of the dose recoverable in the urine of humans (0.3–4.4%) (Chiccarelli et al 1986). It is also possible that mitoxantrone may form glutathione and glucuronide conjugates and these may represent an important detoxification pathway for the drug (Wolf et al 1986).

In patients with reduced hepatobiliary function decreased doses of the drug may be necessary (Savaraj et al 1982), although patients with only liver function test elevations may be excluded (Chlebowski et al 1989). Specific guidelines for such dose adjustments await clarification, but may follow a nomogram reported for doxorubicin based on elevated serum bilirubin levels and poor performance status. For patients with poor performance status and serum bilirubins of 1.5 to 3.0 mg/dL, 50% of the dose is recommended, and for a bilirubin above 3.0 mg/dL, 25% of the dose (Weiss 1989). Alternatively, Chlebowski et al (1989) have suggested giving full-dose therapy at 14 mg/m^2 to patients with moderate bilirubinemia (>1.3 but <3.5 mg/dL) and 8 mg/m^2 for patients with severe hyperbilirubinemia (>3.5 mg/dL).

■ Side Effects and Toxicity

The dose-limiting toxic effect of mitoxantrone is myelosuppression, which can manifest as pancytopenia but more commonly involves only leukopenia (Shenkenberg and Von Hoff 1986). The nadir for leukocyte suppression ranges between 10 and 14 days, with recovery complete by day 21. The degree of myelosuppression is related to the amount of prior therapy (including prior mitoxantrone therapy), the degree of bone marrow involvement with tumor, and the performance status of the patient. A mild anemia may occur in some patients although erythrocytes are not generally affected acutely by this drug. Thrombocytopenia occurs less commonly than granulocytopenia and relatively few patients develop platelet counts below 100,000/mL. Leukopenia is also the dose-limiting toxic effect for a 14-day continuous infusion (Kreisle et al 1991).

The most frequent acute toxic effects are nausea, vomiting, and stomatitis (Crossley 1984). Fortunately, these effects are usually mild in severity. Mitoxantrone produces nausea, vomiting, or both in approximately 43% of patients but it is severe in less than 1% of patients. Indeed, at least 40% of patients may have no nausea or vomiting during treatment with this agent. Mucositis tends to be mild to moderate with an every-3-week schedule, but can become more prominent when daily × 3 schedules are used as in ANLL. Less than 10% of patients on the every-3-week schedule develop serious mucositis; however, this increases substantially with multiple daily dosing schedules. Diarrhea from mitoxantrone is uncommon and no patients have reported severe dehydration as a result of diarrhea. Abdominal pain and constipation are also infrequent.

Alopecia is similarly infrequent in patients receiving mitoxantrone, and on the single-dose schedule used in breast cancer, less than 30% of patients experience moderate to severe hair loss. The selective loss of only gray hair has also been reported (Arlin et al 1988).

Phlebitis is also extremely uncommon with this drug, and although there are two case reports of extravasation necrosis, the majority of extravasations of mitoxantrone usually result in a blue discoloration of the skin which fades slowly (Dorr 1990).

One of the major long-term dose-limiting effects of mitoxantrone is cardiac toxicity, which ranges from transient electrocardiographic changes to severe congestive heart failure. This is typically associated with high cumulative doses. In patients who have not received prior anthracycline therapy or mediastinal radiation, the cumulative cardiotoxic dose limit for mitoxantrone is reported to be 160 mg/m^2 (Shenkenberg and Von Hoff 1986). Patients who have previously received anthracycline therapy, including doxorubicin and daunomycin, should not receive greater than 120 mg/m^2 mitoxantrone. Diagnostic indications for halting mitoxantrone therapy include endomyocardial biopsy with evidence of characteristic changes of anthracycline-induced cardiomyopathy and/or a significant (≥20%) drop in the nuclear ejection fraction (Benjamin et al 1984).

■ Special Applications

Intrathecal Administration. Investigationally, mitoxantrone has been given by intrathecal administration. Doses of 2 mg twice a week were diluted in cerebrospinal fluid (La Porte et al 1985). This therapy is not generally recommended as paraplegia and local nerve demyelinization have been reported (Zuiable et al 1985).

Intraperitoneal Administration. Mitoxantrone has been administered intraperitoneally to patients with advanced ovarian and colon cancer using a dose range of 1 to 23 mg/m^2 (Hall et al 1989). These investigational treatments were well tolerated and none of the patients experienced severe abdominal pain, nausea, or vomiting or significant leukopenia; however, although cellular pharmacology studies show that while high intraperitoneal drug exposures are possible, deep drug penetration into ovarian tumor masses is not achieved. This may seriously limit the efficacy of this experimental regimen.

Intrapleural Administration. In one study, mitoxantrone was administered by intrapleural instillation to control malignant pleural effusions from breast cancer (Alberts et al 1985a,b). No severe side effects were noted and effusions were well controlled.

Hepatic Artery Infusion. Patients with hepatocellular carcinoma have been given mitoxantrone as a 24-hour continuous hepatic artery infusion. Doses of 6 or 10 mg/m^2/d were given for 3 consecutive days and were repeated at 4-week intervals (Shepherd et al 1987). The drug was diluted into 1 L of normal saline without heparin. Partial responses were noted in 6 of 23 patients, with a median duration of 20 weeks. Toxicity included mild nausea and vomiting, moderate alopecia, and granulocytopenia in about one third of patients. Mild thrombocytopenia was noted in less than 10% of patients.

REFERENCES

Alberts DS, Peng Y-M, Bowden GT, Dalton WS, Mackel C. Pharmacology of mitoxantrone: Mode of action and pharmacokinetics. *Invest New Drugs*. 1985a;**3**:101–107.

Alberts DS, Peng Y-M, Leigh S, Davis TP, Woodward DL.

Disposition of mitoxantrone in cancer patients. *Cancer Res.* 1985b;**45**:1879–1884.

Allegra JC, Woodcock T, Woolf S, et al. A randomized trial comparing mitoxantrone with doxorubicin in patients with stage IV breast cancer. *Invest New Drugs.* 1985;**3**: 153–161.

Arlin Z, Feldman E, Mittelman A, et al. High dose short course mitoxantrone (M) with high dose cytarabine (HIDAC) is safe effective therapy for acute lymphoblastic leukemia (ALL). *Proc Am Soc Clin Oncol.* 1991;**10**:223.

Arlin ZA, Friedland ML, Atamer MA. Selective alopecia with mitoxantrone (letter). *N Engl J Med.* 1988;**310**:1464.

Arlin ZA, Silver R, Cassileth P, et al. Phase I–II trial of mitoxantrone in acute leukemia. *Cancer Treat Rep.* 1985;**69**:61–64.

Benjamin RS, Chawla SP, Ewer MS, et al. Evaluation of mitoxantrone cardiac toxicity by nuclear angiography and endomyocardial biopsy (abstract). *Proc Am Soc Clin Oncol.* 1984;**3**:40.

Bowden GT, Roberts R, Alberts DS, Peng Y-M, Garcia D. Comparative molecular pharmacology in leukemic L1210 cells of the anthracene anticancer drugs mitoxantrone and bisantrene. *Cancer Res.* 1985;**45**:4915–4920.

Chiccarelli FS, Morrison JA, Cosulich DB, et al. Identification of human urinary mitoxantrone metabolites. *Cancer Res.* 1986;**46**:4858–4861.

Chlebowski RT, Bulcavage L, Henderson IC, et al. Mitoxantrone use in breast cancer patients with elevated bilirubin. *Breast Cancer Res Treat.* 1989;**14**:267–274.

Cowan JD, Osborne CK, Neidhart JA, Von Hoff DD, Costanzi JJ, Vaughn CB. A randomized trial of doxorubicin, mitoxantrone and bisantrene in advanced breast cancer (a Southwest Oncology Group study). *Invest New Drugs.* 1985;**3**:149–152.

Crespi MD, Ivanier SE, Genovese J, Baldi A. Mitoxantrone affects topoisomerase activities in human breast cancer cells. *Biochem Biophys Res Commun.* 1986;**136**:521–528.

Cress AE, Roberts RA, Bowden GT, Dalton WS. Modification of keratin by the chemotherapeutic drug mitoxantrone. *Biochem Pharmacol.* 1988;**37**(15):3043–3046.

Crossley RJ. Clinical safety and tolerance of mitoxantrone. *Semin Oncol.* 1984;**11**(3, suppl 1):54–58.

Dorr RT. Antidotes to vesicant drug extravasations. *Blood Rev.* 1990;**4**(1):1–21.

Durr FE. Biologic and biochemical effects of mitoxantrone. *Semin Oncol.* 1984;**11**(3, suppl 1):3–10.

Dutcher JP, Wiernik PH, Strauman JJ, Spielvogel A, Dukart G. Mitoxantrone (MITOX) and cytosine arabinoside (ARA-C) in acute non-lymphocytic leukemia (ANLL) and blast crisis of chronic myelogenous leukemia (CML-B) (abstract). *Proc Am Soc Clin Oncol.* 1985;**4**:170.

Ehninger G, Weible KH, Heidemann EG, Waller HD. Mitoxantrone and cyclophosphamide in patients with advanced breast cancer. *Cancer Treat Rep.* 1984;**68**:1283–1284.

Fisher GR, Patterson LH. DNA strand breakage by peroxidase-activated mitoxantrone. *J Pharm Pharmacol.* 1991;**43**:65–68.

Hall C, Dougherty WJ, Lebish IJ, Brock PG, Man A. Warning against use of intrathecal mitoxantrone. *Lancet.* 1989;**1**:734.

Heinemann V, Murray D, Walters R, Meyn RE, Plunkett W. Mitoxantrone-induced DNA damage in leukemia cells is enhanced by treatment with high-dose arabinosylcytosine. *Cancer Chemother Pharmacol.* 1988;**22**:205–210.

Kaminer LS, Choi KE, Daley KM, Larson RA. Continuous infusion mitoxantrone in relapsed acute nonlymphocytic leukemia. *Cancer.* 1990;**65**:2619–2623.

Kharasch ED, Novak RF. Inhibition of microsomal oxidative drug metabolism by 1,4-bis{2-[(2-hydroxyethyl)-amino]-ethylamino}-9,10-anthracenedione diacetate, a new antineoplastic agent. *Mol Pharmacol.* 1982;**22**:471–478.

Kolodziejczyk P, Reszka K, Lown JW. Enzymatic oxidative activation and transformation of the antitumor agent mitoxantrone. *Free Radicals Biol Med.* 1988;**5**:13–25.

Kreisle WH, Alberts DS, List AF, et al. A phase I trial of 14-day continuous intravenous infusion mitoxantrone. *Anti-Cancer Drugs.* 1991;**2**:251–259.

Landys K, Borgstrom S, Anderson T, Noppa H. Mitoxantrone as a first-line treatment of advanced breast cancer. *Invest New Drugs.* 1985;**3**:133–137.

La Porte JP, Godefroy W, Verny A, Gorin NC, Maiman A, Duhamel G. Intrathecal mitozantrone. *Lancet.* 1985;**2**: 160.

Lown JW, Hanstock CC, Bradley RD, Scraba DG. Interactions of the antitumor agents mitoxantrone and bisantrene with deoxyribonucleic acids studied by electron microscopy. *Mol Pharmacol.* 1983;**25**:178–182.

Murdock KC, Child RG, Fabio PF, et al. Antitumor agents. I. 1,4-Bis[(aminoalkyl)amino]-9,10-anthracenediones. *J Med Chem.* 1979;**22**:1024–1030.

Paciucci PA, Ohnuma T, Cuttner J, Silver RT, Holland JF. Mitoxantrone in patients with acute leukemia in relapse. *Cancer Res.* 1983;**43**:3919–3922.

Savaraj N, Lu K, Manuel V, Loo TL. Pharmacology of mitoxantrone in cancer patients. *Cancer Chemother Pharmacol.* 1982;**8**:113–117.

Shenkenberg TD, Von Hoff DD. Mitoxantrone: A new anticancer drug with significant clinical activity. *Ann Intern Med.* 1986;**105**:67–81.

Shepherd FA, Evans WK, Blackstein ME, et al. Hepatic arterial infusion of mitoxantrone in the treatment of primary hepatocellular carcinoma. *J Clin Oncol.* 1987;**5**(4): 635–640.

Stewart JA, McCormack JJ, Krakoff IH. Clinical and clinical pharmacologic studies of mitoxantrone. *Cancer Treat Rep.* 1982;**66**:1327–1331.

Traganos F, Evenson DP, Staiano-Coico L, Darzynkiewicz Z, Melamed MR. Action of dihydroxyanthraquinone on cell cycle progression and survival of a variety of cultured mammalian cells. *Cancer Res.* 1980;**40**:671–681.

Trissel LA, Fulton B, Tramont SM. Visual compatibility of ondansetron with chemotherapeutic agents, antibiotics, and other selected drugs during simulated Y-site injection (abstract #P-468R). In: *25th Annual ASHP Midyear Clinical Meetings and Exhibit, Las Vegas, Nevada;* 1990.

Vietti TJ, Steuber CP, Kim TH, et al. Mitoxantrone in children with advanced malignant disease. In: Rozencweig M, et al, eds. *New Anticancer Drugs: Mitoxantrone and Bisantrene.* New York: Raven Press; 1983:93.

Weiss RB. Mitoxantrone: Its development and role in clinical practice. *Oncology.* 1989;3(6):135–141.

Wolf CR, MacPherson JS, Smyth JF. Evidence for the metabolism of mitoxantrone by microsomal glutathione transferases and 3-methylcholanthrene-inducible glucuronosyl transferases. *Biochem Pharmacol.* 1986;35(9): 1577–1581.

Yap H-Y, Blumenschein GR, Schell FC, Buzdar AU, Valdivieso M, Bodey GP. Dihydroxyanthracenedione: A promising new drug in the treatment of metastatic breast cancer. *Ann Intern Med.* 1981;95:694–697.

Yap H-Y, Esparza L, Blumenschein GR, Hortobagyi GN, Bodey GP. Combination chemotherapy with cyclophosphamide, mitoxantrone and 5-fluorouracil in patients with metastatic breast cancer. *Cancer Treat Rev.* 1983;10(suppl B):53–55.

Zuiable A, Maitland J, Nandi A, Clink HM, Powles RL. Intrathecal mitoxantrone for resistant leukaemia (letter). *Lancet.* 1985;2:1060–1061.

Monocyte/Macrophage Colony-Stimulating Factor

■ Other Names

Recombinant human macrophage colony-stimulating factor; rhM-CSF; CSF-1; monocyte CSF; human urinary colony-stimulating factor.

■ Chemistry

Natural human monocyte/macrophage colony-stimulating factor (M-CSF) is a glycoprotein with a molecular weight of 85,000 (Motoyoshi et al 1978, Ralph et al 1986). The native protein is heavily *N*-glycosylated and exists as two homologous subunits, each with a molecular weight of about 42,000. The gene for M-CSF is located in a single copy on the long arm (q 33) of chromosome 5 (Nienhuis et al 1985). The human M-CSF gene has 10 exons and 9 introns. Messenger RNA splicing is believed to produce at least three different protein forms of about 265, 55, and 438 amino acids. These are termed M-CSFα, M-CSFβ and M-CSFγ, respectively (Cosman et al 1988). Because of variable *N*-glycosylation at two sites, molecular weights can range from 36,000 to 90,000. There are secreted and membrane-anchored forms of M-CSF, although the former appears to be a precursor to the secreted form.

The structure of human M-CSF differs from that of CSF-1 by the presence of a unique additional 65-amino-acid-long sequence from amino acids 150 to 214 (the carboxy terminus of human M-CSF). Up to amino acid 149 the molecules are identical. These additional amino acids may explain the unique ability of human M-CSF to stimulate monocyte production of granulocyte CSF (G-CSF) and granulocyte-macrophage CSF (GM-CSF) without the addition of lipopolysacharide needed by CSF-1 (Motoyoshi et al 1989).

The last 75 amino acids (aa) of M-CSFα, M-CSFβ, and M-CSFγ are identical and include a 23-aa hydrophobic transmembranal domain and a 36-aa cytoplasmic domain (Cerretti et al 1988). There are seven common cysteine residues in the three pro-

```
Ala Pro Met Thr Gln Thr Thr Pro Leu Lys Thr Ser Trp Val Asp Cys Ser Asn
Met Ile Asp Glu Ile Ile Thr His Leu Lys Gln Pro Pro Leu Pro Leu Leu Asp
Phe Asn Asn Leu Asn Gly Glu Asp Gln Asp Ile Leu Met Glu Asn Asn Leu Arg
Arg Pro Asn Leu Glu Ala Phe Asn Arg Ala Val Lys Ser Leu Gln Asp Ala Ser
Ala Ile Glu Ser Ile Leu Lys Asn Leu Leu Pro Cys Leu Pro Leu Ala Thr Ala
Ala Pro Thr Arg His Pro Ile His Ile Lys Asp Gly Asp Trp Asn Glu Phe Arg
Arg Lys Leu Thr Phe Tyr Leu Lys Thr Leu Glu Asn Ala Gln Ala Gln Gln Thr
Thr Leu Ser Leu Ala Ile Phe
```

Amino acid sequence of macrophage colony-stimulating factor

teins along with a common 32-aa signal sequence. The secreted form of M-CSF is a homodimer with a subunit molecular weight of 22,000 or 28,000 (Cerretti et al 1988).

The recombinant human M-CSF produced by Cetus Corporation in *Escherichia coli* is a nonglycosylated homodimeric protein linked by inter- and intramolecular disulfide bonds. The potency is listed at more than 1×10^7 U/mg of protein using a hematopoietic bioassay. In contrast, the purified human urinary CSF used in Japanese trials is more closely related to CSF-1 and has produced some biologic effects not seen with human M-CSF (Motoyoshi et al 1986b). The latter preparations are manufactured by the Green Cross Corporation or Morinaya Milk Industry. These products have a specific activity of 1.4×10^8 U/mg of protein in a standard mouse assay system (Motoyoshi 1987).

■ Antitumor Activity

Monocyte colony stimulating factor does not possess antitumor activity per se. Rather it is a hematopoietic growth factor that acts on monocyte precursors and mature monocytes (Das and Stanley 1982, Stanley et al 1983). In the mouse, M-CSF stimulates macrophages to produce a variety of regulatory proteins including tumor necrosis factor (Warren and Ralph 1986), plasminogen activator (Lin and Gordon 1979), prostaglandins (Kurland et al 1979), interleukin-1 (Moore et al 1980), oxygen free radicals (Wing et al 1985), interferon (Fleit and Rabinovitch 1981), ferritin (Broxmeyer et al 1985), and G-CSF (Metcalf and Nicola 1985). Cells exposed to M-CSF also have enhanced resistance to viral infections (Lee and Warren 1987) and have stimulated yeast killing activity (Karbassi et al 1987).

Immunologic Activity. Human M-CSF also stimulates peripheral blood mononuclear cells (PBMCs) which can result in both indirect immunologic actions (Wing et al 1985) and direct cytotoxic actions against human tumor cell targets (Sampson-Johannes and Carlino 1988). When tested against WEHI-164 cells resistant to natural killer cells, M-CSF produced cytotoxic effects in direct proportion to the amount of tumor necrosis factor produced by the PBMCs (Sampson-Johannes and Carlino 1988); however, M-CSF also stimulates tumoricidal activity in murine P-815 mastocytoma cells resistant to tumor necrosis factor. Cytotoxic activity has been observed in mice bearing B-16 melanoma cells and in human Tu-5 sarcoma cells in vitro (Ralph and Nakoinz 1987). Other studies show that human M-CSF can stimulate human monocytes to express cytotoxic activity against a variety of malignant cells including myeoblast lines K-562, HL-60, and Raji cells (Motoyashi and Takaku 1990).

Antifungal Activity. Perhaps more importantly, M-CSF has shown consistent antifungal activity in patients with refractory fungal infections (O'Neill et al., 1992). Thus, M-CSF has cleared intracerebral and other soft tissue fungal infections that had been resistant to other classic antifungal medications. In patients with fungal infections following autologous bone marrow transplantation (ABMT), M-CSF is associated with enhanced survival, particularly in patients with a Karnofsky performance status greater than 30% (Nemunaitis et al 1992). In a Phase I trial of M-CSF in bone marrow transplant patients with invasive fungal infections, 6 out of 12 evaluable patients had resolution of their infection (Nemunaitis et al 1991). The majority of fungal organisms in this trial were candida species, followed by aspergillus.

Leukemic Cell Differentiation. Human urinary M-CSF or CSF-1 can also induce differentiation in leukemic blasts, leading to reduced leukemic colony growth in vitro. This has been related to the generation of adherent cells with macrophage/monocyte characteristics during cell passage in vitro (Miyauchi et al 1988). Direct stimulatory effects of M-CSF on neutrophils, eosinophils, or megakaryocytes has not been observed. Monocytes thus appear to be the primary targets of M-CSF stimulation, and this includes PBMCs, promonocytes, and large vacuolated macrophage-like cells (Oster et al 1990). Of interest, megakaryocyte numbers may increase in the bone marrow and peripheral blood platelet counts may decrease after each course of M-CSF therapy (Nemunaitis et al 1991).

Anticancer Trials in Humans. Phase II clinical trials with human M-CSF have been performed in Japan in patients with hematologic, urogenital, and gynecologic malignancies receiving cytotoxic chemotherapy (Motoyoshi et al 1986a, 1989). In patients with malignant lymphoma, solid tumors, or lymphoma, partially purified human urinary M-CSF reduced the days of neutropenia (< 2000 granulocytes) by about 3 days (Motoyoshi et al 1986a). There was also a slight effect on platelet count recovery in this trial. A similar, more rapid recovery in leukocyte and neutrophil counts was obtained in patients undergoing high-dose chemotherapy and bone marrow transplantation (Masaoka et al 1988). Of interest, the M-CSF-treated group also had a much lower relapse rate. M-CSF has been an effective myelostimulatory agent in patients developing prolonged neutropenia after receiving aggressive chemotherapy for acute myelogenous leukemia (Motoyoshi and Takaku 1990).

Phase I studies of Cetus Corporation recombinant human M-CSF in the United States have reported increased natural killer cell activity (Zamkoff et al 1991), and partial responses in leiomyosarcoma (Redman et al 1991). One complete response in a patient with renal cell carcinoma has been reported in a Phase I trial of M-CSF involving 23 patients with a variety of metastatic cancers (Sanda et al 1992). There is also one report of improved bone architecture following short-term M-CSF therapy involving 7 patients with infantile osteoporosis (Wang et al 1992). This therapy was well-tolerated, but its short duration may have limited the overall efficacy.

■ Mechanism of Action

Monocyte/macrophage colony-stimulating factor exerts its biologic effects after specific binding to its membrane receptor. The M-CSF receptor is a 165-kDa protein encoded by the c-fms proto-oncogene (Paietta et al 1990, Sherr et al 1985). Cellular sources of M-CSF include monocytes (Oster et al 1989), granulocytes (Lindemann et al 1989), and endothelial cells and fibroblasts (Sieff et al 1987). Much of the antitumor activity of M-CSF is indirect and relates to other cytokines secreted from affected monocytes. These cytotoxic mediators include interleukin-1 and tumor necrosis factor, which are known to have both direct cytotoxic and potent immunostimulatory activities (Warren and Ralph 1986). The tumoricidal activity against WEHI-164 cells is, however, antibody *independent* and thus M-CSF cytotoxicity may not always require an intact immune system. Furthermore, monkey PBMCs exposed to M-CSF have "increased expression of Ia antigen, LFA3, CD16, and CD14 and are able to mediate antibody-independent, cell-mediated cytotoxicity against melanoma and neuroblastoma targets" (Oster et al 1990). Antitumor activity may be increased under low oxygen tension (Broxmeyer et al 1990), or following cytotoxic chemotherapy (Rosenfeld et al 1990).

It appears that there is a common secreted form of M-CSF that is homologous if not identical to M-CSFα. This soluble form of M-CSF can circulate widely to act as a monocyte-specific hematopoietic hormone. The larger membranal form of M-CSF may thus act as a precursor to the soluble form and/or a marker for cell–cell interactions.

■ Availability and Storage

The Cetus-supplied material is investigationally available in vials containing 2.0 mg/mL recombinant human M-CSF in 1.2 mL of solution (2.4 mg total). This solution also contains 12 mg of mannitol in a sodium citrate buffer at a pH of 7.0. No bacteriostatic agent is added. The frozen liquid is recommended to be stored at −20°C or colder. After thawing, the solution is stable at room temperature for at least 24 hours; however, because of the lack of a bacteriostatic agent, use within 4 to 8 hours of thawing is recommended. Vials with particulates should be discarded, and as with all protein solutions, vigorous shaking is contraindicated.

■ Preparation for Use, Stability, and Admixture

Frozen vials are thawed at room temperature and the appropriate dose is withdrawn using aseptic technique. For the Cetus-supplied material, it is recommended that the recombinant human M-CSF be added to a solution containing 0.25% (w/v) human serum albumin (final concentration). This would involve the addition of 1 mL of a 25% albumin solution to each 100 mL of infusate. For infusion solutions, typically 0.9% Sodium Chloride for Injection, USP is used; other admixtures are not recommended. The use of infusion filters is also not recommended because of possible adsorption or binding to the filter surface. Admixture with other solutions is not recommended. Daily doses have typically been diluted into 500 mL of saline (Motoyoshi and Takaku 1990).

■ Administration

Human M-CSF has usually been administered as a brief intravenous infusion over 1 to 2 hours daily (Masaoka et al 1988, Motoyoshi and Takaku 1990). An infusion volume of 50 to 100 mL is common. In U.S. studies, Cetus-supplied recombinant human M-CSF has been administered as a rapid daily intravenous infusion over 15 minutes (Zamkoff et al 1991, Redman et al 1991).

■ Dosage

Human M-CSF is in early phase clinical testing and thus the maximally tolerated dose (MTD) levels are not known. In phase I trials in Japan, daily M-CSF doses of 8×10^6 U were administered for 7 consecutive days (Motoyoshi and Takaku 1990). In children with chronic neutropenia, doses of human urinary CSF of 6×10^8 U/m^2/d were administered for 7 consecutive days (Komiyama et al 1988). For bone marrow transplantation doses of 2×10^5 U/kg were administered to children up to a maximum of 8×10^6 U (Motoyoshi et al 1982, 1986b). For cancer patients receiving standard chemotherapy regimens, a daily dose of 2 to 4×10^6 U was used to augment hematopoietic recovery. This 5-day regimen was started 24 hours after chemotherapy had finished (Motoyoshi et al 1986a).

Phase I studies of Cetus Corporation recombinant human M-CSF have evaluated doses up to 33,000 µg/m^2 (Zamkoff et al 1991). The MTD is not known, but the drug appears to be well tolerated at doses up to 1100 µg/m^2 as an intravenous infusion every 8 hours × 5 days, with a day's rest between cycles (Redman et al 1991). With higher doses of human M-CSF ≥ 3690 µg/m^2), prolonging the infusion to 1 hour has lessened acute respiratory distress in a few patients experiencing this uncommon toxic effect (Zamkoff et al 1991). Severe opthalmologic abnormalities were found to be dose-limiting at M-CSF doses of 30,000 to 100,000 µg/m^2/d in a US Phase I trial in cancer patients (Sandra et al 1992). These doses were administered every 8 hours for 7 days, followed by a 7 to 10 day rest period.

■ Pharmacokinetics

In rats given 0.1, 1.0, or 10 mg/kg of Cetus M-CSF, plasma half-lives of 39, 60, and 74 minutes were described. In monkeys, half-lives of 81 to 85 minutes were described. The volume of distribution in both species approximated plasma volume, or 58 mL/kg in rats and 40 mL/kg in monkeys. In normal subjects, peak levels of urinary human M-CSF varied between 565 and 923 U/mL. The M-CSF disappearance rate was slow, with an apparent plasma half life of over 24 hours (Motoyoshi and Takaku 1990). A half-life value of about 8 days was apparent in this trial. The average serum level of urinary M-CSF activity in humans was 7 ± 3 U/0.1 mL serum *prior* to M-CSF infusion. It reached a "steady-state" level of 30 ± 16 U/0.1 mL on day 4 after initiation of the M-CSF 7-day dosing regimen (Motoyoshi and Takaku 1990).

Cetus-supplied recombinant human M-CSF has produced dose-dependent half-lives in human cancer patients (Zamkoff et al 1991). Similar dose-dependent serum half-lives were described in another phase I trial; however, after 5 days of continued daily dosing, the serum half lives decreased by 50%, suggesting a saturable clearance mechanism (Redman et al 1991). Similar results are described by Sanda et al (1992). The table below summarizes these findings.

■ Side Effects and Toxicity

Fever and chills are the primary clinical toxic effects of urinary-derived M-CSF. Fever over 38°C is the most frequent toxic effect reported, occurring in 32% of patients (Motoyoshi et al 1986a). The development of fever and chills sometimes limits therapy. A skin rash is reported in 95% of patients in one trial (Meisenberg et al 1992). Hypotension and chills have been described in 13 and 5% of patients, respectively. Other effects include palpitations, malaise, and headache, described in 2.6% of patients (Motoyoshi and Takaku 1990). These effects have not been described with the Cetus-supplied recombinant human M-CSF from *E. coli*.

Toxic effects in healthy volunteers include fever, itching, diaphoresis, and mild hypotension (Motoyoshi et al 1982). Liver enzymes and renal function do not change following human urinary-derived M-CSF therapy; however, human M-CSF may significantly reduce serum cholesterol (Motoyoshi and Takaku 1990). Similar effects have been noted with other hematopoietic colony stimulating factors.

SERUM HALF-LIVES OF CETUS CORPORATION HUMAN MONOCYTE/MACROPHAGE COLONY STIMULATING FACTOR IN CANCER PATIENTS

Dose (µg/m^2 as a 15-minute IV infusion)	Serum Half-life (min)	Reference
180	19.8	Zamkoff et al 1991
330	25	Redman et al 1991
1100	84	
≥ 3,690	204	Zamkoff et al 1991
10,000	3.5 to 4.2 hours	Sanda et al 1992

*Half-lives may decrease with repeated daily dosing (Redman et al 1991, Sanda et al 1992).

Phase I trials of Cetus Corporation human M-CSF have described consistent decreases in the platelet count, with thrombocytopenia to less than 100,000 noted in 10% of patients (Zamkoff et al 1991, Sanda et al 1992, Nemunaitis et al 1991). Fever, headache, and myalgias were observed in 35, 20, and 10% of patients, respectively, but were mild in all instances. Effects observed only at the higher dosages (> 11,000 µg/m^2) included ocular burning and photophobia and dyspnea with chest discomfort and wheezing (Zamkoff et al 1991). The latter reactions were easily managed with epinephrine and diphenhydramine, and did not preclude the administration of second doses at a slower (1-hour) infusion rate (Zamkoff et al 1991). With high dose therapy using Cetus recombinant human M-CSF (> 10,000 µg/m^2), severe ocular and ophthalmologic effects are described (Sanda et al 1992). These transient changes include ocular or periorbital inflammation, and occasional result in iridocyclitis. This was well controlled with homatropine (Sanda et al 1992). Scleritis, migraines, and severe photophobia were reported in a few patients. There were no visual abnormalities noted. Minor conjunctival erythema was observed in a larger number of patients, but always resolved within 24 hours.

The Cetus form of human M-CSF is also associated with significant decreases in serum cholesterol and triglycerides (Zamkoff et al 1991). Macrophages stimulated by cytokines such as M-CSF appear to express reduced numbers of receptors for low density lipoproteins (LDLs), the primary carriers of cholesterol (Fogelman et al 1983). As a result of stimulation, there is a reduction in both the influx of cholesterol and in the activity of 3-hydroxy-3-methylglutaryl-coenzyme A, the rate-limiting enzyme in cholesterol synthesis (Fogelman et al 1982). The overall net effect is to transiently, but significantly, reduce circulating cholesterol levels during times of M-CSF elevation. Peripheral blood monocyte counts are increased about two- to threefold at doses above 1100 µg/m^2 (Redman et al 1991); however, an increase in monocyte antitumor cytotoxicity in vitro was not reported.

REFERENCES

Broxmeyer HE, Cooper S, Lu L, et al. Enhanced stimulation of human bone marrow macrophage colony formation in vitro by recombinant human macrophage colony-stimulating factor in agarose medium and at low oxygen tension. *Blood*. 1990;**76**(2):323–329.

Broxmeyer H, Juliano L, Waheed A, Shadduck A. Release from mouse macrophages of acidic isoferritins that suppress hematopoietic progenitor cells is induced by purified L cell colony stimulating factor and suppressed by human lactoferrin. *J Immunol*. 1985;**136**:3224.

Cerretti DP, Wignall J, Anderson D, et al. Human macrophage colony stimulating factor: Alternative RNA and protein processing from a single gene. *Mol Immunol*. 1988;**25**:761.

Cosman D, Wignall J, Anderson D, et al. Human macrophage colony stimulating factor (M-CSF): alternate RNA splicing generates three different proteins that are expressed on the cell surface and secreted. *Behring Inst Mitt*. 1988;**83**:15–26.

Das S, Stanley E. Structure-function studies of a colony stimulating factor (CSF-1). *J Biol Chem*. 1982;**257**:136–139.

Fleit H, Rabinovitch M. Interferon induction in marrow-derived macrophages: regulation by T-cell conditioned medium. *J Cell Physiol*. 1981;**108**:347.

Fogelman AM, Seager J, Groopman JE, et al. Lymphokines secreted by an established lymphocyte line modulate receptor-mediated endocytosis in macrophages derived from human monocytes. *J Immunol*. 1983;**151**(5):2368–2373.

Fogelman AM, Seager J, Habeland ME, et al. Lymphocyte-conditioned medium protects human monocyte-macrophages from cholesteryl ester accumulation. *Proc Natl Acad Sci USA*. 1982;**79**:922.

Karbassi A, Becker JM, Foster JS, et al. Enhanced killing of *Candida albicans* by murine macrophages treated with macrophage colony-stimulating factor: Evidence for augmented expression of mannose receptors. *J Immunol*. 1987;**139**:417–421.

Komiyama A, Ishiguro A, Kubo T, et al. Increases in neutrophil counts by purified human, urinary colony-stimulating factor in chronic eutropenia of childhood. *Blood*. 1988;**71**(1):41–45.

Kurland J, Pelus L, Ralph R, et al. Induction of prostaglandin E synthesis in normal and neoplastic macrophages: role for colony stimulating factor(s) distinct from effects of myeloid progenitor cell proliferation. *Proc Natl Acad Sci USA*. 1987;**76**:2306.

Lee M, Warren M. CSF-1-induced resistance to viral infection in murine macrophages. *J Immunol*. 1987;**138**:3019–3023.

Lin H, Gordon S. Secretion of plasminogen activator by bone marrow-derived mononuclear phagocytes and its enhancement by colony stimulating factor. *J Exp Med*. 1979;**150**:231.

Lindemann A, Riedel D, Oster W, et al. GM-CSF induces cytokine secretion by polymorphonuclear neutrophils. *J Clin Invest*. 1989;**83**:1308–112.

Masaoka T, Motoyoshi K, Takaku F, et al. Administration of human urinary colony stimulating factor after bone marrow transplantation. *Bone Marrow Transplant*. 1988;**3**:121–127.

Meisenberg B, Affronti M, Ross M, et al. Recombinant human macrophage colony-stimulating factor (rhM-CSF) after high-dose chemotherapy (HDC) with autologous bone marrow support (ABMS). *Blood.* 1992;**80**(10 Suppl 1):417a.

Metcalf D, Nicola N. Synthesis by mouse peritoneal cells of G-CSF, the differentiation inducer for myeloid leukemia cells: Stimulation by endotoxin, M-CSF and multi-CSF. *Leukemia Res.* 1985;**9**:35.

Miyauchi J, Wang C, Kelleher CA, et al. The effects of recombinant CSF-1 on blast cells of acute myeloblastic leukemia in suspension culture. *J Cell Physiol* 1988;**135**: 55–62.

Moore R, Oppenheim J, Farrar J, et al. Production of lymphocyte activating factor (Interleukin-1) by macrophages activated with colony stimulating factors. *J Immunol.* 1980;**125**:1302.

Motoyoshi K. Purification, gene cloning and clinical application of human monocyte specific colony-stimulating factor. *Acta Haematol Jpn.* 1987;**50**:1557–1564.

Motoyoshi K, Ishizaka Y, Miura Y, Takaku F. Clinical application of partially purified human urinary colony-stimulating factor. *Immunobiol.* 1986b;**172**:205–212.

Motoyoshi K and Takaku E. Human monocytic colony-stimulating factor (hM-CSF), Phase I/II clinical studies. In: Mertelsman R, Hermann F, eds. *Hematopoietic Growth Factors in Clinical Applications.* New York: Marcel Dekker; 1990;161–175.

Motoyoshi K, Takaku F, Kusumoto K, et al. Phase I and early phase II studies on human urinary colony stimulating factor. *Jpn J Med.* 1982;**21**:187–191.

Motoyoshi K, Takaku E, Maekawa T. Protective effect of partially purified human urinary colony stimulating factor on granulocytopenia after anticancer chemotherapy. *Exper Hematol.* 1986a;**14**:1069–1075.

Motoyoshi K, Takaku F, Mizoguchi H, et al. Purification and some properties of colony-stimulating factor from normal human urine. *Blood.* 1978;**52**:1012–1020.

Motoyoshi K, Yoshida K, Hatake K, et al. Recombinant and native human urinary colony-stimulating factor directly augments granulocytic and granulocyte-macrophage colony-stimulating factor production of human peripheral blood monocytes. *Exp Hematol.* 1982;**17**:68–71.

Nemunaitis J, Meyers JD, Buckner CD, et al. Phase I trial of recombinant human macrophage colony-stimulating factor in patients with invasive fungal infections. *Blood.* 1991;**78**(4):907–913.

Nemunaitis J, Shannon-Dorcy K, Buckner CD, et al. Long term follow up of phase I/II trial bone marrow transplant (BMT) patients with invasive fungal infection who received recombinant human macrophage colony-stimulating factor (rhM-CSF). *Blood.* 1992;**80**(10 suppl 1):292.

Nienhuis AW, Bunn JF, Turner TH, et al. Expression of the human C-FMS protoncogene in hematopoietic cells and its deletion in the (5q⁻)-syndrome. *Cell.* 1985;42:421–425.

O'Neill C, Wynne D, Ando D. Combined use of rM-CSF and antifungal therapy in immuncompromised patients with invasive fungal infections. *Blood.* 1992;**80**(10 Suppl 1):989.

Oster W, Lindemann A, Mertelsmann R, Herrmann F. Production of macrophage-, granulocyte-, granulocyte-macrophage- and multi-colony-stimulating factor by peripheral blood cells. *Eur J Immunol.* 1989;**19**:543–547.

Oster W, Mertel S, Mann R, Hermann F. Regulation of cell function by hematopoietic growth factors. In: Mertelsman R, Hermann F, eds. *Hematopoietic Growth Factors in Clinical Applications.* New York: Marcel Dekker; 1990;30–31.

Paietta E, Racevskis J, Stanley ER, et al. Expression of the macrophage growth factor, CSF-1 and its receptor c-fms by a Hodgkin's disease-derived cell line and its variants. *Cancer Res.* 1990;**50**:2049–2055.

Ralph P, Nakoinz I. Stimulation of macrophage tumoricidal activity by the growth and differentiation factor CSF-1. *Cell Immunol.* 1987;**105**:270–279.

Ralph P, Warren MK, Nakoinz I, et al. Biological properties and molecular biology of the human macrophage growth factor, CSF-1. *Immunobiol.* 1986;**172**:194–204.

Redman B, Flaherty L, Chou TH, et al. Phase I trial of recombinant macrophage-colony stimulating factor (M-CSF) by rapid intravenous (IV) infusion in patients with cancer. *Proc Am Soc Clin Oncol.* 1991;**10**:98.

Rosenfeld CS, Evans C, Shadduck RK. Human macrophage colony-stimulating factor induces macrophage colonies after L-phenylalanine methylester treatment of human marrow. *Blood.* 1990;**76**(9):1783–1787.

Sampson-Johannes A, Carlino J. Enhancement of human monocyte tumoricidal activity by recombinant M-CSF. *J Immunol.* 1988;**141**:3680–3686.

Sanda MG, Yang JC, Topalian SL, et al. Intravenous administration of recombinant human macrophage colony-stimulating factor to patients with metastatic cancer: A phase I study. *J Clin Oncol.* 1992;**10**(10):1643–1649.

Sherr CJ, Rettenmier CW, Sacca R, et al. The C-FMS proto-oncogene product is related to the receptor for the mononuclear phagocyte growth factor CSF-1. *Cell.* 1985;**41**:665–676.

Sieff CA, Schickwann T, Faller V. Interleukin-1 induces cultured human endothelial cell production of granulocyte-macrophage colony-stimulating factor. *J Clin Invest.* 1987;**79**:48–51.

Stanley E, Guilberty L, Tushinsky R, et al. CSF-1, a mononuclear phagocyte lineage-specific hemopoietic growth factor. *J Cell Biochem.* 1983;**21**:151.

Wang W, Morris S, Vilmer E, et al. Treatment of osteopetrosis with macrophage colony-stimulating factor (M-CSF). *Blood.* 1992;**80**(10 Suppl 1):249a.

Warren MK, Ralph P. Macrophage growth factor CSF-1 stimulates human monocyte production of interferon, tumor necrosis factor and colony stimulating activity. *J Immunol.* 1986;**137**:2281–2285.

Wing E, Ampel A, Waheed A, Shudduck R. Macrophage colony-stimulating factor (M-CSF) enhances the capacity of murine macrophages to secret oxygen reduction products. *J Immunol.* 1985;**135**:2052.

Zamkoff K, Hudson J, Groves E, et al. A phase I trial of recombinant macrophage colony stimulating factor, human (rM-CSF), by rapid intravenous infusion in patients were refractory malignancy. *Proc Am Soc Clin Oncol.* 1991;**10**:93.

Nabilone

■ Other Names

Cesamet®, LY-109514 (Eli Lilly and Company).

■ Chemistry

Structure of nabilone

The complete chemical name of nabilone is 3-(1,1-dimethylheptyl)-6,6a,7,8,10,10a-hexahydro-1-hydroxy-6,6-dimethyl-9H-dibenzo[b,d]pyran-9-one. Nabilone is a chemically synthesized relative of marijuana, or Δ^9-tetrahydrocannabinol (THC), having a molecular weight of 372. It differs from THC by the presence of a ketone instead of a methyl group at position 9 of the C ring only. It is therefore technically not a tetrahydrocannabinol.

■ Antitumor Activity

Nabilone is not an antineoplastic, but rather is an antiemetic. Nabilone has been found to be effective in reducing the nausea and vomiting associated with various cancer chemotherapy regimens (Herman et al 1977, 1979). In a phase I trial nabilone, at doses of 2 mg three times a day, was found effective in reducing chemotherapy-induced nausea and vomiting in 10 of 13 cancer patients (Herman et al 1977). In the follow-up phase II trial nabilone produced a response rate of about 80% versus a 36% response rate in the same patients receiving oral prochlorperazine in a double-blind, randomized fashion (Herman et al 1979). Patients receiving 5-day cisplatin regimens appeared to be most resistant to the antiemetic effects of the drug. Steele et al (1979) confirmed the antiemetic efficacy of nabilone in cancer patients receiving a variety of agents including dactinomycin, streptozocin, mechlorethamine, dacarbazine, and low-dose (45–60 mg/m^2) cisplatin. When compared with placebo, nabilone was significantly more effective (Jones et al 1982, Wada et al 1982, Levitt 1982). High-dose (> 60 mg/m^2) cisplatin therapy, again, was relatively unresponsive to nabilone effects.

Since those early reports, a number of randomized studies of nabilone versus other regimens have been conducted, particularly in patients receiving platinum-containing combinations. The largest of these studies are summarized in the table on page 742. As can be seen, in a study by Cunningham et al (1988), patients receiving nabilone + prochlorperazine for prophylaxis of carboplatin-induced emesis preferred that regimen over the combination of metoclopramide + dexamethasone (which was more effective and preferred for cisplatin-induced emesis).

There is also evidence that dexamethasone added to nabilone increases the antiemetic effect and may attenuate the hypertension that can be seen with nabilone alone (Niiranen and Mattson 1987). The addition of domperidone to nabilone does not appear to improve the antiemetic efficacy (Liang et al 1985). Of particular note is the rather impressive single-agent activity of nabilone in preventing chemotherapy-induced emesis in children (Chan et al 1987, Dalzell et al 1986).

■ Mechanism of Action

Nabilone is still under investigation for use as an antiemetic agent. This follows anecdotal evidence that smoking marijuana decreases the nausea and vomiting associated with anticancer agents (Sallen et al 1975) and that oral forms of THC cause the same physiologic effects (Weil et al 1968). The exact mechanism of antiemetic action remains to be defined. Tolerance to therapeutic effects as well as untoward effects has been seen after 3 days in animals and humans (Lemberger and Rowe 1975).

■ Availability and Storage

Nabilone was investigationally available from Eli Lilly and Company (Indianapolis, Indiana). It was supplied in 1- and 2-mg capsules, which should be stored in tight containers at room temperature. Because of long-term animal toxicity, nabilone will probably not reach commercial status.

RANDOMIZED TRIALS OF NABILONE

Agent Used	% of Patients With a Reduction in Nausea and Vomiting	Reference
Nabilone + prochlorperazine versus	19*	Cunningham et al 1988
metoclopramide + dexamethasone	32	
Nabilone versus prochlorperazine	Nabilone significantly superior	Ahmedzai et al 1983
Nabilone[†] versus metoclopramide	No difference[‡]	Priestman et al 1987
Nabilone versus	47	Niiranen and Mattson 1987
nabilone + dexamethasone	63	
Nabilone[§] versus	70	Chan et al 1987
prochlorperazine	30	
Nabilone versus prochlorperazine	Nabilone significantly superior	Niiranen and Mattson 1985
Nabilone versus	60	Niederle et al 1985
alizapride	30	

*However, patients who received carboplatin preferred nabilone + prochlorperazine (see text).
[†]For radiation-induced nausea.
[‡]Incidence and severity of adverse reactions greater for nabilone group.
[§]Trial in children.

■ Preparation for Use, Stability, and Admixture

No stability data are available.

■ Administration

See Dosage.

■ Special Precautions

Continuous seizure activity and sudden death have been noted in dogs receiving more than 0.5 mg/kg/d. These effects have not been noted in patients. The sedation and drowsiness produced by this drug may preclude a patient from driving or engaging in other dangerous activities requiring an alert and responsive sensorium. Patients can sometimes experience significant postural hypotension while on this drug and should be advised accordingly. They should also be advised about such disconcerting psychologic effects as hallucinations, euphoria, and rare paranoid reactions.

■ Drug Interactions

None are known.

■ Dosage

The maximally effective dose of nabilone for antiemesis has not been firmly established; however, the phase I test by Herman et al (1977) defined an effective, safe dose of 1 to 2 mg given three times daily or every 8 hours throughout the chemotherapy regimen. Single doses of 5 mg have produced orthostatic hypotension (without electrocardiographic changes). It is suggested that induction of enzymes after apparently ineffective initial doses may augment effects from subsequent doses. This, however, remains to be established. Dosing in THC studies has shown that the dosing interval is very important to achieve an effect. Thus, enhanced efficacy was seen when doses were given on a rigid, frequent schedule or often enough "to maintain a slight high." This was usually every 4 hours (Sallen et al 1975). Efficacy may also depend on "pretreatment" with nabilone for several hours before chemotherapy. Although tolerance after repeated dosing is also possible, it was not demonstrated in antiemetic studies in animals. This concurs with observations in humans.

■ Pharmacokinetics

Peak blood levels after oral doses have been seen 30 minutes after ingestion, and the oral absorption of nabilone is good. An initial plasma half-life of 2 hours has been reported for the parent compound (Rubin et al 1977). The rapid plasma clearance is apparently explained by avid tissue uptake and subsequent rapid metabolism. The half-lives for nabilone metabolites are significantly prolonged at more than 20 hours. Circulating metabolites are primarily isomeric carbinols formed by reduction at the 9-position ketone. Nabilone appears to be rapidly metabolized in the liver, and the responsible liver enzymes may be induced by initial doses. Long-term marijuana smokers show accelerated drug clearance evidenced by a half-life of 28 hours versus 52 hours for new users. It is not known whether smoking marijuana induces a more rapid clearance of nabilone. The drug and its metabolites are eliminated through biliary excretion. Thus, Rubin et al (1977) showed that most of nabilone is eliminated in the feces ($\simeq$65%), with only about 20% eliminated in the urine. The prolonged clinical effects and the short half-life of the intact nabilone strongly suggest that much of the drug's action is mediated by the various reduced metabolites. It is not known which form(s) is pharmacologically most active.

■ Side Effects and Toxicity

The predominant side effects of nabilone as used in the antiemetic trials have been anticholinergic in nature. These include somnolence and dry mouth noted in more than 80% of patients. Dizziness and decreased coordination were noted in about 70% of patients (Herman et al 1979). Approximately half the patients receiving nabilone also experienced mildly blurred vision and/or decreased coordination. Drowsiness and sedation can be expected to some degree in most patients.

There appear to be common toxic effects for both nabilone and prochlorperazine, with a quantitatively greater number seen with nabilone. A few serious central nervous system reactions have been described after nabilone (Herman et al 1979). These include (1) a drug-induced psychosis with visual hallucinations and concurrent marked feelings of depersonalization and (2) visual hallucinations alone or with paranoia (one case each) and severe lethargy (also one case). Relaxation, a central nervous system effect, is commonly reported; however, true euphoria is only rarely seen. The euphoric and slightly dissociative feelings may be an unpleasant sensation to some patients, especially the elderly. Prior counseling is advised as the dissociative feelings may persist for 2 to 3 days after the drug is discontinued. Several anticipated side effects proved to be uncommon, including euphoria or depression (each seen in only about 20% of patients) and tachycardia (noted in only 11% of patients).

Orthostatic hypotension has been produced by large doses (5 mg) in humans and is not associated with electrocardiographic changes. The hypotension has usually been noted on the second day of administration, with resolution generally by the fourth day. In a phase II study, severe hypotension occurred only once with the initial drug dose (Herman et al 1979).

Unfortunately, more recent long-term toxicity studies in laboratory animals have uncovered serious side effects which can be lethal. A number of dogs treated with more than 0.5 mg/kg/d continuously developed seizure activity, which in a few was associated with sudden death. The exact mechanism of this toxicity is unknown and specific anatomic lesions have not yet been isolated. Earlier autopsy studies in animals did not reveal hematologic, chemical, or histologic aberrations in any major organ system. The human studies have so far similarly not revealed any abnormalities in blood chemistries, electrocardiogram, or hematologic status caused by the drug.

■ Special Applications

Other beneficial effects documented in humans besides antiemesis include reduction in anxiety and reduction of intraocular pressure in open-angle glaucoma. No significant bronchial changes were observed in one preliminary nabilone study in asthmatic patients.

REFERENCES

Ahmedzai S, Carlyle DL, Calder IT, Moran F. Antiemetic efficacy and toxicity of nabilone, a synthetic cannabinoid in lung cancer chemotherapy. *Br J Cancer.* 1983;**48**(5):657–663.

Chan MS, Correia JA, MacLeod SM. Nabilone versus prochlorperazine for control of cancer chemotherapy-induced emesis in children: A double-blind, crossover trial. *Pediatrics.* 1987;**79**(6):946–952.

Cunningham D, Bradley CJ, Forrest GJ, et al. A randomized trial of oral nabilone and prochlorperazine compared to intravenous metoclopramide and dexamethasone in the treatment of nausea and vomiting induced by chemotherapy regimens containing cisplatin or cisplatin analogues. *Eur J Cancer Clin Oncol.* 1988;**24**(4):685–689.

Dalzell AM, Bartlett H, Lilleyman JS. Nabilone: An alternative antiemetic for cancer chemotherapy. *Arch Dis Child.* 1986;**61**(5)502–505.

Herman TS, et al. Nabilone: A potent antiemetic cannabinol with minimal euphoria. *Biomedicine.* 1977;**27**:331–334.

Herman TS, Einhorn LH, Jones SE, et al. Superiority of nabilone over prochlorperazine as an antiemetic in patients receiving cancer chemotherapy. *N Engl J Med.* 1979;**300**(23):1295–1297.

Jones SE, Durant JR, Greco FA, et al. A multi-institutional phase III study of nabilone vs chemotherapy-induced nausea and vomiting. *Cancer Treat Rev.* 1982;**9**:45–48.

Lemberger L, Rowe H. Clinical pharmacology of nabilone, a cannabinol derivative. *Clin Pharmacol Ther.* 1975;**18**(G):720–726.

Levi H. Nabilone vs placebo in the treatment of chemotherapy-induced nausea and vomiting in cancer patients. *Cancer Treat Rev.* 1982;**9**:49–53.

Liang R, Harper P, Rogers H. Double-blind cross over study of the antiemetic efficacy of nabilone + domperidone vs nabilone (meeting abstract). In *3rd European Conference on Clinical Oncology and Cancer Nursing;* 1985:39.

Niederle N, Schutte J, Krischke W, Schmidt CG. Prospective randomized study comparing the antiemetic efficacy of nabilone versus alizapride in nonseminomatous testicular cancer patients receiving cisplatin therapy (meeting abstract). In *3rd European Conference on Clinical Oncology and Cancer Nursing;* 1985:38.

Niiranen A, Mattson K. A cross-over comparison of nabilone and prochlorperazine for emesis induced by cancer chemotherapy. *Am J Clin Oncol.* 1985;**8**(4):336–340.

Niiranen A, Mattson K. Antiemetic efficacy of nabilone and dexamethasone: A randomized study of patients with lung cancer receiving chemotherapy. *Am J Clin Oncol.* 1987;**10**(4):325–329.

Priestman SG, Priestman TJ, Canney PA. A double-blind randomized cross-over comparison of nabilone and metoclopramide in the control of radiation-induced nausea. *Clin Radiol.* 1987;**38**(5):543–544.

Rubin A, Lemberger L, Warrick P, Crabtree RE, Sullivan H, et al. Physiologic disposition of nabilone, a cannabinol derivative in man. *Clin Pharmacol Ther.* 1977;**22**(1):85–91.

Sallen SE, Ziaberg NE, Frei E III. Antiemetic effect of Δ^9-tetrahydrocannabinol in patients receiving cancer chemotherapy. *N Engl J Med.* 1975;**293**:795–797.

Steele N, Braun D, O'Hehir M, Young C. Double-blind comparison of the antiemetic effects of nabilone and prochlorperazine on chemotherapy-induced emesis (abstract C-189). *Proc Am Assoc Cancer Res ASCO.* 1979;**20**:337.

Wada JK, Bogbon DL, Gunnel JC, et al. Double-blind, randomized, crossover trial of nabilone vs placebo in cancer chemotherapy. *Cancer Treat Rev.* 1982;**9**:39–44.

Weil AT, Zinberg NE, Nelsen JM. Clinical and psychological effects of marijuana in man. *Science.* 1968;**162**:1234–1242.

Nafoxidine

■ Other Names

NSC-70735; pyrrolidine; U-11; 110A.

■ Chemistry

Structure of nafoxidine hydrochloride

Nafoxidine was synthesized by Upjohn Laboratories in the early 1960s as an antifertility agent. Additional studies showed it to have activity against an estrogen dependent rodent mammary carcinoma. Nafoxidine is 1-{2-[P-(3,4-dihydro-6-methoxy-2-phenyl-*l*-naphthyl)phenoxy]ethyl}pyrrolidine. Its molecular weight is 462.02 and its empiric formula $C_{29}H_{31}O_2N \cdot HCl$. Nafoxidine is soluble in water to less than 1 mg/mL and is soluble in alcohol (150–200 mg/mL), chloroform (200–300 mg/mL), and octane (12–30 mg/mL).

■ Antitumor Activity

Nafoxidine has been reported to have activity in patients with breast carcinoma (Bloom and Boesen 1974, Heuson et al 1972, 1975, European Organization for Research and Treatment of Cancer 1972, Engelsman et al 1973) and hypernephroma (a 16% response rate) (Paladine et al 1979, Stolbach et al 1981).

■ Mechanism of Action

Nafoxidine probably acts as a competitive inhibitor of estrogen binding at target tissues. It manifests its antiestrogenic effects by competing with estrogens for cytoplasmic estrogen binding sites or receptors, thus reducing the formation of receptor–estrogen complexes. These complexes in estrogen target tissues are thought to migrate to nuclear sites, where estrogenic action is exerted. Nafoxidine bound to estrogenic receptors appears to have a small intrinsic estrogenic activity but much less than that of the receptor–estradiol complex.

■ Availability and Storage

Nafoxidine was supplied by the National Cancer Institute as oral tablets containing 60 mg of nafoxidine hydrochloride with inert ingredients: spray-dried lactose, starch, magnesium stearate, sodium benzoate, and dioctyl sodium sulfosuccinate. The compound is no longer available.

■ Preparation for Use, Stability, and Admixture

The 60-mg tablets were stable at room temperature for at least 2 years.

■ Administration

Nafoxidine was given orally in either single or divided daily doses.

■ Special Precautions

It was recommended that patients protect themselves from direct sunlight and wear sunglasses to minimize photosensitivity toxicity.

■ Drug Interactions

None are known.

■ Dosage

The usual daily dose of nafoxidine was 180 to 360 mg either given as a single dose or, more commonly, divided into three or four equal portions spaced throughout the day.

■ Pharmacokinetics

No data have been reported for this agent.

■ Side Effects and Toxicity

Dermatitis has been reported in over 50% of treated individuals and consists of dryness of the skin with scaliness and sometimes pruritus. This reaction generally but not always lasts as long as therapy is continued. Its severity is probably related to dose and sunlight exposure in that it is usually worse in the summer months. Increased hair loss has been reported in about 10% of those treated.

Lenticular cataracts have been rarely reported and may be related to the photosensitization effect of the drug. In addition, Paladine et al (1979) reported severe conjunctiva sicca with daily nafoxidine in hypernephroma patients.

Gastrointestinal toxicity consists of nausea. Vomiting is only rarely described. Other side effects include lowering of serum cholesterol and hypercalcemia.

REFERENCES

Bloom HJG, Boesen E. Antiestrogens in treatment of breast cancer: Value of nafoxidine in 52 advanced cases. *Br Med J.* 1974;**2:**7–10.

Engelsman E, Persijn JP, Korsten CB, and Cleton FJ. Oestrogen receptor in human breast cancer tissue and response to endocrine therapy. *Br Med J.* 1973;**2:**750–752.

European Organization for Research and Treatment of Cancer. Breast cancer group clinical trial of nafoxidine, an oestrogen antagonist in advanced breast cancer. *Eur J Cancer.* 1972;**8:**387–389.

Heuson JC, Coune A, Staguet M. Clinical trial of nafoxidine, an antioestrogen in advanced breast cancer. *Eur J Cancer.* 1972;**8:**387–389.

Heuson JC, Engelsman E, Blonk-Van Der Wijst J, et al. Comparative trial of nafoxidine and ethinyloestradiol in advanced breast cancer: An EORTC study. *Br Med J.* 1975;**2:**711–713.

Paladine W, Longacre D, Hemings P, Harper G. Nafoxidine, an antiestrogen in hypernephroma (abstract C-3). *Proc Am Assoc Cancer Res ASCO.* 1979;**20:**293.

Stolbach LL, Bess CB, Hall T, Horton J. Treatment of renal carcinoma: A phase III randomized trial of oral medroxy-progesterone (Provera), hydroxyurea, and nafoxidine. *Cancer Treat Rep.* 1981;**65**(7/8):689–692.

Neocarzinostatin

■ Other Names

NCS; zinostatin; NSC-157365; neocarzinostatin K.

■ Chemistry

Neocarzinostatin is a large macromolecular polypeptide antibiotic (molecular weight 10,700). It is a culture broth isolate from *Streptomyces carzinostaticus* (var. F_{41}) first isolated in 1957. Ishida et al (1965) in Japan later purified the drug and described some of the physicochemical and biologic properties.

Chemically, neocarzinostatin is the first polypeptide antibiotic with a defined amino acid sequence. In addition, the precise structure is also known (Meinhofer et al 1972). The drug is an acidic, single-chain polypeptide of 109 amino acid residues. It has an unusual abundance of alanine (the N-terminal amino acid), glycine, serine, and threonine. Asparagine is the C-terminal amino acid. Notably deficient are histidine and methionine residues; however, two disulfide bridges are present, allowing for crosslinking (Samy et al 1974). In nature, the drug occurs as a tightly folded structure which is thereby highly resistant to enzymatic digestion (Ishida et al 1965).

■ Antitumor Activity

In animal tumor systems, neocarzinostatin has demonstrated non-schedule-dependent activity against L-1210 leukemia, Ehrlich ascites sarcoma, and B-16 melanoma (Legha et al 1976). Resistant murine leukemias are also sensitive to the drug. Large clinical trials of neocarzinostatin in Japan reported substantial activity in both solid tumors (notably pancreatic cancer) and leukemia (Ketsueki 1974, Yagisawa 1975, Masaoka et al 1977). Phase I clinical trials in the United States suggested dose-dependent activity for leukemia (McKelvey et al 1978, 1981, Rivera et al 1978) and possible activity against hepatoma (Griffin et al 1978).

The drug has not been demonstrated to have any significant clinical activity in patients with malignant melanoma, non-small cell lung cancer, small cell lung cancer, hepatoma, bladder cancer, or prostate cancer (Von Hoff et al 1984, Ettinger et al 1983, Creech et al 1984, Natale et al 1980, Falkson et al 1980, 1984). Satake et al (1985) reported one complete regression in a patient with renal cell carcinoma; no other responses were observed in this trial.

■ Mechanism of Action

Several mechanisms are postulated for neocarzinostatin antitumor activity. Initial studies demonstrated selective inhibition of DNA synthesis (Ono et al 1966). Sawada et al (1974) subsequently demonstrated inhibition of thymidine incorporation into DNA. With high doses of neocarzinostatin in vitro, free DNA bases are produced, whereas at intermediate doses, both single and double DNA strand scission may occur (Beerman and Goldberg 1977);

```
Ala-Ala-Pro-Thr-Ala-Thr-Val-Thr-Pro-Ser-Ser-Gly-Leu-Ser-Asp-Gly-Thr-Val-Val-Lys-Val-Ala-Gly-Ala-Gly-
            5                   10                  15                  20                  25

Leu-Gln-Ala-Gly-Thr-Ala-Tyr-Asp-Val-Gly-Gln-Cys-Ala-Ser-Val-Asn-Thr-Gly-Val-Leu-Trp-Asn-Ser-Val-Thr-
            30                  35                  40                  45                  50

Ala-Ala-Gly-Ser-Ala-Cys-Asx-Pro-Ala-Asn-Phe-Ser-Leu-Thr-Val-Arg-Arg-Ser-Phe-Glu-Gly-Phe-Leu-Phe-Asp-
            55                  60                  65                  70                  75

Gly-Thr-Arg-Trp-Gly-Thr-Val-Asx-Cys-Thr-Thr-Ala-Ala-Cys-Gln-Val-Gly-Leu-Ser-Asp-Ala-Ala-Gly-Asp-Gly-
            80                  85                  90                  95                  100

Glu-Pro-Gly-Val-Ala-Ile-Ser-Phe-Asn
            105
```

Amino acid sequence of neocarzinostatin

however, the major cytotoxic effect of the drug appears to involve not DNA degradation but interference with DNA template activity (Tsuro et al 1971). More recent observations suggest a possible role for disruption of cell membrane function (Lazarus et al 1977) and/or inhibition of specific cell surface immunoglobin reactions, effects similar to those produced by the microtubular poisons colchicine and vinblastine (Ebina and Ishida 1975).

Bhuyan et al (1972) have shown that cytotoxicity was limited to those cells in G_1, G_2, and M phases of the cell cycle. Furthermore, they confirmed that cell cycle progression is halted by the drug in G_2 without perturbing S phase. Thus, overall, neocarzinostatin arrests cells in the G_2 phase of the cycle.

■ Availability and Storage

Neocarzinostatin is an investigational agent provided by the National Cancer Institute and available in 2000-U (2-mg) ampules for injection. It is supplied as a clear, colorless solution containing, per milliliter, 1000 U neocarzinostatin in 0.015 M acetic acid–sodium acetate buffer, pH 5.0. When stored under refrigeration as recommended (below 4°C), the aqueous drug is stable for at least 2 years. The compound is both hygroscopic and light sensitive. Therefore, it should always remain in the original amber ampule protected from light until used. At room temperature, intact vials retain their potency for several weeks if protected from direct light. Kohno et al (1974), however, documented relatively slow decomposition with storage at room temperature (22–25°C): approximately 10% loss of potency over an 8-month period.

■ Preparation for Use, Stability, and Admixture

Pharmaceutically, neocarzinostatin powder is hygroscopic and thermally unstable at room temperature (Kohno et al 1974). It is also inactivated by natural and ultraviolet light. Additionally, the drug is known to be water soluble and lipid insoluble. The compound is assayed biologically by relative antibacterial activity in *Sarcina lutea*, and concentration is expressed in units (1 U = 1 mg).

Neocarzinostatin ampules, 2000 U/ampule, are usually diluted to a final concentration of 2 to 5 U/mL in either D5W or Normal Saline for Injection, USP. If protected from light, either solution retains chemical potency for at least 24 hours. Because of the extreme light sensitivity, drug syringes for intravenous push administration should optimally be wrapped with foil or light-occlusive material and used immediately after reconstitution. Exposed to sunlight, concentrated (500–4500 U/mL) neocarzinostatin solutions have been documented to lose 50 to 70% antibacterial potency in less than 3 minutes.

Neocarzinostatin is relatively acid stable with an optimal pH for stability ranging between 4.5 and 5.5. Above pH 6.6, degradation is significantly enhanced. Legha et al (1976) report that the drug is stable in solutions of amino acids, sugars, or organic salts but would be inactivated in solutions containing reducing and/or proteolytic substances. Thus, with proper light precautions, all standard infusion solutions may be used for administration.

■ Administration

Neocarzinostatin is most often given as a rapid intravenous infusion over 10 to 20 minutes. Animal toxicity studies have documented local inflammation and necrosis with subcutaneous or intramuscular injections. Therefore, these routes are definitely contraindicated for clinical trials in humans.

Because of the potential for serious local necrosis with extravasation of the drug, only new, unquestionably patent venipuncture sites should be used. A 5- to 10-mL flush of normal saline before and after drug administration is recommended to respectively confirm vein patency and flush any remaining drug from the administration tubing.

Ohnuma et al (1977) studied neocarzinostatin given as a 2-hour infusion or as a continuous infusion for as long as 120 hours. Toxicity with the latter method appeared to be quantitatively reduced and qualitatively favored myelosuppression. Thus, continuous infusions appear to allow the safe use of substantially higher total doses of the drug (see Dosage).

■ Special Precautions

Neocarzinostatin can produce severe local tissue necrosis if extravasation occurs. Therefore, extravasation of the drug must be prevented. The drug is antigenic and produces a high incidence of anaphylactic reactions following repeated injections. Therefore, resuscitative facilities and medical personnel should be readily available during treatments with this agent.

■ Drug Interactions

Neocarzinostatin has variably shown synergism with cytarabine and daunomycin in L-1210 murine leukemia (Fujimoto et al 1974).

■ Dosage

In Japanese studies of neocarzinostatin in leukemia, the dosing schedule was 0.04 to 0.06 mg/kg (1.5 to 2.25 mg/m^2)/d × 15 days (Masaoka et al 1974, Kitajima et al 1975). Courses were repeated in 7- to 10-day intervals depending on the resolution of toxicity. In patients with solid tumors, the daily dose ranged from 2 to 6 mg (average 3 mg) given for 15 to 20 days (Ishida et al 1975). These courses were then repeated at 10- to 20-day intervals. Ishi and Nakamura (1974) used similar total doses given continuously on alternative days.

American phase I investigations by Griffen et al (1978) determined a maximally tolerated dose of 2250 U/m^2/d × 5 given each day as a rapid intravenous injection. In the pediatric study by Rivera et al (1978) a dose range of 3000 to 4500 U/m^2/wk was administered as a slow (10-minute) injection. This was the recommended range for phase II trials in acute leukemia in which activity was suggested.

Ohnuma et al (1977) studied neocarzinostatin given either by continuous infusion or as a 2-hour infusion. For continuous infusions, the maximally tolerated dose was 4500 U/m^2/d × 5 for solid tumors and 6000 U/m^2/d × 5 for patients with acute leukemia. Thus, toxicity appears to be significantly different with continuous drug administration, allowing the use of substantially higher total doses.

■ Pharmacokinetics

Comis et al (1979) described the pharmacokinetics of neocarzinostatin in humans. Basically, two kinetic phases were described: a short initial distribution phase (half-life, 10.5 minutes) unaffected by renal function and a longer secondary elimination phase markedly affected by renal function. In patients with creatinine clearances above 40 mL/min, this elimination half-life varied from 40 to 90 minutes (mean, 73 minutes). With a creatinine clearance (CrCl) below 40 mL/min, the elimination half-life appeared markedly prolonged: 4 hours with a CrCl of 25 mg/min and 7 hours with a CrCl of 15 mL/min (data from only one patient each). The mean elimination half-life in this group (CrCl < 40 mL/min) was approximately 3.7 hours. Dosage reductions of 50% were recommended in the latter group by Hall et al (1983).

Hall and colleagues (1983) found that the drug was eliminated in a multiphasic manner. Mean plasma half-lives were (α) 0.50 and (β) 7.7 hours. The mean plasma clearance was 32.4 mL/min with an apparent volume of distribution of 19.3 L/mL.

In the blood, neocarzinostatin appears to be neither protein bound nor degraded. In humans, the volume of drug distribution is 12 L, or 16% of total body weight. The drug has not been detectable in pleural and peritoneal effusions (Comis et al 1979).

Neocarzinostatin appears to be excreted primarily in the urine. Urinary excretion data show total drug recovery by 24 hours, with slower recovery for patients with renal impairment. Significant metabolism or hepatobiliary excretion was not observed in the study of Comis et al. They also observed that the drug may be found immunochemically intact in the urine. Thus, glomerular filtration appears to be the singular method of drug elimination.

Otsuka et al (1989) found that neocarzinostatin penetrates brain tumor tissue after a bolus injection. They showed that cerebrospinal fluid concentrations of neocarzinostatin are about 16% of simultaneous plasma concentrations.

■ Side Effects and Toxicity

Neocarzinostatin has demonstrated a wide spectrum of clinical toxic effects. Historically, there is some difficulty in interpreting the early studies with neocarzinostatin because the dose varied so widely in the Japanese studies and because the early American formulation by Bristol Laboratories (NSC-69856) constituted a relatively crude preparation. There is also the suggestion by Ohnuma et al (1977) that toxicity is quantitatively reduced with continuous drug infusions.

The typical acute toxic reaction, occurring with the initial short infusion of the drug, consists of a single episode of shaking chills. The onset is rapid, within 0.5 to 1 hour of administration. This may be accompanied by fever, tachycardia, and/or cyanosis (rigor). Rivera et al (1978) noted that the reactions were transient and that patients usually responded to intravenous antihistamines. Griffen et al (1978) additionally documented a prophylactic benefit of 50 mg (IV) of diphenhydramine in adults.

Hypersensitivity reactions of an anaphylactoid

nature are reported in about 3 to 5% of patients. The typical symptoms include wheezing, facial edema, and hypotension. To date, these reactions have always abated with prompt intravenous epinephrine and hydrocortisone. Griffen et al (1978) have successfully re-treated a patient after such an episode using intravenous hydrocortisone prophylaxis.

Gastrointestinal toxicity appears to be mild with this drug. Usually only transient episodes of anorexia or vomiting occur.

Hematologic toxicity appears to be unpredictable with neocarzinostatin. The incidence of serious myelosuppression is low, occurring in about 25% of cases. There is a suggestion of a dose–response relationship with the myelosuppression (Aneha et al 1974). Again, the continuous-infusion study of Ohnuma et al (1977) is of significance in that myelotoxicity became the predominate dose-limiting effect. This contrasts with studies using short infusions wherein the acute reactions described are the more prominent toxic features.

Significant thrombocytopenia (platelet count < 100,000/mm^3) was rare in the Japanese reports. The overall incidence was about 14% (Ishi and Nakamura 1974). Phase I studies in the United States have demonstrated a greater significance of this toxicity. Griffen et al (1978) noted prolonged thrombocytopenia with both repeated courses and in patients previously treated with other marrow-suppressive drugs.

Dermatologic toxicity is limited to a mild skin rash noted in 4% of Japanese patients studied. Interestingly, attempts to scratch test with neocarzinostatin to predict anaphylaxis or other severe hypersensitivity reactions have not been successful. Two episodes of serious drug extravasation were reported by Griffen et al (1978). The severe cutaneous ulcerations produced by neocarzinostatin eventually required skin grafting in both cases.

Although slight hepatic and renal toxic effects are reported in the Japanese studies, significant defects in these organ systems have not been observed in the phase I American investigations. Other rare neocarzinostatin toxic effects have included headache, fatigue, and a possible drug-induced interstitial pneumonitis (Griffen et al 1978, Weiss and Muggia 1980, Natale et al 1980, Calvo et al 1981).

■ Special Applications

Besides antitumor activity, the compound has demonstrated potent antibiotic action against certain gram-positive bacteria including *Staphylococcus aureus* and *Sarcina lutea,* the biologic assay organism (Ishida et al 1965). Recently, a congener of neocarzinostatin, called SMANCS (copoly[styrene] maleic acid-conjugated neocarzinostatin) has been shown to have superior in vitro activity. The compound is undergoing phase II testing in Japan (Oda et al 1989, Koono and Maeda 1988).

REFERENCES

Aneha T, Kikuchi K, Kanno H. Administration of antineoplastic agent of high molecular weight, neocarzinostatin, in cases of gastric cancer. *Jpn J Clin Med.* 1974; **32:**870–874.

Beerman TA, Goldberg IH. Characterization of DNA strand breakage *in vitro* by the antitumor protein neocarzinostatin. *Biochemistry.* 1977;**16:**486–493.

Bhuyan BK, Scheidt LG, Fraser TJ. Cell cycle phase specificity of antitumor agents. *Cancer Res.* 1972;**32:**398–407.

Calvo DB III, Legha SS, McKelvey EM, Bodey GP, Dail DH. Zinostatin-related pulmonary toxicity (letter). *Cancer Treat Rep.* 1981;**65**(1/2):165–167.

Comis RL, Griffen TW, Raso V, Ginsberg SJ. Pharmacokinetics of the protein antitumor antibiotic neocarzinostatin after bolus injection in humans. *Cancer Res.* 1979; **39:**757–761.

Creech RH, Tritchler D, Ettinger DS, et al. Phase II study of PALA, amsacrine, teniposide, and zinostatin in small cell lung carcinoma (EST 2479). *Cancer Treat Rep.* 1984;**68**(9):1183–1184.

Ebina T, Ishida N. Inhibition of formation of microtubular paracrystals in He-La-S3 cells by neocarzinostatin. *Cancer Res.* 1975;**35:**3705–3709.

Ettinger DS, Day R, Ferraro JA, et al. A randomized phase II study of *m*-AMSA (NSC-249992) and neocarzinostatin (NSC-157365) in non-small cell bronchogenic carcinoma. An Eastern Cooperative Group study. *Am J Clin Oncol.* 1983;**6**(2):167–170.

Falkson G, MacIntyre JM, Schutt AJ, et al. Neocarzinostatin versus *m*-AMSA or doxorubicin in hepatocellular carcinoma. *J Clin Oncol.* 1984;**2**(6):581–584.

Falkson G, Von Hoff D, Klaassen D, et al. A phase II study of neocarzinostatin (NSC-157365) in malignant hepatoma. An Eastern Cooperative Oncology Group pilot study. *Cancer Chemother Pharmacol.* 1980;**4**(1):33–36.

Fujimoto S, Inagaki J, Hirokoshi N. Antitumor effects of neocarzinostatin in L1210 mouse leukemia. *Cancer Chemother.* 1974;**5:**850–860.

Griffen TW, Comis RL, Lokich JJ, Blum RH, Canellos GP. Phase I and preliminary phase II study of neocarzinostatin. *Cancer Treat Rep.* 1978;**62**(12):2019–2025.

Hall SW, Knight J, Broughton A, Benjamin RS, McKelvey E. Clinical pharmacology of the anticancer polypeptide neocarzinostatin. *Cancer Chemother Pharmacol.* 1983; **10**(3):200–204.

Ishi K, Nakamura K. Cooperative studies on pancreatic cancer by using neocarzinostatin. *Cancer Chemother Tokyo.* 1974;**1**:433–439.

Ishida N, Ishi K, Kitajima K, Hirati K, Kikuchi M. Clinical evaluation of antitumor protein neocarzinostatin. *Prog Chemother.* 1975;**3**:927–940.

Ishida N, Miyazaki K, Kumagai K, Rikimaru M. Neocarzinostatin, an antitumor antibiotic of high molecular weight, isolation, physiochemical properties and biological activities. *J Antibiot (Tokyo).* 1965;**18**:68–76.

Ketsueki R. Treatment of acute leukemia with neocarzinostatin. *Jpn J Clin Hematol.* 1974;**15**:1309–1316.

Kitajima K, Nagao T, Takahashi I, et al. Cooperative studies on the effects of neocarzinostatin against acute leukemia. *Clin Rep.* 1975;**9**:180–189.

Kohno M, Haneda I, Koyama Y, Kucki M. Studies on the stability of antitumor protein neocarzinostatin. *Jpn J Antibiot.* 1974;**27**:708–724.

Koono T, Maeda H. Targeting cancer chemotherapy using lipoidal as a carrier of anticancer drugs for hepatocellular carcinoma. *Ganto Kasaku Ryoho.* 1988;**4**(pt 2-1):1043–1050.

Lazarus H, Raso V, Samy TSA. *In vitro* inhibition of human leukemic cells (CCRF/CEM) by agarose-immobilized neocarzinostatin. *Cancer Res.* 1977;**37**:3731–3736.

Legha S, Von Hoff DD, Rozencweig M, Abraham D, Slavik M, Muggia M. Neocarzinostatin (NSC-157365) a new cancerostatic compound. *Oncology.* 1976;**33**:265–270.

Masaoka T, Hasegawa Y, Yoshitake J, et al. Mode of decrease of leukemic cells and leukocytes during neocarzinostatin treatment. *Cancer Treat Rep.* 1977;**61**: 73–75.

McKelvey EM, Burgess MA, McCredie KB, Gerald PB. Neocarzinostatin: A phase I clinical trial. *Proc Am Assoc Cancer Res ASCO.* 1978;**19**:186.

McKelvey EM, Murphy W, Zander A, Bodey GP. Neocarzinostatin: Report of a phase II clinical trial. *Cancer Treat Rep.* 1981;**65**(7/8):699–701.

Meinhofer J, Maeda H, Glaser CB, Kivimizu K. Primary structure of the antitumor protein neocarzinostatin. *Science.* 1972;**178**:875–876.

Natale RB, Agoda A, Watson RC, Stover DE. Phase II trial of neocarzinostatin in patients with bladder and prostatic cancer: Toxicity of a five-day iv bolus schedule. *Cancer.* 1980;**45**(11):2836–2842.

Oda T, Sato F, Yamamoto H, Akasi M, Maeda H. Cytotoxicity of SMANCS in comparison with other anticancer agents against various cells in culture. *Anticancer Res.* 1989;**9**(2):261–265.

Ohnuma T, Nogeire C, Cuttner J, Holland JF. Initial clinical studies with neocarzinostatin (NCS). *Proc Am Assoc Cancer Res ASCO.* 1977;**18**:332.

Ono Y, Watanabe Y, Ishida N. Mode of action of neocarzinostatin inhibition of DNA synthesis and degradation of DNA in *Sarcina iutea. Biochim Biophys Acta.* 1966; **199**:46–58.

Otsuka T, Matsukado Y, Uemura S, et al. Pharmacokinetics of neocarzinostatin in patients with malignant glioma. Quantitative analysis of tissue concentration. *Neurol Med Chir (Tokyo).* 1989;**29**(6):471–475.

Rivera G, Howarth C, Aur RJA, Pratt CB. Phase I study of neocarzinostatin in children with cancer. *Cancer Treat Rep.* 1978;**62**(12):2015–2107.

Samy TSA, Atreyi M, Maeda H, Mainhota J. Selective tryptophan oxidation in the antitumor protein neocarzinostatin and effects on conformation and biological activity. *Biochemistry.* 1974;**1**:1007–1013.

Satake I, Tari K, Yamamoto M, Nishimura H. Neocarzinostatin-induced complete regression of metastatic renal cell carcinoma. *J Urol.* 1985;**133**(1):87–89.

Sawada H, Tatsumi K, Sasada M, Shirakawa S, Nakamura T, Wakisaka G. Effect of neocarzinostatin on DNA synthesis in L1210 cells. *Cancer Res.* 1974;**34**:3341–3346.

Tsuro T, Satoh H, Ukita T. Effect of the antitumor antibiotic neocarzinostatin on DNA synthesis *in vitro. J Antibiot (Tokyo).* 1971;**24**:423–429.

Von Hoff DD, Amato DA, Kaufman JH, Falkson G, Cunningham TJ. Randomized trial of chlorozotocin, neocarzinostatin, or methyl-CCNU in patients with malignant melanoma. *Am J Clin Oncol.* 1984;**7**(2):135–139.

Weiss RB, Muggia FM. Cytotoxic drug-induced pulmonary disease: Update 1980. *Am J Med.* 1980;**68**(2):259–266.

Octreotide Acetate

■ Other Names

Sandostatin® (Sandoz Pharmaceuticals Corporation); SMS 201-995.

■ Chemistry

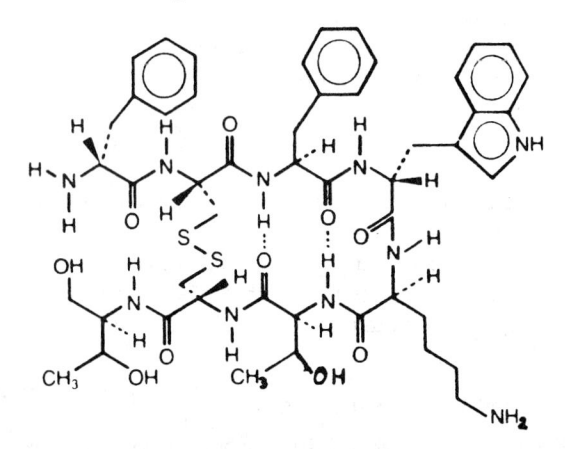

Structure of octreotide acetate

Octreotide is a cyclic octapeptide with the chemical name D-phenylalanyl-L-cysteinyl-L-phenylalanyl-D-tryptophyl-L-lysyl-L-threonyl-N-[2-hydroxy-1-(hydroxymethyl)propyl]-L-cysteinamide, cyclic(2→7) disulfide,[R-(R*,R*)] acetate saH. A disulfide linkage at the two cysteines (positions 2 and 7) cyclizes the otherwise linear molecule. The molecular weight of the free peptide is 1019.3 and the molecular formula $C_{40}H_{66}N_{10}O_{10}S_2$. Octreotide is a synthetic, D-amino acid-substituted derivative of the natural tetradecapeptide somatostatin, a hypothalamic releasing factor inhibitor (Pless et al 1986). As such, it is more active than somatostatin because of blocked enzymatic degradation (Bauer et al 1982) and enhanced binding affinity at the somatostatin receptor.

■ Antitumor Activity

Octreotide is used to suppress the secretory symptoms of neuroendocrine tumors of the gut. This includes palliation of the severe diarrhea and flushing associated with the malignant carcinoid syndrome (Kvols et al 1986) and the profuse watery diarrhea associated with vasoactive intestinal peptide tumors (VIPomas, also known as the pancreatic cholera syndrome) (Santangelo et al 1985, Maton et al 1985, Kraenzlin et al 1985). In the treatment of VIPomas, octreotide also improves certain electrolyte abnormalities such as hypokalemia, excess chloride secretion, and acidosis. There is also a suggestion of VIPoma tumor mass regression after long-term octreotide therapy (Santangelo et al 1985).

Response rates of over 72% are reported in metastatic carcinoid and the carcinoid syndrome (Kvols et al 1986). A decrease of more than 50% in urinary 5-hydroxyindoleacetic acid (5-HIAA, a serotonin breakdown product) is used as the objective indicator of octreotide response in this disease. Importantly, responses can be very prolonged with octreotide and include patients previously treated with surgery, hepatic artery ligation, and/or chemotherapy (5-fluorouracil, doxorubicin, dacarbazine, or streptozocin). Most of the improvements occur during the first month of therapy and remain relatively constant thereafter (Kvols and Buck 1987).

Patients with VIPomas of the pancreatic islet cell experience sudden intense secretory diarrhea and electrolyte disorders, principally a loss of sodium chloride and bicarbonate. Profound hypokalemia and gastric achlorhydria can ensue because of the excess secretion of vasoactive intestinal polypeptide (VIP) from multiple tumor masses in the gut and pancreas. Octreotide improves diarrhea within the first 2 weeks of therapy (Santangelo et al 1987). Other biochemical effects clear at about the same time. Response rates up to 89% have been observed in early VIPoma trials. Long-term responses can be obtained in VIPomas even though circulating VIP levels are not continually suppressed (Anderson and Bloom 1986). Actual VIPoma tumor regression is also sometimes noted following octreotide (Schally 1988).

Octreotide is active in a variety of amine precursor uptake and decarboxylation (APUD) tumors (Dunne and Kutz 1988). These include glucagonomas, insulinomas, gastrinomas, and tumors involving growth hormone-releasing factor (Marbach et al 1985). Endocrine symptoms respond rapidly in association with a fall in circulating tumor peptides.

Acromegaly is also effectively managed by chronic octreotide therapy (Bloom 1987a, Yen et al 1974) without any evidence of the tachyphylaxis seen in rats treated chronically with somatostatin (Lamberts 1987). In addition, octreotide can inhibit pancreatic and breast cancers in experimental animal models (Schally 1988). Human breast cancers are also directly inhibited in vitro (Setyono-Han et al 1987); however, in humans with metastatic pancreatic, gastric, or colorectal cancer, octreotide reduces somatomedin or insulin-like growth factor I after 8 to 13 weeks without inducing objective antitumor responses (Klijn et al 1987).

■ Mechanism of Action

Octreotide mimics somatostatin, a hypothalamic peptide that naturally inhibits the release of a variety of endocrine polypeptide hormones including growth hormone, secretin, motilin, pancreatic polypeptide, glucagon, gastric inhibitory peptide, and insulin (Bloom 1987b). Like somatostatin, octreotide induces a marked suppression of the growth hormone response to hypoglycemia without affecting the adrenocorticotropin or cortisol responses (Lightman et al 1986). Somatostatin has been identified in the D cells of the pancreatic islets (Luft et al 1984), in the D cells of the stomach and intestine (Polak et al 1975), and in the central nervous system, heart, eye, thyroid, thymus, and skin (Dunne and Kutz 1988). Receptors for somatostatin (and octreotide) are similarly distributed widely but are concentrated in the gut. In the rat pituitary, octreotide displaces somatostatin from a subset of about 75% of the high-affinity binding sites, K_D = 0.74 nM (Pless et al 1986). In patients with acromegaly as a result of pituitary adenomas, the K_D for somatostatin receptors in excised pituitaries varied from 0.24 to 1.48 nM, with a β_{max} or binding site concentration of 103 to 1058 fmol/mg of protein (Reubin and Landolt 1984).

In APUD tumors, octreotide suppresses exocrine and endocrine pancreatic function and inhibits the secretion of gut peptides. In this regard, octreotide is approximately 45 times more potent than somatostatin, the natural exocrine inhibitor released from the hypothalamus (Bauer et al 1982). The increased potency relates both to prolonged stability of octreotide, a result of the D-amino acid substitutions, and to a slower "off rate" from the somatostatin receptor (Bauer et al 1982). Activity appears to be enhanced further by subcutaneous administration (Pless et al 1986). There is also some evidence for direct inhibitory action on tumor cells expressing somatostatin receptors (Setyono-Han et al 1987). In human MCF-7 breast cancer cells, high-affinity, saturable somatostatin binding sites have been identified. Furthermore, growth inhibition by octreotide was defined by bell-shaped curves, with maximal inhibition achieved at a 10 nM concentration (Setyono-Han et al 1987).

■ Availability and Storage

Octreotide is commercially available as the acetate salt in ampules containing either 0.05, 0.1, or 0.5 mg/mL of solution (Sandostatin®, Sandoz Pharmaceuticals Corporation, East Hanover, New Jersey). In addition to the acetate, each milliliter of solution also contains 2 mg glacial acetic acid, 2 mg sodium acetate trihydrate, and 7 mg sodium chloride to provide a buffered solution at a pH of about 4.2. A patient home administration kit containing alcohol swabs and an ampule opener is also available. The ampules are stored under refrigeration but can be stored at room temperature for the day of use.

■ Preparation for Use, Stability, and Admixture

The ampule is snapped open and the correct volume of octreotide is aspirated aseptically into a syringe. A filter needle may also be used to withdraw the dose to reduce the likelihood of glass particle contamination. All solutions should be visually inspected and discarded if particulates or discoloration is observed. Prolonged storage of opened ampules is not recommended as no antibacterial agent is present. Admixture with any other medication is also not recommended. Doses should be used immediately after preparation.

■ Administration

Octreotide is administered by subcutaneous injection into areas of body fat (thigh, arm, abdomen). As with insulin therapy, the injection site should be rotated frequently to avoid local site irritation. Multiple injections at the same site over a short period are not recommended. In emergency settings, octreotide can also be administered as an intravenous bolus.

The drug is usually administered two or three times daily to provide for more continuous suppression of peptide hormone release.

■ Dosage

The initial subcutaneous dose is 50 μg given once or twice daily. Dosing is titrated over the first 2 weeks to a range of 100 to 600 μg/d in two or three fractions. Adjustments are based on symptom suppression, primarily diarrhea. Doses above 450 μg are generally not needed although intravenous bolus injections of up to 1000 μg have been well tolerated in healthy volunteers. Patients aged 1 to 83 years have received octreotide without toxicity or special dosing considerations. In pediatric patients, doses of 1 to 10 μg/kg have been well tolerated; however, patients with severe renal dysfunction requiring hemodialysis may require lower octreotide doses because of impaired drug clearance (Sandoz Pharmaceuticals Corporation 1988).

■ Drug Interactions

Octreotide can cause transient hypo- or hyperglycemia and could therefore alter the response to other drugs used to control blood sugar. These would include insulin, diazoxide, sulfonylureas, and beta blockers. Octreotide has also been reported to decrease the blood levels of orally administered cyclosporine, leading to renal transplant rejection in a single patient. This was possibly due to the effect of octreotide on fluid and nutrient absorption. The oral absorption of other drugs may be similarly affected by octreotide. Decreased absorption of dietary fats could theoretically lead to low levels of fat-soluble vitamins. This can be monitored by a 72-hour fecal fat test and determination of serum β-carotene levels.

Pharmacokinetics

The bioavailability of a subcutaneous octreotide injection is about 100% (range, 80–135%), with peak concentrations achieved 0.4 hours after dosing. Clearance of the drug is relatively rapid but much slower than that of somatostatin (see table below). Thus, octreotide has a much longer plasma half-life of 1.5 hours as a result of blocked catabolism of the protein (see table).

In healthy volunteers there is a proportional increase in the area under the plasma concentration curve (AUC) with subcutaneous drug doses up to 400 μg. For doses of 50, 100, 200, and 400 μg the mean $AUC_{(0-)}$ values for octreotide were 320, 650, 1500, and 3100 ng/mL/min, respectively (Kutz et al 1986). Peak drug levels of 2.4, 4.4, 10.6, and 23.5 ng/mL were reported for the same four dose levels, respectively (Kutz et al 1986). There is some suggestion that clearance is reduced by 66% with high doses of 600 μg/d compared with doses of 150 μg/d.

About 65% of the drug is bound to plasma proteins, primarily to lipoprotein and, to a lesser extent, albumin. There is negligible uptake into erythrocytes. Octreotide is slowly catabolized to inactive peptide fragments but about 32% of a dose is excreted unchanged into the urine. Thus, patients with severe renal insufficiency requiring dialysis have markedly reduced clearance from 10 L/h (or 166 mL/min) to 4.5 h (75 mL/min). The effect of hepatic dysfunction on drug clearance is unknown.

Side Effects and Toxicity

The primary toxic effect of octreotide is gastrointestinal upset, principally nausea (8%), abdominal pain (9%), and loose stools (4–6%). Diarrhea may occur in about 7% of patients. Rare gastrointestinal side effects include constipation, flatulence, rectal spasms, and a "bloated" stomach sensation. Documented fat malabsorption is reported in less than 3% of patients. Jaundice and/or liver enzyme elevation is also rare.

Local site reactions include pain in 7.5% of patients. A local wheal or erythema at the injection site is reported in about 1% of patients. Other rare integumentary effects include hair loss, skin flaking or thinning, pruritus, rash, and bruising or bleeding from a superficial wound.

Cardiovascular reactions are rare. They include dizziness, hypertension, thrombophlebitis, orthostatic hypotension, palpitation or chest pain, and congestive heart failure, which is exceedingly uncommon. Flushing is described in 1.4% of patients but edema is noted in only 1% of patients.

Rare central nervous system effects include anxiety, anorexia, depression, hyperesthesia, decreased libido, nervousness and shaking, syncope, insomnia, and tremor.

Endocrine side effects include hypo- or hyperglycemia in 1 to 2% of patients each. Rare endocrine effects include galactorrhea and hypothyroidism associated with a low total and free thyroxine value without an elevation in thyroid-stimulating hormone. These findings suggest a hypothalamic-pituitary dysfunction produced by octreotide. Fasting plasma glucagon levels are known to fall following somatostatin in insulin-dependent diabetics (Gerich et al 1974); however, this can be used therapeutically as an adjunct to insulin to reduce postprandial hyperglycemia.

REFERENCES

Anderson JV, Bloom SR. Neuroendocrine tumors of the gut: Long-term therapy with the somatostatin analogue SMS 201-995. *Scand J Gastroenterol.* 1986;**21**(suppl 119):115–128.

CLINICAL PHARMACOKINETICS OF OCTREOTIDE COMPARED WITH SOMATOSTATIN

	Renal Function	Plasma Half-life (h) α	Plasma Half-life (h) β	Volume of Distribution	Clearance (L/h)	Peak Time, SC (min)
Octreotide*	Normal	0.2	1.5	13.6	10	30
	Impaired	—	—	—	4.5	—
Somatostatin[†]	Normal	—	0.001–0.05 (1–3 min)	—	—	—

*Sandostatin® Package Insert and Kutz et al 1986.
[†]Sheppard et al 1979.

Bauer W, Briner U, Doepfner W, et al. SMS 201-995: A very potent and selective octapeptide analogue of somatostatin with prolonged action. *Life Sci.* 1982;**31**:1133–1140.

Bloom SR. Acromegaly. *Am J Med.* 1987a;**82**(suppl 5B):88–91.

Bloom SR. Somatostatin analogue treatment of endocrine tumors. In: Klijn JGM, Paridaens R, Foekens JA, eds. *Hormonal Manipulation of Cancer: Peptides, Growth Factors, and New (Anti) Steroidal Agents.* New York: Raven Press; 1987b:451–457.

Dunne MJ, Kutz K. Somatostatin analogues in cancer treatment. In: Stoll BA, ed. *Endocrine Management of Cancer.* Basel: Karger; 1988:65–79.

Gerich JE, Lorenzi M, Schneider V, et al. Effects of somatostatin on plasma glucose and glucagon levels in human diabetes mellitus: Pathophysiologic and therapeutic implications. *N Engl J Med.* 1974;**291**:544–547.

Klijn JGM, Setyono-Han B, Bakker GH, et al. Effects of somatostatin analog (Sandostatin®) treatment in experimental and human cancer. In: Klijn JGM, Paridaens R, Foekens JA, eds. *Hormonal Manipulation of Cancer: Peptides, Growth Factors, and New (Anti) Steroidal Agents.* New York: Raven Press; 1987:459–468.

Kraenzlin ME, Ching JLC, Wood SM, et al. Long term treatment of a VIPoma with a somatostatin analog resulting in remission of symptoms and possible shrinkage of metastases. *Gastroenterology.* 1985;**88**:185–187.

Kutz K, Nuesch E, Rosenthaler J. Pharmacokinetics of SMS 201-995 in healthy subjects. *Scand J Gastroenterol.* 1986;**21**(suppl 119);65–72.

Kvols LK, Buck M. Chemotherapy of metastatic carcinoid and islet cell tumors. *Am J Med.* 1987;**82**(suppl 5B):77–83.

Kvols LK, Moertel CG, O'Connell MJ, et al. Treatment of the malignant carcinoid syndrome: Evaluation of a long-acting somatostatin analogue. *N Engl J Med.* 1986;**315**:663–666.

Lamberts SWJ. Somatostatin analog treatment of pituitary tumors. In: Klijn JGM, Paridaens R, Foekens JA, eds. *Hormonal Manipulation of Cancer: Peptides, Growth Factors, and New (Anti) Steroidal Agents.* New York: Raven Press; 1987:441–450.

Lightman SL, Fox P, Dunne MJ. The effect of SMS 201-995, a long-acting somatostatin analogue, on anterior pituitary function in healthy male volunteers. *Scand J Gastroenterol.* 1986;**21**(suppl 119):84–95.

Luft R, Efendic S, Hokfelt T, et al. Immunohistochemical evidence for localization of somatostatin-like immunoreactivity in a cell population of the pancreatic islets. *Med Biol.* 1984;**52**:428–430.

Marbach P, Neufeld M, Pless J. Clinical applications of somatostatin analogs. In: Patel YC, Tannenbaum GS, eds. *Somatostatin.* New York: Plenum Press; 1985:339–353.

Maton P, O'Dorisio TM, Howe BA, et al. Effect of a long-acting somatostatin analog (SMS-201-995) in a patient with pancreatic cholera. *N Engl J Med.* 1985;**312**:17–21.

Pless J, Bauer W, Briner U, et al. Chemistry and pharmacology of SMS 201-995, a long-acting octapeptide analogue of somatostatin. *Scand J Gastroenterol.* 1986;**21**:54–64.

Polak JM, Pearse AGE, Grimelius L, et al. Growth hormone release-inhibiting hormone in gastrointestinal and pancreatic D-cells. *Lancet.* 1975;**1**:.1220–1222.

Reubin JC, Landolt AJ. High density of somatostatin receptors in pituitary tumors from acromegalic patients. *J Clin Endocrinol Metab.* 1984;**59**:1148–1151.

Sandoz Pharmaceuticals Corporation. *Sandostatin® (Octreotide Acetate/Sandoz): Stopping Symptoms Through the Power of Inhibition.* Pharmacy Fact Sheet PA-15 11/88. East Hanover, NJ: Sandoz; 1988.

Santangelo WC, Dueno MI, Krejs GJ. Pseudopancreatic cholera syndrome: Effect of a synthetic somatostatin-analogue, SMS 201-995. *Am J Med.* 1987;**82**(suppl 5B):84–87.

Santangelo WC, O'Dorisio TM, Kim JG, et al. Pancreatic cholera syndrome: Effect of a synthetic somatostatin analog on intestinal water and ion transport. *Ann Intern Med.* 1985;**103**:363–367.

Schally A. Oncological applications of somatostatin analogs. *Cancer Res.* 1988;**48**:6977–6985.

Setyono-Han B, Henkelman MS, Foekens JA, Klijn JGM. Direct inhibitory effects of somatostatin (analogues) in the growth of human breast cancer cells. *Cancer Res.* 1987;**47**:1566–1570.

Sheppard M, Shapiro B, Pimstone B, et al. Metabolic clearance and plasma half-disappearance time of exogenous somatostatin in man. *J Clin Endocrinol Metab.* 1979;**48**:50–53.

Yen SSC, Siler TM, DeVane GW. Effect of somatostatin in patients with acromegaly: Suppression of growth hormone, prolactin, insulin and glucose levels. *N Engl J Med.* 1974;**290**:935–938.

Ormaplatin

■ Other Names

NSC-363812; tetraplatin.

■ Chemistry

Structure of ormaplatin

Ormaplatin is a second-generation platinum analog with the chemical name tetrachloro (*d*, *l*-trans)-1,2-diaminocyclohexane platinum(IV) (Anderson et al 1986). The molecular formula is $C_6H_{14}Cl_4N_2Pt$ and the molecular weight 451.09. It is supplied as the racemic mixture of L-*trans*-(*S,S*), diaminecyclohexane-D-*trans*-(*R,R*), and *cis* enantiomers, each having slightly different cytotoxic potencies (Kido et al 1992).

Antitumor Activity

Ormaplatin demonstrated equal or greater cytotoxic activity than cisplatin in L-1210 murine leukemia (Rahman et al 1988). In addition, ormaplatin demonstrated consistent activity in cisplatin-resistant forms of L-1210 leukemia studied both in vitro (Harrap et al 1987, Orr et al 1989) and in vivo (De-Koning et al 1988, Wilkoff et al 1987, Anderson et al 1986). The drug is active in other preclinical tumor models including murine P-388 leukemia, B-16 melanoma, and M-5076 sarcoma (Anderson et al 1986) and human 8226 myeloma (Kendall et al 1989). Murine plasmacytomas are also sensitive to the drug (Harrap et al 1987), as are human ovarian cancer cells in vitro (Kendall et al 1989, Behrens et al 1987). The mouse tumors colon-38 and pancreas-02 are sensitive to ormaplatin, wherein cisplatin has little activity.

In vitro, the *d-trans-(R,R)* isomer of ormaplatin is sixfold more cytotoxic than racemic ormaplatin. This is followed by the *l-trans* isomer and cisplatin in descending order of magnitude. This difference in cytotoxic potency appears to be a result of the enhanced uptake of the *R,R* isomer, which facilitates greater total platinum binding to DNA (Kido et al 1992). In a spheroid tumor cell model, ormaplatin was able to penetrate well to kill hypoxic and quiescent tumor cells in the spheroid core (Li et al 1989, Bhuyan et al 1991, Durand 1989).

Mechanism of Action

Ormaplatin is believed to bind to DNA and interrupt cell division in a manner similar to that of cisplatin (Blatter et al 1984). Chemical reduction of ormaplatin to diaminocyclohexane platinum(II) (PtDACH) appears to be required for part or all of the cytotoxic activity (Gibbons et al 1989a,b). This can be mediated by a variety of reducing agents, especially glutathione and other protein and nonprotein sulfhydryls (Eastman 1987). Unless reduced, ormaplatin will not react with supercoiled DNA (Blatter et al 1984, 1985). Besides PtDACH, other active transformation products may also produce cytotoxic effects from ormaplatin.

Formation of PtDACH from ormaplatin has been shown to occur in tissue culture medium (Gibbons et al 1989a,b) and in rat plasma (Chaney et al 1989). About 70 to 80% of intra- or extracellular ormaplatin reduction is mediated by sulfhydryls (Chaney et al 1989). Extracellular ascorbic acid and ferric ions can also mediate this conversion (Blatter et al 1984, 1985), and ascorbate additionally enhances platinum complexation with guanosine monophosphate (Van Der Veer et al 1986). The platinum moiety in ormaplatin will also bind to 9-methylguanine, but not to other methylated bases (Choi et al 1988).

The cytotoxicity and DNA lesions caused by related platinum(IV) compounds like ormaplatin differ from those induced by cisplatin. Platinum(IV) compounds induce DNA strand breakage and DNA–protein crosslinks (Panneerselvam et al 1989) and are more easily taken up by cells than is cisplatin (platinum[II]) (Razaka et al 1986). In addition, the aquation of ormaplatin is 15-fold slower than with cisplatin and is not a prerequisite for protein binding (Leroy and Thompson 1989).

Other pharmacologic effects of ormaplatin include immunosuppression, noted by reduced primary response to alloantigens (Smith et al 1986); inhibition of protein kinase C (Ho et al 1989); and noncompetitive inhibition of choline acetyltransferase activity (Ho et al 1987).

Availability and Storage

Ormaplatin is investigationally available from the National Cancer Institute in vials containing 50 mg of yellow lyophilized ormaplatin powder, 45 mg sodium chloride, and 500 mg of Mannitol, USP. The intact vials are stored at room temperature.

Preparation for Use, Stability, and Admixture

Each vial is reconstituted with 10 mL of Sterile Water for Injection, USP, with a resultant pH of 3.3 to 5.3. Ormaplatin may also be reconstituted in 5% dextrose. These solutions are stable at room temperature for at least 24 hours. The stability of ormaplatin is directly related to the chloride ion content of the admixture: at a sodium chloride concentration of 0.018% the stability time of ormaplatin (> 90% remaining) is 6 hours (Cheung et al

1987). There is also little likelihood for hemolysis with ormaplatin in the blood at concentrations up to 5 mg/mL. Ormaplatin does not form plasma protein precipitates.

■ Administration

It is recommended that ormaplatin be diluted in at least 250 mL of normal saline for intravenous administration over 30 minutes. Patients should receive prehydration (5% dextrose in 0.45% saline infused at 100 mL/h for 4 hours) along with aggressive antiemetic prophylaxis before ormaplatin is administered.

■ Dosage

Based on the murine LD_{10} of 10.44 mg/m^2/d × 5 days, the starting human dose in phase I trials was 1 mg/m^2/d × 5 days (one-tenth the maximally tolerated dose in mice). In the initial phase I clinical trial, the maximally tolerated dose was 90 mg/m^2 IV every 28 days in heavily pretreated patients (Christian et al 1992). Recommended doses for phase II trials are not yet available.

■ Pharmacokinetics

Preclinical pharmacokinetic studies in rats have demonstrated peak free plasma platinum levels of 5.8 μg/mL following an intravenous ormaplatin dose of 3 mg/kg. The levels of platinum were comparable to those from an equivalent cisplatin dose over the period from 2 to 24 hours after dosing (Kelly et al 1986). The plasma elimination of total platinum was bisphasic, with half-lives of 23.2 minutes for the α phase and 29.1 hours for the β phase. The concentration × time product was 36.7 μg·h·mL^{-1} with a steady-state volume of distribution of 8.11 L. Total plasma clearance was 0.021 L/h. Corresponding free platinum pharmacokinetics following ormaplatin comprised half-lives of 10.9 minutes (α) and 7.4 hours (β), an AUC of 9.5 mg·h·mL, a volume of distribution of 1.58 L, and a clearance of 0.162 L/h. Like cisplatin, ormaplatin is known to bind tightly to plasma proteins (Leroy and Thompson 1989) and to concentrate in the kidneys, liver, and spleen. The urinary excretion of platinum over 24 hours in the rat averaged 28 to 38% of an ormaplatin dose (Rahman et al 1988). Thus, ormaplatin pharmacokinetics in preclinical models is similar to that of cisplatin.

In humans, ormaplatin exhibits a biphasic elimination pattern. The initial half-life was about 30 minutes, whereas the terminal half-life was unspecified at several hours (Christian et al 1992).

■ Side Effects and Toxicity

Target organs for toxicity in rodents included lymphoid tissues, thymus gland, bone marrow, stomach, gastrointestinal tract, kidneys, liver, and testes. Renal lesions were observed in rats and dogs and involved generalized degeneration, hypertrophy of the tubular epithelium in the medulla and cortex, papillary necrosis, development of hyaline-like droplet degeneration, and necrotic degeneration in the medulla. Most effects were reversible on drug discontinuance. However, severe and possible-cumulative peripheral neuropathy has clouded further development of this agent. This neuropathy tends to be moderate to severe and does not decrease once dosing is discontinued.

Overall, ormaplatin is similar to cisplatin in that nephrotoxicity and, to a lesser degree, myelosuppression are anticipated toxic effects. The drug is strongly mutagenic in both the Ames assay and the unscheduled DNA synthesis assay (Razaka et al 1986).

In heavily pretreated cancer patients, the dose-limiting toxic effect is myelosuppression, principally thrombocytopenia (Christian et al 1992). Neutropenia is typically less common and rarely dose limiting. Nausea and vomiting are common unless prophylactic antiemetic regimens are used. Sensory peripheral neuropathy was seen after a cumulative dose of 225 mg/m^2 was delivered (five cycles of ormaplatin therapy). Renal dysfunction was observed in two patients in the phase I study: one with progressive bladder cancer and one who received cisplatin therapy previously. Other occasional toxic effects included serum glutamic–oxalacetic transaminase elevation, diarrhea, malaise, fatigue, and anorexia (Christian et al 1992).

REFERENCES

Anderson WK, Quagliato DA, Haugwitz RD, et al. Synthesis, physical properties, and antitumor activity of tetraplatin and related tetrachloroplatinum(IV) stereoisomers of 1,2-diaminocyclohexane. *Cancer Treat Rep.* 1986;**70**(8):997–1002.

Behrens BC, Hamilton TC, Masuda H, et al. Characterization of a *cis*-diamminedichloroplatinum(II)-resistant human ovarian cancer cell line and its use in evaluation of platinum analogues. *Cancer Res.* 1987;**47**(2):414–418.

Bhuyan BK, Folz SJ, DeZwaan J, et al. Cytotoxicity of tetraplatin and cisplatin for human and rodent cell lines cultured as monolayers and multicellular spheroids. *Cancer Commun.* 1991;**3**(2):1–7.

Blatter EE, Vollano JF, Krishnan BS, et al. Interaction of the antitumor agents cis,cis,trans Pt IV (NH$_3$)$_2$Cl$_2$OH$_2$ and cis,cis,trans Pt IV [(CH$_3$)$_2$CHNH$_2$]$_2$Cl$_2$(OH)$_2$ and their reduction products with PM2 DNA. *Biochemistry.* 1984;**23**:4817–4820.

Blatter EE, Vollano JF, Krishnan BS, et al. Platinum(IV) antitumor agents. In: *Molecular Basis of Cancer.* Part B: *Macromolecular Recognition, Chemotherapy, and Immunology.* New York: Alan R. Liss; 1985:1985–1991.

Chaney SG, Kaun-Till G, Poma A, Holbrook DJ. Biotransformations of tetraplatin in rat plasma. *Proc Am Assoc Cancer Res.* 1989;**30**:470.

Cheung Y-W, Cradock JC, Vishnuvajjala BR, et al. Stability of cisplatin, iproplatin, carboplatin, and tetraplatin in commonly used intravenous solutions. *Am J Hosp Pharm.* 1987;**44**(1):124–130.

Choi H-K, Terzis A, Stevens RC, et al. Reaction products of a new anticancer agent, Pt(IV)(cyclohexyldiamine)Cl$_4$ with guanosine and 9-methylguanine: Nucleobase and a nucleoside. *Biochem Biophys Res Commun.* 1988;**156**(3):1120–1124.

Christian MC, Kohn E, Sarosy G, et al. Phase I and pharmacologic study of ormaplatin (OP)/tetraplatin. *Proc Am Soc Clin Oncol.* 1992;**11**:117.

DeKoning TF, Aristoff PA, Houchens DP, et al. Biological evaluation of tetraplatin and its stereoisomers. *Proc Am Assoc Cancer Res.* 1988;**29**:340.

Durand RE. Distribution and activity of antineoplastic drugs in a tumor model. *J Natl Cancer Inst.* 1989;**81**:146–152.

Eastman A. Glutathione-mediated activation of anticancer platinum(IV) complexes. *Biochem Pharmacol.* 1987;**36**(23):4177–4178.

Gibbons G, Chaney SG, Holbrook DJ. Intracellular biotransformations of tetraplatin in the L1210 cell line. *Proc Am Assoc Cancer Res.* 1989a;**30**:461.

Gibbons GR, Wyrick S, Chaney SG. Rapid reduction of tetrachloro(d,l-trans)1,2-diaminocyclohexaneplatinum (IV)(tetraplatin) in RPMI 1640 tissue culture medium. *Cancer Res.* 1989b;**49**(6):1402–1407.

Harrap KR, Jones M, Goddard PM, et al. New platinum drugs: Requirement for new screening models. *Proc Am Assoc Cancer Res.* 1987;**28**:315.

Ho BT, Feiffer R, Tansey LW, et al. Inhibition of brain choline acetyltransferase by tetraplatin. *Brain Res Bull.* 1987;**19**(2):283–285.

Ho BT, Phan CP, Lin JR, et al. Inhibition of protein kinase C by tetraplatin. *Proc Am Assoc Cancer Res.* 1989;**30**:470.

Kelly A, Roh JK, Wessells H, et al. Comparative pharmacokinetics of tetraplatin (NSC-363812) and CDDP in rats. *Proc Am Assoc Cancer Res.* 1986;**27**:290.

Kendall D, Alberts D, Peng Y-M. Activity of tetraplatin isomers against cisplatin sensitive and resistant human tumor cell lines. *Proc Am Assoc Cancer Res.* 1989;**30**:469.

Kido Y, Khokhar AR, Siddik ZH. Relative cytotoxicity, uptake and total DNA binding of tetraplatin isomers in L1210 and A2780 cells. *Proc Am Assoc Cancer Res.* 1992;**33**:540.

Leroy AF, Thompson WC. Binding kinetics of tetrachloro-1,2-diaminocyclohexaneplatinum(IV) (tetraplatin) and cis-diamminedichloroplatinum(II) at 37°C with human plasma proteins and with bovine serum albumin. Does aquation precede protein binding? *J Natl Cancer Inst.* 1989;**81**(6):427–436.

Li LH, Bhuyan BK, Wallace TL. Comparison of cytotoxicity of agents on monolayer and spheroid systems. *Proc Am Assoc Cancer Res.* 1989;**30**:612.

Orr RM, O'Neill CF, Murrer BA, et al. Evaluation of novel platinum II and platinum IV ammine/amine complexes using L1210 sublines resistant to cisplatin or tetraplatin. *Proc Am Assoc Cancer Res.* 1989;**30**:509.

Panneerselvam M, Rahman A, Lombardi VT. Molecular mechanisms of resistance of human ovarian cancer cells to cisplatin and tetraplatin. *Proc Am Assoc Cancer Res.* 1989;**30**:523.

Rahman A, Roh JK, Wolpert-Defilippes MK, et al. Therapeutic and pharmacological studies of tetrachloro(d,l-trans)1,2-diaminocyclohexane platinum(IV)(tetraplatin), a new platinum analogue. *Cancer Res.* 1988;**48**(7):1745–1752.

Razaka H, Salles B, Villani G, et al. Toxicity, mutagenicity and induction of recA protein in *Escherichia coli* treated with cis-diamminedichloroplatinum(II) and cis-diamminetetrachloroplatinum(IV). *Chem–Biol Interact.* 1986;**60**(2):207–215.

Smith JW, Neefe J, Orantes D, et al. Immunotoxicity of tetraplatinum in comparison with cis-platinum (CDDP) and carboplatin (CBDCA) in mice. *Proc Am Assoc Cancer Res.* 1986;**27**:290.

Van Der Veer JL, Peters AR, Reeddijk J. Reaction products from platinum(IV) amine compounds and 5'-GMP are mainly bis(5'-GMP)platinum(II)amine adducts. *J Inorg Biochem.* 1986;**26**(issue II):137–142.

Wilkoff LJ, Dulmadge EA, Trader MW, et al. Evaluation of trans-tetrachloro-1,2-diaminocyclohexane platinum(IV) in murine leukemia L1210 resistant and sensitive to cis-diamminedichloroplatinum(II). *Cancer Chemother Pharmacol.* 1987;**20**:96–100.

Oxaliplatin

■ Other Names

API-395 (Axion Pharmaceuticals, United States); NCU-001 (Nagoya City University, Japan); NSC-266046 (National Cancer Institute); RB-1670 (Roger Bellon Laboratories, France); RP-54780 (Rhône-Poulenc Pharmaceuticals, France); 1-OHP; JM-83 (Johnson Mathey, United Kingdom); CAS-61825-94-3.

■ Chemistry

Structure of oxaliplatin

The complete chemical name of oxaliplatin is [(1R,2R)-1,2-cyclohexanediamine-N,N'][oxalato(2-)-O,O']platinum(II). The oxalato ligands act as leaving groups in contrast to the chloride leaving groups in cisplatin. Oxaliplatin has a molecular weight of 397.3 and the molecular formula $C_{18}H_{14}N_2O_4P_t$. The drug is slightly soluble (7.9 mg/mL) in water (Kidani 1989). It is also slightly soluble in methanol (2.1 mg/mL) and in dimethylformamide (9.0 mg/mL). It is insoluble in hexane. Oxaliplatin has a melting point of 260°C. Aqueous solutions in saline exhibit a chemical half-life of 11.2 hours compared with over 1 week for solutions in water (Kidani 1989).

■ Antitumor Activity

Oxaliplatin is active against a number of human and murine tumor cell lines in vitro, including L-1210 mouse leukemia cells resistant to cisplatin (Kraker and Moore 1988). The drug has more potent cytotoxic effects than cisplatin against human HT-29 colon cancer cells (Pendyala et al 1991). It is roughly equipotent to cisplatin in several other human cells including HT144 and SK-MEL-2 melanomas, K562 erythroleukemia, MCF-7 breast cancer, A2780 ovarian cancer, RF4 bladder cancer, and several gliomas (Pendyala et al 1991). Drug concentrations that inhibited 50% of cell growth ranged from 0.17 to 29 µM in these studies. In a P-388 mouse leukemia cell line developed for resistance to cisplatin, oxaliplatin demonstrated cross-resistance (Kraker and Moore 1988).

Oxaliplatin is active in murine tumor models including B-16 melanoma, colon-26 and colon-38, L-1210 leukemia (both parental and cisplatin-resistant), AKR and P-388 leukemias, Lewis lung cancer, MA-16 mammary carcinoma, and M-5076 fibrosarcoma (Tashiro et al 1989). Oxaliplatin has been shown to have greater than additive effects when combined with cisplatin and carboplatin when administered to mice bearing L-1210 leukemia (Mathé et al 1989) (see Drug Interactions).

European phase II trials reported activity for oxaliplatin most consistently in advanced colorectal carcinoma (Levi et al 1991, 1992a,b). In colorectal cancer patients relapsing after 5-fluorouracil, response rates of 43 to 58% are described using chronomodulated infusions of oxaliplatin with 5-fluorouracil and leucovorin (Levi et al 1992a,b). In 29 patients resistant to 5-fluorouracil, 3 partial responses were described (Levi et al 1991). Responses were also observed in cisplatin-resistant ovarian cancer and melanoma. In advanced or recurrent head and neck cancer a 12% response rate was reported by Degarden et al (1991). By use of a chronomodulated infusion (peak rate at 1600 hours down to zero at 0400 hours), oxaliplatin produced a 17% response rate in previously treated patients with breast cancer (Caussanel et al 1990). This same oxaliplatin chronomodulatory schedule produced a 58% response rate when combined with 5-fluorouracil and folinic acid in patients with metastatic colorectal cancer (Levi et al 1992a,b).

■ Mechanism of Action

Oxaliplatin complexes with DNA in a fashion similar to cisplatin. Both agents appear to bind to repeating deoxyguanosines d(GpG) in a single DNA strand (Boudny et al 1992, Inagaki and Kidani 1986). Other DNA adducts formed by oxaliplatin include intrastrand crosslinks at adenine–guanine d(ApG) sites and interstrand crosslinks with guanosines of opposing DNA strands $(dG)_2$ (Jennerwein et al 1989). With oxaliplatin, the nonleaving cyclohexane moiety is projected into the major groove, roughly perpendicular to the helical DNA structure. This conformation reduces steric hindrance found with the related agent, tetraplatin (ormaplatin).

The kinetics of oxaliplatin reaction with DNA is more rapid than with either cisplatin or carboplatin. These other platinum-containing agents react slowly with DNA because of a biphasic process involving the initial rapid loss of one chloride or carboxylato group, transient aquation of the platinum ligand site, and, then, the formation of one stable ligand with DNA. This is followed by the slower loss of the second leaving group and the formation of DNA intra- and intercrosslinks. This process peaks at approximately 12 hours for cisplatin (Kohn 1981) and over 24 hours for carboplatin (Micetich et al 1985). With oxaliplatin, the formation of adducts at d(GpG) and (dG)$_2$ sites is near complete within 15 minutes (Jennerwein et al 1989). Adducts with d(ApG) form more slowly, over a 2-hour period. As a result of this binding, DNA replication and transcription into RNA are blocked, leading to cell death. These effects are not known to be cell cycle (phase) specific.

Availability and Storage

Oxaliplatin is investigationally available through Debiopharm, Inc, Lausanne, Switzerland, and from Axion Pharmaceuticals, Inc, San Francisco, California. The drug is supplied as a lyophilized white powder in 50- and 100-mg amber glass vials containing 450 and 900 mg lactose, respectively. The vials are stored at room temperature (15–30°C) and are chemically stable for 3 years after manufacture. No preservative is included in the vials.

Preparation for Use, Stability, and Admixture

The 50- and 100-mg vials are reconstituted with 25 and 50 mL of Sterile Water for Injection, USP, respectively. The resulting 2 mg/mL solution is chemically stable for 1 week either at room temperature or under refrigeration; however, because of the lack of a preservative, clinical use within 4 hours of reconstitution is recommended.

For infusion therapy, the initial oxaliplatin solution is diluted into D5W up to a final volume of 500 mL. The drug *should not be mixed with any sodium chloride-containing solutions because of instability*. It is also unstable in tris(hydroxymethyl)aminomethane buffer and at an alkaline pH. Direct admixture with leucovorin is not recommended because of incompatibility with certain leucovorin formulations. There is also a potential for binding between platinum and aluminum in intravenous administration sets and needles. Therefore, aluminum-containing needles and infusion sets should not be used with oxaliplatin.

Administration

Oxaliplatin is administered intravenously either as a short infusion in 500 mL of 5% dextrose (Mathé et al 1989) or as a prolonged (5-day) continuous infusion with chronopharmacologic-based flow rate adjustments (Levi et al 1992a, Caussanel et al 1990).

A 12-hour sinusoidal daily infusion scheme was used in several trials. The oxaliplatin infusion rate peaked at 1600 hours (4:00 PM) and was followed by a 12-hour sinusoidal continuous infusion of 5-fluorouracil and folinic acid (Levi et al 1992a,b).

Dosage

The recommended dosage for phase II trials using a short intravenous infusion is 135 mg/m^2 every 3 weeks (Extra et al 1990). For the chronomodulated trials with 5-fluorouracil and leucovorin, the starting oxaliplatin dose was 25 mg/m^2/d (125 mg/m^2 total) as a 5-day continuous intravenous infusion every 3 weeks (see Administration for flow rate parameters). Doses were then escalated by 25 mg/m^2 per course according to individual patient tolerance (Caussanel et al 1990). For phase II trials of this schedule, the recommended dose was 35 mg/m^2/d × 5 or 175 mg/m^2 per course (Caussanel et al 1990).

Drug Interactions

Experimental synergy has been reported for oxaliplatin and 5-fluorouracil in mice bearing L-1210 leukemia (Mathé et al 1989). Similar results were found for oxaliplatin combined with carboplatin in mice bearing B-16 melanoma, Lewis lung cancer, and C26 colon carcinoma (Mathé et al 1989). Further studies showed that the simultaneous administration of oxaliplatin and carboplatin produced curative effects in mice bearing L-1210 leukemia. Of interest, these effects were not produced with the simultaneous combination of carboplatin with cisplatin (Mathé et al 1989).

Pharmacokinetics

Oxaliplatin disposition is similar to that of other platinum-containing agents. Approximately 35 to 50% of a dose is recovered in the urine as different platinum-containing species. Only about 9% of the dose is recovered in the urine as free platinum. The elimination of platinum from the plasma compartment is biphasic. There is a short initial distribution phase of about 15 minutes. The terminal half-life of total platinum-containing species in the plasma has varied from 23 to 39 hours, with the longer half-lives associated with longer oxaliplatin infusion times. Most of the dose (85–88%), is bound to plasma proteins and about 50% of the platinum in the bloodstream is bound to red blood cells. Like cisplatin, the half-life of free platinum in the bloodstream is approximately 100 minutes following oxaliplatin administration.

Drug distribution studies in rabbits show that the highest levels of platinum are found (in descending order) in kidney, spleen, bladder, blood cells, stomach, bile, and small intestine (Kidani 1989). Comparable studies in humans have not been performed.

■ Side Effects and Toxicity

Oxaliplatin produces dose-limiting peripheral neuropathy as well as moderate to severe nausea and vomiting. Mild leukopenia and mild to moderate degrees of thrombocytopenia are typical. The incidence and severity of both neutropenia and paresthesias may be increased by continuous-infusion therapy, particularly if constant-rate infusions are used instead of the chronomodulated method (Caussanel et al 1990). Renal and/or hepatic toxic effects are not reported for oxaliplatin (Mathé et al 1986). The lack of nephrotoxicity represents a considerable difference from other platinum-containing antitumor agents.

Sensory neuropathies with oxaliplatin are characterized by paresthesias of the hands and feet and occasionally the lips. These dysthesias are increased by exposure to cold, including the ingestion of cold food or beverage, which may cause pharyngeal paresthesias. Symptom intensity tends to be cumulative with repeated courses of oxaliplatin. In rare patients, cumulative neurotoxicity can lead to ataxia; however, in contrast to cisplatin and ormaplatin, neurotoxic symptoms of oxaliplatin usually resolve within a week of stopping therapy. Occasionally, longer recovery periods are required. Fortunately, no permanent effects have been observed with oxaliplatin in contrast to the sensory neuropathy associated with cisplatin. With oxaliplatin, up to 60% of patients in phase I studies have experienced a moderate degree of sensory neuropathy; however, some of these patients were previously exposed to cisplatin, although neurotoxic effects are not thought to be synergistic between the two agents. Electromyograms of patients with oxaliplatin neuropathy have shown a significant decrease in sensory nerve conduction with no decrease in motor nerve conduction velocity.

Nausea and vomiting with oxaliplatin are common and, in some patients, may be severe. Therefore, aggressive antiemetic prophylaxis is required for all patients receiving oxaliplatin. In unprotected patients, the duration of emesis has ranged from 1 to 2 days. Severe emesis occurred in over half of study populations, although there was no clear association with the dose given.

Cardiac toxicity, which was seen in preclinical, high-dose acute toxicology studies, has not been observed with oxaliplatin. Similarly, no alopecia or ototoxicity is reported for oxaliplatin. The drug is also nonmutagenic in Ames assays using *Salmonella typhimurium* strains TA-98 and TA-100.

REFERENCES

Boudny V, Vrána O, Gaucheron F, et al. Biophysical analysis of DNA modified by 1,2-diaminocyclohexane platinum(II) complexes. *Nucleic Acids Res.* 1992;**20**(2):267–272.

Caussanel J-P, Levi F, Brienza S, et al. Phase I trial of 5-day continuous venous infusion of oxaliplatin at circadian rhythm-modulated rate compared with constant rate. *J Natl Cancer Inst.* 1990;**82**:1046–1050.

Degarden M, Krakowski J, Conroy T, et al. Phase II trial of oxaliplatin (1-OHP) in locoregionally advanced (LRA), recurrent (R) or metastatic (M) head and neck squamous cell cancer (H+NSCC). Preliminary results (abstract 349). *Eur J Cancer.* 1991;**26**(suppl):1183.

Extra JM, Espie M, Calvo F, et al. Phase I study of oxaliplatin in patients with advanced cancer. *Cancer Chemother Pharmacol.* 1990;**25**:299–303.

Inagaki K, Kidani Y. Differences in binding of (1,2-cydohexane)platinum(II) isomers with d(GpG). *Inorg Chem.* 1986;**25**:1–3.

Jennerwein MM, Eastman A, Khokhar A. Characterization of adducts produced in DNA by isomeric 1,2-diaminocyclohexaneplatinum(II) complexes. *Chem–Biol Interact.* 1989;**70**:39–49.

Kidani Y. Oxaliplatin. *Drugs Future.* 1989;**14**(6):529–532.

Kohn KW. Molecular mechanisms of cross-linking by alkylating agents and platinum complexes. In: Sartorelli AC, Lazo JS, Bertino JR, eds. *Molecular Actions and Targets for Cancer Chemotherapeutic Agents.* Bristol-Myers Cancer Symposia, vol 2. New York: Academic Press; 1981:3–16.

Kraker AJ, Moore CW. Accumulation of *cis*-diamminedichloroplatinum(II) and platinum analogues by platinum-resistant murine leukemia cells in vitro. *Cancer Res.* 1988;**48**:9–13.

Levi F, Brienza S, Focan C, et al. A phase II chronopharmacological trial of oxaliplatin (1-OHP) against metastatic colorectal cancer. *Proc Am Assoc Cancer Res.* 1991;**32**:185.

Levi F, Brienza S, Misset JL, et al. Circumvention of clinical resistance of metastatic colorectal cancer to 5-fluorouracil (5-FU) with circadian-rhythm modulated venous chemotherapy. *Proc Am Soc Clin Oncol.* 1992a;**11**:171.

Levi F, Misset J-L, Brienza S, et al. A chronopharmacologic phase II clinical trial with 5-fluorouracil, folinic acid, and oxaliplatin using an ambulatory multichannel programmable pump. *Cancer.* 1992b;**69**(4):893–900.

Mathé G, Kidani Y, Segiguchi M, et al. Oxalato-platinum or 1-OHP, a third-generation platinum complex: An experimental and clinical appraisal and preliminary comparison with *cis*-platinum and carboplatinum. *Biomed Pharmacother.* 1989;**43**:237–250.

Mathé G, Kidani Y, Triana K, et al. A phase I trial of *trans*-1-diaminocyclohexane oxalato-platinum (1-OHP). *Biomed Pharmacother.* 1986;**40**:372–376.

Micetich KC, Barnes D, Erickson LC. A comparative study of the cytotoxicity and DNA-damaging effects of *cis*-(diammino)(1,1-cyclobutanedicarboxylato)-platinum(II) and *cis*-diamminedichloroplatinum(II) on L1210 cells. *Cancer Res.* 1985;**45**:4043–4047.

Pendyala L, Creagen PJ, Shah G, Molnar MV, Grandjean EM. In vitro cytotoxicity studies of oxaliplatin in human tumor cell lines. *Proc Am Assoc Cancer Res.* 1991;**32**:410.

Tashiro T, Kawada Y, Sakurai Y, et al. Antitumor activity of a new platinum complex, oxalato (*trans*-l-1,2-diaminocyclohexane)platinum(II): New experimental data. *Biomed Pharmacother.* 1989;**43**:251–260.

Paclitaxel

■ Other Names

Taxol® (Bristol-Myers Squibb and Mead Johnson Company); NSC- 125973.

■ Chemistry

Structure of paclitaxel

Paclitaxel is a diterpene plant product derived from the needles and bark of the western yew, *Taxus brevifolia* (Wani et al 1971). It has a molecular weight of 853.9, is poorly soluble in water, and has the empiric formula $C_{47}H_{51}NO_{14}$. The complete chemical name is tax-11-en-9-one, 5β, 20-epoxy-1, 2α, 4, 7β, 13α-hexahydroxy-,4,10-diacetate-2-benzoate 13-β-(benzoylamino)-α-hydroxybenzenepropionate.

■ Antitumor Activity

Paclitaxel is highly active in numerous preclinical tumor models (Rose et al 1992). At the present time paclitaxel has completed phase I studies and is still undergoing phase II testing. Phase II studies have been significantly delayed by drug supply problems. Despite those supply problems, paclitaxel has had documented antitumor activity against a number of malignancies.

In phase I studies paclitaxel produced objective responses in patients with gastric cancer, ovarian cancer, adenocarcinoma of unknown primary (Wiernik et al 1987b; Donehower et al 1987), malignant melanoma (Wiernik et al 1987a), non-small cell lung cancer (Donehower et al 1987, Brown et al 1991), and acute leukemia (Rowinsky et al 1988a).

Phase II studies have shown that paclitaxel has quite remarkable antitumor activity in patients with refractory ovarian cancer. In a study by McGuire et al (1989) a 30% response rate was noted in heavily pretreated patients refractory to platinum-containing regimens. Paclitaxel is also active in the treatment of patients with metastatic breast cancer. A 56% response rate with 12% complete responses is reported in 25 patients who had relapsed on at least one prior regimen of chemotherapy (Holmes et al 1992). Einzig et al (1988b) reported an 18% response rate in patients with metastatic melanomas. A 24% response rate is described in patients with previously untreated non-small cell lung cancer (Murphy et al 1993). There was one complete responder among the 25 evaluable patients in this trial. The drug has not had activity in patients with renal cell carcinoma (Einzig et al 1988a); however, paclitaxel was active in vitro against human bladder tumor cells (Rangel and Niell 1992). Of interest is that one may be able to detect whether or not paclitaxel will be effective for the patient based on in vitro effects of paclitaxel on the patient's blast cells (Rowinsky et al 1988b).

■ Paclitaxel-Containing Combinations

Paclitaxel + Filgrastim. A 24-hour infusion of paclitaxel (250 mg/m^2) every 21 days was combined with 5 µg/kg filgrastim (G-CSF) given subcutaneously on days 3 to 10 (Seidman et al 1992). The overall response rate in 26 evaluable patients was 62% and included one complete responder. This combination is also active in ovarian cancer, but appears to require higher doses of filgrastim to increase paclitaxel dose intensity (Sarosy et al 1992a). The response rate to dose-intensive paclitaxel with filgrastim was 50% in 38 evaluable patients with recurrent ovarian cancer (Sarosy et al 1992b).

Paclitaxel + Doxorubicin + Filgrastim. Paclitaxel + doxorubicin + filgrastim has been evaluated in previously untreated patients with metastatic breast cancer. Unexpectedly severe stomatitis and/or neutropenia was produced at paclitaxel and doxorubicin doses of 160 and 60 mg/m^2, respectively (Holmes et al 1992). Although the combination was active (2/7 partial responses) lower doses are currently being studied (see Dosage).

Paclitaxel + Cisplatin. Paclitaxel + cisplatin has been evaluated in patients with advanced solid tumor malignancies, including some patients refractory to cisplatin-containing regimens. The maximally tolerated doses (MTDs) were 50 to 70% that of each agent given alone. In combination, the MTDs were 135 mg/m^2 for paclitaxel and 75 mg/m^2 for cisplatin, each administered intravenously every 3 weeks. Although synergistic neurotoxicity was observed, this combination was active, producing response rates of 23% in ovarian cancer, 38% in non-small cell lung cancer, and 100% in two breast cancer patients (Donehower and Rowinsky 1992). Responses have also been observed in patients with melanoma (Rowinsky et al 1991a).

Paclitaxel + Cisplatin + Filgrastim. Paclitaxel + Cisplatin + Filgrastim is also active in patients with non-small cell lung cancer, head and neck cancer, and esophageal cancer (Forastiere et al 1992). The dose-limiting toxic effects included neuropathy, myalgias, and nephropathy in decreasing frequency (Forastiere et al 1992). A range of paclitaxel doses (135 to 350 mg/m^2) was evaluated with a fixed cisplatin dose of 75 mg/m^2. These regimens produced mean plasma paclitaxel levels of 0.43 to 2.34 µM (Forastiere et al 1992). Neuropathy was dose limiting at paclitaxel doses of 300 mg/m^2 with 75 mg/m^2 of cisplatin and filgrastim. The recommended dose for phase II studies has been suggested to be 100 mg/m^2 cisplatin, 250 mg/m^2 paclitaxel, and 10 to 20 µg/kg/d filgrastim after chemotherapy (Forastiere et al 1992).

■ Mechanism of Action

Paclitaxel acts as a unique mitotic spindle poison (Schiff et al 1979, Schiff and Horwitz 1980, Fuchs and Johnson 1978). In a manner contrary to that of known mitotic spindle inhibitors such as colchicine and podophyllotoxin (both of which inhibit mitotic spindle formation), paclitaxel promotes assembly of microtubules and stabilizes them against depolymerization (Schiff et al 1979). This induces bundles of stable microtubules and blocks cell cycle traverse in mitosis (Schiff and Horwitz 1980). Paclitaxel also prevents transition from G_0 phase to S phase by blocking cellular response to protein growth factors such as epidermal growth factor. Recent studies using a photoaffinity-labeled palitaxel analog show that paclitaxel binds selectively to the β subunit of tubulin (Rao et al 1992). In this regard, paclitaxel may mimic the activity of GTP, which is an endogenous regulator of tubulin function. The binding of paclitaxel to tubulin is stoichiometric and reversible with a binding constant of 0.9 µmol/L (Parness and Horwitz 1981).

Neutrophil functions inhibited by paclitaxel include chemotaxis, migration, polarization, and killing of phagocytosed microorganism (Roberts et al 1982). Blast transformation of lymphocytes is not altered. Paclitaxel also diminishes cell receptors for and secretion of tumor necrosis factor α. Other specialized cellular secretory functions blocked by paclitaxel include catecholamine release from the adrenal medulla and protein secretion from rat hepatocytes (Rowinsky et al 1990). Paclitaxel may additionally mediate apoptosis as noted by DNA fragmentation in the presence of an intact plasma membrane (Sullivan et al 1992).

The enhanced polymerization of microtubules results in an inability of cells to replicate (Schiff et al 1979).

■ Availability and Storage

Paclitaxel is available from Bristol Myers Squibb Company (Princeton, New Jersey) formulated as a concentrated sterile solution containing 60 mg/mL in a 5-mL ampule (30 mg per ampule) in a mixture of 50% polyoxyethylated castor oil, Cremophor EL®, and 50% dehydrated alcohol, USP. The contents must be diluted as required before use. The intact vials should be stored under refrigeration (2–8°C).

■ Preparation for Use, Stability, and Admixture

Paclitaxel infusion concentrations of 0.6 and 0.03 mg/mL may be obtained by diluting the 300-mg ampule solution with 50 or 1000 mL of 0.9% NaCl for injection or 5% dextrose for injection, respectively. Paclitaxel is usually reconstituted in 50 mL of D5W. *Only glass bottles should be used for paclitaxel administration.* This avoids the problem of leaching the plasticizer DHEP from polyvinyl chloride containers exposed to Cremophor-containing solutions (National Cancer Institute 1990). All solutions exhibit a slight haze which is common to all products containing nonionic surfactants. Paclitaxel solutions diluted to a concentration of 0.6 mg/mL should be used within 24 hours of reconstitution. Paclitaxel solutions diluted to a concentration of 0.03 mg/mL (1 ampule in 1 L) are chemically stable and physically acceptable for up to 24 hours. Using a turbidometric assay, paclitaxel (1.2 mg/mL) was found to be physically compatible with several agents diluted in 5% dextrose for 4 hours at room temperature. These include carboplatin, cimetidine, cisplatin, cyclophosphamide, cytarabine, dexamethasone, diphenhydramine, doxorubicin, etoposide, fluorouracil, haloperidol, lorazepam, methotrexate, metoclopramide, prochlorperazine, ranitidine, and vancomycin (Trissel and Bready 1992).

■ Administration

Paclitaxel is administered by intravenous infusion only. The typical period is 24 hours. Shorter infusion times of 3 to 6 hours are associated with an increased incidence of hypersensitivity reactions and cardiotoxicity, principally bradycardia (see Dosage for typical infusion schedules). To prevent leaching of plasticizer from polyvinyl chloride surfaces, paclitaxel solutions should optimally be infused in glass or polyolefin containers using polyethylene-lined nitroglycerin tubing sets.

A small number of fibers (within acceptable levels of USP Particulate Matter Text) have been observed. Therefore, in-line filtration with a 0.2 -μm filter (Ivex-2®, Abbott Laboratories) is necessary. This does not lower the concentration of the solution. Solutions exhibiting excessive particulate formation or precipitation should not be used.

If the 6-hour infusion is used for patients with solid tumors, the infusion must be administered in a standard protocol. During the first 30 minutes of the 6-hour infusion drug should be delivered at a rate of 42 mL/h (21 mL total). If no adverse effects occur (see below), the rate for the last 5.5 hours of infusion can be increased to 180 mL/h (3 mL/min).

In other phase II studies the 24-hour infusion schedule has been recommended. If that schedule is used, the elaborate steps just outlined do not need to be followed.

■ Special Precautions

Anaphylactic-like hypersensitivity reactions with paclitaxel have been reported by a large number of investigators in from 3 to 28% of patients receiving the drug (Wiernik et al 1987a,b; Rowinsky et al 1988b; Brown et al 1991; Donehower et al 1987; Grem et al 1987; Kris et al 1986). These reactions consist of bronchospasm, dyspnea stridor, facial flushing, periorbital swelling, and hypotension.

Severe hypersensitivity reactions have been seen with first or later infusions. It is unsettled as to whether or not premedication is absolutely necessary for avoiding hypersensitivity. Current evidence indicates that prolongation of the infusion (to ≥ 6 hours) plus premedication with dexamethasone + diphenhydramine + cimetidine (Wiernik et al 1987b) will minimize this adverse effect. One specific pretreatment regimen calls for 20 mg dexamethasone orally 14 and 7 hours before the start of each paclitaxel infusion. In addition, 50 mg diphenhydramine and 50 mg ranitidine (or 300 mg cimetidine) are administered intravenously 30 minutes before the infusion (Wiernik et al 1987b, McGuire et al 1989).

Some (but not all) patients who have had a hypersensitivity reaction to the agent have been able to be retreated with paclitaxel after premedication.

■ Drug Interactions

Paclitaxel produces additive cytotoxicity in experimental tumor models when combined with a number of other cytotoxic agents. In ovarian cancer cells, paclitaxel and doxorubicin are additive, whereas the combination of paclitaxel and vitamin D are synergistic at high paclitaxel:vitamin D concentration ratios (Saunders et al 1992).

In contrast to these results, paclitaxel produced less than additive cytotoxicity with doxorubicin, etoposide, and amsacrine in human MCF-7 breast cancer cells and in A-549 lung cancer cells (Hahn et al 1992).

There is sequence-dependent cytotoxicity with cisplatin. The optimal sequence involves paclitaxel given before cisplatin in resistant L-1210 cells in vitro (Citardi et al 1990). The combination of paclitaxel, which polymerizes microtubules, and estramustine phosphate, which causes depolymerization of microtubules, produces greater than additive effects in human prostate cancer cells in vitro (Speicher et al 1992). This combination also increased the percentage of cells in S phase by an unknown mechanism.

Paclitaxel can sensitize radioresistant ovarian cancer cells to the cytotoxic effects of ionizing radiation in vitro (Steren et al 1992).

Resistance to paclitaxel's cytotoxic effects in vitro can be reversed by calcium channel blockers such as pimozide and nimodipine (Racker et al 1986). It is also possible that paclitaxel's lipophilic diluent, Chremophor EL, can reverse paclitaxel resistance (Chervinsky et al 1992). This is believed to result from disruption of the membrane domains of the multidrug resistance (MDR) efflux pump, P-glycoprotein. Other experimental modulators of paclitaxel-induced MDR include cyclosporin A and dipyridamole (Chervinsky et al 1991). In vitro modulators of paclitaxel resistance include quinidine, cyclosporin A, quinine, and verapamil, in descending order of potency (Lehnert et al 1992).

In contrast, glutathione (GSH) depletion can reduce the antitumor activity of paclitaxel in human MCF-7 breast cancer cells and A-549 lung cancer cells in vitro (Liebmann et al 1992). Depletion of GSH was accomplished by exposure of cells to 5 mM L- buthionine sulfoximine (see *Buthionine Sulfoximine*) prior to paclitaxel.

The total body clearance of paclitaxel may also be altered by concomitant drug therapy with cisplatin. In a phase I trial of this combination, paclitaxel clearance was reduced by 30% if cisplatin was administered immediately prior to paclitaxel (Rowinsky et al 1991a).

■ Dosage

At present there are no hard and fast dosages or schedules that can be recommended for routine use; however, the recommendation in the new package insert is 135 mg/m^2 administered intravenously over 24 hours every 3 weeks. Phase II activity in patients with ovarian cancer has also been routinely observed with a dose of 175 to 250 mg/m^2 as a 24-hour continuous infusion administered every 3 weeks (McGuire et al 1989).

Paclitaxel has been given in many different schedules to patients with solid tumors (see table). In patients with acute leukemia, doses involve 250 to 390 mg/m^2 as a 24-hour infusion repeated every 14 days (depending on day 14 marrow results) (Rowinsky et al 1988a).

Dose reductions are recommended in heavily pretreated patients to prevent excessive myelotoxicity (Donehower et al 1987). Dose adjustments are not recommended in patients with renal dysfunction but may be necessary in patients with hepatobiliary dysfunction characterized by increased serum bilirubin levels; however, specific dosing guidelines are not yet available.

Dose-intensive paclitaxel therapy has been explored in patients with ovarian cancer given concurrent filgrastim (G-CSF) subcutaneously. A paclitaxel dose of 250 mg/m^2 every 3 weeks was used (dose intensity of 83 mg/m^2/wk (Sarosy et al 1992b). Severe peripheral neurotoxicity prevented dose escalation to 300 mg/m^2 every 3 weeks (dose intensity of 100 mg/m^2/wk). The dose of filgrastim was increased to 20 µg/kg/d for the higher-dose-intensity paclitaxel regimens.

Paclitaxel Dose/Schedule	Reference
135–250 mg/m^2* as a 24-hour continuous infusion every 3 weeks	Ohnuma et al 1985, Wiernik et al 1987a
212–225 mg/m^2 as a 6-hour infusion every 3 weeks	Brown et al 1991, Donehower et al 1987
30 mg/m^2 as a 1-hour infusion daily × 5 days every 4 weeks	Grem et al 1987, Legha et al 1986
30 mg/m^2 as a 6-hour infusion daily × 5 days every 3 weeks	Grem et al 1987

*High-dose range involves filgrastim · paclitaxel.

Pharmacokinetics

Paclitaxel's disposition from the plasma appears to follow a biphasic elimination pattern (see table below). Approximately 97.5% of the drug is bound to plasma proteins (Brown et al 1991). Peak plasma levels correlated with the 24-hour infusion dose: 0.56 µmol/L for 200 mg/m^2, 0.88 µmol/L for 250 mg/m^2, and 0.94 µmol/L for a 275 mg/m^2 dose (Wiernik et al 1987b). These doses produced mean AUC of 9.74 mg/L·h, 12.7 mg/L·h and 12.4 mg/L·h, respectively. Clearance of the drug is rapid and is not due to urinary excretion. Instead, hepatic extraction and biliary secretion probably account for the majority of paclitaxel elimination; however, no major metabolites have been identified yet in the plasma. Renal excretion has accounted for 4.3 to 8.2% of the administered paclitaxel (Brown et al 1991; Wernik et al 1987b, Grem et al 1987). Cerebrospinal fluid paclitaxel levels have been undetectable (Rowinsky et al 1988a).

Side Effects and Toxicity

Hypersensitivity reactions to paclitaxel typically occur within 10 minutes of starting a drug infusion. Reactions are neither dose related nor dependent on prior paclitaxel exposure. These reactions probably relate to histamine release mediated by the Chemophor EL diluent (Weiss et al 1990). Clinical features include dyspnea with or without bronchospasm and approximately 41% had hypotension. About 20% of patients will also experience angioedema manifested as laryngeal stridor, epiglottic swelling, or periorbital edema. About three fourths of patients develop urticaria, flushing, and/or an erythematous rash. Rarely reported features include abdominal or extremity pain.

The incidence of these effects is dramatically lessened with prolonged infusions greater than 6 hours. Pretreatment with dexamethasone and H$_1$ and H$_2$ antihistamines prevented repeat hypersensitivity reactions in 11 of 27 patients, 5 receiving a 6-hour paclitaxel infusion and 11 receiving a 24-hour paclitaxel infusion (Weiss et al 1990). The predictive efficacy of intradermal scratch tests using 0.1 mL of undiluted paclitaxel solution is not established (Weiss et al 1990). In addition to the hypersensitivity reactions (discussed under Special Precautions), the dose-limiting toxic effect of paclitaxel has been myelosuppression. This is noted by leukopenia, specifically, granulocytopenia. Leukopenic nadirs occur a mean of 10 days after dosing, with recovery by a mean of 15 days (Legha et al 1986, Brown et al 1991). Neutropenia does not appear to be cumulative, but is increased in heavily pretreated patients who received myelosuppressive or radiation therapy. Anemia and thrombocytopenia are rarely significant with paclitaxel.

In other studies, a peripheral neuropathy manifested by numbness and tingling, pain, impairment of fine motor skills, and difficulty ambulating with loss of deep tendon reflexes has been dose limiting. This toxic effect may be related in severity to pharmacokinetic drug retention with large areas under the concentration × time curve (Brown et al 1991, Wiernik et al 1987a,b). The neuropathy is typically reversible when the agent is discontinued. Symptom resolution usually improves several months after paclitaxel is discontinued (Rowinsky et al 1990). The most common complaint is burning pain in the feet. It is often associated with hyperesthesias.

CLINICAL PHARMACOKINETICS OF PACLITAXEL

		Half-life (h)			Volume of Distribution (L/m^2)	
Schedule	Reference	α	β	Plasma Clearance (L/h/m^2)	Central	Steady State
6-h infusion every 3 weeks	Brown et al 1991	0.49 ± 0.3	4.3 ± 2.5	13.9 ± 6.1	19.17 ± 5.8	48.55 ± 17.9
6-h infusion every 3 weeks	Wiernik et al 1987	0.32	8.6	6*	—	60
24-h infusion	Wiernik et al 1987a	0.27	3.9	23.5	—	182
6-h infusion	Longnecker et al 1987	0.26	6.4	15.18	8.6	67

*Total body clearance.

Physical exams typically reveal distal sensory loss and decreased deep tendon reflexes. The findings suggest axonal degeneration and demyelination. Transient paralytic ileus is rarely described. Transient myalgias and arthralgias have been described in high-dose paclitaxel regimens.

Cardiac side effects have been occasionally associated with brief infusions of paclitaxel in patients without prior cardiac risk factors. Asymptomatic bradycardia is reported in 29% of ovarian cancer patients in one trial (McGuire et al 1989). Bradycardia is typically transient, but it has rarely been associated with progressive bradyarrhythmias leading to heart block during paclitaxel infusions. Ventricular tachycardia is rarely reported and typically very brief (Rowinsky et al 1991b). Chest pains during paclitaxel infusion are rarely described, but one fatal myocardial infarction has been reported.

Other nonhematologic toxic effects include mucositis, diarrhea, dysgeusia, nausea, and vomiting. Alopecia is nearly complete in most patients. Flulike symptoms such as arthralgias, myalgias, fever, rash, headache, and fatigue are described along with rash, and phlebitis (Brown et al 1991; Wiernik et al 1987a,b; Legha et al 1986; Donehower et al 1987).

■ Special Applications

Intraperitoneal administration of paclitaxel has been evaluated in patients with refractory ovarian cancer (Markman et al 1991). The maximally tolerated paclitaxel dose by this route is 175 mg/m^2 in 1 to 2 L of fluid. At higher doses, abdominal pain is dose limiting. Toxic effects include mild bone marrow suppression, allergic reactions, and mild to moderate abdominal pain. Paclitaxel levels in ascites fluid reached 19 to 88 μM within 6 to 24 hours of instillation. The mean half-life in the peritoneal compartment was 73 hours and clearance averaged 0.42 L/m^2/d (Markman et al 1992). This shows that intraperitoneal paclitaxel is cleared extremely slowly. These levels were 150- to 800-fold higher than simultaneously measured plasma levels. Nonetheless, the plasma compartment still experienced significant (cytotoxic) drug exposures (0.05–0.86 μmol/L) (Markman et al 1992). It remains to be seen whether this approach enhances the antitumor efficacy of paclitaxel. In a phase I trial responses were noted in 2 of 25 patients who experienced complete disappearance of ascites with concomitant major reductions in CA-125 levels (Markman et al 1992).

REFERENCES

Brown T, Havlin K, Weiss G, et al. A phase I trial of Taxol (NSC-125975) given by a 6 hour intravenous infusion. *J Clin Oncol.* 1991;**9**:1261–1267.

Chervinsky S, Brecher ML, Baker RM, et al. Cromophor-El (a solvent for cyclosporine-A) reverses multidrug resistance in C1300 neuroblastoma. *Proc Am Assoc Cancer Res.* 1991;**32**:377.

Chervinsky DS, Brecher ML, Hoelcle MJ. Cremophor-El reverses Taxol cross resistance in murine C1300 multidrug resistant neuroblastoma cells. *Proc Am Assoc Cancer Res.* 1992;**33**:477.

Citardi MJ, Rowinsky EK, Schaefer KL, et al. Sequence-dependent cytotoxicity between cisplatin (C) and the antimicrotubule agents Taxol (T) and vincristine (V). *Proc Am Assoc Cancer Res.* 1990;**31**:410.

Donehower RC, Rowinsky EK. The clinical development of taxol. In: *ASCO Educational Book, American Society of Clinical Oncology 28th Annual Meeting,* San Diego, CA, May 17–19: 1992:102–106.

Donehower RC, Rowinsky EK, Grochow LB, Longnecker SM, Ettinger DS. Phase I trial of Taxol in patients with advanced cancer. *Cancer Treat Rep.* 1987;**71**:1171–1177.

Einzig AI, Gorowski E, Sasloff J, Wiernik PH. Phase II trial of Taxol in patients (pts) with renal cell carcinoma. *Proc Am Assoc Cancer Res.* 1988a;**29**:222.

Einzig AI, Trump DL, Sasloff J, Gorowski E, Dutcher J, Wiernik D. Phase II pilot study of Taxol in patients with malignant melanoma. *Proc Am Soc Clin Oncol.* 1988b;**7**:249.

Forastiere AA, Rowinsky E, Chaudry V, et al. Phase I trial of taxol (T) and cisplatin (C) + G-CSF in solid tumors. *Proc Am Soc Clin Oncol.* 1992;**11**:117.

Fuchs D, Johnson R. Cytologic evidence that Taxol, an antineoplastic agent from *Taxus brevifolia,* acts as a mitotic spindle poison. *Cancer Treat Rep.* 1978;**62**:1219.

Grem JL, Tutsch KD, Simon KJ, et al. Phase I study of Taxol administered as a short i.v. infusion daily for 5 days. *Cancer Treat Rep.* 1987;**71**:1179–1184.

Hahn SM, Liebmann JE, Goldspiel BR, et al. Taxol in combination with doxorubicin (Dox), etoposide (VP-16), and m-AMSA: Possible antagonism in vitro. *Proc Am Assoc Cancer Res.* 1992;**33**:441.

Holmes FA, Frye D, Valero V, et al. Phase I study of taxol (T) and doxorubicin (D) with G-CSF in patients (PT) without prior chemotherapy (CT) for metastatic breast cancer (MBC). *Proc Am Soc Clin Oncol.* 1992;**11**:60.

Kris MG, O'Connell JP, Gralla RJ, et al. Phase I trial of Taxol given as a 3-hour infusion every 21 days. *Cancer Treat Rep.* 1986;**70**:605–607.

Legha SJ, Tenney DM, Krakoff IR. Phase I study of Taxol using a 5-day intermittent schedule. *J Clin Oncol.* 1986;**4**:762–766.

Lehnert M, Emerson S, Dalton WS, et al. Reversal of resistance to taxol and taxotere in a human myeloma cell line model of MDR1. *Proc Am Assoc Cancer Res.* 1992;**33**:481.

Liebmann JE, Hahn SM, Mitchell JB, et al. Glutathione depletion by buthionine sulfoximine antagonizes taxol cytotoxicity. *Proc Am Assoc Cancer Res.* 1992;**33**:423.

Longnecker SM, Donehower RC, Cates, et al. High performance liquid chromatographic assay for Taxol in human plasma and urine and pharmacokinetics in a phase I trials. *Cancer Treat Rep.* 1987;**71**:53–59.

Markman M, Rowinsky E, Hakes T, et al. Phase I study of taxol administered by the intraperitoneal (IP) route: A GOG trial. *Proc Am Soc Clin Oncol.* 1991;**10**:185.

Markman M, Rowinsky E, Hakes T, et al. Phase I trial of intraperitoneal taxol: A Gynecologic Oncology Group study. *J Clin Oncol.* 1992;**10**(9):1485–1491.

McGuire WP, Rowinsky EK, Rosenheim NB, Ettinger DS, Armstrong DK, Donehower RL. Taxol: A unique antineoplastic agent with significant activity in advanced epithelioid neoplasms. *Ann Intern Med.* 1989;**111**:273–279.

Murphy WK, Fossella FV, Winn RJ, et al. Phase II study of taxol in patients with untreated advanced non-small-cell lung cancer. *J Natl Cancer Inst.* 1993;**85**(5):384–388.

National Cancer Institute. *NCI Investigational Drugs.* NIH Publication 91-2141. Bethesda, MD: Department of Health and Human Services; 1990:151–153.

Ohnuma T, Zimet AS, Coffey VA, Holland JF, Greenspan EM. Phase I study of Taxol in a 24-hour infusion schedule. *Proc Am Assoc Cancer Res.* 1985;**26**:167.

Parness J, Horwitz SB. Taxol binds to polymerized tubulin in vitro. *J Cell Biol.* 1981;**91**:479–487.

Plowman J, Dykes DJ, Waud WR, et al. Response of murine tumors and human tumor xenografts to Taxol (NSC-125973) in mice. *Proc Am Assoc Cancer Res.* 1992;**33**:514.

Racker E, Wu LT, Destcott D. Use of slow CA^{2+} channel blockers to enhance inhibition by taxol of growth of drug-sensitive and -resistant Chinese hamster ovary cells. *Cancer Treat Rep.* 1986;**70**(2):275–278.

Rangel C, Niell HB. The activity of taxol in human bladder tumor cell lines (HBTCL). *Proc Am Assoc Cancer Res.* 1992;**33**:488.

Rao S, Band Horwitz S, Ringel I. Direct photoaffinity labeling of tubulin with taxol. *J Natl Cancer Inst.* 1992;**84**:785–788.

Roberts RL, Nath J, Friedman MM, et al. Effects of Taxol on human neutrophils. *J Immunol.* 1982;**129**:2134–2141.

Rose WC, Crosswell AR, Casazza AM. Preclinical antitumor evaluation of Taxol. *Proc Am Assoc Cancer Res.* 1992;**33**:518.

Rowinsky EK, Burke PJ, Karp JE, Ettinger DS, Tucker RW, Donehower RC. Phase I study of Taxol in refractory adult acute leukemia. *Proc Am Assoc Cancer Res.* 1988a;**29**:215.

Rowinsky EK, Cazenave LA, Donehower RC. Taxol: A novel investigational antimicrotubule agent. *J Natl Cancer Inst.* 1990;**82**:1247–1259.

Rowinsky EK, Donehower RC, Jones RJ, Tucker RW. Microtubule changes and cytotoxicity in leukemia cell lines treated with Taxol. *Cancer Res.* 1988b;**48**:4093–4100.

Rowinsky E, Gilbert M, McGuire W, et al. Sequences of Taxol & cisplatin: A phase I and pharmacologic study. *J Clin Oncol.* 1991a;**9**:1692–1703.

Rowinsky EK, McGuire WP, Guarneieri T, Fisherman JS, Christian MC, Donehauer RC. Cardiac disturbances during the administration of Taxol. *J Clin Oncol.* 1991b;**9**:1704–1712.

Sarosy G, Bicher A, Kohn E, et al. Patterns of G-CSF (G) usage in ovarian cancer patients receiving dose intense Taxol (T). *Proc Am Assoc Cancer Res.* 1992a;**33**:222.

Sarosy G, Kohn E, Link C, et al. Taxol dose intensification (D.I.) in patients with recurrent ovarian cancer. *Proc Am Soc Clin Oncol.* 1992b;**11**:226.

Saunders DE, Christensen C, LoRusso PM, et al. Inhibition of ovarian carcinoma cells by Taxol combined with vitamin D and Adriamycin. *Proc Am Assoc Cancer Res.* 1992;**33**:442.

Schiff P, Fant J, Horwitz S. Promotion of microtubule assembly in vitro by Taxol. *Nature.* 1979;**277**:665.

Schiff PB, Horwitz SB. Taxol stabilizes microtubules in mouse fibroblast cells. *Proc Natl Acad Sci USA.* 1980;**77**:1561–1565.

Seidman A, Reichman B, Crown J, et al. Activity of taxol with recombinant granulocyte colony stimulating factor (GCSF) as first chemotherapy (C) of patients (PTS) with metastatic breast cancer (MBC). *Proc Am Soc Clin Oncol.* 1992;**11**:59.

Speicher LA, Barone L, Tew KD. The antimicrotubule agents Taxol and estramustine: Effective cytotoxic combination for prostate carcinoma cell lines. *Proc Am Assoc Cancer Res.* 1992;**33**:439.

Steren A, Sevin BU, Perras J, et al. Radiosensitization by Taxol of a human ovarian cancer cell line. *Proc Am Assoc Cancer Res.* 1992;**33**:552.

Sullivan FJ, Hahn SM, Cook JA, et al. Taxol mediated apoptosis in Chinese hamster V79 cells. *Proc Am Assoc Cancer Res.* 1992;**33**:509.

Trissel LA, Bready BB. Turbidimetric assessment of the compatibility of taxol with selected other drugs during simulated Y-site injection. *Amer J Hosp Pharm.* 1992;**49**:1716–1719.

Wani MC, Taylor HL, Wall ME, Coggon P, McPhail AT. Plant antitumor agents. VI. The isolation and structure of Taxol, a novel antileukemic and antitumor agent from *Taxus brevifolia.* *J Am Chem Soc.* 1971;**93**:2325–2327.

Weiss RB, Donehower RC, Wiernik PH, et al. Hypersensitivity reactions from Taxol. *J Clin Oncol.* 1990;**8**(7):1263–1268.

Wiernik PH, Schwartz EL, Einzig A, Strauman JJ, Lipton RB, Dutcher JP. Phase I trial of Taxol given as a 24-hour infusion every 21 days: Responses observed in metastatic melanoma. *J Clin Oncol.* 1987a;**5**:1232–1239.

Wiernik PH, Schwartz EL, Strauman JJ, Dutcher JP, Lipton RB, Paietta E. Phase I clinical and pharmacokinetics study of Taxol. *Cancer Res.* 1987b;**47**:2486–2493.

PALA

Other Names
NSC-224131.

Chemistry

$$HO-\underset{\underset{O}{\parallel}}{C}-\underset{\underset{CH_2-\underset{\underset{O}{\parallel}}{C}-OH}{|}}{CH}-NH-\underset{\underset{O}{\parallel}}{C}-CH_2-\underset{\underset{OH}{|}}{\overset{\overset{O}{\parallel}}{P}}-OH \quad \cdot 2\,Na$$

Structure of PALA

PALA is a highly charged tetravalent hydrophobic antimetabolite. The chemical name is N-(phosphonoacetyl)-disodium L- aspartic acid. It was originally synthesized by Collins and Stark (1971) in follow-up to the suggestion by Pauling (1948) that analogs of transition-state nucleotide intermediates might comprise highly specific antimetabolites. Thus, PALA represents a specific and potent transition-state inhibitor of aspartate transcarbamylase, an enzyme required at an early step of de novo pyrimidine nucleotide biosynthesis. It has a molecular weight of 299 and the empiric formula $C_6H_8NNa_2O_8P$.

Antitumor Activity

In animal tumor screening studies, PALA has demonstrated relatively greater effects in solid tumors, somewhat uncharacteristic for an antimetabolite. Johnson et al (1976) described apparently non-schedule-dependent antitumor efficacy in the Lewis lung murine cancer model and in mice bearing intraperitoneal B-16 melanoma. It was much less effective in Ridgeway osteogenic sarcoma and against L-1210 or P-388 intraperitoneal leukemias in mice.

In phase I studies responses were noted in patients with ovarian cancer, melanoma, and sarcoma (Valdivieso et al 1979, Gralla et al 1979, Erlichman et al 1979).

In phase II studies the drug has not produced significant antitumor activity in patients with small cell lung cancer (Creech et al 1984), cervical cancer (Muss et al 1984), non-small cell lung cancer (Casper et al 1980, Ettinger et al 1984, Creagen et al 1981a), sarcoma (Kurzrock et al 1984, Bramwell et al 1982), ovarian cancer (Muss et al 1984), lymphoma (Muggia et al 1984), renal cell carcinoma (Earhart et al 1983, Natale et al 1982), melanoma (Kleeburg et al 1982), breast cancer (Paridaens et al 1982, Taylor et al 1982), bladder cancer (Natale et al 1982), head and neck cancer (Creagan et al 1981b), and colon cancer (Rubin et al 1981, Van Echo et al 1980, Carroll et al 1980).

Mechanism of Action

PALA blocks de novo pyrimidine synthesis at a very early step: the condensation of N-carbamoyl aspartate from carbamoyl phosphate and aspartate (Grem et al 1988). As noted earlier, PALA is a specific transition-state inhibitor of transferase (aspartate transcarbamylase [or ATCase]). PALA is a competitive inhibitor of carbamoyl phosphate binding to ACTase. The drug is bound 1000 times more tightly than is the normal substrate. The K_i (binding constant) for PALA with mammalian ACTase is approximately 1×10^{-8} M (Hoogenraad 1974). The blockade in pyrimidine synthesis leads to significant depletion of UTP, CTP, dCTP, dTTP, and dGTP pools (Moyer and Handschumacher 1979); however, phosphoribosyl pyrophosphate (PRPP) levels may increase after PALA. In tumor tissues, UTP and CTP may be selectively depleted. Uridine is known to reverse PALA's antiproliferative effects (Johnson 1977).

In animals it was noted initially that the specific activity of ATCase could be directly correlated to drug sensitivity (Johnson et al 1976). Reports in patients, however, found no correlation for ATCase activity and tumor type or tumor response (Valdivieso et al 1979). Tsuboi et al (1977) were also able to confirm the selective inhibition of pyrimidine biosynthesis by PALA in transplanted murine colonic cancer cells. In this model an exogenous pyrimidine supply completely prevented the cellular growth-inhibitory effects of PALA.

PALA has demonstrated relative schedule-independent cytotoxic activity. This implies non-cell cycle phase-specific antitumor action, an unusual attribute for an antimetabolite drug.

Most resistant tumor cells possess enhanced levels of ACTase and other enzymes involved in de novo pyrimidine synthesis (Jayaram et al 1979). The increase in enzyme levels may be caused by amplification of the genes coding for ACTase and other enzymes involved in early pyrimidine synthesis (Wahl et al 1979). Alternatively, altered ACTase enzymes may be found in resistant cells (Jayaram et al 1979). These studies suggest that cellular resistance to

PALA is facile and can occur by a variety of mechanisms, predominated by an increase in target ACTase enzyme levels.

■ Availability and Storage

PALA is available as an investigational agent from the National Cancer Institute as the disodium salt 100 mg/mL in 10-mL ampules, with sodium hydroxide added to adjust the pH to 6.5 to 7.5 in Sterile Water for Injection, USP. It is currently recommended that ampules be stored under refrigeration (2–8°C).

■ Preparation for Use, Stability, and Admixture

PALA should be diluted to a concentration of 1 mg/mL in either isotonic saline or dextrose solution. When diluted according to these guidelines, it is chemically stable for at least 2 weeks at room temperature.

■ Administration

Phase I studies were conducted using the schedules listed in the table below. As yet there is no preferred dose and schedule of PALA. The most commonly used dose in phase II clinical trials has been 2.5 g/d × 2 days as a 60-minute intravenous infusion repeated every 2 weeks.

■ Special Precautions

PALA inhibits the de novo pyrimidine biosynthesis pathways and should be used with great caution in patients receiving nucleosides.

■ Drug Interactions

The combination of 5-fluorouracil (5-FU) and PALA has been shown to be synergistic in vitro and in vivo. Treatment with PALA is supposed to increase the activation of 5-FU by inhibiting the normal pathway of *de novo* pyrimidine biosynthesis and by deleting competing nucleotides, specifically UTP and CTP (Laster et al 1979). In addition, the enhanced levels of PRPP would favor activation of 5-FU to FdUMP. Casper et al (1983) performed a phase I study and determined that a PALA dose of 25 mg/m^2 was effective in inhibiting pyrimidine biosynthesis. Erlichman et al (1982) described similar findings. PALA does not alter 5-FU clearance but does produce additional mucositis and diarrhea. This tends to compromise the dose of 5-FU, and several randomized trials have shown activity for the combination (Ardalan et al 1988), but no advantage for PALA/5-FU compared with 5-FU alone (O'Dwyer et al 1990). The table on page 770 summarizes the most recent studies. An excellent review by O'Dwyer (1990) has recently been published.

A three-drug regimen consisting of PALA, 5-FU, and thymidine has shown activity in patients with colorectal cancer. A 27% response rate was reported with PALA 4 g/m^2 followed in 24 hours by 15 g thymidine and 200 mg/m^2 5-FU (O'Connell et al 1984). In this combination, thymidine is used to increase 5-FU incorporation into RNA.

PALA has also been used with cytarabine to try to decrease cytidine pools and to increase deoxycytidine kinase activity and thereby enhance the acti-

CLINICAL DOSE SCHEDULES AND DOSE-LIMITING TOXIC EFFECTS OF PALA

Schedule	Dose Range (mg/m^2)	Dose-Limiting Toxic Effects	Recommended Dose (mg/m^2)	Reference
30-min infusion weekly	900–6750/course	Diarrhea, skin rash	3750–4500/wk	Gralla et al 1980
5-d continuous infusion	750–9000/course	Diarrhea, mucositis, skin rash	9000/course	Ervin et al 1980
24-h IV continuous	500–10,500/24 h	Vesication and bullae, mucositis	8700/24 h	Hart et al 1980
120-h IV continuous	4000–8700 total dose	—	6500/120 h	
Daily × 5	100–1250/d	Diarrhea, nausea	1250	Kovach et al 1979
Single dose	800–15,000	—	6000 every 3 wk	Valdivieso et al 1980
Daily × 5, 8, or 10	—	—	1 g/m^2/d × 5 d every 2 wk	Valdivieso et al 1980

vation of cytarabine to Ara-CTP. In vitro, PALA does increase cytarabine accumulation (Grant et al 1982). In leukemia patients, the PALA/5-FU combination does not produce significantly enhanced response rates (Blumenreich et al 1981, Plunkett et al 1987).

Dipyridamole has also been combined with PALA to block nucleoside transport and thereby inhibit salvage pathways for uridine and cytidine (Chan et al 1986); however, this combination was only moderately active in patients with soft tissue sarcoma (Markman et al 1987).

Ardalan et al (1988) conducted a randomized trial of high-dose 5-FU in vitro with or without PALA. Ataxia and myelsuppression were dose limiting. The maximally tolerated dose for 5-FU in either arm was 2600 mg/m². In this trial the dose of PALA, 250 mg/m², was administered over 15 minutes 24 hours before the 5-FU. In the single-agent 5-FU arm there were 4 partial responses in 19 patients, whereas in the combination arm there were 2 complete and 11 partial responses in 19 patients.

Mann et al (1985) have completed a randomized trial of PALA versus 5-FU versus PALA + 5-FU in women with metastatic breast cancer. They found that PALA + 5-FU was superior to PALA alone. They did not answer whether the combination was superior to 5-FU.

There is in vitro evidence of synergism between PALA and cytidine (Chan and Howell 1989). It is likely this strategy of using a noncytotoxic nucleoside to increase the activity of antimetabolites will be tested clinically.

The combination of PALA and dipyridamole (an inhibitor of nucleoside transport) has already been evaluated in a phase I trial, with 4 objective responses reported in 65 patients (Markman et al 1987, Chan et al 1986). This combination has been ineffective in patients with sarcoma (Baselga et al 1990).

PALA has also been combined with L-alanosine without any discernible benefit (Morton et al 1987, O'Connell et al 1983).

■ Dosage

A variety of doses of single-agent PALA have been used. The most commonly used dose in phase II trials has been 2.5 g/m²/d × 2 days as a 60-minute in-

CLINICAL TOXIC EFFECTS OF PALA

Tumor Type	Phase	Drug/Dose	Toxic Effect	Number of Responses/ Number Evaluable (%)	Reference
Pancreas	II	PALA 250 mg/m² + IV 5-FU* 2600 mg/m²/24-h infusion 24 h after PALA weekly	Severe leukopenia	1/21 (5%)	Morrell et al 1991
Gastric and colorectal	II	PALA† + thymidine + 5-FU	Leukopenia	9/36 (25%) 7/21 (33%)	Windschitl et al 1990
Colorectal	II	PALA + thymidine + 5-FU	Leukopenia, neurologic	10/37 (27%)	O'Connell et al 1984
Colorectal	I and II	PALA 250 mg/m² IV + 5-FU 2600–3250 mg/m²/24-h infusion 24 h after PALA weekly	Leukopenia, gastrointestinal, neurologic	16/37 (43%)	O'Dwyer et al 1990b
Various	I	PALA + methotrexate + 5-FU two different schedules	Mucositis, diarrhea	0/6 (every other week) 1/4 weekly	Kemeny et al 1989, 1990
Colorectal	II	PALA + 5-FU†	Skin rash, gastrointestinal, neurologic	9/51	Muggia et al 1987

*5-FU, 5-fluorouracil.
†Please see reference for doses and schedule.

CLINICAL PHARMACOKINETICS OF PALA

Schedule	Peak	Half-Life (h) α	Half-Life (h) β	Steady-State Volume of Distribution (mL/kg)	(mL/kg/min)	Reference
Single dose	—	—	5.3	309	1.60	Loo et al 1980
Single dose	—	0.93	4.82 ± 1.49	—	—	Erlichman et al 1980
Single dose (1 h)	4.9 to 9×10^{-4} M	—	—	—	1.43 ± 13	Lankelma et al 1981

travenous infusion repeated every 2 weeks (Kleeberg et al 1982, Bramwell et al 1982, Paridaens et al 1982). Other schedules have included 1500 mg/m²/d × 5 days repeated every 3 weeks (Taylor et al 1982).

■ Pharmacokinetics

The table above is a synopsis of the pharmacokinetics (two-compartment model) of PALA.

Pharmacologic studies have indicated rapid renal excretion of PALA (equivalent to glomerular filtration), with 70% of the unmetabolized drug excreted in 24 hours (Erlichman 1980, Loo et al 1980). Moore and colleagues (1982) have demonstrated that tissues taken from patients treated with PALA have decreased pyrimidine nucleotides. Aspartate transcarbamylase was inhibited in the tissues. PALA concentrations have also been measured in tears (Lankelma et al 1981). The drug has been shown to be transported into brain tumor tissue. The extent of uptake reached 12 to 40% of concurrent plasma levels (Stewart et al 1980).

■ Side Effects and Toxicity

Dose-limiting side effects of PALA in phase I clinical trials include skin rash, diarrhea, and mucositis (Grem et al 1988; Ervin et al 1979). Nausea and vomiting and myelosuppression are mild and not typically dose limiting. Paresthesias and rare seizures are also reported in a small percentage of patients (Gralla et al 1980). Other types of neurotoxic effects are sporadically described. These include headaches, lethargy, and confusion. Ataxia is noted with 24-hour continuous infusions of PALA (Grem et al 1988).

The mucocutaneous toxicity of PALA can include severe mucositis and erythema leading to peeling of the hands and feet. If moderate mucositis or diarrhea occurs, PALA dosing should be temporarily discontinued. For severe diarrhea, intravenous hydration should be instituted.

■ Special Applications

PALA has been used to treat patients with psoriasis with some success (Doyle et al 1984, Earhart et al 1981).

REFERENCES

Ardalan B, Singh O, Silberman H. A randomized phase I and II study of short-term infusion of high-dose fluorouracil with or without N-(phosphonacetyl)-L-aspartic acid in patients with advanced pancreatic and colorectal cancers. *J Clin Oncol.* 1988;**6**(6):1053–1058.

Baselga J, Magill GB, Curley T, Casper ES. Phase II trial of PALA + dipyridamole in patients with metastatic soft tissue sarcoma. *Proc Am Assoc Cancer Res.* 1990;**31**:200.

Blumenreich M, Andreeff M, Chou T-C, et al. Kinetic and biochemical modulation of pyrimidine antimetabolites in therapy of acute leukemia. *Proc Am Assoc Cancer Res.* 1981;**22**:193.

Bramwell V, Van Oosterom A, Mouridsen HT, et al. N-(Phosphonacetyl)-L-aspartate (PALA) in advanced soft tissue sarcoma: A phase II trial of the EORTC soft tissue sarcoma group. *Eur J Cancer Clin Oncol.* 1982;**18**(1):81–84.

Carroll DS, Gralla RJ, Kemeny NE. Phase II evaluation of N-(phosphonacetyl)-L-aspartic acid (PALA) in patients with advanced colorectal carcinoma. *Cancer Treat Rep.* 1980;**64**(2/3):349–351.

Casper ES, Gralla RJ, Kelsen DP, Houghton A, Golbey RB, Young CW. Phase II evaluation of N-(phosphonacetyl)-L-aspartic acid (PALA) in patients with non-small cell carcinoma of the lung. *Cancer Treat Rep.* 1980;**64**(4/5):705–707.

Casper ES, Vale K, Williams L, Martin D, Young CW. Phase I and clinical pharmacological evaluation of biochemical modulation of 5-fluorouracil with N-(phosphonacetyl)-L-aspartic acid. *Cancer Res.* 1983;**43**:2324–2329.

Chan TC, Howell SB. Unexpected synergy between N-phosphonacetyl-L-aspartate and cytidine against human tumor cells. *Eur J Cancer Clin Oncol.* 1989;25(4): 721–727.

Chan TC, Markman, Cleary S, Howell SB. Plasma uridine changes in cancer patients treated with the combination of dipyridamole and N-phosphonacetyl-L-aspartate. *Cancer Res.* 1986;46(6):3168–3172.

Collins KD, Stark GR. Aspartate transcarbamylase interaction with the transition state analog N-(phosphonacetyl)-L-aspartate. *J Biol Chem.* 1971;246:6599–6605.

Creagan ET, Eagan RT, Fleming TR, et al. Phase II evaluation of PALA in patients with metastatic lung cancer. *Cancer Treat Rep.* 1981;65(3/4):356–357.

Creagan ET, Nichols WC, O'Fallon Jr. Phase II evaluation of PALA in patients with advanced head and neck cancer. *Cancer Treat Rep.* 1981;65(9/10):827–829.

Creech RH, Tritchler D, Ettinger DS, et al. Phase II study of PALA, amsacrine, teniposide, and zinostatin in small cell lung carcinoma (EST 2579). *Cancer Treat Rep.* 1984;68(9):1183–1884.

Doyle JA, Perry JO, Rubin J, Moertel CG. Treatment of psoriasis with N-phosphonacetyl-L-apartate. *J Am Acad Dermatol.* 1984;10(1):21–24.

Earhart RH, DeConti RC, Rubin J, Ohnuma T. Response of psoriasis to N-phosphonacetyl-L-apartate (letter). *Lancet.* 1981;1:1257–1258.

Earhart RH, Elson PJ, Rosenthal SN, Hahn RG, Slayton RE. Phase II study of PALA and AMSA in advanced renal cell carcinoma. *Am J Clin Oncol.* 1983;5:555–560.

Erlichman C. An overview of the clinical pharmacology of N-phosphonacetyl-L-aspartate (PALA), a new antimetabolite. *Recent Results Cancer Res.* 1980;74:65–71.

Erlichman C, Donehower RC, Speyer JL, Klecker R, Chabner BA. Phase I–phase II trial of N-phosphonacetyl-L-aspartic acid given by intravenous infusion and 5-fluorouracil given by bolus injection. *J Natl Cancer Inst.* 1982;68(2):227–231.

Erlichman C, Strong JM, Chabner BA. Application of a simple competitive protein-binding assay technique to the pharmacokinetics of N-(phosphonacetyl)-L-aspartate in humans. *Cancer Res.* 1980;40(6):1902–1906.

Erlichman C, Strong J, Wiernik P, et al. Phase I trial of PALA (N-phosphonacetyl-L-aspartate). *Proc Am Assoc Cancer Res ASCO.* 1979;20:314.

Ervin TJ, Blum RH, Canellos GP. N-phosphonacetyl L-aspartate (PALA), phase I trial. *Proc Am Assoc Cancer Res ASCO.* 1979;20:200.

Ervin TJ, Blum RH, Meshad MW, Kufe DW, Johnson RK, Canellos GP. Phase I trial of N-(phosphonacetyl)-L-aspartic acid (PALA). *Cancer Treat Rep.* 1980;64(10/11): 1067–1071.

Ettinger DS, Tritchler D, Earhart R, Creech RH. Phase II study of PALA and PCNU in the treatment of non-small cell lung cancer (EST 2580): An Eastern Cooperative Oncology Group study. *Cancer Treat Rep.* 1984;68(10):1297–1298.

Gralla RJ, Casper ES, Golbey RB, Young EW. Phase I and preliminary phase II studies with N-(phosphonacetyl)-L-aspartic acid (PALA). *Proc Am Assoc Cancer Res ASCO.* 1979;20:115.

Gralla RJ, Casper ES, Natale RB, Yagoda A, Young CW. Phase I trial of PALA. *Cancer Treat Rep.* 1980;64(12): 1301–1305.

Grant A, Rauscher F, Cadman E. Differential effect of N-(phosphonacetyl)-L-aspartate on 1-β-D-arabinofuranosylcytosine metabolism and cytotoxicity in human leukemia and normal bone marrow progenitors. *Cancer Res.* 1982;42:4007–4013.

Grem JL, King SA, O'Dwyer PJ, et al. Biochemistry and clinical activity of N-(phosphonacetyl)-L-aspartate: A review. *Cancer Res.* 1988;48:4441–4454.

Hart RD, Ohnuma T, Holand JF. Initial clinical study with N-(phosphonacetyl)-L-aspartic acid (PALA) in patients with advanced cancer. *Cancer Treat Rep.* 1980;64(4/5): 617–624.

Hoogenraad NJ. Reaction mechanism of aspartate transcarbamylase from mouse spleen. *Arch Biochem Biophys.* 1974;161:76–82.

Jayaram HN, Cooney DA, Vistica DT, et al. Mechanisms of sensitivity of resistance of murine tumors to N-(phosphonacetyl)-L-aspartate (PALA). *Cancer Treat Rep.* 1979;63:1291–1302.

Johnson RK. Reversal of toxicity and antitumor activity of N-(phosphonacetyl)-L-aspartate by uridine or carbamyl-dl-aspartate in vivo. *Biochem Pharmacol.* 1977;26:81–84.

Johnson RK, Inouye T, Goldin A, Stark GR. Antitumor activity of N-(phosphonacetyl)-L-aspartic acid, a transition-state inhibitor of aspartate transcarbamylase. *Cancer Res.* 1976;36:2720–2725.

Kemeny NE, Schneider A, Martin DS. Phase I trial of PALA, methotrexate, fluorouracil, leucovorin, and uridine rescue in patients with advanced cancer. The use of uridine to decrease fluorouracil toxicity. *Cancer Invest.* 1990;8(2):263–264.

Kemeny N, Schneider A, Martin DS, Colofiore J, Sawyer RC, Derby S, Salvia B. Phase I trial of N-(phosphonacetyl)-L-aspartate, methotrexate, and 5-fluorouracil with leucovorin rescue in patients with advanced cancer. *Cancer Res.* 1989;49(16):4636–4639.

Kleeberg UR, Mulder JH, Rumke P, Thomas D, Rozencweig M. N-(Phosphonacetyl)-L-aspartate (PALA) in advanced malignant melanoma: A phase II trial of the EORTC Malignant Melanoma Cooperative Group. *Eur J Clin Oncol.* 1982;18:723–726.

Kovach JS, Schutt AJ, Moertel CG, O'Connel MJ. Phase I study of N-(phosphonacetyl)-L-aspartic acid (PALA). *Cancer Treat Rep.* 1979;63(11/12):1909–1912.

Kurzrock R, Yap BS, Plaser C, et al. Phase II evaluation of PALA in patients with refractory metastatic sarcomas. *Am J Clin Oncol.* 1984;4:305–307.

Lankelma J, Penders PG, Leyva A, et al. Concentrations of N-(phosphonacetyl)-L-aspartate (PALA) in plasma and tears in man. *Eur J Cancer Clin Oncol.* 1981;11:1199–204.

Laster WR, Shabel FM. Collateral sensitivity of P-388/ARA-C and P-388/5-FU to N-(phosphonacetyl)-L-aspartate (PALA). *Proc Am Assoc Cancer Res ASCO.* 1979;**20**:95.

Loo TL, Freidman J, Moore EC, Vadivieso M, Marti Jr, Stewart D. Pharmacological disposition of N-(phosphonacetyl)-L-aspartate in humans. *Cancer Res.* 1980;**40**(1):86–90.

Mann GB, Hortobagyi GN, Buzdar AU, Yap HY Valdivieso M. A comparative study of PALA, PALA plus 5-FU, and 5-FU in advanced breast cancer. *Cancer.* 1985;**56**(6):1320–1324.

Markman M, Chan TC, Cleary S, Howell SB. Phase I trial of combination therapy of cancer with N-phosphonacetyl-L- aspartic acid and dipyridamole. *Cancer Chemother Pharmacol.* 1987;**19**(1):80–83.

Moore EC, Friedman J, Valdivieso M, et al. Aspartate carbamoyltransferase activity, drug concentrations, and pyrimidine nucleotides in tissue from patients treated with N-(phosphonacetyl)-L-aspartate. *Biochem Pharmacol.* 1982;**31**(20):3317–3321.

Morrell LM, Bach A, Richman SP, Goodman P, Fleming TR, MacDonald JS. A phase II multi-institutional trial of low-dose N-(phosphonacetyl)-L-aspartate and high-dose 5-fluorouracil as a short term infusion in the treatment of adenocarcinoma of the pancreas. A Southwest Oncology Group study. *Cancer.* 1991;**67**(2):363–366.

Morton RF, Creasan ET, Cullinan SA, et al. Phase II studies of single-agent cimetidine and the combination N-phosphonacetyl-L-aspartate (NSC-224131) plus L-alanosine (NSC-153353) in advanced malignant melanoma. *J Clin Oncol.* 1987;**5**(7):1078–1082.

Moyer JD, Handschumacher RE. Selective inhibition of pyrimidine synthesis and depletion of nucleotide pools by N-(phosphonacetyl)-L-aspartate. *Cancer Res.* 1979;**39**:3089–3094.

Muggia FM, Camacho FJ, Kaplan BH, et al. Weekly 5-fluorouracil combined with PALA: Toxic and therapeutic effects in colorectal cancer. *Cancer Treat Rep.* 1987;**71**(3):253–256.

Muggia FM, Tsiatis AA, O'Connell MJ, Glick JH, Opfell RW, Coren A. Phase II trial of PALA in lymphoma: An Eastern Cooperative Oncology Group study. *Cancer Treat Rep.* 1984;**68**(3):551–553.

Muss HB, Bundy B, DiSaia PJ, Stehman FB, Beecham J. PALA (NSC- 224131) in advanced carcinoma of the cervix. A phase II study of the Gynecologic Oncology Group. *Am J Clin Oncol.* 1984;**6**:741–744.

Muss HB, Slavik M, Bundy B, Stehman FB, Creasman WT. A phase II study of PALA (NSC-224131) in patients with advanced ovarian carcinoma. A Gynecologic Oncology Group study. *Am J Clin Oncol.* 1984;**3**:257–260.

Natale RB, Yagoda A, Kelsen DP, Gralla RJ, Watson RC. Phase II trial of PALA in hypernephroma and urinary bladder cancer. *Cancer Treat Rep.* 1982;**66**(12):2091–2092.

O'Connell MJ, Moertel CG, Rubin J, Hahn RG, Kvols LK, Schutt AJ. Clinical trial of sequential N-phosphonacetyl-L- aspartate, thymidine, and 5-fluorouracil in advanced colorectal carcinoma. *J Clin Oncol.* 1984;**2**(10):1133–1138.

O'Connell MJ, Rubin J, Schutt AJ, Moertel CG, Kvols LK. Clinical trial of PALA and L-alanosine in advanced colorectal carcinoma. *Cancer Treat Rep.* 1983;**67**(12):1141–1142.

O'Dwyer PJ. Biochemical modulation of 5-flurouracil by PALA. *Cancer Invest.* 1990;**8**(2):261–262.

O'Dwyer PJ, Paul AR, Walczak J, Weiner LM, Litwin S, Comis RL. Phase II study of biochemical modulation of fluorouracil by low-dose PALA in patients with colorectal cancer. *J Clin Oncol.* 1990;**8**(9):1497–1503.

Paridaens R, Mouridsen HT, Palshof T, et al. N-(Phosphonacetyl)-L-aspartate (PALA) in advanced breast cancer: A phase II trial of the EORTC Breast Cancer Cooperative Group. *Eur J Cancer Clin Oncol.* 1982;**18**(1):67–70.

Pauling L. Chemical achievement and hope for the future. *Am Scientist.* 1948;**36**:51–58.

Plunkett W, Adams T, Keating M. Modulation of ara-CTP metabolism in leukemia cells during high-dose ARA-C (HD ARA-C) therapy by thymidine and PALA. *Proc Am Soc Clin Oncol.* 1987;**6**:30.

Rubin J, Purvis J, Britell JC, Hahn RG, Moertel CG, Schutt AJ. Phase II study of PALA in advanced large bowel carcinoma. *Cancer Treat Rep.* 1981;**65**(3/4):335–336.

Stewart DJ, Leavens M, Friedman J, et al. Penetration of N-(phosphonacetyl)-L-aspartate into human central nervous system and intracerebral tumor. *Cancer Res.* 1980;**40**(9):3163–3166.

Taylor SG IV, Davis TE, Falkson G, Keller AM. PALA in advanced breast cancer. A phase II pilot study by the ECOG. *Am J Clin Oncol.* 1982;**5**(6):627–629.

Tsuboi KK, Edmunds HN, Kwong LK. Selective inhibition of pyrimidine biosynthesis and effect on proliferative growth of colon cancer cells. *Cancer Res.* 1977;**37**:3080–3087.

Valdivieso M, Moore EC, Burgess AM, et al. Phase I clinical study of N-(phosphonacetyl)-L-aspartic acid (PALA). *Cancer Treat Rep.* 1980;**64**(2/3):285–292.

Valdivieso M, Moore EC, Loo TL, Bodey GP, Freireich EJ. Phase I clinical study of N-(phosphonacetyl)-L-aspartate (PALA, NSC-224131). *Proc Am Assoc Cancer Res ASCO.* 1979;**20**:187.

Van Echo DA, Diggs CH, Scoltock M, Wiernik PH. Phase II evaluation of N-(phosphonacetyl)-L-aspartic acid (PALA) in metastatic adenocarcinoma of the colon or rectum. *Cancer Treat Rep.* 1980;**64**(2/3)339–342.

Wahl GM, Padgett RA, Stark GR. Gene amplification causes overproduction of the first three enzymes of UMP synthesis in N-(phosphonacetyl)-L-aspartate-resistant hamster cells. *J Biol Chem.* 1979;**254**:8679–8689.

Wiley RG, Gralla RJ, Casper ES, Kemeny N. Neurotoxicity of the pyrimidine synthesis inhibitor N-phosphonoacetyl-L-aspartate. *Ann Neurol.* 1982;**12**(2):175–183.

Windschitl HE, O'Connell MJ, Wieand HS, et al. A clinical trial of biochemical modulation of 5-fluorouracil with N-phosphonoacetyl-L-aspartate and thymidine in advanced gastric and anaplastic colorectal cancer. *Cancer.* 1990;**66**(5):853–856.

Pentostatin

■ Other Names

2'-Deoxycoformycin; dCF; NSC-218321, co-vidarabine, Nipent® (Parke-Davis).

■ Chemistry

Structure of pentostatin

Pentostatin, known chemically as (R)-3-(2-deoxy-β-D-*erythro*-pentofuramosyl)-3,6,7,8-tetrahydroimidazo[4,5[*d*][1,3]diazepin-8-ol, was originally isolated from a strain of *Streptomyces antibioticus*. The molecular formula is $C_{11}H_{16}N_4O_4$ and the molecular weight is 268.27. Pentostatin has a seven-membered ring system and thereby differs from the normal 6-member ring-containing purine transition-state intermediates involved in the conversion of adenosine to inosine. The off-white lyophilized powder is freely soluble in water.

■ Antitumor Activity

Pentostatin is most effective in malignancies derived from lymphocytic cells including hairy cell leukemia, chronic lymphocytic leukemia, mycosis fungoides, acute lymphoblastic leukemia (Koller et al 1979), lymphoblastic lymphoma, and adult T-cell leukemia (O'Dwyer et al 1988). In hairy cell leukemia, overall response rates of 90% are reported, with 50 to 60% complete responses (Johnston et al 1986, 1988, Kraut et al 1986). Several patients failing interferon alfa have also responded to pentostatin (Spiers et al 1987, Foon et al 1986). In one trial, durable complete remissions were obtained in 10 of 11 patients with hairy cell leukemia resistant to interferon alfa (Blick et al 1990). All of these patients had complete remissions, which have lasted from 10 to 30 months without any further therapy (median, 18 months at time of publication) (Blick et al 1990). Similarly, Ho et al (1989) have reported an overall response rate of 79%, with 33% complete responses in 33 patients treated with pentostatin after relapsing on interferon alfa.

In chronic lymphocytic leukemia up to 20% of patients, most who were heavily pretreated, have responded to pentostatin (Grever et al 1985). Patients with prolymphocytic, T cell-derived leukemia have also responded to this agent in a pilot trial (Galton et al 1974). In addition, up to 40% of patients with advanced mycosis fungoides have responded to pentostatin in phase II trials (O'Dwyer et al 1988).

Interestingly, pentostatin is active in patients with adult T-cell leukemias/lymphomas associated with regional outbreaks of the human immunodeficiency virus I (Lofters et al 1988). In acute lymphocytic leukemia in adults, highly toxic dose levels were needed for activity (Smyth et al 1985), thereby obviating a significant role for pentostatin in this disease.

■ Mechanism of Action

Pentostatin is an irreversible inhibitor of the enzyme adenosine deaminase (ADA). ADA regulates intracellular adenosine levels by mediating the hydrolytic deamination of adenosine and deoxyadenosine (see figure). Of interest, a genetic ADA deficiency is associated with severe combined immunodeficiency disease (SCID), which is characterized by impaired B- and T-lymphocyte function, hypogammaglobulinemia, lymphopenia, and numerous systemic infections (Meuwissen et al 1975).

ADA levels are normally highest in lymphatic tissues and in circulating T cells over B cells (Ganeshaguru et al 1981). Leukemic blast cells in the bone marrow also have elevated ADA levels.

The K_i for ADA inhibition by pentostatin is 2.5×10^{-12} M (Agarwal et al 1977). Following ADA inhibition by pentostatin, deoxyribose nucleosides (but not adenosine) accumulate intracellularly. Lymphocytes and erythrocytes are thought to be selectively damaged by pentostatin because of their higher deoxynucleoside kinase (phosphorylation) activities (Carson et al 1977). The subsequent buildup of deoxyadenosine and its phosphorylated congeners, especially deoxy-ATP (Cohen et al 1978), thereby inhibits DNA synthesis, probably by blocking ribonucleotide reductase (Henderson and Smith 1981) (see figure on page 775).

In addition to the buildup of toxic metabolites, ATP is also depleted by pentostatin (Koller and

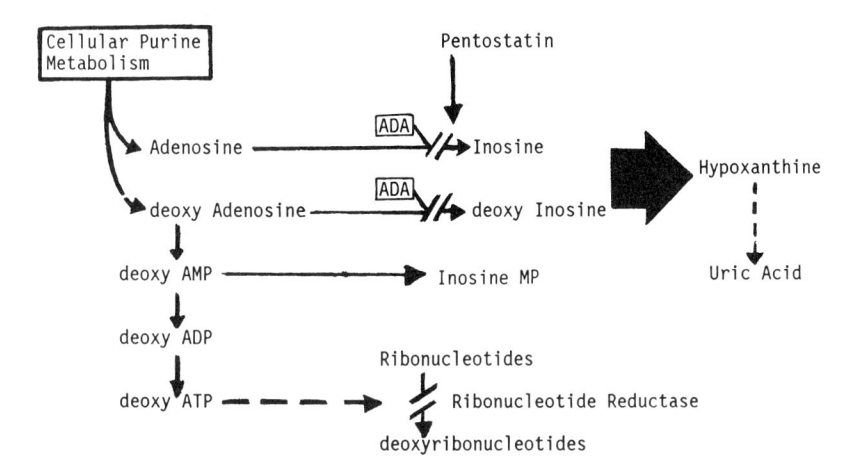

Inhibition of purine metabolism by pentostatin. Inhibition of adenosine deaminase (ADA) by pentostatin leads to a buildup of deoxyadenosine and deoxyadenosine triphosphates. The formation of deoxyribonucleotides is also inhibited by a blockade of ribonucleotide reductase.

Mitchell 1983). Other proposed mechanisms of action for pentostatin include depletion of nicotinamide adenine dinucleotide (NAD) to possibly block DNA repair (Seto et al 1985), inhibition of RNA transcription, direct incorporation of deoxy-ATP into DNA, inhibition of S-adenosylhomocysteine hydrolase, and induction of DNA strand breaks (O'Dwyer et al 1988).

■ Availability and Storage

Pentostatin is commercially available from Parke-Davis (Morris Plains, New Jersey) in 10-mg vials as a lyophilized powder (Nipent®). Mannitol (50 mg) and sodium hydroxide (to adjust pH) are included in this formulation. Storage of the intact vials under refrigeration is recommended (National Cancer Institute 1987).

■ Preparation for Use, Stability, and Admixture

Pentostatin 10-mg vials are reconstituted with 5 mL of Sodium Chloride for Injection, USP. This yields a pale yellow solution of pH 6.7 to 8.7. This solution is chemically stable at room temperature for 72 hours (about 2–4% decomposition). Dilutions of the 10-mg pentostatin vial contents in 500 mL of 0.9% Sodium Chloride for Injection, USP, or Lactated Ringer's Injection, USP, are stable for at least 48 hours at room temperature (0–4% degradation). The drug is also compatible with polyvinyl chloride-type plastics and does not adsorb significantly to such container surfaces. Pentostatin degradation is more rapid in 5% Dextrose Injection, USP, resulting in 2% decomposition in 24 hours and up to 8 to 10% decomposition after 48 hours of storage at room temperature (National Cancer Institute 1987). Under refrigeration, however, pentostatin solutions in 5% dextrose or 0.9% sodium chloride are chemically stable for over 4 days. Pentostatin (0.4 mg/mL) solutions are physically stable for 4 hours with ondansetron (1 mg/mL) (Trissel et al 1990).

■ Administration

Pentostatin is administered intravenously, typically as a short (20–30 minutes) infusions in 50 to 100 mL of isotonic solution. Infusion solutions include 5% dextrose in water and 0.9% sodium chloride. Bolus administration of pentostatin over 1 to 2 minutes has also been used. Although prior protocols have recommended the addition of sodium bicarbonate, (10–44.6 mEq) to the infusion solution for each dose to prolong stability (Koller and Mitchell 1984), this is generally not necessary for short intravenous infusions over no longer than 30 minutes. Pentostatin has also been administered as a continuous 24-hour infusion for periods up to 72 hours (Murphy et al 1984).

■ Special Precautions

As pentostatin is eliminated primarily by the kidney, adequate renal function must be ensured prior to each drug administration. Patients with elevated serum creatinine or blood urea nitrogen should receive reduced doses. Pentostatin also produces significant immunosuppression, often manifested by herpes simplex and herpes zoster, skin infections, and other opportunistic infections. Patients with severe preexisting infections should not receive this agent.

■ Dosage

The tolerable and maximally active dose level of pentostatin is approximately 4 to 5 mg/m²/wk, given for 3 consecutive weeks (O'Dwyer et al 1988, Johnston et al 1988). In phase I studies, a few patients tolerated pentostatin doses up to 30 mg/m²/d × 5 days, but in other trials, this dose has been fatal (O'Dwyer et al 1988). Interpatient tolerance to pentostatin varies greatly and at high dose levels, renal and neurologic toxicity can be severe. In a study in acute lymphocytic leukemia and lymphoma, 10% of patients died from pentostatin toxicity after receiving doses of 10 mg/m²/d × 5 days (Smyth et al 1985). Typically, pentostatin dosing is limited to 3 consecutive weeks with 1 to 2 weeks off therapy to prevent possibly cumulative nephrotoxicity and especially lethargy.

Pharmacodynamic studies of pentostatin use in cancer patients show that adenosine deaminase inhibition in peripheral lymphocytes is maximal (80–90%) after single doses of 4 mg/m² (Grever et al 1981). Thus, the value of higher pentostatin doses is not established in hairy cell leukemia (Kraut et al 1986).

Because up to 90% of pentostatin may be eliminated in the urine, significant dose reductions are necessary in patients with impaired renal function. Presently, no prospectively validated dosing algorithms are available for pentostatin use in patients with compromised renal function. A standard kinetic formula (Anderson et al 1976) was used to generate the dose reduction suggestions found in the table above. These guidelines were based on the following assumptions: a urinary "fraction excreted" for pentostatin of 73% (range 50–96%) and a "normal" creatinine clearance of 120 mL/min. As with any nephrotoxic drug, pentostatin dosing in the patient with renal insufficiency must be very cautiously approached.

■ Drug Interactions

By blocking adenosine deaminase activity pentostatin can augment the toxicity of other nucleoside antimetabolites, including cytarabine (Plunkett et al 1979). Indeed, pentostatin was originally evaluated as a potentiator of the antiviral drug vidarabine (adenine arabinoside), and in combination with pentostatin, vidarabine has increased antiviral and toxic effects (Plunkett et al 1984). Conversely, there is anecdotal evidence that allopurinol may enhance the toxicity of pentostatin and this combination should probably be avoided (personal communication, M. Grever, National Cancer Institute, Bethesda, MD). Both drugs produce skin rashes when used alone and in combination. One case of fatal hypersensitivity vasculitis is reported. Pentostatin is also not recommended to be combined with fludarabine in patients with chronic lymphocytic leukemia. Severe and occasionally fatal pulmonary toxicity has been reported in this setting.

SUGGESTED PENTOSTATIN DOSE ADJUSTMENTS IN PATIENTS WITH IMPAIRED RENAL FUNCTION

Serum Creatinine* (mL/min)	% of Normal Pentostatin Dose
≥ 120	100
100	80
80	70
60	59
40	42
< 20	None[†]

*Not prospectively validated; assumes urinary excretion of 73% of dose and normal creatinine clearance of 120 mL/min (formula of Anderson et al 1976).
[†]Pentostatin is nephrotoxic and dosing in severe renal insufficiency is contraindicated.

■ Pharmacokinetics

Pentostatin pharmacokinetics have been extensively studied by Malspeis et al (1984) and others in phase I clinical trials (see table). Pentostatin assays have most often used spectrophotometric determinations of the conversion of adenine to inosine. Following a rapid intravenous infusion of doses ranging from 0.25 mg/kg/d to 2 to 10 mg/m²/d, pentostatin exhibits a first-order, two-compartment elimination pattern (see table on the top of page 777).

These results show that urinary excretion is the predominant route of pentostatin elimination. The drug does not appear to be bound to tissues or red blood cells. Only about 4% of the drug is bound to plasma proteins. Drug accumulation was also not apparent between dosing intervals. The metabolism

PLASMA PHARMACOKINETICS OF PENTOSTATIN IN ADULTS

Half-life		Volume of Distribution (L/m²)		Urinary Excretion (% Dose)	Clearance (ml/min/m²)		Study
α (min)	β (h)	Steady State	β Phase				
8.7*	4.9	20 ± 5.3	23 ± 6.2	96 ± 12	52 ± 17		Malspeis et al 1984
30–85	5–15	NR†	NR	32–48	NR	NR	Smyth et al 1980
NR	4.9–6.4	NR	NR	50–82	NR	NR	Major et al 1981

*Values are expressed as means, means ± SD, or ranges.
†NR, not reported.

of pentostatin has not been described and most of a dose is apparently excreted intact in the urine; however, increased deoxyadenosine levels may be associated with toxicity (Schneider et al 1980) although not all studies have shown this (O'Dwyer et al 1988).

The table below shows that plasma levels in the range 1 to 5 µM are achievable following tolerable doses of pentostatin. In this regard it is important to recall that the lower dose ranges of 0.25 mg/kg and 4 mg/m² achieve near-maximal inhibition of ADA activity in peripheral blood lymphocytes (see Dosage).

■ Side Effects and Toxicity

The dose-limiting toxic effects of pentostatin include renal dysfunction which can lead to acute renal failure, neurologic toxicity manifested by lethargy, and, rarely, hematologic toxicity manifested by reversible granulocytopenia. These effects are both dose and schedule dependent. The toxic effects are also clearly correlated with pretreatment renal function and performance status.

Renal Toxicity. At high dose levels (>5 mg/m²/d) pentostatin produces renal tubular toxicity manifested by elevations in serum creatinine. If the drug is not discontinued and/or if patients have preexisting renal insufficiency and/or poor performance status, renal toxicity can proceed to acute renal failure. (See Dosage Section for suggestions on dose reductions for mild to moderate renal insufficiency.) Continuous prolonged daily dosing may produce cumulative renal toxic effects at high dose levels. At low dose levels (< 5 mg/m²/d), only 5% of patients will have reversible creatinine elevations that do not proceed to frank renal failure. Adequate hydration and avoidance of other known nephrotoxic agents (such as aminoglycoside antibiotics) are highly recommended.

Hematologic Toxicity. At dose levels of 5 mg/m²/d or less, myelosuppression affecting both granulocytes and platelets may occasionally be dose limiting. The median day of the granulocyte nadir after a consecutive 3-day dosing regimen is reported to be day 15 (Johnston et al 1988). Severe granulocytopenia and thrombocytopenia have occurred only in patients with impaired bone marrow reserve as a result of prior therapy and/or tumor involvement of the marrow.

Lymphocytopenia is an anticipated sequela of pentostatin administration. Fever and infection are also routinely seen, especially with the second or third courses of therapy in patients with hairy cell leukemia (Johnston et al 1988). Both B and T lymphocytes, especially CD4+ cells, are suppressed by pentostatin (Kraut et al 1990). The recovery of CD4+

PENTOSTATIN PLASMA LEVELS IN ADULTS

Study	Dose	Plasma Level (µM)
Malspeis et al 1984	2–10 mg/m²	1.5–4.7
Smyth et al 1980	0.25 mg/kg	0.01–0.1
Major et al 1981	10–30 mg/m²	0.01
Venner et al 1981	0.25 mg/kg (30-min infusion)	1.5
	1 mg/kg (1 h after infusion)	4.7

(helper T cells) may be prolonged and incomplete in some hairy cell leukemia patients treated with pentostatin (Steis et al 1991). In some cases, CD4+ cells had not recovered to pretreatment levels 30 to 40 months after the end of treatment. Skin test reactivity and natural killer cell function may variably remain intact (Kraut et al 1990), but severe systemic infections, primarily pneumonia, can occur (O'Dwyer et al 1986). Causative organisms included gram-positive and gram-negative bacteria; fungi, principally *Candida*; and disseminated herpes zoster varicella (O'Dwyer et al 1986). Over 60% of these infections were fatal in phase I-treated patients. The recovery of dose-related immunosuppression occurs slowly over several months once therapy is halted (Kraut et al 1990). Skin infections (both bacterial and viral) are also common. Herpes simplex and zoster infections may be anticipated in these settings. The early use of antibiotics and the delay of therapy to allow for resolution of herpes infections may help to mitigate severe complications.

Neurologic Toxicity. Pentostatin produces dose-dependent lethargy and fatigue which rarely progress to frank coma. Seizures have also been described following dose-intensive regimens. Lethargy is seen even in patients with good renal function, but it may be lessened by limiting courses to 3 consecutive days and by increasing the interval between pentostatin courses to 2 weeks (O'Dwyer et al 1988). Neurologic toxicity is rarely dose limiting at pentostatin doses of 5 mg/m^2 or less.

Skin and Integument Toxicity. In addition to bacterial and viral (herpes zoster and simplex) infections, pentostatin routinely produces dry skin. A rash has also been reported in patients with hairy cell leukemia. Pentostatin is not reported to be a vesicant if extravasated.

Conjunctival Toxicity. Keratoconjunctivitis is described in some patients receiving pentostatin. This is typically reversible and glucocorticosteroid eye drops are usually not needed. There is also no clear association of conjunctivitis with dose or schedule (O'Dwyer et al 1988).

Gastrointestinal Toxicity. Nausea and vomiting of mild to moderate severity can occur in patients receiving pentostatin. This toxic effect has been easily controlled with antiemetics and is never dose limiting nor prolonged in duration.

Rare Toxic Effects. A few patients treated with high doses of pentostatin have experienced reversible hepatitis manifested by elevation of serum glutamic–oxalacetic and glutamic–pyruvic transaminases. Interstitial/alveolar pulmonary infiltrations have also been described in two patients treated for diagnoses of hairy cell leukemia. These latter cases were characterized by hypoxia and respiratory insufficiency. Following empiric antibiotics and supportive care, both patients recovered after several days. Pulmonary edema, hypotension, and death have been observed following high-dose therapy of patients with lymphoproliferative disorders (Koller and Mitchell 1983). Of interest, these and other major organ toxic effects were associated with high ratios of deoxy-ATP/ATP (> 1.5) monitored in red blood cells. Fatal cerebral edema has also been reported in a single hairy cell leukemia patient who received three doses of 4 mg/m^2 pentostatin every other week.

REFERENCES

Agarwal RP, Spector T, Parks RE. Tight-binding inhibitors. IV. Inhibition of adenosine deaminases by various inhibitors. *Biochem Pharmacol.* 1977;**26**:359–367.

Anderson RJ, Gambertoglio JG, Schrier RW. *Clinical Use of Drugs in Renal Failure.* Springfield, Ill: Charles C Thomas; 1976.

Blick M, Lepe-Zuniga JL, Doig R, Quesada JR. Durable complete remissions after 2'-deoxycoformycin treatment in patients with hairy cell leukemia resistant to interferon alpha. *Am J Hematol.* 1990;**33**:205–209.

Carson DA, Kaye J, Seegmiller JE. Lymphospecific toxicity in adenosine deaminase deficiency and purine nucleoside phosphorylase deficiency: Possible role of nucleoside kinase(s). *Proc Natl Acad Sci USA.* 1977;**74**:5677–5681.

Cohen A, Hirschhorn R, Horowitz SD, et al. Deoxyadenosine triphosphate as a potentially toxic metabolite in adenosine deaminase deficiency. *Proc Natl Acad Sci USA.* 1978;**75**:472–476.

Foon KA, Nakano GM, Loller CA, et al. Response to 2'-deoxycoformycin after failure of interferon-alpha in non-splenectomized patients with hairy cell leukemia. *Blood.* 1986;**68**:297–300.

Galton DA, Goldman JM, Wiltshaw W, et al. Prolymphocytic leukemia. *Br J Haematol.* 1974;**27**:7–23.

Ganeshaguru K, Lee N, Llewellin P, et al. Adenosine deaminase concentrations in leukemia, and lymphoma: Relation to cell phenotypes. *Leukemia Res.* 1981;**5**:215–222.

Grever MR, Leiby JM, Kraut EH, et al. Low-dose deoxycoformycin in lymphoid malignancy. *J Clin Oncol.* 1985;**3**:1196–1201.

Grever MR, Siaw MF, Jacob WF, et al. The biochemical and clinical consequences of 2'-deoxycoformycin in refractory lymphoproliferative malignancy. *Blood.* 1981;**57**:406–417.

Henderson JF, Smith CM. Mechanisms of deoxycoformycin toxicity in vivo. In: Tattersall MHN, Fox RM, eds. *Nucleosides and Cancer Treatment.* Orlando, FL: Academic Press; 1981:208–217.

Ho AD, Thaler J, Mandelli F, et al. Response to pentostatin in hairy-cell leukemia refractory to interferon-alpha. *J Clin Oncol.* 1989;**7**(10):1533–1538.

Johnston JB, Eisenhauer E, Corbet WEN, et al. Efficacy of 2'-deoxycoformycin in hairy-cell leukemia: A study of the National Cancer Institute of Canada Clinical Trials Group. *J Natl Cancer Inst.* 1988;**80**:765–769.

Johnston JB, Glazer RI, Pigh L, et al. The treatment of hairy cell leukemia with 2'-deoxycoformycin. *Br J Hematol.* 1986;**63**:525–534.

Koller CA, Mitchell BS. Alterations in erythrocyte adenine nucleotide pools resulting from 2'-deoxycoformycin therapy. *Cancer Res.* 1983;**43**;1409–1414.

Koller CA, Mitchell BS. Erythrocyte adenosine triphosphate and deoxyadenosine triphosphate measurements predict toxicity following 2'-deoxycoformycin therapy. *Cancer Treat Symp.* 1984;**2**:67–74.

Koller CA, Mitchell BS, Grever MR, et al. Treatment of acute lymphoblastic leukemia with 2'-deoxycoformycin: Clinical and biochemical consequences of adenosine deaminase inhibition. *Cancer Treat Rep.* 1979;**63**:1949–1952.

Kraut EH, Bouroncle BA, Grever MR. Low-dose deoxycoformycin in the treatment of hairy cell leukemia. *Blood.* 1986;**68**:1119–1122.

Kraut EH, Neff JC, Bouroncle BA, et al. Immunosuppressive effects of pentostatin. *J Clin Oncol.* 1990;**8**:848–855.

Lofters W, Campbell M, Gibbs WN, et al. 2'-Deoxycoformycin therapy in adult T-cell leukemia/lymphoma. *Cancer.* in press

Major PP, Agarwal RP, Kufe DW. Clinical pharmacology of deoxycoformycin. *Blood.* 1981;**58**:91–96.

Malspeis L, Weinrib AB, Staubus AE, et al. Clinical pharmacokinetics of 2'-deoxycoformycin. *Cancer Treat Symp.* 1984;**2**:7–15.

Meuwissen JJ, Pollara B, Pickering RJ. Combined immunodeficiency associated with adenosine deaminase deficiency. *J Pediatr.* 1975;**86**:169–181.

Murphy SB, Sinkule JA, Rivera G. Phase I–II clinical and pharmacodynamic study of effects of 2'-deoxycoformycin administered by continuous infusion in children with refractory acute lymphoblastic leukemia. *Cancer Treat Symp.* 1984;**2**:55–61.

National Cancer Institute. *NCI Investigational Drugs— Pentostatin: Pharmaceutical Data.* NIH Publication 88-2141. Bethesda, MD: U.S. Department of Health and Human Services; 1987:100.

O'Dwyer PJ, Spiers ASD, Marsoni S. Association of severe and fatal infections and treatment with pentostatin. *Cancer Treat Rep.* 1986;**70**:1117–1120.

O'Dwyer PJ, Wagner B, Leyland-Jones B, Wittes RE, et al. 2'- Deoxycoformycin (pentostatin) for lymphoid malignancies. *Ann Intern Med.* 1988;**108**:733–743.

Plunkett W, Alexander L, Chubb S, et al. Biochemical basis of the increased activity of 9-β-D-arabinofuranosyladenine in the presence of inhibitors of adenosine deaminase. *Cancer Res.* 1979;**39**:3655–3660.

Plunkett W, Feun LG, Benjamin RS, et al. Modulation of vidarabine metabolism by 2'-deoxycoformycin for therapy of acute leukemia. *Cancer Treat Symp.* 1984;**2**:23–28.

Schneider R, Korngold C, Vale K, et al. Clinical and pharmacologic investigation of deoxycoformycin (abstract). *Proc Am Assoc Cancer Res.* 1980;**21**;185.

Seto S, Carrera CJ, Kubota M, et al. Mechanism of deoxyadenosine and 2-chlorodeoxyadenosine toxicity to nondividing human lymphocytes. *J Clin Invest.* 1985;**75**:377–383.

Smyth JF, Paine RM, Jackman AL, et al. The clinical pharmacology of the adenosine deaminase inhibitor 2'-deoxycoformycin. *Cancer Chemother Pharmacol.* 1980;**5**:93–101.

Smyth JF, Prentice HG, Proctor S, Hoffbrand AV. Deoxycoformycin in the treatment of leukemias and lymphomas. *Ann NY Acad Sci.* 1985;**451**:123–128.

Spiers AS, Moore D, Cassileth PA, et al. Remissions in hairy-cell leukemia with pentostatin (2'-deoxycoformycin). *N Engl J Med.* 1987;**316**:825–830.

Steis RG, Urba WJ, Kopp WC, et al. Kinetics of recovery of CD4+ T cells in peripheral blood of deoxycoformycin-treated patients. *J Natl Cancer Inst.* 1991;**83**(22):1678–1679.

Trissel LA, Fulton B, Tramonte SM. Visual compatibility of ondansetron with chemotherapeutic agents, antibiotics, and other selected drugs during simulated Y-site injection (abstract #P- 468R). In: *25th Annual ASHP Midyear Clinical Meetings and Exhibit, Las Vegas, Nevada;* 1990.

Venner PM, Glazer RI, Blatt J, et al. Levels of 2'-deoxycoformycin, adenosine, and deoxyadenosine in patients with acute lymphoblastic leukemia. *Cancer Res.* 1981;**41**:4508–4511.

Piperazinedione

■ Other Names

Crystalline antibiotic; Actinomycete Fermentation Product; Merck Compound 593A; NSC-135758.

■ Chemistry

Structure of piperazinedione

The chemical name for the compound is 2,5-piperazinedione-3,6-bis(5-chloro-2-piperidyl)-dihydrochloride. It is a natural fermentation product produced by *Streptomyces grisealates* (Gitterman et al 1970) and has a molecular weight of approximately 422, a melting point in the range of 219 to 230°C, and the empiric formula $C_{14}H_{22}Cl_2N_4O_2 \cdot 2HCl$.

■ Antitumor Activity

In animal systems piperazinedione has demonstrated antitumor activity against Ehrlich ascites tumor, Taper liver tumor, and Walker 256 carcinosarcoma (Tarnowski et al 1973), as well as against L-1210 murine leukemia (Schabel et al 1976).

Relatively poor activity has been described for piperazinedione in numerous phase I and II clinical trials. La Gasse et al (1979) and Douglass et al (1979) reported no significant activity for the drug in various gynecologic malignancies (uterine sarcomas, vulvar and endometrial carcinoma) or in colorectal carcinoma, respectively. Ovarian cancer also appears to be minimally responsive to piperazinedione, with an objective response rate of only 3% including no complete responses (Thigpen et al 1984). Another trial also reported no responses for piperazinedione in colorectal cancer (Douglass et al 1985). Jones et al (1977) could detect no significant activity for the drug in myelomas and in non-Hodgkin's lymphoma. They did, however, observe a few partial responses primarily in refractory Hodgkin's disease. In the phase I study by Currie et al (1979) only one partial response was noted in a child with Hodgkin's disease. No responses were seen in refractory adult patients.

Similarly negative results have accumulated for piperazinedione used in advanced malignant melanoma (Al-Sarraf et al 1978), metastatic renal carcinoma (Pasmantier et al 1977), and metastatic breast carcinoma (Palmer et al 1977). A low response rate of 13 to 14% was described in cervical carcinoma (Thigpen et al 1983, 1986). Benjamin et al (1979) reported some utility for the drug in chronic myelogenous leukemia and possibly as a marrow-ablative drug for bone marrow transplantation. The combination of piperazinedione and total-body irradiation reduced blasts in 14 patients with chronic myelogenous leukemia, with 6 reverting back to the chronic phase lasting 3 to 14 months (Vellekoop et al 1986). A low order of activity was noted in various solid tumors and acute myelogenous leukemia in this study.

■ Mechanism of Action

The main mechanism of action of piperazinedione is thought to involve alkylation, ultimately causing inhibition of DNA synthesis (Brockman et al 1976, Wheeler et al 1976). Inhibition of the incorporation of several nucleotides into DNA also has been demonstrated. In addition, the drug has shown activity in certain neoplasms resistant to other alkylating agents and to some antimetabolites (Schabel et al 1976). Overall there appear to be several possible cytotoxic mechanisms of action. Similar to other alkylators, the drug seems to delay cell progression through G_2 phase, but its action is not truly cell cycle phase specific (Wheeler et al 1976).

■ Availability and Storage

The drug was investigationally available from the National Cancer Institute in 10-mL vials containing 5 mg piperazinedione and 30 mg mannitol. The drug was supplied as an off-white lyophilized powder. Dry, unopened vials should be stored under refrigeration (4–10°C) and are stable for at least 18 months (at room temperature or under refrigeration). This agent is not currently available.

■ Preparation for Use, Stability, and Admixture

Piperazinedione is dissolved in 2 to 5 mL of Sterile Water for Injection, USP. With 5 mL of diluent the drug solution will have a pH between 3.0 and 4.0, and each milliliter will contain 1 mg piperazinedione and 6 mg mannitol. These solutions decompose slowly on standing but are chemically stable for at least 24 hours. No bacteriostatic agent is included; therefore, reconstituted vials should ideally be discarded if not used within 8 hours.

■ Administration

Piperazinedione is usually administered intravenously in 100 mL of normal saline over at least 10 minutes. D5W has also been used as a diluent. Only patent intravenous sites should be used, with extra care taken to avoid extravasation. Infiltration of the drug may be expected to cause some necrosis and pain. The intravenous site should be flushed with 5 to 10 mL of normal saline or D5W before and after the infusion to ensure vein patency and to flush remaining drug from the tubing, respectively.

■ Dosage

Piperazinedione is generally given as a single dose every 3 weeks. Typically, single doses of 12 to 15 mg/m^2 are repeated every 3 to 4 weeks for solid tumors (Gottlieb et al 1975). In acute leukemia, single doses of 25 to 30 mg/m^2 have been given. Zander et al (1979) have reported marrow-ablative doses of 25 mg/m^2 given on the sixth and fifth days before radiation and bone marrow transplantation. Consecutive-day schedules have employed 3 mg/m^2/d for 5 days in solid tumors and 5 mg/m^2/d for 5 days for leukemia. The phase I study of Currie et al (1979) confirmed the utility of single intravenous doses of the same total amount as given in the daily (×5) regimen. Thus, the phase II study dose of 12 mg/m^2 used for breast cancer (Palmer et al 1977), renal cancer (Pasmantier et al 1977), melanoma (Al-Sarraf et al 1978), and lymphoma (Jones et al 1977) appears safe. With compromised bone marrow reserve, liver function, or kidney function, lower doses must be used. Benjamin et al (1979) recommended 9 mg/m^2 for patients with extensive prior therapy, prior treatment with nitrosoureas, and abnormal liver function tests; 12 mg/m^2 for patients with prior therapy; 15 mg/m^2 for previously untreated patients; and 24 to 36 mg/m^2 for patients with acute leukemia.

■ Pharmacokinetics

A pharmacokinetic study in a single human patient indicated a biphasic disappearance of radioactive piperazinedione from the plasma: 30 minutes and 3 hours for the first and second phases, respectively. The intact drug also appeared to be rapidly converted to a metabolite of unknown composition. Total radioactivity, however, continued to be excreted for several days.

■ Side Effects and Toxicity

Dose-related myelosuppression appears to be the selective and dose-limiting hematologic toxic effect (Folk et al 1974, Al-Sarraf et al 1978). It usually becomes significant at doses of 12 mg/m^2 and above, with little or no toxicity seen at doses below 5 mg/m^2. Thrombocytopenia generally appears after granulocytopenia. The nadir for leukopenia occurs on days 13 to 21 with recovery by week 4; however, the major toxic effect is thrombocytopenia which tends to be prolonged (Douglass et al 1985). Both have extremely variable onset, nadir, and duration. The degree of thrombocytopenia may be quite unpredictable. These toxic effects may extend as long as 30 days after the dose. Benjamin et al (1979) noted severe marrow aplasia with several deaths in their series.

Currie et al (1979) have compared typical nadirs for daily-dose versus single-dose regimens for both leukopenia and thrombocytopenia; the median nadir in adults occurred approximately on day 18 with recovery by day 34 (daily dose) versus day 14 and day 28 for the single-dose regimen. The latter was identical for children treated in a single-dose fashion. Another interesting finding in this study was that the severity of hematologic suppression did not affect the marrow recovery time.

Jones et al (1977) have additionally noted that Hodgkin's disease patients (who tend to be younger) appear to tolerate the hematologic insult from piperazinedione much better than other patients. For some patients profound and persistent leukopenia and thrombocytopenia occurred. Thus, for patients with Hodgkin's disease, the nadir blood counts and recovery following 12 mg/m^2 drug were on day 14 and day 21, respectively. This compares with nadirs occurring 1 to 2 weeks after identical doses given in other patients in this study, including those with multiple myeloma and non-Hodgkin's lymphoma.

Gastrointestinal toxicity includes nausea and vomiting, reported in about 20% of patients, usually only at doses above 10 mg/m^2. Elevated liver function parameters (serum glutamic–oxalacetic transaminase, partial thromboplastin time) have been especially associated with daily and weekly dosing schedules.

A worsening of preexisting poor renal function has been noted and neurologic toxicity was described in one phase II study (Douglass et al 1985). Piperazinedione is also a potent vesicant and, if extravasated, can cause severe soft tissue damage. This has resulted in the need for limb amputation in one reported extravasation of part of a 12 mg/m^2 dose in the antecubital fossa of a 59-year-old patient (Brenner et al 1980).

REFERENCES

Al-Sarraf M, Thigpen T, Groppe CW, et al. Piperazinedione in patients with advanced malignant melanoma: A Southwest Oncology Group study. *Cancer Treat Rep.* 1978;**62**:1101–1103.

Benjamin RS, Keating MJ, Valdivieso M, et al. Phase I–II study of piperazinedione in adults with solid tumors and acute leukemia. *Cancer Treat Rep.* 1979;**63**(6):939–943.

Brenner DE, Aisner J, Wiernik PH. Severe skin necrosis produced by piperazinedione extravasation. *Cancer Treat Rep.* 1980;**64**(12):1392–1394.

Brockman RW, Shaddix SC, Williams M, et al. Studies with 2,5-piperazinedione,3,6-bis(5-chloro-2-piperidyl)-dihydrochloride. II. Effects on macromolecular synthesis on cell culture and evidence for alkylating activity. *Cancer Treat Rep.* 1976;**60**:1317–1324.

Currie V, Woodcock T, Tan C, et al. Phase I evaluation of piperazinedione in patients with advanced cancer. *Cancer Treat Rep.* 1979;**63**(1):73–76.

Douglass HO Jr, Kaufman J, Engstrom PF, et al. Single agent chemotherapy of advanced colorectal cancer with KRF-159, YOSHI-864 or methotrexate (MTX), piperazinedione, CCNU L-PAM or actinomycin D (abstract C-596). *Proc Am Assoc Cancer Res ASCO.* 1979;**20**:434.

Douglass HO Jr, MacIntyre JM, Kaufman J, et al. Eastern Cooperative Oncology Group phase II studies in advanced measurable colorectal cancer. I. Razoxane, Yoshi-864, piperazinedione, and lomustine. *Cancer Treat Rep.* 1985;**69**(5):543–545.

Folk RM, Peters AC, Pavkov KL, et al. Preclinical toxicologic evaluation of 2,5-piperazinedione, 3,6-bis(5-chloro-2-piperidyl)-dihydrochloride (NSC-135758) in dogs and monkeys. *Cancer Chemother Rep Part 3.* 1974;**5**(1):37–41.

Gitterman CO, Rickes EL, Wolf DE, et al. The human tumor–egg host system. IV. Discovery of a new antitumor agent compound 593A. *J Antibiot.* 1970;**23**:305–310.

Gottlieb JA, Freireich EJ, Bodey GP, et al. Preliminary clinical evaluation of piperazinedione (P) a new crystalline antibiotic. *Proc Am Assoc Cancer Res ASCO.* 1975;**16**:86.

Jones SE, Tucker WG, Haut A, et al. Phase II trial of piperazinedione in Hodgkin's disease, non-Hodgkin's lymphoma and multiple myeloma, a Southwest Oncology Group study. *Cancer Treat Rep.* 1977;**61**:1617–1621.

La Gasse L, Thigpen T, Morrison F. Phase II trial of piperazinedione in treatment of advanced endometrial carcinoma, uterine sarcoma and vulvar carcinoma (abstract C-400). *Proc Am Assoc Cancer Res ASCO.* 1979;**20**:388.

Palmer RL, Samal BA, Vaughn CB, et al. Phase II evaluation of piperazinedione in metastatic breast carcinoma. *Cancer Treat Rep.* 1977;**61**:1711–1712.

Pasmantier MW, Coleman M, Kennedy BJ, et al. Piperazinedione in metastatic renal carcinoma. *Cancer Treat Rep.* 1977;**61**:1731–1732.

Schabel FM Jr, Trader MW, Laster WR Jr, et al. Studies with 2,5-piperazinedione, 3,6-bis(5-chloro-2-piperidyl)-dihydrochloride. III. Biochemical and therapeutic effects in L-1210 leukemias sensitive and resistant to alkylating agents: Comparison with melphalan, cyclophosphamide, and BCNU. *Cancer Treat Rep.* 1976;**60**:1325–1333.

Tarnowski GS, Schmid FA, Hutchison DJ, et al. Chemotherapeutic effects of compound 593A (NSC-135758) on mouse leukemias and some transplanted animal tumors. *Cancer Chemother Rep.* 1973;**57**:21–27.

Thigpen JT, Blessing JA, Arseneau JC, Homesley HD. Phase II trial of piperazinedione (NSC-135758) in the treatment of advanced or recurrent carcinoma of the ovary. A Gynecologic Oncology Group study. *Am J Clin Oncol.* 1984;**7**:261–263.

Thigpen JT, Blessing JA, Fowler WC Jr, Hatch K. Phase II trials of cisplatin and piperazinedione as single agents in the treatment of advanced or recurrent non-squamous cell carcinoma of the cervix: A Gynecologic Oncology Group study. *Cancer Treat Rep.* 1986;**70**(9):1097–1100.

Thigpen JT, Blessing J, Homesley HD, Adcock LL. Phase II trial of piperazinedione (NSC-135758) in the treatment of advanced or recurrent squamous cell carcinoma of the cervix. A Gynecologic Oncology Group study. *Am J Clin Oncol.* 1983;**6**:423–426.

Vellekoop L, Zander AR, Kantarjian HM, et al. Piperazinedione, total body irradiation, and autologous bone marrow transplantation in chronic myelogenous leukemia. *J Clin Oncol.* 1986;**4**(6):906–911.

Wheeler GP, Bono VH, Bowden BJ, et al. Studies with 2,5-piperazinedione, 3,6-bis(5-chloro-2-piperidyl)-dihydrochloride. I. Cell kinetic and biologic effects in cultured L-1210, human epidermoid No. 2, and adenocarcinoma 755 cells. *Cancer Treat Rep.* 1976;**60**:1307–1316.

Zander A, Spitzer G, Verma D, Vellekoop L, et al. Autologous bone marrow transplantation in acute leukemia in relapse (abstract C-481). *Proc Am Assoc Cancer Res ASCO.* 1979;**20**:408.

Pipobroman

■ Other Names

Vercyte®; A-8103; NSC-25154.

■ Chemistry

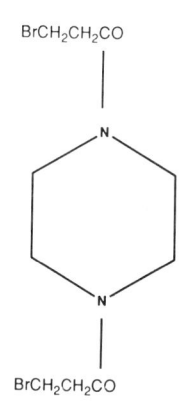

Structure of pipobroman

Pipobroman, 1,4-bis(3-bromopropionyl)piperazine, occurs as a white crystalline powder and is only slightly soluble in water and alcohol.

■ Antitumor Activity

Pipobroman has been used in the treatment of polycythemia vera (Monto et al 1964, Anonymous 1967a,b), Brusumolino et al 1984) and chronic granulocytic leukemia. Up to 92% of patients with polycythemia vera have achieved hematologic remissions.

■ Mechanism of Action

Pipobroman is classified as a polyfunctional alkylating agent. Its precise antineoplastic action is unknown. Pipobroman does not appear to exert its cytotoxic effects during any specific phase of the cell cycle and is therefore cell cycle phase nonspecific.

■ Availability and Storage

Pipobroman was available in 10- and 25-mg grooved tablets and could be stored at room temperature.

■ Administration

Pipobroman is administered only in divided daily doses. There are no data suggesting whether absorption is altered with foods. As pipobroman may cause nausea and vomiting in some individuals, premedication with antiemetics may be of value.

■ Special Precautions

Acute leukemia can be seen in patients with polycythemia vera. The impact of pipobroman on the incidence of acute leukemia is uncertain. The latest reported study indicates that the actuarial risk of acute leukemia is 6% at 5 years and 9% at 7 years from time of diagnosis while the patients with polycythemia are on pipobroman. One must, however, remember that the risk of developing leukemia of patients with polycythemia who do not receive treatment is also substantial.

■ Drug Interactions

None are known.

■ Dosage

The initial dose of pipobroman is 1 mg/kg daily, increasing to a maximum of 3 mg/kg daily at 30-day intervals until the desired hematologic response is achieved. Maintenance doses thereafter range from 0.1 to 0.2 mg/kg/d (Brusumolino et al 1984, Monto et al 1964).

■ Pharmacokinetics

No studies have been reported.

■ Side Effects and Toxicity

Pipobroman produces dose-dependent bone marrow suppression with leukopenia, thrombocytopenia, and anemia. If anemia occurs rapidly, associated with increased bilirubin and reticulocytosis, a hemolytic process may be occurring, in which case the drug should be discontinued.

Gastrointestinal distress in the form of nausea, vomiting, abdominal cramps, and diarrhea may also occur. If abdominal disturbances cannot be adequately controlled, the drug may have to be discontinued. Skin rash has also been reported.

■ Special Applications

None are reported.

REFERENCES

Anonymous. Pipobroman (Vercyte). A new antineoplastic drug. *Med Lett Drugs Ther*. 1967a;9:27.
Anonymous. Evaluation of two antineoplastic agents,

pipobroman (Vercyte) and thioguanine. *JAMA.* 1967b; **200**:619–620.

Brusumolino F, Salvaneschi L, Canevari A, Bernasconi C. Efficacy trial of pipobroman in polycythemia vera and incidence of acute leukemia. *J Clin Oncol.* 1984;**2**:558–561.

Monto RW, Tenpas A, Battle JD, Rohn RJ, Louis J, Louis NB. A-8103 in polycythemia. *JAMA.* 1964;**190**:833–836.

Pirarubicin

■ Other Names

THP-Adriamycin®.

■ Chemistry

Structure of pirarubicin

This anthracycline is a derivative of doxorubicin containing a tetrahydropyranyl group at the 4'-position of the amino sugar. The chemical name is (2"R)-4'-O-tetrahydropyranyl doxorubicin (Umezawa et al 1987) and the molecular weight of the compound is 665. Pirarubicin was originally synthesized by Umezawa in 1979 (Umezawa et al 1979) to follow up on the activity of natural O-hemiacetal and glycosidic derivatives of daunorubicin known as baumycin A1, A2, B1, and B2 (Komiyama et al 1977).

■ Antitumor Activity

Pirarubicin produces antitumor effects superior to those of doxorubicin in a variety of murine tumor models. These include L-1210 and P-388 leukemia, colon-38 cancer, Lewis lung carcinoma, and B-16 melanoma (Tsuruo et al 1982, Umezawa et al 1987). The drug was eightfold cross-resistant in a murine L-5178Y lymphoblast cell line developed for 33-fold resistance to doxorubicin (Umezawa et al 1987).

Significant clinical response rates have been observed in Japanese phase II trials using pirarubicin as a single agent, in some cases as the initial therapy for patients with a variety of solid tumors. The response rates (complete + partial) include 19% in head and neck cancer, 13% in gastric cancer, 21% in breast cancer, 22% in bladder cancer, 30% in renal, pelvic, and ureter cancer, 27% in ovarian cancer, and 24% in uterine cancer (Majima and Ohta 1987). A few partial responses were also noted in colorectal cancer, prostate cancer, sarcoma, and mesothelioma.

Because of the single-agent activity in untreated patients with ovarian cancer a follow-up study with pirarubicin and cisplatin was performed in France. The clinical and pathologic complete response rates were 52 and 33%, respectively. When the complete response rates are combined with partial response rates of 12%, the overall response rate to pirarubicin in ovarian cancer was 64% (Levi et al 1990). Of interest, greater dose intensity and slightly higher response rates were achieved in this study when pirarubicin was given early in the morning and cisplatin in the late afternoon (Levi et al 1990).

Broad phase II studies of pirarubicin have also been performed by the clinical screening group of the EORTC. This group reported response rates of 6% in head and neck cancer, 33% in cervical cancer, and 20% in endometrial cancer (Schneider et al 1990). In a follow-up study in head and neck cancer a 31% response rate (mostly partial responses) was described in 16 evaluable patients (Sridhar et al 1990). A 33% response rate is reported in malignant mesothelioma (Sridhar et al 1992). In contrast to the earlier reports, however, no responses were observed in 26 patients with ovarian cancer, although 19 had received heavy prior therapy including anthracyclines. The drug was also inactive in soft tissue sarcoma and malignant melanoma, with only one response each noted in 13 colorectal cancer patients (8%) and 23 renal cell carcinoma patients (4%) (Schneider et al 1990). Marginal activity (15%, complete responses + partial responses) was also observed in small cell lung carcinoma (Kleisbauer et al 1990), in prostate cancer (1 partial response/12 patients [Rapoport and Falkson 1992]), and in a variety of acute leukemias (response range of 5–15% [Majima and Ohta 1987]). Pirarubicin combined with 5-fluorouracil infusions in breast cancer produced a response rate of 50% (Chevallier et al 1990). This is similar to partial response rates of 31 to 53%

for pirarubicin used as a single agent in breast cancer (Scheithauer et al 1990, Waldman et al 1990).

Pirarubicin is active in hematologic malignancies. The response rate in acute leukemia was 33% (7/21) when pirarubicin was used as a single agent. Three of these patients achieved a complete response (Yamada et al 1987). In 20 patients with malignant lymphomas (primarily non-Hodgkin's lymphoma), there were two complete responses and five partial responses which appeared to be dose dependent (Yamada et al 1987).

■ Mechanism of Action

Pirarubicin appears to accumulate in tumor cells more rapidly than doxorubicin (Umezawa et al 1987). Drug distribution studies in L-5178Y cells show that both doxorubicin and pirarubicin concentrate mainly in the nucleus rather than the cytoplasm (Umezawa et al 1987); however, the compound does not appear to break down intracellularly into doxorubicin.

Pirarubicin inhibits synthesis of both DNA and RNA, ostensibly by intercalation between base pairs in the DNA helix. DNA synthesis appears to be inhibited to a greater extent than RNA synthesis. Both effects occur at lower drug concentrations than with doxorubicin, suggesting that pirarubicin is more potent than doxorubicin at inhibiting polynucleotide synthesis (Umezawa et al 1987); however, both drugs appear to equally inhibit *Escherichia coli* RNA polymerase activity in vitro. And, the affinities of both drugs for calf thymus DNA are equal. Thus, the potency difference in inhibiting macromolecule synthesis may relate to a greater cellular uptake for pirarubicin over doxorubicin.

In addition to inhibiting DNA and RNA synthesis by intercalation, it is also likely that like doxorubicin, pirarubicin produces protein-linked DNA strand breaks by inhibiting the activity of DNA topoisomerase II enzymes.

■ Availability and Storage

Pirarubicin is investigationally supplied in vials containing 10 and 20 mg of powdered drug. The bulk material has been produced from fermentation by the Kyowa Hakko Kogyo Company, Ltd, in Japan. It has subsequently been distributed as a pharmaceutical formulation for investigational trials sponsored by Hoffman-La Roche Inc in the United States and, more recently, by Laboratoire Roger Bellon in France. The vials are stored at room temperature and contain approximately 3% doxorubicin by weight (Miller and Schmidt 1987).

■ Preparation for Use, Stability, and Admixture

Pirarubicin vials are reconstituted in 5 to 10 mL of Sterile Water for Injection, USP. This solution is stable at room temperature and in light for 24 hours (Miller and Schmidt 1987). At $-20°C$ and in the dark, the solution is chemically stable for at least 1 month.

■ Administration

Pirarubicin is most often given as a brief intravenous injection over 5 to 10 minutes.

■ Special Precautions

Care should be taken to prevent extravasation as the drug can produce soft tissue necrosis, although pirarubicin is less potent in this regard than doxorubicin pirarubicin (Dantchev et al 1979).

■ Dosage

The most common dosing schedule for pirarubicin is 40 to 60 mg/m^2 IV every 28 days (Majima and Ohta 1987). Another schedule involves a dose of 25 mg/m^2/d for three consecutive doses given every 3 to 4 weeks (Schneider et al 1990). Leukemia and lymphoma schedules have involved doses ranging from 13 to 34 mg/m^2/d for 3 to 5 days (Yamada et al 1987). In combination with 5-fluorouracil in breast cancer, the recommended phase II doses were 40 mg/m^2 for pirarubicin and 650 to 750 mg/m^2/d × 5 for 5-fluorouracil (Chevallier et al 1990). As a single agent in breast cancer, a dose of 70 mg/m^2 every 3 weeks was well tolerated (Scheithauer et al 1990).

■ Pharmacokinetics

Pharmacokinetic studies of pirarubicin disposition reveal a triphasic elimination pattern. The initial (distribution) half-life in the plasma was 0.78 minute (Majima and Ohta 1987). The terminal elimination half-life for pirarubicin is about 13 hours, which is more rapid than that for doxorubicin (see table on top of page 786). The bulk of the drug is eliminated in the bile, accounting for 20% of a dose after 48 hours. A large part of the drug is excreted as doxorubicin and other metabolites in the bile. Relatively little drug, about 4 to 6% of a dose, is recovered in the urine (Miller and Schmidt 1987). Pirarubicin is metabolized to doxorubicin, pirarubi-

PIRARUBICIN PHARMACOKINETICS

Dose (mg/m²)	Peak Plasma Level (ng/mL)	AUC (ng/mL·h)	Plasma Half-life α (min)	Plasma Half-life β (min)	Plasma Half-life γ (h)	Total Clearance (L/m²·h)	Volume of Distribution (L/m²)
30	375	230	1.0	20	10	130	1963
40	500	353	1.4	17	13	114	2160
50	549	419	1.6	16	14	120	2476
60	1524	625	1.3	20	14	100	2105
70	1811	687	1.4	23	14	109	1914
Mean	—	—	1.4	19	13	115	2124

Data from Miller and Schmidt 1987.

cinol, and doxorubicinol. The major metabolite is doxorubicin, which has a long terminal half-life of 33 hours (Miller and Schmidt 1987). The terminal half-life of the metabolite pirarubicinol was 21 hours compared with 59 hours for doxorubicinol (see table below). The alcoholic metabolites of pirarubicin are not extensively excreted in the urine; however, about 11% of the total doxorubicin formed from pirarubicin is excreted in the urine. By comparison of the areas under the plasma concentration time curve (AUC), it is apparent that following a dose of pirarubicin, there is a two- to threefold greater exposure to the metabolite doxorubicin than to the intact parent molecule pirarubicin. The cumulative exposure to doxorubicinol is slightly less than that of the parent, pirarubicin. The AUC for pirarubicinol is about half that of the parent following intravenous bolus dosing (see second table) (Miller and Schmidt 1987).

These pharmacokinetic studies also showed that pirarubicin rapidly concentrates in blood cells in a dose-dependent fashion. The cumulative drug exposure in this compartment ranged from three- to sixfold higher than in the plasma compartment; however, the elimination half-lives of drug from packed blood cells were identical to those in the plasma (Miller and Schmidt 1987).

■ Side Effects and Toxicity

The major dose-limiting toxic effect of pirarubicin is leukopenia, which is noted in 73% of patients (Majima and Ohta 1987). Thrombocytopenia also occurs in up to 14% of patients, but it is usually much less severe. A variety of gastrointestinal toxic effects also occur, including anorexia (37% overall incidence), mild nausea and vomiting in up to 30% of patients, and stomatitis in only about 5% of pa-

PHARMACOKINETICS OF PIRARUBICIN METABOLITES

Dose (mg/m²)	Metabolite*	Peak Plasma Level (ng/mL)	AUC (ng/mL·h)	Plasma Half-life α (min)	Plasma Half-life β (h)	Cumulative Urinary Excretion (%)
30	Dox	93	250	3.5	27	10.6
	Pirol	5	180	—	20	0.4
	Doxol	2	146	—	42	0.2
50	Dox	148	1040	5.4	33	14.4
	Pirol	6	232	—	23	0.5
	Doxol	3	327	—	69	0.2
70	Dox	155	2193	6.6	35	11.1
	Pirol	5	243	—	25	0.5
	Doxol	5	438	—	61	0.6
Mean	Dox	—	—	5.8	31	11.1
	Pirol	—	—	—	21	0.4
	Doxol	—	—	—	59	0.4

*Dox, doxorubicin; Pirol, pirarubicinol; doxol, doxorubicinol.
Data from Miller and Schmidt 1987.

tients. Other occasional toxic effects include malaise (19%), fever (7%), diarrhea (3%), and alopecia (5%). Some of the nonmyelosuppressive toxic effects have been much more common in European and U.S. trials. For instance, when pirarubicin was given as a single agent in breast cancer, doses of 70 mg/m² produced alopecia in 73% of patients and nausea and vomiting in 70% (Scheithauer et al 1990).

The nadir for leukopenia is 13 days, with recovery by day 22 (Yamada et al 1987). Importantly, the degree of myelosuppression did not appear to be cumulative even in patients with hematologic malignancies (Yamada et al 1987).

Several preclinical studies have reported significantly less cardiotoxicity for pirarubicin compared with doxorubicin (Umezawa et al 1987, Dantchev et al 1979). This has recently been verified in patients receiving pirarubicin (Benjamin et al 1990). In this trial, low endomyocardial biopsy scores were observed after patients had received cumulative pirarubicin doses of 500 to 870 mg/m². A 6% incidence of congestive heart failure was reported after a cumulative dose of 500 mg/m² was administered, and a 14% incidence at cumulative doses of 590 to 870 mg/m². This latter figure includes a patient with preexisting heart disease. If excluded, the congestive heart failure incidence (based on an ejection fraction < 50%) is only 2% at 390 mg/m² and 6% at cumulative pirarubicin doses of 590 to 870 mg/m² (Benjamin et al 1990).

REFERENCES

Benjamin RS, Fenoglio C, Hortobagyi GN, et al. Cardiotoxicity of pirarubicin. *Proc Am Assoc Cancer Res*. 1990;**31**:178.

Chevallier B, Fumoleau P, Monnier A, Kerbrat P, Roche H, Herait P. Combination of pirarubicin (P) and continuous IV infusion of 5-fluorouracil (CI5FU) in metastatic breast cancer (MBC). A cooperative phase II, dose finding study. *Proc Am Soc Clin Oncol*. 1990;**9**:41.

Dantchev D, Paintrand M, Hayat M, Bourut C, Mathe G. Low heart and skin toxicity of a tetrahydropyranyl derivative of Adriamycin (THP-ADM) as observed by electron and light microscopy. *J Antibiot*. 1979;**32**(10):1085–1086.

Kleisbauer JP, Taytard A, Vergeret J, et al. Pirarubicin (P) phase II study in metastatic small-cell lung carcinoma (SCLC) without prior chemotherapy. *Proc Am Assoc Cancer Res*. 1990;**31**:197.

Komiyama T, Matsuzaway, Oki T, et al. Baumycins, new antitumor antibiotics related to daunomycin. *J Antibiot*. 1977;**30**:619–627.

Levi F, Benavides M, Chevelle C, et al. Chemotherapy of advanced ovarian cancer with 4'-O-tetrahydropyranyl doxorubicin and cisplatin: A rnadomized phase II trial with an evaluation of circadian timing and dose-intensity. *J Clin Oncol*. 1990;**8**(4):705–714.

Majima H, Ohta K. Clinical studies of (2″R)-4'- O-tetrahydropyranyl Adriamycin (THP). *Biomed Pharmacother*. 1987;**41**:237–243.

Miller AA, Benvenuto JA. Limited sampling strategy for pirarubicin. *Proc Am Assoc Cancer Res*. 1990;**31**:382.

Miller AA, Schmidt CG. Clinical pharmacology and toxicity of 4'-O-tetrahydropyranyladriamycin. *Cancer Res*. 1987;**47**:1461–1465.

Rapoport BL, Falkson G. Phase II clinical study of pirarubicin in hormone resistant prostate cancer. *Invest New Drugs*. 1992;**10**:119–121.

Scheithauer W, Samonigg H, Depisch D, et al. Pirarubicin (4'-O-tetrahydropyranil-Adriamycin) for treatment of advanced breast cancer. *Invest New Drugs*. 1990;**8**:207–210.

Schneider M, Fumoleau P, Cappelaere P, et al. Phase II pirarubicin (THP-ADM): A study of the Clinical Screening Group (CSG) of the E.O.R.T.C./Updated results. *Proc Am Assoc Cancer Res*. 1990;**31**:207.

Sridhar KS, Doria R, Hussein AM, et al. Activity and toxicity of 4'-O-tetrahydropyranyladriamycin (pirarubicin) in malignant mesothelioma. *Proc Am Soc Clin Oncol*. 1992;**11**:356.

Sridhar KS, Hussein AM, Barmann A, et al. Phase II study of Q3 week IV bolus pirarubicin (4'-O-tetrahydropyranyladriamycin) in head & neck carcinoma (H & N Ca). *Proc Am Soc Clin Oncol*. 1990;**9**:179.

Tsuruo T, Iida H, Tsukagoshi S, Sakurai Y. 4'-O-Tetrahydropyranyladriamycin as a potential new antitumor agent. *Cancer Res*. 1982;**42**:1462–1467.

Umezawa K, Kunimoto S, Takeuchi T. Experimental studies of new anthracyclines: Aclacinomycin, THP-adriamycin and ditrisarubicins. *Biomed Pharmacother*. 1987;**41**:206–213.

Umezawa H, Takahashi Y, Kinoshita M, et al. Tetrahydropyranyl derivatives of daunomycin and adriamycin. *J Antibiot*. 1979;**32**:1082–1084.

Waldman S, Sridhar KS, Richman S, et al. Phase II trial of pirarubicin (P) in advanced breast CA (BC). *Proc Am Soc Clin Oncol*. 1990;**9**:50.

Yamada K, Shirakawa S, Ohno R, et al. A phase II study of (2″R)-4'-O-tetrahydropyranyladriamycin (THP) in hematological malignancies. *Invest New Drugs*. 1987;**5**:299.

Piritrexim

■ Other Names
BW 301; 301U74; PTX.

■ Chemistry

Structure of piritrexim

Piritrexim is a lipid-soluble folate antagonist designed to enter the cell rapidly by passive diffusion (Grivsky et al 1980). It is a competitive inhibitor of dihydrofolate reductase and inhibits the growth of methotrexate-resistant cells. The complete chemical name is 2,4-diamino-6-(2,5-dimethoxybenzyl)-5-methyl-pyrido[2,3-d] pyrimidine.

■ Antitumor Activity

In phase I studies, responses have been noted in patients with melanoma, bladder cancer, malignant fibrous histiocytoma, and gallbladder cancer (Feun et al 1991, Weiss et al 1989, Arbuck et al 1987). These initial phase I studies have been summarized by Laszlo et al 1987.

Piritrexim has been reported to have activity in patients with advanced metastatic melanoma (30% response rate) when used at a dose of 25 mg three times daily × 5 days for 3 weeks of a 4-week cycle (Clendeninn et al 1989, Feun et al 1991). The drug has also been reported to have some activity in patients with head and neck cancer (Uen et al 1988). A response rate of 20% was recently described in heavily pretreated patients with head and neck cancer (Degardin et al 1992). Oral piritrexim had minor activity in patients with advanced soft tissue sarcoma. One of 12 patients with leiomyosarcoma responded in this trial (Schiesel et al 1992).

In other phase II studies, the drug has been found to be inactive or to have limited activity in patients with non-small cell lung cancer (Kris et al 1987, Kirsch et al 1986) and in patients with advanced sarcoma (Carabasi et al 1988). Of great interest have been the three partial responses in four patients with bladder cancer refractory to MVAC who were treated with piritrexim (Clendeninn et al 1991).

■ Mechanism of Action

Piritrexim is an inhibitor of dihydrofolate reductase. Its lipid solubility produces rapid transport by simple passive diffusion into the cell. Additionally, its entry is not temperature sensitive. Furthermore, even very high levels of calcium/leucovorin do not interfere with piritrexim uptake. The lack of any effect on piritrexim uptake by folic acid fits the same pattern as seen with metoprine and DDMP, two other lipid-soluble antifols.

Piritrexim also differs from methotrexate in the rate of drug disappearance from exposed cells once they are placed in drug-free medium. Complete reversal of the inhibition of uridine incorporation into DNA occurs promptly when methotrexate is removed from the medium, whereas, in contrast, only partial recovery from the inhibition caused by piritrexim or metoprine occurs (Duch et al 1982).

■ Availability and Storage

Piritrexim Capsules. Piritrexim is an off-white, odorless powder provided as the isethionate salt in white opaque capsules having no identifying marking. Capsules of 100-mg potency contain 139.2 mg of piritrexim isethionate. The capsules should be stored at 15 to 30°C (59–86°F).

Piritrexim Injection. Piritrexim is provided as the isethionate salt in amber glass ampules containing 10 mL of a solution of 8 mg/mL piritrexim free base (equivalent to 11 mg/mL of the isethionate salt) dissolved in propylene glycol/water for injection (1:1, v/v).

■ Preparation for Use, Stability, and Admixture

Piritrexim Capsules. Under conditions at 50°C, satisfactory physical stability and chemical potency have been observed. Following storage at 50°C for 2 months, assay results were 100% of the initial value for the 100-mg-potency capsule. This storage study is ongoing.

Piritrexim Injection. Immediately prior to intravenous administration, piritrexim isethionate injection is diluted with sterile D5W to provide a final concentration not to exceed 0.25 mg/mL free base

PHASE I TRIAL PERFORMED WITH PIRITREXIM

Schedule	Route	Dose Range Explored (mg/m²)	Dose-Limiting Toxic Effect	Recommended Phase II Dose	Reference
Daily × 21 every 28 d	PO	25–100 mg	Myelosuppression	None	Feun et al 1991
5 of 7 d × 21 d every 28 d	PO	—	Myelosuppression	25 mg three times daily × 5 d	Feun et al 1991
Daily to tolerance	PO	—	Myelosuppression	None	Feun et al 1991
Weekly × 4	IV	44–530	Thrombocytopenia	—	Weiss et al 1989
24-h infusion weekly × 3 every 4 wk	IV	250–450	Myelosuppression Mucositis	—	Arbuck et al 1987
Twice daily × 5 every 21 d*	PO	140–290	Myelosuppression Mucositis	140 mg/m²	Adamson et al 1990

*Pediatric population.

(equivalent to 0.35 mg/mL isethionate salt). The concentration should in no circumstances exceed 0.36 mg/mL free base. It is recommended that the standard dose of 150 mg/m² be placed in 1500 mL of D5W, as long as the concentration is less than 0.25 mg/mL. This should be infused over at least 6 hours, unless the investigator feels the patient is able to tolerate a more rapid infusion.

It is suggested that the American Society of Hospital Pharmacists' recommendations for handling cytotoxic drugs be followed.

In a dilution range of 1/40 to 1/400 (0.2 to 0.02 mg/mL) piritrexim isethionate injection is physically and chemically compatible with D5W for up to 24 hours when stored at 25 or 5°C. Therefore, storage of piritrexim isethionate injection dilution from 1/40 to 1/400 with D5W at either refrigeration or room temperature for up to 24 hours is acceptable.

Piritrexim is to be infused by means of a constant-rate infusion pump. Solutions should be filtered through a 0.22-µm membrane filter as they are being administered (or they may be filtered at time of preparation).

■ Administration

See details in preceding section.

■ Special Precautions

Nothing over and above the usual precautions is required.

■ Drug Interactions

Piritrexim is not antagonized by leucovorin calcium.

■ Dosage

As outlined in the following table above, a number of phase I trials have been performed with piritrexim. As can be seen from the table, the doses have been administered by both oral and intravenous routes. The preferred schedule appears to be

PHARMACOKINETICS OF PIRITREXIM

Schedule	Route	β Half-life (h)	Bioavailability	Total Body Clearance (mL/min/m²)	Reference
Weekly × 4	IV	5.61 ± 2.38	—	136–173	Weiss et al 1989
	PO	5.72 ± 2.04	75 ± 56%		
24-h infusion weekly	IV*	5.5	—	164	Arbuck et al 1987
Single dose	IV and PO[†]	3.7	—	246	Woolley et al 1991
Various	PO	3.6	—	—	Feun et al 1991

*Steady-state plasma levels at 12 h of 2.0 µg/mL.
[†]C_{max} was 0.4 µg/mL; T_{max} was 1.4 h.

25 mg three times daily × 5 days for 3 weeks of a 4-week cycle (Clendeninn et al 1989, Feun et al 1991).

■ Pharmacokinetics

The table on page 789 summarizes the pharmacokinetic data on piritrexim. Most of the studies have used a competitive protein binding assay (Woolley et al 1989).

In a pediatric trial, steady-state plasma levels at 140 mg/m^2 averaged 5.3 ± 0.84 μM and occurred at a median of 1.5 hours after the oral dose. The mean AUC was 18.1 ± 2.3 $\mu M \cdot h$. Absolute bioavailability (compared with a single intravenous dose) was 35 and 93% in two different patients (Adamson et al 1990). Finally, Woolley et al (1991) used [^{14}C] piritrexim in patients with advanced cancer. By 96 hours, 68% of the dose was recovered (57% in urine, 11% in feces). Less than 40% of the dose was recovered unchanged.

■ Side Effects and Toxicity

The usual dose-limiting toxic effect of piritrexim has been myelosuppression (includes anemia and thrombocytopenia). Occasionally, mucositis has also been dose limiting (Feun et al 1991, Adamson et al 1990, Weiss et al 1989, Arbuck et al 1987). Other toxic effects include nausea and vomiting, stomatitis, anorexia, diarrhea, skin rash, and, very occasionally elevation of liver transaminases (Feun et al 1991, Adamson et al 1990, Weiss et al 1989, Arbuck et al 1987). Moderate to severe peripheral venous phlebitis has been noted after intravenous infusion (Weiss et al 1989, Arbuck et al 1987).

■ Special Applications

Piritrexim has been explored for treatment of toxoplasmosis in patients with acquired immunodeficiency syndrome (McCabe and Oster 1989) and in patients with *Pneumocystis carinii* pneumonia (Rosowky et al 1989).

REFERENCES

Adamson PC, Balis FM, Miser J, et al. Pediatric phase I trial and pharmacokinetic study of piritrexim administered orally on a five-day schedule. *Cancer Res.* 1990;**50**(15): 4464–4467.

Arbuck SG, Clendeninn NJ, Douglass HO Jr, et al. Phase I trial of piritrexim (BW 301U) administered by 24-hour IV infusion (meeting abstract). *Proc Am Soc Clin Oncol.* 1987;**6**:47.

Carabasi M, Magill GB, Casper ES, Marks L, Cheng EW. A phase II trial of oral piritrexim (PTX) (BW 301) for advanced sarcomas in adults (meeting abstract). *Proc Am Soc Clin Oncol.* 1988;**7**:276.

Clendeninn NJ, Collier MA, Feun LG, Robinson WA. Prolonged low-dose administration of piritrexim (PTX), a better way to deliver an antifolate (meeting abstract)? In: *Sixth NCI–EORTC Symposium on New Drugs in Cancer Therapy, Amsterdam;* 1989;A461:464.

Clendeninn NJ, Savaraj N, Benedetto P, et al. Compassionate use of oral piritrexim in advanced bladder cancer: An effective drug after progression on MVAC chemotherapy? *Proc Am Assoc Cancer Res.* 1991;**32**(186):1110.

Degardin M, Domenge CH, Cappelaere P, et al. Phase II piritrexim (PTX) study in recurrent and/or metastatic head and neck cancer (HNC). *Proc Am Soc Clin Oncol.* 1992;**11**:244.

Duch DS, Edelstein MP, Bowers SW, Nichol CA. Biochemical and chemotherapeutic studies on 2,4-diamino-6-(2,5-dimethoxybenzyl)-5-methyl-pyrido[2,3-*d*]pyrimidine (BW 301U), a novel lipid soluble inhibitor of dihydrofolate reductase. *Cancer Res.* 1982;**42**(10):3987–3994.

Feun LG, Savaraj N, Benedetto P, et al. Phase I trial of piritrexim capsules using prolonged, low-dose oral administration for the treatment of advanced malignancies. *J Natl Cancer Inst.* 1991;**83**(1):51–55.

Grivsky EM, Lee S, Sigel CW, Duch DS, Nichol CA. Synthesis and antitumor activity of 2,4-diamino-6-(2,5-dimethoxybenzyl)-5-methylpyroido[2,3-*d*]pyrimidine. *J Med Chem.* 1980;**23**(3):327–329.

Kirsch J, Gralla RJ, Kris MG, Burke MT, Kelsen DP, Heelan RT. Phase II study of oral BW 301-U in non-small cell lung cancer (meeting abstract). *Proc Am Assoc Cancer Res.* 1986;**27**:184.

Kris MG, Gralla RJ, Burke MT, et al. Phase II trial of oral piritrexim (BW301U) in patients with stage III non-small cell lung cancer. *Cancer Treat Rep.* 1987;**71**(7/8): 763–764.

Laszlo J, Brenchman WD Jr, Morgan E, et al. Initial clinical studies of piritrexim. *NCI Monogr.* 1987;**5**:121–125.

McCabe RE, Oster S. Current recommendations and future prospects in the treatment of toxoplasmosis. *Drugs.* 1989;**38**(6):973–987.

Rosowky A, Freisheim JH, Hynes JB, et al. Tricyclic 2,4-diaminopyrimidines with broad antifolate activity and the ability to inhibit *Pneumocystis carinii* growth in cultured human lung fibroblasts in the presence of leucovorin. *Biochem Pharmacol.* 1989;**38**(16):2677–2684.

Schiesel JD, Carabasi M, Magill G, et al. Oral piritrexim—A phase II study in patients with advanced soft tissue sarcoma. *Invest New Drugs.* 1992;**10**:97–98.

Uen WC, Hauang AT, Clendeninn NJ, Craig J, Spaulding M. Phase II piritrexim study in squamous head and neck cancer (meeting abstract). *Proc Am Assoc Cancer Res.* 1988;**29**:208.

Weiss GR, Sarosy GA, Shenkenberg TD, et al. A phase I clinical and pharmacological study of weekly intravenous infusion of piritrexim (BW301U). *Eur J Cancer Clin Oncol.* 1989;**25**(12):1867–1873.

Woolley D, DeAngelis D, Liao S, et al. The disposition of ^{14}C-piritrexim in advanced cancer patients. *Proc Am Assoc Cancer Res.* 1991;**32**(346):2053.

Woolley JL Jr, Ringstad JL, Sigel CW. Competitive protein binding assay for piritrexim. *J Pharm Sci.* 1989;**78**(9):749–752.

Piroxantrone Hydrochloride

■ Other Names

Oxantrazole hydrochloride; anthrapyrazole dihydrochloride; NSC-349174.

■ Chemistry

Structure of piroxantrone hydrochloride

Piroxantrone is an anthrapyrazole structurally related to mitoxantrone. Similar substitutions on the anthracenyl nucleus include the hydroxyethylaminoethyl side chain, and the parahydroxyl groups on the third ring. The quinone structure on the middle ring system of mitoxantrone is modified on anthrapyrazole to form part of the pyrazole ring of piroxantrone (Showalter et al 1987). The complete chemical name is 5-[(3-aminopropyl)amino]-7,10-dihydroxy-2-[2-[(2-hydroxyethyl)amino]ethyl]-anthra[1,9-cd]pyrazol-6(2H)-one dihydrochloride. The molecular formula is $C_{21}H_{25}N_5O_4 \cdot 2HCl$ and the formula weight 484.4.

■ Antitumor Activity

Piroxantrone and other anthrapyrazoles demonstrated good activity in preclinical antitumor screens in mice (Leopold et al 1985, Burchenal et al 1985). Sensitive tumors included B-16 melanoma, L-1210 and P-388 leukemias, and mammary MX-1 xenografts. There appears to be partial cross-resistance between piroxantrone and doxorubicin in a P-388 leukemia cell line that was 51-fold resistant to doxorubicin and cross-resistant to numerous other agents including amsacrine, vinblastine, and trimetrexate (Klohs et al 1986). Of interest, verapamil was able to reverse this resistance pattern when combined with piroxantrone. In contrast, some mammary carcinomas resistant to doxorubicin have remained sensitive to piroxantrone in vitro (Leopold et al 1985, Burchenal et al 1985, Sebolt et al 1985, Miller et al 1984). Piroxantrone is not cross-resistant with cytarabine, methotrexate, 6-thioguanine, cisplatin, 5-fluorouracil, and tiazofurin (Burchenal et al 1985).

In phase I clinical trials, disease stabilization was observed in patients with colon, renal, and ovarian cancer (1 each) (Hantel et al 1990). Two objective responses in breast and melanoma were observed in another phase I trial in 30 evaluable patients with a variety of solid tumors (Ames et al 1990). The drug was inactive in renal cell carcinoma (Allen et al 1992).

■ Mechanism of Action

Piroxantrone intercalates between the stacked base pairs in DNA with a binding affinity similar to that of mitoxantrone (Fry et al 1985). This preferentially inhibits the synthesis of DNA over that of RNA. Protein synthesis is unimpaired unless very high concentrations are used. Based on the inhibition of DNA synthesis in logarithmically growing L-1210 leukemia cells, piroxantrone is approximately fourfold more potent than doxorubicin.

Piroxantrone also induces protein-linked DNA strand breaks characteristic of topoisomerase II inhibition (Fry et al 1985); however, the concentration of piroxantrone needed to induce comparable DNA double-strand breaks is twice that of doxorubicin. This suggests that intercalation and impaired DNA synthesis by template inhibition constitute the primary mechanisms of action for piroxantrone (Showalter et al 1987).

A major difference from doxorubicin is the reduced rate of oxygen free radical generation with piroxantrone (Fry et al 1985). There is also evidence that piroxantrone can actually inhibit doxorubicin- or iron-stimulated lipid peroxidation in rabbit hepatic microsomes (Frank and Novak 1986). Less

NADPH oxidation is also produced by piroxantrone compared with doxorubicin (Frank and Novak 1987). These biochemical differences may relate to the lack of a quinone moiety in the anthrapyrazole structure of piroxantrone. Importantly, cardiotoxicity may be similarly reduced in piroxantrone as a result of this structure–activity relationship (Fagan et al 1984).

■ Availability and Storage

Piroxantrone is investigationally available from Warner Lambert Company as a lyophilized 50-mg red powder in 10-mL glass vials. Mannitol 50 mg is present as an excipient. The intact vials are stored in the freezer at −10 to −20°C. At room temperature, however, one lot of vials has been stable for 3 years. The vials are not stable at 50°C (National Cancer Institute 1990).

■ Preparation for Use, Stability, and Admixture

The 50-mg vials are reconstituted with 2.4 mL of Sterile Water for Injection, USP. This yields a red-colored solution containing 20 mg of piroxantrone and 20 mg of mannitol at a pH of 4.6. Further dilution into D5W or 0.9% sodium chloride to a concentration of 0.1 mg/mL provides a solution that is stable for at least 4 days at room temperature (25°C); however, because of the lack of an antibacterial agent, use within 8 hours of reconstitution is recommended.

■ Administration

Piroxantrone is administered by brief intravenous infusion, typically over 1 hour (Hantel et al 1990). Care should be taken to avoid extravasation, as the compound is known to be a local irritant in humans and is a documented vesicant in animal models (Clarke et al 1989). Increasing the final infusate volume from 50 to 300 mL in one study was felt to reduce phlebitis at the infusion site (Ames et al 1990).

■ Dosage

The recommended dose for phase II clinical trials is 150 mg/m^2 (Hantel et al 1990) or 160 mg/m^2 (Ames et al 1990). A 3-week treatment interval was common to both trials. The maximally tolerated dose was reported to be 190 mg/m^2 IV every 3 weeks.

Preliminary trials suggest that piroxantrone dose intensity may be doubled when combined with either filgrastim (G-CSF) (Savarese et al 1992) or sargramostim (GM-CSF) (Bayer et al 1992).

CLINICAL PHARMACOKINETICS OF PIROXANTRONE

Dose (mg/m^2)	Volume of Distribution (L) Central	Volume of Distribution (L) Steady State	Peak Level (μmol/L)	Half-life (min) α	Half-life (min) β	Clearance (L/min/m^2)	AUC (μmol/min/L)
Hantel et al 1988, 1990							
30	1.9	NR*	2.65	1.5	NR		110
45	7.2	NR	2.51	3.3	NR		100
90	8.9	21.4	4.95	2.6	16.1		210
120	8.5	19.3	7.57	2.8	17.8		430
150	10.2	33.0	7.54	3.7	19.8		480
190	9.6	20.3	13.70	5.0	32.1		690
Mean (30–190)	8.3	23.4		3	19		
40–160							
Ames et al 1990		(L/m^2)	(μg/mL)	—	30	1.29	(μg·min/mL)
30		NR					43
45		1.27–1.80	0.4				31
90		0.8–1.32	1.5				87
120		1.06–1.50	1.6				95
140		0.9–1.99	2.2				114
160		1.10–1.51	2.0				126

*NR, not reported.

Pharmacokinetics

Piroxantrone is rapidly eliminated from the plasma in a biphasic pattern (Ames et al 1990, Hantel et al 1988). The table on the opposite page summarizes the pharmacokinetics for 1-hour piroxantrone infusions administered at doses ranging from 45 to 160 mg/m² (Ames et al 1990). As anticipated, very little intact drug, 5.3% of a dose, was eliminated in the urine over 48 hours. The mean total body clearance was 684 mL/min/m². Part of this apparently avid metabolism may involve rapid drug degradation in human plasma (half-life of 30 minutes) (Ames et al 1990).

The very rapid degradation and biphasic drug clearance seen in humans contrast with the pharmacokinetics of piroxantrone in mice and that of most other polycyclic DNA intercalators. More sensitive assays may be needed to definitively rule out the presence of a more prolonged terminal half-life (Frank et al 1987). At pH 4.5, about 40% of piroxantrone is bound to plasma proteins. Binding studies at physiologic pH were hampered by poor drug stability.

Side Effects and Toxicity

The major dose-limiting effect of piroxantrone is myelosuppression noted primarily by leukopenia. The white blood cell nadirs occurred between days 7 and 14 and typically resolved completely by 3 weeks (Hantel et al 1990). Thrombocytopenia is both less severe and less common with piroxantrone.

Minimal nonhematologic toxic effects include mild nausea and vomiting and rare alopecia. Mucositis was noted only at the maximally tolerated dose of 190 mg/m² (Hantel et al 1990); however, vein irritation was very common, and in one trial 6 of 30 patients developed sclerosis in the injected vein (Hantel et al 1990). This effect may be enhanced with more concentrated drug dilutions, and experimentally, extravasation can lead to skin ulceration (Clarke et al 1989).

The drug was not cardiotoxic in animals (Frank et al 1989); however, cardiac dysrhythmias have rarely been observed in patients treated under National Cancer Institute-sponsored protocols (Ames et al 1990). These include premature ventricular contractions and a Mobitz type I heart block in one patient each; however, continuous cardiac monitoring during the infusion period did not reveal any cardiac rhythm disturbances in one trial (Ames et al 1990). Thus far, there is no consistent evidence of reduced cardiac ejection fractions at cumulative piroxantrone doses up to 1030 mg/m² (Ames et al 1990).

REFERENCES

Allen A, Wolf M, Crawford ED, et al. Phase II evaluation of piroxantrone in renal cell carcinoma. A Southwest Oncology Group study. *Invest New Drugs.* 1992;**10**:129–132.

Ames MM, Loprinzi CL, Collis JM, et al. Phase I and clinical pharmacological evaluation of piroxantrone hydrochloride (oxantrazole). *Cancer Res.* 1990;**50**:3905–3909.

Bayer RA, Benson AB, Locker GY, et al. Phase I trial of dose intensification (DI) of piroxantrone (PRX) and GM-CSF in patients with advanced cancer. *Proc Am Soc Clin Oncol.* 1992;**11**:133.

Burchenal JH, Pancoast T, Elslager E. Anthrapyrazole and amsacrine analogs in mouse and human leukemia in vitro and in vivo. *Proc Am Assoc Cancer Res.* 1985;**26**:224.

Clarke BV, Harwood KV, Donehower R. Local toxicity of piroxantrone: An anthrapyrazole with irritant and vesicant properties similar to those of doxorubicin. *J Natl Cancer Inst.* 1989;**81**(17):1331–1332.

Fagan MA, Hacker MP, Newman RA. Cardiotoxic potential of substituted anthra(1,9-cd)pyrazole- 6(2H)ones(anthrapyrazoles) as assessed by the fetal mouse heart organ culture. *Proc Am Assoc Cancer Res.* 1984;**27**:302.

Frank P, Novak RF. Effects of anthrapyrazole antineoplastic agents on lipid peroxidation. *Biochem Biophys Res Commun.* 1986;**140**(3):797–807.

Frank P, Novak RF. Superoxide production and NADPH utilization by anthrapyrazole antineoplastic agents. *Proc Am Assoc Cancer Res.* 1987;**28**:269.

Frank SK, Mathiesen DA, Szurszewski M, et al. Preclinical pharmacology of the anthrapyrazole analog oxantrazole (NSC-349174, piroxantrone). *Cancer Chemother Pharmacol.* 1989;**23**:213–218.

Frank SK, Mathiesen DA, Whitefield LR, et al. High performance liquid chromatographic assay for the experimental anticancer agent oxantrazole. *J Chromatogr.* 1987;**419**:225–232.

Fry DW, Boritzki TJ, Besserer JA, et al. In vitro DNA strand scission and inhibition of nucleic acid synthesis in L1210 leukemia cells by a new class of DNA complexers, the anthra(1,9-cd)-pyraxol-6(2H)-ones (anthrapyrazoles). *Biochem Pharmacol.* 1985;**34**(19):3499–3508.

Hantel A, Donehower RC, Rowinsky EK, et al. Phase I study and pharmacodynamics of piroxantrone (NSC-349174), a new anthrapyrazole. *Cancer Res.* 1990;**50**:3284–3288.

Hantel A, Noe DA, Grochow LB, et al. A phase I and pharmacokinetic study of oxantrazole (OAZ). *Proc Am Assoc Cancer Res.* 1988;**7**:66.

Klohs WD, Steinkampf RW, Havlick MJ, et al. Resistance

to anthrapyrazoles and anthracyclines in multidrug-resistant P388 murine leukemia cells: Reversal by calcium blockers and calmodulin antagonists. *Cancer Res.* 1986;**46**:4352–4356.

Leopold WR, Nelson JM, Plowman J, et al. Anthrapyrazoles, a new class of intercalating agents with high-level, broad spectrum activity against murine tumors. *Cancer Res.* 1985;**45**:5532–5539.

Miller BE, Jackson RC, Heppner GH. Comparison of the effect of PD111815, a substituted anthra[1,9-cd]-pyrazole-6(2H)-one, on mouse mammary tumor subpopulations differentially sensitive to doxorubicin. *Proc Am Assoc Cancer Res.* 1984;**25**:301.

National Cancer Institute. Piroxantrone (NSC-349174). In: *NCI Investigational Drugs: Pharmaceutical Data.* NIH Publication 91–2141. Washington, DC: U.S. Department of Health and Human Services; 1990:132–135.

Savarese D, Berg S, Denicoff A, et al. Phase I/pharmacokinetic study of piroxantrone and granulocyte colony-stimulating factor (G-CSF). *Proc Am Assoc Cancer Res.* 1992;**33**:244.

Sebolt JS, Havlick MJ, Hamelehle KL, et al. Establishment of Adriamycin-resistant mammary adenocarcinoma 16/C in vitro and its sensitivity to the anthrapyrazoles CI-942 and CI-937. *Proc Am Assoc Cancer Res.* 1985;**26**:339.

Showalter HD, Johnson JL, Hofteizer JM, et al. Anthrapyrazole anticancer agents: Synthesis and structure–activity relationships against murine leukemias. *J Med Chem.* 1987;**30**:121–131.

PIXY-321

■ Other Names

GM-CSF/IL-3 fusion protein.

■ Chemistry

PIXY-321 is a fusion protein composed of interleukin-3 (IL-3) and granulocyte–macrophage colony-stimulating factor (GM-CSF). The latter protein is modified at position 23 (leucine for arginine) to preclude cleavage by yeast proteases. Other changes in the GM-CSF protein include the following substitutions to delete two N-glycosylation sites: aspartic acid for asparagine at position 27, and glutamic acid for threonine at position 39. In the IL-3 portion of the molecule, aspartic acid is substituted for asparagine at positions 15 and 70.

The complete PIXY-321 molecule has 271 amino acids. The two component proteins are joined by a short peptide bridge consisting of nine glycines and two serines. This yields a "flexible linker" sequence which allows for separate receptor binding by each component protein domain. The molecular weight of the molecule is about 35,000 ± 3000 (Williams and Park 1991).

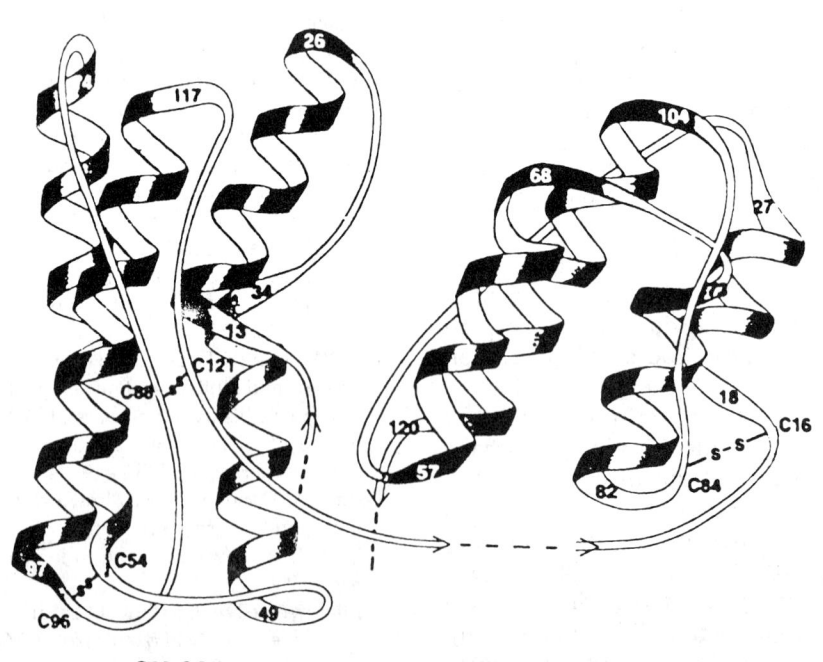

Structure of PIXY-321

The PIXY-321 glycoprotein is produced by recombinant DNA techniques using a yeast expression system (Saccharomyces cerevisiae.) The expression vector for the fusion protein was constructed using the entire GM-CSF coding sequence, sequences encoding the linker, and the full coding region of IL-3 (Williams and Park 1991). Transcription was directed by the promoter for alcohol dehydrogenase II. An α-factor leader sequence is present that directs the secretion of the complete molecule. Circular dichroism studies show that the molecule adopts the expected α-helical structure based on modeling of GM-CSF and IL-3 as four helix bundles (Curtis et al 1991).

■ Antitumor Activity

The basis for PIXY-321 development was the observation that human IL-3 followed by GM-CSF produces synergistic hematopoietic stimulation in primates (Donahue et al 1988). Simultaneous GM-CSF/IL-3 administration appeared to be superior in myelosuppressed primates (MacVittie et al 1991). This suggested that the two molecules worked cooperatively at the cellular level and that a single fusion protein might have enhanced stimulatory activity.

PIXY-321 produces hematopoietic effects in primates characteristic of both GM-CSF and IL-3 (D. E. Williams, unpublished). This includes the rapid GM-CSF-like stimulation of neutrophils and the slow IL-3-like stimulation of platelets (Williams and Park 1991). The function of neutrophils is also enhanced by PIXY-321 in vitro (Young et al 1991). In vitro clonogenic assays of human bone marrow cells have demonstrated that PIXY-321 has a higher specific activity than GM-CSF and/or IL-3 and stimulates erythroid progenitor cells (BFU-E), multilineage myeloid cells (CFU-GEMM), and granulocyte–macrophage progenitor cells (CFU-GM) (Curtis et al 1991). PIXY-321 can also stimulate leukemic myeloid cell lines such as AML-193 that are solely dependent on GM-CSF for proliferation. In these assays, PIXY-321 routinely demonstrates hematopoietic stimulation severalfold greater than that obtained with either IL-3 or GM-CSF used alone or in combination (Curtis et al 1991).

PIXY-321 can also stimulate colony formation by normal human hematopoietic precursors from bone marrow treated with 4-hydroperoxycyclophosphamide. In this model, the level of stimulation for PIXY-321 was greater than that with either IL-3 or GM-CSF (Hami et al 1991). Potential clinical applications of PIXY-321 include the stimulation of bone marrow recovery following chemotherapy, the reversal of myelosuppression from genetic disorders, and use as an aid in reengraftment following bone marrow transplantation. Importantly, human lymphoma cell lines do not show stimulation by PIXY-321. PIXY-321 is active in nonhuman primates and stimulates the broad myeloid progenitors noted in vitro (Curtis et al 1991). Trials in human cancer patients are just beginning.

In early-phase clinical trials, PIXY-321 has produced dose-dependent reductions in neutropenia and thrombocytopenia following standard-dose chemotherapy combinations in patients with breast cancer (Jakubowski et al 1992), ovarian cancer (Runowicz et al 1992), and sarcoma (Vadhan-Raj et al 1992). A 14-day course of daily PIXY-321 following CyADIC chemotherapy in sarcoma patients reduced both the duration of neutropenia (by 3 days) and the number of patients becoming thrombocytopenic. In addition, the hematocrit is maintained in patients receiving PIXY-321 doses greater than 500 µg/m^2 (Vadhan-Raj et al 1992). Similar benefits are described in breast cancer patients receiving PIXY-321 after thiotepa and doxorubicin (Jakubowski et al 1992) and in ovarian cancer patients receiving cyclophosphamide and carboplatin (Runowicz et al 1992). A 2-hr IV infusion of PIXY-321 accelerated both platelet and granulocyte recovery after autologous bone marrow transplantation (Vose et al 1993).

■ Mechanism of Action

In vitro studies demonstrate that PIXY-321 binds to cells expressing specific cell surface receptors for either IL-3 or GM-CSF. In some cell lines such as KG1, there is normally competition between binding of GM-CSF and IL-3. PIXY 321 binds to KG1 cells with affinity comparable to that of GM-CSF and with an affinity 10-fold higher than that of IL-3. HL-60 promyelocytic leukemia cells express a single class of high-affinity GM-CSF receptors (about 240 per cell). In these cells, the binding affinity of PIXY-321 was 5.9×10^{-9} M, compared with 6.2×10^{-9} M for GM-CSF (Williams and Park 1991). Conversely, human JM-1 cells express a single class of high-affinity IL-3 receptors, (about 160/cell). In these cells PIXY-321 binding affinity was 4.3×10^{-9} M, compared with 3.5×10^{-9} M for purified human IL-3 (Williams and Park 1991).

Only human hematopoietic cells, PIXY-321 produces 10- to 20-fold greater colony stimulation than

GM-CSF (Curtis et al 1991, Williams and Park 1991). With AML-193 cells the specific activity of PIXY-321 was 1.81×10^6 U/mg, with a unit defined as the amount of growth factor required to stimulate one-half maximal [^{3}H]-thymidine incorporation by the AML-193 cell line. Thus, the intrinsic hematopoietic synergy seen with PIXY-321 in certain cell lines may relate to the presence of heterogeneous receptors that are capable of binding both GM-CSF and IL-3 (Park et al 1989a,b).

■ Availability and Storage

PIXY-321 is investigationally available from Immunex Corporation in vials containing 500 µg of lyophilized white powdered drug with 40 mg of mannitol, 10 mg of sucrose, and 1.2 mg of tromethamine (Tris) buffer. The drug is stored under refrigeration until reconstituted.

■ Preparation for Use, Stability, and Admixture

Each 500-µg vial is reconstituted with 1.0 mL of Bacteriostatic Sterile Water for Injection containing 0.9% benyl alcohol, USP. This results in a clear solution containing 500 µg/mL PIXY-321 with a pH of 7.4. The solution is stable for 7 days at 4°C after reconstitution. For intravenous infusion doses, human serum albumin (0.1%) should be added to the final infusate to reduce surface adsorption of the protein. The diluted solution should be used within 24 hr and should not be frozen following reconstitution. The solution should not be filtered prior to use.

■ Administration

In initial trials, PIXY-321 was administered subcutaneously, and intravenously.

■ Dosage

Phase I clinical trials in cancer patients receiving cytotoxic chemotherapy combinations have evaluated a range of PIXY-321 doses up to 1000 µg/m²/d for 14 days. For reference, cynomolgus monkeys have been given daily injections of up to 800 µg/kg. In humans, all PIXY-321 doses are initiated 24 hours after the administration of cytotoxic chemotherapy.

Phase I trials in chemotherapy patients have reported good tolerance but minimal hematopoietic stimulation at daily doses up to 500 µg/m². At higher doses of 750 and 1000 µg/m², there is significant improvement in both neutropenia and thrombocytopenia following standard-dose cytotoxic chemotherapy treatments for sarcoma (Vadhan-Raj et al 1992), ovarian cancer (Runowicz et al 1992), and breast cancer (Jakubowski et al 1992).

PHARMACOKINETICS OF INTRAVENOUS PIXY-321 IN MONKEYS

Parameter	Dose (µg/kg/d × 21)		
	100	400	800
AUC (µg/mL/min)	8.7	75.3	129.7
Half-life (min)			
α	2.8	7.9	5.9
β	19.7	52.0	39.7
Clearance (mL/min)	12	5.4	6.4
Steady-state volume of distribution (mL)	161	58	61
Peak level (µg/mL)	2.79	16.0	17.2

■ Pharmacokinetics

In rhesus monkeys given 30 to 100 µg/kg PIXY-321 by an intravenous bolus, the average elimination half-life was 38 minutes. In cynomolgus monkeys (*Macaca fascicularis* PIXY- 321 pharmacokinetics was evaluated at three dose levels (see table above). These results show that the drug is rapidly eliminated from the plasma with a terminal half-life of 19 to 52 minutes. The mean residence time was about 11 minutes. With subcutaneous administration, significantly lower plasma levels and cumulative exposures (AUC) were obtained (see table below). These data suggest that about 30% of the subcutaneous dose is available systemically compared with the comparable intravenous dose in the monkeys. Human pharmacokinetic data is currently unavailable.

■ Side Effects and Toxicity

PIXY-321 has had limited trials in humans and thus comprehensive toxicity data are not yet available; however, as this drug is a fusion protein of IL-3 and GM-CSF, some representative toxic effects from

PHARMACOKINETICS OF SUBCUTANEOUS PIXY-321 IN MONKEYS

Parameter	Dose (µg/kg/d × 21)	
	400	800
AUC (µg/mL/min)	19.3	38.2
Peak level (ng/mL)	45.3	87
Time to peak (min)	4.3	3.6
β half-life (h)	2.2	6.9

both component proteins were anticipated. There appears to be no flulike syndrome with PIXY-321 like that seen with high-dose GM-CSF (Antman et al 1988) and with IL-3 at all dose levels (Kurzrock et al 1991).

The only common side effect is an erythematous skin reaction at the site of subcutaneous injection (Vadhan-Raj et al 1992). Fever is typically of a low grade and is noted in only a few patients (Jakubowski et al 1992). Histamine levels and platelet aggregation studies appear to remain normal. Thus, transient local erythema is the only consistent side effect of PIXY-321 at doses up to 500 µg/m² (Runowicz et al 1992, Vadhan-Raj et al 1992, Jakubowski et al 1992).

REFERENCES

Antman KS, Griffin JD, Ellias A, et al. Effect of recombinant human granulocyte–macrophage colony-stimulating factor on chemotherapy-induced myelosuppression. *N Engl J Med.* 1988;**319**(10):593–598.

Broxmeyer HE, Benninger L, Cooper S, et al. Effects of treatment of patients with sarcoma with PIXY-321 (a genetically engineered GM-CSF/IL-3 fusion protein) on proliferation kinetics of bone marrow and blood myeloid progenitor cells. *Blood.* 1992;**80**(10, suppl 1):87a.

Curtis BM, Williams DE, Broxmeyer HE, et al. Enhanced hematopoietic activity of a human GM-CSF/IL-3 fusion protein. *Proc Natl Acad Sci USA.* 1991;**88**:5809–5813.

Donahue RE, Seehra J, Metzger M, et al. Human IL-3 and GM- CSF act synergistically in stimulating hematopoiesis in primates. *Science.* 1988;**241**:1820–1822.

Hami LS, Shpall EJ, Johnston CF, et al. The effect of PIXY-321 on 4-hydroperoxy-cyclophosphamide (4-HC)-purged and CD34+ positively selected bone marrow. Accepted for presentation, III International Symposium on Bone Marrow Transplantation Purging and Processing, sponsored by the Leukemia Society of America, San Diego, CA; October 1991.

Jakubowski A, Raptis G, Gilewski T, et al. A phase I/II trial of PIXY-321 (PIXY) in patients (PTS) with metastatic breast cancer receiving doxorubicin and thiotepa. *Blood.* 1992;**80**(10, suppl 1):88a.

Kurzrock R, Talpaz M, Estrov Z, et al. Phase I study of recombinant human interleukin-3 in patients with bone marrow failure. *J Clin Oncol.* 1991;**9**(7):1241–1250.

MacVittie TJ, Monroy RL, Farese AM, et al. Cytokine therapy in canine and primate models of radiation-induced marrow aplasia. *Behring Inst Mitt.* 1991;**90**:1–13.

Park LS, Friend D, Price V, et al. Heterogeneity in human interleukin-3 receptors: A subclass that binds human granulocyte/macrophage colony stimulating factor. *J Biol Chem.* 1989a;**264**:5420–5427.

Park LS, Waldron PE, Friend D, et al. Interleukin-3, GM-CSF, and G-CSF receptor expression on cell lines and primary leukemia cells: Receptor heterogeneity and relationship to growth factor responsiveness. *Blood.* 1989b;**74**:56–65.

Runowicz CD, Mandeli J, Speyer J, et al. Phase I/II study of PIXY321 after cyclophosphamide and carboplatin in the treatment of patients with advanced-stage ovarian cancer. *Blood.* 1992;**80**(1)suppl:88a.

Vadhan-Raj S, Papadopoulos N, Burgess A, et al. PIXY-321 (GM-CSF/IL-3 fusion protein) reduces chemotherapy (CT)-induced multilineage myelosuppression in patients with sarcoma. *Blood.* 1992;**80**(10, suppl 1):249a.

Vose JM, Anderson J, Blerman PJ, Garrison L, et al: Initial trial of PIXY321 (GM-CSF/IL-3 fusion protein) following high-dose chemotherapy and autologous bone marrow transplantation (ABMT) for lymphoid malignancy. *Proc Amer Soc Clin Oncol.* 1993;**12**:366.

Williams DE, Park LS. Hematopoietic effects of a granulocyte–macrophage colony-stimulating factor/interleukin-3 fusion protein. *Cancer.* 1991;**67**:2705–2707.

Young CE, McIlheran SM, Vadhan-Raj S, et al. Interleukin-3/granulocyte–macrophage colony-stimulating factor fusion protein effects on human neutrophil function. *Clin Res.* 1991;**39**:445a.

Plicamycin

■ Other Names

Aureolic acid; aurelic acid; Mithracin® (Miles Inc); PA-144; NSC-24559; mithramycin; mitramycin.

■ Chemistry

Plicamycin is an antibiotic isolated from *Streptomyces plicatus*. The brilliant yellow crystalline drug is slightly water soluble. It has a high molecular weight and complex structure consisting of two sugar chains linked to a polycyclic chromophobic group (Rao et al 1960, 1962). Structurally, it resembles chromomycin A_3 and has the empiric formula $C_{52}H_{76}O_{24}$.

■ Antitumor Activity

Plicamycin has its greatest antitumor activity in disseminated embryonal cell carcinoma of the testis or germ cell tumor. (Kennedy 1970a,b, Hescock et al 1989). Its major clinical use, however, is in the treatment of hypercalcemia of malignancy unresponsive to other methods of treatment (Godfrey 1971, Perlia et al 1970). Slayton et al (1971) found breast and kidney cancer patients to be more responsive to the calcium-lowering effects than myeloma, lung, and head and neck cancer patients.

Structure of plicamycin

Plicamycin has some minor antitumor activity in patients with glioblastoma multiforme (Kennedy et al 1965), in patients with hypernephromas, and, occasionally, in those with breast, thyroid, and stomach cancers (Kofman and Eisenstein 1963).

Recently the drug has been found to cause differentiation of chronic myelogenous leukemia blasts (Sampi et al 1987, Callahan et al 1987). Plicamycin is thought to act through the inhibition of messenger RNA synthesis (Kennedy 1970b).

■ Mechanism of Action

Plicamycin possesses a cytotoxic action similar to that of dactinomycin. This is thought to involve adlineation, in which the drug binds primarily to the outside of the DNA molecule (usually by ionic forces) and thereby interrupts DNA-directed RNA synthesis (Yarbro et al 1965). Plicamycin has been found to selectively inhibit transcription of G–C-containing DNA. Intercalation of drug directly into DNA also appears to occur.

The drug demonstrates a consistent calcium-lowering effect not related to the tumoricidal sensitivity of the particular neoplasm to plicamycin. The drug also acts on osteoclasts and blocks the action of parathyroid hormone (Ryan et al 1970). This action is not as rapid as the response to calcitonin (Cochran et al 1970) although the fall in serum calcium begins within hours of injection. It should be remembered that this is accomplished by doses only a fraction of those that can be effective in sensitive tumors. Slayton et al (1971) have thus carefully described the steady fall in serum calcium over the 48 hours following injection. There are associated concomitant decreases in serum inorganic phosphate and 24-hour calcium excretion.

Parsons et al (1967) first noted that plicamycin could block the hypercalcemic effects of high-dose vitamin D. Zull et al (1966) were able to demonstrate that RNA synthesis inhibitors, including dactinomycin, were able to effectively block the pharmacologic effects of vitamin D in vitro. Thus, although structurally somewhat dissimilar, plicamycin and dactinomycin appear to share common non-cell cycle phase-specific mechanisms of action. Of great recent interest is the finding that plicamycin can inhibit transcriptional activity of a transfected human *c-myc* gene (Ray et al 1990).

■ Availability and Storage

Plicamycin is commercially available from Miles Inc, Elkhart, Indiana (Mithracin®), in vials containing 2500 µg of drug with 100 mg of mannitol and disodium phosphate sufficient to result in a pH of 7 when diluted with sterile water. The intact vials are stable for 2 years after manufacture if stored under refrigeration.

■ Preparation for Use, Stability, and Admixture

To reconstitute each vial, 4.9 mL of sterile water for injection is added using only gentle shaking. This should result in a slightly yellow but clear solution with a concentration of 500 µg/ml and a pH of 6.3 to 7.0. D5W is not recommended as an initial diluent because of the acid-unstable nature of the drug. At pH less than 5 some of the drug may hydrolyze (however, stability problems have not been observed when reconstituted drug is added to large-volume D5W solutions). Plicamycin also readily chelates divalent cations (especially iron); therefore any such admixture (eg, with trace element solutions) should be avoided. After reconstitution, the solution is stable for 48 hours under refrigeration. When one vial is diluted with 1000 mL of D5W, the resultant solution is stable for 24 hours at room temperature.

■ Administration

The manufacturer's recommended administration technique is to give the drug as an intravenous infusion over 4 to 7 hours diluted into 1000 mL of D5W. This may avoid the higher incidence of severe gastrointestinal side effects thought to be associated with a rapid intravenous push of the drug (Godfrey 1971). Clinically, a short intravenous infusion (over 20–30 minutes) is often used. Antiemetics before administration may be beneficial in either case. The drug can cause local tissue irritation and damage if delivered outside the vein. Vein patency should be tested before infusion with 5 to 10 mL of D5W or normal saline. If signs of local reaction occur during infusion, another intravenous site should be selected and used for the remainder of drug delivery.

■ Special Precautions

The agent can cause a severe coagulopathy (see Side Effects and Toxicity).

■ Drug Interactions

None are known.

■ Dosage

The dosage used in the past for the treatment of patients with testicular tumors was 25 to 30 µg/kg daily for 8 to 10 days. In the treatment of hypercalcemic conditions secondary to cancer, 25 µg/kg for 3 to 4 days has been recommended An alternate dosing schedule, however, is recommended: 25 to 50 µg/kg IV on alternate days for three to eight doses or until toxicity manifests. In fact, for sensitive animal tumors, greater durations of antitumor effects were observed when the drug was given on alternate days versus continuous daily dosing.

Because of the highly toxic nature of this drug, minimal doses are recommended, especially in the treatment of hypercalcemia when the primary tumor will require other cytotoxic chemotherapy. The duration of action of a single plicamycin dose is 7 to 10 days, with peak effectiveness reached within 72 hours. Therefore, single weekly doses have been successful in managing hypercalcemia resulting from widespread metastatic disease (Ajlouni and Rosenfeld 1974). *Significant hazard is present with this drug if the correct microgram (µg) dosing recommendation is confused with the incorrect milligrams (mg).*

■ Pharmacokinetics

Twenty-five percent of the radioactivity of a labeled dose of plicamycin is excreted in the urine at 2 hours, 40% by 15 hours. Also, the drug appears to distribute well across the blood–brain barrier, and cerebrospinal fluid levels are equivalent to simultaneous plasma levels of drug 4 to 6 hours after an intravenous dose. Distribution of the drug to Kupffer cells in the liver, formed bone surfaces, and renal tubular cells has been shown in animals (*Hospital Formulary* 1970). Unfortunately, pharmacokinetic data with more recent techniques are not available.

■ Side Effects and Toxicity

The major toxic consideration for plicamycin is hemorrhage secondary to a combination of drug-induced thrombocytopenia and simultaneous drug-induced decreases in clotting factors II, V, VII, and X (Kennedy 1970a,b, Currerri and Ansfield 1960). Documented dysfibrinogenemia secondary to plicamycin has also been described (Ashby and Lazarchick 1986). This syndrome may ensue rapidly and is typically heralded by epistaxis, ecchymoses, a facial flushing, and prolonged coagulation times. It should be remembered that the hemorrhagic diathesis may occur even in the absence of significant blood count depression. Epistaxis and facial flushing, therefore, are clear indications to discontinue the agent, at least temporarily. An acquired platelet defect has also been described and was documented by abnormal bleeding times and platelet aggregation (because of ADP) as well as decreased platelet ADP stores (Ahr et al 1978). Overall, classic bone marrow depression is generally mild, producing generally mild leukopenia with more significant thrombocytopenia. The drug does not appear to be especially immunosuppressive.

Gastrointestinal effects include nausea, anorexia, vomiting, and diarrhea. Kennedy (1970a) noted significant individual variation and also suggested tolerance to the gastrointestinal effects with repeated doses. In one study, chlorpromazine (Thorazine®) appeared to be the most effective antiemetic (Kennedy 1970a). No description of use of more recently available antiemetics has been reported. Other gastrointestinal effects included the production of a metallic taste in the mouth in a few patients and stomatitis in 15% of patients. Alopecia appears to be an infrequent complication.

Central nervous system toxicity usually manifests as increasingly severe headache, irritability, akethesia, and finally lethargy.

A characteristic dermatologic reaction is seen in about a third of patients. There is a progressive blushing of the face with eventual thickening and coarsening of skin folds and facial features. Papular excoriations may be noted. With drug discontinuance the reaction subsides, although marked hyperpigmentation and transient desquamation may result.

Both hepatic function and renal function may be affected by plicamycin and direct organ toxicity is highly probable. Two liver enzymes, serum glutamic–oxalacetic transaminase and lactic dehydrogenase, are sharply and transiently elevated by the drug in about 11% of patients (Green and Donehower 1984). Margileth et al (1973) have described a patient who developed multiple arterial occlusions after receiving the drug. According to Kennedy (1970a), a continuing elevation of lactic dehydrogenase with repeated doses is an indication for discontinuance. Prothrombin times are significantly elevated in about 20% of patients treated with high antitumor doses. Kennedy (1970a) anecdotally suggested some advantage for either therapeutic or prophylactic phytonadione on days of mithramycin administration or given orally between treatment courses. The efficacy of this maneuver is unknown.

Proteinuria and increased serum creatinine and urea nitrogen are seen as are lowered serum levels of phosphate, magnesium, potassium, and calcium (Fillastre et al 1974). There is a suggestion that renal toxicity is cumulative with the drug; it appeared to be unrelated to age in Kennedy's study (1970a). In patients who become azotemic the creatinine clearance usually remains abnormal for weeks or months after therapy. Underlying renal impairment may accentuate the nephrotoxicity of the agent (Benedetti et al 1983).

There is the documented potential for producing symptomatic hypocalcemia with this drug, wherein a relative insensitivity to vitamin D may occur. On the other hand, after discontinuation of plicamycin, a light and transient "rebound" hypercalcemia can ensue. It typically lasts only 2 to 4 days.

■ **Special Applications**

Plicamycin can be used to treat Paget's disease-associated hypercalcemia (Ralston et al 1985).

REFERENCES

Ahr DJ, Scialla SJ, Kimball DB. Acquired platelet dysfunction following mithramicin therapy. *Cancer*. 1978;**41**: 448–454.

Ajlouni K, Rosenfeld PS. Treatment of hypercalcemia. *Drug Ther*. 1974:103–111.

Ashby MA, Lazarchick J. Acquired dysfibrinogenemia secondary to mithramycin toxicity. *Am J Med Sci*. 1986; **292**(1):53–55.

Benedetti RG, Heilman KJ, 3d, Gabow PA. Nephrotoxicity following single dose mithramycin therapy. *Am J Nephrol*. 1983;**5**:277–278.

Callahan M, Wall S, Askin F, Dianey D, et al. Granulocytic sarcoma presenting as pulmonary nodules and lymphadenopathy. *Cancer*. 1987;**60**(8):1902–1904.

Cochran M, Peacock M, Sachs G, et al. Renal effect of calcitonin. *Br Med J*. 1970;**1**:135–137.

Curreri AR, Ansfield FJ. Mithramycin—Human toxicology and preliminary therapeutic investigation. *Cancer Chemother Rep*. 1960;16:22.

Fillastre JP, Maitrot J, Canonne MA, et al. Renal function and alterations in plasma electrolyte levels in normocalcaemic and hypercalcaemic patients with malignant diseases, given an intravenous infusion of mithramycin. *Chemotherapy*. 1974;**20**:280–295.

Godfrey TE. Mithramycin for hypercalcemia of malignant disease. *Calif Med*. 1971;**115**:1–4.

Green L, Donehower RC. Hepatic toxicity of low doses of mithramycin in hypercalcemia. *Cancer Treat Rep*. 1984;**11**:1379–1381.

Hescock H Jr, Parker M, Wang TY, Ballinger R, Balducci L. Metastatic carcinoma of unknown primary: Complete response to second-line treatment with plicamycin. *Am J Med Sci*. 1989;**298**(1):34–37.

Hospital Formulary. Washington, DC: American Society of Hospital Pharmacists; 1970.

Kennedy BJ. Metabolic and toxic effects of mithramycin during tumor therapy. *Am J Med.* 1970a;**49**:494–503.

Kennedy BJ. Mithramycin therapy in advanced testicular neoplasms. *Cancer.* 1970b;**26**:755–766.

Kennedy BJ, Griffen WO, Lober P. The specific effect of mithramycin on embryonal carcinoma of the testis. *Cancer.* 1965;**18**:1631.

Kofman S, Eisenstein R. Mithramycin in the treatment of disseminated cancer. *Cancer Chemother Rep.* 1963;**32**:77–81.

Margileth DA, Smith FE, Lane M. Sudden arterial occlusion associated with mithramycin therapy. *Cancer.* 1973;**31**:708–712.

Miller DM, Polansky DA, Thomas SD, et al. Rapid communication: Mithramycin selectively inhibits transcription of G–C containing DNA. *Am J Med Sci.* 1987;**294**(5): 388–394.

Parsons V, Baum M, Self M. Effect of mithramycin on calcium and hydroxyproline metabolism in patients with malignant disease. *Br Med J.* 1967;**1**:474–479.

Perlia CP, Gubisch NJ, Wolter J, Edelberg D, Dederick MM, Taylor SG. Mithramycin treatment of hypercalcia. *Cancer.* 1970;**25**:389–394.

Ralston SH, Gardner MD, Dryburgh FJ, Jenkins AS, Cowan RA, Boyle IT. Comparison of aminohydroxypropylidine diphosphonate, mithramycin, and corticosteroids/calcitonin in treatment of cancer-associated hypercalcaemia. *Lancet.* 1985;**2**:907–910.

Rao KV, Cullen WP, Sobin BA. Mithramycin: Antibiotic with antitumor properties. *Proc Am Assoc Cancer Res.* 1960;**3**:143.

Rao KV, Cullen WP, Sobin BA. New antibiotic with antitumor properties. *Antibiot Chemother.* 1962;**12**:182.

Ray R, Thomas S, Miller DM. Mithramycin selectively inhibits the transcriptional activity of a transfected human c-myc gene. *Am J Med Sci.* 1990;**300**(4):203–208.

Ryan WG, Schwartz TB, Perlia CP. Effects of mithramycin on Paget's disease of bone. *Ann Intern Med.* 1970;**70**:549

Sampi K, Hozumi M, Kumai R, Honma Y, Sakurai M. Differentiation of blasts from patients in myeloid crisis of chronic myelogenous leukemia by in-vivo and in-vitro plicamycin treatment. *Leukemia Res.* 1987;**11**(12):1089–1092.

Slayton RE, Schnider BL, Eliase E, Horton J, Perlia CP. New approach to the treatment of hypercalcemia: The effect of short term treatment with mithramycin. *Clin Pharmacol Ther.* 1971;**12**(5):833–837.

Yarbro JW, Wolhein M, Kennedy BJ. Differential inhibition of RNA synthesis by mithramycin. *Clin Res.* 1965;**13**:341.

Zull JE, Czarnowska-Misztal E, DeLuca HF. On the relationship between vitamin D action and actinomycin-sensitive processes. *Proc Natl Acad Sci USA.* 1966;**55**:177–184.

Porfimer Sodium

■ Other Names

Photofrin®, Photofrin II® (QLT Phototherapeutics, Lederle Laboratories); dihematoporphyrin ether; DHE; NSC-603062.

■ Chemistry

Porfimer sodium is a photosensitizer derived from the heme molecule hematoporphyrin. It is the active (photosensitizing) component of hematoporphyrin derivative (HPD). In the first isolation step, hematoporphyrin is acetylated to the monoacetate, diacetate, and unchanged forms, all of which are inactive. Subsequent exposure to dilute alkali or acid hydrolyzes the acetate groups on two hematoporphyrins to yield an ethyl ether hematoporphyrin

Structure of porfimer sodium

dimer which is active. The commercial product is chemically designated bis-1-[3-(1-hydroxyethyl)-porphyrin-8-yl]ethyl ether (Dougherty 1986), Dougherty et al 1984). The common name for this material is dihematoporphyrin ether (DHE). This material tends to self-associate in aqueous solution even if albumin is present. The self-aggregation property of DHE in tissues may explain the drug's prolonged retention in vivo; however, the aggregate forms of hematoporphyrins do not generate singlet oxygen molecules and therefore are not photodynamically active in tissues (Dougherty 1986).

■ Antitumor Activity

Early clinical reports described antitumor efficacy for a crude hematoporphyrin derivative and visible red light (600–700 nm) for the local treatment of regional chest wall recurrences of breast cancer (Dougherty et al 1979). This drug–light combination was also active in malignant melanoma, mycosis fungoides, chondrosarcoma, and angiosarcoma (Dougherty et al 1978). These early clinical data have been summarized by Dougherty (1986) to show that cutaneous and subcutaneous tumor response rates without recurrence are maintained for up to 1 year in most types of cancer. Activity was also reported in the treatment of stage I superficial squamous cell carcinoma of the lung with 6 of 19 complete responses in one study (Cortese and Kinsey 1984) and 8 of 13 complete responses in another trial (Hayata et al 1984). In this setting, repeat bronchoscopy 3 days after photodynamic therapy is useful to remove debris and excess secretions and to determine if a repeat treatment is necessary to remove any residual tumor (Balchum et al 1984).

In these studies, tumor sizes varied considerably and the light source was typically a 630-nm laser delivering total light energy doses of 20 to 120 J/cm^2 at a dose rate of 15 to 100 mW/cm^2 (Dougherty 1986). The HPD was injected 3 days prior to the laser light therapies. Light from the 630-nm laser was typically delivered through a 200- or 400-μm quartz filter. In some cases of lung cancer, photodynamic therapy was used to debulk tumors as an adjunct to more definitive surgery (Hayata et al 1984).

Photodynamic therapy has also been used to treat cancer of the esophagus, and some palliative responses are obtained even in patients with advanced disease (McCaughan et al 1984); however, complete responses are not possible with photodynamic therapy in esophageal cancer. In contrast, complete responses are noted in early-stage bladder cancer patients with transitional-cell carcinoma (Benson et al 1983, Hisazumi et al 1983, 1984, Shumaker et al 1985). Whole-bladder light energy is delivered endoscopically at doses ranging from 35 to 100 J/cm^2 48 to 72 hours after HPD or DHE treatments. Patients with carcinoma in situ may obtain complete responses for up to 1 year following whole-bladder photodynamic therapy. For example, Prout et al (1987) describe complete eradication of all bladder tumors in 9 of 19 patients (47%) with carcinoma in situ. The overall response rate was 74%, but in 10 patients, 13 tumor sites could not be eradicated. Responses were dependent on superficial tumor size and light dose. Complete tumor ablation was possible with tumors less than 2 cm in diameter.

Photodynamic therapy may also be active in the prophylactic management of bladder cancer (Nseyo et al 1990a). A recent randomized trial reported that 39% of patients recurred after photodynamic therapy compared with 81% in the observation arm (Dugan et al 1991). The median time to recurrence was 13 months with photodynamic therapy versus 3 months in the control group.

Smaller series also report high response rates to photodynamic therapy in localized gynecologic tumors. These include primary vaginal carcinoma (Soma et al 1982) and recurrent vaginal carcinoma (Ward et al 1982).

Locally accessible head and neck cancers can be highly responsive to photodynamic therapy with either porfimer or HPD. Complete response rates of 30% have been maintained for up to 1 year following treatment of localized, accessible lesions with HPD (Wile et al 1982, 1984). Palliative responses are also obtained in a number of patients. Light therapy is given 2 to 3 days after HPD or DHE is administered. Other tumors responsive to photodynamic therapy include glioblastoma (McCulloch et al 1984) and other malignant brain tumors (Laws et al 1981) and, finally, intraocular tumors such as malignant melanoma and retinoblastoma (Murphree et al 1983, Bruce 1984).

■ Mechanism of Action

Hematoporphyrin derivatives act as a photosensitizer in tissues exposed to penetrating light at wavelengths greater than 600 nm. In tissues, the wavelength maximum for optimal light absorption by

HPD is 630 nm, compared with 620 nm for HPD in aqueous solution (Dougherty 1986). Light delivered by a laser acts to direct the activation process to a specific site. The cytotoxic photodynamic reaction requires oxygen which undergoes oxidation to a variety of toxic free radical species (Foote 1984).

The hematoporphyrin-based molecules absorb light energy and are thereby converted to an excited electronic state. They rapidly convert back to their ground state by yielding a hydrogen or electron (type I reaction) or by directly transferring the energy to a ground-state oxygen molecule yielding a singlet oxygen radical (Type II reaction) (Foote 1984). The singlet oxygen and other resultant oxygen free radicals (including superoxide) are very short-lived and react proximally with cell membranes, nucleic acids, proteins, and enzymes. Oxidation of these important cellular constituents leads to cell death. Membrane blebs become evident and red blood cells extravasate into the affected area (Bugelski et al 1981). These histologic reactions have all been shown to involve singlet oxygen (Weishaupt et al 1976).

Recent evidence also suggests that cytokines may be expressed locally following photodynamic therapy and that, in bladder cancer, at least part of the cytotoxic effect is mediated immunologically (Nseyo et al 1990b). This was noted by high urinary levels of interleukin-1, interleukin-2, and tumor necrosis factor α following photodynamic therapy. Of interest, a similar mechanism is believed to operate with intravesical bacillus Calmette–Guérin therapy of bladder cancer.

In tumor tissues, the vascular stroma (macrophages, mast cells, and fibroblasts) are initially most affected by photodynamic therapy. Binding of porfimer to low-density lipoproteins and to the vascular endothelium of tumor cells is an important component of cytotoxicity with photodynamic therapy. This may act to localize drug within the tumor vasculature, and some studies suggest preferential retention of hematoporphyrins in malignant tissues compared with comparable normal tissues.

Hyperthermia is synergistic with photodynamic therapy, possibly by blocking the repair of sublethal damage (Waldow and Dougherty 1984).

■ Availability and Storage

Porfimer sodium is investigationally available from QLT Phototherapeutics of Canada, and Lederle Laboratories, Wayne, New Jersey. It has also been available for studies through the National Cancer Institute. The drug is supplied in glass vials containing 75 mg of sterile freeze-dried powder. No other excipients or preservatives are present in this formulation. The unreconstituted vials are stored in the dark, under refrigeration (2–8°C).

■ Preparation for Use, Stability, and Admixture

Porfimer is reconstituted by the addition of 30 mL of 5% Dextrose for Injection, USP, to each 75-mg vial. This yields a solution containing 2.5 mg/mL. Sodium chloride solutions should not be used for porfimer reconstitution. The reconstituted drug is chemically stable out of light for 24 hours at room temperature; however, because of the lack of a preservative, use within 4 hours of reconstitution is recommended.

■ Administration

Porfimer sodium is administered intravenously over a 3- to 5-minute period as a slow intravenous push. Care should be taken to avoid extravasation as the drug may cause local tissue reactions, especially if the tissues may be exposed to light. Doses of porfimer are typically infused 2 to 3 days prior to laser therapy to allow for adequate distribution and uptake of the photosensitizer into tissues.

■ Dosage

The usual dose of porfimer ranges from 1.5 to 3 mg/kg as an intravenous bolus injection. The most common dose is 2 mg/kg given 48 hours prior to localized light therapy of the tumor.

■ Special Precautions

Patients must be advised to avoid exposure to direct sunlight or heat (ie, hair dryers) for 30 days after porfimer injection. Precautions should also be taken to avoid extravasation as the drug may produce severe local tissue toxicity in sun-exposed areas.

■ Pharmacokinetics

By the use of fluorescence detection, the serum half-life of HPD and porfimer has been estimated at 10 hours (Potter and Mang 1984). In animals, tissue distribution of radiolabeled HPD is generally complete 24 hours after injection (Evensen et al 1984). Several HPD components are found in tissues including polymeric forms, some with covalent linkage (Evensen et al 1984).

In mice, the hematoporphyrin components tend to concentrate in the liver, kidney, and spleen over tumor. Tissues with concentrations lower than those in tumor include skin, heart, muscle, and brain (Evensen et al 1984). In the kidney, HPD components concentrate in the proximal convoluted tubules. Uptake into kidney cells appears to be mediated partially via pinocytosis (Evensen et al 1984). The liver also takes up a large amount of drug (Gomer and Dougherty 1979), possibly via pinocytosis and phagocytosis and by a specific carrier linked to hemopexin (Müller-Eberhard and Morgan 1975). Experimentally, the porphyrins also have a high affinity for embryonic and regenerating tissues (Figge et al 1948) and for growing bone (Barker et al 1970).

In the bloodstream, porphyrins are bound to albumin and hemopexin (Müller-Eberhard and Morgan 1975). The drug molecules are known to be phagocytosed by reticuloendothelial system cells and achieve high concentrations in lysosomes (Swartzendruber et al 1971).

■ Side Effects and Toxicity

The primary side effect of porfimer is excessive skin photosensitization, which may last 4 to 6 weeks following injection. Severe sunburn has resulted in some individuals and patients must be advised to avoid direct sunlight. This includes protection of the eyes from direct sun rays and remaining indoors, away from strong fluorescent or incandescent lighting such as a medical or dental examining lamp. The use of sunscreens should be recommended but is not a proven alternative for strict sunlight avoidance. Patients treated with porfimer should also avoid cone or helmet-type hair dryers, as heat is known to produce a synergistic photodynamic effect with hematoporphyrin derivatives. There may also be synergistic or additive skin toxicity with radiation therapy.

Patients receiving intravesical photodynamic therapy may develop severe bladder irritation after light application. This is noted by dysuria, suprapubic abdominal discomfort, urinary frequency, and nocturia. Unlike other intravesical therapies, bladder contraction (reduction in bladder capacity) appears to be less prominent with photodynamic therapy. Bleeding and sloughing of necrotic tissue may rarely occur.

Superficial tumor sites typically ulcerate and then scabs form. Mild erythema is usually present in normal tissue adjacent to the treated area. Occasionally, these may break down and slowly heal. Allergic reactions to HPD are described and have been effectively treated with diphenhydramine (Dougherty et al 1979). Temperature elevations are rarely reported with HPD therapy. Porfimer does not alter hematologic indices. Liver and renal enzymes are similarly unaffected (Dougherty et al 1978). No other long-term complications are reported.

REFERENCES

Balchum OJ, Doiron DR, Huth GC. Photoradiation therapy of endobronchial lung cancers employing the photodynamic action of hematoporphyrin derivative. *Lasers Surg Med.* 1984;**4**:13–30.

Barker DS, Henderson RW, Storey E. The in vivo localization of porphyrins. *Br J Exp Pathol.* 1970;**51**:628–638.

Benson RC Jr, Kinsey JH, Cortese DA, et al. Treatment of transitional cell carcinoma of the bladder with hematoporphyrin derivative phototherapy. *J Urol.* 1983;**130**:1090–1095.

Bruce RA. An approach to the treatment of ocular malignant melanomas. In: Doiron DR, Gomer CJ, eds. *Porphyrin Localization and Treatment of Tumors.* New York: Alan R. Liss; 1984:777–784.

Bugelski PJ, Porter CW, Dougherty TJ. Autoradiographic distribution of hematoporphyrin derivative in normal and tumor tissue of the mouse. *Cancer Res.* 1981;**41**:4606–4612.

Cortese DA, Kinsey JH. Hematoporphyrin derivative phototherapy in the treatment of bronchogenic carcinoma. *Chest.* 1984;**86**:8–13.

Dougherty TJ. Photosensitization of malignant tumors. *Semin Surg Oncol.* 1986;**2**:24–37.

Dougherty TJ, Kaufman JE, Goldfarb A, et al. Photoradiation therapy for the treatment of malignant tumors. *Cancer Res.* 1978;**38**:2628–2635.

Dougherty TJ, Lawrence G, Kaufman JH, et al. Photoradiation in the treatment of recurrent breast carcinoma. *J Natl Cancer Inst.* 1979;**62**:231–237.

Dougherty TJ, Potter WR, Weishaupt KR. The structure of the active component of hematoporphyrin derivative. In: Doiron DR, Gomer CJ, eds. *Porphyrin Localization and Treatment of Tumors.* New York: Alan R. Liss; 1984:301–314.

Dugan M, Crawford Ed, Nseyo UO, et al. A randomized trial of photodynamic therapy (PDT) after transurethral resection (TURBT) for superficial bladder papillary bladder cancer (SBC): A randomized trial. *Proc Am Soc Clin Oncol.* 1991;**10**:173.

Evensen JF, Moan J, Hindar A, et al. Tissue distribution of

³H-hematoporphyrin derivative and its main components, ⁶⁷Ga and ¹³¹I-albumin, in mice bearing Lewis lung carcinoma. In: Doiron DR, Gomer CJ, eds. *Porphyrin Localization and Treatment of Tumors.* New York: Alan R. Liss; 1984:541–562.

Figge FHJ, Weiland GS, Manganiello LOJ. Cancer detection and therapy. Affinity of neoplastic embryonic and traumatized regenerating tissues for porphyrins and metalloporphyrins. *Proc Soc Exp Biol Med.* 1948;**68**:640–641.

Foote C. Mechanisms of photooxygenation. In: Doiron DR, Gomer CJ, eds. *Porphyrin Localization and Treatment of Tumors.* New York: Alan R. Liss; 1984:3–18.

Gomer CJ, Dougherty TJ. Determination of [³H]- and [¹⁴C]hematoporphyrin derivative distribution in malignant and normal tissue. *Cancer Res.* 1979;**39**:146–151.

Hayata Y, Kato H, Konaka C, et al. Photoradiation therapy with hematoporphyrin derivative in early and stage 1 lung cancer. *Chest.* 1984;**86**:169–177.

Hisazumi H, Misaki T, Miyoshi N. Photoradiation therapy of bladder tumors. *J Urol.* 1983;**130**:685–687.

Hisazumi H, Myoshi N, Naito K, et al. Whole bladder wall photoradiation therapy for carcinoma in situ of the bladder: A preliminary report. *J Urol.* 1984;**131**:884–887.

Laws ER Jr, Cortese DA, Kinsey JH, et al. Photoradiation therapy in the treatment of malignant brain tumors. A phase I (feasibility) study. *Neurosurgery.* 1981;**9**:672–678.

McCaughan JS Jr, Hicks W, Laufman L, et al. Palliation of esophageal malignancy with photoradiation therapy. *Cancer.* 1984;**54**:2905–2910.

McCulloch GAJ, Forbes IJ, Lee KS, et al. Phototherapy in malignant brain tumors. In: Doiron DR, Gomer CJ, eds. *Porphyrin Localization and Treatment of Tumors.* New York: Alan R. Liss; 1984:709–717.

Müller-Eberhard U, Morgan WT. Porphyrin-binding proteins in serum. *Ann NY Acad Sci.* 1975;**244**:624–650.

Murphree AL, Doiron DR, Gomer CJ, et al. Hematoporphyrin derivative photoradiation treatment of ophthalmic tumors. Presented at The Clayton Foundation Symposium on Porphyrin Localization and Treatment of Tumors, Santa Barbara, CA, April 24–28, 1983 (abstract).

Nseyo UO, et al. Photodynamic therapy in the prophylactic management of bladder cancer. Abstract presentation, Western Section AUA, Monterey, CA, September 30–October 4, 1990a.

Nseyo UO, Whalen RK, Duncan MR, et al. Urinary cytokines following photodynamic therapy for bladder cancer: A preliminary report. *Urology.* 1990b;**36**:167–171.

Potter WR, Mang TS. Photofrin II levels by in vivo fluorescence photometry. In: Doiron DR, Gomer CJ, eds. *Porphyrin Localization and Treatment of Tumors.* New York: Alan R. Liss; 1984:177–186.

Prout GR Jr, Lin C-W, Benson R Jr, et al. Photodynamic therapy with hematoporphyrin derivative in the treatment of superficial transitional-cell carcinoma of the bladder. *N Engl J Med.* 1987;**317**:1251–1255.

Shumaker B, Lutz MD, Haas G, et al. Diagnosis and treatment of carcinoma-in-situ of the urinary bladder with hematoporphyrin derivative and laser phototherapy. *Lasers Med Surg.* 1985;**5**:194.

Soma H, Akiya K, Nutahara S, et al. Treatment of vaginal carcinoma with laser photoirradiation following administration of haematoporphyrin derivative. Report of a case. *Ann Chir Gynaecol.* 1982;**71**:133–136.

Swartzendruber DC, Nelson B, Hayes RL. Gallium-67 localization in lysosomal-like granules of leukemic and nonleukemic marine tissue. *J Natl Cancer Inst.* 1971;**46**:941–952.

Waldow SM, Dougherty TJ. Interaction of hyperthermia and photoradiation therapy. *Radiat Res.* 1984;**97**:380–385.

Ward BG, Forbes IJ, Cowled PA, et al. The treatment of vaginal recurrences of gynecologic malignancy with phototherapy following hematoporphyrin derivative pretreatment. *Am J Obstet Gynecol.* 1982;**142**:356–357.

Weishaupt KR, Gomer CJ, Dougherty TJ. Identification of singlet oxygen as the cytotoxic agent in photo-inactivation of a murine tumor. *Cancer Res.* 1976;**36**:2326–2329.

Wile AG, Dahlman A, Burns RG. Laser photoradiation therapy of cancer following hematoporphyrin sensitization. *Lasers Surg Med.* 1982;**2**:163–168.

Wile AG, Movotny J, Mason GR, et al. Photoradiation therapy for head and neck cancer. In: Doiron DR, Gomer CJ, eds. *Porphyrin Localization and Treatment of Tumors.* New York: Alan R. Liss; 1984:681–691.

Prednimustine

■ Other Names

Leo 1031; EORTC 1502; INN; NSC-134087, Stereocyt®.

■ Chemistry

Structure of prednimustine

Prednimustine is an ester conjugate of chlorambucil and prednisolone. The molecular weight is about 665. It was originally synthesized in 1969 at the AB

Leo Research Laboratories in Sweden (Konyves and Kristensson 1971). The complete chemical name is 11β,17,21-trihydroxypregna-1,4-diene-3,20-dione 21-{4-[p-[bis(2-chloroethyl)amino]phenyl]butyrate}. Prednimustine is thus a steroidal alkylating agent with the mustard moiety conjugation at the C-21 position of the steroidal nucleus.

■ Antitumor Activity

Prednimustine has shown experimental antitumor results superior to those of chlorambucil in Walker-256 carcinosarcoma (increased ED_{50} and LD_{50}), carcinogen (DMBA)-induced mammary carcinoma, and L-1210 leukemia (23 times more active on leukemic versus normal bone marrow stem cells) (Konyves et al 1975, Evenaar et al 1973).

In clinical trials the compound has demonstrated activity in chronic lymphocytic leukemia (CLL) (Aungst et al 1974, Brandt et al 1975) and in lymphocytic lymphoma (Moller et al 1975). In CLL and well-differentiated lymphocytic lymphoma, an intermittent high-dose schedule was more active than a continuous low-dose regimen (Idestrom et al 1982). Although one pilot study suggested activity in acute leukemia (Brandt and Konyves 1979), a follow-up trial could not detect any significant activity in acute nonlymphocytic leukemia or in refractory anemia with excess blasts (Gandara et al 1982). More recently Brandt and Konyves (1979) reported a few remissions induced by prednimustine as a single agent or with vincristine in adult acute leukemia. Interestingly, this report confirmed the relative lack of significant toxicity for normal bone marrow cells, first suggested by Evenaar et al (1973). Mattsson et al (1978) have recently confirmed the efficacy of the drug in the treatment of various non-Hodgkin's lymphomas.

An older study detected activity for prednimustine in advanced, metastatic breast carcinoma (Freckman et al 1964). This was more recently confirmed by Konyves et al (1975). In a randomized breast cancer trial of prednimustine on an intermittent or continuous dosing regimen, either regimen produced a 21% response rate. This was superior to the response rate of 11% obtained with a combination of prednisolone and chlorambucil (Lober et al 1983). Combinations of prednimustine with methotrexate, tamoxifen, and 5-fluorouracil (Boesen and Mouridsen 1982) or of prednimustine with mitoxantrone and 5-fluorouracil (Samonigg et al 1991) are active as first- and second-line therapy for patients with advanced breast cancer. Response rates were 75 and 45% in the two trials, respectively.

In a phase II study, Johnsson et al (1979) additionally reported a 38% response rate for prednimustine in advanced ovarian carcinoma. An identical 35% response rate was reported for prednimustine combined with hexamethylmelamine, 5-fluorouracil, and cisplatin, compared with a 28% response rate for prednimustine alone (Leonard et al 1989). Advanced (stage D) prostatic carcinoma is also responsive to prednimustine (Mittelman et al 1977, Catane et al 1978). The objective response rate was 24% in this trial (Mittelman et al 1977).

Clinical studies have corroborated a similar spectrum of both action and toxicity for prednimustine and more typical alkylating agents; however, several investigators have clinically noted a relative lack of cross-resistance to classic alkylating agents. As would be expected, prednimustine also possesses some corticosteroid (prednisolone-like) activity. This implies that slow tapering of the dose or the use of replacement corticosteroid may be necessary on discontinuance of therapy.

■ Mechanism of Action

The cytotoxic mechanism of action for prednimustine involves alkylation of DNA, probably in a fashion similar to that seen with the component alkylating agent chlorambucil. This process, mediated through the bischloroethyl side chain, ultimately involves the transfer of alkyl groups to and subsequent crosslinking of DNA.

Despite the qualitative similarity to chlorambucil and prednisolone, prednimustine's biologic effects are quantitatively different than those produced by an equimolar mixture of the parent conjugates. Suggested explanations for the observed differences include different lipid solubility characteristics and altered uptake patterns across biologic membranes favoring prednimustine. Nonetheless, it is still unclear why animal studies consistently demonstrate a higher therapeutic ratio for prednimustine. Equally unclear is whether these differences are also present in humans.

■ Availability and Storage

Prednimustine is available from the AB Leo Company Inc, Helsingborg, Sweden. It is supplied as 8- and 20-mg tablets. These may be stored at room temperature and are stable for several years from manufacture.

Administration

Prednimustine tablets are administered orally. Daily doses are generally divided into three to four portions.

Dosage

In various non-Hodgkin's lymphomas, Mattsson et al (1978) used a median induction dose of 25 mg/m^2/d) (range, 11–42 mg/m^2/d). These doses were administered on a continuous daily basis until disease progression or severe toxicity ensued. In contrast, Moller et al (1975) occasionally used doses up to 80 mg/d, with 40 mg being the most common dose. Both regimens were continued until relapse occurred, typically after several months to over 1 year. In CLL, Brandt et al (1975) recommended initial daily therapy with 8 to 16 mg/d continuously to reduce white blood counts to the desired range, and then 6 to 8 mg/d as maintenance therapy. In CLL a continuous low-dose regimen, 20 mg orally twice daily, was equivalent to an intermittent high-dose regimen of 100 mg orally twice daily for 3 consecutive days, repeated every 2 weeks (Idestrom et al 1982).

In advanced ovarian carcinoma 3- to 28-day induction regimens were successfully employed by Johnnsson et al (1979). When combined with hexamethylmelamine, 5-fluorouracil, and cisplatin, prednimustine was used at a dose of 15 mg/m^2 orally on days 2 and 15. Dosing was repeated monthly (Leonard et al 1989). The doses in this study were 50 mg/m^2/d divided into four fractions. In other solid tumor studies continuous daily dosing regimens were used for various doses. For example, the dose in breast carcinoma varied from 2 to 100 mg/d (Konyves et al 1975) and from 40 mg/m^2/d continuously to 160 mg/m^2/d × 5, repeated every 3 weeks (Lober et al 1983). In combination with methotrexate, 5-fluorouracil, and tamoxifen, tolerable prednimustine doses were 100 mg/m^2/d, repeated at 4-week intervals (Boesen and Mouridsen 1982). A similar schedule of 110 mg/m^2/d × 5 was reported for prednimustine combined with mitoxantrone and 5-fluorouracil in advanced breast cancer (Samonigg et al 1991).

Pharmacokinetics

In animal studies, a significant portion of the orally ingested drug is excreted unchanged in the feces. In four, fairly healthy study patients, a range of 1 to 35% of a dose was recovered unchanged in the feces (Konyves et al 1975); however in two severely ill study patients, each with hepatic metastases, fecal excretion of unchanged drug amounted to 47 to 55% of the dose. Another trial reported no detection of prednimustine, chlorambucil, or phenylacetic mustard in the plasma of six patients given a single 20-mg oral dose (Newell et al 1983). When a higher 100-mg oral dose was administered to patients with breast cancer, prednisolone levels and AUC values are about half those from a comparable dose of prednisolone (Sayed et al 1981). Maximum prednisolone levels following prednimustine ranged from 17 to 35 µg/dL in this study. This suggests that prednimustine is about 50% bioavailable, but whether hyrolysis to prednisolone occurs in vivo is not known. Another trial with radiolabeled drug demonstrated 40 to 60% label recovery in the urine by 72 hours. No intact prednimustine was measured in the plasma. Prednimustine metabolites had an apparent plasma half-life of 8 hours. The half-life for total radioactivity in the plasma was 10 days (Gaver et al 1983). Similar results were reported using a more specific high-performance liquid chromatography assay: no intact free prednimustine was measured in the plasma; however, the bioavailability of the chlorambucil and phenylacetic acid mustard fragments were 25 and 40%, respectively, of those obtained from the same dose of oral chlorambucil (Oppitz et al 1989). These studies suggest that following oral administration, prednimustine undergoes rapid and extensive presystemic degradation to its component drug moieties. Part of this hydrolysis is mediated by plasma esterases (Hartley-Asp et al 1986).

Side Effects and Toxicity

The most frequent side effect of prednimustine is myelosuppression. It is characterized by dose-dependent leukopenia and thrombocytopenia. Following drug discontinuation, the blood counts generally recover over a relatively long period of 3 to 6 weeks. Konyves et al (1975) noted that occasionally blood counts may continue to fall for 2 to 3 weeks after drug discontinuance. The myelosuppression from prednimustine is almost always reversible. All side effects appear to be greater with continuous daily oral dosing schemes rather than with acute high-dose intermittent regimens (Idestrom et al 1982).

Nausea and vomiting appear to be transient and mild with prednimustine. In addition, mucositis has not been encountered with the drug. Moller et al (1975), however, have described a mild cyclical diarrheal syndrome with prednimustine.

Steroidal side effects with prednimustine have consisted primarily of mild edema and an increase in plasma glucose (Gandara et al 1987); however, a few patients in these studies have developed diabetes, gastritis, hypertension, and myocardial infarction (in a previously hypertensive patient). In addition, a number of patients have reported psychologic changes such as confusion and euphoria as well as marked decreases in a general sense of well-being (Konyves et al 1975).

Alopecia appears to be both infrequent and mild with prednimustine. Other uncommon reactions have included a slight fever, urticaria, and rashes. Infiltrations of the drug have not produced significant local toxicity.

REFERENCES

Aungst CW, Mittelman A, Murphy GP. Treatment of chronic lymphocytic leukemia and lymphosarcoma with a new chlorambucil ester of prednisone (sic) (Leo-1031). *J Surg Oncol.* 1974;7:457–461.

Boesen E, Mouridsen HT. Prednimustine in combination with methotrexate and 5-FU (PMF): A pilot study. *Cancer Treat Rep.* 1982;66:281–283.

Brandt L, Konyves I. Prednimustine (Stereocyt®) in adult acute myeloid leukemia (abstract C-130). *Proc Am Assoc Cancer Res ASCO.* 1979;20:322.

Brandt L, Konyves I, Moller TR. Therapeutic effect of Leo 1031, an alkylating corticosteroid ester, in lymphoproliferative disorders. I. Chronic lymphocytic leukemia. *Acta Med Scand.* 1975;197:317–322.

Catane R, Kaufman I, Mittelman A, et al. Prednimustine therapy of advanced prostatic cancer. *Br J Urol.* 1978;50:29–32.

Evenaar AH, Wins EHR, van Putten LM. Cell killing effectiveness of an alkylating steroid (Leo 1031). *Eur J Cancer.* 1973;9:773–778.

Freckman HA, Fry HL, Mendez FL, Maurer ER. Chlorambucil–prednisolone therapy for disseminated breast carcinoma. *JAMA.* 1964;189:111–118.

Gandara DR, George CB, Ries CA, et al. Treatment of refractory chronic lymphocytic leukemia with prednimustine: A phase II study using strict response criteria. *Cancer Chemother Pharmacol.* 1987;19:165–168.

Gandara DR, Ries CA, Schiff SA, et al. A phase II study of prednimustine in acute non-lymphocytic leukemia, smouldering leukemia, and refractory anemia with excess blasts. *Cancer Chemother Pharmacol.* 1982;9:10–12.

Gaver RC, Deeb G, Pittman KA, et al. Disposition of orally administered ^{14}C-prednimustine in cancer patients. *Cancer Chemother Pharmacol.* 1983;11:139–143.

Hartley-Asp B, Gunnarsson PO, Liljekvist J. Cytotoxicity and metabolism of prednimustine, chlorambucil and prednisolone in a Chinese hamster cell line. *Cancer Chemother Pharmacol.* 1986;16:85–90.

Idestrom K, Kimby E, Bjorkholm M, et al. Treatment of chronic lymphocytic leukaemia and well-differentiated lymphocytic lymphoma with continuous low- or intermittent high-dose prednimustine versus chlorambucil/prednisolone. *Eur J Cancer Clin Oncol.* 1982;18:1117–1123.

Johnsson JE, Trope C, Mattson W, et al. Phase II study of LEO 1031 (prednimustine) in advanced ovarian carcinoma. *Cancer Treat Rep.* 1979;63:421–424.

Konyves I, Kristensson S. Novel corticosteroid esters with alkylating properties. Communication at XIV Scandinavian Congress of Chemistry. *Umea Proc.* 1971:187.

Konyves I, Nordenskjold B, Forshell GP, et al. Preliminary clinical and absorption studies with prednimustine in patients with mammary carcinoma. *Eur J Cancer.* 1975;11:841–844.

Leonard RCF, Smart GE, Livingstone JRB, et al. Randomised trial comparing prednimustine with combination chemotherapy in advanced ovarian carcinoma. *Cancer Chemother Pharmacol.* 1989;23:105–110.

Lober J, Mouridsen HT, Christiansen IE, et al. A phase III trial comparing prednimustine (LEO 1031) to chlorambucil plus prednisolone in advanced breast cancer. *Cancer.* 1983;52:1570–1576.

Mattsson W, von Eyben F, Turesson I, Wahlby S. Prednimustine (NSC-134807, Leo 1031) treatment of lymphocytic and lymphocytic–histiocytic lymphomas. *Cancer.* 1978;41:112–115.

Mittelman A, Catane R, Murphy GP. New steroidal alkylating agents in advanced stage D carcinoma of the prostate. *Cancer Treat Rep.* 1977;61:307–310.

Moller TR, Brandt L, Konyves I, Lindberg G. Therapeutic effect of Leo 1031, an alkylating corticosteroid ester, in lymphoproliferative disorders. *Acta Med Scand.* 1975;197:323–327.

Newell DR, Calvert AH, Harrap KR. Studies on the pharmacokinetics of chlorambucil and prednimustine in man. *Br J Clin Pharmacol.* 1983;15:253–258.

Oppitz M, Musch E, Malek M, et al. Studies on the pharmacokinetics of chlorambucil and prednimustine in patients using a new high-performance liquid chromatographic assay. *Cancer Chemother Pharmacol.* 1989;23:208–212.

Samonigg H, Stoger H, Kasparek A-K, et al. Prednimustine combined with mitoxantrone and 5-fluorouracil for first and second-line chemotherapy in advanced breast cancer. *Cancer Chemother Pharmacol.* 1991;27:477–480.

Sayed A, Van Hove W, Vermeulen A. Prednisolone plasma levels after oral administration of prednimustine. *Oncology.* 1981;38:351–355.

Procarbazine

Other Names

Matulane® (Roche Laboratories); ibenzmethyzin; NSC-77213.

Chemistry

Structure of procarbazine

Chemically, procarbazine is N-methylhydrazine or ibenzymethyl hydrazine; the complete chemical name is N-isopropyl-α-(2-methylhydrazino)-p-toluamide hydrochloride. The drug is water soluble and slightly soluble in alcohol. It is unstable in water or aqueous solutions as a result of autoxidation to a large number of products including hydrogen peroxide. It has a molecular weight of 257.6. At room temperature it exists as a pale white to yellow crystalline substance.

Antitumor Activity

Procarbazine is mainly used in combination with other drugs in the treatment of lymphomas (Stolinsky et al 1970) and has little activity in solid tumors except brain cancer (Martz et al 1963, Samuels et al 1967). Major activity is observed in Hodgkin's disease (Mathe et al 1963, Brunner and Young 1965, Deconti 1971) especially in the combination regimen MOPP, wherein procarbazine is combined cyclically with mechlorethamine, vincristine, and prednisone (DeVita et al 1970). Other responsive malignancies include non-Hodgkin's lymphomas (Livingston and Carter 1970), malignant melanoma (Luce 1972, Carmo-Pereira et al 1984), multiple myeloma (Moon and Edmonson 1970), bronchogenic carcinomas (Samuels et al 1969), and brain tumor (Kumar et al 1974, Gutin et al 1975). The drug appears to lack activity in acute leukemia (Humphrey et al 1973).

Procarbazine has been used to treat polycythemia vera (Martin and Schubert 1966) and lupus erythematosus or graft-versus-host disease (Sullivan et al 1981).

Mechanism of Action

Procarbazine is a prodrug that forms numerous reactive intermediates following microsomal metabolism. There is evidence that several metabolites have cytotoxic activity and overall metabolic/activation pathways are complex (Averbuch 1990). Berneis et al (1963) originally described in vitro depolymerization of DNA by procarbazine-produced hydrogen peroxide. This end product was thought to result from the autoxidation of procarbazine spontaneously in solution; however, Weinkam and Shiba (1978) recently described three pathways of metabolic activation of the drug. They were able to show that following autoxidation to the azo derivative azoprocarbazine, metabolic hydroxylation to at least two cytotoxic azoxy isomers also occurred. This metabolism can be mediated by chemical decomposition and/or via microsomal enzymes. Further chemical reactions ultimately produce highly reactive free radicals including hydrogen peroxide, formaldehyde, and hydroxide radicals.

Another end product is the methyldiazonium ion $CH_3N^+\equiv N$ capable of monofunctional alkylation of DNA. A methyl or N-isopropylbenzamide free radical may also be capable of covalent binding to DNA (Moloney et al 1985). These unstable end products possibly contribute to the cytotoxic activity of the compound. Prough and Tweedie (1979) have recently confirmed the major role of the microsomal P450 enzyme fraction in this metabolic oxidation and subsequent activation of procarbazine.

Chromosomal breakage is observed after procarbazine (Therman 1972). This activity could relate to several products of oxidative breakdown of the parent compound. Macromolecular synthesis of DNA, RNA, and protein is also inhibited by procarbazine (Gale et al 1967, Sartorelli and Tsunamura 1966). These effects are delayed in onset by 12 to 24 hours for RNA and protein inhibition. In contrast, DNA synthesis occurs within several hours and, if not lethal to the cell, is repaired by 8 to 24 hours (Gutterman et al 1969). Procarbazine also inhibits the normal methylation of transfer RNA (Revel and Littauer 1966).

Ultimate interactions with DNA produce alterations characteristic of ionizing radiation and the classic bifunctional alkylating agents (Reed 1971). In experimental animal tumor models, however, procarbazine does not demonstrate cross-resistance with alkylating agents. Kreis (1971) has alternatively proposed that procarbazine causes abnormal selective transmethylation of the N-7 guanine on transfer RNA. This type of lesion could thus inhibit proper RNA synthesis, thereby inhibiting DNA synthesis.

Cytologic studies have shown that the drug suppresses mitosis by prolonging interphase. Thus, procarbazine appears to be somewhat cell cycle phase specific, with marked cytotoxic activity in S and G_2 phases (Rutishauser and Bollag 1963). As with many other neoplastic agents, procarbazine has known mutagenic and carcinogenic potential (Kelly et al 1964, Chaube and Murphy 1969, Zbinden and Maier 1983).

■ Availability and Storage

Procarbazine is commercially available as the hydrochloride salt in 50-mg ivory- to yellow-colored capsules. Crystalline procarbazine was also previously available investigationally as a sterile solution for injection.

Every precaution should be taken to avoid contact of the drug with any moisture before administration because the drug can decompose if exposed to atmospheric oxygen and moisture. The stated expiration dates should be observed; however, the encapsulated form is generally stable at room temperature for at least 2 years.

Bruce and Boehlert (1978) have recently reported on the stability characteristics of procarbazine capsules. The primary procarbazine degradation products observed were N-(1-methylethyl)-4-{[(2-methylamino)hydrazo]methyl}benzamide and N-(1-methylethyl)-4-{[(2-methylazo)methyl}benzamide. In this study the typical concentration range for these and two other minor degradation products found in procarbazine capsules was 0.1 to 0.5% after 4.5 years of storage. Thus, the oral form of the drug as supplied by the manufacturer appears to be quite stable.

■ Preparation for Use, Stability, and Admixture

Chabner et al (1973) have reported on high-dose infusions of procarbazine wherein doses were diluted immediately before use. In this study intravenous procarbazine doses were reconstituted into 25 to 50 mL of D5W. Sterile Water for Injection, USP, and normal saline may also be used. Inasmuch as autoxidation of drug in solution can occur rapidly, all doses for parenteral administration should be prepared immediately before use. In aqueous solution, procarbazine decomposes rapidly in a metal-catalyzed oxidation to azoprocarbazine with the liberation of hydrogen peroxide (Prough and Tweedie 1987, Weinkam and Shiba 1978).

In ultraviolet light, procarbazine solutions slowly isomerize to the inactive hydrazone, N-isopropyl-p-formylbenzamide methylhydrazone. This subsequently hydrolyzes to produce methylhydrazine and N-isopropyl-p-formylbenzamide. Any remainder should also be carefully discarded to avoid unnecessary human exposure to this known carcinogen. Because of stability problems, use of the investigational injection is not being pursued further.

■ Administration

Before oral or parenteral administration it is advisable to ascertain whether any contraindicated drugs are concurrently being taken by the patient. Ethanol, sympathomimetic drugs (ephedrine, isoproterenol, epinephrine, etc), tricyclic antidepressants (imipramine, amitriptyline, etc), heavy intake foods tyramine-containing foods (dark beer, cheese, bananas, etc), and possibly barbiturates should be avoided during therapy with this drug.

In the intravenous procarbazine study by Chabner et al (1973) all doses were diluted in 50 to 100 mL of D5W and slowly infused over a 10- to 15-minute period.

■ Dosage

In the MOPP combination for Hodgkin's disease, the procarbazine dose is 100 mg/m^2/d orally for 14 days (DeVita et al 1970).

The dosage range for procarbazine as a single agent is continuous daily doses of 50 to 200 mg/d given for 10 to 20 days (usually 2 weeks). For convenience, each dose should be calculated to the nearest 50 mg. Some reports recommend that initial daily doses be low (50–100 mg) and sequentially increased each day. This may minimize nausea and vomiting, seen frequently at the beginning of therapy. The total daily dose may be given at a single time or in divided fractions throughout the day. The latter regimen may cause less acute toxicity. Continuous low-dose regimens of 50 to 100 mg/d are reported but are not recommended because of a substantially increased risk of drug-induced carcinogenesis with long-term exposure. With compromised renal status, a blood urea nitrogen above 40 mg/100 mL and/or a serum creatinine above 2.0 mg/100 mL, or depressed hepatic function (total bilirubin > 3.0 mg/100 mL), doses should be substantially reduced.

For intravenous regimens, Chabner et al (1973) used intermittent infusions of high doses of procarbazine. The safe dosage range in this program was 300 to 1000 mg/m^2. Doses larger than 1 g/m^2 were associated with very severe gastrointestinal and central nervous system toxicity.

■ Special Precautions

See Drug Interactions.

■ Drug Interactions

Concurrent use of the following drugs and foods is not recommended and might result in the consequences noted in the table.

The proposed explanation for some of these interactions involves inhibition of monoamine oxidase (MAO), an enzyme that acts to degrade neurotransmitters and other sympathomimetic agents. Inhibition of MAO by procarbazine (DeVita et al 1965) tends to augment or amplify the effects of exogenous doses of sympathomimetic drugs as well as endogenous amines such as tyramine, a sympathomimetic amino acid contained in certain foods. Also, because the tricyclic antidepressants such as amitriptyline act to release stored natural sympathetic amines from neurons, the same net effect of augmentation (synergism) may be seen with concurrent procarbazine.

Procarbazine is reported by the manufacturer to have a degree of disulfiram (Antabuse®)-like activity and therefore concurrent alcohol ingestion could induce severe gastrointestinal toxicity. The manufacturer also reports possible synergism (increased central nervous system depression) with barbiturates, antihistamines, narcotics, hypotensive agents, and phenothiazines. Concurrent dosing should be done cautiously.

Although there is a definite theoretical concern with these interactions, for most, neither animal studies nor clinical cases have been reported to confirm or disprove their clinical significance. Exceptions are the potentiation of barbiturate-induced narcosis by procarbazine, which was elegantly studied in mice (Lee and Lucier 1975), and the scattered anecdotal reports of alcohol intolerance in patients receiving procarbazine.

Shiba and Weinkam (1983) have demonstrated another potentially significant drug interaction in mice that could increase the metabolic activation of procarbazine. In their study, pretreatment of mice with phenobarbital or phenytoin significantly increased the in vivo cytotoxic activity of procarbazine. Their study further demonstrated greater cytotoxic activity for the azoxy metabolites of the drug and suggested that microsomal enzyme induction was the mechanism of interaction. The pretreatment with methylprednisolone in this study produced no alterations in procarbazine metabolism or in cytotoxicity.

INTERACTIONS OF PROCARBAZINE WITH CERTAIN DRUGS AND FOODS

Drug	Possible Result of Interaction
Ethanol Mixed drinks, beer, cough/cold preparations, etc	Severe gastrointestinal toxicity, nausea, vomiting, visual disturbances, headache
Sympathomimetics Ephedrine, epinephrine, isoproterenol	

Antidepressants
  Tricyclics—imipramine, amitriptyline, etc
  Monoamine oxidase inhibitors—pargylline
	Hypertensive crisis, tremor, excitation, cardiac palpitations, angina (clinically important reactions are not common)

Tyramine-rich foods Dark beer, cheese, wine, bananas, etc	

Central nervous system depressants
  Narcotic analgesics—morphine meperidine, etc
  Antihistamines—diphenhydramine, etc
  Phenothiazines—chlorpromazine, etc
  Hypotensives—methyldopa, clonidine, etc
  Barbiturates—hexobarbital
	Additive central nervous system depression (respiratory depression)

Data from Warren and Bender 1977.

Pharmacokinetics

After oral administration, the drug appears to be rapidly and completely absorbed from the gastrointestinal tract and quickly equilibrates between the blood and the central nervous system (Schwartz et al 1967). Peak cerebrospinal fluid levels occur 30 to 90 minutes after either oral or parenteral administration. Procarbazine appears to be rapidly metabolized in humans, with a 7- to 10-minute half-life of intact drug after parenteral administration of radiolabeled procarbazine. Isotopically labeled procarbazine was found to distribute highly into liver, kidney, intestine, and skin (Schwartz et al 1967). There is some suggestion that chronic dosing may increase the concentrations of azoprocarbazine by either metabolic induction or delayed clearance (Shiba and Weinkam 1982). After 24 hours up to 70% of a dose is recovered in the urine (Oliverio et al 1964). The major fraction present is N-isopropyl-terephthalmic acid although more than 5% of the urine fraction exists as unchanged drug.

Overall, both liver biotransformation and renal excretion play significant roles in drug and metabolite clearance.

Side Effects and Toxicity

Hematologic effects include protracted myelosuppression, principally thrombocytopenia. The nadir of thrombocytopenia is usually about 4 weeks; white and red blood cells may decrease after platelets and typically resolve in about 4 to 6 weeks. The effect on erythrocytes may involve oxidative hemolysis by the drug (Sponzo et al 1974). Of note, myelosuppression is conspicuously absent when procarbazine is administered intravenously as a single large bolus or as five daily injections (Chabner et al 1973). Oral procarbazine can also cause hemolysis in patients with glucose-6-phosphate dehydrogenase deficiency.

Dose-related pancytopenia is thus the most common dose-limiting toxic effect. Gastrointestinal complaints include nausea, vomiting, and diarrhea; however, tolerance to the continued administration of procarbazine usually develops in a few days. Rarer gastrointestinal toxic effects include anorexia and protracted diarrhea which, if present, may indicate the need for reduced doses or cessation of therapy. Stomatitis is usually not a problem.

A flulike syndrome of fever, chills, sweating, lethargy, and myalgias and arthralgias may occur with procarbazine. Fortunately, it is generally limited to initial therapy.

Dermatologic reactions are rare but have also been described. These include alopecia, pruritis, and allergic drug rash (in about 3% of patients). The rash may be prevented with future doses if small doses (eg, 20 mg) of prednisone are also given. Glovsky et al (1976) have reported a recurrent but manageable hypersensitivity reaction to procarbazine which was associated with angioedema, urticaria, and a precipitous drop in serum complement.

Central nervous system toxicity may result from the distribution of procarbazine and its active metabolites into the cerebrospinal fluid. A wide variety of symptoms have been attributed to procarbazine, including paresthesias, neuropathies, dizziness, ataxia, and headache (Weiss et al 1974). These reactions probably relate to inhibition of monoamine oxidase enzymes in the central nervous system (DeVita et al 1965) or to the depletion of pyridoxal phosphate stores (Chabner et al 1969). Particularly distressing to the patient are frequent nightmares, depression, insomnia, nervousness, and hallucinations, which occur in up to 30% of patients and may be dose limiting for some. Counseling about these effects should be given before treatment. Tremors, coma, and convulsions are less common but require immediate cessation of therapy.

With a high-dose, intermittent procarbazine infusion regimen, Chabner et al (1973) in fact found various central nervous system toxic effects to be dose limiting over relatively mild hematologic suppression. Mann and Hutchison (1967) have reported a single severe manic reaction related to procarbazine use in a Hodgkin's disease patient.

Ophthalmic toxic effects have been rarely noted and include nystagmus, diplopia, papilledema, photophobia, and retinal hemorrhages.

Other toxic effects include a rare pulmonary condition, which is probably allergic in nature (Jones et al 1972). Lokich and Maloney (1972) reported apparently hypersensitivity-based procarbazine reactions in two additional patients: one with pneumonitis and one with allergic dermatitis. Immunosuppressive actions such as reduced antibody formation may predispose patients to infections (Liske 1973).

Azoospermia and the cessation of menses are almost universally produced with high-dose procarbazine (Sherins and DeVita 1965). In the majority of patients these effects do significantly improve once the drug is discontinued. Experimentally, the administration of antioxidants prevents spermatotoxicity without compromising anticancer effects (Horstman et al 1987).

In rodents, procarbazine significantly reduces plasma pyridoxal phosphate (Chabner et al 1969). In humans, however, exogenous pyridoxine supplementation has not been beneficial in ameliorating any procarbazine toxicity.

As with many other antineoplastic drugs, procarbazine has demonstrated potent teratogenic and carcinogenic potential in experimental animals (Carter 1971, Chaube and Murphy 1969, Kelley et al 1964, Zbinden and Maier 1983). Nonlymphocytic leukemias and adenocarcinomas appear to predominate in exposed animals. There is also a strong potential for teratogenic effects in humans. Nonetheless, there are at least three case reports of normal infants delivered of procarbazine-treated patients (Dun 1970, Gautier and Teste 1969, Wells et al 1968).

REFERENCES

Averbuch SD. Nonclassic alkylating agents. In: Chabner B, Collins J, eds. *Cancer Chemotherapy: Principles and Practice*. Philadelphia, PA: JB Lippincott; 1990:314–322.

Berneis K, Kofler M, Bollag W, et al. The degradation of deoxyriboneucleic acid by new tumor inhibiting compounds: The intermediate formation of hydrogen peroxide. *Experientia (Basel)*. 1963;**19**:132–133.

Bruce GL, Boehlert JP. Separation and quantitation of possible degradation products of procarbazine hydrochloride in its dosage form. *J Pharm Sci*. 1978;**67**(3):424–426.

Brunner KW, Young CW. A methylhydrazine derivative in Hodgkin's disease and other malignant neoplasms: Therapeutic and toxic effects studied in 51 patients. *Ann Intern Med*. 1965;**63**:69–86.

Carmo-Pereira J, Costa FO, Henriques E. Combination cytotoxic chemotherapy with procarbazine, vincristine, and lomustine in disseminated malignant melanoma: 8 years follow-up. *Cancer Treat Rep*. 1984;**68**:1211–1214.

Carter SK, ed. *Proceedings of the Chemotherapy Conference on Procarbazine (Matulane: NSC-77213): Development and Application*. Washington, DC: U.S. Government Printing Office; 1971.

Chabner BA, DeVita VJ, Considine N, et al. Plasma pyridoxal phosphate depletion by the carcinostatic procarbazine. *Proc Soc Exp Biol Med*. 1969;**132**:1119–1122.

Chabner BA, Sponzi R, Hubbard S, et al. High-dose intermittent intravenous infusion of procarbazine (NSC-77213). *Cancer Chemother Rep*. 1973;**57**:361–363.

Chaube S, Murphy ML. Fetal malformation produced in rats by N-isopropyl-α-(2-methylhydrazine)-p-toluamide hydrochloride (procarbazine). *Teratology*. 1969;**2**:23–32.

DeConti RC. Procarbazine in the management of Hodgkin's disease. *JAMA*. 1971;**215**:927–930.

DeVita VT, Hahn MA, Oliverio VT. Monoamine oxidase inhibition by a new carcinostatic agent, N-isopropyl-α-(2-methylhydrazino)-p-toluamide (MIH). *Proc Soc Exp Biol Med*. 1965;**120**:561–565.

DeVita VT, Serpick AA, Carbone PP. Combination chemotherapy in the treatment of advanced Hodgkin's disease. *Ann Intern Med*. 1970;**73**:881–895.

Dun EG. Procarbazine in pregnancy. *Lancet*. 1970;**2**:984.

Gale GR, Simpson JG, Smith AB. Studies of the mode of action of N-isopropyl-alpha-(2-methylhydrazino)-p-toluamide. *Cancer Res*. 1967;**27**:1186–1191.

Gautier J, Teste M. Apropos de deux cas de grossesse survenant au cours d'une maladie de Hodgkin. *Rev Med Tours*. 1969;**3**:759–766.

Glovsky MM, Braunwald J, Opele G, Alenty A. Hypersensitivity to procarbazine associated with angioedema, urticaria, and low serum complement activity. *J Allergy Clin Immunol*. 1976;**57**(2):134–140.

Gutin PH, Wilson CB, Kumar AR, et al. Phase II study of procarbazine, CCNU, and vincristine combination chemotherapy in the treatment of brain tumors. *Cancer*. 1975;**35**:1398–1404.

Gutterman J, Huang AT, Hochstein P. Studies on the mode of action of N-isopropyl-alpha-(2-methylhydrazine)-p-toluamide. *Proc Soc Exp Biol Med*. 1969;**130**:797–802.

Horstman MG, Meadows GG, Yost GS. Separate mechanisms for procarbazine spermatotoxicity and anticancer activity. *Cancer Res*. 1987;**47**:1547–1550.

Humphrey GB, Komp D, Morgan S. An evaluation of procarbazine (NSC-77213) in the treatment of acute leukemia (letter). *Cancer Chemother Rep*. 1973;**57**(4):371.

Jones SE, Moore M, Blank N, et al. Hypersensitivity to procarbazine (Matulane®) manifested by fever and pleuropulmonary reaction. *Cancer*. 1972;**29**:498–500.

Kelly MG, O'Gara GW, Gadehar K, et al. Carcinogenic activity of a new antitumor agent, N-isopropyl-δ-(2-methylhydrazino)-p-toluamide, hydrochoride (NSC-77213). *Cancer Chemother Rep*. 1964;**39**:77–80.

Kreis W. Mechanism of action of procarbazine. (see Carter [1971], pp 35–44.)

Kumar ARV, Renaudin J, Wilson CB, et al. Procarbazine hydrochloride in the treatment of brain tumors. *J Neurosurg*. 1974;**40**:365–371.

Lee IP, Lucier GW. The potentiation of barbiturate-induced narcosis by procarbazine. *J Pharmacol Exp Ther*. 1975;**196**(3):586–593.

Liske R. A comparative study of the action of cyclophosphamide and procarbazine on the antibody production in mice. *Clin Exp Immunol*. 1973;**15**:271–280.

Livingston RB, Carter SK. *Single Agents in Cancer Chemotherapy*. New York: IFI/Plenum Data Corp; 1970:318–336.

Lokich JJ, Maloney WC. Allergic reaction to procarbazine. *Clin Pharmacol Ther*. 1972;**13**:573–574.

Luce JK. Chemotherapy of malignant melanoma. *Cancer*. 1972;**30**:1604–1615.

Mann AM, Hutchison JL. Manic reaction associated with procarbazine hydrochloride therapy of Hodgkin's disease. *Can Med Assoc J*. 1967;**97**:1350–1353.

Martin H, Schubert JCF. Diezytostatische Behardlung der Polycythaema vera mit einem Methylbenzylhydrazi. *Derivat Dtsch Med Wochensehr*. 1966;**91**:55–57.

Martz G, D'Allessandri A, Keel HJ, et al. Preliminary clinical results with a new anti-tumor agent Ro4–6467 (NSC- 77213). *Cancer Chemother Rep*. 1963;**33**:5–14.

Mathe G, Schweisguth O, Schneider M, et al. Methyl hydrazine in the treatment of Hodgkin's disease. *Lancet*. 1963;**2**:1077–1080.

Moloney SJ, Wiebkin P, Cummings SW, et al. Metabolic activation of the terminal N-methyl group of N- isopropyl-alpha-(2-methylhydrazino)-p-toluamide hydrochloride (procarbazine). *Carcinogenesis*. 1985;**6**:397–401.

Moon JH, Edmonson JH. Procarbazine (NSC-77213) and multiple myeloma. *Cancer Chemother Rep*. 1970;**54**:245–248.

Oliverio VT, Denham C, Devita VT, Kelly MG. Some pharmacologic properties of a new antitumor agent N- isopropyl-δ-(2-methylhydrazino)-p-toluamide, hydrochloride (NSC-77213). *Cancer Chemother Rep*. 1964;**42**:1–7.

Prough RA, Tweedie DJ. Procarbazine. In: Powis G, Prough RA, eds. *Metabolism and Action of Anti-cancer Drugs*. London: Taylor & Francis; 1987:29–47.

Reed D. Metabolism and mechanism of action of procarbazine. (See Carter [1971], pp 45–56.)

Revel M, Littauer U. The coding properties of methyl deficient phenylalanine transfer RNA from *Escherichia coli*. *J Mol Biol*. 1966;**15**:389–394.

Rutishauser A, Bollag W. Cytological investigations with a new class of cytotoxic agent: Methylhydrazine derivatives. *Experientia*. 1963;**19**:131–132.

Samuels ML, Leary WV, Alexanian R, et al. Clinical trials with N-isopropyl-(2-methylhydrazino)-p-toluamide hydrochloride in malignant lymphoma and other disseminated neoplasia. *Cancer*. 1967;**20**:1187–1194.

Samuels M, Leary W, Howe C. Procarbazine (NSC-77213) in the treatment of advanced bronchogenic carcinoma. *Cancer Chemother Rep*. 1969;**53**:135–145.

Sartorelli AC, Tsunamura S. Studies on the biochemical mode of action of a cytotoxic methylhydrazine derivative, N-isopropyl-alpha-(2-methylhydrazino)-p-toluamide. *Mol Pharmacol*. 1966;**2**:275–283.

Schwartz DE, Bollag W, Obrecht P. Distribution and excretion studies of procarbazine in animals and man. *Arzneim Forsch*. 1967;**17**:1389–1393.

Sherins RJ, DeVita VT. Effect of drug treatment for lymphoma on male reproductive capacity. Studies of men in remission after therapy. *Ann Intern Med*. 1965;**63**:69–86.

Shiba DA, Weinkam RJ. Quantitative analysis of procarbazine, procarbazine metabolites and chemical degradation products with application to pharmacokinetic studies. *J Chromatogr*. 1982;**229**:397–407.

Shiba DA, Weinkam RJ. The in vivo cytotoxic activity of procarbazine and procarbazine metabolites against L1210 ascites leukemia cells in CDF_1 mice and the effects of pretreatment with procarbazine, phenobarbital, diphenylhydantoin, and methylprednisolone upon in vivo procarbazine activity. *Cancer Chemother Pharmacol*. 1983;**11**:124–129.

Sponzo RW, Arseneau J, Canellos GP. Procarbazine-induced oxidative haemolysis: Relationship to in vivo red cell survival. *Br J Hematol*. 1974;**27**:587–595.

Stolinsky DC, Solomon J, Pugh RP, et al. Procarbazine HCl in Hodgkin's disease, reticulum cell sarcoma, and lymphosarcoma. *Cancer*. 1970;**26**:984–990.

Sullivan KM, Shulman HM, Storb R, et al: Chronic graft-versus-host disease in 52 patients: Adverse natural course and successful treatment with combination immunosuppression. *Blood*. 1981;**57**:267–276.

Therman E. Chromosome breakage by 1-methyl-2-benzylhydrazine in mouse cancer cells. *Cancer Res*. 1972;**32**:1133–1136.

Warren RD, Bender RA. Drug interactions with antineoplastic agents. *Cancer Treat Rep*. 1977;**61**(7):1231–1241.

Weinkam RJ, Shiba DA. Metabolic activation of procarbazine. *Life Sci*. 1978;**22**(11):937–946.

Weiss HD, Walker MD, Wiernik PH. Neurotoxicity of commonly used antineoplastic agents. *N Engl J Med*. 1974;**291**:127–133.

Wells JH, Marshall JR, Carbone PP. Procarbazine therapy for Hodgkin's disease in early pregnancy. *JAMA*. 1968;**205**(13):119–121.

Zbinden G, Maier P. Single dose carcinogenicity of procarbazine in rats. *Cancer Lett*. 1983;**21**:155–161.

Progestins

■ Other Names

Megestrol acetate—Megace® (Bristol-Myers Oncology Division); Provera; medroxyprogestrone acetate—Provera® (The Upjohn Company); hydroxyprogesterone caproate—Prodrox (Legere) 250®.

■ Chemistry

Structure of megestrol acetate

Structure of medroxyprogesterone acetate

Structure of hydroxyprogesterone caproate

The progestins are steroidal compounds related structurally to the natural hormone progesterone.

■ Antitumor Activity

An excellent review of megestrol acetate has been published by Schacter et al (1989). Progestins are useful in advanced, well-differentiated renal cell, endometrial, and breast carcinomas. Approximately one third of patients with recurrent or advanced adenocarcinoma of the endometrium will respond to progestational therapy (Kelley and Baker 1960, Kennedy 1968, Sherman 1969, Reifenstein 1971, Waterman and Benson 1967). Kneale and Evans (1969) further defined that response to progestins was poor in poorly differentiated tumors.

As breast cancers also contain progestin receptors (Horwitz and McGuire 1975), it is not surprising that occasional advanced breast carcinomas will sometimes respond to progestational therapy (Stoll 1969, Muggia et al 1968, Bonomi et al 1988, Carpenter 1988). Megestrol acetate and medroxyprogesterone acetate have been compared in a randomized trial in patients with advanced breast cancer (given as second hormonal treatment after tamoxifen) (Willemse et al 1990). The investigators noted that medroxyprogesterone acetate was more effective in the treatment of bone metastasis but had more progestational agent-related side effects.

In another important trial Lundgren et al (1989) compared megestrol acetate and aminoglutethimide. Response rates to the two agents were similar and there was no difference in survival; however, side effects were more frequent in the aminoglutethimide-treated group. A similar study by Canney et al (1988) reported similar findings.

DeLena et al (1979) have shown that high-dose medroxyprogesterone acetate (1000–1500 mg/d IM) can produce objective remissions in about a third of postmenopausal women with resistant breast cancer. These results are not superior to those obtained with conventional oral doses.

Another definitive study was conducted by Muss et al (1988) and the Piedmont Oncology Group. Patients were randomized to receive either megestrol acetate or tamoxifen. Response rates were the same; however, time to progression and overall survival were better for the tamoxifen-treated group. Furthermore, it should be recalled that after withdrawal of progestational agents, breast cancer can shrink as a result of a withdrawal response (Nowakowski et al 1986).

Rarely, hypernephromas will also respond to progestins with clearing of distant metastatic foci (Bloom and Wallace 1964, Kelley and Baker 1970, Kjaer 1988); however, objective response rates to progestins are usually less than 15% in patients with renal cell carcinoma. In a randomized study by Steineck et al (1990) no difference was found in response or survival of patients receiving medroxyprogesterone versus interferon alfa-2a.

The progestational agents have been explored in a number of other tumor types. Only 3 of 29 patients with hormonal-refractory prostate cancer responded to megestrol acetate (Patel et al 1990); none of 22 did so in another series (Daniel et al 1990). Bonomi et al (1985) reported responses in 11 of 33 patients treated with megestrol acetate. Of interest are recent data indicating that megestrol acetate + diethylstilbestrol at 0.1 mg/d was superior to diethylstilbestrol alone because of fewer side effects (Venner et al 1988).

Megestrol acetate has been proposed as a treatment for meningiomas because of the finding of progesterone receptors in the tumor. Unfortunately, no response has been reported in a trial of megestrol acetate in nine patients with meningiomas (Grunberg and Weiss 1990). On the basis of a pilot study, Creagan et al (1989) have suggested that megestrol acetate be used as adjuvant treatment for malignant melanoma. That pilot study requires confirmation.

Sikic et al (1986) documented a small (8%) but definite activity for high-dose (800 mg/d, taper to 400 mg/d) megestrol acetate in patients with advanced ovarian cancer. This has also been noted by Geisler (1985). Other groups (Greenwald et al 1989, Veenhof et al 1987, Belinson et al 1987) have not demonstrated antitumor activity. Pulmonary lymphangiomyomatosis also responds to the drug (Hughes and Hodder 1987).

■ Role in Cancer Cachexia

Aisner et al (1988) suggested that megestrol acetate could be used to treat cancer-associated cachexia. The table below summarizes the reported randomized trials. As can be seen in that table, megestrol acetate at doses of 480 to 1600 mg/d can improve appetite and quality of life and produce real weight (muscle mass) gain. In addition, megestrol acetate has been used for treatment of cachexia in patients with human immunodeficiency virus infection (Furth 1989, Von Roenn et al 1988).

■ Mechanism of Action

The exact biochemical mechanism of progestin antitumor activity is not well known. Progestins typically have mild glucocorticoid activity and significant antiestrogenic effects. Some of the antiestrogenic effects are mediated by enhanced metabolism of estrogen to inactive forms following progestin therapy. Progestins induce the enzyme 17-hydroxysteroid dehydrogenase, which oxidizes estradiol to the less potent form, estrone. Progestins also activate estrogen sulfotransferase, which catalyzes sulfation of estrogens to less active conjugates (Murad and Kuret 1990). Experimental models of antitumor effects for progestins show that specific cell cytosol acceptor proteins (receptors) are required for the antitumor effects. In such breast cancer cells, progestins have demonstrated direct growth- inhibitory effects in vitro (Allegra and Kiefer 1985). Progestins suppress gonadotropin secretion, and estrogen levels also fall in a dose-dependent fashion following medroxyprogesterone acetate use in breast cancer patients (Blossey et al 1984). Recent evidence indicates that progestational agents can decrease the levels of estrone sulfate and estradiol (Lundgren et al 1990). This of course could be a mechanism for the observed antitumor activity of these agents in patients with breast cancer (Lundgren et al 1990). Progestins decrease the density of estrogen receptors, which could thereby de-

CONTROLLED STUDIES OF MEGESTROL ACETATE FOR NUTRITIONAL SUPPORT

Study	Dose (mg/d)	Conclusion	Toxic Effect
Bruera et al 1990	480	Increased appetite Increased weight Increased muscle mass Increased well-being	Edema, nausea
Loprinzi et al 1990	800	Increased appetitie Increased weight Decreased nausea + emesis	Mild edema
Tchekmedyian et al 1990	1600	Increased appetitie Increased prealbumin Increased quality of life	Hypoglycemia Dyspnea Deep-vein thrombosis

prive a hormonally dependent tumor of its estrogenic stimulation. Insulin receptors are decreased following progestins. Overall, these effects lead to a cytostatic type of inhibition which requires continuous drug exposure for the growth-suppressive effect. The progestins probably act locally on hormonally sensitive cells, which constitute only a small proportion of commonly presenting, potentially sensitive neoplasms. Progestins normally promote the differentiation and maintenance of endometrial tissue. All three synthetic derivatives used in cancer therapy also have very slight catabolic activities. The growth-inhibitory effects of progestins are not cell cycle phase specific but may be maximal in the G_1 phase of dividing cells.

■ Availability and Storage

The table below details the preparations available.

■ Preparation for Use, Stability, and Admixture

Hydroxyprogesterone caproate may crystallize on storage at low temperatures. It may be redissolved by heating in boiling water. Otherwise, the manufacturer's recommendations for the agents should be followed.

■ Administration/Special Precautions

The manufacturer's recommendations should be followed. The injectable forms should be used with caution in patients sensitive to the carriers (sesame or castor oil [hydroxyprogesterone] polyethylene glycol [medroxyprogesterone]). Injectables are intended for intramuscular use only.

■ Drug Interactions

The slight degree of weight gain induced by megestrol acetate has not been shown to significantly change the volume of distribution of any other drug. To date, no other drug interactions have been described for megestrol acetate when used in cancer patients; however, medroxyprogesterone acetate is reported to potentially alter the mixed-function oxidase system of the liver (Camaggi et al 1985, Hedly et al 1985, Rautio et al 1979, Sotaniemi et al 1978). Therefore, the effects of megestrol acetate were compared with those of medroxyprogesterone acetate in breast cancer patients given antipyrine, digitoxin, and warfarin as marker drugs for hepatic metabolism (Lundgren et al 1986). This study reported no significant differences in the clearance of antipyrine and digitoxin; however, the clearance of warfarin decreased by 35% when megestrol acetate was simultaneously administered. The clinical significance of this decrease in warfarin clearance was not established. Megestrol also increased the half-life of warfarin by 71% (Lundgren et al 1986). These results differ from those of prior studies with medroxyprogesterone acetate wherein antipyrine clearance was depressed (Rautio et al 1979). Overall, the results suggest that megestrol acetate does not significantly alter hepatic metabolism of other drugs, in contrast to high-dose medroxyprogesterone acetate.

PROGESTINS AVAILABLE

Drug	Preparations Available	Dose	Comment
Medroxyprogesterone acetate Provera® (PO) Provera® (IM) (The Upjohn Company, Kalamazoo, Michigan)	Tablets: 2.5, 10 mg Injection: 100 mg/mL and 400-mg aqueous (depot) suspension	400–800 mg IM or PO twice weekly	Use with caution in patients with liver disease (all agents)
Hydroxyprogesterone caproate—Prodrox (Legere) 250®		2–5 g IM weekly to remission, then 1 g IM weekly maintenance	Some patients may be sensitive to the oil carrier
Megestrol acetate—Megace® (Bristol-Myers Oncology Division, Princeton, New Jersey)	Tablets 40 mg 160 mg (investigational)*	40 mg PO daily up to 40 mg PO qid (320mg/d maximum)	Few reported side effects

*See Gaver et al 1986.

Dosage

The usual dose ranges are reported in the last table. The standard dose of megestrol acetate in breast cancer and endometrial cancer is 40 mg orally four times a day. Administration of the total 160-mg daily dose at one time appears to be comparable to administration of the four daily fractions in terms of efficacy and side effects (Carpenter and Peterson 1985). Doses of megestrol acetate have varied considerably in patients with renal cell carcinoma. Daily doses with roughly equipotent antitumor activity in this disease range from 60 mg/d (Paine et al 1970), to 50 mg/m^2/d (Hahn et al 1979), to 640 mg/d (Paladine et al 1979). In advanced breast cancer, high-dose megestrol (800 mg/d) produced superior response rates and survival compared with standard doses (Muss et al 1990). Other considerations include the need for initially high doses to achieve control and the use of lower "maintenance" dosing on a regular basis as long as remission continues. Treatment must be continued for at least 2 to 3 months before assuming therapeutic failure. Doses should be reduced in the presence of liver failure.

For possible doses used for treatment of cancer-associated cachexia refer to the table on page 816. This, however, is still an area of active investigation and the precise dose recommendations for this use have not yet been determined.

Pharmacokinetics

Natural progestins are rapidly inactivated. Natural progesterone is highly protein bound (>95%) and has a blood half-life of less than 20 minutes. Like glucocorticosteroids, progestins are carried in the bloodstream bound to transcortin, also called corticosteroid-binding globulin. A large percentage of a dose is stored in fat. After oral dosing, about 70% is extracted by the liver in the first pass. Most of a dose is excreted as various conjugates. The synthetic compounds are similarly handled; therefore, slow-release (intramuscular depot) formulations are often employed. They are metabolized in the liver and excreted partially in the urine. Megestrol appears to have the shortest duration of classic progesterone activity (1 to 3 days), followed by hydroxyprogesterone at 8 to 14 days, and finally medroxyprogesterone (oral, 16 days, intramuscular depot, 4 to 6 weeks). Medroxyprogesterone acetate (Provera®) and megestrol acetate (Megace®) have the advantage of good oral bioavailability.

The half-lives of medroxyprogesterone in the plasma are 1.4 hours (α) and 59 hours (β-phase) (Pannuti et al 1982); however, there is a wide range of steady-state drug concentrations achieved after a standard dose. Following a dose of 1000 mg/m^2/d the median steady-state plasma concentration was 51 ng/mL with a very wide range of 10 to 269 ng/mL (Etienne et al 1992). And, breast cancer patients who developed medroxyprogesterone side effects (45/229) tended to have higher median plasma levels (81 ng/mL) compared with nontoxic patients (32 ng/mL). Furthermore, responding patients in this trial also had significantly higher median steady-state levels of 65 ng/mL compared with median levels of 46 ng/mL in nonresponding patients. In contrast, hepatic dysfunction did not significantly alter median plasma levels of medroxyprogesterone (Etienne et al 1992).

Sensitive methods to detect megestrol acetate have recently become available (Dikkeschei et al 1990). There are large interpatient differences in serum concentrations in patients receiving oral megestrol acetate (Dikkeschei et al 1990). In normal volunteers given oral doses of 20, 40, 80, or 200 mg, peak plasma levels (2–3 hours after drug administration) were 89, 190, 209, and 465 ng/mL. The serum half-life appeared to be biphasic with a terminal half life of 15 to 20 hours (Canetta et al 1983). A mean plasma half-life of 33 to 38 hours was reported by Gaver et al (1986). Metabolites identified in the urine included conjugated and unconjugated 20-hydroxy and 6-hydroxy species, whereas biliary metabolites were exclusively conjugated (Canetta et al 1983).

Relative to the 40-mg commercial tablets (Megace®), the 160-mg investigational tablets had 97% or greater bioavailability. The time to peak plasma level was 2.5 to 2.8 hours (Gaver et al 1986). Mean peak plasma levels following a single 160-mg oral dose were 89 ng/mL for the regular formulation and 134 ng/mL for a micronized formulation. The AUCs following these doses were 1980 and 2474 ng/mL · h, respectively. With four daily oral doses of 40 mg each (160 mg total) the time to a peak plasma level of 107 ng/mL averaged 14.5 hours. The AUC for this schedule was 2249 ng/mL · (Gaver et al 1986). With high-dose megestrol acetate therapy, mean serum levels are approximately 600 and 400 ng/mL for oral daily doses of 800 and 400 mg, respectively (Sikic et al 1986).

Side Effects and Toxicity

Progestins are extremely well-tolerated antitumor agents in the usual large doses. Occasionally, there can be acute local hypersensitivity with transient dyspneic reactions to the oil carriers in the intramuscular preparations. Some of this may be caused by an oil embolism if any part of the dose is inadvertently given intravenously. With high-dose intramuscular therapy, gluteal abscess can occur (DeLena et al 1979). The other acute serious complication is hypercalcemia, which may be noted in breast cancer patients with bony metastases during the first 2 weeks of therapy.

Mild fluid retention and body weight gain are commonly encountered but are usually not clinically significant. A Cushing's syndrome induced by daily medroxyprogesterone acetate (400 mg/d) is also described (Siminoski et al 1989).

Occasionally, some degree of alopecia can occur. Liver function abnormalities may also be encountered, and the dose should probably be reduced in patients with hepatic disease.

If progestins are combined with estrogens, nausea, vomiting, cramps, backache, and vaginal bleeding may occur. Megestrol appears to have a lower incidence of reported adverse effects than other hormonal agents (eg, androgens, estrogens). Jaundice and intrahepatic cholestasis have been reported following high-dose megestrol acetate (Foitl et al 1989).

Birth defects have occasionally been reported in offspring of mothers exposed to medroxyprogesterone acetate during pregnancy; however, large epidemiologic studies have not been able to confirm that the agent caused congenital abnormalities in offspring of women who received the agent (Yovich et al 1988).

Special Applications

As noted earlier, megestrol acetate has been used as an appetite stimulant. (Please refer to Role in Cancer Cachexia.) Megestrol acetate has also been used for the treatment of endometriosis with some success (Schlaff et al 1990).

Progestins have been shown to experimentally modulate drug resistance in tumor cells that express the P-glycoprotein (Fleming et al 1992). In L-1210 mouse leukemia cells, progesterone reverses multidrug resistance induced by mitomycin-C (Dorr and Liddil 1991). This follows reports that the gene regulating multidrug resistance is expressed at high levels in the secretory epithelium of gravid mouse uterus (Arceci et al 1988). Progesterone is a substrate for P-glycoprotein and can displace vinblastine binding in membrane vesicles from multidrug-resistant murine macrophages (Huang-Yang et al 1988); however, progesterone was not able to sensitize multidrug-resistant human acute leukemic myeloblasts to daunorubicin in vitro (Ross et al 1992). Thus, the clinical significance of progesterone modulation of the multidrug resistance phenomenon is not established.

REFERENCES

Aisner J, Tchekmedyian NS, Tait N, et al. Studies of high-dose megestrol acetate: Potential applications in cachexia. *Semin Oncol.* 1988;**15**(2, suppl 1):68–75.

Allegra JC, Kiefer SM. Mechanisms of action of progestational agents. *Semin Oncol.* 1985;**12**(suppl 2):3–5.

Arceci RJ, Croop JM, Horwitz SB, et al. The gene encoding multidrug resistance is induced and expressed at high levels during pregnancy in the secretory epithelium of the uterus. *Proc Natl Acad Sci USA.* 1988;**85**:4350–4354.

Belinson JL, McClure M, Badger G. Randomized trial of megestrol acetate vs. megestrol acetate/tamoxifen for the management of progressive or recurrent epithelial ovarian carcinoma. *Gynecol Oncol.* 1987;**28**(2):151–155.

Bloom HJ, Wallace DM. Hormones and the kidney. *Br Med J.* 1964;**2**(5407):476–480.

Blossey HC, Wander HE, Koebberling J, et al. Pharmacokinetic and pharmacodynamic basis for the treatment of metastatic breast cancer with high-dose medroxyprogesterone acetate. *Cancer.* 1984;**54**:1208–1215.

Bonomi P, Gale M, Von Roenn J, et al. Quantitative estrogen and progesterone receptor levels related to progression-free interval in advanced breast cancer patients treated with megestrol acetate or tamoxifen. *Semin Oncol.* 1988;**15**(2, suppl 2):26–33.

Bonomi P, Pessis D, Bunting N, et al. Megestrol acetate used as primary hormonal therapy in stage D prostatic cancer. *Semin Oncol.* 1985;**12**(1, suppl 1):36–39.

Bruera E, Macmillan K, Kuehn N, et al. A controlled trial of megestrol acetate on appetite, caloric intake, nutritional status, and other symptoms in patients with advanced cancer. *Cancer.* 1990;**66**(6):1279–1282.

Camaggi CM, Strocchi E, Canova N, et al. Medroxyprogesterone acetate (MAP) and tamoxifen (TMX) plasma levels after simultaneous treatment with low TMX and high MAP doses. *Cancer Chemother Pharmacol.* 1985;**14**:229–231.

Canetta R, Florentine S, Hunter H, et al. Megestrol acetate. *Cancer Treat Rev.* 1983;**10**:141–157.

Canney PA, Priestman TJ, Griffiths T, et al. Randomized

trial comparing aminoglutethimide with high-dose medroxyprogesterone acetate in therapy for advanced breast carcinoma. *J Natl Cancer Inst.* 1988;**80**(14):1147–1151.

Carpenter JT Jr. Progestational agents in the treatment of breast cancer. *Cancer Treat Res.* 1988;**39**:147–156.

Carpenter JT Jr, Peterson L. Use of megestrol acetate in advanced breast cancer on a single-daily-dose schedule. *Semin Oncol.* 1985;**12**(1):40–42.

Creagan ET, Ingle JN, Schutt AJ, et al. A prospective, randomized controlled trial of megestrol acetate among high-risk patients with resected malignant melanoma. *Am J Clin Oncol.* 1989;**23**(2):152–155.

Daniel F, MacLeod PM, Tyrrell CJ. Megestrol acetate in relapsed carcinoma of prostate. *Br J Urol.* 1990;**65**(3):275–277.

DeLena M, Brambilla C, Valagussa P, et al. High-dose medroxyprogesterone acetate in breast cancer resistant to endocrine and cytotoxic therapy. *Cancer Chemother Pharmacol.* 1979;**2**:175–180.

Dikkeschei LD, Wolthers BG, de Ruyter-Buitenhuis AW, et al. Determination of megestrol acetate and cyproterone acetate in serum of patients with advanced breast cancer by high-performance liquid chromatography. *J Chromatogr.* 1990;**529**:145–154.

Dorr RT, Liddil JD. Modulation of mitomycin C-induced multidrug resistance in vitro. *Cancer Chemother Pharmacol.* 1991;**27**:290–294.

Etienne MC, Milano G, Frenay M, et al. Pharmacokinetics and pharmacodynamics of medroxyprogesterone acetate in advanced breast cancer patients. *J Clin Oncol.* 1992;**10**:1176–1182.

Fleming GF, Amato JM, Agresti M, et al. Megestrol acetate reverses multidrug resistance and interacts with P-glycoprotein. *Cancer Chemother Pharmacol.* 1992;**29**:445–449.

Foitl DR, Hyman G, Lefkowitch JH. Jaundice and intrahepatic cholestasis following high-dose megestrol acetate for breast cancer. *Cancer.* 1989;**63**(3):438–439.

Furth PA. Megestrol acetate and cachexia associated with human immunodeficiency virus (HIV) infection (letter). *Ann Intern Med.* 1989;**10**(8):667–668.

Gaver RC, Pittman KA, Reilly CM, et al. Evaluation of two new megestrol acetate tablet formulations in humans. *Biopharm Drug Dispos.* 1986;**7**(1):35–46.

Geisler HE. The use of high-dose megestrol acetate in the treatment of ovarian adenocarcinoma. *Semin Oncol.* 1985;**12**(1, suppl 1):20–22.

Greenwald ES, Taylor CD, Vogl S. Study of high dose megestrol acetate (MA) for previously treated patients with ovarian cancer (meeting abstract). *Proc Ann Meet Am Soc Clin Oncol.* 1989;**8**:A154.

Grunberg SM, Weiss MH. Lack of efficacy of megestrol acetate in the treatment of unresectable meningioma. *J Neurooncol.* 1990;**8**(1):61–65.

Hahn RG, Bauer M, Wolter J, et al. Phase II study of single agent therapy with megestrol acetate, VP-16-213, cyclophosphamide and dianhydrogalactitol in advanced renal cell cancer. *Cancer Treat Rep.* 1979;**63**:513–515.

Hedly DW, Christie M, Weatherby RP, et al. Lack of correlations between plasma concentration of medroxyprogesterone acetate, hypothalamic–pituitary function and tumour response in patients with advanced breast cancer. *Cancer Chemother Pharmacol.* 1985;**14**:112–115.

Horwitz KB, McGuire WL. Specific progesterone receptors in human breast cancer. *Steroids.* 1975;**25**:497–505.

Huang-Yang C-P, DePinho SG, Greenberger LM, et al. Progesterone interacts with P-glycoprotein in multidrug-resistant cells and in the endometrium of gravid uterus. *J Biol Chem.* 1989;**264**(2):782–788.

Hughes E, Hodder RV. Pulmonary lymphangiomyomatosis complicating pregnancy. A case report. *J Reprod Med.* 1987;**32**(7):553–557.

Kelley RM, Baker WH. Clinical observations on the effect of progesterone in the treatment of metastatic endometrial carcinoma. In: Pincus G, Vollmer E, eds. *Biological Activities of Steroids in Relation to Cancer.* New York: Academic Press; 1960:447–455.

Kelley RM, Baker WH. Progestational agents in the treatment of carcinoma of the genitourinary tract. In: Sturgis S, Taymore M, eds. *Progress in Gynecology.* New York: Grune & Stratton; 1970:362–375.

Kennedy BJ. Progestogens in the treatment of carcinoma of the endometrium. *Surg Gynecol Obstet.* 1968;**127**:103–114.

Kjaer M. The role of medroxyprogesterone acetate (MAP) in the treatment of renal adenocarcinoma. *Cancer Treat Rev.* 1988;**15**(3):195–209.

Kneale B, Evans J. Progestogen therapy for advanced carcinoma of the endometrium. *Med J Aust.* 1969;**2**:1101–1104.

Loprinzi CL, Ellison NM, Schaid DJ, et al. Controlled trial of megestrol acetate for the treatment of cancer anorexia and cachexia. *J Natl Cancer Inst.* 1990;**82**(13):1127–1132.

Lundgren S, Gundersen S, Klepp R, et al. Megestrol acetate versus aminoglutethimide for metastatic breast cancer. *Breast Cancer Res Treat.* 1989;**14**(2):201–206.

Lundgren S, Kvinnsland S, Utaaker E, et al. Effect of oral high-dose progestins on the disposition of antipyrine, digitoxin, and warfarin in patients with advanced breast cancer. *Cancer Chemother Pharmacol.* 1986;**18**:270–275.

Lundgren S, Linning PE, Utaaker E, et al. Influence of progestins on serum hormone levels in postmenopausal women with advanced breast cancer—I. General findings. *J Steroid Biochem.* 1990;**36**(1/2):99–104.

Muggia FM, Cassileth PA, Ochoa M Jr, et al. Treatment of breast cancer with medroxyprogesterone acetate. *Ann Intern Med.* 1968;**68**:328–337.

Murad F, Kuret JA. Estrogens and progestins. In: Gilman AG, Rall TW, Nies AS, Taylor P, eds. *The Pharmacologic Basis of Therapeutics.* New York: Pergamon Press; 1990:1397–1401.

Muss HB, Case LD, Capizzi RL, et al. High- versus standard-dose megestrol acetate in women with advanced breast cancer: A phase III trial of the Piedmont Oncology Association. *J Clin Oncol.* 1990;**8**(11):1797–1805.

Muss HB, Wells HB, Paschold EH, et al. Megestrol acetate versus tamoxifen in advanced breast cancer: 5-year analysis—A phase III trial of the Piedmont Oncology Association. *J Clin Oncol.* 1988;**6**(7):1098–1106.

Nowakowski V, Bonomi P, Anderson KM, et al. Evaluation of rebound regression after withdrawal of megestrol acetate in a select group of breast cancer patients (meeting abstract). *Breast Cancer Res Treat.* 1986;**8**(1):82.

Paine CH, Wright FW, Ellis F. The use of progestogen in the treatment of metastatic carcinoma of the kidney and uterine body. *Br J Cancer.* 1970;**14**:277.

Paladine W, Longacre D, Hemmings P, et al. Nafoxidine, an anti-estrogen in hypernephroma. *Proc Am Assoc Cancer Res ASCO.* 1979;**20**:293.

Pannuti F, Camaggi CM, Strocchi E, et al. Medroxyprogesterone acetate (MAP) relative bioavailability after single high-dose administration in cancer patients. *Cancer Treat Rep.* 1982;**66**:2043–2049.

Patel SR, Kvols LK, Hahn RG, et al. A phase II randomized trial of megestrol acetate and dexamethasone in the treatment of hormally refractory advanced carcinoma of the prostate. *Cancer.* 1990;**66**(4):655–658.

Rautio A, Kauppila AJ, Tuimala RJ, et al. Antipyrine metabolism and liver function in patients treated with high dose medroxyprogesterone. *Biomedicine.* 1979;**31**:135–138.

Reifenstein EC Sr. Hydroxyprogesterone caproate therapy in advanced endometrial cancer. *Cancer.* 1971;**27**:485–502.

Ross D, Wooten P, Ordóñez JV, et al. *mdr*[1] expression and effects of cyclosporin-A, verapamil and progesterone on daunorubicin cytotoxicity in blast cells from acute myelogenous leukemia patients. *Proc Am Assoc Cancer Res.* 1992;**33**:475.

Schacter L, Rozencweig M, Canetta R, et al. Megestrol acetate: Clinical experience. *Cancer Treat Rev.* 1989;**16**(1):49–63.

Schlaff WD, Dugoff L, Damewood MD, et al. Megestrol acetate for treatment of endometriosis. *Obstet Gynecol.* 1990;**75**(4):646–648.

Sherman AI. Hormonal aspects of endometrial cancer. In: Kistner RW, ed. *New Concepts in Gynecological Oncology.* Chicago: Year Book Medical Publishers; 1969.

Sikic BI, Scudder SA, Ballon SC, et al. High-dose megestrol acetate therapy of ovarian carcinoma: A phase II study by the Northern California Oncology Group. *Semin Oncol.* 1986;**13**(4, suppl 4):26–32.

Siminoski K, Goss P, Drucker DJ. The Cushing syndrome induced by medroxyprogesterone acetate. *Ann Intern Med.* 1989;**111**(9):758–760.

Sotaniemi EA, Hynnynen T, Alquist J, et al. Effect of medroxyprogesterone on the liver function and drug metabolism of patients with primary biliary cirrhosis and chronic active hepatitis. *J Med.* 1978;**9**:117–128.

Steineck G, Strander H, Carbin BE, et al. Recombinant leukocyte interferon alpha-2a and medroxyprogesterone in advanced renal cell carcinoma. A randomized trial. *Acta Oncol.* 1990;**29**(2):155–162.

Stoll BA. Hormone management of advanced breast cancer. *Br Med J.* 1969;**2**:293–297.

Tchekmedyian NS, Hariri L, Siau J, et al. Megestrol acetate in cancer andrexia and weight loss (meeting abstract). *Proc Ann Meet Am Soc Clin Oncol.* 1990;**9**:A336.

Veenhof CH, van der Burg ME, van Oosterom AT, et al. High-dose megestrol acetate in advanced ovarian cancer: A phase II study (meeting abstract). In: *ECCO-4, Fourth European Conference on Clinical Oncology and Cancer Nursing;* 1987:214.

Venner PM, Klotz PG, Klotz LH, et al. Megestrol acetate plus minidose diethylstilbestrol in the treatment of carcinoma of the prostate. *Semin Oncol.* 1988;**15**(2, suppl 1):62–67.

Von Roenn JH, Murphy RL, Weber KM, et al. Megestrol acetate for treatment of cachexia associated with human immunodeficiency virus (HIV) infection. *Ann Intern Med.* 1988;**109**(10):840–841.

Waterman EA, Benson RC. Medroxyprogesterone therapy in advanced endometrial adenocarcinoma. *Obstet Gynecol.* 1967;**30**:626–634.

Willemse PH, van der Ploeg E, Sleijfer DT, et al. A randomized comparison of megestrol acetate (MA) and medroxyprogesterone acetate (MPA) in patients with advanced breast cancer. *Eur J Cancer.* 1990;**26**(3):337–343.

Yovich JL, Turner SR, Draper R. Medroxyprogesterone acetate therapy in early pregnancy has no apparent fetal effects. *Teratology.* 1988;**38**(2):135–144.

Pyrazofurin

■ Other Names

Lilly XW 8791-AMX; PRZF; Pyrazomycin®; NSC-143095; compound 47599.

■ Chemistry

Structure of pyrazofurin

Pyrazofurin is a carbon-linked pyrimidine nucleoside isolated from the fermentation broth of *Streptomyces andidus*. It has a molecular weight of 235 and the empiric formula $C_9H_{13}N_3O_6$ (Williams et al 1969). The complete chemical name is 4-hydroxy-3-β-ribofuranosylpyrazole-5-carboxamide.

■ Antitumor Activity

In experimental animal systems pyrazofurin has demonstrated broad spectrum antiviral activity (Streightoff et al 1969) as well as antitumor activity against lymphomas, sarcomas, plasma cell myelomas, mammary carcinomas, and certain sarcomas (Sweeney et al 1973). The drug enhances the experimental antitumor activity of azacitidine in murine P-388 and L-1210 leukemias and in colon-26 carcinoma (Chiuten et al 1979).

In contrast, the clinical antitumor experience in humans has not been positive. Although preliminary positive reports by Ohnuma and Holland (1977) and Cadman et al (1978) described a few responses in advanced breast cancer, mycosis fungoides, and acute myelogenous leukemias, later reports were less favorable. In patients failing fluoropyrimidine therapy for advanced colorectal carcinoma, pyrazofurin produced no objective responses (Creagan et al 1977, Carrol et al 1979). Similarly, no responses were noted in 27 patients with various metastatic sarcomas (Gralla et al 1978, also see Cormier et al 1980). Vogler and Trulock (1978) observed little activity for pyrazofurin in refractory acute myelogenous leukemia, as did Budman et al (1977) in malignant melanoma. A weekly regimen of pyrazofurin was inactive in various solid tumors including tumors of the lung, colon, breast, and pancreas (Cummings et al 1979). In multiple myeloma only 2 of 14 patients responded to pyrazofurin after relapsing on standard cytotoxic agents (Lake-Lewin et al 1979).

Combinations including pyrazofurin have shown little improvement over standard antileukemic drugs (Kaplan et al 1982). This has been reported for pyrazofurin combined with cytarabine (Kaplan et al 1982) or with azacitidine (Martelo et al 1981). Pyrazofurin alone or in combination with trifluorothymidine was similarly inactive in patients with refractory non-Hodgkin's lymphoma (Warrell et al 1979).

■ Mechanism of Action

Pyrazofurin is an antipyrimidine nucleoside that blocks DNA replication by inhibition of the enzyme orotic acid decarboxylase. This blocks the de novo pathway of pyrimidine synthesis. Biochemical studies have demonstrated greater than 95% inhibition of orotic acid metabolism 24 hours after bolus dosing, with more than 30% inhibition 9 days after dosing (Cadman et al 1978). For antitumor activity the compound must first be phosphorylated to the nucleotide form, which selectively inhibits DNA synthesis (Moyer et al 1982). The synthesis of RNA is only slightly inhibited by pyrazofurin and serum uridine levels are not affected by the drug (Karle et al 1981). Nonetheless, uridine can reverse the growth-inhibitory effects of pyrazofurin and the related antimetabolite PALA (Johnson 1977). Partial protection from pyrazofurin cytotoxicity is provided by thymidine and deoxycytidine (Moyer et al 1982). In vitro, pyrazofurin is much more potent than PALA at depleting cellular pools of the deoxynucleotides cytidine, thymidine, and guanosine. In contrast, the pool of deoxyadenosine triphosphate actually increases after pyrazofurin (Moyer et al 1982).

In human hepatoma cell lines pyrazofurin has demonstrated cell cycle phase specificity for early G_1 and S phases (Lui et al 1979). In addition, the drug was cytotoxic only for cell populations in the logarithmic growth phase. It was inactive against plateau-phase cell populations. Pyrazofurin-induced depletion of the cellular pool of cytidine triphosphate was also documented, and the authors further suggested that pyrazofurin toxicity rescue with uridine or cytidine may be possible.

■ Availability and Storage

Lyophilized pyrazofurin is investigationally available in 300-mg, 10-mL vials adjusted to pH 7.4 with either sodium hydroxide or hydrochloric acid. It is recommended that the vials be stored under refrigeration. In this form they are stable for at least 1 year.

■ Preparation for Use, Stability, and Admixture

Pyrazofurin (300-mg vial) is initially reconstituted with 10 mL normal saline, resulting in a 30 mg/mL solution of pH 7.0 to 8.0. This initial solution is stable for 30 days under refrigeration and 48 hours at room temperature.

The initial solution is usually further diluted in either normal saline or D5W without loss of stability. Dilution in lactated Ringer's injection, however, results in markedly diminished stability and is not recommended. For prolonged refrigerated storage (beyond 8 hours), the use of a bacteriostatic diluent is highly recommended.

■ Administration

Pyrazofurin can be locally irritating; therefore only intravenous administration of the product in either D5W or normal saline is recommended. As such the drug has been given by rapid intravenous (bolus) injection and as a continuous infusion over 1 to 6 days. Creagan et al (1977) used a short 1.5-hour infusion of pyrazofurin diluted into 100 mL of normal saline. It is imperative that vein patency be ensured with this drug, and a flush of 5 to 10 mL before and after drug administration is recommended. The use of preexisting venipuncture sites should be avoided.

■ Dosage

Ohnuma and Holland (1977) have studied pyrazofurin administered as a prolonged infusion. Their recommended dose was 250 mg/m^2 as an intravenous bolus or a 24-hour continuous infusion every 2 to 3 weeks. A dose of 100 mg/m^2 as an intravenous bolus weekly also produced only mild toxicity. A 5- day bolus regimen of 50 mg/m^2/d (with azacitidine) was tolerable in patients with refractory leukemia. Higher doses in this trial produced severe dermatitis and mucositis (Martelo et al 1981). Large infusion doses (up to 1500 mg/m^2) produce severe mucocutaneous toxicity and are probably excessive (Ohnuma and Holland 1977). In the negative phase I and II solid tumor investigations, weekly doses of 100 to 200 mg/m^2 (3–5 mg/kg) were satisfactorily tolerated. The acute leukemia study of Vogler and Trulock (1978) was equally disappointing in that the dose of 45 mg/m^2/d × 5 days produced unacceptable toxicity, necessitating dose reduction to the recommended 30 mg/m^2/d as an intravenous bolus for 5 consecutive days. In this study, courses were repeated at 2-week intervals. Overall then, both the optimal dose and indeed the antitumor efficacy of the compound remain largely undefined.

■ Drug Interactions

Cadman and associates (1978) suggested synergism for pyrazofurin combined with azacitidine in leukemic cells. Williams et al (1979) corroborated this finding in the laboratory, although synergistic toxicity occurred even when additive antitumor effects were not achieved. Similar effects were observed in a clinical trial that demonstrated substantial skin and mucous membrane toxicity for the combination of pyrazofurin and azacitidine (Martelo and Broun 1979). Unfortunately, the combination of pyrazofurin and azacitidine was not more active than azacitidine alone in patients with refractory leukemia (Martelo et al 1981).

■ Pharmacokinetics

Pyrazofurin pharmacokinetics has been measured by a gas chromatographic procedure in nine patients with a variety of advanced solid tumors (Ohnuma et al 1977). The mean early-phase half-life was 10 minutes and ranged from 1.74 to 33 minutes. A more prolonged second phase of elimination had an estimated half-life of 2.5 and 3.5 hours in two patients. Mean peak plasma levels following a single intravenous bolus injection of 100 to 300 mg/m^2 ranged from 3.09 to 18.1 µg/mL. At the 250 mg/m^2 dose recommended for phase II studies, mean peak plasma levels were 5.25 ± 0.78 µg/mL. The volume of distribution for pyrazofurin in the central compartment was approximately 60% of body weight. About 4 to 12% of a dose was recovered as parent drug in the urine over 2 to 10 days after dosing. Following pyrazofurin administration, the urinary excretion of orotidine and orotic acid increased considerably. This fraction tended to be larger after a 24-hour continuous infusion compared with the intravenous bolus.

■ Side Effects and Toxicity

The major dose-limiting toxic effects of pyrazofurin have consisted of severe mucocutaneous ulceration and hematologic depression. Ohnuma and Holland (1977) noted a spectrum of mucosal lesions including oral pain, cheilosis, erythema, and frank ulceration or bullous eruption. Typically, reactions were maximal 3 to 7 days after administration and generally resolved over the ensuing week. Erosive lesions were common, especially in body areas in close contact with clothing, whereas the erythematous, maculopapular, nonpruritic dermatitis could occur anywhere. In this regard, there was substantial local synergy at previous radiation therapy port sites. There is eventual healing, even when actual skin desquamation occurs (Vogler and Trulock 1978).

Pyrazofurin hematologic toxicity also exhibits a dose–response relationship and toxicologic synergy with prior radiotherapy. Depression of all formed blood elements is possible. Thus, anemia, leukopenia, and significant thrombocytopenia may occur. The latter two features are usually restricted to previously irradiated patients (Ohnuma and Holland 1977). In one trial, the mean drop in hemoglobin levels was 3.2 g/dL (Carroll et al 1979).

In colorectal carcinoma Creagan et al (1977) noted diarrhea, stomatitis, and dermatitis along with a mild to moderate leukopenia (nadir, 12 days average; mean duration, 6 days) after 240 mg/m^2 given at 3- to 4-week intervals. A patient developing severe sun sensitivity is also described in this report. The thrombocytopenic nadir in this study occurred on day 13, with a mean 11-day duration (range, 6–21 days). Gralla et al (1978) have additionally confirmed another common hematologic problem with pyrazofurin: a normochronic, normocytic anemia usually noted 1 to 2 weeks after commencing therapy. Depressed red blood cell survival appears to be a reproducible phenomenon with this drug.

Nausea and vomiting were noted by Gralla and Creagan but were curiously rare in the initial report of Ohnuma and Holland (1977). Finally, alopecia does not appear to be a problem with pyrazofurin.

REFERENCES

Budman D, Currie V, Wittes R. Phase II trial of pyrazofurin in malignant melanoma. *Cancer Treat Rep.* 1977;**6**(5):1733–1734.

Cadman EC, Dix DE, Handschumacher RE. Clinical, biological, and biochemical effects of pyrazofurin. *Cancer Res.* 1978;**38**:682–688.

Carroll DS, Kemeny NE, Gralla RJ. Phase II evaluation of pyrazofurin in patients with advanced colorectal carcinoma. *Cancer Treat Rep.* 1979;**63**(1):139–140.

Chiuten DF, Muggia FM, Johnson RK. Antitumor activity of pyrazofurin in patients with 5-azacytidine against murine P388 and L1210 leukemias and colon carcinoma 26. *Cancer Treat Rep.* 1979;**63**:1857–1862.

Cormier WJ, Hahn RG, Edmonson JH, Eagan RT. Phase II study in advanced sarcoma: Randomized trial of pyrazofurin versus combination cyclophosphamide, doxorubicin, and *cis*-dichlorodiammineplatinum(II) (CAP). *Cancer Treat Rep.* 1980;**64**:655–658.

Creagan ET, Rubin J, Moertel CG, et al. Phase II study of pyrazofurin in advanced colorectal carcinoma. *Cancer Treat Rep.* 1977;**61**(3):491–493.

Cummings FJ, Stoller RG, Kaplan HG, Calabresi P. Clinical trial of weekly pyrazofurin. *Cancer Treat Rep.* 1979;**63**:1363–1365.

Gralla RJ, Sordillo PR, Magill GB. Phase II evaluation of pyrazofurin in patients with metastatic sarcoma. *Cancer Treat Rep.* 1978;**62**(10):1573–1574.

Johnson RK. Reversal of toxicity and antitumor activity of *N*-(phosphonacetyl)-L-aspartate by uridine or carbamoyl-DL-aspartate in vivo. *Biochem Pharmacol.* 1977;**26**:81–84.

Kaplan HG, Appelbaum FR, Cheever MA, et al. Treatment of refractory acute nonlymphocytic leukemia with a combination of pyrazofurin and cytarabine. *Cancer Treat Rep.* 1982;**66**:1397–1398.

Karle JM, Anderson LW, Dietrick DP. Effect of inhibitors of the de novo pyrimidine biosynthetic pathway on serum uridine levels in mice. *Cancer Res.* 1981;**41**:4952–4955.

Lake-Lewin D, Myers J, Lee BJ, Young CW. Phase II trial of pyrazofurin in patients with multiple myeloma refractory to standard cytotoxic therapy. *Cancer Treat Rep.* 1979;**63**(8):1403–1404.

Lui MS, Olah E, Tzeng D, Weber G. Cytochemical mechanism of action of pyrazofurin (abstract 248). *Proc Am Assoc Cancer Res ASCO.* 1979;**20**:62.

Martelo OJ, Broun G. Pyrazofurin (PF) and azacytidine (AZA) in refractory acute leukemia (AL) (abstract C-254). *Proc Am Assoc Cancer Res ASCO.* 1979;**20**:352.

Martelo OJ, Broun GO Jr, Petruska PJ. Phase I study of pyrazofurin and 5-azacytidine in refractory adult acute leukemia. *Cancer Treat Rep.* 1981;**65**:237–239.

Moyer JD, Smith PA, Levy EJ. Kinetics of *N*-(phosphonacetyl)-L-aspartate and pyrazofurin depletion of pyrimidine ribonucleotide and deoxyribonucleotide pools and their relationship to nucleic acid synthesis in intact and permeabilized cells. *Cancer Res.* 1982;**42**:4525–4531.

Ohnuma T, Holland JF. Initial clinical study with pyrazofurin. *Cancer Treat Rep.* 1977;**61**(3):389–394.

Ohnuma T, Roboz J, Shapiro ML, et al. Pharmacological and biochemical effects of pyrazofurin in humans. *Cancer Res.* 1977;**37**:2043–2049.

Streightoff FJ, Nelson JD, Cline JC, et al. Antiviral activity of pyrazomycin. In: *Proceedings of the 9th Conference on Antimicrobial Agents and Chemotherapy, Washington, DC*; 1969:8.

Sweeney MJ, Davis FA, Gutowski GE, et al. Experimental antitumor activity of pyrazomycin. *Cancer Res.* 1973;**33**:2619–2623.

Vogler WR, Trulock PD. (Southeastern Cancer Study Group). Phase I study of pyrazofurin in refractory acute myelogenous leukemia. *Cancer Treat Rep.* 1978;**62**(10):1569–1571.

Warrell RP Jr, Currie V, Kempin S, Young C. Phase II trial of pyrazofurin, alone and in combination with trifluorothymidine, in non-Hodgkin's lymphoma. *Cancer Treat Rep.* 1979;**63**(8):1423–1425.

Williams RH, Gerzon K, Hoehn M, et al. Pyrazomycin a novel carbon-linked nucleoside (abstract MICR 38). In: *Proceedings of the 158th American Chemical Society National Meeting, New York*; 1969.

Williams CJ, Swan A, Al-Atia G, Whitehouse JAM. Synergistic antitumor activity and toxicity of pyrazofurin (PZ) and 5-azacytidine (Acacyd) (abstract 226). *Proc Am Assoc Cancer Res ASCO.* 1979;**20**:56.

Razoxane

■ Other Names

ICRF-159; NSC-129943.

■ Chemistry

$$\begin{array}{c} \text{CO-CH}_2 \\ / \\ \text{HN} \\ \backslash \\ \text{CO-CH}_2 \end{array} \text{N-CH}_2\text{-N} \begin{array}{c} \text{CH}_2\text{-CO} \\ / \\ \text{NH} \\ \backslash \\ \text{CH}_2\text{-CO} \end{array}$$

Structure of razoxane

Razoxane is chemically 4,4'-(1-methyl-1,2-ethanediyl)bis-2,6-piperazinedione, a white to off-white crystalline solid with a molecular weight of 268. It has a melting point of 237 to 239°C and is soluble only to 1 g in 1000 mL of water. Razoxane is thus a nonpolar bisdiketopiperazine derivative of the complexing agent ethylenediaminetetraacetic acid (EDTA). It was originally synthesized by Creighton et al (1969).

■ Antitumor Activity

In animal models razoxane has shown marked activity against L-1210 murine leukemia (Venditti 1971) and was active in preventing metastatic pulmonary metastases in carcinogen-sensitive mice (Salsbury et al 1970). In humans, some antitumor activity was noted primarily in acute leukemias (Hellmann 1970, Mathe et al 1970), non-Hodgkin's lymphoma, and refractory Hodgkin's disease (Flannery et al 1978, Corder et al 1984a, O'Connell et al 1980, Hellmann et al 1969). Other investigators have not found significant antitumor activity in patients with acute leukemia (Bakowski et al 1979). Results of clinical trials of razoxane in a variety of solid tumors, including colorectal carcinoma, non-small cell lung cancer, nonsquamous cell carcinoma of the cervix, ovarian cancer, renal cell carcinoma, cervical cancer, gastric cancer, breast cancer, head and neck cancer, and sarcoma have, however, generally been disappointing (Gastrointestinal Tumor Study Group 1985, Douglass et al 1985, Paul et al 1980, Wheeler et al 1984, Conroy et al 1984a,b, Shah et al 1982, Creech et al 1979, Krasnow et al 1982, Borden et al 1982, Natale et al 1983, Homesley et al 1986a, Brubaker et al 1986; Bellet et al 1973, Marciniak et al 1975). The drug has been inactive in combination with cisplatin for the treatment of patients with cervical cancer (Bonomi et al 1988). It has also been inactive when combined with 5-fluorouracil for patients with colorectal cancer (O'Connell et al 1987, Windschitl et al 1983).

There is some evidence that adjuvant treatment of patients with Dukes' stage C adenocarcinoma of the colon may prolong the time to recurrence of their disease (Gilbert et al 1986). The drug has activity in patients with both nonepidemic Kaposi's sarcoma (Olweny et al 1980) and epidemic (acquired immunodeficiency syndrome [AIDS]-related) Kaposi's sarcoma (Hymes 1987).

■ Mechanism of Action

This compound and others related to it were originally developed and studied for their ability to chelate divalent cations. Despite this, the antitumor activity of razoxane probably does not depend on chelation and does not alkylate DNA. Recent mechanistic studies with other structurally related bisdioxopiperazines suggest that these agents do not interact directly with DNA. Rather, they appear to inhibit DNA topoisomerase II enzymes (Tanabe et al 1991, Ishida et al 1991). Enzyme inhibition occurs at an early step that precludes formation of the "cleavable complexes" as seen after other topoisomerase II inhibitors such as etoposide. The precise mechanism is not fully understood; however, razoxane does inhibit DNA synthesis and blocks tritiated thymidine incorporation in a pattern similar to that of irradiation and classic alkylating agents (Creighton and Hellmann 1970, Sharpe et al 1970). The compound appears to effectively arrest mitosis when given during the premitotic and early mitotic phases of cell growth, G_2 and M phases (Hellmann and Field 1970). Razoxane may thus be considered cell cycle phase specific for G_2 and M phases.

Salsbury et al (1970) have additionally shown that razoxane experimentally inhibits the tumor metastasis process apparently by what LeServe and Hellmann (1972) have called *normalization* of tumor blood vessels. This corroborates the earlier experimental observation of Hellmann and Burrage (1969) that the development of malignant pulmonary metastases in mice could be prevented by razoxane. Thus, the prevention of characteristic tumor neovascularization may account for some of the apparent solid tumor cytotoxicity of the compound but would not explain the slight antileukemic activity noted in certain animal models.

■ Availability and Storage

Razoxane (ICRF-159) is investigationally available from the National Cancer Institute in 50-, 250-, and 500-mg off-white, scored tablets. In addition to the drug, the tablets contain the following inert ingredients: microcrystalline cellulose, polyvinylpyrrolidone, alginic acid, and magnesium stearate. The drug may be stored at room temperature (22–25°C) and is stable for at least 2 years. Repta et al (1976) have additionally described the development of a soluble enantiomer of razoxane called ICRF-187 suitable for an investigational injectable formulation.

■ Administration

See Dosage. The compound is an oral agent.

■ Special Precautions

There is some evidence that treatment with razoxane may be associated with an increased incidence of acute myelogenous leukemia (Baglin et al 1987, Gilbert et al 1986, Bhavnani and Wolstenholme 1987, Caffrey et al 1985). This was first described in patients receiving long-term oral therapy for psoriasis (Joshi et al 1981, Horton et al 1984). Some of these patients had previously received methotrexate and had received cumulative razoxane doses of 43 to 450 g by over 9- to 80-month treatment periods. Acute myelomonocytic leukemias are also described in three patients receiving 5-fluorouracil and razoxane for colon or pancreatic carcinomas over 18 to 31 months of therapy. Acute myelocytic leukemia was noted 5 to 9 months after the discontinuation of razoxane therapy. An inversion of chromosome 16 in bone marrow cells was noted in one psoriasis patient who developed acute myelocytic leukemia after receiving 1 year of cyclophosphamide followed by a 2.5-year course of oral razoxane therapy (Baglin et al 1987). The causal relationship and true incidence of razoxane-induced secondary carcinogenesis, if any, are not established. Nonetheless, patient consent forms should reflect this possibility.

■ Drug Interactions

Razoxane in animal tumor systems has been synergistic with a number of other agents including cyclophosphamide, 5-fluorouracil, and doxorubicin (Wampler et al 1974). Additionally, the drug may be effective in preventing anthracycline-induced cardiotoxicity in experimental animals (Herman et al 1972). (See also *Dexrazoxane*). The mechanism may involve intracellular iron chelation by razoxane. This thereby prevents the formation of cardiotoxic chelates between anthracyclines and iron (Hasinoff 1989). According to Wang and Finch (1979) maximal (complete) prophylaxis is possible only by giving razoxane 48 hours before daunomycin. In their study the effect did not relate either to altered daunomycin metabolism (by aldo-keto reductase or reductive glycosidase) or to reduced DNA complex formation capability. At this time, however, this preclinical intriguing interaction has yet to be confirmed clinically for razoxane.

■ Dosage

The recommended total dose from Creaven et al (1973) is 3 g/m^2 given in divided doses every 6 hours for 1 day, once per week for 6 weeks. In patients with solid tumors, Bellet et al (1973) reported maximally tolerated doses of 1 g/m^2/d given at 8-hour intervals for 3 successive days. It has been shown that intestinal absorption may reach a maximum at about 3 g/m^2 (Creaven et al 1973). The divided regimens are thought to enhance drug absorption and therefore drug efficacy (Creaven et al 1974, Venditti 1971). Liesmann et al (1981) have recommended 800 to 1500 mg/m^2 daily × 5 in their phase I schedule. The most commonly employed dose in phase II trials has been 1.5 g/m^2 weekly (Homesley et al 1986a,b).

■ Pharmacokinetics

There are no recent clinical pharmacology studies with razoxane.

After large doses of razoxane (ICRF-159) are given orally, only part of the dose may be absorbed. It appears that a dose is relatively well absorbed up to a tentative maximum of 3 g/m^2 (Creaven et al 1973). Peak plasma concentrations are attained in about 3 hours. The drug appears to concentrate in the liver and kidney, with less drug accumulation in lung, muscle, and tumor. Very little drug penetrates into the brain. The drug appears to be excreted by the kidneys and bile. There is also possible significant enterohepatic circulation in the initial phase of drug distribution which lasts about 25 minutes (Field et al 1971). The slower secondary phase is thought to represent clearance of a metabolite. None of the metabolites of razoxane has been found to be active. One human study showed razoxane to have a plasma half-life of 3.5 hours. Peak plasma levels of approximately 3.8 µg/mL were achieved 2 hours after an oral dose of 3 g/m² (Sadee et al 1975).

■ Side Effects and Toxicity

The principal toxic effect is leukopenia. It is usually mild to moderate (mean nadir of 1–16 days), with recovery in about 8 additional days (Bellet et al 1973). Thrombocytopenia is also usually mild and transient.

A slight fall in hematocrit (>5%) is seen in about 11% of patients treated. Gastrointestinal side effects occur in about 40% of patients. These effects consist of nausea, vomiting, and diarrhea, and occasional mucositis. Significant alopecia has been reported to occur in most patients. Some patients may also exhibit an unusual acneiform papular dermatitis on the trunk, face, and extremities (Marciniak et al 1975).

As noted under Special Precautions, razoxane has been associated with the development of acute leukemia (Baglin et al 1987, Gilbert et al 1986).

■ Special Applications

Razoxane has been used as a radiation sensitizer. In two studies, its use with radiation therapy has been associated with enhanced toxicity and reduced survival (Newman et al 1985, Corder et al 1984b). No benefit was noted in other randomized trials (Belloni et al 1983). The drug has also been used to treat psoriasis with some success (Atherton et al 1980).

REFERENCES

Atherton DJ, Wells RS, Laurent MR, Williams YF. Razoxane (ICRF 159) in the treatment of psoriasis. *Br J Dermatol.* 1980;**102**(3):307–317.

Baglin TP, Galvin GP, Pollock A. Therapy-related acute nonlymphocytic leukemia with inversion of chromosome 16 and a sustained remission. *Cancer Genet Cytogenet.* 1987;**27**(1):167–169.

Bakowski MT, Prentice HG, Liste TA, Malpas JS, McElwair TJ, Powles RL. Limited activity of ICRF-159 in advanced acute leukemia. *Cancer Treat Rep.* 1979;**63**(1):127–129.

Bellet RE, Mastrangelo MJ, Dixon LM, Yarbro JW. Phase I study of ICRF-159 (NSC-129943) in human solid tumors. *Cancer Chemother Rep.* 1973;**57**:185–189.

Belloni C, Mangioni C, Bortolozzi G, et al. ICRF 159 plus radiation versus radiation therapy alone in cervical carcinoma. A double-blind study. *Oncology.* 1983;**40**(3):181–185.

Bhavnani M, Wolstenholme RJ. Razoxane and acute promyelocytic leukaemia (letter). *Lancet.* 1987;**2**:1085.

Bonomi P, Yordan E, Blessing JA. Phase I trial of cisplatin and razoxane (ICRF-159, NSC #119875) in advanced squamous cell carcinoma of the cervix. A Gynecologic Oncology Group pilot study. *Am J Clin Oncol.* 1988;**11**(1):1–2.

Borden EC, Ash A, Enterline HT, et al. Phase II evaluation of dibromodulcitol, ICRF-159, and maytansine for sarcomas. *Am J Clin Oncol.* 1982;**5**(4):417–420.

Brubaker LH, Vogel CL, Einhorn LH, Birch R. Treatment of advanced adenocarcinoma of the kidney with ICRF-187: A Southeastern Cancer Study Group trial. *Cancer Treat Rep.* 1986;**70**(7):915–916.

Caffrey EA, Daker MG, Horton JJ. Acute myeloid leukaemia after treatment with razoxane. *Br J Dermatol.* 1985;**113**(2):131–134.

Conroy JF, Blessing JA, Kessinger A, Homesley HD. Phase II trial of razoxane in the management of recurrent adenocarcinoma of the ovary: A Gynecologic Oncology Group study. *Cancer Treat Rep.* 1984a;**68**(2):439–440.

Conroy JF, Lewis GC Jr, Blessing JA, Mangan C, Hatch K, Wilbanks G. ICRF-159 (razoxane) in patients with advanced squamous cell carcinoma of the uterine cervix. A Gynecologic Oncology Group study. *Am J Clin Oncol.* 1984b;**7**(2):131–133.

Corder MP, McFadden DB, Bell SJ. A trial of razoxane (ICRF-159) in patients with prior therapy for Hodgkin's lymphoma. *Cancer.* 1984a;**54**(8):1496–1498.

Corder MP, Tewfik HH, Clamon GH, et al. Radiotherapy plus razoxane for advanced limited extent carcinoma of the lung. *Cancer.* 1984b;**53**(9):1852–1856.

Creaven PJ, Allen LM, Alford DA. Bioavailability of the antineoplastic drug ICRF-159 in relation to clinical toxicity. In: *Proceedings of the 15th National Meeting of the APHA Academy of Pharmaceutical Sciences;* 1973:96.

Creaven PJ, Cohen MH, Hansen HH, Selawry OS, Taylor SG. Phase I clinical trial of a single-dose and two weekly schedules of ICRF-159 (NSC-129943). *Cancer Chemother Rep.* 1974;**58**:393–400.

Creech RH, Engstrom PF, Harris DT, Catalano RB, Bellet RE. Phase II study of ICRF-159 in refractory metastatic breast cancer. *Cancer Treat Rep.* 1979;**63**:111–114.

Creighton AM, Hellmann GD. Biochemical studies on growth-inhibitor bisdioxopiperazines. I. Effect on DNA, RNA and protein synthesis in mouse-embryo fibroblasts. *Int J Cancer.* 1970;**5**:47–54.

Creighton AM, Hellmann K, Whitecross S. Antitumor activity in a series of bisdiketopiperazines. *Nature.* 1969;**222**:384–385.

Douglass HO Jr, MacIntyre JM, Kaufman J, Von Hoff D, Engstrom PF, Klaassen D. Eastern Cooperative Oncology Group phase II studies in advanced measurable colorectal cancer. I. Razoxane, Yoshi-864, piperazinedione, and lomustine. *Cancer Treat Rep.* 1985;**69**(5):543–545.

Field EO, Mauro E, Hellmann K. Blood clearance of ICRF-159 (NSC-129943). *Cancer Chemother Rep.* 1971;**55**:527–530.

Flannery EP, Corder MP, Sheehan WW, Pajak TF, Bateman JR. Phase II study of ICRF-159 in non-Hodgkin's lymphomas. *Cancer Treat Rep.* 1978;**62**(3):465–467.

Gastrointestinal Tumor Study Group. Phase II trials of hexamethylmelamine, dianhydrogalactitol, razoxane, and beta-2'-deoxythioguanosine as single agents against advanced measurable tumors of the pancreas. *Cancer Treat Rep.* 1985;**69**(6):713–716.

Gilbert JM, Hellmann K, Evans M, et al. Randomized trial of oral adjuvant razoxane (ICRF 159) in resectable colorectal cancer: Five-year follow-up. *Br J Surg.* 1986;**73**(6):446–450.

Hasinoff BB. The interaction of the cardioprotective agent ICRF-187 ((+)-1,2-bis(3,5-dioxopiperazinyl-1-yl)propane); its hydrolysis product (ICRF-198); and other chelating agents with the Fe(III) and Cu(II) complexes of Adriamycin. *Agents Actions.* 1989;**26**:378–390

Hellmann K. Further clinical experiences with ICRF-159. In: Mathe G, ed. *Advances in the Treatment of Acute (Blastic) Leukemias.* New York: Springer-Verlag; 1970:52–53.

Hellmann K, Burrage K. Control of malignant metastases by ICRF-159. *Nature.* 1969;**224**:273–275.

Hellmann K, Field EO. Effect of ICRF-159 on the mammalian cell cycle: Significance for its use in cancer chemotherapy. *J Natl Cancer Inst.* 1970;**44**:539–543.

Hellmann K, Newton K, Whitmore D, Hanham IWF, Bond JV. Preliminary clinical assessment of ICRF-159 in acute leukemia and lymphosarcoma. *Br Med J.* 1969;**1**:822–824.

Herman EH, Mhatre RM, Lee IP, Waravdekar VS. Prevention of the cardiotoxic effects of Adriamycin and daunomycin in the isolated dog heart. *Proc Soc Exp Biol Med.* 1972;**140**:234–239.

Homesley HD, Blessing JA, Berman M. ICRF-159 (razoxane) in patients with advanced nonsquamous cell carcinoma of the cervix. A Gynecologic Oncology Group study. *Am J Clin Oncol.* 1986a;**9**(4):325–326.

Homesley HD, Blessing JA, Conroy J, Hatch K, DiSaia PJ, Twiggs LB. ICRF-159 (razoxane) in patients with advanced adenocarcinoma of the endometrium. A Gynecologic Oncology Group study. *Am J Clin Oncol.* 1986b;**9**(1):15–17.

Horton JJ, Caffrey EA, Clark KGA, McDonald DM, Wells RS, Daker MG. Leukaemia in psoriatic patients treated with razoxane (letter). *Br J Dermatol.* 1984;**110**:663.

Hymes KB. Kaposi's sarcoma in AIDS. In: Wormser GP, Stahl RE, Battone EJ, eds. *AIDS, Acquired Immune Deficiency Syndrome, and Other Manifestations of HIV Infection.* Park Ridge, NJ: Noyes; 1987:747–766.

Ishida R, Miki T, Narita T, et al. Inhibition of intracellular topoisomerase II by antitumor bis(2,6-dioxopiperazine) derivatives: Mode of cell growth inhibition distinct from that of cleavable complex-forming type inhibitors. *Cancer Res.* 1991;**51**:4909–4916.

Joshi R, Smith B, Philips RH, et al. Acute myelomonocytic leukaemia after razoxane therapy. *Lancet.* 1981;**2**:1343–1344.

Krasnow S, Bunn PA Jr, Ihde DC, et al. ICRF-159 in advanced gastric cancer. Absence of activity. *Am J Clin Oncol.* 1982;**5**(6):635–639.

LeServe AW, Hellmann K. Metastases and the normalization of tumor blood vessels by ICRF-159: A new type of drug action. *Br Med J.* 1972;**1**:597–601.

Liesmann J, Belt R, Haas C, Hoogstraten B. Phase I evaluation of ICRF-187 (NSC-169780) in patients with advanced malignancy. *Cancer.* 1981;**47**(8):1959–1962.

Marciniak TA, Moertel CG, Schutt AJ, Hann RG, Reitemeier RJ. Phase II study of ICRF-159 (NSC-129943) in advanced colorectal carcinoma. *Cancer Chemother Rep.* 1975;**59**(4):761–763.

Mathe G, Amiel JL, Hayat M. Preliminary data on acute leukemia treatment with ICRF-159. In: Mathe G, ed. *Advances in the Treatment of Acute (Blastic) Leukemias.* New York: Springer-Verlag; 1970:54–55.

Natale RB, Wheeler RH, Liepman MK, Sauder A, Bricker L. Phase II trial of ICRF-187 in non-small cell lung cancer. *Cancer Treat Rep.* 1983;**67**(3):311–313.

Newman CE, Cox R, Ford CH, Johnson JR, Jones DR, Wheaton M. Reduced survival with radiotherapy and razoxane compared with radiotherapy alone for inoperable lung cancer in a randomized double-blind trial. *Br J Cancer.* 1985;**51**(5):731–732.

O'Connell MJ, Begg CB, Silverstein MN, Glick JH, Oken MM. Randomized clinical trial comparing two dose regimens of ICRF-159 in refractory malignant lymphomas. *Cancer Treat Rep.* 1980;**64**(12):1355–1358.

O'Connell MJ, Schutt AJ, Moertel CG, Rubin J, Hahn RG, Scott M. A randomized clinical trial of combination chemotherapy in advanced colorectal cancer. *Am J Clin Oncol.* 1987;**10**(4):320–324.

Olweny CL, Sikyewunda W, Otim D. Further experience with razoxane (ICRF-159; NSC-129943) in treating Kaposi's sarcoma. *Oncology.* 1980;**37**(3):174–176.

Paul AR, Catalano RB, Engstrom PF. Phase III study of ICRF-159 versus 5-FU in the treatment of advanced metastatic colorectal carcinoma. *Cancer Treat Rep.* 1980;**64**(10/11):1047–1949.

Repta AJ, Baltezor MJ, Bansal PC. Utilization of an enantiomer as a solution to a pharmaceutical problem: Application to solubilization of 1,2-di(-4-piperazine-2,6-dione) propane. *J Pharm Sci.* 1976;**65**(2):238–242.

Sadee W, Staroscik J, Finn C, et al. Determination of (±)-1,2-bis(3,5-dioxopiperazinyl)propane plasma levels in rats, rabbits, and humans by GLC and mass fragmentography. *J Pharm Sci.* 1975;**64**(6):998–1001.

Salsbury AJ, Burrage K, Hellmann K. Inhibition of metastatic spread by ICRF-159: Selective deletion of a malignant characteristic. *Br Med J.* 1970;**4**:344–346.

Shah MK, Engstrom PF, Catalano RB, Paul AR, Bellet RE, Creech RH. Phase II trial of razoxane (ICRF-159) in patients with squamous cell carcinoma of the head and neck previously exposed to systemic chemotherapy. *Cancer Treat Rep.* 1982;**66**(3):557–558.

Sharpe HBA, Field EO, Hellmann K. Mode of action of the cytostatic agent "ICRF-159." *Nature.* 1970;**226**:524–525.

Tanabe K, Ikegami Y, Ishida R, et al. Inhibition of topoisomerase II by antitumor agents bis(2,6-dioxopiperazine) derivatives. *Cancer Res.* 1991;**51**:4903–4908.

Venditti JM. Treatment schedule dependency of experimentally active antileukemic (L-1210) drugs. *Cancer Chemother Rep Part 3.* 1971;**2**:35–59.

Wampler GL, Speckhart VJ, Regelson W. Phase I clinical study of Adriamycin–ICRF-159 combination and other ICRF-159 drug combinations. *Proc Am Soc Clin Oncol.* 1974;**15**:189.

Wang GM, Finch M. Studies on the mechanism of razoxane induced reduction of daunomycin toxicity. *Proc Am Assoc Cancer Res ASCO.* 1979;**20**:23.

Wheeler RH, Bricker LJ, Natale RB, Baker SR. Phase II trial of ICRF-187 in squamous cell carcinoma of the head and neck. *Cancer Treat Rep.* 1984;**68**(2):427–428.

Windschitl H, Scott M, Schutt A, et al. Randomized phase II studies in advanced colorectal carcinoma: A North Central Cancer Treatment Group study. *Cancer Treat Rep.* 1983;**67**(11):1001–1008.

Sargramostim

■ Other Names

Granulocyte–macrophage colony-stimulating factor; GM-CSF; Leukine® (yeast-derived, Immunex); Prokine® (Hoechst-Roussel Pharmaceuticals); Leukomax® (*E. coli*-derived, Schering Corporation).

■ Chemistry

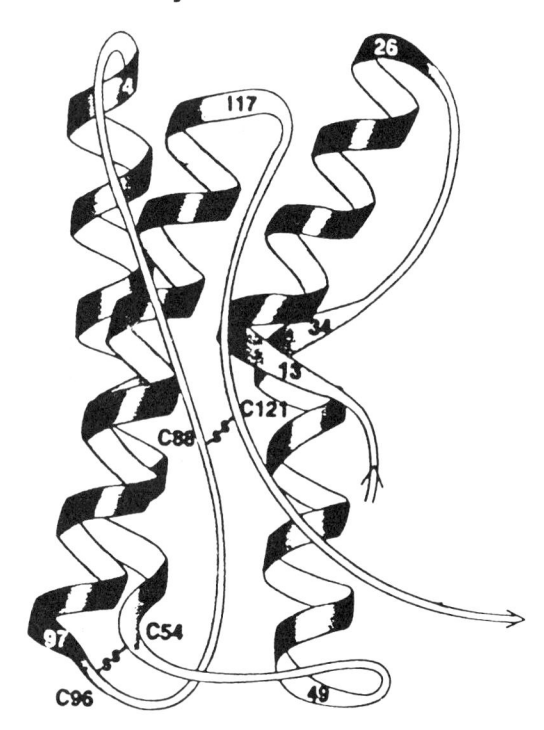

Structure of sargramostim

Sargramostim is a natural human protein produced by recombinant DNA techniques using as host organisms yeast (*Saccharomyces cerevisiae*—Leukine®, Prokine®), the bacterium *Escherichia coli* (Leukomax®), or Chinese hamster ovary cells (original product from Sandoz Pharmaceuticals, not marketed). The mature protein contains 120 to 127 amino acids and two internal cysteine–cysteine disulfide bridges which help maintain the appropriate tertiary structure. There are two arginine-linked glycosylation sites which are variably glycosylated in the yeast-derived preparation. The molecular weight varies with the individual sargramostim products from 14,000 to 35,000. The Immunex product Leukine® can exist in three molecular species having masses of 19,500, 16,800, and 15,500. The Leukine® preparation differs from native sargramostim by the substitution of leucine at position 23 and by a different carbohydrate (glycosylation) makeup. It has a specific activity of approximately 5×10^7 U/mg of protein. The mammalian cell-derived material (Sandoz Pharmaceuticals/Genetics Institute) has a specific activity of 5.4×10^6 U/mg of glycoprotein, with 1 unit equal to the amount needed to stimulate half-maximal incorporation of [^{3}H]thymidine in sensitive leukocytes (Antman et al 1988).

■ Antitumor Activity

Bone Marrow Transplantation and High-Dose Chemotherapy. Yeast-derived sargramostim is officially approved by the U.S. Food and Drug Administration to accelerate bone marrow recovery in patients with non-Hodgkin's lymphoma (NHL), acute lymphoblastic leukemia (ALL) and Hodgkin's disease undergoing autologous bone marrow transplantation (BMT). A variety of marrow-ablative high-dose chemotherapy/radiation therapy regimens have been used with sargramostim in patients with solid tumors (Brandt et al 1988) and lymphoid malignancies (Nemunaitis et al 1988, Kersey et al 1987, Blazar et al 1989). Sargramostim also increases the number of circulating pluripotential stem cells, allowing for stem cell harvesting by leukopheresis (Gianni et al 1989).

Neutropenia of Standard Chemotherapy. Sargramostim has been used to reduce the severity and duration of neutropenia following standard myelosuppressive chemotherapy regimens without autologous bone marrow transplantation (see table). Chemotherapy regimens evaluated with sargramostim include the MAID regimen (mesna, doxorubicin [Adriamycin®], ifosfamide, dacarbazine) used in patients with soft tissue sarcoma (Antman et al 1988) and high-dose single agents such as cyclophosphamide in patients with breast cancer or non-Hodgkin's lymphoma (Gianni et al 1990). Tachyphylaxis to repeated courses of sargramostim with cyclophosphamide and doxorubicin has been reported (Hoekman et al 1991). The reason for the apparent loss of myeloproliferative activity of sargramostim with repeated cycles of chemotherapy in this trial is not known. It has also been investigationally combined with cytarabine in patients with poor-prognosis, newly diagnosed acute leukemia (Estey et al 1990).

Myelodysplasia. In myelodysplasia, sargramostim appears to provide significant improvement in peripheral blood counts, primarily neutrophils, eosinophils, and monocytes. Platelets and, in some patients, reticulocytes and mature red blood cells are occasionally elevated (Vadhan-Raj et al 1987). These latter effects generally require more prolonged sargramostim regimens. Importantly, sargramostim does not appear either to block or to accelerate myeloid disease transformation to a blast phase or progression to frank acute leukemia (Antin et al 1988, Thompson et al 1989, Ganser et al 1989, Vadham-Raj et al 1989). Indeed, a pilot study suggests that sargramostim and low-dose cytarabine can effectively control leukemic cell proliferation and increase numbers of mature myeloid cells in the bone marrow and peripheral blood following chemotherapy (Ganser and Hoelzer 1990).

CLINICAL STUDIES COMBINING SARGRAMOSTIM WITH CHEMOTHERAPY

Cancer Type	Chemotherapy Drugs	Dose (μg/kg/d)	Route	Duration (d)	Reference
Sarcoma	MAID: mesna, doxorubicin, ifosfamide, dacarbazine	4–64	IV, continuous infusion	7	Antman et al 1988
Non-Hodgkin's lymphoma, breast	Cyclophosphamide	5.5	IV, continuous infusion	14	Gianni et al 1990
Small cell lung	Carboplatin, etoposide	5–15	SC bolus	7–21	Morstyn et al 1989
Acute leukemia, resistant	Various	6.1	IV, continuous	≥ 8	Buchner et al 1988

Aplastic Anemia. Finally, sargramostim may also have important stimulatory activity in aplastic anemia (Vadhan-Raj et al 1988). As in myelodysplasia, not all patients respond, and improvements in peripheral blood counts are lost rapidly on drug discontinuance. The level of increase in leukocytes is not as great as in myelodysplasia, and there is usually little improvement in platelet or red blood cell counts (Antin 1990).

Effects on Tumor Cells. Fortunately, sargramostim does not stimulate solid tumor growth in vitro (Salmon and Liu 1989, Foulke et al 1990), but does stimulate some myeloid malignancies; however, this may be used therapeutically to enhance leukemia sensitivity to chemotherapy (Estey et al 1990). Conversely, sargramostim does not appear to have major antiproliferative effects on solid tumor cells in vitro (Foulke et al 1990), although some human small cell lung cancer cell lines may be inhibited by a differentiative mechanism (Yamashita et al 1989).

■ Mechanism of Action

Sargramostim acts to stimulate granulocyte and monocyte proliferation through an interaction with cell surface receptors with a molecular weight of 48,000. There are approximately 500 to 800 sargramostim binding sites on terminally differentiated neutrophils (DiPersio et al 1988). The binding constant for these high affinity sites is about 30 pmol. On monocytes, there are approximately 150 receptor binding sites per cell (Griffin 1989). Some malignant myeloid cell types may also have a second category of low affinity ($K_D = 1$ nM) or nonsaturable binding sites (Griffin 1989). Binding of sargramostim to its receptor results in downregulation as a result of internalization of the receptor–ligand complex.

Following receptor binding a second messenger is activated by sargramostim. This signal transduction step does not appear to involve calcium influx or protein kinase C, but instead may involve coupling to a pertussis toxin-sensitive G-protein (McColl et al 1989). There is also rapid activation of ornithine decarboxylase which is a positive regulator of macromolecular synthesis. Ultimately, bone marrow progenitor cells are stimulated to differentiate into myeloid and monocyte precursors which are then further stimulated to proliferate (Mayer et al 1987). Some megakaryocytic series cells have receptors for sargramostim (Mazur et al 1987), but enhanced platelet production in vivo is usually negligible. Indeed, platelet counts may be transiently depressed following sargramostim, especially if given after high-dose radiotherapy; however, increases in platelet counts have been observed in patients treated with sargramostim and cyclophosphamide (Gianni et al 1990) and carboplatin (Edmonson et al 1989). In myelodysplasia, platelet counts can be variably depressed or slightly increased by sargramostim.

The increase in circulating leukocytes is biphasic following sargramostim. The initial increase peaks after 4 to 5 days and a second increase occurs over the ensuing 5 days. There is, however, an initial drop in leukocyte levels in the peripheral blood 30 minutes after sargramostim administration. This occurs because of rapid induction of the Mo1 leukocyte adhesion antigen (CD11c) on the surface of myelocytes (Arnaout et al 1986). This causes a subpopulation of affected cells to adhere irreversibly to vascular endothelium, primarily in the lungs (Herrmann et al 1989).

In granulocytes, sargramostim induces accelerated depolarization and enhanced generation of the oxygen free radicals superoxide (O_2^-) and hydrogen peroxide (H_2O_2), which are necessary for bacterial killing by neutrophils. The enhancement in respiratory burst extends to eosinophils but not to adherent monocytes (Nathan 1989). The viability of mature eosinophils and neutrophils is increased 6 to 9 hours by sargramostim (Lopez et al 1986). In addition, phagocytic activity for bacteria is increased in neutrophils, (Fleishmann et al 1986, Cannistra et al 1988). In eosinophils, cytotoxicity (Cannistra et al 1988) and leukotriene synthesis are enhanced by sargramostim (Silberstein et al 1986).

In macrophages, sargramostim enhances the release of hydrogen peroxide and the killing of *Leishmania* and trypanosomes (Reed et al 1987). Many of these effects are mediated by tumor necrosis factor (TNF)-dependent mechanisms (Cannistra et al 1987). A large number of other cytokines are also released from myelomonocytic cells following sargramostim exposure. Many of these secreted proteins are potent mediators of inflammation and local cytotoxicity including TNF and interleukin-1 (IL-1) (Wing et al 1989). Other hematopoietic proteins released following sargramostim include interleukin-6 (B-cell growth factor) (Cicco et al 1990), granulocyte colony-stimulating factor (G-CSF) (Lindeman et al 1989), and monocyte/macrophage colony-stimulating factor (M-CSF) (Horiguchi et al 1987). In addition, the antigen-presenting activity of macrophages is enhanced by sargramostim, leading to increased primary antibody responses (Morrisey et al 1987).

■ Availability and Storage

Several different lyophilized formulations of sargramostim are investigationally available and one commercial formulation of yeast-derived material is currently available in the United States (see table below). For all of these preparations, storage under refrigeration is recommended.

■ Preparation for Use, Stability, and Admixture

Leukine®, Prokine® (Yeast-Derived Sargramostim). All of the sargramostim preparations are reconstituted with Sterile Water for Injection, USP (unpreserved). The vials may also be reconstituted with 1 mL bacteriostatic water for injection (0.9% benzyl alcohol or 0.012% propylparaben and 0.12% methylparaben). The yeast-derived preparation (Leukine®) is reconstituted with 1.0 mL of sterile water to yield a clear isotonic solution at a pH of 7.4 ± 0.3. Further dilutions in 0.9% sodium chloride should include 0.1% (v/v) human serum albumin to reduce adsorption of the protein to the surface of the container. The recommended procedure is to add 1 mg albumin/mL saline or 1 mL of 5% albumin solution per 50 mL of 0.9% sodium chloride solution. The vials do not contain a bacterial preservative and, therefore, multiple use is not recommended. Vials should be discarded within 6 hours of reconstitution, although the protein is chemically stable for at least 30 days at room temperature and under refrigeration (2–8°C). Vigorous agitation of the vials is not recommended to avoid breakdown of the protein.

For admixture studies, sargramostim was diluted into 0.9% sodium chloride in 50-mL polyvinyl chloride bags to a concentration of either 6 µg/mL (containing 0.1% human serum albumin) or 15 µg/mL, without albumin. Secondary additives that were visually compatible with the GM-CSF solutions (no visible haze or precipitation) included ceftazidime, dopamine, fentanyl citrate, intravenous gamma globulin, heparin sodium, and a total parenteral nutrition solution containing 10% amino acids and 25.0% dextrose (Matsuura 1992). The 6 µg/mL sargramostim solution formed a haze with vancomycin hydrochloride, suggesting incompatibility with either GM-CSF or albumin. Therefore, direct admixture of GM-CSF with vancomycin is not recommended.

Leukomax® (*E. coli*-derived GM-CSF). The Schering-supplied preparation derived from *E. coli* can be reconstituted with Sterile Water for Injection, USP, or, for prolonged stability, bacteriostatic sterile water containing 0.9% benzyl alcohol, methylparaben, or propylparaben. For subcutaneous injections a small dilution volume of 0.25 mL/700-µg vial is acceptable. Reconstituted solutions are stable for 24 hours in water or 28 days in bacteriostatic water. These solutions are compatible with Becton-Dickinson syringes and can be frozen at temperatures of −20 to −10°C. To minimize drug adsorption, the manufacturer recommends that only small final infusion volumes be used: 25 mL for the 400-µg vial, 50 mL for the 700-µg vial, and 100 mL for the 2100-µg vial. The Schering product is reported to be incompatible

FORMULATIONS OF RECOMBINANT HUMAN SARGRAMOSTIM

Trade Name	Manufacturer	Host Cells for rDNA	Lyophilized Powder Vial Sizes (µg)	Glycosylation
Leukine®	Immunex Corporation Seattle, Washington	Yeast (*Saccharomyces cerevisiae*)	250, 500	Variable
Prokine®	Hoechst-Roussel Pharmaceuticals Somerville, New Jersey	Yeast (*S. cerevisiae*)	250, 500	Variable
Leukomax®	Schering Corporation Kenilworth, New Jersey	Bacteria (*Escherichia coli*)	400, 700	None
(Unmarketed)	Sandoz Pharmaceuticals/Genetics Institute East Hanover, New Jersey	Mammalian (Chinese hamster ovary)	—	Variable

with the Port-A-Cath infusion system but it can be administered through Travenol solution administration sets or through the Kendall-McGaw Accu-Pro® Mini-Drop nitroglycerin administration set.

■ Administration

Most doses of sargramostim are administered by infusion, which appears to preclude the local site reactions seen with subcutaneous injections. Nonetheless, sargramostim is active by the subcutaneous route, and in some studies slightly greater hematopoietic effects have been observed (Lieschke et al 1990). Continuous-infusion sargramostim has also been used and this method may further increase the hematopoietic effects of the agent (Gianni et al 1990). Conversely, a rash and first-dose hypoxia/hypotensive reaction may be more common with intravenous doses (Lieschke et al 1990).

■ Dosage

A wide variety of sargramostim doses have been used in its different clinical applications (see table below). The current dose recommended in high-dose chemotherapy/autologous bone marrow transplantation is 250 µg/m^2/d for 21 consecutive days starting 24 hours after marrow reinfusion. Lower doses of 125 µg/m^2/d for shorter periods of 7 to 14 days are used following standard-dose chemotherapy regimens. For any postchemotherapy applications, an interval of not less than 24 hours is recommended to allow clearance of all cancer drugs and resolution of their acute myelosuppressive effects before sargramostim is administered. This delay in dosing is recommended to prevent sargramostim-induced enhanced susceptibility of normal bone marrow cells to the cytotoxic effects of chemotherapy. For high-dose chemotherapy followed by autologous bone marrow transplant, a 3-week treatment duration is recommended to enhance engraftment, whereas shorter courses are adequate to reduce febrile neutropenia following standard-dose chemotherapy. For patients with diseases characterized by primary bone marrow failure, chronic low-dose daily therapy appears to be required to effectively increase peripheral blood counts. Thus, brief courses of sargramostim in the setting of myelodysplasia, aplastic anemia, or acquired immunodeficiency syndrome (AIDS)-induced neutropenia, provide only modest and transient hematopoietic responses.

■ Drug Interactions

Acute leukemic myeloblasts may constitutively express sargramostim (Young et al 1987), and cell processing techniques such as E-rosetting and T-cell depletion increase this expression (Kaufmann et al 1988). Nonetheless, this property has been exploited to increase the sensitivity of leukemic blast cells to cytarabine in vitro (Bhalla et al 1988, Cannistra et al 1989, Karp et al 1990). Leukemic blast cells preincubated with sargramostim formed higher levels of cytarabine triphosphate, the active nucleotide form of the drug (Bhalla et al 1988). The retention of cytarabine nucleotide is also increased in vitro following sargramostim (Karp et al 1990). These effects were not seen in normal bone marrow myeloblasts (Bhalla et al 1988). Sargramostim also increases the

DOSES OF SARGRAMOSTIM FOR DIFFERENT CLINICAL APPLICATIONS

Clinical Application	Dose (µg/m^2/d)	Initiation (days after chemotherapy)	Duration (d)	Route of Administration	Reference
High-dose chemotherapy/ bone marrow transplantation	250	1	21	2-h infusion	Brandt et al 1988
Febrile neutropenia of myelosuppressive chemotherapy	5–6 µg/kg	1	7–14	Continuous IV infusion, subcutaneous injection	Antman et al 1988
Myelodysplasia	30–120	—	14–21 (repeated cycles)	12-h continuous IV infusion	Antin et al 1988
Aplastic anemia	120–240	—	14–21 (repeated cycles)	12-h infusion, continuous IV infusion	Antin 1990
AIDS-associated neutropenia	4–8 µg/kg	—	6 mo	SC injection	Groopman et al 1987

percentage of leukemic blast cells in S phase, which further enhances cytarabine cytotoxicity (Cannistra et al 1989).

Cytarabine followed by sargramostim (*E. coli*, Schering) has been used in 12 patients with poor-prognosis, newly diagnosed acute myelocytic leukemia (Estey et al 1990). Early leukemic relapse was observed in only one of eight evaluable patients, which is similar to early relapse rates without a colony-stimulating factor. This suggests that the combination can be safely evaluated in larger controlled clinical trials.

■ Pharmacokinetics

In humans, the elimination of sargramostim appears to follow two phases (see table). The longer apparent half-life for subcutaneously administered doses suggests that absorption from the subcutaneous site may be both dose dependent and rate limiting for sargramostim. The nonglycosylated product from *E. coli* produces biphasic half-lives of 0.24 to 1.18 hours and 0.62 to 9.07 hours following an intravenous bolus and intravenous infusion, respectively (Cebon et al 1990). Of interest, clearance of sargramostim ranged from 3 to 32 L/h and was greatest for doses less than 3 µg/kg given subcutaneously. Clearance of drug was slowest following an intravenous infusion over 2 hours, which produced very high peak plasma concentrations of up to 24 ng/mL. This suggests that there may be a saturable mechanism of drug elimination and/or that bioavailability differs considerably for the two administration methods. Very little if any sargramostim is excreted intact in the urine, although catabolism to inactive fragments in the renal tubules may constitute a major route of elimination. In one trial, only 0.001 to 0.2% of immunoreactive sargramostim appeared in the urine (Cebon et al 1990).

In preclinical studies, there was a correlation between the degree of N-linked glycosylation and delayed drug clearance. This produced longer plasma half-lives of human sargramostim in rats (Donahue et al 1986).

■ Side Effects and Toxicity

Dose-dependent toxic effects are produced by sargramostim, with moderate to severe effects noted at doses above 16 µg/kg/d (Brandt et al 1988). Severe dose-limiting effects were noted at doses of 32 µg/kg and especially 64 µg/kg/d. These high-dose effects include pericarditis, fluid retention, and venous thromboses (Brandt et al 1988). The fluid retention with high doses appears to result from a capillary leak syndrome similar to that seen with interleukin-2. At lower daily doses, toxic effects include a flulike syndrome characterized by lethargy, malaise, and fever. Headache is also sometimes described. The onset of fever directly follows the administration of sargramostim by 60 to 90 minutes and temperatures are rarely above 38.5°C. Drug-induced fevers have a short duration of about 1 to 4 hours in contrast to the brisk onset continual fevers of an infectious etiology.

A first-dose cardiopulmonary effect may occur in some patients. It is characterized by hypoxia and hypotension and is more common with 2-hour infusions than subcutaneous injections (Lieschke et al 1989a). Symptoms include flushing, musculoskeletal pain, dyspnea, and nausea. Tachycardia, hypotension, and arterial oxygen desaturation are also

PRELIMINARY HUMAN PHARMACOKINETICS FOR SARGRAMOSTIM

Preparation (Manufacturer)	Route	Dose (µg/kg)	Half-life α (min)	Half-life β (h)	Time to Peak (h)	Peak Plasma Concentration (ng/mL)	AUC (ng/mL·h)
E. coli	IV	10	17.7	1.5	—	> 50	—
(Schering)	SC	3	—	10–15	3.8	3.6	21.4
	SC	10	—	10–15	6.3	16.2	78.7
Yeast	IV infusion over 2 h	250 µg/m²	12–17	2	—	22	—
(Immunex)	SC	125 µg/m²	—	12–15	2	0.35–3.9	—

Data from Cebon et al 1988 and Leukine® (Sargramostim) Formulary Monograph, Immunex Corporation, 1991.

observed. Dyspnea tended to be especially problematic in patients with coexistent pulmonary diseases such as small cell lung cancer (Lieschke and Morstyn 1990). This effect may be caused by enhanced expression of the Mo1 leukocyte adhesion antigen, resulting in the permanent entrapment of some leukocytes on pulmonary capillary endothelium.

Bone pain is a common side effect of sargramostim. It manifests as a dull aching pain in the flank and in the long bones in children. The pain is typically easily managed with nonsteroidal anti-inflammatory agents. Pain intensity peaks just prior to the two waves of neutrophil release from the bone marrow (at 1–2 hours and 12–24 hours, respectively).

Mild local reactions at subcutaneous injection sites occur in about one third of patients (Lieschke et al 1989b). The sites appear reddened and inflamed but do not progress to open ulcers. Reactions are probably due to the local release of interleukin-1 and TNF from macrophages activated and/or recruited locally by sargramostim. A generalized rash has also been seen in some patients.

At high doses, thromboses at the tip of venous catheters are described (Antman et al 1988). Severe sequelae are rare and include pulmonary embolism and effusions of the peritoneum or pericardia. Other occasional toxic effects include hypoalbuminemia and elevations in alkaline phosphatase and γ-glutamyl transpeptidase (Lieschke and Morstyn 1990).

Neutrophil chemotaxis or migration may be impaired following sargramostim as a result of increased cellular rigidity and adhesiveness (Arnaout et al 1986). In one study circulating neutrophils produced under sargramostim stimulation had an impaired ability to diapedese out of the vascular system into a peripheral site of inflammation, in this case the artificial "skin window" model (Peters et al 1988). The clinical significance of this finding is not established.

REFERENCES

Antin JH. Use of recombinant human granulocyte–macrophage colony-stimulating factor in the treatment of aplastic anemia. In: Mertelsmann R, Herrmann F, eds. *Hematopoietic Growth Factors in Clinical Applications.* New York/Basel: Marcel Dekker; 1990:279–289.

Antin JH, Smith BR, Holmes W, Rosenthal DS. Phase I/II study of recombinant human granulocyte–macrophage colony-stimulating factor in aplastic anemia and the myelodysplastic syndrome. *Blood.* 1988;**72**:705–713.

Antman KS, Griffin JD, Ellias A, et al. Effect of recombinant human granulocyte–macrophage colony-stimulating factor on chemotherapy-induced myelosuppression. *N Engl J Med.* 1988;**319**:593–598.

Arnaout MA, Wang EA, Clark SC. Human recombinant granulocyte–macrophage colony-stimulating factor increases cell–cell adhesion and surface expression of adhesion-promoting surface glycoproteins on mature granulocytes. *J Clin Invest.* 1986;**7**:597–601.

Bhalla K, Birkhofer M, Arlin Z, et al. Effect of recombinant GM-CSF on the metabolism of cytosine arabinoside in normal and leukemic human bone marrow cells. *Leukemia.* 1988;**2**:810–813.

Blazar BR, Kersey JH, McGlave PB, et al. In vivo administration of recombinant human granulocyte/macrophage colony-stimulating factor in acute lymphoblastic leukemia patients receiving purged autografts. *Blood.* 1989;**73**:849–857.

Brandt SJ, Peters WP, Atwater SK, et al. Effect of recombinant human granulocyte–macrophage colony-stimulating factor on hematopoietic reconstitution after high-dose chemotherapy and autologous bone marrow transplantation. *N Engl J Med.* 1988;**318**:869–876.

Buchner T, Hiddeman W, Zuhlsdorf M. Human recombinant granulocyte–macrophage colony stimulating factor (GM-CSF) treatment of patients with acute leukemia in aplasia and at high risk of death. *Behring Inst Mitt.* 1988;**83**:308–312.

Cannistra SA, Groshek P, Griffin JD. Granulocyte–macrophage colony-stimulating factor enhances the cytotoxic effects of cytosine arabinoside in acute myeloblastic leukemia and in the myeloid blast crisis phase of chronic myeloid leukemia. *Leukemia.* 1989;**3**:328–334.

Cannistra SA, Rambaldi A, Spriggs DR, et al. Human granulocyte–macrophage colony-stimulating factor induces expression of the tumor necrosis factor genes by the U937 cell line and by normal human monocytes. *J Clin Invest.* 1987;**79**:1720–1728.

Cannistra SA, Socinski MA, Groshek P, et al. In vivo administration of human granulocyte–monocyte colony stimulating factor (GM-CSF) enhances monocyte tumoricidal activity (abstract). *Proc Am Soc Clin Oncol.* 1988;**7**:167.

Cebon JS, Bury RW, Lieschke GJ, et al. The effects of dose and route of administration on the pharmacokinetics of granulocyte–macrophage colony-stimulating factor. *Eur J Cancer.* 1990;**26**(10):1064–1069.

Cebon J, Dempsey P, Fox R, et al. Pharmacokinetics of human granulocyte–macrophage colony-stimulating factor using a sensitive immunoassay. *Blood.* 1988;**72**:1340–1347.

Cicco NA, Lindemann A, Content J, et al. Inducible production of interleukin-6 by human polymorphonuclear neutrophils: Role of granulocyte–macrophage colony-stimulating factor and tumor necrosis factor-alpha. *Blood.* 1990;**75**(10):2049–2052.

DiPersio J, Billing P, Kaufman S. Characterization of the

human granulocyte–macrophage colony stimulating factor (GM-CSF) receptor. *J Biol Chem.* 1988;**263**:1834–1841.

Donahue RE, Wang EA, Kaufman RJ, et al. Effects of N-linked carbohydrate on the in vivo properties of human GM-CSF. *Cold Spring Harbor Symp Quant Biol.* 1986;**51**:685–692.

Edmonson JH, Long HJ, Jeffries JA, et al. Amelioration of chemotherapy-induced thrombocytopenia by GM-CSF: Apparent dose and schedule dependency. *J Natl Cancer Inst.* 1989;**81**:1510–5112.

Estey EH, Dixon D, Kantarjian M, et al. Treatment of poor-prognosis, newly diagnosed acute myeloid leukemia with ara-C and recombinant human granulocyte–macrophage colony-stimulating factor. *Blood.* 1990;**75**:1766–1769.

Fleishmann J, Golde DW, Weisbart RH. Granulocyte–macrophage colony-stimulating factor enhances phagocytosis of bacteria by human neutrophils. *N Engl J Med.* 1986;**314**:361–363.

Foulke RS, Marshall MH, Trotta PP, Von Hoff DD. In vitro assessment of the effects of granulocyte–macrophage colony-stimulating factor on primary human tumors and derived lines. *Cancer Res.* 1990;**50**:6264–6267.

Ganser A, Hoelzer D. Hematopoietic growth factors in clinical applications. In: Mertelsmann R, Herrmann F, eds. *GM-CSF/Ara-C in Myelodysplastic Syndromes.* New York/Basel: Marcel Dekker; 1990:255–277.

Ganser A, Volers B, Greher J, et al. Recombinant human granulocyte–macrophage colony-stimulating factor in patients with myelodysplastic syndromes—A phase I/II trial. *Blood.* 1989;**73**:31–37.

Gianni AM, Bregni M, Siena S, et al. Recombinant human granulocyte–macrophage colony-stimulating factor reduces hematologic toxicity and widens clinical applicability of high-dose cyclophosphamide treatment in breast cancer and non-Hodgkin's lymphoma. *J Clin Oncol.* 1990;**8**:768–778.

Gianni AM, Siena S, Bregni M, et al. Granulocyte–macrophage colony-stimulating factor to harvest circulating haemopoietic stem cells for autotransplantation. *Lancet.* 1989;**1**:580–585.

Griffin JD. Hematopoietins in oncology: Factoring out myelosuppression. *J Clin Oncol.* 1989;**7**:151–155.

Groopman JE, Mitsuyasu RT, DeLeo MJ, et al. Effect of recombinant human granulocyte–macrophage colony-stimulating factor on myelopoiesis in the acquired immunodeficiency syndrome. *N Engl J Med.* 1987;**317**: 593–598.

Herrmann F, Schulz G, Lindemann A, et al. Hematopoietic responses in patients with advanced malignancy treated with recombinant human granulocyte–macrophage colony-stimulating factor. *J Clin Oncol.* 1989;**7**:159–167.

Hoekman K, Wagstaff J, van Groeningen CJ, et al. Effects of recombinant human granulocyte–macrophage colony-stimulating factor on myelosuppression induced by multiple cycles of high-dose chemotherapy in patients with advanced breast cancer. *J Natl Cancer Inst.* 1991;**83**(21):1546–1553.

Horiguchi J, Warren MK, Kufe D. Expression of the macrophage-specific colony stimulating factor in human monocytes treated with granulocyte–macrophage colony stimulating factor. *Blood.* 1987;**61**:1259.

Karp JE, Burke PJ, Donehower RC. Effects of rhGM-CSF on intracellular ara-C pharmacology in vitro in acute myelocytic leukemia: Comparability with drug-induced humoral stimulatory activity. *Leukemia.* 1990;**4**:553–556.

Kaufman DC, Baer MR, Gao XZ, et al. The granulocyte–macrophage colony-stimulating factor (GM-CSF) gene is inducible in acute myelocytic leukemia (AML). *Proc Am Assoc Cancer Res.* 1988;**29**:55.

Kersey JH, Weisdorf D, Nesbit ME, et al. Comparison of autologous and allogeneic bone marrow transplantation for treatment of high-risk refractory acute lymphoblastic leukemia. *N Engl J Med.* 1987;**317**:461.

Lieschke GJ, Cebon J, Morstyn G. Characterization of the clinical effects of the first dose of granulocyte–macrophage colony-stimulating factor. *Blood.* 1989a;**74**:2634–2643.

Lieschke GJ, Maher D, Cebon J, et al. Effects of bacterially synthesized recombinant human granulocyte–macrophage colony stimulating factor in patients with advanced malignancy. *Ann Intern Med.* 1989b;**110**:357–364.

Lieschke GJ, Maher D, O'Connor M, et al. Phase I study of intravenously administered bacterially synthesized granulocyte–macrophage colony-stimulating factor and comparison with subcutaneous administration. *Cancer Res.* 1990;**50**:606–614.

Lieschke GJ, Morstyn G. Role of G-CSF and GM-CSF in the prevention of chemotherapy-induced neutropenia. In: Mertelsmann R, Herrmann F, eds. *Hematopoietic Growth Factors in Clinical Applications.* New York/Basel: Marcel Dekker; 1990:191–223.

Lindeman A, Oster W, Ziegler-Heitbrock HWL. Recombinant granulocyte–macrophage colony stimulating factor induces monokine secretion by polymorphonuclear leukocytes. *J Clin Invest.* 1989;**83**:1308–1312.

Lopez AF, Williamson DJ, Gamble JR. Recombinant human granulocyte–macrophage colony stimulating factor stimulates in vitro mature human neutrophil and eosinophil function, surface receptor expression, and survival. *J Clin Invest.* 1986;**78**:1220–1228.

Matsuura G. Visual compatibility of sargramostim (GM-CSF) during simulated Y-site administration with selected agents. *Hosp Pharm.* 1992;**27**:200, 202, 209.

Mayer P, Lam C, Obenaus H, et al. Recombinant human GM-CSF induces leukocytosis and activates peripheral blood polymorphonuclear neutrophils in nonhuman primates. *Blood.* 1987;**70**:206–213.

Mazur EM, Cohen JL, Wong GG, et al. Modest stimulatory effect of recombinant human GM-CSF on colony growth from peripheral blood human megakaryocyte progenitor cells. *Exp Hematol.* 1987;**15**:1128–1133.

McColl SR, Kreis C, DiPersio JF. Involvement of guanine nucleotide binding proteins in neutrophil activation and priming by GM-CSF. *Blood.* 1989;**73**:588–591.

Morrisey PJ, Bressler L, Park LS. Granulocyte–macrophage colony-stimulating factor augments the primary antibody response by enhancing the function of antigen-presenting cells. *J Immunol.* 1987;**139**:1113–1117.

Morstyn G, Lieschke GJ, Scherdau W. Clinical experience with human granulocyte colony-stimulating factor and granulocyte macrophage colony stimulating factor. *Semin Hematol.* 1989;**26**:9–13.

Nathan CF. Respiratory burst in adherent human neutrophils: Triggering by colony stimulating factors CSF-GM and CSF-G. *Blood.* 1989;**73**:301–306.

Nemunaitis J, Singer JW, Buckner CD, et al. Use of recombinant human granulocyte–macrophage colony-stimulating factor in autologous marrow transplantation for lymphoid malignancies. *Blood.* 1988;**72**:834–836.

Peters WP, Stuart A, Affronti ML, et al. Neutrophil migration is defective during recombinant human granulocyte–macrophage colony-stimulating factor infusion after autologous bone marrow transplantation in humans. *Blood.* 1988;**72**:1310–1315.

Reed SG, Nathan CF, Phil DL. Recombinant granulocyte/macrophage colony stimulating factor activates macrophages to inhibit *Trypanosoma cruzi* and release hydrogen peroxide: Comparison with interferon gamma. *J Exp Med.* 1987;**166**:1734–1739.

Salmon SE, Liu R. Effects of granulocyte–macrophage colony-stimulating factor on in vitro growth of human solid tumors. *J Clin Oncol.* 1989;**7**:1346–1350.

Silberstein DS, Owen WF, Gasson JC. Enhancement of human eosinophil cytotoxicity and leukotriene synthesis by biosynthetic (recombinant) granulocyte–macrophage colony-stimulating factor. *J Immunol.* 1986;**137**:3290–3294.

Thompson JA, Lee DJ, Kidd P, et al. Subcutaneous granulocyte–macrophage colony-stimulating factor in patients with myelodysplastic syndrome: Toxicity, pharmacokinetics, and hematologic effects. *J Clin Oncol.* 1989;**7**:629–637.

Vadhan-Raj S, Broxmeyer HE, Spitzer G, et al. Stimulation of nonclonal hematopoiesis and suppression of the neoplastic clone after treatment with recombinant human granulocyte–macrophage colony-stimulating factor in a patient with therapy-related myelodysplastic syndrome. *Blood.* 1989;**74**:1491–1498.

Vadhan-Raj S, Buescher S, Broxmeyer HE, et al. Stimulation of myelopoiesis in patients with aplastic anemia by recombinant human granulocyte–macrophage colony-stimulating factor. *N Engl J Med.* 1988;**319**:1628–1634.

Vadhan-Raj S, Keating M, LeMaistre A, et al. Effects of recombinant human granulocyte–macrophage colony-stimulating factor in patients with myelodysplasia syndromes. *N Engl J Med.* 1987;**317**:1545.

Wing EJ, Magee DM, Whiteside TL, et al. Recombinant human granulocyte/macrophage colony-stimulating factor enhances monocyte cytotoxicity and secretion of tumor necrosis factor α and interferon in cancer patients. *Blood.* 1989;**73**:643–646.

Yamashita Y, Nara N, Aoki N. Antiproliferative and differentiative effect of granulocyte–macrophage colony-stimulating factor on a variant human small cell lung cancer cell line. *Cancer Res.* 1989;**49**:5334–5338.

Young DC, K Wagner, Griffin JD. Constitutive expression of the granulocyte–macrophage colony-stimulating factor gene in acute myeloblastic leukemia. *J Clin Invest.* 1987;**79**:100–106.

Semustine

■ Other Names

Methyl-CCNU; MeCCNU; NSC-95441.

■ Chemistry

Structure of semustine

Semustine differs from lomustine only by the presence of a methyl group (rather than a hydroxyl) in the *para* position of the cyclohexyl ring. Like lomustine and carmustine, semustine is quite lipid soluble. Chemically, semustine is 1-(2-chloroethyl)-3-(4-methylcyclohexyl)-1-nitrosourea. Semustine possesses an asymmetric structure which originally facilitated pharmacokinetic studies and is more readily formulated as an oral preparation. Of the three nitrosoureas, semustine is the most lipid soluble followed by lomustine and carmustine. It has a molecular weight of 248 and the empiric formula $C_{10}H_{18}ClN_3O_2$.

■ Antitumor Activity

In preclinical animal tumor screening studies semustine demonstrated activity highly superior to that of the other, commercially available compounds, carmustine and lomustine, in the Lewis lung carcinoma model (Wasserman et al 1975). It was also effective in B-16 melanoma and both intraperitoneally and intracerebrally implanted L-1210 leukemia. According to Schabel (1973) semustine had the greatest activity in a number of solid tumors (including Lewis lung) and quantitatively was only half as toxic as the other nitrosoureas in animals. In a combined preclinical/clinical study, Emanuel et al (1974) found semustine to be effective against several animal tumors with acceptable toxicity and responsiveness to carcinoma of the lung and Hodgkin's disease.

In the clinical review by Wasserman et al (1975) the following response rates were noted for semustine used as a single agent: brain (27%), Hodgkin's disease (26%), non-Hodgkin's lymphomas (18%). Tumors with response rates below 15% include melanoma (12%), lung cancer (10%), breast cancer (4%), colorectal cancer (11%), head and neck cancer (11%), renal cell carcinoma (0%), and cervical cancer (13%). Even in the responsive (> 15%) tumors, semustine consistently demonstrated less antitumor effectiveness than the other, commercially available nitrosoureas.

The initial excitement with semustine was its use in combination chemotherapy with 5-fluorouracil (5-FU) or with 5-FU + vincristine for the treatment of advanced colorectal carcinoma (Moertel et al 1976, Baker et al 1976a,b, Falkson and Falkson 1976); however, with further study these higher response rates were not confirmed (Lokich et al 1977, Moertel 1978, Kemeny et al 1977). The combination of 5-FU + semustine + vincristine + streptozotocin has also been used (Kemeny et al 1988). To date, however, it has not been definitely shown to be superior to single-agent 5-FU (Buroker et al 1984, Weltz et al 1983). In summary, semustine appears to add little to 5-FU alone for the treatment of advanced colorectal cancer.

Of greater interest, however, has been the use of semustine in combination with 5-FU for the *adjuvant* treatment of colorectal cancer. The results, however, are conflicting. An Eastern Cooperative Oncology Group study has shown that 5-FU + semustine is not superior to 5-FU alone for adjuvant treatment of colon cancer (Mansour et al 1989). A Southwest Oncology Group study of 5-FU + semustine versus a surgical control group demonstrated the beneficial effect for the chemotherapy (Panettierre et al 1988). Likewise, the National Surgical Adjuvant Breast and Large Bowel Program (NSABP, Protocol C-01) demonstrated that the combination 5-FU + semustine + vincristine improved disease-free survival and overall survival (over a control of surgery alone) for patients with colon cancer (Wolmark et al 1988). The Veterans' Administration Surgical Oncology Group demonstrated a survival advantage for patients receiving 5-FU + semustine versus observation alone; however, that advantage was only seen in patients with one to four positive nodes in the resected specimen (Higgins et al 1984). And, for patients with rectal cancer, the NSABP demonstrated improvement in disease-free survival and overall survival by treatment with 5-FU + semustine + vincristine versus a control of surgery alone (Fisher et al 1988). In contrast, the Gastrointestinal Tumor Study Group (1984) reported no effect for 5-FU + semustine ± MER-BCG on recurrence-free survival or survival of patients with Dukes' stage B_2, C_1, or C_2 colon cancer. Finally, the Radiation Therapy Oncology Group was not able to demonstrate a benefit from treatment with 5-FU + semustine + irradiation versus irradiation alone for patients with residual, inoperable, or locally recurrent carcinoma of the rectum (Rominger et al 1985).

In summary, there is limited evidence to indicate a role for the use of 5-FU + semustine for patients with colorectal cancer. And, as detailed later, any possible benefit to the use of 5-FU + semustine must be balanced with the human leukemogenic effect of the semustine. Furthermore, more effective and safe 5-FU combinations with leucovorin or levamisole constitute currently recommended treatment for patients with colorectal carcinoma.

A number of studies have included semustine in the adjuvant treatment of gastric cancer. The Eastern Cooperative Oncology Group (ECOG) found no benefit for treatment with surgery + 5-FU + semustine versus surgery alone (Engstrom et al 1985). Similarly, the Italian Gastrointestinal Tumor Study Group (1988) found no difference in survival for patients given 5-FU + semustine after surgery versus surgery alone. And in the Veterans' Administration Study Group study, surgery + 5-FU + semustine gave no improvement in survival versus surgery alone (Higgins et al 1983). In contrast, the Gastrointestinal Study Group reported that adjuvant 5-FU + semustine improved both time to recurrence and survival versus surgery alone (Douglass et al 1984). Thus, there is as yet no consensus on the appropriateness of the 5-FU + semustine used for the adjuvant treatment of patients with gastric cancer.

■ Mechanism of Action

Semustine probably behaves similarly to the related nitrosourea compound lomustine. The principal action resembles alkylation; however, as with the other nitrosoureas there is usually not complete cross-resistance with classic alkylating agents. The cytotoxic effect involves several active metabolites which are produced in part by microsomal mixed function oxidases. Overall, the alkylation of a variety of cellular macromolecules by semustine results in the inhibition of synthesis of both DNA and RNA (Kann et al 1974, Wheeler and Alexander 1974). Carbamoylation of protein is one of the observed processes accounting for the cellular growth inhibition and possibly a blockade in DNA repair. Although there may be slight G_2-phase arrest and increased activity in S phase, the agent does not appear to be cytotoxic in any particular phase of the dividing cell cycle (nonphase specific) (Tobey and Crissman 1975).

■ Availability and Storage

Semustine is investigationally available from the National Cancer Institute in 100-mg (brown and black), 50-mg (brown), and 1-mg (white) hard gelatin capsules. Mannitol, magnesium stearate, and colloidal silicon dioxide (inert ingredients) are also present. Storage of the drug under refrigeration is recommended but not absolutely essential. Exposures of semustine to temperatures above 9°F (32.2°C) is to be avoided. The drug may be stored in the freezer. Prolonged exposure to moisture should be avoided as the drug is hygroscopic.

■ Preparation for Use, Stability, and Admixture

The appropriate dose should be dispensed to the nearest 10 mg. Because of delayed myelosuppressive toxicity, probably no more than a single treatment should be dispensed at one time. Again, all doses should be protected from excess heat and moisture. Capsules in intact bottles are stable for 3 years if refrigerated, 1 year at room temperature, and 30 days at temperatures greater than 40°C.

■ Administration

All doses of semustine are intended for oral administration. Taking the drug on an empty stomach may help to lessen the severity of nausea and vomiting, but individual patient sensitivity or preference should be observed. Several investigators recommended that alcohol be avoided for a short period after taking this drug. When semustine is taken on an empty stomach, absorption is relatively complete, usually after 30 to 60 minutes. Thus, vomiting after this time usually will not significantly reduce drug efficacy. Other drugs that might cause vomiting should optimally be given at least 2 hours after semustine. This will allow the drug to be absorbed before the nausea and vomiting produced by a second agent.

■ Special Precautions

A number of studies had hinted that semustine might be a leukemogenic agent (Panettiere et al 1988, Engstrom et al 1985, Gastrointestinal Study Group 1984). A retrospective study by Boice et al (1983) appears to have confirmed that semustine is indeed leukemogenic.

■ Drug Interactions

None are known.

■ Dosage

The dosage range for semustine has been reported to be 125 to 200 mg/m^2 given no more frequently than every 6 weeks. Often an extended period of observation without further nitrosourea treatment (6–10 weeks) may be necessary to allow for resolution of myelosuppression, which is characteristically delayed. Dosage reduction is thus indicated for patients with compromised bone marrow status and probably also for patients with severe liver impairment. No specific dose reduction schemes have been promulgated. It should be noted that with repeated doses, myelosuppression tends to be cumulative.

■ Pharmacokinetics

As with the other nitrosourea compounds, semustine undergoes considerable biotransformation, partially by microsomal enzymes (Hill et al 1975). After an oral dose, peak, plasma levels occur within 1 to 6 hours. Up to 60% of a given dose can be retrieved in the urine as metabolites after 48 hours. Some of these metabolites are active and have much longer half-lives in the blood than the parent compound (Sponzo et al 1973).

Because of its low molecular weight and high lipid solubility, this agent and/or its metabolites readily cross the blood–brain barrier. Cerebrospinal fluid levels of some of these metabolites approximate simultaneously measured plasma levels, suggesting a role for this agent in brain and other central nervous system tumors. Sponzo et al (1973) have noted that absolute cerebrospinal fluid drug levels are 15 to 30% of recurrent plasma levels.

Metabolism appears to be at least partially mediated by microsomal enzyme systems. Thus, bil-

Side Effects and Toxicity

The dose-limiting hematologic toxic effect for semustine is a protracted myelosuppression (Sieber and Adamson 1974). The nadir for thrombocytopenia usually occurs 4 weeks after an oral dose but can occur as long as 8 weeks after dosing (Young et al 1973). Depression of both white and red cells usually occurs later than the decrease in platelets. Resolution of bone marrow effect may not occur until after 4 to 10 weeks have elapsed. Myelosuppression may thus be cumulative with subsequent dosing. Some oncologists routinely reduce the second or third dose by 25 to 50% to prevent cumulative myelosuppression.

The gastrointestinal side effects of nausea and vomiting commonly occur 4 to 6 hours after administration and are occasionally followed by a lingering sensation of anorexia. Antiemetics have been used with varying degrees of success.

Renal and hepatic toxic effects are seen infrequently. These usually resolve without affecting the treatment course and usually manifest only as abnormalities in liver function tests or as a rise in the blood urea nitrogen, respectively. Delayed hepatocellular damage, however, has been dose limiting in some animal studies. Renal toxicity has also been noted, especially in monkeys. An acute central nervous system toxicity presenting as a metabolic encephalopathy has been reported (Schein 1969).

Rare pulmonary fibrosis has been described with semustine (Block et al 1990).

Special Applications

There are none.

REFERENCES

Ahmann DL. Nitrosoureas in the management of disseminated malignant melanoma. *Cancer Treat Rep.* 1976;60:747–751.

Baker LH, Talley RW, Matter R, et al. Phase III comparison of the treatment of advanced gastrointestinal cancer with bolus weekly 5-FU vs methyl-CCNU plus bolus weekly 5-FU: A Southwest Oncology Group study. *Cancer.* 1976a;38:1–7.

Baker LH, Vaitkevicius EG. Gastrointestinal Committee of the Southwest Oncology Group. Randomized prospective trial comparing 5-fluouracil (NSC-19893) to 5-fluorouracil and methyl-CCNU (NSC-95441) in advanced gastrointestinal cancer. *Cancer Treat Rep.* 1976b;60:733–737.

Block M, Lachowiez RM, Rios C, Hirschl S. Pulmonary fibrosis associated with low-dose adjuvant methyl-CCNU. *Med Pediatr Oncol.* 1990;18(3):256–260.

Boice JD Jr, Greene MH, Killen JY Jr, et al. Leukemia and preleukemia after adjuvant treatment of gastrointestinal cancer with semustine (methyl-CCNU). *N Engl J Med.* 1983;309(18):1079–1084.

Buroker T, Moertel C, Gleming T, et al. A randomized comparison of 5-FU containing drug combinations with 5-FU alone in advanced colorectal carcinoma (meeting abstract). *Proc Annu Meet Am Soc Clin Oncol.* 1984;3:138.

Douglass HD Jr, Stablein DM, Bruckner HW, et al. Long term follow-up of gastric cancer adjuvant therapy: The Gastrointestinal Tumor Study Group experience (meeting abstract). In: *Fourth International Conference on the Adjuvant Therapy of Cancer;* 1984:61.

Emanual NM, Vermel EM, Ostrovskaya LA, Korman NP. Experimental and clinical studies of the anti-tumor activity of 1-methyl-1-nitrosourea (NSC-23909). *Cancer Chemother Rep.* 1974;58:135–148.

Engstrom PF, Lavin PT, Douglass HD Jr, Brunner KW. Postoperative adjuvant 5-fluorouracil plus methyl CCNU therapy for gastric cancer patients. Eastern Cooperative Oncology Group study (EST 3275). *Cancer.* 1985;55(9):1868–1873.

Falkson G, Falkson HC. Fluorouracil, methyl-CCNU and vincristine in cancer of the colon. *Cancer.* 1976;38:1468–1470.

Fisher B, Wolmark N, Rockette H, et al. Postoperative adjuvant chemotherapy or radiation therapy for rectal cancer: Results from NSABP protocol R-01. *J Natl Cancer Inst.* 1988;80(1):21–29.

Gastrointestinal Tumor Study Group. Adjuvant therapy of colon cancer—Results of a prospectively randomized trial. *N Engl J Med.* 1984;310(12):737–743.

Higgins GA Jr, Amadeo JH, McElhinney J, McCaughan JJ, Keehn RJ. Efficacy of prolonged intermittent therapy with combined 5-fluorouracil and methyl-CCNU following resection for carcinoma of the large bowel. A Veterans Administration Surgical Oncology Group report. *Cancer.* 1984;53(1):1–8.

Higgins GA, Amadeo JH, Smith DE, Humphrey EW, Keehn RJ. Efficacy of prolonged intermittent therapy with combined 5-FU and methyl-CCNU following resection for gastric carcinoma. A Veterans Administration Surgical Oncology Group report. *Cancer.* 1983;52(6):1105–1012.

Hill DI, Kirk MC, Struck RF. Microsomal metabolism of nitrosoureas. *Cancer Res.* 1975;35:296–301.

Italian Gastrointestinal Tumor Study Group. Adjuvant treatments following curative resection for gastric cancer. *Br J Surg.* 1988;**75**(11):1100–1104.

Kann HE Jr, Kohn KW, Wilderlife L. Effects of 1, 3-bis(2-chloroethyl)-1-nitrosourea and related compounds on nuclear RNA metabolism. *Cancer Res.* 1974;**34**:1982–1988.

Kemeny N, Reichman B, Geller N, Hollander P. Implementation of the group sequential methodology in a randomized trial in metastatic colorectal carcinoma. *Am J Clin Oncol.* 1988;**11**(1):66–72.

Kemeny N, Yagoda A, Golbey R. Randomized study of 2 different schedules of methyl CCNU (Me CCNU), 5-fluorouracil (5-FU), and vincristine (VCR) for metastatic colorectal carcinoma. *Proc Am Assoc Cancer Res ASCO.* 1977;**18**:336.

Lokich JJ, Skarin AT, Mayer RJ, Frei E III. Lack of effectiveness of combined 5-fluorouracil and methyl-CCNU therapy in advanced colorectal cancer. *Cancer.* 1977;**40**:2792–2796.

Mansour E, Ryan L, Lerner H, et al. Lack of effectiveness of 5-FU and methyl CCNU as compared to 5-FU for adjuvant therapy in colon cancer: A randomized trial of the Eastern Cooperative Oncology Group (ECOG) (EST2276) (meeting abstract). *Proc Annu Meet Am Soc Clin Oncol.* 1989;**8**:115.

Moertel CG. Chemotherapy of gastrointestinal cancer. *N Engl J Med.* 1978;**299**(19):1049–1052.

Moertel CG, Sahutt AJ, Reitemeier RJ, Hahn RG. Therapy for gastrointestinal cancer with the nitrosoureas alone and in drug combination. *Cancer Treat Rep.* 1976;**60**(6):729–732.

Panettiere FJ, Goodman PJ, Costanzi JJ, et al. Adjuvant therapy in large bowel adenocarcinoma: Long-term results of a Southwest Oncology Group study. *J Clin Oncol.* 1988;**6**(6):947–954.

Rominger CJ, Gunderson LL, Gelber RD, Conner N. Radiation therapy alone or in combination with chemotherapy in the treatment of residual or inoperable carcinoma of the rectum and rectosigmoid or pelvic recurrence following colorectal surgery. Radiation Therapy Oncology Group study (76-16). *Am J Clin Oncol.* 1985;**8**(2):118–127.

Schabel FM. Historical development and future promise of the nitrosoureas as anticancer agents. *Cancer Chemother Rep.* 1973;**4**(Pt 3):3–6.

Schein PS. Methyl-1-nitrosourea depression of brain nicotinamide adenine dinucleotide in the production of neurological toxicity. *Proc Soc Exp Biol Med.* 1969;**131**:517–520.

Sieber SM, Adamson RH. Potential hazards associated with the use of 1-methyl-1 nitrosourea (NSC-23909). *Cancer Chemother Rep.* 1974;**58**:617–618.

Sponzo RW, DeVita VT, Oliverio VT. Physiologic disposition of 1-(2-chloroethyl)-3-cyclohexyl-1-nitrosourea (CCNU) and 1-(2-chloroethyl)-3-(4-methylcyclohexyl)-1-nitrosourea (MeCCNU) in man. *Cancer.* 1973;**31**:1154–1159.

Tobey RA, Crissman HA. Comparative effects of three nitrosourea derivatives on mammalian cell cycle progression. *Cancer Res.* 1975;**35**:460–470.

Wasserman TH, Slavik M, Carter SK. Methyl CCNU in clinical cancer therapy. *Cancer Treat Rev.* 1975;**1**:251.

Weltz MD, Perry DJ, Blom J, Butler WM. Methyl-CCNU, 5-fluorouracil, vincristine, and streptozocin (MCF-STREP) in metastatic colo-rectal carcinoma. *J Clin Oncol.* 1983;**1**(2):135–137.

Wheeler GP, Alexander JA. Duration of inhibition of synthesis of DNA in tumors and host tissues after single doses of nitrosoureas. *Cancer Res.* 1974;**34**:1957–1964.

Wolmark N, Fisher B, Rockette H, et al. Postoperative adjuvant chemotherapy or BCG for colon cancer: Results from NSABP protocol R-01. *J Natl Cancer Inst.* 1988;**80**(1):30–36.

Young RC, Walker MD, Canellos GP, Schein PS, Chabner BA, DeVita VT. Initial clinical trials with methyl CCNU 1-(2-chloroethyl)-3-(4-methyl cyclohexyl)-1-nitrosourea (Me CCNU). *Cancer.* 1973;**31**:1164–1169.

Spirogermanium

Other Names

SG; NSC-192965; spirogermanium HCl.

Chemistry

Structure of spirogermanium

Spirogermanium is a germanium-containing aza-spirane with a molecular weight of 414 and the empiric formula $C_{17}H_{36}GeN_2 \cdot HCl$. The full chemical name is 8,8-diethyl-N,N-dimethyl-2-aza-8-germa-spiro[4.5]decane-2-propanamine dihydrochloride. It is a white powder that is freely soluble in water and 95% ethanol. The drug had antitumor activity in animals bearing Walker-256, mammary adenocarcinoma, and prostatic carcinoma. A good review article on the compound was published by Slavik et al (1983).

■ Antitumor Activity

In phase I studies the drug induced a response in one patient with chronic lymphocytic lymphoma (CLL) (Wooley et al 1979). In phase II studies the drug has had some activity in heavily pretreated patients with Hodgkin's (2 partial responses in 9 patients) and non-Hodgkin's (2 complete response in 38 patients) lymphoma (Sessa et al 1989, Boros et al 1986). Others have not demonstrated that activity (Eisenhauer et al 1985b). Falkson and Falkson (1983) found a response rate of 25% in women with refractory breast cancer. The drug has been inactive in patients with small cell lung cancer (Ettinger et al 1990); non-small cell lung cancer (Lad et al 1989, Dhingra et al 1986, Ettinger et al 1989); melanoma (Alavi et al 1989, Eisenhauer et al 1985a); colon cancer (Pandya et al 1988); colorectal carcinoma (Ajani et al 1986); prostate cancer (Saiers et al 1987a, Dexeus et al 1986); renal cell carcinoma (Schulman et al 1984, Saiers et al 1987b); glioblastoma multiforme (Goodwin et al 1987); cervical cancer (Brenner et al 1985); ovarian cancer (Weiselberg et al 1982, Brenner et al 1983, Kavanagh et al 1985); and breast cancer (Kuebler et al 1984, Falkson and Falkson 1983, Budman et al 1982b, Pinnamaneni et al 1984). Trope et al (1981) reported an 11% response rate for spirogermanium in patients with refractory ovarian cancer.

■ Mechanism of Activity

The antitumor activity of spirogermanium appears to be via an inhibition of protein synthesis (Kanematsu and Kada 1978). Mirabelli et al (1989) noted that spirogermanium can also affect macrophage function.

■ Availability and Storage

Spirogermanium is supplied by the Division of Cancer Treatment, National Cancer Institute, for injection in 10-mL vials containing 10 mg/mL spirogermanium with sodium chloride 9 mg and sodium hydroxide and/or hydrochloric acid to adjust to pH 5.0 to 6.0 in Sterile Water for Injection, USP. The intact vials should be stored at room temperature.

The compound is also available as an investigational oral compound.

■ Preparation for Use, Stability, and Admixture

For administration by slow intravenous infusion, further dilution in 0.9% Sodium Chloride, USP, is recommended. The intravenous solution should be used only if the solution is sparkling clear. The intact vials are stable for at least 2 years at room temperature.

■ Administration

The initial schedule of administration was a single dose administered every 6 weeks. At doses of 50 mg/m^2 or greater, burning at the injection site and transient central nervous system toxicity (euphoria, dysmetria, nystagmus) were noted (Woolley et al 1979). More prolonged infusions over 15 to 30 minutes allowed the administration of doses of 80 to 120 mg/m^2 without toxicity (at a rate of 1–2 mg/min).

Legha et al (1983) demonstrated that 150 mg/m^2 spirogermanium could be given as a constant intravenous infusion for 30 days.

The oral formulation of the drug is given daily at a dose of 200 mg (Harvey et al 1990).

■ Special Precautions

Three cases of pulmonary toxicity possibly associated with spirogermanium have been reported (see Side Effects and Toxicity).

■ Drug Interactions

None are known.

■ Dosage

The most commonly used schedule in phase II trials has been as an intravenous infusion three times per week for 2 weeks, two times per week for the next 2 weeks, and then weekly. The doses have ranged from 80 to 120 mg/m^2 (Budman et al 1982a, Lad et al 1989, Sessa et al 1989, Vogelzang et al 1985). Other doses given have included 150–200 mg/m^2/d × 5 repeated every 14 days. Legha and colleagues (1983) demonstrated that spirogermanium could be given as a continuous infusion at a dose of 150 mg/m^2/d × 30 days. The dose recommended for the oral schedule is 200 mg/d (Harvey et al 1990).

■ Pharmacokinetics

In one reported study of the pharmacokinetics of spirogermanium in humans, elimination from the plasma was rapid. The mean plasma half-life was 8.8 ± 3.4 minutes, the mean systemic clearance was 5.5 ± 3.4 L/min·m^2, and the volume of distribution at steady state was 67.2 ± 49.9 L/m^2. The steady-state plasma concentration was 349 ± 299 mg/mL. No evidence of drug accumulation was noted. Enterohepatic circulation of the drug was suggested (Hutson et al 1986).

In contrast to the rapid half-life, Larsson et al (1980) reported a two-compartment model for the drug with a terminal elimination phase half-life of 60 to 200 minutes. The initial (distribution) half-life was 10 to 20 minutes. Their data suggested a 2- to 3-day interval between doses.

■ Side Effects and Toxicity

Dose-limiting toxic effects on the bolus schedule have involved central neurotoxicity manifested by dizziness, euphoria, nystagmus, lethargy, and visual distortion. These signs and symptoms were completely reversible. As noted earlier, doses could be escalated to 80 to 120 mg/m^2 by prolonging the infusion to deliver 1 to 2 mg/min. Burning at the site of injection was also noted at the higher doses (Woolley et al 1979, 1984, Lad et al 1989, Sessa et al 1989). As noted under Special Precautions, three cases of presumed pulmonary toxicity consisting of dyspnea and interstitial infiltration have been reported (after cumulative doses of 2.5 to 12g). One patient improved after treatment with 60 mg/d prednisone (Dixon et al 1984).

The oral form of spirogermanium produces nausea and vomiting as dose-limiting toxic effects (Harvey et al 1990). In addition, some patients receiving the oral formulation developed elevations in liver transaminases.

■ Special Applications

Spirogermanium has been proposed as an agent to treat rheumatoid arthritis (Mirabelli et al 1988). It has also been used to treat experimental *Trypanosoma cruzi* (Tanowitz et al 1987) and malaria (Mrema et al 1983).

REFERENCES

Ajani JA, Faintuch JS, McClure RK, Levin B, Boman BM, Krakoff IH. Phase II study of spirogermanium in patients with advanced colorectal carcinoma. *Invest New Drugs.* 1986;**4**(4):383–385.

Alavi JB, Schoenfeld D, Skeel RT, Kirkwood R, Tsung L, Marsh JC. Phase II trial of spirogermanium and vindesine in malignant glioma. *Am J Clin Oncol.* 1989;**2**(1):8–10.

Boros L, Tsiatis AA, Neiman RS, Mann RB, Blick JH. Phase II Eastern Cooperative Oncology Group study of spirogermanium in previously treated lymphoma. *Cancer Treat Rep.* 1986;**70**(7):917–918.

Brenner DE, Jones HW, Rosenshein NB, et al. Phase II evaluation of spirogermanium in advanced ovarian carcinoma. *Cancer Treat Rep.* 1983;**67**(2):193–194.

Brenner DE, Rosenshein NB, Dilon M, et al. Phase II study of spirogermanium in patients with advanced carcinoma of the cervix. *Cancer Treat Rep.* 1985;**69**(4):457–458.

Budman DR, Schulman P, Vinciguerra V, Desnan TJ. Phase I trial of spirogermanium given by infusion in a multiple-dose schedule. *Cancer Treat Rep.* 1982a;**66**(1):173–175.

Budman DR, Ginsberg S, Perry M, et al. Phase II trial of spirogermanium in breast adenocarcinoma: A Cancer and Leukemia Group B study. *Cancer Treat Rep.* 1982b;**6**(8):1667–1668.

Dexeus FH, Logothetis C, Samuels ML, Hossan B. Phase II study of spirogermanium in metastatic prostate cancer. *Cancer Treat Rep.* 1986;**70**(9):1129–1130.

Dhingra HM, Umsawasdi T, Chiuten DF, et al. Phase II study of spirogermanium in advanced (extensive) non-small cell lung cancer. *Cancer Treat Rep.* 1986;**70**(5):673–674.

Dixon C, Hagemeister F, Legha S, Bodey GP. Pulmonary toxicity associated with spirogermanium. *Cancer Treat Rep.* 1984;**68**(6):907–908.

Eisenhauer E, Kerr I, Bodurtha A, et al. A phase II study of spirogermanium in patients with metastatic malignant melanoma. An NCI Canada Clinical Trials Group study. *Invest New Drugs.* 1985a;**3**(3):303–305.

Eisenhauer E, Quirt I, Connors JM, Maroun J, Skillings J. A phase II study of spirogermanium as second line therapy in patients with poor prognosis lymphoma. An NCI Canada Clinical Trials Group study. *Invest New Drugs.* 1985b;**3**(3):307–310.

Ettinger DS, Finkelstein DM, Donehower RC, et al. Phase II study of N-methylformamide, spirogermanium, and 4-demethoxydaunorubicin in the treatment of non-small cell lung cancer (EST 3583): An Eastern Cooperative Oncology Group study. *Med Pediatr Oncol.* 1989;**17**(3):197–201.

Ettinger DS, Finkelstein DM, Abeloff MD, et al. Phase II study of N-methylformamide (NSC-3051) and spirogermanium (NSC-192965) in the treatment of advanced small cell lung cancer. *Invest New Drugs.* 1990;**8**(2):183–185.

Falkson G, Falkson HC. Phase II trial of spirogermanium for treatment of advanced breast cancer. *Cancer Treat Rep.* 1983;**67**(2):189–190.

Goodwin JW, Crowley J, Tranum B, et al. Phase II trial of spirogermanium in central nervous system tumors: A Southwest Oncology Group study. *Cancer Treat Rep.* 1987;**71**(1):99–100.

Harvey J, McFadden M, Smith FP, Joubert L, Schein PS. Phase I study of oral spirogermanium. *Invest New Drugs.* 1990;**8**(1):53–56.

Hutson P, Evrard M, Cobleish M, Lad T, McGuire SP,

Cichock G. Pharmacokinetic and pharmacodynamic studies of spirogermanium (SG) in advanced non-small cell lung cancer (NSCLC) (meeting abstract). *Proc Am Soc Clin Oncol.* 1986;**5**:38.

Kanematsu K, Kada T. Mutagencity of metal compounds (abstract). *Mutat Res.* 1978;**53**:207–208.

Kavanagh JJ, Saul PB, Copeland LJ, Gershenson DM, Krakoff IH. Continuous-infusion spirogermanium for the treatment of refractory carcinoma of the ovary: A phase II trial. *Cancer Treat Rep.* 1985;**69**(1):139–140.

Kuebler JP, Tormey DC, Harper GR, Change YC, Khandekar JD, Falkson G. Phase II study of spirogermanium in advanced breast cancer. *Cancer Treat Rep.* 1984;**68**(1):1515–1516.

Lad TE, Bloush RR, Evrard M, et al. Phase II trial of spirogermanium in advanced non-small cell lung cancer. An Illinois Cancer Council study. *Invest New Drugs.* 1989;**7**(2/3):223–224.

Larsson H, Trope C, Mattson W, Orbett B. Clinical pharmacokinetics of intravenously administered spirogermanium. *Proc Am Soc Clin Oncol.* 1980;**21**:334.

Legha SS, Ajani JA, Bodey GP. Phase I study of spirogermanium given daily. *J Clin Oncol.* 1983;**1**(5):331–336.

Mirabelli CK, Badger AM, Sung CP, et al. Pharmacological activities of spirogemanium and other structurally related azaspiranes: Effects on tumor cell and macrophage functions. *Anticancer Drug Des.* 1989;**3**(4):231–242.

Mirabelli CK, Sung CP, Picker DH, Barnard C, Hydes P, Badger AM. Effect of metal containing compounds on superoxide release from phorbol myristate acetate stimulated murine peritoneal macrophages: Inhibition by auranofin and spirogermanium. *J Rheumatol.* 1988;**15**(7):1064–1069.

Mrema JE, Slavik M, Davis J. Spirogermanium: A new drug with antimalarial activity against chloroquine-resistant *Plasmodium falciparum*. *Int J Clin Pharmacol Ther Toxicol.* 1983;**21**(4):167–171.

Pandya KJ, Kramar A, Asbury RF, Haller DG. A phase II study of spirogermanium in advanced large bowel cancer. An Eastern Cooperative Oncology Group study. *Am J Clin Oncol.* 1988;**11**(4):496–498.

Pinnamaneni K, Yap HY, Lesha SS, Blemenschein GR, Bodey GP. Phase II study of spirogermanium in the treatment of metastatic breast cancer. *Cancer Treat Rep.* 1984;**68**(9):1197–1198.

Saiers JH, Blumenstein B, Slavik M, Costanzi JH, Crawford ED. Phase II study of spirogermanium in advanced adenocarcinoma of the prostate: A Southwest Oncology Group study. *Cancer Treat Rep.* 1987a;**1**(12):1305–1306.

Saiers JH, Slavik M, Stephens RL, Crawford ED. Therapy for advanced renal cell cancer with spirogermanium: A Southwest Oncology Group study. *Cancer Treat Rep.* 1987b;**71**(2):207–208.

Schulman P, Davis RB, Rafla S, Green M, Henderson E. Phase II trial of spirogermanium in advanced renal cell carcinoma: A Cancer and Leukemia Group B study. *Cancer Treat Rep.* 1984;**68**(1):1305–1306.

Sessa C, Ten Bokkel Huinik W, Clavel M, et al. A phase II study of spirogermanium in patients with advanced malignant lymphoma. *Invest New Drugs.* 1989;**7**(2/3):219–222.

Slavik M, Blanc O, Davis J. Spirogemanium: A new investigational drug of novel structure and lack of bone marrow toxicity. *Invest New Drugs.* 1983;**1**(3):225–234.

Tanowitz HB, Brennessel DJ, Baum SG, Salso MP, Braunstein V, Wittner M. *Trypanosoma cruzi*: Inhibition by spirogermanium hydrochloride. *Exp Parasitol.* 1987;**64**(1):57–63.

Trope C, Mattsson W, Gynning I, Johnsson JE, Sigurdsson K, Orbert B. Phase II study of spirogermanium in advanced ovarian malignancy. *Cancer Treat Rep.* 1981;**65**(1/2):119–120.

Vogelzang NJ, Gesme DH, Kennedy BJ. A phase II study of spirogermanium in advanced human malignancy. *Am J Oncol.* 1985;**8**(4):341–344.

Weiselberg L, Budman DR, Schulman P, Vinciguerra V, Desnan TJ, Pasmantier M. Phase II trial of spirogermanium in advanced epithelial carcinoma of the ovary. *Cancer Treat Rep.* 1982;**66**(8):1675–1676.

Woolley PV, Ahlgren JD, Byrne PJ, Priego VM, Schein PS. A phase I trial of spirogermanium administered on a continuous infusion schedule. *Invest New Drugs.* 1984;**2**(3):305–309.

Woolley PV, Maguire P, Fox P, Hoth D, Slavik M, Schein P. Studies with the antitumor agent spirogermanium. *Proc Am Assoc Cancer Res.* 1979;**20**:436.

Spiromustine

■ Other Names

Spirohydantoin mustard; NSC-172112.

■ Chemistry

Structure of spiromustine

Spiromustine was rationally developed as an agent that would cross the blood–brain barrier (Peng et al 1975). Structurally, it is a combination of a nitrogen mustard alkylating agent and a derivative of the anticonvulsant 5,5-diphenylhydantoin. The drug penetrates the blood–brain barrier so well in dogs that the concentration of free drug in the cerebrospinal fluid is comparable to the concentration of free drug in the plasma (Plowman et al 1977).

Chemically, spiromustine is 1,3-diazaspiro-(4,5)decane-2,4-dione, 3-[2-[bis(2 chloroethyl)amino]-ethyl]—Spirohydantoin Mustard. It has a molecular weight of 336.3 and the empiric formula $C_{14}H_{23}Cl_2N_3O_2$. Spiromustine is a water-insoluble solid that rapidly hydrolyzes in aqueous solution. The water solubility alone is less than 10 µg/mL. The compound is soluble in N,N-dimethylacetamide (>300 mg/mL).

Antitumor Activity

Spiromustine has had documented activity in phase I trials in patients with gliomas (Curt et al 1985) and in three patients with metastases to the brain (gastric cancer, small cell carcinoma of the lung, and renal cell carcinoma) (Brown et al 1986).

The severe neurotoxicity noted with spiromustine has precluded all but one published phase II clinical trial. Prados et al (1987) conducted a phase II trial of the agent in 15 evaluable patients with recurrent malignant gliomas. All had had prior surgery, radiotherapy, and treatment with a nitrosourea. The dose and schedule used was 3 mg/m² twice a week with 2- to 4-day intervals between doses, for 3 consecutive weeks. No objective responses were noted.

Mechanism of Action

Spiromustine is thought to exert its antitumor effect by crosslinking DNA. The agent is not cell cycle specific (Deen et al 1979, Shoemaker et al 1983).

Availability and Storage

Spiromustine is available from the National Cancer Institute as a duo-pak containing one 10-mL vial of sterile spiromustine 60 mg in dry form and one ampule (with 1 mL) of sterile N,N-dimethylacetamide (DMA) for use as a solvent. The package containing intact vials and ampules should be stored under refrigeration (28°C).

Preparation for Use, Stability, and Admixture

The preparation for use is somewhat complicated. One milliliter of the sterile DMA is added to the vial containing the 60 mg of spiromustine. The resultant solution contains 60 mg/mL drug. The appropriate dose of spiromustine is then added to a 100-mL bottle of Intralipid® (fat emulsion 10%, Cutter) with constant swirling. The use of a Vortex® mechanical mixer to create this swirling is recommended. (See Fortner et al [1975] for details.) The drug should be added into the midst of the swirling Intralipid® using a 22-gauge, 3.5-in. spinal needle. The emulsion–drug mixture should be administered within 60 minutes. The mixture should *never* be added to aqueous solutions. Spiromustine is extremely unstable in aqueous media.

It should also be remembered that contact of undiluted DMA solvent with plastic items should be avoided. Glass syringes are recommended.

The stability of the drug in the intact vials has not been reported. When prepared in the Intralipid® emulsion, spiromustine decomposes rapidly, with 10% decomposition in 45 to 54 minutes. Therefore, administration of the emulsion admixture should be completed within this period and should not exceed 60 minutes.

One final point is that solubility of spiromustine is sufficiently poor that a 1 mg/mL concentration of the drug in the Intralipid® emulsion should not be exceeded.

Administration

A total of nine phase I trials have explored a variety of schedules. The results of those phase I trials in terms of recommended doses are detailed in the table on the top of page 846.

In each of the trials, central nervous system reactions constituted the dose-limiting toxic effect. Pretreatment with physostigmine ameliorated some of the neurotoxic effects (see Side Effects and Toxicity). The most reasonable dose and schedule appears to be 6 mg/m² per week × 3 weeks followed by a 1-week rest period, then repeated. Pretreatment with 2 mg of physostigmine by slow infusion prior to administration of spiromustine is recommended, with repeated doses of physostigmine every 60 to 90 minutes as needed (Brown et al 1986).

Special Precautions

Spiromustine can cause severe neurotoxic effects (see Side Effects and Toxicity).

Drug Interactions

None are known.

PHASE I TRIAL RESULTS

Schedule	Maximally Tolerated Dose (mg/m²)	Recommended Phase II Dose (mg/m²)	Comments	Reference
Once every 3 wk	6	—		Pazdur et al 1987
Weekly × 3, rest 2 wk	3	—		Pazdur et al 1987
IV bolus every 4 h × 3 every 28 d	12.5	—	Physostigmine reversed toxic effects	Curt et al 1985
Daily × 3, every 28 d	Too toxic	—		Brown et al 1986
IV every other day × 3 every 28 d	Too toxic	—		Brown et al 1986
Weekly × 3 every 28 d	6 (8 with physostigmine)	6		Brown et al 1986
1-h infusion every 4 wk	6	—		Sigman et al 1984
Daily × 5	4.8 mg/m²/d	—		Sigman et al 1984
IV bolus once weekly × 3 every 28 d	9.5 mg/m²/wk	—	With physostigmine pediatric trial	Heideman et al 1988

■ Dosage

As mentioned earlier, the most reasonable dose/schedule for spiromustine is probably 6 mg/m² per week × 3 weeks (Brown et al 1986). The published phase II trial dose in patients with recurrent gliomas was 3 mg/m² twice a week with 2- to 4-day intervals between doses for 3 consecutive weeks. Also as noted earlier, both of these schedules require the concomitant administration of physostigmine (Prados et al 1987).

■ Pharmacokinetics

The pharmacokinetic studies are summarized in the table below. Methods to determine plasma level are isotope dilution mass spectroscopy (Curt et al 1985) and gas chromatography with thermionic detection (Heideman et al 1988).

The compound is highly protein bound. Cerebrospinal fluid levels averaged 4.7% of the plasma levels. This is surprising and demonstrates that despite its lipophilicity, the drug does not reach high levels in the cerebrospinal fluid.

■ Side Effects and Toxicity

The dose-limiting toxic effect of spiromustine was a central nervous system syndrome characterized by xerostomia, mydriasis, lethargy, disorientation, delerium, confusion, and hallucinations. These effects are clearly related to dose, cumulative, and reversible (usually within 48 hours). Electroencephalograms show diffuse slowing. Cerebrospinal fluid examinations showed only minor protein elevations in one patient. The central nervous system effects were ameliorated somewhat by pretreatment with physostigmine (see doses under Administration).

Other toxic effects noted include nausea and

SUMMARY OF PHARMACOKINETIC STUDIES

Schedule	Plasma Level Peak	Half-life (min) α	Half-life (min) β	Total Body Clearance (mL/min/m²)	Reference
IV bolus every 4 h × 3 every 28 d	> 200 ng/mL	1	13	—	Curt et al 1985
IV bolus weekly × 3 every 28 d	—	1.6 ± 0.7	15.9 ± 8.3	2131 ± 732	Heideman et al 1988

vomiting and, very occasionally, grade 2 leukopenia (Brown et al 1986, Heisman et al 1988, Simon et al 1984, Sigman et al 1984, Curt et al 1985, Pazdur et al 1987).

■ Special Applications

None are known.

REFERENCES

Brown TD, Ettinger DS, Donehower RC. A phase I trial of spirohydantoin mustard (NSC-172112) in patients with advanced cancer. *J Clin Oncol.* 1986;**4**:1270–1276.

Curt GA, Kelley JA, Kufta CV, et al. A phase I and pharmacokinetic study of spiromustine in CNS malignancy. *Proc Am Soc Clin Oncol.* 1985;**4**:C124.

Deen DF, Hoshino T, Williams ME, Nomura K, Bartle PM. Response of 9L tumor cells in vitro to spirohydontoin mustard. *Cancer Res.* 1979;**39**:4336–4340.

Fortner CL, Grove WR, Bowie D, Walker M. Fat emulsion vehicle for intravenous administration of an aqueous insoluble drug. *Am J Hosp Pharm.* 1975;**32**:582–584.

Heideman RL, Kelley JA, Packer RJ, et al. A pediatric phase I and pharmacokinetic study of spirohydantoin mustard. *Cancer Res.* 1988;**48**:2292–2295.

Pazdur R, Redman BG, Corbett T, Phillips M, Baker LH. Phase I trial of spiromustine (NSC-172112) and evaluation of toxicity and schedule in a murine model. *Cancer Res.* 1987;**47**:4213–4217.

Peng GW, Marquez VE, Driscoll JS. Potential central nervous system antitumor agent hydantoin derivatives. *J Med Chem.* 1975;**18**:846–849.

Plowman J, Lakings DB, Owens ES, Adamson RH. Initial studies on the penetration of spirohydantoin mustard into the cerebrospinal fluid of dogs. *Pharmacology.* 1977;**15**:359–366.

Prados M, Rodriguez L, Seager M, Silver P, Levin V. Phase II study of spirohydantoin mustard for the treatment of recurrent malignant gliomas. *Cancer Treat Rep.* 1987;**71**:1105–1106.

Shoemaker DD, O'Dwyer PJ, Marsoni S, Plowman J, Davignon JP, Davis RD. *Invest New Drugs.* 1983;**1**:303–308.

Sigman LM, Van Echo DA, Egorin MJ, et al. Phase I trial of spiromustine (NSC-172112). *Proc Am Soc Clin Oncol.* 1984;**25**:C-119.

Simon S, McSherry JW, Krakoff IH, Stewart JA. Spiromustine (spirohydantoin mustard; NSC-172112): A phase I trial. *Proc Am Soc Clin Oncol.* 1984;**25**:C-111.

Streptonigrin

■ Other Names

Bruneomycin; rufocromomycin; Nigrin®; NSC-45383; BA-163; PC-501.

■ Chemistry

Structure of streptonigrin

Streptonigrin is an antibiotic isolated from *Streptomyces flocculus*. Its complete chemical name is 5-amino-6-(7-amino-5,8-dihydro-6-methoxy-5,8-dioxo-2-quinolyl)-4-(2-hydroxy-3,4-dimethoxyphenyl)-3-methylpicolinic acid. It has the empiric formula $C_{25}H_{22}N_4O_8$ and a molecular weight of 506. The compound was isolated by Rao and Cullen (1960) and the structure determined by Rao et al in 1963. Streptonigrin is structurally similar to mitomycin-C by possessing the aminoquinone moiety. It is one of a group of substituted 5,8-quinoline quinones with antineoplastic activity.

■ Antitumor Activity

Streptonigrin exhibits a broad spectrum of antineoplastic activity in a variety of animal tumors, including Ridgeway and Wagner osteogenic sarcomas, Lewis lung carcinoma, and several transplanted human tumors (Oleson et al 1961, Reilly and Sugiura 1961).

In human cancers the drug has shown its greatest activity in Hodgkin's and non-Hodgkin's lymphomas. It is often combined with vincristine and prednisone in histiocytic varieties (Carter 1968). Some activity has also been demonstrated in squamous cell carcinomas of the uterine cervix and of the head and neck, adenocarcinoma of the breast, and gastrointestinal tumors (Moertel and Reitmeier 1967). A preliminary study additionally showed activity in localized melanoma (by regional perfusion) and orally in the management of the cutaneous lymphoma mycosis fungoides (Harris et al 1965).

■ Mechanism of Action

Lown and Sim (1976) determined that the cytotoxic mechanism of streptonigrin involves single-strand cleavage of DNA. This process appears to first require reductive activation of the compound to generate reactive hydroxyl and superoxide ions. Free radical scavengers can completely inhibit the DNA-breaking reaction. A stable nitroxide free radical with superoxide dismutase activity (Tempol) can block streptonigrin cytotoxicity in vitro (Krishna et al 1992). More recently, streptonigrin has been shown to interfere with DNA topoisomerase II enzymes to form strand breaks. This was mediated by the formation of a cleavable complex between DNA strands and topoisomerase II (Yamashita et al 1990). Beside DNA strand scission, several cellular metabolic respiratory enzymes are sensitive to the free radicals produced by the drug. This may account for some of the drug's cytotoxicity. The DNA scission from streptonigrin also appears to be similar to that produced by superoxide radical generation from the xanthine–xanthine oxidase reaction.

The cytotoxic process is probably cell cycle nonspecific but may be maximal in G_2 and S phases.

■ Availability and Storage

Streptonigrin was previously available investigationally from the National Cancer Institute as 0.2-mg capsules (also containing lactose, starch, and stearic acid) and as a 0.5-mg kit for injection, which includes 2.5 mL special diluent (10% dimethylsulfoxide [DMSO], 10% ethanol, 2.2% 0.05 M citric acid, and 77.8% 0.1 M disodium phosphate). Both may be stored at room temperature and protected from light before use. This agent is no longer available in the United States.

■ Preparation for Use, Stability, and Admixture

When the 2.5 mL diluent is aseptically added to the 0.5-mg vial, the resultant concentration is 0.2 mg/mL. This may be added to D5W or normal saline for infusion. The drug is light sensitive and should be protected when continuous (24-hour) infusions are used. The drug is probably stable for at least 24 hours but should optimally be used within 8 hours of reconstitution.

Admixture data are currently unavailable.

■ Administration

It is sometimes recommended that two oral doses be taken over 0.5 hour along with an antiemetic to prevent nausea and vomiting.

The parenteral formulation has been administered intravenously, cautiously as a bolus injection through a running intravenous line. Moertel and Reitmeier (1967), Sullivan et al (1963), and Harris et al (1965) evaluated continuous, 24-hour intravenous infusions over several days and suggested that less hematologic toxicity may result with this method. The latter group also evaluated intraarterial and isolated (regional) perfusions of the drug (see Special Applications). For intravenous use it is recommended that vein patency be tested with 5 to 10 mL of saline or D5W before drug administration.

■ Special Precautions

Streptonigrin is a vesicant and must not be delivered outside the vein as infiltration may lead to serious tissue necrosis. The use of light protection is recommended for solutions to be used in continuous infusions.

■ Dosage

Oral doses in preliminary studies have usually been 1.0 mg/m^2/wk for 4 to 6 consecutive weeks. The optimal dose of streptonigrin has not been established. Harris et al (1965), however, suggested that an adequate total dose of oral streptonigrin is 5 mg, given as 0.2 to 0.4 mg (one to two capsules) daily until toxicity occurred.

For intravenous applications, doses of 5 to 7 µg/kg/d for up to 6 consecutive days have been recommended (McCracken and Aboody 1965, Moertel and Reitmeier 1967). These are then repeated at 4- to 6-week intervals.

■ Side Effects and Toxicity

The usual dose-limiting toxic effect of streptonigrin is unpredictable and severe bone marrow depression. Animal studies have confirmed human observations that the compound can be highly toxic and has a narrow therapeutic margin. (The LD$_{50}$ in dogs is only 4 to 5 µg/kg/d × 10 days [Hackethal et al 1961].)

The nadir for leukopenia following streptonigrin is delayed, occurring up to 4 weeks after initiation. Blood counts may remain depressed for several weeks. Reversal is apparently more prompt after oral dosing, although gastrointestinal side effects are more prominent. Thrombocytopenia also occurs and roughly parallels the course of leukopenia.

Nausea and vomiting are relatively common, especially with oral dosing, and the symptoms are not often adequately controlled with antiemetics. A number of patients have developed severe, prolonged symptoms following streptonigrin. Hackethal et al (1961) noted variable degrees of anorexia, weight loss, and diarrhea. Stomatitis, however, was rare.

In primates given streptonigrin, Hackethal et al (1961) reported extensive hemorrhages in heart tissues, glomerulonephritis, and focal necrosis of both kidney and hepatic tissues. In humans, azotemia has been noted rarely, along with a flapping tremor and toxic psychosis. This may corroborate some of the unusual animal toxic effects noted earlier.

Other side effects noted by Harris et al (1965) include alopecia, allergic reaction, and tongue pigmentation (in one patient each).

Fever is common, occurring in roughly a third of patients. It usually begins on the second to fourth day of consecutive daily dosing.

Serious necrosis can occur with drug infiltration. In animals given subcutaneous and intraperitoneal injections, severe fat necrosis with inflammation and significant ascites were followed by serious peritoneal adhesions.

■ Special Applications

Harris et al (1965) evaluated intraarterial streptonigrin infusions in nine patients. Doses were 7 µg/kg/d for 5 days, but only transient responses were produced, and this route was not recommended for further investigation. This study group also evaluated the isolation–perfusion technique in three patients with cervical carcinomas. The total dosage used was 35 µg/kg; two questionable objective and three subjective responses were noted. Neither route is recommended at this time.

REFERENCES

Carter SK. *Streptonigrin—A Review Chemotherapy Fact Sheet*. Washington, DC: National Cancer Institute, Program Analysis Branch; 1968.

Hackethal CA, Golbey RB, Jan CTC, et al. Clinical observations on effects of streptonigrin in patients with neoplastic disease. *Antibiot Chemother*. 1961;**11**:178–183.

Harris MN, Medrek TJ, Golomb FM, et al. Chemotherapy with streptonigrin in advanced cancer. *Cancer.* 1965;**18**:49–57.

Krishna MC, Hahn SM, DeGraff W, et al. Modulation of doxorubicin (ADR) and streptonigrin (STN) cytotoxicity in Chinese hamster V79 cells by a stable nitroxide free radical, Tempol (TP). *Proc Am Assoc Cancer Res*. 1992;**33**:509.

Lown JW, Sim SK. Studies related to antitumor antibiotics. VIII. Cleavage of DNA by streptonigrin analogues and the relationship to antineoplastic activity. *Can J Biochem*. 1976;**54**:446–452.

McCracken S, Aboody A. Continuous intravenous infusion of streptonigrin (NSC-45383) in patients with bronchial carcinoma. *Cancer Chemother Rep*. 1965;**46**:23–26.

Moertel CG, Reitmeier RJ. Evaluation of streptonigrin (NSC-45383) by continuous intravenous infusion in the treatment of advanced gastrointestinal cancer. *Cancer Chemother Rep*. 1967;**51**:73–76.

Oleson JJ, Calderella LA, Mios KJ, et al. Effects of streptonigrin on experimental tumors. *Antibiot Chemother*. 1961;**11**:158–164.

Rao KV, Bieman K, Woodward RB. Structure of streptonigrin. *J Am Chem Soc*. 1963;**85**:2532–2533.

Rao KV, Cullen WP. Streptonigrin antitumor substance. I. Isolation and characterization. *Antibiot Annu*. 1960;**7**:950–953.

Reilly HG, Sugiura K. An antitumor spectrum of streptonigrin. *Antibiot Chemother*. 1961;**11**(3):174–177.

Sullivan RD, Miller E, Zurek WZ, Rodrigues FR. Clinical effects of prolonged (continuous) infusion of streptonigrin (NSC-45383) in advanced cancer. *Cancer Chemother Rep*. 1963;**33**:27–40.

Wilson WL, Labra C, Barrist E. Preliminary observations on the use of streptonigrin as an antitumor agent in human beings. *Antibiot Chemother*. 1961;**11**:147–150.

Yamashita Y, Kawada S, Fujii N, Nakano H. Induction of mammalian DNA topoisomerase II dependent DNA cleavage by antitumor antibiotic streptonigrin. *Cancer Res*. 1990;**50**:581–584.

Streptozocin

■ Other Names

Streptozotocin; SZN; NSC-85998; U-9889; Zanosar® (The Upjohn Company).

■ Chemistry

Structure of streptozocin

Streptozocin is a naturally occurring nitrosourea related structurally to semustine and lomustine. Chemically, the drug is 2-deoxy-2-(3-methyl-3-nitrosoureido)-D-glucopyranose. It has a molecular weight of 265 and the empiric formula $C_8H_{15}N_3O_7$. This drug is derived from *Streptomyces achromogenes* variety 128 (White 1963) and has broad-spectrum antibacterial properties as well as antitumor activity.

Similar to the other nitrosoureas, it possesses relatively good lipid solubility, but the lyophilized drug is also water soluble. The molecule does not, however, possess the chloroethyl side chain(s) present in the other nitrosoureas. These side chains are thought to be involved in the alkylation process. Streptozocin also contains a glucose moiety not present in the other compounds. The glucose moiety is believed to contribute to reduced myelotoxicity, specificity for pancreatic islet cells, and the drug's much slower reactivity toward DNA compared with other nitrosoureas.

■ Antitumor Activity

In preclinical animal tumor screening studies streptozocin demonstrated significant antitumor effects against L-1210 murine leukemia, sarcoma-180, Walker carcinosarcoma, and Ehrlich carcinoma.

Streptozocin has shown clinically significant antitumor activity in both beta and nonbeta pancreatic islet cell tumors (Carter et al 1971, Murray-Lyon et al 1968, Schein et al 1973a–c, Broder and Carter 1973) and malignant carcinoid (Feldman et al 1972). It is equally active in non-insulin secreting pancreatic islet cell tumors, with an overall response rate of approximately 36% (Moertel et al 1980). Activity has been reported in non-small cell lung cancer, squamous cell carcinoma of the oral cavity, synovial sarcoma, adenocarcinoma of the gallbladder (Stolinsky et al 1972), malignant Zollinger–Ellison tumors (Ruffner 1976), and Hodgkin's disease. Nonbeta cell pancreatic tumors (Verner–Morrison syndrome) may also respond (Gagel et al 1976). The table summarizes the streptozocin-sensitive tumors in humans (Weiss 1982).

Negative clinical responses have been reported for streptozocin used in sarcoma (Chang and Wiernik 1975), small cell bronchogenic carcinoma

CLINICAL RESPONSES TO STREPTOZOCIN (REFERENCES)

Sensitive Tumors	Tumors Sensitive To Streptozocin-Containing Combinations

Pancreatic islet cell tumors
  Gastrinomas (Stadil et al 1976)
  ACTHoma (Walter et al 1973)
  Parathormonona (DeWys et al 1973)
  Somatostatinoma (Pipeleers et al 1979)
  Glucagonomas (Danforth et al 1976)
  Seroninoma (Schein et al 1974)
  VIPoma (Kahn et al 1975)
	Hodgkin's disease (Schein et al 1974, Levi et al 1977)
	
	Colon carcinoma (Kemeny et al 1980, Horton et al 1975)

Carcinoid tumors (Moertel et al 1971, Moertel 1975, Chernicoff et al 1979)	Hepatoma (Falkson et al 1978) Pancreatic ductal carcinoma (Moertel et al 1977, Wiggans et al 1978)

Data from Weiss 1982.

(Bunn et al 1978), small cell anaplastic carcinoma of the lung (Kane et al 1978), renal cell carcinoma (Licht and Garnick 1987), and the combination chemotherapy of metastatic breast cancer (Band et al 1977). When streptozocin was combined with 5-fluorouracil, Seligman et al (1977) noted an objective response rate of 25.5% in patients with several types of advanced gastrointestinal carcinomas. A similar low response rate is described in metastatic renal cell carcinoma (Licht and Garnick 1987). Streptozocin has also been used with a variety of other agents in active regimens. These include combinations with mitomycin-C + 5-fluorouracil in advanced pancreatic cancer (Gastrointestinal Tumor Study Group 1986) and streptozocin + doxorubicin + bleomycin + vincristine in patients with recurrent Hodgkin's disease (Vinciguerra et al 1986) (see table).

■ Mechanism of Action

Streptozocin undergoes spontaneous decomposition to yield a methylcarbonium ion which can form DNA–DNA (interstrand) crosslinks. The glucose moiety on streptozocin may decrease this activity. Streptozocin has been shown to selectively inhibit DNA synthesis without significantly affecting RNA or protein synthesis (Heineman and Howard 1965). Some isocyanate is also formed from streptozocin decomposition and this produces carbamoylation of proteins, primarily, but not exclusively, to lysine residues in protein (Heal et al 1979); however, carbamoylating activity does not correlate with the antitumor activity of any of the nitrosoureas (Panasci et al 1977). Thus, inhibition of DNA synthesis by alkylation remains the primary cytotoxic mechanism.

Streptozocin alkylation of DNA (Bennet and Pegg 1981) has been used to explain the ability of the drug to sensitize resistant cells to other nitrosoureas (Futscher et al 1989). This activity may be mediated by inactivation of the enzyme O^6-alkylguanine transferase, a DNA repair protein that removes DNA alkyl adducts from the O^6-position of guanine (Day et al 1980).

Streptozocin also affects several key enzymatic sites in the glyconeogenesis pathway (Katzen et al 1970). The drug has been shown to selectively inhibit the synthesis of pyridine nucleotides in mouse liver (Schein et al 1973b). The diabetogenic effect of streptozocin is the direct result of irreversible damage to the pancreatic beta cell, causing degranulation and loss of normal insulin secretory function (Arison et al 1967, Junod et al 1967). This is now known to be due to reduced uptake and synthesis of NAD within the cell (Schein et al 1973b). Indeed, NAD replenishment can correct this defect in experimental mouse models. Also, the addition of NAD can block the diabetogenic effects without altering antitumor activity. Kawashima et al (1978) have also shown that a single streptozocin injection may slowly produce hypertension in rats. Interestingly, this occurs after the maximal hyperglycemic effect has occurred. Histologic examination after high doses in this study showed pancreatic cell degranulation and necrosis with vacuolization and deposition of periodic acid/Schiff reagent-positive materials in the proximal renal tubules.

At drug levels lower than those necessary for DNA synthesis inhibition, streptozocin can inhibit the progression of cells out of G_2 phase; however, the drug is active in all phases of the cell cycle (Bhuyan et al 1970).

■ Availability and Storage

Streptozocin is commercially available in 1-g vials for injection (Zanosar®, The Upjohn Company, Kalamazoo, Michigan). These vials should be stored under refrigeration and protected from light. They are stable for at least 3 years if refrigerated and 1 year at room temperature. The pH is adjusted to 3.8 to 4.2 with 220 mg citric acid and sodium hydroxide.

■ Preparation for Use, Stability, and Admixture

The manufacturer recommends adding 9.5 mL of either normal saline or Sterile Water for Injection, USP, to the 1-g vial. This provides a 100 mg/mL solution stable for 2 days at room temperature (longer under refrigeration and if protected from light); however, because the solution contains no preservative it is recommended that any unused portion be discarded after 8 hours. Streptozocin is reported to be physically compatible with 1 mg/mL ondansetron for 4 hours (Trissel et al 1990).

■ Administration

Streptozocin has been given (1) by intravenous infusion (in D5W or normal saline) over 6 hours, (2) as a short infusion in 100 to 200 mL of D5W over 10 to 15 minutes, and (3) as a rapid intravenous bolus injection. With the bolus administration, however, many patients will complain of an intense perivenous burning sensation. This may extend some distance up the arm from the site of a rapid injection. Thus, the use of the short infusion (30–45 minutes) may eliminate or reduce this painful sequela.

■ Special Precautions

Vein patency should be checked before injection with a 5- to 10-mL flush of either normal saline or D5W. The same procedure should be used after drug administration to flush any remaining drug solution from the tubing and the vein proximal to the venipuncture area. Aggressive pretreatment with antiemetics is strongly recommended to prevent nausea and vomiting, which are often severe.

Adequate hydration is also recommended to prevent acute renal tubule toxicity from active metabolites. Streptozocin is directly toxic to the kidneys and doses should be lowered in patients with preexisting renal disease. The drug is also diabetogenic, and a marked hypoglycemic effect may occur. Intravenous dextrose should be available during the administration of streptozocin to counter an immediate release of insulin with hypoglycemia. However, the drug has been given safely to diabetic patients without serious sequalae.

■ Dosage

As a single agent streptozocin has been given as six consecutive weekly doses of 1.0 to 1.5 g/m^2 followed by a 4-week observation period. In other protocols using streptozocin–drug combinations, doses of 1.0 g/m^2 or 500 mg/m^2 for 5 consecutive days have been employed followed by 4- to 6-week observation periods, respectively.

■ Drug Interactions

Because of the marked diabetogenic effects, numerous potentially significant hyperglycemic drug interactions are possible. One example is the combined use of corticosteroids with streptozocin. Koranyi and Gero (1979) have recently suggested that phenytoin (Dilantin®) pretreatment can protect the pancreatic beta cell from streptozocin cytotoxicity; however, this might simultaneously abrogate the therapeutic effect in patients with islet cell tumors. In another experimental trial, local hyperthermia did not enhance streptozocin activity (Marmor and Hahn 1979).

Experimentally, several biochemical approaches may be able to modulate streptozocin-induced diabetes. These include nicotinamide (Schein et al 1967) and 3-O-methylglucose, a nontoxic, nonmetabolized analog of glucose (Wick et al 1976). Streptozotocin may also increase the sensitivity of resistant cells to the effects of other nitrosoureas by inactivating the DNA repair enzyme O^6-alkylguanine transferase (Futscher et al 1989). This may thereby "sensitize" resistant tumor cells to other DNA-reactive anticancer agents.

■ Pharmacokinetics

Streptozocin has a pharmacokinetic pattern similar to that of the other nitrosoureas (carmustine and lomustine). After rapid bolus intravenous injection, unchanged drug is rapidly cleared from the plasma (half-life, 35 minutes), and no intact drug is found in the plasma 3 hours after injection; however, streptozocin metabolites persist in the plasma longer than 24 hours after injection. Metabolites identified from radiolabelled drug studies have demonstrated a triphasic plasma clearance with a short initial phase (half-life, 6 minutes), an intermediate phase (half-life, 3.5 hours), and a prolonged terminal phase (half-life, 40 hours). These drug metabolites cross into the cerebrospinal fluid at varying rates and to varying extents but are still detectable in the cerebrospinal fluid 24 hours after injection. Good tumor tissue penetration has also been documented. In addition, the drug metabolites appear to concentrate to some extent in the liver and kidney. Fifteen percent of the total administered dose is recovered in the urine and less than 1% in the feces. Metabolite elimination by exhalation has been documented but the extent to which it impacts on metabolism is unknown. At least three metabolites have been detected in the urine (Adolphe et al 1975, 1977).

■ Side Effects and Toxicity

Severe gastrointestinal effects including nausea and vomiting can occur with streptozocin. These toxic effects have been dose limiting in several studies. Parenterally, orally, and rectally administered antiemetics are often inadequate at preventing these side effects. These gastrointestinal toxic effects may get progressively worse over the 5-day course of therapy (Lokich et al 1973). Duodenal ulcers caused by streptozocin have also been reported (DuPriest et al 1975).

When given as a single agent, streptozocin does not appear to produce substantial myelosuppressive toxicity. Myelosuppression occurs in approximately 20% of patients. This effect is generally mild; however, when streptozocin is combined with other nitrosoureas or cytotoxic agents, a synergistic effect on hematologic toxicity is observed (Lokich et al 1973). This may relate to a drug–drug metabolic interaction or competition for binding or transport sites. For example, enhanced thrombocytopenia noted with concomitant carmustine administration can be both severe and prolonged.

Nephrotoxicity is often dose limiting when streptozocin is used alone. Usually, transient proteinurea and azotemia are seen; however, permanent tubular damage has been noted. The earliest sign of renal damage is hypophosphatemia. Toxicity has been likened to that occurring with type I glycogen storage disease characterized by glucose-6-phosphate dehydrogenase deficiency (G6PD), and the two conditions may be interrelated. Intraaortic administration increases morbidity and mortality and may relate to augmented drug delivery to the kidneys. A clear dose-dependent relationship has not yet been documented between streptozocin administration and nephrotoxicity.

Sadoff (1970) noted that the kidney was the major organ of drug toxicity and, in a phase I, trial observed various renal tubular defects ranging from azotemia (in half the patients) to a fulminant Fanconi's syndrome. Anuria occurred in 2 of 18 patients, producing one fatality and one survivor after 2 weeks of peritoneal dialysis. In this study hypophosphatemia invariably occurred after the first or second injection. Other common defects included renal glycosuria (80% of patients), acetonuria in 28%, and renal tubular acidosis in 10 of 18 patients. The last toxic effect included hyperchloremic acidosis (urine pH > 7.0) and aminoaciduria. More recently, Myerowitz et al (1978) have reported renal biopsy findings in a patient with streptozocin nephrotoxicity. Biopsy demonstrated a tubulointerstitial nephritis, with cellular nodules observed in the glomeruli. At autopsy both kidneys were small with atrophic cortices. Each demonstrated substantial interstitial fibrosis and tubular atrophy, with numerous renal cortical spindle cell nodules.

Thus, renal toxicity occurs frequently, in from 45 to 65% of patients (Broder and Carter 1973). It usually involves mild proteinuria, glycosuria, and hypophosphatemia, although, occasionally, irreversible azotemia may ensue. According to the review by Myerowitz et al, ten deaths from renal toxicity have been documented in various studies.

The mechanism for streptozocin-induced nephrotoxicity is most likely due to the urinary excretion of approximately 10 to 20% of intact active drug. It is thus not surprising that streptozocin has also caused or induced various renal neoplasms in experimental animals (Rakieten et al 1968, Arison and Feudale 1967). Furthermore, because of its close structural similarity to the nitrosamines (well-known carcinogens), streptozocin has experimentally induced other tumors in animals (Sibay and Hayes 1969, Berman et al 1973).

Hepatotoxicity has been observed after streptozocin administration. It is generally mild and transient, and is characterized by painless jaundice with elevations of serum glutamic–oxalacetic transaminase, alkaline phosphatase, and bilirubin after the second week of therapy.

Streptozocin has been documented to alter glucose metabolism in some individuals, and this is probably related to its effects on pancreatic beta cells. Diabetic patients have received the drug without serious sequelae. After a dose of streptozocin in patients with insulimona (a tumor of pancreatic beta cells), there is generally a progressive elevation of fasting blood sugar and a decrease in serum insulin levels. Acutely, there may be a burst of insulin release immediately after injection, with resultant acute lowering of blood sugars. This may require emergency glucose repletion.

Although streptozocin appears to cause mild aberrations of glucose metabolism in some patients (Sadoff 1972), this is neither a uniform nor a predictable side effect and if it occurs, is usually transient.

Streptozocin can produce immediate burning pain in the vein for drug administration. This may be more severe with short infusions (< 15 to 20 minutes) (DuPriest et al 1975). In some sensitive patients, pretreatment with 5 mL of a 50/50 mixture of 1% lidocaine and normal saline or D5W may be of benefit in preventing pain or inflammation. Direct admixture data are not available, and mixture is therefore not advised.

As with other nitrosoureas, long-term therapy may predispose patients to a risk of second malignancies. One case of acute leukemia has been described in a 69-year-old man who received a cumulative dose of 67 g of streptozocin over 28 months (Green and Anderson 1981).

■ Special Applications

Continuous Intravenous Infusion. Seibert et al (1979) evaluated the continuous intravenous infusion of streptozocin (0.5–1.0 g/d × 5) in a phase I study. The average dose of streptozocin in this study was 3300 mg/m². Neither renal dysfunction or myelosuppression was observed. Significant toxicity included severe nausea and vomiting in three patients (with gastrointestinal cancer) and confusion, lethargy, and depression in five patients, each without prior central nervous system complaints. There were 2 responses in 10 patients with previously treated non-Hodgkin's lymphomas. In this study central nervous system toxicity appeared to be dose limiting over the usual, renal, hepatic, and gastrointestinal toxicity.

Intraperitoneal Therapy. Streptozocin has been administered intraperitoneally in a single patient with advanced ovarian cancer (Panasci et al 1982). A dose of 1 g was administered intraperitoneally six times within a 3-week period. There was no nausea, vomiting, or renal toxicity. The half-life of streptozocin in the peritoneal space was 61 minutes, with a volume of distribution of 3 L. The half-life of unchanged streptozocin in peritoneal fluid was 42 minutes. Plasma drug levels were always less than 1 to 10% of the simultaneous intraperitoneal drug level. In another trial using 1 g IP dosing, the AUC for streptozocin in the intraperitoneal cavity was 183 mM·min with peak levels of 1.9 mM (Goel et al 1991). Clearance averaged 19 mL/min in 10 patients. The corresponding plasma values were much lower, with a mean peritoneal AUC/plasma AUC of 6.4.

Intraarterial Therapy. Streptozocin has also been administered into the hepatic arteries of two patients with metastatic islet cell tumors (Kahn et al 1975). The patients received three to five doses of 1.5 g streptozocin over 35 to 60 minutes. Plasma drug concentrations following intraarterial administration were 50% of levels reported when the same dose was given intravenously. Approximately 25% of the dose was recovered in the urine after intraarterial therapy compared with 38% after intravenous therapy. Both patients responded favorably to intraarterial streptozocin, with major symptomatic improvements in diarrhea lasting at least 12 months (Kahn et al 1975).

REFERENCES

Adolphe AB, Glasofer ED, Troetel WM, et al. Fate of streptozotocin (NSC-85998) in patients with advanced cancer. *Cancer Chemother Rep.* 1975;**59**(3):547–556.

Adolphe AB, Glasofer ED, Troetel WM, et al. Preliminary pharmacokinetics of streptozotocin, an antineoplastic antibiotic. *J Clin Pharmacol.* 1977;**17**:379–388.

Arison RN, Ciaccio EI, Glitzer MS, et al. Light and electron microscopy of lesions in rats rendered diabetic with streptozotocin. *Diabetes.* 1967;**16**:51–56.

Arison RN, Feudale E. Induction of renal tumors by streptozotocin in rats. *Nature.* 1967;**214**:1254–1255.

Band PR, Canellos GP, Sears M, et al. Phase II trial with bleomycin, CCNU and streptozotocin in patients with metastatic cancer of the breast. *Cancer Treat Rep.* 1977;**61**(7):1365–1367.

Bennet R, Pegg AE. Alkylation of DNA in rat tissues following administration of streptozotocin. *Cancer Res.* 1981;**41**:2786–2790.

Berman LD, Hayes JA, Sibay TM. Effect of streptozotocin on Chinese hamsters (*Cricetulus griseus*). *J Natl Cancer Inst.* 1973;**51**:1287–1294.

Bhuyan BK, Scheidt LG, Fraser TJ. Cell cycle specificity of several antitumor agents. *Proc Am Assoc Cancer Res.* 1970;**11**:8.

Broder LE, Carter SK. Pancreatic islet cell carcinoma. II. Results of therapy with streptozotocin in 52 patients. *Ann Intern Med.* 1973;**79**:108–118.

Bunn PA Jr, Ihde DC, Cohen MH, et al. Streptozotocin in advanced small cell bronchogenic carcinoma: An ineffective nonmyelosuppressive agent. *Cancer Treat Rep.* 1978;**62**(3):479–481.

Carter SK, Broder L, Freidman M. Streptozotocin and metastatic insulinoma. *Ann Intern Med.* 1971;**74**:445–461.

Chang P, Wiernik PH. Combination chemotherapy with Adriamycin and streptozotocin. I. Clinical results in patients with advanced sarcoma. *Clin Pharmacol Ther.* 1975;**20**:605–610.

Chernicoff D, Bukowski RM, Groppe CW Jr, et al. Combination chemotherapy for islet cell carcinoma and metastatic carcinoid tumors with 5-fluorouracil and streptozotocin. *Cancer Treat Rep.* 1979;**63**:795–796.

Danforth DN, Triche T, Doppman JL, et al. Elevated plasma proglucagon-like component with a glucagon-secreting tumor. Effect of streptozotocin. *N Engl J Med.* 1976;**295**:242–245.

Day R, Ziolkowski C, Scudiero D, et al. Defective repair of alkylated DNA by human tumour and SV-40 transformed human cell strains. *Nature.* 1980;**288**:724–727.

DeWys WD, Stoll R, Au W, et al. Effects of streptozotocin on an islet cell carcinoma with hypercalcemia. *Am J Med.* 1973;**55**:671–676.

DuPriest RW, Huntington MC, Massay WH, et al. Streptozotocin therapy in 22 cancer patients. *Cancer.* 1975;**35**:358–376.

Falkson G, Moertel CG, Lavin P, et al. Chemotherapy studies in primary liver cancer. A prospective randomized trial. *Cancer.* 1978;**42**:2149–2156.

Feldman JM, Quickel KE Jr, Mareck RL, Lebovitz HE. Streptozotocin treatment of metastatic carcinoid tumors. *South Med J.* 1972;**65**:1325–1330.

Futscher BW, Micetich KC, Barnes DM, et al. Inhibition of a specific DNA repair system and nitrosourea cytotoxicity in resistant human cancer cell. *Cancer Commun.* 1989;**1**(1):65–73.

Gagel RF, Costanza ME, DeLellis RA, et al. Streptozocin-treated Verner–Morrison syndrome. *Arch Intern Med.* 1976;**136**:1429–1435.

Gastrointestinal Tumor Study Group. Phase II studies of drug combinations in advanced pancreatic carcinoma: Fluorouracil plus doxorubicin plus mitomycin-C and two regimens of streptozotocin plus mitomycin-C plus fluorouracil. *J Clin Oncol.* 1986;**4**:1794–1798.

Goel R, McClay EF, Kirmani S, et al. Pharmacokinetic study of intraperitoneal streptozotocin. *Proc Am Assoc Cancer Res.* 1991;**32**:173.

Green MR, Anderson RE. Acute myelocytic leukemia following prolonged streptozotocin therapy. *Cancer.* 1981;**47**:1963–1965.

Heal JM, Fox PA, Schein PS. Effect of carbamoylation on the repair of nitrosourea-induced DNA alkylation damage in L1210 cells. *Cancer Res.* 1979;**39**:82–89.

Heinemann B, Howard AJ. Effect of compounds with both antitumor and bacteriophage-inducing activities on *E. coli* nucleic synthesis. *Antimicrob Agents Chemother.* 1965;**5**:488–492.

Horton J, Mittelman A, Taylor SG III, et al. Phase II trials with procarbazine (NSC-77213), streptozotocin (NSC-85998), 6-thioguanine (NSC-752), and CCNU (NSC-79037) in patients with metastatic cancer of the large bowel. *Cancer Chemother Rep.* 1975;**59**:333–340..

Junod A, Lamber AE, Orci L, et al. Studies of the diabetogenic action of streptozotocin. *Proc Soc Exp Biol Med.* 1967;**126**:201–205.

Kahn CR, Levy AG, Gardner JD, et al. Pancreatic cholera: Beneficial effects of treatment with streptozotocin. *N Engl J Med.* 1975;**292**(18):941–945.

Kane RC, Bernath AM, Cashdollar RR. Phase II trial of streptozotocin for small cell anaplastic carcinoma of the lung. *Cancer Treat Rep.* 1978;**62**(3):477–478.

Katzen HM, Soderman DD, Wiley CE. Multiple forms of hexokinase. *J Biol Chem.* 1970;**245**(16):4081–4096.

Kawashima H, Igarashi T, Nakajima Y, et al. Chronic hypertension induced by streptozotocin in rats. *Arch Pharmacol.* 1978;**305**:123–126.

Kemeny N, Yagoda A, Braun D, et al. Therapy for metastatic colorectal carcinoma with a combination of methyl CCNU, 5- fluorouracil, vincristine and streptozotocin (MOF-Strep). *Cancer.* 1980;**45**:876–881.

Koranyi L, Gero L. Influence of diphenylhydantoin on the effect of streptozotocin (letter). *Br Med J.* 1979;**1**:127.

Levi JA, Wiernik PH, Diggs CH. Combination chemotherapy of advanced previously treated Hodgkin's disease with streptozotocin, CCNU, Adriamycin, and bleomycin. *Med Pediatr Oncol.* 1977;**3**:33–40.

Licht JD, Garnick MB. Phase II trial of streptozocin in the treatment of advanced renal cell carcinoma. *Cancer Treat Rep.* 1987;**71**(1):97–98.

Lokich JJ, Chawla PL, Frei E. 1,3-Bis-(2-chloroethyl)-1-nitrosourea and streptozotocin chemotherapy. *Clin Pharmacol Ther.* **17**:374–378.

Marmor JB, Hahn GM. Effects of four nitrosoureas with local hyperthermia on primary tumor and lung metastases (abstract 271). *Proc Am Assoc Cancer Res ASCO.* 1979;**20**:67.

Moertel CG. Clinical management of advanced gastrointestinal cancer. *Cancer.* 1975;**36**:675–682.

Moertel CG, Douglas HO, Hanley J, et al. Treatment of advanced adenocarcinoma of the pancreas with combinations of streptozotocin plus 5-fluorouracil and streptozotocin plus cyclophosphamide. *Cancer.* 1977;**40**:605–608.

Moertel CG, Hanley JA, Johnson LA. Streptozocin alone compared with streptozocin plus fluorouracil in the treatment of advanced islet-cell carcinoma. *N Engl J Med.* 1980;**303**(21):1189–1194.

Moertel CG, Reitmeier RJ, Schutt AJ, Hahn RG. Phase II study of streptozotocin (NSC-85998) in the treatment of advanced gastrointestinal cancer. *Cancer Chemother Rep.* 1971;**55**:303–307.

Murray-Lyon IM, Eddleston ALWF, Williams R, et al. Treatment of multiple-hormone-producing malignant islet cell tumor with streptozotocin. *Lancet.* 1968;**2**:895–898.

Myerowitz RL, Sartiano GP, Cavallo T. Nephrotoxic and cytoproliferative effects of streptozotocin. *Cancer.* 1978;**38**:1550–1555.

Panasci LC, Fox PA, Schein PS. Structure–activity studies of methylnitrosourea antitumor agents with reduced murine bone marrow toxicity. *Cancer Res.* 1977;**37**:3321–3328.

Panasci LC, Skalski V, St-Germain J, et al. Pharmacology and toxicity of IP streptozocin in ovarian cancer: A case report. *Cancer Treat Rep.* 1982;**66**(7):1595–1596.

Pipeleers D, Somers G, Gepts W, et al. Plasma pancreatic hormone levels in a case of somatostatinoma: Diagnostic and therapeutic implications. *J Clin Endocrinol Metab.* 1979;**49**:572–579.

Rakieten N, Gordon BS, Cooney DA, et al. Renal tumorigenic action of streptozotocin (NSC-85998) in rats. *Cancer Chemother Rep.* 1968;**52**:563–567.

Ruffner BW. Chemotherapy for malignant Zollinger–Ellison tumors. *Arch Intern Med.* 1976;**136**:1032–1034.

Sadoff L. Nephrotoxicity of streptozocin (NSC-85998). *Cancer Chemother Rep.* 1970;**54**:457–459.

Sadoff L. Patterns of intravenous glucose tolerance and insulin response before and after treatment with streptozotocin (NSC-85998). *Cancer Chemother Rep.* 1972;**56**:61–69.

Schein P, Kahn R, Gorden P, et al. Streptozotocin for malignant insulinomas and carcinoid tumor. Report of eight cases and review of the literature. *Arch Intern Med.* 1973a;**132**:555–561.

Schein PS, Cooney DA, McMenamin MG, et al. Streptozotocin diabetes—Further studies on the mechanism of depression of nicotinamide adenine dinucleotide concentrations in mouse pancreatic islets and liver. *Biochem Pharmacol.* 1973b;**22**:2625–2631.

Schein PS, Cooney DA, Vernon MC. The use of nicotinamide to modify the toxicity of streptozotocin diabetes without loss of antitumor activity. *Cancer Res.* 1967;**27**(pt 1):2324–2332.

Schein PS, McMenamin M, Anderson T. 3-(Tetra acetyl glucopyranos-2-yl)-1-(2-chloroethyl)-2-nitrosourea, an antitumor agent with modified bone marrow toxicity. *Cancer Res.* 1973c;**33**;2005–2009.

Schein PS, O'Connell MJ, Blom J, et al. Clinical antitumor activity and toxicity of streptozotocin (NSC-85998). *Cancer.* 1974;**34**:993–1000.

Seibert K, Golub G, Smiledge P, Nystrom JS. Continuous streptozotocin infusion: A phase I study. *Cancer Treat Rep.* 1979;**63**:2035–2037.

Seligman M, Bukowski RM, Groppe CW, et al. Chemotherapy of metastatic gastrointestinal neoplasms with 5-fluorouracil and streptozotocin. *Cancer Treat Rep.* 1977;**61**(7):1375–1377.

Sibay TM, Hayes JA. Potential carcinogenic effect of streptozotocin. *Lancet.* 1969;**2**:912.

Stadil F, Stage G, Rehfeld JF, et al. Treatment of Zollinger–Ellison syndrome with streptozotocin. *N Engl J Med.* 1976;**294**:1440–1442.

Stolinsky DC, Sadoff L, Braunwald J, Bateman JR. Streptozotocin in the treatment of cancer-phase II study. *Cancer.* 1972;**30**:61–67.

Trissel LA, Fulton B, Tramonte SM. Visual compatibility of ondansetron with chemotherapeutic agents, antibiotics, and other selected drugs during simulated Y-site injection (abstract #P-468R). In: *25th Annual ASHP Midyear Clinical Meetings and Exhibit, Las Vegas, Nevada;* 1990.

Vinciguerra V, Propert KJ, Coleman M, et al. Alternating cycles of combination chemotherapy for patients with recurrent Hodgkin's disease following radiotherapy. A prospectively randomized study by the Cancer and Leukemia Group B. *J Clin Oncol.* 1986;**4**(6):838–846.

Walter RM, Ensinck JW, Ricketts H, et al. Insulin and ACTH production by a streptozotocin responsive islet cell carcinoma. *Am J Med.* 1973;**55**:667–670.

Weiss RB. Streptozocin: A review of its pharmacology, efficacy, and toxicity. *Cancer Treat Rep.* 1982;**66**(3):427–438.

White FR. Streptozotocin. *Cancer Chemother Rep.* 1963;**30**:49–53.

Wick M, Rossini A, Glynn D. Reduction of streptozotocin (Sz) toxicity by 3-O-methylglucose (3-O-MG) with enhancement of antitumor activity in L-1210 leukemia (abstract 431). *Proc Am Assoc Cancer Res ASCO.* 1976;**17**:108.

Wiggans RG, Woolley PV, MacDonald JS, et al. Phase II trial of streptozotocin, mitomycin-C, and 5-fluorouracil (SMF) in the treatment of advanced pancreatic cancer. *Cancer.* 1978;**41**:387–391.

Sulofenur

■ Other Names

Diarylsulfonylurea; DSU; LY-186641.

■ Chemistry

Structure of sulofenur

Sulofenur is one of a number of diarylsulfonylureas, a novel class of antitumor agents. These were originally synthesized at Eli Lilly Laboratories as intermediates in the development of a potential herbicide. The compound has a molecular weight of 350.83 and the empiric formula $C_{16}H_{15}ClN_2O_3S$. The complete chemical name is N-(5-indanylsulfonyl)-N'-4-(chlorophenyl)urea. The compound has broad-spectrum antitumor activity as well as curative potential for human colon cancer growing in nude mice (Grindey et al 1986, 1987).

■ Antitumor Activity

In preclinical studies, sulofenur exhibited broad antitumor activity against several mouse tumors. These include adenocarcinoma-755, M-5 ovarian carcinoma, C6 colon carcinoma, C3H mammary carcinoma, Lewis lung carcinoma, and Madison lung carcinoma (Grindey et al 1987). The drug was also active in nude mice bearing human colon cancer xenografts (Houghten et al 1983).

Sulofenur is just completing phase I studies. To date, responses have been noted in patients with refractory ovarian cancer, head and neck cancer, and refractory seminoma (Taylor et al 1989, Burris et al 1990; Armand et al 1989). Sulofenur was inactive in advanced non-small cell lung carcinoma (Munshi et al 1991). Similarly, a Canadian National Cancer Institute trial reported no responses to sulofenur in previously untreated patients with either small cell carcinoma of the lung (9 patients) or renal cell carcinoma (18 patients) (Weinerman et al 1991). Sulofenur was also inactive in previously untreated patients with advanced colorectal carcinoma (Herrmann et al 1991). In patients with previously treated ovarian cancer, sulofenur produced an 11% response rate on a 14-day schedule and a 17% response rate on a 21-day schedule (Alberts et al 1990).

■ Mechanism of Action

The mechanism of action for this agent is unknown. Of note, the agent does not inhibit synthesis of DNA, RNA, or protein and has no cell cycle specificity (Grindey et al 1987). In Chinese hamster ovary cells, cytotoxicity is highly dependent on serum concentrations used during drug exposure. The 50% inhibitory concentration is 57 μM in serum-containing medium and only 2 μM in albumin-free medium. Cell death was noted morphologically by the loss of microvilli, with death occurring 4 to 6 hours after exposure to high drug concentrations (Boder et al 1992). At lower drug concentrations, cells progressed through several generations, with death occurring after 24 to 36 hours. Surviving cells were observed to have disrupted actin-based functions evidenced by multinucleations and inhibited cytokinesis. Another cell culture study detected an early drug effect at increasing intracellular calcium levels. Later events involved mitochondrial dysfunction, noted just prior to cell death (Trump et al 1992). Cellular and mitochondrial swelling was noted in these cells and it is possible that cells undergo apoptosis, or programmed cell death, in response to sulofenur. This is based on preliminary observations of increased calcium and endonuclease activity resulting in DNA degradation.

■ Availability and Storage

Sulofenur is available from Eli Lilly Laboratories, Indianapolis, Indiana. The drug is provided as opaque white capsules in strengths of 5, 25, 100, and 250 mg. The compound can be stored at room temperature.

■ Preparation for Use, Stability, and Admixture

Sulofenur is administered in an oral dosage form and no preparation is necessary. The agent is stable for at least 1 year at room temperature. It is suggested that the Occupational Safety and Health Administration's guidelines for the handling of cytotoxic drugs, as outlined in the *American Journal of Hospital Pharmacy* 1980;**43**:1143, be followed.

■ Administration

Sulofenur is administered in an oral form. The agent should be given on an empty stomach (nothing to eat or drink for 1 hour before), and nothing other than water should be allowed for 30 minutes after drug administration.

■ Special Precautions

Because of the hemolytic anemia noted with the drug, patients with a glucose-6-phosphate dehydrogenase deficiency or with a history of or ongoing hemolysis (positive direct or indirect Coombs) should not be given sulofenur. In addition, patients with a history of hypersensitivity to sulfa compounds should not receive the agent. Of particular interest is that sulofenur can cause interference in the measurement of serum creatinine by the Jaffe reaction. An enzymatic technique on a solid support appears to be interference free (Bonnay et al 1989).

■ Drug Interactions

Sulofenur has produced clinically significant hypoprothrombinemia when administered concurrently with warfarin (Fossella et al 1991). This was due to displacement of warfarin from protein binding sites, resulting in a fourfold increase in unbound (free) warfarin concentration (Fossella et al 1991). Sulofenur should therefore not be combined with warfarin.

■ Dosage

The optimal dosage and schedule are still under investigation. Kuttesch et al (1988) used a weekly schedule and reached a maximally tolerated dose of 1950 mg/m^2 as a single dose. Taylor et al (1989) administered the agent daily for 7 days and achieved a maximally tolerated dose of 1200 mg/m^2/d × 7 days. Brown et al (1989a,b) used a daily × 21 schedule and a single dose every 3 weeks schedule. Maximally tolerated doses were 630 mg/m^2/d × 21 and 2550 mg/m^2, respectively. Armand et al (1989) explored the daily × 14 every 21 days schedule. Hemolytic anemia was noted at the 900 mg/m^2 dose level. Burris et al (1990) reported a daily × 5 with a 2-day rest followed by daily × 5 and 2 days off again schedule. The maximally tolerated dose on that schedule was 1080 mg/m^2. This schedule appeared to be the best tolerated.

■ Pharmacokinetics

The table on page 858 describes the salient features of the pharmacology of the agent. Overall, the disposition of sulofenur in plasma best fits a one- or two-compartment model. Sulofenur is highly protein bound (>99% in human plasma). Two metabolites (a hydroxy and a keto) have been found in the serum (Taylor et al 1989, Kuhn et al 1988, Burris et al

PHARMACOKINETICS OF SULOFENUR

Schedule	Reference	β Half-life (h)	Clearance (mL/min/m^2)	AUC (μg·h/mL)	Steady State Volume of Distribution
Daily × 7	Taylor et al 1989	30.1 (harmonic mean)	2.04	8883	12.62 ± 7.00
Daily × 5, 2-d rest	Burris et al 1990	—	—	3938	—
Daily × 21	Brown et al 1989a	—	—	4372	—
Every 3 wk	Brown et al 1989b	40	—	1.9	—

1990). A correlation between dose and decreases in hemoglobin and increases in methemoglobin has been described (Taylor et al 1989, Burris et al 1990).

■ Side Effects and Toxicity

Dose-limiting toxic effects of sulofenur have included methemoglobinemia, anemia, and red cell hemolysis (Taylor et al 1989, Brown et al 1989a, Burris et al 1990). In general, the degree of both anemia and methemoglobinemia was dose related. The degree of methemoglobinemia can be quite impressive. In some studies methylene blue (1 mg/kg) has been used and caused a rapid resolution of the methemoglobinemia (Taylor et al 1989). The degree of methemoglobinemia appears to be least with the daily × 5 2 day off schedule of administration (Burris et al 1990).

The anemia noted with the agent was associated with biochemical changes suggesting hemolysis (increased lactic dehydrogenase, increased bilirubin, increased reticulocyte count, and decreased haptoglobin). Peripheral blood smears revealed degmacytes ("rat bite" cells) (Taylor et al 1989).

Reversible hepatotoxicity has been reported in two patients with elevations of transaminases, alkaline phosphatase, and bilirubin (Taylor et al 1989, Burris et al 1990).

Of interest is that this agent has not caused hypoglycemia, alopecia, granulocytopenia, or gastrointestinal disturbances.

■ Special Applications

None are known.

REFERENCES

Alberts D, Taylor C, Matias B, et al. Phase II trial of sulofenur (LY186641) in patients with previously treated, advanced ovarian cancer. In: *UICC Meeting, Hamburg, West Germany, August 21*; 1990.

Armand JP, Recondo G, Gouyette A, et al. Phase I and pharmacokinetic study of LY 186641 administered daily for 2 weeks every 21 days. *Proc Am Soc Clin Oncol.* 1989;**8**:77.

Boder GB, Grindey GB, Schultz RM. Acute and chronic effects of the sulfonylurea sulofenur (LY186641) on cells in culture. *Proc Am Assoc Cancer Res.* 1992;**33**:509.

Bonnay M, Gouyette A, Chabot G, Recondo G, Belehradek M, Armand JP. Flavone outer and (LM975) and LY186641: Opposite interferences on creatinine assay with alkaline picrate. *Invest New Drugs.* 1989;**7**:458.

Brown T, O'Rourke T, Craig J, et al. Orally administered LY186641: A phase I clinical and pharmacologic study on a daily × 21 schedule. *Proc Am Soc Clin Oncol.* 1989a;**8**:70.

Brown T, O'Rourke T, Craig J, et al. Phase I experience with LY 186641: An oral sulfonylurea administered once every three weeks or daily for 21 days. *Invest New Drugs.* 1989b;**7**:455.

Burris H, Brown T, O'Rourke T, et al. LY186641: Amelioration of toxicity with an alternate schedule of administration. *Proc Am Soc Clin Oncol.* 1990;**9**:86(A335).

Fossella FV, Lippman SM, Seitz DE, et al. Hypoprothrombinemia from coadministration of sulofenur (LY 186641) and warfarin: Report of three cases. *Invest New Drugs.* 1991;**9**:357–359.

Grindey GB, Boder GB, Grossman CS, et al. Further development of diarylsulfamylureas as novel anti-cancer drugs. *Proc Am Assoc Cancer Res.* 1987;**28**:309.

Grindey GB, Boder GB, Harper RW, et al. Identification of diarylsulfamylureas as novel antitumor agents. *Proc Am Assoc Cancer Res.* 1986;**27**:277.

Herrmann R, Hennig FW, Neuhaus P, Rochlitz CF, Gogler H, Nasseri M, Ermisch S. Sulofenur (LY 186641) in colorectal cancer (CRC), a priming agent for 5 fluorouracil (FU)? *Proc Am Soc Clin Oncol.* 1991;**10**:A449.

Houghton JA, Houghton PJ. Human drug sensitivity testing in vitro. In: Hill BT, Dendy PP (eds). The Xenograftas an Intermediate Model System. San Diego, CA: Academic Press. 1983;179–200.

Kuhn J, Craig J, Havlin K, et al. Phase I clinical and pharmacokinetic evaluation of oral LY186641 administered on a single dose Q21d schedule. *Proc Am Soc Clin Oncol.* 1988;**7**:60.

Kuttesch J, Hainsworth J, Satterlee W, Hamilton M, Grindey G, Hande K. Pharmacokinetics of N-[[(4- chlorophenyl)amino]carbonyl-2, 3-dihydro-1H-indene-5-sulfonamide (LY186641). *Proc Am Soc Clin Oncol.* 1988;7:63.

Munshi NC, Seitz DE, Fossella F, et al. Phase II study of sulofenur (LY 186641), a novel antineoplastic agent, in advanced non-small cell lung cancer. *Proc Am Assoc Cancer Res.* 1991;32:189.

Taylor CW, Alberts DS, Ketcham MA, et al. Clinical pharmacology of a novel diarylsulfamylurea antitumor agent. *J Clin Oncol.* 1989;7:1733–1740.

Trump BF, Jain PT, Phelps PC, et al. Effects of sulofenur LY186641 on intracellular ionized calcium $(Ca^{2+})_i$ in colon carcinoma cells. *Proc Am Assoc Cancer Res.* 1992;33:30.

Weinerman B, Shepherd F, Eisenhauer E, et al. NCI Canada phase II studies of sulofenur (S) in untreated small cell lung (SCCL) and renal (RCC) cancers. *Proc Am Soc Clin Oncol.* 1991;10:251.

Suramin Sodium

■ Other Names

Antrypol®; Germanin®; Bayer 205; Fourneau 309; belganyl, Naphuride Sodium®, Naganol®.

■ Chemistry

Suramin's chemical name is 8,8'-[carbonylbis[imino-3,1-phenylenecarbonylimino(4-methyl-3, 1-phenylene)carbonylimino]]bis-1,3,5-naphthalenetrisulfonic acid. The trisodium salt has excellent water solubility (> 10% w/v) but is only sparingly soluble in 95% ethanol. It is insoluble in more lipophilic organic solvents including benezene, ether, petroleum ether, and chloroform. It is also chemically stable to boiling (Hawking 1978). The flocculent powder appears white or pink and will absorb water if exposed directly to the atmosphere. The molecular formula is $C_{51}H_{34}N_6Na_6O_{23}S_6$ and the molecular weight 1429.21. The compound was originally discovered in 1917 by O. Dressel and R. Kothe (Dressel 1961).

■ Antitumor Activity

Suramin is best known as an antitrypanosomal agent and has been used for decades to treat certain African parasitic infections such as Rhodesian and Gambian trypanosomiasis (Hawking 1978). It also has activity against immature forms of some filarial worms including *Onchocerca volvulus*. Antiviral activity for suramin in vitro was described by De Clercq in 1979. The compound appears to inhibit reverse transcriptase in RNA tumor viruses (De Clercq 1979). It can also block the human T-lymphotropic virus type III (acquired immunodeficiency syndrome [AIDS]) retrovirus in vitro (Broder et al 1985) and has been shown to protect human T lymphocytes from infection by the AIDS virus (Mitsuya et al 1984); however, it does not appear to be highly effective at affecting the clinical course of AIDS in patients (Levine et al 1986, Kaplan et al 1987, Broder et al 1985). In a clinical trial of suramin in AIDS patients with Kaposi's sarcoma, detectable viral titers decreased when suramin was administered (Broder et al 1985). Importantly, a few patients with lymphoma or Kaposi's sarcoma in this study had minor antitumor responses.

A follow-up study of suramin was performed in 13 cancer patients: 8 with adrenal carcinoma, 4 with renal cancer, and 1 with adult T-cell leukemia/lymphoma (Stein et al 1989). Four partial responses were observed in two patients with adrenal cancer, one patient with renal cell carcinoma, and one patient with T-cell leukemia/lymphoma. In another trial, the response rate to suramin was very low: only 1 partial response in 26 patients with renal cell cancer (Motzer et al 1992).

Antitumor activity has been observed in hor-

Structure of suramin sodium

monally refractory prostate cancer (Myers et al 1990). In 15 patients with measurable disease, 6 patients (40%) had significant reductions in tumor mass. Antitumor responses were noted in 3 of 6 patients. In 20 prostate cancer patients with bone disease, significant pain relief occurred in 14 of 20 (70%) patients. Prostate-specific antigen levels dropped substantially in over 50% of patients with normalization in 4 of 20; however, prostate cancer patients with bone disease respond poorly to suramin if serum androgens are elevated, especially if dihydroepiandrostenedione (DHEA) is increased (Myers et al 1990). A 54% response rate in prostate cancer was recently reported in patients with bone-only disease (Tkaczuk et al 1992). Plasma suramin levels may need to be maintained above 200 μg/mL to obtain responses in patients with D_2 hormone-refractory prostate cancer (Kelly et al 1992).

There is experimental evidence for significant synergy for suramin combined with tumor necrosis factor α and doxorubicin in prostate carcinoma in vitro (see Drug Interactions). Antitumor activity in vitro has also been observed in lymphomas (Spigelman et al 1987) and in fresh human tumors isolated from patients with malignant melanoma, multiple myeloma, and ovarian cancer (Salmon et al 1990). In addition, activity has been observed in human sarcoma cell lines (Hargis et al 1990) and in rhabdomyosarcoma cells in vitro (Minniti et al 1992).

In cisplatin-refractory advanced ovarian carcinoma, three of five patients receiving two or more courses have achieved a partial response in a pilot study (Alberts et al 1991). The overall response rate in 18 heavily pretreated ovarian cancer patients was 20%. Greater activity has been reported in prostate cancer, with objective responses observed in 4 of 8 patients (50%) (Armand et al 1991), in 6 of 16 patients (43%) in a continuous-infusion trial (Ahmann et al 1991), and in 4 of 4 evaluable patients in another trial using an initial infusion loading dose and subsequent brief infusion doses to maintain plasma levels in the range of 300 μg/mL (Eisenberger et al 1991). Another prostate cancer trial used a similar individualized infusion/maintenance dosing regimen and objective responses were observed in 6 of 16 (37%) patients (Iversen et al 1991).

■ Mechanism of Action

Suramin produces diverse biologic effects, each of which may contribute to the antitumor effect. First, the drug inactivates an array of normal cellular enzymes. This is believed to involve drug binding to free cationic amino acid residues near the active site of the enzymes (Williamson 1970). Enzymes thus inhibited (50% inhibitory concentrations) include hyaluronidase (10^{-6} to 10^{-7} M), urease (10^{-4} M), hexokinase (10^{-4} to 10^{-5} M), and RNA polymerase (10^{-5} M) (Waring 1965). Various lysosomal enzymes are also inhibited by suramin accumulation in lysosomes (Smeesters and Jaques 1968). Cellular ATP metabolism is affected by suramin because of inhibition of ATP synthesis (Calcaterra et al 1988). Suramin inhibits ATPases (Fortes et al 1973) and several enzymes involved with phosphorylation and dephosphorylation (Rodnight 1970). The effects on RNA and subsequently DNA synthesis, as well as inhibition of mitochondrial oxidative enzymes, may account for the trypanostatic effects of suramin. In human prostate cancer cell lines, suramin also inhibits mitochondrial function (Rago et al 1992a). This leads to impaired mitochondrial retention of rhodamine-123 and the uncoupling of cellular oxygen consumption. Importantly, these effects were observed in vitro at clinically relevant suramin concentrations (Rago et al 1992a).

Suramin can also bind to several tumor growth factors including platelet-derived growth factor (PDGF) (Hosang 1985, Garrett et al 1984), epidermal growth factor (EGF), transforming growth factor β (TGF-β (Betsholtz et al 1986, Coffey et al 1987), and insulin-like growth factor 1 (IGF-1) (Pollak and Richard 1990). By avidly binding to these growth factors, suramin deprives the tumor cell of hormonal stimulation, thereby inhibiting tumor cell growth. In rhabdomyosarcoma cells suramin inhibits the specific binding of insulin-like growth factor II which interrupts an autocrine growth stimulation pathway (Minniti et al 1992). Whether this cytostatic type of growth inhibition invariably leads to actual tumor cell cytolysis is unclear. Suramin may also inhibit second-messenger enzymes involved in signal transduction for some of the protein growth factors such as protein kinase C type I to III activity (Mahoney et al 1990).

Suramin increases tyrosine phosphorylation, which could halt intracellular signaling from growth-related protein hormones (McLellan et al 1992). This may be caused by inhibition of protein tyrosine phosphatase activity (Berggren et al 1992). Recent evidence suggests that suramin may inhibit DNA topoisomerase II enzymes without stabilizing the "cleavable" complex, as is seen with other topoisomerase II inhibitors (Larsen et al 1991). Suramin also blocks DNA synthesis by inhibiting DNA polymerases. This action requires very low drug concentrations of 8 to 36 µM (IC$_{50}$) for DNA polymerases alpha and sigma, respectively (Jindal et al 1990). Eukaryotic DNA polymerase C was relatively insensitive to the drug.

An alternative biologic explanation for suramin's antitumor effect involves increases in tissue glycosaminoglycan levels, especially heparan and dermatan sulfate (Horne et al 1988). This is mediated by inhibition of the lysosomal enzyme iduronate sulfatase, which normally breaks down glycosaminoglycans. In animals, the increase in specific glycosaminoglycans by suramin can lead to a lysosomal storage disease similar to Hunter's syndrome (Constantopoulos et al 1980). The increase in tissue glycosaminoglycans following suramin can also produce anticoagulation, inhibition of tumor angiogenesis (Folkman and Klagsbrun 1987), and the induction of normal cellular differentiation (Fujita et al 1987). Suramin is known to localize to vascular endothelial cells and this may explain some of its activity as a powerful inhibitor of angiogenesis (Jamis-Dow et al 1991). All of these novel effects may contribute to the unique antitumor activity of suramin.

■ Availability and Storage

Suramin sodium is investigationally available from FBA Pharmaceuticals, Division of Mobay Corporation, New York City, a Bayer U.S.A. company. The product is supplied under the auspices of the National Cancer Institute in clear glass vials containing 1 g of lyophilized sodium suramin. The vials can be stored at room temperature but should be protected from light.

■ Preparation for Use, Stability, and Admixture

Suramin sodium vials are reconstituted with 10 mL of Sterile Water for Injection, USP, yielding a 100 mg/mL clear solution. Doses for infusion can be diluted further using either D5W or 0.9% sodium chloride. At a concentration of 10 mg/mL, suramin solutions in saline or dextrose are stable for at least 2 weeks at room temperature and under ultraviolet lighting conditions.

It is reported that the slightly acidic solution of suramin can precipitate with basic drugs such as pentamidine (Hawking 1978). Suramin may thus be physically incompatible with a variety of basic drugs and direct admixtures should be avoided.

■ Administration

In AIDS trials, suramin was administered as a series of six weekly intravenous injections given over 20 minutes (Broder et al 1985; Kaplan et al 1987). To increase the dose intensity of suramin, recent trials in cancer patients have used continuous intravenous infusions (Stein et al 1989) (See Dosage for specific administration regimens.)

■ Special Precautions

A test dose of suramin is sometimes recommended prior to the initial bolus or infusion dose of the drug. The intravenous test dose of up to 200 mg is used to elicit a rare acute complication of the drug that involves circulatory collapse with nausea, vomiting, and shock (Duke and Anderson 1972). The reported incidence of this reaction is 1 in every 2000 to 4500 patients (Apted 1970). It may relate to a very rapid intravenous injection of the drug when used in patients with trypanosomiasis.

Suramin may displace other highly protein-bound drugs and can require supplemental vitamin K and glucocorticosteroid therapy (see Drug Interactions).

■ Dosage

In vitro antitumor studies suggest that suramin levels of 200 to 225 µg/mL are required for growth-inhibitory effects (Stein et al 1989, Salmon et al 1990). To achieve these levels, doses of up to 350 mg/m²/d have been given by continuous intravenous infusion (Stein et al 1989). In the induction phase, a daily dose of 350 mg/m²/d is given by continuous intravenous infusion until a plasma level of 280 to 300 µg/mL is achieved. Thereafter, the weekly infusion rate during the induction course is adjusted on the basis of the plasma suramin level (see table on page 862). Once a steady-state level of 280 µg/mL or greater is achieved, suramin is then discontinued for 2 months to observe for antitumor response. Subsequent cycles of therapy are given at 2-month intervals.

New strategies for suramin dosing include the use of an intravenous-infusion loading course followed by intermittent brief infusion "maintenance" doses (Eisenberger et al 1991). The precise doses for this type of schedule are aimed at maintaining plasma suramin levels between 150 and 300 µg/mL (Reyno et al 1992). Other schedules are currently under development and will probably require strict individualization based on limited sampling models with Bayesian feedback (Iversen et al 1991). More

SURAMIN INFUSION NOMOGRAM

Suramin Level (µg/mL)	Infusion Rate (mg/m²/d)
0 (Initiation)	350
0–149	425
150–199	350
200–240	262
241–279	200
> 280	0

Data from Myers et al 1990.

recently, this group has described responses in prostate cancer patients who maintained a suramin concentration above 200 µg/mL for 7 weeks using weekly bolus doses adjusted by an adaptive control algorithm (Kelly et al 1992). And, from the experience in AIDS patients it is clear that repetitive weekly doses of 1 to 1.5 g can be safely administered for periods up to 24 consecutive weeks (Kaplan et al 1987).

■ Drug Interactions

Because of the high degree of protein binding, suramin may displace other highly bound drugs. This is especially crucial with agents such as aspirin and nonsteroidal anti-inflammatory drugs. These highly bound drugs could produce severe bleeding complications if displaced by suramin, which itself causes bleeding by binding to various circulating clotting factors (Stein et al 1989). It is therefore recommended that vitamin K be administered to patients receiving suramin. In addition, suramin causes necrosis of the adrenal gland after several courses of therapy. This mandates the administration of glucocorticosteroids with mineralocorticoid activity to patients receiving this drug beyond an initial course of therapy.

Suramin has been shown to have synergistic antitumor activity with tumor necrosis factor α (TNF-α) and doxorubicin (Fruehauf et al 1990). The human prostate cancer cell lines LNCaP (testosterone dependent) and PC-3 (testosterone independent) were respectively threefold and sevenfold more sensitive to suramin in the presence of doxorubicin. PC-3 cells were resistant to TNF-α, and suramin did not sensitize these cells; however, the TNF-sensitive LNCaP cells demonstrated a synergistic increase in TNF sensitivity in the presence of clinically achievable suramin concentrations. Synergy was also reported for suramin and doxorubicin in human breast cancer cell lines in vitro (Favoni et al 1991). The mechanism(s) for the observed synergy is unclear. The combination of suramin prior to the topoisomerase I inhibitor camptothecin was also synergistic in vitro (Lopez et al 1992).

In breast cancer cells, suramin is reported to block the antiproliferative effects of hydroxytamoxifen and doxorubicin (Berthois et al 1992). In contrast, suramin was most effective in multidrug-resistant breast cancer cells, suggesting a selective toxicity mechanism (Berthois et al 1992).

■ Pharmacokinetics

Suramin exhibits a slow overall elimination as a result of the very high degree of protein binding in the blood and tissues. In antiretroviral trials with AIDS patients, peak suramin levels following six 1-g bolus doses averaged about 150 µg/mL (Broder et al 1985). The half-life of suramin in these patients ranged from 44 to 54 days (Collins et al 1986). Suramin levels were determined using reverse-phase high-performance liquid chromatography with a gradient type of elution (Klecker and Collins 1985).

These studies also showed that 99.7 to 99.8% of the drug was bound to proteins in the circulation. Thus, the low total body clearance of about 0.5 mL/min was due primarily to renal elimination of the small unbound (free) fraction of the drug in the plasma. Drug distribution studies have shown that compared with plasma, genitourinary tissues tend to accumulate suramin (Rago et al 1992b,c). Levels in prostate tissues 1.5 weeks after a 6-g course of suramin were 85 ± 19 µg/g, compared with 41 µg/mL in the plasma. Muscle levels of suramin are less than those in plasma. After a dose of 17 g given over 10 weeks, suramin levels (µg/g) varied in different tissues: 276 in testis, 174 in lung, 148 in kidney, 131 in prostate, 112 in fat, 78 in liver, 44 in heart and pancreas, 32 in muscle, and 16 in brain (Rago et al 1992b).

Pharmacokinetic analyses of suramin disposition in prostate cancer patients show similar clearance patterns but with a much shorter terminal elimination half-life (see table) (Forrest et al 1990). It is clear that small changes in renal function or protein binding can produce substantial changes in the terminal half-life of suramin. Furthermore, the use of a two-compartment model for suramin appears to fit the data best (Lieberman et al 1990). Monitoring the disposition of the test dose can be used to plan individual infusion programs (Hutson et al 1991).

Suramin appears to penetrate the blood–brain barrier poorly. A cancer patient who developed

MEAN SURAMIN PHARMACOKINETICS IN PROSTATE CANCER PATIENTS*

	Mean	SE
Half-life (d)		
α	1.4	0.4
β	21.8	3.2
Clearance (L/d/m^2)		
Total	0.52	0.04
Distributive phase	1.6	0.3
Steady-state volume of distribution (L/m^2)	13.4	1.3

*Means and SEs from 111 observations.
Data from Forrest et al 1990.

postviral Guillain–Barré syndrome during suramin treatment had a cerebrospinal fluid suramin level of 3 µg/mL compared with a simultaneous plasma level of 350 µg/mL (Stein et al 1989). Thus, cerebrospinal fluid levels of suramin are less than 1% of the simultaneous plasma concentration.

Pharmacodynamic studies suggest that current infusion regimens can produce plasma concentration × time products (AUCs) of 9187 to 13,465 mg·day/L (Iversen et al 1991, Alberts et al 1991). These are at least five times greater than the median IC$_{50}$ AUCs needed for inhibitory activity against fresh human tumor cells in vitro (Alberts et al 1991). In contrast, neurotoxic effects appear to be related to peak concentrations above 300 µg/mL (Kilbourn et al 1991).

■ Side Effects and Toxicity

Preclinical studies of acute high doses of suramin in primates showed hyperemic swollen intestines, degenerating kidney tubules, an atrophic spleen, and peripheral blood lymphocytopenia and anemia (Gibson et al 1977). Intoxicated animals developed hemorrhages and chronic diarrhea and appeared emaciated. When used as an antitrypanosomal agent, suramin produced a range of rare, immediate reactions. These include nausea and vomiting (which is lessened by slowing the rate of injection), shock and loss of consciousness, colic, urticaria, and a slight temperature increase (Hawking 1978). A fever can become more prominent over the ensuing 24 hours. Other late reactions (after 3–24 hours) include photophobia and lacrimation, abdominal distention, and cutaneous hyperesthesia of the soles or palms. This is rarely followed by desquamation (Hawking 1978). Chronic toxic effects in patients treated for trypanosomal infections include albuminuria, exfoliative dermatitis, stomatitis, and general weakness. It is also clear that chronic suramin therapy is highly toxic to the adrenal gland, resulting in degenerative necrosis after several months of therapy.

Toxic effects in cancer patients consistently involve proteinuria of up to 2 g/d (Stein et al 1989). A concomitant elevation in the serum creatinine occurs in about 60% of patients, although other nephrotoxic predisposing factors were also present in these patients. Elevation of liver function enzymes (serum glutamic–oxalacetic and glutamic–pyruvic transaminases) was noted in 8 of 15 patients, and a rash was described in 6 of 15 (40%) of patients. Fever and rash are much less common with infusions of suramin than with the older intravenous bolus dosing method; however, suramin infusions do produce myelotoxicity in about one third of patients (Stein et al 1989). In one study this manifested as thrombocytopenia (< 75,000/mL) in 4 of 15 patients and leukopenia (< 2000/mL) in 3 of 15 patients.

A more common toxic effect was a drug-induced coagulopathy seen in 11 of 15 patients. This was characterized by an elevated thrombin time, prothrombin time, and partial thromboplastin time; however, frank hemorrhage occurred in only four patients and was not a factor in the one treatment-related death (presumed sepsis) (Stein et al 1989). Of interest, one patient showed a reasonable correlation between a high suramin level and the elevation in the thrombin time test, which occurred just prior to attaining a partial response (Stein et al 1989).

Adrenal insufficiency was noted in only three patients in this trial, but this low incidence is probably related to the relatively short duration of treatment. An unusual ocular toxic effect, vortex keratopathy, was also described in 5 of 15 patients in this trial (Stein et al 1989). Visual symptoms, however, were noted in only two patients. They included photophobia, tearing, and blurred vision. Symptomatic patients were treated with artificial tears but were nonetheless incapacitated for 2 weeks. Ophthalmologic biopsies were compatible with an accumulation of glycosaminoglycans in lysosomes in the eye.

Suramin may also inhibit the immune system, leading to an increased incidence of infection in treated patients. Staphylococcal infections were most common in one survey (Senderowicz et al 1991). In some studies, catheter infections were seen with a high frequency (Senderowicz et al 1991, Alberts et al 1991). This may be mediated by suramin-induced lysosomal dysfunction in macrophages (Warr and Jakab 1983). One study was unable to show a defect in neutrophil superoxide generation or zymosan particle ingestion (Senderowicz et al 1991). In mice, suramin is known to reduce delayed-type hypersensitivity and can decrease natural killer monocyte cytotoxic effects mediated by TNF-α (Zhang et al 1988).

Suramin produces peripheral neuropathy typically after high cumulative doses or acutely when extremely elevated blood levels are achieved. In some cases this may be the dose-limiting toxic effect. Proximal muscle weakness 1 to 2 weeks following exposure to levels greater than 300 μg/mL has been described (Kilbourn et al 1991). This syndrome appears to be distinct from the peripheral neuropathy noted in other trials. The muscle weakness may be caused by decreased cytochrome C oxidase activity in muscle tissues (Rago et al 1992b). Mitochondrial morphology is also abnormal and sarcolemma collections suggest a toxic mitochondrial myopathy as the cause of the painful muscle weakness (Rago et al 1992b).

Other toxic effects reported with suramin include hyperamylasemia, hypophosphatemia, and atrial fibrillation. In one case, transient, uneventful fibrillation developed after the patient had been off the drug for 2 weeks. In the other instance, atrial fibrillation with a rapid ventricular response developed during a second course of suramin therapy at a serum concentration of about 150 μg/mL.

REFERENCES

Ahmann FR, Schwartz J, Dorr R, Salmon S. Suramin in hormone resistant metastatic prostate cancer: Significant anticancer activity but unanticipated toxicity. *Proc Am Soc Clin Oncol.* 1991;**10**:178.

Alberts D, Miranda E, Dorr R, et al. Phase II and pharmacokinetic (PK) and human tumor cloning assay (HTCA) study of suramin in advanced ovarian cancer. *Proc Am Soc Clin Oncol.* 1991;**10**:187.

Apted FIC. In: Mulligan HW, ed. *The African Trypanosomiases.* London: Allen & Unwin; 1970:684.

Armand JP, Bonnay M, Gandia D, et al. Phase I–II suramin (SRM) study in advanced cancer patients (pts). *Proc Am Assoc Cancer Res.* 1991;**32**:175.

Berggren M, Abraham R, Powis G. Inhibition of protein tyrosine phosphatase by the anticancer drugs gallium nitrate and suramin. *Proc Am Assoc Cancer Res.* 1992;**33**:86.

Berthois Y, Dong X-F, Martin P-M, et al. Antagonism by suramin of the growth-inhibitory effect of hydroxytamoxifen and doxorubicin in human MCF-7 breast cancer cells. *J Natl Cancer Inst.* 1992;**84**:1438–1439.

Betsholtz C, Johnsson A, Heldin C-H, Westermark B. Efficient reversion of simian sarcoma virus-transformation and inhibition of growth factor-induced mitogenesis by suramin. *Proc Natl Acad Sci USA.* 1986;**83**:6440–6444.

Broder S, Yarchoan R, Collins JM, et al. Effects of suramin on HTLV-III/LAV infection presenting as Kaposi's sarcoma or AIDS-related complex: Clinical pharmacology and suppression of virus replication in vivo. *Lancet.* 1985;**2**:627–630.

Calcaterra NB, Vicario LR, Roveri OA. Inhibition by suramin of mitochondrial ATP synthesis. *Biochem Pharmacol.* 1988;**37**(13):2521–2527.

Coffey R, Leof E, Shipley G, et al. Suramin inhibition of growth factor receptor binding and mitogenicity in AKR-2B cells. *J Cell Phys.* 1987;**132**:143–148.

Collins JM, Klecker RW, Yarchosn R, et al. Clinical pharmacokinetics of suramin in patients with HTLV-III/LAV infection. *J Clin Pharmacol.* 1986;**67**:666–671.

Constantopoulos G, Rees S, Cragg B, et al. Experimental animal model for mucopolysaccharidosis: Suramin-induced glycosaminoglycan and sphingolipid accumulation in the rat. *Proc Natl Acad Sci USA.* 1980;**77**:3700–3704.

De Clercq E. Suramin: A potent inhibitor of the reverse transcriptase of RNA tumor viruses. *Cancer Lett.* 1979;**8**:9–22.

Dressel J. The discovery of germanin by Oskor Dressel and Richard Cothe. Translated by R.E. Oesper. *J Chem Ed.* 1961;**38**:620.

Duke BOL, Anderson J. Onchocerciasis and its treatment. *Trop Doctor.* 1972;**2**:107–114.

Eisenberger M, Jodrell D, Sinibaldi V, et al. Preliminary evidence of anti-tumor activity against prostate cancer (PrCa) observed in a phase I trial with suramin. *Proc Am Soc Clin Oncol.* 1991;**10**:168.

Favoni RE, Rosso R, Pirani P, et al. Synergistic activity of suramin and doxorubicin on human breast cancer cell lines. *Proc Am Assoc Cancer Res.* 1991;**32**:384.

Folkman J, Klagsbrun M. Angiogenic factors. *Science.* 1987;**235**;442–447.

Forrest A, Scher HI, Tong W, Smart-Curley T, Vasquez J, Petrylak D. Development of an adaptive control algorithm for suramin (SUR) (abstract #284). *Proc Am Soc Clin Oncol.* 1990;**9**:73.

Fortes PA, Ellory JC, Lew VL. Suramin: A potent ATPase inhibitor which acts on the inside surface of the sodium pump. *Biochim Biophys Acta.* 1973;**318**:262–272.

Fruehauf JP, Myers CE, Sinha BK. Synergistic activity of suramin with tumor necrosis factor α and doxorubicin on human prostate cancer cell lines. *J Natl Cancer Inst.* 1990;**82**:1206–1209.

Fujita M, Spray D, Choi H, et al. Glycosaminoglycans and proteoglycans induce gap junction expression and restore transcription of tissue-specific mRNAs in primary liver cultures. *Hepatology.* 1987;**7**:1S–9S.

Garrett J, Coughlin S, Niman H, et al. Blockade of autocrine stimulation in simian sarcoma virus transformed cells reverses down-regulation of platelet-derived growth factor receptors. *Proc Natl Acad Sci USA.* 1984;**81**:7466–7470.

Gibson DW, Duke BO, Connor DH. Histopathological studies on suramin toxicity in a chimpanzee. *Tropenmed Parasitol.* 1977;**28**(3):387–405.

Hargis JB, Danesi R, Myers C, La Rocca R. Suramin activity in human sarcoma cell lines (abstract #2433). *Proc Am Assoc Cancer Res.* 1990;**31**:410.

Hawking F. Suramin: With special reference to onchocerciasis. *Adv Pharmacol Chemother.* 1978;**15**:289–322.

Horne M, Stein CA, LaRocca RV, et al. Circulating glycosaminoglycan anticoagulants associated with suramin treatment. *Blood.* 1988;**71**:273–279.

Hosang M. Suramin binds to platelet-derived growth factor and inhibits its biological activity. *J Cell Biochem.* 1985;**29**:265–273.

Hutson P, Arzoomanian R, Tombes MB, et al. Test dose guided rapid IV suramin infusions with weekly IV maintenance doses. *Proc Am Soc Clin Oncol.* 1991;**10**:99.

Iversen J, Scher H, Motzer R, et al. Suramin (SUR): Impact of individualized pharmacokinetic (PK) dosing on outcome in patients with prostatic cancer (PC) and renal cell carcinoma (RCC). *Proc Am Soc Clin Oncol.* 1991;**10**:103.

Jamis-Dow CA, Weiss GH, Merino MJ, et al. Suramin selectively localizes to vascular endothelial cells: A possible basis for the antiangiogenesis activity of suramin. *Proc Am Assoc Cancer Res.* 1991;**32**:83.

Jindal HK, Anderson CW, Davis RG, Vishwanatha JK. Suramin affects DNA synthesis in HeLa cells by inhibition of DNA polymerases. *Cancer Res.* 1990;**50**:7754–7757.

Kaplan LD, Wolfe PR, Volberding PA, et al. Lack of response to suramin in patients with AIDS and AIDS-related complex. *Am J Med.* 1987;**82**:615–620.

Kelly WK, Scher HI, Bajorin DF, et al. Phase I trial of suramin in patients with advanced cancer. *Proc Am Assoc Cancer Res.* 1992;**33**:530.

Kilbourn R, Dexeus F, Amato R, et al. Clinical pharmacology of suramin administered by IV bolus injection in patients with refractory prostate cancer. *Proc Am Soc Clin Oncol.* 1991;**10**:112.

Klecker R, Collins J. Quantitation of suramin by reverse-phase ion-pairing high-performance liquid chromatography. *J Liq Chromatogr.* 1985;**8**:1685–1696.

Larsen AK, Lelievre S, Bojanowski K, et al. Suramin is an inhibitor of DNA topoisomerase II. *Proc Am Assoc Cancer Res.* 1991;**32**:338.

Levine A, Gill P, Cohen J, et al. Suramin antiviral therapy in the acquired immunodeficiency syndrome. *Ann Intern Med.* 1986;**105**:32–37.

Lieberman R, Katzper M, Cooper M, et al. Nonmem (NM) population (POP) pharmacokinetic (PK) analysis and Bayesian (BAY) forecasting (FOR) during suramin (SUR) therapy in prostate cancer: One versus two-compartment PK models (abstract #262). *Proc Am Soc Clin Oncol.* 1990;**9**:68.

Lopez R, Viriziuela J, Smitskamp-Wilms E, et al. Schedule dependent synergistic effect of suramin and camptothecin in vitro. *Proc Am Soc Clin Oncol.* 1992;**11**:126.

Mahoney CW, Azzi A, Huang K-P. Effects of suramin, an anti-human immunodeficiency virus reverse transcriptase agent, on protein kinase C. *J Biol Chem.* 1990;**265**(10):5424–5428.

McLellan CA, Myers CE, Sartor O. Suramin increases tyrosine phosphorylation in prostate cancer cell lines. *Proc Am Assoc Cancer Res.* 1992;**33**:273.

Minniti C, Horowitz M, Craig C, et al. Inhibition of an autocrine growth pathway in rhabdomyosarcoma (RMS) by suramin: Development of a phase II study. *Proc Am Soc Clin Oncol.* 1992;**11**:366.

Mitsuya H, Popovic M, Yarchoan R, Matsushita S, Gallo RC, Broder S. Suramin protection of T cells in vitro against infectivity and cytopathic effect of HTLV-III. *Science.* 1984;**226**:172–174.

Motzer RJ, Nanus DM, Scher HI, et al. A phase II trial of suramin in patients with advanced renal cell carcinoma. *Proc Am Assoc Cancer Res.* 1992;**33**:220.

Myers CE, LaRocca R, Stein C, et al. Treatment of hormonally refractory prostate cancer with suramin. *Proc Am Soc Clin Oncol.* 1990;**9**:133.

Pollak M, Richard M. Suramin interferes with the binding of insulin-like growth factor I (IGF-I) to human osteosarcoma cells and blocks IGF-I stimulated proliferation (abstract #206). *Proc Am Soc Clin Oncol.* 1990;**9**:54.

Rago R, Brazy P, Wilding G. Tetrazolium conversion, rhodamine 123 retention, and oxygen consumption to quantitate suramin's inhibition of respiration. *Proc Am Assoc Cancer Res.* 1992a;**33**:510.

Rago R, Suffit R, Miles J, et al. Suramin (SUR) weakness due to Fanconi's syndrome and mitochondrial myopathy supports disruption of mitochondria or energy balance as mechanism of activity. *Proc Am Soc Clin Oncol.* 1992b;**11**:114.

Rago R, Tutsch K, Pomplun M, et al. Human plasma and tissue levels of suramin. *Proc Am Assoc Cancer Res.* 1992c;**33**:429.

Reyno L, Sinibaldi V, Eisenberger M, et al. Phase I trial of intermittent IV bolus suramin (SUR) utilizing adaptive control with feedback (ACF) dosing. *Proc Am Soc Clin Oncol.* 1992;**11**:130.

Rodnight R. The effect of chemical agents on the turnover of the bound phosphate associated with the sodium-and-potassium ion-stimulated adenosine triphosphatase in ox brain microsomes. *Biochem J.* 1970;**120**:1–13.

Salmon SE, Liu R, Alberts DS, et al. Predicted antitumor activity of suramin in ovarian cancer and metastatic melanoma (abstract #263). *Proc Am Soc Clin Oncol.* 1990;**9**:68.

Senderowicz A, Scher H, Gordon M, et al. Infectious complications of suramin in patients with genitourinary tumors. *Proc Am Assoc Cancer Res.* 1991;**32**:203.

Smeesters C, Jaques PJ. Influence of injected suramin on enzymic equipment of rat liver lisosomes in vivo. Proc Int Congr Cell Biol, 12th, 1968 Excerpta Med Found Int Congr Ser No 166, Abstract No. 143, p. 82.

Spigelman Z, Dowers A, Kennedy S, et al. Antiproliferative effects of suramin on lymphoid cells. *Cancer Res.* 1987;**47**:4696–4698.

Stein CA, LaRocca RV, Thomas R, McAtee N, Myers CE. Suramin: An anticancer drug with a unique mechanism of action. *J Clin Oncol.* 1989;**7**(4):499–508.

Tkaczuk K, Eisenberger M, Sinibaldi V, et al. Activity of suramin (Su) in prostate cancer (PC) observed in a phase I trial. *Proc Am Soc Clin Oncol.* 1992;**11**:201.

Waring MJ. The effects of antimicrobial agents on ribonucleic acid polymerase. *Mol Pharmacol.* 1965;**1**:1–13.

Warr G, Jakab G. Lung macrophage defense responses during suramin induced lysosomal dysfunction. *Exp Mol Pathol.* 1983;**38**:193–207.

Williamson J. Review of chemotherapeutic and chemoprophylactic agents. In: Mulligan HW, ed. *The African Trypanosomiases.* London: Allen & Unwin; 1970:125–221.

Zhang HX, Sozzani S, D'Allessandro F, et al. Modulation by suramin of NK and monocytic cell-mediated cytotoxicity in human and murine cells. *Int J Immunopharmacol.* **10**:695–707.

Tamoxifen

Other Names

Nolvadex® (ICI Pharma); Tam; NSC-180973; ICI-46474.

Chemistry

Structure of tamoxifen

Tamoxifen is a nonsteroidal antiestrogenic analog of clomiphene. Chemically, it is a *trans* isomer of triphenylethylene. The complete chemical name of the compound is 2,2-(4-(1,2-diphenyl-1-butenyl)-phenoxy)-N,N-dimethylethylamine:citrate (1:1). The commercial product is supplied as the citrate salt. The molecular formula of tamoxifen (base) is $C_{26}H_{29}NO$ and the molecular weight 371.5. The citrate adds a $C_6H_8O_7$ moiety of molecular weight 192.12 to the formulation.

Antitumor Activity

In laboratory rats, tamoxifen can inhibit the growth of established dimethylbenzanthracene (DMBA)-induced mammary cancers (Jordan 1974, Nicholson and Golder 1975) and the development of new tumors in response to the same carcinogenic stimulus (Jordan 1974, 1984). Thus, Jordan et al (1977) were able to effectively inhibit DMBA-induced tumorigenesis using long-term prophylactic tamoxifen.

Clinically, tamoxifen is active in a number of solid tumors (see table on the opposite page). In human studies the established major indication for tamoxifen is advanced breast cancer, optimally in postmenopausal patients with estrogen receptor(ER)-positive tumors (Kiang and Kennedy 1977). Glick et al (1979, 1982) reported that tamoxifen was relatively inactive in renal cell carcinoma and only marginally effective in advanced prostate cancer patients (Glick et al 1980). A Southwest Oncology Group report (Al-Sarraf et al 1981) has also described minimal activity for low-dose tamoxifen in advanced renal cell cancer. In this study of 49 renal cell patients there were 2 partial responses and 14 patients had disease improvement or stabilization. Tamoxifen is also active in endometrial cancer (Swenerton et al 1979). In this small preliminary trial, there were 3 of 10 partial responders. Other unpublished trials conducted by Bonte et al and Hald et al have noted response rates of 27% with some complete responders. The duration of response ranged from 9 to 46 months in these trials.

Because of the occasional isolation of estrogen receptor tissue in melanomas (Fisher et al 1976), in pancreatic tissues (Sandberg et al 1973), and in large bowel tumors (McClendon et al 1977, Alford et al 1979), a number of clinical trials in solid tumors were initiated. Investigations with tamoxifen have shown limited activity for single-agent tamoxifen in melanoma (Meyskens and Voakes 1980, Masiel et al 1980, Creagan et al 1980, Nesbit et al 1979). More recent studies suggest that high-dose tamoxifen combined with dacarbazine and carmustine produces a

CLINICAL RESPONSE RATES TO TAMOXIFEN IN METASTATIC CANCER

Cancer Type	Tamoxifen (mg/d)	Other Drugs (mg/m^2)	Objective Response Rate*	Reference
Breast	20	None	45%	Taylor et al 1986
Endometrial	20	None	30%	Swenerton et al 1980
Melanoma	20	None	0–12%	Creagan et al 1980, Meyskens and Voakes 1980
	40	Carmustine (150)	43	Berd et al 1991
	160	Dacarbazine (220/d × 3)	47	
Prostate, stage D	20	None	7%	Glick et al 1982
Renal cell	20	None	6.3%	Al-Sarraf et al 1981

*Includes complete and partial responses only.

complete response rate of up to 27% in patients with metastatic melanoma (Berd et al 1991).

Nonetheless, advanced breast cancer is the principal clinical indication for tamoxifen. Overall, the response rate to low-dose tamoxifen as a single agent in this disease ranges from 20 to 70% and is highly dependent on estrogen receptor levels. The drug is also effective in advanced male breast cancer (Aisner et al 1979). As with other hormonal agents used in female breast cancer, tamoxifen appears most effective in patients who are postmenopausal 5 or more years. In this setting tamoxifen produces remission durations ranging from several months to over 2 years. Response rates to tamoxifen are noted in patients failing other hormonal manipulations, but response rates are progressively lower (Ward 1977, Manni et al 1976, Kiang and Kennedy 1977), especially in those tumors with estrogen receptor protein contents greater than 10 fmol/mg of protein (Brule 1976, Kiang and Kennedy 1977, Lerner et al 1976, Morgan et al 1976, Manni et al 1976). For reference, McGuire et al (1978) have suggested that the highest responses may be possible in tumors containing more than 100 fmol of estrogen receptor per milligram of cytosol protein.

Long-term adjuvant tamoxifen may also be useful in lymph node-negative breast cancer (Tormey and Jordan 1984); however, a recent interim report in 3538 postmenopausal women suggests that tamoxifen does not lessen the risk of developing breast cancer in the opposite breast (Andersson et al 1991). In contrast, a retrospective review of 133 randomized trials showed that tamoxifen lowered the risk of cancer developing in the contralateral breast by 39% (Early Breast Cancer Trialists' Collaborative Group 1992). A slightly increased risk of endometrial cancer may also limit this therapeutic approach. Nonetheless, tamoxifen reduces annual recurrence rates by 25% and mortality by 17% in patients with early breast cancer. Thus, tamoxifen appears to prevent the onset of metastatic disease when used prophylactically in patients with early breast cancer.

Some patients with negative or low estrogen receptor levels are responsive to tamoxifen (Brule 1976). Heuson (1976) also noted good response rates in premenopausal patients (partial response rates of 20 and 33%, respectively). Whether tamoxifen is clinically superior to ovariectomy or ovarian radiation is unclear. The drug is active in estrogen receptor-positive premenopausal women who wish to avoid surgery or radiation therapy (Sunderland and Osborne 1991), but escalated tamoxifen doses may be needed in premenopausal patients to continually suppress high endogenous estrogen levels in some responding patients (Manni and Pearson 1980). Similar dose escalations may occasionally be helpful in relapsing postmenopausal patients with metastatic disease (Manni and Arafah 1981); however, reinduction of response is not always possible with such dose escalation (Stewart et al 1982).

The dominant site of disease also appears to be a response factor in breast cancer. Visceral disease, especially liver metastases, is typically less responsive to tamoxifen (Lerner et al 1976, Morgan et al 1976) than soft tissue disease followed by bony disease (Kiang and Kennedy 1977).

Because of a lack of significant hematologic toxicity, tamoxifen is often combined with other cytotoxic chemotherapeutic agents. As would be anticipated, overall response rates are slightly improved with no increase in toxicity due to tamoxifen. This has perhaps been best documented for tamoxifen combined with cyclophosphamide, methotrexate, and 5-fluorouracil (Bonadonna's "CMF" regimen) (Morgan et al 1976, Cocconi et al 1979). Indeed, tamoxifen therapy for advanced breast cancer may be more efficacious than initial CMF therapy (Priestman et al 1977). This is especially true in postmenopausal women with metastatic disease (Taylor et al 1986). Then, if patients relapse on tamoxifen, they may still be effectively treated with CMF doses adjusted on the basis of renal dysfunction (Taylor et al 1986). Tamoxifen is also highly effective when used as an adjuvant therapy in postmenopausal women with positive lymph node involvement (Early Breast Cancer Trialists' Collaborative Group 1992). Survival is improved by approximately 8% with tamoxifen in such patients with positive lymph nodes.

Besides cytotoxic drugs, tamoxifen has been combined with a number of other hormonal drugs and/or surgical manipulations. The combination of tamoxifen plus fluoxymesterone appears to be clinically active with an increased response rate of 45% versus 28% for tamoxifen alone (Tormey et al 1976). Lerner and Marcovitz (1979) demonstrated salvage of nearly 60% of tamoxifen failures using this two-drug combination; however, in stage IV disease, tamoxifen is superior to fluoxymesterone (Westerberg 1980). And, in another study, combined treatment with tamoxifen and medroxyprogesterone acetate provided no better therapy than tamoxifen alone (Mouridsen et al 1979).

■ Mechanism of Action

Tamoxifen is an estrogen antagonist with a nonsteroidal triphenylethylene type of structure similar to that of the antiestrogen clomiphene. The drug blocks estrogen receptors in most but not all hormonal tissues. In strict pharmacologic terms, it could therefore be classified and is thusly classified as a mixed estrogen antagonist/agonist. Cell culture studies of human breast cancer demonstrate that tamoxifen levels 10,000-fold greater than those of estradiol suppress both estrogen-stimulated growth and progesterone receptor induction. Furthermore, this effect is readily reversible at lower levels of the antiestrogen (Horwitz and McGuire 1978).

Tamoxifen does not block estrogen receptor (ER) synthesis nor is degradation accelerated (Jordan 1984). Indeed, ER levels are upregulated two- to fourfold by tamoxifen (Kiang et al 1989). Instead, tamoxifen binds to the ER and induces a conformational change therein. This complex can bind to DNA but subsequent transcription of RNA (expression of estrogen-dependent genes) is blocked or significantly altered (Furr and Jordan 1984). Tamoxifeninduced antitumor effects are cell cycle (phase) specific, with maximal activity in mid-G_2 phase (Sutherland et al 1986). The drug also causes rapidly cycling breast cancer cells to shift to a slower cycling type of cell. These effects lead to a cytostatic type of growth inhibition with an increase in overall cell cycle transit times. At high concentrations a block in G_1 phase correlates with direct cytotoxicity. Overall, however, tamoxifen appears to produce cytostatic effects in hormonally responsive tumor tissues.

In cell cultures, tamoxifen has also been shown to induce the secretion of transforming growth factor β (TGF-β), which is associated with inhibitory activity for several types of epithelial cells, including breast cancers (Knabbe et al 1987).

The direct estrogen-antagonistic properties of tamoxifen include blockade of thymidine incorporation, DNA polymerase activity, synthesis of the estrogen-specific 52,000-molecular-weight protein (Swain and Lippman 1990), and calmodulin synthesis (Lerner and Jordan 1990). Tamoxifen also reduces the estrogen-dependent polyamine synthesis enzyme ornithine decarboxylase. This lowers cellular polyamine levels and leads to growth inhibition, which can be reversed by exogenous putrescine (Thomas et al 1989). Tamoxifen also lowers plasma levels of the peptide hormone insulin-like growth factor I (IGF-I) in breast cancer patients (Colletti et al 1989). This protein stimulates cell replication, protein synthesis, and thymidine incorporation into DNA (Clemmons and Van Wyk 1984). Thus, the 50% decrease in plasma IGF-I levels induced by tamoxifen may mediate some of the drug's antitumor activity in breast cancer patients.

By contrast, in some tissues tamoxifen can act like a pure estrogenic substance. Such estrogenic effects are noted in the vaginal epithelium (Ferrazzi et al 1977) and in the skeletal bones of postmenopausal women with advanced breast cancer treated with tamoxifen (Turken et al 1989).

■ Availability and Storage

Tamoxifen is commercially available from ICI Pharma, Wilmington, Delaware, as round, white tablets of 15.2 mg tamoxifen citrate (equivalent to 10 mg of tamoxifen). These can be stored at room temperature and should be protected from heat and light.

■ **Special Precautions**

In premenopausal patients it may be prudent to suggest barrier forms of contraception because, initially, short-term tamoxifen therapy can effectively induce ovulation (Klopper and Hall 1971, Macourt 1974).

■ **Dosage**

The most commonly used clinical schedule is 10 mg orally twice a day or 20 mg once daily on a continuous basis. In most studies the total daily dose ranges from 20 to 80 mg. Doses up to 100 mg/m^2 twice a day have been employed, although toxicity (especially retinopathy) may be much greater at these higher dose levels (Tormey et al 1976). There is not yet conclusive evidence of greater benefit at higher doses, although some relapsing patients may respond to higher daily tamoxifen doses to overcome endogenous estrogen concentrations (Manni and Arafah 1981). Premenopausal patients may similarly require higher tamoxifen doses to overcome endogenous estrogen concentrations (Manni and Pearson 1980).

Tormey et al (1976) have reported a dosing study using a range of 2 to 120 mg/m^2 twice daily. This group concluded that tamoxifen was more effective and less toxic at daily doses less than 12 mg/m^2. From a number of studies, however, the efficacy of low daily doses of tamoxifen (10–20 mg) would seem to be well established. In addition, the need for continuous dosing does seem well founded in that disease control is typically lost rapidly on drug discontinuance. A significant difference for once daily versus more frequent administration does not appear to be established. Thus, once-a-day dosing of tamoxifen is rational.

In contrast, pharmacokinetic studies have suggested that a loading dose regimen of high-dose tamoxifen may be used to rapidly achieve steady-state antitumor tamoxifen levels (Fabian and Sternson 1979, Wilkinson et al 1982). In the former report a 20 to 80 mg/m^2 dose of tamoxifen was given twice daily for 7 days followed by 20 mg/m^2/d continuously as maintenance. Mean peak blood levels after a singe (acute) oral dose were approximately 16 ng/mL 6 hours after dosing (average half-life 9–12 hours), and steady-state levels (approximately 194 ng/mL) were not reached until after 4 weeks of daily doses of 20 mg/m^2. Of interest, all responders had steady-state tamoxifen levels above 150 ng/mL and the median time to response was 6 weeks (2 weeks beyond attainment of steady state). With a 40 mg/m^2 twice daily loading course, steady-state levels (> 225 ng/mL) were attained in 1 week. The average tamoxifen half-life on chronic dosing was 5.5 days, but the range was highly variable at 3 to 21 days. Another group recommended a simpler loading dose comprising an initial (day 1 only) dose of 100 mg/m^2 followed by 20 mg daily. This dose rapidly achieved mean blood levels of 150 ng/mL in 12 of 12 breast cancer patients (Wilkinson et al 1982). The efficacy of the suggested loading dose regimen remains to be clinically substantiated.

■ **Drug Interactions**

Tamoxifen has been used successfully with a number of other hormonal agents, including fluoxymesterone (Lerner and Marcovitz 1979, Tormey et al 1976), and with the antiprolactins levodopa, bromocriptine, and levodopa–carbidopa (Ward 1975, 1977). Combined therapy was ineffective with medroxyprogesterone acetate (Mouridsen et al 1979) (see Antitumor Activity). In an experimental combination with insulin, tamoxifen showed antitumor efficacy. A possible explanation for this effect is the decreased levels of estrogen receptors observed in insulin-treated human breast cell cultures (Butler et al 1979).

Other in vitro studies have shown that the cytotoxic drugs vincristine, doxorubicin, melphalan, and 5-fluorouracil can reduce estrogen binding capacity in MCF-7 breast cancer cells (Clarke et al 1986). The clinical significance of this observation, if any, is unknown. Tamoxifen may also attenuate the cytotoxic activity of the anticancer agents 5-fluorouracil and doxorubicin (Hug et al 1985). Of interest, this effect was observed in vitro on ER-positive and ER-negative tumor cells. Tamoxifen may also potentiate the mild hepatotoxicity induced by chronic allopurinol therapy (Shah et al 1982).

Finally, tamoxifen has been shown to modulate the multidrug resistance (MDR) phenomenon in tumor cells treated with natural-product antineoplastic agents (Ramu et al 1984). Importantly, tamoxifen doses of 150 mg/m^2 twice daily do achieve the plasma concentration of 5 μM required for reversal of the MDR phenotype in vitro (Trump et al 1991). In this trial, the combination of high-dose tamoxifen and vinblastine (1.5 mg/m^2/d × 5 days)

CLINICAL PHARMACOKINETICS OF TAMOXIFEN*

Tamoxifen Species	Time To Peak (h) or Absorption	Mean Half-life (Range) α (h)	Mean Half-life (Range) β (d)	Time To Steady State (wk of daily dosing)	Mean Steady-State Level+ (ng/mL)	Reference
Parent	6	4–14	7 (3–21)	16	262	Fabian et al 1981
N-Desmethyl metabolite	—	—	(10–14)	8	200–300	Fabian et al 1981, Jordan et al 1983
Metabolite Y	—	—	20 (approx)	25 (approx)	6–60	Jordan et al 1983

*Based on doses of 10 mg twice daily.

was tolerable and no increase in myelotoxicity or neurotoxicity was observed.

■ Pharmacokinetics

In women given radiolabeled drug, Fromson et al (1973a,b) noted that the majority of radioactivity appeared in the feces over several days to weeks. The urine contained only small levels of observed radioactivity. Most of a single dose was eliminated as a conjugated moiety. Approximately 30% of the radiolabel was eliminated as a hydroxylated metabolite or as unchanged drug. Peak radioactivity from 0.3 mg/kg doses of tamoxifen occurred after 4 to 7 hours. These correlated with peak blood levels of 0.06 to 0.14 mg/mL, 20 to 30% of which was unchanged drug. An initial half-life of 7 to 14 hours was followed by secondary plateau peaks occurring 4 or more days later. These secondary peaks (prolonged blood levels) are believed to result from enterohepatic circulation, probably of drug metabolites. Studies by Fromson et al (1973a,b) have shown that about 75% of total radioactivity is recovered in the feces as conjugates of tamoxifen metabolites.

A number of more recent investigations using specific assays have provided contrasting results (see table). Adam et al (1979) have described six tamoxifen metabolites from bile or feces, with the primary metabolite identified as N-desmethyltamoxifen. There are at least five different tamoxifen metabolites with varying degrees of estrogen antagonist activity (see table). Most of these metabolites have mixed estrogen agonist/antagonist activities like tamoxifen, based on the hormonal tissue studied (Kemp et al 1983). Of interest, metabolite E (identified only in dog bile) is a pure estrogen agonist, whereas the N-oxide metabolite seen in all species is a pure antagonist in MCF-7 breast cancer cells (Bates et al 1982). These metabolites are formed by hepatic microsomal cytochrome P450 activity. Biliary secretion of conjugates appears to mediate most of the drug's elimination. Very little drug is excreted in the urine.

The pharmacokinetics of the N-desmethyl metabolite of tamoxifen shows that significant accumulation is possible with standard daily dosing schemes. The acute level of N-desmethyltamoxifen after 10 mg of tamoxifen was only 2.5 ng/mL,

HORMONAL ACTIVITY OF TAMOXIFEN METABOLITES

Metabolite	Metabolite Abbreviation	Relative Estrogen Receptor Binding Potency*	Estrogenic Effects in Rodent Tissues
Tamoxifen	—	6	Antagonist in breast and uterus, agonist in bone
4-Hydroxytamoxifen	B	280	Antagonist/partial agonist
Tamoxifen N-oxide	—	6	Pure antagonist (MCF-7 human breast cells)
N-Desmethyltamoxifen	X	4	Antagonist/partial agonist
Tamoxifen primary alcohol	Y	0.5	Antagonist/partial agonist
Tamoxifen phenol+	E	3	Pure estrogen agonist

*17 β-Estradiol binding = 100. Numbers greater than 100 indicate more potent binding. Numbers less than 100 indicate less potent binding.
+Seen in dog bile only, formed by loss of tamoxifen basic side chain.
Data from Jordan et al 1983.

whereas the chronic level after 21 days of 10 mg twice daily ranged from 86 to 224 ng/mL. Thus, metabolite levels may be 0.71 to 2.3 times concurrent tamoxifen levels and, therefore, probably account for a large portion of the drug's pharmacologic activity (Jordan et al 1983).

Wilkinson and Ribeiro (1979) have described acute and chronic biphasic drug elimination patterns. After 10 mg tamoxifen a peak of 15 to 25 ng/mL was obtained, with decay over a (terminal) 35 ± 16-hour mean half-life. With chronic administration (10 mg twice daily for 3 weeks) a dosing interval "valley" level of 113 ng/mL, compared with a peak level of approximately 150 ng/mL, occurred about 3 hours after ingestion. The terminal half-life was 107 hours, suggesting perhaps a third and very prolonged elimination phase for intact drug. Thus, similarly dosed clinical regimens should produce steady-state tamoxifen levels ranging from 80 to 200 ng/mL.

Patients with renal dysfunction do not accumulate tamoxifen (Sutherland et al 1984); however, tamoxifen levels and related metabolites do increase in patients with liver obstruction (DeGregorio et al 1989). In a single patient, tamoxifen and N-desmethyltamoxifen levels of 750 to 1000 ng/mL, respectively, were obtained in a jaundiced patient receiving 20 mg of tamoxifen daily (DeGregorio et al 1989). These levels are much higher than those obtained in historical patients with normal hepatobiliary function.

■ Side Effects and Toxicity

Tamoxifen rarely causes myelosuppression. It has been inconclusively implicated in causing slight and transient thrombocytopenia (Cole et al 1971, Morgan et al 1976) and leukopenia (Tormey et al 1976, Lerner et al 1976). Reduced hemoglobin has also been described rarely (Tormey et al 1976).

Tamoxifen can induce menopausal symptoms in premenopausal patients. Symptoms including hot flashes, nausea, and occasionally vomiting are observed in less than 25% of patients. These are usually not dose limiting and tolerance tends to develop rapidly.

Other gynecologic problems such as vaginal bleeding and menstrual irregularities may occur infrequently. In addition, skin rashes, pruritus vulvae, dizziness, headache, and depression may occur. Other general reactions include lassitude, headache, leg cramps, dizziness, slight peripheral edema, and a distaste for food. Reduction of dosage can sometimes ameliorate several adverse reactions without loss of disease control.

Some patients may experience an acute "flare" of their breast cancer symptoms (Veldhuis and Santen 1979). Signs include an increase in bone pain along with hypercalcemia in patients with bony disease and a flare of any local soft tissue disease (Veldhuis 1978). This is seen only during initial therapy (Tormey et al 1976); however, the reactions can necessitate additional analgesics for a brief period. The acute flare reactions are rare and are probably due to the slight estrogenic activity of the drug in bone (Reddel and Sutherland 1984). On many occasions these reactions have been associated with a subsequent antitumor response. In patients with soft tissue disease, lesions may indurate, redden, and enlarge, or new lesions may occur. Careful observation of the patient during these flares is important lest hypercalcemia or a serious exacerbation of the breast cancer be neglected. Tamoxifen flare has also been reported in a patient with advanced endometrial cancer (Brooks and Lippman 1985). The symptom in this case was acute abdominal pain, which subsided after 5 days of continued tamoxifen therapy. The initial nature of the tamoxifen flare should be kept in mind as similar reactions after the first month of therapy almost certainly represent disease progression.

High-dose tamoxifen has resulted in a few cases of severe retinopathy which are primarily paramacular. The edema can cause a significant decrease in visual acuity. Affected patients were receiving very high doses (> 200 mg/d) for prolonged periods of over a year (Kaiser-Kupfer and Lippman 1978). Similar retinopathy was reported by McKeown et al (1981). Reversible ocular toxicity has also been reported in a 42-year-old patient receiving low-dose tamoxifen. Symptoms included bilateral optic disc swelling, retinal hemorrhages, and visual impairment 3 weeks after starting tamoxifen at a dose of 10 mg twice daily (Ashford et al 1988). Fortunately, all symptoms resolved rapidly on drug discontinuance.

As might be expected, however, premenopausal patients may develop greater toxic reactions from the antiestrogenic effects of tamoxifen (Morgan et al 1976). Sexually active premenopausal patients treated with tamoxifen may be more likely to become pregnant, as the drug is known to induce ovulation (Tajima et al 1977, Klopper and Hall 1971, Senior et al 1978). Tamoxifen-induced lactation is also reported in a premenopausal patient (Favis et al 1979). Long-term adjuvant tamoxifen may also increase the incidence of endometrial carcinoma in breast cancer patients (Andersson et al 1991).

A few cases of pulmonary emboli have been inconclusively associated with tamoxifen (Lerner et al 1976). In larger and higher-dose studies, however, this side effect is not mentioned. Jordan et al (1987) found that long-term tamoxifen does consistently depress antithrombin III levels but only by about 10% in postmenopausal patients. There was also an increase in sex hormone-binding globulin, which could help to further the antiestrogenic effects of the drug. Overall, the degree of antithrombin III depression found in this trial does not connote serious risk for thromboembolic disorders with tamoxifen.

Tamoxifen can cause a slight hypertriglyceridemia (Rossner and Wallgren 1984). This is similar to known effects of estrogens on plasma lipoprotein levels (Kissebah et al 1973). In most patients, triglyceride levels are rarely elevated above normal limits. Furthermore, in patients with normal triglycerides and elevated cholesterol levels, tamoxifen actually lowered low-density lipid cholesterol levels (Rossner and Wallgren 1984); however, in patients who are slightly hyperlipidemic prior to starting tamoxifen, significant lipemia may result when tamoxifen is administered (Brun et al 1986). A low activity of lipoprotein lipase and hepatic triglyceride lipase may explain the amplified increase in very low density lipids, triglycerides, and cholesterol. Fortunately, all effects on lipids are rapidly lost on drug discontinuance (Brun et al 1986).

Cholestatic liver damage has been rarely described with tamoxifen (Blackburn et al 1984). Occasionally, liver enzymes may increase slightly while on therapy and tamoxifen reportedly enhanced allopurinol-induced hepatotoxicity in one case (Shah et al 1982). There is also one case report of peliosis hepatis with chronic tamoxifen therapy (Loomus et al 1985). Although hepatic tumors have been described in rats given high doses of tamoxifen (5–35 mg/kg/d) chronically, hepatic tumors have not been reported in humans receiving standard doses and the clinical relevance of the rat data is not established (Andersson et al 1991). There is currently a controversy over whether tamoxifen increases the incidence of endometrial cancer. Two adjuvant tamoxifen trials in Britain demonstrated no increased risk (Stewart and Knight 1989, Ribeiro and Swindell 1988), whereas two Danish trials reported increased odds ratios of 6.4 (Andersson et al 1991) and 3.3 (Andersson et al 1991). Thus, overall it is not clear if long-term tamoxifen poses any carcinogenic risk, although careful ongoing follow-up is required for endometrial cancer. Finally, tamoxifen does not decrease bone mineralization as had been hypothesized. In contrast, clinical studies suggest that tamoxifen actually increases bone mineralization in the spine as a result of estrogenic action on bone tissues (Turken et al 1989). This confirms the findings of decreased bone resorption with tamoxifen in rats treated with tamoxifen (Turner et al 1987).

REFERENCES

Adam HK, Patterson JS, Kamp JF, et al. The metabolism of tamoxifen in man (abstract 190). *Proc Am Assoc Cancer Res ASCO.* 1979;**20**:47.

Aisner J, Ross DD, Wiernik PH. Tamoxifen in advanced male breast cancer. *Arch Intern Med.* 1979;**139**:480–481.

Alford TC, Do HM, Geelhoed GW, et al. Steroid hormone receptors in human colon cancers. *Cancer.* 1979;**43**:980–984.

Al-Sarraf M, Eyre H, Bonnet J, et al. Study of tamoxifen in metastatic renal cell carcinoma and the influence of certain prognostic factors: A Southwest Oncology Group study. *Cancer Treat Rep.* 1981;**65**:447–451.

Andersson M, Storm HH, Mouridsen HT. Incidence of new primary cancers after adjuvant tamoxifen therapy and radiotherapy for early breast cancer. *J Natl Cancer Inst.* 1991;**83**(14):1013–1017.

Ashford AR, Donev I, Tiwari RP, Garrett TJ. Reversible ocular toxicity related to tamoxifen therapy. *Cancer.* 1988;**61**:33–35.

Bates DJ, Foster AB, Griggs LJ, et al. Metabolism of tamoxifen N-oxide. *Biochem Pharmacol.* 1982;**31**:2823–2827.

Berd D, McLaughlin CJ, Hart E, et al. Short course, high-dose tamoxifen (TAM) with cytotoxic chemotherapy for metastatic melanoma (abstract). *Proc Am Soc Clin Oncol.* 1991;**10**:291.

Blackburn AM, Amiel SA, Millis RR, et al. Tamoxifen and liver damage. *Br Med J.* 1984;**289**:288–289.

Brooks BJ Jr, Lippman ME. Tamoxifen flare in advanced endometrial carcinoma. *J Clin Oncol.* 1985;**3**:222–223.

Brule G. Co-operative clinical study of 178 patients treated with "Nolvadex." The Hormonal Control of Breast Cancer. In: *Proceedings of a Symposium in Manchester, 9th June;* 1976:35.

Brun LD, Gagne C, Rousseau C, et al. Severe lipemia induced by tamoxifen. *Cancer.* 1986;**57**:2123–2126.

Butler WB, Kelsey WH, Goran N. Role of insulin in modifying the response of the human breast cancer cell line MCF-7 to anti-estrogens (abstract 1001). *Proc Am Assoc Cancer Res ASCO.* 1979;**20**:247.

Clarke R, Morwood J, van den Berg HW, et al. Effect of cytotoxic drugs on estrogen receptor expression and response to tamoxifen in MCF-7 cells. *Cancer Res.* 1986;**46**:6116–6119.

Clemmons DR, Van Wyk JJ. Factors controlling blood concentration of somatomedin C. *Clin Endocrinol Metab.* 1984;**13**:113–143.

Cocconi G, De Lisi V, Boni C, et al. Chemotherapy (CMF) vs combination of hormonal and chemotherapy (CMF plus tamoxifen) in metastatic breast cancer (abstract C-45). *Proc Am Assoc Cancer Res.* 1979;**20**:302.

Cole MP, Jones CTA, Todd IDH. The treatment of advanced carcinoma of the breast with the antioestrogenic agent tamoxifen (ICI 46.474)—A series of 96 patients. *Adv Antimicrob Antineoplast Chemother.* 1971;**2**:529–531.

Colletti RB, Roberts JD, Devlin JT, Copeland KC. Effect of tamoxifen on plasma insulin-like growth factor I in patients with breast cancer. *Cancer Res.* 1989;**49**:1882–1884.

Creagan ET, Ingle JN, Green SJ, et al. Phase II study of tamoxifen in patients with disseminated malignant melanoma. *Cancer Treat Rep.* 1980;**64**:199–201.

DeGregorio MW, Wiebe VJ, Venook AP, Holleran WM. Elevated plasma tamoxifen levels in a patient with liver obstruction. *Cancer Chemother Pharmacol.* 1989;**23**:194–195.

Early Breast Cancer Trialists' Collaborative Group. Systemic treatment of early breast cancer by hormonal, cytotoxic, or immune therapy. *Lancet.* 1992;**339**:1–15.

Fabian C, Sternson L. Tamoxifen (TAM) blood levels following initial and chronic dosing in patients with breast cancer: Correlation with clinical data (abstract C-145). *Proc Am Assoc Cancer Res ASCO.* 1979;**20**:326.

Fabian C, Sternson L, El-Serafi M, et al. Clinical pharmacology of tamoxifen in patients with breast cancer: Correlation with clinical data. *Cancer.* 1981;**48**:876–882.

Favis GR, Alavi JB, Glick JH. Lactation from tamoxifen (letter). *Ann Intern Med.* 1979;**90**(6):993–994.

Ferrazzi E, Carter G, Mattarazzo R, Fiorentino M. Oestrogen-like effect of tamoxifen on vaginal epithelium (letter). *Br Med J.* 1977;**1**:1351–1352.

Fisher RL, Nifeld ME, Lippman ME. Estrogen receptors in new malignant melanoma. *Lancet.* 1976;**2**:337.

Fromson JH, Pearson S, Bramah S. The metabolism of tamoxifen (ICI 46.474): Part I in laboratory animals. *Xenobiotica.* 1973a;**3**:693–709.

Fromson JM, Pearson S, Bramah S. The metabolism of tamoxifen (ICI 46.474): Part II in female patients. *Xenobiotica.* 1973b;**3**:711–714.

Furr BA, Jordan VC. The pharmacology and clinical uses of tamoxifen. *Pharmacol Ther.* 1984;**25**:127–205.

Glick J, Wein A, Negendank W, et al. Tamoxifen in metastatic prostate and renal cancer (abstract C-81). *Proc Am Assoc Cancer Res ASCO.* 1979;**20**:311.

Glick JH, Wein A, Padavic K, et al. Tamoxifen in refractory metastatic carcinoma of the prostate. *Cancer Treat Rep.* 1980;**64**:813–818.

Glick JH, Wein A, Padavic K, et al. Phase II trial of tamoxifen in metastatic carcinoma of the prostate. *Cancer.* 1982;**49**:1367–1372.

Heuson JC. Current overview of EORTC clinical trials with tamoxifen. *Cancer Treat Rep.* 1976;**60**:1463–1466.

Horwitz KB, McGuire WI. Estrogen control of progesterone receptor in human breast cancer. Correlation with nuclear processing of estrogen receptor. *J Biol Chem.* 1978;**253**(7):2223–2228.

Hug V, Hortobagyi GN, Drewinko B, Finders M. Tamoxifen-citrate counteracts the antitumor effects of cytotoxic drugs in vitro. *J Clin Oncol.* 1985;**3**:1672–1677.

Jordan VC. Antitumor activity of the antiestrogen CI 46,474 (tamoxifen) in the dimethylbenzanthracene (DMBA)-induced rat mammary carcinoma model (abstract). *J Steroid Biochem.* 1974;**5**:354.

Jordan VC. Biochemical pharmacology of antiestrogen action. *Pharmacol Rev.* 1984;**36**:245–276.

Jordan VC, Bain RR, Brown RR, et al. Determination and pharmacology of a new hydroxylated metabolite of tamoxifen observed in patient sera during therapy for advanced breast cancer. *Cancer Res.* 1983;**43**:1446–1450.

Jordan VC, Collings MM, Rowsby L, Prestwich G. A monohydroxylated metabolite of tamoxifen with potent anti-oestrogenic activity. *J Endocrinol.* 1977;**75**:306–316.

Jordan VC, Fritz NF, Tormey DC. Long-term adjuvant therapy with tamoxifen: Effects on sex hormone binding globulin and antithrombin III. *Cancer Res.* 1987;**47**:4517–4519.

Kaiser-Kupfer MI, Lippman ME. Tamoxifen retinopathy. *Cancer Treat Rep.* 1978;**62**(3):315–320.

Kemp JV, Adam HK, Wakeling AE, et al. Identification and biological activity of tamoxifen metabolites in human serum. *Biochem Pharmacol.* 1983;**32**:2045–2052.

Kiang DT, Kennedy BJ. Tamoxifen (antiestrogen) therapy in advanced breast cancer. *Ann Intern Med.* 1977;**87**:687–690.

Kiang DT, Kollander RE, Thomas T, Kennedy BJ. Up-regulation of estrogen receptors by nonsteroidal antiestrogens in human breast cancer. *Cancer Res.* 1989;**49**:5312–5316.

Kissebah AH, Harrigan P, Wynn V. Mechanism of hypertriglyceridemia associated with contraceptive steroids. *Horm Metab Res.* 1973;**5**:184–190.

Klopper A, Hall M. New synthetic agent for the induction of ovulation: Preliminary trials in women. *Br Med J.* 1971;**1**:152–154.

Knabbe C, Lippman ME, Wakefield L, et al. Evidence that TGFβ is a hormonally regulated negative growth factor in human breast cancer. *Cell.* 1987;**48**:417–428.

Lerner LJ, Jordan VC. Development of antiestrogens and their use in breast cancer: Eighth Cain Memorial Award Lecture. *Cancer Res.* 1990;**50**:4177–4189.

Lerner HJ, Marcovitz E. Treatment of advanced breast cancer with tamoxifen (TAM) and fluoxymesterone (abstract 319). *Proc Am Assoc Cancer Res ASCO.* 1979;**20**:79.

Lerner HJ, Pand PR, Israel L, Leung BS. Phase I study of

tamoxifen: Report of 74 patients with stage IV breast cancer. *Cancer Treat Rep.* 1976;**60**:1431–1435.

Loomus G, Aneja P, Bohta RA. A case of peliosis hepatis in association with tamoxifen therapy. *Am J Clin Pathol.* 1985;**80**:881–883.

Macourt DC. A new synthetic agent for the induction of ovulation. *Med J Aust.* 1974;**1**:631–632.

Manni A, Arafah BM. Tamoxifen-induced remission in breast cancer by escalating the dose to 40 mg daily after progression on 20 mg daily: A case report and review of the literature. *Cancer.* 1981;**48**:873–875.

Manni A, Pearson OH. Antiestrogen-induced remissions in premenopausal women with stage IV breast cancer. Effects on ovarian function. *Cancer Treat Rep.* 1980;**64**:779–785.

Manni A, Trujillo J, Marshall JS, Pearson OH. Antioestrogen-induced remissions in stage IV breast cancer. *Cancer Treat Rep.* 1976;**60**:1445–1450.

Masiel A, Buttrick P, Bitran J. Tamoxifen in the treatment of malignant melanoma. *Cancer Treat Rep.* 1980;**60**:531–532.

McClendon JE, Appleby D, Claudon DB, et al. Colonic neoplasma tissue estrogen receptor and carcino-embryonic antigen. *Arch Surg.* 1977;**112**:240.

McGuire WL, Horwitz KB, Zava DT, et al. Hormones in breast cancer: Update 1978. *Metab Clin Exp.* 1978;**27**:487.

McKeown CA, Swartz M, Blom J, Maggiano JM. Tamoxifen retinopathy. *Br J Ophthalmol.* 1981;**65**:177–179.

Meyskens FL Jr, Voakes JB. Tamoxifen in metastatic malignant melanoma. *Cancer Treat Rep.* 1980;**64**:171–173.

Morgan LR, Schein PS, Woolley PV, et al. Therapeutic use of tamoxifen in advanced breast cancer: Correlation with biochemical parameters. *Cancer Treat Rep.* 1976;**60**:1437–1443.

Mouridsen HT, Ellemann K, Mattsson W, et al. Therapeutic effect of tamoxifen versus tamoxifen combined with medroxyprogesterone acetate in advanced breast cancer in postmenopausal women. *Cancer Treat Rep.* 1979;**63**(2):171–175.

Nesbit RA, Woods RL, Tattersal MHN, et al. Tamoxifen in malignant melanoma. *N Engl J Med.* 1979;**301**:1241–1242.

Nicholson RI, Golder MP. The effect of synthetic antioestrogens on the growth and biochemistry of rat mammary tumours. *Eur J Cancer.* 1975;**11**:571–579.

Priestman T, Baum M, Jones V, Forbes J. Comparative trial of endocrine versus cytotoxic treatment in advanced breast cancer. *Br J Med.* 1977;**1**:1248–1250.

Ramu A, Glaubiger D, Fuks Z. Reversal of acquired resistance to doxorubicin in P388 murine leukemia cells by tamoxifen and other triparanol analogues. *Cancer Res.* 1984;**44**:4392–4395.

Reddel RR, Sutherland RL. Tamoxifen stimulation of human breast cancer cell proliferation in vitro: A possible model for tamoxifen tumour flare. *Eur J Cancer Clin Oncol.* 1984;**20**(11):1419–1424.

Ribeiro G, Swindell R. The Christie Hospital adjuvant tamoxifen trial—Status at 10 years. *Br J Cancer.* 1988;**57**:601–603.

Rossner S, Wallgren A. Serum lipoproteins and proteins after breast cancer surgery and effects of tamoxifen. *Atherosclerosis.* 1984;**52**:239–346.

Sandberg AA, Kirdani RY, Vardalsis MJ, Murphy GP. Estrogen receptor protein of pancreas. *Steroids.* 1973;**22**:259.

Senior BE, Cawood MI, Oakev RF, et al. A comparison of the effects of clomiphene and tamoxifen treatment on the concentrations of oestradiol and progesterone in the peripheral plasma of infertile women. *Clin Endocrinol.* 1978;**8**(5):381–389.

Shah KA, Levin J, Rosen N, et al. Allopurinol hepatotoxicity potentiated by tamoxifen. *NY State J Med.* 1982;**82**:1745–1746.

Stewart JF, Minton MJ, Rubens RD. Trial of tamoxifen at a dose of 40 mg daily after disease progression during tamoxifen therapy at a dose of 20 mg daily. *Cancer Treat Rep.* 1982;**66**(6):1445–1446.

Stewart H, Knight GM. Tamoxifen and the uterus and endometrium. *Lancet.* 1989;**1**:375–376.

Sunderland MC, Osborne CK. Tamoxifen in premenopausal patients with metastatic breast cancer: A review. *J Clin Oncol.* 1991;**9**:1283–1297.

Sutherland RL, Reddel RR, Murphy LC, et al. Effects of antiestrogens on cell cycle progression. In: Jordan VC, ed. *Estrogen/Antiestrogen Action and Breast Cancer Therapy.* Madison: University Wisconsin Press; 1986:265–281.

Sutherland CM, Sternson LA, Muchmore JH, et al. Effect of impaired renal function on tamoxifen. *J Surg Oncol.* 1984;**27**:222–223.

Swain SM, Lippman ME. Endocrine therapies of cancer. In: Chabner BA, Collins JM, eds. *Cancer Chemotherapy: Principles and Practice.* Philadelphia: JB Lippincott; 1990:59–109.

Swenerton KD. Treatment of advanced endometrial adenocarcinoma with tamoxifen. *Cancer Treat Rep.* 1980;**64**(6/7):805–811.

Swenerton KD, White GW, Boyes DA. Treatment of advanced endometrial carcinoma with tamoxifen (letter). *N Engl J Med.* 1979;**301**(2):105.

Tajima C, Tamaski Y, Takamizawa H. Trials of tamoxifen for the induction of ovulation. *Acta Obstet Gynaecol Jpn.* 1977;**29**:57–62.

Taylor SG, Gelman RS, Falkson G, Cummings FJ. Combination chemotherapy compared to tamoxifen as initial therapy for stage IV breast cancer in elderly women. *Ann Intern Med.* 1986;**104**:455–461.

Thomas T, Trend B, Butterfield JR, et al. Regulation of ornithine decarboxylase gene expression in MCF-7 breast cancer cells by antiestrogens. *Cancer Res.* 1989;**49**:5852–5857.

Tormey DC, Jordan VC. Long term tamoxifen adjuvant therapy in node-positive breast cancer: A metabolic and pilot clinical study. *Breast Cancer Res Treat.* 1984;**4**:297–302.

Tormey DC, Simon RM, Lippman ME, et al. Evaluation of tamoxifen dose in advanced breast cancer: A progress report. *Cancer Treat Rep.* 1976;**60**:1451–1459.

Trump DL, Smith DC, Schold SC, et al. High dose tamoxifen and five day continuous infusion vinblastine: A phase I trial of an inhibitor of the MDR-1 phenotype (abstract). *Proc Am Soc Clin Oncol.* 1991;**10**:96.

Turken S, Siris E, Seldin D, et al. Effects of tamoxifen on spinal bone density in women with breast cancer. *J Natl Cancer Inst.* 1989;**81**(14):1086–1088.

Turner RT, Wakely GK, Hannon KS, et al. Tamoxifen prevents the skeletal effects of ovarian deficiency in rats. *J Bone Mineral Res.* 1987;**2**:449–456.

Veldhuis JD. Tamoxifen and hypercalcemia. *Ann Intern Med.* 1978;**89**:1013.

Veldhuis JD, Santen RJ. Tamoxifen flare (letter). *JAMA.* 1979;**241**(23):2506–2507.

Ward HWC. Clinical experience with anti-hormone therapy. In: *Proceedings of a Symposium on Hormonal Control of Breast Cancer, Alderley Park, 24 September;* 1975:53.

Ward HWC. Combined anti-prolactin and anti-oestrogen therapy for breast carcinoma. *Clin Oncol.* 1977;**3**:91–95.

Westerberg H. Tamoxifen and fluoxymesterone in advanced breast cancer: A controlled clinical trial. *Cancer Treat Rep.* 1980;**64**:117–121.

Wilkinson P, Ribeiro G. Tamoxifen citrate pharmacokinetics in patients with metastatic breast cancer (abstract C-71). *Proc Am Assoc Cancer Res ASCO.* 1979;**20**:309.

Wilkinson PM, Ribeiro GG, Adam HK, et al. Tamoxifen (Nolvadex) therapy—Rationale for loading dose followed by maintenance dose for patients with metastatic breast cancer. *Cancer Chemother Pharmacol.* 1982;**10**:33–35.

Taxotere

■ Other Names

RP-56976; NSC-628503, docetaxel.

■ Chemistry

Structure of taxotere

Because of supply problems with paclitaxel (currently available by sacrificing the tree bark of *Taxus brevifolia*), a program was begun at Rhône-Poulenc Rorer Pharmaceuticals Inc. to work on hemisynthesis of taxotere using a starting material of natural 10-deacetyl baccatin III extracted from the leaves of *Taxus baccata L.* (Mangatal et al 1989, Lavelle et al 1989, Denis et al 1990). Taxotere has the molecular weight 807.9 and the formula $C_{43}H_{53}NO_{14}$. The full chemical name is 4-acetoxy-2α-benzoyloxy-β,20-epoxy-1β,7β,10β-trihydroxy-9-oxotax-11-en-13α-yl-(2R,3s)-3-*tert*.-butoxycarbamido-2-hydroxy-3-phenyl-propionate.

■ Antitumor Activity

Taxotere has documented antitumor activity in a wide variety of in vivo preclinical models. It is more active than taxol in human tumor cell lines in vitro (Aapro et al 1992). Taxotere is also broadly active in human tumor xenografts in nude mice.

The compound has been found inactive against P-388 resistant to doxorubicin, MA16/C adenocarcinoma, and the M5076 sarcoma (Lavelle et al 1989, Bissery et al 1990, 1991, Ringel and Horwitz 1991). Taxotere has been found to be superior to taxol in the B-16 melanoma model. It is also active in vivo when combined with cisplatin, doxorubicin, or vincristine (Bissery et al 1992).

In initial clinical trials, taxotere has produced clinical responses in patients with breast cancer, ovarian cancer, non-small cell lung cancer, and pancreatic cancer (Burris et al 1993a). Ovarian cancer appears to be consistently sensitive to taxotere (Extra et al 1991). In large ongoing trials taxotere has shown impressive activity in patients with breast cancer (with and without prior chemotherapy) and in patients with non-small cell lung cancer (Seidman et al 1993, Trudeau et al 1993, Huinink Ten Bokkel et al 1993, Fumoleau et al 1993, Burris et al 1993b, Rigas et al 1993).

■ Mechanism of Action

Taxotere does not inhibit synthesis of DNA, RNA, or protein (Riou et al 1992). Preliminary data indicate that taxotere has a mechanism of action similar to that of taxol but with differential effects on tau binding sites and on microtubule-associated proteins (Fromes et al 1992). Taxotere enhances microtubule assembly and inhibits the depolymerization of tubulin (Barasoain et al 1991). In this regard, it is more potent than taxol. As with taxol, this can lead to bundles of microtubules in the cell, leading to an inability of the cell to divide (Ringel et al 1991). Cell cycle traverse is halted in M phase.

■ Availability and Storage

Taxotere is available as an investigational agent from Rhone-Poulenc Rorer Pharmaceuticals Inc Central Research, Collegeville, Pennsylvania, as a solution for intravenous administration following appropriate dilutions. The drug is currently supplied as a 1- or 5-mL concentrated sterile solution of 15 mg/mL in 50% polysorbate 80/Tween® 80 and 50% dehydrated alcohol. Taxotere should be stored at 4°C. The vials should be protected from light.

■ Preparation for Use, Stability, and Admixture

Drug handling precautions for cytostatic drugs should be followed. Avoid contact or inhalation. The appropriate amount of taxotere should be drawn up and added just prior to use to the appropriate amount of D5W. The maximum taxotere concentration in the D5W solution should never exceed 0.3 mg/mL to ensure a maximum solvent concentration of 2%. For that reason the maximum dosage of taxotere that can be diluted in 500 mL of D5W is 150 mg.

If the total dose to be administered to the patient increases over 150 mg, taxotere must be diluted in a larger volume of D5W.

The appropriate amount of drug from the vial should be placed in 500 mL of D5W for infusion. No in-line filtration or light protection is required during the infusion.

Once diluted, taxotere is stable for at least 8 hours over a range of concentrations of 5 mg in 250 mL (0.02 mg/mL) to 500 mg in 500 mL (1 mg/mL).

■ Administration

The recommended dose and schedule for taxotere have not been worked out. Schedules being tested in phase I studies include a single dose every 28 days, a 6-hour infusion every 28 days, a 24-hour infusion every 21 days, 1-hour infusion daily × 5 every 21 days, and 1-hour infusions on days 1 and 8 every 28 days. Further patient accrual on the preceding studies should define the most dose-intensive schedule.

■ Special Precautions

In initial clinic trials with taxotere severe but reversible neutropenia has been noted (Extra et al 1991). An anaphylactic-like reaction consisting of shortness of breath, rash, anxiety, and difficulty breathing has also been noted. Patients have been re-treated after appropriate premedications: dexamethasone 20 mg IV at 14 and 7 hours before taxotere, and diphenhydramine 50 mg and ranitidine 50 mg, both 30 minutes before taxotere. Of great interest is that the episodes have not recurred with pretreatment.

■ Drug Interactions

Like taxol, taxotere has been shown to have experimental radiosensitizing effects in vitro (Choy et al 1992). Experimental multidrug resistance to taxol can be reversed in vitro by quinidine, cyclosporin A, quinine, and verapamil, in descending order of potency (Lehnert et al 1992).

■ Dosage

The recommended taxotere dose as a 1-hour infusion for 5 days every 21 days was 12 mg/m^2/d (Pazdur et al 1992). The dose recommended for phase II studies of a 6-hour infusion every 21 days was 100 mg/m^2 for good-risk patients and 80 mg/m^2 for poor-risk patients (Burris et al 1993a). The maximally tolerated dose for a 24-hour infusion every 3 weeks is 90 mg/m^2 (Bissett et al 1992). The recommended dose for phase II studies with this schedule is not reported.

■ Pharmacokinetics

A 6-hour taxotere infusion at doses of 5 to 100 mg/m^2 produces average peak plasma levels of 38 to 1090 ng/mL (Irvin et al 1992). Drug elimination from the plasma is biexponential with a mean harmonic terminal half-life of approximately 3.3 hours (Bruno et al 1992). Urinary excretion of taxotere was minimal (see table on the opposite page).

Although there is considerable variability in pharmacokinetics between different patients, the AUCs appear to correlate with granulocyte nadirs (Pazdur et al 1992).

■ Side Effects and Toxicity

Toxic effects noted in phase I trials with taxotere to date have included dose-limiting neutropenia. Thrombocytopenia has also been noted but is less frequent. There have been reports of anaphylactic-

MEAN CLINICAL PHARMACOKINETICS OF TAXOTERE

Dose (mg/m²)	Infusion Time (h)	Reference	Half-life α (min)	Half-life β (h)	Volume of Distribution (L/m²)	Clearance (L/h/m²)	AUC (μg·h/mL)
16	1	Pazdur et al 1992	7.4	3.4	95.6	35.8	0.475
40–100	6	Irvin et al 1992	—	3.2	36.6*	17.7	1.8–10.8
55	1	De Valeriola et al 1992	—	—	72*	28	2.09

*Volume of distribution at steady state.

like reactions in a few patients. These reactions have even been noted in a few patients on the first course of treatment with taxotere. After pretreatment with diphenhydramine and dexamethasone the patients have been able to be re-treated without difficulty. Other toxic effects noted include phlebitis, a transient maculopapular violaceous rash, and alopecia. Recently, a drug-associated edema has been reported. This includes pleural effusions and peripheral edema. The mechanism for this edema is unclear. Methods to prevent the edema are being explored. Neurologic toxic effects have not been problematic in the phase I trials (Burris et al 1993a). Similarly, cardiac toxic effects have not been noted in preliminary studies (Pazdur et al 1992).

■ Special Applications

None are known.

REFERENCES

Aapro M, Braakhuis B, et al. Superior activity of taxotere (Ter) over taxol (Tol) in vitro. EORTC CASSG Group. *Proc Am Assoc Cancer Res.* 1992;**33**:516.

Barasoain I, de Ines C, Diaz F, et al. Interaction of tubulin and cellular microtubules with taxotere (RP 56976), a new semisynthesic analog of taxol. *Proc Am Assoc Cancer Res.* 1991;**32**:329.

Bissery MC, Bayssas M, Lavelle F. Preclinical evaluation of intravenous taxotere (RP 56976, NSC 628503), a taxol analog. *Proc Am Assoc Cancer Res.* 1990;**31**:417.

Bissery MC, Renard A, Montay G, Bayssas M, Lavelle F. Taxotere: Antitumor activity and pharmacokinetics in mice. *Proc Am Assoc Cancer Res.* 1991;**32**:401.

Bissery MC, Vrignaud P, Bayssas M, et al. In vivo evaluation of taxotere (RP56976, NSC628503) in combination with cisplatinum, doxorubicin, or vincristine. *Proc Am Assoc Cancer Res.* 1992;**33**:443.

Bissett D, Setanoians A, Cassidy J, et al. Phase I and pharmacokinetics study of taxotere (RP56976) administered as a 24 hour infusion. *Cancer.* **53**:523–527.

Bruno R, Vergniol JC, Montay G, et al. Clinical pharmacology of taxotere (RP56976) given as 1–2 hr infusion every 2–3 weeks. *Proc Am Assoc Cancer Res.* 1992;**33**:261.

Burris H, Irvin R, Kuhn J, et al. A phase I clinical trial of taxotere administered as either a 2 hour or a 6 hour intravenous infusion. *J Clin Oncol.* 1993a;**11**:950–958.

Burris H, Eckardt J, Fields S, et al. Phase II trials of taxotere in patients with non-small cell lung cancer. *Proc Am Soc Clin Oncol.* 1993;**12**:335

Choy H, Rodriguez F, Wilcox B, et al. Radiation sensitizing effects of taxotere (RP 56976). *Proc Am Assoc Cancer Res.* 1992;**33**:500.

Denis TN, Correa A, Greene AF. An improved synthesis of the taxol side chain and of RP 56976. *J Org Chem.* 1990;**55**:1957–1959.

De Valeriola D, Brassinne C, Piccart M, et al. Phase I pharmacokinetic (PK) study of taxotere (T) (RP56976, NSC628503) administered as a weekly infusion. *Proc Am Assoc Cancer Res.* 1992;**33**:261.

Extra JM, Rousseau F, Bourhis J, Dieras V, Marty M. Phase I trial of taxotere (RP 56976, NSC 628503). *Proc Am Assoc Cancer Res.* 1991;**32**:205.

Fromes Y, Gounon P, Bissery MC, et al. Differential effects of taxol and taxotere (RP56976, NSC628503) on Tau and MAP2 containing microtubules. *Proc Am Assoc Cancer Res.* 1992;**33**:511.

Fumoleau P, Chevallier B, Kerbrat P, et al. First line chemotherapy with taxotere (T) in advanced breast cancer (ABC): A phase II study of the EOTRC Clinical Screening Group (CSG). *Proc Am Soc Clin Oncol.* 1993;**12**:56.

Harrison SD Jr, Dykes DJ, Shepherd RV, et al. Response of human tumor xenografts to taxotere. *Proc Am Assoc Cancer Res.* 1992;**33**:526.

Huinink Ten Bokkel WW, Van Oosterom AT, Piccart M. Taxotere in advanced breast cancer: A phase II trial of the EORTC Clinical Trials Group. *Proc Am Soc Clin Oncol.* 1993;**12**:70.

Irvin RJ, Burris H, Eckardt J, et al. Pharmacokinetics of a 6 hr taxotere infusion (RP56976, NSC 628503). *Proc Am Soc Clin Oncol.* 1992;**11**:108.

Lavelle F, Fizames C, Gueritte-Voegelein F, Guenard D, Potier P. Experimental properties of RP 56976, a taxol derivative. *Proc Am Assoc Cancer Res.* 1989;**30**:566.

Lehnert M, Emerson S, Dalton WS, et al. Reversal of resistance to taxol and taxotere in a human myeloma cell line model of MDR1. *Proc Am Assoc Cancer Res.* 1992;**33**:481.

Mangatal L, Adeline M-T, Guenard D, Gueritte-Voegelein F, Potier P. Application of the vicinal oxyamination reaction with asymmetric induction to the hemisynthesis of taxol and analogues. *Tetrahedron.* 1989;**45**:4177–4190.

Pazdur R, Newman RA, Newman BM, et al. Phase I trial of taxotere (RP56976). *Proc Am Soc Clin Oncol.* 1992; **11**:111.

Rigas JR, Francis PA. Phase II trial of taxotere in non-small cell lung cancer. *Proc Am Soc Clin Oncol.* 1993;**12**:336.

Ringel I, Horwitz SB. Studies with RP 56976 (taxotere): A semisynthetic analogue of taxol. *J Natl Cancer Inst.* 1991;**83**:288–291.

Riou JF, Naudin A, Lavelle F. Cellular activities of taxotere. *Proc Am Assoc Cancer Res.* 1992;**33**:525.

Seidman AD, Hudis C, Crown JPA, et al. Phase II evaluation of taxotere (RP56976, NSC 628503) as initial chemotherapy for metastatic breast cancer. *Proc Am Soc Clin Oncol.* 1993;**12**:63.

Trudeau ME, Eisenhauer E, Lofters W. Phase II study of taxotere as first line chemotherapy for metastatic breast cancer (MBC). A National Cancer Institute of Canada Clinical Trials Group (NCIC CTG) study. *Proc Am Soc Clin Oncol.* 1993;**12**:64.

Tegafur

■ Other Names

FT-207; NSC-148958; Ftorafur.

■ Chemistry

Structure of tegafur

Chemically tegafur is 5-fluoro-1-(tetrahydro-2-furyl)-uracil or N_1-(2'-furanidyl)-5-fluorouracil. It is supplied as the racemic mixture of R and S isomers. The drug is chemically similar to 5-fluorodeoxyuridine except that it has no hydroxymethyl group. Thus, tegafur is basically 5-fluorouracil linked to a furan ring dehydroxylated ribose sugar. The drug has a molecular weight of 200.16 and a pK_a of 7.8. It is reported to hydrolyze in acid medium (pH 1.2–2.0) and in the presence of heat (80°C) to release 5-fluorouracil. Thus, it is more stable in a slightly alkaline medium.

■ Antitumor Activity

Tegafur was synthesized in the Soviet Union in 1966. Since that time it has demonstrated antitumor activity in melanoma, hepatoma, and lung cancer in animals. Antitumor effects have also been reported in preliminary Japanese studies (Hatori et al 1973) and studies in the Soviet Union (Blokhina et al 1972, Karev et al 1972, Smolyanskaya and Trigarinov 1972). In phase I studies performed in the United States antitumor activity has been observed in advanced colorectal adenocarcinomas (Smart et al 1975, Valdivieso et al 1976).

Single-agent partial response rates in colorectal carcinoma range from 4 to 11%, with a 7% response rate reported in head and neck cancer (Friedman and Ignoffo 1980) (see table). The combination of tegafur with doxorubicin and mitomycin-C has produced partial response rates in 15 to 20% of previously treated and untreated gastric cancer patients (Woolley et al 1979). Similar combinations in pancreatic and biliary tract cancer produced response rates of 0 to 25%. Only one of seven patients with gallbladder cancer treated with tegafur achieved an objective response (Hall et al 1979). When tegafur was combined with semustine and mitomycin-C in colorectal cancer, response rates of 14 to 27% were described (as reviewed by Friedman and Ignoffo 1980). A recent randomized trial of adjuvant mitomycin-C with oral tegafur revealed only a minor increase in progression-free intervals and sur-

CLINICAL ANTITUMOR ACTIVITY OF TEGAFUR

	Other Drugs	Response Rate (%)*
Colorectal cancer	None	4–11
Colorectal cancer	Mitomycin-C ± semustine	14–27
Head and neck cancer	None	7
Gastric cancer	Doxorubicin, mitomycin-C ± carmustine	20
Pancreas	Doxorubicin, carmustine	0–25
Colorectal cancer	None (oral tegafur)	29
Breast cancer	None (oral tegafur)	40
Gall bladder	Doxorubicin, carmustine	30

*Primarily partial responses (≥ 50% tumor shrinkage) except for 1 of 7 complete responses in gallbladder cancer.

vival in patients with stage II gastric cancer (Cirera et al 1992). The drug is also active orally, producing partial responses in 6 of 21 colorectal cancer patients and in 3 of 7 breast cancer patients (Ansfield et al 1983).

■ Mechanism of Action

Tegafur may act as a transport form or prodrug of 5-fluorouracil. On cleavage of the pseudonucleoside bond, a free sugar moiety and 5-fluorouracil are liberated. The basic activity of the drug is that of an antipyrimidine that is essentially identical to 5-fluorouracil (Meiren and Belousova 1972). A single daily injection of tegafur may thus approximate a continuous infusion of 5-fluorouracil through the slow metabolic breakdown of tegafur to 5-fluorouracil (see Pharmacokinetics).

Sayed and Sadee (1983) have shown that there are two major pathways for tegafur activation. Oxidation of the C-5' position produces 5-fluorouracil and succinaldehyde. This conversion is mediated by microsomal cytochrome P450 enzymes. In an alternate pathway, soluble enzymes mediate cleavage of the N-1 to C-2' bond in tegafur to yield 5-fluorouracil. This is immediately metabolized to α-hydroxybutyrolactone or the equivalent acid (Sayed and Sadee 1983). There is also some evidence that tegafur metabolites other than 5-fluorouracil may mediate some of the toxic effects of the drug (Harrison et al 1979).

Once liberated, 5-fluorouracil acts to inhibit thymidylate synthetase after conversion to 5-fluorodeoxyuridylate monophosphate (FdUMP). This ultimately halts DNA synthesis. 5-Fluorouracil can also block RNA synthesis by incorporation of 5-fluorouracil triphosphate into RNA. (For a complete review see the *5-Fluorouracil* monograph.) Tegafur is a cell cycle phase-specific agent with the most marked cytotoxic effects expressed in S (DNA synthesis) phase.

■ Availability and Storage

Tegafur is available investigationally as a lyophilized caked powder in 500-mg glass vials. Each vial also contains 250 mg of anhydrous sodium carbonate (4.7 mEq of sodium per vial). The vials may be stored at room temperature. Storage at room temperature affords stability for at least 6 months. The drug has also been investigationally available as 500-mg tablets for oral use. These, too, may be stored at room temperature, protected from light.

■ Preparation for Use, Stability, and Admixture

Intact vials can be reconstituted with 9.7 mL of Sterile Water for Injection, USP, yielding a 50 mg/1 mL solution (25 mg/1 mL of sodium carbonate) at a pH of 8.2 to 9.2. This solution is chemically stable for at least 96 hours at room temperature or under refrigeration. Further dilutions into 250 to 500 mL of D5W are also stable. Because the lyophilized form contains no preservative, the vials should not be used in a multidose fashion. The unused portion of any vial should be discarded within 8 hours of initial entry.

■ Administration

Doses of tegafur can be infused in 100 to 500 mL of D5W over 1 hour or longer periods. The patient should be in a recumbent position if possible to minimize problems of dizziness during the infusion. D5W in normal saline has also been used successfully as an infusion vehicle.

■ Dosage

Doses of tegafur have ranged from 1 to 3 g/m^2/d for five consecutive days. More commonly, doses of 2 g/m^2/d are used initially and adjusted course to course by 0.25 to 0.5 g/m^2/d increments commensurate with toxicity and clinical effects. High-dose regimens of 3 to 5 g/m^2 were evaluated by Hall et al (1977). Moderate to severe central nervous system toxic effects occurred in some patients given doses greater than 4 g/m^2. Doses need adjustment in the presence of severe liver dysfunction and when signs of neurologic toxicity are noted. Intravenous doses may be repeated at 2- to 3-week intervals. Oral tegafur dosing information is preliminary: initial researchers have used (1) 500 mg twice daily, escalating 500 mg/d every other day to toxicity (Morgan et al 1979); (2) 1 to 2 g/d × 5 days (Weeth 1979); (3) 1 g per dose in the pharmacologic study of Diasio et al (1979). These doses were relatively well tolerated in these patients.

With repeated intravenous injections, the drug is erratically and relatively poorly tolerated. Weeth (1979) used fractionated monthly bolus injections (0.5-, 2-, and 8-hour infusions) without significant success as individual daily dose limits remained 0.5 to 1.0 g/d. In contrast, the 1- to 2-g daily oral dose used in this study was substantially better tolerated, which suggests a possible role for continuous daily dosing. Ansfield et al (1979) have thus used fractionated oral doses of 1.5 to 1.75 g/d × 5 without evidence of severe toxicity and with preliminary evidence of therapeutic activity. An oral dose of 500 to

750 mg/m² twice daily for 5 days was recommended in a review of the U.S. clinical experience (Friedman and Ignoffo 1980).

■ Drug Interactions

Because of the extensive metabolism of tegafur, drugs that alter microsomal enzymes may interact with tegafur. In mice, the enzyme inducers phenobarbital and 3-methylcholanthrene enhance central nervous system toxicity and lethality from tegafur (Belitsky et al 1981). The opposite effect was noted with the combination of tegafur and SKF-525, a drug known to block microsomal enzymes. In this instance, SKF-525 blocked tegafur toxicity in mice. The coadministration of uracil has also been shown to block the central nervous system and cardiac toxicity of tegafur in mice (Yamamoto et al 1984). The mechanism of inhibition was presumed to involve a blockade in 5-fluorouracil breakdown to α-fluoro-β-alanine. Uracil also increases the experimental antitumor effects of tegafur, possibly by enhancing drug uptake into a variety of tissues including tumors (Fujii et al 1979). Cytosine similarly enhanced experimental tegafur antitumor effects to a lesser extent (Fujii et al 1979).

■ Pharmacokinetics

Tegafur is extensively metabolized to 5-fluorouracil in vivo (Horwitz et al 1975). The release of 5-fluorouracil from this metabolic transformation appears to be rather slow. In mice, the drug distributes to tumor cells, spleen, thymus, kidney, pancreas, skin, stomach, and lung. Metabolites found in the urine in rat studies were primarily tegafur and α-fluoro-β-alanine (Cohen 1975). Metabolic products of tegafur's major metabolite, 5-fluorouracil, are reviewed under 5-*Fluorouracil.* Generally, they are excreted about 10 to 30% in the urine and 60 to 80% via the lungs as carbon dioxide.

Preliminary pharmacokinetic studies in humans demonstrate a median half-life of 18.6 hours for tegafur versus 30 minutes for 5-fluorouracil (Lu et al 1975). Results of a more recent investigation by Au et al (1979) demonstrate biphasic tegafur plasma decay with a median terminal phase half-life of 9.3 hours (range, 6–16 hours). The half-life was longest in those patients with severe liver dysfunction. Total plasma clearance of the drug approximated 50 mL/kg/h in one study (Hills et al 1977), whereas the volume of distribution appears to range from 0.4 to 0.8 L/kg (Au et al 1979). This latter group reported 5-fluorouracil levels less than 5% of tegafur levels and additionally isolated a number of hydroxylated tegafur intermediate metabolites from the urine.

Studies of oral tegafur by a number of investigators have shown excellent oral absorption for the investigational 500-mg tablets (Diasio et al 1979, Weeth 1979, Morgan et al 1979). Diasio et al further determined that plasma levels peaked approximately 2 hours after ingestion and were relatively sustained with the oral dosage form. Areas under the plasma concentration × time curves were equivalent for oral and intravenous doses in this study. Byfield et al (1985) showed that mean serum 5-fluorouracil levels were 3 to 13 ng/mL on days 2, 3, and 4 following an oral tegafur dose of 1 g/m². The day 4 levels of 5-fluorouracil increased to 70, 73, and 273 ng/mL with oral tegafur doses of 1.5, 2.0, and 2.5 g/m², respectively. At the highest dose, the 5-fluorouracil levels were equivalent to those produced by a continuous 5-fluorouracil infusion of 17.5 mg/kg/24 h (Byfield et al 1985). At a dose of 5 g/m², mean serum 5-fluorouracil levels of 2 μg/mL or greater are reduced for over 50 hours (Loo et al 1978). Furthermore, the major metabolite, dehydrotegafur, was consistently present at about 10 times the levels of 5-fluorouracil.

Another pharmacokinetic trial compared oral and intravenous tegafur in cancer patients (Anttila et al 1983). Oral absorption was complete and no significant first-pass metabolism was apparent. Total serum clearance was 69 mL/h·kg with a volume of distribution of 0.66 L/kg. The distribution and elimination half-lives were 1 and 7.6 hours, respectively. Human urinary metabolites of tegafur include *trans*-3'- and *cis*-4'-hydroxytegafur (Benvenuto et al 1979).

As stated earlier, there are two distinct metabolic activation pathways for tegafur (Au and Sadee 1980) (see Mechanism of Action). The R isomer of tegafur is preferentially cleaved at the N_1–C_2' position to form 5-fluorouracil and γ-butyric lactone by soluble (nonmicrosomal) enzymes (Au and Sadee 1981). In contrast, less of the 4'-hydroxylated metabolites are produced by microsomal enzymes. The preferred conformation of the glycoside is α-L-4'-hydroxy or β-L-4'-hydroxide. Thus, little tegafur is metabolized to the natural β-D configuration. No glucuronide or sulfate conjugates of the hydroxylated metabolites were observed. Metabolism of tegafur may also be affected by drugs that alter hepatic enzymes (see Drug Interactions).

Preliminary data have indicated that tegafur readily crosses the blood–brain barrier, achieving central nervous system levels 75% of those in the plasma. This may explain some of the dose-limiting central nervous system toxic effects.

■ Side Effects and Toxicity

Tegafur produces significant gastrointestinal and central nervous system toxic effects (Valdivieso et al 1976). The frequency of severe nausea and vomiting appears to increase with increasing single doses, especially beyond the 2.0 g/m^2/d level. Esophagitis and mucositis have also been noted in the second week of treatment but are usually mild and transient (2–4 days). Moderate diarrhea has been noted in only a few patients; however, nausea and vomiting may occasionally persist beyond the last day of a 5-day intravenous injection regimen. Toxicity with oral tegafur involves primarily gastrointestinal effects, principally nausea and vomiting, which can be severe at doses greater than 1.5 g/m^2/d for 2 to 3 weeks (Dindogru et al 1980).

Acute central nervous system toxic effects have consisted of restlessness, agitation, and confusion lasting several hours after administration. A delayed form of central nervous system toxicity involving ataxia and dizziness can occur up to 5 to 10 days after cessation of therapy. Frank coma has also been observed with tegafur. Severe dose-limiting central nervous system toxicity has been described along with gastrointestinal toxicity in patients with advanced gastrointestinal cancer wherein no antitumor efficacy was obtained. A cumulative dose of 25 g/m^2 has been correlated with increased risk of toxic effects.

Hematologic toxicity has been infrequent at most doses used. It appears to be virtually eliminated with chronic daily dosing (Ansfield et al 1979). This corroborates the observation that continuous-infusion 5-fluorouracil is less myelosuppressive than equivalent doses given by rapid injection (Siefert et al 1975). Myelotoxicity with oral tegafur is typically mild to moderate, although severe thrombocytopenia is produced in 30% of patients (Ansfield et al 1983). In this regard, oral tegafur toxicity appears to approximate that of continuous-infusion 5-fluorouracil.

Another common toxic effect is weakness, seen after successive courses or large single intravenous doses (> 2 g/m^2/d). Fever and chills are described in 8% of patients (Valdivieso et al 1976). These instances occurred immediately after injection and lasted 2 to 3 hours without serious sequelae. Some observers have noted postural hypotension after rapid injections of tegafur, and for this reason frequent blood pressure determinations should be obtained during infusions.

REFERENCES

Ansfield FJ, Kallas G, Singson I. Phase I–II clinical studies with IV and oral ftorafur, a preliminary report. *Proc Am Assoc Cancer Res.* 1979;**20**:349.

Ansfield FJ, Kallas GJ, Singson JP. Phase I–II studies of oral tegafur (ftorafur). *J Clin Oncol.* 1983;**1**(2):107–110.

Anttila MI, Sotaniemi EA, Kairaluoma MI, et al. Pharmacokinetics of ftorafur after intravenous and oral administration. *Cancer Chemother Pharmacol.* 1983;**10**:150–153.

Au JL, Wu AT, Friedman MA. Pharmacokinetics and metabolism of ftorafur in man. *Cancer Treat Rep.* 1979;**63**:343–350.

Au JL-S, Sadee W. Activation of ftorafur (R,S-1-(tetrahydro-2-furanyl)-5-fluorouracil) to 5-fluorouracil and γ-butyrolactone. *Cancer Res.* 1980;**40**:2814–2819.

Au JL-S, Sadee W. Stereoselective metabolism of ftorafur (R,2–1-tetrahydro-2-furanyl)-5-fluorouracil). *Cancer Chemother Pharmacol.* 1981;**7**:55–59.

Belitsky GA, Bukhman VM, Konopleva IA. Changes in toxic and antitumor properties of ftorafur by induction or inhibition of the microsomal enzymes activity. *Cancer Chemother Pharmacol.* 1981;**6**:183–187.

Benvenuto JA, Liehr JG, Winkler T, et al. Human urinary metabolites of 1-(tetrahydro-2-furanyl)-5-fluorouracil (ftorafur). *Cancer Res.* 1979;**39**:3199–3201.

Blokhina NG, Vozny EK, Garin AM. Results of treatment of malignant tumors with ftorafur. *Cancer.* 1972;**30**:390–392.

Byfield JE, Hornbeck CL, Frankel SS, et al. Relevance of the pharmacology of oral tegafur to its use as a 5-FU prodrug. *Cancer Treat Rep.* 1985;**69**:645–652.

Cirera L, Cardona T, Batiste E, et al. Randomized trial of adjuvant chemotherapy vs control in stage III gastric cancer. *Proc Am Soc Clin Oncol.* 1992;**11**:160.

Cohen AM. The disposition of ftorafur in rats after intravenous administration. *Drug Metab Dispos.* 1975;**3**:303–308.

Diasio RB, Hunter HL, LaBudde JA, Mayol RF. Pharmacologic study of oral ftorafur: Potential for improved oral delivery of 5-fluorouracil (abstract C-455). *Proc Am Assoc Cancer Res ASCO.* 1979;**20**:401.

Dindogru A, Vaitkevicius VK, Young JD, et al. Pharmacologic studies and phase I evaluation of oral ftorafur (FTF). *Proc Am Assoc Cancer Res.* 1980;**21**:167.

Friedman MA, Ignoffo RJ. A review of the United States clinical experience of the fluoropyrimidine, ftorafur (NSC-148958). *Cancer Treat Rev.* 1980;**7**:205–213.

Fujii S, Kitano S, Ikenaka K, Shirasaka T. Effect of coadministration of uracil or cytosine on the antitumor activity of clinical doses of 1-(2-tetrahydrofuryl)-5-fluorouracil and level of 5-fluorouracil in rodents. *Gann.* 1979;**70**:209–214.

Hall SW, Benjamin RS, Murphy WK, et al. Adriamycin, BCNU, ftorafur chemotherapy of pancreatic and biliary tract cancer. *Cancer.* 1979;**44**:2008–2013.

Hall SW, Valdivieso M, Benjamin RS. Intermittent high single-dose ftorafur: Phase I clinical trial with a pharmacologic–toxicity correlation. *Cancer Treat Rep.* 1977;**61**(8): 1495–1498.

Harrison SD Jr, Denine EP, Giles HD. Evidence for toxicologic activity of ftorafur independent of conversion to 5-fluorouracil. *Cancer Treat Rep.* 1979;**63**(8):1389–1391.

Hatori T, Furue H, Furukawa K. Clinical experiences with FT-207. *Jpn J Cancer Clin.* 1973;**19**(1):50–53.

Hills EB, Godefroi VC, O'Leary IA, et al. GLC determination of ftorafur in biological fluids. *J Pharm Sci.* 1977;**66**:1497–1499.

Horwitz J, Burke B, Hills E, et al. Clinical disposition of 5-fluorouracil administered by rapid injection, oral ingestion, and slow infusion. *Proc Am Assoc Cancer Res.* 1975;**16**:109.

Karev NI, Blokhina NG, Vozny EK, Pershin MP. Experience with ftorafur treatment in breast cancer. *Neoplasma.* 1972;**19**:347–350.

Loo TL, Benjamine RS, Lu K, et al. Metabolism and disposition of Baker's antifolate (NSC-139105), ftorafur (NSC-148958), and dichlorallyl lawsone (NSC-125771) in man. *Drug Metab Rev.* 1978;**8**(1):137–150.

Lu K, Loo TI, Benvenuto JA, et al. Pharmacologic disposition and metabolism of ftorafur (abstract 150). *Pharmacologist.* 1975;**17**:202.

Meiren D, Belousova A. On the mechanism of action of ftorafur, a new antineoplastic agent. *Bopr Med Khim.* 1972;**18**(3):288–293.

Morgan LR, Browder H, Carter RD. Oral ftorafur: A feasibility study (abstract C-439). *Proc Am Assoc Cancer Res ASCO.* 1979;**20**:397.

Sayed YM, Sadee W. Metabolic activation of *R,S*-1-(tetrahydro-2-furanyl)-5-fluorouracil (ftorafur) to 5-fluorouracil by soluble enzymes. *Cancer Res.* 1983;**43**:4039–4044.

Siefert P, Baker L, et al. Comparison of continuously infused 5-fluorouracil with bolus injection in treatment of patients with colorectal adenocarcinoma. *Cancer.* 1975;**36**:123–138.

Smart CR, Townsend LB, Rusho WJ, et al. Phase I study of ftorafur, an analog of 5-fluorouracil. *Cancer.* 1975;**36**:103–106.

Smolyanskaya AZ, Trigarinov OA. The biological activity of the antitumor antimetabolite "ftorafur." *Neoplasma.* 1972;**19**:341–345.

Valdivieso M, Bodey GP, Gottlieb JA, et al. Clinical evaluation of ftorafur (pyrimidine-deoxyribose *N*-2'-furanidyl-5-fluorouracil). *Cancer Res.* 1976;**36**:1821–1824.

Weeth JB. Ftorafur: Oral tablet trial follows intravenous phase I study (abstract C-64). *Proc Am Assoc Cancer Res ASCO.* 1979;**20**:307.

Woolley PV, MacDonald JS, Smythe T, et al. A phase 2 trial of ftorafur, Adriamycin and mitomycin-C (FAM 2) in advanced gastric adenocarcinoma. *Cancer.* 1979;**44**: 1211–1214.

Yamamoto J, Haruno A, Yoshimura Y, et al. Effect of coadministration of uracil on the toxicity of tegafur. *J Pharm Sci.* 1984;**73**(2):212–214.

Teniposide

■ Other Names

NSC-122819; VM-26; thenylidene-Lignan P; Vumon® (Bristol Myers).

■ Chemistry

Structure of teniposide

Podophyllin resin derivatives have been used as medicaments for over 250 years (Kelly and Hartwell 1954b). In 1861 Bentley reported cytotoxic activity for podophyllin which in a latter report was very useful as topical solution in oil for treating condyloma acuminatum (Kaplan 1942).

Teniposide is a semisynthetic podophyllotoxin derived from the root of *Podophyllum peltatum* (the May apple or mandrake) (Kelly and Hartwell 1954a). It represents a crystalline derivative of α-peltatin, one of numerous cytotoxic compounds present in podophyllin. Teniposide has the empiric formula of $C_{32}H_{32}O_{13}S$ and the molecular weight 656. The complete chemical name is 4'-demethyl-epipodophyllotoxin 9-(4,6-*O*-2-thenylidene-β-D-glucopyranoside). Teniposide is insoluble in water so the preparation for clinical use is dissolved in a mixture of organic (lipid) solvents containing Cremophor EL (polyethoxylated castor oil).

Several reviews have been written on teniposide (Holthuis 1988, Dombernowsky and Hansen 1988, Rivera 1988, O'Dwyer et al 1984).

■ Antitumor Activity

The table below summarizes the single-agent activity reported with teniposide. The drug may be useful for treatment of brain metastases in patients with small cell lung cancer (Giaccone et al 1988).

Teniposide has been used successfully in combination regimens to treat children with relapsed acute lymphocytic leukemia (see table on top of the page). The combinations noted in that table have been reported. Unfortunately, despite the fact that these combinations are active, teniposide has not been approved by the Food and Drug Administration because its contribution to the success of the combinations is unclear (Grem et al 1988).

■ Mechanism of Action

Teniposide is an inhibitor of topoisomerase II (Lonn et al 1989). It does not bind to DNA but rather inhibits the strand-passing and DNA ligase activities of topoisomerase II enzymes in the cell nucleus. This leads to protein-associated DNA double-strand breaks, which presumably halt the cell division (Chen et al 1984). The drug is phase specific with action in late S and early G_2 phases of the cell cycle (Misra and Roberts 1975).

TENIPOSIDE COMBINATION THERAPY IN ACUTE LYMPHOCYTIC LEUKEMIA

Combination	Response Rate (%)	Reference(s)
Teniposide + methotrexate	17	Ochs et al 1991
Teniposide + cytarabine	48–79	Ochs et al 1990, Rivera et al 1986, Rivera et al 1980

■ Availability and Storage

Teniposide is investigationally available from Bristol-Myers Oncology Division, Evansville, Indiana, in 10 mg/mL, 5-mL ampules. Each milliliter of clear, light yellow solution contains teniposide 10 mg, benzyl alcohol 30 mg, N,N-demethyl acetamide 60 mg, Cremophor EL® (purified) 500 mg, maleic acid to adjust pH to 5.1, and absolute alcohol to a total volume of 1 mL (Rozencweig et al 1977). Before mixing, the intact vials are stable for about 4 years from the date of manufacture when stored at room temperature.

CLINICAL ANTITUMOR ACTIVITY OF TENIPOSIDE

Tumor Type	Response Rate (%)	Reference
Endometrial	9	Muss et al 1991
Colon	0	Oishi et al 1990, Locker et al 1986
Kaposi's sarcoma (AIDS related)	50	Schwartsmann et al 1990
Small cell lung (AIDS related)	0, 5, 29, 34	Tummarello et al 1989, 1990, Giaccone et al 1988b, Bork et al 1986, Creech et al 1984, Pedersen et al 1984
Non-small cell lung	17	Giaconne et al 1987
Ovary	0–12	Van der Burg et al 1987, Muss et al 1986
Bladder	5–7	Qazi et al 1982, Oishi et al 1987
Cervix	4–22	Pfeiffer et al 1990, Muss et al 1990
Breast	0–5	Boas et al 1990, Cox et al 1988, Tirelli et al 1984b
Lymphoma		
Cutaneous T cell	40	Sorio et al 1987
Non-Hodgkin's	22, 43	Tirelli et al 1984a
Chronic myelogenous leukemia	0	Zagonel et al 1986
Multiple myeloma	28	Tirelli et al 1985
Renal	2	Oishi et al 1987

Preparation for Use, Stability, and Admixture

Teniposide is supplied as a nonaqueous solution and must be diluted with at least 5 equivalent vol (preferably 10–20 vol) of diluent. Both sodium chloride and D5W have been used as diluents. Teniposide, however, is structurally similar to etoposide, which is physically incompatible with D5W. It is therefore suggested that special scrutiny for precipitation be carried out if D5W is used as the diluent.

After dilution, teniposide is physically stable for at least 4 hours at room temperature and for at least 6 hours if further diluted with 50 to 100 mL of normal saline. Hydrocortisone (50 mg hemisuccinate) and heparin (5000 U) have been directly added to teniposide solutions in normal saline without apparent problems in at least one European study (Pavone-Macaluso et al 1976). The efficacy of this procedure in reducing local irritation is not known. Compatibility data on other admixtures are similarly unavailable.

Administration

Teniposide should be given by intravenous infusion only. It should not be given by the intravenous push technique because it may precipitate severe hypotension. The drug should, therefore, be administered over at least 45 minutes to decrease the potential for hypotension.

Extravasation should also be avoided. A 5- to 10-mL flush of normal saline before drug administration should be given to check vein patency. After drug administration, an additional 5- to 10-mL flush is recommended to help ensure that all residual drug has been washed from the tubing.

Drug Interactions

Preclinical data suggested that teniposide enhanced the intracellular accumulation of methotrexate. In patients receiving simultaneous teniposide and methotrexate the late plasma levels of methotrexate were lower, suggesting a clinical interaction between the two agents (Rodman et al 1990).

The use of vincristine in combination with teniposide appears to induce a more severe peripheral neurotoxicity than use of vincristine alone (Griffiths et al 1986).

Dosage

Many doses and schedules have been used for treatment of patients with solid tumors. Some of the most common regimens follow:

- 45–60 mg/m^2/d × 5 every 21 days (Bork et al 1986, Cox et al 1988, Oishi et al 1990, Mathe et al 1974)
- 120–160 mg/m^2 on days 1, 3, and 5 every 21 days (Giaccone et al 1988a,b, 1987)
- 100 mg/m^2 on days 1 and 2 every 3 weeks (van der Burg et al 1987)
- 100 mg/m^2/wk (Muss et al 1990, 1991, Dombernowsky et al 1972)

In children, Bleyer et al (1979) started at 130 mg/m^2/wk and after 3 to 6 weeks escalated to 150 and 180 mg/m^2, respectively, (if neutropenia is allowed).

In patients with acute lymphocytic leukemia, a typical regimen would include 165 mg/m^2 teniposide twice a week × 4 weeks and 300 mg/m^2 cytosine arabinoside on the same schedule (Rivera et al 1980). Recently, teniposide (plus other agents) has been escalated in patients with small cell lung cancer using hematopoietic growth factors (Noda et al 1991). Teniposide could be escalated up to 120 mg/m^2/d × 5. The recommended dose was 100 mg/m^2/d × 5.

Pharmacokinetics

Allen and Creaven (1975) have studied the human pharmacokinetics of both teniposide and etoposide, and some significant differences are readily apparent. Teniposide plasma-decay kinetics tended to be triphasic, demonstrating the presence of both a "shallow" and a "deep" peripheral compartment. The drug is apparently highly protein bound to albumin (99.4%) without direct evidence of specific binding to DNA. It is also highly metabolized (86%). The mean steady-state volume of distribution in that study was approximately 28.5% of body weight, with a mean central compartment volume of 3.5 L. The mean overall clearance of teniposide was 16 mL/min. Overall, teniposide was eliminated much more slowly than etoposide, which has a renal clearance six times larger than that of teniposide. Approximate mean half-lives for the three phases of teniposide elimination in this report were 45 minutes, 4 hours, and 20 hours for the final phase (Allen and Creaven 1975). In another report by this group (Creaven and Allen 1975) urinary elimination appeared to account for about 40% of an administered dose 72 hours after injection. Approximately 80% of this fraction was metabolite. Fecal drug recovery amounted to only less than 10% of the dose, and cerebrospinal fluid drug levels were less than 1% of simultaneous peak plasma levels. Thus, teniposide does not appear to efficiently penetrate the normal blood–brain barrier. In one patient who had received prior cranial surgery and irradiation, however, cerebrospinal fluid levels were about 27% of those in the plasma.

Most of teniposide is metabolized in humans, although a substantial fraction is ultimately eliminated in the urine. In addition, the drug has a long terminal elimination phase, ranging from 11 to 39 hours (average ~ 20 hours), and patients with the longer terminal half-lives tend to experience greater hematologic toxic effects.

There is an excellent review on the more recent pharmacokinetics of teniposide (Clark and Slevin 1987). Most studies show a biexponential decay following intravenous administration of the drug. Only 5 to 20% of teniposide can be accounted for by excretion (Holthuis et al 1987). Most of the urinary fraction is metabolites. Only about 8.8 to 13.9% of a dose is excreted in the urine intact. The table below summarizes the clinical pharmacokinetics of teniposide. Low concentrations of teniposide can be detected in saliva, duodenal fluid, and cerebrospinal fluid (Holthuis et al 1987). Teniposide was detected in postmortem tissues from one of four patients receiving drug a median of 8 days before dying. In this patient, the highest concentrations (ng/g) were found in spleen (1643), prostate (1380), heart (1037), large bowel (242), liver (177), and pancreas (131) (Stewart et al 1992).

Pharmacokinetic studies performed after intraperitoneal administration of teniposide have shown that total exposure for the peritoneal cavity averaged 10-fold greater than that of plasma (Canal et al 1989a). In comparative kinetic studies of intrapleural versus intravenous administration of teniposide, intrapleural administration produced higher intrapleural drug levels (Montaldo et al 1990).

The clearance of teniposide may vary considerably from patient to patient. In children with recurrent hematologic or solid tumors, teniposide doses of 300 to 750 mg/m^2 as a 72-hour continuous infusion produced clearance values ranging from 3.7 to 43.8 mL/min/m^2 (Rodman et al 1987). Importantly, responders had lower mean clearance of 12.1 mL/min/m^2 compared with a clearance of 21.3 mL/min/m^2 in nonresponders. This variation in clearance led to a four- to sixfold variation in systemic drug exposures. Responses were noted in patients achieving a steady-state plasma concentration of more than 12 mg/L (Rodman et al 1991).

Teniposide given into the pericardial sac in patients with malignant pericardial effusion has produced intrapericardial levels 15 to 21 times the plasma levels with responses of the patients' disease (Figoli et al 1987). Two of the three treated patients had no reaccumulation of fluid for 2 and 5 months after treatment. The half-life of intrapericardial drug elimination was biphasic, with a terminal half life ranging from 9 to 16 hours. Peak drug levels in the pericardial fluid were about 195 µg/mL.

■ Side Effects and Toxicity

Hematologic toxic effects are the typical dose-limiting consequences of intravenous teniposide (Muggia et al 1971). In this regard, leukopenia tends

CLINICAL PHARMACOKINETICS OF TENIPOSIDE

Dose and Schedule	Steady-State Concentration (µg/mL)	α	β	γ	Steady-State Volume of Distribution	Clearance (mL/min/m^2)	Reference
300–750 mg/m^2 as 72-h infusion							
Responders	15.2	—	12.4	—	11.4	12.1	Rodman et al 1987
Nonresponders	6.2	—	6.6	—	8.6	21.3	Rodman et al 1987
70–180 mg/m^2, single dose	—	—	—	—	13.2–24.7	5.8–10.2	Holthuis 1988
165 mg/m^2 over 30–60 min	—	—	—	—	7.9 ± 4.0	13.8 ± 6	Holthuis et al 1987
100–150 mg/m^2 over 1 h	—	—	6.9 ± 0.9	—	—	15.6 ± 2.0	D'Incalci et al 1985

to predominate although thrombocytopenia is also observed. Neither toxic effect has been consistently shown to be cumulative. The range for leukopenic nadirs is 3 to 14 days, generally occurring in about 1 week. Heavy prior irradiation and/or chemotherapy necessitate substantial dosage reduction. With biweekly doses of about 1 to 3 mg/kg, a cumulative dose of 250 to 500 mg was required to produce significant bone marrow toxicity (Dombernowsky et al 1972). Cerny et al (1988) have documented that elderly patients with small cell lung cancer can be particularly sensitive to the myelosuppressive effects of the drug.

Hypotension has also been a problem with teniposide, but only after rapid intravenous push administration. With administration over periods longer than 30 minutes, hypotension is rare. Delayed hypotension and cardiac toxicity have not been described for teniposide.

Significant hepatic and renal toxicity has not been reported. Alopecia is rarely reported (Muggia et al 1971) and is readily reversible once the patient is off therapy (Dombernowsky et al 1972).

Chemical phlebitis at the injection site was also universally noted by Dombernowsky et al (1972). This reaction is commonly described for podophyllum derivatives (Vaitkevicius and Reed 1966). Similar local reactions, commonly thought to be caused by the solvent, have been described following intraperitoneal injection wherein severe abdominal pain may be produced (Dombernowsky et al 1972).

Severe skin rashes have been described in patients receiving teniposide in a high-dose (1 g/m^2) regimen (de Vries et al 1986). An immune hemolytic anemia with renal failure has been described for the drug (Habibi et al 1982).

Severe hypertension secondary to teniposide administration has been described (Shimizu et al 1987). O'Dwyer et al (1986) have reported that (depending on the method of detection) the incidence of hypertension reactions to teniposide ranged from 3.6 to 6.5%. The reactions were most common in patients with brain tumors or neuroblastoma.

Recently, Kellie et al (1991) have reported that children with acute lymphocytic leukemia receiving teniposide have a 52% chance of hypersensitivity reaction to the agent. This is characterized by urticaria, angioedema, flushing, rashes, or hypotension occurring some time during the course of treatment. With hydrocortisone and diphenhydramine pretreatment, there was no evidence of increasing symptom severity on rechallenge and no deaths occurred. There is evidence the hypersensitivity may be caused by the polyethoxylated caster oil (Cremophor EL) vehicle (Siddal et al 1989); however, Nolte et al (1988) have shown hypersensitivity reactions are due to teniposide-induced degranulation of basophils. Pediatric patients with neuroblastoma may experience a higher incidence of allergic reactions to teniposide (14/105 patients) versus pediatric patients with leukemias or lymphoid malignancies (2/82 patients) (Hayes et al 1985). Importantly, repeat reactions in neuroblastoma patients were not prevented by pretreatment with hydrocortisone and diphenhydramine.

There is also a suggestion from the literature that teniposide may be associated with secondary leukemia (Kreissman et al 1990). Recently, weekly or biweekly teniposide and/or etoposide as part of maintenance therapy for acute lymphocytic leukemia in children have been associated with an increased risk (12%) of developing secondary acute myelogenous leukemia (Pui et al 1991). The prolonged schedule involving weekly or biweekly dosing was felt to contribute substantially to the increased leukemogenic risk compared with the 1.6% risk with therapy every 2 weeks during remission induction only. Epipodophyllotoxin-induced secondary leukemias tend to lack a myelodysplastic phase and involve monoblasts or myelomonoblasts and translocation of the long arm of chromosome 11 (11q23) (Pui et al 1989).

■ Special Applications

Intravesicular Administration. Pavone-Macaluso et al (1975, 1976) have successfully used local bladder instillations of teniposide in patients with multiple or diffuse superficial papillary tumors. For these applications, 50-mg doses of teniposide were diluted to 30 mL with sterile water for injection or normal saline and administered over 1 hour on 5 consecutive days. Courses were repeated at monthly intervals for 6 months. Regression of lesions occurred in three of six patients with two long-term responders (>1 year). This method was also used successfully as chemoprophylactic therapy to prevent recurrence in 10 other patients (Pavone-Macaluso et al 1976).

About a third of patients developed a severe chemical cystitis. This was noted after the first instillation and tended to become progressively more severe with each repeated course. Hematologic toxicity was not observed with this experimental regimen.

Intrapericardial Administration. Teniposide has been investigationally administered at a dose of 50 mg/m^2 (Figoli et al 1987). This prevented further fluid accumulation in two of three treated patients (see Pharmacokinetics also).

REFERENCES

Allen LM, Creaven PJ. Comparison of the human pharmacokinetics of VM-26 and VP-16, two antineoplastic epipodophyllotoxin glucopyranoside derivatives. *Eur J Cancer.* 1975;**11**:697–707.

Bleyer WA, Krivit W, Chard RL, Hammond D. Phase II study of VM-26 in acute leukemia, neuroblastoma, and other refractory childhood malignancies: A report from the Children's Cancer Study group. *Cancer Treat Rep.* 1979;**63**:977–981.

Boas J, Rasmussen D, Hansen OP, Engelholm SA, Dombernowsky P. Phase II study of teniposide in advanced breast cancer. *Cancer Chemother Pharmacol.* 1990;**25**(6):463–464.

Bork E, Hansen M, Dombernowsky P, Hansen SW, Pedersen AG, Hansen HH. Teniposide (VM-26), an overlooked highly active agent in small-cell lung cancer. Results of a phase II trial in untreated patients. *J Clin Oncol.* 1986;**4**(4):524–527.

Canal P, Bugat R, Chatelut E, et al. A phase I/pharmacokinetic study of intraperitoneal teniposide (VM 26). *Eur J Cancer Clin Oncol.* 1989a;**25**(5):815–820.

Canal YP, Chatelut E, Bugat R, De Biasi J, Houin G. Pharmacokinetic model for intraperitoneal administration of drugs: Application to teniposide in humans. *J Pharm Sci.* 1989b;**78**(5):389–392.

Cerny T, Pedrazzini A, Joss RA, Brunner KW. Unexpected high toxicity in a phase II study of teniposide (VM-26) in elderly patients with untreated small cell lung cancer (SCLC). *Eur J Cancer Clin Oncol.* 1988;**24**(11):1791–1794.

Chen GL, Yang L, Rowe TC, et al. Nonintercalative antitumor drugs interfere with the breakage–reunion reaction of mammalian DNA topoisomerase II. *J Biol Chem.* 1984;**259**(21):13560–13566.

Chiuten DF, Bennett JM, Creech RH, et al. VM-26, a new anticancer drug with effectiveness in malignant lymphoma: An Eastern Cooperative Oncology Group study (EST 1474). *Cancer Treat Rep.* 1979;**63**(1):7–11.

Clark PI, Slevin ML. The clinical pharmacology of etoposide and teniposide. *Clin Pharmacokinet.* 1987;**12**(4):223–252.

Cox EB, Vogel CL, Carpenter JR Jr, Raney M. Phase II evaluation of teniposide (VM-26) in metastatic breast carcinoma. A Southwestern Cancer Study Group trial. *Invest New Drugs.* 1988;**6**(1):37–39.

Creaven PJ, Allen LM. PTG, a new antineoplastic epipodophyllotoxin. *Clin Pharmacol Ther.* 1975;**18**:227–233.

Creech RH, Tritchler D, Ettinger DS, et al. Phase II study of PALA, amsacrine, teniposide, and zinostatin in small cell lung carcinoma. *Cancer Treat Rep.* 1984;**68**(9):1183–1184.

Dahl GV, Rivera GK, Look AT, et al. Teniposide plus cytarabine improves outcome in childhood acute lymphoblastic leukemia presenting with a leukocyte count greater than or equal to 100 × 10(9)/L. *J Clin Oncol.* 1987;**5**(7):1015–1021.

De Vries EG, Mulder NH, Postmus PE, Vriesendorp R, Willemse PH, Sleijfer DT. High-dose teniposide for refractory malignancies: A phase I study. *Cancer Treat Rep.* 1986;**70**(5):595–598.

D'Incalci M, Rossi C, Sessa C, et al. Pharmacokinetics of teniposide in patients with ovarian cancer. *Cancer Treat Rep.* 1985;**69**(1):73–77.

Dombernowsky P, Hansen HH. The epipodophyllotoxin derivatives VM26 and VP16: Experimental and clinical aspects. *Eur J Haematol.* 1988;**48**(suppl):49–57.

Dombernowsky P, Nissen N, Larsen V. Clinical investigation of a new podophyllum derivative, epipodophyllotoxin, 4′-demethyl-9-(4,6-O-2-thenylidene-β-D-glucopyranoside) NSC-122819, in patients with malignant lymphomas and solid tumors. *Cancer Chemother Rep.* 1972;**56**:71–82.

Figoli F, Zanette ML, Tirelli U, et al. Pharmacokinetics of VM 26 given intrapericardially or intravenously in patients with malignant pericardial effusion. *Cancer Chemother Pharmacol.* 1987;**20**(3):239–242.

Giaccone G, Donadio M, Bonardi GM, Testore F, Calciati A. Teniposide (VM-26): An effective treatment for brain metastases of small cell carcinoma of the lung. *Eur J Cancer Clin Oncol.* 1988a;**24**(4):629–631.

Giaccone G, Donadio M, Ferrati P, et al. Teniposide in the treatment of non-small cell lung carcinoma. *Cancer Treat Rep.* 1987;**71**(1):83–85.

Giaccone G, Donalio M, Bonardi G, Testore F, Calciati A. Teniposide in the treatment of small-cell lung cancer: The influence of prior chemotherapy. *J Clin Oncol.* 1988b;**6**(8):1264–1270.

Grem JL, Hoth DF, Leyland-Jones B, King SA, Ungerleider RS, Wittes RE. Teniposide in the treatment of leukemia: A case study of conflicting priorities in the development of drugs for fatal diseases. *J Clin Oncol.* 1988;**6**(2):351–379.

Griffiths JD, Stark RJ, Ding JC, Cooper IA. Vincristine neurotoxicity enhanced in combination chemotherapy including both teniposide and vincristine. *Cancer Treat Rep.* 1986;**70**(4):519–521.

Habibi B, Lopez M, Serdaru M, et al. Immune hemolytic anemia and renal failure due to teniposide. *N Engl J Med.* 1982;**306**(18):1091–1093.

Hayes FA, Abromowitch M, Green AA. Allergic reactions to teniposide in patients with neuroblastoma and lymphoid malignancies. *Cancer Treat Rep.* 1985;**69**(4):439–441.

Holthuis JJ. Etoposide and teniposide. Bioanalysis, metabolism and clinical pharmacokinetics. *Pharm Weekbl (Sci.)* 1988;**10**(3):101–116.

Holthuis JJ, de Vries LG, Postmus PE, et al. Pharmacokinetics of high-dose teniposide. *Cancer Treat Rep.* 1987;**71**(6):599–603.

Kaplan IW. Condylomata acuminata. *New Orleans M & SJ.* 1942;**94**:388–390.

Kellie SJ, Crist WM, Pui CH, et al. Hypersensitivity reactions to epipodophyllotoxins in children with acute lymphoblastic leukemia. *Cancer.* 1991;**67**(4):1070–1075.

Kelly M, Hartwell J. The biological effects and chemical composition of podophyllin. A review. *J Natl Cancer Inst.* 1954a;**14**:967–1010.

Kelly M, Hartwell JL. Podophyllum. A review. *J Natl Cancer Inst.* 1954b;**14**:647.

Kreissman SG, Gelber RD, Sallan SE, Leavitt P, Cohen HJ. Secondary acute myeloid leukemia (AML) in children treated for acute lymphoblastic leukemia (ALL) (meeting abstract). *Proc Am Soc Clin Oncol.* 1990;**9**:219.

Locker GY, Lanzotti V, Khandekar JD, et al. Phase II trial of teniposide in previously treated and untreated patients with advanced colorectal carcinoma: An Illinois Cancer Council trial. *Cancer Treat Rep.* 1986;**70**(2):307–308.

Lonn U, Lonn S, Nylen U, Winblad G. Altered formation of DNA in human cells treated with inhibitors of DNA topoisomerase II (etoposide and teniposide). *Cancer Res.* 1989;**49**(22):6202–6207.

Mathe G, Schwarzenberg L, Pouillart P, et al. Two epipodophyllotoxin derivatives, VM 26 and VP 16213, in the treatment of leukemias, hematosarcomas, and lymphomas. *Cancer.* 1974;**34**:985–992.

Misra NC, Roberts D. Inhibition by 4′-demethylepipodophyllotoxin 9-(4,6-O-2-thenylidene-β-D-glucopyranoside) of human lymphoblast cultures in G_2 phase of the cell cycle. *Cancer Res.* 1975;**35**:99–105.

Montaldo PG, Figoli F, Zanette ML, et al. Pharmacokinetics of intrapleural versus intravenous etoposide (VP 16) and teniposide (VM 26) in patients with malignant pleural effusion. *Oncology.* 1990;**47**(1):55–61.

Muggia F, Selawry O, Hansen H. Clinical studies with a new podophyllotoxin derivative epipodophyllotoxin, 4′-demethyl-9-(4,6-O-2-thenylidene-β-D-glucopyranoside) NSC-122819. *Cancer Chemother Rep.* 1971;**55**:575–581.

Muss H, Bundy BN, DiSaia PJ, Twiggs LB. Teniposide in epithelial ovarian carcinoma: A phase II trial of the Gynecologic Oncology Group. *Cancer Treat Rep.* 1986;**70**(10):1231–1232.

Muss HB, Bundy BN, Adcock L. Teniposide (VM-26) in patients with advanced endometrial carcinoma. A phase II trial of the Gynecologic Oncology Group. *Am J Clin Oncol.* 1991;**14**(1):36–37.

Muss HB, Bundy BN, Given FT, Stehman FB. Teniposide (VM-26) in patients with nonsquamous-cell carcinoma of the cervix. A phase II trial of the Gynecologic Oncology Group. *Am J Clin Oncol.* 1990;**13**(2):117–118.

Noda K, Eguchi K, Nakada K, et al. Dose escalation study of VM-26 with DCCP and RH G-CSF in patients with small cell lung cancer (SCLC). *Proc Am Soc Cancer Oncol.* 1991;**10**:263.

Nolte H, Carstensen H, Hertz H. VM-26 (teniposide)-induced hypersensitivity and degranulation of basophils in children. *Am J Pediatr Hematol Oncol.* 1988;**10**(4):308–312.

O'Dwyer PJ, Alonso MT, Leyland-Jones B, Marsoni S. Teniposide: A review of 12 years of experience. *Cancer Treat Rep.* 1984;**68**(12):1455–1466.

O'Dwyer PJ, King SA, Fortner CL, Leyland-Jones B. Hypersensitivity reactions to teniposide (VM-26): An analysis. *J Clin Oncol.* 1986;**4**(8):1262–1269.

Ochs J, Rivera GK, Pollock BH, Buchanan G, Crist W, Freeman AI. Teniposide (VM-26) and continuous infusion cytosine arabinoside leukemia. A Pediatric Oncology Group pilot study. *Cancer.* 1990;**66**(8):1671–1677.

Ochs J, Rodman J, Abromowitch M, et al. A phase II study of combined methotrexate and teniposide infusions prior to reinduction therapy in relapsed childhood acute lymphoblastic leukemia: A Pediatric Oncology Group study. *J Clin Oncol.* 1991;**9**(1):139–144.

Oishi N, Berenberg J, Blumenstein BA, et al. Teniposide in metastatic renal and bladder cancer: A Southwest Oncology Group study. *Cancer Treat Rep.* 1987;**71**(12):1307–1308.

Oishi N, Fleming TR, Laufman L, et al. VM-26 in colorectal carcinoma: A Southwest Oncology Group study. *Invest New Drugs.* 1990;**8**(1):93–95.

Pavone-Macaluso M, Caramia G, Rizzo FP, Messana V. Preliminary evaluation of VM-26, a new epipodophyllotoxin derivative, in the treatment of urogenital tumours. *Eur Urol.* 1975;**1**:53–56.

Pavone-Macaluso M, EORTC. Genito-urinary tract co-operative group: Single-drug chemotherapy of bladder cancer with Adriamycin, VM-26, or bleomycin. *Eur Urol.* 1976;**2**:138–141.

Pedersen AG, Bork E, Osterlind K, Dombernowsky P, Hensen HH. Phase II study of teniposide in small cell carcinoma of the lung. *Cancer Treat Rep.* 1984;**68**(10):1289–1291.

Pfeiffer P, Cold S, Bertelsen K, Panduro J, Sandberg E, Rose C. Teniposide in recurrent or advanced cervical carcinoma: A phase II trial in patients not previously treated with cytotoxic therapy. *Gynecol Oncol.* 1990;**37**(2):230–233.

Pui C-H, Behm FG, Raimondi SC, et al. Secondary acute myeloid leukemia in children treated for acute lymphoid leukemia. *N Engl J Med.* 1989;**321**:136–142.

Pui C-H, Ribeiro RC, Hancock ML, et al. Acute myeloid leukemia in children treated with epipodophyllotoxins for acute lymphoblastic leukemia. *N Engl J Med.* 1991;**325**:1682–1687.

Qazi R, Elson P, Khadekar JD. Phase II evaluation of VM-26 in patients with metastatic transitional cell carcinoma of the urinary tract: An Eastern Cooperative Oncology Group study. *Cancer Treat Rep.* 1982;**66**(2):405–406.

Rivera G, Dahl GV, Bowman WP, Avery TL, Wood A, Aur RJ. VM-26 and cytosine arabinoside combination chemotherapy for initial induction failures in childhood lymphocytic leukemia. *Cancer.* 1980;**46**(8):1727–1730.

Rivera GK. The epipodophyllotoxin teniposide in therapy for childhood acute lymphocytic leukemia. *J Clin Oncol.* 1988;**6**(2):191–193.

Rivera GK, Buchanan G, Boyett JM, et al. Intensive retreatment of childhood acute lymphoblastic leukemia in first bone marrow relapse. A Pediatric Oncology Group study. *N Engl J Med.* 1986;**315**(5):273–278.

Rodman JH, Abromowitch M, Sinkule JA, Hayes FA, Rivera GK, Evans WE. Clinical pharmacodymanics of continuous infusion teniposide: Systemic exposure as a determinant of response in a phase I trial. *J Clin Oncol.* 1987;**5**(7):1007–1014.

Rodman JH, Sunderland M, Kavanagh RL, et al. Pharmacokinetics of continuous infusion of methotrexate and teniposide in pediatric cancer patients. *Cancer Res.* 1990;**50**(14):4267–4271.

Rodman JH, Sunderland M, Kavanagh RL, et al. Pharmacokinetics of continuous infusion of methotrexate and teniposide in pediatric cancer patients. *J Clin Oncol.* 1991;**9**(1):139–144.

Rozencweig M, Von Hoff DD, Henney JE, Muggia FM. VM-26 and VP-16–213: A comparative analysis. *Cancer.* 1977;**40**:334–342.

Schwartsmann G, Spinz E, Kronfeld M, et al. Phase II study of teniposide (VM-26) in patients with AIDS-related Kaposi's sarcoma (meeting abstract). *Proc Am Soc Clin Oncol.* 1990;9:210.

Shimizu H, Frankel LS, Culbert SJ. Severe hypertensive reactions to teniposide (VM-26) in infants with congenital leukemia. *Am J Pediatr Hematol Oncol.* 1987;**9**(3):239–241.

Siddal DJ, Martin J, Nunn AJ. Anaphylactic reactions to teniposide. *Lancet.* 1989;**1**:394.

Sinkule JA, Stewart CF, Crom WR, Melton ET, Dahl GV, Evans WE. Teniposide (VM-26) disposition in children with leukemia. *Cancer Res.* 1984;**44**(3):1235–1237.

Sorio R, Tirelli U, Zagonel V, et al. Teniposide (VM-26) in cutaneous T-cell lymphoma (CTCL): A phase II study (meeting abstract). In: *Fourth European Conference on Clinical Oncology and Cancer Nursing, Nov 1–4, 1987, Madrid.* Fed Eur Cancer Soc; 1987:269.

Stewart D, Grewaal D, Goel R, et al. Human autopsy tissue etoposide (E) and teniposide (T). *Proc Am Soc Clin Oncol.* 1992;**11**:129.

Tirelli U, Carbone A, Crivellari D, et al. A phase II trial of teniposide (VM26) in advanced non-Hodgkin's lymphoma, with emphasis on the treatment of elderly patients. *Cancer.* 1984a;**54**(3):393–396.

Tirelli U, Carbone A, Zagoni V, et al. Phase II study of teniposide (VM-26) in multiple myeloma. *Am J Clin Oncol.* 1985;**8**(4):329–331.

Tirelli U, Franchin G, Crivellari D, et al. Phase II study of VM 26 in extensively pretreated breast cancer. *Am J Clin Oncol.* 1984b;**7**(5):451–452.

Tummarello D, Guidi F, Di Furia L, Gramazio A, Menichetti E, Cellerino R. A phase II study with teniposide (VM26) in patients with progressed or relapsed small cell lung cancer (SCLC). *J Chemother.* 1989;**1**(1):64–67.

Tummarello D, Guidi F, Torresi U, Dazzi C, Cellerino R. Teniposide (VM26) as second-line treatment for small cell lung cancer. *Anticancer Res.* 1990;**10**(2A):397–399.

Vaitkevicius VK, Reed ML. Clinical studies with podophyllum compounds SPI-77 (NSC-72274) and SPG-827 (NSC-42076). *Cancer Chemother Rep.* 1966;**50**:565–571.

Van der Burg ME, ten Bokkel Huinink WW, Vriesendorp R, et al. Teniposide (VM-26) in patients with advanced refractory ovarian cancer: A phase II study of the Netherlands Joint Study Group for Ovarian Cancer. *Eur J Cancer Clin Oncol.* 1987;**23**(7):997–998.

Zagonel V, Tirelli U, Veronesi A, et al. Teniposide is not effective in chronic lymphocytic leukemia. *Blut.* 1986;**52**(1):59–61.

Terephthalamidine

■ Other Names

NSC-57155; terephthalamidine derivative; symetamine.

■ Chemistry

Structure of terephthalamidine

Terephthalamidine is the derivative of a class of antitumor agents, the phthalanilides, introduced in 1962. The phthalanilides were described by Hirt and Berchtold (1962) and were regarded as "phosphatide blockers." These agents were shown to have potent activity against a broad spectrum of murine leukemias and lymphomas (Burchenal 1964).

Terephthalamidine has a molecular weight of 426. It is soluble in water (>40 mg/mL), moderately soluble in dimethylsulfoxide (11 mg/mL), and poorly soluble (<1 mg/mL) in ethanol, dimethylacetamide, butanol, and chloroform. The complete chemical name is N',N''-bis[p-(methylamidino)phenyl]terephthalamidine tetrahydrochloride.

■ Antitumor Activity

In the early 1960s two compounds in the series of the phthalanilides were selected for clinical trial. These included NSC-35843 and NSC-57155. In phase I clinical trials, NSC-35843 caused nausea and vomiting, and reversible paralysis of lateral and upward gaze and palpebral muscle weakness (2- to 4-hour infusion). When NSC-57155 was given as a 24-hour infusion, there was no paralysis but reversible nystagmus and transient blurring of vision with diplopia were noted (Louis et al 1962, Lyman et al 1962). Phase I–II trials with the 24-hour continuous infusion in children with lymphoma showed that the agent was safe up to 8 mg/kg/d × 3 to 18 days and showed some antitumor activity (Oettgen et al 1963). In phase I trials with NSC-57155, infusions of 1.2 mg/kg/d × 42 days were well tolerated; however, in one patient at a dose of 1.6 mg/kg/d for 24 days, ophthalmoplegia, bulbar signs, shock, and death were noted (Louis et al 1963). Of note, a patient in this study with metastatic seminoma had a complete regression of all tumor, and a patient with Hodgkin's disease had a transient improvement; however, trials with both NSC-35843 and NSC-57155 (also known as terephthalamidine and symetamine) were discontinued in the mid-1960s largely because of the unusual toxic effects.

In 1982 the National Cancer Institute set up a special group of investigators to review antineoplastic agents tested in the 1960s that might have been inadequately studied. One of the agents they recommended for another evaluation was NSC-57155 (terephthalamidine). The group felt the compound should be reevaluated for three reasons: (1) Preclinically, the agent was very active against leukemias, including those with acquired resistance to clinically active agents. (2) The agent had activity in the M-5076 sarcoma, a more recent addition to the NCI tumor screen (Johnson et al 1983). (3) The clinical trials performed in the 1960s were felt to be inadequate.

■ Mechanism of Action

The mechanism of action of terephthalamidine is uncertain. In vitro the phthalanilides form ionic complexes with many biologic components, including nucleic acids, proteins, and lipids. At the biochemical level, studies of leukemia cells, either in culture or in mice, have indicated that the phthalanilides inhibit the synthesis of DNA, RNA, protein, and lipids (Kensler 1963; Rogers et al 1954). The unique intracellular distribution of drug (as lipid complexes from the nuclear and mitrochondrial fractions) suggest that the physiologic site of drug activity is probably in the nucleus and mitochondria through an effect on phospholipid–histone–DNA equilibrium (Yesair et al 1967).

■ Availability and Storage

Terephthalamidine is supplied for authorized investigational studies under the auspices of the National Cancer Institute, Maryland. The compound is formulated as a freeze-dried powder containing 250 mg of drug as the anhydrous base. The vials should be stored under refrigeration (2–8°C).

■ Preparation for Use, Stability, and Admixture

The drug is currently undergoing phase I clinical trials; therefore the optimal method for use is unknown. In the phase I trial as a 120-hour continuous infusion, the full daily dose is diluted in 450 mL of normal saline in a polyvinyl chloride bag and infused over 24 hours by use of an infusion pump. Fresh drug needs to be made up every 24 hours of infusion.

■ Administration

As noted earlier, terephthalamidine is now undergoing phase I clinical trials with a 120-hour continuous infusion repeated every 21 days. Based on the clinical toxic effects noted in prior phase I trials the current phase I trials with this agent started at 14 mg/m^2/d (only 4% of the dose that caused ophthalmoplegia in the initial clinical trials). Dose-limiting inanition, weakness, and severe weight loss have been encountered.

■ Special Precautions

As noted earlier, 1.6 mg/kg/d × 24 days (infusions) was associated with ophthalmoplegia.

■ Drug Interactions

None are known.

■ Dosage

At this point in the redevelopment of terephthalamidine no dosage recommendations can be made.

Pharmacokinetics

Very limited pharmacokinetic studies were conducted with terephthalamidine in humans in 1965 (two patients). The half-life after intravenous infusion of 1 mg/kg ^{14}C-labeled terephthalamidine was approximately 45 minutes (Kreis et al 1965). Forty-nine percent of [^{14}C]-terephthalamidine was excreted in urine within 6 days. In mice receiving an intravenous dose of 2.4 mg/kg, the drug analyzed by high-performance liquid chromatography was eliminated biexponentially with a terminal half-life of 22 minutes (Waud and Hill 1988). Additional clinical pharmacology parameters are being measured in the ongoing phase I trial with the agent.

Side Effects and Toxicity

In the early studies of terephthalamidine in the 1960s, infusions of 1.2 mg/kg/d × 42 days were well tolerated; however, at 1.6 mg/kg/d for 24 days, one patient developed ophthalmoplegia, bulbar signs, shock, and death. Toxic effects, which have now been reported on the 120-hour continuous-infusion phase I trial of the agent, include severe anorexia, extreme weight loss, and weakness. The etiology of these severe side-effects is unknown.

REFERENCES

Burchenal JH. Present status of the terephthalanilides. II. Studies on the mechanism of antileukemic action. In: Plattner PA, ed. *Chemotherapy of Cancer.* Amsterdam: Elsevier; 1964:234–239.

Hirt R, Berchtold R. Biophysical studies with synthetic lecithins as a road to new chemotherapeutic agents. *Cancer Chemother Rep.* 1962;**18**:5–7.

Johnson RK, Faurette LF, Clement JJ, Burchenal JH. Detailed evaluation of NSC-57155 in tumor bearing mice. *Proc Am Assoc Cancer Res.* 1983;**23**:325.

Kensler CJ. Chemotherapeutic activity of phthalanilidine: An approach to anticancer therapy? *Cancer Chemother Rep.* 1963;**23**:1353–1363.

Kreis W, Ellison R, Lyman MS, Burchenal JH. Clinical investigation of the physiologic disposition of a phthalanilidine (NSC-38280) and a phthalanilidine derivative (NSC-57155) in 7 patients. *Cancer Res.* 1965;**25**:402–407.

Louis J, Taylor HG, Sutow WW, Bergsagel DE, Griffith KM. Phase I evaluation of 4′, 4″-di-2-imidazolin-2-yltereph-thalmilide dihydrochloride (NSC-35843). *Cancer Chemother Rep.* 1962;**23**:51–54.

Louis J, Taylor HG, Sutow WW, Lyman MS, Burchenal JH. Phase I evaluation of terephthalamidine (N^1,N^{11}-bio-p-(N^1-methylamidinophenyl)tetrahydrochloride) (NSC-57155). *Proc Am Assoc Cancer Res.* 1963;**4**:40.

Lyman M, Wollner N, Ellison RR, et al. Effects of NSC 38280 in man. *Proc Am Assoc Cancer Res.* 1962;**3**:340.

Oettgen HF, Clifford P, Burchenal TH. Malignant lymphoma involving the jaw in African children. Treatment with 2-chloro-4′,4″-di-2-imidazolin-2-ylterephthalamide dihydroxychloride. *Cancer Chemother Rep.* 1963;**27**: 45–54.

Rogers WI, Yesair DW, Wodinsky I, Mahoney AJ Jr, Sivak A, Kensler CJ. Intracellular localization and effects of 2-chloro-r′-4′-di(2-imidazolin-2-yl)terephthala-nilidine (NSC60339) in liver, kidney and P388 leukemia. *Proc Am Assoc Cancer Res.* 1954;**5**:54.

Waud WR, Hill DL. High-performance liquid chromatographic determination of terephthalanilidine in plasma. *J Chromatogr.* 1988;**425**(1):220–226.

Yesair DW, Rogers WI, Baronolosky PE, Wodinsky I, Thayer PS, Kensler CJ. Relationship of uptake and binding of an antileukemic phthalanilidine to its biochemical and chemotherapeutic effects of P388 lymphocytic leukemia cells. *Cancer Res.* 1967;**27**:314–321.

Teroxirone

Other Names

Henkel's compound; triazinetrione triepoxide; α-TGI; NSC-296934.

Chemistry

Structure of teroxirone

Teroxirone is a triepoxide-containing agent with the molecular formula $C_{12}H_{15}N_5O_6$ and the molecular weight 297.3. Chemically, teroxirone is α-triglycidyl-S-triazinetrione. Two isomers of teroxirone were initially isolated by Henkel Cie (Budnowski 1968), but the α isomer was selected for development because of increased water solubility and preclinical antitumor activity (Spreafico et al 1980).

Antitumor Activity

Teroxirone showed constant antitumor activity in L-1210 and P-388 murine leukemias (Attassi et al 1980,

Spreafico et al 1980). The drug also had activity against B-16 melanoma and was most effective when given by multiple-day schedules compared with single-day or intermittent schedules. In L-1210 leukemia, daily treatment for 5 or 9 days increased life span by a maximum of 650% compared with control mice (Spreafico et al 1980).

In contrast, no antitumor responses were observed in a phase I trial in 53 patients with advanced carcinoma (Rubin et al 1987). Similar largely negative results have been described in phase I trials conducted in Europe (Cavalli et al 1981; Hansen et al 1981).

■ Mechanism of Action

Teroxirone is an alkylating agent that can produce crosslinks between DNA strands or between DNA and proteins (Ames et al 1985). This activity follows opening of the epoxide rings to yield unstable electrophilic carbonium ions. Crosslinking activity for teroxirone has been demonstrated in murine L-1210 leukemia cells and in human lung A-204 rhabdomyosarcoma cells (Ames et al 1985). In vitro cytotoxicity from teroxirone can be blocked by the addition of rat liver microsomes with the release of epoxide hydrolysis products. This suggests that the epoxide moieties on teroxirone mediate cytotoxicity and that microsomal metabolism diminishes the alkylating activity by hydrolyzing the three epoxides on the molecule.

■ Availability and Storage

Initial European trials used a teroxirone formulation that dissolved in water only after vigorous shaking (Hansen et al 1981). The U.S. formulation of teroxirone dissolved more readily. It was investigationally available from the National Cancer Institute and was supplied in 20-mL vials. Each vial contained 100 mg of lyophilized teroxirone and mannitol. The intact vials were recommended to be stored under refrigeration (2–8°C) (National Cancer Institute 1987).

■ Preparation for Use, Stability, and Admixture

The 100-mg vials were reconstituted with 10 mL of Sterile Water for Injection, USP, to yield a solution containing 10 mg/mL of teroxirone at a pH of 6.0 to 8.0. In buffer systems, solutions of teroxirone at pH 3 to 9.7 were stable at 25°C for 4 hours with approximately 2 to 5% decomposition (National Cancer Institute 1987).

■ Administration

Teroxirone is administered intravenously. Bolus injections of large doses have been associated with severe, dose-limiting thrombophlebitis and are therefore not generally recommended. To reduce the severe phlebitis seen in early trials, the infusion solution was changed to 1 part drug (in sterile water) with 6 parts 5% dextrose in half-normal saline. The infusion times were also doubled from 10 minutes to 20 minutes. Occasionally, a portion of the dose was administered into peripheral veins on opposite arms to lessen the severe acute phlebitis and vein blistering (Rubin et al 1987).

■ Dosage

The recommended dose for phase II studies was 375 mg/m^2/d × 5 consecutive days (Rubin et al 1987). This dose is repeated at 5-week intervals.

■ Pharmacokinetics

Teroxirone is rapidly eliminated from the plasma following a brief intravenous infusion (see table). Peak levels of drug are achieved immediately after injection and average 46 µg/mL following infusions of 1500 mg/m^2 given at 25 mg/min and 1000 mg/m^2 given at 45 mg/min.

Teroxirone is metabolized to inactive species when incubated in human blood or rat liver microsomes. Decomposition at 37°C averaged 50% after 1 hour in whole blood and 10% after 1 hour in plasma. There does not appear to be a requirement for NADPH in the metabolic inactivation of teroxirone. It is dependent on the presence of functional microsomal enzymes (Ames et al 1984). Incubation of teroxirone with hepatic but not lung microsomes results in the loss of antitumor activity as well as the production of epoxide hydrolysis products. A portion of this inactivation can be blocked by the addi-

PHARMACOKINETICS OF TEROXIRONE IN HUMANS*

Plasma half-life	1.4 min
Total body clearance	5.7 L/min
Total volume of distribution	12.9 L

*Rapid intravenous infusion of 140 to 500 mg/m^2 over 3 to 10 minutes in nine adult cancer patients (Ames et al 1984).

tion of an inhibitor of epoxide hydrase, cyclohexene oxide.

In rabbits, teroxirone was not well absorbed orally and the elimination half-life was rapid (< 5 minutes) (Ames et al 1984). Little intact drug was renally excreted; however, up to 65% of total drug radiolabel was recovered in the urine over 24 hours (Ames et al 1984).

■ Side Effects and Toxicity

In U.S. studies myelosuppression was the major dose-limiting toxic effect with 5-day dosing schedules (Ames et al 1984). Leukopenia was noted in about 80% of courses. Thrombocytopenia was more infrequent, noted in about 30% of courses (Rubin et al 1987).

When teroxirone was administered as a single agent, severe phlebitis was encountered without significant myelosuppression. With large single doses, cutaneous blistering occurred over the vein used for infusion. This same toxic effect was also prominent in European studies with teroxirone (Hansen et al 1981). This toxic effect was only partially lessened by further dilution of the drug or with slowed intravenous infusion rates (Rubin et al 1987). Typically, mild erythema or superficial pigmentation occurred over the veins. Occasionally, complete occlusion of the vein has occurred.

Other nonhematologic toxic effects include moderate nausea and vomiting, mild stomatitis, and occasional diarrhea.

REFERENCES

Ames MM, Gretsch SK. DNA–DNA and DNA–protein crosslink formation by the experimental antitumor agent teroxirone (NSC-296934) in murine L1210 leukemia and human A204 rhabdomyosarcoma cell lines (abstract #829). *Proc Am Assoc Cancer Res.* 1985;**26**:211.

Ames MM, Kovach JS, Rubin J. Pharmacological characterization of teroxirone, a triepoxide antitumor agent, in rats, rabbits, and humans. *Cancer Res.* 1984;**44**:4151–4156.

Attassi G, Spreafico F, Dumont P, et al. Antitumoral effect in mice of a new triepoxide derivative: 1,3,5-Triglycidyl-S-triazinetrione (NSC-296934). *Eur J Cancer.* 1980;**16**:1561–1567.

Budnowski M. Preparation and properties of the diasteroisomers 1,3,5-triglycidyl-S-triazine-triones. *Agnew Chem Int Ed Engl.* 1968;**7**:827–828.

Cavalli F, Kaplan S, Varini M, Joss R. Phase I trial of α-1,3,50-triglycidyl-S-triazinetrione (TGT, NSC-296934). *Proc Am Assoc Cancer Res.* 1981;**22**:191.

Hansen HH, Dombernowsky P, Piccart M, et al. Phase I clinical trials with α-1,3,5-triglycidyl-S-triazinetrione (TGT) (NSC-296934) (abstract 49). In: *Program and Abstracts, Third NCI–EORTC Symposium on New Drugs in Cancer Therapy, Institut Jules Bordet, Brussels, Belgium, October 1 to 17, 1981.*

National Cancer Institute. Teroxirone. In: *NCI Investigational Drugs: Pharmaceutical Data.* NIH Publication 88-2141, rev. Washington, DC: U.S. Department of Health and Human Services; 1987:133–135.

Rubin J, Kovach JS, Ames MM, et al. Phase I study of two schedules of teroxirone. *Cancer Treat Rep.* 1987;**71**(5):489–492.

Spreafico F, Atassi G, Filippeschi S, et al. A characterization of the activity of α-1,3,5-triglycidyl-S-triazinetrione, a novel antineoplastic compound. *Cancer Chemother Pharmacol.* 1980;**5**:103–108.

Thioguanine

■ Other Names

6-TG; Tabloid® brand thioguanine (Burroughs Wellcome Company).

■ Chemistry

Structure of 6-thioguanine

Thioguanine is a chemical analog of naturally occurring purines and differs from 6-mercaptopurine only by the presence of a 2-position amino group. Its molecular weight is 167.2. The drug is reported to be water insoluble and occurs as a yellow crystalline powder. The complete chemical name is 2-amino-1,7-dihydro-6H-purine-6-thione.

■ Antitumor Activity

Activity has been demonstrated in acute non-lymphocytic and lymphocytic leukemias most often in combination with cytarabine (Lewis et al 1977, Valeriote et al 1976, Armitage et al 1976). The drug is also active in chronic myelogenous leukemia (Spiers et al 1975). Minor activity was observed in patients with advanced colorectal carcinoma given high-dose infusions of thioguanine (Konits et al 1982, Presant et al 1980, Kovach et al 1986). A similar low response rate to high-dose infusions is described in multiple myeloma (Edelstein et al 1990). The drug appears to be inactive in metastatic breast cancer (Pandya et al 1980), non-small cell lung cancer (Lyss et al 1990), and recurrent or metastatic squamous cell carcinoma of the head and neck (Kruter et al 1992).

There appear to be no significant differences with respect to indications or efficacy between thioguanine and mercaptopurine, with the important exception that thioguanine can be used without dose reduction when given concurrently with allopurinol (Rundles et al 1963). The use and major toxic effects are likewise similar, and the two drugs are mutually cross-resistant (Nelson et al 1975).

■ Mechanism of Action

Thioguanine acts similarly to 6-mercaptopurine as a purine-based antimetabolite (Grindey 1979). Because of its similarity to natural purines (hypoxanthine, guanine, and adenine), the drug substitutes for natural purine bases in nucleotide synthesis reactions which are thereafter inhibited. Free (intact) drug is not pharmacologically active. Thioguanine is metabolized by the enzyme hypoxanthine–guanine phosphoribosyltransferase to a nucleotide form that inhibits a number of reactions in de novo RNA and DNA synthesis. Thioguanine is known to inhibit one of the earliest enzymatic reactions in purine nucleotide synthesis, namely, phosphoribosylpyrophosphate amidotransferase activity (Grindey 1979). Although the thioguanylate metabolite of thioguanine is a poor substrate for guanylate kinase, it is nonetheless phosphorylated to the triphosphate form, which is incorporated into DNA in the place of guanosine triphosphate. Indeed, Le Page and Whitecar (1971) found that after 5 days of daily dosing, the DNA guanine content is almost entirely replaced by thioguanine. Incorporation of drug into DNA after single doses is very slight, verifying the schedule dependence of this antimetabolite.

The cytotoxic activity of thioguanine is specific primarily to S phase of the dividing cell cycle. Le Page and Whitecar (1971) also described enhanced induction of sensitive cells into S phase following continuous exposure to thioguanine for 5 days.

■ Availability and Storage

Thioguanine is commercially available from Burroughs Wellcome Company (Research Triangle Park, North Carolina). It is supplied in 40-mg tablets that can be stored at room temperature.

An injectable form is available investigationally from Burroughs Wellcome. It is supplied as 75-mg lyophilized powder in a 10-mL vial, which also contains sodium hydroxide in a sufficient quantity to produce the sodium salt of thioguanine. The intact vials should be stored under refrigeration (2–8°C). The vials are stable for at least 4 years under refrigeration and 2 years at room temperature.

■ Preparation for Use, Stability, and Admixture

The 75-mg vial should initially be diluted with 5 mL of Sodium Chloride for Injection, USP. Each milliliter of the resultant solution will contain 15 mg 6-thioguanine and have a pH of 10 to 12. This solution is stable for at least 24 hours under refrigeration. If the reconstituted drug is stored at room temperature, a precipitate may form. The injectable form of thioguanine contains no antibacterial preservatives and can have a high pH of 11.2. Sodium bicarbonate (0.5 mEq/75 mg) can lower the pH to reduce phlebitis during infusions (Kovach et al 1986); however, the addition of bicarbonate reduces the stability of the thioguanine solution to approximately 8 hours.

For intravenous administration this solution may be further diluted with D5W or normal saline. The diluted solution is stable for 24 hours either at room temperature or under refrigeration (Trissel et al 1985).

■ Administration

Thioguanine is administered orally between meals, if possible, to facilitate complete absorption. The total daily dose can be taken at one time.

The injectable form should be given intravenously over 5 to 30 minutes in at least 250 mL of D5W or normal saline. The injection site should initially be flushed with 5 to 10 mL normal saline to ensure venous patency. Although 6-thioguanine is not a vesicant, pain and phlebitis during brief (5-minute) infusions can be common and may relate to the pH of the intravenous formulation. In one trial, 0.5 mEq of sodium bicarbonate was added for each 75 mg of drug to lower the final pH to 9.2 (Kovach et al 1986). Large doses have been administered intravenously over 4 hours (Edelstein et al 1990). A continuous infusion over 5 days has also been evaluated (Kruter et al 1992).

■ Dosage

The standard clinical dose is 2 to 2.5 mg/kg/d for both children and adults. In the absence of serious toxicity the dose may be increased to 3 mg/kg. The total daily dose should be calculated to the nearest 20 mg (one-half tablet). Unlike mercaptopurine and azathioprine, the dose of thioguanine does not need to be reduced with concurrent allopurinol therapy. Doses may need to be reduced for liver or renal dysfunction, although criteria for adjustment have not been established. In general the daily dose can be titrated to the desired hematologic effects.

High-dose intermittent therapy for solid tumors has been studied at initial doses of 700 mg/m^2 IV and 1.4 g/m^2 PO, given every 3 weeks (Presant et al 1980). An intravenous infusion dose of 1 g/m^2 every 3 weeks was studied in myeloma patients (Edelstein et al 1990). A tolerable continuous-infusion dose in head and neck cancer was 35 mg/m^2/d × 5 days, repeated every 5 weeks (Kruter et al 1992).

Because of poor and highly variable oral bioavailability in leukemia patients, doses should probably be adjusted to achieve some degree of leukopenia as a marker of drug absorption (Krakoff et al 1961).

■ Pharmacokinetics

Pharmacologic studies in humans using radioactively labeled thioguanine (125 mg/m^2) have demonstrated biphasic drug elimination (see table) (Lu et al 1982, Konits et al 1982). After 24 hours, 65 to 85% of labeled drug is excreted in the urine. Initially, intact drug is excreted but subsequently metabolites (principally 6-thioxanthines) predominate (Elion et al 1960). In humans, LePage and Whitecar (1971) noted 24-hour urinary excretion of 41 to 81% of an intravenous dose compared with 24 to 64% of an oral dose. One hour after injection, 70% of radioactive drug is found in the plasma as intact thioguanine, 13% as thioxanthine, 11% as thiouric acid, and 1% each as methylthioguanine and methylthioxanthine. By 13 hours, this distribution changes significantly: methylthioguanine 34%, thiouric acid 24%, methylthioxanthine 12%, thioxanthine 10%, and thioguanine 2% (Le Page and Whitecar 1971).

PHARMACOKINETICS OF THIOGUANINE IN HUMANS

	Study	
	Lu et al 1982	Konits et al 1982
Plasma half-life		
α (min)	40	3
β (h)	28.9	5.9
Volume of distribution (mL/kg)	148	NL*
Total body clearance (mL/kg/min)	0.74	NL
Urinary excretion (% dose)		
5 h	54	NL
24 h	75	NL

*NL, not listed.
Data from Lu et al 1982, using radiolabeled thioguanine, and Konits et al 1982, using a more specific high-performance liquid chromatography assay.

Oral thioguanine is poorly absorbed (Denes and Presant 1979), with maximal blood levels (drug and metabolites) after oral doses achieved 10 to 12 hours after ingestion.

Early urinary elimination recovery studies suggested that about 20 to 30% of thioguanine is absorbed from the tablet dosage form (Elion et al 1962). In another study, only about 10% of a dose was absorbed (LePage and Whitecar 1971). Plasma concentrations with oral doses vary up to 30-fold in leukemia patients.

Oral thioguanine in mice did not appear to cross the blood–brain barrier.

Methylation of thioguanine constitutes the major form of drug detoxification. This reaction is not affected by allopurinol as are the major detoxication reactions with mercaptopurine and azathioprine.

■ Drug Interactions

The mercaptopurine metabolite methylmercaptopurine riboside has been shown to stabilize intracellular pools of thioguanylate, the active metabolite of thioguanine (Nelson and Parks 1972). The combination has been used to sensitize resistant cells to thioguanine-induced cytotoxicity in vitro. Other potential approaches to enhance thiopurine activation involve augmenting the intracellular levels of phosphoribosylpyrophosphate by using metabolic inhibitors such as methotrexate, azaserine, and 6-diazo-5-oxo-L-norleucine (DON) (Grindey 1979).

Thioguanine may also increase the soft tissue

toxicity of busulfan. Esophageal varices were reported in 12 of 330 patients receiving thioguanine and busulfan for maintenance treatment of chronic myelogenous leukemia (Key et al 1987). Subsequent liver biopsies were performed in four patients, all of whom showed evidence of nodular regenerative hyperplasia.

Thioguanine also increases the experimental therapeutic activity of chloroethyl nitrosoureas such as nimustine (Fujimoto et al 1977), carmustine, and PCNU (*N*-(2-chloroethyl)-*N'*-(2,6-dioxo-3-piperidyl)-*N*-nitrosourea)(Wang et al 1991). This positive interaction may result from enhanced alkylation by nitrosoureas at the S^6-position of thioguanine residues incorporated into the DNA strand (Bodell 1986). Also, S^6-alkylguanine adducts are not repaired as readily as O^6 adducts by the enzyme O^6-alkylguanine transferase (Yarosh et al 1986).

■ Side Effects and Toxicity

Myelosuppression is the major dose-limiting hematologic toxic effect. It is characterized by leukopenia, which generally precedes the onset of thrombocytopenia. Anemia occurs to a lesser extent. With chronic daily dosing, bone marrow suppression may persist for several days after termination of the drug. With intravenous doses myelosuppression may be approximately 2.5-fold greater than with similar oral doses (Denes and Presant 1979).

Acute gastrointestinal toxic effects are infrequent but include nausea, vomiting, and anorexia. Stomatitis and severe diarrhea generally necessitate dosage reduction. Esophageal varices were described in patients receiving busulfan and thioguanine for chronic myelogenous leukemia (Key et al 1987).

Hepatic toxicity in the form of jaundice has been noted in a few patients. Baseline liver function studies and periodic monitoring of hepatic function are recommended, especially in patients with preexisting liver dysfunction. Fatal hepatic veno-occlusive disease (Budd–Chiari syndrome) has been reported in two patients with acute leukemia (Griner et al 1976). A case of reversible hepatic veno-occlusive disease is also reported in a 23-year-old leukemic patient treated for 10 months with maintenance 6-thioguanine therapy (Gill et al 1982).

Some patients have noted a loss of vibratory sensation and an unsteady gait while taking 6-thioguanine. A rash is only rarely reported but nasal congestion and rhinorrhea may be common with high-dose regimens using intravenous thioguanine (Konits et al 1982).

Crystalluria with elevation of serum creatinine is also described in patients receiving thioguanine infusions (Konits et al 1982). Presant et al (1980) have described transient renal dysfunction manifested by increases in blood urea nitrogen and serum creatinine. The drug crystals which precipitate in the renal parenchyma are composed primarily of acid-insoluble thioguanine and 6-thiouric acid (Konits et al 1982). In such high-dose studies, renal dysfunction can be both serious and permanent (Konits et al 1982).

Although thioguanine has not been a potent mutagen in vitro, there are some case reports of teratogenicity when combined with other agents. The combination of cytarabine and thioguanine produced fetal trisomy C in one case (Maurer et al 1971). In contrast, treatment with the same regimen in week 26 of gestation was associated with delivery of a normal infant (Raich and Curet 1975). Spontaneous abortion has been observed in leukemic patients who received thioguanine-containing multidrug regimens during pregnancy (Zuazu et al 1991); however, the relative contribution of 6-thioguanine to these outcomes is not known.

■ Special Applications

Thioguanine has been administered intraperitoneally to 25 patients with advanced ovarian cancer. The recommended dose for phase II studies is 744 mg/m^2/48 h (Zimm et al 1988). This dose was infused continuously through a Tenckhoff catheter using a portable programmable infusion pump. The infusion rate was 1 L/24 h. The infusion solution was 0.9% sodium chloride buffered to a pH of 9.0 to 9.5 with sterile sodium bicarbonate.

The dose-limiting toxic effect of intraperitoneal thioguanine was granulocytopenia. There was no evidence of chemical peritonitis and emesis was observed in only four patients (Zimm et al 1988). Anorexia during the infusion was reported in most patients. Six patients developed photosensitivity reactions within 24 hours of starting intraperitoneal thioguanine. One patient achieved a partial response; there were four minor responses. All of the responses occurred in patients with small-volume intraperitoneal disease (< 2-cm lesion diameters).

Thioguanine levels in the peritoneal fluid were markedly elevated over those in the plasma. The mean steady-state intraperitoneal level was 1970 μmol/L compared with a plasma level of 1.1 μmol/L following an intraperitoneal dose of 744 mg/m² (Zimm et al 1988). The half-life of drug in the intraperitoneal compartment ranged from 0.8 to 1.2 hours. Overall, this study suggests that intraperitoneal thioguanine is clinically tolerable and achieves significantly elevated local drug exposure in the intraperitoneal space.

REFERENCES

Armitage JO, Burns CP. Maintenance of remission in adult acute nonmyeloblastic leukemia using intermittent courses of cytosine arabinoside (NSC-752). *Cancer Treat Rep.* 1976;**60**(5):585–589.

Bodell WJ. Investigation of 6-thiodeoxyguanosine alkylation products and their role in the potentiation of BCNU cytotoxicity. In: Singer B, Bartsch H, eds. *The Role of Cyclic Nucleic Acid Adducts in Carcinogenesis and Mutagenesis.* Lyon: International Agency for Research on Cancer; 1986:147–154.

Denes A, Presant C. 6-Thioguanine (TG): A phase I study of intermittent oral (p.o.) and intravenous (i.v.) therapy in solid tumors (ST). *Proc Am Assoc Cancer Res ASCO.* 1979;**20**:107.

Edelstein MB, Crowley JJ, Valeriote FA, et al. A phase II study of intravenous 6-thioguanine (NSC-752) in multiple myeloma. *Invest New Drugs.* 1990;**8**:83–86.

Elion GB, Callahan SW, Hitchings GH, Rundles W. The metabolism of 2-amino-6-(1-methyl-4-nitro-5-imidazolyl)thiol purine (B.W. 57-323) in man. *Cancer Chemother Rep.* 1960;**8**:47–52.

Elion GB, Callahan SW, Hitchings GH, et al. Experimental, clinical and metabolic studies of thiopurines. *Cancer Chemother Rep.* 1962;**16**:197–202.

Fujimoto S, Inagaki J, Horikoshi N, Hoshino A. Combination chemotherapy of 6-thioguanine with various antitumor agents against murine leukemia L-1210. *Gann.* 1977;**68**:543–552.

Gill RA, Onstad GR, Cardamone JM, et al. Hepatic veno-occlusive disease caused by 6-thioguanine. *Ann Intern Med.* 1982;**96**:58–60.

Grindey GB. Clinical pharmacology of the 6-thiopurines. *Cancer Treat Rev.* 1979;**6**:19–25.

Griner PF, Elbadawi A, Packman CH. Veno-occlusive disease of the liver after chemotherapy of acute leukemia. *Ann Intern Med.* 1976;**85**:578–582.

Key NS, Kelly PMA, Emerson PM, et al. Oesophageal varices associated with busulphan–thioguanine combination therapy for chronic myeloid leukaemia. *Lancet.* 1987;**2**:1050–1052.

Konits PH, Egorin MJ, Van Echo DA, et al. Phase II evaluation and plasma pharmacokinetics of high-dose intravenous 6-thioguanine in patients with colorectal carcinoma. *Cancer Chemother Pharmacol.* 1982;**8**:199–203.

Kovach JS, Rubin J, Creagan ET, et al. Phase I trial of parenteral 6-thioguanine given on 5 consecutive days. *Cancer Res.* 1986;**46**:5959–5962.

Krakoff IH, Ellison RR, Tan CTC. Clinical evaluation of thioguanosine. *Cancer Res.* 1961;**21**:1015–1018.

Kruter F, Eisenberger M, Sinibaldi V, et al. Phase II trial of 5 day continuous intravenous infusion of 6-thioguanine in patients with recurrent and metastatic squamous cell carcinoma of the head and neck. *Invest New Drugs.* 1992;**10**:89–91.

Le Page GA, Whitecar JP. The pharmacology of 6-thioguanine in man. *Cancer Res.* 1971;**31**:1627–1631.

Lewis JP, Unman JW, Marshall GJ, Pajak TF, Bateman JR. Randomized clinical trial of cytosine arabinoside and 6-thioguanine in remission induction and consolidation of adult nonlymphocytic acute leukemia. *Cancer.* 1977;**39**(4):1387–1396.

Lu K, Benvenuto JA, Bodey GP, et al. Pharmacokinetics and metabolism of β-2'-deoxythioguanosine and 6-thioguanine in man. *Cancer Chemother Pharmacol.* 1982;**8**:119–123.

Lyss AP, Vokes EE, Goutsou M, et al. Cisplatin/5-FU/leucovorin (PFL) or intravenous 6-thioguanine (6TG) in advanced non-small cell lung cancer (NSCLC): A randomized phase II study. *Proc Am Soc Clin Oncol.* 1990;**9**:239.

Maurer LH, Forcier RJ, McIntyre OR. Fetal group C trisomy after cytosine arabinoside and thioguanine. *Am Intern Med.* 1971;**75**:809–810.

Nelson JA, Carpenter JW, Rose LM. Mechanisms of action of 6-thioguanine, 6-mercaptopurine, and 8-azaguanine. *Cancer Res.* 1975;**35**(10):2872–2878.

Nelson JA, Parks RE Jr. Biochemical mechanisms for the synergism between 6-thioguanine and 6-(methylmercapto)purine ribonucleoside in sarcoma 180 cells. *Cancer Res.* 1972;**32**:2034–2041.

Pandya KJ, Tormey DC, Davis TE, et al. Phase II trial of 6-thioguanine in metastatic breast cancer. *Cancer Treat Rep.* 1980;**64**:191–192.

Presant CA, Denes AE, Klein L, et al. Phase I and preliminary phase II observations of high-dose intermittent 6-thioguanine. *Cancer Treat Rep.* 1980;**64**:1109–1113.

Raich PC, Curet LB. Treatment of acute leukemia during pregnancy. *Cancer.* 1975;**36**:861–862.

Rundles RW, Wyngaarden GH, Hitchings GH, et al. Effects of a xanthine oxidase inhibitor on thiopurine metabolism, hyperuricemia and gout. *Trans Assoc Am Physicians.* 1963;**76**:126.

Spiers AS, Kaur J, Galton DAG, Goldman JM. Thioguanine as primary treatment for chronic granulocytic leukemia. *Lancet.* 1975;**1**:829–833.

Trissel LA, et al. *NCI Investigational Drugs: Pharmaceutical Data.* Bethesda, MD: National Cancer Institute, Department of Health and Human Services; 1985.

Valeriote F, Vietti T, Edelstein M. Combined effect of cytosine arabinoside and thiopurines. *Cancer Treat Rep.* 1976;**60**(12):1925–1934.

Wang AM, Elion GB, Friedman HS, et al. Positive therapeutic interaction between thiopurines and alkylating drugs in human glioma xenografts. *Cancer Chemother Pharmacol.* 1991;**27**:278–284.

Yarosh DB, Hurst-Calderone S, Babich MA, Day RS III. Inactivation of O^6-methylguanine-DNA methyltransferase and sensitization of human tumor cells to killing by chloroethyl nitrosourea by O^6-methylguanine as a free base. *Cancer Res.* 1986;**46**:1663–1668.

Zimm S, Cleary SM, Horton CN, et al. Phase I/pharmacokinetic study of thioguanine administered as a 48-hour continuous intraperitoneal infusion. *J Clin Oncol.* 1988;**6**:696–700.

Zuazu J, Julia A, Sierra J, et al. Pregnancy outcome in hematologic malignancies. *Cancer.* 1991;**67**:703–709.

Thiotepa

■ Other Names

Thio-Tepa; thio-TEPA; TESPA; TSPA (**but not** TEPA); CL 8206 (Lederle Laboratories); triethylenethiophosphoramide; NSC-6396.

■ Chemistry

Structure of thiotepa

Chemically, thiotepa is 1,1′,1″-phosphinothioylidynetrisaziridine, an ethylenimine-type compound. The molecular weight is 189.2 and the molecular formula $C_6H_{12}N_3PS$. The drug is relatively nonpolar and freely soluble in water (19 g/100 mL at 25°C). It is also freely soluble in ethanol and is soluble in ether, benzene, and chloroform. It can be extracted from aqueous solutions with toluene, ethyl acetate, diethyl ether, and hexane in decreasing order of efficiency (Cohen et al 1984).

■ Antitumor Activity

Thiotepa has activity in a variety of tumors including Hodgkin's disease and leukemia (Shay et al 1953) and breast cancer and ovarian cancer (Ultmann et al 1957; Greenspan 1975). In the treatment of metastatic bladder carcinoma, its use has largely been replaced by other alkylating agents used in combinations such as MAID (mesna, doxorubicin, ifosfamide, dacarbazine). In contrast, it is active as a topical bladder irrigation for multiple superficial papillary tumors of the bladder (National Bladder Cancer Collaborative Group A 1977, Burnand et al 1976, Pavone-Macaluso 1976). Intravesical drug may also be useful as an adjuvant to local surgery of bladder tumors (Boyd and Burnard 1975). Thiotepa is active in the control of malignant effusions in various body cavities, for example, pericardial, pleural, peritoneal (Anderson and Brincker 1968). The drug is active intrathecally in the treatment of carcinomatous meningitis (Jones and Swinney 1961, Veenema et al 1969). Edwards et al (1973) have recently found the drug to be ineffective in patients with malignant gliomas. Likewise, little therapeutic advantage was described for intraperitoneal thiotepa (Wadler et al 1989). Limited activity was described in the treatment of essential thrombocythemia for a combination of thiotepa and chlorambucil (Case 1984).

Solid tumor response rates to standard doses in breast cancer range from 17% (Miller 1961) to 81% (Arthur 1968). One particularly active combination is the VATH regimen containing vinblastine, doxorubicin (Adriamycin®), thiotepa, and halotestin. A partial response rate of 52% is reported for this combination in postmenopausal patients who were refractory to other regimens (Perloff et al 1978). In advanced ovarian cancer single-agent response rates range from less than 10% for intravenous thiotepa (Wallach et al 1970) to 34% for intraperitoneal thiotepa (Villasana and Bloedorn 1968). Thiotepa-containing multidrug combinations have been associated with response rates of 47 to 56% in ovarian cancer (Kottmeir 1968, Bruckner et al 1985).

(See Special Applications for results with intracavitary, intrathecal, and high-dose bone marrow transplantation regimens.)

■ Mechanism of Action

Thiotepa acts as a polyfunctional alkylating agent and is pharmacologically similar to nitrogen mustard; however, thiotepa is not a vesicant and can be administered by any parenteral route or directly into a tumor-bearing area. The active alkylating radicals are the ethylenimine moieties, which are metabolically produced in vivo. Thus, thiotepa is not cell cycle phase specific. The cellular uptake of thiotepa is biphasic and is characterized by a rapid initial cell association phase of 10 seconds and a second linear uptake phase which lasts about 5 hours (Egorin et al 1990).

Experimental studies in murine colon tumors suggest that the primary metabolite, triethylenephosphoramide (TEPA), constitutes the majority of the drug's solid tumor activity (Phillips et al 1988). In this study the highly differentiated MAC-26 tumor was much more sensitive to thiotepa than were the poorly differentiated MAC-15A or MAC-13 tumors (Phillips et al 1988).

Recent information suggests that thiotepa functions largely as a prodrug, with subsequent activation of the three aziridine groups on the molecule (Egorin and Snyder 1990). A proposed sequential activation scheme involves hydrolysis of the phosphorus–nitrogen bonds to yield hydroxylated thiotepa with the liberation of reactive aziridine moieties. This may ultimately yield inactive ethanolamine residues, which may be incorporated into phosphatidylethanolamine. The metabolic activation of thiotepa to cytotoxic species may be mediated in part by microsomal cytochrome P450 enzymes in a process dependent on both oxygen and NADPH (Teicher et al 1989). Of further interest, this study also showed that the metabolite TEPA was markedly less cytotoxic than the parent molecule in human MCF breast cancer cells (Teicher et al 1989). Thiotepa was also more cytotoxic toward euoxic tumor cells in vitro compared with hypoxic cells (see Drug Interactions for Fluosol DA effect).

■ Availability and Storage

Thiotepa is available from Lederle Laboratories (Pearl River, New York) in 15-mg vials of white crystalline drug along with 80 mg of NaCl and 50 mg of $NaHCO_3$ (for tonicity) per vial. The intact vials must be stored under refrigeration at 2 to 8°C (35 to 46°F).

■ Preparation for Use, Stability, and Admixture

Initially, each vial should be reconstituted with 1.5 mL of Sterile Water for Injection, USP. This results in a 5 mg/0.5 mL hypertonic solution. Acidic diluents should not be used. The solution may be clear to slightly opaque; denser-appearing solutions should be discarded.

An isotonic solution containing 1 mg/mL can be prepared by diluting the vial with 15 mL of Sterile Water for Injection, USP. Solutions so prepared are chemically stable for 5 days when stored in the refrigerator. As no preservatives are added, any unused portion optimally should be discarded after 24 hours.

Thiotepa is reported to be physically compatible with 5% Dextrose in Water, USP; Normal Saline, USP; dextrose/saline combinations; Ringer's injection; and lactated Ringer's injection. Thiotepa is known to be compatible with procaine 2%, epinephrine HCl 1:1000, or both when used for local (intratumoral) injections.

Stability in urine has been investigated in light of the intravesical use of the drug (Cohen et al 1984). Thiotepa was found to be more stable at 22°C than 37°C and at pH 6 to 7 than 4 to 5.5; however, alkylating activity was maintained for several hours under all conditions.

■ Administration

Thiotepa may be given by many parenteral routes; however, the intravenous push and intracavitary routes are the ones most commonly encountered (see table). For intravenous push doses, the initial isotonic solution described earlier is given as a rapid bolus injection. Because the drug is not a vesicant, pain or phlebitis is not anticipated. Intravenous infusion, intramuscular, and subcutaneous doses of

THIOTEPA DOSES FOR DIFFERENT ROUTES OF ADMINISTRATION

Dose	Frequency (wk)	Route	Dilution
0.3–0.4 mg/kg	3–4	IV push	10–20 mL saline or 5% dextrose
15–35 mg/m^2	3–4	IV infusion × 48 h	1 L/d
60 mg	Weekly × 4	Intravesical	30–60 mL saline
0.8 mg/kg	Once	Intraperitoneal	1.8–2.0 L
0.6–0.8	Once	Intracavitary (pleural, pericardial)	20 mL saline or dextrose
10–15 mg	3–4	Intrathecal	3–5 mL lactated Ringer's injection

thiotepa may be used but offer no advantages over an intravenous bolus injection. Intracavitary doses generally require further dilution so that larger volumes may be instilled. Generally, volumes of 10 to 20 mL are used for intrapleural and pericardial doses, diluted in isotonic saline. Intraperitoneal delivery requires larger volumes (see Special Applications). Frequent patient repositioning after instillation can maximize distribution of the drug.

■ Intravesical Administration

Bladder instillations are generally prepared with 60 mg of drug diluted into 30 to 60 mL of Sterile Water for Injection, USP. The solution is placed by catheter and retained for 2 hours for maximum effect. To maximize contact area the patient may be repositioned at 15-minute intervals. Treatment can be repeated in 4 weeks if toxic effects have resolved. Thiotepa has also been administered as a continuous intravenous infusion over 48 hours (Kreis et al 1983).

Alternatively, Burnand et al (1976) have used a single treatment of 90 mg in 100 mL sterile water instilled into the bladder with a syringe. The solution was retained for 15 minutes while the patient was lying in the left lateral position, then the right lateral position for 15 minutes before the bladder was emptied and the catheter removed. This therapy was not repeated unless follow-up cystoscopy showed recurrence.

Intrathecal Administration. Intrathecal doses of from 1 to 10 mg/m^2 have been given at concentrations of 1 to 5 mg/mL. The usual adult intrathecal dose is 15 mg diluted in 3 to 5 mL of Lactated Ringer's Injection, USP. This solution is reported to approximate the ionic content of the cerebrospinal fluid (Cradock et al 1978). Intrathecal volumes of up to 20 mL have been well tolerated in adults and may facilitate optimal drug distribution within the central nervous system (Gutin et al 1976).

■ Dosage

A variety of dosing schedules are used for thiotepa (see table on page 899). Doses are generally 0.5 mg/kg repeated at 1- to 4-week intervals. Another schedule calls for 6 mg/m^2 IM or IV (0.2 mg/kg) daily for 4 days, repeated every 2 to 4 weeks. In a continuous-infusion regimen, a dose of 15 to 35 mg/m^2 has been administered over 48 hours (Kreis et al 1983).

A recent phase I trial of intravenous thiotepa without bone marrow transplantation has reported the maximal tolerated dose to be 65 mg/m^2 given as a 10-minute infusion every 3 to 4 weeks (O'Dwyer et al 1991). Unfortunately, this dose could not be escalated further with the use of sargramostim (see Drug Interactions)

■ Drug Interactions

Thiotepa can decrease pseudocholinesterase levels. This might result in an enhanced or exaggerated effect from concomitant skeletal muscle relaxants like succinylcholine (Zsigmond and Robins 1972). When thiotepa was combined with sargramostim, it was not possible to significantly elevate thiotepa doses because of severe and cumulative platelet toxicity (O'Dwyer et al 1992).

■ Pharmacokinetics

Early studies with radiolabeled thiotepa suggested rapid clearance of drug from the plasma with no intact drug recovered in the urine (Nadkarni et al 1959). Oral drug absorption was erratic and incomplete (Mellett et al 1962). Studies with a specific assay in mice showed that unlabeled thiotepa was rapidly cleared from the plasma and widely distributed, although liver levels were consistently lower than levels in other tissues (Egorin et al 1984). Thiotepa is only minimally bound to plasma proteins, less than 40% (McDermott et al 1984).

Clinical pharmacokinetic studies have confirmed the preclinical data. At standard intravenous doses of 12 mg/m^2, thiotepa plasma levels declined in a rapid, biphasic manner (Cohen et al 1986). Urinary excretion accounted for a relatively small fraction of drug and metabolite elimination.

The table on the opposite page summarizes the pharmacokinetics of thiotepa following standard and high-dose regimens used with bone marrow transplantation. With standard doses of 12 mg/m^2, urinary excretion of thiotepa and TEPA and alkylating activity accounted for 1.5, 4.2, and 23.5% of the dose, respectively (Cohen et al 1986). TEPA rapidly reached a level of about 0.1 mg/mL which remained relatively constant for more than 4 hours after dosing. Indeed, 2 hours after drug administration, TEPA levels exceeded those of thiotepa. The conversion of thiotepa to TEPA is believed to involve oxidative desulfuration; however, the combined total of TEPA and thiotepa does not account for all of the plasma alkylating activity. Some of the ethyleneamine moieties liberated by metabolism of the aziridines may be ultimately hydrolyzed to ethanolamine, which is incorporated into phosphatidylethanolamine (Egorin et al 1990). Thus there may be other active metabolites of thiotepa that contribute to the antitumor activity of the drug. Of interest, at intermediate dose levels of 30 to 75 mg/m^2, thiotepa exhibited a dose-dependent decrease in clearance with increasing dose (O'Dwyer et al 1991). The half-life changed from 51.6 to 212 minutes over the dose range. Again, the TEPA half-life of 3 to 21 hours was considerably longer than that of thiotepa. As a result, the AUC for TEPA was 5- to 10-fold higher than the AUC for thiotepa (O'Dwyer et al 1991).

With high-dose thiotepa, similar pharmacokinetics is observed and there is no consistent evidence for metabolic saturation at doses up to 4.8 mg/kg (Ackland et al 1988). At the highest dose levels evaluated (6–7 mg/kg), however, the plasma AUC value increased over fourfold from the AUC obtained at the 4.8 mg/kg dose (see table). One explanation may be the presence of moderate liver dysfunction in several patients treated at these higher levels (Ackland et al 1988). As with the lower doses, very little thiotepa or metabolite was excreted in the urine. The cumulative exposure to TEPA represented only 13 to 14% of the thiotepa AUC, which is less than that observed in the low-dose studies. Finally, the concomitant use of cyclophosphamide (Ackland et al 1988) does not appear to alter the pharmacokinetics of high-dose thiotepa when used alone (Lazarus et al 1987).

Intraventricular thiotepa pharmacokinetics has been studied in patients with meningeal carcinomatoses given intrathecal doses of 10 mg (Grochow et al 1982, Strong et al 1986). The half-lives of thiotepa in the cerebrospinal fluid were 20 minutes and 8 hours for the α and β phases, respectively (Grochow et al 1982). A longer half-life of 14 hours was reported in patients with a cerebrospinal fluid outflow block. The cerebrospinal fluid drug level 30 minutes after intrathecal injection ranged from 20 to 200 µg/mL and was more than 0.1 µg/mL even after 10 hours. In another study, a single patient displayed total body clearance of intrathecal thiotepa of 518 mL/min, with a ventricular clearance of 1.8 mL/min (Strong et al 1986). In this patient the mean cerebrospinal fluid AUC was 5470 µg/min/mL compared with 20 µg/min/mL in the plasma. Following intraventricular dosing, the AUC for lumbar cerebrospinal fluid was only 5% that in ventricular space. Levels achieved in the ventricles were over 100-fold greater than those in the plasma following standard intravenous doses. The low AUC in lumbar cerebrospinal fluid indicates poor drug distribution out of the ventricular space. Other experimental findings show poor penetration of thiotepa into deep parenchymal brain tissue (Blasberg et al 1975).

■ Side Effects and Toxicity

The dose-limiting toxic effect of intravenous thiotepa is myelosuppression. Myelosuppression may also occur after intravesical thiotepa, but has rarely been fatal (Bruce and Edgcomb 1967). The myelosuppressive effect is additive with radiation and/or other cytotoxic agents, especially other alkylating agents. Leukopenia has a short nadir of 7 to 10 days with a typically brisk recovery. The platelet nadir is about 3 weeks (Hagen 1991). This allows re-

CLINICAL PHARMACOKINETICS OF THIOTEPA

IV Dose	Half-life (min) α	Half-life (min) β	Volume of Distribution	Peak Plasma Level (µg/mL)	Total Body Clearance (mL/min/m^2)	Plasma AUC (g/mL·min)	Reference
12 mg/m^2	7.7	125	0.25 L/kg	1–2	186	106	Cohen et al 1986
30–75 mg/m^2	6–12	78–134	47–72 L/m^2	—	315–780	3–14.2 µM·min × 10^2	O'Dwyer et al 1991
20 mg	24	114	0.8 L/kg	0.5	177	66	Hagen et al 1988
30 mg	23	110	0.7 L/kg	0.7	175	109	Hagen 1991
15–35 mg/m^2*	—	—	—	0.05–0.12 µM*	—	—	Kreis et al 1983
1.8 mg/kg						319	
3.6 mg/kg	5–15	160	1.6 L/kg	—	195 (mL/h/kg)	540	Ackland et al 1988
4.8 mg/kg							
6–7 mg/kg						2304	

*Continuous intravenous infusion over 48 hours.

peat dosing in 3 to 4 weeks, even in combination myelosuppressive regimens (Perloff et al 1978). Thrombocytopenia can occasionally be delayed in onset and recovery. Of interest, TEPA reportedly produces more myelosuppression than thiotepa (Humphrey and Hitchcock 1957). Myelosuppression from intravesical thiotepa is dose related and is characterized primarily by thrombocytopenia (Hollister and Coleman 1980). There is also a positive correlation between thiotepa exposure following 60- and 80-mg doses and the degree of myelosuppression (Hagen 1991). Thus, patients with higher thiotepa AUCs experienced greater percentage reductions in both platelet and leukocyte counts. No such correlations were observed with the active metabolite TEPA (Hagen 1991).

Acute toxic effects are rarely severe and include nausea, vomiting, dizziness, and headache. Allergic reactions such as hives and bronchoconstriction have been reported but are rare (Donegan 1974).

Paresthesias have occurred when hypertonic solutions are administered intrathecally (Colhoun et al 1978). Renal failure is reported in a single case by Schellhammer (1973). It appeared to be caused by an extensive bladder reaction that led to partial ureteral obstruction following four uneventful 60-mg bladder instillations.

Toxic effects other than myelosuppression observed with intravesical therapy include urinary frequency and urgency, dysuria, rare chemical cystitis, and rash. Leukemia has rarely been associated with long-term intravesical thiotepa therapy (Carey and Long 1977, Easton and Poon 1983).

As with many alkylating agents, acute nonlymphocytic leukemia is reported following intravenous thiotepa (Zarrabi and Rosner 1979). Other second cancers are also described, including a second breast cancer in 36 of 633 breast cancer patients (5.7%) and other solid tumors in 40 of 633 patients (6.3%) (Chan et al 1977). The rate of developing non-small cell lung cancer following thiotepa appears to be low. For example, only 13 of 5455 patients with ovarian cancer developed non-small cell lung cancer following exposure to multiple alkylating agents including thiotepa (Reimer et al 1977).

■ Special Applications

Locally Administered Intracavitary Administration. Initially, doses of 60 mg are used in adults for control of malignant peritoneal or pleural effusions (Anderson and Brincker 1968). Doses of 45 mg may be used in patients with chronic renal impairment, cardiovascular disease, or poor performance status. Generally, the clinical response to intracavitary thiotepa has been of short duration.

Doses should not be repeated more frequently than at 1-week intervals.

Intravesical (Urinary) Bladder Administration. Doses of 60 mg are instilled into the bladder and retained more than 2 hours. This can be repeated at 1- to 4-week intervals. Second and third doses should be administered in relation to the degree of hematologic depression present.

Bone Marrow Transplant Administration. High-dose thiotepa has been shown to be clinically active in bone marrow transplantation regimens when used alone (Herzig et al 1987, Wolff et al 1987, Lazarus et al 1987) or in combination with cyclophosphamide (Eder et al 1988, Williams et al 1987) or mitoxantrone and etoposide (Dunphy et al 1989). The pharmacologic rationale for its use in this setting involves limited extramedullary (nonmarrow) toxicity and an experimental dose–response effect that does not plateau at high drug concentrations (Teicher et al 1990). Responsive diseases include a variety of refractory cancers, such as lymphomas (Bitran et al 1990), cancer of the breast (Lazarus et al 1987, Antman et al 1990), and, rarely, malignant melanoma (Wolff et al 1987), colon carcinoma (Fay et al 1987), and pediatric solid tumors (Saarinen et al 1989). In refractory lymphomas an overall response rate of 57% is described (Bitran et al 1990). Of interest, 27% of these responses involved complete disease remissions. One of the major explanations for the relative clinical efficacy of high-dose thiotepa in autologous bone marrow transplantation (ABMT) regimens is that compared with other alkylating agents, relatively little toxicity occurs in nonmyelopoietic tissues. This yields a high multiple for the dose of thiotepa when combined with autologous bone marrow rescue. The highest thiotepa dose that does not require ABMT is 180 mg/m^2. With ABMT the maximally tolerated dose is 900 to 1125 mg/m^2, with the lower dose used in combination chemotherapy regimens (Wolff et al 1990).

In patients with refractory lymphomas various doses of intravenous thiotepa (500 mg/m^2) have been administered with high-dose cyclophosphamide, 6 g/m^2, and carboplatin, 800 mg/m^2 (Antman et al 1990). An 81% response rate with this regimen was described in patients with refractory breast cancer (Antman et al 1990). In another trial, thiotepa doses were 1.8 and 3.6 mg/kg, representing a 6- to 12-fold escalation over standard intravenous doses (Williams et al 1986). In refractory solid tumors a dose–response relationship has been described for single-agent thiotepa doses of 180 to 1125 mg/m^2 (about 70 times the conventional dose) (Brown et al 1986). An unusual toxic effect of high-dose therapy is a general "bronzing" or hyperpigmentation of skin, especially occluded skin sites. Other extramedullary toxic effects of high-dose thiotepa include liver transaminase and bilirubin elevations and dose-dependent central nervous system effects. Central nervous system effects include inappropriate behavior, confusion, and somnolence. A 5% incidence is reported at 900 mg/m^2 and 15% at higher doses (Wolff et al 1990). Overall, mucositis and esophagitis are the dose-limiting nonhematologic effects of high-dose therapy (Wolff et al 1990).

Intrathecal Administration. Doses of from 1 to 10 mg/m^2 (body surface area) administered once or twice weekly have been administered in cases of documented malignant central nervous system disease such as leptomeningeal cancer (Gutin et al 1976). The commonly used dose is 15 mg.

Intraperitoneal Administration. Doses of 0.8 mg/kg have been instilled intraperitoneally in a volume of 1.8 to 2.0 L; however, because of good systemic bioavailability, this route of drug administration does not allow for major dose escalations over standard intravenous doses. Another recent trial has evaluated intraperitoneal thiotepa doses ranging from 30 to 60 mg/m^2 (Wadler et al 1989). At 50 mg/m^2, grade III myelosuppression was produced, but there was no nausea, vomiting, or alopecia. The loss of thiotepa from the peritoneal cavity was biexponential, with mean half-lives of 0.26 and 2.1 hours. The rate of thiotepa systemic absorption from the intraperitoneal space was 90 mL/min. The AUC for thiotepa in the intraperitoneal space ranged from 7 to 34 µg/mL · h. Systemic AUCs from these intraperitoneal doses ranged from 0.95 to 7.7 µg/mL·h, yielding a small intraperitoneal AUC/systemic AUC ratio (or pharmacokinetic advantage) of 4.3, and the active metabolite TEPA appeared rapidly in the plasma. These features suggest that intraperitoneal thiotepa may not provide a major improvement over standard systemic therapy.

REFERENCES

Ackland SP, Choi KE, Ratain MJ, et al. Human plasma pharmacokinetics of thiotepa following administration of high-dose thiotepa and cyclophosphamide. *J Clin Oncol.* 1988;**6**:1192–1196.

Anderson AP, Brincker H. Intracavitary thio-TEPA in malignant pleural and peritoneal effusions. *Acta Radiol [Ther] (Stockh).* 1968;**7**:369–378.

Antman K, Eder JP, Elias A, et al. High-dose thiotepa alone and in combination regimens with bone marrow support. *Semin Oncol.* 1990;**17**(1, suppl 3):33–38.

Arthur K. Some aspects of chemotherapy in breast carcinomatosis. *Clin Radiol.* 1968;**19**:351–356.

Bitran JD, Williams SF, Moormeier J, Mick R. High-dose combination chemotherapy with thiotepa and autologous hematopoietic stem cell reinfusion in the treatment of patients with relapsed refractory lymphomas. *Semin Oncol.* 1990;**17**(1, suppl 3):39–42.

Blasberg R, Patlak CS, Fenstermacher JD. Intrathecal chemotherapy: Brain tissue profiles after ventriculocisternal perfusion. *J Pharmacol Exp Ther.* 1975;**195**:73–83.

Boyd PJR, Burnard KG. Proceedings: Adjuvant intravesical thio-TEPA and bladder tumor recurrence. *Br J Surg.* 1975;**62**(2):162.

Brown R, Herzig R, Fay J, et al. A phase I–II study of high-dose N, N'N"-triethylenethiophosphoramide (thiotepa) and autologous bone marrow transplantation (AMT) for refractory malignancies. *Proc Am Soc Clin Oncol.* 1986;**5**:127.

Bruce DW, Edgcomb JH. Pancytopenia and generalized sepsis following treatment of cancer of the bladder with instillations of triethylene thiophosphoramide. *J Urol.* 1967;**97**:482–485.

Bruckner HW, Dinse GE, Davis TE, et al. A randomized comparison of cyclophosphamide, Adriamycin, and 5-fluorouracil with triethylenethiophosphoramide and methotrexate, both as sequential and as fixed rotational treatment in patients with advanced ovarian cancer. *Cancer.* 1985;**55**:26–40.

Burnand KG, Boyd PJR, Mayo ME, et al. Single dose intravesical thio-TEPA as an adjuvant to cystodiathermy in the treatment of transitional cell bladder carcinoma. *Br J Urol.* 1976;**48**(1):55–59.

Carey RW, Long JC. Case 28-1977. Presentation of a case. *N Engl J Med.* 1977;**297**:102–107.

Case DC Jr. Therapy of essential thrombocythemia with thiotepa and chlorambucil. *Blood.* 1984;**63**:51–54.

Chan PYM, Sadoff L, Winkley JH. Second malignancies following first breast cancer in prolonged thiotepa adjuvant chemotherapy. In: Salmon SE, Jones SE, eds. *Adjuvant Therapy of Cancer.* Amsterdam: Elsevier; 1977:597–607.

Cohen BE, Egorin MJ, Kohlhepp EA, et al. Human plasma pharmacokinetics and urinary excretion of thiotepa and its metabolites. *Cancer Treat Rep.* 1986;**70**:859–864.

Cohen BE, Egorin MJ, Nayar MSB, Gutierrez PL. Effects of pH and temperature on the stability and decomposition of N, N', N"-triethylenethiophosphoramide in urine and buffer. Cancer Res. 1984;44:4312–4316.

Colhoun EH, Rylett BJ. Further facts about neuromuscular blockades by nitrogen mustard and by thio-TEPA (letter). Anesthesiology. 1978;48(5):381.

Cradock JC, Kleinman LM, Rahman A. Evaluation of some pharmaceutical aspects of intrathecal methotrexate sodium, cytarabine and hydrocortisone sodium succinate. Am J Hosp Pharm. 1978;35:402–406.

Donegan WL. Extended surgical adjuvant thiotepa for mammary carcinoma. Arch Surg. 1974;109:187–192.

Dunphy F, Hortobagy G, Buzdar A, et al. High response rate following chemotherapy failure in metastatic breast cancer using high-dose mitoxantrone/etoposide/thiotepa and autologous marrow support. Proc Am Assoc Cancer Res. 1989;30:251.

Easton DJ, Poon MA. Acute nonlymphocytic leukemia following bladder instillations with thiotepa. Can Med Assoc J. 1983;129:578–579.

Eder JP, Antman K, Elias A, et al. Cyclophosphamide and thiotepa with autologous bone marrow transplantation in patients with solid tumors. J Natl Cancer Inst. 1988;80:1221–1226.

Edwards MS, Levin VA, Seager ML, et al. Phase II evaluation of thio-TEPA for treatment of central nervous system tumors. Cancer Treat Rep. 1973;63(8):1419–1421.

Egorin MJ, Akman SR, Gutierrez PL. Plasma pharmacokinetics and tissue distribution of thiotepa in mice. Cancer Treat Rep. 1984;68:1265–1268.

Egorin MJ, Snyder SW. Characterization of nonexchangeable radioactivity in L1210 cells incubated with [^{14}C]thiotepa: Labeling of phosphatidylethanolamine. Cancer Res. 1990;50:4044–4049.

Egorin MJ, Snyder SW, Wietharn BE. Effects of ethanolamine and choline on thiotepa cellular accumulation and cytotoxicity in L1210 cells. Cancer Res. 1990;50:4322–4327.

Fay JW, Herzig RH, Herzig GP, Wolff SN. Treatment of metastatic colon carcinoma with intensive thiotepa and autologous marrow transplantation. In: Herzig GP, ed. High-Dose Thiotepa and Autologous Marrow Transplantation: Advances in Cancer Chemotherapy. New York: John Wiley & Sons; 1987:31–34.

Greenspan EM. Comparison of regression induction with triethylene thiophosphoramide or methotrexate in bulky stage IIIb ovarian carcinoma. Natl Cancer Inst Monogr. 1975;42:173–182.

Grochow LB, Grossman S, Garrett S, et al. Pharmacokinetics of intraventricular thiotepa (TT) in patients with meningeal carcinomatosis. Proc Am Soc Clin Oncol. 1982;1:19.

Gutin PH, Weiss HD, Wiernik PH, Walker MD. Intrathecal N,N',N"-triethylenethiophosphoramide (Thio-TEPA [NSC 6396]) in the treatment of malignant meningeal disease: Phase I–II study. Cancer. 1976;38:1471–1475.

Hagen B. Pharmacokinetics of thio-TEPA and TEPA in the conventional dose-range and its correlation to myelosuppressive effects. Cancer Chemother Pharmacol. 1991;27:373–378.

Hagen B, Walstad RA, Nilsen OG. Pharmacokinetics of thio-TEPA at two different doses. Cancer Chemother Pharmacol. 1988;22:356–358.

Herzig RH, Fay JW, Herzig GP, et al. Phase I–II studies with high-dose thiotepa and autologous marrow transplantation in patients with refractory malignancies. In: Herzig GP, ed. High-Dose Thiotepa and Autologous Marrow Transplantation: Advances in Cancer Chemotherapy. New York: John Wiley & Sons; 1987:17–23.

Hollister D Jr, Coleman M. Hematologic effects of intravesicular thiotepa therapy for bladder carcinoma. JAMA. 1980;244:2065–2067.

Humphrey EW, Hitchcock CR. Biological effects of the phosphoramides in patients with advanced cancer. Cancer. 1957;10:231–238.

Jones HC, Swinney J. Thiotepa in the treatment of tumors of the bladder. Lancet. 1961;2:615–618.

Kottmeir HL. Treatment of ovarian carcinomas with thio-TEPA. Clin Obstet Gynecol. 1968;11:428–438.

Kreis W, Budman D, Vinciguerra V, et al. Phase I continuous infusion of triethylenethiophosphoramide (thiotepa) over 48 hours. Proc Am Assoc Cancer Res. 1983;24:140.

Lazarus HM, Reed MD, Spitzer TR, et al. High-dose i.v. thiotepa and cryopreserved autologous bone marrow transplantation for therapy of refractory cancer. Cancer Treat Rep. 1987;71:689–695.

McDermott BJ, Double JA, Bibby MC, et al. Methodology for assay of thiotepa in plasma and initial pharmacokinetic studies. Br J Cancer. 1984;50:261.

Mellett LB, Hodgson PE, Woods LA. Absorption and fate of C^{14}-labeled N,N',N"-triethylenethiophosphoramide (thio-TEPA) in humans and dogs. J Lab Clin Med. 1962;60(5):818–825.

Miller A. Thiotepa in carcinoma of breast treated by bilateral adrenalectomy and oophorectomy. Br Med J. 1961;1:619–621.

Nadkarni MV, Trams EG, Smith PK. Preliminary studies on the distribution and fate of TEM, TEPA, and Myleran in the human. Cancer Res. 1959;19:713–718.

National Bladder Cancer Collaborative Group A. The role of intravesical thio-TEPA in the management of superficial bladder cancer. Cancer Res. 1977;37(8, pt 2):2916–2917.

O'Dwyer PJ, LaCreta F, Engstrom PF, et al. Phase I/pharmacokinetic reevaluation of thioTEPA. Cancer Res. 1991;51:3171–3176.

O'Dwyer PJ, LaCreta FP, Schilder R, et al. Phase I trial of thiotepa in combination with recombinant human granulocyte–macrophage colony-stimulating factor. J Clin Oncol. 1992;10(8):1352–1358.

Pavone-Macaluso M. Permeability of the bladder mucosa

to thio-TEPA, Adriamycin and daunomycin in men and rabbits. *Urol Res.* 1976;**4**(1):9–13.

Perloff M, Hart RD, Holland JF. Vinblastine, Adriamycin, thiotepa, and halotestin (VATH): Therapy for advanced breast cancer refractory to prior chemotherapy. *Cancer.* 1978;**42**:2534–2537.

Phillips RM, Bibby MC, Double JA. Experimental correlations of in vitro drug sensitivity with in vivo responses to thiotepa in a panel of murine colon tumors. *Cancer Chemother Pharmacol.* 1988;**21**:168–172.

Reimer RR, Hoover R, Fraumeni JF Jr, et al. Acute leukemia after alkylating-agent therapy of ovarian cancer. *N Engl J Med.* 1977;**297**:177–181.

Saarinen VM, Hovi L, Makiperna A. High dose thiotepa with autologous bone marrow rescue in pediatric solid tumors. *Proc Am Soc Clin Oncol.* 1989;**8**:303.

Schellhammer PF. Renal failure associated with the use of thio-TEPA. *J Urol.* 1973;**110**:498–501.

Shay H, Zarafonetis C, Smith N, et al. Treatment of leukemia with triethylene thiophosphoramide (thio-TEPA): Preliminary results in experimental and clinical leukemia. *Arch Intern Med.* 1953;**92**:628–645.

Strong JM, Collins JM, Lester C, Poplack DG. Pharmacokinetics of intraventricular and intravenous N,N',N"-triethylenethiophosphoramide (thiotepa) in rhesus monkeys and humans. *Cancer Res.* 1986;**46**:6101–6104.

Teicher BA, Holden SA, Eder JP, et al. Preclinical studies relating to the use of thiotepa in the high dose setting alone and in combination. *Semin Oncol.* 1990;**1**(suppl 3):18–32.

Teicher BA, Waxman DJ, Holden SA, et al. Evidence for enzymatic activation and oxygen involvement in cytotoxicity and antitumor activity of N,N',N"-triethylenethiophosphoramide. *Cancer Res.* 1989;**49**: 4996–5001.

Ultmann JE, Hyman GA, Crandall C, et al. Triethylenethiophosphoramide (thio-TEPA) in the treatment of neoplastic disease. *Cancer.* 1957;**10**(5):902–911.

Veenema RJ, Dean AL, Uson AC, et al. Thiotepa bladder instillations: Therapy and prophylaxis for superficial bladder tumors. *J Urol.* 1969;**101**:711–715.

Villasanta U, Bloedorn FG. Operation, external irradiation, radioactive isotopes, and chemotherapy in treatment of metastatic ovarian malignancies. *Am J Obstet Gynecol.* 1968;**102**:531–536.

Wadler S, Egorin MJ, Zuhowski EG, et al. Phase I clinical and pharmacokinetic study of thiotepa administered intraperitoneally in patients with advanced malignancies. *J Clin Oncol.* 1989;**7**(1):132–139.

Wallach RC, Kabako W, Blinick G, et al. Thiotepa chemotherapy for ovarian carcinoma. Influence of remission and toxicity on survival. *Obstet Gynecol.* 1970;**35**:278–286.

Williams SF, Bitran JD, Kaminer L, et al. A phase I–II study of bialkylator chemotherapy, high-dose thio-TEPA, and cyclophosphamide with autologous bone marrow reinfusion in patients with advanced cancer. *J Clin Oncol.* 1987;**5**:260–265.

Williams S, Bitran J, Ratain M, et al. A phase I–II study of bialkylator chemotherapy (BACT) with high-dose thiotepa (TT) and cytoxan and autologous bone marrow reinfusion in patients with refractory lymphoma and disseminated carcinoma. *Proc Am Soc Clin Oncol.* 1986; **5**:141.

Wolff SN, Herzig RH, Fay JW, et al. High-dose N,N',N"-triethylenethiophosphoramide (thiotepa) with autologous bone marrow transplantation: Phase I studies. *Semin Oncol.* 1990;**17**(1, suppl 3):2–6.

Wolff SN, Herzig RH, Herzig GP, et al. High-dose thiotepa with autologous bone marrow transplantation for metastatic malignant melanoma. In: Herzig GP, ed. *High-Dose Thiotepa and Autologous Marrow Transplantation: Advances in Cancer Chemotherapy.* New York: John Wiley & Sons; 1987:25–28.

Zarrabi MH, Rosner F, Grunwald HW, et al. Chronic lymphocytic leukemia terminating in acute leukemia. *NY State Med J.* 1991;**79**:1072–1075.

Zsigmond EK, Robins G. The effect of a series of anticancer drugs on plasma cholinesterase activity. *Can Anaesth Soc J.* 1972;**19**:75.

Thymidine Injection

■ Other Names

TdR; NSC-21548; 2,4-(1H, 3H)-pyrimidinedione.

■ Chemistry

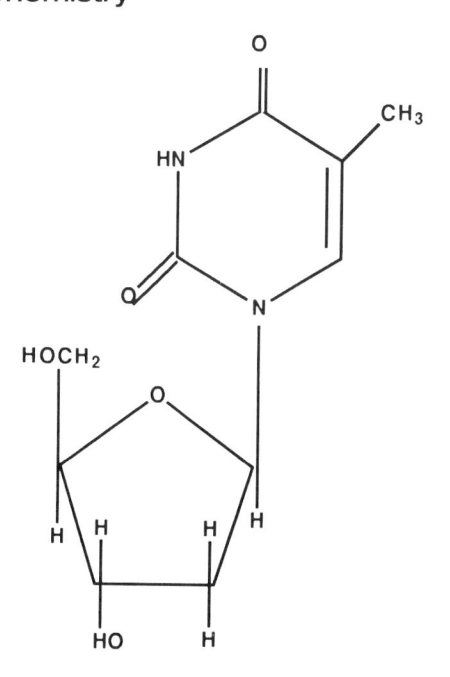

Structure of thymidine

Thymidine is a naturally occurring deoxyribonucleoside which is commercially produced by direct chemical synthesis or is derived from animal sources. The molecular weight is 242.2 and the empiric formula $C_{10}H_{14}N_2O_5$. The complete chemical name is 1-(2-deoxy-β-D-ribofuranosyl)-5-methyluracil.

■ Antitumor Activity

When used alone in animal systems in large doses, thymidine has demonstrated selective cytoxicity for neoplastic cells over normal host cells (Lee et al 1977a,b). Lee et al (1979) also demonstrated antitumor activity for high-dose thymidine in heterotransplanted human tumors in nude mice (including typically resistant melanoma, lung, and breast cancers).

Bruno et al (1981) and Schornagel et al (1982) have published excellent reviews on the use of thymidine in clinical oncology. By itself, thymidine has not been shown to have any significant antitumor activity against solid tumors in humans. In a phase I–II clinical trial with thymidine alone, Chiuten et al (1980) observed minimal objective clinical responses (including a less than partial response in one melanoma patient) and clearing of leukemia cells in the peripheral blood and a reduction in hepatosplenomegaly in three patients with nonlymphocytic leukemia. Woodcock et al (1979) also observed clearing of peripheral blasts in two leukemic patients treated with high-dose thymidine but were similarly unable to produce complete responses characterized by marrow hypocellularity. Kufe et al (1980) have described the antitumor activity of thymidine in patients with T-cell leukemia and with acute myelocytic leukemia. They have also reported responses in two of three patients with mycosis fungoides (Kufe et al 1981).

In experimental in vitro and in vivo tumor systems, high-dose thymidine alters the toxicity of several chemotherapeutic antimetabolites including methotrexate (Ensminger and Frei 1977, Tattersall et al 1975) and 5-fluorouracil (Kirkwood and Frei 1978, Martin et al 1978, Vogel et al 1979). Grossie et al (1979) were able to show significant antitumor synergism for thymidine combined with the fluorinated pyrimidine ftorafur in P-388 murine leukemia. In murine breast cancer (Martin and Stolfi 1977, Sawyer et al 1979) and in murine colon cancer, thymidine treatment before 5-fluorouracil appears to moderately increase antitumor effects (70% increase).

In a small number of patients with head and neck cancer treated with thymidine and high-dose methotrexate, Leyva et al (1979) were able to effectively reduce high-dose methotrexate toxicity; however, no antitumor effects were demonstrable in the 10 patients studied. Ensminger and Frei (1977) did note minimal responses for a similar combination used in four advanced cancer patients (two colon cancers, one breast cancer, and one renal carcinoma). Thymidine has been reported by others to prevent methotrexate toxicity in patients (Ensminger and Frei 1977, Howell et al 1978, 1980); however, this use has not been widely practiced because of the investigational nature of the thymidine.

Woodcock et al (1980) reported responses in 2 of 18 patients treated with the combination 5-fluorouracil + thymidine. Of interest, the patients had been refractory to 5-fluorouracil-containing combinations. Buroker and colleagues (1984) reported on the results of a randomized trial of 5-fluorouracil alone (500 mg/m^2/d × 5 every 5 weeks) versus 5-fluorouracil (300 mg/m^2) + thymidine (45 g every 4 weeks) in patients with advanced previously untreated colorectal carcinoma. The thymidine did not significantly increase the response rate or the survival of those patients.

■ Mechanism of Action

An excellent overview of thymidine's mechanism of action has been published by Martin et al (1980). Thymidine levels are normally low in the blood (Hughes et al 1973). In these circumstances thymidine is selectively incorporated into the cellular DNA distributed throughout body tissues. Thus small injections of exogenous thymidine are either rapidly excreted or catabolized primarily in the liver (Cleaver 1967). From mouse studies the observed plasma half-life of small thymidine doses is short, ranging from 5 to 10 minutes (Hughes et al 1973). It is similarly evanescent in the plasma of humans (Ensminger and Frei 1977). Therefore, large bolus doses or continuous infusions are used to effect high extracellular thymidine concentrations. This leads to alterations in intracellular nucleotide pool concentrations within 1 to 2 minutes (Bjursell and Reichard 1973). The available thymidine can be rapidly incorporated into newly synthesized DNA; however, for direct thymidine cytotoxicity via DNA synthesis inhibition, massive thymidine levels (0.5–2.0 mM) are necessary, at least in in vitro cell culture systems (Cleaver 1967). These cytotoxic levels can be achieved in vivo only with doses upward of 64 to 128 g/m^2/d IV (Ensminger and Frei 1978).

The major cytotoxic effect of high-dose thymidine is mediated through elevation of thymidine triphosphate (dTTP) levels intracellularly (O'Dwyer et al 1987). The primary lesion is believed to involve inhibition of ribonucleotide reductase (Reichard 1978).Thymidine-induced cytotoxicity can be reversed by deoxycytidine triphosphate (dCTP) (Egan et al 1981), suggesting that dCTP depletion is a key part of thymidine's mechanism of action (Fox et al 1980). Direct DNA damage and blocked DNA repair have also been postulated to explain thymidine's enhancement of alkylating agent damage (Meuth and Green 1974). These latter effects may lead to enhanced mutagenesis in cells exposed to thymidine (Peterson et al 1978). Overall, however, the primary cytotoxic mechanism appears to be inhibition of ribonucleotide reductase. This process is cell cycle phase specific for late G_1 and early S phase.

Other major antitumor applications for low-dose thymidine involve toxicity-altering interactions with antimetabolites, mediated through the alterations in intracellular nucleotide pools. Because the half-life of thymidine is very short, there is substantial benefit to continuous thymidine infusion whereby a constant extracellular thymidine gradient may be maintained. This facilitates the enhanced cytotoxic actions of the fluoropyrimidine and folate antagonists (see Drug Interactions).

■ Availability and Storage

Thymidine is investigationally available from the National Cancer Institute, Bethesda, Maryland, as a 3% injectable solution in 0.6% sodium chloride. Thus, each 500-mL bottle contains 15 g of thymidine (3 g/100 mL) with 103 mEq sodium/500 mL. The solution is approximately isotonic (300 mosmol) and has a final pH of 4.5 to 7.5. The bottles should be stored at room temperature. Refrigeration is not recommended as precipitation of crystals may occur.

■ Preparation for Use, Stability, and Admixture

The investigational solution is supplied ready for intravenous administration. Stored at room temperature it is chemically stable for at least 2 years; however, it is recommended that only clear solutions with intact vacuum be used. Admixture with other drugs should be avoided as compatibility data are not available. Thymidine solutions may be run through an in-line filter. The bottle as supplied also requires a self-venting administration set.

■ Administration

Thymidine solutions are intended for intravenous administration, either as a short infusion or by continuous infusion over several days. The latter method may maximize the pharmacologic effects of the drug (Ensminger and Frei 1977). Earlier reports of thymidine used for nonneoplastic indications reference intramuscular administration (Butterworth and Perez-Santiago 1956) of low doses as ineffective over high intravenous doses (Killman 1964).

■ Special Precautions

None are known.

■ Drug Interactions

Methotrexate Interaction. With methotrexate, Ensminger and Frei (1977) have demonstrated that continuous-infusion thymidine can protect against methotrexate toxicity and actually increase the maximally tolerated dose of the antifole by 20- to 60-fold. Substantial animal work further suggests a necessary purine interaction with thymidine to prevent methotrexate gastrointestinal toxicity (Straw et al 1976). Proper sequencing of thymidine and methotrexate also appears to be important in preventing methotrexate toxicity. Thus, Jackson (1979) has demonstrated that thymidine given before methotrexate (and continued throughout) rescues cells from both antithymidylate and antipurine methotrexate effects. When thymidine was given after methotrexate, only antithymidylate effects were reversed. Bone marrow cytokinetic studies with thymidine and methotrexate have generally shown no significant changes in mitotic labeling indexes (Ensminger and Frei 1977).

5-Fluorouracil Interaction. With 5-fluorouracil, an opposite trend appears to be in effect: combined thymidine–5-fluorouracil therapy lowered the minimal toxic dose to one-third that when 5-fluorouracil is used alone. In addition, the dose-limiting toxic effect changed from gastrointestinal problems to myelosuppression. In previous in vitro cell culture studies it has been noted that both thymidine and 5-fluorouracil are similarly transported into cells, phosphorylated, and catabolized (Fink et al 1956, Chaudhuri et al 1958). One mechanism for the pyrimidine interaction may relate to the observed prolongation of 5-fluorouracil levels by thymidine, with apparent inhibition of catabolism of 5-fluoro-2'-deoxy-β-uridine (5-FUDR), the active metabolite (Cooley et al 1979) (see Pharmacokinetics). Fried et al (1979) have observed that the cellular kinetic changes produced by thymidine and 5-fluorouracil are essentially the same as with thymidine alone, causing cells to accumulate in late S phase and at the G_2/M junction. Mendelsohn and Howell (1981) have documented that thymidine inhibits progression of T-cell lymphoma cells through S phase. For direct cytotoxicity, of course, thymidine requires active DNA synthesis and is thus a classic S phase-specific antimetabolite.

Cisplatin Interaction. Thymidine and cisplatin have also been described as synergistic in vitro. A phase I clinical trial of the combination has been reported in preliminary form. Cisplatin appears to significantly affect the renal clearance of thymidine and its in vivo metabolite thymine (Schilsky 1985).

■ Dosage

The optimal dose of thymidine for either antitumor or drug interaction effects is not known. In the first instance in vitro cell culture studies have determined that very high concentrations, in the millimolar range, are required to effect inhibition of DNA synthesis (Cleaver 1967). It may be possible to achieve these concentrations clinically with peripheral intravenous infusion of 64 to 128 g/m^2/d or with hepatic artery infusions of 16 to 32 g/m^2/d (Ensminger and Frei 1978). Woodcock et al (1979) have also described a requirement for high doses, 45 to 90 g/m^2/d to produce plasma levels of 0.45 to 3.33 mM, and Chiuten et al (1980), in a single-agent phase I–II study, used 75 g/m^2/d × 5 days to produce 1 to 3 mM levels.

In ameliorating methotrexate toxicity the most commonly employed dose is 8.0 g/m^2/d for several days (usually during and for 1–2 days after methotrexate infusion) (Creaven et al 1979, Leyva et al 1979, Ensminger and Frei 1977). Howell et al (1979), however, have reported that the minimum effective thymidine dose for methotrexate infusions (3 g/m^2/d) is approximately 1 g/m^2/d. Because near-complete methotrexate rescue was produced with doses that only marginally elevated serum thymidine levels, Howell et al (1980) suggested that there is a very steep dose–response curve for thymidine-induced methotrexate marrow rescue. They further suggest that thymidine doses greater than 1 g/m^2/d may somewhat obscure the selective methotrexate toxicity reversal pattern of thymidine.

When combined with fluorinated pyrimidines, low-dose thymidine lowers the minimally toxic dose of the antimetabolite. Thus, when Vogel et al (1979) used concurrent thymidine infusions of 8 g/m^2/d × 5.5 days, the minimally toxic dose of 5-fluorouracil was reduced to approximately one-third of 5-fluorouracil used alone. High doses of thymidine combined with fluorinated pyrimidines would therefore be expected to produce unacceptably severe toxicity, as was seen in the study of Vogel et al.

■ Pharmacokinetics

Ensminger and Frei (1977) have described the disposition of relatively low dose (8 g/m^2/d) infusions of thymidine. The median steady-state thymidine level during the infusion was 1.5 μM, compared with a pretreatment level of 0.19 μM. Following a pulse dose and discontinuance of the infusion, plasma levels rapidly declined with a half-life of 8 to 10 minutes. Cerebrospinal fluid thymidine levels equaled simultaneous blood levels after 2 hours of constant infusion. In this study less than 2% of intact thymidine was recovered in the urine, but on refrigeration, urine specimens precipitated out thymine crystals. To produce millimolar thymidine levels, much higher doses must be employed (see table).

In vivo, thymidine is metabolized to the free base thymine, which is inactive. Zaharko et al (1979) have suggested that thymidine elimination kinetics is altered with time of infusion. Thus, after 30 minutes of high-dose (94 mg/kg/h) thymidine infusion the thymidine and thymine half-lives were 10 and

THYMIDINE INFUSION SCHEDULES AND PHARMACOKINETICS

Reference	Thymidine Infusion Dose (g/m^2/d)	Mean Steady-State Thymidine Level (mM)
Chiuten et al 1980	75 × 5	1–3
Zaharko et al 1979	90	2
Woodcock et al 1979	40–90	0.45–3.3
Kufe et al 1980	75 × 5	1–2

35 minutes, respectively. After 8 hours of infusion the apparent thymidine and thymine half-lives were greatly increased (slowed elimination) at 80 and 235 minutes, respectively. Woodcock et al (1979) have also suggested saturability of thymidine excretion pathways. Thus, they noted distinct variations in thymidine half-lives with different dose levels: 7.5 minutes at 2 g/m², 32 minutes at 5 g/m², 47 minutes at 10 g/m², and 106 minutes at 30 g/m². Patients receiving the highest thymidine doses in this study (120 g/d) excreted up to 35% of the dose as intact thymidine and 25% as thymine. Urinary levels of the major metabolite, β-aminoisobutyric acid, were also very high in this study.

A number of studies have addressed possible thymidine alteration of methotrexate disposition. Creaven et al (1979) describe apparently prolonged methotrexate pharmacokinetics when 2 g/m²/d methotrexate is combined with calcium leucovorin and thymidine 8 g/m²/d. Methotrexate elimination was either biphasic or triphasic in this study (half-lives: 5, 20–30, and 40–180 hours producing mean steady-state levels of approximately 4.4×10^{-5} M). With cessation of the infusion these levels declined over 4 to 7 days to the purported nontoxic range of 1 to 2×10^{-8} M. The minor 7-hydroxymethotrexate metabolite found in the urine amounted to only 3% of the dose in this study and thus is apparently insignificant (Ensminger and Frei 1977).

With 5-fluorouracil, concurrent thymidine also appears to prolong drug elimination. In dogs Cooley et al (1979) have shown that thymidine increases the 5-fluorouracil half-life from 40 (normal) to 90 minutes. This occurs in addition to the enhancement of plasma levels of the active metabolite 5-FUDR. Urinary 5-fluorouracil recovery actually appeared to increase by 50%, probably reflecting thymidine-induced inhibition of 5-FUDR catabolism. In patients, concurrent thymidine + 5-fluorouracil administration reduced the plasma clearance of 5-fluorouracil (Au et al 1982).

■ Side Effects and Toxicity

In the high-dose phase I–II trial of five daily bolus doses, Chiuten et al (1980) reported that hematologic suppression appeared to predominate. Leukopenia and anemia occurred in over half the patients, significant thrombocytopenia in about a third. The nadir for myelosuppression occurred on day 7 and ranged from 900 to 3800 cells/mm³ (average, 2500/mm³). The median thrombocytopenic nadir occurred on about day 6 and ranged from 28,000 to 136,000 (average, 97,500).

Almost 90% of the patients in this study developed some nausea, vomiting, and anorexia. Diarrhea occurred in two thirds of patients and indigestion was reported in about a fourth of patients.

Central nervous system toxicity was also common in this study, with somnolence occurring in 89% of patients. At least two thirds of patients developed severe headaches while receiving the drug. Over half of patients also experienced visual hallucinations and about a quarter reported noticeable impairment of memory (Chiuten et al 1980).

Renal, hepatic, and allergic toxic effects were not encountered. Alopecia did not occur (Chiuten et al 1980). Woodcock et al (1979), however, did note that one patient with very high thymidine levels developed a slight alopecia and also demonstrated an observable therapeutic response to the drug.

■ Special Applications

Ensminger and Frei (1978) have successfully used hepatic artery infusions of thymidine (16–32 g/m²/d) in patients with metastatic colon cancer. These doses were well tolerated and produced selectively higher hepatic levels (into the potentially cytotoxic 0.5–2.0 mM range) than very high dose peripheral intravenous infusions of 64 to 128 g/m²/d in the same patients. Hepatic artery access was maintained via 5% dextrose solution with 1 U/mL heparin added. This study showed that the hepatic extraction of thymidine was very efficient (at low doses of 8 g/m²/d) with extraction ratios of 0.77 to 0.91. With higher intravenous doses of 16 to 32 g/m²/d, hepatic extraction became less efficient, with extraction ratios ranging from 0.6 to 0.4, respectively. This was reduced further to less than 0.2 at 128 g/m²/d. Antitumor efficacy for these procedures, however, is still not known.

REFERENCES

Au JL, Rustum YM, Ledesma EJ, Mittelman A, Creaven PJ. Clinical pharmacological studies of concurrent infusion of 5-fluorouracil and thymidine in treatment of colorectal carcinomas. *Cancer Res.* 1982;**42**(7):2930–2937.

Bjursell G, Reichard P. Effects of thymidine on deoxyribonucleoside triphosphate pools and deoxyribonucleic acid synthesis in Chinese hamster ovary cells. *J Biol Chem.* 1973;**248**:3904–3909.

Bruno S, Poster DS, Bono VH, Macdonald JS, Kubota TT.

High-dose thymidine in clinical oncology. *Cancer Treat Rep.* 1981;**65**(1/2):57–63.

Buroker T, Moertel C, Fleming T, et al. A randomized comparison of 5FU containing drug combinations with 5FU alone in advanced colorectal carcinomas. *Proc Am Soc Clin Oncol.* 1984;**3**:138.

Butterworth CE, Perez-Santiago. An evaluation of thymidine in treatment of tropical sprue. *Proc Soc Exp Biol Med.* 1956;**92**:762–763.

Chaudhuri N, Mukherjee K, Heidelberger C. Studies on fluorinated pyrimidines. VII. The degradative pathway. *Biochem Pharmacol.* 1958;**1**:328–342.

Chiuten DF, Wiernik PH, Zaharko DS, Edwards L. Phase I–II and clinical pharmacokinetics study of high dose thymidine given by continuous intravenous infusion. *Cancer Res.* 1980;**40**:818–822.

Cleaver J. *Thymidine Metabolism and Cell Kinetics.* Amsterdam: North Holland; 1967:54–94.

Cooley J, Furlong NB, Loo TL. Pharmacokinetics of 5-fluorouracil in combination with thymidine in the dog. *Proc Am Assoc Cancer Res ASCO.* 1979;**29**:161.

Creaven PJ, Zakrzewski SF, Kinahan J, Mittleman A. Methotrexate (MTX) pharmacokinetics and metabolism in patients receiving prolonged high dose MTX infusion with thymidine (TdR) and leucovorin CF. *Proc Am Assoc Cancer Res ASCO.* 1979;**20**:381–383.

Egan EM, Sargent C, Rosowsky A, et al. Rescue of thymidine cytotoxicity in L1210 ascites by elevated endogenous levels of deoxycytidine. *Cancer Treat Rep.* 1981;**65**: 853–860.

Ensminger WD, Frei E III. The prevention of methotrexate toxicity by thymidine infusion in humans. *Cancer Res.* 1977;**37**:1857–1863.

Ensminger WD, Frei E III. High dose intravenous and hepatic artery infusions of thymidine. *Clin Pharmacol Ther.* 1978;**24**(5):610–615.

Fink K, Cline RE, Henderson RB, Fink RM. Metabolism of thymine (methyl-C^{14} or -2- C^{14}) by rat liver in vitro. *J Biol Chem.* 1956;**221**:425.

Fox RM, Tripp EH, Tattersall MHN. Mechanism of deoxycytidine rescue of thymidine toxicity in human T-leukemic lymphocytes. *Cancer Res.* 1980;**40**:1718–1721.

Fried J, Perez AG, Doblin JM. Effects of thymidine (TdR) and/or 5-fluorouracil (t-FU) on survival and growth kinetics of the La cells (abstract 484). *Proc Am Assoc Cancer Res ASCO.* 1979;**20**:120.

Grossie VB Jr, Wengrovitz PS, Farquhar D, Loo TL. Combination chemotherapy of ftorafur (FT) with thymidine (TdR) against P-388 murine leukemia (abstract 679). *Proc Am Assoc Cancer Res ASCO.* 1979;**20**:168.

Howell SB, Ensminger WD, Krishan A, Frei E III. Thymidine rescue of high dose methotrexate in humans. *Cancer Res.* 1978;**38**:325–330.

Howell SB, Herbst K, Boss G, Frei E III. Thymidine (TDR) rescue of methotrexate (MTX) in man. *Proc Am Assoc Cancer Res ASCO.* 1979;**20**:72.

Howell SB, Herbst K, Boss GR, Frei E III. Thymidine requirements for the rescue of patients treated with high dose methotrexate. *Cancer Res.* 1980;**40**:1824–1829.

Hughes WL, Christine M, Stollar B. A radioimmunoassay for measurement of serum thymidine. *Anal Biochem.* 1973;**55**:468–478.

Jackson RC. Thymidine rescue from methotrexate toxicity: Sequence-dependent biochemical effects (abstract 289). *Proc Am Assoc Cancer Res ASCO.* 1979;**20**:72.

Killman S. Erythropoietic response to thymidine in pernicious anaemia. *Acta Med Scand.* 1964;**175**:489–497.

Kirkwood JM, Frei E III. 5-Fluorouracil (FU) with thymidine (TdR): A phase I study. *Proc Am Assoc Cancer Res ASCO.* 1978; **19**:635.

Kufe DW, Beardsley P, Karp D, et al. High-dose thymidine infusions in patients with leukemia and lymphoma. *Blood.* 1980;**55**(4):580–589.

Kufe DW, Wick MM, Moschella S, Major P. Effect of high-dose thymidine infusions in patients with mycosis fungoides. *Cancer.* 1981;**48**(7):1513–1516.

Lee SS, Giovanella BC, Stehlin JS. Effect of excess thymidine on the growth of human melanoma cells transplanted in thymus deficient nude mice. *Cancer Lett.* 1977a;**3**:209–214.

Lee SS, Giovanella BC, Stehlin JS. Selective lethal effect of thymidine on human and mouse tumor cells. *J Cell Physiol.* 1977b;**92**:401–406.

Lee SS, Giovanella BC, Stehlin JS, Brunn JC. Further studies on the long term effects of high dose thymidine infusion (TdR) on human tumors heterotransplanted in nude mice (abstract 945). *Proc Am Assoc Cancer Res ASCO.* 1979;**20**:234.

Leyva A, Weiss R, Schornagel JH, Pinedo HM. Plasma levels of pyrimidines and purines during methotrexate (MTX)–thymidine (TdR) treatment. *Proc Am Assoc Cancer Res ASCO.* 1979;**20**:250.

Martin DS, Stolfi RL. Thymidine (TdR) enhancement of antitumor activity of 5-fluorouracil (FU) against advanced murine CD8F$_1$ breast carcinoma. *Proc Am Assoc Cancer Res ASCO.* 1977;**18**:126.

Martin DS, Stolfi RL, Sawyer RC, et al. An overview of thymidine. *Cancer.* 1980;**45**(5, suppl):1117–1128.

Martin DS, Stolfi RL, Spiegelman S. Striking augmentation of the in vitro anticancer activity of 5-fluorouracil (FU) by combination with pyrimidine nucleosides: An RNA effect. *Proc Am Assoc Cancer Res ASCO.* 1978;**19**:882.

Mendelsohn J, Howell SB. Thymidine (TDR) as a potential chemotherapeutic agent: Cytokinetic studies. *Acta Pathol Microbiol Scand [A].* 1981;**274**:509–510.

Meuth M, Green H. Alterations leading to increased ribonucleotide reductase in cells selected for resistance to deoxynucleoside. *Cell.* 1974;**3**:367–374.

O'Dwyer PJ, King SA, Hoth DF, et al. Role of thymidine in biochemical modulation: A review. *Cancer Res.* 1987;**47**: 3911–3919.

Peterson AR, Landolph JR, Peterson H, Heidelberger C. Mutagenesis of Chinese hamster cells facilitated by thymidine and deoxycytidine. *Nature.* 1978;**276**:508–510.

Reichard P. From deoxynucleotides to DNA synthesis. *Fed Proc.* 1978;**37**:9–14.

Sawyer R, Nayak R, Speigelman S, Martin D. Mechanism

of action of 5-fluorouracil (FU) in the chemotherapy of the murine mammary tumor. *Proc Am Assoc Cancer Res ASCO.* 1979;**20**:263.

Schilsky R. Phase I clinical and pharmacologic study of thymidine (TDR) and cisplatin (DDP) in patients with advanced cancer (meeting abstract). *Proc Am Assoc Cancer Res.* 1985;**26**:152.

Schornagel JH, Leyva A, Pinedo HM. Is there a role for thymidine in cancer chemotherapy? *Cancer Treat Rev.* 1982;**9**(4):331–352.

Straw J, Talbot D, Taylor GA, Harrap K. Effects of thymidine (TdR) and/or purines on the reversibility of methotrexate (MTX) toxicity in mice. *Proc Am Assoc Cancer Res.* 1976;**17**:115.

Tattersall M, Brown B, Frei E III. The reversal of methotrexate toxicity by thymidine with maintenance of antitumor effects. *Nature.* 1975;**253**:198–200.

Vogel SJ, Presant CA, Ratkin GA, Klahr C. Phase I study of thymidine plus 5-fluorouracil infusions in advanced colorectal carcinoma. *Cancer Treat Rep.* 1979;**63**(1):1–5.

Woodcock T, Damin L, O'Hehir MO, Hansen H, Andreef M, Young C. Early clinical and pharmacokinetic evaluation of thymidine therapy in patients with advanced cancer. *Proc Am Assoc Cancer Res ASCO.* 1979;**20**:114.

Woodcock TM, Martin DS, Damin LA, Kemeny NE, Young CW. Combination clinical trials with thymidine and fluorouracil: A phase I and clinical pharmacologic evaluation. *Cancer.* 1980;**45**(5, suppl):1135–1143.

Zaharko DS, Bolten BJ, Giovanella BC, Stehlin JC. Thymidine and thymine measurements in biological fluids. *Proc Am Assoc Cancer Res ASCO.* 1979;**20**:62.

Tiazofurin

■ Other Names

TCAR; riboxamide; NSC-286193.

■ Chemistry

Structure of tiazofurin

Tiazofurin is a novel synthetic C-nucleoside that is structurally related to the potent antiviral agent ribovirin (Witkowski et al 1972, Roberts et al 1987). It has a molecular weight of 206.27, is water soluble (250 mg/mL), and has the empiric formula $C_9H_{12}N_2O_5S$. Although originally designed as a new antiviral agent, tiazofurin later proved to be more interesting as a possible antineoplastic agent. The complete chemical name is 2-β-D-ribofuranosyl-thiazole-4-carboxamide.

■ Antitumor Activity

Tiazofurin has not been shown to have phase II clinical activity against any solid tumors in humans. More specifically, the compound has been inactive against squamous cell carcinoma of the head and neck in patients previously untreated with chemotherapy (Dimery et al 1987) and against malignant melanoma in patients previously untreated with chemotherapy (Goldberg and Ahlgren 1988). The substantial toxicity of this agent has precluded additional phase II studies.

Interest in tiazofurin has been rejuvenated by reports by Tricot and colleagues (1989a,b) that tiazofurin had activity in patients with refractory acute myeloid leukemia. They used a 1-hour infusion of tiazofurin with escalations up to total doses of 23,650 mg/m^2 given over a 13-day period. They observed responses without bone marrow hypoplasia. The agent was felt to be acting as a differentiating agent. Overall, in 17 patients reported, there were 5 complete responses and 2 hematologic improvements. All five patients with chronic myelogenous leukemia blast crisis were noted to have reentered the chronic phase of their disease (Tricot et al 1989a,b). Toxic effects were substantial with pleuropericarditis and somnolence; however, these results are clearly worthy of follow-up study.

Of importance in the studies by Tricot et al, assays of inosine-5'-monophosphate dehydrogenase activities and GTP concentrations in leukemia cells were used to monitor the effect of tiazofurin and adjust drug dosage. This was based on the work of Jayaram and colleagues (1986, 1988), who noted that leukemia cells were more sensitive to tiazofurin than were normal marrow cells. Additional trials using tiazofurin for treatment of patients with acute leukemia should include that important biochemical monitoring.

Mechanism of Action

Tiazofurin is metabolized to thiazole-4-carboxamide adenine dinucleotide, an analog of NAD. This anabolite potentially inhibits inosine-5′-monophosphate (IMP), dehydrogenase which results in depletion of intracellular guanine nucleotide pools and cell death (Cooney et al 1982, Jayaram et al 1982). Lui and colleagues (1984) have found that antitumor activity against hepatoma 3924A in rats depends on a decrease in guanine triphosphate (GTP) and, in particular, a sustained depletion of guanine nucleotide pools. Melink et al (1990) have noted that in patients with solid tumors, tiazofurin is rarely able to maintain adequate depletion of guanine nucleotide pools before serious toxicity (pleuropericarditis) intervenes.

Availability and Storage

Tiazofurin is available from the National Cancer Institute formulated as a freeze-dried dosage form in 10-mL flint vials that contain 1000 mg tiazofurin. The intact vials should be stored under refrigeration.

Preparation for Use, Stability, and Admixture

The intact dosage form is to be reconstituted with 4.6 mL of Sterile Water for Injection, USP, and yields a clear colorless solution containing 200 mg of tiazofurin per milliliter of solution at pH 6.0 to 7.5. The reconstituted solution is hypertonic (calculated approximately 1200 mosmol/kg) and may be further diluted with Sodium Chloride Injection, USP, or 5% Dextrose in Water, USP. At 1 mg/mL tiazofurin, the drug was stable in these intravenous fluids for at least 1 week at room temperature. The intact dosage form was undergoing a 4-year shelf-life surveillance study. Pending results of this evaluation, refrigeration is recommended for storage (O'Dwyer et al 1984).

Administration

Tiazofurin has been given as a continuous infusion for 5 days, daily × 5 by bolus injection, in single doses every 3 to 4 weeks, weekly, and daily as a 1-hour/infusion until the disappearance of blasts in patients with acute leukemia (Melink et al 1985, 1990, Batist et al 1985, Trump et al 1985, Currie et al 1985). The drug is given intravenously. No episodes of extravasation necrosis have been reported with tiazofurin.

Special Precautions

As will be noted later, a substantial pleuropericarditis consisting of pleural discomfort and chest pain has been noted at high doses of the agent. In addition, severe neurologic toxic effects have been noted including hemiparesis, actual blindness, and obtundation (see Side Effects and Toxicity).

Drug Interactions

None are reported; however, allopurinol is given with tiazofurin to prevent the hyperuricemia noted at higher doses. Administration of allopurinol also elevates the serum concentration of hypoxanthine, which can completely inhibit the activity of hypoxanthine–guanine phosphoribosyltransferase, the salvage enzyme of guanylate synthesis (Tricot et al 1989a).

Dosage

At present, there are no recommended doses for additional phase II trials because of the inactivity and substantial toxicity of tiazofurin. For patients with leukemia, the dosages of tiazofurin are adjusted based on biochemical measurements of IMP dehydrogenase activity and GTP in leukemic cells. (Tricot et al 1989b). It is recommended that the literature be consulted before embarking on phase II trials in patients with acute leukemia.

Pharmacokinetics

The pharmacokinetic parameters for tiazofurin are summarized in the table on the opposite page.

The total urine excretion has ranged from 15 to 5%. (Melink et al 1985, Roberts et al 1987, Trump et al 1985).

Cerebrospinal fluid was obtained from two patients receiving 550 and 1100 mg/m^2/d × 5. Cerebrospinal fluid concentrations were 19.9 and 18.5 mM, respectively, or 42 and 37% of the concurrent plasma levels (Balis et al 1985). The drug can penetrate brain tumors but does not appear to be actively concentrated in the tumor cells (Green et al 1986).

Alonso et al (1984) have documented a relationship between renal dysfunction and the degree of myelosuppression.

Side Effects and Toxicity

When tiazofurin is administered by daily × 5 continuous infusion or as a single dose, severe unpredict-

CLINICAL PHARMACOKINETICS OF TIAZOFURIN

Schedule	Reference	Half-life (h) α	β	γ	Plasma Clearance (L/h/m^2)	Volume of Distribution (L/m^2) Central	Steady State
Daily × 5 every 28 d in adults	Melink et al 1985	0.11	7.56	—	Biphasic	14.23 ± 7.89	30.03 ± 10.32
Daily × 5 every 21 d in children	Balis et al 1985	0.12	1.6	5.5	Triphasic	—	29.3 ± 7.6
Daily × 5 every 21 d	Green et al 1986	0.13	5.60	—	3.73 ± 1.99	14.56 ± 6.49	33.7 ± 11.37
Daily × 5 continuous infusion:	Batist et al 1985	—	7.7	—	4.2 ± 0.96	—	—
Daily × 5 every 21 d	Roberts et al 1987	0.26	4.18	—	5.85 ± 1.90	—	42.9 ± 17.2
Daily × 5 continuous infusion	Trump et al 1985	0.50	8.0	—	3.72 ± 0.96	15.5 ± 8.2	34.3 ± 8.4
Daily × 5 continuous infusion	Raghaven et al 1986	—	—	—	1.74 ± 0.24	—	—

able central nervous system toxic effects can be seen. These include confusion, obtundation, hemiparesis, cortical blindness, headaches, and irritability (Batist et al 1985, Balis et al 1985, Currie et al 1985, Raghaven et al 1986, Trump et al 1985).

On the daily × 5 (bolus) schedule, dose-limiting pleuropericarditis is noted. This presents as a viral-like illness (Melink et al 1985). Similar toxic effects were noted on the weekly administration schedule (Melink et al 1990). In one case, a fatal cardiomyopathy occurred (Roberts et al 1987). Other toxic effects have included impressive elevations in creatine phosphokinase MM bands, myalgias, conjunctivitis, hyperuricemia, and nausea and vomiting. Myelosuppression has been infrequent and occasionally related to renal insufficiency, probably causing decreased urinary excretion of the agent (Balis et al 1985, Alonso et al 1984).

Magnetic resonance imaging scans of the brain in patients receiving biochemically monitored doses of tiazofurin have demonstrated extensive changes, suggesting ischemia (Rippe et al 1988). This effect is rapidly reversed on discontinuation of the drug.

■ Special Applications

An area incompletely explored is the use of tiazofurin plus other agents (suggested by animal tumor synergism studies) (Harrison et al 1986). These have not been used because of the severe systemic toxicities of tiazofurin.

REFERENCES

Alonso MT, O'Dwyer PJ, Leyland-Jones B, Ellenberg SS. Tiazofurin: Myelosuppression at low doses relates to nephrotoxicity. *Proc Am Soc Clin Oncol.* 1984;3:35.

Balis FM, Lange BJ, Packer RJ, et al. Pediatric phase I trial and pharmacokinetic study of tiazofurin (NSC-286193). *Cancer Res.* 1985;45:5169–5172.

Batist G, Klecker RW, Jayaram HN, et al. Phase I and pharmacokinetic study of tiazofurin (9TCAR, NSC-286193) administered by continuous infusion. *Investi New Drugs.* 1985;3:349–357.

Cooney DA, Jayaram HN, Gebeyeu G, et al. The conversion of 2-β-D-ribofuranosylthiazole-4-carboxamide to an analog of NAD with IMP dehydrogenase-inhibiting properties. *Biochem Pharmacol.* 1982;31:2133–2136.

Currie VE, Budman D, Hancock C, et al. Phase I and clinical pharmacologic evaluation of tiazofurin (TCAR) by an intermittent schedule. *Proc Am Assoc Cancer Res.* 1985;22:188.

Dimery IW, Neidham JA, McCarthy K, Krakhoff IH, Hang WK. Phase II trial of tiazofurin in recurrent squamous cell carcinoma of the head and neck. *Cancer Treat Rep.* 1987;71:425–426.

Goldberg R, Ahlgren J. Treatment of metastatic malignant melanoma (MMM) with tiazofurin: A phase II study: *Proc Am Soc Clin Oncol.* 1988;7:253.

Green RM, Stewart DJ, Maroun JA. Clinical pharmacology of tiazofurin (2-β-D-ribofuranosylthiazole-4-carboxamide, NSC-286193). *Invest New Drugs.* 1986;4:387–394.

Harrison SD, O'Dwyer PJ, Trades MW. Therapeutic synergism of tiazofurin and selected antitumor drugs against sensitive and resistant P388 leukemia in mice. *Cancer Res.* 1986;46:3396–3400.

Jayaram HN, Dion RL, Glazer RI, et al. Initial studies on the mechanism of action of a new oncologic thiazole nucleoside, 2-β-D-ribofuranosylthiazole-4-carboxamide, (NSC-286193). *Biochem Pharmacol.* 1982;**31**:2371–2380.

Jayaram HN, Lapis E, Calderan CM, Tricot GJ, Hoffman R, Weber G. Biochemistry of a predictive test to select leukemia patients sensitive to tiazofurin treatment. *Proc Am Assoc Cancer Res.* 1988;**29**:16.

Jayaram HN, Pillwein K, Nichols CR, Hoffman R, Weber G. Selective sensitivity to tiazofurin of human leukemic cells. *Biochem Pharmacol.* 1986;**35**:2029–2032.

Lui MS, Faderan MA, Liepnieks JJ, et al. Modulation of IMP dehydrogenase activity and guanylate metabolism by tiazofurin (2-β-D-ribofuranosylthiazole-4-carboxamide). *J Biol Chem.* 1984;**259**:5078–5082.

Melink TJ, Sarosy G, Hanauske AR, et al. Phase I trial and biochemical evaluation of tiazofurin administered on a weekly schedule. *Selective Cancer Ther.* 1990;**6**:51–61.

Melink TJ, Von Hoff DD, Kuhn JG, et al. Phase I evaluation and pharmacokinetics of tiazofurin (2-β-D-ribofuranosylthiazole-4-carboxamide, NSC-286193). *Cancer Res.* 1985;**45**:2859–2865.

O'Dwyer PJ, Shoemaker DD, Jayaram HN, et al. Tiazofurin: A new antitumor agent. *Invest New Drugs.* 1984;**2**:79–84.

Raghaven D, Bishop J, Sampson D, et al. Phase I and pharmacokinetic study of tiazofurin (NSC-286193) administered by 5-day continuous infusion. *Cancer Chemother Pharmacol.* 1986;**16**:160–164.

Rippe DJ, Edwards MK, Schrodt JF, Rosnanno JR, D'Amaris PG, Boyko OR. Reversible cerebral lesions associated with tiazofurin usage, MR demonstration. *J Computer Assisted Tomogr.* 1988;**12**(6):1078–1081.

Roberts JD, Stewart JA, McCormack JJ, et al. Phase I trial of tiazofurin administered by IV bolus daily for 5 days, with pharmacokinetic evaluation. *Cancer Treat Rep.* 1987;**71**:141–149.

Tricot GJ, Jayaram HN, Lapis E, et al. Biochemically directed therapy of leukemia with tiazofurin, a selective blocker of inosine 5′-phosphate dehydrogenase activity. *Cancer Res.* 1989a;**49**:3696–3701.

Tricot GJ, Jayaram HN, Nichols CR, et al. Hematologic and biochemical action of tiazofurin (NSC-286193) in a case of refractory acute myeloid leukemia. *Cancer Res.* 1989b;**47**:4988–4991.

Trump DL, Tutsch KD, Koeller JM, Tormey DC. Phase I clinical study with pharmacokinetic analysis of 2-β-D-ribofuranosyl-thiazole-4-carboxamide, (NSC-286193) administered as a five day infusion. *Cancer Res.* 1985;**45**:2853–2858.

Witkowski JT, Robins RK, Sidwell RW, Simm CN. Design synthesis and broad spectrum antiviral activity of 1-D-ribofuranosyl-1,2,4-triazole-3-carboxamide and related nucleosides. *J Medchem.* 1972;**15**:1150–1154.

Topotecan

■ Other Names

SKF 104864; 10-dimethylaminomethyl-9-hydroxy-camptothecin; NSC-609699.

■ Chemistry

Structure of topotecan

Topotecan is a semisynthetic analog of camptothecin that incorporates a stable basic side chain at the 9-position of the A-ring of 10-hydroxycamptothecin (see figure). The basic side chain of topotecan affords increased aqueous solubility to the compound without requiring hydrolysis of the E-ring lactone. The compound has a molecular weight of 457.9 (the HCl salt) (the free base is 421.53) and the empiric formula $C_{23}H_{23}N_3O_5 \cdot HCl$. Chemically, topotecan is (S)-10-[(dimethylamino)methyl]-4-ethyl-4,9-dihydroxy-1H-pyrano[3′,4′ : 6,7]indolizino[1,2-b]quinoline-3,14-(4H,12H)-dione.

Topotecan was synthesized because clinical trials with a similar compound (sodium camptothecin) showed clinical activity in the late 1960s. In phase I trials of sodium camptothecin involving approximately 50 patients, objective responses were noted in patients with colorectal carcinoma, non-small cell lung cancer, gastric cancer, melanoma, and acute nonlymphocytic leukemia (Gottlieb et al 1970, Muggia et al 1972, Creaven et al 1972). In the initial phase II trials with the agent, 2 partial responses were noted in 61 patients with colorectal cancer (Moertel et al 1972) and no responses were noted in 15 patients with melanoma (Gottlieb and Luce 1972). Additional phase II studies with sodium camptothecin were limited because of unpredictable and severe myelosuppression, gastrointestinal toxicity, and hemorrhagic cystitis. Alopecia was also noted. Clinical trials with sodium camptothecin were eventually discontinued because of these unpredictable toxic effects (myelosuppression and cystitis); however, interest in the camptothecin derivatives has remained high because of the responses noted in the early studies (Von Hoff et al 1977).

Camptothecin is isolated from *Camptotheca acuminata,* an ornamental tree found in the Peoples Republic of China. As the toxic effects of this agent were felt to be caused by its poor aqueous solubility, Kingsbury et al (1989) synthesized topotecan, which had increased aqueous solubility and an intact E-ring lactone, the active portion of the drug. It also retained its antitumor activity in vivo (Tuhnjun et al 1989).

Compared with sodium camptothecin, topotecan has increased hydrophilicity and is water soluble at an acidic pH. Therefore, topotecan is expected to have decreased potential for bladder toxicity.

■ Antitumor Activity

Topotecan has a very broad spectrum of antitumor activity in a variety of in vivo animal models. Topotecan has comparable antitumor activity when administered orally, intravenously, intraperitoneally, and subcutaneously. Topotecan produced over a 95% increase in life span (ILS) at its maximally tolerated dose (MTD) in the following intraperitoneally implanted murine tumor models: P-388 leukemia, L-1210 leukemia, B-16 melanoma, B-16 melanoma/F10 subline, and M-5076 reticulum cell sarcoma. It is active in B-16 melanoma refractory to sodium camptothecin. In addition, the agent is quite active against human tumor colony-forming cells (Burris et al 1990).

Topotecan is still an investigational agent undergoing phase I/II clinical trials. Nonetheless, in these early trials, responses have been noted in patients with non-small cell lung cancer, ovarian cancer, and esophageal cancer (Recondo et al 1991, Rowinsky et al 1991, Wall et al 1990, 1991, Sirott et al 1991).

Additional phase II trial information is necessary to determine the spectrum of antitumor activity of this compound.

■ Mechanism of Action

Like camptothecin, topotecan is a specific inhibitor of topoisomerase I (Kingsbury et al 1989). Cellular pharmacology studies have shown that the compound is a more selective inhibitor of topoisomerase I than is sodium camptothecin. It has been established unequivocally that the biologic activity of these compounds is due solely to inhibition of topoisomerase I, which causes single-strand breaks in DNA. This results in lethal DNA damage during the course of DNA replication. Topoisomerase I has been demonstrated to be intimately involved in DNA replication as it relieves the torsional strain introduced ahead of the moving replication fork.

Against the purified enzyme, camptothecin is three- to fourfold more potent as an inhibitor of topoisomerase I than is topotecan. Both compounds inhibit the enzyme by an identical mechanism; they stabilize the covalent complex of enzyme and strand-cleaved DNA which is an intermediate of the catalytic mechanism. The compounds have no binding affinity for either DNA or topoisomerase I, but bind with measurable affinity to the enzyme–DNA complex. Stabilization of the "cleavable complex" by camptothecin and topotecan is completely analogous to the inhibition of topoisomerase II by the epipodophyllotoxin glycosides and various intercalators.

Neither camptothecin nor topotecan has any effect on topoisomerase II. The stabilization of the topoisomerase I "cleavable complex" by camptothecin or topotecan is readily reversible. It has been demonstrated by high-performance liquid chromatography and nuclear magnetic resonance techniques that topotecan (and presumably camptothecin) undergoes a pH-dependent hydrolysis of the E-ring lactone (see figure on page 916).

The slow reaction kinetics indicates that only the closed lactone form of the drug is active at stabilizing the topoisomerase I-cleaved DNA complex. This observation provides some rationale for the observed high degree of activity of topotecan at low pH. Tumor cells, particularly hypoxic cells prevalent in solid neoplasms, have reduced intracellular pH (Wike-Hooley et al 1985). At pH below 7.0, the closed form of topotecan predominates and more than 80% of the lactone is presented at pH 6.0. Thus, in such cells, the drug will be more effective inhibiting topoisomerase I than in cells having higher intracellular pH. This also provides a rationale for enhancing the activity of topotecan by modulating intracellular pH in tumor cell populations. The hydrolysis of the E-ring lactone at alkaline pH also likely has a major impact on the pharmacokinetics of topotecan, as will be discussed further later.

pH-dependent hydrolysis of topotecan

■ Availability and Storage

The lyophilized formulation of topotecan is investigationally supplied by the Division of Cancer Treatment, National Cancer Institute, Bethesda, Maryland. It is manufactured by Smith Kline, Beecham Laboratories and is supplied as an injection in 5-mg vials (as the base) with 100 mg of mannitol. The pH is adjusted to 3.0 with HCl/NaOH. The lyophilized powder is light yellow in color. The intact vials should be stored under refrigeration (2–8°C).

■ Preparation for Use, Stability, and Admixture

A 5-mg vial is reconstituted with 2 mL of Sterile Water for Injection, USP. This yields a solution containing 2.5 mg of topotecan as the base and 50 mg of Mannitol, USP/mL.

A shelf-life surveillance study of the intact vials is ongoing. The single-use lyophilized dosage form contains no antibacterial preservatives, and it is advised that the reconstituted solution be discarded 8 hours after initial entry. To ensure stability and solubility of topotecan for infusions in the clinic, the drug should be diluted with D5W. This is particularly pertinent when one considers the slow conversion of topotecan to the E-ring hydrolyzed carboxylate which occurs at physiologic pH. At equilibrium, the ratio of open-ring form to lactone is greater than 4:1 at pH 7.0. Hydrolysis of the lactone will not occur if the drug is kept in an acid environment. It is entirely likely that some of the unpredictability in the toxicity seen in clinical trials of sodium camptothecin may have resulted from lack of control over infusion of the drug formulation so that the lactone form of camptothecin, which is 10-fold more toxic than sodium camptothecin in mice, may have formed prior to injection. This may have been exacerbated by the virtual aqueous insolubility of the lactone form of camptothecin. Topotecan, preformulated as the E-ring hydrolyzed sodium salt, retains activity in mice as it will equilibrate with the active closed form in vivo. The open form is three- to fourfold less potent in vivo, possibly because of an observed increase in clearance.

■ Administration

Topotecan is administered intravenously. As the compound is still undergoing phase I trials, the optimal method of administration has not yet been determined. Options for administration studied have so far included a 30-minute infusion every 3 weeks, a 30-minute infusion daily × 5 every 3 weeks, a 24-hour infusion every 3 weeks, a 120-hour infusion every 3 weeks, and a 72-hour infusion repeated every 3 weeks.

■ Special Precautions

The pH of the infusion solution must be as acidic as possible (D5W) to maintain topotecan in its active form. Topotecan can cause severe myelosuppression.

■ Drug Interactions

Filgrastim administered concurrently with topotecan resulted in enhanced neutropenia and thrombocytopenia (Rowinsky et al 1992). The administration of filgrastim after topotecan was superior to concurrent administration at lessening neutropenia. Nonetheless, 5 µg/kg filgrastim does not allow for a significant dose escalation of topotecan on the daily ×5 schedule (Rowinsky et al 1992, Murphy et al 1992).

Hyperthermia does not enhance the experimental cytotoxic activity of topotecan in FSaII fibrosarcoma cells in vitro (Herman et al 1992).

The combination of topotecan with the topoisomerase II inhibitor etoposide results in synergistic growth inhibition in human tumor colony-forming assays in vitro (Anzai et al 1992a). The optimal ratio of etoposide to topotecan was 0.2 in this experimental cell culture study. Synergistic cytotoxicity is also reported for topotecan and 2'-deoxy-5-azacytidine in five human tumor cell lines in vitro (Anzai et al 1992b).

■ Dosage

The table below outlines the schedules and doses used in phase I studies. At the time of this writing these are active studies and the final recommended doses may change.

The dose-limiting toxic effect in the preceding studies has been myelosuppression (mostly neutropenia). The dose-limiting toxic effect of neutropenia prevented escalation of topotecan doses above 2.5 mg/m^2/d × 5 days (Rowinsky et al 1992). A 3-day continuous infusion schedule has also been recommended as a means of increasing topotecan dose intensity. Doses up to 1.6 mg/m^2/d have been evaluated in this regimen (Eckardt et al 1992).

■ Pharmacokinetics

Topotecan undergoes pH-dependent reversible hydrolysis of the lactone ring, yielding the open carboxylate form (see figure on the opposite page). Only the lactone form is active as an inhibitor of topoisomerase I. The quantitation of the lactone and carboxylate forms is determined by a specific and sensitive (2 ng/mL) reverse-phase high-performance liquid chromatography (HPLC) assay with a fluorometric detection technique (Kuhn et al 1990, Tong et al 1991). Using a rapid HPLC method for the lactone form, investigators have observed that the pharmacokinetic data fit a two-compartment model (Sirott et al 1991, Rowinsky et al 1991, Wall et al 1991, Kuhn et al 1990). The lactone form is the predominant form during the infusion but inactive hydrolysis products may form with 50% conversion to the open ring form within 15 minutes of infusion (Kuhn et al 1990). Preliminary pharmacokinetic data have been obtained on the various schedules (see table on page 918).

Renal excretion appears to be the major route of elimination (Wall et al 1991, Kuhn et al 1990). Renal clearance accounts for 70% of the drug's clearance (Rowinsky et al 1991). Preliminary studies using a thermal spray/mass spectrometry technique for urine indicate demethylatation as a possible metabolic pathway (Recondo et al 1991).

■ Side Effects and Toxicity

In all schedules tested to date, the dose-limiting toxic effect has been neutropenia (Sirott et al 1991, Wall et al 1990, 1991, Rowinsky et al 1991, Recondo

TOPOTECAN DOSES IN CLINICAL TRIALS

Schedule	Range of Doses (mg/m^2/d)	Recommended Phase II Dose	Reference
30-min infusion every 3 wk	2.5–22.5	17.5	Wall et al 1990, 1991
30-min infusion daily × 5 every 3 wk	0.5–2.5	1.5 with escalation to 2.0	Rowinsky et al 1991, Sirott et al 1991
24-h infusion every 3 wk	1.9–5.0	4.0	Recondo et al 1991
	0.5–2.0	1.5	Haas et al 1992
	2.5–10.5	8 h*	Ten Bokkel Huinink et al 1992
	3–7.5	5.5*	Cole et al 1992
(in children)	1–2	1.5	Haas et al 1992

*Maximally tolerated dose.

CLINICAL PHARMACOLOGY STUDIES OF TOPOTECAN

Schedule	Dose (mg/m²)	AUC (ng·min/mL)	Steady-State Volume of Distribution	Half-life (min) α	Half-life (min) β	Clearance (mL/min/m²)	Peak Plasma Level (Lactone)	Comments	Reference
30-min infusion daily × 5	1.5	1473* (1212–1719)	186* (125–257)	9* (2.6–16.6)	103	2080† (1221–2459)	NR‡	Lactone form	Sirott et al 1991
30-min infusion	15	NR			186		417 ng/mL	Lactone form	Wall et al 1991
30-min infusion	1.5–2	NR	20.7 (day 1) 40.3 (day 5)	3.3	80	630	15–209 nmol/L	Lactone form	Rowinsky et al 1991
24-h infusion	8.4	NR	NR	120	480	NR	20 ng/mL	—	Ten Bokkel Huinink et al 1992
24-h infusion	3–7.5	NR	NR	NR	144	441	6.4–30.7 nM	Parent (topotean)	Cole et al 1992

*Mean
†Median
‡NR, not reported.

et al 1991). Thrombocytopenia and anemia have also been noted. Other toxic effects include mild nausea and vomiting in one third of patients, fever of 101°F or greater in one third of patients, occasional diarrhea, and mild flulike symptoms.

Hemorrhagic cystitis, a dose-limiting toxic effect of camptothecin, has not been observed; however, microscopic hematuria has been seen in 12% of patients (Wall et al 1991, Recondo et al 1991).

■ Special Applications

Although only studied in preclinical models, topotecan may be radiation sensitized (Battern et al 1990).

REFERENCES

Anzai H, Frost P, Abbruzzese JL. Synergistic cytotoxicity with combined inhibition of topoisomerase (Topo) I and II. *Proc Am Assoc Cancer Res.* 1992a;**33**:431.

Anzai H, Frost P, Abbruzzese JL. Synergestic cytotoxicity with 2'-deoxy-5-aracytidine and topotecan in vitro and in vivo. *Cancer Res.* 1992b;**52**:2180–2185.

Battern MB, Hofmann GA, McCabe FL, Johnson RK. Synergistic killing by ionizing radiation and topoisomerase I inhibitor SK&F 104864. *Proc Am Assoc Cancer Res.* 1990;**31**:436.

Burris H, Kuhn J, Johnson R, Von Hoff D. SKF 104864: Preclinical studies of a new topoisomerase I inhibitor. *Proc Am Assoc Cancer Res.* 1990;**31**:431.

Cole D, Blaney S, Balis F, et al. A phase I and pharmacokinetic study of topotecan in pediatric patients. *Proc Am Soc Clin Oncol.* 1992;**11**:116.

Creaven PJ, Allen LM, Muggia FM. Plasma camptothecin (NSC-100880) levels during a 5-day course of treatment: Relation to dose and toxicity. *Cancer Chemother Rep.* 1972;**56**:573–578.

Eckardt J, Burris H, Kuhn J, et al. Phase I and pharmacokinetic trial of continuous infusion topotecan in patients with refractory solid tumors. *Proc Am Soc Clin Oncol.* 1992;**11**:138.

Gottlieb JA, Guarino AM, Call JB, et al. Preliminary pharmacologic and clinical evaluation of camptothecin sodium (NSC-100880). *Cancer Chemother Rep.* 1970;**54**:461–470.

Gottlieb JA, Luce LK. Treatment of malignant melanoma with camptothecin (NSC-100880). *Cancer Chemother Rep.* 1972;**56**:103–105.

Haas NB, LaCreta FP, Walczak J, et al. Phase I/pharmacokinetic trial of topotecan on a weekly 24-hour infusional schedule. *Proc Am Assoc Cancer Res.* 1992;**33**:523.

Herman TS, Khandakar V, Korbut T, et al. Cytotoxicity, tumor cell survival and tumor growth delay with camptothecin or topotecan under hyperthermic conditions alone or with cisplatin. *Proc Am Assoc Cancer Res.* 1992;**33**:499.

Kingsbury WD, Hertzberg RP, Beuhm TC, et al. Clinical synthesis and structure–activity relationships related to SKF 104864, a novel water-soluble analog of camptothecin. *Proc Am Assoc Cancer Res.* 1989;**30**:622.

Kuhn J, Burris S, Wall J, et al. Pharmacokinetics of the topoisomerase I inhibitor SK&F104864. *Proc Am Soc Clin Oncol.* 1990;**9**:70.

Moertel CG, Schutt AJ, Reitemeier RJ, Hahn RG. Phase II study of camptothecin (NSC-100880) in the treatment of advanced gastrointestinal cancer. *Cancer Chemother Rep.* 1972;**56**:95–101.

Muggia FM, Creaven PJ, Hansen HH, et al. Phase I clinical trial of weekly and daily treatment with camptothecin (NSC-100880): Correlation with preclinical studies. *Cancer Chemother Rep.* 1972;**56**:515–521.

Murphy B, Saltz L, Sirott M, et al. Granulocyte-colony stimulating factor (G-CSF) does not increase the maximum tolerated dose (MTD) in a phase I study of topotecan (T). *Proc Am Soc Clin Oncol.* 1992;**11**:139.

Recondo C, Abbruzzese J, Newman B, et al. A phase I trial of topotecan (TOPO) administered by a 24 hour infusion. *Proc Am Assoc Cancer Res.* 1991;**32**:206.

Rowinsky E, Grochow L, Hendricks C, et al. Phase I and pharmacologic study of topotecan (SK&F104864): A novel topoisomerase I inhibitor. *Proc Am Soc Clin Oncol.* 1991;**10**:93.

Rowinsky E, Sartorius S, Grochow L, et al. Phase I & pharmacologic study of topotecan, an inhibitor of topoisomerase I, with granulocyte colony-stimulating factor (G-CSF): Toxicologic differences between concurrent & post-treatment G-CSF administration. *Proc Am Soc Clin Oncol.* 1992;**11**:116.

Sirott MN, Saltz L, Young C, et al. Phase I and clinical pharmacologic study of intravenous topotecan. *Proc Am Soc Clin Oncol.* 1991;**10**:104.

Ten Bokkel Huinink WW, Rodenhuis S, Beijnen J. Phase I study of the topoisomerase I inhibitor topotecan (SK&F 104864-A). *Proc Am Soc Clin Oncol.* 1992;**11**:110.

Tong W, Saltz L, Sirott M, et al. Rapid HPLC assay for topotecan. *Proc Am Assoc Cancer Res.* 1991;**32**:433.

Tuhnjun RK, McCabe L, Fancetto LF, et al. SKF104864, a water soluble analog of camptothecin with broad-spectrum activity in preclinical tumor models. *Proc Am Assoc Cancer Res.* 1989;**30**:623.

Von Hoff DD, Rozencweig M, Soper WT, et al. Commentary: Whatever happened to NSC ———? *Cancer Treat Rep.* 1977;**81**:759–768.

Wall D, Burris H, Rudriguez G, et al. Phase I trial of topotecan (SK&F104864) in patients with refractory solid tumors. *Proc Am Soc Clin Oncol.* 1991;**10**:98.

Wall D, Harlin K, Burris H, et al. Phase I study of SK&F104864, a novel topoisomerase I inhibitor. *Proc Am Soc Clin Oncol.* 1990;**9**:86.

Wike-Hooley JL, Van Den Berg AP, Van Der Zee J, Reinhold HS. Human tumor pH and its variation. *Eur J Cancer Clin Oncol.* 1985;**7**:785–791.

Toremifene

■ Other Names

Toremifene; Fc-1157a.

■ Chemistry

Structure of toremifene

Toremifene is a triphenylethylene derivative related to tamoxifen that has potent antiestrogenic activity in both in vitro and in vivo models (Kallio et al 1986, Kangas et al 1986). The complete chemical name is 4-chloro-1,2-diphenyl-1-{4-[2-(N,N-dimethylamino)-ethoxy]phenyl}-1-butene. As tamoxifen has not only an antiestrogenic effect but also estrogenic effects, the question has been whether those estrogenic effects are harmful. Toremifene was designed to have improved antiestrogenic effects and less of an estrogenic effect (Zaccheo et al 1986).

■ Antitumor Activity

Toremifene has been documented to have antitumor activity in patients with advanced estrogen receptor (ER)-positive breast cancer. In 46 postmenopausal women with ER-positive breast cancer (without prior hormonal or cytotoxic therapy), Valavaara and colleagues (1988) found that toremifene at a dose of 60 mg per day resulted in 17% complete and 26% partial response rates. Median response durations ranged from 15.5 to 21.6 months. Soft tissue and visceral masses appeared to respond equally well. Bone metastases appeared to respond less favorably. Of note is that levels of ERs and progesterone receptors measured on the primary or metastatic breast lesions did not appear to correlate with response. Higher doses of the drug are currently being explored.

■ Mechanism of Action

Toremifene is believed to work because of its ability to compete with estrogen for estrogen binding sites. The agent was developed because it appears to have less intrinsic estrogenic activity than does tamoxifen. In rat DMBA models, toremifene is synergistic with progestational agents, whereas tamoxifen is not. Of note is that toremifene has demonstrated antitumor activity against the ER-negative uterine sarcoma in mice, indicating the drug may have some cytotoxic effects not mediated via the antiestrogenic activities (Kangas et al 1986). Toremifene also manifests a dose-dependent antitumor effect seen only at high concentrations of tamoxifen.

In ER-negative human breast cancer cells, toremifene produces a dose-dependent cell cycle arrest in G_0–G_1, reducing the number of cells entering S phase (Wiebe et al 1992).

■ Availability and Storage

Toremifene is available as an investigational agent from Adria Laboratories, Columbus, Ohio. Toremifene is supplied as tablets of 10, 20, 60, and 200 mg, with 50 or 100 tablets per bottle.

■ Preparation for Use, Stability, and Admixture

No preparation for use is necessary. The shelf-life at room temperature is 3 years.

■ Administration

The optimal dose of toremifene has not yet been established. In the only phase II study reported to date, an oral dose of 60 mg per day was used (Valavaara et al 1988). The drug should be given once each morning prior to breakfast, as a single dose on an empty stomach.

■ Special Precautions

To date, none have been necessary.

■ Drug Interactions

Toremifene can modulate multidrug resistance (MDR) in tumor cells that express the P-glycoprotein (DeGregorio et al 1989). Doxorubicin resistance can be overcome in nude mice bearing multidrug-resistant human breast cancer cells (Baker et al 1992). The modulating activity is shared by the major toremifene metabolites, N-desmethyltoremi-

STEADY-STATE LEVELS OF TOREMIFINE AND MAJOR TOREMIFENE METABOLITES

Daily Dose (mg)	Mean Steady-State Level (μg/mL)		
	Toremifene	Desmethyltoremifene	4-Hydroxytoremifene
10	0.14	0.47	—
20	0.28	0.99	—
40	0.31	1.35	—
60	0.88	3.06	—
200	1.41	5.94	0.44
400	3.45	11.9	0.89

*Data from DeGregorio et al 1989.

fene and 4-hydroxytoremifene. This activity is not related to antiestrogenic activity, but can be achieved at pharmacologic dose levels (Wiebe et al 1992).

■ Dosage

See Administration.

■ Pharmacokinetics

In female volunteers, the drug is well absorbed after oral administration after doses from 3 to 680 mg. Peak serum levels are recorded in 4 hours. The elimination half-life for the drug is approximately 5 days (Wiebe et al 1990). The pharmacokinetics was not dose dependent. At a dose of 60 mg/d, a steady state was reached in 6 weeks. The mean steady-state concentration is 0.6 μg/mL. There is a dose-dependent increase in steady-state levels of parent drug and the major metabolites which are probably active (see table). The time to steady state is also dose dependent: 1 week at greater than 200 mg/d and 3 weeks at doses less than 60 mg/d. Most of the drug is excreted in the feces (70%) over 2 weeks with an apparent enterohepatic circulation. The primary metabolites in patients include the N-desmethyl, deaminohydroxy, and 4-hydroxy derivatives of toremifene. These metabolites are active at reversing multidrug resistance to doxorubicin in vitro (Wiebe et al 1992). Toremifene is nearly 100% bound to serum proteins (albumin) (Wiebe et al 1990).

■ Side Effects and Toxicity

Phase I experience with the compound has only been published in abstract form (Kivinen and Maenpaa 1986). In normal volunteers, the drug was well tolerated at doses up to 460 mg/d as a single oral dose or orally daily for 5 consecutive days. When administered daily for 5 days at doses of 220 to 680 mg, toremifene caused a modest decrease in antithrombin III blood levels and a moderate decrease in serum follicle-stimulating hormone and luteinizing hormone levels. At 680 mg/d, one patient reported vertigo and a second reported vertigo and nausea.

In phase II studies at a dose of 60 mg daily, the side effects were characterized as mild and transient (Valavaara et al 1988). Sweating/hot flashes were the most common symptoms reported, with one patient experiencing tremors. Other toxic effects (in 2 or 3 of the 36 patients) included leukopenia, nausea, sleep disturbance, anorexia, epigastric pain, and muscle stiffness.

■ Special Applications

None are reported.

REFERENCES

Baker J, Wiebe S, Koester V, et al. Toremifene (Tor) enhances doxorubicin (Dox) accumulation, inhibits protein kinase-C (PKC) activity, increases PKC message, and enhances cytotoxicity in a tumor-bearing multidrug resistant nude mouse model. *Proc Am Soc Clin Oncol.* 1992;**11**:109.

DeGregorio MW, Ford JM, Benz CC, et al. Toremifene:Pharmacologic and pharmacokinetic basis of reversing multidrug resistance. *J Clin Oncol.* 1989;7(9):1359–1364.

Kallio S, Kangas L, Blanco G, et al. A new triphenylethylene compound, Fc-1157a. *Cancer Chemother Pharmacol.* 1986;**17**:103–108.

Kangas L, Nieminen A-L, Blanco G, et al. A new triphenylethylene compound, Fc-11578a. II. Antitumor effects. *Cancer chemother Pharmacol.* 1986;**17**:109–113.

Kivinen S, Maenpaa J. Effect of toremifene on clinical, hematological, and hormonal parameters in different dose levels in phase I study (Abstract 2994). *Int Cancer Congress, Budapest.* 1986:778.

Valavaara R, Pyrhonen S, Heikkinen M, et al. Toremifene, a new antiestrogenic compound, for treatment of advanced breast cancer. Phase II study. *Eur J Cancer Clin Oncol.* 1988;**24**:785–790.

Wiebe VJ, Benz CC, Shemano I, et al. Pharmacokinetics of toremifene and its metabolites in patients with advanced breast cancer: A multicenter phase I pharmacokinetic trial. *Cancer Chemother Pharmacol.* 1990;**25**:247–251.

Wiebe V, Koester S, Lindberg M, et al. Toremifene and its metabolites enhance doxorubicin accumulation in estrogen receptor negative multidrug resistant human breast cancer cells. *Invest New Drugs.* 1992;**10**:63–71.

Zaccheo T, Ornati G, diSalle E. Antiestrogenic and antitumor properties of the new triphenylethylene derivative toremifene in the rat (abstract 2996). *Int Cancer Congress, Budapest.* 1986:778.

Tretinoin

■ Other Names

All-*trans*-retinoic acid; tRA; Ro 1–5488 (Roche Laboratories); Retin-A® (Ortho Pharmaceutical Corporation).

■ Chemistry

Structure of tretinoin®

All-*trans*-retinoic acid (3,7-dimethyl-9-(2,6,6-trimethyl-1-cyclohexen-1-yl)-2,4,6,8-nonatetraenoic acid) is a natural retinoid metabolite of retinol (vitamin A). The all-*trans* molecule is the naturally occurring form of retinoic acid formed from the breakdown of β-carotene by enterocytes (Napoli 1986). Retinoic acid may also be formed from the metabolism of retinol and retinaldehyde by NAD aldehyde dehydrogenases (Lee et al 1990).

trans-Retinoic acid (tRA) is highly lipophilic and has a molecular weight of 300.42. The molecular formula is $C_{20}H_{28}O_2$.

■ Antitumor Activity

In preclinical studies, tRA can induce normal differentiation in a variety of malignant cell lines, especially myeloblastic leukemia cells (Breitman et al 1980, 1981, 1983, Koeffler and Amatruda 1985). Other tumor cell lines sensitive to tRA in vitro include neuroblastoma (Sidell 1982, Sidell et al 1983), teratocarcinoma (Strickland and Mahdavi 1978, Dmitrovsky et al 1990), and melanoma (Lotan and Lotan 1980, Meyskens and Fuller 1980).

The differentiating effects of tRA can be additive or synergistic in vitro with a wide number of other agents including cytotoxic drugs such as cytarabine (Hassan and Rees 1988), polar solvents such as dimethylsulfoxide (Breitman and He 1990), and cytokines such as interferon gamma (Peck and Bollag 1991, Hemmi and Breitman 1987) or alfa (Higuchi et al 1991, Peck and Bollag 1991), tumor necrosis factor and both filgrastim and sargramostim (Peck and Bollag 1991, Hemmi et al 1989, Santini et al 1989, Colombat et al 1991). (See Drug Interactions for a more complete listing).

trans-Retinoic acid also induces direct growth inhibition without differentiation in a wide variety of malignant cell types (see table on opposite page). This growth inhibitory activity requires retinoic acid receptors (Robertson et al 1991) and is significantly greater for tRA compared with *cis*-retinoic acid (cRA) (Crouch and Helman 1991). In human tumor colony-forming assays of various solid tumor types, only about 10 to 20% of individual cancers were sensitive to tRA in vitro (Cowan et al 1983). In contrast, there is nearly universal differentiation of acute promyelocytic leukemia cells to normal myelocytes following tRA exposure.

A large number of clinical trials have been performed with tRA in patients with hematologic malignancies, particularly acute promyelocytic leukemia (APL), or the M3 leukemia subtype in the FAB classification system (as reviewed by Stone and Mayer 1990). This disease is associated with a characteristic chromosomal translocation between the long arm of chromosome 15 and the region of the long arm of chromosome 7 coding for the nuclear retinoic acid receptor α (Larson et al 1984) (see Mechanism of Action). tRA produces high complete remission rates in APL of up to 95 to 100% (Warrell et al 1991, Chen et al 1991, Castaigne et al 1990, Menger et al 1988). Importantly, tRA therapy is not associated with the consumptive coagulopathy associated with cytotoxic agents in APL. Indeed, fi-

GROWTH INHIBITION OF HUMAN TUMOR CELLS BY TRANS-RETINOIC ACID IN VITRO

Tumor Type	Reference
Acute myelogenous leukemia	Lawrence et al 1987, Findley et al 1986
Neuroblastoma	Sidell et al 1983, Reynolds et al 1991
Breast carcinoma	Marth et al 1986, Fontana 1987, Lotan 1979, LaCroix and Lippman 1980, Halter et al 1988
Lung cancer, small cell and non-small cell	Doyle et al 1989, Munker et al 1987
Melanoma	Lotan 1979
Chondrosarcoma, osteosarcoma	Thein and Lotan 1982
Prostate cancer	Peehl et al 1991
Rhabdomyosarcoma	Crouch et al 1990
Squamous cell carcinoma	Jetten et al 1990, Sacks et al 1989

Data from Smith et al 1992.

brinogen levels normalize in most patients receiving tRA. Responses to oral tRA are obtained gradually over a 1- to 2-month period of treatment. Unfortunately, these responses are not long-lived and the cells retain the t(15:17) translocation despite continued tRA therapy. Remission durations range from 2 to 13+ months (Castaigne et al 1990) and may actually be decreased with maintenance cytotoxic chemotherapy regimens that include continued tRA therapy (Chen et al 1991). This contrasts with reports of enhanced remission duration for maintenance regimens that alternate cytotoxic chemotherapy courses with tRA (Sun et al 1990).

Acute myelogenous leukemia blast cells are only partially responsive to tRA therapy. A complete response was observed in 1 of 41 pediatric patients (Bell et al 1991). Limited experience with the cRA isomer suggests its activity is similarly poor in acute myelogenous leukemia when used as a single agent in an elderly population (Hoffman and Robinson 1988) or in combination with low-dose cytarabine (Kramer et al 1991). (See *Isotretinoin* monograph).

Topical tRA produces partial or complete regression of basal cell carcinoma in most patients (Epstein 1986). Topical cRA is similarly effective in this disease (Sankowski et al 1987). Experimentally, topical tRA is occasionally active in local control of malignant melanoma (Levine and Meyskens 1980) and at reducing cervical intraepithelial dysplasia (Surwit et al 1982). In another pilot trial, topical tRA gel was effective at reducing the size of cutaneous lesions in seven of eight patients with AIDS-related Kaposi's sarcoma (Bonhomme et al 1991).

■ Mechanism of Action

trans-Retinoic acid is one of several natural retinoids that have diverse differentiating effects on cells. These effects include a role in normal morphogenesis, hematopoiesis, and immune function. Retinoid effects are mediated via two types of retinoic acid cytosolic receptors, CRABP-I and CRABP-II, which are distinct from those for retinol (Chytil and Ong 1984). The binding proteins appear to mediate the transfer of tRA from the cytosol to the nucleus (Takase et al 1986). The CRABPs may also act as a cytosolic storage site for retinoic acid as noted by the loss of retinoic acid activity when CRABPs are overexpressed (Boylan and Gudas 1991). Although CRABP may be required for normal morphogenesis during embryologic development, they are not absolutely required for the differentiating (antitumor) effects of retinoids in myeloid leukemia cells (Breitman et al 1983).

In the nucleus there are three types of retinoic acid receptors (RARs α, β, and γ) which are members of the steroid–thyroid type of nuclear receptors (Petkovich et al 1987). The nuclear RARs control gene transcription by directly interacting with DNA sequences termed *retinoic acid response elements*. These elements regulate the transcription of a number of genes involved in cellular growth inhibition and differentiation (Smith et al 1992). These include the genes for laminin, a cytoskeletal protein, growth hormone, transglutaminase, osteocalcin, the genes for other retinoid response elements such as RAR-β and RABP-II, and promoter genes for a variety of embryonal proteins (as reviewed by Smith et al 1992).

Of interest, the chromosomal breakpoint in

APL cells occurs at the region of chromosome 17 associated with the first intron for RAR-α (Borrow et al 1990). This results in the expression of abnormal messenger RNA transcripts for RAR-α in patients with APL (Miller et al 1990). APL patients entering complete remission show markedly decreased levels of aberrant RAR-α with tRA therapy (Warrell et al 1991).

At a cellular level, retinoic acid affects morphogenesis by controlling limb bud development (Tickle et al 1982). Unfortunately this property creates a powerful teratogenic potential for exogenous retinoids when used in pregnant females.

Retinoid effects on immune function and normal hermatopoiesis have been extensively studied. Retinoic acid is known to enhance both humoral antibody responses to different antigens (Jurin and Tannock 1972), and T-lymphocyte proliferation and activation (Eccles 1985). There is also evidence of enhanced phagocytosis by macrophages (Dillehay et al 1988), augmentation of interleukin-2 receptors on thymocytes (Sidell and Ramsdell 1988), and an increase in interleukin-2-induced tumor-infiltrating lymphocytes (Lin and Chu 1990).

The hematopoietic differentiating effect of retinoic acid is observed at concentrations as low as 10 to 30 nmol/L, but typically much higher levels of 100 to 1000 nmol/L are required (Breitman et al 1980, Sidell and Ramsdell 1988). In HL-60 promyelocytic leukemia cells, retinoic acid treatment for 4 days causes cells to attain most morphologic features of normal mature granulocytes, except secondary granule formation (Koeffler and Amatruda 1985, Imaizumi and Breitman 1987). Functionally, these retinoic acid-treated cells increase superoxide anion formation associated with normal antibacterial potential. Growth is also inhibited commensurate with the differentiating effect (Breitman et al 1980). These same retinoid effects are noted in leukemia cells from patients with APL (Breitman et al 1981, Flynn et al 1986).

The differentiating activity of retinoic acid in lymphoid cancer cells as well as in solid tumors may relate to the production of transforming growth factor β (TGF-β) (Smith et al 1992). TGF-β includes a family of proteins that are potent inhibitors of epithelial cell growth, including lung trachea, breast, ovary, skin, prostate, and lymphoid/myeloid cell types. Cell death from retinoic acid-induced TFG-β may be in turn mediated by apoptosis, or programmed cell death. This normal cell-suicide process is believed to involve the activation of endogenous endonucleases by Ca^{2+} or Mg^{2+}, leading to DNA degradation followed by cell death. The causal link between retinoic acid, TFG-β, and apoptosis is thus far limited to events in embryogenesis; however, it may nonetheless be involved in mediating some of the antitumor effects of tRA, especially in epithelial cells.

■ Availability and Storage

All-*trans*-retinoic acid has been investigationally supplied in 10-mg soft gelatin capsules from Roche Laboratories, Nutley, New Jersey, and from Second Shanghai Medical University, Shanghai, China. The capsules are stored at room temperature and should be protected from light.

A topical solution of β-tRA, tretinoin (Retin-A®), is commercially available from Ortho Pharmaceutical Corporation, Dermatological Division, Raritan, New Jersey. It is supplied as a 0.05% (w/v) solution or gel and a 0.05 or 0.1% (w/v) hydrophilic cream. The cream base contains stearic acid, isopropyl myristate polyoxyl 40 stearate, stearyl alcohol, xantham gum, sorbic acid, and butylated hydroxytoluene (BHT) as an antioxidant. The gel formulation also contains BHT, 90% alcohol (w/w), and hydroxypropyl cellulose. The liquid formulation contains BHT, polyethylene glycol 400, and 55% (w/v) alcohol.

■ Administration

In APL, tRA is administered orally. For malignant melanoma, the drug has been investigationally applied topically (Levine and Meyskens 1980). In this trial, one drop of 0.05% β-tRA solution (Retin-A®) was applied topically to each lesion once daily for up to 12 weeks. The site was covered with occlusive tape (Blenderm®) after each application (Levine and Meyskens 1980). An investigational collagen sponge delivery device was used to treat cervical dysplasia with β-tRA in one trial (Surwit et al 1982). A topical 1% gel formulation of β-tRA has also been used to treat cutaneous lesions in patients with Kaposi's sarcoma (Bonhomme et al 1991).

■ Dosage

The most common dose in APL is 45 mg/m²/d, with the daily dose split into two fractions administered in the morning and 6 hours later (Warrell et al 1991). Oral doses of APL are administered daily for up to 90 days (Castaigne et al 1990). Trials in China have used fixed doses of 60 to 80 mg/d given continuously until a complete remission is obtained (Chen et al 1991). A higher dose range of 45 to 100 mg/m²/d does not appear to produce any higher response rate in APL (Meng-er et al 1988). Maintenance doses of tRA are rarely used. They are given after a complete response is obtained and doses have ranged from 20 to 30 mg/m²/d (Meng-er et al 1988). A pilot study in children with refractory hematologic malignancies has recommended a tRA dose of 60 mg/m²/d (Smith et al 1992).

■ Drug Interactions

Synergistic or additive differentiating effects in vitro have been described for a number of tRA combinations. The table below summarizes the tRA combinations that have been examined in human AML or HL-60 leukemic cells in vitro. These combinations appear to increase the sensitivity of AML cells to the differentiating effects of tRA. In addition, the concentrations of tRA required for differentiation are lowered when combinations are used. This has been noted both for cytotoxic agents such as cytarabine (Chomienne et al 1986) and for a diverse group of cytokines including filgrastim, sargramostim, tumor necrosis factor α, and interferons alfa and gamma (see table). Clinical trials to evaluate these combinations are currently underway. The goals of these trials are to prolong remission durations significantly and use lower and less toxic tRA doses.

■ Pharmacokinetics

trans-Retinoic acid, derived from dietary retinol, is normally found in the body at concentrations of approximately 10 to 20 nmol/mL (Napoli et al 1985). These physiologic levels are highly bound nonspecifically to albumin. About 95% of tRA is bound in the plasma, with only trace amounts found in high-density or low-density lipoproteins (Muindi et al 1992).

Following a single oral tRA dose of 45 mg/m², peak plasma levels of approximately 347 ng/mL (approximately $10^{-6}M$) are achieved within 1 to 2 hours. The median time to a peak of 0.4 µg/mL was 90 minutes in another pharmacokinetic study of oral

TRANS RETINOIC ACID DRUG COMBINATIONS SHOWING ENHANCED DIFFERENTIATING ACTIVITY IN HUMAN LEUKEMIC CELLS IN VITRO

Agents Combined with tRA	Cell Type	Reference
Polar solvents		
Dimethylsulfoxide		Breitman and He 1990
Hexamethylene bisacetamide (HMBA)		Breitman and He 1990
Dimethylformamide + dactinomycin	AML*	Hassan and Rees 1990
Cytotoxic agents		
Cytarabine + HMBA	AML	Hasan and Rees 1988, Chomienne et al 1986
	AML	Hassan and Rees 1989
Tiazofurin	HL-60 promyelocytes	Yamaji et al 1990
Azacitidine	HL-60 promyelocytes	Dore et al 1990
Cytokines		
Interferon gamma	U-937 monoblasts	Gullberg et al 1985
	Breast cancer	Marth et al 1986
	HL-60	Peck and Bollag 1991, Hemmi and Breitman 1987
Interferon alfa	Neuroblastoma	Higuchi et al 1991
	HL-60, U-937	Peck and Bollag 1991
	Squamous bladder cancer	Recondo et al 1991
Tumor necrosis factor + interferon gamma	HL-60	Tobler et al 1987, Peck and Bollag 1991
	HL-60	Trinchieri et al 1987
Filgrastim	HL-60, U-937	Peck and Bollag 1991, Santini et al 1989, Columbat et al 1991
Sargramostim	HL-60	Hemmi et al 1989

*Acute myelogenous leukemia.

all-*trans*-retinoic acid (Lefebvre et al 1991). The half-life of tRA in the plasma is 48 minutes (compared with 12–14 hours for cRA). Another trial reported a serum half-life ranging from 17 to 77 minutes with a median of 30 minutes (Lefebvre et al 1991). Elimination appears to be monophasic (Muindi et al 1992). The only metabolite detected in plasma or urine is 4-oxo-all-*trans*-retinoic acid, which is present in the urine as the glucuronide conjugate (Muindi et al 1992). Only 1% of the dose of retinoic acid is excreted in the urine and is recovered as the glucuronide. In the plasma, about 10% of the total retinoic acid is present as the 4-oxo-glucuronide conjugate. No retinoic acid was detected in cerebrospinal fluid of patients experiencing intracranial hypertension on retinoic acid therapy (Muindi et al 1992).

In 12 of 15 patients, detectable levels of cRA indicated significant isomerization of tRA to cRA (Lefebvre et al 1991). This trial also reported that failure to respond was associated with low peak plasma tRA levels of less than 0.5 μg/mL and with high clearance values of more than 200 L/h. In responding patients, clearance values tended to range from 24 to 106 L/h (Lefebvre et al 1991).

Continuous daily therapy with tRA in mice leads to significant reductions in steady-state plasma concentrations (Creech-Kraft et al 1991, Kalin et al 1981). The mechanism for enhanced clearance of tRA levels with continued dosing is not known but may include reduced systemic availability by intestinal and hepatic metabolism (Roberts et al 1979). Alternatively, tRA levels may decrease as a result of induction of hepatic metabolism by cytochrome P450 enzymes which mediate conversion of tRA to the 4-oxo metabolite (Roberts et al 1980, Leo et al 1984).

Pharmacokinetic studies in rhesus monkeys have demonstrated that the plasma elimination of tRA doses of 45 mg/m^2 may involve three distinct phases. These include a brief initial exponential decline, a secondary plateau in elimination, and a final brisk exponential decline in drug levels (Adamson et al 1992). This elimination pattern suggests a capacity-limited (saturable) kinetic process with a Michaelis–Menten constant (K_m) of 3.2 μM for early (capacity-limited) elimination. As this is near the peak plasma levels achieved after tRA doses of 45 mg/m^2, the pharmacokinetics of tRA may be dose dependent (Adamson et al 1992). Glucuronidation of tRA in mice has also been reported to be dose dependent (Swanson et al 1981).

■ Side Effects and Toxicity

The most common side effect of tRA is headache. This generally occurs several hours after ingestion. The headaches are usually manageable with mild analgesics, although immediate dose reduction is required for patients experiencing severe headache as a result of pseudotumor cerebri (intracranial hypertension). Lumbar punctures, high-dose glucocorticosteroids, and narcotic analgesics are required to treat this emergent condition which is more common in children given high-dose tRA. Dizziness and vomiting may be associated with severe headaches from chronic high-dose (> 80 mg/m^2/d) tRA therapy (Smith et al 1992).

trans-Retinoic acid also produces dry skin and mucous membranes in up to 90% of patients. This is accompanied by erythema, xerostomia, desquamation of skin, and cheilitis (lip inflammation) which can be treated with liberal applications of topical emollients. Rarely, scrotal and/or penile ulcerations have been observed. Occular manifestations of tRA toxicity include dryness of the eyes and blepharoconjunctivitis with occasional corneal ulcerations.

Bone pain occurs in about 10 to 20% of patients, particularly during early remission induction therapy. This can become intense enough to require short-term narcotic analgesics. Chronic retinoid use can lead to arthralgias and myalgias, and in children, premature closure of the epiphyses is described. Chronic use of tRA can also cause spinal ligament calcification and osteoporosis (Kilcoyne 1988).

Metabolic effects of tRA include hypertriglyceridemia and, to a lesser degree, hypercholesterolemia. These effects do not generally lead to any serious toxic sequelae but could be additive with any preexisting conditions.

Hepatic toxic effects of tRA typically involve transient elevations of serum bilirubin, alkaline phosphatase, and serum transaminases. These elevations slowly resolve once therapy is halted and do not lead to permanent hepatic injury.

All retinoids are teratogens and, therefore, tRA should not be used in pregnant females. Limb bud malformations, microcephaly, and palpebral aplasia with exophthalmia are most commonly observed in experimental teratogenesis studies in rodents (Willhite and Shealy 1984, Geelen 1979, Cahen 1964).

Hematologic effects of tRA in APL patients usually involve leukocytosis (white blood cell count > 20,000/mm^3). This is seen in up to 40% of patients and may be part of a constellation of symptoms called the "retinoic acid syndrome." This syndrome is observed in 10 to 20% of APL patients during remission induction of therapy and may be associated with a positive clinical response to tRA therapy. Symptoms of the retinoic acid syndrome include a high fever, respiratory distress with radiographic evidence of diffuse pulmonary infiltrates, pleural or pericardial effusions, and occasionally impaired myocardial contractility and hypotension. This is the most serious reaction seen with tRA therapy of APL and may require endotracheal intubation and mechanical ventilation to prevent serious consequences of progressive hypoxemia. Care must be taken to differentiate this life-threatening syndrome from uncomplicated leukocytosis. Patients expiring from the retinoic acid syndrome as a result of multiorgan failure typically have autopsy evidence of extensive infiltration of myeloid cells in the lungs, skin, kidney, liver, and lymph nodes. Treatment of the syndrome with a short course of high-dose corticosteroids may be very effective. A recommended regimen calls for dexamethasone 10 mg IV every 12 hours for 3 or more days at an early point in the development of the syndrome (ie, at the appearance of unexplained fever and dyspnea) (Warrell 1992). One group suggests that retinoid therapy may be continued through the syndrome, whereas French researchers discontinue tRA and immediately institute full-dose cytotoxic chemotherapy.

REFERENCES

Adamson PC, Balis FM, Smith MA, et al. Dose-dependent pharmacokinetics of all-*trans*-retinoic acid. *J Natl Cancer Inst.* 1992;**84**:1332–1335.

Bell B, Findley H, Krischer J, et al. Phase II study of 13-*cis*-retinoic acid in pediatric patients with acute non-lymphocytic leukemia—A Pediatric Oncology Group Study. *J Immunother.* 1991;**10**:77–83.

Bonhomme L, Fredj G, Averous S, et al. Topical treatment of epidemic Kaposi's sarcoma with all-*trans*-retinoic acid. *Ann Oncol.* 1991;**2**:234–235.

Borrow J, Goddard AD, Sheer D, et al. Molecular analysis of acute promyelocytic leukemia breakpoint cluster region on chromosome 17. *Science.* 1990;**249**:1577–1580.

Boylan J, Gudas L. Overexpression of the cellular retinoic acid binding protein-I (CRABP-I) results in a reduction in differentiation-specific gene expression in F9 teratocarcinoma cells. *J Cell Biol.* 1991;**112**:965–979.

Breitman T, Collins S, Keene B. Terminal differentiation of human promyelocytic leukemic cells in primary culture in response to retinoic acid. *Blood.* 1981;**57**:1000–1004.

Breitman T, He R. Combinations of retinoic acid with either sodium butyrate, dimethylsulfoxide, or hexamethylene bisacetamide synergistically induce differentiation of the human myeloid leukemia cell line HL60. *Cancer Res.* 1990;**50**:6268–6273.

Breitman T, Keene B, Hemmi H. Retinoic acid-induced differentiation of fresh human leukaemia cells and the human myelomonocytic leukaemia cell lines, HL-60, U-937, and THP-1. *Cancer Surv.* 1983;**2**:261–291.

Breitman T, Selonic S, Collins S. Induction of differentiation of the human promyelocytic leukemia cell line (HL-60) by retinoic acid. *Proc Natl Acad Sci USA.* 1980;**77**:2936–2940.

Cahen RL. Evaluation of the teratogenicity of drugs. *Clin Pharmacol Ther.* 1964;**5**:480–514.

Castaigne S, Chomienne C, Daniel MT, et al. All-*trans* retinoic acid as a differentiation therapy for acute promyelocytic leukemia. I. Clinical results. *Blood.* 1990;**76**:1704–1709.

Chen Z-X, Xue Y-Q, Tao R-F, et al. A clinical and experimental study on all-*trans* retinoic acid-treated acute promyelocytic leukemia patients. *Blood.* 1991;**78**:1413–1419.

Chomienne C, Balitrand N, Degos L, et al. 1-β-D-Arabinofuranosyl cytosine and all-*trans* retinoic acid in combination accelerates and increases monocyte differentiation of myeloid leukemic cells. *Leukemia Res.* 1986;**10**:631–636.

Chytil F, Ong D. Cellular retinoid-binding proteins. In: Sporn M, Roberts A, Goodman D, eds. *The Retinoids.* Orlando, FL: Academic Press; 1984;**2**:90–125.

Colombat P, Santini V, Delwel R, et al. Primary human acute myeloblastic leukaemia: An analysis of in vitro granulocytic maturation following stimulation with retinoic acid and G-CSF. *Br J Haematol.* 1991;**79**:382–389.

Cowan J, Von Hoff D, Dinesman A, et al. Use of a human tumor cloning system to screen retinoids for antineoplastic activity. *Cancer.* 1983;**51**:92–96.

Creech-Kraft J, Slikker W, Bailey J, et al. Plasma pharmacokinetics and metabolism of 13-*cis* and all-*trans*-retinoic acid in the cynomolgus monkey and the identification of 13-*cis* and all-*trans* retinoyl-beta-glucuronides: A comparison to one human case study with isotretinoin. *Drug Metab Dispos.* 1991;**19**:317–324.

Crouch G, El-Badry O, Helman L. All-*trans* retinoic acid inhibition of cell growth in human rhabdomyosarcoma cell lines is not directly mediated through IGF-II. *Proc Am Assoc Cancer Res.* 1990;**31**:29.

Crouch G, Helman L. All-*trans*-retinoic acid inhibits the growth of human rhabdomyosarcoma cell lines. *Cancer Res.* 1991;**51**:4882–4887.

Dillehay D, Walia A, Lamon E. Effects of retinoids on macrophage function and Il-1 activity. *J Leuk Biol.* 1988;**44**:353–360.

Dmitrovsky E, Moy D, Miller W, et al. Retinoic acid causes a decline in TGF-α expression, cloning efficiency, and tumorigenicity in a human embryonal cancer cell line. *Oncogene Res.* 1990;**5**:233–239.

Dore B, Momparler L, Momparler R. Modification of the *c-myc* expression and differentiation in HL-60 myeloid leukemic cells by 5-aza-2′-deoxycytidine and retinoic acid. *Proc Am Assoc Cancer Res.* 1990;**31**:424.

Doyle L, Giangiulo D, Hussain A, et al. Differentiation of human variant small cell cancer cell lines to a classic morphology by retinoic acid. *Cancer Res.* 1989;**49**:6745–6751.

Eccles S. Effects of retinoids on growth and dissemination of malignant tumours: Immunological considerations. *Biochem Pharmacol.* 1985;**34**:1599–1610.

Epstein J. All-*trans*-retinoic acid and cutaneous cancers. *J Am Acad Dermatol.* 1986;**15**:772–778.

Findley H, Steuber C, Ruymann F, et al. Effect of retinoic acid on myeloid antigen expression and clonal growth of leukemic cells from children with acute nonlymphocytic leukemia—A Pediatric Oncology Group study. *Leukemia Res.* 1986;**10**:43–50.

Flynn P, Miller J, Weisdorf D, et al. Retinoic acid treatment of acute promyelocytic leukemia: In vitro and in vivo observations. *Blood.* 1986;**62**:1211–1217.

Fontana J. Interaction of retinoids and tamoxifen on the inhibition of human mammary carcinoma cell proliferation. *Exp Cell Biol.* 1987;**55**:136–144.

Geelen JA. Hypervitaminosis A induced teratogenesis. *CRC Crit Rev Toxicol.* 1979;**6**:351–375.

Gullberg U, Nilsson E, Einhorn S, et al. Combinations of interferon-γ and retinoic acid or 1α, 25-dihydroxycholecalciferol induce differentiation of the human monoblast leukemia cell line U-937. *Exp Hematol.* 1985;**13**:675–679.

Halter S, Fraker L, Adcock D, et al. Effect of retinoids on xenotransplanted human mammary carcinoma cells in athymic mice. *Cancer Res.* 1988;**48**:3733–3736.

Hassan H, Rees J. Retinoic acid alone and in combination with cytosine arabinoside induces differentiation of human myelomonocytic and monoblastic leukaemic cells. *Hematol Oncol.* 1988;**6**:39–45.

Hassan H, Rees J. Triple combination of retinoic acid + low concentration of cytosine arabinoside + hexamethylene bisacetamide induces differentiation of human AML blasts in primary culture. *Hematol Oncol.* 1989;**7**:429–440.

Hassan H, Rees J. Triple combination of retinoic acid plus actinomycin D plus dimethylformamide induces differentiation of human acute myeloid leukaemic blasts in primary culture. *Cancer Chemother Pharmacol.* 1990;**26**:26–30.

Hemmi H, Breitman T. Combinations of recombinant human interferons and retinoic acid synergistically induce differentiation of the human promyelocytic leukemia cell line HL-60. *Blood.* 1987;**69**:501–507.

Hemmi H, Nakamura T, Shimizu Y, et al. Identification of components of differentiation-inducing activity of human T-cell lymphoma cells by induction of differentiation in human myeloid leukemia cells. *J Natl Cancer Inst.* 1989;**81**:952–956.

Higuchi T, Hannigan G, Malkin D, et al. Enhancement by retinoic acid and dibutyryl cyclic adenosine 3′:5′-monophosphate of the differentiation and gene expression of human neuroblastoma cells induced by interferon. *Cancer Res.* 1991;**51**:3958–3964.

Hoffman S, Robinson W. Use of differentiation-inducing agents in the myelodysplastic syndrome and acute nonlymphocytic leukemia. *Am J Hematol.* 1988;**28**:124–127.

Imaizumi M, Breitman T. Retinoic acid-induced differentiation of the human promyelocytic leukemia cell line, HL-60, and fresh human leukemia cells in primary culture: A model for differentiation inducing therapy of leukemia. *Eur J Haematol.* 1987;**38**:289–302.

Jetten A, Kim J, Sacks P, et al. Inhibition of growth and squamous-cell differentiation markers in cultured human head and neck squamous carcinoma cells by β-all-*trans* retinoic acid. *Int J Cancer.* 1990;**45**:195–202.

Jurin M, Tannock I. Influence of vitamin A on immunological response. *Immunology.* 1972;**23**:283–287.

Kalin J, Starling M, Hill D. Disposition of all-*trans* retinoic acid in mice following oral doses. *Drug Metab Dispos.* 1981;**9**:196–201.

Kilcoyne R. Effects of retinoids in bone. *J Am Acad Dermatol.* 1988;**19**:212–216.

Koeffler H, Amatruda T. The effect of retinoids on haemopoiesis—Clinical and laboratory studies. In: Nugent J, Clark S, eds. *Retinoids, Differentiation, and Disease.* London: Ciba Foundation; 1985:252–273.

Kramer Z, Boros L, Wiernik P, et al. 13-*cis*-Retinoic acid in the treatment of elderly patients with acute myeloid leukemia. *Cancer.* 1991;**67**:1484–1486.

LaCroix A, Lippman M. Binding of retinoids to human breast cancer cell lines and their effects on cell growth. *J Clin Invest.* 1980;**65**:586–591.

Larson RA, Kondo K, Vardiman JW, et al. Evidence for a 15;17 translocation in every patient with acute promyelocytic leukemia. *Am J Med.* 1984;**76**:827–841.

Lawrence H, Conner K, Kelly M, et al. *cis*-Retinoic acid stimulates the clonal growth of some myeloid leukemia cells in vitro. *Blood.* 1987;**69**:302–307.

Lee M-O, Dockham P, Sladek N. Identification of human liver aldehyde dehydrogenases that catalyze the oxidation of retinaldehyde to retinoic acid. *Pharmacologist.* 1990;**32**:156.

Lefebvre P, Thomas G, Gourmel B, et al. Pharmacokinetics of oral all-*trans* retinoic acid in patients with acute promyelocytic leukemia. *Leukemia.* 1991;**5**:1054–1058.

Leo M, Iida S, Lieber C. Retinoic acid metabolism by a system reconstituted with cytochrome P-450. *Arch Biochem Biophys.* 1984;**234**:305–312.

Levine N, Meyskens FL. Topical vitamin-A-acid therapy for cutaneous metastatic melanoma. *Lancet.* 1980;**2**:224–226.

Lin T, Chu T. Enhancement of murine lymphokine-activated killer cell activity by retinoic acid. *Cancer Res.* 1990;**50**:3013–3018.

Lotan R. Different susceptibilities of human melanoma and breast carcinoma cell lines to retinoic acid-induced growth inhibition. *Cancer Res.* 1979;**39**:1014–1019.

Lotan R, Lotan D. Stimulation of melanogenesis in a human melanoma cell line by retinoids. *Cancer Res.* 1980;**40**:3345–3350.

Marth C, Daxenbichler G, Dapunt O. Synergistic antiproliferative effect of human recombinant interferons and retinoic acid in cultured breast cancer cells. *J Natl Cancer Inst.* 1986;**77**:1197–1202.

Meng-er H, Yu-chen Y, Shu-rong C, et al. Use of all-*trans* retinoic acid in the treatment of acute promyelocytic leukemia. *Blood.* 1988;**72**:567–572.

Meyskens F, Fuller B. Characterization of the effects of different retinoids on the growth and differentiation of human melanoma cell lines and selected subclones. *Cancer Res.* 1980;**40**:2194–2196.

Miller WH Jr, Warrell RP Jr, Frankel SR, et al. Novel retinoic acid receptor-alpha transcripts in acute promyelocytic leukemia responsive to all-*trans*-retinoic acid. *J Natl Cancer Inst.* 1990;**82**:1932–1933.

Muindi JRF, Frankel SR, Huselton C, et al. Clinical pharmacology of oral all-*trans* retinoic acid in patients with acute promyelocytic leukemia. *Cancer Res.* 1992;**52**:2138–2142.

Munker M, Munke R, Saxton R, et al. Effect of recombinant monokines, lymphokines and other agents on clonal proliferation of human lung cancer cell lines. *Cancer Res.* 1987;**47**:4081–4085.

Napoli J. Retinol metabolism in LLC-PK1 cells. *J Biol Chem.* 1986;**261**:13592–13597.

Napoli J, Pramanik B, Williams J, et al. Quantification of retinoic acid by gas-liquid chromatography–mass spectrometry: total versus all-*trans* retinoic acid in human plasma. *J Lipid Res.* 1985;**26**:387–392.

Peck R, Bollag W. Potentiation of retinoid-induced differentiation of HL-60 and U937 cell lines by cytokines. *Eur J Cancer.* 1991;**27**:53–57.

Peehl D, Wong S, Stamey T. Cytostatic effects of suramin on prostate cancer cells cultured from primary tumors. *J Urol.* 1991;**145**:624–630.

Petkovich M, Brand N, Krust A, et al. A human retinoic acid receptor which belongs to the family of nuclear receptors. *Nature.* 1987;**330**:444–450.

Recondo G, RG K, Logothetis C. Evidence for synergistic antitumor effect of 5-fluorouracil (5-FU) with alpha-interferon and 5-FU with 13-*cis* retinoic acid or 4-hydroxyphenylretinamide in human transitional cell carcinoma cell lines. *Proc Am Assoc Cancer Res.* 1991;**32**:341.

Reynolds C, Kane D, Einhorn P, et al. Response of neuroblastoma to retinoic acid in vitro and in vivo. In: Evans A, D'Angio G, Knudson A, et al, eds. *Advances in Neuroblastoma Research.* New York: Liss; 1991;**3**:203–211.

Roberts A, Lamb L, Sporn M. Metabolism of all-*trans* retinoic acid in hamster liver microsomes: Oxidation of 4-hydroxy- to 4-keto-retinoic acid. *Arch Biochem Biophys.* 1980;**199**:374–383.

Roberts A, Nichols M, Newton D, et al. In vitro metabolism of retinoic acid in hamster intestine and liver. *J Biol Chem.* 1979;**245**:6296–6302.

Robertson K, Mueller L, Collins S. Retinoic acid receptors in myeloid leukemia: Characterization of receptors in retinoic acid-resistant K-562 cells. *Blood.* 1991;**77**:340–347.

Sacks P, Oke V, Amos B, et al. Modulation of growth, differentiation, and glycoprotein synthesis by β-all-*trans* retinoic acid in a multicellular tumor spheroid model for squamous carcinoma of the head and neck. *Int J Cancer.* 1989;**44**:926–933.

Sankowski A, Janik P, Jeziorska M, et al. The results of topical application of 13-*cis*-retinoic acid on basal cell carcinoma. A correlation of the clinical effect with histopathological examination and serum retinol level. *Neoplasma.* 1987;**34**:485–489.

Santini V, Delvel R, Lowenberg B. Terminal granulocytic maturation in acute myeloid leukemia (AML). *Exp Hematol.* 1989;**17**:646.

Sidell N. Retinoic acid-induced growth inhibition and morphologic differentiation of human neuroblastoma cells in vitro. *J Natl Cancer Inst.* 1982;**68**:589–593.

Sidell N, Altman A, Haussler M, et al. Effects of retinoic acid (RA) on the growth and phenotypic expression of several human neuroblastoma cell lines. *Exp Cell Res.* 1983;**148**:21–30.

Sidell N, Ramsdell R. Retinoic acid upregulates interleukin-2 receptors on activated human thymocytes. *Cell Immunol.* 1988;**115**:299–309.

Smith MA, Parkinson DR, Cheson BD, et al. Retinoids in cancer therapy. *J Clin Oncol.* 1992;**10**:839–864.

Stone R, Mayer R. The unique aspects of acute promyelocytic leukemia. *J Clin Oncol.* 1990;**8**:1913–1921.

Strickland S, Mahdavi V. The induction of differentiation in teratocarcinoma stem cells by retinoic acid. *Cell.* 1978;**15**:393–403.

Sun G, Huang M, Chen S, et al. The study on post-induction remission therapies in complete remission patients with APLK induced by all-*trans* retinoic acid. *Chin J Hematol.* 1990;**11**:402–410.

Surwit EA, Graham V, Droegemueller W, et al. Evaluation of topically applied *trans*-retinoic acid in the treatment of cervical intraepithelial lesions. *Am J Obstet Gynecol.* 1982;**143**:821–823.

Swanson BN, Frolik CA, Zaharevitz DW, et al. Dose-dependent kinetics of all-*trans*-retinoic acid in rats. *Biochem Pharmacol.* 1981;**30**:107–113.

Takase S, Ong D, Chytil F. Transfer of retinoic acid from its complex with cellular retinoic acid-binding protein to the nucleus. *Arch Biochem Biophys.* 1986;**247**:328–334.

Thein R, Lotan R. Sensitivity of cultured human osteosarcoma and chondrosarcoma cells to retinoic acid. *Cancer Res.* 1982;**42**:4771–4775.

Tickle C, Alberts B, Wolpert L, et al. Local application of retinoic acid to the limb bud mimics the action of the polarizing region. *Nature.* 1982;**296**:564–565.

Tobler A, Munker R, Heitjan D, et al. In vitro interaction of recombinant tumor necrosis factor alpha and all-*trans*-retinoic acid with normal and leukemic hematopoietic cells. *Blood.* 1987;**70**:1940–1946.

Trinchieri G, Rosen M, Perussia B. Retinoic acid cooperates with tumor necrosis factor and immune interferon in inducing differentiation and growth inhibition of the human promyelocytic leukemic cell line HL-60. *Blood.* 1987;**69**:1218–1224.

Warrell RR. All trans retinoic acid. In: *American Society of Clinical Oncology Educational Book, 28th Meeting, San Diego, CA, May 17–19,* 1992;107–112.

Warrell RP Jr, Frankel SR, Miller WH Jr, et al. Differentiation therapy of acute promyelocytic leukemia with tretinoin (all-*trans* retinoic acid). *N Engl J Med.* 1991;**324**:1385–1393.

Willhite CC, Shealy YF. Amelioration of embryotoxicity by structural modification of the terminal group of cancer chemopreventive retinoids. *J Natl Cancer Inst.* 1984;**72**:689–695.

Yamaji Y, Natsumeda Y, Nagai M, et al. Synergistic action of tiazofurin (TR) and retinoic acid (RA) on differentiation in HL-60 leukemic cells. *Proc Am Assoc Cancer Res.* 1990;**31**:424.

Trifluoperazine Hydrochloride

■ Other Names

Stelazine® (SmithKline Beecham Pharmaceuticals).

■ Chemistry

Structure of trifluoperazine hydrochloride

Trifluoperazine hydrochloride is a phenothiazine derivative belonging to the piperazine group. It has a molecular weight of 407.49 and the molecular formula $C_{21}H_{24}F_3N_3$-S. The compound is freely soluble in water. The complete chemical name is 10-[3-(4-methylpiperazin-1-yl)propyl]-2-(trifluoromethyl)-10H-phenothiazine.

■ Antitumor Activity

Trifluoperazine hydrochloride has not been used in clinical oncology for its antitumor activity but rather for its purported ability to modulate drug resistance in patient's tumors. Trifluoperazine is one of the most potent inhibitors of calmodulin (Ganapathi and Grabowski 1983).

Although calmodulin inhibitors have been shown to have cytotoxic activity (Hart et al 1986), the greatest interest in trifluoperazine hydrochloride has been in its ability to enhance the cytotoxicity of doxorubicin and daunorubicin (Ganapathi et al 1984a,b) (see later).

In an attempt to capitalize on the preclinical findings, Miller and colleagues (1988) conducted a phase I–II clinical trial of trifluoperazine hydrochloride plus doxorubicin. Both patients with acquired (previous response with relapse) resistance to doxorubicin and patients with intrinsic (no previous response) resistance to doxorubicin were treated. Trifluoperazine was administered orally in divided doses (every 6 hours) starting 24 hours before doxorubicin and continuing for 6 consecutive days with dose escalation from 20 to 100 mg/d. Doxorubicin was administered as a 96-hour infusion at a dose of 60 mg/m² on days 2 to 5. The maximally tolerated dose of trifluoperazine was 60 mg/d, with the dose-limiting toxic effect being extrapyramidal effects. The investigators found no changes in the toxicity of doxorubicin. The recommended doses for phase II trials were trifluoperazine 15 mg orally four times per day on days 1 to 6 and doxorubicin 60 mg/m² as a continuous infusion on days 2 to 5.

Of great interest in the preceding study is that 6 partial responses and 1 complete response were noted in 36 evaluable patients (19% response rate). Seven of the twenty-one patients with acquired resistance responded, whereas none of the 15 patients with intrinsic resistance responded. The seven responses were noted in two patients with breast cancer, two patients with non-Hodgkin's lymphoma, and one patient each with sarcoma, ovarian cancer, and small cell lung cancer (the one complete response). Clearly, this interesting lead needs to be followed up with additional studies.

Mechanism of Action

In vitro model systems have documented that resistance to doxorubicin can be on the basis of the resistant cell extruding the intracellular doxorubicin, leading to a lack of accumulation of the drug within the resistant cells (Inabu et al 1979). A variety of calcium channel blockers and calmodulin inhibitors have been shown to inhibit the active efflux of doxorubicin (Tsuruo et al 1982, Ganapathi and Grabowski 1983, Ganapathi et al 1984a,b). Ganapathi et al (1983, 1984a) have documented that the calmodulin inhibitor trifluoperazine, at a concentration of 5 µM, can enhance the cytotoxicity of doxorubicin. Of note is that trifluoperazine was even more effective at improving the cytotoxicity of daunorubicin.

Of additional interest is the finding that calmodulin inhibitors such as trifluoperazine can also cause enhanced bleomycin-induced DNA damage and cytotoxicity (Lazo et al 1985).

Availability and Storage

Trifluoperazine (Stelazine®) is a product of SmithKline Beecham Pharmaceuticals, Philadelphia, Pennsylvania. It is available in six dosage forms for oral and for parenteral administration. For the clinical trial reported earlier, the oral form was used. Tablets are available in sizes of 1, 2, 5, and 10 mg. Inactive ingredients in the tablets consist of cellulose, croscarmellose sodium, FD&C Blue No. 2, FD&C Yellow No. 6, gelatin, lactose, magnesium stearate, talc, titanium dioxide, and trace amounts of other inactive ingredients. The tablets should be stored at room temperature (15–30°C [59–86°F]) and protected from moisture. No refrigeration is required.

Preparation for Use, Stability, and Admixture

No preparation for use is necessary. The tablets are stored under previously stated conditions.

Administration

The use of trifluoruperazine hydrochloride to enhance the cytotoxicity of doxorubicin in patients whose tumors are resistant to that agent is an investigational use. The doses and methods of administration of trifluoperazine hydrochloride and doxorubicin used in these investigational studies were outlined earlier (Miller et al 1988).

Special Precautions

As noted earlier, the use of trifluoperazine hydrochloride for reversal of resistance of a patient's tumor to doxorubicin is an investigational use requiring an IND and should not be part of routine clinical practice.

Drug Interactions

When doxorubicin was used in combination with trifluoperazine the plasma levels of doxorubicin did not appear to be affected (Miller et al 1988); however, that conclusion was based on comparisons to levels of doxorubicin when the drug was given alone in other studies (Legha et al 1982).

Dosage

See Antitumor Activity.

Pharmacokinetics

Miller and colleagues (1988) have noted that in their phase I–II study of trifluoperazine+doxorubicin, the concentration of trifluoperazine varied from 4.16 to 19.04 µg/mL (for patients receiving 20–40 mg daily) and from 39.46 to 129.83 µg/mL (for patients receiving 60–80 mg of trifluoperazine). It is of note that the plasma concentrations achieved in these patients were 10- to 100-fold *lower* than those used in vitro (1.64 µg/mL). It is conceivable that tumor tissue levels of trifluoperazine were higher than the plasma levels achieved in patients; however, it is worrisome that higher trifluoperazine levels (closer to those used in vitro) were not achievable in the phase I–II study of trifluoperazine + doxorubicin (Miller et al 1988).

Side Effects and Toxicity

The product insert for Stelazine® should be consulted for the extensive listing of side and toxic effects of the agent; however, for the use of the agent to putatively reverse resistance to doxorubicin, the toxic effects consisted of mild to moderate sedation. Other toxic effects were motor restlessness or akathisias, which improved with diphenhydramine. Severe extrapyramidal side effects were noted in 4 of 36 patients (Miller et al 1988).

Toxic effects of the combination ascribable to doxorubicin included leukopenia, thrombocytopenia, nausea, vomiting, and mucositis. Six patients had a decrease in resting left ventricular ejection fraction 15% or more of the baseline value, but most of the patients had received significant amounts of prior doxorubicin (Miller et al 1988).

REFERENCES

Ganapathi R, Grabowski D. Enhancement of sensitivity to Adriamycin in resistant P388 leukemia by the calmodulin inhibitor trifluoperazine. *Cancer Res.* 1983;**43**:3696–3699.

Ganapathi R, Grabowski D, Rouse W. Differential effect of the calmodulin inhibitor trifluoperazine on cellular accumulation, retention, and cytotoxicity of anthracyclines in doxorubicin (Adriamycin)-resistant P388 mouse leukemia cells. *Cancer Res.* 1984a;**44**:5056–5061.

Ganapathi R, Grabowski D, Turinic R, Valenzuela R. Correlation between potency of calmodulin inhibitors and effect on cellular levels and cytotoxic activity of doxorubicin (Adriamycin) in resistant P388 mouse leukemia cells. *Eur J Cancer Clin Oncol.* 1984b;**20**:799–806.

Hart WN, Lazo JS. Calmodulin: A potential target for cancer chemotherapeutic agents. *J Clin Oncol.* 1986;**4**:994–1012.

Inabu M, Kobayashi H, Sakurai Y, Johnson RK. Active efflux of daunorubicin and Adriamycin in sensitive and resistant sublines of P388 leukemia. *Cancer Res.* 1979;**39**:2200–2203.

Lazo JS, Hait WN, Kennedy KA, Braun ID, Meandzija B. Enhanced bleomycin-induced DNA damage and cytotoxicity with calmodulin antagonists. *Proc Am Assoc Cancer Res.* 1985;**26**:326.

Legha SJ, Benjamin RS, MacKay B, et al. Reduction of doxorubicin cardiotoxicity by prolonged continuous intravenous infusion. *Ann Intern Med.* 1982;**96**:133–139.

Miller RL, Bukowski RM, Budd GT, et al. Clinical modulation of doxorubicin resistance by the calmodulin-inhibitor, trifluoperazine: A phase I/II trial. *J Clin Oncol.* 1988;**6**:880–888.

Tsuruo T, Iida H, Tsu Kaqoshi S, Sakurai Y. Increased accumulation of vincristine and Adriamycin in drug-resistant P388 tumor cells following incubation with calcium antagonists and calmodulin inhibitors. *Cancer Res.* 1982;**42**:4730–4733.

Trifluridine

■ Other Names

F3TDR; NSC-75520.

■ Chemistry

Structure of trifluridine

Trifluridine has a molecular weight of 296 and the empiric formula $C_{10}H_{11}F_3N_2O_5$. It is one of a series of fluorinated pyrimidines isolated by Heidelberger et al (1965). It shares some structural similarity to ftorafur and floxuridine. The chemical name is 2′-deoxy-5-(trifluoromethyl)uridine.

■ Antitumor Activity

Trifluridine has shown activity in neuroblastoma (Helson 1975).

■ Mechanism of Action

Trifluridine is believed to act similarly to floxuridine. As such it must initially be phosphorylated to the nucleotide form. It may then falsely substitute for the normal pyrimidine base deoxyuridylate to inhibit the enzyme thymidylate synthetase. This leads to deprivation of the essential DNA nucleotide, thymidine. DNA synthesis and subsequent cellular division are thereby halted in S phase. Though they are similar in nature, the exact kinetics of trifluridine inhibition of thymidylate synthetase differ from those of the active floxuridine nucleotide (floxuridine phosphate).

■ Availability and Storage

Trifluridine was investigationally available from the National Cancer Institute as a lyophilized powder in 200-mg vials. The vials may be stored at room temperature.

■ Preparation for Use, Stability, and Admixture

To each 200-mg vial, 8 mL of Sterile Water for Injection, USP, is added to yield a solution of pH 4.5 to 5.5. This solution should be used within 8 hours of reconstitution; however, the drug is probably chemically stable for much longer.

■ Administration

Trifluridine has been administered as a 15-minute intravenous infusion.

■ Dosage

Recommended phase II doses for this agent have not been reported. In combination with other agents, however, doses of 45 mg/kg/d for 1 to 5 days have been used. The dose range in these studies was 40 to 80 mg/kg/d.

■ Pharmacokinetics

Trifluridine is metabolized differently from the other fluorinated pyrimidines. Studies of radiolabeled drug in mice have shown that (1) relatively little radioactive carbon is exhaled; (2) the pyrimidine ring is not metabolically degraded and the nucleoside is cleaved to the pyrimidine base 5-carboxyuracil; and (3) roughly 50% of a dose (measured as total radioactivity) is excreted in the urine in 24 hours (Heidelberger et al 1965). A small amount of drug penetrates into the central nervous system, and the drug exhibits relative localization in tumor and spleen in mice. Human drug disposition studies have not been performed.

■ Side Effects and Toxicity

In animal studies, hematopoietic, renal, and hepatic function is altered by the drug. In humans the most common toxic effects are vomiting, chills, and fever of 103 to 104°F. The latter two symptoms are not generally seen unless doses greater than 20 mg/kg are used. The use of intravenous hydrocortisone 5 minutes before trifluridine administration can alleviate these symptoms.

Hematologic suppression is also produced with trifluridine and is mildly additive to other myelosuppressive agents. Lymphocyte, platelet, and white blood cell suppression has been noted when trifluridine is used in combination with cyclophosphamide and vincristine.

REFERENCES

Heidelberger C, Booha J, Kampschroer B. Fluorinated pyrimidines. XXIV. In vivo metabolism of 5-trifluoromethyluracil-2-C^{14}- and 5-trifluoromethyl-2'deoxyuridine. *Cancer Res.* 1965;**25**(3):377–381.

Heidelberger C, Parson DG, Remy DC. The synthesis of 5-trifluoromethyluracil and 5-trifluoromethyl 2-deoxyridine. *J Am Chem Soc.* 1962;**84**:35, 97–98.

Helson L. Management of disseminated neuroblastoma. *CA.* 1975;**25**(5):265–277.

Trimetrexate

■ Other Names

NSC-352122 (glucuronate); NSC-249008; TMQ; JB-11; TMTX.

■ Chemistry

Structure of trimetrexate

Trimetrexate is a 2,4-diaminoquinazoline folate analog supplied for injection as the glucuronate salt (Warner-Lambert Company). The complete chemical name is 6-(((3,4,5-trimethoxyphenyl)amino) methyl)-5-methyl-2,4-quinazolinediamine-D-glucuronic acid salt. The molecular weight is 564 and the molecular formula $C_{19}H_{23}N_5O_3 \cdot C_6H_{10}O_7$. The powdered glucuronate salt is greenish yellow to tan. The compound is more lipophilic than methotrexate but still has good water solubility of more than 50 mg/mL.

■ Antitumor Activity

In preclinical tumor models, trimetrexate has shown therapeutic activity in L-1210 and P-388 leukemia, B-16 melanoma, CD8F1 mammary carcinoma, colon-26, and colon-38 (Lin and Bertino 1987). Trimetrexate was inactive in human lung, mammary, and colon xenografts in mice. Good activity was observed in human tumor colony-forming assays performed in a variety of solid tumors including colon cancer, lung cancer, and breast cancer (Latham et al 1984). Trimetrexate also has activity against protozoal infections and was originally synthesized as an antimalarial agent (Elslager and Davoll 1974). In vitro antiprotozoal activity has been observed in *Pneumocystis carinii* (Allegra et al 1986) and in *Toxoplasma gondii* (Kovacs et al 1986).

In phase I clinical studies, 3 of 16 responses (1 complete) were noted in colorectal cancer (Lin and Bertino 1987). Minor responses were seen in several patients with esophageal cancer (1), breast cancer (3), and adenocarcinoma of the lung (1) (Fanucchi et al 1987). Preliminary analyses from ongoing phase II trials indicate that single-agent trimetrexate is moderately active (15–20% objective response rates) in breast, non-small cell lung, and head and neck cancer. Median response duration in non-small cell lung cancer was 9.5 weeks (Fossella et al 1992). A 10% response rate is described in esophageal cancer (Brown et al 1992). Responses of brief duration were noted in children with recurrent acute lymphoblastic leukemia (Pappo et al 1990). The drug was also inactive in cervical cancer and in pancreatic cancer (Shiomoto et al 1992).

■ Mechanism of Action

Like methotrexate, trimetrexate is a potent inhibitor of the enzyme dihydrofolate reductase (DHFR) in bacteria, protozoa, animals, and humans (Bertino et al 1979). This agent depletes reduced intracellular folates. This results in inhibition of the enzymatic conversion of uridylate to thymidine, blocking DNA synthesis. The lack of reduced folates produced by trimetrexate also leads to inhibition of several of other 1-carbon transfer reactions, especially those involving formyl-transferases (Lin and Bertino 1987). This effect can lead to impaired nucleotide synthesis and inhibition of synthesis of both RNA and DNA.

There are several mechanistic differences between methotrexate and trimetrexate. At high drug concentrations, both agents are antagonized by leucovorin; however, trimetrexate cytotoxicity is also blocked by thymidine. At higher concentrations, thymidine must be combined with hypoxanthine to block trimetrexate activity. In contrast, this combination does not block high cytotoxicity from concentrations of methotrexate (Broome et al 1982). The uptake mechanism of trimetrexate also differs substantially from that of methotrexate. Because of its quinazoline-based structure, trimetrexate does not interact with the reduced folate transport system used by both methotrexate and leucovorin (Kamen et al 1984, Diddens et al 1983). Two cellular influx mechanisms for trimetrexate have been suggested: (1) simple passive diffusion, and (2) facilitated transport by a saturable, temperature- and sulfhydryl-sensitive system (Lin and Bertino 1987).

Trimetrexate is also not polyglutamated inside cells, which normally aids in maintaining methotrexate intracellular concentrations. Nonetheless, cellular drug levels 10 to 100-fold higher than methotrexate are achieved with trimetrexate. This may explain some of the enhanced cytotoxicity seen with trimetrexate.

Resistance to trimetrexate may occur by different mechanisms from methotrexate. This is particularly true for transport-mediated resistance (Kamen et al 1984, Bertino et al 1985). Furthermore, trimetrexate activity may be unaffected in cells resistant to methotrexate because of polyglutamation defects (Cowan and Jolivet 1984); however, other forms of antifol resistance may apply, including increased DHFR expression by genetic amplification or other processes (Diddens et al 1983). Cells expressing the multidrug resistance phenotype may also express collateral resistance to trimetrexate (Arkin et al 1989, Klohs et al 1986). Interestingly, verapamil appears to partially restore trimetrexate sensitivity in multidrug-resistance cells (Klohs et al 1986).

■ Availability and Storage

Trimetrexate glucuronate is investigationally supplied by the Warner-Lambert Company, Ann Arbor, Michigan, in 6-mL vials containing 25 mg of lyophilized powder. The intact vials are stored at room temperature for at least 24 months (National Cancer Institute, 1983).

■ Preparation for Use, Stability, and Admixture

Each 25-mg vial is reconstituted with 1.9 to 2.0 mL of Sterile Water for Injection, USP. Each milliliter will then contain 12.5 mg of drug at a pH of 3.5 to 5.5. Doses for infusion may be further diluted to a concentration of 0.1 mg/mL in D5W. This solution is stable for 48 hours at room temperature or under refrigeration. Trimetrexate solutions are not sensitive to light but may precipitate at a pH above 5.0 to 6.0. Trimetrexate is incompatible with sodium chloride or other saline-containing solutions.

■ Administration

Trimetrexate is typically administered as a brief intravenous infusion in dextrose (0.1 mg/mL) over 5 to 30 minutes. Longer infusion times and/or the use of more dilute solutions are felt to reduce some toxic effects including central nervous system effects seen in mice and phlebitis seen in early clinical trials. Trimetrexate has also been administered as a continuous infusion for 24 hours (Allegra et al 1990) or for 5 days (Bishop et al 1989, Reece et al 1987).

■ Dosage

A variety of dosing administration schedules have been evaluated with trimetrexate (see table below). There is significantly enhanced toxicity with more frequent drug administrations (schedule dependence). Thus, for either a continuous 5-day infusion or a 5-day bolus schedule, much lower daily trimetrexate doses are tolerated. For example, the maximally tolerated 5-day dose is in the range 6.8 to 8 mg/m^2/d (Stewart et al 1988), compared with a single monthly bolus dose of 220 mg/m^2 (Grochow et al 1989). Patient re-treatment with trimetrexate has generally been possible at 3-week intervals on any dosing schedule.

Patients with reduced liver function, noted by increased bilirubin and reduced albumin levels, may require lower trimetrexate doses. In such patients impaired clearance and increased toxicity have been described (Fanucchi et al 1987). Renal dysfunction can also increase toxicity, presumably by decreasing drug clearance (Ho et al 1986).

■ Drug Interactions

Trimetrexate is synergistic in vitro with carboxypeptidase G, which enzymatically depletes cellular folates (Lin and Bertino 1987). Trimetrexate is also synergistically active in combination with either fluorouracil, vincristine, thioguanine, doxorubicin, and especially cyclophosphamide (Leopold et al 1986). Trimetrexate resistance mediated by the MDR mechanism can be partially reversed by concomitant verapamil (Klohs et al 1986). In certain antiprotozoal applications, trimetrexate was synergistic when combined with sulfadiazine (Kovacs et al 1986).

■ Pharmacokinetics

The table on page 936 summarizes the pharmacokinetics of trimetrexate given by different infusion schedules. The drug exhibits either a two- or three-compartment disposition pattern. Terminal half-lives of 10 to 16 hours are described when the drug is measured by either a specific high-performance liquid chromatography (HPLC) assay or by inhibition of the DHFR enzyme. The mean volume of distribution is about 24 L/m^2, which approximates total body water. Mean total body clearance is ap-

MAXIMALLY TOLERATED DOSING SCHEDULES FOR IV TRIMETREXATE

Daily Dose (mg/m^2)	Infusion Method (Time)	Repeat Doses/Course	Repeat Cycle (d)	Reference
110	Brief (5–10 min)	Weekly × 3	28	Balis et al 1987
220	Brief (15–30 min)	None	28	Grochow et al 1989
150	Continuous (24 h)	None	28	Allegra et al 1990
8	Brief (10 min)	Daily × 5	21	Stewart et al 1988
8	Continuous (24 h)	Daily × 5	21	Bishop et al 1989
6.8	Continuous (24 h)	Daily × 5	21	Rosen et al 1986
4.0	Daily bolus	Daily × 9	28	Jolivet et al 1986

CLINICAL PHARMACOKINETICS OF TRIMETREXATE BY HPLC ASSAY

Plasma Concentration (Time After Dose)	Method of IV Administration	Dose (mg/m²)	Terminal Half-life (h)	Total Body Clearance (mL/min/m²)	Volume of Distribution (L/m²)	Urinary Recovery (% Dose)	AUC (μM·h)	Reference
—	Bolus	120	16.4	28	25	9 (24 h)	—	Lin et al 1987
—	Bolus	50–155	11–18	33	33	16	—	Fanucchi et al 1987
0.3–3.1 μM (24 h)	Bolus (children)	35–145	7.6	40	12	13	64–309	Balis et al 1987
9.5–61 μmol/L (1 h)	Bolus	175–220	17–18	36.5	32.4	—	416	Grochow et al 1989
34–316 ng/mL/h (steady state)	Infusion (5 d)	5–60	14.5	29	—	22.5	67	Reece et al 1987
1.1–14.7 μM (peak)	Bolus	3–15	6–10	21	21	10–20	2–50	Stewart et al 1988
8.3 μM (end of 200-mg infusion)	Infusion (24 h)	16–220	13	32	27	6	—	Allegra et al 1990

proximately 33 mL/min/m², which suggests that nonrenal, probably hepatic, clearance is the primary route of drug elimination. Renal clearance accounts for only about 10% of total body clearance of drug.

Two polar metabolites of trimetrexate have been identified by HPLC analyses of patient plasma. Both are O-demethylated glucuronide conjugates at the 4-position of the phenoxymethyl ring (Tong et al 1985, McCormack et al 1986). These metabolites can bind to DHFR in vitro and are thus probably active in vivo. The DHFR assay on urine specimens also shows higher drug levels than the HPLC assay. Thus, some active metabolites may be excreted in the urine.

Urinary recovery of unchanged trimetrexate ranges from 10 to 20% of a dose (see first table), whereas fecal recovery accounts for less than 10% (Lin et al 1987). Unfortunately the drug does not distribute well into the central nervous system, with cerebrospinal levels only 1 to 2% those in the plasma (Balis et al 1987, Allegra et al 1990). This may partially relate to high binding (> 98%) of trimetrexate to human plasma proteins (Fanucchi et al 1987).

■ Side Effects and Toxicity

The major dose-limiting toxic effect of trimetrexate is myelosuppression, primarily leukocytopenia. With a single intravenous bolus injection, the nadir occurs at 6 to 8 days, with recovery by days 12 to 14 (Weir et al 1982, Lin et al 1987). Thrombocytopenia is generally less profound with nadirs at 10 to 15 days after administration (Lin et al 1987; Fanucchi et al 1987). In contrast, with more frequent administration schedules, thrombocytopenia is dose-limiting (Jolivet et al 1986) and is occasionally fatal (Fanucchi et al 1987). Anemia also occurs with more frequent trimetrexate dosing schedules. None of the myelosuppressive effects appear to be cumulative.

Gastrointestinal toxic effects include mild to moderate nausea and vomiting, mucositis, and transient liver enzyme elevations (Lin et al 1987, Balis et al 1987, Grochow et al 1989).

Local reactions have commonly been described with a trimetrexate dose of 150 mg/m² or greater (Weiss et al 1986). Phlebitis has been particularly troublesome, but may be lessened somewhat by dilution and/or slowing of the infusion. Erythema and pain at the injection site are common even in patients receiving infusions through central venous access devices (Allegra et al 1990). A generalized erythematous, maculopapular rash is also common at high doses (Lin and Bertino 1987). These rashes generally present on the neck and upper chest 4 to 5 days after starting the drug. They can be intensely pruritic but usually begin to remit 7 to 10 days after onset (Weiss et al 1986). Skin biopsies of involved areas may show lymphohistiocytic infiltrates, including eosinophils in a perivascular and interstitial distribution. Treatment with corticosteroids and antihistamines does not prevent these reactions (Allegra et al 1990). Hyperpigmentation at the injection site is also seen with trimetrexate and there may be synergy with skin toxicity at prior irradiation sites (Allegra et al 1990, Stewart et al 1988).

Generalized, immediate hypersensitivity reactions are described in about 2% of patients receiving trimetrexate (Grem et al 1990). The immediate reaction involves hypotension and a loss of consciousness. Other symptoms include facial flushing; a flulike syndrome with myalgias, fever, and malaise; bronchospasm; periorbital edema; and difficulty in swallowing (Lin et al 1987, Grochow et al 1989). Rechallenge invariably reproduces these side effects.

Nephrotoxic effects may also occur and this can increase the likelihood of more severe systemic toxicity (Lin and Bertino 1987); however, the elevations in serum creatinine are usually transient.

Two retrospective studies have evaluated potential predictors of severe or life-threatening toxic effects from trimetrexate. Drug administration schedules with a greater likelihood of causing severe myelosuppression, mucositis, and hepatic problems were the daily × 5 and weekly × 3 schedules (Grem et al 1988). The total dose delivered also correlated to greater toxicity, whereas performance status and prior therapy were not strong predictors of toxicity. Strong correlates of severe toxicity included baseline albumin of 3.5 g/dL or less and pretreatment protein levels of 6.0 g/dL or less (Grem et al 1988). Low protein levels and the presence of metastatic liver disease were identified as predictors of toxicity in another study (Eisenhauer et al 1988).

REFERENCES

Allegra CJ, Drake J, Swan J, et al. Preliminary results of a phase I–II trial for the treatment of *Pneumocystis carinii* pneumonia (PCP) using a potent lipid-soluble dihydrofolate reductase (DHFR) inhibitor, trimetrexate (TMTX). In: *Program and Abstracts of the 26th Interscience Conference on Antimicrobial Agents and Chemotherapy,* 1986:224.

Allegra CJ, Jenkins J, Weiss RB, et al. A phase I and pharmacokinetic study of trimetrexate using a 24-hour continuous-infection schedule. *Invest New Drugs.* 1990;**8:** 159–166.

Arkin H, Ohnuma T, Kamen BA, et al. Multidrug resistance in a human leukemic cell line selected for resistance to trimetrexate. *Cancer Res.* 1989;**49:**6556–6561.

Balis FM, Patel R, Luks E, et al. Pediatric phase I trial and pharmacokinetic study of trimetrexate. *Cancer Res.* 1987;**47:**4973–4976.

Bertino JR, Mini E, Sawicki WL. Effects of trimetrexate on human leukemia cells from patients sensitive and resistant to methotrexate (MTX). *Proc Am Soc Clin Oncol.* 1985;**4:**44.

Bertino JR, Sawiski WL, Moroson BA, et al. 2,4-Diamino-5-methyl-6-[(3,4,5-trimethoxyanilino) methyl]quinazoline (TMQ), a potent nonclassical folate antagonist inhibitor-1. *Biochem Pharmacol.* 1979;**28:**1983–1987.

Bishop JF, Raghavan D, Olver IN, et al. A phase I study of trimetrexate (NSC 352122) administered by 5-day continuous intravenous infusion. *Cancer Chemother Pharmacol.* 1989;**24:**246–250.

Broome MG, Johnson RK, Evans SF, et al. Leucovorin reversal studies with TMQ and a triazine antifol, in comparison with methotrexate. *Proc Am Assoc Cancer Res.* 1982;**23:**178.

Brown T, Fleming T, Tangen C, et al. A phase II trial of trimetrexate in the treatment of esophageal cancer: A Southwest Oncology Group trial. *Proc Am Soc Clin Oncol.* 1992;**11:**166.

Cowan KH, Jolivet JJ. A methotrexate-resistant human breast cancer cell line with multiple defects, including diminished formation of methotrexate polyglutamates. *J Biol Chem.* 1984;**257:**10793–10800.

Diddens H, Niethammer D, Jackson RC. Patterns of cross-resistance to the antifolate drugs trimetrexate, metoprine, homofolate and CB 3717 in human lymphoma and osteosarcoma cells resistant to methotrexate. *Cancer Res.* 1983;**43:**5286–5292.

Eisenhauer EA, Zee BC, Pater JL, Walsh WR. Trimetrexate: Predictors of severe or life-threatening toxic effects. *J Natl Cancer Inst.* 1988;**80:**1318–1322.

Elslager EF, Davoll J. Synthesis of fused pyrimidines as folate antagonists. In: Castle RN, Townsend LB, eds. *Lectures in Heterocyclic Chemistry.* Orem, UT: Hetero; 1974;**2:**s97–s133.

Fanucchi MP, Walsh TD, Fleisher M, et al. Phase I and clinical pharmacology study of trimetrexate administered weekly for three weeks. *Cancer Res.* 1987;**47:**3303–3308.

Fossella FV, Winn R, Holoyo P, et al. Phase II study of trimetrexate (TMTX) for non-small cell lung cancer (NSCLC). *Proc Am Soc Clin Oncol.* 1992;**11:**305.

Grem JL, Ellenberg SS, King SA, Shoemaker DD. Correlates of severe or life-threatening toxic effects from trimetrexate. *J Natl Cancer Inst.* 1988;**80:**1313–1318.

Grem JL, King SA, Costanza ME, Brown TD. Hypersensitivity reactions to trimetrexate. *Invest New Drugs.* 1990;**8:**211–213.

Grochow LB, Noe DA, Ettinger DS, Donehower RC. A phase I trial of trimetrexate glucuronate (NSC 352122) given every 3 weeks: Clinical pharmacology and pharmacodynamics. *Cancer Chemother Pharmacol.* 1989;**24:** 314–320.

Ho DHW, Covington WP, Legha S, et al. Clinical pharmacology of trimetrexate. *Proc Am Assoc Cancer Res.* 1986;**27:**173.

Jolivet J, Landry L, Pinard M-F, et al. Daily bolus × 9 trimetrexate (TMTX): A phase I clinical, pharmacokinetic and pharmacodynamic study. *Proc Am Assoc Cancer Res.* 1986;**27:**174.

Kamen BA, Eibl B, Cashmore A, Bertino J. Uptake and efficacy of trimetrexate (TMQ, 2,4-diamino-5-methyl-6-[3,4,5-trimethoxyanilino)methyl]quinazoline), a nonclassical antifolate in methotrexate-resistant leukemia cells in vitro. *Biochem Pharmacol.* 1984;**33:**1697–1699.

Klohs WD, Steinkampf RW, Besserer JA, et al. Cross resistance of pleiotropically drug resistant P388 leukemia cells to the lipophilic antifolates trimetrexate and BW 310U. *Cancer Lett.* 1986;**31:**253–260.

Kovacs JA, Allegra CJ, Swan JC, et al. Trimetrexate and BW 301, two lipid-soluble antifolates, exert potent antitoxoplasma effects. In: *Program and Abstracts of the 26th Interscience Conference of Antimicrobial Agents and Chemotherapy;* 1986:298.

Latham B, Von Hoff DD, Elslager E. Use of a human tumor cloning system to evaluate analogs of methotrexate and mitoxantrone. *Cancer Treat Rep.* 1984;**68:**733–738.

Leopold WR, Dykes DD, Griswold DP Jr. Therapeutic synergy of trimetrexate (CI-898) in combination with doxorubicin, Cytoxan, 6-thioguanine, 5-fluorouracil, vincristine or cisplatin against P388 leukemia. *Proc Am Assoc Cancer Res.* 1986;**27:**253.

Lin JT, Bertino JR. Trimetrexate: A second generation folate antagonist in clinical trial. *J Clin Oncol.* 1987;**5:**2032–2040.

Lin JT, Cashmore AR, Baker M, et al. Phase I studies with trimetrexate: Clinical pharmacology, analytical methodology and pharmacokinetics. *Cancer Res.* 1987;**47:**609–616.

McCormack JJ, Webster LK, Tong WP, et al. Studies of a metabolite of trimetrexate. *Proc Am Assoc Cancer Res.* 1986;**27:**256.

National Cancer Institute. *Clinical Brochure for Trimetrexate Glucuronate.* Bethesda, MD: NCI; November 1983.

Pappo A, Dubowy R, Ravindranath Y, et al. Phase II trial of trimetrexate in the treatment of recurrent childhood acute lymphoblastic leukemia: A Pediatric Oncology Group Study. *J Natl Cancer Inst.* 1990;**82:**1641–1642.

Reece PA, Morris RG, Bishop JF, et al. Pharmacokinetics of trimetrexate administered by five-day continuous infusion to patients with advanced cancer. *Cancer Res.* 1987;**47:**2996–2999.

Rosen M, Ohnuma T, Zimet A, et al. Phase I study of trimetrexate (TMTX, TMQ, JB-11) glucuronate in a 5-day infusion schedule. *Proc Am Assoc Cancer Res.* 1986;**27**:172.

Shiomoto GM, Kuo S, Wade J, et al. Phase II study of trimetrexate glucuronate in the treatment of advanced carcinoma of the pancreas. *Proc Am Soc Clin Oncol.* 1992;**11**:184.

Stewart JA, McCormack JJ, Tong W, Low JB, et al. Phase I clinical and pharmacokinetic study of trimetrexate using a daily × 5 schedule. *Cancer Res.* 1988;**48**:5029–5035.

Tong WP, Stewart JA, McCormack JJ, et al. Metabolism of 2,4-diamino-5-methyl-6-(3,4,5-trimethoxyanilino)methylquinazoline (trimetrexate, TMQ) in man. *Proc Am Soc Clin Oncol.* 1985;**4**:31.

Warner-Lambert Research Group. Studies on cellular resistance and membrane transport with the quinazoline antifolate, trimetrexate. Minutes of the Phase I Working Group Meeting and Biochemical Modulators Advisory Group Meeting, Washington, DC, November 19–20, 1984, 127–131.

Weir EC, Cashmore AR, Dreyer RN, et al. Pharmacology and toxicity of a potent "nonclassical" 2,4-diamino quinazoline folate antagonist, trimetrexate, in normal dogs. *Cancer Res.* 1982;**42**:1696–1702.

Weiss RB, James WD, Major WB, et al. Skin reactions induced by trimetrexate, an analog of methotrexate. *Invest New Drugs.* 1986;**4**:159–163.

Tumor Necrosis Factor

■ Other Names

Tumor necrosis factor-α (macrophage-derived); tumor necrosis factor-β (lymphocyte derived); TNF; recombinant tumor necrosis factor (human); NSC-606515; rhTNF (recombinant human TNF).

■ Chemistry

In 1975 Carswell and colleagues reported that mice treated with bacillus Calmette–Guérin and endotoxin had necrosis of their previously implanted Meth A sarcomas. Of note was that the cause of the tumor regression was a host factor they named *tumor necrosis factor* (TNF). The molecule consists of 157 amino acids and has a molecular weight of approximately 17,000.

Two forms of TNF have been isolated; TNF-α (macrophage-derived) and TNF-β (lymphocyte-derived) (Aggarwal et al 1984, 1985). The genes for both forms of TNF have been cloned and a recombinant form of human TNF-α was scaled up for clinical trials (Pennica et al 1984, Shirai et al 1985, Gray et al 1984).

```
         1                         10                              20
        val arg ser ser ser arg thr pro ser asp lys pro val ala his val val ala asn pro gln ala glu gly
                         30                              40
        gln leu gln trp leu asn arg arg ala asn ala leu leu ala asn gly val glu leu arg asp asn gln leu
                 50                              60                     *   70
        val val pro ser glu gly leu tyr leu ile tyr ser gln val leu phe lys gly gln gly cys pro ser thr his
                         80                              90
        val leu leu thr his thr ile ser arg ile ala val ser tyr gln thr lys val asn leu leu ser ala ile lys
                100   *                          110                             120
        ser pro cys gln arg glu thr pro glu gly ala glu ala lys pro trp tyr glu pro ile tyr leu gly gly val
                         130                             140
        phe gln leu glu lys gly asp arg leu ser ala glu ile asn arg pro asp tyr leu asp phe ala glu ser
                 150
        gly gln val tyr phe gly ile ile ala leu
```

Proposed amino acid sequence for human tumor necrosis factor. The two cysteines are identified (by asterisks) to show the site of a disulfide bond. *Redrawn from Goeddel et al 1986.*

Recombinant TNF has been tested in a variety of preclinical systems. Substantial antitumor activity has been documented against murine and human tumors growing in vitro and in vivo (Sugarman et al 1985, Balkwill et al 1986, 1990, Harauaka et al 1984). TNF has excellent antitumor activity when the agent is given intratumorally into human xenografts growing in nude mice (Balkwill et al 1986). In addition to an antitumor effect there is also evidence that TNF-α may be involved in the cachexia of malignancy (Oliff et al 1987, Lowry and Muldauer 1990, Tracey et al 1988, Balkwill et al 1987). At present, however, there are few data indicating that tumors in mice can produce TNF-a at high enough concentrations to be responsible for weight loss in patients (Socher et al 1988, Lowry and Muldauer 1990).

Tumor necrosis factor has been found to have a variety of other biologic activities. It is able to induce cytokines including interleukin-1, interferon beta, interleukin-6, granulocyte–macrophage colony-stimulating factor, granulocyte colony-stimulating factor, macrophage colony-stimulating factor, platelet-derived growth factor, and prostaglandins (Balkwill et al 1990). In patients, recombinant human TNF has been found to significantly reduce natural killer cell activity, TNF and interleukin-1 production capacity, and proliferative responses to concanavalin A (Kist et al 1988). TNF has also been implicated in the genesis of cancer-associated hypercalcemia (Johnson et al 1989).

Many fine reviews of TNF have recently been completed and should be used by readers interested in further details (Balkwill et al 1990, Lowry and Muldauer 1990, Frei and Spriggs 1989).

■ Antitumor Activity

After 7 years of clinical study there is, as yet, no indication that TNF has any consistent antitumor activity in humans. Only occasional responses have been noted in phase I trials, including patients with small cell lung cancer, renal cell carcinoma, lymphoma, and pancreatic cancer (Chapman et al 1987, Selby et al 1987, Trump et al 1988, Creagan et al 1988). Of interest is the recent report by Raeth et al (1991) who noted significant clinical activity for TNF given intraperitoneally in patients with ascites secondary to refractory ovarian cancer and other tumors.

Phase II studies in patients with colorectal cancer have found no responses in 14 evaluable patients (previously treated with one prior treatment regimen) (Kemeny et al 1990) and one partial response in 17 patients with refractory colorectal cancer (Abbruzzese and Levin 1989).

Aboulafia et al (1989) have found no activity in five patients with AIDS-related Kaposi's sarcoma. Figlin et al (1988) found no activity for the compound in 14 patients with advanced renal cell carcinomas and 11 patients with advanced malignant melanomas.

It is likely that future clinical explorations for TNF will be in use in combinations with other cytokines (eg, interferon gamma, interleukin-2) (Retsas et al 1989, Salmon et al 1987) and in combination with conventional cytotoxic agents (such as the topoisomerase II inhibitors (Cottman et al 1989).

■ Mechanism of Action

At present, the mechanism of action of TNF is unknown. Proposed mechanisms of action include activation of phospholipase A_2, activation of lysosomes, activation of serine proteases, and generation of superoxides (Balkwill et al 1990). Of interest is that TNF does not appear to be directly toxic to the tumor cells, and antitumor activity is noted only when the tumor is vascularized. In mice, TNF is thought to act by effects on the vasculature (intravascular deposition of fibrin) and a stimulation of a T-cell mediated immune response (Palladino et al 1987, Havell et al 1988, Nawroth et al 1988).

It is now known that the cytotoxicity of TNF is probably mediated by a receptor and the receptor ligand is internalized (Tsujimoto et al 1985); however, further information regarding signal transduction following the internalization event is lacking (Frei and Spriggs 1989).

■ Availability and Storage*

Tumor necrosis factor has been made by a number of manufacturers. One of the materials used in trials sponsored by the National Cancer Institute has been provided by the Cetus Corporation, Emeryville, California, as either a lyophilized product or a frozen liquid product. For the lyophilized product, each vial contains approximately 0.3 mg recombinant TNF. (Refer to vial label for *exact* mg.) When reconstituted with 1.2 mL Sterile Water for Injection, USP, or Sodium Chloride Injection, USP, the solution contains *approximately* 0.25 mg recombinant TNF per milliliter. (Refer to the specifications accompanying each lot for the *exact* mg/mL.) In addi-

*Adapted from CetusChiron Corporation's Investigators Brochure.

tion to recombinant TNF, the solution contains 1.5% mannitol and 0.5% sucrose in sodium citrate buffer. There is no bacteriostatic agent. The pH after reconstitution is between 6.2 and 6.8. The vials should be stored at 2 to 8°C.

For the frozen liquid product, each vial contains approximately 0.3 mg recombinant TNF in 1.2 mL of solution. The approximate recombinant TNF concentration is 0.25 mg/mL. (Refer to the vial label for the exact mg/mL.) In addition to recombinant TNF, the solution contains 1% mannitol in sodium phosphate buffer. There is no bacteriostatic agent. The pH of the solution is between 7.2 and 7.8. The frozen liquid should be stored at −20°C or colder.

■ Preparation for Use, Stability, and Admixture

Lyophilized Product. For the lyophilized product the reconstitution procedure includes two steps:

1. Remove the flip-off plastic cap and swab the area of the stopper with antiseptic.
2. Aseptically inject 1.2 mL of either Sterile Water for Injection, USP, or Sodium Chloride Injection, USP, into the vial. To mix, swirl gently until the recombinant TNF is dissolved. *Do not shake.*

The expiration date is indicated on the vial and carton label. After reconstitution, the solution is stable at room temperature but should be used within 4 hours for sterility considerations.

For the frozen liquid product, the thawing procedure includes removing the vials from the freezer and allowing them to thaw at room temperature. A warm water bath or other technique should not be used to accelerate thawing. The product should not be shaken.

The expiration date is indicated on the vial and carton label. After thawing, the solution is stable at room temperature but should be used within 4 hours for sterility considerations. Agitation of thawed vials should be avoided because this may result in the formation of proteinaceous particles. Vials noted to contain such particles should not be used. Thawed solution may be refrozen one time.

Note: See Special Precautions for additional dilution instructions.

Intravenous Infusion Solution. Genentech, Inc, has also supplied recombinant TNF for National Cancer Institute use. They recommend the following procedure.

Recombinant TNF can be administered intravenously in a solution of normal (physiologic) saline containing human serum albumin (HSA) at a concentration of 2 mg/mL. HSA must be added to the normal saline before the recombinant TNF to prevent adherence of recombinant TNF to the intravenous infusion apparatus. This solution is run out through the attached intravenous tubing before the recombinant TNF is added. Only normal saline should be used for intravenous infusion of recombinant TNF.

The following procedure is recommended for the preparation of intravenous infusions of recombinant TNF:

1. Add HSA at a final concentration of 2 mg/mL to a plastic intravenous bag containing 50 mL of normal saline (30-minute intravenous infusions) of 100 mL of normal saline (4-hour intravenous infusions). Alternatively, a 150-mL-size Travenol Buretrol may be used in place of the plastic intravenous bag. Fifty milliliters of normal saline (30-minute intravenous infusions) or 100 mL normal saline (4-hour intravenous infusions) should be added to the Buretrol followed by the HSA at 2 mg/mL. For 24-hour intravenous infusions, a 20-mL-size Travenol Autosyringe may be used with up to 20 mL normal saline and HSA at 2 mg/mL.
2. Gently swirl and invert the bag to ensure adequate mixing and coating of the surface. *Do not shake.*
3. Add recombinant TNF at the prescribed dose and, again, gently swirl and invert the bag. *Do not shake.*

■ Administration

Because TNF is still an investigational agent no most appropriate dose or schedule has been established. The doses and schedules used in phase I studies are outlined in the table on page 942 and are discussed under Dosage. Although systemic side effects might be decreased with subcutaneous administration, the local inflammatory effects at the injection site are quite severe (Chapman et al 1987). Feinberg and colleagues (1988) have reported no apparent differences in clinical toxic effects for a 30-minute versus a 4-hour infusion.

Pretreatment with intravenous methylprednisolone (200–500 mg) 2 hours before TNF and

PHASE I TRIALS OF TUMOR NECROSIS FACTOR

Schedule	Route	Dose Range	Dose-Limiting Toxic Effects	Dose Recommended for Phase II Trials	Reference
2 Days, repeat every 2 wk	IV	9×10^3 to 9×10^5 U/m^2 (4–400 µg/m^2)	Hypotension, abnormal liver function tests, leukopenia	6×10^5 U/m^2	Selby et al 1987*
Twice weekly × 4 wk	Alternate SC and IV	1–200 µg/m^2 IV 5–250 µg/m^2 SC	Inflammation at SC site, fever, rigors, fatigue	50 µg/m^2 SC None given for IV	Chapman et al 1987†
Every 3 wk	IV	$1–48 \times 10^4$ U/m^2	Hypotension	48×10^4/U/m^2	Creaven et al 1987*
Daily × 5 every 2–3 wk	IV IV	5–200 µg/m^2	Hypotension, phlebitis, rigors	150 µg/m^2	Creagan et al 1988
Daily × 5 every 2 wk	IV 30 min IV 4 h	5–250 µg/m^2/d	Constitutional symptoms, hypotension	200 µg/m^2	Feinberg et al 1988†
Single dose 3 times/wk	IV Intratumor	$0.1–5 \times 10^6$ U $0.1–2 \times 10^6$	Constitutional symptoms, hypotension	2×10^6 Unknown	Taguchi 1988‡
3 Times/wk	IV	5–250 µg/m^2	Hypotension, systemic symptoms	250 µg/m^2	Trump et al 1988
Daily × 5 every other week	IV (15 min)	2–200 µg/m^2	Hypotension, hemorrhagic gastritis	160 µg/m^2	Krigel et al 1988

*Recombinant human tumor necrosis factor from Asahi Chemical Industry Company.
†Recombinant human tumor necrosis factor Genentech, Inc, South San Francisco, California.
‡Recombinant human tumor necrosis factor Kyowa Hakko Co. Ltd., Tokyo, Japan and Takeda Chemical Ind., Osaka, Japan.

oral indomethacin has been reported by Selby and colleagues (1987) to drastically reduce the rigors, fevers, tachycardia, and hypertension associated with administration of TNF. Other investigators have found meperidine hydrochloride given to patients with severe rigors can control the rigors.

■ Special Precautions§

Because proteins such as recombinant TNF can adhere to the walls of bottles and tubing, recombinant TNF should be administered in a solution containing 0.25% serum albumin. One way to accomplish this is to add the specified dose of recombinant TNF solution to 100 mL of Sodium Chloride Injection, USP, to which 1 mL of 25% Normal Serum Albumin (Human), USP, has been added. Dilutions in other solutions or mixture with other drugs should be avoided.

Because of the general tendency of proteins to adhere to surfaces, both unnecessary dilution of the recombinant TNF solution and use of infusion filters should be avoided.

■ Drug Interactions

The methylxanthine hemorheologic agent pentoxifylline {1-(5-oxohexyl)-3,7-dimethylxanthine [Trental®, Hoescht-Roussel Pharmaceuticals]} has been shown to alter endogenous TNF-α production (Han et al 1990). This effect appears to be mediated by inhibition of synthesis of TNF-α messenger RNA (Han et al 1990). Pentoxifylline has been used clinically to treat the complications of bone marrow transplantation which have previously been associated with elevated levels of TNF-α (Bianco et al 1991). Pentoxifylline is not recommended for use in antitumor trials with TNF-α.

■ Dosage

The table outlines the dose range and schedule of TNF used in phase I trials as well as the dose-limiting toxic effects. As can be seen in that table, there are a large number of schedules as well as dosages. At this point, no specific dose or schedule recommendations are possible.

§Adapted from CetusChiron Corporation's Investigators Brochure.

Pharmacokinetics

Traditional pharmacokinetic parameters for TNF are difficult to find in the published literature. Chapman et al (1987) noted that the highest serum level was 80 ng/mL after an injection of 200 µg/m². No TNF was detectable in a 4-hour sample. The terminal phase of elimination suggested a half-life of 20 minutes. They were barely able to detect serum levels of TNF after a subcutaneous dose of 250 µg/m² (peak level of 0.14 ng/mL).

Feinberg and colleagues (1988) measured serum TNF levels in patients receiving more than 100 µg/m². Peak serum levels exceeding 10 ng/mL were observed 30 minutes after infusion. No cumulative effects on plasma levels (day 5 versus day 1) have been observed by Chapman et al (1987) or Feinberg et al (1988). Creagan and colleagues (1988) noted that plasma levels were too low for detection at doses of 20×10^6 u/m². At higher doses, however, TNF plasma clearance ranged from 7.43 to 32.46 L/h with an AUC of 11,706 to 91,506 U/h·L. The half-life ranged from 0.20 to 0.72 hours. The data were variable but suggested nonlinear pharmacokinetics for the agent.

Selby et al (1987) noted that the median half-life of TNF was 17 minutes (range, 8–61 minutes). There was great variability between patients. The pharmacokinetics was nonlinear. Maximum serum concentrations ranged from 2.1 to 583 U/mL. The AUCs ranged from 364 to 45,712 U/mL·min, the clearance ranged from 49.5 to 457 mL/min, and the volume of distribution ranged from 2.59 to 7.3 L.

The reason for the nonlinear kinetics of TNF is unclear, but it may be saturation of a clearance mechanism with higher doses of the agent.

Side Effects and Toxicity

Almost all trials with recombinant TNF-α have described hypotension (Krigel et al 1988, Selby et al 1987, Creagan et al 1988, Chapman et al 1987); rigors (Krigel et al 1988, Trump et al 1988, Chapman et al 1987, Creagan et al 1988), which appear 10 minutes into infusion and do not appear dose related; fatigue (Chapman et al 1987); fever (Feinberg et al 1988, Krigel et al 1988); mild granulocytopenia (Feinberg et al, 1988, Creaven et al 1987); increased fibrin split products (Krigel et al 1988, Chapman et al 1987); increased serum triglycerides (supposedly from inhibition of lipoprotein lipase) (Krigel et al 1988, Feinberg et al 1988); decreased serum cholesterol and decreased high- and low-density lipoproteins (Krigel et al 1988). Other less common toxic effects include acute superficial hemorrhagic gastritis (Krigel et al 1988); nausea and vomiting (Feinberg et al 1988); peripheral cyanosis (Krigel et al 1988); hypertension, usually associated with rigors (Selby et al 1987, Chapman et al 1987); phlebitis (Creagan et al 1988); diarrhea (Selby et al 1987); monocytopenia (Trump et al 1988); relative eosinophilia (Creagan et al 1988); transient increases in liver function tests (Feinberg et al 1988); decreases in serum transferrin levels (Krigel et al 1988); acute angina (Feinberg et al 1988); mild hypercalcemia (Selby et al 1987); and severe inflammation at subcutaneous injection sites (Chapman et al 1987).

Also of note is that administration of TNF is associated with a significant decrease in serum levels of zinc and a rise in plasma cortisol and C-reactive protein (Chapman et al 1987).

Retinal vein thrombosis has been reported in one phase II trial with the agent (Kemeny et al 1990). Of particular interest is the lack of detectable antibodies against TNF in serum before or after treatment (Chapman et al 1987, Feinberg et al 1988).

As noted earlier, prophylactic acetaminophen can prevent fevers and meperidine can control rigors (Krigel et al 1988). Ibuprofen does not appear to affect the symptoms (Trump et al 1988, Creagen et al 1988).

REFERENCES

Abbruzzese J, Levin B. Treatment of advanced colorectal cancer. *Hematol Oncol Clin North Am.* 1989;**3**:135–153.

Aboulafia D, Miles S, Saks S, Mitsuyasu. Intravenous recombinant tumor necrosis factor in the treatment of AIDS-related Kaposi's sarcoma. *J Acquired Immune Defic Syndr.* 1989;**2**:54–58.

Aggarwal BB, Moffat B, Harkins RN. Human lymphotoxin: Production by a lymphoblastoid cell line, purification and initial characterization. *J Biol Chem.* 1984;**259**:686–691.

Aggarwal BB, Moffat B, Harkins RN. Human lymphotoxin: Production by a macrophage cell line, purification and initial characterization. *J Biol Chem.* 1985;**259**:686.

Balkwill F, Burke F, Talbot D, et al. Evidence for tumor necrosis factor/cachectin production in cancer. *Lancet.* 1987;**2**:1229–1232.

Balkwill FR, Lee A, Aldan G. Human tumor xenografts treated with recombinant human tumor necrosis factor alone or in combinations with interferon. *Cancer Res.* 1986;**46**:3990–3993.

Balkwill FR, Naylor MS, Malk S. Tumour necrosis factor as an anticancer agent. *Eur J Cancer.* 1990;**26**:641–644.

Bianco JA, Appelbaum FR, Nemunaitis J, et al. Phase I–II

trial of pentoxifylline for the prevention of transplant-related toxicities following bone marrow transplantation. *Blood.* 1991;**78**(5):1205–1211.

Carswell EA, Old LJ, Kassel RJ, Green S, Fiore N, Williamson B. An endotoxin-induced serum factor that causes necrosis of tumors. *Proc Natl Acad Sci USA.* 1975;**72**:3666–3670.

Chapman PB, Lester TJ, Casper ES, et al. Clinical pharmacology of recombinant human tumor necrosis factor in patients with advanced cancer. *J Clin Oncol.* 1987;**5**:1942–1951.

Cottman FD, Green LM, Godwin A, Ware CF. Cytotoxicity mediated by tumor necrosis factor in variant subclones of the ME-180 cervical carcinoma line: Modulation by specific inhibitors of DNA topoisomerase II. *J Cell Biochem.* 1989;**39**:95–105.

Creagen ET, Kovach JS, Moertel CH, Frytak S, Kvols LK. A phase I clinical trial of recombinant human tumor necrosis factor. *Cancer.* 1988;**62**:2467–2471.

Creaven PJ, Plager JE, Dupere S, et al. Phase I clinical trial of recombinant human tumor necrosis factor. *Cancer Chemother Pharmacol.* 1987;**20**:137–144.

Feinberg B, Kurzrock R, Talpaz M, Blick M, Saks S, Gutterman JU. A phase I trial of intravenously-administered recombinant tumor necrosis factor-alpha in cancer patients. *J Clin Oncol.* 1988;**6**:1328–1334.

Figlin R, de Kernian J, Sarna G, Moldauwer N, Saks S. Phase II study of recombinant tumor necrosis factor (RNTF) in patients with metastatic renal cell carcinoma (RCCA) and malignant melanoma (MM). *Proc Am Soc Clin Oncol.* 1988;**7**:A652.

Frei E III, Spriggs D. Tumor necrosis factor: Still a promising agent. *J Clin Oncol.* 1989;**7**:291–294.

Goeddel DV, Aggarwal BB, Gray PW, et al. Tumor necrosis factors: Gene structure and biological activities. *Cold Spring Harbor Symp Quant Biol.* 1986;**1**:597–609.

Gray PW, Aggarwal BB, Benton CV, et al. Cloning and expression of cDNA for human lymphotoxin, a lymphokine with tumour necrosis activity. *Nature.* 1984;**312**:721.

Han J, Thompson P, Beutler B. Dexamethasone and pentoxifylline inhibit endotoxin-induced cachectin/tumor necrosis factor synthesis at separate points in the signaling pathway. *J Exp Med.* 1990;**172**:391.

Harauaka K, Satomi N, Sakurai A. Antitumor activity of murine tumor necrosis factor (TNF) against transplanted murine tumors and heterotransplanted human tumors in nude mice. *Int J Cancer.* 1984;**34**:263–267.

Havell EA, Fiers W, Norton RJ. The antitumor formation of TNF against an established murine sarcoma is indirect, immunologically dependent and limited by severe toxicity. *J Exp Med.* 1988;**167**:1067–1085.

Johnson RA, Boyce BF, Mundy GR, Roodman GD. Tumors producing human tumor necrosis factor induced hypercalcemia and osteoclastic bone resorption in nude mice. *Endocrinology.* 1989;**124**:1424–1427.

Kemeny N, Childs B, Larchian W, Rosado K, Kelsen D. A phase II trial of recombinant tumor necrosis factor in patients with advanced colorectal carcinoma. *Cancer.* 1990;**66**:659–663.

Kist A, Ho AD, Rath U, et al. Decrease of natural killer cell activity and monokine production in deoxyplarol blood of patients treated with recombinant tumor necrosis factor. *Blood.* 1988;**72**:344–348.

Krigel R, Padavic K, Ottery F, Rudolf A, Camis D. Metabolic changes in patients treated in a phase I trial of recombinant tumor necrosis factor (RTNF). *Proc Am Assoc Cancer Res.* 1988;**29**:432.

Lowry SF, Muldauer LL. Tumor necrosis factor and other cytokines in the pathogenesis of cancer cachexia. *Principle Pract Oncol Updates.* 1990;**8**:1–12.

Nawroth PD, Handley G, Matsueda R, et al. Tumor necrosis factor cachectin-induced intravascular fibrin formation in meth A fibrosarcomas. *J Exp Med.* 1988;**168**:637–647.

Oliff A, Defeo-Jones D, Boyer M, et al. Tumors secreting human TNF/cachectin induce cachexia in mice. *Cell.* 1987;**50**:555–563.

Palladino MA Jr, Shalaby MR, Kramer SM, et al. Characterization of the antitumor activities of human tumor necrosis factor alpha and the comparison with other cytokines: Induction of tumor-specific immunity. *J Immunol.* 1987;**138**:4023–4032.

Pennica D, Nedwin G, Hayflick J, et al. Human tumour necrosis factor: Precursor structure, expression and homology to lymphotoxin. *Nature.* 1984;**312**:724–729.

Raeth U, Schmid H, Karck U, Kempeni J, Schlick E, Kaufmann M. Phase II trial of recombinant human tumor necrosis factor-alpha (RHUTNF) in patients with malignant ascites from ovarian carcinomas and non-ovarian tumors with intraperitoneal spread. *Proc Annu Meet Am Soc Clin Oncol.* 1991;**10**:A610.

Retsas S, Leslie M, Bottomley D. Intralesional tumor necrosis factor combined with interferon gamma in metastatic melanoma. *Br Med J.* 1989;**298**:1290–1291.

Salmon SE, Young L, Scuderi P, Clark B. Antineoplastic effect of tumor necrosis factor alone and in combination with gamma interferon on tumor biopsies in clonogenic assay. *J Clin Oncol.* 1987;**5**:1816–1821.

Selby P, Hobbs S, Viner C, et al. Tumor necrosis factor in man in clinical and biological observations. *Br J Cancer.* 1987;**56**:803–808.

Shirai T, Yamaguchi H, Ito H, Todd C, Wallace B. Cloning and expression in *Escherichia coli* of the gene for human tumour necrosis factor. *Nature.* 1985;**313**:803–806.

Socher SH, Martinez D, Craig JB, Kuhn JG, Oliff A. Tumor necrosis factor not detectable in patients with clinical cancer cachexia. *J Natl Cancer Inst.* 1988;**80**:595–598.

Sugarman BT, Aggarwal BB, Hass PE, Figari IS, Palladino MA, Shepard HM. Recombinant tumor necrosis factor-alpha: Effects on normal and transformed cells in vitro. *Science.* 1985;**230**:943–945.

Taguchi T. Phase I study of recombinant human tumor necrosis factor(rHa-TNF:PT-050). *Cancer Detect Prev.* 1988;**12**:561–572.

Tracey KJ, Wei HE, Manogue KR, et al. Cachectin/tumor necrosis factor induces cachexia, anemia, and inflammation. *J Exp Med.* 1988;**167**:1211–1227.

Trump DL, Remick SC, Alberti D, et al. A clinical trial of recombinant tumor necrosis factor (RTNF) administered three times weekly (abstract 648). *Proc Am Soc Clin Oncol.* 1988;**7**:168.

Tsujimoto M, Yip YF, Vilcek J. Tumor necrosis factor: Specific binding and internalization in sensitive and resistant cells. *Proc Natl Acad Sci USA.* 1985;**82**:7626–7630.

Uracil Mustard*

■ Other Names

U-8344 (The Upjohn Company); NSC-34462.

■ Chemistry

Structure of uracil mustard

Uracil mustard 5-[bis(2-chloroethyl)amino]uracil occurs as an off-white crystalline powder. It is soluble in water (1 mg/mL) and alcohol (7.5 mg/mL).

■ Antitumor Activity

Uracil mustard is active in a variety of preclinical tumor models including Walker-256 carcinoma, S-91 melanoma, L-1210 leukemia, sarcoma-180, and a variety of lymphomas (Lane and Kelly 1960, Lytle and Petering 1959). Minor responses have also been noted in human leukemia and lymphoma (Kennedy and Theologides 1961). Activity in lymphomas and chronic leukemias and in a few patients with ovarian cancer was described by Shanbrom et al (1960).

Uracil mustard has also been used in the treatment of essential thrombocythemia (Shamasunder et al 1980, Robertson 1970).

■ Mechanism of Action

Uracil mustard is a polyfunctional alkylating agent and hence is not cell cycle phase specific. The drug binds covalently to DNA to inhibit DNA synthesis and thereby induce cell death.

■ Availability and Storage

The drug was investigationally available from the Upjohn Company Research Laboratories, Kalamazoo, Michigan. It was supplied as 1-mg capsules and may be stored at room temperature. Ampules containing 5 mg powdered drug were also available (Lane et al 1960).

■ Administration

Uracil mustard is given orally. Because nausea and vomiting are common, some authors recommend that the dose be administered before bedtime, hoping the patient may sleep through the nausea.

■ Dosage

Various dosing schedules have been used. One method initiates therapy at doses of 1 to 2 mg/d until the desired hematologic effect is obtained. Another, more common dosing schedule involves a dose of 3 to 5 mg/d for the first 7 days, followed by 1 mg/d until the desired hematologic effect is obtained. Single weekly oral doses of 6 to 20 mg were successfully used by Lane et al (1960). Intravenous doses ranged from 5 mg three times per week or 0.4 mg/kg per week as a single infusion (Lane et al 1960). Continuous daily treatment with 1 mg/d has been used if the patient achieves a response. Some authors recommend 1 week without treatment ("rest period") after every 3 weeks of continuous therapy. Doses of 1 to 2 mg/d were administered for 14 days to patients with essential thrombocytosis (Shamasunder et al 1980).

■ Side Effects and Toxicity

Myelosuppression is dose related. Leukopenia and thrombocytopenia are more frequent, but anemia may also occur. Maximum depression of the bone marrow may not be manifested until 2 to 4 weeks after discontinuance of the drug. If radiotherapy or other antineoplastic drugs are used in conjunction with uracil mustard, significant myelosuppression may be observed; therefore, doses should be reduced in this circumstance.

---

*This monograph is included for reference only; initial trials have not supported the need for further clinical investigation of this compound.

Gastrointestinal toxic effects, including anorexia, nausea, vomiting, and diarrhea, can be frequent. Pruritis, dermatitis, alopecia, and abnormal skin pigmentation have been reported. Drug-induced neurologic symptoms include nervousness, mental cloudiness, and depression. Hepatotoxicity has been reported rarely. Alopecia and jaundice caused by uracil mustard have not been observed (Shanbrom et al 1960).

REFERENCES

Kennedy BJ, Theologides A. Uracil mustard, a new alkylating agent for oral administration in the management of patients with leukemia and lymphoma. *N Engl J Med.* 1961;**264**:790–793.

Lane M, Kelley M. The antitumor activity of 5-bis-(2'-chloroethyl)-aminouracil (uracil mustard). *Cancer Res.* 1960a;**20**:511–517.

Lane M, Lipowska B, Hal TC, Colsky J. A preliminary report: Observations on the clinical pharmacology of 5-[bis(2-chloroethyl)amino]uracil (uracil mustard; NSC-34462). *Cancer Chemother Rep.* 1960b;**9**:31–36.

Lytle DA, Petering HG. 5-Bis(2'-chloroethyl)aminouracil: New antitumor agent. *J Natl Cancer Inst.* 1959;**23**:153–162.

Robertson JH. Uracil mustard in the treatment of thrombocythemia. *Blood.* 1970;**35**:288–297.

Shamasunder HK, Gregory SA, Knospe WH. Uracil mustard in the treatment of thrombocytosis. *JAMA.* 1980;**244**:1454–1455.

Shanbrom E, Miller S, Haar H, Opfell R. Therapeutic spectrum of uracil-mustard, a new oral antitumor drug. *JAMA.* 1960;**174**:1702–1705.

Vinblastine Sulfate

■ Other Names

Vincaleukoblastine; VLB; NSC-49842; Velban® (Eli Lilly and Company); Velbe® (Eli Lilly and Company).

■ Chemistry

Structure of vinblastine

Vinblastine is the sulfate salt of an alkaloid isolated from *Vinca rosea* (periwinkle). It is structurally related to vincristine, another alkaloid isolated from the same plant. Vinblastine sulfate is freely soluble in water and occurs as a white crystalline powder. The empiric formula is $C_{46}H_{58}N_4O_9 \cdot H_2SO_4$.

■ Antitumor Activity

Vinblastine is approved for use in patients with Hodgkin's disease, non-Hodgkin's lymphoma, testicular carcinoma, histiocytosis X, choriocarcinomas, and breast cancer (Frei et al 1961, Carter 1974, Hammond et al 1973, Smart et al 1964, Hertz et al 1960, Bonadonna et al 1975, Einhorn and Donohue 1977, Yap et al 1979). In addition, the agent has shown antitumor activity in bladder cancer, renal cell carcinoma, and chronic myelocytic leukemia in blast crisis (Gomez and Sokal 1979). Of course, in most instances the drug is used in combination regimens for all of the preceding diseases (eg, Bonadonna et al 1975, Navarro et al 1989). Vinblastine has been used in combination with mitomycin-C and cisplatin in the treatment of patients with non-small cell lung cancer (Dillman et al 1986, DiMaggio et al 1988, Kalman et al 1983, Kris et al 1985). In addition, the agent has been found to have activity in acquired immunodeficiency syndrome (AIDS)-related Kaposi's sarcoma (Krown et al 1986).

■ Mechanism of Action

Vinblastine binds to tubulin. That binding inhibits microtubule assembly which inhibits mitotic spindle formation. This causes an accumulation of cells in metaphase (Noble and Beer 1968, Owellen et al 1975, 1977).

Vinblastine is considered cell cycle phase specific for mitosis; however, the cytotoxic effect probably occurs in S phase and is only expressed in M phase. At high doses, direct effects may be noted in S and G_1 phases. Vinblastine may thus be assumed to have stathmokinetic effects similar to those of vincristine.

■ Availability and Storage

Vinblastine sulfate is commercially available in rubber-stoppered vials containing 10 mg of vinblastine sulfate as a lyophilized drug (Velban®, Eli Lilly and Company, Indianapolis, Indiana). It should be stored under refrigeration and protected from light before mixing.

Preparation for Use, Stability, and Admixture

The solution for administration is usually prepared by adding 10 mL of sodium chloride for injection (which may be preserved with either phenols or benzyl alcohol) to the 10-mg vial. The use of other solutions is not generally recommended. The resultant solution has a concentration of 1.0 mg/mL and a pH of 3.5 to 5. Solutions prepared with preserved sodium chloride injection may be stored in the refrigerator (protected from light) for 30 days without significant loss of potency. Vinblastine (0.12 mg/mL) is physically compatible for 4 hours with ondansetron (1 mg/mL) in D5W (Trissel et al 1990).

Administration

Vinblastine is usually given by the intravenous push technique, with the total dose being delivered over about 1 minute. This is usually accomplished by slowly pushing the dose through the injection site of a running intravenous infusion. Alternately, the drug may be given directly into the vein. If this method is followed, the "double-needle" technique should be used (ie, do not use the same needle to withdraw the dose from the vial that is used for the direct injection into the vein). Vinblastine is very irritating and should not be given intramuscularly or subcutaneously. It is therefore recommended that vein patency be checked before drug administration by flushing with a small quantity of normal saline or D5W. After the dose has been given, the site should again be flushed to ensure that all of the drug has been delivered into the vein. If extravasation should occur, refer to the Special Precautions section.

Vinblastine has been used as a 5-day continuous infusion of 1.5 to 2 mg/m^2/d (Yap et al 1979). Each day's dose may be diluted in a liter of D5W or normal saline, which is then administered over 24 hours.

Special Precautions

Extravasation must be avoided. If extravasation occurs, administration of the remaining drug must be stopped immediately. Different techniques have been employed to minimize the local reaction. The manufacturer recommends local injection of hyaluronidase and application of heat to the area to dispose of the drug. It is possible that heat may aggravate a local reaction. Dorr and Alberts (1985) favor injection of a corticosteroid into the infiltration site along with sodium chloride to dilute the drug. Only minor tissue damage has occurred when vinblastine extravasation has been treated with 50 to 500 mg hydrocortisone sodium succinate. This is followed by cold compresses to minimize spread of the reaction.

Liver disease may alter the elimination of vinblastine and necessitate a dosage reduction. Neurotoxicity may be more frequent in patients with underlying neurologic problems or those who are weak or cachectic at the start of treatment. Alopecia may possibly be decreased if a tourniquet or ice bag is placed just below the hair line around the scalp during drug administration and for a short time thereafter. Controversy exists regarding this procedure, as the reduced blood flow to the scalp may spare not only the hair follicle but also metastatic disease in this area, thus reducing the efficacy of therapy. This technique obviously is not indicated if vinblastine is administered by continuous infusion.

Drug Interactions

Like vincristine, vinblastine increases the cellular uptake of methotrexate by some malignant cells; however, its propensity to do this appears to be less than with vincristine (Zager et al 1973).

Samuels and co-workers (Samuels and Howe 1970, Samuels et al 1975) have additionally suggested that therapeutic synergism in patients with testicular cancer could occur by sequential administration of vinblastine before a continuous infusion of bleomycin. The rationale is that the cell synchronization of tumor cells by vinblastine (in the late G_2 or early M phase) would facilitate enhanced cell-kill with bleomycin, which is G_2 phase specific. Although interesting mechanistically, clinical results documenting a significant degree of synergism are lacking. Bolin et al (1983) have described a patient who had decreased plasma phenytoin levels, which were felt to be caused by administration of intravenous vinblastine.

Dosage

Vinblastine has been given by several different dosing schemes. The dose varies depending on the protocol being followed, the condition of the patient, other drugs or radiation being used, and individual patient response. Usually the drug is given no more frequently than once every week. The dosage range is 0.1 to 0.5 mg/kg/wk (4.0–20 mg/m^2). Patients are customarily started at a low dose of 8 mg/m^2 (as a single agent) and worked up in 0.05 mg/kg increments depending on the degree of resulting leukopenia. Yap et al (1979) found that doses of 1.5 to 1.7 mg/m²/d for 5 days by continuous infusion usually produced only mild to moderate myelosuppression, but doses of 2 mg/m²/d for 5 days produced severe (life threatening) myelosuppression.

■ Pharmacokinetics

As can be seen in the table, after intravenous administration, vinblastine is rapidly cleared from the plasma and concentrated in various tissues. The apparent volume of distribution for the central compartment is quite large (three to four times blood volume). This is in contrast to vincristine and vindesine which approximate total body water in distribution. There is a triphasic vinblastine elimination pattern, with average half-lives of 25 minutes, 53 minutes, and 19 to 25 hours, respectively (Owellen et al 1977, Nelson 1982). The drug is also known to localize in platelet and leukocyte fractions of whole blood (Owellen and Hartke 1975). Radiolabeled drug study has shown that urinary elimination will recover about 33% of the total vinblastine radioactivity with 21% appearing in the stool, both after 72 hours (Owellen and Hartke 1975). A large portion of the radiolabel was retained in the body: 73% of a dose 6 days after dosing. Apparently, insufficient amounts of the drug pass the blood–brain barrier to produce an effective concentration in the central nervous system. Vinblastine is partially metabolized to deacetyl vinblastine, which is more active on a weight basis (Owellen et al 1977). Vinblastine is partially metabolized in the liver. Most drug is therefore ultimately excreted intact in the bile or the urine. Toxicity may, however, be increased if obstructive liver disease is present, and doses should be greatly reduced.

Following continuous vinblastine infusions Lu et al (1979) have described both extended terminal half-lives and high steady-state drug levels: 1µg/mL at 1 mg/m²/d (terminal half-life, 28 days); 3 µg/mL at 1.7 mg/m²/d (terminal half-life, 3 days); and 6 µg/mL at 2 mg/m²/d (terminal half-life, 6 days).

■ Side Effects and Toxicity

The major toxic effect of vinblastine is a dose-related bone marrow depression. Interestingly, this is more frequent and severe than with the close structural analog vincristine. Leukopenia occurs with a nadir of 4 to 10 days, with recovery occurring over another 7 to 14 days. Because of the relatively predictable nadir it may be possible to cautiously administer vinblastine as often as every 10 days up to every week. The duration of leukopenia is also apparently dose related, and vinblastine will usually produce thrombocytopenia; however, serious platelet depressions with commonly used doses are generally infrequent.

Erythrocytes are usually only slightly depressed. Myelosuppression is usually mild at doses of 1.5 to 1.7 mg/m²/d by the 5-day continuous infusion regimen, but becomes severe if the dose is increased to 2 mg/m²/d × 5 days.

In general, vinblastine is well tolerated. Nausea and vomiting occur rarely and are at least partially responsive to antiemetics. Gastrointestinal symptoms (which may be related to neurotoxicity) include constipation, adynamic ileus, and abdominal pain especially when high doses are used (eg, > 20 mg). These side effects are rarely seen with doses less than 10 mg. Prophylactic stool softeners may be helpful in preventing constipation.

Neurotoxicity associated with vinblastine occurs less frequently than with vincristine and is

PHARMACOKINETICS OF VINBLASTINE

Schedule	Half-life (h) α	Half-life (h) β	Half-life (h) γ	Clearance (L/kg/h)	Volume (L/kg) Central Compartment	Volume (L/kg) Distribution	Reference
Bolus (7–14 mg)	0.062 ± 0.04	1.64 ± 0.34	24.8 ± 7.5	0.740 ± 0.319	0.696 ± 0.482	27.3 ± 14.9	Nelson 1982
Bolus (0.167–0.2 mg/kg)	0.065 ± 0.02	0.88 ± 0.22	19.5 ± 1.08	—	—	—	Owellen et al 1977

most frequently observed in patients on prolonged therapy or in those receiving high individual doses. Symptoms include paresthesias, peripheral neuropathy, depression, headache, malaise, jaw pain, urinary retention, tachycardia, orthostatic hypotension, and convulsions. Vocal cord paralysis (Brook and Schreiber 1971) and cranial nerve paralysis have also been reported.

Other side effects include a reversible and mild alopecia, rashes, and photosensitivity reactions (Breza et al 1975). Stomatitis, which can occasionally become severe, is also reported. Transient hepatitis has been reported on the continuous infusion regimen.

Vinblastine solution is topically irritating and has caused corneal irritation when inadvertently splashed in the eyes (McClendon and Bron 1978). Precautions should be employed by all persons working with the drug.

There have been several reports of a Raynaud's phenomenon associated with vinblastine and/or bleomycin in patients with testicular cancer. The reaction consists of delayed presentation of a cold feeling in the hands with physical evidence of cyanosis (Teutsch et al 1977). Ginsberg et al (1977) demonstrated a case of vinblastine-associated syndrome of inappropriate antidiuretic hormone secretion, previously thought to occur only with vincristine.

Also, although there are reports of normal infants delivered from vinblastine-treated patients (Armstrong et al 1964, Lacher 1964), the drug is well documented as a teratogen in humans (Cohlan and Kitay 1965). Thus, as with most anticancer drugs, usage in pregnancy is strongly contraindicated.

General muscle and tumor pain are commonly experienced by a number of patients receiving vinblastine, especially in high doses (Stark and Fletcher 1966, Lucas and Huang 1977). The tumor pain is described as intense stinging or burning and is abrupt in onset (1–3 minutes), lasting from 20 minutes to 3 hours. Parenteral narcotics and the substitution of vincristine have been described as beneficial in some cases.

■ Special Applications

Vinblastine has been used along with cisplatin as an intraarterial form of treatment for patients with breast cancer metastases in the liver. The toxic effects noted included paralytic ileus, leukopenia, syndrome of inappropriate antidiuretic hormone secretion, arterial thrombus, and occlusion (Fraschini et al 1987, 1988). Intralesional vinblastine has been used with some success in patients with Kaposi's sarcoma (Newman 1988).

Vinblastine solution (0.2 mg/mL) has also been injected directly into oral lesions in patients with kaposis sarcoma (Epstein 1993). Under local anesthesia, doses of 0.1 mL injected per 0.5 cm of lesion surface area were administered at total doses up to 4 mL (0.8 mg). Tumor shrinkage > 50% was achieved in 74% of patients with a median response duration of 3.5 months. Side effects included pain, numbness, and ulceration which both resolved rapidly.

REFERENCES

Armstrong JG, Dyke RW, Fouts PJ, Jansen CJ. Delivery of a normal infant during the course of oral vinblastine sulfate therapy for Hodgkin's disease. *Ann Intern Med.* 1964;**61**:106–112.

Bolin P, Riva R, Albani F, et al. Decreased phenytoin level during antineoplastic therapy: A case report. *Epilepsia.* 1983;**24**:75–78.

Bonadonna G, Zucali R, Monfardini S, DeLena M, Uslenghi C. Combination chemotherapy of Hodgkin's disease with Adriamycin, bleomycin, vinblastine and imidazole carboxamide versus MOPP. *Cancer.* 1975;**36**:252–259.

Breza TS, Halprin KM, Taylor JR. Photosensitivity reaction to vinblastine. *Arch Dermatol.* 1975;**111**:1168–1179.

Brook J, Schreiber W. Vocal cord paralysis: A toxic reaction to vinblastine (NSC-49842) therapy. *Cancer Chemother Rep.* 1971;**55**:591–593.

Carter SK. The chemical therapy of breast cancer. *Semin Oncol.* 1974;**1**:131–141.

Cohlan SW, Kitay D. The teratogenic effect of vincaleukoblastine in the pregnant rat. *J Pediatr.* 1965;**66**:541–544.

Dillman RO, Seagren SL, Propert K, Kreisman H, Eaton WL, Green MR. Complete responses in regional stage III non-small cell lung cancer (NSCLC) with vinblastine (VLB) and cisplatinum (CDDP) (meeting abstract). *Proc Ann Meet Am Soc Clin Oncol.* 1986:5.

DiMaggio JJ, Kris MG, Gralla RJ, et al. Dose intensity versus toxicity trial in non-small cell lung cancer (NSCLC) with MVP (mitomycin + vinblastine (V)+ cisplatin (P) (meeting abstract). *Proc Ann Meet Assoc Cancer Res.* 1988:29.

Dorr RT, Alberts DS. Vinca alkaloid skin toxicity: Antidote and drug disposition studies in the mouse. *J Natl Cancer Inst.* 1985;**74**:113–120.

Einhorn LH, Donohue J. cis-Diamminedichloroplatinum, vinblastine and bleomycin combination chemotherapy in disseminated testicular cancer. *Ann Intern Med.* 1977;**87**:293–298.

Epstein JB: Treatment of oral Kaposi's sarcoma with intralesional vinblastine. *Cancer.* 1993;**71**:1722–1725.

Fraschini G, Charnsangavej C, Carrasco CH, Buzdar AU, Jabboury KW, Hortobagyi GN. Percutaneous hepatic arterial infusion of cisplatin–vinblastine for refractory breast carcinoma metastatic to the liver. *Am J Clin Oncol.* 1988;**11**(1):34–38.

Fraschini G, Fleishman G, Wallace S, Hortobagyi G. Percutaneous hepatic arterial infusion (HAI) of cisplatin (C) and vinblastine (V), as single agents or in combination (C + V) for breast cancer (BC) metastatic to the liver (meeting abstract) *Proc Ann Meet Am Soc Clin Oncol.* 1987;**6**:64.

Frei E III, Franzino A, Schnider BI, et al. Clinical studies of vinblastine. *Cancer Chemother Rep.* 1961;**12**:125–129.

Ginsberg SJ, Comis RL, Fitzpatrick AV. Vinblastine and inappropriate ADH secretion (letter). *N Engl J Med.* 1977;**296**(16):941.

Gomez GA, Sokal JE. Use of vinblastine in the terminal phase of chronic myelocytic leukemia. *Cancer Treat Rep.* 1979;**63**(8):1385–1387.

Hammond CB, Borcet LG, Tyrey L, et al. Treatment of metastatic trophoblastic disease: Good and poor prognosis. *Am J Obstet Gynecol.* 1973;**115**:451–457.

Hertz R, Lipsett MB, Moy RH. Effect of vincaleukoblastine on metastatic choriocarcinoma and related trophoblastic tumors in women. *Cancer Res.* 1960;**20**:1050–1053.

Kalman LA, Kris MG, Gralla RJ, et al. Vinca alkaloid and cisplatin combination therapy in non-small cell lung cancer (NSCLC): Results of a randomized trial with a comparison of methods of response assessment in 109 patients. (meeting abstract). *Proc Ann Meet Am Soc Clin Oncol.* 1983:2.

Kris MG, Gralla RJ, Kalman LA, et al. Randomized trial comparing vindesine plus cisplatin with vinblastine plus cisplatin in patients with non-small cell lung cancer with an analysis of methods of response assessment. *Cancer Treat Rep.* 1985;**69**(4):387–395.

Krown SE, Gold JW, Real FX, et al. Interferon alpha-PA +/− vinblastine (VLB) in AIDS-associated Kaposi's sarcoma (KS/AIDS): Therapeutic activity, toxicity and effects on HTLV-III/LAV viremia (meeting abstract). *J Interferon Res.* 1986;**6**(suppl 1):3.

Lacher MJ. Use of vinblastine sulfate to treat Hodgkin's disease during pregnancy. *Ann Intern Med.* 1964;**61**:113–115.

Lu K, Yap HY, Watts S, Loo TL. Comparative clinical pharmacology of vinblastine (VLB) in patients with advanced breast cancer: Single versus continuous infusion. *Proc Am Assoc Cancer Res ASCO.* 1979;**20**:371.

Lucas VS, Huang AT. Vinblastine-related pain in tumors. *Cancer Treat Rep.* 1977;**61**(9):1735–1736.

McClendon BF, Bron AJ. Corneal toxicity from vinblastine solution. *Br J Ophthalmol.* 1978;**62**:97–99.

Navarro M, Bellmunt J, Balana C, Colomer R, Jolis L, del Campo JM. Mitomycin-C and vinblastine in advanced breast cancer. *Oncology.* 1989;**46**(3):137–142.

Nelson RL. The comparative clinical pharmacology and pharmacokinetics of vindesine, vincristine, and vinblastine in human patients with cancer. *Med Pediatr Oncol.* 1982;**10**:115–127.

Newman SB. Treatment of epidemic Kaposi's sarcoma (KS) with intralesional vinblastine injection. *Proc Ann Meet Soc Clin Oncol.* 1988;**7**:5.

Noble RL, Beer CT. Experimental observations concerning the mode of action of vinca alkaloids. In: Shedden WIH, ed. *The Vinca Alkaloids in the Chemotherapy of Malignant Disease.* Alburcham, England: John Sherratt and Sons; 1968:4–11.

Owellen RJ, Hartke CA. The pharmacokinetics of 4-acetyl tritium vinblastine in two patients. *Cancer Res.* 1975;**35**:975–980.

Owellen RJ, Hartke CA, Hains FO. Pharmacokinetics and metabolism of vinblastine in humans. *Cancer Res.* 1977;**37**:2597–2602.

Samuels ML, Howe CD. Vinblastine in the management of testicular cancer. *Cancer.* 1970;**25**:1009–1017.

Samuels ML, Johnson DE, Holoye PY. Continuous intravenous bleomycin (NSC-125066) therapy with vinblastine (NSC-49842) in stage II testicular neoplasia. *Cancer Chemother Rep.* 1975;**59**:563–570.

Smart CR, Rochlin DB, Nahum AM, Silva A, Wagner D. Clinical experience with vinblastine sulfate (NSC-49842) in squamous cell carcinoma and other malignancies. *Cancer Chemother Rep.* 1964;**34**:31–45.

Stark DB, Fletcher WS. Severe tumor pain with intravenous injection of vinblastine sulfate (NSC-49842). *Cancer Chemother Rep.* 1966;**50**(5):281–282.

Stutzman L. Current status of treatment of lymphomas. *South Med J.* 1975;**68**:908–913.

Teutsch C, Lipton A, Harvey HA. Raynaud's phenomenon as a side effect of chemotherapy with vinblastine and bleomycin for testicular carcinoma. *Cancer Treat Rep.* 1977;**61**:925–926.

Trissel LA, Fulton B, Tramonte SM. Visual compatibility of ondansetron with chemotherapeutic agents, antibiotics, and other selected drugs during simulated Y-site injection (abstract #P-468R). In: *24th Annual ASHP Midyear Clinical Meetings and Exhibit, Las Vegas, Nevada;* 1990.

Yap H, Blumenschein GR, Hortobagyi GN, Tashima CK, Loo TL. Continuous 5-day infusion vinblastine (VLB) in treatment of refractory advanced breast cancer. *Proc Am Assoc Cancer Res ASCO.* 1979;**20**:334.

Zager RF, Frisby SA, Oliverio VT. The effects of antibiotics and cancer chemotherapeutic agents on the cellular transport and antitumor activity of methotrexate in L1210 murine leukemia. *Cancer Res.* 1973;**33**:1670–1676.

Vincristine Sulfate

■ Other Names

22-Oxovincaleukoblastine; NSC-67574; LCR; VCR; Oncovin® (Eli Lilly and Company).

■ Chemistry

Structure of vincristine sulfate

Vincristine is the sulfate salt of a dimeric alkaloid isolated from the plant *Catharanthus rosea* (the periwinkle plant). It is structurally similar to vinblastine, another alkaloid isolated from the same plant. Both vinca alkaloids are formed from two multiringed units, vindoline and catharanthine, which are linked by a carbon–carbon bond. Vincristine sulfate occurs as freely water-soluble, colorless crystals. The empiric formula is $C_{46}H_{56}N_4O_{10} \cdot H_2SO_4$ and the molecular weight 923.

■ Antitumor Activity

Vincristine has broad-spectrum antitumor activity in human cancer (Holland et al 1973). Interestingly, the activity of this drug in several of the animal tumor screening systems such as L-1210 leukemia was poor because of the brief duration of treatment. The major clinical indication for vincristine is in acute lymphoblastic leukemia (Bohannon et al 1963), usually in combination with prednisone, occasionally with asparaginase and an anthracycline such as daunorubicin or doxorubicin (Karon et al 1966, Haggard et al 1968, Mauer and Simone 1976). It has also been used in (1) breast carcinoma (eg, in CMF-VP, the Cooper Regimen) (Cooper 1969); (2) sarcomas, including Ewing's sarcoma and rhabdomyosarcoma; (3) Wilms' tumor with radiation and dactinomycin (Vietti et al 1970); (4) Hodgkin's disease (eg, in the MOPP regimen); (5) in neuroblastoma alone (James and George 1964) or with cyclophosphamide (Sawitsky et al 1970); and, finally, (6) non-Hodgkin's lymphomas (eg, the BACOP or CHOP regimens).

Vincristine has minor activity in treating idiopathic and secondary forms of thrombocytopenia (Ahn et al 1974). Vincristine is also active when administered by intravenous infusion over several days. This has been observed both in hematologic malignancies such as multiple myeloma (Jackson et al 1985) and in solid tumors such as breast cancer and non-small cell carcinoma of the lung (Jackson et al 1981). Some of the responses to vincristine infusions were obtained in patients refractory to conventional doses administered as bolus injections every 3 to 4 weeks.

■ Mechanism of Action

The mechanism of action of vincristine has traditionally been attributed to mitotic inhibition causing an arrest of cell division in metaphase. Metaphase arrest is due to reversible binding between the drug and a common pair of sites on each subunit protein (α, β) of tubulin. This produces a halt in the assembly of microtubules in S phase (Noble and Beer 1968). The depolymerized tubulin proteins do not allow for assembly of the mitotic spindle and cell division is halted in the metaphase stage of mitosis (Frei et al 1964). The binding affinities (K_D) of vincristine for soluble and crystaline tubulin are 0.1 and 4 μM, respectively (Wilson et al 1978).

Some cells may be only temporarily arrested in mitosis, producing a cell cycle block (stathmokinesis). If drug concentrations fall below a critical threshold, cells can "escape" vincristine lethality and successfully divide.

Other pharmacologic effects noted at extremely high vincristine concentrations include decreased protein and RNA synthesis, altered lipid synthesis, and blocked uptake of glutamic acid (Bender and Chabner 1982).

Vincristine is considered a cell cycle phase-specific agent for mitosis; however, because the drug binds to tubulin in S phase, RNA and DNA synthesis may also be interrupted, probably by the effects on the DNA-directed RNA polymerase system (Creasey 1968).

Vincristine appears to induce a form of multidrug resistance (MDR) characterized by decreased drug accumulation as a result of enhanced efflux (Sirotnak et al 1986); the presence of a 180,000 molecular weight membrane P-glycoprotein (Beck et al 1979); cross-resistance with other natural product anticancer agents (especially anthracyclines); and complete or partial reversal of resistance with calcium channel antagonists, cyclosporin A, phenothiazines, and other noncytotoxic lipophilic agents (Tsuruo et al 1983). Another mechanism of vincristine resistance involves cellular mutations in α and β tubulin proteins that have enhanced stability against depolymerization.

■ Availability and Storage

Vincristine sulfate is commercially available in 1- and 5-mg rubber stoppered vials (Oncovin®, Eli Lilly and Company, Indianapolis, Indiana). The 1-mg vial also contains 10 mg lactose and the 5-mg vial, 50 mg lactose. Both the 1- and 5-mg vials of vincristine are packaged with a 10-mL ampule of bacteriostatic sodium chloride for injection, preserved with 0.9% benzyl alcohol.

Before dilution, vincristine should be stored under refrigeration. At room temperature, the undiluted drug is stable for at least 6 months. Vincristine must be protected from light, even in the crystalline form, to prevent degradation.

■ Preparation for Use, Stability, and Admixture

When the 1-mg vial is diluted with 10 mL of the diluent, the resultant concentration is 100 µg (0.1 mg/mL). When the 5-mg vial is diluted with 10 mL of this diluent, the resultant concentration is 500 µg (0.5 mg/mL). Solutions thus prepared may be stored under refrigeration for 15 days without significant loss of potency; however, vincristine must be protected from light to prevent deterioration.

Vincristine is also physically compatible with a large number of other anticancer agents. These include bleomycin, cisplatin, cyclophosphamide, cytarabine, doxorubicin, 5-fluorouracil, leucovorin, methotrexate, mitomycin-C, and vinblastine (McCrae and King 1976, Cohen et al 1985, Beijnen et al 1986). Vincristine (0.05 mg/mL in D5W) is physically stable for 4 hours with ondansetron 1 mg/mL (Trissel et al 1990). Vincristine is also stable in polyvinyl chloride infusion containers (Benvenuto et al 1981).

■ Administration

Vincristine sulfate is usually given by the intravenous push technique, with the entire dose being administered over almost 1 minute. This may be accomplished by injection of the drug directly into a vein, by the double-needle technique (use of a different needle for reconstitution and direct injection), or directly into the injection site of an intravenous infusion. Alternatively, vincristine may be further diluted in 50 mL of D5W or normal saline and administered over about 15 minutes, although this may increase the likelihood of a severe local reaction if the drug extravasates during an unattended infusion in a peripheral vein. It is therefore recommended that central venous access be used if available and, if not, that the vein patency be checked by prior administration of about 5 to 10 mL of normal saline or D5W. The infusion line should be similarly flushed after the drug is administered to ensure that the entire drug has been delivered into the vein.

Prolonged infusions of vincristine are performed for 1 to 5 days with the daily dose diluted into 250 to 500 mL. Alternatively, the total infusion dose can be delivered in a more concentrated solution by portable infusion pump. Vincristine has been infused continuously with doxorubicin over a 96-hour period (Barlogie et al 1984). *Warning:* Vincristine is highly neurotoxic and must *not* be administered intrathecally.

■ Special Precautions

Liver disease may alter the elimination of vincristine. This may necessitate a dosage modification in patients with elevated serum bilirubin levels (specific dose reduction guidelines have not been promulgated).

Neurotoxicity may be more frequent or severe in patients with underlying neurologic problems and those with lymphoma (Watkins and Griffin 1978).

Extravasation must be avoided. If extravasation occurs, administration of the remaining drug must be stopped immediately. The manufacturer recommends local injection of 150 U hyaluronidase in 1 mL saline and application of mild heat to the area to disperse the drug.

■ Dosage

Vincristine has been given in many different dosing regimens and with many other drugs. Most commonly, the dose in children and adults does not exceed 2 mg given every week. One report suggests that children can tolerate higher doses (mg/m^2) than adults (Kaufman et al 1976). This, however, has not been confirmed in a rigorous study design or retrospective review. In adults the dose generally ranges from 0.4 to 1.4 mg/m^2, given not more frequently than every week (the lower doses may be given twice weekly under special conditions). Some inadvertent overdoses given intravenously have been surprisingly well tolerated (Berenson 1971) but have caused myelosuppression (rather than neurotoxicity) as the major feature of overdosage (Kaufman et al 1976).

The recommended maximal vincristine intravenous infusion dose is 0.5 mg/m^2/d for 5 days (Jackson et al 1981). Lower doses of 0.25 mg/m^2/d may be advisable for patients with poor performance status or preexisting neurologic symptoms (Jackson et al 1985). When vincristine is infused continuously with doxorubicin for 96 hours, a dose of 0.4 mg/d (about 0.23 mg/m^2) is recommended (Barlogie et al 1984).

■ Drug Interactions

The stathmokinetic effect (cell cycle arrest) of vincristine may theoretically be used advantageously in combination with a drug such as bleomycin. Bleomycin has been demonstrated to be most effective in M and G$_2$ phases of the cell cycle. Vincristine can temporarily cause a striking increase in the population of cells in mitosis, with maximum effects noted after 6 to 12 hours. On the basis of these data, sequential therapy, first with vincristine (to synchronize the tumor cells) and then with bleomycin 6 to 12 hours later, is theoretically logical. A kinetically based synergistic response has been demonstrated in some animal tumors (Barranco and Humphrey 1971). Clearly, "cell synchronization" is probably not clinically effective in humans, but it has been attempted in lung cancer (Livingston et al 1973).

The neurotoxicity of vincristine may also be additive with that of other drugs acting on the peripheral nervous system (Hilderbrand and Kevis 1971).

Vincristine appears to increase the cellular uptake of methotrexate by malignant cells. This principle has been applied in high-dose methotrexate therapy. The clinical relevance of this interaction is not established. Tejada and Zubrod (1979) reported a 2.5-fold increase in methotrexate levels in cerebrospinal fluid when vincristine was given intravenously 23 hours after high-dose methotrexate therapy was initiated. The effect lasted approximately 3 hours.

Vincristine resistance associated with P-glycoprotein expression can be reversed in vitro with a variety of calcium channel blocking agents such as verapamil (Tsuruo et al 1983). These noncytotoxic modulators may also be useful clinically to reverse vincristine resistance.

A variety of potential pharmacologic antagonists have been purported to reverse vinca alkaloid toxicity. There is currently little evidence that some of these agents are effective. Thus, despite an early positive report of the use of high-dose leucovorin (Grush and Morgan 1979), a follow-up trial showed no antidotal efficacy for leucovorin (Thomas et al 1982). In contrast, there is good preclinical evidence that low concentrations of glutamic acid, ornithine, citrulline, and arginine can completely inhibit vinca alkaloid cytotoxicity in vitro (Johnson et al 1960). There is also one positive prospective clinical trial of the use of glutamic acid (500 mg orally three times daily) to prevent vincristine neurotoxicity (Jackson et al 1988). Conversely, it may be advisable to avoid the simultaneous infusion of vincristine with amino acid solutions such as in hyperalimentation formulations (Bender and Chabner 1982). There is also a report that low doses of the dopamine (D$_2$) receptor inhibitor metoclopramide (Reglan®, 10–20 mg IV every 4–6 hours) can reverse the symptoms of vincristine-induced paralytic ileus in cancer patients (Garewal and Dalton 1985).

■ Pharmacokinetics

After injection, vincristine is rapidly distributed to body tissues and bound to the formed blood elements (especially red blood cells and platelets). The elimination of the drug appeared to be triphasic in one human study (see table on page 954) (Bender et al 1977). Over 50% of the drug is cleared within the first 20 minutes of injection. The primary means of elimination is hepatic extraction, with secretion into the bile and feces. One third of an administered dose may be found in the feces within the first 24 hours; two thirds, within 72 hours. About 12 and 37% of the dose is excreted in the urine in 72 hours in adults and children, respectively (see table). The reason for the relative difference in urinary clearance for adults and children is unknown.

Several pharmacokinetic factors indicate that the slow elimination of vincristine is due to avid tissue binding (Donigan and Owellen 1973): (1) the

VINCRISTINE PHARMACOKINETICS IN HUMANS

Population (N)	Dose	Drug Analysis Method*	Peak	Half-life (min) α	β	γ	Recovery (%) Feces	Bile	Urine	Reference
Adults (4)	2 mg	HPLC, radiolabel	4 μM	0.8	7	164	69	—	12	Bender et al 1977
Adult (1) with biliary T-tube	0.5 mg	HPLC, radiolabel	30 nM (plasma) 600 nM (bile)	—	—	—	3	28	26	Jackson et al 1978
Children (4)	1.3–2 mg/m^2	RIA	0.3 μM	2.6	41	1531	—	—	37	Sethi and Kimball 1981

*HPLC, high-performance liquid chromatography; RIA, radioimmunoassay; radiolabel, [^{3}H-]vincristine.

large plasma clearance at 146 mL/min/1.73 m^2; (2) the large volume of distribution at steady state (215 L/1.73 m^2); (3) a low elimination rate constant from tissues to plasma; and (4) the long biologic half-life of over 24 hours (Sethi and Kimball 1981). Overall, this leads to large systemic drug exposures in both adults and children, with an area under the plasma concentration × time curve (AUC) of about 28 μM · min following standard doses (Sethi and Kimball 1981).

In both feces and urine, about half of the dose is recovered in the form of metabolites. Jackson et al (1978) found biliary excretion to be the primary pathway for drug elimination. In a patient with a biliary T-tube, they recovered 76% of a radiolabeled dose after 72 hours, with metabolites rapidly appearing in the bile (46% of the 2-hour recovery). Patients with obstructive liver disease may therefore be more susceptible to the toxic effects of vincristine.

One pharmacokinetic study has confirmed a correlation between the cumulative dose, the grade of neurotoxicity, and the AUC of vincristine in the plasma (Desai et al 1982). In this trial, low-grade neurotoxicity was observed when cumulative vincristine doses were 2 mg/m^2 for a 2-month period. These doses produced an AUC of 18 to 19 ng/mL · h. In contrast, grade 2 neurotoxicity was associated with a cumulative dose and AUC of 4.3 mg/m^2 and 77 ng/mL · h, respectively. And grade 3 neurotoxicity was observed in six patients with a cumulative 2-month dose and AUC of 4 mg/m^2 and 183 ng/mL·h, respectively (Desai et al 1982). The only factor that correlated with high AUCs for vincristine and the subsequent development of severe neurotoxicity was elevated serum alkaline phosphatase levels prior to dosing.

Vincristine does not appear to cross into the central nervous system and has been found to be extremely destructive when given intrathecally to animals (Schochet et al 1968).

■ **Side Effects and Toxicity**

Neurotoxic effects constitute the common dose-limiting toxicity with vincristine (Weiden and Wright 1972, Sandler et al 1969). Jaw pain (probably a trigeminal neuralgia) may occur in some patients but is usually limited to high doses of drug. Mild analgesics may be of benefit. Fever has been described in children receiving vincristine maintenance therapy for leukemia and lymphoma. Fevers of 38 to 39°C typically occur 6 to 24 hours after drug injection. They were associated with fatigue and anorexia and could proceed for 2 to 3 days (longer in courses without concurrent glucocorticosteroids) (Ishii et al 1988). Seizures have rarely been noted in children (Johnson et al 1973). Shepherd et al (1978) described a case of accidental intrathecal administration of vincristine in a 5½-year-old.

Constipation and paralytic ileus (also symptoms of peripheral neurotoxicity) are common and are frequently associated with abdominal pain. Stool softeners, mild laxatives, enemas, and metoclopramide (see Drug Interactions) may be helpful. The ileus will reverse itself on temporary discontinuance of the drug. Bladder atony as a result of the drug is reported (Gottlieb and Cuttner 1971).

At the usual doses, vincristine is much less toxic to the bone marrow than vinblastine and most other antineoplastic drugs. Thus, vincristine is included at full dose in many myelosuppressive drug combinations. If bone marrow depression occurs, it is usually mild.

Other rare side effects include central nervous system depression, cranial nerve paralysis, and a syndrome of inappropriate secretion of antidiuretic hormone (SIADH), which results in hyponatremia (Suskind et al 1972, Slater et al 1969, Robertson et al 1973, Cutting 1971).

There are rare single case reports of ocular complications (Albert et al 1967), including transient cortical blindness (Byrd et al 1981), drug-induced or drug-associated orthostatic hypotension (Carmichael et al 1970), and ataxia–athetosis in a child (Carpentieri and Lockhart 1978).

It is well known that cisternal injection of vincristine in animals inevitably leads to ascending paralysis and death (Wisniewski et al 1968). Inadvertent intrathecal injection of vincristine is uniformly fatal and must be avoided at all costs (Shepherd et al 1978, Gaidys et al 1983, Bain et al 1991, Solimando and Wilson 1982). In human patients given accidental intrathecal injections the clinical course proceeds rapidly from headache and backache (day 1) to generalized muscle weakness and loss of deep tendon reflexes (day 2), apnea (day 5), loss of brain wave activity (days 7–9), and death (day 12) (Shepherd et al 1978). Rapid washout of vincristine from the cerebrospinal fluid has delayed but not prevented this fulminant lethal course (Shepherd et al 1978, Gaidys et al 1983). Special pharmacy labeling of all vincristine syringes has been recommended to prevent the iatrogenic tragedy of intrathecal vincristine (Solimando and Wilson 1982).

Vincristine produces severe soft tissue necrosis if inadvertently extravasated (James and George 1964). Occasionally, vinca alkaloid extravasation symptoms may be delayed several hours (Dorr and Jones 1979) but usually pain and swelling are immediate. Although corticosteroids have anecdotally been reported to be effective (Bellone 1981, Choy 1979) in animal models, they either increase vinca skin toxicity (Dorr and Alberts 1985) or have no antidotal activity (Harrison et al 1983). The most effective local antidotes in a quantitative mouse skin toxicity model include the spreading factor enzyme, hyaluronidase, and the topical application of mild heating (Dorr and Alberts 1985). Clinical recommendations involve the injection of 150 U hyaluronidase in 3 mL saline directly into the site after evacuation of any entrapped fluid. Warm compresses may be optionally added afterward with care to avoid significant compression of the site.

REFERENCES

Ahn YS, Harrington WJ, Seelman RC, et al. Vincristine therapy of idiopathic and secondary thrombocytopenias. *N Engl J Med.* 1974;**291**:376–380.

Albert DM, Wong VG, Henderson ES. Ocular complications of vincristine therapy. *Arch Ophthalmol.* 1967;**78**: 709–713.

Bain PG, Lantos PL, Djurovic V, et al. Intrathecal vincristine: A fatal chemotherapeutic error with devastating central nervous system effects. *J Neurol.* 1991;**238**:230–234.

Barlogie B, Smith L, Alexanian R. Effective treatment of advanced multiple myeloma refractory to alkylating agents. *N Engl J Med.* 1984;**310**:1353–1356.

Barranco SC, Humphrey RM. The effects of bleomycin on survival and cell progression in Chinese hamster cells in vitro. *Cancer Res.* 1971;**31**:1218–1223.

Beck WT, Mueller TJ, Tanzer LR. Altered surface membrane glycoproteins in vinca alkaloid-resistant human leukemic lymphoblasts. *Cancer Res.* 1979;**39**:2070–2076.

Beijnen JH, Neef C, Meuwissen OJAT, et al. Stability of intravenous admixtures of doxorubicin and vincristine. *Am J Hosp Pharm.* **43**:3022–3027.

Bellone JD. Treatment of vincristine extravasation (letter). *JAMA.* 1981;**245**:343.

Bender R, Castle M, Margileth D, et al. The pharmacokinetics of [^{3}H] vincristine in man. *Clin Pharmacol Ther.* 1977;**22**(4):430–438.

Bender RA, Chabner BA. Tubulin binding agents. In: Chabner B, ed. *Pharmacologic Principles of Cancer Treatment.* Philadelphia: WB Saunders; 256–268.

Benvenuto JA, Anderson RW, Kerkof K, et al. Stability and compatibility of antitumor agents in glass and plastic containers. *Am J Hosp Pharm.* 1981;**38**:1914–1918.

Berenson MP. Recovery after inadvertent massive overdosage of vincristine (NSC-67574). *Cancer Chemother Rep.* 1971;**55**:525–526.

Bohannon RA, Miller DG, Diamond HD. Vincristine in the treatment of lymphomas and leukemias. *Cancer Res.* 1963;**23**:613–621.

Byrd RL, Rohrbaugh TM, Raney RB Jr, et al. Transient cortical blindness secondary to vincristine therapy in childhood malignancies. *Cancer.* 1981;**47**:37–40.

Carmichael SM, Eagleton L, Ayes CR, et al. Orthostatic hypotension during vincristine therapy. *Arch Intern Med.* 1970;**126**:290–293.

Carpentieri U, Lockhart LH. Atoxia and athetosis as side effects of chemotherapy with vincristine in non-Hodgkin's lymphoma. *Cancer Treat Rep.* 1978;**62**(4):561–562.

Choy DS. Effective treatment of inadvertent intramuscular administration of vincristine (letter). *JAMA.* 1979;**241**: 695.

Cohen MH, Johnston-Early A, Hood MA, et al. Drug precipitation with IV tubing: A potential hazard of chemotherapy administration. *Cancer Treat Rep.* 1985;**69**:1325–1326.

Cooper R. Combination chemotherapy in hormone-resistant breast cancer (abstract). *Proc Am Assoc Cancer Res.* 1969;**10**:15.

Creasey WA. Modifications in biochemical pathways produced by the vinca alkaloids. *Cancer Chemother Rep.* 1968;**52**:501.

Cutting HO. Inappropriate secretion of antidiuretic hormone secondary to vincristine therapy. *Am J Med.* 1971;**51**:269–271.

Desai ZR, Van den Berg HW, Bridges JM, et al. Can severe vincristine neurotoxicity be prevented? *Cancer Chemother Pharmacol.* 1982;**8**:211–214.

Donigan DW, Owellen RJ. Interaction of vinblastine, vincristine and colchicine with serum proteins. *Biochem Pharmacol.* 1973;**22**:2113–2119.

Dorr RT, Alberts DS. Vinca alkaloid skin toxicity: Antidote and drug disposition studies in the mouse. *J Natl Cancer Inst.* 1985;**74**:113–120.

Dorr RT, Jones SE. Inapparent infiltrations associated with vindesine administration. *Med Pediatr Oncol.* 1979;**6**:285–288.

Frei E III, Whang J, Scoggins RB, et al. The stathmokinetic effect of vincristine. *Cancer Res.* 1964;**24**:1918–1925.

Gaidys WG, Dickerman JD, Walters CL, et al. Intrathecal vincristine. Report of a fatal case despite CNS washout. *Cancer.* 1983;**52**:799–801.

Garewal HS, Dalton WS. Metoclopramide in vincristine-induced ileus. *Cancer Treat Rep.* 1985;**69**(11):1309–1311.

Gottlieb RJ, Cuttner J. Vincristine-induced bladder atony. *Cancer.* 1971;**28**:674–675.

Gottschalk PG, Dyck PJ, Kiely JM. Vinca alkaloid neuropathy: Nerve biopsy studies in rats and in man. *Neurology.* 1968;**18**:875–882.

Grush OC, Morgan SK. Folinic acid rescue for vincristine toxicity. *Clin Toxicol.* 1979;**14**(1):71–78.

Haggard ME, Fernbach DJ, Holcomb TM, et al. Vincristine in acute leukemia of childhood. *Cancer.* 1968;**22**:438–444.

Harrison B, Godefroid R, SunWoo Y, et al. Histopathological evolution of vincristine (VCR) skin toxicity and treatment with local dexamethasone (DXM) (abstract). *Proc Am Soc Clin Oncol.* 1983;**2**:86.

Hildebrand J, Kevis Y. Additive toxicity of vincristine and other drugs for the peripheral nervous system. *Acta Neurol Belg.* 1971;**71**:486–491.

Holland JF, Scharlau C, Gailani S, et al. Vincristine treatment of advanced cancer: A cooperative study of 393 cases. *Cancer Res.* 1973;**33**:1258–1264.

Ishii E, Hara T, Mizuno Y, et al. Vincristine-induced fever in children with leukemia and lymphoma. *Cancer.* 1988;**61**:660–662.

Jackson DV, Case LD, Pope EK, et al. Single agent vincristine by infusion in refractory multiple myeloma. *J Clin Oncol.* 1985;**3**(11):1508–1512.

Jackson DV, Castle MC, Bender RA. Biliary excretion of vincristine. *Clin Pharmacol Ther.* 1978;**24**(1):101–107.

Jackson DV Jr, Sethi VS, Spurr CL, et al. Intravenous vincristine infusion: Phase I trial. *Cancer.* 1981;**48**:2559–2564.

Jackson DV, Wells HB, Atkins JN, et al. Amelioration of vincristine neurotoxicity by glutamic acid. *Am J Med.* 1988;**84**:1016–1022.

James DH, George P. Vincristine in children with malignant solid tumors. *J Pediatr.* 1964;**64**:534–541.

Johnson FL, Bernstein ID, Hartman JR, et al. Seizures associated with vincristine sulfate therapy. *J Pediatr.* 1973;**82**:699–702.

Johnson IS, Wright HF, Svoboda GH, et al. Antitumor principles derived from *Vinca rosea* Linn. I. Vincaleukoblastine and leurosine. *Cancer Res.* 1960;**20**:1016–1022.

Karon M, Freireich EJ, Frei E III, et al. The role of vincristine in the treatment of childhood acute leukemia. *Clin Pharmacol Ther.* 1966;**77**:332–339.

Kaufman IA, Khung FH, Koenig HM, et al. Overdosage with vincristine. *J Pediatr.* 1976;**89**(4):671–674.

Livingston RB, Bodey GP, Gottlieb HA, et al. Kinetic scheduling of vincristine (NSC-125066) and bleomycin (NSC-125066) in patients with lung cancer and other malignant tumors. *Cancer Chemother Rep Part 1.* 1973;**57**:219–224.

Mauer AM, Simone JV. The current status of the treatment of childhood acute lymphoblastic leukemia. *Cancer Treat Rev.* 1976;**3**:17–41.

McRae MP, King JC. Compatibility of antineoplastic, antibiotic, and corticosteroid drugs in intravenous admixtures. *Am J Hosp Pharm.* 1976;**33**:1010–1013.

Noble RL, Beer CJ. Experimental observations concerning the mode of action of vinca alkaloids. In: Shedden WIH, ed. *The Vinca Alkaloids in the Chemotherapy of Malignant Disease.* Alburcham, England: John Sherratt and Sons; 1968:4–11.

Robertson GL, Bhoopalam N, Zelkowitz LJ. Vincristine neurotoxicity and abnormal secretion of antidiuretic hormone. *Arch Intern Med.* 1973;**132**:717–720.

Sandler SG, Tobin W, Henderson ES. Vincristine induced neuropathy: A clinical study of fifty leukemic patients. *Neurology.* 1969;**19**:367–374.

Sawitsky A, Desposito F, Treat C, et al. Vincristine and cyclophosphamide therapy in generalized neuroblastoma: A collaborative study. *Am J Dis Child.* 1970;**119**:308–313.

Schochet SS, Lampert PW, Earle KM. Neuronal changes induced by intrathecal vincristine sulphate. *J Neuropathol Exp Neurol.* 1968;**27**:645–658.

Sethi VS, Kimball JC. Pharmacokinetics of vincristine sulfate in children. *Cancer Chemother Pharmacol.* 1981;**6**:111–115.

Shepherd DA, Steuber CP, Starling KA, et al. Accidental intrathecal administration of vincristine. *Med Pediatr Oncol.* 1978;**5**:85–88.

Sirotnak FM, Yang C-H, Mines LS, et al. Markedly altered membrane transport and intracellular binding of vincristine in multidrug-resistant Chinese hamster cells selected for resistance to vinca alkaloids. *J Cell Physiol.* 1986;**126**:266–274.

Slater LM, Wainer RA, Serpick AA. Vincristine neurotoxicity with hyponatremia. *Cancer*. 1969;**23**:122–125.

Solimando DA, Wilson JP. Prevention of accidental intrathecal administration of vincristine sulfate. *Hosp Pharm*. 1982;**17**:540–542.

Suskind RM, Brusilow SW, Zehr J. Syndrome of inappropriate secretion of antidiuretic hormone produced by vincristine toxicity (with bioassay of ADH level). *J Pediatr*. 1972;**81**:90–92.

Tejada F, Zubrod CG. Vincristine effect on methotrexate cerebrospinal fluid concentration. *Cancer Treat Rep*. 1979;**63**(1):143–145.

Thomas LL, Braat PC, Somers R, et al. Massive vincristine overdose: Failure of leucovorin to reduce toxicity. *Cancer Treat Rep*. 1982;**66**:1967–1969.

Trissel LA, Fulton B, Tramonte SM. Visual compatibility of ondansetron with chemotherapeutic agents, antibiotics, and other selected drugs during simulated Y-site injection (abstract #P-468R). In: *25th Annual ASHP Midyear Clinical Meetings and Exhibit, Las Vegas, Nevada;* 1990.

Tsuruo T, Iida H, Nojiri M, et al. Circumvention of vincristine and Adriamycin resistance in vitro and in vivo by calcium influx blockers. *Cancer Res*. 1983;**43**:2905–2910.

Vietti TJ, Sullivan MP, Haggard ME, et al. Vincristine sulfate and radiation therapy in metastatic Wilms' tumor. *Cancer*. 1970;**25**:12–20.

Watkins SM, Griffin JP. High incidence of vincristine-induced neuropathy in lymphomas. *Br Med J*. 1978;**1**:610–612.

Weiden PL, Wright SE. Vincristine neurotoxicity. *N Engl J Med*. 1972;**286**:1369–1370.

Wilson L, Morse NC, Bryan J. Characterization of acetyl-³H-labelled vinblastine binding to vinblastine–tubulin crystals. *J Mol Biol*. 1978;**121**:255–268.

Wisniewski H, Shelanski ML, Terry RD. Effects of mitotic spindle inhibitors on neurotubules and neurofilaments in anterior horn cells. *J Cell Biol*. 1968;**38**:224–229.

Vindesine

■ Other Names

Eldisine; desacetylvinblastine amide; deacetylvinblastine carboxamide; DVA; Lilly CT-3231.

■ Chemistry

Structure of vindesine

Vindesine is a vinca alkaloid with a chemistry similar to that of the commercially available alkaloids, vinblastine and vincristine. The drug is a synthetic derivative of vinblastine with a molecular weight of 851 as the sulfate salt. The empiric formula is $C_{43}H_{55}N_5O_7 \cdot H_2SO_4$. Vindesine structurally differs from vinblastine primarily by a carboxamide group in place of a methyl ester. The complete chemical name is 3-(aminocarbonyl)-O⁴-deacetyl-3-de(methoxycarbonyl)vinkaleukablastine.

■ Antitumor Activity

In preclinical systems vindesine had a wider spectrum of activity than vincristine or vinblastine (Sweetney et al 1974, Todd et al 1976). Vindesine was not as neurotoxic as vincristine in animals. Overall, the agent appears to have its greatest clinical utility in combinations for the treatment of non-small cell lung cancer (NSCLC). Numerous other tumors are also responsive to vindesine.

In phase I clinical trials, vindesine exhibited antitumor activity in several tumor types (partial responses) including acute leukemia, melanoma, non-small cell lung cancer, and renal cell carcinoma (Currie et al 1976, Bodey and Freireich 1976, Dyke and Nelson 1977, Kiwit 1977, Tan 1977, Wong et al 1977).

The table on the top of page 958 details some of the phase II activity for the agent. In a study by Yau et al (1985), intermittent bolus vindesine was com-

PHASE II ACTIVITY OF VINDESINE

Tumor Type	Range of Response Rates (%)	Reference
ALL, CML*	63	Mathe et al 1978, Bayssas et al 1979
Lymphoma	55	Bayssas et al 1979
Breast cancer	0–11, 29	Hansen and Brincker 1984, Smith et al 1978, Amoroso et al 1989
Melanoma	12, 16, 20, 30	Nelimark et al 1983, Quagliana et al 1984, Smith et al 1978, Retsas et al 1979
Head and neck	0–20	Haas et al 1983, Sledge et al 1984, Vogl et al 1984
Esophagus	11, 13, 27	Lizuka et al 1989, Kelsen et al 1979, Bezwoda et al 1984
Mesothelioma	0–4	Kelsen et al 1983, Boutin et al 1987
Germ cell tumors	12	Reynolds et al 1979
Glioma	4	Alavi et al 1989
Non-small cell lung	0, 10, 12, 22, 23, 25	Luedke et al 1983, 1990, Johnson et al 1990, Sorensen et al 1987, Postmus et al 1987, Jewkes et al 1983
Prostate	19	Jones et al 1983
Small cell lung	0, 5, 33	Morgan 1986, Fuks et al 1982, Chang et al 1984
Multiple myeloma	13	Salvagno et al 1985
Cervix	0–30	Rhomberg 1986, Kavanagh et al 1985
Renal	0	Fossa et al 1983
Sarcoma	0–3	Yap et al 1983, Sordillo et al 1981
Colon	0–6	Pazdur et al 1982, Diaz and Rubio and Martin-Jimenez 1984, Saiers et al 1982
Gastric	0	Kenny et al 1983

*ALL, acute lymphocytic leukemia; CML, chronic myelogenous leukemia.

pared with continuous-infusion vindesine. There were no differences in response rates.

The greatest use of vindesine in recent years has been in combination with other agents. This is particularly true for patients with lung cancer. The table on the top of the opposite page summarizes some of those combination studies.

The most impressive randomized trial incorporating vindesine was the National Cancer Institute of Canada trial in which patients with advanced NSCLC were randomized to receive best supportive care versus vindesine (+) platinum versus cyclophosphamide (+) doxorubicin (+) platinum. In that study, survival was the best (12 weeks' advantage) for the vindesine + platinum arm of the study. The cost per year of life gained on the vindesine + platinum was approximately $15,000 (Jaakkimainen et al 1990). A similar study of cisplatin + vindesine versus supportive care in NSCLC was conducted by Woods et al (1990). It showed a 28% response rate in the chemotherapy arm patients but no improvement in survival. Toxicity was also rated as a "frequently severe." In a direct comparison trial of cisplatin + vindesine versus cisplatin + vinblastine in patients with NSCLC there were no differences in response rates or survival times (Kris et al 1985a). Thus, vindesine does not yet appear to produce a truly unique therapeutic impact in NSCLC, but it is clearly active in platinum-containing combinations.

Of particular note in combination chemotherapy is the finding that vindesine and prednisone or prednisolone have induced complete responses in up to 38% of patients with chronic myelogenous leukemia in blast crisis (Jehn and Mezger 1985, Lemoine et al 1985).

In randomized trials, vindesine has not been shown to increase the response rate for the malignancies shown in the table on the bottom of the opposite page.

■ Mechanism of Action

Vindesine appears to act similarly to the other vinca alkaloids. Cell death probably occurs by disruption of the microtubular spindle structure through binding to tubulin, the subunit protein of microtubules. The effect is schedule (cell cycle) dependent, with marked activity evident in the metaphase portion of mitosis. This mitotic arrest-type activity has been termed a *stathmokinetic effect*, and either cell death or cell cycle synchronization may occur. Besides the microtubular-mediated metaphase arrest, other potentially cytotoxic aberrations caused by the vinca derivatives include alterations in neurotubules (Schochet et al 1968) and inhibition of axoplasmic transport (Ochs 1974).

COMBINATION STUDIES USING VINDESINE

Combination	Tumor Type	Range of Response Rates (%)	Reference
Vindesine + platinum	Non-small cell lung	10, 12, 16, 19, 25, 39, 44	Gralla et al 1981, Fuks et al 1985, Ruckdeschel et al 1986, Casper et al 1989, Tourani et al 1990, Hainsworth et al 1989, Harvey et al 1987, Shinkai et al 1986
Vindesine + platinum + ifosfamide	Non-small cell lung	20, 48	Honda et al 1990, Rosell et al 1990
Vindesine + mitomycin-C	Non-small cell lung	29	Kris et al 1985b
Vindesine + mitomycin-C + platinum	Non-small cell lung	26, 41	Joss et al 1990, Miller et al 1986, Rosell et al 1990
Vindesine + etoposide + platinum	Non-small cell lung	24, 40, 56	Klastersky et al 1983, Hainsworth et al 1989, Vokes et al 1989
Vindesine + mitomycin-C + hexamethylmelamine	Non-small cell	34	Bonomi et al 1986
Vindesine + mitomycin-C	Non-small cell	23, 58	Sculier et al 1986, Main et al 1986
Vindesine + platinum + bleomycin	Non-small cell	48	Bakker et al 1986
Vindesine + mitomycin-C	Breast	14, 16–26	Lyss et al 1989, Di Costanzo et al 1986
Vindesine + mitomycin-C + mitoxantrone	Breast	33	Belpomme et al 1987
Vindesine + medroxy progesterone	Breast	28	Falkson and Falkson 1986
Vindesine + platinum	Head and neck	52	Tellez-Bernal et al 1990
Vindesine + platinum + mitomycin-C	Head and neck	63	Leyvraz et al 1987
Vindesine + platinum + dacarbazine	Melanoma	38	Verschraegen et al 1988, Ringborg et al 1990, Pectasides et al 1989
Vindesine + bleomycin + dacarbazine	Melanoma	32	Mulder et al 1989
Vindesine + bleomycin + dacarbazine + actinomycin D	Melanoma	33	Mulder et al 1986
Vindesine + lomustine + bleomycin	Lymphoma	57	Lennard et al 1989
Vindesine + platinum + bleomycin	Esophagus	24, 47	Dinwoodie et al 1986, Roth et al 1988
Vindesine + platinum + mitoguazone	Esophagus	41	Kelsen et al 1986

RANDOMIZED TRIALS WITH VINDESINE SHOWING NO ADVANTAGES WITH VINDESINE ARM

Tumor Type	Randomization	Reference
Breast cancer	Epirubicin vs epirubicin + vindesine	Nielson et al 1990
Non-small cell lung cancer	Vindesine + radiation therapy versus radiation therapy alone	Johnson et al 1990
	Vindesine + platinum versus etoposide + platinum	Dhingra et al 1985
Soft tissue sarcomas	Doxorubicin + vindesine versus doxorubicin alone	Borden et al 1990
Prostate	Vindesine plus diethylstilbestrol versus diethylstilbestrol	Cervellino et al 1990
Melanoma	Vindesine plus dacarbazine versus dacarbazine	Ringborg et al 1989
	Vindesine plus procarbazine plus lomustine versus dacarbazine + procarbazine + lomustine	Carmo-Pereira et al 1986

Availability and Storage

Vindesine is available as an investigational agent from Eli Lilly and Company (Indianapolis, Indiana) as 10 mg of lyophilized drug in glass ampules. Refrigerated storage is required. Each vial also contains 50 mg of mannitol and sodium hydroxide and/or sulfuric acid to adjust pH. A separate 10-mL normal saline diluent is included, preserved with 0.9% benzyl alcohol and hydrochloic acid and/or sodium hydroxide to adjust pH.

Preparation for Use, Stability, and Admixture

Each 10-mg ampule is reconstituted with 10 mL of the provided diluent or Normal Saline, USP. This solution is chemically stable for at least 2 weeks under refrigeration. Admixture compatibility data are not available, thus, the admixture of vindesine with antibiotics or other drugs is not recommended. Vindesine injection, however, is compatible with most infusion solutions including normal saline and 5% dextrose. The compound in the unopened glass ampule is stable for 1 year at refrigeration temperature.

Administration

Vindesine may be administered as a slow intravenous push into the tubing of a new free-flowing intravenous line, directly into the vein (using double-needle technique), or directly by small-gauge butterfly set. In each case, vein patency must be ensured as the drug is a painful vesicant if delivered outside the vein. A 10-mL normal saline flush is recommended before and after administration to test vein patency and to flush any remaining drug from the tubing, respectively. Because of occasional delayed or inapparent infiltration and the inherent irritative nature of the drug, a number of investigators now recommend that 50 to 100 mL of fluid be given before and after drug injection (Dorr and Jones 1979). Vindesine has also been given by continuous intravenous infusion over 48 hours (Mathe et al 1978, Holland et al 1979) or 96 hours (Bensmaine et al 1992).

Special Precautions

This drug should not be given concomitantly with another vinca alkaloids such as vincristine and vinblastine because of the potential for cumulative neurotoxicity. Patients probably require lowered doses or less frequent administration if liver function is abnormal or if maximal doses of other vinca alkaloids have recently been given. There is evidence suggesting that cumulative neurotoxicity may be possible with vindesine.

Drug Interactions

Vindesine has been shown to increase the apparent plasma clearance of methotrexate (Lena et al 1984). Vindesine also decreases the hydroxylation of methotrexate (Bore et al 1986). Tubiana et al (1985) noted that vindesine did not affect cerebrospinal fluid levels of methotrexate. An interaction between vindesine + etoposide and warfarin (increased prothrombin time) has also been described.

Dosage

The dosage recommendations from phase I studies were for 2.0 mg/m^2 IV every week (Currie et al 1976, Blum and Dawson 1976) or 4.0 mg/m^2 IV every 10 to 14 days (Bodey and Freireich 1976). The most common dose used in the ongoing phase II investigations is 3.0 mg/m^2 every week for 2 to 3 weeks of a 28-day cycle. Mathe et al (1978) alternately use 2.0 mg/m^2 given on 2 consecutive days and repeated weekly. Reynolds et al (1979) have successfully used daily doses of 1.3 mg/m^2 for 5 to 7 days, repeated every 3 weeks. The addition of filgrastim 2 µg/kg/d subcutaneously prevented neutropenia from a vindesine–cisplatin combination in patients with NSCLC. Although doses of vindesine (3 mg/m^2 on days 1 and 8) were not escalated, filgrastim allowed the treatment cycle to be reduced from 28 to 21 days (Mori et al 1992).

Pharmacokinetics

Pharmacokinetically, vindesine appears to behave in a manner similar to the other vinca alkaloids. These drugs show triphasic elimination, primarily by metabolism and biliary excretion (Nelson et al 1976, Owellen et al 1977). Urinary excretion of vindesine accounts for only 13% of total drug eliminated. Blood levels after intravenous bolus dosing demonstrate a short initial distribution phase of about 3 minutes. This is followed by a secondary half-life of about 100 minutes. As with the other vincas, a third, prolonged phase of more than 20 hours is also noted. This elimination profile is significantly more prolonged than that of either vincristine or vinblastine and suggests that drug accumulation with repeated dosing is possible. The very large volumes of distribution (58 L for the second phase and 600 L for the third phase), the decreased renal clearance, and the prolonged serum half-lives suggest that extensive tissue binding and delayed drug elimination may occur. Jackson et al (1984) have noted that excretion averaged 8 to 11%. Cersosimo et al (1983) noted a triphasic elimination pattern with a terminal half-life of 24.2 hours. Elimination was felt to be primarily through hepatic metabolism.

Rahmani et al (1985), using a continuous infusion of vindesine, noted that plasma concentrations reached a steady state after about 30 hours. Steady-state concentrations ranged from 4 to 15 µg/mL. In relating pharmacokinetic parameters to toxicity, Ohnuma et al (1985) noted that the rate of elimination and/or the AUC, rather than peak serum level, played a role in the degree of hematologic toxicity.

■ Side Effects and Toxicity

Bone marrow suppression is the usual dose-limiting toxic effect seen with weekly or bimonthly dosing. Neutropenia appears to predominate significantly over thrombocytopenia with usual doses (Currie et al 1976, Smith et al 1978, Reynolds et al 1979, Bodey and Freireich 1976). Vindesine hematologic toxicity appears to be rapid, producing brief nadirs. The platelet count was more likely to rise than fall in a number of studies. Of interest are continued reports of significant thrombocytosis produced by biweekly vindesine (3 mg/m^2) in patients with various metastatic malignancies (Rossof et al 1979). This occurred in 45% of patients and was independent of leukopenia. Mathe et al (1978), however, recorded more severe platelet depressions, possibly accounting for three deaths in their study. Jumean et al (1979) have reported ineffective erythropoiesis induced by vindesine. Characteristic changes included megaloblastic red cell hyperplasia, reticulocytopenia, anisocytosis, and poikilocytosis.

Neurotoxicity, similar to that noted with vincristine, becomes dose limiting to varying degrees at lower doses (Smith et al 1978, Casper et al 1979, Kelsen et al 1979). In addition, total dose-limiting cumulative neurotoxicity is suggested by the pharmacokinetic data. Neurotoxicity manifests initially as distal paresthesias, proximal muscle weakness, and loss of deep tendon reflexes without any concomitant electroneurologic changes. Cortical blindness has been described (Heran et al 1990). Abdominal cramping is common with infrequent constipation, hoarseness, and sometimes severe transient jaw pain. Paralytic ileus has rarely been dose limiting (Bayssas et al 1979); however, this toxic effect has been reported to be lethal (Rossof et al 1979, Kanoh 1989). The peripheral paresthesias clinically resemble vincristine neurotoxicity, with symptoms developing after three to four courses. It is typically mild and not particularly progressive. Interestingly, neurotoxicity was not predicted from preclinical toxicity screening in large animals. Urinary retention and postural hypotension have been noted but are apparently rare (Rossof et al 1979). Obrist et al (1979) similarly describe neurotoxic effects in about 40% of patients, including symptoms of fatigue, myalgia, vertigo, diarrhea, skin and gastric pains, tinnitus, and rarely tremor.

Gastrointestinal toxic effects other than the above neurologic manifestations includes occasional nausea, vomiting, and diarrhea. The incidence and severity of these reactions are generally low with vindesine.

In a number of series, the major toxic effect of the drug has been alopecia. It has affected over 80 to 90% of patients, being total in about one fourth of these (Retsas et al 1979). Dyke et al (1979) described a progressive type of alopecia in their review.

Other toxic effects include cellulitis and phlebitis at the injection site. Mild stomatitis has been seen in both adults and children receiving the drug. An erythematous maculopapular rash is reported (Smith et al 1978) along with non-infection-related fever occurring in about half of patients within 48 hours of administration. Myalgias are also observed during this period.

Infiltration of vindesine is infrequent and may be delayed in presentation. It more commonly occurs on initial therapy in patients with poor veins. Treatment of infiltration has included topical application of ice and local infiltration of hydrocortisone. There has generally been good resolution; however, the ulcers formed may be painful. They take weeks to resolve (Dorr and Jones 1979). Inapparent infiltrations have also been noted by others (Rossof et al 1979).

Interstitial (possibly drug-induced) pneumonitis has been reported from combinations of doxorubicin + vindesine (Isawa et al 1989), vindesine + radiation therapy (Bott et al 1986), and mitomycin-C + vindesine (Luedke et al 1985, Kris et al 1984).

Of note is one recent study in which 14 patients received vindesine for periods of 1 to 7 years without evidence of cumulative toxicity (Rhomberg et al 1990).

A patient who was allergic to vincristine sulfate (skin and cardiovascular) has been reported to be able to be treated with vindesine without sequelae (Gassel et al 1984).

Of final interest is a report by Peng et al (1991) who noted that vindesine, vincristine, and vinblastine were tightly bound to alpha and beta globulins. They speculate that inadvertent intrathecal administration of the vinca alkaloids might be treated with injection of the globulins into the intrathecal space.

One patient who received an overdose of vindesine (10 times the normal dose) survived with maximal supportive care including leucovorin, citrulline, arginine, and ornithine (Fiorentino et al 1982).

■ Special Applications

None are known.

REFERENCES

Alavi JB, Schoenfeld D, Skeel RT, Kirkwood R, Tsung L, Marsh JC. Phase II trial of spirogermanium and vindesine in malignant glioma. *Am J Clin Oncol.* 1989;**12**(1):8–10.

Amoroso D, Bertelli G, Pronzato P, et al. Continuous venous infusion of vindesine in metastatic breast cancer: Experience with a subcutaneously implanted system and portable pump. *Anticancer Res.* 1989;**9**(1):141–143.

Bakker W, van Oosterom AT, Aaronson NK, van Bruekelen FJ, Bin MC, Hermans J. Vindesine, cisplatin, and bleomycin combination chemotherapy in non-small cell lung cancer: Survival and quality of life. *Eur J Cancer Clin Oncol.* 1986;**22**(8):963–970.

Bayssas M, Gouveia J, de Vassal F, et al. Phase II clinical trials with vindesine for remission induction in leukemias and lymphomas. Apparent absence of cross resistance with vincristine. *Proc Am Assoc Cancer Res ASCO* 1979;**20**(192):48.

Belpomme D, Heritier F, Gisselbrecht C, et al. Long duration of response with vindesine–mitoxantrone–mitomycin (VMMc) combination chemotherapy in metastatic breast cancer: A pilot phase II study. *Cancer Treat Rep.* 1987;**71**(9):845–847.

Bensmaine A, Tellez-Bernal E, Guillot T, et al. CDDP, 5-FU, leucovorin and vindesine (PFLV) by CI in locally advanced HNSCC: No change in therapeutic index. *Proc Am Soc Clin Oncol.* 1992;**11**:245.

Bezwoda WR, Berman DP, Weaving A, Nissenbaum M. Treatment of esophageal cancer with vindesine: An open trial. *Cancer Treat Rep.* 1984;**68**(5):783–785.

Blum RH, Dawson DM. Vindesine (V)—phase I study of a vinca alkaloid. *Proc Am Assoc Cancer Res ASCO.* 1976;**17**(429):109.

Bodey GP, Freireich EJ. Initial clinical studies of vindesine (desacetyl vinblastine amide sulfate). *Proc Am Assoc Cancer Res.* 1976;**17**(510):128.

Bonomi PD, Pazdur R, Stolbach L, Mason B, Ettinger D. Phase II trial of mitomycin, vindesine, and hexamethylamelamine in metastatic non-small cell bronchogenic carcinoma. *Cancer Treat Rep.* 1986;**70**(12):1447–1448.

Borden EC, Amato DA, Edmonson JH, Ritch PS, Shiraki M. Randomized comparison of doxorubicin and vindesine to doxorubicin for patients with metastatic soft-tissue sarcomas. *Cancer.* 1990;**66**(5):862–867.

Bore P, Lena N, Imbert AM, et al. Methotrexate–vindesine association in head and neck cancer: Modification of methotrexate's hydroxylation in the presence of vindesine. *Cancer Chemother Pharmacol.* 1986;**17**(2):171–176.

Bott SJ, Stewart FM, Prince-Fiocco MA. Interstitial lung disease associated with vindesine and radiation therapy for carcinoma of the lung. *South Med J.* 1986;**79**(7):894–896.

Boutin C, Irisson M, Guerin JC, et al. Phase II trial of vindesine in malignant pleural mesothelioma. *Cancer Treat Res.* 1987;**71**(2):205–206.

Carmo-Pereira J, Costa FD, Henriques E. Cytotoxic chemotherapy of disseminated cutaneous malignant melanoma—A prospective and randomized clinical trial of procabazine, vindesine and lomustine versus procarbazine, DTIC and lomustine. *Eur J Cancer Clin Oncol.* 1986;**22**(12):1435–1439.

Casper ES, Gralla RJ, Golbey RB. Vindesine (DVA) and cis-dichlorodiammineplatinum II (DDP) combination chemotherapy in non-small cell lung cancer. *Proc Am Assoc Cancer Res ASCO.* 1979;**20**:337(C-190).

Cersosimo RJ, Bromer R, Licciardello JT, Hong WK. Pharmacology, clinical efficacy and adverse effects of vindesine sulfate, a new vinca alkaloid. *Pharmacotherapy.* 1983;**3**(5):259–274.

Cervellino JC, Araujo CE, Pirisi C, Podskubka O, Morera E. Combined hormonal therapy with high-dose diethylstilbestrol diphosphate (DES-DP) intravenous infusion plus vindesine (VND) for the treatment of advanced prostatic carcinoma: A controlled study. *J Surg Oncol.* 1990;**43**(4):250–253.

Chang AYC, Witte RS, Tormey DC, Ramirez G, Evaluation of vindesine in patients with refractory small cell lung cancer. *Cancer Treat Rep.* 1984;**68**(11):1407–1408.

Currie V, Wong P, Tan R, Krakoff I. Preliminary clinical studies of desacetyl vinblastine amide sulfate (DVA) and new vinca alkaloid. *Proc Am Assoc Cancer Res ASCO.* 1976;**17**(694):174.

Dhingra HM, Valdivieso M, Carr DT, et al. Randomized trial of three combinations of cisplatin with vindesine and/or VP-16–213 in the treatment of advanced non-small cell lung cancer. *J Clin Oncol.* 1985;**3**(2):176–183.

Diaz-Rubio E, Martin-Jimenez M. Vindesine in the treatment of advanced colorectal cancer: A phase II study. *Cancer Treat Rep.* 1984;**68**(3):555–556.

Di Costanzo F, Gori S, Tonato M, et al. Vindesine and Mitomycin C in chemotherapy: Refractory advanced breast cancer. *Cancer.* 1986;**57**(5):904–907.

Dinwoodie WR, Bartolucci AA, Lyman GH, Velez-Garcia E, Martelo OJ, Sarma PR. Phase II evaluation of cisplatin, bleomycin, and vindesine in advanced squamous cell carcinoma of the esophagus: A Southwestern Cancer Study Group trial. *Cancer Treat Rep.* 1986;**70**(2):267–270.

Dorr RT, Jones SE. Inapparent infiltrations associated with vindesine administration. *Med Pediatr Oncol.* 1979;**6**:285–288.

Dyke RW, Nelson RL. Phase I anti-cancer agents. Vindesine (desacetyl vinblastine amide sulfate). *Cancer Treat Rev.* 1977;**4**:135–142.

Dyke RW, Nelson RL, Brade WP. Vindesine: A short review of preclinical and first clinical data. *Cancer Chemother Pharmacol.* 1979;**2**:229–232.

Falkson HC, Falkson G. High-dose medroxyprogesterone acetate in combination with vindesine in advanced breast cancer. *Eur J Cancer Clin Oncol.* 1986;**22**(12):1511–1514.

Fiorentino MV, Slvagno L, Sileni CV, et al. Vindesine overdose. *Cancer Treat Rep.* 1982;**66**:1247–1248.

Fossa SD, Denis L, van Oosterom AT, de Pauw M, Stoter G. Vindesine in advanced renal cancer. A study of EORTC Genito-urinary Tract Cancer Cooperative Group. *Eur J Cancer Clin Oncol.* 1983;**19**(4):473–475.

Fuks JZ, Aisner J, Carney DN, et al. A phase II trial of vindesine in patients with refractory small-cell carcinoma of the lung. *Am J Clin Oncol.* 1982;**5**(1):49–52.

Fuks JZ, Patel H, Van Echo DA, Hornedo J, Aisner J. Vindesine and high dose cisplatin in the treatment of advanced non-small cell lung cancer. *Med Pediatr Oncol.* 1985;**13**(2):73–77.

Gassel WD, Gropp C, Havemann K. Acute allergic reaction due to vincristine sulfate. A case report. *Oncology.* 1984;**41**(6):403–405.

Gralla RJ, Casper ES, Kelsen DP, et al. Cisplatin and vindesine combination chemotherapy for advanced carcinoma of the lung: A randomized trial investigating two dosage schedules. *Ann Intern Med.* 1981;**95**(4):414–420.

Haas CD, Fabian CJ, Stephens RL, Kish J. Vindesine in head and neck cancer. A Southwest Oncology Group phase II pilot study. *Invest New Drugs.* 1983;**1**(4):339–340.

Hainsworth JD, Johnson DH, Hande KR, Greco FA. Chemotherapy of advanced non-small lung cancer: A randomized trial of three cis-platin-based chemotherapy regimens. *Am J Clin Oncol.* 1989;**12**(4):245–249.

Hansen PV, Brincker H. Vindesine in the treatment of metastatic breast cancer. *Eur J Cancer Clin Oncol.* 1984;**20**(10):1221–1225.

Harvey VJ, Slevin ML, Cheek SP, et al. A randomized trial comparing vindesine and cisplatinum to vindesine and methotrexate in advanced non-small cell lung carcinoma. *Eur J Cancer Clin Oncol.* 1987;**23**(11):1615–1619.

Heran F, Defer G, Brugieres P, Brenot F, Gaston A, Degos JD. Cortical blindness during chemotherapy: Clinical, CT, and MR correlations. *J Comput Assist Tomogr.* 1990;**14**(2):262–266.

Holland JF, Adrejczuk A, Greenspan E. Initial clinical and pharmacological studies with vindesine: i.v. bolus versus 24-hrs infusion. *Proc Am Assoc Cancer Res ASCO.* 1979;**20**(186):46.

Honda R, Fujita A, Ingue Y, Asakawa M, Suzuki A. Cisplatin, ifosfamide and vindesine in the chemotherapy of non-small cell lung cancer: A combination phase II study. *Cancer Chemother Pharmacol.* 1990;**26**(5):373–376.

Isawa T, Ono R, Motomiya M, Tamahashi N. Fatal acute interstitial pneumonia induced by low-dose doxorubicin and vindesine. *Tohoku J Exp Med.* 1989;**158**(2):149–154.

Jaakkimainen L, Goodwin PJ, Pater J, Warde P, Murray N, Rapp E. Counting the costs of chemotherapy in a National Cancer Institute of Canada randomized trial in non-small cell lung cancer. *J Clin Oncol.* 1990;**8**(8):1301–1309.

Jackson DV Jr, Sethi VS, Long TR, Muss HB, Spurr CL. Pharmacokinetics of vindesine bolus and infusion. *Cancer Chemother Pharmacol.* 1984;**13**(2):114–119.

Jehn U, Mezger J. Treatment of chronic myeloid leukemia blast crisis with vindesine and prednisone. *Cancer Treat Rep.* 1985;**69**(4):445–448.

Jewkes J, Harper PG, Tobias JS, Geddes DM, Souhami RL, Spiro SG. Comparison of vincristine and vindesine in the treatment of inoperable non-small cell bronchial carcinoma. *Cancer Treat Rep.* 1983;**67**(12):1119–1121.

Johnson DH, Einhorn LH, Bartolucci A, et al. Thoracic radiotherapy does not prolong survival in patients with locally advanced, unresectable non-small cell lung cancer. *Ann Intern Med.* 1990;**113**(1):33–38.

Jones WG, Fossa SD, Denis L, et al. An EORTC phase II study of vindesine in advanced prostate cancer. *Eur J Cancer Clin Oncol.* 1983;**19**(5):583–588.

Joss RA, Burki K, Dalquen P, et al. Combination chemotherapy with mitomycin, vindesine and cisplatin for non-small cell lung cancer. Association of antitumor activity with initial tumor burden and treatment center. *Cancer.* 1990;**65**(11):2426–2434.

Jumean HG, Camitta B, Holcengerg J, Hodach A. Desacetyl vinblastine amide sulfate induced ineffective erythropoiesis. *Cancer.* 1979;**44**(1):64–68.

Kanoh I. Fatal paralytic ileus following vindesine chemotherapy in a patient with myeloma-associated amyloidosis (letter). *Eur J Haematol.* 1989;**42**(1):108.

Kavanagh JJ, Saul PB, Gershenson DM, Copeland LJ, Wharton JT. Continuous-infusion vindesine in refractory carcinoma of the cervix: A phase II trial. *Cancer Treat Rep.* 1985;**69**(11):1317–1318.

Kelsen D, Gralla R, Cheng E, Martini N. Vindesine in the treatment of malignant mesothelioma: A phase II study. *Cancer Treat Rep.* 1983;67(9):821–822.

Kelsen DP, Bains M, Golbey R, Woodcock T. Vindesine in the treatment of esophageal carcinoma (abstract C-193). *Proc Am Assoc Cancer Res ASCO.* 1979;20:338.

Kelsen DP, Fein R, Coonley C, Heelan R, Bains M. Cisplatin, vindesine, and mitoguazone in the treatment of esophageal cancer. *Cancer Treat Rep.* 1986;70(2):255–259.

Kenny JB, Scarffe JH, Maley WV. Phase II trial of vindesine in advanced gastric cancer. *Cancer Treat Rep.* 1983;67(1):89–90.

Kiwit W. Phase II study of vindesine in childhood advanced malignancies. In: *Proceedings of the 10th International Congress of Chemotherapy, Zurich;* 1977: abstract 642.

Klastersky J, Sculier JP, Nicaise C, et al. Combination chemotherapy with cisplatin, etoposide, and vindesine in non-small cell lung carcinoma: A clinical trial of the EORTC lung cancer working party. *Cancer Treat Rep.* 1983;67(7):727–730.

Kris MG, Gralla RJ, Kalman LA, et al. Randomized trial comparing vindesine plus cisplatin with vinblastine plus cisplatin in patients with non-small cell lung cancer, with an analysis of methods of response assessment. *Cancer Treat Rep.* 1985a;69(4):387–395.

Kris MG, Gralla RJ, Kelson DP, et al. Trial of vindesine plus mitomycin in stage-3 non-small cell lung cancer. An active regimen for outpatient treatment. *Chest.* 1985b;87(3):368–372.

Kris MG, Pablo D, Gralla RJ, Burke MT, Prestifilippo J, Lewin D. Dyspnea following vinblastine or vindesine administration in patients receiving mitomycin plus vinca alkaloid combination therapy. *Cancer Treat Rep.* 1984;68(7/8):1029–1031.

Lemoine F, Najman A, Laporte JP, Gorin NC, Duhamel G. Vindesine–prednisone in the treatment of blast crisis on chronic myeloid leukemia. *Cancer Treat Rep.* 1985;69(2):203–204.

Lena N, Imbert AM, Pignon T, et al. Methotrexate-vindesine association in the treatment of head and neck cancer. Influence of vindesine on methotrexate's pharmacokinetic behavior. *Cancer Chemother Pharmacol.* 1984;12:120–124.

Lennard AL, Proctor SJ, Dawson AA. Lomustine, vindesine and bleomycin (LVB) used in the treatment of relapsed advanced Hodgkin's disease. A prospective study on behalf of the East of Scotland and Newcastle Lymphoma Group (ESNLG). *Hematol Oncol.* 1989;7(1):77–86.

Leyvraz S, Barrelet L, Savary M, Bernasconi S. Combination of mitomycin, vindesine, and cisplatin in the treatment of head and neck squamous cell carcinoma. *Cancer Treat Rep.* 1987;71(1):81–82.

Lizuka T, Kakegawa T, Ide H, et al. A phase II study of vindesine in the treatment of esophageal carcinoma. Japanese Esophageal Oncology Group. *Jpn J Clin Oncol.* 1989;19(4):380–383.

Luedke D, McLaughlin TT, Daughaday C, et al. Mitomycin C and vindesine associated pulmonary toxicity with variable clinical expression. *Cancer.* 1985;55(3):542–545.

Luedke DW, Einhorn L, Omur GA, et al. Randomized comparison of two combination regimens versus minimal chemotherapy in non-small cell lung cancer: A Southwestern Cancer Study Group trial. *J Clin Oncol.* 1990;8(5):886–891.

Luedke DW, Luedke SL, Petruska P, Brown GO, Leavitt J, Schlueter J. A randomized prospective study of vindesine versus doxorubicin and cyclophosphamide in the treatment of epidermoid lung cancer. *Cancer.* 1983;51(5):778–782.

Lyss AP, Luedke SL, Einhorn L, Luedke DW, Raney M. Vindesine and mitomycin C in metastatic breast cancer. A Southwestern Cancer Study Group trial. *Oncology.* 1989;46(6):357–359.

Main J, Clark RA, Hutcheon A. Vindesine and mitomycin C in inoperable non-small cell lung cancer. *Eur J Cancer Clin Oncol.* 1986;22(8):983–985.

Mathe G, Misset JL, de Vassal F, et al. Phase II clinical trial with vindesine for remission induction in acute leukemia, blastic crisis of chronic myeloid leukemia, lymphosarcoma and Hodgkins's disease: Absence of cross-resistance with vincristine. *Cancer Treat Rep.* 1978;62(5):805–809.

Miller TP, Vance RB, Ahman FR, Rodney SR. Extensive non-small cell lung cancer treated with mitomycin, ciplatin, and vindesine (MiPE): A Southwest Oncology Group study. *Cancer Treat Rep.* 1986;70(9):1101–1104.

Morgan DA. Efficacy and tolerability of vindesine in the treatment of small-cell lung cancer. A phase II study. *Cancer Chemother Pharmacol.* 1986;18(2):172–173.

Mori K, Saitou Y, Tominaga K. Phase I/II study of recombinant human G-CSF (rG-CSF) in patients receiving chemotherapy of 5 day continuous infusion of cisplatin (Pi) vindesine (V) for non-small cell lung cancer. *Proc Am Soc Clin Oncol.* 1992;11:307.

Mulder NH, Sleijfer DT, de Vries EG, Schraffordt Koops H, Samson MJ, Willemse PH. Phase II study of bleomycin, dacarbazine (DTIC) and vindesine in disseminated malignant melanoma. *J Cancer Res Clin Oncol.* 1989;115(1):93–95.

Mulder NH, Sleijfer DT, Smit JM, De Vries EG, Willemse PH, Koops HS. Phase II study of bleomycin, actinomycin D, DTIC and vindesine in disseminated malignant melanoma. *Eur J Cancer Clin Oncol.* 1986;22(7):879–881.

Nelimark RA, Peterson BA, Vosika GJ, Conroy JA. Vindesine for metastatic malignant melanoma. Phase II trial. *Am J Clin Oncol.* 1983;6(5):561–564.

Nelson RL, Root MA, Dyke RW, Ahmadzai S. Pharmacokinetics of desacetyl vinblastine amide (vindesine) in man (abstract 118). *Proc Am Assoc Clin Res.* 1976;17:30.

Nielson D, Dombernowsky P, Skovgaard T, et al. Epirubicin or epirubicin and vindesine in advanced breast cancer. A phase II study. *Ann Oncol.* 1990;**1**(4):275–280.

Obrist R, Paravicini U, Hartmann D, Nagel GA, Obrect JP. Vindesine: A clinical trial with special reference to neurological side effects. *Cancer Chemother Pharmacol.* 1979;**2**:233–237.

Ochs S. Trophic functions of the neuron. Three mechanisms of neurotropic interactions. Systems of material transport in nerve fibers (axoplasmic transport) related to nerve function and trophic control. *Ann NY Acad Sci.* 1974;**228**:202–223.

Ohnuma T, Norton L, Andrejczuk A, Holland JF. Pharmacokinetics of vindesine given as an intravenous bolus and 24-hour infusion in humans. *Cancer Res.* 1985;**45**(1):464–469.

Owellen RJ, Root MA, Hains FO. Pharmacokinetics of vindesine and vincristine in humans. *Cancer Res.* 1977;**37**:2603–2607.

Pazdur R, Rossof AH, Chandra G, Bonmi PD, Slayton RE, Woltr J. Vindesine: Phase II evaluation in colon cancer and description of its platelet stimulating activity. *Cancer Chemother Pharmacol.* 1982;**9**(1):41–44.

Pectasides D, Yianniotis H, Alevizakos N, et al. Treatment of metastatic malignant melanoma with dacarbazine, vindesine and cisplatin. *Br J Cancer.* 1989;**60**(4):627–629.

Peng Y-S, Peng Y-M, Dalton WS, Alberts DS, Dyke RW. Binding of vincristine, vinblastine and vindesine to human α & β-globulins, δ-globulins, albumin and serum in vitro. *Proc Am Soc Clin Oncol.* 1991;**32**(1955):329.

Postmus PE, Mulder NH, Schipper DL, de Vries EG. Twice weekly Vindesine, a phase II study in lung cancer. *J Cancer Res Clin Oncol.* 1987;**113**(1):99–100.

Quagliana JM, Stephens RL, Baker LH, Costanzi JJ. Vindesine in patients with metastatic malignant melanoma: A Southwest Oncology Group study. *J Clin Oncol.* 1984;**2**(4):316–319.

Rahmani R, Kleisbauer JP, Cano JP, Martin M, Barbet J. Clinical pharmacokinetics of vindesine infusion. *Cancer Treat Rep.* 1985;**69**(7/8):839–844.

Rapp E, Pater JL, Curmier Y, et al. Chemotherapy can prolong survival in patients with advanced non-small cell lung cancer—a report of a Canadian multicenter randomized trial. *J Clin Oncol.* 1988;**6**:633–641.

Retsas S, Newton KA, Wetbury G. Vindesine as a single agent in the treatment of advanced malignant melanoma. *Cancer Chemother Pharmacol.* 1979;**2**:257–260.

Reynolds TF, Cvitkovic E, Golbey RB, Young CW. Phase II trial of vindesine (DVA) in patients with germ cell tumors. *Proc Am Assoc Cancer Res ASCO.* 1979;**20**:338.

Rhomberg W, Eiter H, Soltesz E, Bohler F. Long-term application of vindesine: Toxicity and tolerance. *J Cancer Res Clin Oncol.* 1990;**116**(6):651–653.

Rhomberg WU. Vindesine for recurrent and metastatic cancer of the uterine cervix: A phase II study. *Cancer Treat Rep.* 1986;**70**(12):1455–1457.

Ringborg U, Jungnelius U, Hansson J, Strander H. Dacarbazine–vindesine–cisplatin in disseminated malignant melanoma. A phase I–II trial. *Am J Clin Oncol.* 1990;**13**(3):214–217.

Ringborg U, Rudenstam CM, Hansson J, Hafstrom L, Stenstam B, Strander H. Dacarbazine versus dacarbazine–vindesine in disseminated malignant melanoma: A randomized phase II study. *Med Oncol Tumor Pharmacother.* 1989;**6**(4):285–289.

Rosell R, Abad-Esteve A, Moreno I, et al. A randomized study of two vindesine plus cisplatin-containing regimens with the addition of mitomycin C or ifosfamide in patients with advanced non-small cell lung cancer. *Cancer.* 1990;**65**(8):1692–1699.

Rossof AH, Chandra G, Wolter J, Showel J. Phase II trial of vindesine (desacetyl vinblastine amide sulfate, VND) in advanced metastatic cancer. *Proc Am Assoc Cancer Res ASCO.* 1979;**20**(588):146.

Roth JA, Pass HI, Flanagan MM, Graeber GM, Rosenberg JC, Steinberg S. Randomized clinical trial of preoperative and postoperative adjuvant chemotherapy with cisplatin, vindesine, and bleomycin for carcinoma of the esophagus. *J Thorac Cardiovasc Surg.* 1988;**96**(2):242–248.

Ruckdeschel JC, Finkelstein DM, Ettinger DS, et al. A randomized trial of the four most active regimens for metastatic non-small-cell lung cancer. *J Clin Oncol.* 1986;**4**(1):721–723.

Saiers JH, Slavik M, McKinney DR. Phase II evaluation of vindesine for patients with advanced colorectal carcinoma. *Cancer Treat Res.* 1982;**66**(3):583–584.

Salvagno L, Paccagnella A, Chiarion Sileni V, et al. Vindesine in plasma cell tumors. Tumor 1985;**71**(6):533–536.

Schochett SS, Jr, Lampert PW, Earle KM. Neuronal changes indiced by intrathecal vincristine sulphate. *J Neuropathol Exp Neurol.* 1968;**27**:645–658.

Sculier JP, Klastersky J, Dumont JP, et al. Combination chemotherapy with mitomycin and vindesine in advanced non-small cell lung cancer: A pilot study by the Lung Cancer Working Party (Belgium). *Cancer Treat Rep.* 1986;**70**(6):773–775.

Shinkai T, Saijo N, Eguchi K, et al. Cisplatin and vindesine combination chemotherapy for non-small cell lung cancer: A randomized trial comparing two dosages of cisplatin. *Jpn J Cancer Res.* 1986;**77**(8):782–789.

Sledge GW Jr, Clark GM, Von Hoff DD. Phase II trial of vindesine in adenocarcinoma of the lung. *Cancer Treat Rep.* 1984;**68**(3):555–556.

Smith IE, Hedley DW, Powles TJ, McElwain TJ. Vindesine: A phase II study in the treatment of breast carcinoma, malignant melanoma, and other tumors. *Cancer Treat Rep.* 1978;**62**(10):1427–1433.

Sordillo PP, Magill GB, Gralla RJ. Phase II evaluation of vindesine sulfate in patients with advanced sarcomas. *Cancer Treat Rep.* 1981;**65**(5/6):515–516.

Sorensen JB, Hansen HH, Dombernowsky P, et al. Chemotherapy for adenocarcinoma of the lung (WHO III): A randomized study of vindesine versus lomustine, cyclophosphamide, and methotrexate versus all four drugs. *J Clin Oncol.* 1987;**5**(8):1169–1177.

Sweetney MJ, Cullinan GJ, Poore GA, Gerzon K. Experimental anti-tumor activity of vinblastine amides. *Proc Am Assoc Cancer Res ASCO.* 1974;**15**:37.

Tan C. Clinical and pharmacokinetic studies of vindesine (DVA) in 35 children with malignant disease. In: *Proceedings of the 10th International Congress of Chemotherapy, Zurich;* 1977: abstract 639.

Tellez-Bernal E, Recondo G, Guillot T, et al. A phase II study of cisplatin and continuous infusion of vindesine in metastatic head and neck squamous cell cancer. *Cancer.* 1990;**66**(4):640–644.

Todd GC, Gibson WR, Morton DM. Toxicology of vindesine (desacetyl-vinblastine amide) in mice, rats and dogs. *J Toxicol Environ Health.* 1976;**1**:843–849.

Tourani JM, Penaud D, Caubarrere I, et al. Cisplatin and vindesine for disseminated non-small cell lung cancer. Results of a prospective trial with 81 patients. *Bull Cancer (Paris).* 1990;**77**(11):1107–1113.

Tubiana N, Lena N, Barbet J, et al. Methotrexate–vindesine association in leukemia: Pharmacokinetic study. *Med Oncol Tumor Pharmacother.* 1985;**2**(2):99–102.

Verschraegen CF, Kleeberg UR, Mulder J, et al. Combination of cisplatin, vindesine, and dacarbazine in advanced malignant melanoma. A phase II Study of the EORTC Malignant Melanoma Cooperative Group. *Cancer.* 1988;**62**(6):1061–1065.

Vogl SE, Camacho FJ, Kaplan BH, O'Donnell MR. Phase II trial of vindesine in advanced squamous cell cancer of the head and neck. *Cancer Treat Rep.* 1984;**68**(3):559–560.

Vokes EE, Bitran JD, Hoffman PC, Ferguson MK, Weichselbaum RR, Golomb HM. Neoadjuvant vindesine, etoposide, and cisplatin for locally advanced non-small cell lung cancer. Final report of a phase II study. *Chest.* 1989;**96**(1):110–113.

Wong PP, Yagoda A, Currie VE, Young CW. Phase II study of vindesine sulphate in the therapy of advanced renal carcinoma. *Cancer Treat Rep.* 1977;**61**:1727–1729.

Woods RL, Williams CJ, Levi J, et al. A randomized trial of cisplatin and vindesine versus supportive care only in advanced non-small cell lung cancer. *Br J Cancer.* 1990;**61**(4):608–611.

Yap BS, Benjamin RS, Plager C, Burgess MA, Papdoupoulos N, Bodey GP. A randomized study on continuous infusion vindesine versus vinblastine in adults with refractory metastatic sarcomas. *Am J Clin Oncol.* 1983;**6**(2):235–238.

Yau JC, Yap YY, Buzdar AU, Hortobagyl GN, Bodey GP, Blumenschein GR. A comparative randomized trial of vinca alkaloids in patients with metastatic breast carcinoma. *Cancer.* 1985;**55**(2):337–340.

Vinorelbine

■ Other Names

Navelbine® (Pierre Fabre Oncologie, France Burroughs Wellcome Company, USA); PM 259.

■ Chemistry

Structure of vinorelbine

Vinorelbine is a semisynthetic vinca alkaloid derivative of vinblastine (Langlois et al 1976). The complete chemical name is 3′,4′-didehydro-4′-deoxy-C5′-noranhydrovinblastine. The name is usually shortened to 5′-noranhydrovinblastine. The molecular formula is $C_{53}H_{66}N_4O_{20}$ and includes the two tartaric acid residues ($C_8H_{12}O_{12}$). The molecular weight is 1079.15 including the two tartaric acids (300.18).

■ Antitumor Activity

Vinorelbine has demonstrated antitumor activity in a number of murine tumors in vivo. These include P-388 leukemia, B-16 melanoma, and L-1210 leukemia. The drug is active in human tumor xenografts in nude mice. Sensitive human xenograft tumors include LC-06 and LX-1 small cell lung cancers, QG-56 non-small cell lung cancer, MX-1 breast cancer, and 4-I-ST gastric cancer (Cros et al 1989). Compared with other vinca alkaloids, vinorelbine had superior activity in vitro against A-2780 human ovarian cancer and human N6 bronchial epidermoid carcinoma. Antitumor activity in a large number of human tumor cell lines is observed at low drug concentrations of 1 to 10 nmol/L (Cros et al 1989).

Vinorelbine has demonstrated significant activity in human cancer in vivo. In metastatic breast cancer, overall response rates of 45% (20% complete) (Canobbio et al 1989) to 51% are reported in previously untreated patients (Lluch et al 1992). As second- or third-line therapy in breast cancer, single-agent vinorelbine as an intravenous push followed by a continuous infusion produced an overall response rate of 30% (Izzo et al 1992). Oral vinorelbine had excellent activity in advanced breast cancer, with objective responses described in 6 of 10 patients (Favre et al 1989). Soft tissue disease responded best in this study. The combination of epirubicin and vinolrelbine produced a 46% overall response rate in patients with advanced breast cancer, about half of whom were previously untreated (Chadjaa et al 1992). In heavily pretreated patients with advanced ovarian cancer, vinorelbine produced an overall response rate of 15%, almost all partial responses (George et al 1989).

A 33% response rate is reported in non-small cell lung cancer (Depierre et al 1989). The median response duration was 34 weeks and eight patients had responses lasting more than 1 year, again regardless of the initial stage of disease. A 65% response rate is reported in non-small cell lung cancer patients receiving vinorelbine and cisplatin, 5-fluorouracil, and leucovorin (de Cremoux et al 1992). A 16% partial response rate is reported in previously treated patients with small cell lung cancer who received vinorelbine as single-agent therapy (Jassem et al 1992).

The drug is active in previously treated patients with Hodgkin's disease, with partial responses observed in some heavily pretreated patients (Marty et al 1989).

■ Mechanism of Action

Like other vinca alkaloids vinorelbine blocks polymerization of microtubules, leading to impaired formation of the mitotic spindle (Bien et al 1989, Fellous et al 1989). This ultimately results in the accumulation of cells in the metaphase portion of mitosis. Vinorelbine is thus cell cycle specific in its cell killing and produces a blockade in cell cycle progression in G_2 and M phases.

On a molecular basis vinorelbine induces tubulin aggregation into spirals and paracrystals. This involves selective binding to the Tau family of microtubule-associated proteins (Fellous et al 1989).

■ Availability and Storage

Vinorelbine is investigationally available as a 10 mg/mL solution in 1- or 5-mL vials of the ditartrate salt (Pierre Fabre Oncologie, Paris, France). It is stored under refrigeration and is stable for at least 2 years. The drug is also investigationally available as a liquid-filled gelatin capsule containing 40 mg vinorelbine for oral administration.

■ Preparation for Use, Stability, and Admixture

Vinorelbine solution is typically diluted into 100 to 250 mL of 0.9% Sodium Chloride for Injection, USP, or 5% Dextrose for Injection, USP. Dilute solutions are stable for at least 24 hours at room temperature.

■ Administration

Vinorelbine sterile solution is typically administered as a brief intravenous infusion over 20 to 30 minutes. The oral capsules are taken on an empty stomach as a single ingestion. A preliminary pharmacokinetic trial has reported no significant effect of food on vinorelbine absorption (Rahmani et al 1989). Because of the need for sedating antiemetics and antidiarrheal agents, dosing of the oral capsules is recommended for bedtime. This may lessen gastrointestinal toxic effects (Lucas et al 1992).

■ Special Precautions

Care should be exercised to avoid extravasation as vinorelbine may cause soft tissue necrosis. Although no studies are available, because vinorelbine is similar to other vinca alkaloids with respect to dosage, hyaluronidase may be useful as a local vinorelbine extravasation antidote. The manufacturer also recommends dose reduction in patients with hepatic insufficiency, but specific guidelines have not been published.

■ Dosage

In phase I clinical trials the maximum tolerated dose of intravenous vinorelbine ranged from 27.5 to 35.4 mg/m^2 per week (Depierre et al 1989). Weekly doses of 30 mg/m^2 are typically administered (George et al 1989). In such settings, a median of seven injections are common (George et al 1989). Drug administration is usually postponed 1 week if full hematologic recovery is not evident prior to dosing. Doses have been further reduced by 25% if treatment was postponed for 3 weeks to allow for hematologic recovery.

A recommended dose for phase II studies of oral vinorelbine capsules in breast cancer was 80 mg/m^2 weekly (Favre et al 1989). As an intravenous push/infusion combination in breast cancer, the recommended dose was 8 mg intravenous push day 1 followed by 8 mg/m^2/d for 4 consecutive days as a continuous intravenous infusion (total dose, 40 mg/m^2 every 3 weeks) (Izzo et al 1992).

■ Pharmacokinetics

Vinorelbine is eliminated slowly from the body as is common with other vinca alkaloids (Krikorian et al 1989). The drug has a large apparent volume of distribution, which is due most likely to extensive tissue binding and up to 80% binding to plasma proteins. The triphasic elimination pattern for vinorelbine is similar to that of vinblastine (see table). Elimination is primarily nonrenal, although only 20% of a radiolabeled dose is recovered in human feces 48 hours after administration. In rats, up to 60% of a dose undergoes hepatic extraction on the "first pass" through the liver (Marty et al 1989). On incubation with human hepatocytes, about 90% of the drug is recovered intact with two minor metabolites noted: vinorelbine-N-oxide and deacetylvinorelbine (Marty et al 1989). In the rat and in primates, high drug concentrations are found in the spleen, liver, kidney, heart, and lungs (Krikorian et al 1989). These tissue concentrations appear to be 3 to 10 times higher than those achieved with other vinca alkaloids.

Orally administered liquid drug has pharmacokinetics similar to that of intravenously administered drug (Rahmani et al 1989). Absorption is rapid, with 80% of the peak plasma level attained within 2 hours of ingestion. Bioavailability averaged about 40% using a radioimmunoassay technique in a few patients (Favre et al 1989). There did not appear to be any drug accumulation with six sequential weekly doses (Rahmani et al 1989). The pharmacokinetics of the liquid-filled capsules has also been studied (Lucas et al 1992). Compared with intravenous dosing, the absolute mean bioavailability of vinorelbine from the capsules was 24%. An oral dose of 100 mg/m^2 produced peak plasma levels of 109 ng/mL 1.6 hours after ingestion. Clearance averaged 5.4 L/h/kg, which was higher than that following an intravenous dose, 1.2 L/h/kg (Lucas et al 1992).

■ Side Effects and Toxicity

In preclinical settings the dose-limiting toxic effect is leukopenia. The compound was mutagenic and embryotoxic but not teratogenic (Marty et al 1989). In phase I clinical trials using a weekly dosing schedule, leukopenia was the dose-limiting toxic effect. Thrombocytopenia was not usually noted except in pretreated ovarian cancer patients. The leukopenia is described as noncumulative and of a short duration (< 7 days) (Marty et al 1989). Significant anemia has been observed in 2% of patients treated in phase II studies. Leukopenia is also the dose-limiting toxic effect of oral vinorelbine (Favre et al 1989). Gastrointestinal toxic effects were mild or absent and only 1 of 19 patients experienced neurotoxic effects with the oral drug delivered as a liquid solution. With the gelatin capsules, nausea, vomiting, and diarrhea are much more common (Lucas et al 1992).

Neurotoxicity, noted by decreased deep tendon reflexes, is reported in 6 to 29% of patients. Constipation is rare (0–17%) and paresthesias are very rare (2–10% of patients); however, prior vinca therapy and/or abdominal radiation can increase the incidence of paresthesias. With the intravenous formulation, emesis of mild severity is reported in only 20% of patients and alopecia in only 25% (Depierre et al 1989). Vinorelbine is a vesicant in a mouse model and experimental lesions can be reduced by hyaluronidase injections into the site.

VINORELBINE PHARMACOKINETICS IN HUMANS

	Mean	SD
Half-life		
α (min)	2–6	—
β (h)	1.9	0.8
γ (h)	40	18
Steady-state volume of distribution (L/kg)	27	19
AUC (ng/mL/h)	2250	—
Clearance (L/kg/h)	0.8	0.53
Urinary elimination (%)	<8–18.20	—

Data from Bore et al 1989 and Marty et al 1989.

REFERENCES

Binet S, Fellous A, Lataste H, et al. In situ analysis of the action of Navelbine® on various types of microtubules using immunoflurorescence. *Semin Oncol.* 1989;**16**:5–8.

Bore P, Rahmani R, van Cantfort J, et al. Pharmacokinetics of a new anticancer drug, Navelbine, in patients. Comparative study of radioimmunologic and radioactive determination methods. *Cancer Chemother Pharmacol.* 1989;**23**:247–251.

Canobbio L, Boccardo F, Pastorino G, et al. Phase-II study of Navelbine® in advanced breast cancer. *Semin Oncol.* 1989;**16**:33–36.

Chadjaa M, Izzo J, May F, et al. Preliminary data on 4′-epiadriamycine (EPI)—Vinorelbine (VNB): A new active combination in advanced breast cancer. *Proc Am Assoc Cancer Res.* 1992;**33**:214.

Cros S, Wright M, Morimoto M, et al. Experimental antitumor activity of Navelbine®. *Semin Oncol.* 1989;**16**:15–20.

De Cremoux H, Monnet I, Azli N, et al. Fluorouracil (FU)/leucovorin (AF)/vinorelbine (VNB)/cisplatin (P) in non-small cell lung cancer (NSCLC): A phase II study. *Proc Am Soc Clin Oncol.* 1992;**11**:303.

Depierre A, Lemarie E, Dabouis G, et al. Efficacy of Navelbine® (NVB) in non-small cell lung cancer (NSCLC). *Semin Oncol.* 1989;**16**(2, suppl 4):26–29.

Favre R, Delgado M, Besenval M, et al. Phase I trial of escalating doses of orally administered Navelbine (NVB): Part II—Clinical results (abstract 246). *Proc Am Soc Clin Oncol.* 1989;**8**:64.

Fellous A, Ohayon R, Vacassin T, et al. Biochemical effects of Navelbine® on tubulin and associated proteins. *Semin Oncol.* 1989;**16**:9–14.

George MJ, Heron JF, Kerbrat P, et al. Navelbine® in advanced ovarian epithelial cancer: A study of the French oncology centers. *Semin Oncol.* **16**(2, suppl 4):30–32.

Izzo J, Toussaint C, Chabot G, et al. High activity and dose intensity (DI) relationship in advanced breast cancer (ABC) with continuous infusion (CIV) of Navelbine (NVB). *Proc Am Soc Clin Oncol.* 1992;**11**:71.

Jassem J, Karnicka-Mlodkowska H, van Pottelsberghe C, et al. EORTC phase II study of Navelbine (NVB) in previously treated patients (PTS) with small cell lung carcinoma (SCLC). *Proc Am Soc Clin Oncol.* 1992;**11**:309.

Krikorian A, Rahmani R, Bromet M, et al. Pharmacokinetics and metabolism of Navelbine®. *Semin Oncol.* 1989;**16**:21–25.

Langlois N, Gueritte F, Langlois Y, et al. Application of a modification of the Polonovski reaction to the synthesis of vinblastine-type alkaloid. *J Am Chem Soc.* 1976;**28**:7017–7024.

Lluch A, Conde G, Casado A. Phase II trial with Navelbine (NVB) in advanced breast cancer (ABC) previously untreated. *Proc Am Soc Clin Oncol.* 1992;**11**:72.

Lucas S, Donehower R, Rowinsky E, et al. Clinical results of a study of the absolute bioavailability (ABA) and pharmacokinetics (PK) of weekly Navelbine (NVB) liquid-filled soft gelatin capsules at full therapeutic doses in patients with solid tumors. *Proc Am Soc Clin Oncol.* 1992;**11**:111.

Marty M, Extra JM, Espie M, et al. Advances in vinca-alkaloids: Navelbine®. *Nouv Rev Fr Hematol.* 1989;**31**:77–84.

Rahmani R, Bore P, Cano JP, et al. Phase I trial of escalating doses of orally administered Navelbine (NVB): Part I—Pharmacokinetics (abstract 289). *Proc Am Soc Clin Oncol.* 1989;**8**:74.

Vinzolidine

■ Other Names

LY-104208 (Eli Lilly and Company); VZL.

■ Chemistry

Structure of vinzolidine

Vinzolidine is a semisynthetic derivative of the vinca alkaloid vinblastine. It differs from vinblastine by the presence of a lipophilic β-chlorethyl side chain and a stiff heterocyclic oxazolidinedione ring at carbon-3 of the vindoline moiety. These modifications make the structure both more rigid and more lipophilic in the domain believed to be important for drug–receptor binding at specific microtubule protein sites (Bender and Chabner 1982). The β-chloroethyl side chain aids in lipophilicity but does not yield any alkylating activity because of the stability of the chloride–carbon bond under physiologic conditions. The chemical name is 3″-(2-chloroethyl)-3-de(methoxycarbonyl)-3-deoxy-2″,4″-dioxospiro[oxazolidine-5″,3-vincaleukoblastine] sulfuric acid salt. The molecular formula is $C_{48}H_{58}ClN_5O_9 \cdot H_2SO_4$ and the formula weight 982.6 (Eli Lilly and Company 1982).

■ Antitumor Activity

In preclinical studies, vinzolidine showed antitumor activity in B-16 melanoma, P-1534 leukemia, Gardner and 6C3HED lymphosarcomas, adenocarcinoma 755, and C3H mammary cancer. It was minimally active in Lewis lung cancer, Ridgeway osteogenic sarcoma, and L-1210 leukemia. The drug was also active in murine mammary carcinoma

(Bissery et al 1988). In fresh human tumors examined in colony-forming assays in vitro, vinzolidine demonstrated broad and schedule-dependent antitumor activity (Takasugi et al 1984b). Sensitive human tumor types included melanoma (48%), lung cancer (48%), breast cancer (40%), renal cancer (33%), and ovarian cancer (24%). A few in vitro responses were noted in two of seven colon specimens, one of three pancreatic cancers, and three of four gastric cancers. Continuous drug exposure was much more effective than a 1-h exposure in this trial.

Oral vinzolidine was also active in early clinical trials in patients with a variety of solid tumors and lymphomas. A single dose every 2 weeks produced one response in a patient with squamous cell lung cancer and two responses in four patients with lymphoma (1 with mycosis fungoides, one with nodular, poorly differentiated lymphoma) (Budman et al 1984). With a daily × 5 regimen, three responses were observed in adenocarcinomas of the lung and pancreas and in metastatic carcinoid (one each) (Takasugi et al 1984a). The overall response rate in this trial was 3/34 complete responses). Of note, a very prolonged remission was achieved in the single patient with pancreatic cancer. Nonresponsive tumors included breast cancer (nine patients), melanoma (five patients), and colon carcinoma (five patients), despite some in vitro evidence of activity in two of the melanoma specimens and in one breast cancer specimen (Takasugi et al 1984a). No antitumor activity was observed in a phase I trial of biweekly intravenous vinzolidine (Budman et al 1990). In contrast, 2 of 11 responses were achieved in patients with Kaposi's sarcoma who were treated orally every 2 weeks (Sarna et al 1985). As in some other trials, however, this study was prematurely halted because of variable, life-threatening myelosuppression (see Pharmacokinetics and Side Effects and Toxicity).

Intravenous vinzolidine is active and has produced responses in 5 of 42 phase I patients with different solid tumors (Taylor et al 1990). Partial responses were observed in breast cancer (1), melanoma (2), and renal cell cancer (2). Unfortunately, erratic myelosuppression was observed even with the intravenous formulation.

■ Mechanism of Action

Vinzolidine arrests cell division in the metaphase portion of mitosis. This leads to an accumulation of cells in late S phase/early mitosis. Vinzolidine appears to bind to tubulin protein subunits in a fashion similar to and competitive with other vinca alkaloids such as vincristine and vinblastine; however, a higher binding affinity for vinzolidine is postulated because of the structural modifications at the vindoline portion of the molecule (see Chemistry). Microtubule formation is inhibited after the drug binds to tubulin and subsequent formation of the mitotic spindle is blocked. This leads to cell death in the metaphase portion of mitosis, prior to cell division (Bender and Chabner 1982).

In vitro studies clearly show a marked improvement in cell killing following continuous drug exposure (Takasugi et al 1984b). Thus, vinzolidine is a cell cycle phase-specific agent with marked schedule dependence favoring prolonged drug exposures. The greater degree of lipophilicity with vinzolidine probably enhances oral bioavailability, but may also increase myelosuppression as a result of increased drug disposition into bone marrow.

■ Availability and Storage

Vinzolidine is investigationally available from Eli Lilly and Company Indianapolis, Indiana, in two formulations: oral capsules and ampules containing 5 or 10 mg of lyophilized sterile powder (Eli Lilly and Company 1982). Oral vinzolidine capsules containing 5, 10, or 20 mg should be kept frozen at −10°C prior to use. Injectable vinzolidine powder is also stored frozen prior to reconstitution.

■ Preparation for Use, Stability, and Admixture

Vinzolidine lyophilized powder for intravenous administration is reconstituted in normal saline to a concentration of 1 mg/mL. Because of limited stability at room temperature, it is recommended that all intravenous doses be reconstituted immediately prior to use. Specific admixture information is not available but the intravenous drug is compatible with standard infusion solutions such as saline and D5W. It is recommended that oral doses dispensed to patients be stored in the home refrigerator (4°C).

■ Administration

Oral vinzolidine capsules are taken on an empty stomach. Large doses, given once every 2 weeks, are administered in three equal fractions each about 6 to 8 hours apart (Budman et al 1984). On a 5-day oral regimen, single daily doses are administered in 6 to 8 oz of water (Takasugi et al 1984a).

Intravenous vinzolidine doses have been given as a direct intravenous bolus injection over 1 to 2 minutes (Taylor et al 1990) or as a rapid intravenous injection over 1 minute through the side port of a freely flowing intravenous infusion (Budman et al 1990). Care should be taken to avoid extravasation as vinzolidine is probably a potent vesicant in soft tissues.

■ Dosage

The maximally tolerated doses of different vinzolidine schedules are summarized in the table below. In dosing this agent it is important to recognize that there has been marked interpatient variability in myelosuppression from standard doses. Thus, careful monitoring and early dosage deescalation are needed to prevent severe toxic effects. Also, patients with marked hepatobiliary dysfunction should probably receive lower doses of vinzolidine, although specific dose adjustments have not been reported.

■ Pharmacokinetics

Vinzolidine is slowly and incompletely absorbed following oral ingestion of the capsules (Kreis et al 1986, 1988). Based on total urinary and fecal recovery of ^{3}H-labeled drug, a bioavailability of about 50% is achieved with the oral capsules. The peak level is achieved about 3 to 4 hours after ingestion, with an absorption half-life of 1 hour (range, 0.66–1.7) (see table on the following page). Following absorption, vinzolidine is slowly eliminated with biphasic half-lives of 10.5 minutes (α) and 172 hours (β). This disposition pattern, studied using ^{3}H-labeled drug, is decidedly longer than the mean terminal half-life of 23 hours described for intravenous vinzolidine by Taylor et al (1990). Vinzolidine's terminal-phase half-life is similar to that of vinblastine, about 25 hours (Nelson et al 1980, 1983); however, the volume of distribution in the central compartment is much higher for vinzolidine, at 76.5 L or 15 to 20 times the blood volume (Taylor et al 1990). Thus, vinzolidine behaves pharmacokinetically like the other vinca alkaloids, which have a large apparent volumes of distribution because of avid binding to extravascular tissues and proteins (Taylor et al 1990).

The primary means of vinzolidine elimination is by the fecal route, which accounts for about 49% of an oral dose (Kreis et al 1986). Most of this fecal excretion is mediated by biliary secretion. Less than 5% of a dose is excreted in the urine. There are several polar metabolites of vinzolidine but their exact structures and activities are not known (Kreis et al 1986). There are also spontaneous breakdown products from vinzolidine incubated in plasma.

When the oral dose is compared with intravenous doses using the area under the plasma concentration × time curve (AUC), there is a roughly linear correlation up to a dose of 0.7 mg/kg or about 28 mg/m^2. At higher oral doses, there is a disproportionate increase in the AUC (Kreis et al 1986, 1988). This suggests that enhanced systemic drug exposure may occur at doses greater than 28 mg/m^2 which is within the range of the maximally tolerated total dose. This could explain some of the erratic toxic effects seen at vinzolidine doses of 30 mg/m^2 and greater.

■ Side Effects and Toxicity

Myelosuppression of variable intensity is the dose-limiting side effect of vinzolidine. Neutropenia is both dose related and reversible, with nadirs at 11

VINZOLIDINE DOSE SCHEDULES

Route	Daily Dose (mg/m^2) Maximally Tolerated	Recommended Good Risk	Recommended Poor Risk[†]	Frequency (d)	Repeat Interval (wk)	Reference
PO	45	35	30	1	2	Budman et al 1984
PO	11*	7*	5*	5*	3	Takasugi et al 1984a
PO	45	30	25	1	2	Sarna et al 1985
IV	9	—	—	1	2	Budman et al 1990
IV	3.5	—	—	3	21	Taylor et al 1990

*60% of the total dose of 35 to 25 mg/m^2 given on day 1 and 10% of the total dose given on days 2 to 5 thereafter after (Koeller et al 1984).
[†]Heavily pretreated patients and/or those with poor performance status.

VINZOLIDINE PHARMACOKINETICS IN HUMANS

Route	Absorption Peak (μg/mL)	Absorption Half-time (h)	Plasma Half-life (h) α	Plasma Half-life (h) β	Volume of Distribution	Clearance	AUC (μg·h/L)	Excretion (% of dose) Fecal	Excretion (% of dose) Urine
PO*	3.5	1.0	10.5	172	6.7 L/kg	0.093 L/kg/h	11.8	49	3.6
IV†	—	—	—	23	76.5 L	40.7 L/min	120	—	—

*Data from Kreiss et al (1986) using single oral doses of 1.5 to 36.5 mg/m^2 ^{3}H-labeled vinzolidine measured after high-performance liquid chromatographic separation from metabolites.
†Data from Taylor et al (1990) using intravenous doses of 3.5 mg/m^2/d × 5 as measured by radioimmunoassay.

days following a single oral dose (Budman et al 1984) and between days 7 and 15 after five daily doses (60% of the total dose given on day 1) (Takasugi et al 1984a). Recovery was usually complete by days 14 and 21, respectively. Thrombocytopenia and anemia are uncommon, occurring in 5% or less of patients (Budman et al 1984). The degree of myelosuppression is erratic and some patients may experience severe granulocytopenia and sepsis following standard oral or intravenous doses of the drug. Thus, the variable myelosuppression with oral vinzolidine is not entirely explainable by the interindividual variations in absorption, as repeated oral drug courses in the same patient produced erratic granulocytopenia. This was not correlated to performance status, prior therapy, and liver and/or renal function (Taylor et al 1990). Unfortunately, erratic myelosuppression from course to course in the same patient is also observed with intravenous vinzolidine (Taylor et al 1990).

The second most common effect of vinzolidine is peripheral neurotoxicity, which is described in about a third of patients (Takasugi et al 1984a). Findings include myalgias, paresthesias, weakness, arthralgia, jaw pain, and paralytic ileus. These symptoms are similar to the neurologic side effects of other vinca alkaloids and are usually cumulative but not dose limiting. With high doses, the syndrome of inappropriate antidiuretic hormone release can occur as noted by hyponatremia.

Gastrointestinal toxic effects are usually of mild to moderate intensity in about 30% of patients at all dose levels. Symptoms include nausea and vomiting, diarrhea, and mucositis. There may also be a direct effect on gastrointestinal mucosa; gastrointestinal bleeding has been documented following vinzolidine (Takasugi et al 1984a). Alopecia of varying intensity is relatively uncommon with vinzolidine.

With intravenous vinzolidine given biweekly, phlebitis was a common problem at all dose levels (Budman et al 1990). In contrast, on a 3-consecutive-day intravenous schedule, venous site reactions were reported in less than 5% of patients (Taylor et al 1990). Vinzolidine is probably a vesicant if inadvertently extravasated. Specific antidote studies are not available.

REFERENCES

Bender RA, Chabner BH. Tubulin binding agents. In: Chabner BA, ed. *Pharmacologic Principles of Cancer Treatment.* Philadelphia: WB Saunders; 1982:256–268.

Bissery MC, White K, Polin L, et al. Murine solid tumor activity of vinzolidine. *Proc Am Assoc Cancer Res.* 1988;**29**:333.

Budman DR, Kreis W, Behr J, et al. Phase I trial of intravenous vinzolidine (LY 104208) given on a biweekly dosing schedule. *Invest New Drugs.* 1990;**8**:269–274.

Budman DR, Schulman P, Marks M, et al. Phase I trial of vinzolidine. *Cancer Treat Rep.* 1984;**68**:979–982.

Eli Lilly and Company. *Vinzolidine: An Investigational New Drug. Information for Clinical Investigators.* 1982: Eli Lilly and Company Document No. AS6111.

Koeller JM, Trump DL, Witte RS, et al. Phase I trial and pharmacokinetics of vinzolidine on a daily × 5 oral schedule. *Proc Am Assoc Cancer Res.* 1984;**25**:163.

Kreis W, Budman DR, Freeman J, et al. Clinical pharmacology studies with IV administered ^{3}H-vinzolidine. *Proc Am Assoc Cancer Res.* 1988;**29**:216.

Kreis W, Budman DR, Schulman P, et al. Clinical pharmacology of vinzolidine. *Cancer Chemother Pharmacol.* 1986;**16**:70–74.

Nelson RL, Dyke RW, Root MA. Comparative pharmacokinetics of vindesine, vincristine and vinblastine in patients with cancer. *Cancer Treat Rev.* 1980;**7**(suppl):17–24.

Nelson RL, Root MA. Clinical pharmacokinetics of vinzolidine, a new orally active vinca alkaloid derivative. *Proc Am Assoc Cancer Res.* 1983;**24**:130.

Sarna G, Mitsuyasu R, Figlin R, et al. Oral vinzolidine as therapy for Kaposi's sarcoma and carcinomas of lung, breast, and colon/rectum. *Cancer Chemother Pharmacol.* 1985;**14**:12–14.

Takasugi BJ, Robertone AB, Salmon SE, et al. Five-day schedule of vinzolidine, an oral vinca alkaloid, in a variety of tumors. *Invest New Drugs*. 1984a;**2**:387–390.

Takasugi BJ, Salmon SE, Nelson RL, et al. Antitumor activity of vinzolidine in the human tumor clonogenic assay and comparison with vinblastine. *Invest New Drugs*. 1984b;**2**:49–53.

Taylor CW, Salmon SE, Satterlee WG, et al. A phase I and pharmacokinetic study of intravenous vinzolidine. *Invest New Drugs*. 1990;**8**:S51–S57.

Yoshi 864

■ Other Names

Improsulfan; NSC-102627.

■ Chemistry

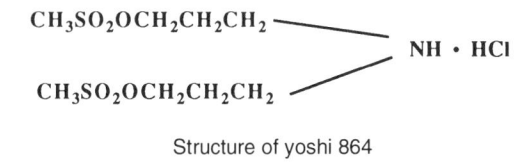

$$CH_3SO_2OCH_2CH_2CH_2\diagdown$$
$$NH \cdot HCl$$
$$CH_3SO_2OCH_2CH_2CH_2\diagup$$

Structure of yoshi 864

Yoshi 864 was first synthesized in Japan by El-Merzabini and Sakurai (1965a,b) in an effort to derive new alkylating agents non-cross-resistant to nitrogen mustard derivatives. Yoshi 864 has a molecular weight of 218 and the empiric formula $C_8H_{19}O_6S_2N \cdot HCl$. It most closely resembles busulfan, both possessing similar methanesulfonyl alkylating groups. The complete chemical name is 3,3'-iminobis-1-propanol dimethanesulfonate (ester) hydrochloride.

■ Antitumor Activity

In phase I trials the agent had activity in patients with chronic myelogeneous leukemia. The drug also induced partial responses in two of five patients with head and neck cancer and one patient with an unknown primary (Hirano et al 1972, Altman et al 1975). Unfortunately, these early findings were never followed up in formal phase II studies. Phase II studies of the agent in patients with colorectal carcinomas and squamous cell carcinoma of the cervix refractory to prior chemotherapy showed no evidence of significant antitumor activity (Douglass et al 1985, Slavik et al 1983).

■ Mechanism of Action

Yoshi 864 probably acts as a bifunctional alkylating agent similar to busulfan. The ultimate cytotoxic effect of the drug appears to involve inhibition of DNA synthesis (Gale et al 1975). It is also occasionally effective in typical alkylator-resistant experimental tumors, especially L-1210 leukemia. Thus, the precise mechanism, which is not known, may well involve alternate explanations to simple alkylation of DNA.

■ Availability and Storage

Yoshi 864 is investigationally available in 10-mL rubber-stoppered glass vials containing 100 mg of lyophilized drug. It is recommended that the intact vials be stored at deep-freeze temperature (−20 to −10°C). Under deep-freeze temperatures the vials are stable for at least 4 years or for at least 2 months if stored under refrigeration. An investigational oral tablet form of the drug, as the tosylate, has also been evaluated.

■ Preparation for Use, Stability, and Admixture

It is recommended that each vial be reconstituted with 5 mL sterile water for injection, forming a 20 mg/mL solution of pH 3.0 to 5.0. This solution is chemically stable for 6 hours either at room temperature or under refrigeration. The drug is similarly stable when further diluted in either normal saline or 5% dextrose injection. Admixture compatibility data are not available for Yoshi 864.

■ Administration

Yoshi 864 is administered intravenously, usually as a slow push. A 5- to 10-mL flush of either normal saline or 5% dextrose solution is recommended before and after drug administration. This may help to pretest vein patency and flush any remaining drug from the tubing or proximal vein lumen. All injections should be closely monitored and performed only through unquestionably patent veins as the drug has slight vesicant properties if infiltrated.

■ Special Precautions

The agent is a vesicant and extreme care should be taken to avoid extravasation.

■ Drug Interactions

None are known.

Dosage

Hirano et al (1972) originally used daily doses of approximately 1 mg/kg up to a total of about 20 mg/kg. In the phase I study of Altman et al (1975), doses ranged from 0.25 to 2.7 mg/kg IV push daily for 5 days. Both responses and hematologic toxicity were first noted at 1.5 mg/kg, and neither significantly increased at doses beyond this amount. The recommended dose for phase II investigations was 2.0 mg/kg/d × 5, repeated every 6 weeks. This was also the dose evaluated in phase II studies (Slavik et al 1983, Douglass et al 1985).

Pharmacokinetics

The disposition of ^{14}C-labeled Yoshi 864 has been studied only in laboratory mice (Glasofer et al 1974). Following intraperitoneal injection, tissues selectively retaining the radiolabel include the heart, the kidney, and the liver. Radioactivity was also noted in the brain within 1 hour of injection. Urinary excretion accounted for the majority of drug elimination, predominantly as unchanged drug and methanesulfonic acid followed by three unidentified metabolites.

Side Effects and Toxicity

The major dose-limiting toxic effect of Yoshi 864 has been myelosuppression. In the phase I study of Altman et al (1975), the median leukopenic nadir was 2500 cells/mm^3 occurring at 4 weeks, whereas the median thrombocytopenic nadir occurred on day 24 with recovery over 1 to 3 weeks. Anemia was insignificant although the hemoglobin fell 1 to 2 g/dL in 11 of 25 courses. Hirano et al (1972) also noted hematologic depression as the sole dose-limiting toxic effect in the chronic daily dosing study. The nadirs in this study, however, tended to occur earlier, at about 10 days. With repeated courses, the hematologic toxic effects tend to become progressively more severe. Nausea and vomiting become significant in courses using high doses (around 2.7 mg/kg). They may persist over a 6- to 12-day period (as in three of seven courses in the study by Altman et al 1975). In the Central Oncology Group study using 2.0 mg/kg, moderate or severe nausea and vomiting were rare with incidences of 3 and 1%, respectively. Diarrhea was noted in only one patient. The second potentially dose-limiting toxic effect of Yoshi 864 is dose-related neurotoxicity. At 2 mg/kg only one of five patients developed somnolence which lasted up to 5 days; however, at 2.7 mg/kg/d, it was both more common and more severe, occurring in four of seven courses with patients sleeping up to 20 h/d (Altman et al 1975). These episodes typically began the third day of the 5-day infusion regimen and lasted 6 to 10 days. A few patients have become reversibly comatose while receiving the drug. There is also a single instance of a mild local reaction to infiltration of the drug. Significant hepatic, renal, and allergic toxic effects are not yet reported for Yoshi 864.

Special Applications

None are known.

REFERENCES

Altman SJ, Fletcher WS, Andrews NC, Wilson WL, Pisher T. Yoshi-864 (NSC-102627) 1-propanol,3'-propanol-3'-iminodi-dimethanesulfonate (ester) hydrochloride a phase I study. *Cancer.* 1975;**35:**1145–1147.

Douglass HO Jr, MacIntyre JM, Kaufman J, Von Hoff DD, Engstrom PF, Klassen D. Eastern Cooperative Oncology Group phase II studies in advanced measurable colorectal cancer. I. Rozoxane, Yoshi-9864, piperazinedione, and lomustine. *Cancer Treat Rep.* 1985;**69:**543–545.

El-Merzabini MM, Sakurai Y. Inhibition of tumor growth by new sulfonic acid esters of aminoglycols. *Gann.* 1965a;**56:**575–587.

El-Merzabini MM, Sakurai Y. A new alkylating antitumor agent effective on experimental tumors resistant to nitrogen mustard. *Gann.* 1965b;**56:**589–598.

Gale GR, Smith AB, Atkins LM. Comparative effects of yoshi-864 and busulfan on certain transplantable murine tumors. *Proc Soc Exp Biol Med.* 1975;**149**(11):98–101.

Glasofer ED, Weiss AJ, Manthei RW. Studies on the disposition of 1-propanol-3,3'-iminodi-dimethanesulfonate. *Pharmacologist.* 1974;**16:**262.

Hirano M, Miura M, Kakizawa H, et al. Effect of two new sulfonic acid esters of aminoglycols on chronic myelogenous leukemia. *Cancer Chemother Rep Part 1.* 1972;**56**(1):47–52.

Slavik M, Moss H, Blessing JA. Phase II clinical study of Yoshi-864 in squamous cell carcinoma of the uterine cervix. *Cancer Treat Rep.* 1983;**67:**395–496.

Zorubicin

■ Other Names

RP 22050; NSC-164011; benzoylhydrazone-daunorubicin (daunorubicin benzoylhydrazone hydrochloride); Rubidazone® (distributed by Rhodia, Inc, and manufactured by Specia, France).

■ Chemistry

Zorubicin is a semisynthetic anthracycline antitumor agent in the class of daunorubicin. It consists of an amino sugar linked to a four-ringed anthracycline chromophore. This anthracycline is related to daunorubicin and can be produced by chemical reaction of benzoylhydrazine with the keto group at carbon 13 of the daunorubicin side chain. The molecular weight of zorubicin is approximately 646.

The glycosidic bond may be unstable in alkaline pH so the drug should probably be maintained at a pH from 3 to 7.

■ Antitumor Activity

Zorubicin has shown substantial activity in acute lymphocytic leukemias with response rates of up to 50% (Jacquillat et al 1966, 1976). A response rate of 57% was reported in previously untreated patients with acute myelocytic leukemia. Benjamin et al (1979b) have shown lower response rates for zorubicin in both acute lymphocytic and myelogenous leukemias. A follow-up trial in heavily pretreated acute myelogenous leukemia patients given zorubicin and azacitidine showed little efficacy for this combination (Peterson et al 1982). Activity was observed in two patients with hairy cell leukemia (Steward et al 1979). There is some evidence that zorubicin is also active in non-Hodgkin's lymphomas (Jacquillat et al 1976). In patients with chronic myelogenous leukemia, zorubicin produced a 29% response rate, but no patients responded in blast cell crisis (Bickers et al 1981). Zorubicin was also active in an intensive four-drug regimen (ROAP) in chronic myelogenous leukemia (Kantarjian et al 1985). A 53% response rate was reported in this trial, with a median duration of response of 6 months. In contrast, activity in solid tumors was disappointing. In pretreated patients with metastatic breast cancer, no significant activity was reported (Legha et al 1979, Ingle et al 1979, Smith et al 1983). Similarly negative results were obtained by Fraile et al (1978) in adenocarcinoma of the colon and advanced squamous cell carcinoma of the lung.

In pediatric patients with various advanced solid and hematologic malignancies, there is little clinical efficacy for zorubicin (Dasgupta et al 1979, Tan et al 1981). Of interest, in a number of these studies, doxorubicin produced some responses. Thus, anthracycline cross-resistance did not appear to explain zorubicin's inactivity. In summary, zorubicin appears to be consistently less active than doxorubicin in patients with solid tumors.

■ Mechanism of Action

Zorubicin acts similarly to the other anthracyclines: it intercalates into the DNA helix with subsequent

Structure of zorubicin

inhibition of DNA and RNA synthesis. Like other anthracyclines, zorubicin induces a cell cycle block at G_2/M interphase (Barlogie et al 1978). There is a preference for inhibiting DNA synthesis over RNA synthesis (Maral 1979); however, the rate of macromolecule inhibition with zorubicin is appreciably slower than that with either daunorubicin or doxorubicin. Zorubicin was also shown to be mutagenic in the Ames bacterial assay (Maral 1979). Unique features of zorubicin include the release of daunorubicin in vivo, reduced conversion to daunorubicinol, and possible activity as a daunorubicin reductase inhibitor.

Zorubicin also probably interferes with topoisomerase II enzymes, leading to protein-linked DNA strand breaks. This activity is maximal in the G_2 phase of the cell cycle.

■ Availability and Storage

Zorubicin was investigationally available through the National Cancer Institute from Rodia, Inc, of France. It was supplied as a lyophilized orange-red powder in 50-mg vials also containing approximately 100 mg of mannitol. Some initial drug batches contained 8 to 12% daunorubicin as an impurity (Trissel 1978). A 4-mL glass ampule of glycine–sodium glycinate buffer was included for each 50 mg of drug to ensure proper pH after initial reconstitution. Both the drug and buffer should be stored in a cool, dry place, preferably at 4°C or less, and protected from direct sunlight.

■ Preparation for Use, Stability, and Admixture

For each 50-mg vial of zorubicin, 4 mL of the buffered glycine–sodium glycinate diluent is initially added to the vial. This yields a 12.5 mg/mL solution which is stable for 8 hours at room temperature of 24 hours under refrigeration. This solution may then be added to either 250 or 500 mL of saline, lactated Ringer's injection, or Normosol-R®. Dextrose should not be added to zorubicin because of possible acid-catalyzed decomposition. The manufacturer has recommended that a final drug concentration of 2 mg/mL not be exceeded.

Even in this final solution there can be a rapid loss of stability. The stability times for zorubicin (50 μg/mL) in 5% dextrose, 0.9% sodium cloride, and lactated Ringer's injection were short at 18 minutes, 2.6 hours, and 3.4 hours, respectively (Poochikian et al 1981). The best infusate for zorubicin was normosol-R® with a stability time of 22 hours. Thus, low pH values such as pH 4.5 in 5% dextrose can dramatically enhance drug decomposition. Heparin may also be incompatible with zorubicin, as is the case with the related anthracyclines, daunomycin and doxorubucin.

■ Administration

The recommended infusion time for zorubicin solutions is 30 minutes to 1 hour. Only new and unquestionably patent venipuncture sites should be used. Extravasation of this drug is likely to be accompanied by extreme pain, tissue sloughing, and necrosis. A 5- to 10-mL flush of D5W or normal saline is recommended both before and after each infusion to ensure vein patency and flush any remaining drug from the tubing. It is further recommended that the infusion not be left unattended and that the patient be instructed to immediately report any change in sensation such as stinging. A change in sensation may hallmark extravasation and the infusion must be immediately halted and the site evaluated. Hydrocortisone has been added to infusions of doxorubicin and daunorubicin to decrease phlebitis and may also be injected into infiltrated areas to minimize tissue damage. Efficacy and drug stability with this admixture are not known.

■ Special Precautions

Fever, chills, and hives have been noted after zorubicin administration. Pretreatment with an intravenous antihistamine such as diphenhydramine and/or hydrocortisone is recommended for all patients. Nonetheless, Dasgupta et al (1979) observed an urticarial skin rash in more than 40% of pediatric patients, sometimes despite diphenhydramine-hydrocortisone pretreatments.

■ Dosage

As a single agent, relatively high doses of 300 to 600 mg/m² have been used in patients with acute leukemias; however, these doses were associated with increased myelotoxicity and some fatalities. Thus, a more prudent dose of 150 to 200 mg/m², repeated in several weeks, was used in combination with other cytotoxic agents. Only patients with good hematologic reserve should receive the 150 to 200 mg/m² dose. With compromised bone marrow reserve, decreased hepato/biliary function, or markedly lowered renal function, the use of lower zorubicin doses is recommended; however, no specific guidelines for dose reduction have been promulgated.

Cumulative doses are recommended not to exceed 3500 mg/m² if zorubicin is the only anthracycline the patient has received. Prior treatment with doxorubicin and/or daunorubicin (150–250 mg/m²) requires a total cumulative dose limit of 1750 mg/m² to minimize the development of cardiotoxicity. Benjamin et al (1979b) noted dose-limiting mucositis at 600 mg/m² and determined an optimal antileukemic dose of 150 mg/m² when used alone or of 200 mg/m² when combined with a 7-day infusion of cytarabine. The recommended phase II solid tumor dose was also 200 mg/m².

■ Pharmacokinetics

Preliminary pharmacologic studies indicate that the drug behaves similarly to daunorubicin. In mice, the drug distributes into the kidney, heart, gastrointestinal tract, spleen, and (slightly) urine; however, the levels of tissue fluorescence were much lower with zorubicin than after daunorubicin (Baurain et al 1979). Fluorescent drug distribution studies in humans have demonstrated urinary elimination of 25% of a dose with an overall plasma half-life (total fluorescence) of approximately 35 hours (Benjamin et al 1976).

Daunorubicin appears to be the major plasma species present after zorubicin injection. The finding of less daunorubicinol after zorubicin than after daunorubicin may be evidence of enzymatic inhibition of daunorubicin reductase by zorubicin (Benjamin et al 1976). If similar to daunorubicin, the liver is most likely the major site for biotransformation of zorubicin. Although biliary excretion of zorubicin accounts for the majority of drug elimination, some renal excretion of the daunorubicin metabolite occurs. Thus, renal elimination still is important for eliminating up to 10 to 20% of a dose of zorubicin.

■ Side Effects and Toxicity

The acute dose-limiting hematologic toxicity of zorubicin is myelosuppression. The nadir for myelosuppression has been reported to occur at a median of 11 days (range, 5–20 days). Aplasia and fatal sepsis occurred in 21% of severely ill patients, with leukemia in one series (Benjamin et al 1979b). Recovery from leukopenia usually requires 21 to 28 days (Kovach et al 1979).

Nonspecific electrocardiographic changes with zorubicin can cause acute cardiotoxic side effects but they are usually transient. Cardiomyopathy (pump failure) has been noted in patients who have received previous anthracyclines, doxorubicin and/or daunorubicin. It presents and is treated similarly to congestive heart failure from other causes. A total cumulative dose of 3500 mg/m² for zorubicin is recommended in patients without prior anthracycline therapy to reduce the incidence of cardiomyopathy. Whether or not zorubicin will produce less cardiotoxicity than other anthracyclines is not established. Of all monitoring methods, serial endomyocardial biopsy appears both most difficult and rewarding. Benjamin et al (1979a) have recently used this grading method in a preliminary study to follow patients on anthracycline therapy. For zorubicin, the recommendation to discontinue therapy was made in two of five patients: one at a cumulative dose of 475 mg/m² (plus 115 mg/m² prior doxorubicin) and the other at a cumulative dose of 1500 mg/m² zorubicin. In a follow-up report, Benjamin et al (1979b) described fatal congestive heart failure in six patients receiving cumulative zorubicin doses of 1050 to 2600 mg/m². All had previously received low-dose anthracycline therapy, however.

The administration of zorubicin frequently causes allergic reactions including fever, chills, and hives. Therefore, pretreatment with an intravenous antihistamine such as diphenhydramine is recommended for all patients. This was noted to alleviate symptoms in some patients. The greater initial incidence of this reaction in early trials may relate to impurities in original lots of drug. There are consistent reports of an urticarial drug rash. In Dasgupta and colleagues' pediatric study, prophylactic diphenhydramine and/or hydrocortisone were not particularly helpful. In a dog model, histamine release was felt to mediate some of the acute cardiovascular toxic effects such as tachycardia as well as the chronic (cumulative-dose) cardiomyopathy (Herman and Young 1979).

Nausea, vomiting, and diarrhea of moderate intensity are common with zorubicin and antiemetic prophylaxis is required in all patients. A severe mucositis can also be common with some dosing regimens (Benjamin et al 1979b).

As with other anthracyclines, zorubicin may be expected to produce serious local tissue destruction if inadvertently extravasated. Characteristically, these ulcers do not heal well and require repeated debridement and local skin grafting. Prevention is imperative but, if zorubicin is extravasated, local ice and topical dimethylsulfoxide are empirically recommended.

Alopecia appears to be less severe with zorubicin than with other anthracyclines. Renal dysfunction has been seen in patients not pretreated with allopurinol because of uric acid nephropathy. There can also be transient hepatic dysfunction following zorubicin treatment. Normal biliary function should be confirmed before dosing, as dysfunction could lead to higher blood levels and prolonged toxicity from zorubicin.

Zorubicin may induce radiation "recall" reactions manifested by skin lesions in previously irradiated sites. The drug will also impart a red color to the urine for several days after administration but this does not signify toxicity. Patients should be so advised.

REFERENCES

Barlogie B, Drewinko B, Benjamine RS, Loo TL. Kinetic response of cultured human lymphoid cells to rubidazone. *J Natl Cancer Inst.* 1978;60:279.

Baurain R, Campeneere DD-D, Trouet A. Distribution and metabolism of rubidazone and daunorubicin in mice. *Cancer Chemother Pharmacol.* 1979;2:37–41.

Benjamin RS, Ewer MS, Mackay B, et al. (1979a) An endomyocardial biopsy study of anthracycline-induced cardiomyopathy—Detection, reversibility and potential amelioration (abstract C-335). *Proc Am Assoc Cancer Res ASCO.* 1979a;20:372.

Benjamin RS, Keating MJ, McCredie KB, et al. Clinical and pharmacologic studies with rubidazone (R) in adults with acute leukemia (AL) (abstract 285). *Proc Am Assoc Cancer Res ASCO.* 1976;17:72.

Benjamin RS, Keating MJ, Swenerton KD, et al. Clinical studies with rubidazone. *Cancer Treat Rep.* 1979b;63:925–929.

Bickers J, Benjamine R, Wilson H, et al. Rubidazone in adults with previously treated acute leukemia and blast cell phase of chronic myelocytic leukemia: A Southwest Oncology Group study. *Cancer Treat Rep.* 1981;65:427–430.

Dasgupta I, Steinherz L, Steinherz P, Tan C. Trial of rubidazone in children with cancer (abstract 631). *Proc Am Assoc Cancer Res ASCO.* 1979;20:156.

Fraile RJ, Samson MK, Buroker TR, et al. Clinical trial of rubidazone in advanced squamous cell carcinoma of the lung and adenocarcinoma of the large intestine. *Cancer Treat Rep.* 1978;62(10):1599–1601.

Herman EH, Young RSK. Acute cardiovascular alterations induced by low doses of Adriamycin, rubidazone, and daunorubicin in the anesthetized beagle dog. *Cancer Treat Rep.* 1979;63:1771–1779.

Ingle JN, Ahmann DL, O'Fallon JR, et al. Randomized phase II trial of rubidazone and Adriamycin in women with advanced breast cancer. *Cancer Treat Rep.* 1979;63:1701–1705.

Jacquillat CL, Boiron M, Weil M, et al. Rubidomycin, a new agent active in the treatment of acute leukemia. *Lancet.* 1966;2:27–28.

Jacquillat CL, Weil M, Gemon-Auclerc MF, et al. Clinical study of rubidazone (22 050 R.P.), a new daunorubicin derived compound, in 170 patients with acute leukemias and other malignancies. *Cancer.* 1976;37:653–659.

Kantarjian HM, Vellekoop L, McCredie KB, et al. Intensive combination chemotherapy (ROAP 10) and splenectomy in the management of chronic myelogenous leukemia. *J Clin Oncol.* 1985;3:192–200.

Kovach JS, Ames MM, Sternad ML, O'Connell MJ. Phase I trial and assay of rubidazone (NSC 164011) in patients with advanced solid tumors. *Cancer Res.* 1979;39:823–828.

Legha SS, Benjamin RS, Buzdar AU, et al. Rubidazone in metastatic breast cancer. *Cancer Treat Rep.* 1979;63(1):135–137.

Maral R. Biological activities of rubidazone. *Cancer Chemother Pharmacol.* 1979;2:31–35.

Peterson BA, Bloomfield CD, Gottlieb AJ, et al. 5-Azacitidine and zorubicin for patients with previously treated acute nonlymphocytic leukemia: A Cancer and Leukemia Group B pilot study. *Cancer Treat Rep.* 1982;66:563–566.

Poochikian GK, Cradock JC, Flora KP. Stability of anthracycline antitumor agents in four infusion fluids. *Am J Hosp Pharm.* 1981;38:483–486.

Smith FE, Gad-el-Mawla N, Tranum B, et al. Phase II evaluation of rubidazone (NSC-164011) in advanced carcinoma of the breast. A Southwest Oncology Group study. *Invest New Drugs.* 1983;1:315–319.

Steward DJ, Benjamine RS, McCredie KB, et al. The effectiveness of rubidazone in hairy cell leukemia (leukemic reticuloendotheliosis). *Blood.* 1979;54:298–304.

Tan CTC, Mitta SK, Steinherz L, Miller DR. Phase I trial of rubidazone (NSC-164011) in children with cancer. *Med Pediatr Oncol.* 1981;9:347–353.

Trissel LA. Pharmaceutical Resources Branch, Developmental Therapeutics Program, Division of Cancer Treatment, National Cancer Institutes, personal communication, March 1978.

Appendices

APPENDIX 1: NOMOGRAM FOR DETERMINATION OF BODY SURFACE AREA FROM HEIGHT AND WEIGHT—ADULTS

$S = W^{0.426} \times H^{0.785} \times 71.84$, or $\log S = \log W \times 0.425 + \log H \times 0.725 + 1.856\ 4$ (S = body surface in cm^2, W = weight in kg, H = height in cm).

From Du Bois D, Du Bois EF. A formula to estimate the approximate surface area if height and weight are known. Arch Intern Med. 1916;17:863–867. Reprinted with permission.

APPENDIX 2: NOMOGRAM FOR DETERMINATION OF BODY SURFACE AREA FROM HEIGHT AND WEIGHT—CHILDREN

$S = W^{0.425} \times H^{0.725} \times 71.84$, or $\log S = \log W \times 0.425 + \log H \times 0.725 + 1.856\,4$ (S = body surface in cm^2, W = weight in kg, H = height in cm).
From Du Bois D, Du Bois EF. A formula to estimate the approximate surface area if height and weight are known. Arch Intern Med. 1916;17:863–867. Reprinted with permission.

APPENDIX 3: FORMULA FOR ESTIMATION OF CREATININE CLEARANCE (CrCl) USING SERUM CREATININE (Cr_s)

Cockcroft and Gault Method

$$\text{Male CrCl (mL/min)} = \frac{(140 - \text{age}) \text{ weight}}{72 \cdot Cr_s}$$

where age is in years, weight is in kilograms, and Cr_s is in mg/dL. For females, the CrCl value is reduced by 15% (multiply male value by 0.85).

Reference: Cockcroft DW, Gault MH. Prediction of creatinine clearance from serum creatinine. Nephron. 1976;16:31–41.

Jelliffe Method

$$\text{CrCl (mL/min)} = \frac{98 - 0.8 \, (\text{age} - 20)}{Cr_s}$$

where age is rounded off to the nearest decade (in years) and values for females are 0.9 times those in males. Serum creatinine is in mg/dL.

Reference: Jelliffe RW. Creatinine clearance: Bedside estimate. Ann Intern Med. 1973;79:604–605.

Measured Urinary Creatinine Clearance

$$\text{CrCl} = [\text{Urine Cr (mg/dL)}/Cr_s \text{ (mg/dL)}] \times [\text{urine volume (mL)/time (min)}]$$

Reference: Rhodes PJ, Rhodes RS, McClelland GH, et al. Evaluation of eight methods for estimating creatinine clearance in men. Clin Pharm. 1987;6:399–406.

Index

110 A (nafoxidine), 744–745
A-8103 (pipobroman), 783–784
Abbott-43818 (leuprolide acetate), 630–633
absolute granulocyte count, 58–59
ABVD regimen, 343–344, 396
5-AC (azacitidine), 209–212
Accutane (isotretinoin), 617–624
ACE regimen, 461
acetaminophen, combination, with interferon alfa, 573t
N-acetyl-aminoglutethimide, pharmacokinetics, 173, 173t
N-acetylamonafide, 177
N-acetylcysteine
  bladder irrigations, 560
  drug interactions
    with cyclophosphamide, 322t, 323
    with doxorubicin, 402t
  in management of doxorubicin extravasation, 112
acetyl-sarcolysin L-leucine (asaley), 200
acivicin, 131–134
  administration, 131–132
  antitumor activity, 131
  availability and storage, 131
  chemistry, 131
  dosage, 132, 132t
  drug interactions, with homoharringtonine, 537
  mechanism of action, 131
  pharmacokinetics, 132, 133t
  precautions with, 132
  preparation, 131
  side effects, 132–133
  stability, 131
  toxicity, 132–133
Aclacinomycin (aclarubicin), 135–140
  as irritant, 110t
Aclacinomycin A (aclarubicin), 135–140
aclarubicin, 135–140
  administration, 136–137
  admixture, 136
  antitumor activity, 135, 136t
  availability and storage, 136

chemistry, 135
dose, 137, 137t
drug interactions, 137
mechanism of action, 135–136
pharmacokinetics, 137, 138t
preparation, 136
side effects, 137–138
special applications, 138
stability, 136
toxicity, 137–138
ACM (aclarubicin), 135–140
acodazole, 140–143
  administration, 141
  admixture, 141
  antitumor activity, 140
  availability and storage, 141
  chemistry, 140
  dosage, 141, 141t
  mechanism of action, 140–141
  pharmacokinetics, 141, 142t
  precautions with, 141
  preparation, 141
  side effects, 142–143
  stability, 141
  toxicity, 142–143
acodazole hydrochloride (acodazole), 140–143
acquired immune deficiency syndrome. See also human immunodeficiency virus
  suramin sodium's activity in, 859
AC regimen, 396
N-[4-(9-acridinylamino)-3-methoxyphenyl]methanesulfonamide (amsacrine), 182–189
acridinylanisidide (amsacrine), 182–189
acrolein, drug interactions, with cyclophosphamide, 323
acronycine, 143–145
  administration, 144
  antitumor activity, 143–144
  availability and storage, 144
  chemistry, 143
  dose, 144
  mechanism of action, 144

pharmacokinetics, 144t, 144–145
side effects, 145
toxicity, 145
ACT-D (dactinomycin), 349–354
Actinomycete Fermentation Product (piperazinedione), 780–782
actinomycin C_1 (dactinomycin), 349–354
Actinomycin D (dactinomycin), 349–354
adenosine, drug interactions, with doxorubicin, 401t
admixtures. See also specific agents
  safe handling of, 124
adoptive immunotherapy, 151
adozelesin, 146–148
  administration, 147
  admixture, 147
  antitumor activity, 146
  availability and storage, 146
  chemistry, 146
  dosage, 147
  drug interactions, 147
  mechanism of action, 146
  pharmacokinetics, 147
  preparation, 147
  side effects, 147–148
  stability, 147
  toxicity, 147–148
ADR-529 (dexrazoxane), 367–371
adrenal corticosteroids, 18t
Adrenaline (epinephrine), 69t–70t
Adria (doxorubicin), 395–416
Adriamycin (doxorubicin), 23–24, 395–416
Adroyd (oxymethalone), 192t
Adrucil (5-fluorouracil), 500–515
AF-1890 (lonidamine), 650–653
alanosine, 148–150
  administration, 149
  admixture, 149
  antitumor activity, 148
  availability and storage, 149
  chemistry, 148
  dosage, 149, 149t
  drug interactions, with PALA, 770
  mechanism of action, 148–149

Page numbers followed by **t** and **f** denote tables and figures, respectively.

alanosine (*cont.*)
  pharmacokinetics, 149
  preparation, 149
  side effects, 149
  stability, 149
  toxicity, 149
L-alanosine (alanosine), 148–150
  drug interactions, with PALA, 770
alcohol, drug interactions
  with diethyldithiocarbamate, 389
  with levamisole, 635
  with *N*-methylformamide, 707
  with procarbazine, 811, 811t
aldesleukin (IL-2), 150–161
  administration, 153–154
  admixture, 153
  antitumor activity, 151t, 151–152
  availability and storage, 152
  capillary leak syndrome with, 158
  chemistry, 150–151
  dosage, 153, 154t
  drug interactions, 153–156, 155t
  flulike syndrome with, 156–158
  mechanism of action, 152
  pharmacokinetics, 156, 157t
  precautions with, 153
  preparation, 153
  side effects, 156–158
  special applications, 159
  stability, 153
  toxicity
    cardiac, 158
    central nervous system, 158
    hematologic, 158
    renal, 158
    skin, 158
aledronate, 47
Alferon N Injection (interferon alfa), 564–582
alizapride, 742t
Alkeran (melphalan), 20, 662–672
alkylating agents, 15–22, 16t
  extravasation, 111t, 113
  mechanism of action, 15–18, 19f
  suspected, 21–22
alkyllysophospholipid (edelfosine), 423–425
allopurinol sodium, 27, 161–166
  administration, 162
  admixture, 162
  as antiparasitic agent, 161
  antitumor activity, 161
  availability and storage, 162
  chemistry, 161
  dosage, 162
  drug interactions, 162–163
    with azathioprine, 214

  with cyclophosphamide, 322, 322t
  with dacarbazine, 345
  with doxorubicin, 401t
  with 5-fluorouracil, 504
  with ifosfamide, 561
  with methotrexate, 696t
  with pentostatin, 776
  with tamoxifen, 870
  with tiazofurin, 912
  mechanism of action, 161–162
  mouthwash, 164
  pharmacokinetics, 163–164
  preparation, 162
  side effects, 164
  special applications, 164
  stability, 162
  suppositories, 164
  toxicity, 164
all-*trans*-retinoic acid (tretinoin), 922–930
allyl alcohol, drug interactions, with doxorubicin, 401t
ALP (edelfosine), 423–425
alpha-interferon (interferon alfa), 564–582
  antibodies, 577
altretamine, 21–22, 166–170
  administration, 71t, 167
  antitumor activity, 166–167
  availability and storage, 167
  chemistry, 166
  dosage, 167
  drug interactions, 167–168
  indications for, 16t
  mechanism of action, 167
  pharmacokinetics, 168t, 168–169
  side effects, 169
  toxicity, 169
AMAP 773 (BWA 773U82), 248–251
AMAP-A (BW 502A 502U83·HCl), 251–252
Amboclorin (chlorambucil), 20
Amen (medroxyprogesterone acetate), 171
amethopterin (methotrexate), 692–705
amifostine (ethiofos), 453–459
  in management of hypercalcemia of malignancy, 50
4-amino-1-β-D-arabinofuranosyl-2(1*H*)-pyrimidinone (cytarabine), 332–340
4-amino-1-β-D-arabinofuranosyl-1,3,5-triazin-2(1)-one (fazarabine), 474–476
p-aminobenzoic acid, drug interactions, with methotrexate, 695
2-amino-4-(*S*-butylsulfonimidoyl)-25-

  butanoic acid (buthionine sulfoximine), 241–248
3-(-aminocarbonyl)-O^4-deacetyl-3-de-(methoxycarbonyl)vinka-leukoblastine (vindesine), 957–966
L-(α*S*,5*S*)-α-amino-3-chloro-4,5-dihydro-5-isoxazolacetic acid (acivicin), 131–134
4-amino-*N*-[5-chloro-2-quinoxalinyl]benzenesulfonamide (chloroquinoxaline sulfonamide), 279–280
2-amino-1,7-dihydro-6*H*-purine-6-thione (6-thioguanine), 893–898
5-amino-2-[2-(dimethylamine)ethyl]-1*H*-benz[de-]isoquinoline-1,3-(2*H*)-dione (amonafide), 175–180
aminoglutethimide, 33–34, 170–175
  administration, 172
  antitumor activity, 171
  availability and storage, 172
  chemistry, 170
  dosage, 172
  drug interactions, 172t, 172
    with corticosteroids, 305
  indications for, 18t
  mechanism of action, 171–172
  pharmacokinetics, 172–173, 173t
  precautions with, 172
  side effects, 173–174
  toxicity, 173–174
aminoglycosides, drug interactions, with gallium nitrate, 522
L-2-amino-3-[(*N*-nitroso)hydroxylamino]propionic acid (alanosine), 148–150
3-(4-aminophenyl)-3-ethyl-2,6-piperidinedione (aminoglutethimide), 170–175
aminophylline, 69t–70t
S-[(3-aminopropyl)amino]-ethanediol, dihydrogen phosphate (ester) (ethiofos), 453–459
4-amino-1-β-D-ribofuranosyl-1,3,5-triazine-2(1*H*)-one (azacitidine), 209–212
amitriptyline, drug interactions, with procarbazine, 811, 811t
amonafide, 175–180
  administration, 176
  antitumor activity, 176
  availability and storage, 176
  chemistry, 175–176
  dosage, 177, 177t
  mechanism of action, 176
  pharmacokinetics, 177, 178t

Page numbers followed by **t** and **f** denote tables and figures, respectively.

precautions with, 176
preparation, 176
side effects, 177
stability, 176
toxicity, 177
amphotericin B, drug interactions
  with carmustine, 269
  with daunorubicin HCl, 358
  with 5-fluorouracil, 504
  with gallium nitrate, 522
  with methotrexate, 696
ampligen, 180–182
  administration, 181
  antihuman immunodeficiency activity, 180
  antitumor activity, 180
  availability and storage, 181
  chemistry, 180
  dosage, 181
  mechanism of action, 181
  pharmacokinetics, 181
  side effects, 181
  toxicity, 181
AMSA (amsacrine), 182–189
m-AMSA (amsacrine), 23–24, 182–189
amsacrine, 23–24, 182–189
  administration, 184–185
  admixture, 184
  antitumor activity, 183t, 183–184
  availability and storage, 184
  chemistry, 182–183
  dosage, 185
  drug interactions, 185
    with eflornithine, 427
  extravasation, management of, 115t
  indications for, 16t
  mechanism of action, 184
  pharmacokinetics, 185–186
  precautions with, 185
  preparation, 184
  side effects, 186–187
  stability, 184
  toxicity, 186–187
  as vesicant, 67t, 112, 113
Amsidine (amsacrine), 23–24, 182–189
anabolic steroids, in regulation of bone remodeling, 38t
Anadrol-50 (oxymethalone), 192t
anaphylaxis, 68–70
  management of, 69t–70t
Anapolon (oxymethalone), 192t
ancitabine (cyclocytidine), 318–319
AndroCyp (testosterone cypionate), 32
androgens, 17t, 32, 189–194
  administration, 191
  admixture, 191
  antitumor activity, 190
  availability and storage, 191, 192t
  chemistry, 189–190
  dosage, 191, 192t

mechanism of action, 190–191
pharmacokinetics, 191
preparation, 191
side effects, 191–193
stability, 191
Android-10 (methyltestosterone), 32
Andro L.A. (testosterone enanthate), 32
Androlan (testosterone propionate), 32
anesthetic
  drug interactions, with *Corynebacterium parvum*, 311
  lipid-soluble, drug interactions, with Fluosol, 517
anguidine, 194–196
  administration, 195
  admixture, 195
  antitumor activity, 195
  availability and storage, 195
  chemistry, 194
  dosage, 195
  mechanism of action, 195
  precautions with, 195
  preparation, 195
  side effects, 196
  special applications, 196
  stability, 195
  toxicity, 196
9,10-anthracenedicarboxaldehyde bis-[(4,5-dihydro-1H-imidazol-2-yl)-hydrazone]dihydrochloride (bisantrene HCl), 224–227
anthracycline, drug interactions
  with dexrazoxane, 369
  with razoxane, 826
anthrapyrazole dihydrochloride (piroxantrone hydrochloride), 791–794
antiadrenal, 18t
antiandrogen, 18t
antibiotics, drug interactions, with methotrexate, 695
anticancer drugs. See also specific agents
  selectivity of, 9–10
anticoagulants, drug interactions, with methotrexate, 695
antidiabetic drugs, oral, drug interactions, with allopurinol sodium, 163
antiestrogen, 18t
antihistamines
  drug interactions, with procarbazine, 811, 811t
  in management of doxorubicin extravasation, 112
antihormonal agents, 18t, 33–34
antimetabolites, 5t, 15, 25–28
  indications for, 17t
  mechanism of action, 4, 26f
antineoplastic agents. See also specific agents

oral, 71t
safe handling of, 60–61, 62t–63t
antipyrene, drug interactions
  with aminoglutethimide, 172
  with progestins, 817
Antril, 589
Antrypol (suramin sodium), 859–866
APE regimen, 461, 692
aphidicolin glycinate, 197–200
  admixture, 198
  antitumor activity, 197
  availability and storage, 198
  chemistry, 197
  dosage, 198
  mechanism of action, 197–198
  pharmacokinetics, 198, 198t, 199t
  preparation, 198
  side effects, 198–199
  stability, 198
  toxicity, 198–199
API-395 (oxaliplatin), 758–761
Aquavene, 84, 85f
Ara-A (vidarabine), 27
  drug interactions, with allopurinol sodium, 163
Ara-AC (fazarabine), 474–476
9-β-D-arabinofuranosyl-2-fluoroadenine 5′-monophosphate (fludarabine phosphate), 495–499
arabinosyl-2-fluoroadenine monophosphate (fludarabine phosphate), 27
Ara-C (cytarabine), 332–340
ara-CMP, 28
ara-CTP, 28
Aredia (pamidronate), in management of hypercalcemia of malignancy, 47–51
arginine, drug interactions, with vincristine sulfate, 953
Aristocort (triamcinolone), 303t
arylmethylaminopropanediol (BW 502A 502U83·HCl), 251–252
arylmethylaminopropanediol (BWA 773U82), 248–251
asaley, 200
  administration, 200
  antitumor activity, 200
  chemistry, 200
  dose, 200
  mechanism of action, 200
  side effects, 200
  toxicity, 200
ascorbate, drug interactions
  with doxorubicin, 401t
  with ifosfamide, 560–561
L-asnase (asparaginase), 201–209
L-ASP (asparaginase), 201–209
asparaginase, 34, 201–209
  administration, 202–203

asparaginase (cont.)
  admixture, 202
  antitumor activity, 201–202
  availability and storage, 202
  chemistry, 201
  covalently conjugated to polyethylene glycol, 201
  dosage, 203–204
  drug interactions, 204, 204t
    with homoharringtonine, 537
    with methotrexate, 695, 696, 697t
  hypersensitivity reactions with, 68
  indications for, 18t
  mechanism of action, 5t, 202
  modified, 206
  pharmacokinetics, 204–205
  precautions with, 203
  preparation, 202
  side effects, 205–206
  special applications, 206
  stability, 202
  toxicity, 205–206
  unit, 201
L-asparaginase (asparaginase), 201–209
L-asparaginase amidohydrolase (asparaginase), 201–209
asparagine rescue, 206
aspirin
  combination, with interferon alfa, 573t
  drug interactions
    with corticosteroids, 305
    with suramin sodium, 862
Asta D 7093 (mesna), 685–689
AT-125 (acivicin), 131–134
aurelic acid (plicamycin), 797–801
aureolic acid (plicamycin), 25, 797–801
Auto Syringe, 90
azacitidine, 28, 209–212
  administration, 210
  admixture, 210
  antitumor activity, 209
  availability and storage, 209–210
  chemistry, 209
  dosage, 210
  drug interactions, 210
    with tretinoin, 925t
  indications for, 17t
  mechanism of action, 209
  pharmacokinetics, 210–211
  preparation, 210
  side effects, 211
  special applications, 211
  stability, 210
  toxicity, 211
5-azacytidine (azacitidine), 28, 209–212, 393
aza-dCTP, 28

azaserine, drug interactions, with 6-thioguanine, 895
azathioprine, 212–215
  administration, 213
  admixture, 213
  antitumor activity, 213
  availability and storage, 213
  chemistry, 212
  dosage, 214
  drug interactions, 214
    with allopurinol sodium, 162
    with dacarbazine, 345
    with diethyldithiocarbamate, 389
  injectable, 213
  mechanism of action, 213
  oral, 213
  pharmacokinetics, 214
  precautions with, 213–214
  preparation, 213
  side effects, 214–215
  stability, 213
  toxicity, 214–215
azidothymidine, combination, with interferon alfa, 573t
aziquone, drug interactions, with eflornithine, 427
aziridine, indications for, 16t
aziridine thiophosphoramide, 20
aziridinyl benzoquinone (diaziquone), 375–380
Azone (1-dodecylazacycloheptan-2-one), 429
AZQ (diaziquone), 375–380

B-1348 (chlorambucil), 275–279
BA-163 (streptonigrin), 847–849
BA-16038 (aminoglutethimide), 170–175
bacillus Calmette-Guérin, 216–219, 309. See also methanol extraction residue of bacillus Calmette-Guérin
  administration, 217
    intraperitoneal, 103
    intrapleural, 104
  antitumor activity, 216
  availability and storage, 217
  chemistry, 216
  drug interactions, 218
  mechanism of action, 216
  pharmacokinetics, 218
  precautions with, 217–218
  preparation, 217
  side effects, 218
  stability, 217
  toxicity, 218

BACON regimen, 228
BACOP regimen, 228, 320, 396, 435–436, 951
BAF [Baker's antifol (soluble)], 219–222
Baker's antifol (soluble), 219–222
  administration, 220
  admixture, 220
  antitumor activity, 219–220
  availability and storage, 220
  chemistry, 219
  dosage, 220
  mechanism of action, 220
  pharmacokinetics, 221
  precautions with, 220
  preparation, 220
  side effects, 221
  stability, 220
  toxicity, 221
barbiturates, drug interactions
  with chlorambucil, 276
  with *Corynebacterium parvum*, 311
  with cyclophosphamide, 322, 322t
  with ifosfamide, 560–561
  with procarbazine, 811, 811t
battery, definition of, 120
Baxter 5- and 7-day infusor pumps, 92, 92f
Bayer 205 (suramin sodium), 859–866
BB-IND 2861 (interleukin-4), 601–605
B-cell growth factor (interleukin-4), 601–605
B-cell stimulatory factor 1 (interleukin-4), 601–605
B-cell stimulatory factor 2 (interleukin-6), 605–609
BCGF [B-cell growth factor (interleukin-4)], 601–605
BCG live (bacillus Calmette-Guérin), 216–219
BCG-MER (methanol extraction residue of bacillus Calmette-Guérin), 689–691
BCNU (carmustine), 9, 267–275
  as irritant, 114
belganyl (suramin sodium), 859–866
Benadryl (diphenhydramine HCl), 69t–70t
benznidazole, drug interactions, with lomustine, 646
benzoylhydrazone-daunorubicin (zorubicin), 975–978
bepridil, drug interactions, with doxorubicin, 401t
beta blockers, drug interactions, with octreotide acetate, 752
Betaseron (interferon beta), 582–585
BHD regimen, 343

Page numbers followed by **t** and **f** denote tables and figures, respectively.

BiCNU (carmustine), 20, 267–275
biologic agents, intraperitoneal administration, 103
bioreductive alkylator, 21
bisantrene hydrochloride, 224–227
   administration, 225
   admixture, 225
   antitumor activity, 224–225
   availability and storage, 225
   chemistry, 224
   dosage, 225, 225t
   drug interactions, 225
   mechanism of action, 225
   pharmacokinetics, 226
   precautions with, 225
   preparation, 225
   side effects, 226
   stability, 225
   toxicity, 226
   as vesicant, 67t
1,4-bis(3-bromopropionyl)piperazine (pipobroman), 783–784
bischlorethylamines, 20
4-[bis(2-chloroethyl)amino]benzenebutyric acid (chlorambucil), 275–279
1,3-bis(2-chloroethyl)-1-nitrosourea (carmustine), 267–275
3-[2-[bis(2-chloroethyl)amino]ethyl]-1,3-diazaspiro[4.5]decane-2,4-dione (spiromustine), 844–847
4-[bis(2-chloroethyl)amino]-L-phenylalanine monohydrochloride (melphalan), 662–672
2-[bis(2-chloroethyl)amino]tetrahydro-2H-1,3,2-oxazaphosphorine 2-oxide monohydrate (cyclophosphamide), 319–332
5-[bis(-2-chloroethyl)amino]uracil (uracil mustard), 945–946
1,4-bis(2'-chloroethyl)-1,4-diazabicyclo[2.2.1]heptane diperchlorate (dabis maleate), 342–343
bischloronitrosourea (carmustine), 267–275
bis-1-[3-(1-hydroxyethyl)-porphyrin-8-yl]ethyl ether (porfimer sodium), 801–805
bisphosphonates, in management of hypercalcemia of malignancy, 47–51
Blenoxane (bleomycin sulfate), 22, 227–236
Bleo (bleomycin sulfate), 227–236
bleomycin sulfate, 10, 22, 227–236
   administration, 229
      intraarterial, 233
      intraperitoneal, 102
      intrapleural, 104
      intratumoral injection, 233
      oral, 234
      topical application, 233
   admixture, 229
   antitumor activity, 228
   availability and storage, 229
   bladder instillation, 233
   chemistry, 227–228
   compatibility with other drugs, 229, 229t
   dosage, 230, 230t
      in renal failure, 230, 230t
   drug interactions, 230–231
      with cisplatin, 289
      with dexrazoxane, 369
      with diethyldithiocarbamate, 389
      with eflornithine, 427, 428t
      with vinblastine sulfate, 947–948
      with vincristine sulfate, 953
   hypersensitivity reactions with, 68
   indications for, 16t
   as irritant, 110t
   for malignant effusions, 233
   mechanism of action, 4, 5t, 228–229
   pharmacokinetics, 230t, 231, 231t
   precautions with, 229–230
   preparation, 229
   resistance, 228–229
   side effects, 231–233
   special applications, 233–234
   stability, 229, 229t
   toxicity, 231–233
BLM² (bleomycin sulfate), 227–236
blood–brain barrier
   penetration of, by drugs, 95–96
   as tumor sanctuary, 95
BM21-0955, 47
BMT. *See* bone marrow transplantation
BMY-28090 (elsamitrucin), 433–434
body surface area, determination, from height and weight, 60
   nomogram for adults, 980
   nomogram for children, 981
bone
   formation, 36–38
   metabolism, regulation of, 35–36
   remodeling, regulation of, 36–38
   resorption, 36–38
bone marrow toxicity, 6
bone marrow transplantation
   autologous
      high-dose carmustine with, 270–272
      high-dose cyclophosphamide with, 326, 327t
      high-dose busulfan and cyclophosphamide with, 239–240
      high-dose etoposide with, 6467
      melphalan with, 668–669, 669t
      thiotepa with, 902–903
Brevicon (ethinyl estradiol), 31
5-bromodeoxyuridine
   drug interactions, with cytarabine, 335
   incorporation, in assay of cell cycle times, 5
Broviac Silastic catheter, 81
bruneomycin (streptonigrin), 847–849
BSA. *See* body surface area
BSF (busulfan), 236–241
BSF-2 (interleukin-6), 605–609
BSF-1 [B-cell stimulatory factor 1 (interleukin-4)], 601–605
BSO (buthionine sulfoximine), 241–248
busulfan, 20, 236–241
   administration, 71t, 237
   antitumor activity, 236
   availability and storage, 237
   chemistry, 236
   dosage, 237
   drug interactions, with 6-thioguanine, 895–896
   high-dose, with cyclophosphamide, with bone marrow transplantation, 239–240
   indications for, 16t
   mechanism of action, 237
   pharmacokinetics, 237–238, 238t
   side effects, 238–239
   special applications, 239–240
   toxicity, 238–239
busulphan (busulfan), 236–241
1,4-butanedioldimethanesulfonate (busulfan), 236–241
buthionine sulfoximine, 241–248
   administration, 244
   admixture, 243
   antitumor activity, 241–242
   availability and storage, 243
   chemistry, 241
   dosage, 244
   drug interactions, 244
      with cyclophosphamide, 322t, 323
      with doxorubicin, 401t
      with paclitaxel, 764
   mechanism of action, 242–243, 243f, 243t
   pharmacokinetics, 244t, 244–245, 245t
   precautions with, 244
   preparation, 243
   side effects, 245–246
   stability, 243
   toxicity, 245–246
L-buthionine sulfoximine, drug interactions
   with amsacrine, 185
   with bleomycin sulfate, 230
   with melphalan, 666
butylated hydroxytoluene, in management of doxorubicin extravasation, 112
BW-57-322 (azathioprine), 212–215

BW 301 (piritrexim), 788–791
BW 502 (BW 502A 502U83·HCl), 251–252
BW 773 (BWA 773U82), 248–251
BWA 770U (crisnatol), 253
BWA 773U82, 248–251, 253
   administration, 249
   admixture, 249
   antitumor activity, 249
   availability and storage, 249
   chemistry, 248–249
   dosage, 250
   drug interactions, 250
   mechanism of action, 249
   precautions with, 249
   preparation, 249
   side effects, 250
   stability, 249
   toxicity, 250
BW 502A 502U83·HCl, 251–252
   administration, 251
   admixture, 251
   antitumor activity, 251
   availability and storage, 251
   chemistry, 251
   dosage, 252
   mechanism of action, 251
   pharmacokinetics, 252
   precautions with, 251–252
   preparation, 251
   side effects, 252
   special applications, 252
   stability, 251
   toxicity, 252
BWA 770U mesylate (crisnatol), 316–318
BW 7U85 mesylate, 253–254
   administration, 253–254
   antitumor activity, 253
   availability and storage, 253
   chemistry, 253
   dosage, 254
   mechanism of action, 253
   pharmacokinetics, 254
   preparation, 253
   side effects, 254
   stability, 253
   toxicity, 254

C. parvum (*Corynebacterium parvum*), 309–314
CACP (cisplatin), 286–298
CADD pump, 90
caffeine, drug interactions
   with carmustine, 269
   with doxorubicin, 401t

CAF regimen, 435, 598
calcitonin
   in calcium homeostasis, 35–36, 37t
   in management of hypercalcemia of malignancy, 43–44, 51
   in regulation of bone remodeling, 38t
calcitriol
   in calcium homeostasis, 35–36, 37t
   in regulation of bone remodeling, 38
calcium
   homeostasis, 35–36
   hormonal regulation of, 35–36, 37t
   serum levels, 35, 36t
calcium channel blockers, drug interactions
   with paclitaxel, 764
   with vincristine sulfate, 953
calcium folinate (leucovorin calcium), 624–630
calcium 5-formyl-5,6,7,8-tetrahydrofolate (leucovorin calcium), 624–630
calusterone, 189, 192t
   antitumor activity, 190
   side effects, 193
CAMP regimen, 692
camptothecin, 915
Camptothecin-11 (CPT-11), 314–316
cancer cachexia, treatment of, 816
capillary leak syndrome, with aldesleukin, 158
caracemide, 245–256
   admixture, 255
   antitumor activity, 255
   availability and storage, 255
   chemistry, 254
   dosage, 255
   mechanism of action, 255
   pharmacokinetics, 256
   preparation, 255
   side effects, 256
   stability, 255
   toxicity, 256
carbamazepine, drug interactions, with mitoguazone, 714
carbamic acid (diaziquone), 375–380
Carbethimer (carbetimer), 257–259
carbetimer, 257–259
   administration, 257
   antitumor activity, 257
   availability and storage, 257
   chemistry, 257
   dosage, 257, 258t
   drug interactions, 257
   mechanism of action, 257
   pharmacokinetics, 257
   preparation, 257
   side effects, 258

   special applications, 258
   stability, 257
   toxicity, 258
carbon tetrachloride, drug interactions
   with cyclophosphamide, 322t, 323
   with Fluosol, 517
carboplatin, 21, 259–267
   administration, 261
      intraperitoneal, 102, 264–265
   admixture, 261
   antitumor activity, 259–260
   availability and storage, 261
   chemistry, 259
   dosage, 261t, 261–262
   drug interactions, 262
      with oxaliplatin, 759
   ethiofos with, 455
   indications for, 16t
   local toxicity, 114
   mechanism of action, 260–261
   modulation, by DDTC, 388
   pharmacokinetics, 262t, 262–263
   preparation, 261
   sargramostim with, 830t
   side effects, 263–264
   special applications, 264–265
   stability, 261
   toxicity, 263–264
carboplatin + cyclophosphamide, 287
carboxyimamidate (carbetimer), 257–259
carboxypeptidase G, drug interactions
   with methotrexate, 696
   with trimetrexate, 935
carcinogenesis, in renewing tissues, 7
Cardioxane (dexrazoxane), 367–371
carmustine, 9, 20, 267–275
   administration, 268–269
      intraarterial, 272
      topical solution, 272
   admixture, 268
   antitumor activity, 267
   availability and storage, 268
   chemistry, 267
   combination, with interferon alfa, 572, 573t
   dosage, 269
   drug interactions, 269
      with eflornithine, 427
      with levamisole, 635
      with lomustine, 646
      with lonidamine, 651
      with 6-thioguanine, 896
   ethiofos with, 455, 455t
   high-dose
      administration, 271
      antitumor activity, 270–271

Page numbers followed by **t** and **f** denote tables and figures, respectively.

with bone marrow transplantation, 270–272
 dose, 271
 pharmacokinetics, 271, 271t
 toxicity, 271–272
indications for, 16t
as irritant, 67t, 110t, 114
mechanism of action, 267–268
pharmacokinetics, 269–270, 270t
preparation, 268
side effects, 270
special applications, 270–272
stability, 268, 269t
toxicity, 270
carnitine, drug interactions, with doxorubicin, 401t
carzelesin, 146
CAS-61825-94-3 (oxaliplatin), 758–761
CAS Registry No. 4891-15-0 (estramustine phosphate), 443–446
CAS Registry No. 10034-93-2 (hydrazine sulfate), 540–543
CAS Registry No. 10318-26-0 (dibromodulcitol), 380–384
catheters, 80t, 80–85
 arterial, 84–85
 Broviac Silastic, 81
 central venous, 80–84, 109
  indwelling Silastic right atrial, 81f, 81–83
   anatomic location for, 81, 81f
   heparin flushing of, 82–83
   single-, double-, and triple-lumen, 82, 82f
  long-term peripherally inserted, 83–84
  potential complications and problems with, 80t
  short-term, 83
 extravasation with. See extravasation
 Groshong, 82f, 82–83
 Hickman, 81–82, 82f
 versus implantable ports, choosing between, 87, 88t
 intraperitoneal, 85, 85f, 100–101
 Intrasil, 84
 Landmark, 84, 84f, 85f
 midline venous, 84
 peripherally inserted (central), 109
 semipermanent, for intraperitoneal chemotherapy, 100
 Tenckhoff intraperitoneal, 85, 85f, 100
CAVEx regimen, 461
CAV regimen, 287, 368
CB 3025 (melphalan), 662–672
CBDCA (carboplatin), 259–267
CBH (dabis maleate), 342–343
CC-1065, 146–147, 147
CCNU (lomustine), 20, 644–649
2-CdA (cladribine), 298–301

CeeNU (lomustine), 20, 644–649
CEF regimen, 435
β cell-activating factor (interleukin-1, alpha and beta), 589–595
cell cycle, 3–4, 4f
 times, 5
cell cycle (phase)-specific drugs, 4, 5t
cell-kill hypothesis, 9
cell proliferation
 in normal tissue, 6, 6f
 in tumors, 6–7
cell survival curves, 3–4, 4f
central nervous system, drug penetration into, 95–96, 96t. See also intrathecal chemotherapy
central venous catheters. See catheters, central venous
cephalothin, drug interactions, with methotrexate, 696t, 696
certification, in oncology nursing, 122–123
Cerubidine (daunorubicin HCl), 23–24, 355–364
Cesamet (nabilone), 741–744
CGP 30694 (edatrexate), 419–422
CGP-32349 (4-hydroxyandrostenedione), 543–545
CGS 16949A (fadrazole), 472–474
CHAD regimen, 166
CHAP regimen, 166
chemotherapy
 administration, 57–94
  ambulatory settings, 60
  checklist for, 64t
  home settings, 60
  intraarterial, 73. See also specific agents
  intraosseous, 70–71. See also specific agents
  intraperitoneal, 73, 98–103. See also specific agents
  intrapleural, 103–104
  intrathecal, 72–73, 95–98. See also specific agents
  intravenous, 61–70
   legal implications for nurses in, 123–125
   methods, 61
  intraventricular, 72–73. See also specific agents
  intravesical (bladder), 73. See also specific agents
  oral, 71t, 71–72
  professional qualifications for, 57–58
  regional, 61, 72–73. See also specific agents
  responsibility for, 57
  settings for, 57
  training programs, 58
 assessment for, 58t, 58–59
 delivery systems, 73–92

classification of, 80t
documentation, 73, 74f–75f, 125–126
dosage, calculation of, 60
drug preparation, precautions with, 60–61, 62t–63t
nonvesicant agents, 109, 110t
preparation of patient and family for, 58–60
routes of administration, 61
systemic, 61
CHIP (iproplatin), 613–617
chloral hydrate, drug interactions, with ifosfamide, 560–561
chlorambucil, 20, 275–279
 administration, 71t, 276
 antitumor activity, 275–276
 availability and storage, 276
 chemistry, 275
 combination, with interferon alfa, 573t
 dosage, 276
 drug interactions, 276
 indications for, 16t
 mechanism of action, 276
 pharmacokinetics, 276–277, 277t
 side effects, 277–278
 toxicity, 277–278
chloramphenicol, drug interactions, with methotrexate, 696t
2-chlorodeoxyadenosine (cladribine), 298–301
2-chloro-2′-deoxy-β-D-adenosine (cladribine), 298–301
3-(2-chloroethyl)-2-[(2-chloroethyl)amino]-tetrahydro-2H-1,3,2-oxazaphosphorine-2-oxide (ifosfamide), 558–563
1-(2-chloroethyl)-3-cyclohexyl-1-nitrosourea (lomustine), 644–649
2-[[[(2-chloroethyl)-nitrosoamino]carbonyl]amino]-2-deoxy-D-glucose (chlorozotocin), 280–284
1-(2-chloroethyl)-3-(4-methylcyclohexyl)-1-nitrosourea (semustine), 837–841
chloroquinoxaline sulfonamide, 279–280
 administration, 280
 antitumor activity, 279
 availability and storage, 279
 chemistry, 279
 dosage, 280
 mechanism of action, 279
 pharmacokinetics, 280
 precautions with, 280
 preparation, 279–280
 side effects, 280
 stability, 279–280
 toxicity, 280

chlorotrianisene (estrogens), 31, 446–451, 448t
  indications for, 17t
  pharmacokinetics, 449
chlorozotocin, 280–284
  administration, 281
  antitumor activity, 281
  availability and storage, 281
  chemistry, 280–281
  dosage, 282
  drug interactions, with lomustine, 646
  mechanism of action, 281
  pharmacokinetics, 282
  precautions with, 281
  side effects, 282
  toxicity, 282
chlorpromazine, drug interactions
  with bleomycin sulfate, 230
  with doxorubicin, 402t
chlorsulfaquinoxaline (chloroquinoxaline sulfonamide), 279–280
CHOP-BLEO regimen, 231
CHOP regimen, 305, 396, 435, 951
chromomycin A_3, 284–286
  administration, 285
  antitumor activity, 284
  availability and storage, 284
  chemistry, 284
  dosage, 285
  mechanism of action, 284
  pharmacokinetics, 285
  precautions with, 285
  preparation, 284–285
  side effects, 285
  special applications, 285
  stability, 284–285
  toxicity, 285
2[(6-chrysenylmethyl)amino]-2-methyl-1,3-propanediol (crisnatol), 316–318
cimetidine, drug interactions
  with altretamine, 168
  with amsacrine, 185
  with carmustine, 269
  with cyclophosphamide, 322t, 323
  with diaziquone, 377
  with doxorubicin, 400, 401t
  with ifosfamide, 561
  with lomustine, 646
  with melphalan, 666
cisplatin, 10, 21, 286–298
  administration, 288–289
    intraarterial, 292
    intraperitoneal, 100, 101–102, 293
    intrapleural, 104
    intravesical, 293

admixture, 288
allergic reactions to, 290–291
antitumor activity, 286–287
  with breast cancer, 287
  with colorectal cancer, 287
  with gastric cancer, 287
  with head and neck cancer, 287
  with non-small cell lung cancer, 286–287
  with osteosarcoma, 287
  with ovarian cancer, 287
  with pediatric brain tumors, 287
  with penile cancer, 287
  with small cell lung cancer, 287
  with untreated bladder cancer, 287
availability and storage, 288
cardiotoxicity, 291–292
chemistry, 286
combination, with interferon alfa, 572, 573t
dosage, 289
drug interactions, 289, 292
  with bleomycin sulfate, 231
  with edatrexate, 420
  with eflornithine, 427
  with etoposide, 464
  with floxuridine, 491–492
  with ifosfamide, 560
  with lonidamine, 651
  with mesna, 686
  with paclitaxel, 764
  with thymidine, 908
emesis with, 291
ethiofos with, 455, 455t
extravasation, management of, 113, 115t
hepatic toxicity, 292
high-dose, 289
hypersensitivity reactions with, 68
with hyperthermia, 293
hypomagnesemia with, 292
indications for, 16t
as irritant, 110t
local toxicity, 292
mechanism of action, 15, 18, 287–288
modulation, by DDTC, 388
myelosuppression with, 292
nephrotoxicity, 291
  modulation of, by sodium thiosulfate, 103
neurotoxicity, 291
ototoxicity, 291
pharmacokinetics, 289–290, 290t
precautions with, 289
preparation, 288
as radiosensitizer, 293
side effects, 290–292

special applications, 292–293
stability, 288
toxicity, 290–292
cisplatin + bleomycin + vinblastine, 286
cisplatin + cyclophosphamide, 287
cisplatin + cytarabine, administration
  intraperitoneal, 102
  intrapleural, 104
cisplatin + cytarabine + bleomycin, intraperitoneal administration, 102
cisplatin + doxorubicin + cyclophosphamide, 287
cisplatin + etoposide, intraperitoneal administration, 103
cisplatin + etoposide + doxorubicin, 287
cisplatin + 5-fluorouracil, 287
cisplatin + methotrexate, 287
cisplatin + vinblastine + radiation therapy, 287
Cisplatyl (cisplatin), 10
citrovorum factor (leucovorin calcium), 624–630
citrulline, drug interactions, with vincristine sulfate, 953
CL 8206 (thiotepa), 898–905
CL-216942 (bisantrene hydrochloride), 224–227
  as vesicant, 67t
CL-232315 (mitoxantrone hydrochloride), 730–735
cladribine, 298–301
  administration, 300
  admixture, 299–300
  antitumor activity, 298–299, 299t
  availability and storage, 299
  chemistry, 298
  dosage, 300
  mechanism of action, 299
  pharmacokinetics, 300
  preparation, 299–300
  side effects, 300
  stability, 299–300
  toxicity, 300
clinical trials, consent in, 121
clodronate, 47
  structure of, 47f
CMF regimen, 692, 695, 868
CMF-VP regimen, 302, 951
COAP regimen, 320
coenzyme Q, drug interactions, with doxorubicin, 401t
colaspase (asparaginase), 201–209
colchicine, resistance to, 11t
colchicine derivatives, 5t

Page numbers followed by **t** and **f** denote tables and figures, respectively.

colony-forming assays, 7
colony-stimulating factors, 6. *See also* granulocyte colony-stimulating factor (filgrastim); granulocyte-macrophage colony-stimulating factor; macrophage colony-stimulating factor; monocyte/macrophage colony-stimulating factor; rhGM-CSF
  drug interactions, with melphalan, 666
  hematopoietic, drug interactions, with melphalan, 666
COMB regimen, 228
COMLA regimen, 692
compliance, with oral therapy, 71–72
compound 47599 (pyrazofurin), 821–824
conjugated estrogens (estrogens), 446–451
  indications for, 17t
consent, 119–121
Cooper regimen, 302
coparvax (*Corynebacterium parvum*), 309–314
copoly[styrene] maleic acid-conjugated neocarzinostatin, 749
COP regimen, 320
corticosteroids, 31, 32–33, 302–309
  administration, 304
  admixture, 304
  antitumor activity, 302
  availability and storage, 303t, 304
  chemistry, 302
  compatibility with other agents, 304, 304t
  dosage, 304–305, 305t
  drug interactions, 305–306
    with aminoglutethimide, 172t, 172
    with cyclophosphamide, 322t, 323
    with melphalan, 666
    with streptozocin, 852
  formulations, 303t
  mechanism of action, 5t, 302–304
  pharmacokinetics, 306, 306t
  preparation, 304
  side effects, 306–307
  stability, 304
  toxicity, 306–307
cortisol (hydrocortisone)
  chemistry, 302
  mechanism of action, 303
Corynebacterium parvum, 309–314
  administration, 310
  admixture, 310
  antitumor activity, 309
  availability and storage, 310
  chemistry, 309
  dosage, 311

  drug interactions, 311
    with dacarbazine, 345
  mechanism of action, 309–310
  precautions with, 310–311
  preparation, 310
  side effects, 311–312
  special applications, 312
  stability, 310
  toxicity, 311–312
Cosmegen (dactinomycin), 23–24, 349–354
co-vidarabine (pentostatin), 774–779
CPM (cyclophosphamide), 319–332
CPT-11 (irinotecan), 314–316
  administration, 314
  antitumor activity, 314
  availability and storage, 314
  chemistry, 314
  dosage, 315
  mechanism of action, 314
  pharmacokinetics, 315
  precautions with, 314–315
  preparation, 314
  side effects, 315
  stability, 314
  toxicity, 315
CQS (chloroquinoxaline sulfonamide), 279–280
cRA (isotretinoin), 617–624
Crasnitin (asparaginase), 201–209
creatinine clearance, estimation of, 982
Cremophor EL, 29
  drug interactions, with paclitaxel, 764
  hypersensitivity reactions caused by, 385–386, 417, 418
crisnatol, 253, 316–318
  administration, 317
  admixture, 316–317
  antitumor activity, 316
  availability and storage, 316
  chemistry, 316
  dosage, 317
  mechanism of action, 316
  pharmacokinetics, 317
  precautions with, 317
  preparation, 316–317
  side effects, 317
  special applications, 317
  stability, 316–317
  toxicity, 317
cromolyn sodium, drug interactions, with doxorubicin, 401t
crystalline antibiotic (piperazinedione), 780–782
CSF-1 (monocyte/macrophage colony-stimulating factor), 735–740
CTX (cyclophosphamide), 319–332
Cyclo-C (cyclocytidine), 318–319
cyclocytidine, 318–319
  administration, 319

  antitumor activity, 318
  availability and storage, 318
  chemistry, 318
  dosage, 319
  mechanism of action, 318
  pharmacokinetics, 319
  preparation, 318–319
  side effects and toxicity, 319
  stability, 318–319
$O^{2,2'}$-cyclocytidine (cyclocytidine), 318–319
2,2'-*O*-cyclocytidine hydrochloride (cyclocytidine), 318–319
[(1*R*,2*R*)-1,2-cyclohexanediamine-*N*,*N*'][oxalato(2-)-*O*,*O*']platinum(II) (oxaliplatin), 758–761
cyclophosphamide, 20, 319–332
  administration, 71t, 321
  admixture, 321
  antitumor activity, 320
  availability and storage, 320–321
  chemistry, 319–320
  combination, with interferon alfa, 572, 573t
  dosage, 321–322
  drug interactions, 322t, 322–323
    with allopurinol sodium, 162–163
    with corticosteroids, 306
    with *Corynebacterium parvum*, 311
    with dibromodulcitol, 381
    with doxorubicin, 401t
    with hexamethylene bisacetamide, 532
    with interferon alfa, 572
    with interleukin-2, 154t, 155–156
    with methotrexate, 696, 697t
    with razoxane, 826
    with trimetrexate, 935
  ethiofos with, 454–455, 455t
  high-dose, 326–328, 327t
    with autologous bone marrow transplantation, 326, 327t
    pharmacokinetics, 327, 328t
    side effects and toxicity, 327–328
  hypersensitivity reactions with, 68
  indications for, 16t
  mechanism of action, 320
  pharmacokinetics, 323–325, 324t
  precautions with, 322
  preparation, 321
  sargramostim with, 830, 830t
  side effects, 20, 325–326
  special applications, 326–328
  stability, 321
  toxicity, 325–326
cyclophosphamide + methotrexate + etoposide, 461
cyclopropyl pyrroloindole antitumor agents, 146

cyclosporine, drug interactions
    with doxorubicin, 401t, 403
    with octreotide acetate, 752
    with paclitaxel, 764
Cycrin (medroxyprogesterone), 31–32
Cyfos (ifosfamide), 20
Cytadren (aminoglutethimide), 33–34, 170–175
cytarabine, 28, 332–340
    administration, 334
        intraperitoneal, 338
        intrathecal, 96, 97, 337–338
    admixture, 333–334
    antitumor activity, 332–333
    availability and storage, 333
    chemistry, 332
    dosage, 334
    drug interactions, 334–335
        with asparaginase, 204, 204t
        with azacitidine, 210
        with eflornithine, 427
        with etoposide, 464
        with floxuridine, 491
        with fludarabine phosphate, 497–498
        with hydroxyurea, 547
        with maytansine, 655
        with methotrexate, 696, 697t
        with mitoxantrone hydrochloride, 732
        with neocarzinostatin, 748
        with PALA, 769–770
        with pentostatin, 776
        with sargramostim, 833–834
        with tretinoin, 925, 925t
    high-dose
        pharmacokinetics, 335–336
        side effects and toxicity, 336–337, 337t
    indications for, 17t
    isolated limb perfusion, 338
    mechanism of action, 5t, 333
    pharmacokinetics, 335–336
    preparation, 333–334
    sargramostim with, 830, 830t
    side effects, 336–337
    special applications, 337–338
    stability, 333–334
    toxicity, 336–337
cytembena, 341–342
    admixture, 341
    antitumor activity, 341
    availability and storage, 341
    chemistry, 341
    dosage, 341
    mechanism of action, 341
    pharmacokinetics, 341

    preparation, 341
    side effects, 341
    special applications, 341
    stability, 341
    toxicity, 341
cytidine, drug interactions, with PALA, 770
Cytosar-U (cytarabine), 28, 332–340
cytosine, drug interactions, with tegafur, 880
cytosine arabinoside (cytarabine), 332–340
    administration, intraperitoneal, 102
cytosine arabinoside + cisplatin + doxorubicin, intraperitoneal administration, 102
cytotoxic agents. See also specific agents
    drug interactions, with interleukin-2, 154t
    safe handling of, 60–61, 62t–63t, 124
Cytoxan (cyclophosphamide), 20, 319–332

dabis maleate, 342–343
    antitumor activity, 342
    chemistry, 342
    mechanism of action, 342
dacarbazine, 10, 21–22, 343–349
    administration, 345
        intraarterial, 347
        intrathecal, 98, 347
        intraventricular, 347
    admixture, 344–345
    antitumor activity, 343–344
    availability and storage, 344
    chemistry, 343
    dosage, 345
    drug interactions, 345
        with interleukin-2, 156
    indications for, 16t
    as irritant, 67t, 110t, 114
    mechanism of action, 344
    pharmacokinetics, 345–346, 346t
    preparation, 344–345
    side effects, 346–347
    special applications, 347
    stability, 344–345
    toxicity, 346–347
DACT (dactinomycin), 349–354
dactinomycin, 23–24, 349–354
    administration, 350
        intraarterial, 353
    admixture, 350
    antitumor activity, 349–350
    availability and storage, 350

    chemistry, 349
    dosage, 350
    drug/therapeutic interactions, 350–351
    extravasation, 111t
        with heat, 352
    indications for, 16t
    isolated limb perfusion, 353
    mechanism of action, 350, 350t
    pharmacokinetics, 351
    precautions with, 350
    preparation, 350
    resistance to, 11t
    side effects, 351–352
    special applications, 352
    stability, 350
    toxicity, 351–352
    as vesicant, 67t, 112
DAG (dianhydrogalactitol), 372–375
danazol, 192t
    antitumor activity, 190
    chemistry, 189
    mechanism of action, 190
    pharmacokinetics, 191
    side effects, 193
Danocrine (danazol), 192t
DAU (deazauridine), 365–367
daunomycin, drug interactions, with neocarzinostatin, 748
daunomycin + cyclocytidine, 318
daunomycin + cytosine arabinoside, 318
Daunomycin HCl (daunorubicin HCl), 355–364
daunorubicin benzoylhydrazone hydrochloride (zorubicin), 975–978
daunorubicin HCl, 23–24, 355–364. See also liposomal daunorubicin
    administration, 357–358
    admixture, 357
    antitumor activity, 355, 356t
    availability and storage, 357
    cardiotoxicity, 361–362, 362t
    chemistry, 355
    compatibility with other agents, 357, 358t
    dermatologic effects, 361
    dosage, 358, 359t
    drug interactions, 358–359
    extravasation, 111t, 112, 361
        management of, 115t
    flare reaction with, 69t
    gastrointestinal effects, 361
    hepatorenal toxicity, 361
    hypersensitivity reactions with, 68
    indications for, 16t
    mechanism of action, 355–357
    myelosuppression with, 360

Page numbers followed by t and f denote tables and figures, respectively.

pharmacokinetics, 359–360, 360t
preparation, 357
resistance, 11t
  modulation, with trifluoperazine hydrochloride, 930
side effects, 360–362
stability, 357
toxicity, 360–362
as vesicant, 67t
DaunoXome (liposomal daunorubicin), 637–639
DBD (dibromodulcitol), 380–384
dCF (pentostatin), 774–779
DCNU (chlorozotocin), 280–284
DDC (diethyldithiocarbamate), 387–390
o,p'-DDD (mitotane), 726–729
4DDM (idarubicin HCl), 551–558
DDP (cisplatin), 286–298
DDTC (diethyldithiocarbamate), 387–390
  drug interactions, with cisplatin, 292
deacetylvinblastine carboxamide (vindesine), 957–966
deazauridine, 365–367
  administration, 366
  admixture, 365–366
  antitumor activity, 365
  availability and storage, 365
  chemistry, 365
  dosage, 366
  drug interactions, 366
  pharmacokinetics, 366
  preparation, 365–366
  side effects, 366
  stability, 365–366
  toxicity, 366
3-deazauridine (deazauridine), 365–367
Decadron (dexamethasone/dexamethasone phosphate), 32–33, 69t–70t, 303t
Deca-Durabolin (nandrolone decanoate), 192t
dedifferentiation, 7
Delalutin (hydroxyprogesterone caproate), 31–32
Delestrogen (estradiol valerate), 448t
Deletestry (testosterone enanthate), 192t
Delta-Cortef (prednisolone sodium succinate), 303t
Deltasone (prednisone), 32–33, 303t
4-demethoxydaunorubicin (idarubicin HCl), 551–558
4'-demethyl-epipodophyllotoxin 9-(4,6-O-ethylidene-β-D-glucopyranoside) (etoposide), 460–472
Demulen (ethinyl estradiol), 31
2'-deoxycoformycin (pentostatin), 27, 774–779
4'-deoxydox (esorubicin), 439–443

4'-deoxydoxorubicin (esorubicin), 439–443
2'-deoxy-5-fluoruridine (floxuridine), 489–495
β-2'-deoxyguanosine, 222–224
  admixture, 222–223
  antitumor activity, 222
  availability and storage, 222
  chemistry, 222
  dosage, 223
  drug interactions, 223
  mechanism of action, 222
  pharmacokinetics, 223
  preparation, 222–223
  side effects, 223
  stability, 223
  toxicity, 223
2-deoxy-2-(3-methyl-3-nitrosoureido)-D-glucopyranose (streptozocin), 850–856
1-(2-deoxy-β-D-ribofuranosyl)-5-methyluracil (thymidine injection), 905–911
2'-deoxy-5-(trifluoromethyl)uridine (trifluridine), 932–933
Depo-Estradiol (estradiol cypionate), 448t
Depo-Medrol (methylprednisolone aacetate), 303t
Depo-Provera (medroxyprogesterone acetate), 31–32, 171
Depo-Testosterone (testosterone cypionate), 192t
DES (diethylstilbestrol), 9, 31, 446–451, 448t
desacetylvinblastine amide (vindesine), 957–966
dexamethasone, 32–33, 69t–70t, 303t
  chemistry, 302
  combination, with interferon alfa, 573t
  compatibility with other agents, 304t
  dosage, 304–305, 305t
  drug interactions, 305
    with aminoglutethimide, 172t, 172
    with daunorubicin HCl, 358
    with interleukin-1, 592–593
    with interleukin-2, 154t, 155
    with methotrexate, 696t
    with mifepristone, 710
    with nabilone, 741
  indications for, 18t
  mechanism of action, 303
  pharmacokinetics, 306, 306t
dexrazoxane, 367–371
  administration, 368–369
  admixture, 368
  antitumor activity, 367–368
  availability and storage, 368
  cardioprotective effect, 369, 370

chemistry, 367
dosage, 369
drug interactions, 369
mechanism of action, 368
pharmacokinetics, 369, 370t
precautions with, 369
preparation, 368
side effects, 369–370
special applications, 369, 370
stability, 368
toxicity, 369–370
dextran sulfate, drug interactions, with mitomycin-C, 720
5% Dextrose Injection, USP, drug interactions, with diaziquone, 377
dFdC (gemcitabine), 524–526
α-DFMO (eflornithine), 425–431, 713, 714
  drug interactions, with amsacrine, 185
DHAC (dihydro-5-azacytidine), 393–395
DHAD (mitoxantrone hydrochloride), 730–735
DHAQ (mitoxantrone hydrochloride), 730–735
DHE (porfimer sodium), 801–805
diacetoxyscipenol (anguidine), 194–196
2,4-diamino-6-(2,5-dimethoxybenzyl)-5-methyl-pyrido[2,3-d]pyrimidine (piritrexim), 788–791
N-[4-[[(2-diamino-6-pteridinyl)methyl]methylamino]benzoyl]-L-glutamic acid (methotrexate), 692–705
diammine [1,1-cyclobutane-dicarboxylato(2-)-O,O']platinum(II), (SP-4-2) (carboplatin), 259–267
cis-diamminedichloroplatinum(II) (cisplatin), 286–298
Dianabol (methandrosteneolone), 192t
dianhydrogalactitol, 372–375
  admixture, 373
  antitumor activity, 372
  availability and storage, 373
  chemistry, 372
  dosage, 373
  mechanism of action, 373
  pharmacokinetics, 373–374
  preparation, 373
  side effects, 374
  stability, 373
  toxicity, 374
dianhydrogalactitol + carmustine, 372
dianhydrogalactitol + cisplatin, 372
dianhydrogalactitol + doxorubicin + cisplatin, 372
dianhydrogalactitol + etoposide, 372
dianhydrogalactitol + etoposide + triazinate, 372
diarylsulfonylurea (sulofenur), 856–859

diaziquone, 375–380
  administration, 377
    intrathecal, 98, 378–379, 379t
    intraventricular, 378, 378t
  admixture, 376
  antitumor activity, 375–376
  availability and storage, 376
  chemistry, 375
  dosage, 377
  drug interactions, 377
  mechanism of action, 376
  pharmacokinetics, 377–378, 378t
  precautions with, 377
  preparation, 376
  side effects, 378
  special applications, 378–379
  stability, 376
  toxicity, 378
diaziquone + carmustine, 376
6-diazo-5-oxo-L-norleucine, drug interactions, with 6-thioguanine, 895
diazoxide, drug interactions, with octreotide acetate, 752
1,6-dibromo-1,6-dideoxy-galactitol (dibromodulcitol), 380–384
dibromodulcitol, 380–384
  administration, 381
  antitumor activity, 380–381
  availability and storage, 381
  chemistry, 380
  dosage, 381–382
  drug interactions, 381
  mechanism of action, 381
  pharmacokinetics, 382
  precautions with, 381
  side effects, 382–383
  stability, 381
  toxicity, 382–383
DIC (dacarbazine), 343–349
dichlondazolic acid (lonidamine), 650–653
1-(2,4-dichlorobenzyl)-1H-indazole-3-carboxylic acid (lonidamine), 650–653
1,1-dichloro-2-(o-chlorophenyl)-2-(p-chlorophenyl)-ethane (mitotane), 726–729
dichlorodihydroxybis(2-propylamine) platinum(V) (iproplatin), 613–617
2,2'-dichloro-N-methyldiethylamine hydrochloride (mechlorethamine hydrochloride), 657–662
dicoumarol, drug interactions, with mitomycin-C, 720
3',4'-didehydro-4'-deoxy-C5'-norhydrovinblastine (vinorelbine), 966–969

didemnin B, 384–387
  administration, 385
  antitumor activity, 385
  availability and storage, 385
  chemistry, 384–385
  dosage, 385–386
  mechanism of action, 385
  pharmacokinetics, 386
  precautions with, 386
  preparation, 385
  side effects, 386
  special applications, 386
  stability, 385
  toxicity, 386
Didronel (etidronate), in management of hypercalcemia of malignancy, 47–50
dienestrol, 31
  indications for, 17t
8,8-diethyl-N,N-dimethyl-2-aza-8-germaspiro[4.5]decane-2-propanamine dihydrochloride (spirogermanium), 841–844
diethyldithiocarbamate, 387–390
  administration, 389
  antitumor activity, 388
  availability and storage, 389
  chemistry, 387–388
  dosage, 389
  drug interactions, 389
    with cisplatin, 292
  as immunorestorative agent, 388
  mechanism of action, 388–389
  pharmacokinetics, 389–390, 390t
  side effects, 390
  toxicity, 390
diethylmaleate, drug interactions, with 4-ipomeanol, 611
diethylstilbestrol, 9, 31, 446–451, 448t
  antitumor activity, 447
  chemistry, 446–447
  dosage, 448
  indications for, 17t
  mechanism of action, 447
  pharmacokinetics, 449
  side effects, 450
difluorodeoxycytidine (gemcitabine), 524–526
2',2'-difluorodeoxycytidine (gemcitabine), 524–526
α-difluoromethylornithine (eflornithine), 425–431, 713, 714
digitalis glycosides, drug interactions, with doxorubicin, 401t
digitoxin, drug interactions, with aminoglutethimide, 172, 172t
diglycoaldehyde, 391–393

  administration, 392
  admixture, 392
  antitumor activity, 391
  chemistry, 391
  dosage, 392
  for hypercalcemia, 392
  mechanism of action, 5t, 391–392
  pharmacokinetics, 392
  precautions with, 392
  preparation, 392
  side effects, 392
  stability, 392
  toxicity, 392
dihematoporphyrin ether (porfimer sodium), 801–805
dihydro-5-azacytidine, 393–395
  administration, 394
  antitumor activity, 393
  availability and storage, 393
  chemistry, 393
  dosage, 394
  mechanism of action, 393
  pharmacokinetics, 394, 394t
  precautions with, 394
  preparation, 393
  side effects, 394
  special applications, 394
  stability, 393–394
  toxicity, 394
5,6-dihydro-5-azacytidine (dihydro-5-azacytidine), 393–395
dihydrofolate reductase, 10
1-{2-[P-(3,4-dihydro-6-methoxy-2-phenyl-1-naphthyl)phenoxy]ethyl}-pyrrolidine (nafoxidine), 744–745
3,12-dihydro-6-methoxy-3,3,12-trimethyl-7H-pyrano-[2,3-C]acridin-7-one (acronycine), 143–145
dihydropteridine deficiency, leucovorin calcium for, 628
1,5-dihydro-4H-pyrazolo[3,4-d]pyrimidin-4-one (allopurinol sodium), 161–166
dihydroxy-anthracenedione dihydrochloride (mitoxantrone hydrochloride), 730–735
1,4-dihydroxy-5,8-bis[(2-[(2-hydroxyethyl)amino]ethyl)-amino]-9,10-anthracenedione dihydrochloride (mitoxantrone hydrochloride), 730–735
diisopyramide, drug interactions, with BW 502A 502U83·HCl, 252
Dilantin (phenytoin), drug interactions with corticosteroids, 305

Page numbers followed by **t** and **f** denote tables and figures, respectively.

with dacarbazine, 345
with streptozocin, 852
10-dimethylaminomethyl-9-hydroxycamptothecin (topotecan), 914–919
dimethylformamide, 705
dimethylformamide + dactinomycin, drug interactions, with tretinoin, 925t
dimethylsulfoxide
 drug interactions
  with doxorubicin, 401t
  with tretinoin, 925t
 in management of doxorubicin extravasation, 112, 115t
 in management of mitomycin-C extravasation, 113–114, 115t, 722
5-(3,3-dimethyl-1-triazeno)imidazole-4-carboxamide (dacarbazine), 343–349
5-(3,3-dimethyl-1-triazenyl)-1*H*-imidazole-4-carboxamide (dacarbazine), 343–349
diphenhydramine HCl, 69t–70t
2,2-(4-(1,2-diphenyl-1-butenyl)phenoxy)-*N,N*-dimethylethylamine:citrate (1:1) (tamoxifen), 866–875
dipyridamole, drug interactions
 with cisplatin, 289
 with cytarabine, 335
 with doxorubicin, 401t
 with floxuridine, 491
 with 5-fluorouracil, 505
 with paclitaxel, 764
 with PALA, 770
4-dm-DNR (idarubicin HCl), 551–558
4-DMDR (idarubicin HCl), 551–558
DMF (dimethylformamide), 705
DMSO (dimethylsulfoxide)
 in management of doxorubicin extravasation, 112, 115t
 in management of mitomycin-C extravasation, 113–114, 115t
DNA-interactive agents, 15–25, 16t–17t
DNA-intercalating agents, 110–113. *See also specific agent*
 extravasation, 111t
DNA minor groove binder, 17t, 25
DNA strand-breakage agent, 16t, 22
docetaxel (taxotere), 29, 875–878
documentation, 73, 74f–75f, 125–126
 computerized, 126
1-dodecylazacycloheptan-2-one, 429
dopamine HCl, 69t–70t
Doriden (glutethimide), 170
Doriden-Sed (glutethimide), 170
dormastonalone propionate, 192t
dose modifying factors for hematopoietic toxicity, with DNA alkylating agents and ethiofos, 454–455, 455t
DOX (doxorubicin), 395–416
DOXOL (doxorubicinol), 404t, 405
doxorubicin, 23–24, 395–416. *See also liposome encapsulated doxorubicin*
 administration, 398–399
  intraarterial, 408–409
  intraperitoneal, 100, 101–102
  intrapleural, 104, 409
  intravenous, 403–405, 404t
 admixture, 397–398
 antitumor activity, 396
 availability and storage, 397, 397t
 bladder instillation, 409–410
 cardiotoxicity, 407t, 407–408
 cell cycle specificity, 397
 chemistry, 395
 combination, with interferon alfa, 573t
 compatibility with other parenteral agents, 398, 398t
 covalent binding, 396
 DNA binding, 396
 dosage, 399t, 399–400, 400t
 drug interactions, 400–403, 401t–403t
  with amsacrine, 185
  with corticosteroids, 306
  with *Corynebacterium parvum*, 311
  with dexrazoxane, 369, 370
  with dibromodulcitol, 381
  with eflornithine, 427
  with interferon alfa, 572
  with lonidamine, 651
  with paclitaxel, 764
  with razoxane, 826
  with suramin sodium, 862
  with tamoxifen, 869
  with trimetrexate, 935
 ethiofos with, 455
 extravasation, 110–111, 111t
  antidotes to, 111–112
  management of, 115t
  reactions, 406
 flare reaction with, 69t
 free radical formation, 396–397
 hypersensitivity reactions with, 68
 indications for, 16t
 inhibition of topoisomerases I and II, 397
 mechanism of action, 4, 5t, 396–397
 metal complexes, 396
 multidrug resistance induced by, 400
 myelosuppression with, 406
 pharmacokinetics, 403–406, 404t
  and age, 406
  alterations in, 405
  and intraarterial administration, 406
  and intraperitoneal administration, 406
 in obesity, 405
 with repeated doses, 405–406
 precautions with, 400
 preparation, 397–398
 radiosensitization with, 408
 resistance, 11t
  modulation, with trifluoperazine hydrochloride, 930
 side effects, 406–408
 special applications, 408–410
 stability, 397–398, 398t
 toxicity, 406–408
 venous flare reactions, 406–407
 as vesicant, 67t
doxorubicin HCl (doxorubicin), 395–416
doxorubicinol, 404t, 405
Drolban (dormastonalone propionate), 192t
drug dosages. *See also specific agents*
 nurse's knowledge of, 125
drug preparation. *See also specific agents*
 safety precautions in, 124–125
drug resistance, 10t, 10–11
 multiple, 11t, 11–12
DSU (sulofenur), 856–859
DTC (diethyldithiocarbamate), 387–390
DTIC (dacarbazine), 10
 as irritant, 114
DTIC-Dome (dacarbazine), 10, 21–22, 343–349
Durabolin (nandrolone phenylpropionate), 192t
DVA (vindesine), 957–966
4'-DXDX (esorubicin), 439–443

echinomycin, 416–418
 administration, 417, 418t
 availability and storage, 417
 chemistry, 416–417
 dosage, 418, 418t
 mechanism of action, 416–417
 pharmacokinetics, 418
 precautions with, 417
 preparation, 417
 side effects, 418
 stability, 417
 toxicity, 418
ECHO regimen, 461
10-Edam (edatrexate), 419–422
EDAP regimen, 461
edatrexate, 419–422
 administration, 420
 admixture, 420
 antitumor activity, 419–420
 availability and storage, 420
 chemistry, 419

edatrexate (cont.)
  dosage, 420
  drug interactions, 420
  mechanism of action, 420
  pharmacokinetics, 420–421, 421t
  preparation, 420
  side effects, 421–422
  special applications, 422
  stability, 420
  toxicity, 421–422
edelfosine, 423–425
  administration, 424
  antitumor activity, 423
  availability and storage, 423–424
  chemistry, 423
  dosage, 424
  mechanism of action, 423
  preparation, 424
  side effects, 424
  stability, 424
  toxicity, 424
education, of patient and family, 59, 59t
eflornithine, 425–431
  admixture, 427
  anti-infective activity, 426
  antitumor activity, 425–426
  availability and storage, 426–427
  chemistry, 425
  chemopreventive activity, 426
  combination, with interferon alfa, 572–574, 573t
  dosage, 427
  drug interactions, 427, 428t
    with amsacrine, 185
    with doxorubicin, 401t
    with mitoguazone, 713, 714
  mechanism of action, 426
  pharmacokinetics, 427–428, 428t
  preparation, 427
  side effects, 428–429
  special applications, 429
  stability, 427
  toxicity, 428–429
Efudex (5-fluorouracil), 500–515
eldesine (vindesine), 957–966
Elipten (aminoglutethimide), 170–175
Elliott's B solution, 431–433, 694
  administration, 432
  admixture, 432
  availability and storage, 432
  chemistry, 431, 432t
  dosage, 432
  mechanism of action, 431–432
  particulate matter in, 432
  preparation, 432
  stability, 432
  use in oncology, 431–432

Elobromol (dibromodulcitol), 380–384
Elrodorm (glutethimide), 170
Elsamicin (elsamitrucin), 433–434
elsamitrucin, 433–434
  administration, 433
  admixture, 433
  antitumor activity, 433
  availability and storage, 433
  chemistry, 433
  dosage, 433
  mechanism of action, 433
  pharmacokinetics, 433–434
  preparation, 433
  side effects, 434
  stability, 433
  toxicity, 434
Elspar (asparaginase), 34, 201–209
Emcyt (estramustine phosphate), 31, 443–446
emetine
  drug interactions, with azacitidine, 210
  resistance to, 11t
endogenous pyrogen (interleukin-1, alpha and beta), 589–595
Endoxan (cyclophosphamide), 319–332
enflurane, drug interactions, with dactinomycin, 351
EORTC 1502 (prednimustine), 805–808
EPEG (etoposide), 460–472
4'-epidoxorubicin (epirubicin), 434–439
4'-epi-DX (epirubicin), 434–439
epinephrine, 69t–70t
epipodophyllotoxin (etoposide), 460–472
  extravasation, management of, 114, 115t
epirubicin, 434–439
  administration, 436
    intraarterial, 438
    intraperitoneal, 438
    intravesical, 438
  admixture, 436
  antitumor activity, 434–436, 435t
  availability and storage, 436
  chemistry, 434
  combination, with interferon alfa, 573t
  dosage, 436
  drug interactions, with lonidamine, 651
  mechanism of action, 436
  pharmacokinetics, 436–437, 437t
  preparation, 436
  side effects, 437–438
  special applications, 438
  stability, 436
  toxicity, 437–438
  as vesicant, 67t, 112
Ergamisol (levamisole), 28, 634–637

Erwinia asparaginase (asparaginase), 201–209
ESO (esorubicin), 439–443
esorubicin, 439–443
  administration, 440
  admixture, 440
  antitumor activity, 440
  availability and storage, 440
  chemistry, 439–440
  dosage, 440
  mechanism of action, 440
  pharmacokinetics, 441, 441t
  preparation, 440
  side effects, 441–442
  stability, 440
  toxicity, 441–442
  as vesicant, 112
Estinyl (ethinyl estradiol), 446–451, 448t
Estrace (estradiol), 31
Estracyte (estramustine phosphate), 443–446
Estraderm (estradiol), 31
estradiol, 31
  indications for, 17t
estradiol benzoate, 448t
estradiol cypionate, 448t
estradiol valerate, 448t
estramustine phosphate, 443–446
  administration, 444
  antitumor activity, 443
  availability and storage, 444
  chemistry, 443
  dosage, 444
  drug interactions, 444
    with paclitaxel, 764
  mechanism of action, 444
  pharmacokinetics, 445
  precautions with, 444
  preparation, 444
  side effects, 445
  toxicity, 445
Estratest (methyltestosterone), 32
estrogens, 17t, 31, 446–451
  admixture, 447, 448t
  antitumor activity, 447
  availability and storage, 447, 448t
  chemistry, 446–447
  dosage, 448t, 448
  indications for, 29, 31
  mechanism of action, 447
  pharmacokinetics, 448–449
  precautions with, 447
  preparation, 447, 448t
  relative potencies, 448, 449t
  side effects, 449–450
  stability, 447, 448t
  toxicity, 449–450

Page numbers followed by **t** and **f** denote tables and figures, respectively.

etanidazole, 451–453
  administration, 452
  antitumor activity, 451
  availability and storage, 452
  chemistry, 451
  dosage, 452
  drug interactions, 452
  mechanism of action, 451–452
  pharmacokinetics, 452
  precautions with, 452
  preparation, 452
  side effects, 452
  special applications, 452–453
  stability, 452
  toxicity, 452
ethanesulfonic acid compound [Baker's antifol (soluble)], 219–222
ethinyl estradiol (estrogens), 31, 446–451, 448t
  chemistry, 446–447
  dosage, 448
  indications for, 17t
ethiofos, 453–459
  administration, 456
  admixture, 456
  antitumor activity, 454–456
  availability and storage, 456
  chemistry, 453–454
  with DNA alkylating agents, 454–455
  dosage, 457
  drug interactions, 457
  in management of hypercalcemia of malignancy, 50
  mechanism of action, 456
  pharmacokinetics, 457
  with platinum-containing agents, 455, 455t
  precautions with, 456
  preparation, 456
  with radiation therapy, 454, 454t
  side effects, 457–458
  stability, 456
  toxicity, 457–458
ethyl alcohol, drug interactions, with methotrexate, 695
10-ethyl-10-deazaaminopterin (edatrexate), 419–422
ethylidene-lignan P (etoposide), 460–472
7-ethyl-10-[4-(1-piperidino)-1-piperidino]barbonyloxycamptothecin (CPT-11), 314–316
Ethyol (ethiofos), 453–459
etidronate
  in management of hypercalcemia of malignancy, 47–50
  structure of, 47f
ET-18-OCH$_3$ (edelfosine), 423–425

etoposide, 24, 459–472
  administration, 71t, 462–463
    intraperitoneal, 466
    intrapleural, 104, 466–467
    intrathecal, 98
    intravenous, 462–463, 464–465
    oral, 463, 465
  admixture, 462
  antitumor activity, 460–461
  availability and storage, 461–462
  chemistry, 459
  dosage, 463t, 463–464
  drug interactions, 464
    with aclarubicin, 137
    with cisplatin, 289
    with methotrexate, 697t
    with topotecan, 917
  extravasation, management of, 114, 115t
  high-dose, 467
    administration, 467–468
  indications for, 17t
  as irritant, 67t, 110t
  mechanism of action, 5t, 461
  pharmacokinetics, 464–465
  precautions with, 463
  preparation, 462
  resistance to, 11t
  sargramostim with, 830t
  side effects, 465–466
  solutions, utility times for, 462, 462t
  special applications, 466–468
  stability, 462
  toxicity, 465–466
Eulexin (flutamide), 33–34, 518–520
Excalibur introducer needle, 83–84, 84f
expert nursing care, 122
extracellular fluid, in regulation of calcium homeostasis, 35–36, 36f
extravasation. See also specific agents
  of alkylating agents, 113
  causes of, 109
  definition of, 66
  detection of, 66–68
  of DNA-intercalating agents, 110–113
  and drug administration technique, 68
  and education and participation of patient, 67
  incidence of, 66, 109
  with intraosseous infusions, 71
  legal implications for nurses, 125
  and location of vein, 67
  pharmacologic management of, 109–115
  and practitioner's knowledge/skills, 67
  and preexisting venous lines, 67–68
  prevention of, 66–68, 109

  risk factors for, 67, 67t
  of vesicants, 111t

FAA (flavone acetic acid), 485–489
FAC regimen, 396
fadrazole, 472–474
  administration, 473
  antitumor activity, 472–473
  availability and storage, 473
  chemistry, 472
  dosage, 473
  mechanism of action, 473
  pharmacokinetics, 473
  side effects, 473
  toxicity, 473
FAM regimen, 500–501, 718
FAMTX regimen, 501
FAP regimen, 501
F-ara-AMP (fludarabine phosphate), 27
Farmorubicin (epirubicin), 434–439
fazarabine, 474–476
  administration, 475
  admixture, 474–475
  antitumor activity, 474
  availability and storage, 474
  chemistry, 474
  dosage, 475
  mechanism of action, 474
  pharmacokinetics, 475
  preparation, 474–475
  side effects, 475
  stability, 474–475
  toxicity, 475
Fc-1157a (toremifene), 920–922
fenretinide, 476–479
  administration, 477
  antitumor activity, 476
  availability and storage, 477
  chemistry, 476
  dosage, 477
  drug interactions, 477
  mechanism of action, 476
  pharmacokinetics, 477, 477t
  side effects, 477–478
  toxicity, 477–478
FI-7701 (epirubicin), 434–439
filgrastim, 454, 479–484
  administration, 481
  admixture, 481
  availability and storage, 481
  biologic activity, 479
  chemistry, 479–480
  dosage, 481
  drug interactions
    with interleukin-3, 598
    with topotecan, 916–917
    with tretinoin, 925, 925t
  mechanism of action, 480–481

filgrastim (cont.)
  pharmacokinetics, 481–482
  precautions with, 481
  preparation, 481
  side effects, 482
  stability, 481
  toxicity, 482
finasteride, 484–485
  administration, 484
  antitumor activity, 484
  availability and storage, 484
  chemistry, 484
  dosage, 485
  mechanism of action, 484
  pharmacokinetics, 485, 485t
  side effects, 485
  toxicity, 485
FLAMP (fludarabine phosphate), 495–498
flavone acetic acid, 485–489
  administration, 486
  antitumor activity, 486
  availability and storage, 486
  chemistry, 485
  dosage, 486
  drug interactions, 486
  mechanism of action, 486
  pharmacokinetics, 486–487, 487t
  precautions with, 486
  preparation, 486
  side effects, 487
  special applications, 488
  stability, 486
  toxicity, 487
floxuridine, 489–495
  administration, 490–491
    circadian-timed, 493
    intracavitary, 493
    intraventricular, 493
  admixture, 490
  antitumor activity, 489
  availability and storage, 490
  chemistry, 489
  dosage, 491
  drug interactions, 491–492
    with methotrexate, 695, 697t
  indications for, 17t
  as irritant, 110t
  mechanism of action, 489–490
  pharmacokinetics, 492
  preparation, 490
  side effects, 492–493
  special applications, 493
  stability, 490
  toxicity, 492–493
Fludara (fludarabine phosphate), 27, 495–498

fludarabine phosphate, 27, 495–498
  administration, 497
    intraperitoneal, 498
  admixture, 497
  antitumor activity, 496
  availability and storage, 497
  chemistry, 495–496
  dosage, 497
  drug interactions, 497–498
    with pentostatin, 776
  indications for, 17t
  mechanism of action, 496–497
  pharmacokinetics, 498
  precautions with, 497
  preparation, 497
  side effects, 498
  special applications, 498
  stability, 497
  toxicity, 498
flulike syndrome, with aldesleukin, 156–158
2-[1-fluor(anthenylmethyl)amino]-2-methyl-1,3-propanediol (BWA 773U82), 248–251
2-fluoro-Ara-AMP (fludarabine phosphate), 495–498
5-fluoro-2,4(1H,3H)-pyrimidine-dione (5-fluorouracil), 500–515
5-fluoro-1-(tetrahydro-2-furyl)-uracil (tegafur), 878–882
5-fluorouracil, 27–28, 500–515, 634
  administration, 502–503
    circadian rhythm considerations, 502–503
    intraarterial, 509
    intracavitary, 510
    intraperitoneal, 101, 509–510
    intrathecal, 508
    topical, 508–509
  admixture, 501–502
  for anal carcinoma, 501
  antitumor activity, 500–501
  availability and storage, 501
  for bladder cancer, 501
  for breast cancer, 501
  cardiotoxicity, 508
  chemistry, 500
  for colorectal cancer, 500–501
  combination, with interferon alfa, 573t
  for condylomata acuminata, 510
  for corns, 510
  dermatologic effects, 507
  dosage, 503
  drug interactions, 503–505
    with allopurinol sodium, 163
    with dibromodulcitol, 381

    with floxuridine, 491
    with hexamethylene bisacetamide, 532
    with homoharringtonine, 537
    with hydroxyurea, 547
    with interferon alfa, 574–575
    with isotretinoin, 620
    with levamisole, 635
    with methotrexate, 695–696, 697t
    with oxaliplatin, 759
    with PALA, 769–770
    with razoxane, 826
    with tamoxifen, 869
    with thymidine, 907–908
    with trimetrexate, 935
  ethiofos with, 455, 455t
  for gastric cancer, 501
  gastrointestinal effects, 507
  and glaucoma surgery, 510
  for head and neck cancer, 501
  indications for, 17t
  infusions, 502
  intravenous push, 502
  as irritant, 110t
  with leucovorin, 626–627, 628
  mechanism of action, 5t, 501
  myelosuppression, 507
  neurotoxicity, 508
  oral administration, 508
  palmar-plantar erythrodysesthesias, 507
  for pancreatic cancer, 501
  personnel exposure to, 508
  pharmacokinetics, 505–507, 506t
  portal vein infusion, 509
  precautions with, 503
  preparation, 501–502
  for psoriasis, 510
  side effects, 507–508
  special applications, 508–510
  stability, 501–502
  for systemic sclerosis, 510
  toxicity, 507–508
  vein toxicity, 507–508
fluorouracil (5-fluorouracil), 500–515
Fluorouracil Injection (5-fluorouracil), 500–515
5-fluorouracil + semustine, 838
5-fluorouracil + semustine + vincristine, 838
5-fluorouracil + semustine + vincristine + streptozotocin, 838
fluoruropyrimidines, combination, with interferon alfa, 573t
Fluosol, 515–518
  administration, 517
  admixture, 517

antitumor activity, 515–516
availability and storage, 516–517
chemistry, 515
dosage and administration, 517
drug interactions, 517
mechanism of action, 516
pharmacokinetics, 517
preparation, 517
side effects, 517–518
solutions, composition of, 515, 516t
stability, 517
toxicity, 517–518
Fluosol/carbogen breathing, 515–516
Fluosol DA (Fluosol), 515–518
fluoxymesterone, 32, 192t
antitumor activity, 190
chemistry, 189
indications for, 17t
flutamide, 33–34, 518–520
administration, 519
antitumor activity, 518
availability and storage, 519
chemistry, 518
dosage, 519
indications for, 18t
mechanism of action, 518–519
pharmacokinetics, 519
side effects, 519–520
toxicity, 519–520
folate antagonists, 25–27
indications for, 17t
Folex (methotrexate), 692–705
folinic acid (leucovorin calcium), 624–630
(6RS)-folinic acid (leucovorin calcium), 624–630
folinic acid rescue, with methotrexate, 25
folinic acid-SF (leucovorin calcium), 624–630
FOMI regimen, 718
5-formyl-FH$_4$ (leucovorin calcium), 624–630
N^5-formyltetrahydrofolate (leucovorin calcium), 624–630
fosfestrol, 448t
Fourneau 309 (suramin sodium), 859–866
FT-207 (tegafur), 878–882
F3TDR (trifluridine), 932–933
Ftorafur (tegafur), 878–882
5-FU (5-fluorouracil), 500–515
FUDR (floxuridine), 489–495
fumaric acid, drug interactions, with mitomycin-C, 720
Fungizone (amphotericin B), drug interactions, with carmustine, 269
N_1-(2′-furanidyl)-5-fluorouracil (tegafur), 878–882

1-(3-furyl)-4-hydroxy-1-pentanone (4-ipomeanol), 609–613

galactitol (dianhydrogalactitol), 372–375
gallium nitrate, 521–523
administration, 521–522
availability and storage, 521
biologic activity, 521
chemistry, 521
dosage, 522
drug interactions, 522
in management of hypercalcemia of malignancy, 44–47, 51
mechanism of action, 521
pharmacokinetics, 522
precautions with, 522
preparation, 521
side effects, 522
special applications, 522
stability, 521
toxicity, 522
Gammaphos (ethiofos), 453–459
Ganite (gallium nitrate), 521–523
G-CSF (filgrastim), 479–484
gemcitabine, 524–526
administration, 525
antitumor activity, 524
availability and storage, 524
chemistry, 524
dosage, 525
mechanism of action, 524
pharmacokinetics, 525, 525t
preparation, 525
side effects, 525–526
stability, 525
toxicity, 525–526
gene amplification, in drug resistance, 10–11
gentamicin, drug interactions, with doxorubicin, 401t
Germanin (suramin sodium), 859–866
glucocorticosteroids
drug interactions, with interleukin-2, 154t, 155
in management of doxorubicin extravasation, 111–112
in management of hypercalcemia of malignancy, 44, 51
in regulation of bone remodeling, 38t
glutamic acid, drug interactions, with vincristine sulfate, 953
glutethimide, 170
GM-CSF (sargramostim), 829–837
GM-CSF/IL-3 fusion protein (PIXY-321), 794–797
Gompertzian model, of tumor growth, 7–9, 8f

gonadotropin-releasing hormone agonists, 33
goserelin acetate, 33, 527–528
administration, 527–528
admixture, 527
antitumor activity, 527
availability and storage, 527
chemistry, 527
dosage, 528
indications for, 18t
mechanism of action, 527
pharmacokinetics, 528, 528t
preparation, 527
side effects, 528
stability, 527
toxicity, 528
granisetron, 291
granulocyte colony-stimulating factor (filgrastim), 479–484
drug interactions
with isotretinoin, 620
with melphalan, 666
in regulation of bone remodeling, 38
granulocyte-macrophage colony-stimulating factor (sargramostim), 829–837
drug interactions
with interleukin-3, 598
with isotretinoin, 620
in regulation of bone remodeling, 38
Groshong catheter, 82f, 82–83
Groshong three-position valve, 82, 83f
growth factors, drug interactions, with interleukin-1, 592–593
growth fraction, 5

HAD (4-hydroxyandrostenedione), 543–545
Halotestin (fluoxymesterone), 192t
halothane, drug interactions
with cyclophosphamide, 323
with dactinomycin, 351
HCM. See hypercalcemia of malignancy
Henkel's compound (teroxirone), 891–893
heparin
drug interactions, with mitoxantrone hydrochloride, 732
flushing catheters with, 82–83
heparin sodium, drug interactions, with daunorubicin HCl, 358
hepsulfam, 529–531
administration, 530
antitumor activity, 529
availability and storage, 529
chemistry, 529
dosage, 530, 530t
drug interactions, 530

hepsulfam (cont.)
  mechanism of action, 529
  pharmacokinetics, 530, 530t
  precautions with, 530
  preparation, 529
  side effects, 530
  special applications, 531
  stability, 529–530
  toxicity, 530–531
1,7-heptanediol bis-sulfamate (hepsulfam), 529–531
1,7-heptanediol sulfamic acid ester (hepsulfam), 529–531
Hexa-CAF regimen, 166
Hexalen (altretamine), 21–22, 166–170
  administration, 71t
hexamethylene bisacetamide, 531–536
  administration, 532
  admixture, 532
  antitumor activity, 531–532
  availability and storage, 532
  chemistry, 531
  dosage, 532
  drug interactions, 532–533
    with tretinoin, 925t
  mechanism of action, 532
  pharmacokinetics, 532t, 532–533
  preparation, 532
  side effects, 534
  special applications, 534
  stability, 532
  toxicity, 534
N,N'-hexamethylene bisacetamide (hexamethylene bisacetamide), 531–536
hexamethylmelamine (altretamine), 22, 166–170
  administration, 71t
N,N,N',N',N'',N''-hexamethyl-1,3,5-triazine-2,4,6-triamine (altretamine), 166–170
Hickman catheter, 81–82, 82f
HMBA (hexamethylene bisacetamide), 531–536
HMM (altretamine), 166–170
HN2 (mechlorethamine hydrochloride), 9, 657–662
Holoxan (ifosfamide), 20, 558–563
homoharringtonine, 536–540
  administration, 537
  admixture, 537
  antitumor activity, 536–537
  availability and storage, 537
  chemistry, 536
  dosage, 537
  drug interactions, 537
  mechanism of action, 537

  pharmacokinetics, 538
  preparation, 537
  side effects, 538
  special applications, 538
  stability, 537
  toxicity, 538
Honvol (fosfestrol), 448t
hormonal agents, 9, 15, 29–34
  indications for, 17t–18t
  mechanism of action, 29–30
  side effects, 31
4-HPR (fenretinide), 476–479
HU (hydroxyurea), 545–551
Huber-point needle, 86, 87f
human immunodeficiency virus, infection, ampligen activity in, 180
human T-lymphotropic virus type III, suramin sodium's activity against, 859
human urinary colony-stimulating factor (monocyte/macrophage colony-stimulating factor), 735–740
HXM (altretamine), 166–170
hyaluronidase
  in management of epipodophyllotoxin extravasation, 114, 115t
  in management of vinca alkaloid extravasation, 114, 115t
hydrazine sulfate, 540–543
  administration, 541
  antitumor activity, 540–541
  availability and storage, 541
  chemistry, 540
  dosage, 541
  drug interactions, 541–542
  mechanism of action, 541
  pharmacokinetics, 542
  side effects, 542
  toxicity, 542
Hydrea (hydroxyurea), 34, 545–551
hydrocortisone
  chemistry, 302
  dosage, 304–305, 305t
  drug interactions
    with interleukin-2, 154t, 155
    with methotrexate, 696t
  indications for, 18t
  pharmacokinetics, 306, 306t
hydrocortisone + aminoglutethimide, 171
hydrocortisone sodium phosphate, 303t
  compatibility with other agents, 304t
hydrocortisone sodium succinate, 69t–70t, 303t
  compatibility with other agents, 304t
  drug interactions, with methotrexate, 696

Hydrocortone (hydrocortisone sodium phosphate), 303t
Hydroxon (hydroxyprogesterone caproate), 31–32
4-hydroxyandrostenedione, 543–545
  admixture, 544
  antitumor activity, 543
  availability and storage, 544
  chemistry, 543
  dosage, 544
  mechanism of action, 543–544
  pharmacokinetics, 544
  preparation, 544
  side effects, 544–545
  stability, 544
  toxicity, 544–545
4-hydroxyandrost-4-ene-3,17-dione (4-hydroxyandrostenedione), 543–545
hydroxycarbamide (hydroxyurea), 545–551
4-hydroxy-cyclophosphamide, drug interactions, with lonidamine, 651
17β-hydroxy-11β-(4-dimethylaminophenyl)-17α-(1-propynl)estra-4,9-dien-3-one (mifepristone), 708–711
2-[(10-(2-hydroxy-ethoxy)-anthracen-9-ylmethyl)amino]-2-methyl-1,3-propanediol (BW 502), 251–252
N-(2-hydroxyethyl)-2-(2-nitro-1-imidazolyl)-acetamide (etanidazole), 451–453
hydroxyl daunorubicin (doxorubicin), 395–416
N-4-hydroxyphenyl-all-trans-retinamide (fenretinide), 476–479
hydroxyprogesterone caproate (progestins), 31–32, 815–821
  antitumor activity, 815–816
  availability and storage, 817t
  chemistry, 815
  dosage, 817t, 818
  indications for, 18t
  pharmacokinetics, 818
  stability, 817
4-hydroxy-3-β-ribofuranosylpyrazole-5-carboxamide (pyrazofurin), 821–824
hydroxyurea, 34, 545–551
  administration, 71t, 546
  admixture, 546
  antitumor activity, 545–546
  availability and storage, 546
  chemistry, 545
  dosage, 547

Page numbers followed by t and f denote tables and figures, respectively.

drug interactions, 547
  with cytarabine, 335
  with interleukin-1, 593
and drug resistance, 548–549
indications for, 18t
mechanism of action, 5t, 546
pharmacokinetics, 547–548
precautions with, 546–547
preparation, 546
for psoriasis, 548
as radiation sensitizer, 546
for sickle cell anemia, 548
side effects, 548
special applications, 548–549
stability, 546
toxicity, 548
hypercalcemia, with estrogens, 449
hypercalcemia of malignancy, 35–53
  clinical features of, 40t, 40–41
  differential diagnosis, 38, 39t
  hematologic, 39–40
  humoral, 39–40
  iatrogenic factors contributing to, 41
  incidence of, 35
  management of, 41–50
    approaches to, 51
    bisphosphonates in, 47–50
    calcitonin in, 43–44, 51
    diuretic-induced calciuresis in, 43, 51
    ethiofos in, 50
    gallium nitrate in, 44–47, 51
    glucocorticoids in, 44, 51
    loop diuretics in, 42–43, 51
    phosphates in, 50
    plicamycin in, 44, 51
    prostaglandin synthesis inhibitors in, 50
    restoration of extracellular volume in, 42, 51
    saline diuresis in, 42–43, 51
  and osteolytic metastases, 39–40
  pathogenesis of, 38–40
  tumors associated with, 35
hyperparathyroidism, primary, 41
hypersensitivity reactions, 68, 69t–70t
hypotensive agents, drug interactions, with procarbazine, 811, 811t

ibenzmethyzin (procarbazine), 809–814
ICI-46474 (tamoxifen), 866–875
ICRF-159 (razoxane), 825–829
  drug interactions
    with daunorubicin HCl, 359
    with doxorubicin, 401t
ICRF-187 (dexrazoxane), 367–371, 400
  drug interactions
    with daunorubicin HCl, 359

with doxorubicin, 401t
ICRF-925, 369
IDA (idarubicin HCl), 551–558
Idamycin (idarubicin HCl), 23–24, 551–558
idarubicin HCl, 23–24, 551–558
  administration, 553
    intravenous, 553–555, 554t
    oral, 555, 555t
  admixture, 552–553
  antitumor activity, 551–552
  availability and storage, 552
  chemistry, 551
  dosage, 553
  drugs compatible with, 553, 553t
  drugs incompatible with, 553, 553t
  indications for, 17t
  mechanism of action, 552
  pharmacokinetics, 553–555, 554t, 555t
  preparation, 552–553
  side effects, 555–556
  stability, 552–553
  toxicity, 555–556
  as vesicant, 112
IFEX (ifosfamide), 20, 558–563
IFN-β_{ser17} (interferon beta), 582–585
ifosfamide, 20, 558–563
  administration, 559
  admixture, 559
  antitumor activity, 558
  availability and storage, 559
  chemistry, 558
  dosage, 560
  drug interactions, 560–561
    with cisplatin, 289
  indications for, 16t
  local toxicity, 114
  mechanism of action, 558–559
  pharmacokinetics, 561
  precautions with, 559–560, 560t
  preparation, 559
  side effects, 20, 561–562
  stability, 559
  toxicity, 561–562
IL-1α (interleukin-1, beta), 589–595
IL-1β (interleukin-1, beta), 589–595
IL-2. See interleukin-2 or aldesleukin
IL-3 (interleukin-3), 595–601
IL-4 (interleukin-4), 601–605
IL-6 (interleukin-6), 605–609
IMI-28 (epirubicin), 434–439
IMI-30 (idarubicin HCl), 551–558
IMI-58 (esorubicin), 439–443
3,3′-iminobis-1-propanol dimethanesulfonate (ester) hydrochloride (yoshi 864), 973–974
Immunex, 598
implantable ports, 80t, 85–87, 109
  versus catheters, choosing between, 87, 88t

extravasation with. See extravasation
intraperitoneal, 85, 86f
intravenous, 85
OmegaPort-AB intraarterial, 85, 85f
potential complications and problems with, 80t
single- and double-port systems, 85
improsulfan (yoshi 864), 973–974
Imuran (azathioprine), 212–215
Imuthiol (diethyldithiocarbamate), 387–390
N-(5-indanylsulfonyl)-N′-4-(chlorophenyl)urea (sulofenur), 856–859
indomethacin
  combination, with interferon alfa, 574t
  drug interactions
    with interferon alfa, 574
    with interleukin-1, 592–593
    with interleukin-2, 154t, 155
infection, with intraperitoneal chemotherapy, 101
infiltration
  extravasation with, 109–115
informed consent, 119–121
Infusaid 400 internal implanted pump, 88–89, 89f, 90t
  filling, 88, 90t
infusion pumps, implantable, 80t
  external, 89–92
  internal, 88–89
INN (prednimustine), 805–808
inosine dialdehyde (diglycoaldehyde), 391–393
Inox (diglycoaldehyde), 391–393
insulin
  drug interactions
    with doxorubicin, 402t
    with octreotide acetate, 752
    with tamoxifen, 869
  in regulation of bone remodeling, 38t
Interfarm (interferon alfa), 564–582
interferon alfa, 564–582
  administration, 570–571
    intralesional, 570–571
    intraperitoneal, 103, 578
    intrapleural, 578
    intrathecal, 98, 578
    intraventricular, 578
    intravesical, 578
    systemic, 570
  admixture, 569–570
  antitumor activity, 565t, 565–567
  antiviral therapy, 567, 568t, 571t, 571–572
  availability and storage, 569, 570t
  chemistry, 564–565
  for chronic myelogenous leukemia, 565t, 566, 571t, 571–572
  dosage, 571t, 571–572

interferon alfa (*cont.*)
  drug interactions, 572–575, 573t–574t
    with cyclophosphamide, 322t, 323
    with doxorubicin, 400, 402t
    with eflornithine, 427, 428t
    with interleukin-2, 154t, 155
    with isotretinoin, 620
    with tretinoin, 925, 925t
  genes and proteins induced by, 568, 569t
  for hairy cell leukemia, 565t, 565–566, 571t, 571–572
  for hematologic malignancy, 565t, 565–566
  infusion systems, 570
  for Kaposi's sarcoma, 565t, 566, 571t, 571–572
  locoregional applications, 566–567, 567t
  for malignant melanoma, 565t, 566, 571t, 571–572
  mechanism of action, 567–569
  for multiple myeloma, 565t, 566, 571t, 571–572
  for non-Hodgkin's lymphoma, 565t, 566
  pharmacokinetics, 575t, 575–576
  precautions with, 571
  preparation, 569–570
  for renal cell carcinoma, 565t, 566, 571t, 571–572
  side effects, 576–577
  for solid tumors, 565t, 566–567, 571t, 571–572
  special applications, 578
  stability, 569–570
  for topical rhinovirus prophylaxis, 578
  toxicity, 576–577
interferon alfa C (interferon alfa), 564–582
interferon alfa-n3 (interferon alfa), 564–582
interferon beta, 582–585
  administration, intraperitoneal, 103
  admixture, 583
  antitumor activity, 582–583
  availability and storage, 583
  chemistry, 582
  combination, with interferon alfa, 573t
  dosage, 583, 584t
  drug interactions
    with cyclophosphamide, 322t, 323
    with interleukin-2, 154t, 155
  mechanism of action, 583
  pharmacokinetics, 583–584
  precautions with, 583
  preparation, 583
  side effects, 584
  special applications, 584
  stability, 583
  toxicity, 584
interferon-β_2 (interleukin-6), 605–609
interferon-β_{ser17} (interferon beta), 582–585
interferon gamma, 585–589
  administration, 586
    intraperitoneal, 103
    intrapleural, 104
  antitumor activity, 585–586
  availability and storage, 586
  chemistry, 585, 586f
  combination, with interferon alfa, 573t
  dosage, 587, 587t
  drug interactions, 586–587
    with interleukin-2, 154t, 155
    with tretinoin, 925, 925t
  mechanism of action, 586
  pharmacokinetics, 587
  preparation, 586
  side effects, 587
  special applications, 587–588
  stability, 586
  toxicity, 587
interleukin-1
  alpha and beta, 589–595
    administration, 592
    admixture, 592
    antitumor activity, 589–591
      animal studies, 590
      clinical trials, 590–591
      in vitro studies, 589–590
    availability and storage, 592
    chemistry, 589
    dosage, 592
    drug interactions, 592–593
    mechanism of action, 591–592
    pharmacokinetics, 593
    preparation, 592
    side effects, 593
    stability, 592
    toxicity, 593
  drug interactions
    with doxorubicin, 402t
    with interleukin-4, 604
    with isotretinoin, 620
interleukin-2 (aldesleukin), 150–161
  administration, intraperitoneal, 103
  drug interactions
    with dacarbazine, 345
    with interleukin-3, 598
    with interleukin-4, 604
  units, 151
interleukin-3, 595–601
  administration, 597
  admixture, 597
  antitumor activity, 596–597
  availability and storage, 597
  chemistry, 595
  dosage, 597
  drug interactions, 598
  mechanism of action, 595–596
  pharmacokinetics, 598, 598t
  preparation, 597
  side effects, 599
  stability, 597
  toxicity, 599
interleukin-4, 601–605
  administration, 603–604
  admixture, 603
  antitumor activity, 601–602
  availability and storage, 603
  chemistry, 601, 602f
  dosage, 604
  drug interactions, 604
    with isotretinoin, 620
  mechanism of action, 603
  pharmacokinetics, 604
  preparation, 603
  side effects, 604
  stability, 603
  toxicity, 604
interleukin-6, 605–609
  admixture, 607
  administration, 607
  antitumor activity, 605–606
  availability and storage, 607
  chemistry, 605, 606f
  dosage, 607
  mechanism of action, 606–607
  pharmacokinetics, 607–608
  precautions with, 607
  preparation, 607
  side effects, 608
  stability, 607
  toxicity, 608
intraarterial chemotherapy, 73. *See also specific agents*
intraosseous chemotherapy, 70–71. *See also specific agents*
intraperitoneal chemotherapy, 73, 98–103. *See also specific agents*
  combination regimens, 102–103
  with investigational drugs, 103
intrapleural chemotherapy, 103–104. *See also specific agents*
  combination, 103–104
  single-agent, 103–104
Intrasil catheter, 84
intrathecal chemotherapy, 72–73, 95–98. *See also specific agents*
  diluent for, 98

Page numbers followed by **t** and **f** denote tables and figures, respectively.

INDEX 1005

intrathecal injection, 98
20% Intravascular Perfluorochemical Emulsion (Fluosol), 515–518
intravenous chemotherapy, 61–70. *See also specific agents*
    legal implications for nurses in, 123–125
    methods, 61
intraventricular chemotherapy, 72–73. *See also specific agents*
intravesical (bladder) chemotherapy, 73. *See also specific agents*
Intron A (interferon alfa), 98, 564–582
Intropin (dopamine HCl), 69t–70t
iododeoxyuridine, 547
IPO (4-ipomeanol), 609–613
4-ipomeanol, 609–613
    administration, 610
    admixture, 610
    antitumor activity, 609–610
    availability and storage, 610
    chemistry, 609
    dosage, 610
    drug interactions, 610–611
    mechanism of action, 610
    pharmacokinetics, 611
    precautions with, 610
    preparation, 610
    side effects, 611–612
    stability, 610
    toxicity, 611–612
iproplatin, 613–617
    administration, 614
    admixture, 614
    antitumor activity, 613–614
    availability and storage, 614
    chemistry, 613
    dosage, 614
    mechanism of action, 614
    pharmacokinetics, 614–616, 615t
    preparation, 614
    side effects, 616
    stability, 614
    toxicity, 616
irinotecan (CPT-11), 314–316
iron chelators, drug interactions, with doxorubicin, 400, 401t
irritants, 66, 67t, 109, 110t, 114
isophosphamide (ifosfamide), 558–563
N-isopropyl-α-(2-methylhydrazino)-p-toluamide hydrochloride (procarbazine), 809–814
isotretinoin, 617–624
    antitumor activity, 618–619
    availability and storage, 620
    chemistry, 617
    dosage, 620, 621t
    drug interactions, 620
    for leukemia and myelodysplastic syndromes, 618–619

    mechanism of action, 619–620
    pharmacokinetics, 620–621
    precautions with, 620
    side effects, 621–622
    for solid tumors, 619
    toxicity, 621–622
IV infusion, 61, 63
IV piggyback, 61
IV push, 61, 63
IV side-arm, 61, 63, 68, 68t

JB-11 (trimetrexate), 933–939
JM-8 (carboplatin), 259–267
JM-9 (iproplatin), 613–617
JM-83 (oxaliplatin), 758–761

Kenacort (triamcinolone), 303t
3-keto-aphidicolin, 198

labeling index, 5–7
    and chemotherapeutic sensitivity, 12t
LAK. *See* lymphokine-activated killer cells
Landmark catheter, 84, 84f, 85f
LCR (vincristine sulfate), 951–957
LED (liposome encapsulated doxorubicin), 639–644
legal issues, for nurses, in chemotherapy administration, 119–128
Leo 1031 (prednimustine), 805–808
L-leucine, drug interactions, with melphalan, 666
leucovorin calcium, 25, 28, 624–630
    administration, 626
    admixture, 626
    antitumor activity, 624–625
    availability and storage, 625–626
    chemistry, 624
    for dihydropteridine deficiency, 628
    dosage, 626–627
    drug interactions
        with edatrexate, 420
        with floxuridine, 491
        with 5-fluorouracil, 504
    intraarterial, with floxuridine, 628–629
    mechanism of action, 625
    modulation of methotrexate neurotoxicity, 97
    pharmacokinetics, 627–628
    precautions with, 626
    preparation, 626
    side effects, 628
    special applications, 628–629
    stability, 626

Leucovorin Calcium for Injection (leucovorin calcium), 624–630
leucovorin calcium tablets (leucovorin calcium), 624–630
leucovorin rescue, 626–627, 627t
    with methotrexate, 25, 692–693, 699t, 699–700
D-Leu^6-des-Gly^{10}-Pro^9-N-ethyl-LHRH (leuprolide acetate), 630–633
leukemia, meningeal, prevention and treatment of, 95–97
Leukeran (chlorambucil), 20, 71t, 275–279
Leukine (sargramostim), 829–837
    preparation, 832, 832t
leukocyte endogenous mediator (interleukin-1, alpha and beta), 589–595
leukocyte interferon, type I (interferon alfa), 564–582
Leukomax (sargramostim), 829–837
    preparation, 832t, 832–833
leuprolide acetate, 33, 630–633
    administration, 632
    admixture, 632
    antitumor activity, 630–631
    availability and storage, 631–632
    chemistry, 630
    dosage, 632
    indications for, 18t
    mechanism of action, 631
    pharmacokinetics, 632
    preparation, 632
    side effects, 632–633
    stability, 632
    toxicity, 632–633
leuprorelin acetate (leuprolide acetate), 630–633
Leustatin (cladribine), 298–301
levamisole, 28, 634–637
    administration, 635
    admixture, 635
    antitumor activity, 634
    availability and storage, 635
    chemistry, 634
    dosage, 635
    drug interactions, 635
        with ethiofos, 457
    mechanism of action, 634–635
    pharmacokinetics, 636
    precautions with, 635
    preparation, 635
    side effects, 636
    stability, 635
    toxicity, 636
levamisole + 5-fluorouracil, 634, 635–636
levamisole hydrochloride (levamisole), 634–637
Levlen (ethinyl estradiol), 31

LI. *See* labeling index
lidocaine, in management of doxorubicin extravasation, 112
LifeCare PCA Plus II, 90, 92f
Lilly 18947, drug interactions, with cyclophosphamide, 323
Lilly CT-3231 (vindesine), 957–966
Lilly XW 8791-AMX (pyrazofurin), 821–824
liposomal daunorubicin, 637–639
  administration, 638
  admixture, 638
  antitumor activity, 637
  availability and storage, 637–638
  chemistry, 637
  dosage, 638
  pharmacokinetics, 638, 638t
  preparation, 638
  side effects, 638–639
  stability, 638
  toxicity, 638–639
liposomal doxorubicin, as irritant, 110t, 112
liposome encapsulated doxorubicin, 639–644
  administration, 641
  admixture, 641
  antitumor activity, 639–640
  availability and storage, 640–641
  chemistry, 639
  clinical activity, 639–640
  dosage, 641
  mechanism of action, 640
  pharmacokinetics, 641–642, 642t, 643t
  preclinical activity, 639–640
  preparation, 641
  side effects, 642–643
  special applications, 643
  stability, 641
  toxicity, 642–643
Litalir (hydroxyurea), 545–551
lomustine, 20, 644–649
  administration, 71t, 645
  admixture, 645
  antitumor activity, 644–645
  availability and storage, 645
  chemistry, 644
  dosage, 645–646
  drug interactions, 646
  indications for, 16t
  mechanism of action, 645
  for mycosis fungoides, 648
  pharmacokinetics, 646–647, 647t
  preparation, 645
  for psoriasis, 647–648
  side effects, 647
  special applications, 647–648

  stability, 645
  toxicity, 647
lonidamine, 650–653
  administration, 651
  antitumor activity, 650t, 650–651
  availability and storage, 651
  chemistry, 650
  dosage, 651–652
  drug interactions, 651
  mechanism of action, 651
  pharmacokinetics, 652
  side effects, 652
  special applications, 652
  toxicity, 652
Lupron (leuprolide acetate), 33, 630–633
Luteinizing hormone-releasing hormone antagonists, 18t, 33
LY-104208 (vinzolidine), 969–973
LY-109514 (nabilone), 741–744
LY-186641 (sulofenur), 856–859
LY 188011 (gemcitabine), 524–526
lymphocyte-activating factor (interleukin-1, alpha and beta), 589–595
lymphokine-activated killer cells, 151–158
Lysodren (mitotane), 33–34, 726–729
  drug interactions, with corticosteroids, 305

MACOP-B regimen, 396
macrophage colony-stimulating factor, in regulation of bone remodeling, 38
MAID regimen, 830, 830t, 898
Maitansine (maytansine), 654–657
  as vesicant, 67t
malpractice, 123, 125, 127
marijuana, 741
Matulane (procarbazine), 21–22, 809–814
maytansine, 654–657
  administration, 655
  antitumor activity, 654
  availability and storage, 654–655
  chemistry, 654
  dosage, 655
  drug interactions, 655
  mechanism of action, 654
  precautions with, 655
  preparation, 655
  side effects, 655–656
  stability, 655
  toxicity, 655–656
  as vesicant, 67t
M-BACOD regimen, 396, 625, 692

MBBA (cytembena), 341–342
McN-R-1967 (fenretinide), 476–479
MCP regimen, 320
MeCCNU (semustine), 71t, 837–841
mechlorethamine hydrochloride, 9, 20, 657–662
  administration, 658
    intracavitary, 660–661
    intralesional, 661
    topical, 661
  admixture, 658
  antitumor activity, 657
  availability and storage, 658
  chemistry, 657
  dosage, 658–659
  drug interactions, 659
  ethiofos with, 454–455, 455t
  extravasation, 111t, 659
    management of, 113, 115t
  hypersensitivity reactions with, 68
  indications for, 16t
  mechanism of action, 15, 18, 19f, 657–658
  pharmacokinetics, 659
  precautions with, 659
  preparation, 658
  side effects, 659–660
  sodium thiosulfate 1/6 solution, preparation, 659
  special applications, 660–661
  stability, 658
  toxicity, 659–660
  as vesicant, 113
medical adrenalectomy, 33, 171
medical castration, 630
medical records, 125–126. *See also* documentation
medphalan, 663
Medrol (methylprednisolone), 32–33, 303t
medroxyprogesterone acetate (progestins), 31–32, 171, 815–821
  antitumor activity, 815–816
  availability and storage, 817t
  chemistry, 815
  dosage, 817t, 818
  drug interactions, 817
    with aminoglutethimide, 172t, 172
  pharmacokinetics, 818
  side effects, 819
medroxyprogesterone caproate, indications for, 18t
Medtronic pump, 88–89, 90t
Megace (megestrol acetate), 31–32, 815–821
megestrol acetate (progestins), 31–32, 815–821

Page numbers followed by **t** and **f** denote tables and figures, respectively.

antitumor activity, 815–816
availability and storage, 817t
chemistry, 815
dosage, 817t, 818
drug interactions, 817
indications for, 18t
mechanism of action, 816–817
in nutritional support, 816, 816t
pharmacokinetics, 818
side effects, 819
special applications, 819
megestrol acetate + diethylstilbestrol, antitumor activity, 816
melphalan, 20, 662–672
  administration, 71t, 664
    intraperitoneal, 102, 669–670
  admixture, 664
  antitumor activity, 663t, 663–664, 664t
  availability and storage, 664
  with bacillus Calmette-Guérin, 663
  with bone marrow transplantation, 668–669, 669t
  chemistry, 662–663
  with cisplatin, 663t
  combination, with interferon alfa, 574t
  with cyclophosphamide, 663
  with dacarbazine, 663
  dosage, 665
  drug interactions, 665–666
    with lonidamine, 651
    with tamoxifen, 869
  with 5-fluorouracil, 663, 663t
  high-dose, 668–669, 669t
    individualization, test dose for, 669
  hypersensitivity reactions with, 68
  indications for, 16t
  intravenous, pharmacokinetics, 666–667, 667t
  mechanism of action, 664
  with methylmelamine, 663t
  with misonidazole, 663
  oral, pharmacokinetics, 667
  pharmacokinetics, 666–667
  with prednisone, 663, 663t
  preparation, 664
  regional perfusion with, 668
  resistance to, 11t
  side effects, 667–668
  special applications, 668–670
  stability, 664, 665
  toxicity, 667–668
  with vinblastine, 663t
  with vincristine, 663, 663t
menadiol sodium diphosphonate (vitamin K$_2$), drug interactions, with hydrazine sulfate, 542
menadione (vitamin K$_3$), drug interactions
  with doxorubicin, 402t
  with hydrazine sulfate, 541–542

menogaril, 673–677
  administration, 674, 674t
  admixture, 674
  antitumor activity, 673, 673t
  availability and storage, 674
  chemistry, 673
  dosage, 674–676, 675t
  as irritant, 110t
  mechanism of action, 674
  pharmacokinetics, 675t, 676
  preparation, 674
  side effects, 676
  stability, 674
  toxicity, 676
  as vesicant, 112
menogarol (menogaril), 673–677
merbarone, 678–680
  administration, 679
  admixture, 678–679
  antitumor activity, 678
  availability and storage, 678
  chemistry, 678
  dosage, 679
  mechanism of action, 678
  pharmacokinetics, 679
  precautions with, 678–679
  preparation, 678
  side effects, 679
  special applications, 679
  stability, 678
  toxicity, 679
MER-BCG (methanol extraction residue of bacillus Calmette-Guérin), 689–691
2-mercaptoethane-sulfonatic acid sodium salt (mesna), 685–689
6-mercaptopurine, 27, 680–685
  administration, 71t, 681
    intrathecal, 98
  admixture, 681
  antitumor activity, 680
  availability and storage, 680–681
  chemistry, 680
  dosage, 681
  drug interactions, 681–682
    with allopurinol sodium, 162
    with asparaginase, 204, 204t
    with dacarbazine, 345
    with methotrexate, 697t
    with 6-thioguanine, 895
  indications for, 17t
  mechanism of action, 5t, 680
  pharmacokinetics, 682t, 682–683
  preparation, 681
  side effects, 683
  special applications, 683–684
  stability, 681
  toxicity, 683
mercaptopurine (6-mercaptopurine), 680–685

Merck Compound 593A (piperazinedione), 780–782
mesna, 20, 685–689
  administration, 686
  admixture, 686
  antitumor activity, 685
  availability and storage, 686
  chemistry, 685
  dosage, 686
  drug interactions, 686–687
    with cyclophosphamide, 322t, 323
    with ifosfamide, 560
  mechanism of action, 685–686
  pharmacokinetics, 687–688, 688t
  preparation, 686
  side effects, 688
  stability, 686
  toxicity, 688
mesna/ifosfamide, dosage and administration, 686, 687t
Mesnex (mesna), 20, 685–689
metallothionein, drug interactions, with corticosteroids, 305
methandrosteneolone, 192t
methanesulfonate ester, indications for, 16t
methanol extraction residue of bacillus Calmette-Guérin, 689–691
  administration, 690
  antitumor activity, 689–690
  availability and storage, 690
  chemistry, 689
  dosage, 690
  mechanism of action, 690
  side effects, 690–691
  toxicity, 690–691
Methosarb (calusterone), 189, 192t
methotrexate, 25–27, 692–705
  administration, 71t, 694
    intraperitoneal, 99, 102
    intrathecal, 96–97, 701
    intrathecal injection, 98
  admixture, 694
  antitumor activity, 692
  with L-asparaginase, 700
  availability and storage, 693–694
  with carboxypeptidase G, 700–701
  chemistry, 692
  dosage, 694t, 694–695
    in renal insufficiency, 695, 695t
  drug interactions, 695–696, 696t, 697t
    with asparaginase, 204, 204t
    with cisplatin, 289
    with cytarabine, 334–335
    with daunorubicin HCl, 358
    with eflornithine, 427
    with etoposide, 464
    with 5-fluorouracil, 504
    with teniposide, 464, 884
    with thymidine, 907

INDEX

methotrexate (cont.)
  with vinblastine sulfate, 947
  with vincristine sulfate, 953
  with vindesine, 959
  with folinic acid rescue, 25
  high-dose, 693, 699–700
    toxicity, 699–700, 700t
  hypersensitivity reactions with, 68
  indications for, 17t
  with leucovorin rescue, 25, 626–627, 627t, 692–693, 699t, 699–700
  leukoencephalopathy, leucovorin calcium for, 629
  mechanism of action, 4, 5t, 692–693
  neurotoxicity, modulation of, with systemic leucovorin, 97
  for nonmalignant conditions, 692
  pharmacokinetics, 697t, 697–698
  preparation, 694
  for psoriasis, 692
    dosage, 695
  resistance, 693
  side effects, 698–699
  special applications, 699–701
  stability, 694
  with thymidine rescue, 700
  toxicity, 698–699
Methotrexate for Injection (methotrexate), 692–705
Methotrexate LPF (methotrexate), 692–705
Methotrexate Tablets (methotrexate), 692–705
N-[(-methylamino)carbonyl]-N-[[(methylamino)-carbonyl]oxy]acetamide (caracemide), 254–256
2α-methylandrostan-17-β-ol-3-one, 190
methyl-CCNU (semustine), 837–841
3-methylcholanthrene, drug interactions
  with 4-ipomeanol, 611
  with tegafur, 879–880
2α-methyldihydrotestosterone, 190
methylene blue, drug interactions, with doxorubicin, 402t
4,4′-(1-methyl-1,2-ethanediyl)-bis(2,6-piperazinedione) (dexrazoxane), 367–371
4,4′-(1-methyl-1,2-ethanediyl)bis-2,6-piperazinedione (razoxane), 825–829
2,2′-(1-methyl-1,2-ethanediylidene)-bis(hydrazinecarboximidamide) (mitoguazone), 711–717
N-methylformamide, 705–708
  administration, 706

  admixture, 706
  antitumor activity, 705–706
  availability and storage, 706
  chemistry, 705
  dosage, 706–707
  drug interactions, 707
  mechanism of action, 706
  pharmacokinetics, 707
  preparation, 706
  side effects, 707
  stability, 706
  toxicity, 707
methyl-GAG (mitoguazone), 711–717
  as irritant, 67t
3-O-methylglucose, drug interactions, with streptozocin, 852
methylglyoxal bis(guanylhydrazone) (mitoguazone), 711–717
N-methyl-N-[4-[(7-methyl-1H-imidazol[4,5-f]-quinolin-9-yl)amino]phenyl]monohydrochloride (acodazole), 140–143
6-(1-[methyl-4-nitro-1H-imidazol-5-yl)thio]-1H-purine (azathioprine), 212–215
2-methyl-N-[4-nitro-3-(trifluoromethyl)phenyl]propanamide (flutamide), 518–520
7-con-O-methylnogarol (menogaril), 673–677
7-(R)-O-methylnogarol (menogaril), 673–677
10-[3-(4-methylpiperazin-1-yl)propyl]-2-(trifluoromethyl)-10H-phenothizine (trifluoperazine hydrochloride), 930–932
methylprednisolone, 32–33, 303t
  chemistry, 302
  compatibility with other agents, 304t
  dosage, 304–305, 305t
  drug interactions, 306
  indications for, 18t
methylprednisolone acetate, 303t
methylprednisolone sodium succinate, 303t
  drug interactions, with methotrexate, 696
  pharmacokinetics, 306, 306t
N-(2-methyl-2-propyl)-3-oxo-4-aza-5α-androst-1-ene-17β-carboxamide (finasteride), 484–485
methyltestosterone, 32, 192t
  indications for, 17t
Meticortelone (prednisolone sodium succinate), 303t
Meticorten (prednisone), 303t

metoclopramide, 742t
  drug interactions, with vincristine sulfate, 953
metoclopramide + dexamethasone, 291, 741, 742t
metoclopramide + dexamethasone + lorazepam, 291
metoclopramide + lorazepam, 291
metoclopramide + methylprednisolone, 291
Mexate (methotrexate), 692–705
MGBG (mitoguazone), 711–717
microangiopathic hemolytic anemia, mitomycin-C-induced, 721
mifepristone, 708–711
  administration, 710
  antitumor activity, 708–709
  availability and storage, 709
  chemistry, 708
  dosage, 710
  drug interactions, 710
  mechanism of action, 709
  pharmacokinetics, 710
  side effects, 710
  toxicity, 710
MIME regimen, 558, 711
mini-infusion, 61
misonidazole, drug interactions
  with lomustine, 646
  with melphalan, 665–666
Mistabron (mesna), 685–689
Misulban (busulfan), 20
Mithracin (plicamycin), 25, 797–801
mithramycin (plicamycin), 25, 797–801
  in management of hypercalcemia of malignancy, 44, 51
mitoguazone, 711–717
  administration, 713–714
  admixture, 713
  antitumor activity, 711–713, 712t
  availability and storage, 713
  chemistry, 711
  dosage, 714
  drug interactions, 714
    with eflornithine, 427, 428t
  as irritant, 67t
  mechanism of action, 713
  pharmacokinetics, 714
  preparation, 713
  side effects, 714
  special applications, 714
  stability, 713
  toxicity, 714
Mitolac (dibromodulcitol), 380–384
mitolactol (dibromodulcitol), 380–384
mitomycin (mitomycin-C), 717–726

Page numbers followed by **t** and **f** denote tables and figures, respectively.

mitomycin-C, 21, 717–726
  administration, 719
    intraarterial, 722–723
    intraperitoneal, 723
    intrapleural, 104, 723
  admixture, 719
  antitumor activity, 718
  availability and storage, 719
  chemistry, 717–718
  dosage, 719–720
  drug interactions, 720
  ethiofos with, 455, 455t
  extravasation, 111t
    management of, 113–114, 115t, 721–722
  indications for, 16t
  mechanism of action, 718–719
  pharmacokinetics, 720t, 720–721
  precautions with, 720
  preparation, 719
  side effects, 721–722
  special applications, 722–723
  stability, 719
  topical bladder instillation, 722
  toxicity, 721–722
  as vesicant, 67t, 113–114
mitotane, 33–34, 726–729
  administration, 727
  admixture, 727
  antitumor activity, 726–727
  availability and storage, 727
  chemistry, 726
  dosage, 727–728
  drug interactions, 727
    with corticosteroids, 305
  indications for, 18t
  mechanism of action, 727
  pharmacokinetics, 728
  precautions with, 727
  preparation, 727
  side effects, 728
  stability, 727
  toxicity, 728
mitoxantrone hydrochloride, 23–24, 730–735
  administration, 731
    intraperitoneal, 102, 733
    intrapleural, 104, 733
    intrathecal, 733
  admixture, 731
  antitumor activity, 730
  availability and storage, 731
  chemistry, 730
  dosage, 731–732
  drug interactions, 732
    with dexrazoxane, 369
  hepatic artery infusion, 733
  indications for, 17t
  as irritant/vesicant, 110t, 112, 113
  mechanism of action, 730–731

  pharmacokinetics, 732
  preparation, 731
  side effects, 732–733
  special applications, 733
  stability, 731
  toxicity, 732–733
mitramycin (plicamycin), 797–801
MOAD regimen, 692
MOB regimen, 228
monoamine oxidase, inhibition, by procarbazine, 811
monocyte CSF (monocyte/macrophage colony-stimulating factor), 735–740
monocyte/macrophage colony-stimulating factor, 735–740
  administration, 737
  admixture, 737
  antitumor activity, 736–737
  availability and storage, 737
  chemistry, 735–736
  dosage, 737–738
  mechanism of action, 737
  pharmacokinetics, 738, 738t
  preparation, 737
  side effects, 738–739
  stability, 737
  toxicity, 738–739
mononuclear cell factor (interleukin-1, alpha and beta), 589–595
MOPP-BLEO regimen, 228
MOPP regimen, 305, 320, 657, 809, 951
6-MP (6-mercaptopurine), 680–685
MSC-241240 (carboplatin), 259–267
MTX (methotrexate), 692–705
Multi CSF (interleukin-3), 595–601
multidrug resistance. See also P-glycoprotein, overexpression
  with topoisomerase II inhibitors, 24–25
Mustargen (mechlorethamine hydrochloride), 9, 20, 657–662
mutagenic agents, 10
Mutamycin (mitomycin-C), 21, 717–726
MVAC regimen, 287, 788
myeloma, and bone, interactions between, 39, 39f
Myleran (busulfan), 20, 236–241
Mylosar (azacitidine), 209–212
Mytosan (busulfan), 20

N-137 (carbetimer), 257–259
nabilone, 741–744
  antiemetic activity, 741, 742t
  availability and storage, 741
  chemistry, 741
  dosage and administration, 742
  mechanism of action, 741
  pharmacokinetics, 742–743

  precautions with, 742
  side effects, 743
  special applications, 743
  toxicity, 743
nabilone + prochlorperazine, 741, 742t
nafcillin, drug interactions, with amsacrine, 185
Nafidamide (amonafide), 175–180
nafoxidine, 744–745
  administration, 745
  antitumor activity, 744
  availability and storage, 745
  chemistry, 744
  dosage, 745
  mechanism of action, 744–745
  precautions with, 745
  side effects, 745
  stability, 745
  toxicity, 745
Naganol (suramin sodium), 859–866
nandrolone decanoate, 192t
nandrolone phenylpropionate, 192t
Naphuride Sodium (suramin sodium), 859–866
narcotics, drug interactions
  with hexamethylene bisacetamide, 532–533
  with procarbazine, 811, 811t
natural interferon alfa-n2 (interferon alfa), 564–582
Navelbine (vinorelbine), 966–969
NCS (neocarzinostatin), 746–750
NCU-001 (oxaliplatin), 758–761
NDC 4-1935-08 (floxuridine), 489–495
NED-137 (carbetimer), 257–259
neocarzinostatin, 746–750
  administration, 747
  admixture, 747
  antitumor activity, 746
  availability and storage, 747
  chemistry, 746
  dosage, 748
  drug interactions, 748
  hypersensitivity reactions with, 68
  mechanism of action, 746–747
  pharmacokinetics, 748
  precautions with, 747
  preparation, 747
  side effects, 748–749
  stability, 747
  toxicity, 748–749
neocarzinostatin K (neocarzinostatin), 746–750
Neoplatin (cisplatin), 10
Neosar (cyclophosphamide), 20, 319–332
Neupogen (filgrastim), 479–484
neuromuscular blockers, drug interactions, with azathioprine, 214
nicotinamide, drug interactions, with streptozocin, 852

Nigrin (streptonigrin), 847–849
nimodipine, drug interactions, with paclitaxel, 764
nimustine, drug interactions, with 6-thioguanine, 896
Nipent (pentostatin), 27, 774–779
nitrogen mustard (mechlorethamine hydrochloride), 20, 657–662
　extravasation, 111t
　indications for, 16t
　mechanism of action, 15, 18, 19f
nitrosoureas, 20–21
　indications for, 16t
　mechanism of action, 15, 18
　side effects, 21
4′-nitro-3′-trifluoromethylisobutyranilide (flutamide), 518–520
nitrous oxide, drug interactions, with cyclophosphamide, 323
NMF (*N*-methylformamide), 705–708
Nolvadex (tamoxifen), 33–34, 866–875
nonsteroidal anti-inflammatory drugs, drug interactions
　with interleukin-2, 154t
　with suramin sodium, 862
nonvesicant agents, 109, 110t
Novantrone (mitoxantrone hydrochloride), 23–24, 730–735
novobiocin, drug interactions, with amsacrine, 185
NSC-102627 (yoshi 864), 973–974
NSC-102816 (azacitidine), 209–212
NSC-104800 (dibromodulcitol), 380–384
NSC-104801 (cytembena), 341–342
NSC-105014-F (cladribine), 298–301
NSC-109229 (*Escherichia coli*) (asparaginase), 201–209
NSC-10924 (ifosfamide), 558–563
NSC-113891 (mesna), 685–689
NSC-116327 (bacillus Calmette-Guérin), 216–219
NSC-116341 (bacillus Calmette-Guérin), 216–219
NSC-118994 (diglycoaldehyde), 391–393
NSC-119875 (cisplatin), 286–298
NSC-122819 (teniposide), 882–889
NSC-123127 (doxorubicin), 395–416
NSC-125066 (bleomycin sulfate), 227–236
NSC-125973 (paclitaxel), 761–767
NSC-126849 (deazauridine), 365–367
NSC-129943 (razoxane), 825–829
NSC-132313 (dianhydrogalactitol), 372–375
NSC-134087 (prednimustine), 805–808
NSC-135758 (piperazinedione), 780–782
NSC-13875 (altretamine), 166–170

NSC-1390 (allopurinol sodium), 161–166
NSC-139105 (Baker's antifol (soluble)), 219–222
NSC-141537 (anguidine), 194–196
NSC-141540 (etoposide), 460–472
NSC-141549 (amsacrine), 182–189
NSC-141633 (homoharringtonine), 536–540
NSC-143095 (pyrazofurin), 821–824
NSC-143769 (methanol extraction residue of bacillus Calmette-Guérin), 689–691
NSC-145668 (cyclocytidine), 318–319
NSC-148958 (tegafur), 878–882
NSC-150014 (hydrazine sulfate), 540–543
NSC-15200 (gallium nitrate), 521–523
NSC-153353 (alanosine), 148–150
NSC-153858 (maytansine), 654–657
NSC-157365 (neocarzinostatin), 746–750
NSC-163501 (acivicin), 131–134
NSC-164011 (zorubicin), 975–978
NSC-167780 (asaley), 200
NSC-169780 (dexrazoxane), 367–371
NSC-172112 (spiromustine), 844–847
NSC-177023 (levamisole), 634–637
NSC-178248 (chlorozotocin), 280–284
NSC-180973 (tamoxifen), 866–875
NSC-182985 (diaziquone), 375–380
NSC-192965 (spirogermanium), 841–844
NSC-197213 (*Corynebacterium parvum*), 309–314
NSC-19893 (5-fluorouracil), 500–515
NSC-209834 (aclarubicin), 135–140
NSC-21548 (thymidine injection), 905–911
NSC-218321 (pentostatin), 774–779
NSC-220537 (*Corynebacterium parvum*), 309–314
NSC-224131 (PALA), 768–773
NSC-234714 (aphidicolin glycinate), 197–200
NSC-24559 (plicamycin), 797–801
NSC-249008 (trimetrexate), 933–939
NSC-249992 (amsacrine), 182–189
NSC-25154 (pipobroman), 783–784
NSC-253272 (caracemide), 245–256
NSC-256439 (idarubicin HCl), 551–558
NSC-256927 (iproplatin), 613–617
NSC-256942 (epirubicin), 434–439
NSC-26271 (cyclophosphamide), 319–332
NSC-264880 (dihydro-5-azacytidine), 393–395
NSC-266046 (oxaliplatin), 758–761
NSC-267469 (esorubicin), 439–443

NSC-269148 (menogaril), 673–677
NSC-26980 (mitomycin-C), 717–726
NSC-27640 (floxuridine), 489–495
NSC-281272 (fazarabine), 474–476
NSC-286193 (tiazofurin), 911–914
NSC-296934 (teroxirone), 891–893
NSC-296961 (ethiofos), 453–459
NSC-301379 (mitoxantrone hydrochloride), 730–735
NSC-301467 (etanidazole), 451–453
NSC-3051 (*N*-methylformamide), 705–708
NSC-3053 (dactinomycin), 349–354
NSC-305884 (acodazole), 140–143
NSC-3088 (chlorambucil), 275–279
NSC-308847 (amonafide), 175–180
NSC-312887 (fludarabine phosphate), 495–498
NSC-32065 (hydroxyurea), 545–551
NSC-325319 (didemnin B), 384–387
NSC-326231 (buthionine sulfoximine), 241–248
NSC-32946 (mitoguazone), 711–717
NSC-329680 (hepsulfam), 529–531
NSC-336628 (merbarone), 678–680
NSC-337766 (bisantrene hydrochloride), 67t, 224–227
NSC-339004 (chloroquinoxaline sulfonamide), 279–280
NSC-34462 (uracil mustard), 945–946
NSC-347512 (flavone acetic acid), 485–489
NSC-349174 (piroxantrone hydrochloride), 791–794
NSC-349348 (4-ipomeanol), 609–613
NSC-352122 (trimetrexate), 933–939
NSC-35843, 890
NSC-3590 (leucovorin calcium), 624–630
NSC-363812 (ormaplatin), 754–757
NSC-38721 (mitotane), 726–729
NSC-403169 (acronycine), 143–145
NSC-409962 (carmustine), 267–275
NSC-45383 (streptonigrin), 847–849
NSC-45388 (dacarbazine), 343–349
NSC-49842 (vinblastine sulfate), 946–950
NSC-526417 (echinomycin), 416–418
NSC-57155 (terephthalamidine), 889–891
NSC-57198 (dabis maleate), 342–343
NSC-58514 (chromomycin A$_3$), 284–286
NSC-603062 (porfimer sodium), 801–805
NSC-606515 (tumor necrosis factor), 939–945
NSC-609699 (topotecan), 914–919

Page numbers followed by **t** and **f** denote tables and figures, respectively.

NSC-620212 (liposome encapsulated doxorubicin), 639–644
NSC-628503 (taxotere), 875–878
NSC-63878 (cytarabine), 332–340
NSC-6396 (thiotepa), 898–905
NSC-67574 (vincristine sulfate), 951–957
NSC-70735 (nafoxidine), 744–745
NSC-71261 (β-2′-deoxyguanosine), 222–224
NSC-740 (methotrexate), 692–705
NSC-750 (busulfan), 236–241
NSC-755 (6-mercaptopurine), 680–685
NSC-75520 (trifluridine), 932–933
NSC-762 (mechlorethamine hydrochloride), 657–662
NSC-77213 (procarbazine), 809–814
NSC-79037 (lomustine), 644–649
NSC-83142 (daunorubicin HCl), 355–364
NSC-85998 (streptozocin), 850–856
NSC-8806 (melphalan), 662–672
NSC-89199 (estramustine phosphate), 443–446
NSC-95441 (semustine), 837–841
NSC-955580 (hexamethylene bisacetamide), 531–536
NSC #V-7 (Elliott's B solution), 431–433
nurses
  certification, 122–123
  in chemotherapy administration
    legal implications for, 119–128
    professional qualifications for, 57–58
    responsibility for, 57
  continuing education of, 125
  expert care provision by, 122
  in informed consent process, 119–121
  as patient advocates, 121
  professional liability insurance for, 126–127
  supervision of, 121–122
nursing practice, overlap with medical practice, 119, 122

1-O-octadecyl-2-O-methyl-rac-glycero-3-phosphocholine (edelfosine), 423–425
octreotide acetate, 750–754
  administration, 752
  admixture, 752
  antitumor activity, 751
  availability and storage, 752
  chemistry, 750–751
  dosage, 752
  drug interactions, 752
  mechanism of action, 751–752
  pharmacokinetics, 753, 753t
  preparation, 752
  side effects, 753
  stability, 752
  toxicity, 753
4-OHA (4-hydroxyandrostenedione), 543–545
1-OHP (oxaliplatin), 758–761
OK-432, administration, intrapleural, 104
OmegaPort-AB intraarterial port, 85, 85f
OmegaPort-PT intraperitoneal port, 85, 86f
OmegaPort venous access port, 85–86, 87f
7-OMEN (menogaril), 673–677
Ommaya reservoir, 72, 72f, 96, 98
ONCC (Oncology Nursing Certification Corporation), 122–123
oncology nurses. See nurses
Oncology Nursing Certification Corporation, 122–123
Oncology Nursing Society
  Cancer Chemotherapy: Guidelines and Recommendations for Nursing Education and Practice, 125
  guidelines
    for documentation, 126
    for nurses in informed consent process, 120
    for professional qualifications for chemotherapy administration, 57–58
Oncovin (vincristine sulfate), 28–29, 951–957
ondansetron, 291
ONS. See Oncology Nursing Society
orange crush (bisantrene hydrochloride), 224–227
  as vesicant, 67t
OraTestryl (oxymethalone), 192t
Oreton (M) (methyltestosterone), 192t
Oreton (testosterone propionate), 192t
Orimeten (aminoglutethimide), 170–175
ormaplatin, 754–757
  administration, 756
  admixture, 755–756
  antitumor activity, 755
  availability and storage, 755
  chemistry, 754–755
  dosage, 756
  mechanism of action, 755
  pharmacokinetics, 756
  preparation, 755
  side effects, 756
  stability, 755–756
  toxicity, 756
ornithine, drug interactions, with vincristine sulfate, 953
Ortho Dienestrol Cream (dienestrol), 31

osteoblasts, 37–38
  agents that act on, 38t
osteoclast-activating factors, 38
osteoclasts, 36–37, 37f, 38
  agents that act on, 38t
osteon, 36
Osteoport, 71, 71f, 87–88
  advantages of, 88, 88t
ouabain, drug interactions, with doxorubicin, 402t
oxaliplatin, 758–761
  administration, 759
  admixture, 759
  antitumor activity, 758
  availability and storage, 759
  chemistry, 758
  dosage, 759
  drug interactions, 759
  mechanism of action, 758–759
  pharmacokinetics, 759–760
  preparation, 759
  side effects, 760
  stability, 759
  toxicity, 760
oxantrazole hydrochloride (piroxantrone hydrochloride), 791–794
oxipurinol, 163–164
4-oxo-2-phenyl-4H-1-benzopyran-8-acetic acid (flavone acetic acid), 485–489
22-oxovincaleukoblastine (vincristine sulfate), 951–957
oxymethalone, 192t

PA-144 (plicamycin), 797–801
paclitaxel, 29, 761–767
  administration, 763
    intraperitoneal, 766
  admixture, 763
  antitumor activity, 761–762
  availability and storage, 763
  chemistry, 761
  dosage, 764
  drug interactions, 764
  indications for, 17t
  mechanism of action, 762–763
  pharmacokinetics, 764–765, 765t
  precautions with, 763
  preparation, 763
  side effects, 765–766
  special applications, 766
  stability, 763
  toxicity, 765–766
paclitaxel + cisplatin, 762
paclitaxel + cisplatin + filgrastim, 762
paclitaxel + doxorubicin + filgrastim, 762

paclitaxel + filgrastim, 762
PALA, 768–773
　administration, 769, 769t
　admixture, 769
　antitumor activity, 768
　availability and storage, 769
　chemistry, 768
　dosage, 770
　drug interactions, 769–770
　mechanism of action, 768–769
　pharmacokinetics, 770, 770t
　precautions with, 769
　preparation, 769
　for psoriasis, 771
　side effects, 770–771
　special applications, 771
　stability, 769
　toxicity, 770–771, 771t
PALA + thymidine, drug interactions, with 5-fluorouracil, 505, 769
L-PAM (melphalan), 662–672
pamidronate
　in management of hypercalcemia of malignancy, 47–51
　structure of, 47f
Pancretec pump, 90
Paraplatin (carboplatin), 21, 259–267
parathyroid hormone
　in calcium homeostasis, 35–36, 37t
　in regulation of bone remodeling, 38t
parathyroid-related peptide, 38–39
Patient's Bill of Rights, 120
PC-501 (streptonigrin), 847–849
PCNU, drug interactions, with 6-thioguanine, 896
PEG-LA (polyethylene glycol–L-asparaginase), 201, 204, 206
penicillin G, drug interactions, with methotrexate, 696t
pentostatin, 27, 774–779
　administration, 775
　admixture, 775
　antitumor activity, 774
　availability and storage, 775
　chemistry, 774
　conjunctival toxicity, 778
　dosage, 776
　　with renal impairment, 776, 776t
　drug interactions, 776
　　with fludarabine phosphate, 498
　gastrointestinal toxicity, 778
　hematologic toxicity, 777–778
　indications for, 17t
　mechanism of action, 774–775
　neurologic toxicity, 778
　pharmacokinetics, 776–777, 777t
　precautions with, 775–776

　preparation, 775
　renal toxicity, 777
　side effects, 777–778
　skin and itegument toxicity, 778
　stability, 775
　toxicity, 777–778
　　rare effects, 778
pentoxyfylline 1-(5-oxohexyl)-3,7-dimethylxanthine, drug interactions, with tumor necrosis factor, 942
Peptichemio, 663, 663t
percentage labeled mitosis, 5, 6
perhexilene maleate, drug interactions, with daunorubicin HCl, 358
peritonitis, chemical, 101–102
Per-Q-Cath, 83f, 83–84, 84f
P-glycoprotein, overexpression, and multiple drug resistance, 11–12, 12f, 24–25, 358, 819, 920
Pharmorubicin (epirubicin), as vesicant, 67t
phenobarbital, drug interactions
　with amsacrine, 185
　with dacarbazine, 345
　with doxorubicin, 402t
　with ethiofos, 457
　with ifosfamide, 560–561
　with 4-ipomeanol, 611
　with lomustine, 646
　with procarbazine, 811, 811t
　with tegafur, 879–880
phenothiazines, drug interactions
　with BW 502A 502U83·HCl, 252
　with *Corynebacterium parvum*, 311
　with doxorubicin, 402t
　with procarbazine, 811, 811t
phenylalanine mustard (melphalan), 662–672
phenytoin, drug interactions
　with corticosteroids, 305
　with dacarbazine, 345
　with ifosfamide, 560–561
　with methotrexate, 695, 696t
　with procarbazine, 811, 811t
　with streptozocin, 852
　with vinblastine sulfate, 948
phosphates, in management of hypercalcemia of malignancy, 50
1,1'1''-phosphinothioylidynetrisaziridine (thiotepa), 898–905
N-(phosphonoacetyl)-disodium L-aspartic acid (PALA), 505, 768–773
Photofrin (porfimer sodium), 801–805
Photofrin II (porfimer sodium), 801–805
phthalanilides, 889–890

pimozide, drug interactions, with paclitaxel, 764
piperazinedione, 780–782
　administration, 781
　admixture, 780–781
　antitumor activity, 780
　availability and storage, 780
　chemistry, 780
　dosage, 781
　mechanism of action, 780
　pharmacokinetics, 781
　preparation, 780–781
　side effects, 781–782
　stability, 780–781
　toxicity, 781–782
2,5-piperazinedione-3,6-bis(5-chloro-2-piperidyl)-dihydrochloride (piperazinedione), 780–782
piperonyl butoxide, drug interactions, with 4-ipomeanol, 610–611
pipobroman, 783–784
　administration, 783
　antitumor activity, 783
　availability and storage, 783
　chemistry, 783
　dosage, 783
　mechanism of action, 783
　precautions with, 783
　side effects, 783
　toxicity, 783
pirarubicin, 784–787
　administration, 785
　admixture, 785
　antitumor activity, 784–785
　availability and storage, 785
　chemistry, 784
　dosage, 786
　mechanism of action, 785
　pharmacokinetics, 785t, 786, 786t
　precautions with, 785
　preparation, 785
　side effects, 786–787
　stability, 785
　toxicity, 786–787
piritrexim, 788–791
　admixture, 788–789
　antitumor activity, 788
　availability and storage, 788
　chemistry, 788
　dosage, 789t, 789–790
　drug interactions, 789
　mechanism of action, 788
　pharmacokinetics, 789t, 790
　for *Pneumocystis carinii* pneumonia, 790
　preparation, 788–789
　side effects, 790

Page numbers followed by **t** and **f** denote tables and figures, respectively.

special applications, 790
stability, 788–789
toxicity, 790
for toxoplasmosis, 790
piroxantrone hydrochloride, 791–794
administration, 792
admixture, 792
antitumor activity, 791
availability and storage, 792
chemistry, 791
dosage, 792
mechanism of action, 791–792
pharmacokinetics, 792t, 793
preparation, 792
side effects, 793
stability, 792
toxicity, 793
PIXY-321, 598, 794–797
administration, 796
antitumor activity, 795
availability and storage, 796
chemistry, 794–795
dosage, 796
mechanism of action, 795–796
pharmacokinetics, 796, 796t
preparation, 796
side effects, 797
stability, 796
toxicity, 797
plasmacytoma growth factor (interleukin-6), 605–609
Platinol (cisplatin), 10, 21, 286–298
platinum (cisplatin), 286–298
platinum complexes, 21
platinum-vinblastine(velban)-BLEO regimen, 228
plicamycin, 25, 797–801
administration, 799
admixture, 799
antitumor activity, 797–798
availability and storage, 798–799
chemistry, 797, 798
dosage, 799
for hypercalcemia, in Paget's disease, 800
indications for, 17t
as irritant, 67t
in management of hypercalcemia of malignancy, 44, 51
mechanism of action, 798
pharmacokinetics, 799
precautions with, 799
preparation, 799
side effects, 799–800
special applications, 800
stability, 799
toxicity, 799–800
PLM. See percentage labeled mitosis
PM 259 (vinorelbine), 966–969
podophyllotoxins, 5t

resistance to, 11t
point mutation, in drug resistance, 10–11
polima (carbetimer), 257–259
polyethylene glycol-L-asparaginase, 201, 204, 206
polymixin B, drug interactions, with 5-fluorouracil, 504
polysorbate 80, drug interactions, with doxorubicin, 402t
POMP regimen, 680
porfimer sodium, 801–805
administration, 803
admixture, 803
antitumor activity, 802
availability and storage, 803
chemistry, 801–802
dosage, 803
mechanism of action, 802–803
pharmacokinetics, 803–804
precautions with, 803
preparation, 803
side effects, 804
stability, 803
toxicity, 804
Port-A-Cath, 100–101
ports. See implantable ports
prednimustine, 805–808
administration, 807
antitumor activity, 806
availability and storage, 806
chemistry, 805–806
dosage, 807
mechanism of action, 806
pharmacokinetics, 807
side effects, 807–808
toxicity, 807–808
prednisolone, 32–33
chemistry, 302
drug interactions, with methotrexate, 696t
indications for, 18t
pharmacokinetics, 306, 306t
prednisolone sodium succinate, 303t
prednisone, 32–33, 303t
chemistry, 302
combination, with interferon alfa, 574t
dosage, 304–305, 305t
drug interactions
with asparaginase, 204, 204t
with interferon alfa, 574
with methotrexate, 696t
with mifepristone, 710
indications for, 18t
mechanism of action, 5t
pharmacokinetics, 306, 306t
Premarin (estrogens), 446–451, 448t
dosage, 448
prenylamine, drug interactions, with doxorubicin, 402t
probenecid, drug interactions

with cisplatin, 289
with methotrexate, 695, 696t
procainamide, drug interactions, with BW 502A 502U83·HCl, 252
procarbazine, 21–22, 809–814
administration, 71t, 810
admixture, 810
antitumor activity, 809
availability and storage, 810
chemistry, 809
dosage, 810–811
drug interactions, 811, 811t
indications for, 16t
mechanism of action, 5t, 809–810
pharmacokinetics, 812
preparation, 810
side effects, 812–813
stability, 810
toxicity, 812–813
prochlorperazine, 742t
drug interactions, with doxorubicin, 402t
prochlorperazine + dexamethasone + lorazepam, 291
Pro-Depo (hydroxyprogesterone caproate), 31–32
Prodox 250 (hydroxyprogesterone caproate), 815–821
professional liability insurance, for nurses, 126–127
progestins, 18t, 31–32, 815–821
administration, 817
antitumor activity, 815–816
availability and storage, 817t
dosage, 817t, 818
drug interactions, 817
indications for, 29
mechanism of action, 816–817
pharmacokinetics, 818
precautions with, 817
preparation, 817
side effects, 819
special applications, 819
stability, 817
toxicity, 819
Progynon B (estradiol benzoate), 448t
Prokine (sargramostim), 829–837
preparation, 832, 832t
Proleukin (aldesleukin), 150–161
ProMACE/MOPP regimen, 460–461
ProMACE regimen, 692
propranolol, drug interactions, with doxorubicin, 402t
Proscar (finasteride), 484–485
prostaglandin synthesis inhibitors, in management of hypercalcemia of malignancy, 50
Provera (medroxyprogesterone), 31–32
Provera (medroxyprogesterone acetate), 171, 815–821

PRZF (pyrazofurin), 821–824
PTHrP. *See* parathyroid-related peptide
PTX (piritrexim), 788–791
pumps. *See* infusion pumps
purine antagonists, 27
    indications for, 17t
Purinethol (6-mercaptopurine), 27, 680–685
puromycin, resistance to, 11t
PVB regimen, 540
pyrazofurin, 821–824
    administration, 823
    admixture, 822–823
    antitumor activity, 822
    availability and storage, 822
    chemistry, 821–822
    dosage, 823
    drug interactions, 823
    mechanism of action, 822
    pharmacokinetics, 823
    preparation, 822–823
    side effects, 823–824
    stability, 822–823
    toxicity, 823–824
    as vesicant, 67t
Pyrazomycin (pyrazofurin), 821–824
    as vesicant, 67t
pyrimidine antagonists, 27–28
    indications for, 17t
2,4-(1*H*,3*H*)-pyrimidinedione (thymidine injection), 905–911
pyrophosphates, 47, 47f
pyrrolidine (nafoxidine), 744–745

Q-Port, 86, 87f
quinidine, drug interactions
    with BW 502A 502U83·HCl, 252
    with paclitaxel, 764
quinine, drug interactions, with paclitaxel, 764
Quinomycin A (echinomycin), 416–418

R 12564 (levamisole), 634–637
radiation recall, 408
radioresistance, with ethiofos therapy, 454, 454t
ranitidine, drug interactions
    with cyclophosphamide, 322t, 323
    with doxorubicin, 400, 402t
razoxane, 825–829
    antitumor activity, 825
    availability and storage, 826

chemistry, 825
dosage, 826
drug interactions, 826
mechanism of action, 825
pharmacokinetics, 826–827
precautions with, 826
for psoriasis, 827
as radiation sensitizer, 827
side effects, 827
special applications, 827
toxicity, 827
RB-1670 (oxaliplatin), 758–761
recombinant gamma interferon (interferon gamma), 585–589
recombinant human interferon alfa-2a (interferon alfa), 564–582
recombinant human interferon alfa-2b (interferon alfa), 564–582
recombinant human interferon beta (interferon beta), 582–585
recombinant human macrophage colony-stimulating factor (monocyte/macrophage colony-stimulating factor), 735–740
recombinant methionyl human granulocyte colony-stimulating factor (filgrastim), 479–484
recombinant tumor necrosis factor (tumor necrosis factor), 939–945
regional drug delivery, 72–73
Reglan (metoclopramide), drug interactions, with vincristine sulfate, 953
respondeat superior, 121
Retin-A (tretinoin), 922–930
13-*cis*-retinoic acid (isotretinoin), 617–624
retinoic acid response elements, 923–924
retinoic acid syndrome, 927
rGIFN (interferon gamma), 585–589
Rheumatrex (methotrexate), 692–705
rhGM-CSF, drug interactions, with cytarabine, 335
rhM-CSF (monocyte/macrophage colony-stimulating factor), 735–740
rhTNF (recombinant human tumor necrosis factor), 939–945
rhuIL3 (interleukin-3), 595–601
1-β-D-ribofuranosyl-2,4(1*H*,3*H*)-pyridinedione (deazauridine), 365–367
2-β-D-ribofuranosylthiazole-4-carboxamide (tiazofurin), 911–914
riboxamide (tiazofurin), 911–914
ricin, drug interactions, with doxorubicin, 402t
Rimso-50 (dimethylsulfoxide), 110–113

$rI_n \cdot r(C_{12}, U)_n$ (ampligen), 180–182
risendronate, 47
r-metHuG-CSF. *See* filgrastim
RMI 71782A (eflornithine), 425–431
RNA, mismatched double-stranded (ampligen), 180–182
Ro 1-5488 (tretinoin), 922–930
Ro 4-3780 (isotretinoin), 617–624
Ro 5-0360 (floxuridine), 489–495
ROAP regimen, 975
Roferon-A (interferon alfa), 98, 564–582
RP 22050 (zorubicin), 975–978
RP-54780 (oxaliplatin), 758–761
RP-56076 (taxotere), 875–878
RU-486 (mifepristone), 708–711
RU-38486 (mifepristone), 708–711
Rubex (doxorubicin), 395–416
Rubidazone (zorubicin), 975–978
rubidomycin HCl (daunorubicin HCl), 355–364
rufocromomycin (streptonigrin), 847–849

salicylates, drug interactions, with methotrexate, 695, 696t
Sandostatin (octreotide acetate), 750–754
L-sarcolysine (melphalan), 662–672
sargramostim, 829–837
    administration, 833
    admixture, 832–833
    antitumor activity, 830t, 830–831
    in aplastic anemia, 831
    availability and storage, 832
    with bone marrow transplantation and high-dose chemotherapy, 830
    chemistry, 829–830
    dosage, 833, 833t
    drug interactions, 833–834
        with thiotepa, 900
        with tretinoin, 925, 925t
    effects on tumor cells, 831
    mechanism of action, 831–832
    in myelodysplasia, 830
    and neutropenia of standard chemotherapy, 830
    pharmacokinetics, 834, 834t
    preparation, 832–833
    side effects, 834–835
    stability, 832–833
    toxicity, 834–835
SDZ IL-E964 (interleukin-3), 595–601
semustine, 837–841
    administration, 71t, 839

Page numbers followed by **t** and **f** denote tables and figures, respectively.

admixture, 839
antitumor activity, 837–838
availability and storage, 839
chemistry, 837
dosage, 839
mechanism of action, 838–839
pharmacokinetics, 839–840
precautions with, 839
preparation, 839
side effects, 840
stability, 839
toxicity, 840
SG (spirogermanium), 841–844
side effects, of chemotherapy. *See also specific agents*
mechanism of, 6
SKF-525, drug interactions, with tegafur, 880
SKF 104864 (topotecan), 914–919
SKF-525A, drug interactions
with cyclophosphamide, 323
with lomustine, 646
SMANCS, 749
SMS 201-995 (octreotide acetate), 750–754
social support, of patient, 59
sodium bicarbonate, in management of doxorubicin extravasation, 112
sodium bromebrate (cytembena), 341–342
sodium camptothecin, 915
sodium 2-mercaptoethanesulfonate (mesna), 20
sodium methotrexate (methotrexate), 692–705
sodium thiosulfate
as antidote
to cisplatin extravasation, 113
to mechlorethamine extravasation, 113
drug interactions, with cisplatin, 292
modulation of cisplatin nephrotoxicity, 103
Solu-Cortef (hydrocortisone sodium succinate), 69t–70t, 303t
Solu-Medrol (methylprednisolone sodium succinate), 303t
somatostatin, pharmacokinetics, 753, 753t
spirogermanium, 841–844
administration, 842
admixture, 842
as antiparasitic agent, 843
antitumor activity, 842
availability and storage, 842
chemistry, 841
dosage, 842
mechanism of action, 842
pharmacokinetics, 842–843

precautions with, 842
preparation, 842
for rheumatoid arthritis, 843
side effects, 843
special applications, 843
stability, 842
toxicity, 843
spirogermanium HCl (spirogermanium), 841–844
spirohydantoin mustard (spiromustine), 844–847
spiromustine, 844–847
administration, 845
admixture, 845
antitumor activity, 845
availability and storage, 845
chemistry, 844–845
dosage, 846, 846t
mechanism of action, 845
pharmacokinetics, 846, 846t
precautions with, 845
preparation, 845
side effects, 846–847
stability, 845
toxicity, 846–847
SR 2508 (etanidazole), 451–453
standards of care, 123–124
stanozolol, 192t
chemistry, 189
stathmokinetic effect, 959
Stelazine (trifluoperazine hydrochloride), 930–932
stem cell concept, applied to tumors, 7, 8f
stem cells, and susceptibility to chemotherapy, 6
Stereocyt (prednimustine), 805–808
steroid hormones
action, 30, 30f
receptors, 30
steroid psychosis, 32
steroid rage, 32
Stilbestrol (diethylstilbestrol), 9, 31
Stilphostrol (fosfestrol), 448t
streptonigrin, 847–849
administration, 848
intraarterial, 849
admixture, 848
antitumor activity, 847–848
availability and storage, 848
chemistry, 847
dosage, 848
mechanism of action, 848
precautions with, 848
preparation, 848
side effects, 848–849
special applications, 849
stability, 848
toxicity, 848–849
streptozocin, 20–21, 850–856

administration, 851–852
intraarterial, 854
intraperitoneal, 854
admixture, 851
antitumor activity, 850t, 850–851
availability and storage, 851
chemistry, 850
continuous intravenous infusion, 853–854
dosage, 852
drug interactions, 852
indications for, 16t
as irritant, 67t
mechanism of action, 851
pharmacokinetics, 852
precautions with, 852
preparation, 851
side effects, 852–853
special applications, 853–854
stability, 851
toxicity, 852–853
streptozotocin (streptozocin), 20, 850–856
drug interactions, with doxorubicin, 400, 402t
succinylcholine, drug interactions
with azathioprine, 214
with cyclophosphamide, 322t, 323
with thiotepa, 900
sulfadiazine, drug interactions, with trimetrexate, 935
sulfamin (hepsulfam), 529–531
sulfasoxazole, drug interactions, with methotrexate, 696t
sulfonylureas, drug interactions, with octreotide acetate, 752
sulofenur, 856–859
administration, 857
antitumor activity, 856–857
availability and storage, 857
chemistry, 856
dosage, 857
drug interactions, 857
mechanism of action, 857
pharmacokinetics, 857–858, 858t
precautions with, 857
preparation, 857
side effects, 858
stability, 857
toxicity, 858
support, of patient and family, 60
suramin sodium, 859–866
administration, 861
admixture, 861
antitumor activity, 859–860
availability and storage, 861
chemistry, 859
dosage, 861–862, 862t
drug interactions, 862
mechanism of action, 860–861

suramin sodium (cont.)
  pharmacokinetics, 862–863, 863t
  precautions with, 861
  preparation, 861
  side effects, 863–864
  stability, 861
  toxicity, 863–864
symetamine (terephthalamidine), 889–891
sympathomimetics, drug interactions, with procarbazine, 811, 811t
SZN (streptozocin), 850–856

Tabloid brand thioguanine (6-thioguanine), 893–898
TACE (chlorotrianisene), 31, 446–451, 448t
  chemistry, 446–447
Tagamet (cimetidine), drug interactions, with carmustine, 269
Tam (tamoxifen), 866–875
tamoxifen, 33–34, 447, 866–875
  antitumor activity, 866–868, 867t
  availability and storage, 868–869
  chemistry, 866
  dosage, 869
  drug interactions, 869–870
    with aminoglutethimide, 172, 172t
    with mifepristone, 710
    with suramin sodium, 862
  indications for, 18t
  mechanism of action, 868
  metabolites, hormonal activity of, 870t, 870–871
  pharmacokinetics, 870t, 870–871
  precautions with, 869
  side effects, 871–872
  toxicity, 871–872
TAP-144 (leuprolide acetate), 630–633
Taxol (paclitaxel), 29, 761–767
  administration, intraperitoneal, 103
  drug interactions, 876
taxotere (docetaxel), 29, 875–878
  administration, 876
  admixture, 876
  antitumor activity, 875
  availability and storage, 876
  chemistry, 875
  dosage, 876
  drug interactions, 876
  mechanism of action, 875–876
  pharmacokinetics, 876, 877t
  precautions with, 876
  preparation, 876
  side effects, 876–877

  stability, 876
  toxicity, 876–877
TCAR (tiazofurin), 911–914
T-cell growth factor (aldesleukin), 150–161
TdR (thymidine injection), 905–911
Teceleukin (interleukin-2), 150–161
tegafur, 878–882
  administration, 879
  admixture, 879
  antitumor activity, 878, 878t
  availability and storage, 879
  dosage, 879
  drug interactions, 880
  mechanism of action, 879
  pharmacokinetics, 880
  preparation, 879
  side effects, 881
  stability, 879
  toxicity, 880–881
tegafur + doxorubicin + carmustine, 878, 878t
tegafur + doxorubicin + mitomycin-C + carmustine, 878, 878t
tegafur + mitomycin-C + semustine, 878, 878t
Tegretol (carbamazepine), drug interactions, with mitoguazone, 714
Tenckhoff intraperitoneal catheter, 85, 85f, 100
teniposide, 882–889
  administration, 884
    intrapericardial, 887
    intravesicular, 886–887
  admixture, 884
  antitumor activity, 883, 883t
  availability and storage, 883
  chemistry, 882
  dosage, 884
  drug interactions, 884
    with methotrexate, 697t
  extravasation, management of, 114, 115t
  hypersensitivity reactions with, 68
  indications for, 17t
  as irritant, 67t, 110t
  mechanism of action, 5t, 883
  pharmacokinetics, 884–885, 885t
  preparation, 884
  side effects, 885–886
  special applications, 886–887
  stability, 884
  toxicity, 885–886
teniposide + cytarabine, 883, 883t
teniposide + methotrexate, 883, 883t
terephthalamidine, 889–891
  administration, 890

  admixture, 890
  antitumor activity, 890
  availability and storage, 890
  chemistry, 889–890
  dosage, 890
  mechanism of action, 890
  pharmacokinetics, 891
  precautions with, 890
  preparation, 890
  side effects, 891
  stability, 890
  toxicity, 891
terephthalamidine derivative (terephthalamidine), 889–891
teroxirone, 891–893
  administration, 892
  admixture, 892
  antitumor activity, 891–892
  availability and storage, 892
  chemistry, 891
  dosage, 892
  mechanism of action, 892
  pharmacokinetics, 892t, 892–893
  preparation, 892
  side effects, 893
  stability, 892
  toxicity, 893
Teslac (testolactone), 192t
TESPA (thiotepa), 898–905
testolactone, 192t
  antitumor activity, 190
  chemistry, 189
testosterone
  chemistry, 189
  indications for, 17t
  pharmacokinetics, 191
testosterone cypionate, 32, 192t
testosterone enanthate, 32, 192t
testosterone propionate, 32, 192t
  chemistry, 189–190
Testred (methyltestosterone), 32
tetrachloro (d,l-trans)-1,2-diaminocyclohexane platinum(IV) (ormaplatin), 754–757
tetracycline, drug interactions, with methotrexate, 696t
tetrahydrocannabinol, 741
4-[5,6,7,8-tetrahydroimidazo[1,5α]-pyridin-5-yl]benzonitrile monohydrochloride (fadrazole), 472–474
(−)-(S)-2,3,5,6-tetrahydro-6-phenylimidazo[2,1-b]thiazole monohydrochloride (levamisole), 634–637
(2″R)-4′-O-tetrahydropyranyl doxorubicin (pirarubicin), 784–787

Page numbers followed by **t** and **f** denote tables and figures, respectively.

tetraplatin (ormaplatin), 754–757
6-TG (thioguanine), 893–898
βTGdr (β-2'-deoxyguanosine), 222–224
α-TGI (teroxirone), 891–893
THC (tetrahydrocannabinol), 741
thenylidene-Liganan P (teniposide), 882–889
theophylline, drug interactions
   with allopurinol sodium, 163
   with aminoglutethimide, 172, 172t
   with carmustine, 269
TheraCys (bacillus Calmette-Guérin), 216–219
Therex 3000 internal implanted pump, 88–89, 89f, 90t
   filling, 88, 91t
Thioguanine, 27, 893–898
   administration, 71t, 894–895
      intraperitoneal, 896–897
   admixture, 894
   antitumor activity, 893–894
   availability and storage, 894
   chemistry, 893
   dosage, 895
   drug interactions, 895–896
      with mitomycin-C, 720
      with trimetrexate, 935
   indications for, 17t
   mechanism of action, 5t, 894
   pharmacokinetics, 895, 895t
   preparation, 894
   side effects, 896
   special applications, 896–897
   stability, 894
   toxicity, 896
thiophosphoramide, 20
   intrathecal administration, 97, 98
thiotepa, 898–905
   administration, 899t, 899–900
      with bone marrow transplant, 902–903
      intracavitary, locally adminsitered, 902
      intraperitoneal, 903
      intrathecal, 96, 903
      intravesical, 899t, 900, 902
   admixture, 899
   antitumor activity, 898
   availability and storage, 899
   chemistry, 898
   dosage, 899t, 900
   drug interactions, 900
   indications for, 16t
   mechanism of action, 898–899
   pharmacokinetics, 900–901, 901t
   preparation, 899
   side effects, 901–902
   special applications, 902–903
   stability, 899
   toxicity, 901–902

Thio-Tepa (thiotepa), 898–905
thio-TEPA (thiotepa), 898–905
Thorazine (chlorpromazine), drug interactions, with bleomycin sulfate, 230
THP-Adriamycin (pirarubicin), 784–787
thymidine
   drug interactions
      with carboplatin, 262
      with cytarabine, 335
      with floxuridine, 491
      with 5-fluorouracil, 504
      with interferon alfa, 574
      with methotrexate, 696t
      with PALA, 505, 769
   hepatic artery infusion, 909
   tritiated, incorporation, in assay of cell cycle times, 5
thymidine injection, 905–911
   administration, 907
   admixture, 907
   antitumor activity, 906
   availability and storage, 907
   chemistry, 905–906
   dosage, 908, 908t
   drug interactions, 907–908
   mechanism of action, 906–907
   pharmacokinetics, 908t, 908–909
   preparation, 907
   side effects, 909
   special applications, 909
   stability, 907
   toxicity, 909
thymidine rescue, with methotrexate, 700
thyroxine, in regulation of bone remodeling, 38t
tiapamil, drug interactions, with daunorubicin HCl, 358
tiazofurin, 911–914
   administration, 912
   admixture, 912
   antitumor activity, 911
   availability and storage, 912
   chemistry, 911
   dosage, 912
   drug interactions, 912
      with tretinoin, 925t
   mechanism of action, 912
   pharmacokinetics, 912, 913t
   precautions with, 912
   preparation, 912
   side effects, 912–913
   special applications, 913
   stability, 912
   toxicity, 912–913
Tice BCG (bacillus Calmette-Guérin), 216–219
TLC-D99 (liposome encapsulated doxorubicin), 639–644

TMQ (trimetrexate), 933–939
TMTX (trimetrexate), 933–939
TNF (tumor necrosis factor), 939–945
tolbutamide, drug interactions, with methotrexate, 696t
topical cooling, in management of doxorubicin extravasation, 112, 115t
topoisomerase II inhibitors, 16t–17t, 22–24
   intercalating, 23–24
   mechanism of action, 22–23
   multidrug resistance with, 24–25
   nonintercalating, 23–24
topotecan, 914–919
   administration, 916
   admixture, 916
   antitumor activity, 915
   availability and storage, 916
   chemistry, 914–915
   dosage, 917, 917t
   drug interactions, 916–917
   mechanism of action, 915–916
   pharmacokinetics, 917
   precautions with, 916
   preparation, 916
   side effects, 917–918
   special applications, 919
   stability, 916
   toxicity, 917–918
toremifene, 920–922
   administration, 920
   admixture, 920
   antitumor activity, 920
   availability and storage, 920
   chemistry, 920
   drug interactions, 920–921
      with doxorubicin, 403
   mechanism of action, 920
   pharmacokinetics, 921, 921t
   preparation, 920
   side effects, 921
   stability, 920
   toxicity, 921
toxicity, of chemotherapy, mechanism of, 6
Toyomycin (chromomycin A$_3$), 284–286
tRA (tretinoin), 922–930
Trental (pentoxyfylline 1-(5-oxohexyl)-3,7-dimethylxanthine), drug interactions, with tumor necrosis factor, 942
tretinoin, 922–930
   administration, 924
   antitumor activity, 922–923, 923t
   availability and storage, 924
   chemistry, 922
   dosage, 924–925
   drug interactions, 925, 925t
   mechanism of action, 923–924

tretinoin (cont.)
  pharmacokinetics, 925–926
  side effects, 926–927
  toxicity, 926–927
triamcinolone, 303t
  chemistry, 302
triazinate [Baker's antifol (soluble)], 219–222
triazinetrione triepoxide (teroxirone), 891–893
tricyclic antidepressants, drug interactions
  with BW 502A 502U83·HCl, 252
  with procarbazine, 811, 811t
triethylenemelamine, 166
  chemistry, 166
triethylene-thiophosphoramide (thiotepa), 20, 898–905
trifluoperazine hydrochloride, 930–932
  administration, 931
  availability and storage, 931
  chemistry, 930
  drug interactions, 931
    with doxorubicin, 400, 402t
  mechanism of action, 931
  modulation of drug resistance, 930
  pharmacokinetics, 931
  precautions with, 931
  side effects, 931–932
  toxicity, 931–932
trifluridine, 932–933
  administration, 933
  admixture, 933
  antitumor activity, 932
  availability and storage, 933
  chemistry, 932
  dosage, 933
  mechanism of action, 932
  pharmacokinetics, 933
  preparation, 933
  side effects, 933
  stability, 933
  toxicity, 933
α-triglycidyl-S-triazinetrione (teroxirone), 891–893
11β,17,21-trihydroxypregna-1,4-diene-3,20-dione 21-4[p[bis(2-chloroethyl)amino]phenyl]butyrate (prednimustine), 805–808
trimethylcolchicinic acid, mechanism of action, 5t
trimetrexate, 933–939
  administration, 935
  admixture, 935
  antitumor activity, 934
  availability and storage, 934–935
  chemistry, 933–934
  dosage, 935, 935t
  drug interactions, 935
  mechanism of action, 934
  pharmacokinetics, 935–937, 936t
  preparation, 935
  side effects, 937
  stability, 935
  toxicity, 937
TSPA (thiotepa), 898–905
tubulin-interactive agents, 15, 28–29
  indications for, 17t
tumor
  cell loss, 5–7
  chemotherapeutic sensitivity
    classification of, 12–13, 13t
    kinetic parameters and, 12t, 12–13
  doubling time, 5–7
    and chemotherapeutic sensitivity, 12t
  growth
    and acquisition of drug resistance, 11, 11f
    cell-kill hypothesis, 9
    Gompertzian model, 7–9, 8f
    models of, 7–9
  growth fraction, and chemotherapeutic sensitivity, 12t
  growth kinetics, 4–7
  stem cell concept, 7, 8f
tumor flare, 32
tumor-infiltrating lymphocyte, 151–152
tumor-inhibitory factor 2 (interleukin-1, alpha and beta), 589–595
tumor lysis syndrome, after intrathecal methotrexate, 97
tumor necrosis factor, 939–945
  administration, 941–942, 942t
  admixture, 941
  antitumor activity, 940
  availability and storage, 940–941
  chemistry, 939–940
  dosage, 942t, 942–943
  drug interactions, 942
    with interleukin-2, 154t, 155
    with isotretinoin, 620
  intravenous infusion solution, 941
  lyophilized product, 941
  mechanism of action, 940
  pharmacokinetics, 943
  precautions with, 942
  preparation, 941
  side effects, 943
  stability, 941
  toxicity, 943
tumor necrosis factor α, 939–945
  drug interactions, with suramin sodium, 862

tumor necrosis factor β, 939–945
tumor necrosis factor + interferon gamma, drug interactions, with tretinoin, 925, 925t
tyramine-rich foods, interactions, with procarbazine, 811, 811t
TZT [Baker's antifol (soluble)], 219–222

U-11 (nafoxidine), 744–745
U-42126 (acivicin), 131–134
U-73975 (adozelesin), 146–148
U-8344 (uracil mustard), 945–946
U-9889 (streptozocin), 850–856
301U74 (piritrexim), 788–791
UCB 3938 (mesna), 685–689
7U85 mesylate (BW 7U85 mesylate), 253–254
uracil mustard, 20, 945–946
  administration, 945
  antitumor activity, 945
  availability and storage, 945
  chemistry, 945
  dosage, 945
  drug interactions, with tegafur, 880
  indications for, 16t
  mechanism of action, 945
  side effects, 945–946
  toxicity, 945–946
uridine, interactions with 5-fluorouracil, 504
urokinase, interactions with mitomycin-C, 720
Uromitexan (mesna), 685–689
uroprotectants. See N-acetylcysteine; mesna

vaccine
  antitumor, interactions with cyclophosphamide, 323
  interactions with dactinomycin, 351
VAC regimen, 396
VAD. See vascular access devices
VAD regimen, 305
vascular access, 73
vascular access devices, 80, 109. See also catheters; implantable ports; infusion pumps
  candidates for, criteria for, 80, 81t
  extravasation with. See extravasation
  flowsheet for, 78f
  monitoring tool for, 79f
VATH regimen, 898
VCAP regimen, 320

Page numbers followed by **t** and **f** denote tables and figures, respectively.

VCR (vincristine sulfate), 951–957
Velban (vinblastine sulfate), 28–29, 946–950
Velbe (vinblastine sulfate), 946–950
venipuncture, 63–66
　attempts, limit on number of, 67
　multiple, 67
VePesid (etoposide), 24, 71t, 460–472
verapamil, drug interactions
　with daunorubicin HCl, 358–359
　with doxorubicin, 402t–403t
　with etoposide, 464
　with paclitaxel, 764
　with trimetrexate, 935
　with vincristine sulfate, 953
Vercyte (pipobroman), 783–784
vesicants, 66, 67t, 109
　administration, 63, 66, 68, 68t
　definition of, 66
　extravasation, 111t
vidarabine, drug interactions
　with allopurinol sodium, 163
　with pentostatin, 776
vinblastine sulfate, 28–29, 946–950
　administration, 947
　　intraarterial, 949
　　intralesional, 949
　admixture, 947
　antitumor activity, 946
　availability and storage, 946
　chemistry, 946
　combination, with interferon alfa, 574t
　dosage, 948
　drug interactions, 947–948
　　with estranustine phosphate, 444
　　with methotrexate, 696
　extravasation, 111t
　　management of, 114, 115t
　indications for, 17t
　mechanism of action, 4, 5t, 946
　pharmacokinetics, 948, 948t
　precautions with, 947
　preparation, 947
　resistance to, 11t
　side effects, 948–949
　special applications, 949
　stability, 947
　toxicity, 948–949
　as vesicant, 67t
vinca alkaloids, 5t, 28–29. *See also* vinblastine; vincristine; vindesine
　extravasation, 111t
　　management of, 114
vincaleukoblastine (vinblastine sulfate), 946–950
vincristine sulfate, 28–29, 951–957
　administration, 952

admixture, 952
antitumor activity, 951
availability and storage, 952
chemistry, 951
dosage, 952–953
drug interactions, 953
　with asparaginase, 204, 204t
　with bleomycin sulfate, 230
　with eflornithine, 427
　with methotrexate, 696, 697t, 698
　with mitomycin-C, 720
　with tamoxifen, 869
　with teniposide, 884
　with trimetrexate, 935
extravasation, 111t
　management of, 114, 115t
indications for, 17t
mechanism of action, 4, 5t, 951–952
pharmacokinetics, 953–954, 954t
precautions with, 952
preparation, 952
resistance, 11t
side effects, 954–955
stability, 952
toxicity, 954–955
as vesicant, 67t
vindesine, 957–966
　administration, 959
　admixture, 959
　antitumor activity, 957–959, 958t, 959t
　availability and storage, 959
　chemistry, 957
　dosage, 959
　drug interactions, 959
　　with eflornithine, 427
　extravasation, 111t
　　management of, 114
　mechanism of action, 958
　pharmacokinetics, 959–960
　precautions with, 959
　preparation, 959
　resistance to, 11t
　side effects, 961–962
　stability, 959
　toxicity, 961–962
　as vesicant, 67t
vindesine + bleomycin + dacarbazine, 959t
vindesine + bleomycin + dacarbazine + actinomycin D, 959t
vindesine + etoposide + platinum, 959t
vindesine + lomustine + bleomycin, 959t
vindesine + medroxyprogesterone, 959t
vindesine + mitomycin-C, 959t
vindesine + mitomycin-C + hexamethylmelamine, 959t
vindesine + mitomycin-C + mitoxantrone, 959t

vindesine + mitomycin-C + platinum, 959t
vindesine + platinum, 959t
vindesine + platinum + bleomycin, 959t
vindesine + platinum + dacarbazine, 959t
vindesine + platinum + ifosfamide, 959t
vindesine + platinum + mitoguazone, 959t
vindesine + platinum + mitomycin-C, 959t
vinorelbine, 966–969
　administration, 967
　admixture, 967
　antitumor activity, 966–967
　availability and storage, 967
　chemistry, 966
　dosage, 967–968
　mechanism of action, 967
　pharmacokinetics, 968, 968t
　precautions with, 967
　preparation, 967
　side effects, 968
　stability, 967
　toxicity, 968
vinzolidine, 969–973
　administration, 970–971
　admixture, 970
　antitumor activity, 969–970
　availability and storage, 970
　chemistry, 969
　dosage, 971, 971t
　mechanism of action, 970
　pharmacokinetics, 971, 972t
　preparation, 970
　side effects, 971–972
　stability, 970
　toxicity, 971–972
Vira-A (vidarabine), drug interactions, with allopurinol sodium, 163
Vitacuff, 82
vitamin A, drug interactions, with carmustine, 269
vitamin D, drug interactions, with paclitaxel, 764
vitamin D$_3$, in regulation of bone remodeling, 38t
vitamin E, drug interactions, with doxorubicin, 403t
vitamin K$_2$, drug interactions, with hydrazine sulfate, 542
vitamin K$_3$, drug interactions, with hydrazine sulfate, 540–542
VLB (vinblastine sulfate), 946–950
VM-26 (teniposide), 882–889
VMCP regimen, 320, 663
VMP regimen, 692

VP-16 (etoposide), 460–472
VP-16-213 (etoposide), 71t, 460–472
VS103 (liposomal daunorubicin), 637–639
Vumon (teniposide), 882–889
VZL (vinzolidine), 969–973

warfarin, drug interactions
   with allopurinol sodium, 163
   with aminoglutethimide, 172t, 172
   with amsacrine, 185
   with doxorubicin, 403t
   with megestrol acetate, 817
   with methotrexate, 695
   with sulofenur, 857
   with vindesine + etoposide, 959
warm compresses
   in management of epipodophyllotoxin extravasation, 114, 115t
   in management of vinca alkaloid extravasation, 114, 115t

Wellcovorin (leucovorin calcium), 624–630
Wellferon (interferon alfa), 564–582
Winstrol (stanozolol), 192t
WR-2721 (ethiofos), 453–459
   drug interactions, with cisplatin, 292
   in management of hypercalcemia of malignancy, 50
Wy-5321 (diglycoaldehyde), 391–393

yoshi 864, 973–974
   administration, 973
   admixture, 973
   antitumor activity, 973
   availability and storage, 973
   chemistry, 973
   dosage, 974
   mechanism of action, 973
   pharmacokinetics, 974
   precautions with, 973
   preparation, 973
   side effects, 974
   stability, 973
   toxicity, 974

Z4942 (ifosfamide), 558–563
Zanosar (streptozocin), 20–21, 850–856
Zinecard (dexrazoxane), 367–371
zinostatin (neocarzinostatin), 746–750
   hypersensitivity reactions with, 68
Zoladex (goserelin acetate), 33, 527–528
zorubicin, 975–978
   administration, 976
   admixture, 976
   antitumor activity, 975
   availability and storage, 976
   chemistry, 975
   dosage, 976–977
   mechanism of action, 975–976
   pharmacokinetics, 977
   precautions with, 976
   preparation, 976
   side effects, 977–978
   stability, 976
   toxicity, 977–978
Zyloprim (allopurinol sodium), 27, 161–166